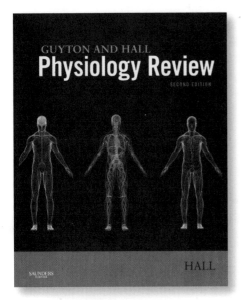
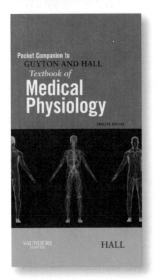

Guyton and Hall
Textbook of Medical Physiology

TWELFTH EDITION

Guyton and Hall
Textbook of Medical Physiology

John E. Hall, Ph.D.

Arthur C. Guyton Professor and Chair
Department of Physiology and Biophysics
Associate Vice Chancellor for Research
University of Mississippi Medical Center
Jackson, Mississippi

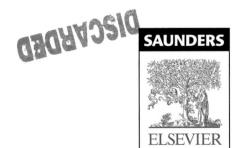

SAUNDERS

ELSEVIER

SAUNDERS
ELSEVIER

1600 John F. Kennedy Blvd.
Ste 1800
Philadelphia, PA 19103-2899

TEXTBOOK OF MEDICAL PHYSIOLOGY

ISBN: 978-1-4160-4574-8
International Edition: 978-0-8089-2400-5

Library of Congress Cataloging-in-Publication Data

Hall, John E. (John Edward), 1946-
  Guyton and Hall textbook of medical physiology / John Hall. – 12th ed.
    p. ; cm.
  Rev. ed. of: Textbook of medical physiology. 11th ed. c2006.
  Includes bibliographical references and index.
  ISBN 978-1-4160-4574-8 (alk. paper)
  1. Human physiology. 2. Physiology, Pathological. I. Guyton, Arthur C. II.
  Textbook of medical physiology. III. Title. IV. Title: Textbook of medical physiology.
    [DNLM: 1. Physiological Phenomena. QT 104 H1767g 2011]
  QP34.5.G9 2011
  612–dc22   2009035327

Publishing Director: William Schmitt
Developmental Editor: Rebecca Gruliow
Editorial Assistant: Laura Stingelin
Publishing Services Manager: Linda Van Pelt
Project Manager: Frank Morales
Design Manager: Steve Stave
Illustrator: Michael Schenk
Marketing Manager: Marla Lieberman

Printed in the United States of America

Last digit is the print number: 9 8 7 6 5 4 3 2

To

My Family

For their abundant support, for their patience and
understanding, and for their love

To

Arthur C. Guyton

For his imaginative and innovative research
For his dedication to education
For showing us the excitement and joy of physiology
And for serving as an inspirational role model

Preface

The first edition of the *Textbook of Medical Physiology* was written by Arthur C. Guyton almost 55 years ago. Unlike most major medical textbooks, which often have 20 or more authors, the first eight editions of the *Textbook of Medical Physiology* were written entirely by Dr. Guyton, with each new edition arriving on schedule for nearly 40 years. The *Textbook of Medical Physiology*, first published in 1956, quickly became the best-selling medical physiology textbook in the world. Dr. Guyton had a gift for communicating complex ideas in a clear and interesting manner that made studying physiology fun. He wrote the book to help students learn physiology, not to impress his professional colleagues.

I worked closely with Dr. Guyton for almost 30 years and had the privilege of writing parts of the 9th and 10th editions. After Dr. Guyton's tragic death in an automobile accident in 2003, I assumed responsibility for completing the 11th edition.

For the 12th edition of the *Textbook of Medical Physiology*, I have the same goal as for previous editions—to explain, in language easily understood by students, how the different cells, tissues, and organs of the human body work together to maintain life.

This task has been challenging and fun because our rapidly increasing knowledge of physiology continues to unravel new mysteries of body functions. Advances in molecular and cellular physiology have made it possible to explain many physiology principles in the terminology of molecular and physical sciences rather than in merely a series of separate and unexplained biological phenomena.

The *Textbook of Medical Physiology*, however, is not a reference book that attempts to provide a compendium of the most recent advances in physiology. This is a book that continues the tradition of being written for students. It focuses on the basic principles of physiology needed to begin a career in the health care professions, such as medicine, dentistry and nursing, as well as graduate studies in the biological and health sciences. It should also be useful to physicians and health care professionals who wish to review the basic principles needed for understanding the pathophysiology of human disease.

I have attempted to maintain the same unified organization of the text that has been useful to students in the past and to ensure that the book is comprehensive enough that students will continue to use it during their professional careers.

My hope is that this textbook conveys the majesty of the human body and its many functions and that it stimulates students to study physiology throughout their careers. Physiology is the link between the basic sciences and medicine. The great beauty of physiology is that it integrates the individual functions of all the body's different cells, tissues, and organs into a functional whole, the human body. Indeed, the human body is much more than the sum of its parts, and life relies upon this total function, not just on the function of individual body parts in isolation from the others.

This brings us to an important question: How are the separate organs and systems coordinated to maintain proper function of the entire body? Fortunately, our bodies are endowed with a vast network of feedback controls that achieve the necessary balances without which we would be unable to live. Physiologists call this high level of internal bodily control *homeostasis*. In disease states, functional balances are often seriously disturbed and homeostasis is impaired. When even a single disturbance reaches a limit, the whole body can no longer live. One of the goals of this text, therefore, is to emphasize the effectiveness and beauty of the body's homeostasis mechanisms as well as to present their abnormal functions in disease.

Another objective is to be as accurate as possible. Suggestions and critiques from many students, physiologists, and clinicians throughout the world have been sought and then used to check factual accuracy as well as balance in the text. Even so, because of the likelihood of error in sorting through many thousands of bits of information, I wish to issue a further request to all readers to send along notations of error or inaccuracy. Physiologists understand the importance of feedback for proper function of the human body; so, too, is feedback important for progressive improvement of a textbook of physiology. To the many persons who have already helped, I express sincere thanks.

A brief explanation is needed about several features of the 12th edition. Although many of the chapters have been revised to include new principles of physiology, the text length has been closely monitored to limit the book size so that it can be used effectively in physiology courses for medical students and health care professionals. Many of the figures have also been redrawn and are in full color. New references have been chosen primarily for their presentation of physiologic principles, for the quality of their own references, and for their easy accessibility. The selected bibliography at the end of the chapters lists papers mainly from recently published scientific journals that can be freely accessed from the PubMed internet site at http://www.ncbi.nlm.nih.gov/sites/entrez/. Use of these references, as well as cross-references from them, can give the student almost complete coverage of the entire field of physiology. The effort to be as concise as possible has, unfortunately, necessitated a more simplified and dogmatic presentation of many physiologic principles than I normally would have desired. However, the bibliography can be used to learn more about the controversies and unanswered questions that remain in understanding the complex functions of the human body in health and disease.

Another feature is that the print is set in two sizes. The material in large print constitutes the fundamental physiologic information that students will require in virtually all of their medical activities and studies.

The material in small print is of several different kinds: first, anatomic, chemical, and other information that is needed for immediate discussion but that most students will learn in more detail in other courses; second, physiologic information of special importance to certain fields of clinical medicine; and, third, information that will be of value to those students who may wish to study particular physiologic mechanisms more deeply.

I wish to express sincere thanks to many persons who have helped to prepare this book, including my colleagues in the Department of Physiology and Biophysics at the University of Mississippi Medical Center who provided valuable suggestions. The members of our faculty and a brief description of the research and educational activities of the department can be found at the web site: http://physiology.umc.edu/. I am also grateful to Stephanie Lucas and Courtney Horton Graham for their excellent secretarial services, to Michael Schenk and Walter (Kyle) Cunningham for their expert artwork, and to William Schmitt, Rebecca Gruliow, Frank Morales, and the entire Elsevier Saunders team for continued editorial and production excellence.

Finally, I owe an enormous debt to Arthur Guyton for the great privilege of contributing to the *Textbook of Medical Physiology,* for an exciting career in physiology, for his friendship, and for the inspiration that he provided to all who knew him.

John E. Hall

Contents

UNIT I

Introduction to Physiology: The Cell and General Physiology

CHAPTER 1

Functional Organization of the Human Body and Control of the "Internal Environment" 3

Cells as the Living Units of the Body 3

Extracellular Fluid—The "Internal Environment" 3

"Homeostatic" Mechanisms of the Major Functional Systems 4

Control Systems of the Body 6

Summary—Automaticity of the Body 9

CHAPTER 2

The Cell and Its Functions 11

Organization of the Cell 11

Physical Structure of the Cell 12

Comparison of the Animal Cell with Precellular Forms of Life 17

Functional Systems of the Cell 18

Locomotion of Cells 23

CHAPTER 3

Genetic Control of Protein Synthesis, Cell Function, and Cell Reproduction 27

Genes in the Cell Nucleus 27

The DNA Code in the Cell Nucleus Is Transferred to an RNA Code in the Cell Cytoplasm—The Process of Transcription 30

Synthesis of Other Substances in the Cell 35

Control of Gene Function and Biochemical Activity in Cells 35

The DNA-Genetic System Also Controls Cell Reproduction 37

Cell Differentiation 39

Apoptosis—Programmed Cell Death 40

Cancer 40

UNIT II

Membrane Physiology, Nerve, and Muscle

CHAPTER 4

Transport of Substances Through Cell Membranes 45

The Lipid Barrier of the Cell Membrane, and Cell Membrane Transport Proteins 45

Diffusion 46

"Active Transport" of Substances Through Membranes 52

CHAPTER 5

Membrane Potentials and Action Potentials 57

Basic Physics of Membrane Potentials 57

Measuring the Membrane Potential 58

Resting Membrane Potential of Nerves 59

Nerve Action Potential 60

Roles of Other Ions During the Action Potential 64

Propagation of the Action Potential 64

Re-establishing Sodium and Potassium Ionic Gradients After Action Potentials Are Completed—Importance of Energy Metabolism 65

Plateau in Some Action Potentials 66

Rhythmicity of Some Excitable Tissues—Repetitive Discharge 66

Special Characteristics of Signal Transmission in Nerve Trunks 67

Excitation—The Process of Eliciting the Action Potential 68

Recording Membrane Potentials and Action Potentials 69

CHAPTER 6

Contraction of Skeletal Muscle 71

Physiologic Anatomy of Skeletal Muscle 71

General Mechanism of Muscle Contraction 73

Molecular Mechanism of Muscle Contraction 74

Energetics of Muscle Contraction 78

Characteristics of Whole Muscle Contraction 79

CHAPTER 7

Excitation of Skeletal Muscle: Neuromuscular Transmission and Excitation-Contraction Coupling 83

Transmission of Impulses from Nerve Endings to Skeletal Muscle Fibers: The Neuromuscular Junction 83

Molecular Biology of Acetylcholine Formation and Release 86

Drugs That Enhance or Block Transmission at the Neuromuscular Junction 86

Myasthenia Gravis Causes Muscle Paralysis 86

Muscle Action Potential 87

Excitation-Contraction Coupling 88

CHAPTER 8

Excitation and Contraction of Smooth Muscle 91

Contraction of Smooth Muscle 91

Nervous and Hormonal Control of Smooth Muscle Contraction 94

UNIT III
The Heart

CHAPTER 9

Cardiac Muscle; The Heart as a Pump and Function of the Heart Valves 101

Physiology of Cardiac Muscle 101

Cardiac Cycle 104

Relationship of the Heart Sounds to Heart Pumping 107

Work Output of the Heart 107

Chemical Energy Required for Cardiac Contraction: Oxygen Utilization by the Heart 109

Regulation of Heart Pumping 110

CHAPTER 10

Rhythmical Excitation of the Heart 115

Specialized Excitatory and Conductive System of the Heart 115

Control of Excitation and Conduction in the Heart 118

CHAPTER 11

The Normal Electrocardiogram 121

Characteristics of the Normal Electrocardiogram 121

Methods for Recording Electrocardiograms 123

Flow of Current Around the Heart during the Cardiac Cycle 123

Electrocardiographic Leads 124

CHAPTER 12

Electrocardiographic Interpretation of Cardiac Muscle and Coronary Blood Flow Abnormalities: Vectorial Analysis 129

Principles of Vectorial Analysis of Electrocardiograms 129

Vectorial Analysis of the Normal Electrocardiogram 131

Mean Electrical Axis of the Ventricular QRS—and Its Significance 134

Conditions That Cause Abnormal Voltages of the QRS Complex 137

Prolonged and Bizarre Patterns of the QRS Complex 137

Current of Injury 138

Abnormalities in the T Wave 141

CHAPTER 13

Cardiac Arrhythmias and Their Electrocardiographic Interpretation 143

Abnormal Sinus Rhythms 143

Abnormal Rhythms That Result from Block of Heart Signals Within the Intracardiac Conduction Pathways 144

Premature Contractions 146

Paroxysmal Tachycardia 148

Ventricular Fibrillation 149

Atrial Fibrillation 151

Atrial Flutter 152

Cardiac Arrest 153

UNIT IV
The Circulation

CHAPTER 14

Overview of the Circulation; Biophysics of Pressure, Flow, and Resistance 157

Physical Characteristics of the Circulation 157

Basic Principles of Circulatory Function 158

Interrelationships of Pressure, Flow, and Resistance 159

CHAPTER 15

Vascular Distensibility and Functions of the Arterial and Venous Systems   **167**
Vascular Distensibility   167
Arterial Pressure Pulsations   168
Veins and Their Functions   171

CHAPTER 16

The Microcirculation and Lymphatic System: Capillary Fluid Exchange, Interstitial Fluid, and Lymph Flow   **177**
Structure of the Microcirculation and Capillary System   177
Flow of Blood in the Capillaries— Vasomotion   178
Exchange of Water, Nutrients, and Other Substances Between the Blood and Interstitial Fluid   179
Interstitium and Interstitial Fluid   180
Fluid Filtration Across Capillaries Is Determined by Hydrostatic and Colloid Osmotic Pressures, as Well as Capillary Filtration Coefficient   181
Lymphatic System   186

CHAPTER 17

Local and Humoral Control of Tissue Blood Flow   **191**
Local Control of Blood Flow in Response to Tissue Needs   191
Mechanisms of Blood Flow Control   191
Humoral Control of the Circulation   199

CHAPTER 18

Nervous Regulation of the Circulation, and Rapid Control of Arterial Pressure   **201**
Nervous Regulation of the Circulation   201
Role of the Nervous System in Rapid Control of Arterial Pressure   204
Special Features of Nervous Control of Arterial Pressure   209

CHAPTER 19

Role of the Kidneys in Long-Term Control of Arterial Pressure and in Hypertension: The Integrated System for Arterial Pressure Regulation   **213**
Renal–Body Fluid System for Arterial Pressure Control   213
The Renin-Angiotensin System: Its Role in Arterial Pressure Control   220
Summary of the Integrated, Multifaceted System for Arterial Pressure Regulation   226

CHAPTER 20

Cardiac Output, Venous Return, and Their Regulation   **229**
Normal Values for Cardiac Output at Rest and During Activity   229
Control of Cardiac Output by Venous Return—Role of the Frank-Starling Mechanism of the Heart   229
Pathologically High or Low Cardiac Outputs   232
Methods for Measuring Cardiac Output   240

CHAPTER 21

Muscle Blood Flow and Cardiac Output During Exercise; the Coronary Circulation and Ischemic Heart Disease   **243**
Blood Flow Regulation in Skeletal Muscle at Rest and During Exercise   243
Coronary Circulation   246

CHAPTER 22

Cardiac Failure   **255**
Circulatory Dynamics in Cardiac Failure   255
Unilateral Left Heart Failure   259
Low-Output Cardiac Failure— Cardiogenic Shock   259
Edema in Patients with Cardiac Failure   259
Cardiac Reserve   261

CHAPTER 23

Heart Valves and Heart Sounds; Valvular and Congenital Heart Defects   **265**
Heart Sounds   265
Abnormal Circulatory Dynamics in Valvular Heart Disease   268
Abnormal Circulatory Dynamics in Congenital Heart Defects   269
Use of Extracorporeal Circulation During Cardiac Surgery   271
Hypertrophy of the Heart in Valvular and Congenital Heart Disease   272

CHAPTER 24

Circulatory Shock and Its Treatment   **273**
Physiologic Causes of Shock   273
Shock Caused by Hypovolemia— Hemorrhagic Shock   274
Neurogenic Shock—Increased Vascular Capacity   279
Anaphylactic Shock and Histamine Shock   280
Septic Shock   280

Physiology of Treatment in Shock 280
Circulatory Arrest 281

UNIT V
The Body Fluids and Kidneys

CHAPTER 25
The Body Fluid Compartments: Extracellular and Intracellular Fluids; Edema 285
Fluid Intake and Output Are Balanced During Steady-State Conditions 285
Body Fluid Compartments 286
Extracellular Fluid Compartment 287
Blood Volume 287
Constituents of Extracellular and Intracellular Fluids 287
Measurement of Fluid Volumes in the Different Body Fluid Compartments—the Indicator-Dilution Principle 287
Determination of Volumes of Specific Body Fluid Compartments 289
Regulation of Fluid Exchange and Osmotic Equilibrium Between Intracellular and Extracellular Fluid 290
Basic Principles of Osmosis and Osmotic Pressure 290
Osmotic Equilibrium Is Maintained Between Intracellular and Extracellular Fluids 291
Volume and Osmolality of Extracellular and Intracellular Fluids in Abnormal States 292
Glucose and Other Solutions Administered for Nutritive Purposes 294
Clinical Abnormalities of Fluid Volume Regulation: Hyponatremia and Hypernatremia 294
Edema: Excess Fluid in the Tissues 296
Fluids in the "Potential Spaces" of the Body 300

CHAPTER 26
Urine Formation by the Kidneys: I. Glomerular Filtration, Renal Blood Flow, and Their Control 303
Multiple Functions of the Kidneys 303
Physiologic Anatomy of the Kidneys 304
Micturition 307
Physiologic Anatomy of the Bladder 307
Transport of Urine from the Kidney Through the Ureters and into the Bladder 308
Filling of the Bladder and Bladder Wall Tone; the Cystometrogram 309
Micturition Reflex 309

Abnormalities of Micturition 310
Urine Formation Results from Glomerular Filtration, Tubular Reabsorption, and Tubular Secretion 310
Glomerular Filtration—The First Step in Urine Formation 312
Determinants of the GFR 314
Renal Blood Flow 316
Physiologic Control of Glomerular Filtration and Renal Blood Flow 317
Autoregulation of GFR and Renal Blood Flow 319

CHAPTER 27
Urine Formation by the Kidneys: II. Tubular Reabsorption and Secretion 323
Renal Tubular Reabsorption and Secretion 323
Tubular Reabsorption Includes Passive and Active Mechanisms 323
Reabsorption and Secretion Along Different Parts of the Nephron 329
Regulation of Tubular Reabsorption 334
Use of Clearance Methods to Quantify Kidney Function 340

CHAPTER 28
Urine Concentration and Dilution; Regulation of Extracellular Fluid Osmolarity and Sodium Concentration 345
Kidneys Excrete Excess Water by Forming Dilute Urine 345
Kidneys Conserve Water by Excreting Concentrated Urine 346
Quantifying Renal Urine Concentration and Dilution: "Free Water" and Osmolar Clearances 354
Disorders of Urinary Concentrating Ability 354
Control of Extracellular Fluid Osmolarity and Sodium Concentration 355
Osmoreceptor-ADH Feedback System 355
Importance of Thirst in Controlling Extracellular Fluid Osmolarity and Sodium Concentration 357
Salt-Appetite Mechanism for Controlling Extracellular Fluid Sodium Concentration and Volume 360

CHAPTER 29
Renal Regulation of Potassium, Calcium, Phosphate, and Magnesium; Integration of Renal Mechanisms for Control of Blood Volume and Extracellular Fluid Volume 361
Regulation of Extracellular Fluid Potassium Concentration and Potassium Excretion 361

Control of Renal Calcium Excretion and Extracellular Calcium Ion Concentration   367

Control of Renal Magnesium Excretion and Extracellular Magnesium Ion Concentration   369

Integration of Renal Mechanisms for Control of Extracellular Fluid   370

Importance of Pressure Natriuresis and Pressure Diuresis in Maintaining Body Sodium and Fluid Balance   371

Distribution of Extracellular Fluid Between the Interstitial Spaces and Vascular System   373

Nervous and Hormonal Factors Increase the Effectiveness of Renal–Body Fluid Feedback Control   373

Integrated Responses to Changes in Sodium Intake   376

Conditions That Cause Large Increases in Blood Volume and Extracellular Fluid Volume   376

Conditions That Cause Large Increases in Extracellular Fluid Volume but with Normal Blood Volume   377

CHAPTER 30

Acid-Base Regulation   379

H^+ Concentration Is Precisely Regulated   379

Acids and Bases—Their Definitions and Meanings   379

Defending Against Changes in H^+ Concentration: Buffers, Lungs, and Kidneys   380

Buffering of H^+ in the Body Fluids   380

Bicarbonate Buffer System   381

Phosphate Buffer System   383

Proteins Are Important Intracellular Buffers   383

Respiratory Regulation of Acid-Base Balance   384

Renal Control of Acid-Base Balance   385

Secretion of H^+ and Reabsorption of HCO_3^- by the Renal Tubules   386

Combination of Excess H^+ with Phosphate and Ammonia Buffers in the Tubule Generates "New" HCO_3^- 388

Quantifying Renal Acid-Base Excretion   389

Renal Correction of Acidosis—Increased Excretion of H^+ and Addition of HCO_3^- to the Extracellular Fluid   391

Renal Correction of Alkalosis—Decreased Tubular Secretion of H^+ and Increased Excretion of HCO_3^- 391

Clinical Causes of Acid-Base Disorders   392

Treatment of Acidosis or Alkalosis   393

Clinical Measurements and Analysis of Acid-Base Disorders   393

CHAPTER 31

Diuretics, Kidney Diseases   397

Diuretics and Their Mechanisms of Action   397

Kidney Diseases   399

Acute Renal Failure   399

Chronic Renal Failure: An Irreversible Decrease in the Number of Functional Nephrons   401

Specific Tubular Disorders   408

Treatment of Renal Failure by Transplantation or by Dialysis with an Artificial Kidney   409

UNIT VI

Blood Cells, Immunity, and Blood Coagulation

CHAPTER 32

Red Blood Cells, Anemia, and Polycythemia   413

Red Blood Cells (Erythrocytes)   413

Anemias   420

Polycythemia   421

CHAPTER 33

Resistance of the Body to Infection: I. Leukocytes, Granulocytes, the Monocyte-Macrophage System, and Inflammation   423

Leukocytes (White Blood Cells)   423

Neutrophils and Macrophages Defend Against Infections   425

Monocyte-Macrophage Cell System (Reticuloendothelial System)   426

Inflammation: Role of Neutrophils and Macrophages   428

Eosinophils   430

Basophils   431

Leukopenia   431

Leukemias   431

CHAPTER 34

Resistance of the Body to Infection: II. Immunity and Allergy   433

Acquired (Adaptive) Immunity   433

Allergy and Hypersensitivity   443

CHAPTER 35

Blood Types; Transfusion; Tissue and Organ Transplantation   445

Antigenicity Causes Immune Reactions of Blood   445

O-A-B Blood Types   445

Rh Blood Types   447

Transplantation of Tissues and Organs   449

CHAPTER 36

Hemostasis and Blood Coagulation 451
Events in Hemostasis 451
Vascular Constriction 451
Mechanism of Blood Coagulation 453
Conditions That Cause Excessive Bleeding in
Humans 457
Thromboembolic Conditions in the
Human Being 459
Anticoagulants for Clinical Use 459
Blood Coagulation Tests 460

UNIT VII

Respiration

CHAPTER 37

Pulmonary Ventilation 465
Mechanics of Pulmonary Ventilation 465
Pulmonary Volumes and Capacities 469
Minute Respiratory Volume Equals Respiratory
Rate Times Tidal Volume 471
Alveolar Ventilation 471
Functions of the Respiratory Passageways 472

CHAPTER 38

**Pulmonary Circulation, Pulmonary Edema,
Pleural Fluid** 477
Physiologic Anatomy of the Pulmonary
Circulatory System 477
Pressures in the Pulmonary System 477
Blood Volume of the Lungs 478
Blood Flow Through the Lungs and Its
Distribution 479
Effect of Hydrostatic Pressure Gradients in
the Lungs on Regional Pulmonary Blood Flow 479
Pulmonary Capillary Dynamics 481
Fluid in the Pleural Cavity 483

CHAPTER 39

**Physical Principles of Gas Exchange;
Diffusion of Oxygen and Carbon Dioxide
Through the Respiratory Membrane** 485
Physics of Gas Diffusion and Gas
Partial Pressures 485
Compositions of Alveolar Air and Atmospheric
Air Are Different 487
Diffusion of Gases Through the Respiratory
Membrane 489
Effect of the Ventilation-Perfusion Ratio on
Alveolar Gas Concentration 492

CHAPTER 40

**Transport of Oxygen and Carbon Dioxide in
Blood and Tissue Fluids** 495
Transport of Oxygen from the Lungs to the
Body Tissues 495
Transport of Carbon Dioxide in the Blood 502
Respiratory Exchange Ratio 504

CHAPTER 41

Regulation of Respiration 505
Respiratory Center 505
Chemical Control of Respiration 507
Peripheral Chemoreceptor System for Control
of Respiratory Activity—Role of Oxygen in
Respiratory Control 508
Regulation of Respiration During Exercise 510
Other Factors That Affect Respiration 512

CHAPTER 42

**Respiratory Insufficiency—Pathophysiology,
Diagnosis, Oxygen Therapy** 515
Useful Methods for Studying Respiratory
Abnormalities 515
Pathophysiology of Specific Pulmonary
Abnormalities 517
Hypoxia and Oxygen Therapy 520
Hypercapnia—Excess Carbon Dioxide in the
Body Fluids 522
Artificial Respiration 522

UNIT VIII

**Aviation, Space, and Deep-Sea Diving
Physiology**

CHAPTER 43

**Aviation, High-Altitude, and
Space Physiology** 527
Effects of Low Oxygen Pressure on the Body 527
Effects of Acceleratory Forces on the Body in
Aviation and Space Physiology 531
"Artificial Climate" in the Sealed Spacecraft 533
Weightlessness in Space 533

CHAPTER 44

**Physiology of Deep-Sea Diving and
Other Hyperbaric Conditions** 535
Effect of High Partial Pressures of Individual
Gases on the Body 535
Scuba (Self-Contained Underwater Breathing
Apparatus) Diving 539
Special Physiologic Problems in Submarines 540
Hyperbaric Oxygen Therapy 540

UNIT IX

The Nervous System: A. General Principles and Sensory Physiology

CHAPTER 45

Organization of the Nervous System, Basic Functions of Synapses, and Neurotransmitters — **543**

General Design of the Nervous System — 543

Major Levels of Central Nervous System Function — 545

Comparison of the Nervous System with a Computer — 546

Central Nervous System Synapses — 546

Some Special Characteristics of Synaptic Transmission — 557

CHAPTER 46

Sensory Receptors, Neuronal Circuits for Processing Information — **559**

Types of Sensory Receptors and the Stimuli They Detect — 559

Transduction of Sensory Stimuli into Nerve Impulses — 560

Nerve Fibers That Transmit Different Types of Signals and Their Physiologic Classification — 563

Transmission of Signals of Different Intensity in Nerve Tracts—Spatial and Temporal Summation — 564

Transmission and Processing of Signals in Neuronal Pools — 564

Instability and Stability of Neuronal Circuits — 569

CHAPTER 47

Somatic Sensations: I. General Organization, the Tactile and Position Senses — **571**

Classification of Somatic Senses — 571

Detection and Transmission of Tactile Sensations — 571

Sensory Pathways for Transmitting Somatic Signals into the Central Nervous System — 573

Transmission in the Dorsal Column–Medial Lemniscal System — 573

Transmission of Less Critical Sensory Signals in the Anterolateral Pathway — 580

Some Special Aspects of Somatosensory Function — 581

CHAPTER 48

Somatic Sensations: II. Pain, Headache, and Thermal Sensations — **583**

Types of Pain and Their Qualities—Fast Pain and Slow Pain — 583

Pain Receptors and Their Stimulation — 583

Dual Pathways for Transmission of Pain Signals into the Central Nervous System — 584

Pain Suppression ("Analgesia") System in the Brain and Spinal Cord — 586

Referred Pain — 588

Visceral Pain — 588

Some Clinical Abnormalities of Pain and Other Somatic Sensations — 590

Headache — 590

Thermal Sensations — 592

UNIT X

The Nervous System: B. The Special Senses

CHAPTER 49

The Eye: I. Optics of Vision — **597**

Physical Principles of Optics — 597

Optics of the Eye — 600

Ophthalmoscope — 605

Fluid System of the Eye—Intraocular Fluid — 606

CHAPTER 50

The Eye: II. Receptor and Neural Function of the Retina — **609**

Anatomy and Function of the Structural Elements of the Retina — 609

Photochemistry of Vision — 611

Color Vision — 615

Neural Function of the Retina — 616

CHAPTER 51

The Eye: III. Central Neurophysiology of Vision — **623**

Visual Pathways — 623

Organization and Function of the Visual Cortex — 624

Neuronal Patterns of Stimulation During Analysis of the Visual Image — 626

Fields of Vision; Perimetry — 627

Eye Movements and Their Control — 627

Autonomic Control of Accommodation and Pupillary Aperture — 631

CHAPTER 52

The Sense of Hearing — **633**

Tympanic Membrane and the Ossicular System — 633

Cochlea — 634

Central Auditory Mechanisms — 639

Hearing Abnormalities — 642

CHAPTER 53

The Chemical Senses—Taste and Smell 645

Sense of Taste 645

Sense of Smell 648

UNIT XI

The Nervous System: C. Motor and Integrative Neurophysiology

CHAPTER 54

Motor Functions of the Spinal Cord; the Cord Reflexes 655

Organization of the Spinal Cord for Motor Functions 655

Muscle Sensory Receptors—Muscle Spindles and Golgi Tendon Organs—And Their Roles in Muscle Control 657

Flexor Reflex and the Withdrawal Reflexes 661

Crossed Extensor Reflex 663

Reciprocal Inhibition and Reciprocal Innervation 663

Reflexes of Posture and Locomotion 663

Scratch Reflex 664

Spinal Cord Reflexes That Cause Muscle Spasm 664

Autonomic Reflexes in the Spinal Cord 665

Spinal Cord Transection and Spinal Shock 665

CHAPTER 55

Cortical and Brain Stem Control of Motor Function 667

Motor Cortex and Corticospinal Tract 667

Role of the Brain Stem in Controlling Motor Function 673

Vestibular Sensations and Maintenance of Equilibrium 674

Functions of Brain Stem Nuclei in Controlling Subconscious, Stereotyped Movements 678

CHAPTER 56

Contributions of the Cerebellum and Basal Ganglia to Overall Motor Control 681

Cerebellum and Its Motor Functions 681

Basal Ganglia—Their Motor Functions 689

Integration of the Many Parts of the Total Motor Control System 694

CHAPTER 57

Cerebral Cortex, Intellectual Functions of the Brain, Learning, and Memory 697

Physiologic Anatomy of the Cerebral Cortex 697

Functions of Specific Cortical Areas 698

Function of the Brain in Communication—Language Input and Language Output 703

Function of the Corpus Callosum and Anterior Commissure to Transfer Thoughts, Memories, Training, and Other Information Between the Two Cerebral Hemispheres 704

Thoughts, Consciousness, and Memory 705

CHAPTER 58

Behavioral and Motivational Mechanisms of the Brain—The Limbic System and the Hypothalamus 711

Activating-Driving Systems of the Brain 711

Limbic System 714

Functional Anatomy of the Limbic System; Key Position of the Hypothalamus 714

Hypothalamus, a Major Control Headquarters for the Limbic System 715

Specific Functions of Other Parts of the Limbic System 718

CHAPTER 59

States of Brain Activity—Sleep, Brain Waves, Epilepsy, Psychoses 721

Sleep 721

Epilepsy 725

Psychotic Behavior and Dementia—Roles of Specific Neurotransmitter Systems 726

Schizophrenia—Possible Exaggerated Function of Part of the Dopamine System 727

CHAPTER 60

The Autonomic Nervous System and the Adrenal Medulla 729

General Organization of the Autonomic Nervous System 729

Basic Characteristics of Sympathetic and Parasympathetic Function 731

Autonomic Reflexes 738

Stimulation of Discrete Organs in Some Instances and Mass Stimulation in Other Instances by the Sympathetic and Parasympathetic Systems 738

Pharmacology of the Autonomic Nervous System 739

CHAPTER 61

Cerebral Blood Flow, Cerebrospinal Fluid, and Brain Metabolism 743

Cerebral Blood Flow 743

Cerebrospinal Fluid System 746

Brain Metabolism 749

UNIT XII

Gastrointestinal Physiology

CHAPTER 62

General Principles of Gastrointestinal Function—Motility, Nervous Control, and Blood Circulation   753

General Principles of Gastrointestinal Motility   753

Neural Control of Gastrointestinal Function—Enteric Nervous System   755

Functional Types of Movements in the Gastrointestinal Tract   759

Gastrointestinal Blood Flow—"Splanchnic Circulation"   759

CHAPTER 63

Propulsion and Mixing of Food in the Alimentary Tract   763

Ingestion of Food   763

Motor Functions of the Stomach   765

Movements of the Small Intestine   768

Movements of the Colon   770

Other Autonomic Reflexes That Affect Bowel Activity   772

CHAPTER 64

Secretory Functions of the Alimentary Tract   773

General Principles of Alimentary Tract Secretion   773

Secretion of Saliva   775

Esophageal Secretion   776

Gastric Secretion   777

Pancreatic Secretion   780

Secretion of Bile by the Liver; Functions of the Biliary Tree   783

Secretions of the Small Intestine   786

Secretion of Mucus by the Large Intestine   787

CHAPTER 65

Digestion and Absorption in the Gastrointestinal Tract   789

Digestion of the Various Foods by Hydrolysis   789

Basic Principles of Gastrointestinal Absorption   793

Absorption in the Small Intestine   794

Absorption in the Large Intestine: Formation of Feces   797

CHAPTER 66

Physiology of Gastrointestinal Disorders   799

Disorders of Swallowing and of the Esophagus   799

Disorders of the Stomach   799

Disorders of the Small Intestine   801

Disorders of the Large Intestine   802

General Disorders of the Gastrointestinal Tract   803

UNIT XIII

Metabolism and Temperature Regulation

CHAPTER 67

Metabolism of Carbohydrates, and Formation of Adenosine Triphosphate   809

Central Role of Glucose in Carbohydrate Metabolism   810

Transport of Glucose Through the Cell Membrane   810

Glycogen Is Stored in Liver and Muscle   811

Release of Energy from Glucose by the Glycolytic Pathway   812

Release of Energy from Glucose by the Pentose Phosphate Pathway   816

Formation of Carbohydrates from Proteins and Fats—"Gluconeogenesis"   817

Blood Glucose   817

CHAPTER 68

Lipid Metabolism   819

Transport of Lipids in the Body Fluids   819

Fat Deposits   821

Use of Triglycerides for Energy: Formation of Adenosine Triphosphate   822

Regulation of Energy Release from Triglycerides   825

Phospholipids and Cholesterol   826

Atherosclerosis   827

CHAPTER 69

Protein Metabolism   831

Basic Properties   831

Transport and Storage of Amino Acids   831

Functional Roles of the Plasma Proteins   833

Hormonal Regulation of Protein Metabolism   835

CHAPTER 70

The Liver as an Organ   837

Physiologic Anatomy of the Liver   837

Hepatic Vascular and Lymph Systems   837

Metabolic Functions of the Liver   839

Measurement of Bilirubin in the Bile as a Clinical Diagnostic Tool   840

CHAPTER 71

Dietary Balances; Regulation of Feeding; Obesity and Starvation; Vitamins and Minerals 843

Energy Intake and Output Are Balanced Under Steady-State Conditions 843

Dietary Balances 843

Regulation of Food Intake and Energy Storage 845

Obesity 850

Inanition, Anorexia, and Cachexia 851

Starvation 852

Vitamins 852

Mineral Metabolism 855

CHAPTER 72

Energetics and Metabolic Rate 859

Adenosine Triphosphate (ATP) Functions as an "Energy Currency" in Metabolism 859

Control of Energy Release in the Cell 861

Metabolic Rate 862

Energy Metabolism—Factors That Influence Energy Output 863

CHAPTER 73

Body Temperature Regulation, and Fever 867

Normal Body Temperatures 867

Body Temperature Is Controlled by Balancing Heat Production and Heat Loss 867

Regulation of Body Temperature— Role of the Hypothalamus 871

Abnormalities of Body Temperature Regulation 875

UNIT XIV

Endocrinology and Reproduction

CHAPTER 74

Introduction to Endocrinology 881

Coordination of Body Functions by Chemical Messengers 881

Chemical Structure and Synthesis of Hormones 881

Hormone Secretion, Transport, and Clearance from the Blood 884

Mechanisms of Action of Hormones 886

Measurement of Hormone Concentrations in the Blood 891

CHAPTER 75

Pituitary Hormones and Their Control by the Hypothalamus 895

Pituitary Gland and Its Relation to the Hypothalamus 895

Hypothalamus Controls Pituitary Secretion 897

Physiological Functions of Growth Hormone 898

Posterior Pituitary Gland and Its Relation to the Hypothalamus 904

CHAPTER 76

Thyroid Metabolic Hormones 907

Synthesis and Secretion of the Thyroid Metabolic Hormones 907

Physiological Functions of the Thyroid Hormones 910

Regulation of Thyroid Hormone Secretion 914

Diseases of the Thyroid 916

CHAPTER 77

Adrenocortical Hormones 921

Synthesis and Secretion of Adrenocortical Hormones 921

Functions of the Mineralocorticoids— Aldosterone 924

Functions of the Glucocorticoids 928

Adrenal Androgens 934

Abnormalities of Adrenocortical Secretion 934

CHAPTER 78

Insulin, Glucagon, and Diabetes Mellitus 939

Insulin and Its Metabolic Effects 939

Glucagon and Its Functions 947

Somatostatin Inhibits Glucagon and Insulin Secretion 949

Summary of Blood Glucose Regulation 949

Diabetes Mellitus 950

CHAPTER 79

Parathyroid Hormone, Calcitonin, Calcium and Phosphate Metabolism, Vitamin D, Bone, and Teeth 955

Overview of Calcium and Phosphate Regulation in the Extracellular Fluid and Plasma 955

Bone and Its Relation to Extracellular Calcium and Phosphate 957

Vitamin D 960

Parathyroid Hormone 962

Calcitonin 966

Summary of Control of Calcium Ion Concentration 966

Pathophysiology of Parathyroid Hormone, Vitamin D, and Bone Disease   967

Physiology of the Teeth   969

CHAPTER 80

Reproductive and Hormonal Functions of the Male (and Function of the Pineal Gland)   973

Physiologic Anatomy of the Male Sexual Organs   973

Spermatogenesis   973

Male Sexual Act   978

Testosterone and Other Male Sex Hormones   979

Abnormalities of Male Sexual Function   984

Erectile Dysfunction in the Male   985

Pineal Gland—Its Function in Controlling Seasonal Fertility in Some Animals   986

CHAPTER 81

Female Physiology Before Pregnancy and Female Hormones   987

Physiologic Anatomy of the Female Sexual Organs   987

Female Hormonal System   987

Monthly Ovarian Cycle; Function of the Gonadotropic Hormones   988

Functions of the Ovarian Hormones—Estradiol and Progesterone   991

Regulation of the Female Monthly Rhythm—Interplay Between the Ovarian and Hypothalamic-Pituitary Hormones   996

Abnormalities of Secretion by the Ovaries   999

Female Sexual Act   1000

Female Fertility   1000

CHAPTER 82

Pregnancy and Lactation   1003

Maturation and Fertilization of the Ovum   1003

Early Nutrition of the Embryo   1005

Function of the Placenta   1005

Hormonal Factors in Pregnancy   1007

Response of the Mother's Body to Pregnancy   1009

Parturition   1011

Lactation   1014

CHAPTER 83

Fetal and Neonatal Physiology   1019

Growth and Functional Development of the Fetus   1019

Development of the Organ Systems   1019

Adjustments of the Infant to Extrauterine Life   1021

Special Functional Problems in the Neonate   1023

Special Problems of Prematurity   1026

Growth and Development of the Child   1027

UNIT XV

Sports Physiology

CHAPTER 84

Sports Physiology   1031

Muscles in Exercise   1031

Respiration in Exercise   1036

Cardiovascular System in Exercise   1038

Body Heat in Exercise   1039

Body Fluids and Salt in Exercise   1040

Drugs and Athletes   1040

Body Fitness Prolongs Life   1041

Index   1043

Introduction to Physiology: The Cell and General Physiology

1. Functional Organization of the Human Body and Control of the "Internal Environment"

2. The Cell and Its Functions

3. Genetic Control of Protein Synthesis, Cell Function, and Cell Reproduction

Functional Organization of the Human Body and Control of the "Internal Environment"

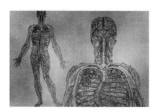 The goal of physiology is to explain the physical and chemical factors that are responsible for the origin, development, and progression of life. Each type of life, from the simple virus to the largest tree or the complicated human being, has its own functional characteristics. Therefore, the vast field of physiology can be divided into *viral physiology, bacterial physiology, cellular physiology, plant physiology, human physiology,* and many more subdivisions.

Human Physiology. In *human physiology,* we attempt to explain the specific characteristics and mechanisms of the human body that make it a living being. The very fact that we remain alive is the result of complex control systems, for hunger makes us seek food and fear makes us seek refuge. Sensations of cold make us look for warmth. Other forces cause us to seek fellowship and to reproduce. Thus, the human being is, in many ways, like an automaton, and the fact that we are sensing, feeling, and knowledgeable beings is part of this automatic sequence of life; these special attributes allow us to exist under widely varying conditions.

Cells as the Living Units of the Body

The basic living unit of the body is the cell. Each organ is an aggregate of many different cells held together by intercellular supporting structures.

Each type of cell is specially adapted to perform one or a few particular functions. For instance, the red blood cells, numbering 25 trillion in each human being, transport oxygen from the lungs to the tissues. Although the red cells are the most abundant of any single type of cell in the body, there are about 75 trillion additional cells of other types that perform functions different from those of the red cell. The entire body, then, contains about 100 trillion cells.

Although the many cells of the body often differ markedly from one another, all of them have certain basic characteristics that are alike. For instance, in all cells, oxygen reacts with carbohydrate, fat, and protein to release the energy required for cell function. Further, the general chemical mechanisms for changing nutrients into energy are basically the same in all cells, and all cells deliver end products of their chemical reactions into the surrounding fluids.

Almost all cells also have the ability to reproduce additional cells of their own kind. Fortunately, when cells of a particular type are destroyed, the remaining cells of this type usually generate new cells until the supply is replenished.

Extracellular Fluid—The "Internal Environment"

About 60 percent of the adult human body is fluid, mainly a water solution of ions and other substances. Although most of this fluid is inside the cells and is called *intracellular fluid,* about one third is in the spaces outside the cells and is called *extracellular fluid.* This extracellular fluid is in constant motion throughout the body. It is transported rapidly in the circulating blood and then mixed between the blood and the tissue fluids by diffusion through the capillary walls.

In the extracellular fluid are the ions and nutrients needed by the cells to maintain cell life. Thus, all cells live in essentially the same environment—the extracellular fluid. For this reason, the extracellular fluid is also called the *internal environment* of the body, or the *milieu intérieur,* a term introduced more than 100 years ago by the great 19th-century French physiologist Claude Bernard.

Cells are capable of living, growing, and performing their special functions as long as the proper concentrations of oxygen, glucose, different ions, amino acids, fatty substances, and other constituents are available in this internal environment.

Differences Between Extracellular and Intracellular Fluids. The extracellular fluid contains large amounts of *sodium, chloride,* and *bicarbonate ions* plus nutrients for the cells, such as *oxygen, glucose, fatty acids,* and *amino acids.* It also contains *carbon dioxide* that is being transported from the cells to the lungs to be excreted, plus other cellular waste products that are being transported to the kidneys for excretion.

The intracellular fluid differs significantly from the extracellular fluid; for example, it contains large amounts of *potassium, magnesium,* and *phosphate ions* instead of the sodium and chloride ions found in the extracellular fluid. Special mechanisms for transporting ions through the cell membranes maintain the ion concentration differences between the extracellular and intracellular fluids. These transport processes are discussed in Chapter 4.

"Homeostatic" Mechanisms of the Major Functional Systems

Homeostasis

The term *homeostasis* is used by physiologists to mean *maintenance of nearly constant conditions in the internal environment.* Essentially all organs and tissues of the body perform functions that help maintain these relatively constant conditions. For instance, the lungs provide oxygen to the extracellular fluid to replenish the oxygen used by the cells, the kidneys maintain constant ion concentrations, and the gastrointestinal system provides nutrients.

A large segment of this text is concerned with the manner in which each organ or tissue contributes to homeostasis. To begin this discussion, the different functional systems of the body and their contributions to homeostasis are outlined in this chapter; then we briefly outline the basic theory of the body's control systems that allow the functional systems to operate in support of one another.

Extracellular Fluid Transport and Mixing System—The Blood Circulatory System

Extracellular fluid is transported through all parts of the body in two stages. The first stage is movement of blood through the body in the blood vessels, and the second is movement of fluid between the blood capillaries and the *intercellular spaces* between the tissue cells.

Figure 1-1 shows the overall circulation of blood. All the blood in the circulation traverses the entire circulatory circuit an average of once each minute when the body is at rest and as many as six times each minute when a person is extremely active.

As blood passes through the blood capillaries, continual exchange of extracellular fluid also occurs between the plasma portion of the blood and the interstitial fluid that fills the intercellular spaces. This process is shown in Figure 1-2. The walls of the capillaries are permeable to most molecules in the plasma of the blood, with the exception of plasma protein molecules, which are too large to readily pass through the capillaries. Therefore, large amounts of fluid and its dissolved constituents *diffuse* back and forth between the blood and the tissue spaces, as shown by the arrows. This process of diffusion is caused by kinetic motion of the molecules in both

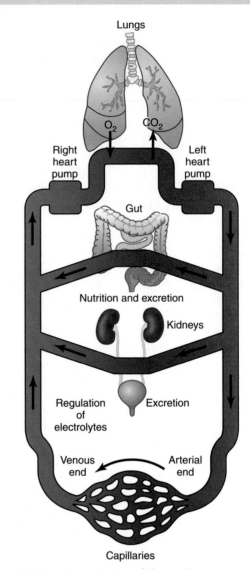

Figure 1-1 General organization of the circulatory system.

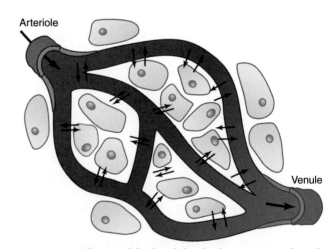

Figure 1-2 Diffusion of fluid and dissolved constituents through the capillary walls and through the interstitial spaces.

the plasma and the interstitial fluid. That is, the fluid and dissolved molecules are continually moving and bouncing in all directions within the plasma and the fluid in the intercellular spaces, as well as through the capillary pores.

Few cells are located more than 50 micrometers from a capillary, which ensures diffusion of almost any substance from the capillary to the cell within a few seconds. Thus, the extracellular fluid everywhere in the body—both that of the plasma and that of the interstitial fluid—is continually being mixed, thereby maintaining homogeneity of the extracellular fluid throughout the body.

Origin of Nutrients in the Extracellular Fluid

Respiratory System. Figure 1-1 shows that each time the blood passes through the body, it also flows through the lungs. The blood picks up oxygen in the alveoli, thus acquiring the *oxygen* needed by the cells. The membrane between the alveoli and the lumen of the pulmonary capillaries, the *alveolar membrane,* is only 0.4 to 2.0 micrometers thick, and oxygen rapidly diffuses by molecular motion through this membrane into the blood.

Gastrointestinal Tract. A large portion of the blood pumped by the heart also passes through the walls of the gastrointestinal tract. Here different dissolved nutrients, including *carbohydrates, fatty acids,* and *amino acids,* are absorbed from the ingested food into the extracellular fluid of the blood.

Liver and Other Organs That Perform Primarily Metabolic Functions. Not all substances absorbed from the gastrointestinal tract can be used in their absorbed form by the cells. The liver changes the chemical compositions of many of these substances to more usable forms, and other tissues of the body—fat cells, gastrointestinal mucosa, kidneys, and endocrine glands—help modify the absorbed substances or store them until they are needed. The liver also eliminates certain waste products produced in the body and toxic substances that are ingested.

Musculoskeletal System. How does the musculoskeletal system contribute to homeostasis? The answer is obvious and simple: Were it not for the muscles, the body could not move to the appropriate place at the appropriate time to obtain the foods required for nutrition. The musculoskeletal system also provides motility for protection against adverse surroundings, without which the entire body, along with its homeostatic mechanisms, could be destroyed instantaneously.

Removal of Metabolic End Products

Removal of Carbon Dioxide by the Lungs. At the same time that blood picks up oxygen in the lungs, *carbon dioxide* is released from the blood into the lung alveoli; the respiratory movement of air into and out of the lungs carries the carbon dioxide to the atmosphere. Carbon dioxide is the most abundant of all the end products of metabolism.

Kidneys. Passage of the blood through the kidneys removes from the plasma most of the other substances besides carbon dioxide that are not needed by the cells.

These substances include different end products of cellular metabolism, such as urea and uric acid; they also include excesses of ions and water from the food that might have accumulated in the extracellular fluid.

The kidneys perform their function by first filtering large quantities of plasma through the glomeruli into the tubules and then reabsorbing into the blood those substances needed by the body, such as glucose, amino acids, appropriate amounts of water, and many of the ions. Most of the other substances that are not needed by the body, especially the metabolic end products such as urea, are reabsorbed poorly and pass through the renal tubules into the urine.

Gastrointestinal Tract. Undigested material that enters the gastrointestinal tract and some waste products of metabolism are eliminated in the feces.

Liver. Among the functions of the liver is the detoxification or removal of many drugs and chemicals that are ingested. The liver secretes many of these wastes into the bile to be eventually eliminated in the feces.

Regulation of Body Functions

Nervous System. The nervous system is composed of three major parts: the *sensory input portion,* the *central nervous system* (or *integrative portion*), and the *motor output portion.* Sensory receptors detect the state of the body or the state of the surroundings. For instance, receptors in the skin apprise one whenever an object touches the skin at any point. The eyes are sensory organs that give one a visual image of the surrounding area. The ears are also sensory organs. The central nervous system is composed of the brain and spinal cord. The brain can store information, generate thoughts, create ambition, and determine reactions that the body performs in response to the sensations. Appropriate signals are then transmitted through the motor output portion of the nervous system to carry out one's desires.

An important segment of the nervous system is called the *autonomic system.* It operates at a subconscious level and controls many functions of the internal organs, including the level of pumping activity by the heart, movements of the gastrointestinal tract, and secretion by many of the body's glands.

Hormone Systems. Located in the body are eight major *endocrine glands* that secrete chemical substances called *hormones.* Hormones are transported in the extracellular fluid to all parts of the body to help regulate cellular function. For instance, *thyroid hormone* increases the rates of most chemical reactions in all cells, thus helping to set the tempo of bodily activity. *Insulin* controls glucose metabolism; *adrenocortical hormones* control sodium ion, potassium ion, and protein metabolism; and *parathyroid hormone* controls bone calcium and phosphate. Thus, the hormones provide a system for regulation that complements the nervous system. The nervous system regulates many muscular and secretory activities of the body, whereas the hormonal system regulates many metabolic functions.

Protection of the Body

Immune System. The immune system consists of the white blood cells, tissue cells derived from white blood cells, the thymus, lymph nodes, and lymph vessels that protect the body from pathogens such as bacteria, viruses, parasites, and fungi. The immune system provides a mechanism for the body to (1) distinguish its own cells from foreign cells and substances and (2) destroy the invader by *phagocytosis* or by producing *sensitized lymphocytes* or specialized proteins (e.g., *antibodies)* that either destroy or neutralize the invader.

Integumentary System. The skin and its various appendages, including the hair, nails, glands, and other structures, cover, cushion, and protect the deeper tissues and organs of the body and generally provide a boundary between the body's internal environment and the outside world. The integumentary system is also important for temperature regulation and excretion of wastes and it provides a sensory interface between the body and the external environment. The skin generally comprises about 12 to 15 percent of body weight.

Reproduction

Sometimes reproduction is not considered a homeostatic function. It does, however, help maintain homeostasis by generating new beings to take the place of those that are dying. This may sound like a permissive usage of the term *homeostasis,* but it illustrates that, in the final analysis, essentially all body structures are organized such that they help maintain the automaticity and continuity of life.

Control Systems of the Body

The human body has thousands of control systems. The most intricate of these are the genetic control systems that operate in all cells to help control intracellular function and extracellular functions. This subject is discussed in Chapter 3.

Many other control systems operate *within the organs* to control functions of the individual parts of the organs; others operate throughout the entire body *to control the interrelations between the organs.* For instance, the respiratory system, operating in association with the nervous system, regulates the concentration of carbon dioxide in the extracellular fluid. The liver and pancreas regulate the concentration of glucose in the extracellular fluid, and the kidneys regulate concentrations of hydrogen, sodium, potassium, phosphate, and other ions in the extracellular fluid.

Examples of Control Mechanisms

Regulation of Oxygen and Carbon Dioxide Concentrations in the Extracellular Fluid. Because oxygen is one of the major substances required for chemical reactions in the cells, the body has a special control mechanism to maintain an almost exact and constant oxygen concentration in the extracellular fluid. This mechanism depends principally on the chemical characteristics of *hemoglobin,* which is present in all red blood cells. Hemoglobin combines with oxygen as the blood passes through the lungs. Then, as the blood passes through the tissue capillaries, hemoglobin, because of its own strong chemical affinity for oxygen, does not release oxygen into the tissue fluid if too much oxygen is already there. But if the oxygen concentration in the tissue fluid is too low, sufficient oxygen is released to re-establish an adequate concentration. Thus, regulation of oxygen concentration in the tissues is vested principally in the chemical characteristics of hemoglobin itself. This regulation is called the *oxygen-buffering function of hemoglobin.*

Carbon dioxide concentration in the extracellular fluid is regulated in a much different way. Carbon dioxide is a major end product of the oxidative reactions in cells. If all the carbon dioxide formed in the cells continued to accumulate in the tissue fluids, all energy-giving reactions of the cells would cease. Fortunately, a higher than normal carbon dioxide concentration in the blood *excites the respiratory center,* causing a person to breathe rapidly and deeply. This increases expiration of carbon dioxide and, therefore, removes excess carbon dioxide from the blood and tissue fluids. This process continues until the concentration returns to normal.

Regulation of Arterial Blood Pressure. Several systems contribute to the regulation of arterial blood pressure. One of these, the *baroreceptor system,* is a simple and excellent example of a rapidly acting control mechanism. In the walls of the bifurcation region of the carotid arteries in the neck, and also in the arch of the aorta in the thorax, are many nerve receptors called *baroreceptors,* which are stimulated by stretch of the arterial wall. When the arterial pressure rises too high, the baroreceptors send barrages of nerve impulses to the medulla of the brain. Here these impulses inhibit the *vasomotor center,* which in turn decreases the number of impulses transmitted from the vasomotor center through the sympathetic nervous system to the heart and blood vessels. Lack of these impulses causes diminished pumping activity by the heart and also dilation of the peripheral blood vessels, allowing increased blood flow through the vessels. Both of these effects decrease the arterial pressure back toward normal.

Conversely, a decrease in arterial pressure below normal relaxes the stretch receptors, allowing the vasomotor center to become more active than usual, thereby causing vasoconstriction and increased heart pumping. The decrease in arterial pressure also raises arterial pressure back toward normal.

Normal Ranges and Physical Characteristics of Important Extracellular Fluid Constituents

Table 1-1 lists some of the important constituents and physical characteristics of extracellular fluid, along with their normal values, normal ranges, and maximum limits without causing death. Note the narrowness of the normal range for each one. Values outside these ranges are usually caused by illness.

Most important are the limits beyond which abnormalities can cause death. For example, an increase in the body temperature of only 11°F (7°C) above normal can lead to a vicious cycle of increasing cellular metabolism that destroys the cells. Note also the narrow range for acid-base balance in the body, with a normal pH value of 7.4 and lethal values only about 0.5 on either side of normal. Another important factor is the potassium ion concentration because whenever it decreases to less than one-third normal, a person is likely to be paralyzed as a result of the nerves' inability to carry signals. Alternatively, if the potassium ion concentration increases to two or more times normal, the heart muscle is likely to be severely depressed. Also, when the calcium ion concentration falls below about one-half normal, a person is likely to experience tetanic contraction of muscles throughout the body because of the spontaneous generation of excess nerve impulses in the peripheral nerves. When the glucose concentration falls below one-half normal, a person frequently develops extreme mental irritability and sometimes even convulsions.

These examples should give one an appreciation for the extreme value and even the necessity of the vast numbers of control systems that keep the body operating in health; in the absence of any one of these controls, serious body malfunction or death can result.

Characteristics of Control Systems

The aforementioned examples of homeostatic control mechanisms are only a few of the many thousands in the body, all of which have certain characteristics in common as explained in this section.

Negative Feedback Nature of Most Control Systems

Most control systems of the body act by *negative feedback*, which can best be explained by reviewing some of the homeostatic control systems mentioned previously. In the regulation of carbon dioxide concentration, a high concentration of carbon dioxide in the extracellular fluid increases pulmonary ventilation. This, in turn, decreases the extracellular fluid carbon dioxide concentration because the lungs expire greater amounts of carbon dioxide from the body. In other words, the high concentration of carbon dioxide initiates events that decrease the concentration toward normal, which is *negative* to the initiating stimulus. Conversely, if the carbon dioxide concentration falls too low, this causes feedback to increase the concentration. This response is also negative to the initiating stimulus.

In the arterial pressure-regulating mechanisms, a high pressure causes a series of reactions that promote a lowered pressure, or a low pressure causes a series of reactions that promote an elevated pressure. In both instances, these effects are negative with respect to the initiating stimulus.

Therefore, in general, if some factor becomes excessive or deficient, a control system initiates *negative feedback*, which consists of a series of changes that return the factor toward a certain mean value, thus maintaining homeostasis.

"Gain" of a Control System. The degree of effectiveness with which a control system maintains constant conditions is determined by the *gain* of the negative feedback. For instance, let us assume that a large volume of blood is transfused into a person whose baroreceptor pressure control system is not functioning, and the arterial pressure rises from the normal level of 100 mm Hg up to 175 mm Hg. Then, let us assume that the same volume of blood is injected into the same person when the baroreceptor system is functioning, and this time the pressure increases only 25 mm Hg. Thus, the feedback control system has caused a "correction" of –50 mm Hg—that is, from

Table 1-1 Important Constituents and Physical Characteristics of Extracellular Fluid

	Normal Value	Normal Range	Approximate Short-Term Nonlethal Limit	Unit
Oxygen	40	35-45	10-1000	mm Hg
Carbon dioxide	40	35-45	5-80	mm Hg
Sodium ion	142	138-146	115-175	mmol/L
Potassium ion	4.2	3.8-5.0	1.5-9.0	mmol/L
Calcium ion	1.2	1.0-1.4	0.5-2.0	mmol/L
Chloride ion	108	103-112	70-130	mmol/L
Bicarbonate ion	28	24-32	8-45	mmol/L
Glucose	85	75-95	20-1500	mg/dl
Body temperature	98.4 (37.0)	98-98.8 (37.0)	65-110 (18.3-43.3)	°F (°C)
Acid-base	7.4	7.3-7.5	6.9-8.0	pH

175 mm Hg to 125 mm Hg. There remains an increase in pressure of +25 mm Hg, called the "error," which means that the control system is not 100 percent effective in preventing change. The gain of the system is then calculated by the following formula:

$$\text{Gain} = \frac{\text{Correction}}{\text{Error}}$$

Thus, in the baroreceptor system example, the correction is –50 mm Hg and the error persisting is +25 mm Hg. Therefore, the gain of the person's baroreceptor system for control of arterial pressure is –50 divided by +25, or –2. That is, a disturbance that increases or decreases the arterial pressure does so only one-third as much as would occur if this control system were not present.

The gains of some other physiologic control systems are much greater than that of the baroreceptor system. For instance, the gain of the system controlling internal body temperature when a person is exposed to moderately cold weather is about –33. Therefore, one can see that the temperature control system is much more effective than the baroreceptor pressure control system.

Positive Feedback Can Sometimes Cause Vicious Cycles and Death

One might ask the question, Why do most control systems of the body operate by negative feedback rather than positive feedback? If one considers the nature of positive feedback, one immediately sees that positive feedback does not lead to stability but to instability and, in some cases, can cause death.

Figure 1-3 shows an example in which death can ensue from positive feedback. This figure depicts the pumping effectiveness of the heart, showing that the heart of a healthy human being pumps about 5 liters of blood per minute. If the person is suddenly bled 2 liters, the amount of blood in the body is decreased to such a low level that not enough blood is available for the heart to pump effectively. As a result, the arterial pressure falls and the flow of blood to the heart muscle through the coronary vessels diminishes. This results in weakening of the heart, further diminished pumping, a further decrease in coronary blood flow, and still more weakness of the heart; the cycle repeats itself again and again until death occurs. Note that each cycle in the feedback results in further weakening of the heart. In other words, the initiating stimulus causes more of the same, which is *positive feedback.*

Positive feedback is better known as a "vicious cycle," but a mild degree of positive feedback can be overcome by the negative feedback control mechanisms of the body and the vicious cycle fails to develop. For instance, if the person in the aforementioned example were bled only 1 liter instead of 2 liters, the normal negative feedback mechanisms for controlling cardiac output and arterial pressure would overbalance the positive feedback and the person would recover, as shown by the dashed curve of Figure 1-3.

Positive Feedback Can Sometimes Be Useful. In some instances, the body uses positive feedback to its advantage. Blood clotting is an example of a valuable use of positive feedback. When a blood vessel is ruptured and a clot begins to form, multiple enzymes called *clotting factors* are activated within the clot itself. Some of these enzymes act on other unactivated enzymes of the immediately adjacent blood, thus causing more blood clotting. This process continues until the hole in the vessel is plugged and bleeding no longer occurs. On occasion, this mechanism can get out of hand and cause the formation of unwanted clots. In fact, this is what initiates most acute heart attacks, which are caused by a clot beginning on the inside surface of an atherosclerotic plaque in a coronary artery and then growing until the artery is blocked.

Childbirth is another instance in which positive feedback plays a valuable role. When uterine contractions become strong enough for the baby's head to begin pushing through the cervix, stretch of the cervix sends signals through the uterine muscle back to the body of the uterus, causing even more powerful contractions. Thus, the uterine contractions stretch the cervix and the cervical stretch causes stronger contractions. When this process becomes powerful enough, the baby is born. If it is not powerful enough, the contractions usually die out and a few days pass before they begin again.

Another important use of positive feedback is for the generation of nerve signals. That is, when the membrane of a nerve fiber is stimulated, this causes slight leakage of sodium ions through sodium channels in the nerve membrane to the fiber's interior. The sodium ions entering the fiber then change the membrane potential, which in turn causes more opening of channels, more change of potential, still more opening of channels, and so forth. Thus, a slight leak becomes an explosion of sodium entering the interior of the nerve fiber, which creates the nerve action potential. This action potential in turn causes electrical current to flow along both the outside and the inside

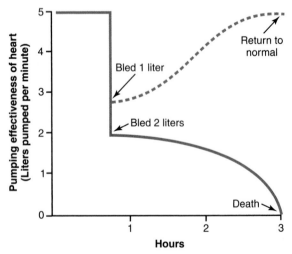

Figure 1-3 Recovery of heart pumping caused by *negative feedback* after 1 liter of blood is removed from the circulation. Death is caused by *positive feedback* when 2 liters of blood are removed.

of the fiber and initiates additional action potentials. This process continues again and again until the nerve signal goes all the way to the end of the fiber.

In each case in which positive feedback is useful, the positive feedback itself is part of an overall negative feedback process. For example, in the case of blood clotting, the positive feedback clotting process is a negative feedback process for maintenance of normal blood volume. Also, the positive feedback that causes nerve signals allows the nerves to participate in thousands of negative feedback nervous control systems.

More Complex Types of Control Systems—Adaptive Control

Later in this text, when we study the nervous system, we shall see that this system contains great numbers of interconnected control mechanisms. Some are simple feedback systems similar to those already discussed. Many are not. For instance, some movements of the body occur so rapidly that there is not enough time for nerve signals to travel from the peripheral parts of the body all the way to the brain and then back to the periphery again to control the movement. Therefore, the brain uses a principle called *feed-forward control* to cause required muscle contractions. That is, sensory nerve signals from the moving parts apprise the brain whether the movement is performed correctly. If not, the brain corrects the feed-forward signals that it sends to the muscles the *next* time the movement is required. Then, if still further correction is necessary, this will be done again for subsequent movements. This is called *adaptive control*. Adaptive control, in a sense, is delayed negative feedback.

Thus, one can see how complex the feedback control systems of the body can be. A person's life depends on all of them. Therefore, a major share of this text is devoted to discussing these life-giving mechanisms.

Summary—Automaticity of the Body

The purpose of this chapter has been to point out, first, the overall organization of the body and, second, the means by which the different parts of the body operate in harmony. To summarize, the body is actually a *social order of about 100 trillion cells* organized into different functional structures, some of which are called *organs*. Each functional structure contributes its share to the maintenance of homeostatic conditions in the extracellular fluid, which is called the *internal environment*. As long as normal conditions are maintained in this internal environment, the cells of the body continue to live and function properly. Each cell benefits from homeostasis, and in turn, each cell contributes its share toward the maintenance of homeostasis. This reciprocal interplay provides continuous automaticity of the body until one or more functional systems lose their ability to contribute their share of function. When this happens, all the cells of the body suffer. Extreme dysfunction leads to death; moderate dysfunction leads to sickness.

Bibliography

Adolph EF: Physiological adaptations: hypertrophies and superfunctions, *Am Sci* 60:608, 1972.

Bernard C: *Lectures on the Phenomena of Life Common to Animals and Plants*, Springfield, IL, 1974, Charles C Thomas.

Cannon WB: *The Wisdom of the Body*, New York, 1932, WW Norton.

Chien S: Mechanotransduction and endothelial cell homeostasis: the wisdom of the cell, *Am J Physiol Heart Circ Physiol* 292:H1209, 2007.

Csete ME, Doyle JC: Reverse engineering of biological complexity, *Science* 295:1664, 2002.

Danzler WH, editor: *Handbook of Physiology, Sec 13: Comparative Physiology*, Bethesda, 1997, American Physiological Society.

DiBona GF: Physiology in perspective: the wisdom of the body. Neural control of the kidney, *Am J Physiol Regul Integr Comp Physiol* 289:R633, 2005.

Dickinson MH, Farley CT, Full RJ, et al: How animals move: an integrative view, *Science* 288:100, 2000.

Garland T Jr, Carter PA: Evolutionary physiology, *Annu Rev Physiol* 56:579, 1994.

Gao Q, Horvath TL: Neuronal control of energy homeostasis, *FEBS Lett* 582:132, 2008.

Guyton AC: *Arterial Pressure and Hypertension*, Philadelphia, 1980, WB Saunders.

Guyton AC, Jones CE, Coleman TG: *Cardiac Output and Its Regulation*, Philadelphia, 1973, WB Saunders.

Guyton AC, Taylor AE, Granger HJ: *Dynamics and Control of the Body Fluids*, Philadelphia, 1975, WB Saunders.

Herman MA, Kahn BB: Glucose transport and sensing in the maintenance of glucose homeostasis and metabolic harmony, *J Clin Invest* 116:1767, 2006.

Krahe R, Gabbiani F: Burst firing in sensory systems, *Nat Rev Neurosci* 5:13, 2004.

Orgel LE: The origin of life on the earth, *Sci Am* 271:76, 1994.

Quarles LD: Endocrine functions of bone in mineral metabolism regulation, *J Clin Invest* 118:3820, 2008.

Smith HW: *From Fish to Philosopher*, New York, 1961, Doubleday.

Tjian R: Molecular machines that control genes, *Sci Am* 272:54, 1995.

9

The Cell and Its Functions

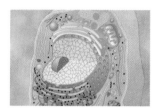

Each of the 100 trillion cells in a human being is a living structure that can survive for months or many years, provided its surrounding fluids contain appropriate nutrients. To understand the function of organs and other structures of the body, it is essential that we first understand the basic organization of the cell and the functions of its component parts.

Organization of the Cell

A typical cell, as seen by the light microscope, is shown in Figure 2-1. Its two major parts are the *nucleus* and the *cytoplasm.* The nucleus is separated from the cytoplasm by a *nuclear membrane,* and the cytoplasm is separated from the surrounding fluids by a *cell membrane,* also called the *plasma membrane.*

The different substances that make up the cell are collectively called *protoplasm.* Protoplasm is composed mainly of five basic substances: water, electrolytes, proteins, lipids, and carbohydrates.

Water. The principal fluid medium of the cell is water, which is present in most cells, except for fat cells, in a concentration of 70 to 85 percent. Many cellular chemicals are dissolved in the water. Others are suspended in the water as solid particulates. Chemical reactions take place among the dissolved chemicals or at the surfaces of the suspended particles or membranes.

Ions. Important ions in the cell include *potassium, magnesium, phosphate, sulfate, bicarbonate,* and smaller quantities of *sodium, chloride,* and *calcium.* These are all discussed in more detail in Chapter 4, which considers the interrelations between the intracellular and extracellular fluids.

The ions provide inorganic chemicals for cellular reactions. Also, they are necessary for operation of some of the cellular control mechanisms. For instance, ions acting at the cell membrane are required for transmission of electrochemical impulses in nerve and muscle fibers.

Proteins. After water, the most abundant substances in most cells are proteins, which normally constitute 10 to 20 percent of the cell mass. These can be divided into two types: *structural proteins* and *functional proteins.*

Structural proteins are present in the cell mainly in the form of long filaments that are polymers of many individual protein molecules. A prominent use of such intracellular filaments is to form *microtubules* that provide the "cytoskeletons" of such cellular organelles as cilia, nerve axons, the mitotic spindles of mitosing cells, and a tangled mass of thin filamentous tubules that hold the parts of the cytoplasm and nucleoplasm together in their respective compartments. Extracellularly, fibrillar proteins are found especially in the collagen and elastin fibers of connective tissue and in blood vessel walls, tendons, ligaments, and so forth.

The *functional proteins* are an entirely different type of protein, usually composed of combinations of a few molecules in tubular-globular form. These proteins are mainly the *enzymes* of the cell and, in contrast to the fibrillar proteins, are often mobile in the cell fluid. Also, many of them are adherent to membranous structures inside the cell. The enzymes come into direct contact with other substances in the cell fluid and thereby catalyze specific intracellular chemical reactions. For instance, the chemical reactions that split glucose into its component parts and then combine these with oxygen to form carbon dioxide and water while simultaneously providing energy for cellular function are all catalyzed by a series of protein enzymes.

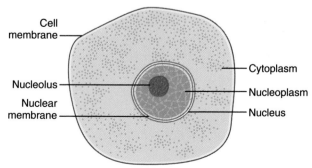

Figure 2-1 Structure of the cell as seen with the light microscope.

Lipids. Lipids are several types of substances that are grouped together because of their common property of being soluble in fat solvents. Especially important lipids are *phospholipids* and *cholesterol,* which together constitute only about 2 percent of the total cell mass. The significance of phospholipids and cholesterol is that they are mainly insoluble in water and, therefore, are used to form the cell membrane and intracellular membrane barriers that separate the different cell compartments.

In addition to phospholipids and cholesterol, some cells contain large quantities of *triglycerides,* also called *neutral fat.* In the *fat cells,* triglycerides often account for as much as 95 percent of the cell mass. The fat stored in these cells represents the body's main storehouse of energy-giving nutrients that can later be dissoluted and used to provide energy wherever in the body it is needed.

Carbohydrates. Carbohydrates have little structural function in the cell except as parts of glycoprotein molecules, but they play a major role in nutrition of the cell. Most human cells do not maintain large stores of carbohydrates; the amount usually averages about 1 percent of their total mass but increases to as much as 3 percent in muscle cells and, occasionally, 6 percent in liver cells. However, carbohydrate in the form of dissolved glucose is always present in the surrounding extracellular fluid so that it is readily available to the cell. Also, a small amount of carbohydrate is stored in the cells in the form of *glycogen,* which is an insoluble polymer of glucose that can be depolymerized and used rapidly to supply the cells' energy needs.

Physical Structure of the Cell

The cell is not merely a bag of fluid, enzymes, and chemicals; it also contains highly organized physical structures, called *intracellular organelles.* The physical nature of each organelle is as important as the cell's chemical constituents for cell function. For instance, without one of the organelles, the *mitochondria,* more than 95 percent of the cell's energy release from nutrients would cease immediately. The most important organelles and other structures of the cell are shown in Figure 2-2.

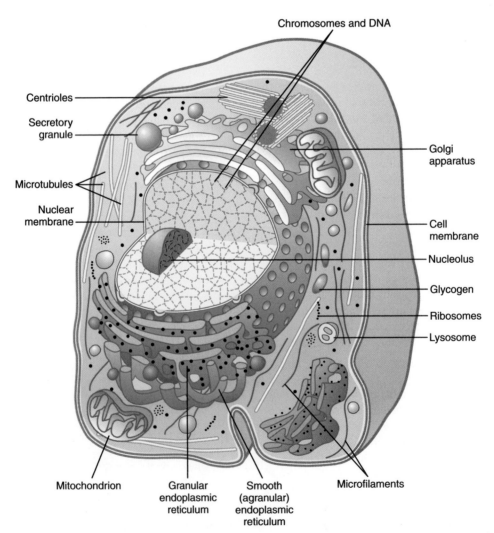

Figure 2-2 Reconstruction of a typical cell, showing the internal organelles in the cytoplasm and in the nucleus.

Membranous Structures of the Cell

Most organelles of the cell are covered by membranes composed primarily of lipids and proteins. These membranes include the *cell membrane, nuclear membrane, membrane of the endoplasmic reticulum,* and *membranes of the mitochondria, lysosomes,* and *Golgi apparatus.*

The lipids of the membranes provide a barrier that impedes the movement of water and water-soluble substances from one cell compartment to another because water is not soluble in lipids. However, protein molecules in the membrane often do penetrate all the way through the membrane, thus providing specialized pathways, often organized into actual *pores,* for passage of specific substances through the membrane. Also, many other membrane proteins are *enzymes* that catalyze a multitude of different chemical reactions, discussed here and in subsequent chapters.

Cell Membrane

The cell membrane (also called the *plasma membrane*), which envelops the cell, is a thin, pliable, elastic structure only 7.5 to 10 nanometers thick. It is composed almost entirely of proteins and lipids. The approximate composition is proteins, 55 percent; phospholipids, 25 percent; cholesterol, 13 percent; other lipids, 4 percent; and carbohydrates, 3 percent.

Lipid Barrier of the Cell Membrane Impedes Water Penetration. Figure 2-3 shows the structure of the cell membrane. Its basic structure is a *lipid bilayer,* which is a thin, double-layered film of lipids—each layer only one molecule thick—that is continuous over the entire cell surface. Interspersed in this lipid film are large globular protein molecules.

The basic lipid bilayer is composed of phospholipid molecules. One end of each phospholipid molecule is soluble in water; that is, it is *hydrophilic.* The other end is soluble only in fats; that is, it is *hydrophobic.* The phosphate end of the phospholipid is hydrophilic, and the fatty acid portion is hydrophobic.

Because the hydrophobic portions of the phospholipid molecules are repelled by water but are mutually attracted to one another, they have a natural tendency to attach to one another in the middle of the membrane, as shown in Figure 2-3. The hydrophilic phosphate portions then constitute the two surfaces of the complete cell membrane, in contact with *intracellular* water on the inside of the membrane and *extracellular* water on the outside surface.

The lipid layer in the middle of the membrane is impermeable to the usual water-soluble substances, such as ions, glucose, and urea. Conversely, fat-soluble substances, such as oxygen, carbon dioxide, and alcohol, can penetrate this portion of the membrane with ease.

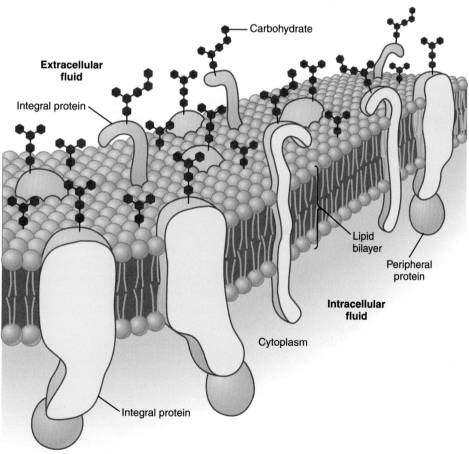

Figure 2-3 Structure of the cell membrane, showing that it is composed mainly of a lipid bilayer of phospholipid molecules, but with large numbers of protein molecules protruding through the layer. Also, carbohydrate moieties are attached to the protein molecules on the outside of the membrane and to additional protein molecules on the inside. (Redrawn from Lodish HF, Rothman JE: The assembly of cell membranes. Sci Am 240:48, 1979. Copyright George V. Kevin.)

The cholesterol molecules in the membrane are also lipid in nature because their steroid nucleus is highly fat soluble. These molecules, in a sense, are dissolved in the bilayer of the membrane. They mainly help determine the degree of permeability (or impermeability) of the bilayer to water-soluble constituents of body fluids. Cholesterol controls much of the fluidity of the membrane as well.

Integral and Peripheral Cell Membrane Proteins. Figure 2-3 also shows globular masses floating in the lipid bilayer. These are membrane proteins, most of which are *glycoproteins*. There are two types of cell membrane proteins: *integral proteins* that protrude all the way through the membrane and *peripheral proteins* that are attached only to one surface of the membrane and do not penetrate all the way through.

Many of the integral proteins provide structural *channels* (or *pores*) through which water molecules and water-soluble substances, especially ions, can diffuse between the extracellular and intracellular fluids. These protein channels also have selective properties that allow preferential diffusion of some substances over others.

Other integral proteins act as *carrier proteins* for transporting substances that otherwise could not penetrate the lipid bilayer. Sometimes these even transport substances in the direction opposite to their electrochemical gradients for diffusion, which is called "active transport." Still others act as *enzymes*.

Integral membrane proteins can also serve as *receptors* for water-soluble chemicals, such as peptide hormones, that do not easily penetrate the cell membrane. Interaction of cell membrane receptors with specific *ligands* that bind to the receptor causes conformational changes in the receptor protein. This, in turn, enzymatically activates the intracellular part of the protein or induces interactions between the receptor and proteins in the cytoplasm that act as *second messengers*, thereby relaying the signal from the extracellular part of the receptor to the interior of the cell. In this way, integral proteins spanning the cell membrane provide a means of conveying information about the environment to the cell interior.

Peripheral protein molecules are often attached to the integral proteins. These peripheral proteins function almost entirely as enzymes or as controllers of transport of substances through the cell membrane "pores."

Membrane Carbohydrates—The Cell "Glycocalyx." Membrane carbohydrates occur almost invariably in combination with proteins or lipids in the form of *glycoproteins* or *glycolipids.* In fact, most of the integral proteins are glycoproteins, and about one tenth of the membrane lipid molecules are glycolipids. The "glyco" portions of these molecules almost invariably protrude to the outside of the cell, dangling outward from the cell surface. Many other carbohydrate compounds, called *proteoglycans*—which are mainly carbohydrate substances bound to small protein cores—are loosely attached to the outer surface of the cell as well. Thus, the entire outside surface of the cell often has a loose carbohydrate coat called the *glycocalyx.*

The carbohydrate moieties attached to the outer surface of the cell have several important functions: (1) Many of them have a negative electrical charge, which gives most cells an overall negative surface charge that repels other negative objects. (2) The glycocalyx of some cells attaches to the glycocalyx of other cells, thus attaching cells to one another. (3) Many of the carbohydrates act as *receptor substances* for binding hormones, such as insulin; when bound, this combination activates attached internal proteins that, in turn, activate a cascade of intracellular enzymes. (4) Some carbohydrate moieties enter into immune reactions, as discussed in Chapter 34.

Cytoplasm and Its Organelles

The cytoplasm is filled with both minute and large dispersed particles and organelles. The clear fluid portion of the cytoplasm in which the particles are dispersed is called *cytosol;* this contains mainly dissolved proteins, electrolytes, and glucose.

Dispersed in the cytoplasm are neutral fat globules, glycogen granules, ribosomes, secretory vesicles, and five especially important organelles: the *endoplasmic reticulum,* the *Golgi apparatus, mitochondria, lysosomes,* and *peroxisomes.*

Endoplasmic Reticulum

Figure 2-2 shows a network of tubular and flat vesicular structures in the cytoplasm; this is the *endoplasmic reticulum.* The tubules and vesicles interconnect with one another. Also, their walls are constructed of lipid bilayer membranes that contain large amounts of proteins, similar to the cell membrane. The total surface area of this structure in some cells—the liver cells, for instance—can be as much as 30 to 40 times the cell membrane area.

The detailed structure of a small portion of endoplasmic reticulum is shown in Figure 2-4. The space inside the tubules and vesicles is filled with *endoplasmic matrix,* a watery medium that is different from the fluid in the cytosol outside the endoplasmic reticulum. Electron micrographs show that the space inside the endoplasmic reticulum is connected with the space between the two membrane surfaces of the nuclear membrane.

Substances formed in some parts of the cell enter the space of the endoplasmic reticulum and are then conducted to other parts of the cell. Also, the vast surface area of this reticulum and the multiple enzyme systems attached to its membranes provide machinery for a major share of the metabolic functions of the cell.

Ribosomes and the Granular Endoplasmic Reticulum. Attached to the outer surfaces of many parts of the endoplasmic reticulum are large numbers of minute granular particles called *ribosomes.* Where these are present, the reticulum is called the *granular endoplasmic reticulum.* The ribosomes are composed of a mixture of RNA and proteins, and they function to synthesize new protein molecules in the cell, as discussed later in this chapter and in Chapter 3.

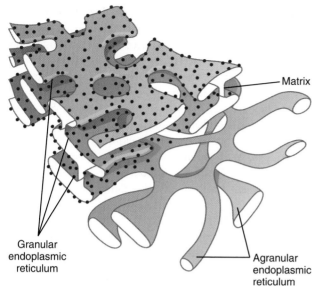

Figure 2-4 Structure of the endoplasmic reticulum. (Modified from DeRobertis EDP, Saez FA, DeRobertis EMF: Cell Biology, 6th ed. Philadelphia: WB Saunders, 1975.)

Agranular Endoplasmic Reticulum. Part of the endoplasmic reticulum has no attached ribosomes. This part is called the *agranular,* or *smooth, endoplasmic reticulum.* The agranular reticulum functions for the synthesis of lipid substances and for other processes of the cells promoted by intrareticular enzymes.

Golgi Apparatus

The Golgi apparatus, shown in Figure 2-5, is closely related to the endoplasmic reticulum. It has membranes similar to those of the agranular endoplasmic reticulum. It is usually composed of four or more stacked layers of thin, flat, enclosed vesicles lying near one side of the nucleus. This apparatus is prominent in secretory cells, where it is located on the side of the cell from which the secretory substances are extruded.

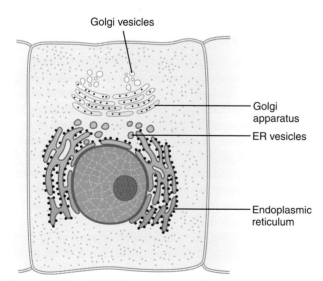

Figure 2-5 A typical Golgi apparatus and its relationship to the endoplasmic reticulum (ER) and the nucleus.

The Golgi apparatus functions in association with the endoplasmic reticulum. As shown in Figure 2-5, small "transport vesicles" (also called endoplasmic reticulum vesicles, or *ER vesicles*) continually pinch off from the endoplasmic reticulum and shortly thereafter fuse with the Golgi apparatus. In this way, substances entrapped in the ER vesicles are transported from the endoplasmic reticulum to the Golgi apparatus. The transported substances are then processed in the Golgi apparatus to form lysosomes, secretory vesicles, and other cytoplasmic components that are discussed later in the chapter.

Lysosomes

Lysosomes, shown in Figure 2-2, are vesicular organelles that form by breaking off from the Golgi apparatus and then dispersing throughout the cytoplasm. The lysosomes provide an *intracellular digestive system* that allows the cell to digest (1) damaged cellular structures, (2) food particles that have been ingested by the cell, and (3) unwanted matter such as bacteria. The lysosome is quite different in different cell types, but it is usually 250 to 750 nanometers in diameter. It is surrounded by a typical lipid bilayer membrane and is filled with large numbers of small granules 5 to 8 nanometers in diameter, which are protein aggregates of as many as 40 different *hydrolase (digestive) enzymes.* A hydrolytic enzyme is capable of splitting an organic compound into two or more parts by combining hydrogen from a water molecule with one part of the compound and combining the hydroxyl portion of the water molecule with the other part of the compound. For instance, protein is hydrolyzed to form amino acids, glycogen is hydrolyzed to form glucose, and lipids are hydrolyzed to form fatty acids and glycerol.

Ordinarily, the membrane surrounding the lysosome prevents the enclosed hydrolytic enzymes from coming in contact with other substances in the cell and, therefore, prevents their digestive actions. However, some conditions of the cell break the membranes of some of the lysosomes, allowing release of the digestive enzymes. These enzymes then split the organic substances with which they come in contact into small, highly diffusible substances such as amino acids and glucose. Some of the specific functions of lysosomes are discussed later in the chapter.

Peroxisomes

Peroxisomes are similar physically to lysosomes, but they are different in two important ways. First, they are believed to be formed by self-replication (or perhaps by budding off from the smooth endoplasmic reticulum) rather than from the Golgi apparatus. Second, they contain oxidases rather than hydrolases. Several of the oxidases are capable of combining oxygen with hydrogen ions derived from different intracellular chemicals to form hydrogen peroxide (H_2O_2). Hydrogen peroxide is a highly oxidizing substance and is used in association with *catalase,* another oxidase enzyme present in large quantities in peroxisomes, to oxidize many substances that might otherwise be poisonous to the cell. For instance, about half the alcohol a person drinks is detoxified by the peroxisomes of the liver cells in this manner.

Secretory Vesicles

One of the important functions of many cells is secretion of special chemical substances. Almost all such secretory substances are formed by the endoplasmic reticulum–Golgi apparatus system and are then released from the Golgi apparatus into the cytoplasm in the form of storage vesicles called *secretory vesicles* or *secretory granules.* Figure 2-6 shows typical secretory vesicles inside pancreatic acinar cells; these vesicles store protein proenzymes (enzymes that are not yet activated). The proenzymes are secreted later through the outer cell membrane into the pancreatic duct and thence into the duodenum, where they become activated and perform digestive functions on the food in the intestinal tract.

Mitochondria

The mitochondria, shown in Figures 2-2 and 2-7, are called the "powerhouses" of the cell. Without them, cells would be unable to extract enough energy from the nutrients, and essentially all cellular functions would cease.

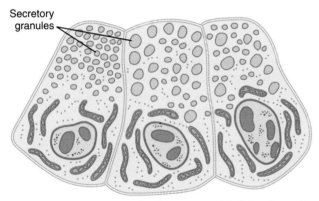

Figure 2-6 Secretory granules (secretory vesicles) in acinar cells of the pancreas.

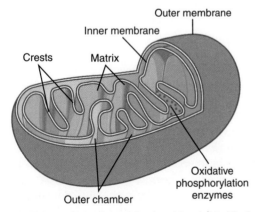

Figure 2-7 Structure of a mitochondrion. (Modified from DeRobertis EDP, Saez FA, DeRobertis EMF: Cell Biology, 6th ed. Philadelphia: WB Saunders, 1975.)

Mitochondria are present in all areas of each cell's cytoplasm, but the total number per cell varies from less than a hundred up to several thousand, depending on the amount of energy required by the cell. Further, the mitochondria are concentrated in those portions of the cell that are responsible for the major share of its energy metabolism. They are also variable in size and shape. Some are only a few hundred nanometers in diameter and globular in shape, whereas others are elongated—as large as 1 micrometer in diameter and 7 micrometers long; still others are branching and filamentous.

The basic structure of the mitochondrion, shown in Figure 2-7, is composed mainly of two lipid bilayer–protein membranes: an *outer membrane* and an *inner membrane.* Many infoldings of the inner membrane form *shelves* onto which oxidative enzymes are attached. In addition, the inner cavity of the mitochondrion is filled with a *matrix* that contains large quantities of dissolved enzymes that are necessary for extracting energy from nutrients. These enzymes operate in association with the oxidative enzymes on the shelves to cause oxidation of the nutrients, thereby forming carbon dioxide and water and at the same time releasing energy. The liberated energy is used to synthesize a "high-energy" substance called *adenosine triphosphate* (ATP). ATP is then transported out of the mitochondrion, and it diffuses throughout the cell to release its own energy wherever it is needed for performing cellular functions. The chemical details of ATP formation by the mitochondrion are given in Chapter 67, but some of the basic functions of ATP in the cell are introduced later in this chapter.

Mitochondria are self-replicative, which means that one mitochondrion can form a second one, a third one, and so on, whenever there is a need in the cell for increased amounts of ATP. Indeed, the mitochondria contain *DNA* similar to that found in the cell nucleus. In Chapter 3 we will see that DNA is the basic chemical of the nucleus that controls replication of the cell. The DNA of the mitochondrion plays a similar role, controlling replication of the mitochondrion.

Cell Cytoskeleton—Filament and Tubular Structures

The fibrillar proteins of the cell are usually organized into filaments or tubules. These originate as precursor protein molecules synthesized by ribosomes in the cytoplasm. The precursor molecules then polymerize to form *filaments.* As an example, large numbers of actin filaments frequently occur in the outer zone of the cytoplasm, called the *ectoplasm,* to form an elastic support for the cell membrane. Also, in muscle cells, actin and myosin filaments are organized into a special contractile machine that is the basis for muscle contraction, as discussed in detail in Chapter 6.

A special type of stiff filament composed of polymerized *tubulin* molecules is used in all cells to construct strong tubular structures, the *microtubules.* Figure 2-8 shows typical microtubules that were teased from the flagellum of a sperm.

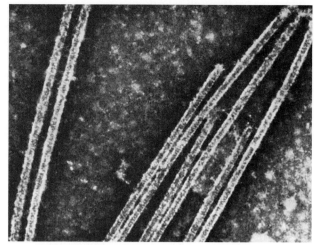

Figure 2-8 Microtubules teased from the flagellum of a sperm. (From Wolstenholme GEW, O'Connor M, and the publisher, JA Churchill, 1967. Figure 4, page 314. Copyright the Novartis Foundation, formerly the Ciba Foundation.)

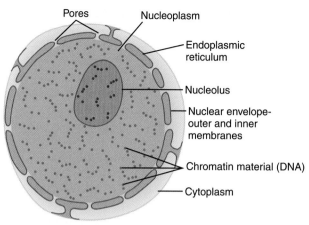

Figure 2-9 Structure of the nucleus.

Another example of microtubules is the tubular skeletal structure in the center of each cilium that radiates upward from the cell cytoplasm to the tip of the cilium. This structure is discussed later in the chapter and is illustrated in Figure 2-17. Also, both the *centrioles* and the *mitotic spindle* of the mitosing cell are composed of stiff microtubules.

Thus, a primary function of microtubules is to act as a *cytoskeleton,* providing rigid physical structures for certain parts of cells.

Nucleus

The nucleus is the control center of the cell. Briefly, the nucleus contains large quantities of DNA, which are the *genes.* The genes determine the characteristics of the cell's proteins, including the structural proteins, as well as the intracellular enzymes that control cytoplasmic and nuclear activities.

The genes also control and promote reproduction of the cell itself. The genes first reproduce to give two identical sets of genes; then the cell splits by a special process called *mitosis* to form two daughter cells, each of which receives one of the two sets of DNA genes. All these activities of the nucleus are considered in detail in the next chapter.

Unfortunately, the appearance of the nucleus under the microscope does not provide many clues to the mechanisms by which the nucleus performs its control activities. Figure 2-9 shows the light microscopic appearance of the *interphase* nucleus (during the period between mitoses), revealing darkly staining *chromatin material* throughout the nucleoplasm. During mitosis, the chromatin material organizes in the form of highly structured *chromosomes,* which can then be easily identified using the light microscope, as illustrated in the next chapter.

Nuclear Membrane

The *nuclear membrane,* also called the *nuclear envelope,* is actually two separate bilayer membranes, one inside the other. The outer membrane is continuous with the endoplasmic reticulum of the cell cytoplasm, and the space between the two nuclear membranes is also continuous with the space inside the endoplasmic reticulum, as shown in Figure 2-9.

The nuclear membrane is penetrated by several thousand *nuclear pores.* Large complexes of protein molecules are attached at the edges of the pores so that the central area of each pore is only about 9 nanometers in diameter. Even this size is large enough to allow molecules up to 44,000 molecular weight to pass through with reasonable ease.

Nucleoli and Formation of Ribosomes

The nuclei of most cells contain one or more highly staining structures called *nucleoli.* The nucleolus, unlike most other organelles discussed here, does not have a limiting membrane. Instead, it is simply an accumulation of large amounts of RNA and proteins of the types found in ribosomes. The nucleolus becomes considerably enlarged when the cell is actively synthesizing proteins.

Formation of the nucleoli (and of the ribosomes in the cytoplasm outside the nucleus) begins in the nucleus. First, specific DNA genes in the chromosomes cause RNA to be synthesized. Some of this is stored in the nucleoli, but most of it is transported outward through the nuclear pores into cytoplasm. Here, it is used in conjunction with specific proteins to assemble "mature" ribosomes that play an essential role in forming cytoplasmic proteins, as discussed more fully in Chapter 3.

Comparison of the Animal Cell with Precellular Forms of Life

The cell is a complicated organism that required many hundreds of millions of years to develop after the earliest form of life, an organism similar to the present-day *virus,* first appeared on earth. Figure 2-10 shows the relative sizes of (1) the smallest known virus, (2) a large virus, (3) a *rickettsia,* (4) a *bacterium,* and (5) a *nucleated cell,* demonstrating that the cell has a diameter about 1000 times that of the smallest virus and, therefore, a volume about

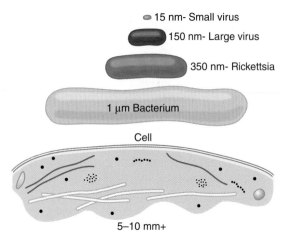

15 nm- Small virus

150 nm- Large virus

350 nm- Rickettsia

1 µm Bacterium

Cell

5–10 mm+

Figure 2-10 Comparison of sizes of precellular organisms with that of the average cell in the human body.

1 billion times that of the smallest virus. Correspondingly, the functions and anatomical organization of the cell are also far more complex than those of the virus.

The essential life-giving constituent of the small virus is a *nucleic acid* embedded in a coat of protein. This nucleic acid is composed of the same basic nucleic acid constituents (DNA or RNA) found in mammalian cells, and it is capable of reproducing itself under appropriate conditions. Thus, the virus propagates its lineage from generation to generation and is therefore a living structure in the same way that the cell and the human being are living structures.

As life evolved, other chemicals besides nucleic acid and simple proteins became integral parts of the organism, and specialized functions began to develop in different parts of the virus. A membrane formed around the virus, and inside the membrane, a fluid matrix appeared. Specialized chemicals then developed inside the fluid to perform special functions; many protein enzymes appeared that were capable of catalyzing chemical reactions and, therefore, determining the organism's activities.

In still later stages of life, particularly in the rickettsial and bacterial stages, *organelles* developed inside the organism, representing physical structures of chemical aggregates that perform functions in a more efficient manner than can be achieved by dispersed chemicals throughout the fluid matrix.

Finally, in the nucleated cell, still more complex organelles developed, the most important of which is the *nucleus* itself. The nucleus distinguishes this type of cell from all lower forms of life; the nucleus provides a control center for all cellular activities, and it provides for exact reproduction of new cells generation after generation, each new cell having almost exactly the same structure as its progenitor.

Functional Systems of the Cell

In the remainder of this chapter, we discuss several representative functional systems of the cell that make it a living organism.

Ingestion by the Cell—Endocytosis

If a cell is to live and grow and reproduce, it must obtain nutrients and other substances from the surrounding fluids. Most substances pass through the cell membrane by *diffusion* and *active transport.*

Diffusion involves simple movement through the membrane caused by the random motion of the molecules of the substance; substances move either through cell membrane pores or, in the case of lipid-soluble substances, through the lipid matrix of the membrane.

Active transport involves the actual carrying of a substance through the membrane by a physical protein structure that penetrates all the way through the membrane. These active transport mechanisms are so important to cell function that they are presented in detail in Chapter 4.

Very large particles enter the cell by a specialized function of the cell membrane called *endocytosis.* The principal forms of endocytosis are *pinocytosis* and *phagocytosis.* Pinocytosis means ingestion of minute particles that form vesicles of extracellular fluid and particulate constituents inside the cell cytoplasm. Phagocytosis means ingestion of large particles, such as bacteria, whole cells, or portions of degenerating tissue.

Pinocytosis. Pinocytosis occurs continually in the cell membranes of most cells, but it is especially rapid in some cells. For instance, it occurs so rapidly in macrophages that about 3 percent of the total macrophage membrane is engulfed in the form of vesicles each minute. Even so, the pinocytotic vesicles are so small—usually only 100 to 200 nanometers in diameter—that most of them can be seen only with the electron microscope.

Pinocytosis is the only means by which most large macromolecules, such as most protein molecules, can enter cells. In fact, the rate at which pinocytotic vesicles form is usually enhanced when such macromolecules attach to the cell membrane.

Figure 2-11 demonstrates the successive steps of pinocytosis, showing three molecules of protein attaching to the membrane. These molecules usually attach to

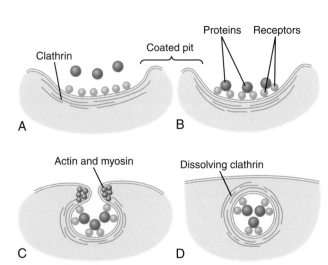

Clathrin

Coated pit

Proteins   Receptors

A   B

Actin and myosin

Dissolving clathrin

C   D

Figure 2-11 Mechanism of pinocytosis.

specialized protein *receptors* on the surface of the membrane that are specific for the type of protein that is to be absorbed. The receptors generally are concentrated in small pits on the outer surface of the cell membrane, called *coated pits.* On the inside of the cell membrane beneath these pits is a latticework of fibrillar protein called *clathrin,* as well as other proteins, perhaps including contractile filaments of *actin* and *myosin.* Once the protein molecules have bound with the receptors, the surface properties of the local membrane change in such a way that the entire pit invaginates inward and the fibrillar proteins surrounding the invaginating pit cause its borders to close over the attached proteins, as well as over a small amount of extracellular fluid. Immediately thereafter, the invaginated portion of the membrane breaks away from the surface of the cell, forming a *pinocytotic vesicle* inside the cytoplasm of the cell.

What causes the cell membrane to go through the necessary contortions to form pinocytotic vesicles is still unclear. This process requires energy from within the cell; this is supplied by ATP, a high-energy substance discussed later in the chapter. Also, it requires the presence of calcium ions in the extracellular fluid, which probably react with contractile protein filaments beneath the coated pits to provide the force for pinching the vesicles away from the cell membrane.

Phagocytosis.

Phagocytosis occurs in much the same way as pinocytosis, except that it involves large particles rather than molecules. Only certain cells have the capability of phagocytosis, most notably the tissue macrophages and some of the white blood cells.

Phagocytosis is initiated when a particle such as a bacterium, a dead cell, or tissue debris binds with receptors on the surface of the phagocyte. In the case of bacteria, each bacterium is usually already attached to a specific antibody, and it is the antibody that attaches to the phagocyte receptors, dragging the bacterium along with it. This intermediation of antibodies is called *opsonization,* which is discussed in Chapters 33 and 34.

Phagocytosis occurs in the following steps:

1. The cell membrane receptors attach to the surface ligands of the particle.

2. The edges of the membrane around the points of attachment evaginate outward within a fraction of a second to surround the entire particle; then, progressively more and more membrane receptors attach to the particle ligands. All this occurs suddenly in a zipper-like manner to form a closed *phagocytic vesicle.*

3. Actin and other contractile fibrils in the cytoplasm surround the phagocytic vesicle and contract around its outer edge, pushing the vesicle to the interior.

4. The contractile proteins then pinch the stem of the vesicle so completely that the vesicle separates from the cell membrane, leaving the vesicle in the cell interior in the same way that pinocytotic vesicles are formed.

Digestion of Pinocytotic and Phagocytic Foreign Substances Inside the Cell—Function of the Lysosomes

Almost immediately after a pinocytotic or phagocytic vesicle appears inside a cell, one or more *lysosomes* become attached to the vesicle and empty their *acid hydrolases* to the inside of the vesicle, as shown in Figure 2-12. Thus, a *digestive vesicle* is formed inside the cell cytoplasm in which the vesicular hydrolases begin hydrolyzing the proteins, carbohydrates, lipids, and other substances in the vesicle. The products of digestion are small molecules of amino acids, glucose, phosphates, and so forth that can diffuse through the membrane of the vesicle into the cytoplasm. What is left of the digestive vesicle, called the *residual body,* represents indigestible substances. In most instances, this is finally excreted through the cell membrane by a process called *exocytosis,* which is essentially the opposite of endocytosis.

Thus, the pinocytotic and phagocytic vesicles containing lysosomes can be called the *digestive organs* of the cells.

Regression of Tissues and Autolysis of Cells.

Tissues of the body often regress to a smaller size. For instance, this occurs in the uterus after pregnancy, in muscles during long periods of inactivity, and in mammary glands at the end of lactation. Lysosomes are responsible for much of this regression. The mechanism by which lack of activity in a tissue causes the lysosomes to increase their activity is unknown.

Another special role of the lysosomes is removal of damaged cells or damaged portions of cells from tissues. Damage to the cell—caused by heat, cold, trauma, chemicals, or any other factor—induces lysosomes to rupture. The released hydrolases immediately begin to digest the surrounding organic substances. If the damage is slight, only a portion of the cell is removed and the cell is then repaired. If the damage is severe, the entire cell is

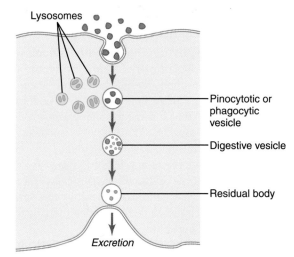

Figure 2-12 Digestion of substances in pinocytotic or phagocytic vesicles by enzymes derived from lysosomes.

digested, a process called *autolysis*. In this way, the cell is completely removed and a new cell of the same type ordinarily is formed by mitotic reproduction of an adjacent cell to take the place of the old one.

The lysosomes also contain bactericidal agents that can kill phagocytized bacteria before they can cause cellular damage. These agents include (1) *lysozyme*, which dissolves the bacterial cell membrane; (2) *lysoferrin*, which binds iron and other substances before they can promote bacterial growth; and (3) acid at a pH of about 5.0, which activates the hydrolases and inactivates bacterial metabolic systems.

Synthesis and Formation of Cellular Structures by Endoplasmic Reticulum and Golgi Apparatus

Specific Functions of the Endoplasmic Reticulum

The extensiveness of the endoplasmic reticulum and the Golgi apparatus in secretory cells has already been emphasized. These structures are formed primarily of lipid bilayer membranes similar to the cell membrane, and their walls are loaded with protein enzymes that catalyze the synthesis of many substances required by the cell.

Most synthesis begins in the endoplasmic reticulum. The products formed there are then passed on to the Golgi apparatus, where they are further processed before being released into the cytoplasm. But first, let us note the specific products that are synthesized in specific portions of the endoplasmic reticulum and the Golgi apparatus.

Proteins Are Formed by the Granular Endoplasmic Reticulum. The granular portion of the endoplasmic reticulum is characterized by large numbers of ribosomes attached to the outer surfaces of the endoplasmic reticulum membrane. As discussed in Chapter 3, protein molecules are synthesized within the structures of the ribosomes. The ribosomes extrude some of the synthesized protein molecules directly into the cytosol, but they also extrude many more through the wall of the endoplasmic reticulum to the interior of the endoplasmic vesicles and tubules, into the *endoplasmic matrix*.

Synthesis of Lipids by the Smooth Endoplasmic Reticulum. The endoplasmic reticulum also synthesizes lipids, especially phospholipids and cholesterol. These are rapidly incorporated into the lipid bilayer of the endoplasmic reticulum itself, thus causing the endoplasmic reticulum to grow more extensive. This occurs mainly in the smooth portion of the endoplasmic reticulum.

To keep the endoplasmic reticulum from growing beyond the needs of the cell, small vesicles called *ER vesicles* or *transport vesicles* continually break away from the smooth reticulum; most of these vesicles then migrate rapidly to the Golgi apparatus.

Other Functions of the Endoplasmic Reticulum. Other significant functions of the endoplasmic reticulum, especially the smooth reticulum, include the following:

1. It provides the enzymes that control glycogen breakdown when glycogen is to be used for energy.

2. It provides a vast number of enzymes that are capable of detoxifying substances, such as drugs, that might damage the cell. It achieves detoxification by coagulation, oxidation, hydrolysis, conjugation with glycuronic acid, and in other ways.

Specific Functions of the Golgi Apparatus

Synthetic Functions of the Golgi Apparatus. Although the major function of the Golgi apparatus is to provide additional processing of substances already formed in the endoplasmic reticulum, it also has the capability of synthesizing certain carbohydrates that cannot be formed in the endoplasmic reticulum. This is especially true for the formation of large saccharide polymers bound with small amounts of protein; important examples include *hyaluronic acid* and *chondroitin sulfate.*

A few of the many functions of hyaluronic acid and chondroitin sulfate in the body are as follows: (1) they are the major components of proteoglycans secreted in mucus and other glandular secretions; (2) they are the major components of the *ground substance* outside the cells in the interstitial spaces, acting as fillers between collagen fibers and cells; (3) they are principal components of the organic matrix in both cartilage and bone; and (4) they are important in many cell activities including migration and proliferation.

Processing of Endoplasmic Secretions by the Golgi Apparatus—Formation of Vesicles. Figure 2-13 summarizes the major functions of the endoplasmic reticulum and Golgi apparatus. As substances are formed in the endoplasmic reticulum, especially the proteins, they are transported through the tubules toward portions of the smooth endoplasmic reticulum that lie nearest the

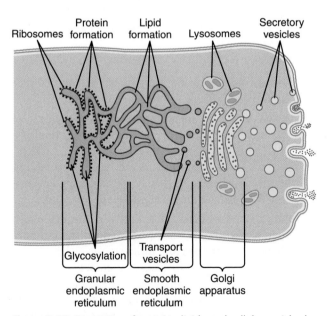

Figure 2-13 Formation of proteins, lipids, and cellular vesicles by the endoplasmic reticulum and Golgi apparatus.

Golgi apparatus. At this point, small *transport vesicles* composed of small envelopes of smooth endoplasmic reticulum continually break away and diffuse to the *deepest layer* of the Golgi apparatus. Inside these vesicles are the synthesized proteins and other products from the endoplasmic reticulum.

The transport vesicles instantly fuse with the Golgi apparatus and empty their contained substances into the vesicular spaces of the Golgi apparatus. Here, additional carbohydrate moieties are added to the secretions. Also, an important function of the Golgi apparatus is to compact the endoplasmic reticular secretions into highly concentrated packets. As the secretions pass toward the outermost layers of the Golgi apparatus, the compaction and processing proceed. Finally, both small and large vesicles continually break away from the Golgi apparatus, carrying with them the compacted secretory substances, and in turn, the vesicles diffuse throughout the cell.

To give an idea of the timing of these processes: When a glandular cell is bathed in radioactive amino acids, newly formed radioactive protein molecules can be detected in the granular endoplasmic reticulum within 3 to 5 minutes. Within 20 minutes, newly formed proteins are already present in the Golgi apparatus, and within 1 to 2 hours, radioactive proteins are secreted from the surface of the cell.

Types of Vesicles Formed by the Golgi Apparatus— Secretory Vesicles and Lysosomes. In a highly secretory cell, the vesicles formed by the Golgi apparatus are mainly *secretory vesicles* containing protein substances that are to be secreted through the surface of the cell membrane. These secretory vesicles first diffuse to the cell membrane, then fuse with it and empty their substances to the exterior by the mechanism called *exocytosis.* Exocytosis, in most cases, is stimulated by the entry of calcium ions into the cell; calcium ions interact with the vesicular membrane in some way that is not understood and cause its fusion with the cell membrane, followed by exocytosis—that is, opening of the membrane's outer surface and extrusion of its contents outside the cell.

Some vesicles, however, are destined for intracellular use.

Use of Intracellular Vesicles to Replenish Cellular Membranes. Some of the intracellular vesicles formed by the Golgi apparatus fuse with the cell membrane or with the membranes of intracellular structures such as the mitochondria and even the endoplasmic reticulum. This increases the expanse of these membranes and thereby replenishes the membranes as they are used up. For instance, the cell membrane loses much of its substance every time it forms a phagocytic or pinocytotic vesicle, and the vesicular membranes of the Golgi apparatus continually replenish the cell membrane.

In summary, the membranous system of the endoplasmic reticulum and Golgi apparatus represents a highly metabolic organ capable of forming new intracellular structures, as well as secretory substances to be extruded from the cell.

Extraction of Energy from Nutrients—Function of the Mitochondria

The principal substances from which cells extract energy are foodstuffs that react chemically with oxygen—carbohydrates, fats, and proteins. In the human body, essentially all carbohydrates are converted into *glucose* by the digestive tract and liver before they reach the other cells of the body. Similarly, proteins are converted into *amino acids* and fats into *fatty acids.* Figure 2-14 shows oxygen and the foodstuffs—glucose, fatty acids, and amino acids—all entering the cell. Inside the cell, the foodstuffs react chemically with oxygen, under the influence of enzymes that control the reactions and channel the energy released in the proper direction. The details of all these digestive and metabolic functions are given in Chapters 62 through 72.

Briefly, almost all these oxidative reactions occur inside the mitochondria and the energy that is released is used to form the high-energy compound *ATP.* Then, ATP, not the original foodstuffs, is used throughout the cell to energize almost all the subsequent intracellular metabolic reactions.

Functional Characteristics of ATP

Adenosine triphosphate

ATP is a nucleotide composed of (1) the nitrogenous base *adenine,* (2) the pentose sugar *ribose,* and (3) three *phosphate radicals.* The last two phosphate radicals are connected with the remainder of the molecule by so-called *high-energy phosphate bonds,* which are represented in the formula shown by the symbol ~. *Under the physical and chemical conditions of the body,* each of these high-energy bonds contains about 12,000 calories of energy per mole of ATP, which is many times greater than the energy stored in the average chemical bond, thus giving rise to the term *high-energy bond.* Further, the high-energy phosphate bond is very labile so that it can be split instantly on demand whenever energy is required to promote other intracellular reactions.

When ATP releases its energy, a phosphoric acid radical is split away and *adenosine diphosphate* (ADP) is formed. This released energy is used to energize virtually many of the cell's other functions, such as synthesis of substances and muscular contraction.

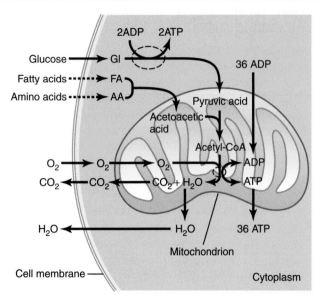

Figure 2-14 Formation of adenosine triphosphate (ATP) in the cell, showing that most of the ATP is formed in the mitochondria. ADP, adenosine diphosphate.

To reconstitute the cellular ATP as it is used up, energy derived from the cellular nutrients causes ADP and phosphoric acid to recombine to form new ATP, and the entire process repeats over and over again. For these reasons, ATP has been called the *energy currency* of the cell because it can be spent and remade continually, having a turnover time of only a few minutes.

Chemical Processes in the Formation of ATP—Role of the Mitochondria. On entry into the cells, glucose is subjected to enzymes in the *cytoplasm* that convert it into *pyruvic acid* (a process called *glycolysis*). A small amount of ADP is changed into ATP by the energy released during this conversion, but this amount accounts for less than 5 percent of the overall energy metabolism of the cell.

About 95 percent of the cell's ATP formation occurs in the mitochondria. The pyruvic acid derived from carbohydrates, fatty acids from lipids, and amino acids from proteins is eventually converted into the compound *acetyl-CoA* in the matrix of the mitochondrion. This substance, in turn, is further dissoluted (for the purpose of extracting its energy) by another series of enzymes in the mitochondrion matrix, undergoing dissolution in a sequence of chemical reactions called the *citric acid cycle,* or *Krebs cycle.* These chemical reactions are so important that they are explained in detail in Chapter 67.

In this citric acid cycle, acetyl-CoA is split into its component parts, *hydrogen atoms* and *carbon dioxide.* The carbon dioxide diffuses out of the mitochondria and eventually out of the cell; finally, it is excreted from the body through the lungs.

The hydrogen atoms, conversely, are highly reactive, and they combine instantly with oxygen that has also diffused into the mitochondria. This releases a tremendous amount of energy, which is used by the mitochondria to convert large amounts of ADP to ATP. The processes of these reactions are complex, requiring the

participation of many protein enzymes that are integral parts of mitochondrial *membranous shelves* that protrude into the mitochondrial matrix. The initial event is removal of an electron from the hydrogen atom, thus converting it to a hydrogen ion. The terminal event is combination of hydrogen ions with oxygen to form water plus the release of tremendous amounts of energy to large globular proteins, called *ATP synthetase,* that protrude like knobs from the membranes of the mitochondrial shelves. Finally, the enzyme ATP synthetase uses the energy from the hydrogen ions to cause the conversion of ADP to ATP. The newly formed ATP is transported out of the mitochondria into all parts of the cell cytoplasm and nucleoplasm, where its energy is used to energize multiple cell functions.

This overall process for formation of ATP is called the *chemiosmotic mechanism* of ATP formation. The chemical and physical details of this mechanism are presented in Chapter 67, and many of the detailed metabolic functions of ATP in the body are presented in Chapters 67 through 71.

Uses of ATP for Cellular Function. Energy from ATP is used to promote three major categories of cellular functions: (1) *transport* of substances through multiple membranes in the cell, (2) *synthesis of chemical compounds* throughout the cell, and (3) *mechanical work.* These uses of ATP are illustrated by examples in Figure 2-15: (1) to supply energy for the transport of sodium through the cell membrane, (2) to promote protein synthesis by the ribosomes, and (3) to supply the energy needed during muscle contraction.

In addition to membrane transport of sodium, energy from ATP is required for membrane transport of potassium ions, calcium ions, magnesium ions, phosphate ions,

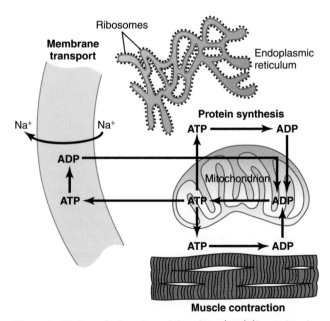

Figure 2-15 Use of adenosine triphosphate (ATP) (formed in the mitochondrion) to provide energy for three major cellular functions: membrane transport, protein synthesis, and muscle contraction. ADP, adenosine diphosphate.

chloride ions, urate ions, hydrogen ions, and many other ions and various organic substances. Membrane transport is so important to cell function that some cells—the renal tubular cells, for instance—use as much as 80 percent of the ATP that they form for this purpose alone.

In addition to synthesizing proteins, cells make phospholipids, cholesterol, purines, pyrimidines, and a host of other substances. Synthesis of almost any chemical compound requires energy. For instance, a single protein molecule might be composed of as many as several thousand amino acids attached to one another by peptide linkages; the formation of each of these linkages requires energy derived from the breakdown of four high-energy bonds; thus, many thousand ATP molecules must release their energy as each protein molecule is formed. Indeed, some cells use as much as 75 percent of all the ATP formed in the cell simply to synthesize new chemical compounds, especially protein molecules; this is particularly true during the growth phase of cells.

The final major use of ATP is to supply energy for special cells to perform mechanical work. We see in Chapter 6 that each contraction of a muscle fiber requires expenditure of tremendous quantities of ATP energy. Other cells perform mechanical work in other ways, especially by *ciliary* and *ameboid motion,* described later in this chapter. The source of energy for all these types of mechanical work is ATP.

In summary, ATP is always available to release its energy rapidly and almost explosively wherever in the cell it is needed. To replace the ATP used by the cell, much slower chemical reactions break down carbohydrates, fats, and proteins and use the energy derived from these to form new ATP. More than 95 percent of this ATP is formed in the mitochondria, which accounts for the mitochondria being called the "powerhouses" of the cell.

Locomotion of Cells

By far the most important type of movement that occurs in the body is that of the muscle cells in skeletal, cardiac, and smooth muscle, which constitute almost 50 percent of the entire body mass. The specialized functions of these cells are discussed in Chapters 6 through 9. Two other types of movement—*ameboid locomotion* and *ciliary movement*—occur in other cells.

Ameboid Movement

Ameboid movement is movement of an entire cell in relation to its surroundings, such as movement of white blood cells through tissues. It receives its name from the fact that amebae move in this manner and have provided an excellent tool for studying the phenomenon.

Typically, ameboid locomotion begins with protrusion of a *pseudopodium* from one end of the cell. The pseudopodium projects far out, away from the cell body, and partially secures itself in a new tissue area. Then the remainder of the cell is pulled toward the pseudopodium. Figure 2-16 demonstrates this process, showing an elon-

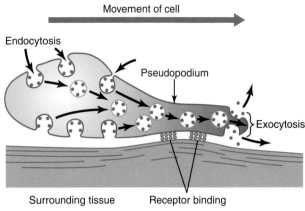

Figure 2-16 Ameboid motion by a cell.

gated cell, the right-hand end of which is a protruding pseudopodium. The membrane of this end of the cell is continually moving forward, and the membrane at the left-hand end of the cell is continually following along as the cell moves.

Mechanism of Ameboid Locomotion. Figure 2-16 shows the general principle of ameboid motion. Basically, it results from continual formation of new cell membrane at the leading edge of the pseudopodium and continual absorption of the membrane in mid and rear portions of the cell. Also, two other effects are essential for forward movement of the cell. The first effect is attachment of the pseudopodium to surrounding tissues so that it becomes fixed in its leading position, while the remainder of the cell body is pulled forward toward the point of attachment. This attachment is effected by *receptor proteins* that line the insides of exocytotic vesicles. When the vesicles become part of the pseudopodial membrane, they open so that their insides evert to the outside, and the receptors now protrude to the outside and attach to ligands in the surrounding tissues.

At the opposite end of the cell, the receptors pull away from their ligands and form new endocytotic vesicles. Then, inside the cell, these vesicles stream toward the pseudopodial end of the cell, where they are used to form still new membrane for the pseudopodium.

The second essential effect for locomotion is to provide the energy required to pull the cell body in the direction of the pseudopodium. Experiments suggest the following as an explanation: In the cytoplasm of all cells is a moderate to large amount of the protein *actin.* Much of the actin is in the form of single molecules that do not provide any motive power; however, these polymerize to form a filamentous network, and the network contracts when it binds with an actin-binding protein such as *myosin.* The whole process is energized by the high-energy compound ATP. This is what happens in the pseudopodium of a moving cell, where such a network of actin filaments forms anew inside the enlarging pseudopodium. Contraction also occurs in the ectoplasm of the cell body, where a preexisting actin network is already present beneath the cell membrane.

Types of Cells That Exhibit Ameboid Locomotion.

The most common cells to exhibit ameboid locomotion in the human body are the *white blood cells* when they move out of the blood into the tissues to form *tissue macrophages.* Other types of cells can also move by ameboid locomotion under certain circumstances. For instance, fibroblasts move into a damaged area to help repair the damage and even the germinal cells of the skin, though ordinarily completely sessile cells, move toward a cut area to repair the opening. Finally, cell locomotion is especially important in development of the embryo and fetus after fertilization of an ovum. For instance, embryonic cells often must migrate long distances from their sites of origin to new areas during development of special structures.

Control of Ameboid Locomotion—Chemotaxis.

The most important initiator of ameboid locomotion is the process called *chemotaxis.* This results from the appearance of certain chemical substances in the tissues. Any chemical substance that causes chemotaxis to occur is called a *chemotactic substance.* Most cells that exhibit ameboid locomotion move toward the source of a chemotactic substance—that is, from an area of lower concentration toward an area of higher concentration—which is called *positive chemotaxis.* Some cells move away from the source, which is called *negative chemotaxis.*

But how does chemotaxis control the direction of ameboid locomotion? Although the answer is not certain, it is known that the side of the cell most exposed to the chemotactic substance develops membrane changes that cause pseudopodial protrusion.

Cilia and Ciliary Movements

A second type of cellular motion, *ciliary movement,* is a whiplike movement of cilia on the surfaces of cells. This occurs in only two places in the human body: on the surfaces of the respiratory airways and on the inside surfaces of the uterine tubes (fallopian tubes) of the reproductive tract. In the nasal cavity and lower respiratory airways, the whiplike motion of cilia causes a layer of mucus to move at a rate of about 1 cm/min toward the pharynx, in this way continually clearing these passageways of mucus and particles that have become trapped in the mucus. In the uterine tubes, the cilia cause slow movement of fluid from the ostium of the uterine tube toward the uterus cavity; this movement of fluid transports the ovum from the ovary to the uterus.

As shown in Figure 2-17, a cilium has the appearance of a sharp-pointed straight or curved hair that projects 2 to 4 micrometers from the surface of the cell. Many cilia often project from a single cell—for instance, as many as 200 cilia on the surface of each epithelial cell inside the respiratory passageways. The cilium is covered by an outcropping of the cell membrane, and it is supported by 11 microtubules—9 double tubules located around the periphery of the cilium and 2 single tubules down

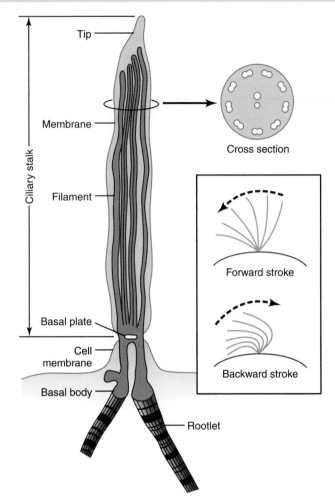

Figure 2-17 Structure and function of the cilium. (Modified from Satir P: Cilia. Sci Am 204:108, 1961. Copyright Donald Garber: Executor of the estate of Bunji Tagawa.)

the center, as demonstrated in the cross section shown in Figure 2-17. Each cilium is an outgrowth of a structure that lies immediately beneath the cell membrane, called the *basal body* of the cilium.

The *flagellum of a sperm* is similar to a cilium; in fact, it has much the same type of structure and same type of contractile mechanism. The flagellum, however, is much longer and moves in quasi-sinusoidal waves instead of whiplike movements.

In the inset of Figure 2-17, movement of the cilium is shown. The cilium moves forward with a sudden, rapid whiplike stroke 10 to 20 times per second, bending sharply where it projects from the surface of the cell. Then it moves backward slowly to its initial position. The rapid forward-thrusting, whiplike movement pushes the fluid lying adjacent to the cell in the direction that the cilium moves; the slow, dragging movement in the backward direction has almost no effect on fluid movement. As a result, the fluid is continually propelled in the direction of the fast-forward stroke. Because most ciliated cells have large numbers of cilia on their surfaces and because all the cilia are oriented in the same direction, this is an effective means for moving fluids from one part of the surface to another.

Mechanism of Ciliary Movement. Although not all aspects of ciliary movement are clear, we do know the following: First, the nine double tubules and the two single tubules are all linked to one another by a complex of protein cross-linkages; this total complex of tubules and cross-linkages is called the *axoneme*. Second, even after removal of the membrane and destruction of other elements of the cilium besides the axoneme, the cilium can still beat under appropriate conditions. Third, there are two necessary conditions for continued beating of the axoneme after removal of the other structures of the cilium: (1) the availability of ATP and (2) appropriate ionic conditions, especially appropriate concentrations of magnesium and calcium. Fourth, during forward motion of the cilium, the double tubules on the front edge of the cilium slide outward toward the tip of the cilium, while those on the back edge remain in place. Fifth, multiple protein arms composed of the protein *dynein,* which has ATPase enzymatic activity, project from each double tubule toward an adjacent double tubule.

Given this basic information, it has been determined that the release of energy from ATP in contact with the ATPase dynein arms causes the heads of these arms to "crawl" rapidly along the surface of the adjacent double tubule. If the front tubules crawl outward while the back tubules remain stationary, this will cause bending.

The way in which cilia contraction is controlled is not understood. The cilia of some genetically abnormal cells do not have the two central single tubules, and these cilia fail to beat. Therefore, it is presumed that some signal, perhaps an electrochemical signal, is transmitted along these two central tubules to activate the dynein arms.

Bibliography

Alberts B, Johnson A, Lewis J, et al: *Molecular Biology of the Cell,* 6th ed, New York, 2007, Garland Science.

Bonifacino JS, Glick BS: The mechanisms of vesicle budding and fusion, *Cell* 116:153, 2004.

Chacinska A, Koehler CM, Milenkovic D, Lithgow T, Pfanner N: Importing mitochondrial proteins: machineries and mechanisms, *Cell* 138:628, 2009.

Cohen AW, Hnasko R, Schubert W, Lisanti MP: Role of caveolae and caveolins in health and disease, *Physiol Rev* 84:1341, 2004.

Danial NN, Korsmeyer SJ: Cell death: critical control points, *Cell* 116:205, 2004.

Dröge W: Free radicals in the physiological control of cell function, *Physiol Rev* 82:47, 2002.

Edidin M: Lipids on the frontier: a century of cell-membrane bilayers, *Nat Rev Mol Cell Biol* 4:414, 2003.

Ginger ML, Portman N, McKean PG: Swimming with protists: perception, motility and flagellum assembly, *Nat Rev Microbiol* 6:838, 2008.

Grant BD, Donaldson JG: Pathways and mechanisms of endocytic recycling, *Nat Rev Mol Cell Biol* 10:597, 2009.

Güttinger S, Laurell E, Kutay U: Orchestrating nuclear envelope disassembly and reassembly during mitosis, *Nat Rev Mol Cell Biol* 10:178, 2009.

Hamill OP, Martinac B: Molecular basis of mechanotransduction in living cells, *Physiol Rev* 81:685, 2001.

Hock MB, Kralli A: Transcriptional control of mitochondrial biogenesis and function, *Annu Rev Physiol* 71:177, 2009.

Liesa M, Palacín M, Zorzano A: Mitochondrial dynamics in mammalian health and disease, *Physiol Rev* 89:799, 2009.

Mattaj IW: Sorting out the nuclear envelope from the endoplasmic reticulum, *Nat Rev Mol Cell Biol* 5:65, 2004.

Parton RG, Simons K: The multiple faces of caveolae, *Nat Rev Mol Cell Biol* 8:185, 2007.

Raiborg C, Stenmark H: The ESCRT machinery in endosomal sorting of ubiquitylated membrane proteins, *Nature* 458:445, 2009.

Ridley AJ, Schwartz MA, Burridge K, et al: Cell migration: integrating signals from front to back, *Science* 302:1704, 2003.

Saftig P, Klumperman J: Lysosome biogenesis and lysosomal membrane proteins: trafficking meets function, *Nat Rev Mol Cell Biol* 10:623, 2009.

Scarpulla RC: Transcriptional paradigms in mammalian mitochondrial biogenesis and function, *Physiol Rev* 88:611, 2008.

Stenmark H: Rab GTPases as coordinators of vesicle traffic, *Nat Rev Mol Cell Biol* 10:513, 2009.

Traub LM: Tickets to ride: selecting cargo for clathrin-regulated internalization, *Nat Rev Mol Cell Biol* 10:583, 2009.

Vereb G, Szollosi J, Matko J, et al: Dynamic, yet structured: the cell membrane three decades after the Singer-Nicolson model, *Proc Natl Acad Sci U S A* 100:8053, 2003.

Genetic Control of Protein Synthesis, Cell Function, and Cell Reproduction

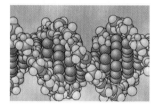

Virtually everyone knows that the genes, located in the nuclei of all cells of the body, control heredity from parents to children, but most people do not realize that these same genes also control day-to-day function of all the body's cells. The genes control cell function by determining which substances are synthesized within the cell—which structures, which enzymes, which chemicals.

Figure 3-1 shows the general schema of genetic control. Each gene, which is a nucleic acid called *deoxyribonucleic acid* (DNA), automatically controls the formation of another nucleic acid, *ribonucleic acid* (RNA); this RNA then spreads throughout the cell to control the formation of a specific protein. The entire process, from *transcription* of the genetic code in the nucleus to *translation* of the RNA code and formation or proteins in the cell cytoplasm, is often referred to as *gene expression*.

Because there are approximately 30,000 different genes in each cell, it is theoretically possible to form a large number of different cellular proteins.

Some of the cellular proteins are *structural proteins*, which, in association with various lipids and carbohydrates, form the structures of the various intracellular organelles discussed in Chapter 2. However, the majority of the proteins are *enzymes* that catalyze the different chemical reactions in the cells. For instance, enzymes promote all the oxidative reactions that supply energy to the cell, and they promote synthesis of all the cell chemicals, such as lipids, glycogen, and adenosine triphosphate (ATP).

Genes in the Cell Nucleus

In the cell nucleus, large numbers of genes are attached end on end in extremely long double-stranded helical molecules of DNA having molecular weights measured in the billions. A very short segment of such a molecule is shown in Figure 3-2. This molecule is composed of several simple chemical compounds bound together in a

regular pattern, details of which are explained in the next few paragraphs.

Basic Building Blocks of DNA. Figure 3-3 shows the basic chemical compounds involved in the formation of DNA. These include (1) *phosphoric acid,* (2) a sugar called *deoxyribose,* and (3) four nitrogenous *bases* (two purines, *adenine* and *guanine,* and two pyrimidines, *thymine* and *cytosine*). The phosphoric acid and deoxyribose form the two helical strands that are the backbone of the DNA molecule, and the nitrogenous bases lie between the two strands and connect them, as illustrated in Figure 3-6.

Nucleotides. The first stage in the formation of DNA is to combine one molecule of phosphoric acid, one molecule of deoxyribose, and one of the four bases to form an acidic nucleotide. Four separate nucleotides are thus formed, one for each of the four bases: *deoxyadenylic, deoxythymidylic, deoxyguanylic,* and *deoxycytidylic acids.* Figure 3-4 shows the chemical structure of deoxyadenylic

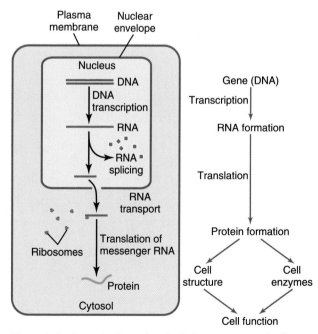

Figure 3-1. General schema by which the genes control cell function.

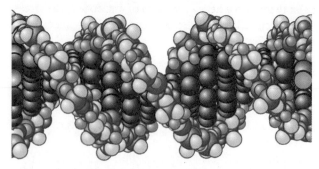

Figure 3-2. The helical, double-stranded structure of the gene. The outside strands are composed of phosphoric acid and the sugar deoxyribose. The internal molecules connecting the two strands of the helix are purine and pyrimidine bases; these determine the "code" of the gene.

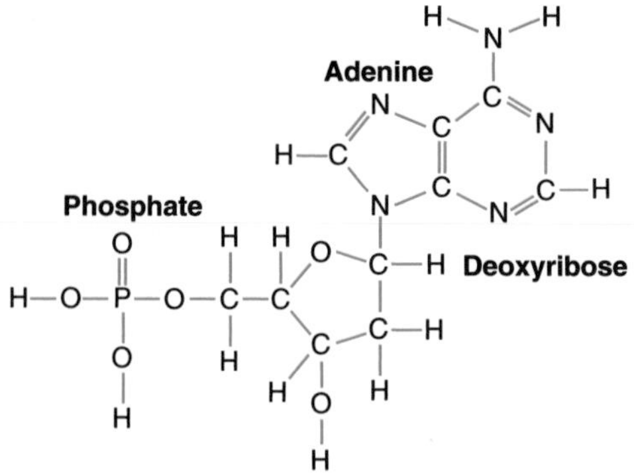

Figure 3-4. Deoxyadenylic acid, one of the nucleotides that make up DNA.

acid, and Figure 3-5 shows simple symbols for the four nucleotides that form DNA.

Organization of the Nucleotides to Form Two Strands of DNA Loosely Bound to Each Other. Figure 3-6 shows the manner in which multiple numbers of nucleotides are bound together to form two strands of DNA. The two strands are, in turn, loosely bonded with each other by weak cross-linkages, illustrated in Figure 3-6 by the central dashed lines. Note that the backbone of

each DNA strand is composed of alternating phosphoric acid and deoxyribose molecules. In turn, purine and pyrimidine bases are attached to the sides of the deoxyribose molecules. Then, by means of loose *hydrogen bonds* (dashed lines) between the purine and pyrimidine bases, the two respective DNA strands are held together. But note the following:

1. Each purine base *adenine* of one strand always bonds with a pyrimidine base *thymine* of the other strand, and

2. Each purine base *guanine* always bonds with a pyrimidine base *cytosine.*

Figure 3-3. The basic building blocks of DNA.

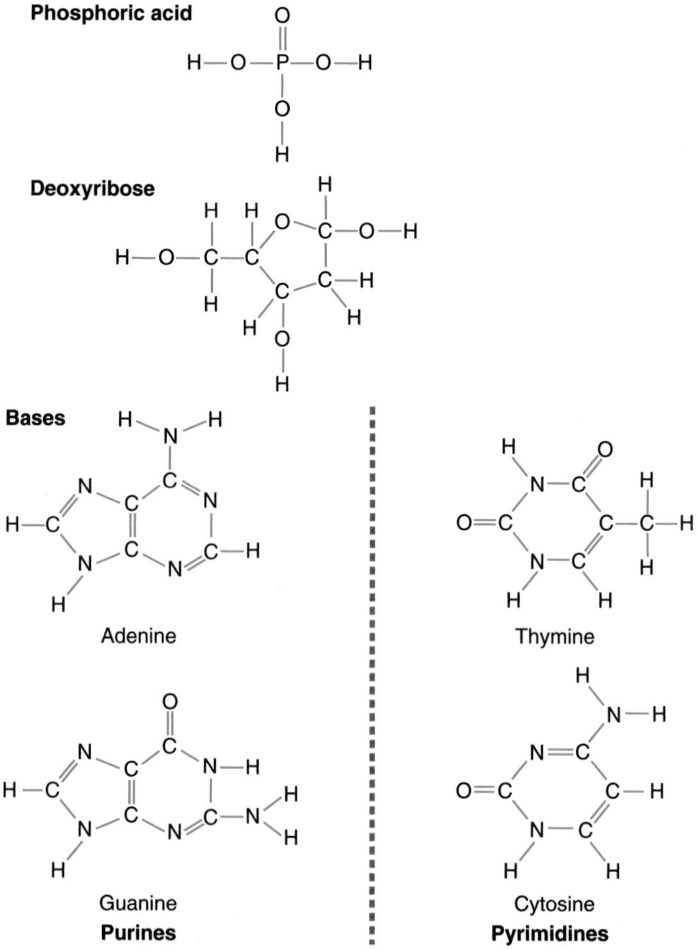

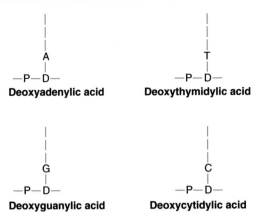

Figure 3-5. Symbols for the four nucleotides that combine to form DNA. Each nucleotide contains phosphoric acid (*P*), deoxyribose (*D*), and one of the four nucleotide bases: *A*, adenine; *T*, thymine; *G*, guanine; or *C*, cytosine.

Thus, in Figure 3-6, the sequence of complementary pairs of bases is CG, CG, GC, TA, CG, TA, GC, AT, and AT. Because of the looseness of the hydrogen bonds, the two strands can pull apart with ease, and they do so many times during the course of their function in the cell.

To put the DNA of Figure 3-6 into its proper physical perspective, one could merely pick up the two ends and

twist them into a helix. Ten pairs of nucleotides are present in each full turn of the helix in the DNA molecule, as shown in Figure 3-2.

Genetic Code

The importance of DNA lies in its ability to control the formation of proteins in the cell. It does this by means of a *genetic code.* That is, when the two strands of a DNA molecule are split apart, this exposes the purine and pyrimidine bases projecting to the side of each DNA strand, as shown by the top strand in Figure 3-7. It is these projecting bases that form the genetic code.

The genetic code consists of successive "triplets" of bases—that is, each three successive bases is a *code word.* The successive triplets eventually control the sequence of amino acids in a protein molecule that is to be synthesized in the cell. Note in Figure 3-6 that the top strand of DNA, reading from left to right, has the genetic code GGC, AGA, CTT, the triplets being separated from one another by the arrows. As we follow this genetic code through Figures 3-7 and 3-8, we see that these three respective triplets are responsible for successive placement of the three amino acids, *proline, serine,* and *glutamic acid,* in a newly formed molecule of protein.

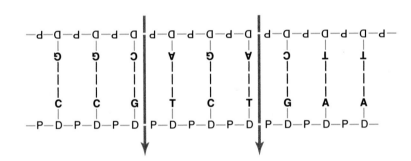

Figure 3-6. Arrangement of deoxyribose nucleotides in a double strand of DNA.

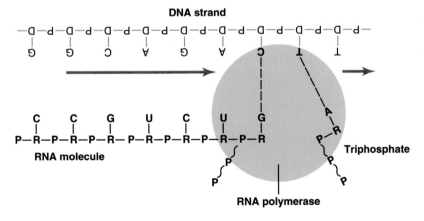

Figure 3-7. Combination of ribose nucleotides with a strand of DNA to form a molecule of RNA that carries the genetic code from the gene to the cytoplasm. The *RNA polymerase* enzyme moves along the DNA strand and builds the RNA molecule.

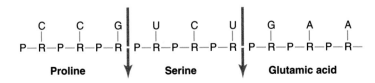

Figure 3-8. Portion of an RNA molecule, showing three RNA "codons"—CCG, UCU, and GAA—that control attachment of the three amino acids, *proline, serine,* and *glutamic acid,* respectively, to the growing RNA chain.

The DNA Code in the Cell Nucleus Is Transferred to an RNA Code in the Cell Cytoplasm—The Process of Transcription

Because the DNA is located in the nucleus of the cell, yet most of the functions of the cell are carried out in the cytoplasm, there must be some means for the DNA genes of the nucleus to control the chemical reactions of the cytoplasm. This is achieved through the intermediary of another type of nucleic acid, RNA, the formation of which is controlled by the DNA of the nucleus. Thus, as shown in Figure 3-7, the code is transferred to the RNA; this process is called *transcription.* The RNA, in turn, diffuses from the nucleus through nuclear pores into the cytoplasmic compartment, where it controls protein synthesis.

Synthesis of RNA

During synthesis of RNA, the two strands of the DNA molecule separate temporarily; one of these strands is used as a template for synthesis of an RNA molecule. The code triplets in the DNA cause formation of *complementary* code triplets (called *codons*) in the RNA; these codons, in turn, will control the sequence of amino acids in a protein to be synthesized in the cell cytoplasm.

Basic Building Blocks of RNA. The basic building blocks of RNA are almost the same as those of DNA, except for two differences. First, the sugar deoxyribose is not used in the formation of RNA. In its place is another sugar of slightly different composition, *ribose,* containing an extra hydroxyl ion appended to the ribose ring structure. Second, thymine is replaced by another pyrimidine, *uracil.*

Formation of RNA Nucleotides. The basic building blocks of RNA form *RNA nucleotides,* exactly as previously described for DNA synthesis. Here again, four separate nucleotides are used in the formation of RNA. These nucleotides contain the bases *adenine, guanine, cytosine,* and *uracil.* Note that these are the same bases as in DNA, except that uracil in RNA replaces thymine in DNA.

"Activation" of the RNA Nucleotides. The next step in the synthesis of RNA is "activation" of the RNA nucleotides by an enzyme, *RNA polymerase.* This occurs by adding to each nucleotide two extra phosphate radicals to form triphosphates (shown in Figure 3-7 by the two RNA nucleotides to the far right during RNA chain formation). These last two phosphates are combined with the nucleotide by *high-energy phosphate bonds* derived from ATP in the cell.

The result of this activation process is that large quantities of ATP energy are made available to each of the nucleotides, and this energy is used to promote the chemical reactions that add each new RNA nucleotide at the end of the developing RNA chain.

Assembly of the RNA Chain from Activated Nucleotides Using the DNA Strand as a Template—The Process of "Transcription"

Assembly of the RNA molecule is accomplished in the manner shown in Figure 3-7 under the influence of an enzyme, *RNA polymerase.* This is a large protein enzyme that has many functional properties necessary for formation of the RNA molecule. They are as follows:

1. In the DNA strand immediately ahead of the initial gene is a sequence of nucleotides called the *promoter.* The RNA polymerase has an appropriate complementary structure that recognizes this promoter and becomes attached to it. This is the essential step for initiating formation of the RNA molecule.

2. After the RNA polymerase attaches to the promoter, the polymerase causes unwinding of about two turns of the DNA helix and separation of the unwound portions of the two strands.

3. Then the polymerase moves along the DNA strand, temporarily unwinding and separating the two DNA strands at each stage of its movement. As it moves along, it adds at each stage a new activated RNA nucleotide to the end of the newly forming RNA chain by the following steps:

   a. First, it causes a hydrogen bond to form between the end base of the DNA strand and the base of an RNA nucleotide in the nucleoplasm.

   b. Then, one at a time, the RNA polymerase breaks two of the three phosphate radicals away from each of these RNA nucleotides, liberating large amounts of energy from the broken high-energy phosphate bonds; this energy is used to cause covalent linkage of the remaining phosphate on the nucleotide with the ribose on the end of the growing RNA chain.

   c. When the RNA polymerase reaches the end of the DNA gene, it encounters a new sequence of DNA nucleotides called the *chain-terminating sequence;* this causes the polymerase and the newly formed RNA chain to break away from the DNA strand. Then the polymerase can be used again and again to form still more new RNA chains.

   d. As the new RNA strand is formed, its weak hydrogen bonds with the DNA template break away, because the DNA has a high affinity for rebonding with its own complementary DNA strand. Thus, the RNA chain is forced away from the DNA and is released into the nucleoplasm.

Thus, the code that is present in the DNA strand is eventually transmitted in *complementary* form to the RNA chain. The ribose nucleotide bases always combine with the deoxyribose bases in the following combinations:

DNA Base	RNA Base
guanine	cytosine
cytosine	guanine
adenine	uracil
thymine	adenine

Four Different Types of RNA. Each type of RNA plays an independent and entirely different role in protein formation:

1. *Messenger RNA* (mRNA), which carries the genetic code to the cytoplasm for controlling the type of protein formed.

2. *Transfer RNA* (tRNA), which transports activated amino acids to the ribosomes to be used in assembling the protein molecule.

3. *Ribosomal RNA,* which, along with about 75 different proteins, forms *ribosomes,* the physical and chemical structures on which protein molecules are actually assembled.

4. *MicroRNA* (miRNA), which are single-stranded RNA molecules of 21 to 23 nucleotides that can regulate gene transcription and translation.

Messenger RNA—The Codons

mRNA molecules are long, single RNA strands that are suspended in the cytoplasm. These molecules are composed of several hundred to several thousand RNA nucleotides in unpaired strands, and they contain *codons* that are exactly complementary to the code triplets of the DNA genes. Figure 3-8 shows a small segment of a molecule of messenger RNA. Its codons are CCG, UCU, and GAA. These are the codons for the amino acids proline, serine, and glutamic acid. The transcription of these codons from the DNA molecule to the RNA molecule is shown in Figure 3-7.

RNA Codons for the Different Amino Acids. Table 3-1 gives the RNA codons for the 22 common amino acids found in protein molecules. Note that most of the amino acids are represented by more than one codon;

Table 3-1. RNA Codons for Amino Acids and for Start and Stop

Amino Acid	RNA Codons					
Alanine	GCU	GCC	GCA	GCG		
Arginine	CGU	CGC	CGA	CGG	AGA	AGG
Asparagine	AAU	AAC				
Aspartic acid	GAU	GAC				
Cysteine	UGU	UGC				
Glutamic acid	GAA	GAG				
Glutamine	CAA	CAG				
Glycine	GGU	GGC	GGA	GGG		
Histidine	CAU	CAC				
Isoleucine	AUU	AUC	AUA			
Leucine	CUU	CUC	CUA	CUG	UUA	UUG
Lysine	AAA	AAG				
Methionine	AUG					
Phenylalanine	UUU	UUC				
Proline	CCU	CCC	CCA	CCG		
Serine	UCU	UCC	UCA	UCG	AGC	AGU
Threonine	ACU	ACC	ACA	ACG		
Tryptophan	UGG					
Tyrosine	UAU	UAC				
Valine	GUU	GUC	GUA	GUG		
Start (CI)	AUG					
Stop (CT)	UAA	UAG	UGA			

CI, chain-initiating; CT, chain-terminating.

also, one codon represents the signal "start manufacturing the protein molecule," and three codons represent "stop manufacturing the protein molecule." In Table 3-1, these two types of codons are designated CI for "chain-initiating" and CT for "chain-terminating."

Transfer RNA—The Anticodons

Another type of RNA that plays an essential role in protein synthesis is called *tRNA* because it transfers amino acid molecules to protein molecules as the protein is being synthesized. Each type of tRNA combines specifically with 1 of the 20 amino acids that are to be incorporated into proteins. The tRNA then acts as a *carrier* to transport its specific type of amino acid to the ribosomes, where protein molecules are forming. In the ribosomes, each specific type of transfer RNA recognizes a particular codon on the mRNA (described later) and thereby delivers the appropriate amino acid to the appropriate place in the chain of the newly forming protein molecule.

Transfer RNA, which contains only about 80 nucleotides, is a relatively small molecule in comparison with mRNA. It is a folded chain of nucleotides with a cloverleaf appearance similar to that shown in Figure 3-9. At one end of the molecule is always an adenylic acid; it is to this that the transported amino acid attaches at a hydroxyl group of the ribose in the adenylic acid.

Because the function of tRNA is to cause attachment of a specific amino acid to a forming protein chain, it is essential that each type of tRNA also have specificity for a particular codon in the mRNA. The specific code in the tRNA that allows it to recognize a specific codon is again a triplet of nucleotide bases and is called an *anticodon*. This is located approximately in the middle of the tRNA molecule (at the bottom of the cloverleaf configuration shown in Figure 3-9). During formation of the protein molecule, the anticodon bases combine loosely by hydrogen

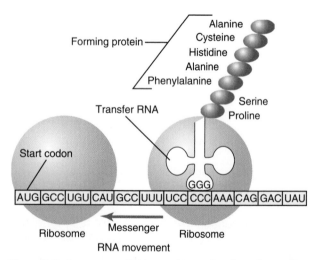

Figure 3-9. A messenger RNA strand is moving through two ribosomes. As each "codon" passes through, an amino acid is added to the growing protein chain, which is shown in the right-hand ribosome. The transfer RNA molecule transports each specific amino acid to the newly forming protein.

bonding with the codon bases of the mRNA. In this way, the respective amino acids are lined up one after another along the mRNA chain, thus establishing the appropriate sequence of amino acids in the newly forming protein molecule.

Ribosomal RNA

The third type of RNA in the cell is ribosomal RNA; it constitutes about 60 percent of the *ribosome*. The remainder of the ribosome is protein, containing about 75 types of proteins that are both structural proteins and enzymes needed in the manufacture of protein molecules.

The ribosome is the physical structure in the cytoplasm on which protein molecules are actually synthesized. However, it always functions in association with the other two types of RNA as well: *tRNA* transports amino acids to the ribosome for incorporation into the developing protein molecule, whereas *mRNA* provides the information necessary for sequencing the amino acids in proper order for each specific type of protein to be manufactured.

Thus, the ribosome acts as a manufacturing plant in which the protein molecules are formed.

Formation of Ribosomes in the Nucleolus. The DNA genes for formation of ribosomal RNA are located in five pairs of chromosomes in the nucleus, and each of these chromosomes contains many duplicates of these particular genes because of the large amounts of ribosomal RNA required for cellular function.

As the ribosomal RNA forms, it collects in the *nucleolus*, a specialized structure lying adjacent to the chromosomes. When large amounts of ribosomal RNA are being synthesized, as occurs in cells that manufacture large amounts of protein, the nucleolus is a large structure, whereas in cells that synthesize little protein, the nucleolus may not even be seen. Ribosomal RNA is specially processed in the nucleolus, where it binds with "ribosomal proteins" to form granular condensation products that are primordial subunits of ribosomes. These subunits are then released from the nucleolus and transported through the large pores of the nuclear envelope to almost all parts of the cytoplasm. After the subunits enter the cytoplasm, they are assembled to form mature, functional ribosomes. Therefore, proteins are formed in the cytoplasm of the cell, but not in the cell nucleus, because the nucleus does not contain mature ribosomes.

MicroRNA

A fourth type of RNA in the cell is *miRNA*. These are short (21 to 23 nucleotides) single-stranded RNA fragments that regulate gene expression (Figure 3-10). The miRNAs are encoded from the transcribed DNA of genes, but they are not translated into proteins and are therefore often called *noncoding RNA*. The miRNAs are processed by the cell into molecules that are complementary to mRNA and act to decrease gene expression. Generation of miRNAs involves special processing of longer primary precursor

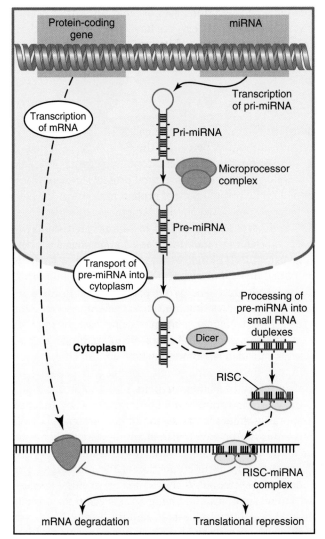

Figure 3-10. Regulation of gene expression by microRNA (miRNA). Primary miRNA (pri-miRNA), the primary transcripts of a gene processed in the cell nucleus by the microprocessor complex to pre-miRNAs. These pre-miRNAs are then further processed in the cytoplasm by *dicer,* an enzyme that helps assemble an RNA-induced silencing complex (RISC) and generates miRNAs. The miR-NAs regulate gene expression by binding to the complementary region of the RNA and repressing translation or promoting degradation of the mRNA before it can be translated by the ribosome.

RNAs called *pri-miRNAs,* which are the primary transcripts of the gene. The pri-miRNAs are then processed in the cell nucleus by the *microprocessor complex* to pre-miRNAs, which are 70 nucleotide stem-loop structures. These pre-miRNAs are then further processed in the cytoplasm by a specific *dicer enzyme* that helps assemble an *RNA-induced silencing complex* (RISC) and generates miRNAs.

The miRNAs regulate gene expression by binding to the complementary region of the RNA and promoting repression of translation or degradation of the mRNA before it can be translated by the ribosome. miRNAs are believed to play an important role in the normal regulation of cell function, and alterations in miRNA function have been associated with diseases such as cancer and heart disease.

Another type of microRNA is *small interfering RNA* (siRNA), also called *silencing RNA* or *short interfering RNA.* The siRNAs are short, double-stranded RNA molecules, 20 to 25 nucleotides in length, that interfere with the expression of specific genes. siRNAs generally refer to synthetic miRNAs and can be administered to silence expression of specific genes. They are designed to avoid the nuclear processing by the microprocessor complex, and after the siRNA enters the cytoplasm it activates the RISC silencing complex, blocking the translation of mRNA. Because siRNAs can be tailored for any specific sequence in the gene, they can be used to block translation of any mRNA and therefore expression by any gene for which the nucleotide sequence is known. Some researchers have proposed that siRNAs may become useful therapeutic tools to silence genes that contribute to the pathophysiology of diseases.

Formation of Proteins on the Ribosomes—The Process of "Translation"

When a molecule of messenger RNA comes in contact with a ribosome, it travels through the ribosome, beginning at a predetermined end of the RNA molecule specified by an appropriate sequence of RNA bases called the "chain-initiating" codon. Then, as shown in Figure 3-9, while the messenger RNA travels through the ribosome, a protein molecule is formed—a process called *translation.* Thus, the ribosome reads the codons of the messenger RNA in much the same way that a tape is "read" as it passes through the playback head of a tape recorder. Then, when a "stop" (or "chain-terminating") codon slips past the ribosome, the end of a protein molecule is signaled and the protein molecule is freed into the cytoplasm.

Polyribosomes. A single messenger RNA molecule can form protein molecules in several ribosomes at the same time because the initial end of the RNA strand can pass to a successive ribosome as it leaves the first, as shown at the bottom left in Figure 3-9 and in Figure 3-11. The protein molecules are in different stages of development in each ribosome. As a result, clusters of ribosomes frequently occur, 3 to 10 ribosomes being attached to a single messenger RNA at the same time. These clusters are called *polyribosomes.*

It is especially important to note that a messenger RNA can cause the formation of a protein molecule in any ribosome; that is, there is no specificity of ribosomes for given types of protein. The ribosome is simply the physical manufacturing plant in which the chemical reactions take place.

Many Ribosomes Attach to the Endoplasmic Reticulum. In Chapter 2, it was noted that many ribosomes become attached to the endoplasmic reticulum. This occurs because the initial ends of many forming protein molecules have amino acid sequences that immediately attach to specific receptor sites on the endoplasmic reticulum; this causes these molecules to penetrate the

Figure 3-11. Physical structure of the ribosomes, as well as their functional relation to messenger RNA, transfer RNA, and the endoplasmic reticulum during the formation of protein molecules. (Courtesy Dr. Don W. Fawcett, Montana.)

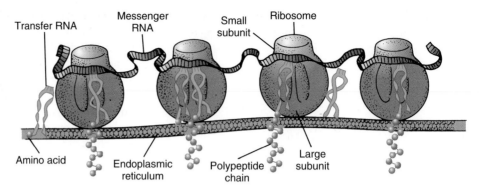

reticulum wall and enter the endoplasmic reticulum matrix. This gives a granular appearance to those portions of the reticulum where proteins are being formed and entering the matrix of the reticulum.

Figure 3-11 shows the functional relation of messenger RNA to the ribosomes and the manner in which the ribosomes attach to the membrane of the endoplasmic reticulum. Note the process of translation occurring in several ribosomes at the same time in response to the same strand of messenger RNA. Note also the newly forming polypeptide (protein) chains passing through the endoplasmic reticulum membrane into the endoplasmic matrix.

Yet it should be noted that except in glandular cells in which large amounts of protein-containing secretory vesicles are formed, most proteins synthesized by the ribosomes are released directly into the cytosol instead of into the endoplasmic reticulum. These proteins are enzymes and internal structural proteins of the cell.

Chemical Steps in Protein Synthesis. Some of the chemical events that occur in synthesis of a protein molecule are shown in Figure 3-12. This figure shows representative reactions for three separate amino acids, AA_1,

AA_2, and AA_{20}. The stages of the reactions are the following: (1) Each amino acid is *activated* by a chemical process in which ATP combines with the amino acid to form an *adenosine monophosphate complex with the amino acid*, giving up two high-energy phosphate bonds in the process. (2) The activated amino acid, having an excess of energy, then *combines with its specific transfer RNA to form an amino acid–tRNA complex* and, at the same time, releases the adenosine monophosphate. (3) The transfer RNA carrying the amino acid complex then comes in contact with the messenger RNA molecule in the ribosome, where the anticodon of the transfer RNA attaches temporarily to its specific codon of the messenger RNA, thus lining up the amino acid in appropriate sequence to form a protein molecule. Then, under the influence of the enzyme *peptidyl transferase* (one of the proteins in the ribosome), *peptide bonds* are formed between the successive amino acids, thus adding progressively to the protein chain. These chemical events require energy from two additional high-energy phosphate bonds, making a total of four high-energy bonds used for each amino acid added to the protein chain. Thus, the synthesis of proteins is one of the most energy-consuming processes of the cell.

Figure 3-12. Chemical events in the formation of a protein molecule.

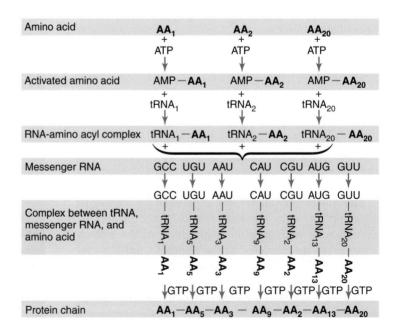

Peptide Linkage. The successive amino acids in the protein chain combine with one another according to the typical reaction:

$$
\begin{array}{l}
\underset{|}{\overset{NH_2}{|}} \; \underset{|}{\overset{O}{\|}} \qquad \quad \overset{H}{\underset{|}{}} \; \overset{R}{\underset{|}{}} \\
R - C - C - OH + H - N - C - COOH \longrightarrow \\[2mm]
\qquad \overset{NH_2}{\underset{|}{}} \; \overset{O}{\underset{|}{\|}} \; \overset{H}{\underset{|}{}} \; \overset{R}{\underset{|}{}} \\
\qquad R - C - C - N - C - COOH + H_2O
\end{array}
$$

In this chemical reaction, a hydroxyl radical (OH^-) is removed from the COOH portion of the first amino acid and a hydrogen (H^+) of the NH_2 portion of the other amino acid is removed. These combine to form water, and the two reactive sites left on the two successive amino acids bond with each other, resulting in a single molecule. This process is called *peptide linkage.* As each additional amino acid is added, an additional peptide linkage is formed.

Synthesis of Other Substances in the Cell

Many thousand protein enzymes formed in the manner just described control essentially all the other chemical reactions that take place in cells. These enzymes promote synthesis of lipids, glycogen, purines, pyrimidines, and hundreds of other substances. We discuss many of these synthetic processes in relation to carbohydrate, lipid, and protein metabolism in Chapters 67 through 69. It is by means of all these substances that the many functions of the cells are performed.

Control of Gene Function and Biochemical Activity in Cells

From our discussion thus far, it is clear that the genes control both the physical and chemical functions of the cells. However, the degree of activation of respective genes must be controlled as well; otherwise, some parts of the cell might overgrow or some chemical reactions might overact until they kill the cell. Each cell has powerful internal feedback control mechanisms that keep the various functional operations of the cell in step with one another. For each gene (approximately 30,000 genes in all), there is at least one such feedback mechanism.

There are basically two methods by which the biochemical activities in the cell are controlled: (1) *genetic regulation,* in which the degree of activation of the genes and the formation of gene products are themselves controlled and (2) *enzyme regulation,* in which the activity levels of already formed enzymes in the cell are controlled.

Genetic Regulation

Genetic regulation, or regulation of *gene expression,* covers the entire process from transcription of the genetic code in the nucleus to the formation or proteins in the cytoplasm.

Regulation of gene expression provides all living organisms the ability to respond to changes in their environment. In animals that have many different types of cells, tissues, and organs, differential regulation of gene expression also permits the many different cell types in the body to each perform their specialized functions. Although a cardiac myocyte contains the same genetic code as a renal tubular epithelia cell, many genes are expressed in cardiac cells that are not expressed in renal tubular cells. The ultimate measure of gene "expression" is whether (and how much) of the gene products (proteins) are produced because proteins carry out cell functions specified by the genes. Regulation of gene expression can occur at any point in the pathways of transcription, RNA processing, and translation.

The Promoter Controls Gene Expression. Synthesis of cellular proteins is a complex process that starts with the transcription of DNA into RNA. The transcription of DNA is controlled by regulatory elements found in the promoter of a gene (Figure 3-13). In eukaryotes, which includes all mammals, the basal promoter consists of a sequence of seven bases (TATAAAA) called the *TATA box,* the binding site for the *TATA-binding protein* (TBP) and several other important *transcription factors* that are collectively referred to as the *transcription factor IID complex.* In addition to the transcription factor IID complex, this region is where transcription factor IIB binds to both the DNA and RNA polymerase 2 to facilitate transcription of the DNA into RNA. This basal promoter is found in all protein-coding genes and the polymerase must bind with this basal promoter before it can begin traveling along the DNA strand to synthesize RNA. The *upstream promoter* is located farther upstream from the transcription start site and contains several binding sites for positive or negative transcription factors that can effect transcription through interactions with proteins bound to the basal promoter. The structure and transcription factor binding sites in the upstream promoter vary from gene to gene to give rise to the different expression patterns of genes in different tissues.

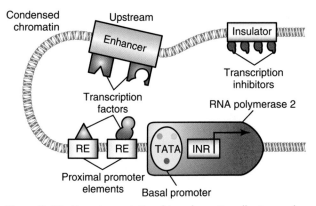

Figure 3-13. Gene transcriptional in eukaryotic cells. A complex arrangement of multiple clustered enhancer modules interspersed with insulator elements, which can be located either upstream or downstream of a basal promoter containing TATA box (TATA), proximal promoter elements (response elements, RE), and Initiator sequences (INR).

Transcription of genes in eukaryotes is also influenced by *enhancers,* which are regions of DNA that can bind transcription factors. Enhancers can be located a great distance from the gene they act on or even on a different chromosome. They can also be located either upstream or downstream of the gene that they regulate. Although enhancers may be located a great distance away from their target gene, they may be relatively close when DNA is coiled in the nucleus. It is estimated that there are 110,000 gene enhancer sequences in the human genome.

In the organization of the chromosome, it is important to separate active genes that are being transcribed from genes that are repressed. This can be challenging because multiple genes may be located close together on the chromosome. This is achieved by chromosomal *insulators.* These insulators are gene sequences that provide a barrier so that a specific gene is isolated against transcriptional influences from surrounding genes. Insulators can vary greatly in their DNA sequence and the proteins that bind to them. One way an insulator activity can be modulated is by *DNA methylation.* This is the case for the mammalian insulin-like growth factor 2 (IGF-2) gene. The mother's allele has an insulator between the enhancer and promoter of the gene that allows for the binding of a transcriptional repressor. However, the paternal DNA sequence is methylated such that the transcriptional repressor cannot bind to the insulator and the IGF-2 gene is expressed from the paternal copy of the gene.

Other Mechanisms for Control of Transcription by the Promoter. Variations in the basic mechanism for control of the promoter have been discovered with rapidity in the past 2 decades. Without giving details, let us list some of them:

1. A promoter is frequently controlled by transcription factors located elsewhere in the genome. That is, the regulatory gene causes the formation of a regulatory protein that in turn acts either as an activator or a repressor of transcription.

2. Occasionally, many different promoters are controlled at the same time by the same regulatory protein. In some instances, the same regulatory protein functions as an activator for one promoter and as a repressor for another promoter.

3. Some proteins are controlled not at the starting point of transcription on the DNA strand but farther along the strand. Sometimes the control is not even at the DNA strand itself but during the processing of the RNA molecules in the nucleus before they are released into the cytoplasm; rarely, control might occur at the level of protein formation in the cytoplasm during RNA translation by the ribosomes.

4. In nucleated cells, the nuclear DNA is packaged in specific structural units, the *chromosomes.* Within each chromosome, the DNA is wound around small proteins called *histones,* which in turn are held tightly together

in a compacted state by still other proteins. As long as the DNA is in this compacted state, it cannot function to form RNA. However, multiple control mechanisms are beginning to be discovered that can cause selected areas of chromosomes to become decompacted one part at a time so that partial RNA transcription can occur. Even then, specific *transcriptor factors* control the actual rate of transcription by the promoter in the chromosome. Thus, still higher orders of control are used for establishing proper cell function. In addition, signals from outside the cell, such as some of the body's hormones, can activate specific chromosomal areas and specific transcription factors, thus controlling the chemical machinery for function of the cell.

Because there are more than 30,000 different genes in each human cell, the large number of ways in which genetic activity can be controlled is not surprising. The gene control systems are especially important for controlling intracellular concentrations of amino acids, amino acid derivatives, and intermediate substrates and products of carbohydrate, lipid, and protein metabolism.

Control of Intracellular Function by Enzyme Regulation

In addition to control of cell function by genetic regulation, some cell activities are controlled by intracellular inhibitors or activators that act directly on specific intracellular enzymes. Thus, enzyme regulation represents a second category of mechanisms by which cellular biochemical functions can be controlled.

Enzyme Inhibition. Some chemical substances formed in the cell have direct feedback effects in inhibiting the specific enzyme systems that synthesize them. Almost always the synthesized product acts on the first enzyme in a sequence, rather than on the subsequent enzymes, usually binding directly with the enzyme and causing an allosteric conformational change that inactivates it. One can readily recognize the importance of inactivating the first enzyme: this prevents buildup of intermediary products that are not used.

Enzyme inhibition is another example of negative feedback control; it is responsible for controlling intracellular concentrations of multiple amino acids, purines, pyrimidines, vitamins, and other substances.

Enzyme Activation. Enzymes that are normally inactive often can be activated when needed. An example of this occurs when most of the ATP has been depleted in a cell. In this case, a considerable amount of cyclic adenosine monophosphate (cAMP) begins to be formed as a breakdown product of the ATP; the presence of this cAMP, in turn, immediately activates the glycogen-splitting enzyme phosphorylase, liberating glucose molecules that are rapidly metabolized and their energy used for replenishment of the ATP stores. Thus, cAMP acts as an enzyme activator for the enzyme phosphorylase and thereby helps control intracellular ATP concentration.

Another interesting instance of both enzyme inhibition and enzyme activation occurs in the formation of the purines and pyrimidines. These substances are needed by the cell in approximately equal quantities for formation of DNA and RNA. When purines are formed, they *inhibit* the enzymes that are required for formation of additional purines. However, they *activate* the enzymes for formation of pyrimidines. Conversely, the pyrimidines inhibit their own enzymes but activate the purine enzymes. In this way, there is continual cross-feed between the synthesizing systems for these two substances, resulting in almost exactly equal amounts of the two substances in the cells at all times.

Summary. In summary, there are two principal methods by which cells control proper proportions and proper quantities of different cellular constituents: (1) the mechanism of genetic regulation and (2) the mechanism of enzyme regulation. The genes can be either activated or inhibited, and likewise, the enzyme systems can be either activated or inhibited. These regulatory mechanisms most often function as feedback control systems that continually monitor the cell's biochemical composition and make corrections as needed. But on occasion, substances from without the cell (especially some of the hormones discussed throughout this text) also control the intracellular biochemical reactions by activating or inhibiting one or more of the intracellular control systems.

The DNA-Genetic System Also Controls Cell Reproduction

Cell reproduction is another example of the ubiquitous role that the DNA-genetic system plays in all life processes. The genes and their regulatory mechanisms determine the growth characteristics of the cells and also when or whether these cells will divide to form new cells. In this way, the all-important genetic system controls each stage in the development of the human being, from the single-cell fertilized ovum to the whole functioning body. Thus, if there is any central theme to life, it is the DNA-genetic system.

Life Cycle of the Cell. The life cycle of a cell is the period from cell reproduction to the next cell reproduction. When mammalian cells *are not inhibited and are reproducing as rapidly as they can,* this life cycle may be as little as 10 to 30 hours. It is terminated by a series of distinct physical events called *mitosis* that cause division of the cell into two new daughter cells. The events of mitosis are shown in Figure 3-14 and are described later. The actual stage of mitosis, however, lasts for only about 30 minutes, so more than 95 percent of the life cycle of even rapidly reproducing cells is represented by the interval between mitosis, called *interphase.*

Except in special conditions of rapid cellular reproduction, inhibitory factors almost always slow or stop the uninhibited life cycle of the cell. Therefore, different cells of the

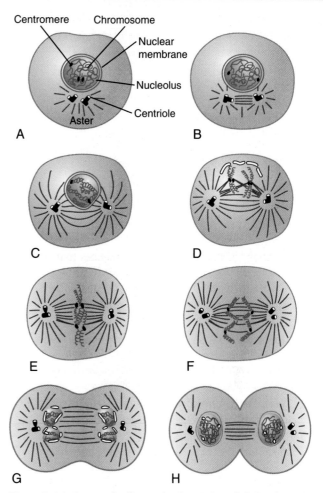

Figure 3-14. Stages of cell reproduction. *A, B,* and *C,* Prophase. *D,* Prometaphase. *E,* Metaphase. *F,* Anaphase. *G* and *H,* Telophase. (From Margaret C. Gladbach, Estate of Mary E. and Dan Todd, Kansas.)

body actually have life cycle periods that vary from as little as 10 hours for highly stimulated bone marrow cells to an entire lifetime of the human body for most nerve cells.

Cell Reproduction Begins with Replication of DNA

As is true of almost all other important events in the cell, reproduction begins in the nucleus itself. The first step is *replication (duplication) of all DNA in the chromosomes.* Only after this has occurred can mitosis take place.

The DNA begins to be duplicated some 5 to 10 hours before mitosis, and this is completed in 4 to 8 hours. The net result is two exact *replicas* of all DNA. These replicas become the DNA in the two new daughter cells that will be formed at mitosis. After replication of the DNA, there is another period of 1 to 2 hours before mitosis begins abruptly. Even during this period, preliminary changes that will lead to the mitotic process are beginning to take place.

Chemical and Physical Events of DNA Replication. DNA is replicated in much the same way that RNA is transcribed in response to DNA, except for a few important differences:

1. Both strands of the DNA in each chromosome are replicated, not simply one of them.

2. Both entire strands of the DNA helix are replicated from end to end, rather than small portions of them, as occurs in the transcription of RNA.

3. The principal enzymes for replicating DNA are a complex of multiple enzymes called *DNA polymerase,* which is comparable to RNA polymerase. It attaches to and moves along the DNA template strand while another enzyme, *DNA ligase,* causes bonding of successive DNA nucleotides to one another, using high-energy phosphate bonds to energize these attachments.

4. Formation of each new DNA strand occurs simultaneously in hundreds of segments along each of the two strands of the helix until the entire strand is replicated. Then the ends of the subunits are joined together by the DNA ligase enzyme.

5. Each newly formed strand of DNA remains attached by loose hydrogen bonding to the original DNA strand that was used as its template. Therefore, two DNA helixes are coiled together.

6. Because the DNA helixes in each chromosome are approximately 6 centimeters in length and have millions of helix turns, it would be impossible for the two newly formed DNA helixes to uncoil from each other were it not for some special mechanism. This is achieved by enzymes that periodically cut each helix along its entire length, rotate each segment enough to cause separation, and then resplice the helix. Thus, the two new helixes become uncoiled.

DNA Repair, DNA "Proofreading," and "Mutation."
During the hour or so between DNA replication and the beginning of mitosis, there is a period of active repair and "proofreading" of the DNA strands. That is, wherever inappropriate DNA nucleotides have been matched up with the nucleotides of the original template strand, special enzymes cut out the defective areas and replace these with appropriate complementary nucleotides. This is achieved by the same DNA polymerases and DNA ligases that are used in replication. This repair process is referred to as *DNA proofreading.*

Because of repair and proofreading, the transcription process rarely makes a mistake. But when a mistake is made, this is called a *mutation.* The mutation causes formation of some abnormal protein in the cell rather than a needed protein, often leading to abnormal cellular function and sometimes even cell death. Yet given that there are 30,000 or more genes in the human genome and that the period from one human generation to another is about 30 years, one would expect as many as 10 or many more mutations in the passage of the genome from parent to child. As a further protection, however, each human genome is represented by two separate sets of chromosomes with almost identical genes. Therefore, one functional gene of each pair is almost always available to the child despite mutations.

Chromosomes and Their Replication

The DNA helixes of the nucleus are packaged in chromosomes. The human cell contains 46 chromosomes arranged in 23 pairs. Most of the genes in the two chromosomes of each pair are identical or almost identical to each other, so it is usually stated that the different genes also exist in pairs, although occasionally this is not the case.

In addition to DNA in the chromosome, there is a large amount of protein in the chromosome, composed mainly of many small molecules of electropositively charged *histones.* The histones are organized into vast numbers of small, bobbin-like cores. Small segments of each DNA helix are coiled sequentially around one core after another.

The histone cores play an important role in the regulation of DNA activity because as long as the DNA is packaged tightly, it cannot function as a template for either the formation of RNA or the replication of new DNA. Further, some of the regulatory proteins have been shown to *decondense* the histone packaging of the DNA and to allow small segments at a time to form RNA.

Several nonhistone proteins are also major components of chromosomes, functioning both as chromosomal structural proteins and, in connection with the genetic regulatory machinery, as activators, inhibitors, and enzymes.

Replication of the chromosomes in their entirety occurs during the next few minutes after replication of the DNA helixes has been completed; the new DNA helixes collect new protein molecules as needed. The two newly formed chromosomes remain attached to each other (until time for mitosis) at a point called the *centromere* located near their center. These duplicated but still attached chromosomes are called *chromatids.*

Cell Mitosis

The actual process by which the cell splits into two new cells is called *mitosis.* Once each chromosome has been replicated to form the two chromatids, in many cells, mitosis follows automatically within 1 or 2 hours.

Mitotic Apparatus: Function of the Centrioles.
One of the first events of mitosis takes place in the cytoplasm, occurring during the latter part of interphase in or around the small structures called *centrioles.* As shown in Figure 3-14, two pairs of centrioles lie close to each other near one pole of the nucleus. These centrioles, like the DNA and chromosomes, are also replicated during interphase, usually shortly before replication of the DNA. Each centriole is a small cylindrical body about 0.4 micrometer long and about 0.15 micrometer in diameter, consisting mainly of nine parallel tubular structures arranged in the form of a cylinder. The two centrioles of each pair lie at right angles to each other. Each pair of centrioles, along with attached *pericentriolar material,* is called a *centrosome.*

Shortly before mitosis is to take place, the two pairs of centrioles begin to move apart from each other. This is caused by polymerization of protein microtubules growing between the respective centriole pairs and actually pushing them apart. At the same time, other microtubules grow radially away from each of the centriole pairs, forming a spiny star, called the *aster,* in each end of the cell. Some of the spines of the aster penetrate the nuclear membrane and help separate the two sets of chromatids during mitosis. The complex of microtubules extending between the two new centriole pairs is called the *spindle,* and the entire set of microtubules plus the two pairs of centrioles is called the *mitotic apparatus.*

Prophase. The first stage of mitosis, called *prophase,* is shown in Figure 3-14*A, B,* and *C.* While the spindle is forming, the chromosomes of the nucleus (which in interphase consist of loosely coiled strands) become condensed into well-defined chromosomes.

Prometaphase. During this stage (see Figure 3-14*D*), the growing microtubular spines of the aster fragment the nuclear envelope. At the same time, multiple microtubules from the aster attach to the chromatids at the centromeres, where the paired chromatids are still bound to each other; the tubules then pull one chromatid of each pair toward one cellular pole and its partner toward the opposite pole.

Metaphase. During metaphase (see Figure 3-14*E*), the two asters of the mitotic apparatus are pushed farther apart. This is believed to occur because the microtubular spines from the two asters, where they interdigitate with each other to form the mitotic spindle, actually push each other away. There is reason to believe that minute contractile protein molecules called *"molecular motors,"* perhaps composed of the muscle protein *actin,* extend between the respective spines and, using a stepping action as in muscle, actively slide the spines in a reverse direction along each other. Simultaneously, the chromatids are pulled tightly by their attached microtubules to the very center of the cell, lining up to form the *equatorial plate* of the mitotic spindle.

Anaphase. During this phase (see Figure 3-14*F*), the two chromatids of each chromosome are pulled apart at the centromere. All 46 pairs of chromatids are separated, forming two separate sets of 46 *daughter chromosomes.* One of these sets is pulled toward one mitotic aster and the other toward the other aster as the two respective poles of the dividing cell are pushed still farther apart.

Telophase. In telophase (see Figure 3-14*G* and *H*), the two sets of daughter chromosomes are pushed completely apart. Then the mitotic apparatus dissolutes, and a new nuclear membrane develops around each set of chromosomes. This membrane is formed from portions of the endoplasmic reticulum that are already present in the cytoplasm. Shortly thereafter, the cell pinches in two, midway between the two nuclei. This is caused by formation of a contractile ring of *microfilaments* composed of *actin* and probably *myosin* (the two contractile proteins of muscle) at the juncture of the newly developing cells that pinches them off from each other.

Control of Cell Growth and Cell Reproduction

We know that certain cells grow and reproduce all the time, such as the blood-forming cells of the bone marrow, the germinal layers of the skin, and the epithelium of the gut. Many other cells, however, such as smooth muscle cells, may not reproduce for many years. A few cells, such as the neurons and most striated muscle cells, do not reproduce during the entire life of a person, except during the original period of fetal life.

In certain tissues, an insufficiency of some types of cells causes these to grow and reproduce rapidly until appropriate numbers of them are again available. For instance, in some young animals, seven eighths of the liver can be removed surgically, and the cells of the remaining one eighth will grow and divide until the liver mass returns to almost normal. The same occurs for many glandular cells and most cells of the bone marrow, subcutaneous tissue, intestinal epithelium, and almost any other tissue except highly differentiated cells such as nerve and muscle cells.

We know little about the mechanisms that maintain proper numbers of the different types of cells in the body. However, experiments have shown at least three ways in which growth can be controlled. First, growth often is controlled by *growth factors* that come from other parts of the body. Some of these circulate in the blood, but others originate in adjacent tissues. For instance, the epithelial cells of some glands, such as the pancreas, fail to grow without a growth factor from the sublying connective tissue of the gland. Second, most normal cells stop growing when they have run out of space for growth. This occurs when cells are grown in tissue culture; the cells grow until they contact a solid object, and then growth stops. Third, cells grown in tissue culture often stop growing when minute amounts of their own secretions are allowed to collect in the culture medium. This, too, could provide a means for negative feedback control of growth.

Regulation of Cell Size. Cell size is determined almost entirely by the amount of functioning DNA in the nucleus. If replication of the DNA does not occur, the cell grows to a certain size and thereafter remains at that size. Conversely, it is possible, by use of the chemical *colchicine,* to prevent formation of the mitotic spindle and therefore to prevent mitosis, even though replication of the DNA continues. In this event, the nucleus contains far greater quantities of DNA than it normally does, and the cell grows proportionately larger. It is assumed that this results simply from increased production of RNA and cell proteins, which in turn cause the cell to grow larger.

Cell Differentiation

A special characteristic of cell growth and cell division is *cell differentiation,* which refers to changes in physical and functional properties of cells as they proliferate in the embryo to form the different bodily structures and organs.

The description of an especially interesting experiment that helps explain these processes follows.

When the nucleus from an intestinal mucosal cell of a frog is surgically implanted into a frog ovum from which the original ovum nucleus was removed, the result is often the formation of a normal frog. This demonstrates that even the intestinal mucosal cell, which is a well-differentiated cell, carries all the necessary genetic information for development of all structures required in the frog's body.

Therefore, it has become clear that differentiation results not from loss of genes but from selective repression of different gene promoters. In fact, electron micrographs suggest that some segments of DNA helixes wound around histone cores become so condensed that they no longer uncoil to form RNA molecules. One explanation for this is as follows: It has been supposed that the cellular genome begins at a certain stage of cell differentiation to produce a regulatory *protein* that forever after represses a select group of genes. Therefore, the repressed genes never function again. Regardless of the mechanism, mature human cells produce a maximum of about 8000 to 10,000 proteins rather than the potential 30,000 or more if all genes were active.

Embryological experiments show that certain cells in an embryo control differentiation of adjacent cells. For instance, the *primordial chorda-mesoderm* is called the *primary organizer* of the embryo because it forms a focus around which the rest of the embryo develops. It differentiates into a *mesodermal axis* that contains segmentally arranged *somites* and, as a result of *inductions* in the surrounding tissues, causes formation of essentially all the organs of the body.

Another instance of induction occurs when the developing eye vesicles come in contact with the ectoderm of the head and cause the ectoderm to thicken into a lens plate that folds inward to form the lens of the eye. Therefore, a large share of the embryo develops as a result of such inductions, one part of the body affecting another part, and this part affecting still other parts.

Thus, although our understanding of cell differentiation is still hazy, we know many control mechanisms by which differentiation *could* occur.

Apoptosis—Programmed Cell Death

The 100 trillion cells of the body are members of a highly organized community in which the total number of cells is regulated not only by controlling the rate of cell division but also by controlling the rate of cell death. When cells are no longer needed or become a threat to the organism, they undergo a suicidal *programmed cell death,* or *apoptosis.* This process involves a specific proteolytic cascade that causes the cell to shrink and condense, to disassemble its cytoskeleton, and to alter its cell surface so that a neighboring phagocytic cell, such as a macrophage, can attach to the cell membrane and digest the cell.

In contrast to programmed death, cells that die as a result of an acute injury usually swell and burst due to loss of cell membrane integrity, a process called cell *necrosis.* Necrotic cells may spill their contents, causing inflammation and injury to neighboring cells. Apoptosis, however, is an orderly cell death that results in disassembly and phagocytosis of the cell before any leakage of its contents occurs, and neighboring cells usually remain healthy.

Apoptosis is initiated by activation of a family of proteases called *caspases.* These are enzymes that are synthesized and stored in the cell as inactive *procaspases.* The mechanisms of activation of caspases are complex, but once activated, the enzymes cleave and activate other procaspases, triggering a cascade that rapidly breaks down proteins within the cell. The cell thus dismantles itself, and its remains are rapidly digested by neighboring phagocytic cells.

A tremendous amount of apoptosis occurs in tissues that are being remodeled during development. Even in adult humans, billions of cells die each hour in tissues such as the intestine and bone marrow and are replaced by new cells. Programmed cell death, however, is normally balanced with the formation of new cells in healthy adults. Otherwise, the body's tissues would shrink or grow excessively. Recent studies suggest that abnormalities of apoptosis may play a key role in neurodegenerative diseases such as Alzheimer's disease, as well as in cancer and autoimmune disorders. Some drugs that have been used successfully for chemotherapy appear to induce apoptosis in cancer cells.

Cancer

Cancer is caused in all or almost all instances by *mutation* or by some other *abnormal activation* of cellular genes that control cell growth and cell mitosis. The abnormal genes are called *oncogenes.* As many as 100 different oncogenes have been discovered.

Also present in all cells are *antioncogenes,* which suppress the activation of specific oncogenes. Therefore, loss or inactivation of antioncogenes can allow activation of oncogenes that lead to cancer.

Only a minute fraction of the cells that mutate in the body ever lead to cancer. There are several reasons for this. First, most mutated cells have less survival capability than normal cells and simply die. Second, only a few of the mutated cells that do survive become cancerous, because even most mutated cells still have normal feedback controls that prevent excessive growth.

Third, those cells that are potentially cancerous are often destroyed by the body's immune system before they grow into a cancer. This occurs in the following way: Most mutated cells form abnormal proteins within their cell bodies because of their altered genes, and these proteins activate the body's immune system, causing it to form antibodies or sensitized lymphocytes that react against the cancerous cells, destroying them. In support of this is the fact that in people whose immune systems have been suppressed, such as in those taking immuno-suppressant drugs after kidney or heart transplantation, the probability of a cancer's developing is multiplied as much as fivefold.

Fourth, usually several different activated oncogenes are required simultaneously to cause a cancer. For instance, one such gene might promote rapid reproduction of a cell line, but no cancer occurs because there is not a simultaneous mutant gene to form the needed blood vessels.

But what is it that causes the altered genes? Considering that many trillions of new cells are formed each year in humans, a better question might be, why is it that all of us do not develop millions or billions of mutant cancerous cells? The answer is the incredible precision with which DNA chromosomal strands are replicated in each cell before mitosis can take place, and also the proofreading process that cuts and repairs any abnormal DNA strand before the mitotic process is allowed to proceed. Yet despite all these inherited cellular precautions, probably one newly formed cell in every few million still has significant mutant characteristics.

Thus, chance alone is all that is required for mutations to take place, so we can suppose that a large number of cancers are merely the result of an unlucky occurrence.

However, the probability of mutations can be increased manyfold when a person is exposed to certain chemical, physical, or biological factors, including the following:

1. It is well known that *ionizing radiation,* such as x-rays, gamma rays, and particle radiation from radioactive substances, and even ultraviolet light can predispose individuals to cancer. Ions formed in tissue cells under the influence of such radiation are highly reactive and can rupture DNA strands, thus causing many mutations.

2. *Chemical substances* of certain types also have a high propensity for causing mutations. It was discovered long ago that various aniline dye derivatives are likely to cause cancer, so workers in chemical plants producing such substances, if unprotected, have a special predisposition to cancer. Chemical substances that can cause mutation are called *carcinogens.* The carcinogens that currently cause the greatest number of deaths are those in cigarette smoke. They cause about one quarter of all cancer deaths.

3. *Physical irritants* can also lead to cancer, such as continued abrasion of the linings of the intestinal tract by some types of food. The damage to the tissues leads to rapid mitotic replacement of the cells. The more rapid the mitosis, the greater the chance for mutation.

4. In many families, there is a strong *hereditary tendency* to cancer. This results from the fact that most cancers require not one mutation but two or more mutations before cancer occurs. In those families that are particularly predisposed to cancer, it is presumed that one or more cancerous genes are already mutated in the inherited genome. Therefore, far fewer additional mutations must take place in such family members before a cancer begins to grow.

5. In laboratory animals, certain types of viruses can cause some kinds of cancer, including leukemia. This usually results in one of two ways. In the case of DNA viruses, the DNA strand of the virus can insert itself directly into one of the chromosomes and thereby cause a mutation that leads to cancer. In the case of RNA viruses, some of these carry with them an enzyme called *reverse transcriptase* that causes DNA to be transcribed from the RNA. The transcribed DNA then inserts itself into the animal cell genome, leading to cancer.

Invasive Characteristic of the Cancer Cell. The major differences between the cancer cell and the normal cell are the following: (1) The cancer cell does not respect usual cellular growth limits; the reason for this is that these cells presumably do not require all the same growth factors that are necessary to cause growth of normal cells. (2) Cancer cells are often far less adhesive to one another than are normal cells. Therefore, they tend to wander through the tissues, enter the blood stream, and be transported all through the body, where they form nidi for numerous new cancerous growths. (3) Some cancers also produce *angiogenic factors* that cause many new blood vessels to grow into the cancer, thus supplying the nutrients required for cancer growth.

Why Do Cancer Cells Kill?

The answer to this question is usually simple. Cancer tissue competes with normal tissues for nutrients. Because cancer cells continue to proliferate indefinitely, their number multiplying day by day, cancer cells soon demand essentially all the nutrition available to the body or to an essential part of the body. As a result, normal tissues gradually suffer nutritive death.

Bibliography

Alberts B, Johnson A, Lewis J, et al: *Molecular Biology of the Cell,* ed 5, New York, 2008, Garland Science.

Aranda A, Pascal A: Nuclear hormone receptors and gene expression, *Physiol Rev* 81:1269, 2001.

Brodersen P, Voinnet O: Revisiting the principles of microRNA target recognition and mode of action, *Nat Rev Mol Cell Biol* 10:141, 2009.

Cairns BR: The logic of chromatin architecture and remodelling at promoters, *Nature* 461:193, 2009.

Carthew RW, Sontheimer EJ: Origins and mechanisms of miRNAs and siRNAs, *Cell* 136:642, 2009.

Castanotto D, Rossi JJ: The promises and pitfalls of RNA-interference-based therapeutics, *Nature* 457:426, 2009.

Cedar H, Bergman Y: Linking DNA methylation and histone modification: patterns and paradigms, *Nat Rev Genet* 10:295, 2009.

Croce CM: Causes and consequences of microRNA dysregulation in cancer, *Nat Rev Genet* 10:704, 2009.

Frazer KA, Murray SS, Schork NJ, et al: Human genetic variation and its contribution to complex traits, *Nat Rev Genet* 10:241, 2009.

Fuda NJ, Ardehali MB, Lis JT: Defining mechanisms that regulate RNA polymerase II transcription in vivo, *Nature* 461:186, 2009.

Hahn S: Structure and mechanism of the RNA polymerase II transcription machinery, *Nat Struct Mol Biol* 11:394, 2004.

Hastings PJ, Lupski JR, Rosenberg SM, et al: Mechanisms of change in gene copy number, *Nat Rev Genet* 10:551, 2009.

Hoeijmakers JH: DNA damage, aging, and cancer, *N Engl J Med* 361:1475, 2009.

Hotchkiss RS, Strasser A, McDunn JE, et al: Cell death, *N Engl J Med* 361:1570, 2009.

Jinek M, Doudna JA: A three-dimensional view of the molecular machinery of RNA interference, *Nature* 457:40, 2009.

Jockusch BM, Hüttelmaier S, Illenberger S: From the nucleus toward the cell periphery: a guided tour for mRNAs, *News Physiol Sci* 18:7, 2003.

Kim VN, Han J, Siomi MC: Biogenesis of small RNAs in animals, *Nat Rev Mol Cell Biol* 10:126, 2009.

Misteli T, Soutoglou E: The emerging role of nuclear architecture in DNA repair and genome maintenance, *Nat Rev Mol Cell Biol* 10:243, 2009.

Moazed D: Small RNAs in transcriptional gene silencing and genome defence, *Nature* 457:413, 2009.

Siller KH, Doe CQ: Spindle orientation during asymmetric cell division, *Nat Cell Biol* 11:365, 2009.

Sims RJ 3rd, Reinberg D: Is there a code embedded in proteins that is based on post-translational modifications? *Nat Rev Mol Cell Biol* 9:815, 2008.

Stappenbeck TS, Miyoshi H: The role of stromal stem cells in tissue regeneration and wound repair. *Science* 324:1666, 2009.

Sutherland H, Bickmore WA: Transcription factories: gene expression in unions?, *Nat Rev Genet* 10:457, 2009.

UNIT II

Membrane Physiology, Nerve, and Muscle

4. Transport of Substances Through Cell Membranes

5. Membrane Potentials and Action Potentials

6. Contraction of Skeletal Muscle

7. Excitation of Skeletal Muscle: Neuromuscular Transmission and Excitation-Contraction Coupling

8. Excitation and Contraction of Smooth Muscle

Transport of Substances Through Cell Membranes

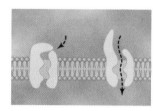

Figure 4-1 gives the approximate concentrations of important electrolytes and other substances in the *extracellular fluid* and *intracellular fluid*. Note that the extracellular fluid contains a large amount of *sodium* but only a small amount of *potassium*. Exactly the opposite is true of the intracellular fluid. Also, the extracellular fluid contains a large amount of *chloride* ions, whereas the intracellular fluid contains very little. But the concentrations of *phosphates* and *proteins* in the intracellular fluid are considerably greater than those in the extracellular fluid. These differences are extremely important to the life of the cell. The purpose of this chapter is to explain how the differences are brought about by the transport mechanisms of the cell membranes.

The Lipid Barrier of the Cell Membrane, and Cell Membrane Transport Proteins

The structure of the membrane covering the outside of every cell of the body is discussed in Chapter 2 and illustrated in Figures 2-3 and 4-2. This membrane consists almost entirely of a *lipid bilayer,* but it also contains large numbers of protein molecules in the lipid, many of which penetrate all the way through the membrane, as shown in Figure 4-2.

The lipid bilayer is not miscible with either the extracellular fluid or the intracellular fluid. Therefore, it constitutes a barrier against movement of water molecules and water-soluble substances between the extracellular and intracellular fluid compartments. However, as demonstrated in Figure 4-2 by the leftmost arrow, a few substances can penetrate this lipid bilayer, diffusing directly through the lipid substance itself; this is true mainly of lipid-soluble substances, as described later.

The protein molecules in the membrane have entirely different properties for transporting substances. Their molecular structures interrupt the continuity of the lipid bilayer, constituting an alternative pathway through the cell membrane. Most of these penetrating proteins, therefore, can function as *transport proteins.* Different proteins function differently. Some have watery spaces all the way through the molecule and allow free movement of water, as well as selected ions or molecules; these are called *channel proteins.* Others, called *carrier proteins,* bind with molecules or ions that are to be transported; conformational changes in the protein molecules then move the substances through the interstices of the protein to the other side of the membrane. Both the channel proteins and the carrier proteins are usually highly selective for the types of molecules or ions that are allowed to cross the membrane.

"Diffusion" Versus "Active Transport." Transport through the cell membrane, either directly through the lipid bilayer or through the proteins, occurs by one of two basic processes: *diffusion* or *active transport.*

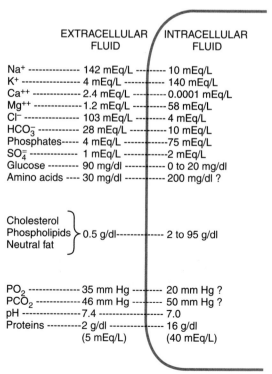

	EXTRACELLULAR FLUID	INTRACELLULAR FLUID
Na⁺	142 mEq/L	10 mEq/L
K⁺	4 mEq/L	140 mEq/L
Ca⁺⁺	2.4 mEq/L	0.0001 mEq/L
Mg⁺⁺	1.2 mEq/L	58 mEq/L
Cl⁻	103 mEq/L	4 mEq/L
HCO₃⁻	28 mEq/L	10 mEq/L
Phosphates	4 mEq/L	75 mEq/L
SO₄⁼	1 mEq/L	2 mEq/L
Glucose	90 mg/dl	0 to 20 mg/dl
Amino acids	30 mg/dl	200 mg/dl ?
Cholesterol Phospholipids Neutral fat	0.5 g/dl	2 to 95 g/dl
PO₂	35 mm Hg	20 mm Hg ?
PCO₂	46 mm Hg	50 mm Hg ?
pH	7.4	7.0
Proteins	2 g/dl (5 mEq/L)	16 g/dl (40 mEq/L)

Figure 4-1 Chemical compositions of extracellular and intracellular fluids.

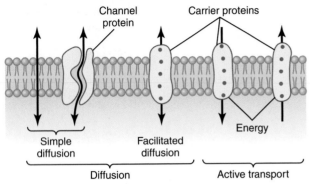

Figure 4-2 Transport pathways through the cell membrane, and the basic mechanisms of transport.

Although there are many variations of these basic mechanisms, diffusion means random molecular movement of substances molecule by molecule, either through intermolecular spaces in the membrane or in combination with a carrier protein. The energy that causes diffusion is the energy of the normal kinetic motion of matter.

By contrast, active transport means movement of ions or other substances across the membrane in combination with a carrier protein in such a way that the carrier protein causes the substance to move against an energy gradient, such as from a low-concentration state to a high-concentration state. This movement requires an additional source of energy besides kinetic energy. Following is a more detailed explanation of the basic physics and physical chemistry of these two processes.

Diffusion

All molecules and ions in the body fluids, including water molecules and dissolved substances, are in constant motion, each particle moving its own separate way. Motion of these particles is what physicists call "heat"—the greater the motion, the higher the temperature—and the motion never ceases under any condition except at absolute zero temperature. When a moving molecule, A, approaches a stationary molecule, B, the electrostatic and other nuclear forces of molecule A repel molecule B, transferring some of the energy of motion of molecule A to molecule B. Consequently, molecule B gains kinetic energy of motion, while molecule A slows down, losing some of its kinetic energy. Thus, as shown in Figure 4-3, a single molecule

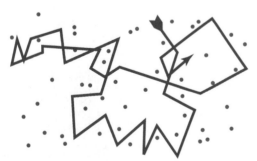

Figure 4-3 Diffusion of a fluid molecule during a thousandth of a second.

in a solution bounces among the other molecules first in one direction, then another, then another, and so forth, randomly bouncing thousands of times each second. This continual movement of molecules among one another in liquids or in gases is called *diffusion.*

Ions diffuse in the same manner as whole molecules, and even suspended colloid particles diffuse in a similar manner, except that the colloids diffuse far less rapidly than molecular substances because of their large size.

Diffusion Through the Cell Membrane

Diffusion through the cell membrane is divided into two subtypes called *simple diffusion* and *facilitated diffusion.* Simple diffusion means that kinetic movement of molecules or ions occurs through a membrane opening or through intermolecular spaces without any interaction with carrier proteins in the membrane. The rate of diffusion is determined by the amount of substance available, the velocity of kinetic motion, and the number and sizes of openings in the membrane through which the molecules or ions can move.

Facilitated diffusion requires interaction of a carrier protein. The carrier protein aids passage of the molecules or ions through the membrane by binding chemically with them and shuttling them through the membrane in this form.

Simple diffusion can occur through the cell membrane by two pathways: (1) through the interstices of the lipid bilayer if the diffusing substance is lipid soluble and (2) through watery channels that penetrate all the way through some of the large transport proteins, as shown to the left in Figure 4-2.

Diffusion of Lipid-Soluble Substances Through the Lipid Bilayer. One of the most important factors that determines how rapidly a substance diffuses through the lipid bilayer is the *lipid solubility* of the substance. For instance, the lipid solubilities of oxygen, nitrogen, carbon dioxide, and alcohols are high, so all these can dissolve directly in the lipid bilayer and diffuse through the cell membrane in the same manner that diffusion of water solutes occurs in a watery solution. For obvious reasons, the rate of diffusion of each of these substances through the membrane is directly proportional to its lipid solubility. Especially large amounts of oxygen can be transported in this way; therefore, oxygen can be delivered to the interior of the cell almost as though the cell membrane did not exist.

Diffusion of Water and Other Lipid-Insoluble Molecules Through Protein Channels. Even though water is highly insoluble in the membrane lipids, it readily passes through channels in protein molecules that penetrate all the way through the membrane. The rapidity with which water molecules can move through most cell membranes is astounding. As an example, the total amount of water that diffuses in each direction through the red cell membrane during each second is about 100 times as great as the volume of the red cell itself.

Other lipid-insoluble molecules can pass through the protein pore channels in the same way as water molecules if they are water soluble and small enough. However, as they become larger, their penetration falls off rapidly. For instance, the diameter of the urea molecule is only 20 percent greater than that of water, yet its penetration through the cell membrane pores is about 1000 times less than that of water. Even so, given the astonishing rate of water penetration, this amount of urea penetration still allows rapid transport of urea through the membrane within minutes.

Diffusion Through Protein Pores and Channels— Selective Permeability and "Gating" of Channels

Computerized three-dimensional reconstructions of protein pores and channels have demonstrated tubular pathways all the way from the extracellular to the intracellular fluid. Therefore, substances can move by simple diffusion directly along these pores and channels from one side of the membrane to the other.

Pores are composed of integral cell membrane proteins that form open tubes through the membrane and are always open. However, the diameter of a pore and its electrical charges provide selectivity that permits only certain molecules to pass through. For example, protein pores, called *aquaporins* or *water channels*, permit rapid passage of water through cell membranes but exclude other molecules. At least 13 different types of aquaporins have been found in various cells of the human body. Aquaporins have a narrow pore that permits water molecules to diffuse through the membrane in single file. The pore is too narrow to permit passage of any hydrated ions. As discussed in Chapters 29 and 75, the density of some aquaporins (e.g., aquaporin-2) in cell membranes is not static but is altered in different physiological conditions.

The protein channels are distinguished by two important characteristics: (1) They are often *selectively permeable* to certain substances, and (2) many of the channels can be opened or closed by *gates* that are regulated by electrical signals *(voltage-gated channels)* or chemicals that bind to the channel proteins *(ligand-gated channels).*

Selective Permeability of Protein Channels.

Many of the protein channels are highly selective for transport of one or more specific ions or molecules. This results from the characteristics of the channel itself, such as its diameter, its shape, and the nature of the electrical charges and chemical bonds along its inside surfaces.

Potassium channels permit passage of potassium ions across the cell membrane about 1000 times more readily than they permit passage of sodium ions. This high degree of selectivity, however, cannot be explained entirely by molecular diameters of the ions since potassium ions are slightly larger than sodium ions. What is the mechanism for this remarkable ion selectivity? This question was partially answered when the structure of a *bacterial potassium channel* was determined by x-ray crystallography. Potassium channels were found to have a *tetrameric*

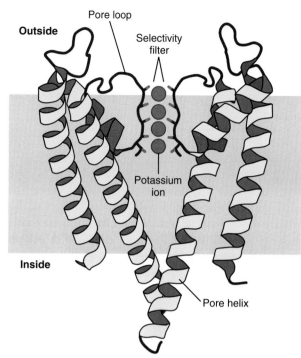

Figure 4-4 The structure of a potassium channel. The channel is composed of four subunits (only two are shown), each with two transmembrane helices. A narrow selectivity filter is formed from the pore loops and carbonyl oxygens line the walls of the selectivity filter, forming sites for transiently binding dehydrated potassium ions. The interaction of the potassium ions with carbonyl oxygens causes the potassium ions to shed their bound water molecules, permitting the dehydrated potassium ions to pass through the pore.

structure consisting of four identical protein subunits surrounding a central pore (Figure 4-4). At the top of the channel pore are *pore loops* that form a narrow *selectivity filter*. Lining the selectivity filter are *carbonyl oxygens*. When hydrated potassium ions enter the selectivity filter, they interact with the carbonyl oxygens and shed most of their bound water molecules, permitting the dehydrated potassium ions to pass through the channel. The carbonyl oxygens are too far apart, however, to enable them to interact closely with the smaller sodium ions, which are therefore effectively excluded by the selectivity filter from passing through the pore.

Different selectivity filters for the various ion channels are believed to determine, in large part, the specificity of the channel for cations or anions or for particular ions, such as Na^+, K^+, and Ca^{++}, that gain access to the channel.

One of the most important of the protein channels, the *sodium channel,* is only 0.3 by 0.5 nanometer in diameter, but more important, the inner surfaces of this channel are lined with amino acids that are *strongly negatively charged*, as shown by the negative signs inside the channel proteins in the top panel of Figure 4-5. These strong negative charges can pull small *dehydrated* sodium ions into these channels, actually pulling the sodium ions away from their hydrating water molecules. Once in the channel, the sodium ions diffuse in either direction according to the usual laws of diffusion. Thus, the sodium channel is specifically selective for passage of sodium ions.

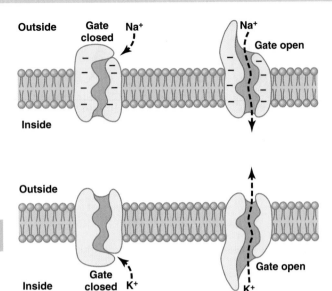

Figure 4-5 Transport of sodium and potassium ions through protein channels. Also shown are conformational changes in the protein molecules to open or close "gates" guarding the channels.

Gating of Protein Channels. Gating of protein channels provides a means of controlling ion permeability of the channels. This is shown in both panels of Figure 4-5 for selective gating of sodium and potassium ions. It is believed that some of the gates are actual gatelike extensions of the transport protein molecule, which can close the opening of the channel or can be lifted away from the opening by a conformational change in the shape of the protein molecule itself.

The opening and closing of gates are controlled in two principal ways:

1. *Voltage gating.* In this instance, the molecular conformation of the gate or of its chemical bonds responds to the electrical potential across the cell membrane. For instance, in the top panel of Figure 4-5, when there is a strong negative charge on the inside of the cell membrane, this presumably could cause the outside sodium gates to remain tightly closed; conversely, when the inside of the membrane loses its negative charge, these gates would open suddenly and allow tremendous quantities of sodium to pass inward through the sodium pores. This is the basic mechanism for eliciting action potentials in nerves that are responsible for nerve signals. In the bottom panel of Figure 4-5, the potassium gates are on the intracellular ends of the potassium channels, and they open when the inside of the cell membrane becomes positively charged. The opening of these gates is partly responsible for terminating the action potential, as is discussed more fully in Chapter 5.

2. *Chemical (ligand) gating.* Some protein channel gates are opened by the binding of a chemical substance (a ligand) with the protein; this causes a conformational or chemical bonding change in the protein molecule that opens or closes the gate. This is called *chemical gating*

or *ligand gating.* One of the most important instances of chemical gating is the effect of acetylcholine on the so-called *acetylcholine channel.* Acetylcholine opens the gate of this channel, providing a negatively charged pore about 0.65 nanometer in diameter that allows uncharged molecules or positive ions smaller than this diameter to pass through. This gate is exceedingly important for the transmission of nerve signals from one nerve cell to another (see Chapter 45) and from nerve cells to muscle cells to cause muscle contraction (see Chapter 7).

Open-State Versus Closed-State of Gated Channels. Figure 4-6*A* shows an especially interesting characteristic of most voltage-gated channels. This figure shows two recordings of electrical current flowing through a single sodium channel when there was an approximate 25-millivolt potential gradient across the membrane. Note that the channel conducts current either "all or none." That is, the gate of the channel snaps open and then snaps closed, each open state lasting for only a fraction of a millisecond up to several milliseconds. This demonstrates the rapidity with which changes can occur during the opening and closing of the protein molecular gates. At one voltage potential, the channel may remain closed all the time or almost all the time, whereas at another voltage level, it may remain open either all or most of the time. At in-between voltages, as shown in the figure, the gates tend to snap open and closed intermittently, giving an average current flow somewhere between the minimum and the maximum.

Patch-Clamp Method for Recording Ion Current Flow Through Single Channels. One might wonder how it is technically possible to record ion current flow through single protein channels as shown in Figure 4-6*A*. This has been achieved by using the "patch-clamp" method illustrated in Figure 4-6*B*. Very simply, a micropipette, having a tip diameter of only 1 or 2 micrometers, is abutted against the outside of a cell membrane. Then suction is applied inside the pipette to pull the membrane against the tip of the pipette. This creates a seal where the edges of the pipette touch the cell membrane. The result is a minute membrane "patch" at the tip of the pipette through which electrical current flow can be recorded.

Alternatively, as shown to the right in Figure 4-6*B*, the small cell membrane patch at the end of the pipette can be torn away from the cell. The pipette with its sealed patch is then inserted into a free solution. This allows the concentrations of ions both inside the micropipette and in the outside solution to be altered as desired. Also, the voltage between the two sides of the membrane can be set at will—that is, "clamped" to a given voltage.

It has been possible to make such patches small enough so that only a single channel protein is found in the membrane patch being studied. By varying the concentrations of different ions, as well as the voltage across the membrane, one can determine the transport characteristics of the single channel and also its gating properties.

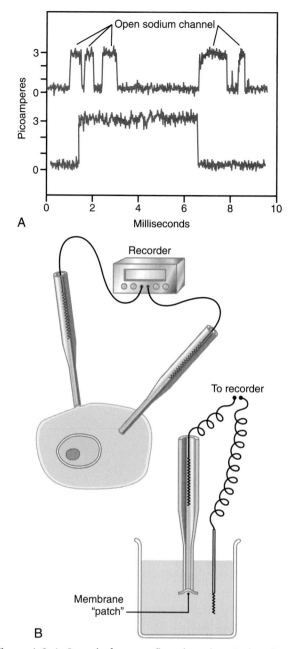

Figure 4-6 *A,* Record of current flow through a single voltage-gated sodium channel, demonstrating the "all or none" principle for opening and closing of the channel. *B,* The "patch-clamp" method for recording current flow through a single protein channel. To the left, recording is performed from a "patch" of a living cell membrane. To the right, recording is from a membrane patch that has been torn away from the cell.

Facilitated Diffusion

Facilitated diffusion is also called *carrier-mediated diffusion* because a substance transported in this manner diffuses through the membrane using a specific carrier protein to help. That is, the carrier *facilitates* diffusion of the substance to the other side.

Facilitated diffusion differs from simple diffusion in the following important way: Although the rate of simple diffusion through an open channel increases proportionately with the concentration of the diffusing substance,

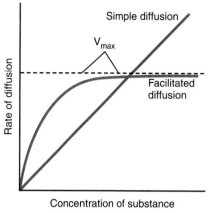

Figure 4-7 Effect of concentration of a substance on rate of diffusion through a membrane by simple diffusion and facilitated diffusion. This shows that facilitated diffusion approaches a maximum rate called the V_{max}.

in facilitated diffusion the rate of diffusion approaches a maximum, called V_{max}, as the concentration of the diffusing substance increases. This difference between simple diffusion and facilitated diffusion is demonstrated in Figure 4-7. The figure shows that as the concentration of the diffusing substance increases, the rate of simple diffusion continues to increase proportionately, but in the case of facilitated diffusion, the rate of diffusion cannot rise greater than the V_{max} level.

What is it that limits the rate of facilitated diffusion? A probable answer is the mechanism illustrated in Figure 4-8. This figure shows a carrier protein with a pore large enough to transport a specific molecule partway through. It also shows a binding "receptor" on the inside of the protein carrier. The molecule to be transported enters the pore and becomes bound. Then, in a fraction of a second, a conformational or chemical change occurs in the carrier protein, so the pore now opens to the opposite side of the membrane. Because the binding force of the receptor is weak, the thermal motion of the attached molecule causes

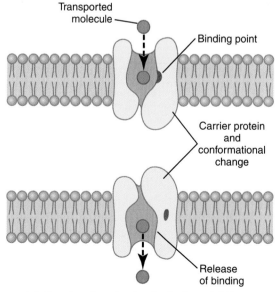

Figure 4-8 Postulated mechanism for facilitated diffusion.

49

it to break away and to be released on the opposite side of the membrane. The rate at which molecules can be transported by this mechanism can never be greater than the rate at which the carrier protein molecule can undergo change back and forth between its two states. Note specifically, though, that this mechanism allows the transported molecule to move—that is, to "diffuse"—in either direction through the membrane.

Among the most important substances that cross cell membranes by facilitated diffusion are *glucose* and most of the *amino acids.* In the case of glucose, at least five glucose transporter molecules have been discovered in various tissues. Some of these can also transport other monosaccharides that have structures similar to that of glucose, including galactose and fructose. One of these, glucose transporter 4 (GLUT4), is activated by insulin, which can increase the rate of facilitated diffusion of glucose as much as 10-fold to 20-fold in insulin-sensitive tissues. This is the principal mechanism by which insulin controls glucose use in the body, as discussed in Chapter 78.

Factors That Affect Net Rate of Diffusion

By now it is evident that many substances can diffuse through the cell membrane. What is usually important is the *net* rate of diffusion of a substance in the desired direction. This net rate is determined by several factors.

Net Diffusion Rate Is Proportional to the Concentration Difference Across a Membrane. Figure 4-9*A* shows a cell membrane with a substance in high concentration on the outside and low concentration on the inside. The rate at which the substance diffuses *inward* is proportional to the concentration of molecules on the *outside* because this concentration determines how many molecules strike the outside of the membrane each second. Conversely, the rate at which molecules diffuse *outward* is proportional to their concentration *inside* the membrane. Therefore, the rate of net diffusion into the cell is proportional to the concentration on the outside *minus* the concentration on the inside, or:

$$\text{Net diffusion} \propto (C_o - C_i)$$

in which C_o is concentration outside and C_i is concentration inside.

Effect of Membrane Electrical Potential on Diffusion of Ions—The "Nernst Potential." If an electrical potential is applied across the membrane, as shown in Figure 4-9*B*, the electrical charges of the ions cause them to move through the membrane even though no concentration difference exists to cause movement. Thus, in the left panel of Figure 4-9*B*, the concentration of *negative* ions is the same on both sides of the membrane, but a positive charge has been applied to the right side of the membrane and a negative charge to the left, creating an electrical gradient across the membrane. The positive charge attracts the negative ions, whereas the negative charge repels them. Therefore, net diffusion

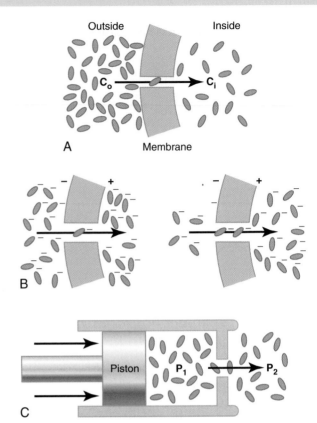

Figure 4-9 Effect of concentration difference (*A*), electrical potential difference affecting negative ions (*B*), and pressure difference (*C*) to cause diffusion of molecules and ions through a cell membrane.

occurs from left to right. After some time, large quantities of negative ions have moved to the right, creating the condition shown in the right panel of Figure 4-9*B*, in which a concentration difference of the ions has developed in the direction opposite to the electrical potential difference. The concentration difference now tends to move the ions to the left, while the electrical difference tends to move them to the right. When the concentration difference rises high enough, the two effects balance each other. At normal body temperature (37°C), the electrical difference that will balance a given concentration difference of *univalent* ions—such as sodium (Na+) ions—can be determined from the following formula, called the *Nernst equation:*

$$\text{EMF (in millivolts)} = \pm 61\log\frac{C_1}{C_2}$$

in which EMF is the electromotive force (voltage) between side 1 and side 2 of the membrane, C_1 is the concentration on side 1, and C_2 is the concentration on side 2. This equation is extremely important in understanding the transmission of nerve impulses and is discussed in much greater detail in Chapter 5.

Effect of a Pressure Difference Across the Membrane. At times, considerable pressure difference develops between the two sides of a diffusible membrane.

This occurs, for instance, at the blood capillary membrane in all tissues of the body. The pressure is about 20 mm Hg greater inside the capillary than outside.

Pressure actually means the sum of all the forces of the different molecules striking a unit surface area at a given instant. Therefore, when the pressure is higher on one side of a membrane than on the other, this means that the sum of all the forces of the molecules striking the channels on that side of the membrane is greater than on the other side. In most instances, this is caused by greater numbers of molecules striking the membrane per second on one side than on the other side. The result is that increased amounts of energy are available to cause net movement of molecules from the high-pressure side toward the low-pressure side. This effect is demonstrated in Figure 4-9*C*, which shows a piston developing high pressure on one side of a "pore," thereby causing more molecules to strike the pore on this side and, therefore, more molecules to "diffuse" to the other side.

Osmosis Across Selectively Permeable Membranes—"Net Diffusion" of Water

By far the most abundant substance that diffuses through the cell membrane is water. Enough water ordinarily diffuses in each direction through the red cell membrane per second to equal about *100 times the volume of the cell itself.* Yet normally the amount that diffuses in the two directions is balanced so precisely that zero net movement of water occurs. Therefore, the volume of the cell remains constant. However, under certain conditions, a *concentration difference for water* can develop across a membrane, just as concentration differences for other substances can occur. When this happens, net movement of water does occur across the cell membrane, causing the cell either to swell or shrink, depending on the direction of the water movement. This process of net movement of water caused by a concentration difference of water is called *osmosis.*

To give an example of osmosis, let us assume the conditions shown in Figure 4-10, with pure water on one side of the cell membrane and a solution of sodium chloride on the other side. Water molecules pass through the cell membrane with ease, whereas sodium and chloride ions pass through only with difficulty. Therefore, sodium chloride solution is actually a mixture of permeant water molecules and nonpermeant sodium and chloride ions, and the membrane is said to be *selectively permeable* to water but much less so to sodium and chloride ions. Yet the presence of the sodium and chloride has displaced some of the water molecules on the side of the membrane where these ions are present and, therefore, has reduced the concentration of water molecules to less than that of pure water. As a result, in the example of Figure 4-10, more water molecules strike the channels on the left side, where there is pure water, than on the right side, where the water concentration has been reduced. Thus, net movement of water occurs from left to right—that is, *osmosis* occurs from the pure water into the sodium chloride solution.

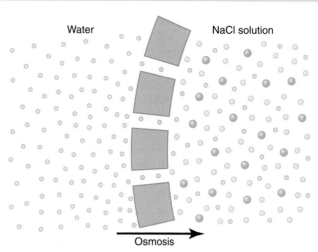

Figure 4-10 Osmosis at a cell membrane when a sodium chloride solution is placed on one side of the membrane and water is placed on the other side.

Osmotic Pressure

If in Figure 4-10 pressure were applied to the sodium chloride solution, osmosis of water into this solution would be slowed, stopped, or even reversed. The exact amount of pressure required to stop osmosis is called the *osmotic pressure* of the sodium chloride solution.

The principle of a pressure difference opposing osmosis is demonstrated in Figure 4-11, which shows a selectively permeable membrane separating two columns of fluid, one containing pure water and the other containing a solution of water and any solute that will not penetrate the membrane. Osmosis of water from chamber B into chamber A causes the levels of the fluid columns to become farther and farther apart, until eventually a pressure difference develops between the two sides of the membrane great enough to oppose the osmotic effect.

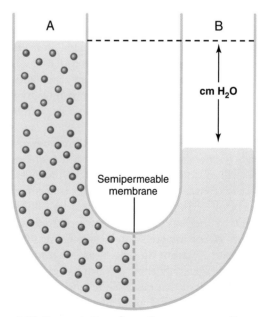

Figure 4-11 Demonstration of osmotic pressure caused by osmosis at a semipermeable membrane.

The pressure difference across the membrane at this point is equal to the osmotic pressure of the solution that contains the nondiffusible solute.

Importance of Number of Osmotic Particles (Molar Concentration) in Determining Osmotic Pressure. The osmotic pressure exerted by particles in a solution, whether they are molecules or ions, is determined by the *number* of particles per unit volume of fluid, *not by the mass* of the particles. The reason for this is that each particle in a solution, regardless of its mass, exerts, on average, the same amount of pressure against the membrane. That is, large particles, which have greater mass (m) than small particles, move at slower velocities (v). The small particles move at higher velocities in such a way that their average kinetic energies (k), determined by the equation

$$k = \frac{mv^2}{2}$$

are the same for each small particle as for each large particle. Consequently, the factor that determines the osmotic pressure of a solution is the concentration of the solution in terms of number of particles (which is the same as its *molar concentration* if it is a nondissociated molecule), not in terms of mass of the solute.

"Osmolality"—The Osmole. To express the concentration of a solution in terms of numbers of particles, the unit called the *osmole* is used in place of grams.

One osmole is 1 gram molecular weight of osmotically active solute. Thus, 180 grams of glucose, which is 1 gram molecular weight of glucose, is equal to 1 osmole of glucose because glucose does not dissociate into ions. If a solute dissociates into two ions, 1 gram molecular weight of the solute will become 2 osmoles because the number of osmotically active particles is now twice as great as is the case for the nondissociated solute. Therefore, when fully dissociated, 1 gram molecular weight of sodium chloride, 58.5 grams, is equal to 2 osmoles.

Thus, a solution that has *1 osmole of solute dissolved in each kilogram of water* is said to have an *osmolality of 1 osmole per kilogram*, and a solution that has 1/1000 osmole dissolved per kilogram has an osmolality of 1 milliosmole per kilogram. The normal osmolality of the extracellular and intracellular fluids is about *300 milliosmoles per kilogram of water.*

Relation of Osmolality to Osmotic Pressure. At normal body temperature, 37°C, a concentration of 1 osmole per liter will cause *19,300 mm Hg* osmotic pressure in the solution. Likewise, *1 milliosmole* per liter concentration is equivalent to *19.3 mm Hg* osmotic pressure. Multiplying this value by the 300 milliosmolar concentration of the body fluids gives a total calculated osmotic pressure of the body fluids of 5790 mm Hg. The measured value for this, however, averages only about 5500 mm Hg. The reason for this difference is that many of the ions in the body fluids, such as sodium and chloride ions, are highly attracted to one another; consequently, they cannot move entirely unrestrained in the fluids and create their full osmotic pressure potential. Therefore, on average, the actual osmotic pressure of the body fluids is about 0.93 times the calculated value.

The Term "Osmolarity." *Osmolarity* is the osmolar concentration expressed as *osmoles per liter of solution* rather than osmoles per kilogram of water. Although, strictly speaking, it is osmoles per kilogram of water (osmolality) that determines osmotic pressure, for dilute solutions such as those in the body, the quantitative differences between osmolarity and osmolality are less than 1 percent. Because it is far more practical to measure osmolarity than osmolality, this is the usual practice in almost all physiological studies.

"Active Transport" of Substances Through Membranes

At times, a large concentration of a substance is required in the intracellular fluid even though the extracellular fluid contains only a small concentration. This is true, for instance, for potassium ions. Conversely, it is important to keep the concentrations of other ions very low inside the cell even though their concentrations in the extracellular fluid are great. This is especially true for sodium ions. Neither of these two effects could occur by simple diffusion because simple diffusion eventually equilibrates concentrations on the two sides of the membrane. Instead, some energy source must cause excess movement of potassium ions to the inside of cells and excess movement of sodium ions to the outside of cells. When a cell membrane moves molecules or ions "uphill" against a concentration gradient (or "uphill" against an electrical or pressure gradient), the process is called *active transport.*

Different substances that are actively transported through at least some cell membranes include sodium ions, potassium ions, calcium ions, iron ions, hydrogen ions, chloride ions, iodide ions, urate ions, several different sugars, and most of the amino acids.

Primary Active Transport and Secondary Active Transport. Active transport is divided into two types according to the source of the energy used to cause the transport: *primary active transport* and *secondary active transport.* In primary active transport, the energy is derived directly from breakdown of adenosine triphosphate (ATP) or of some other high-energy phosphate compound. In secondary active transport, the energy is derived secondarily from energy that has been stored in the form of ionic concentration differences of secondary molecular or ionic substances between the two sides of a cell membrane, created originally by primary active transport. In both instances, transport depends on *carrier proteins* that penetrate through the cell membrane, as is true for facilitated diffusion. However, in active transport, the carrier protein functions differently from the carrier in facilitated diffusion because it is capable of imparting energy to the transported substance to move it against the electrochemical gradient. Following are some examples of primary active transport and secondary active transport, with more detailed explanations of their principles of function.

Primary Active Transport

Sodium-Potassium Pump

Among the substances that are transported by primary active transport are sodium, potassium, calcium, hydrogen, chloride, and a few other ions.

The active transport mechanism that has been studied in greatest detail is the *sodium-potassium (Na⁺-K⁺)* pump, a transport process that pumps sodium ions outward through the cell membrane of all cells and at the same time pumps potassium ions from the outside to the inside. This pump is responsible for maintaining the sodium and potassium concentration differences across the cell membrane, as well as for establishing a negative electrical voltage inside the cells. Indeed, Chapter 5 shows that this pump is also the basis of nerve function, transmitting nerve signals throughout the nervous system.

Figure 4-12 shows the basic physical components of the Na⁺-K⁺ pump. The *carrier protein* is a complex of two separate globular proteins: a larger one called the α subunit, with a molecular weight of about 100,000, and a smaller one called the β subunit, with a molecular weight of about 55,000. Although the function of the smaller protein is not known (except that it might anchor the protein complex in the lipid membrane), the larger protein has three specific features that are important for the functioning of the pump:

1. It has three *receptor sites for binding sodium ions* on the portion of the protein that protrudes to the inside of the cell.

2. It has two *receptor sites for potassium ions* on the outside.

3. The inside portion of this protein near the sodium binding sites has ATPase activity.

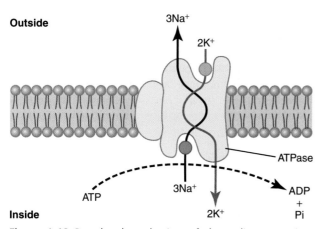

Figure 4-12 Postulated mechanism of the sodium-potassium pump. ADP, adenosine diphosphate; ATP, adenosine triphosphate; Pi, phosphate ion.

When two potassium ions bind on the outside of the carrier protein and three sodium ions bind on the inside, the ATPase function of the protein becomes activated. This then cleaves one molecule of ATP, splitting it to adenosine diphosphate (ADP) and liberating a high-energy phosphate bond of energy. This liberated energy is then believed to cause a chemical and conformational change in the protein carrier molecule, extruding the three sodium ions to the outside and the two potassium ions to the inside.

As with other enzymes, the Na⁺-K⁺ ATPase pump can run in reverse. If the electrochemical gradients for Na⁺ and K⁺ are experimentally increased enough so that the energy stored in their gradients is greater than the chemical energy of ATP hydrolysis, these ions will move down their concentration gradients and the Na⁺-K⁺ pump will synthesize ATP from ADP and phosphate. The phosphorylated form of the Na⁺-K⁺ pump, therefore, can either donate its phosphate to ADP to produce ATP or use the energy to change its conformation and pump Na⁺ out of the cell and K⁺ into the cell. The relative concentrations of ATP, ADP, and phosphate, as well as the electrochemical gradients for Na⁺ and K⁺, determine the direction of the enzyme reaction. For some cells, such as electrically active nerve cells, 60 to 70 percent of the cells' energy requirement may be devoted to pumping Na⁺ out of the cell and K⁺ into the cell.

The Na⁺-K⁺ Pump Is Important For Controlling Cell Volume. One of the most important functions of the Na⁺-K⁺ pump is to control the volume of each cell. Without function of this pump, most cells of the body would swell until they burst. The mechanism for controlling the volume is as follows: Inside the cell are large numbers of proteins and other organic molecules that cannot escape from the cell. Most of these are negatively charged and therefore attract large numbers of potassium, sodium, and other positive ions as well. All these molecules and ions then cause osmosis of water to the interior of the cell. Unless this is checked, the cell will swell indefinitely until it bursts. The normal mechanism for preventing this is the Na⁺-K⁺ pump. Note again that this device pumps three Na⁺ ions to the outside of the cell for every two K⁺ ions pumped to the interior. Also, the membrane is far less permeable to sodium ions than to potassium ions, so once the sodium ions are on the outside, they have a strong tendency to stay there. Thus, this represents a net loss of ions out of the cell, which initiates osmosis of water out of the cell as well.

If a cell begins to swell for any reason, this automatically activates the Na⁺-K⁺ pump, moving still more ions to the exterior and carrying water with them. Therefore, the Na⁺-K⁺ pump performs a continual surveillance role in maintaining normal cell volume.

Electrogenic Nature of the Na⁺-K⁺ Pump. The fact that the Na⁺-K⁺ pump moves three Na⁺ ions to the exterior for every two K⁺ ions to the interior means that a net of one positive charge is moved from the interior of the cell to the exterior for each cycle of the pump. This creates positivity outside the cell but leaves a deficit of positive ions inside the cell; that is, it causes negativity on the inside. Therefore, the Na$^+$-K$^+$ pump is said to be *electrogenic* because it creates an electrical potential across the cell membrane. As discussed in Chapter 5, this electrical potential is a basic requirement in nerve and muscle fibers for transmitting nerve and muscle signals.

Primary Active Transport of Calcium Ions

Another important primary active transport mechanism is the *calcium pump.* Calcium ions are normally maintained at extremely low concentration in the intracellular cytosol of virtually all cells in the body, at a concentration about 10,000 times less than that in the extracellular fluid. This is achieved mainly by two primary active transport calcium pumps. One is in the cell membrane and pumps calcium to the outside of the cell. The other pumps calcium ions into one or more of the intracellular vesicular organelles of the cell, such as the sarcoplasmic reticulum of muscle cells and the mitochondria in all cells. In each of these instances, the carrier protein penetrates the membrane and functions as an enzyme ATPase, having the same capability to cleave ATP as the ATPase of the sodium carrier protein. The difference is that this protein has a highly specific binding site for calcium instead of for sodium.

Primary Active Transport of Hydrogen Ions

At two places in the body, primary active transport of hydrogen ions is important: (1) in the gastric glands of the stomach and (2) in the late distal tubules and cortical collecting ducts of the kidneys.

In the gastric glands, the deep-lying *parietal cells* have the most potent primary active mechanism for transporting hydrogen ions of any part of the body. This is the basis for secreting hydrochloric acid in the stomach digestive secretions. At the secretory ends of the gastric gland parietal cells, the hydrogen ion concentration is increased as much as a millionfold and then released into the stomach along with chloride ions to form hydrochloric acid.

In the renal tubules are special *intercalated cells* in the late distal tubules and cortical collecting ducts that also transport hydrogen ions by primary active transport. In this case, large amounts of hydrogen ions are secreted from the blood into the urine for the purpose of eliminating excess hydrogen ions from the body fluids. The hydrogen ions can be secreted into the urine against a concentration gradient of about 900-fold.

Energetics of Primary Active Transport

The amount of energy required to transport a substance actively through a membrane is determined by how much the substance is concentrated during transport. Compared with the energy required to concentrate a substance 10-fold, to concentrate it 100-fold requires twice as much energy, and to concentrate it 1000-fold requires three times as much energy. In other words, the energy

required is proportional to the *logarithm* of the degree that the substance is concentrated, as expressed by the following formula:

$$\text{Energy (in calories per osmole)} = 1400 \log \frac{C_1}{C_2}$$

Thus, in terms of calories, the amount of energy required to concentrate 1 osmole of a substance 10-fold is about 1400 calories; or to concentrate it 100-fold, 2800 calories. One can see that the energy expenditure for concentrating substances in cells or for removing substances from cells against a concentration gradient can be tremendous. Some cells, such as those lining the renal tubules and many glandular cells, expend as much as 90 percent of their energy for this purpose alone.

Secondary Active Transport—Co-Transport and Counter-Transport

When sodium ions are transported out of cells by primary active transport, a large concentration gradient of sodium ions across the cell membrane usually develops—high concentration outside the cell and low concentration inside. This gradient represents a storehouse of energy because the excess sodium outside the cell membrane is always attempting to diffuse to the interior. Under appropriate conditions, this diffusion energy of sodium can pull other substances along with the sodium through the cell membrane. This phenomenon is called *co-transport;* it is one form of *secondary active transport.*

For sodium to pull another substance along with it, a coupling mechanism is required. This is achieved by means of still another carrier protein in the cell membrane. The carrier in this instance serves as an attachment point for both the sodium ion and the substance to be co-transported. Once they both are attached, the energy gradient of the sodium ion causes both the sodium ion and the other substance to be transported together to the interior of the cell.

In *counter-transport,* sodium ions again attempt to diffuse to the interior of the cell because of their large concentration gradient. However, this time, the substance to be transported is on the inside of the cell and must be transported to the outside. Therefore, the sodium ion binds to the carrier protein where it projects to the exterior surface of the membrane, while the substance to be counter-transported binds to the interior projection of the carrier protein. Once both have bound, a conformational change occurs, and energy released by the sodium ion moving to the interior causes the other substance to move to the exterior.

Co-Transport of Glucose and Amino Acids Along with Sodium Ions

Glucose and many amino acids are transported into most cells against large concentration gradients; the mechanism of this is entirely by co-transport, as shown in Figure 4-13. Note that the transport carrier protein has two binding sites on its exterior side, one for sodium and one

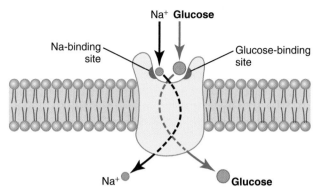

Figure 4-13 Postulated mechanism for sodium co-transport of glucose.

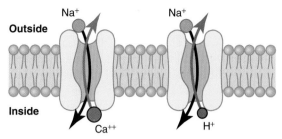

Figure 4-14 Sodium counter-transport of calcium and hydrogen ions.

for glucose. Also, the concentration of sodium ions is high on the outside and low inside, which provides energy for the transport. A special property of the transport protein is that a conformational change to allow sodium movement to the interior will not occur until a glucose molecule also attaches. When they both become attached, the conformational change takes place automatically, and the sodium and glucose are transported to the inside of the cell at the same time. Hence, this is a *sodium-glucose co-transport* mechanism. Sodium-glucose co-transporters are especially important mechanisms in transporting glucose across renal and intestinal epithelial cells, as discussed in Chapters 27 and 65.

Sodium co-transport of the amino acids occurs in the same manner as for glucose, except that it uses a different set of transport proteins. Five *amino acid transport proteins* have been identified, each of which is responsible for transporting one subset of amino acids with specific molecular characteristics.

Sodium co-transport of glucose and amino acids occurs especially through the epithelial cells of the intestinal tract and the renal tubules of the kidneys to promote absorption of these substances into the blood, as is discussed in later chapters.

Other important co-transport mechanisms in at least some cells include co-transport of chloride ions, iodine ions, iron ions, and urate ions.

Sodium Counter-Transport of Calcium and Hydrogen Ions

Two especially important counter-transport mechanisms (transport in a direction opposite to the primary ion) are *sodium-calcium counter-transport* and *sodium-hydrogen counter-transport* (Figure 4-14).

Sodium-calcium counter-transport occurs through all or almost all cell membranes, with sodium ions moving to the interior and calcium ions to the exterior, both bound to the same transport protein in a counter-transport mode. This is in addition to primary active transport of calcium that occurs in some cells.

Sodium-hydrogen counter-transport occurs in several tissues. An especially important example is in the *proximal tubules* of the kidneys, where sodium ions move

from the lumen of the tubule to the interior of the tubular cell, while hydrogen ions are counter-transported into the tubule lumen. As a mechanism for concentrating hydrogen ions, counter-transport is not nearly as powerful as the primary active transport of hydrogen ions that occurs in the more distal renal tubules, but it can transport extremely *large numbers of hydrogen ions,* thus making it a key to hydrogen ion control in the body fluids, as discussed in detail in Chapter 30.

Active Transport Through Cellular Sheets

At many places in the body, substances must be transported all the way through a cellular sheet instead of simply through the cell membrane. Transport of this type occurs through the (1) intestinal epithelium, (2) epithelium of the renal tubules, (3) epithelium of all exocrine glands, (4) epithelium of the gallbladder, and (5) membrane of the choroid plexus of the brain and other membranes.

The basic mechanism for transport of a substance through a cellular sheet is (1) *active transport* through the cell membrane *on one side* of the transporting cells in the sheet, and then (2) either *simple diffusion* or *facilitated diffusion* through the membrane *on the opposite side* of the cell.

Figure 4-15 shows a mechanism for transport of sodium ions through the epithelial sheet of the intestines, gallbladder, and renal tubules. This figure shows that the epithelial cells are connected together tightly at the luminal pole by means of junctions called "kisses." The brush border on the luminal surfaces of the cells

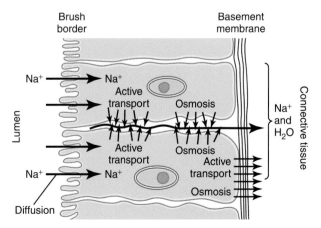

Figure 4-15 Basic mechanism of active transport across a layer of cells.

is permeable to both sodium ions and water. Therefore, sodium and water diffuse readily from the lumen into the interior of the cell. Then, at the basal and lateral membranes of the cells, sodium ions are actively transported into the extracellular fluid of the surrounding connective tissue and blood vessels. This creates a high sodium ion concentration gradient across these membranes, which in turn causes osmosis of water as well. Thus, active transport of sodium ions at the basolateral sides of the epithelial cells results in transport not only of sodium ions but also of water.

These are the mechanisms by which almost all the nutrients, ions, and other substances are absorbed into the blood from the intestine; they are also the way the same substances are reabsorbed from the glomerular filtrate by the renal tubules.

Throughout this text are numerous examples of the different types of transport discussed in this chapter.

Bibliography

Agre P, Kozono D: Aquaporin water channels: molecular mechanisms for human diseases, *FEBS Lett* 555:72, 2003.

Ashcroft FM: From molecule to malady, *Nature* 440:440, 2006.

Benos DJ, Stanton BA: Functional domains within the degenerin/epithelial sodium channel (Deg/ENaC) superfamily of ion channels, *J Physiol* 520:631, 1999.

Benziane B, Chibalin AV: Frontiers: skeletal muscle sodium pump regulation: a translocation paradigm, *Am J Physiol Endocrinol Metab* 295:E553, 2008.

Biel M, Wahl-Schott C, Michalakis S, Zong X: Hyperpolarization-activated cation channels: from genes to function, *Physiol Rev* 89:847, 2009.

Blaustein MP, Zhang J, Chen L, et al: The pump, the exchanger, and endogenous ouabain: signaling mechanisms that link salt retention to hypertension, *Hypertension* 53:291, 2009.

Bröer S: Amino acid transport across mammalian intestinal and renal epithelia, *Physiol Rev* 88:249, 2008.

DeCoursey TE: Voltage-gated proton channels: what's next? *J Physiol* 586:5305, 2008.

DeCoursey TE: Voltage-gated proton channels and other proton transfer pathways, *Physiol Rev* 83:475, 2003.

DiPolo R, Beaugé L: Sodium/calcium exchanger: influence of metabolic regulation on ion carrier interactions, *Physiol Rev* 86:155, 2006.

Drummond HA, Jernigan NL, Grifoni SC: Sensing tension: epithelial sodium channel/acid-sensing ion channel proteins in cardiovascular homeostasis, *Hypertension* 51:1265, 2008.

Gadsby DC: Ion channels versus ion pumps: the principal difference, in principle, *Nat Rev Mol Cell Biol* 10:344, 2009.

Jentsch TJ, Stein V, Weinreich F, Zdebik AA: Molecular structure and physiological function of chloride channels, *Physiol Rev* 82:503, 2002.

Kaupp UB, Seifert R: Cyclic nucleotide-gated ion channels, *Physiol Rev* 82:769, 2002.

King LS, Kozono D, Agre P: From structure to disease: the evolving tale of aquaporin biology, *Nat Rev Mol Cell Biol* 5:687, 2004.

Kleyman TR, Carattino MD, Hughey RP: ENaC at the cutting edge: regulation of epithelial sodium channels by proteases, *J Biol Chem* 284:20447, 2009.

Mazzochi C, Benos DJ, Smith PR: Interaction of epithelial ion channels with the actin-based cytoskeleton, *Am J Physiol Renal Physiol* 291:F1113, 2006.

Peres A, Giovannardi S, Bossi E, Fesce R: Electrophysiological insights into the mechanism of ion-coupled cotransporters, *News Physiol Sci* 19:80, 2004.

Russell JM: Sodium-potassium-chloride cotransport, *Physiol Rev* 80:211, 2000.

Shin JM, Munson K, Vagin O, Sachs G: The gastric HK-ATPase: structure, function, and inhibition, *Pflugers Arch* 457:609, 2009.

Tian J, Xie ZJ: The Na-K-ATPase and calcium-signaling microdomains, *Physiology (Bethesda)* 23:205, 2008.

Membrane Potentials and Action Potentials

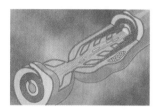

Electrical potentials exist across the membranes of virtually all cells of the body. In addition, some cells, such as nerve and muscle cells, are capable of generating rapidly changing electrochemical impulses at their membranes, and these impulses are used to transmit signals along the nerve or muscle membranes. In other types of cells, such as glandular cells, macrophages, and ciliated cells, local changes in membrane potentials also activate many of the cells' functions. The present discussion is concerned with membrane potentials generated both at rest and during action by nerve and muscle cells.

Basic Physics of Membrane Potentials

Membrane Potentials Caused by Diffusion

"Diffusion Potential" Caused by an Ion Concentration Difference on the Two Sides of the Membrane. In Figure 5-1A, the potassium concentration is great *inside* a nerve fiber membrane but very low *outside* the membrane. Let us assume that the membrane in this instance is permeable to the potassium ions but not to any other ions. Because of the large potassium concentration gradient from inside toward outside, there is a strong tendency for extra numbers of potassium ions to diffuse outward through the membrane. As they do so, they carry positive electrical charges to the outside, thus creating electropositivity outside the membrane and electronegativity inside because of negative anions that remain behind and do not diffuse outward with the potassium. Within a millisecond or so, the potential difference between the inside and outside, called the *diffusion potential*, becomes great enough to block further net potassium diffusion to the exterior, despite the high potassium ion concentration gradient. In the normal mammalian nerve fiber, *the potential difference required is about 94 millivolts, with negativity inside the fiber membrane.*

Figure 5-1B shows the same phenomenon as in Figure 5-1A, but this time with high concentration of sodium ions *outside* the membrane and low sodium *inside*. These ions are also positively charged. This time, the membrane is highly permeable to the sodium ions but impermeable to all other ions. Diffusion of the positively charged sodium ions to the inside creates a membrane potential of opposite polarity to that in Figure 5-1A, with negativity outside and positivity inside. Again, the membrane potential rises high enough within milliseconds to block further net diffusion of sodium ions to the inside; however, this time, in the mammalian nerve fiber, *the potential is about 61 millivolts positive inside the fiber.*

Thus, in both parts of Figure 5-1, we see that a concentration difference of ions across a selectively permeable membrane can, under appropriate conditions, create a membrane potential. Later in this chapter, we show that many of the rapid changes in membrane potentials observed during nerve and muscle impulse transmission result from the occurrence of such rapidly changing diffusion potentials.

Relation of the Diffusion Potential to the Concentration Difference—The Nernst Potential. The diffusion potential level across a membrane that exactly opposes the net diffusion of a particular ion through the membrane is called the *Nernst potential* for that ion, a term that was introduced in Chapter 4.

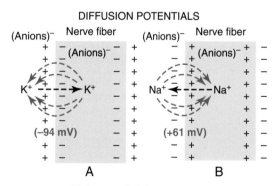

Figure 5-1 *A,* Establishment of a "diffusion" potential across a nerve fiber membrane, caused by diffusion of potassium ions from inside the cell to outside through a membrane that is selectively permeable only to potassium. *B,* Establishment of a "diffusion potential" when the nerve fiber membrane is permeable only to sodium ions. Note that the internal membrane potential is negative when potassium ions diffuse and positive when sodium ions diffuse because of opposite concentration gradients of these two ions.

The magnitude of this Nernst potential is determined by the *ratio* of the concentrations of that specific ion on the two sides of the membrane. The greater this ratio, the greater the tendency for the ion to diffuse in one direction, and therefore the greater the Nernst potential required to prevent additional net diffusion. The following equation, called the *Nernst equation,* can be used to calculate the Nernst potential for any univalent ion at normal body temperature of 98.6°F (37°C):

$$\text{EMF (millivolts)} = \pm 61 \times \log \frac{\text{Concentration inside}}{\text{Concentration outside}}$$

where EMF is electromotive force.

When using this formula, it is usually assumed that the potential in the extracellular fluid outside the membrane remains at zero potential, and the Nernst potential is the potential inside the membrane. Also, the sign of the potential is positive (+) if the ion diffusing from inside to outside is a negative ion, and it is negative (–) if the ion is positive. Thus, when the concentration of positive potassium ions on the inside is 10 times that on the outside, the log of 10 is 1, so the Nernst potential calculates to be –61 millivolts inside the membrane.

Calculation of the Diffusion Potential When the Membrane Is Permeable to Several Different Ions

When a membrane is permeable to several different ions, the diffusion potential that develops depends on three factors: (1) the polarity of the electrical charge of each ion, (2) the permeability of the membrane *(P)* to each ion, and (3) the concentrations *(C)* of the respective ions on the inside *(i)* and outside *(o)* of the membrane. Thus, the following formula, called the *Goldman equation,* or the *Goldman-Hodgkin-Katz equation,* gives the calculated membrane potential on the *inside* of the membrane when two univalent positive ions, sodium (Na⁺) and potassium (K⁺), and one univalent negative ion, chloride (Cl⁻), are involved.

$$\text{EMF (millivolts)}$$
$$= -61 \times \log \frac{C_{Na_i^+}P_{Na^+} + C_{K_i^+}P_{K^+} + C_{Cl_o^-}P_{Cl^-}}{C_{Na_o^+}P_{Na^+} + C_{K_o^+}P_{K^+} + C_{Cl_i^-}P_{Cl^-}}$$

Let us study the importance and the meaning of this equation. First, sodium, potassium, and chloride ions are the most important ions involved in the development of membrane potentials in nerve and muscle fibers, as well as in the neuronal cells in the nervous system. The concentration gradient of each of these ions across the membrane helps determine the voltage of the membrane potential.

Second, the degree of importance of each of the ions in determining the voltage is proportional to the membrane permeability for that particular ion. That is, if the membrane has zero permeability to both potassium and chloride ions, the membrane potential becomes entirely dominated by the concentration gradient of sodium ions alone, and the resulting potential will be equal to the Nernst potential for sodium. The same holds for each of the other two ions if the membrane should become selectively permeable for either one of them alone.

Third, a positive ion concentration gradient from *inside* the membrane to the *outside* causes electronegativity inside the membrane. The reason for this is that excess positive ions diffuse to the outside when their concentration is higher inside than outside. This carries positive charges to the outside but leaves the nondiffusible negative anions on the inside, thus creating electronegativity on the inside. The opposite effect occurs when there is a gradient for a negative ion. That is, a chloride ion gradient from the *outside to the inside* causes negativity inside the cell because excess negatively charged chloride ions diffuse to the inside, while leaving the nondiffusible positive ions on the outside.

Fourth, as explained later, the permeability of the sodium and potassium channels undergoes rapid changes during transmission of a nerve impulse, whereas the permeability of the chloride channels does not change greatly during this process. Therefore, rapid changes in sodium and potassium permeability are primarily responsible for signal transmission in neurons, which is the subject of most of the remainder of this chapter.

Measuring the Membrane Potential

The method for measuring the membrane potential is simple in theory but often difficult in practice because of the small size of most of the fibers. Figure 5-2 shows a small pipette filled with an electrolyte solution. The pipette is impaled through the cell membrane to the interior of the fiber. Then another electrode, called the "indifferent electrode," is placed in the extracellular fluid, and the potential difference between the inside and outside of the fiber is measured using an appropriate voltmeter. This voltmeter is a highly sophisticated electronic apparatus that is capable of measuring small voltages despite extremely high resistance to electrical flow through the tip of the micropipette, which has a lumen diameter usually less than 1 micrometer and a resistance more than a million ohms. For recording rapid *changes* in the membrane potential during transmission of nerve impulses, the microelectrode is connected to an oscilloscope, as explained later in the chapter.

The lower part of Figure 5-3 shows the electrical potential that is measured at each point in or near the nerve fiber membrane, beginning at the left side of the figure and

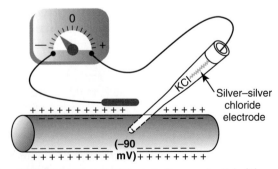

Figure 5-2 Measurement of the membrane potential of the nerve fiber using a microelectrode.

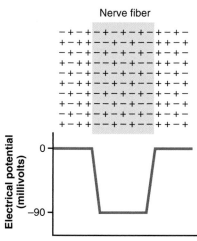

Figure 5-3 Distribution of positively and negatively charged ions in the extracellular fluid surrounding a nerve fiber and in the fluid inside the fiber; note the alignment of negative charges along the inside surface of the membrane and positive charges along the outside surface. The lower panel displays the abrupt changes in membrane potential that occur at the membranes on the two sides of the fiber.

passing to the right. As long as the electrode is outside the nerve membrane, the recorded potential is zero, which is the potential of the extracellular fluid. Then, as the recording electrode passes through the voltage change area at the cell membrane (called the *electrical dipole layer*), the potential decreases abruptly to –90 millivolts. Moving across the center of the fiber, the potential remains at a steady –90-millivolt level but reverses back to zero the instant it passes through the membrane on the opposite side of the fiber.

To create a negative potential inside the membrane, only enough positive ions to develop the electrical dipole layer at the membrane itself must be transported outward. All the remaining ions inside the nerve fiber can be both positive and negative, as shown in the upper panel of Figure 5-3. Therefore, an incredibly small number of ions must be transferred through the membrane to establish the normal "resting potential" of –90 millivolts inside the nerve fiber; this means that only about 1/3,000,000 to 1/100,000,000 of the total positive charges inside the fiber must be transferred. Also, an equally small number of positive ions moving from outside to inside the fiber can reverse the potential from –90 millivolts to as much as +35 millivolts within as little as 1/10,000 of a second. Rapid shifting of ions in this manner causes the nerve signals discussed in subsequent sections of this chapter.

Resting Membrane Potential of Nerves

The resting membrane potential of large nerve fibers when not transmitting nerve signals is about –90 millivolts. That is, the potential *inside the fiber* is 90 millivolts more negative than the potential in the extracellular fluid on the outside of the fiber. In the next few paragraphs, the transport properties of the resting nerve membrane for sodium and potassium and the factors that determine the level of this resting potential are explained.

Active Transport of Sodium and Potassium Ions Through the Membrane—The Sodium-Potassium (Na⁺-K⁺) Pump. First, let us recall from Chapter 4 that all cell membranes of the body have a powerful Na⁺-K⁺ pump that continually transports sodium ions to the outside of the cell and potassium ions to the inside, as illustrated on the left-hand side in Figure 5-4. Further, note that this is an *electrogenic pump* because more positive charges are pumped to the outside than to the inside (three Na⁺ ions to the outside for each two K⁺ ions to the inside), leaving a net deficit of positive ions on the inside; this causes a negative potential inside the cell membrane.

The Na⁺-K⁺ pump also causes large concentration gradients for sodium and potassium across the resting nerve membrane. These gradients are the following:

$$\text{Na}^+ \text{ (outside): 142 mEq/L}$$

$$\text{Na}^+ \text{ (inside): 14 mEq/L}$$

$$\text{K}^+ \text{ (outside): 4 mEq/L}$$

$$\text{K}^+ \text{ (inside): 140 mEq/L}$$

The ratios of these two respective ions from the inside to the outside are

$$\text{Na}^+_{inside}/\text{Na}^+_{outside} = 0.1$$

$$\text{K}^+_{inside}/\text{K}^+_{outside} = 35.0$$

Leakage of Potassium Through the Nerve Membrane. The right side of Figure 5-4 shows a channel protein, sometimes called a *"tandem pore domain," potassium channel,* or *potassium (K⁺) "leak" channel,* in the nerve membrane through which potassium can leak even in a resting cell. The basic structure of potassium channels was described in Chapter 4 (Figure 4-4). These K⁺ leak channels may also leak sodium ions slightly but are far more permeable to potassium than to sodium, normally about 100 times as permeable. As discussed later, this differential in permeability is a key factor in determining the level of the normal resting membrane potential.

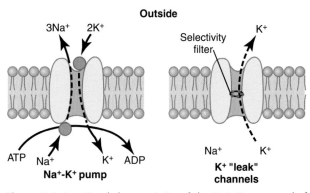

Figure 5-4 Functional characteristics of the Na⁺-K⁺ pump and of the K⁺ "leak" channels. ADP, adenosine diphosphate; ATP, adenosine triphosphate. The K⁺ "leak" channels also leak Na⁺ ions into the cell slightly, but are much more permeable to K⁺.

Origin of the Normal Resting Membrane Potential

Figure 5-5 shows the important factors in the establishment of the normal resting membrane potential of −90 millivolts. They are as follows.

Contribution of the Potassium Diffusion Potential.
In Figure 5-5*A*, we make the assumption that the only movement of ions through the membrane is diffusion of potassium ions, as demonstrated by the open channels between the potassium symbols (K⁺) inside and outside the membrane. Because of the high ratio of potassium ions inside to outside, 35:1, the Nernst potential corresponding to this ratio is −94 millivolts because the logarithm of 35 is 1.54, and this multiplied by −61 millivolts is −94 millivolts. Therefore, if potassium ions were the only factor causing the resting potential, the resting potential

inside the fiber would be equal to −94 millivolts, as shown in the figure.

Contribution of Sodium Diffusion Through the Nerve Membrane.
Figure 5-5*B* shows the addition of slight permeability of the nerve membrane to sodium ions, caused by the minute diffusion of sodium ions through the K⁺-Na⁺ leak channels. The ratio of sodium ions from inside to outside the membrane is 0.1, and this gives a calculated Nernst potential for the inside of the membrane of +61 millivolts. But also shown in Figure 5-5*B* is the Nernst potential for potassium diffusion of −94 millivolts. How do these interact with each other, and what will be the summated potential? This can be answered by using the Goldman equation described previously. Intuitively, one can see that if the membrane is highly permeable to potassium but only slightly permeable to sodium, it is logical that the diffusion of potassium contributes far more to the membrane potential than does the diffusion of sodium. In the normal nerve fiber, the permeability of the membrane to potassium is about 100 times as great as its permeability to sodium. Using this value in the Goldman equation gives a potential inside the membrane of −86 millivolts, which is near the potassium potential shown in the figure.

Contribution of the Na⁺-K⁺ Pump.
In Figure 5-5*C*, the Na⁺-K⁺ pump is shown to provide an additional contribution to the resting potential. In this figure, there is continuous pumping of three sodium ions to the outside for each two potassium ions pumped to the inside of the membrane. The fact that more sodium ions are being pumped to the outside than potassium to the inside causes continual loss of positive charges from inside the membrane; this creates an additional degree of negativity (about −4 millivolts additional) on the inside beyond that which can be accounted for by diffusion alone. Therefore, as shown in Figure 5-5*C*, the net membrane potential with all these factors operative at the same time is about −90 millivolts.

In summary, the diffusion potentials alone caused by potassium and sodium diffusion would give a membrane potential of about −86 millivolts, almost all of this being determined by potassium diffusion. Then, an additional −4 millivolts is contributed to the membrane potential by the continuously acting electrogenic Na⁺-K⁺ pump, giving a net membrane potential of −90 millivolts.

Nerve Action Potential

Nerve signals are transmitted by *action potentials*, which are rapid changes in the membrane potential that spread rapidly along the nerve fiber membrane. Each action potential begins with a sudden change from the normal resting negative membrane potential to a positive potential and then ends with an almost equally rapid change back to the negative potential. To conduct a nerve signal, the action potential moves along the nerve fiber until it comes to the fiber's end.

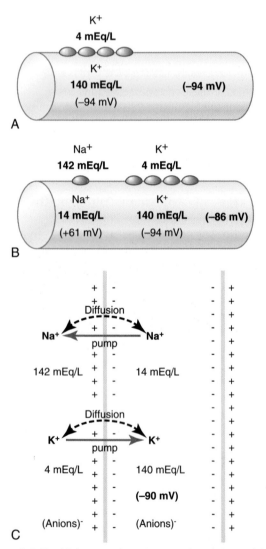

Figure 5-5 Establishment of resting membrane potentials in nerve fibers under three conditions: *A,* when the membrane potential is caused entirely by potassium diffusion alone; *B,* when the membrane potential is caused by diffusion of both sodium and potassium ions; and *C,* when the membrane potential is caused by diffusion of both sodium and potassium ions plus pumping of both these ions by the Na⁺-K⁺ pump.

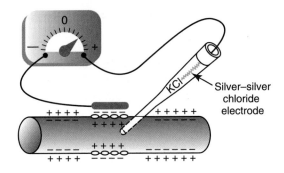

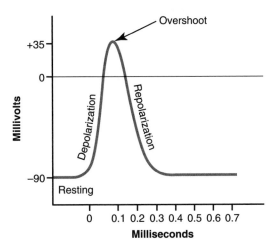

Figure 5-6 Typical action potential recorded by the method shown in the upper panel of the figure.

neurons, the potential merely approaches the zero level and does not overshoot to the positive state.

Repolarization Stage. Within a few 10,000ths of a second after the membrane becomes highly permeable to sodium ions, the sodium channels begin to close and the potassium channels open more than normal. Then, rapid diffusion of potassium ions to the exterior re-establishes the normal negative resting membrane potential. This is called *repolarization* of the membrane.

To explain more fully the factors that cause both depolarization and repolarization, we will describe the special characteristics of two other types of transport channels through the nerve membrane: the voltage-gated sodium and potassium channels.

Voltage-Gated Sodium and Potassium Channels

The necessary actor in causing both depolarization and repolarization of the nerve membrane during the action potential is the *voltage-gated sodium channel*. A *voltage-gated potassium channel* also plays an important role in increasing the rapidity of repolarization of the membrane. *These two voltage-gated channels are in addition to the Na^+-K^+ pump and the K^+ leak channels.*

Voltage-Gated Sodium Channel—Activation and Inactivation of the Channel

The upper panel of Figure 5-7 shows the voltage-gated sodium channel in three separate states. This channel has two *gates*—one near the outside of the channel called the *activation gate*, and another near the inside called the

The upper panel of Figure 5-6 shows the changes that occur at the membrane during the action potential, with transfer of positive charges to the interior of the fiber at its onset and return of positive charges to the exterior at its end. The lower panel shows graphically the successive changes in membrane potential over a few 10,000ths of a second, illustrating the explosive onset of the action potential and the almost equally rapid recovery.

The successive stages of the action potential are as follows.

Resting Stage. This is the resting membrane potential before the action potential begins. The membrane is said to be "polarized" during this stage because of the −90 millivolts negative membrane potential that is present.

Depolarization Stage. At this time, the membrane suddenly becomes permeable to sodium ions, allowing tremendous numbers of positively charged sodium ions to diffuse to the interior of the axon. The normal "polarized" state of −90 millivolts is immediately neutralized by the inflowing positively charged sodium ions, with the potential rising rapidly in the positive direction. This is called *depolarization*. In large nerve fibers, the great excess of positive sodium ions moving to the inside causes the membrane potential to actually "overshoot" beyond the zero level and to become somewhat positive. In some smaller fibers, as well as in many central nervous system

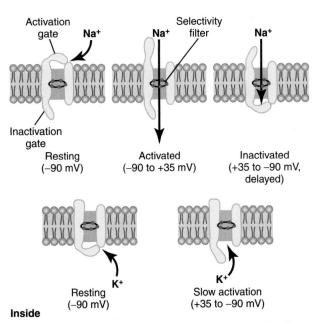

Figure 5-7 Characteristics of the voltage-gated sodium (*top*) and potassium (*bottom*) channels, showing successive activation and inactivation of the sodium channels and delayed activation of the potassium channels when the membrane potential is changed from the normal resting negative value to a positive value.

61

inactivation gate. The upper left of the figure depicts the state of these two gates in the normal resting membrane when the membrane potential is −90 millivolts. In this state, the activation gate is closed, which prevents any entry of sodium ions to the interior of the fiber through these sodium channels.

Activation of the Sodium Channel. When the membrane potential becomes less negative than during the resting state, rising from −90 millivolts toward zero, it finally reaches a voltage—usually somewhere between −70 and −50 millivolts—that causes a sudden conformational change in the activation gate, flipping it all the way to the open position. This is called the *activated state;* during this state, sodium ions can pour inward through the channel, increasing the sodium permeability of the membrane as much as 500- to 5000-fold.

Inactivation of the Sodium Channel. The upper right panel of Figure 5-7 shows a third state of the sodium channel. The same increase in voltage that opens the activation gate also closes the inactivation gate. The inactivation gate, however, closes a few 10,000ths of a second after the activation gate opens. That is, the conformational change that flips the inactivation gate to the closed state is a slower process than the conformational change that opens the activation gate. Therefore, after the sodium channel has remained open for a few 10,000ths of a second, the inactivation gate closes, and sodium ions no longer can pour to the inside of the membrane. At this point, the membrane potential begins to recover back toward the resting membrane state, which is the repolarization process.

Another important characteristic of the sodium channel inactivation process is that the inactivation gate will not reopen until the membrane potential returns to or near the original resting membrane potential level. Therefore, it is usually not possible for the sodium channels to open again without first repolarizing the nerve fiber.

Voltage-Gated Potassium Channel and Its Activation

The lower panel of Figure 5-7 shows the voltage-gated potassium channel in two states: during the resting state (left) and toward the end of the action potential (right). During the resting state, the gate of the potassium channel is closed and potassium ions are prevented from passing through this channel to the exterior. When the membrane potential rises from −90 millivolts toward zero, this voltage change causes a conformational opening of the gate and allows increased potassium diffusion outward through the channel. However, because of the slight delay in opening of the potassium channels, for the most part, they open just at the same time that the sodium channels are beginning to close because of inactivation. Thus, the decrease in sodium entry to the cell and the simultaneous increase in potassium exit from the cell combine to speed the repolarization process, leading to full recovery of the

resting membrane potential within another few 10,000ths of a second.

Research Method for Measuring the Effect of Voltage on Opening and Closing of the Voltage-Gated Channels—The "Voltage Clamp." The original research that led to quantitative understanding of the sodium and potassium channels was so ingenious that it led to Nobel Prizes for the scientists responsible, Hodgkin and Huxley. The essence of these studies is shown in Figures 5-8 and 5-9.

Figure 5-8 shows an experimental apparatus called a *voltage clamp,* which is used to measure flow of ions through the different channels. In using this apparatus, two electrodes are inserted into the nerve fiber. One of these is to measure the voltage of the membrane potential, and the other is to conduct electrical current into or out of the nerve fiber. This apparatus is used in the following way: The investigator decides which voltage he or she wants to establish inside the nerve fiber. The electronic portion of the apparatus is then adjusted to the desired voltage, and this automatically injects either positive or negative electricity through the current electrode at whatever rate is required to hold the voltage, as measured by the voltage electrode, at the level set by the operator. When the membrane potential is suddenly increased by this voltage clamp from −90 millivolts to zero, the voltage-gated sodium and potassium channels open and sodium and potassium ions begin to pour through the channels. To counterbalance

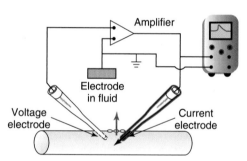

Figure 5-8 "Voltage clamp" method for studying flow of ions through specific channels.

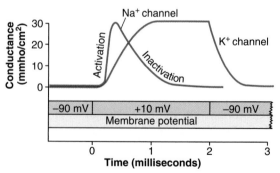

Figure 5-9 Typical changes in conductance of sodium and potassium ion channels when the membrane potential is suddenly increased from the normal resting value of −90 millivolts to a positive value of +10 millivolts for 2 milliseconds. This figure shows that the sodium channels open (activate) and then close (inactivate) before the end of the 2 milliseconds, whereas the potassium channels only open (activate), and the rate of opening is much slower than that of the sodium channels.

the effect of these ion movements on the desired setting of the intracellular voltage, electrical current is injected automatically through the current electrode of the voltage clamp to maintain the intracellular voltage at the required steady zero level. To achieve this, the current injected must be equal to but of opposite polarity to the net current flow through the membrane channels. To measure how much current flow is occurring at each instant, the current electrode is connected to an oscilloscope that records the current flow, as demonstrated on the screen of the oscilloscope in Figure 5-8. Finally, the investigator adjusts the concentrations of the ions to other than normal levels both inside and outside the nerve fiber and repeats the study. This can be done easily when using large nerve fibers removed from some invertebrates, especially the giant squid axon, which in some cases is as large as 1 millimeter in diameter. When sodium is the only permeant ion in the solutions inside and outside the squid axon, the voltage clamp measures current flow only through the sodium channels. When potassium is the only permeant ion, current flow only through the potassium channels is measured.

Another means for studying the flow of ions through an individual type of channel is to block one type of channel at a time. For instance, the sodium channels can be blocked by a toxin called *tetrodotoxin* by applying it to the outside of the cell membrane where the sodium activation gates are located. Conversely, *tetraethylammonium ion* blocks the potassium channels when it is applied to the interior of the nerve fiber.

Figure 5-9 shows typical changes in conductance of the voltage-gated sodium and potassium channels when the membrane potential is suddenly changed by use of the voltage clamp from −90 millivolts to +10 millivolts and then, 2 milliseconds later, back to −90 millivolts. Note the sudden opening of the sodium channels (the activation stage) within a small fraction of a millisecond after the membrane potential is increased to the positive value. However, during the next millisecond or so, the sodium channels automatically close (the inactivation stage).

Note the opening (activation) of the potassium channels. These open slowly and reach their full open state only after the sodium channels have almost completely closed. Further, once the potassium channels open, they remain open for the entire duration of the positive membrane potential and do not close again until after the membrane potential is decreased back to a negative value.

Summary of the Events That Cause the Action Potential

Figure 5-10 shows in summary form the sequential events that occur during and shortly after the action potential. The bottom of the figure shows the changes in membrane conductance for sodium and potassium ions. During the resting state, before the action potential begins, the conductance for potassium ions is 50 to 100 times as great as the conductance for sodium ions. This is caused by much greater leakage of potassium ions than sodium ions through the leak channels. However, at the onset of the action potential, the sodium channels instantaneously become activated and allow up to a 5000-fold increase in

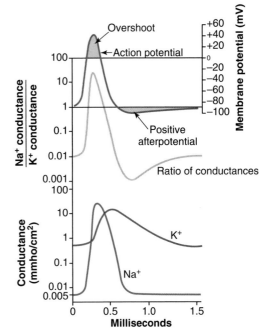

Figure 5-10 Changes in sodium and potassium conductance during the course of the action potential. Sodium conductance increases several thousand-fold during the early stages of the action potential, whereas potassium conductance increases only about 30-fold during the latter stages of the action potential and for a short period thereafter. (These curves were constructed from theory presented in papers by Hodgkin and Huxley but transposed from squid axon to apply to the membrane potentials of large mammalian nerve fibers.)

sodium conductance. Then the inactivation process closes the sodium channels within another fraction of a millisecond. The onset of the action potential also causes voltage gating of the potassium channels, causing them to begin opening more slowly a fraction of a millisecond after the sodium channels open. At the end of the action potential, the return of the membrane potential to the negative state causes the potassium channels to close back to their original status, but again, only after an additional millisecond or more delay.

The middle portion of Figure 5-10 shows the ratio of sodium conductance to potassium conductance at each instant during the action potential, and above this is the action potential itself. During the early portion of the action potential, the ratio of sodium to potassium conductance increases more than 1000-fold. Therefore, far more sodium ions flow to the interior of the fiber than do potassium ions to the exterior. This is what causes the membrane potential to become positive at the action potential onset. Then the sodium channels begin to close and the potassium channels begin to open, so the ratio of conductance shifts far in favor of high potassium conductance but low sodium conductance. This allows very rapid loss of potassium ions to the exterior but virtually zero flow of sodium ions to the interior. Consequently, the action potential quickly returns to its baseline level.

Roles of Other Ions During the Action Potential

Thus far, we have considered only the roles of sodium and potassium ions in the generation of the action potential. At least two other types of ions must be considered: negative anions and calcium ions.

Impermeant Negatively Charged Ions (Anions) Inside the Nerve Axon. Inside the axon are many negatively charged ions that cannot go through the membrane channels. They include the anions of protein molecules and of many organic phosphate compounds, sulfate compounds, and so forth. Because these ions cannot leave the interior of the axon, any deficit of positive ions inside the membrane leaves an excess of these impermeant negative anions. Therefore, these impermeant negative ions are responsible for the negative charge inside the fiber when there is a net deficit of positively charged potassium ions and other positive ions.

Calcium Ions. The membranes of almost all cells of the body have a calcium pump similar to the sodium pump, and calcium serves along with (or instead of) sodium in some cells to cause most of the action potential. Like the sodium pump, the calcium pump transports calcium ions from the interior to the exterior of the cell membrane (or into the endoplasmic reticulum of the cell), creating a calcium ion gradient of about 10,000-fold. This leaves an internal cell concentration of calcium ions of about 10^{-7} molar, in contrast to an external concentration of about 10^{-3} molar.

In addition, there are *voltage-gated calcium channels*. Because calcium ion concentration is more than 10,000 times greater in the extracellular than the intracellular fluid, there is a tremendous diffusion gradient for passive flow of calcium ions into the cells. These channels are slightly permeable to sodium ions and calcium ions, but their permeability to calcium is about 1000-fold greater than to sodium under normal physiological conditions. When they open in response to a stimulus that depolarizes the cell membrane, calcium ions flow to the interior of the cell.

A major function of the voltage-gated calcium ion channels is to contribute to the depolarizing phase on the action potential in some cells. The gating of calcium channels, however, is slow, requiring 10 to 20 times as long for activation as for the sodium channels. For this reason they are often called *slow channels*, in contrast to the sodium channels, which are called *fast channels*. Therefore, the opening of calcium channels provides a more sustained depolarization, whereas the sodium channels play a key role in initiating action potentials.

Calcium channels are numerous in both cardiac muscle and smooth muscle. In fact, in some types of smooth muscle, the fast sodium channels are hardly present; therefore, the action potentials are caused almost entirely by activation of slow calcium channels.

Increased Permeability of the Sodium Channels When There Is a Deficit of Calcium Ions. The concentration of calcium ions in the extracellular fluid also has a profound effect on the voltage level at which the sodium channels become activated. When there is a deficit of calcium ions, the sodium channels become activated (opened) by a small increase of the membrane potential from its normal, very negative level. Therefore, the nerve fiber becomes highly excitable, sometimes discharging repetitively without provocation rather than remaining in the resting state. In fact, the calcium ion concentration needs to fall only 50 percent below normal before spontaneous discharge occurs in some peripheral nerves, often causing *muscle "tetany."* This is sometimes lethal because of tetanic contraction of the respiratory muscles.

The probable way in which calcium ions affect the sodium channels is as follows: These ions appear to bind to the exterior surfaces of the sodium channel protein molecule. The positive charges of these calcium ions in turn alter the electrical state of the sodium channel protein itself, in this way altering the voltage level required to open the sodium gate.

Initiation of the Action Potential

Up to this point, we have explained the changing sodium and potassium permeability of the membrane, as well as the development of the action potential itself, but we have not explained what initiates the action potential.

A Positive-Feedback Cycle Opens the Sodium Channels. First, as long as the membrane of the nerve fiber remains undisturbed, no action potential occurs in the normal nerve. However, if any event causes enough initial rise in the membrane potential from −90 millivolts toward the zero level, the rising voltage itself causes many voltage-gated sodium channels to begin opening. This allows rapid inflow of sodium ions, which causes a further rise in the membrane potential, thus opening still more voltage-gated sodium channels and allowing more streaming of sodium ions to the interior of the fiber. This process is a positive-feedback cycle that, once the feedback is strong enough, continues until all the voltage-gated sodium channels have become activated (opened). Then, within another fraction of a millisecond, the rising membrane potential causes closure of the sodium channels and opening of potassium channels and the action potential soon terminates.

Threshold for Initiation of the Action Potential. An action potential will not occur until the initial rise in membrane potential is great enough to create the positive feedback described in the preceding paragraph. This occurs when the number of Na$^+$ ions entering the fiber becomes greater than the number of K$^+$ ions leaving the fiber. A sudden rise in membrane potential of 15 to 30 millivolts is usually required. Therefore, a sudden increase in the membrane potential in a large nerve fiber from −90 millivolts up to about −65 millivolts usually causes the explosive development of an action potential. This level of −65 millivolts is said to be the *threshold* for stimulation.

Propagation of the Action Potential

In the preceding paragraphs, we discussed the action potential as it occurs at one spot on the membrane. However, an action potential elicited at any one point on an excitable membrane usually excites adjacent portions of the membrane, resulting in propagation of the action

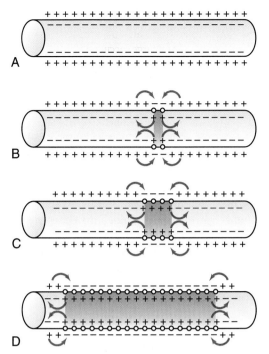

Figure 5-11 Propagation of action potentials in both directions along a conductive fiber.

All-or-Nothing Principle. Once an action potential has been elicited at any point on the membrane of a normal fiber, the depolarization process travels over the entire membrane if conditions are right, or it does not travel at all if conditions are not right. This is called the *all-or-nothing principle,* and it applies to all normal excitable tissues. Occasionally, the action potential reaches a point on the membrane at which it does not generate sufficient voltage to stimulate the next area of the membrane. When this occurs, the spread of depolarization stops. Therefore, for continued propagation of an impulse to occur, the ratio of action potential to threshold for excitation must at all times be greater than 1. This "greater than 1" requirement is called the *safety factor* for propagation.

Re-establishing Sodium and Potassium Ionic Gradients After Action Potentials Are Completed—Importance of Energy Metabolism

The transmission of each action potential along a nerve fiber reduces slightly the concentration differences of sodium and potassium inside and outside the membrane because sodium ions diffuse to the inside during depolarization and potassium ions diffuse to the outside during repolarization. For a single action potential, this effect is so minute that it cannot be measured. Indeed, 100,000 to 50 million impulses can be transmitted by large nerve fibers before the concentration differences reach the point that action potential conduction ceases. Even so, with time, it becomes necessary to re-establish the sodium and potassium membrane concentration differences. This is achieved by action of the Na$^+$-K$^+$ pump in the same way as described previously in the chapter for the original establishment of the resting potential. That is, sodium ions that have diffused to the interior of the cell during the action potentials and potassium ions that have diffused to the exterior must be returned to their original state by the Na$^+$-K$^+$ pump. Because this pump requires energy for operation, this "recharging" of the nerve fiber is an active metabolic process, using energy derived from the adenosine triphosphate (ATP) energy system of the cell. Figure 5-12 shows that the nerve fiber produces excess heat during recharging, which is a measure of energy expenditure when the nerve impulse frequency increases.

A special feature of the Na$^+$-K$^+$ ATPase pump is that its degree of activity is strongly stimulated when excess sodium ions accumulate inside the cell membrane. In fact, the pumping activity increases approximately in proportion to the third power of this intracellular sodium concentration. That is, as the internal sodium concentration rises from 10 to 20 mEq/L, the activity of the pump does not merely double but increases about eightfold. Therefore, it is easy to understand how the "recharging" process of the nerve fiber can be set rapidly into motion whenever the concentration differences of sodium and potassium ions across the membrane begin to "run down."

potential along the membrane. This mechanism is demonstrated in Figure 5-11. Figure 5-11*A* shows a normal resting nerve fiber, and Figure 5-11*B* shows a nerve fiber that has been excited in its midportion—that is, the midportion suddenly develops increased permeability to sodium. The arrows show a "local circuit" of current flow from the depolarized areas of the membrane to the adjacent resting membrane areas. That is, positive electrical charges are carried by the inward-diffusing sodium ions through the depolarized membrane and then for several millimeters in both directions along the core of the axon. These positive charges increase the voltage for a distance of 1 to 3 millimeters inside the large myelinated fiber to above the threshold voltage value for initiating an action potential. Therefore, the sodium channels in these new areas immediately open, as shown in Figure 5-11*C* and *D,* and the explosive action potential spreads. These newly depolarized areas produce still more local circuits of current flow farther along the membrane, causing progressively more and more depolarization. Thus, the depolarization process travels along the entire length of the fiber. This transmission of the depolarization process along a nerve or muscle fiber is called a *nerve* or *muscle impulse.*

Direction of Propagation. As demonstrated in Figure 5-11, an excitable membrane has no single direction of propagation, but the action potential travels in all directions away from the stimulus—even along all branches of a nerve fiber—until the entire membrane has become depolarized.

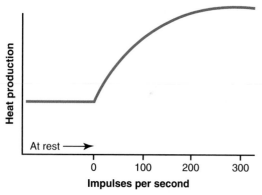

Figure 5-12 Heat production in a nerve fiber at rest and at progressively increasing rates of stimulation.

Plateau in Some Action Potentials

In some instances, the excited membrane does not repolarize immediately after depolarization; instead, the potential remains on a plateau near the peak of the spike potential for many milliseconds, and only then does repolarization begin. Such a plateau is shown in Figure 5-13; one can readily see that the plateau greatly prolongs the period of depolarization. This type of action potential occurs in heart muscle fibers, where the plateau lasts for as long as 0.2 to 0.3 second and causes contraction of heart muscle to last for this same long period.

The cause of the plateau is a combination of several factors. First, in heart muscle, two types of channels enter into the depolarization process: (1) the usual voltage-activated sodium channels, called *fast channels*, and (2) voltage-activated calcium-sodium channels, which are slow to open and therefore are called *slow channels*. Opening of fast channels causes the spike portion of the action potential, whereas the prolonged opening of the slow calcium-sodium channels mainly allows calcium ions to enter the fiber, which is largely responsible for the plateau portion of the action potential as well.

A second factor that may be partly responsible for the plateau is that the voltage-gated potassium channels are slower than usual to open, often not opening much until the end of the plateau. This delays the return of the membrane potential toward its normal negative value of −80 to −90 millivolts.

Rhythmicity of Some Excitable Tissues—Repetitive Discharge

Repetitive self-induced discharges occur normally in the heart, in most smooth muscle, and in many of the neurons of the central nervous system. These rhythmical discharges cause (1) the rhythmical beat of the heart, (2) rhythmical peristalsis of the intestines, and (3) such neuronal events as the rhythmical control of breathing.

Also, almost all other excitable tissues can discharge repetitively if the threshold for stimulation of the tissue cells is reduced low enough. For instance, even large nerve fibers and skeletal muscle fibers, which normally are highly stable, discharge repetitively when they are placed in a solution that contains the drug veratrine or when the calcium ion concentration falls below a critical value, both of which increase sodium permeability of the membrane.

Re-excitation Process Necessary for Spontaneous Rhythmicity. For spontaneous rhythmicity to occur, the membrane even in its natural state must be permeable enough to sodium ions (or to calcium and sodium ions through the slow calcium-sodium channels) to allow automatic membrane depolarization. Thus, Figure 5-14 shows that the "resting" membrane potential in the rhythmical control center of the heart is only −60 to −70 millivolts. This is not enough negative voltage to keep the sodium and calcium channels totally closed. Therefore, the following sequence occurs: (1) some sodium and calcium ions flow inward; (2) this increases the membrane voltage in the positive direction, which further increases membrane permeability; (3) still more ions flow inward;

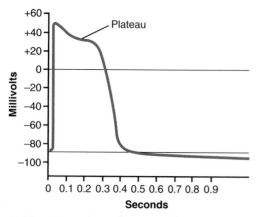

Figure 5-13 Action potential (in millivolts) from a Purkinje fiber of the heart, showing a "plateau."

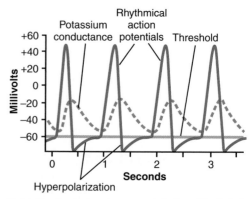

Figure 5-14 Rhythmical action potentials (in millivolts) similar to those recorded in the rhythmical control center of the heart. Note their relationship to potassium conductance and to the state of hyperpolarization.

and (4) the permeability increases more, and so on, until an action potential is generated. Then, at the end of the action potential, the membrane repolarizes. After another delay of milliseconds or seconds, spontaneous excitability causes depolarization again and a new action potential occurs spontaneously. This cycle continues over and over and causes self-induced rhythmical excitation of the excitable tissue.

Why does the membrane of the heart control center not depolarize immediately after it has become repolarized, rather than delaying for nearly a second before the onset of the next action potential? The answer can be found by observing the curve labeled "potassium conductance" in Figure 5-14. This shows that toward the end of each action potential, and continuing for a short period thereafter, the membrane becomes more permeable to potassium ions. The increased outflow of potassium ions carries tremendous numbers of positive charges to the outside of the membrane, leaving inside the fiber considerably more negativity than would otherwise occur. This continues for nearly a second after the preceding action potential is over, thus drawing the membrane potential nearer to the potassium Nernst potential. This is a state called *hyperpolarization*, also shown in Figure 5-14. As long as this state exists, self-re-excitation will not occur. But the increased potassium conductance (and the state of hyperpolarization) gradually disappears, as shown after each action potential is completed in the figure, thereby allowing the membrane potential again to increase up to the *threshold* for excitation. Then, suddenly, a new action potential results and the process occurs again and again.

Special Characteristics of Signal Transmission in Nerve Trunks

Myelinated and Unmyelinated Nerve Fibers. Figure 5-15 shows a cross section of a typical small nerve, revealing many large nerve fibers that constitute most of the cross-sectional area. However, a more careful look reveals many more small fibers lying between the large ones. The large fibers are *myelinated*, and the small ones are *unmyelinated*. The average nerve trunk contains about twice as many unmyelinated fibers as myelinated fibers.

Figure 5-16 shows a typical myelinated fiber. The central core of the fiber is the *axon*, and the membrane of the axon is the membrane that actually conducts the action potential. The axon is filled in its center with *axoplasm*, which is a viscid intracellular fluid. Surrounding the axon is a *myelin sheath* that is often much thicker than the axon itself. About once every 1 to 3 millimeters along the length of the myelin sheath is a *node of Ranvier.*

The myelin sheath is deposited around the axon by Schwann cells in the following manner: The membrane of a Schwann cell first envelops the axon. Then the Schwann cell rotates around the axon many times, laying down multiple layers of Schwann cell membrane containing the lipid substance *sphingomyelin.* This substance is an excellent electrical insulator that decreases ion flow through the membrane about 5000-fold. At the juncture between each two successive

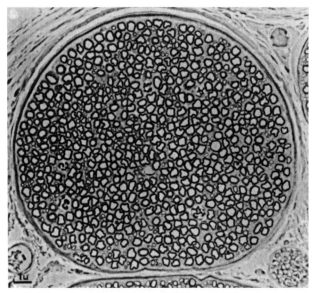

Figure 5-15 Cross section of a small nerve trunk containing both myelinated and unmyelinated fibers.

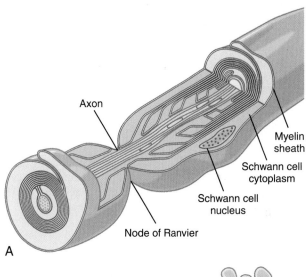

A

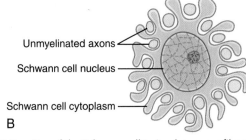

B

Figure 5-16 Function of the Schwann cell to insulate nerve fibers. *A*, Wrapping of a Schwann cell membrane around a large axon to form the myelin sheath of the myelinated nerve fiber. *B*, Partial wrapping of the membrane and cytoplasm of a Schwann cell around multiple unmyelinated nerve fibers (shown in cross section). (*A*, Modified from Leeson TS, Leeson R: Histology. Philadelphia: WB Saunders, 1979.)

Schwann cells along the axon, a small uninsulated area only 2 to 3 *micro*meters in length remains where ions still can flow with ease through the axon membrane between the extracellular fluid and the intracellular fluid inside the axon. This area is called the *node of Ranvier.*

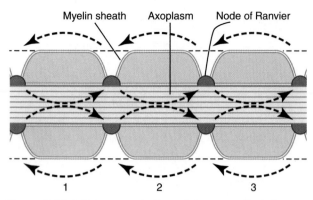

Myelin sheath   Axoplasm   Node of Ranvier

1   2   3

Figure 5-17 Saltatory conduction along a myelinated axon. Flow of electrical current from node to node is illustrated by the arrows.

"Saltatory" Conduction in Myelinated Fibers from Node to Node. Even though almost no ions can flow through the thick myelin sheaths of myelinated nerves, they can flow with ease through the nodes of Ranvier. Therefore, action potentials occur *only at the nodes.* Yet the action potentials are conducted from node to node, as shown in Figure 5-17; this is called *saltatory conduction.* That is, electrical current flows through the surrounding extracellular fluid outside the myelin sheath, as well as through the axoplasm inside the axon from node to node, exciting successive nodes one after another. Thus, the nerve impulse jumps along the fiber, which is the origin of the term "saltatory."

Saltatory conduction is of value for two reasons. First, by causing the depolarization process to jump long intervals along the axis of the nerve fiber, this mechanism increases the velocity of nerve transmission in myelinated fibers as much as 5- to 50-fold. Second, saltatory conduction conserves energy for the axon because only the nodes depolarize, allowing perhaps 100 times less loss of ions than would otherwise be necessary, and therefore requiring little metabolism for re-establishing the sodium and potassium concentration differences across the membrane after a series of nerve impulses.

Still another feature of saltatory conduction in large myelinated fibers is the following: The excellent insulation afforded by the myelin membrane and the 50-fold decrease in membrane capacitance allow repolarization to occur with little transfer of ions.

Velocity of Conduction in Nerve Fibers. The velocity of action potential conduction in nerve fibers varies from as little as 0.25 m/sec in small unmyelinated fibers to as great as 100 m/sec (the length of a football field in 1 second) in large myelinated fibers.

Excitation—The Process of Eliciting the Action Potential

Basically, any factor that causes sodium ions to begin to diffuse inward through the membrane in sufficient numbers can set off automatic regenerative opening of the sodium channels. This can result from *mechanical* disturbance of the membrane, *chemical* effects on the membrane, or passage of *electricity* through the membrane. All these are used at different points in the body to elicit nerve or muscle

action potentials: mechanical pressure to excite sensory nerve endings in the skin, chemical neurotransmitters to transmit signals from one neuron to the next in the brain, and electrical current to transmit signals between successive muscle cells in the heart and intestine. For the purpose of understanding the excitation process, let us begin by discussing the principles of electrical stimulation.

Excitation of a Nerve Fiber by a Negatively Charged Metal Electrode. The usual means for exciting a nerve or muscle in the experimental laboratory is to apply electricity to the nerve or muscle surface through two small electrodes, one of which is negatively charged and the other positively charged. When this is done, the excitable membrane becomes stimulated at the negative electrode.

The cause of this effect is the following: Remember that the action potential is initiated by the opening of voltage-gated sodium channels. Further, these channels are opened by a decrease in the normal resting electrical voltage across the membrane. That is, negative current from the electrode decreases the voltage on the outside of the membrane to a negative value nearer to the voltage of the negative potential inside the fiber. This decreases the electrical voltage across the membrane and allows the sodium channels to open, resulting in an action potential. Conversely, at the positive electrode, the injection of positive charges on the outside of the nerve membrane heightens the voltage difference across the membrane rather than lessening it. This causes a state of hyperpolarization, which actually decreases the excitability of the fiber rather than causing an action potential.

Threshold for Excitation, and "Acute Local Potentials." A weak negative electrical stimulus may not be able to excite a fiber. However, when the voltage of the stimulus is increased, there comes a point at which excitation does take place. Figure 5-18 shows the effects of successively applied stimuli of progressing strength. A weak stimulus at point A causes the membrane potential to change from −90 to −85 millivolts, but this is not a sufficient change for the automatic regenerative processes of the action potential to develop. At point B, the stimulus is greater, but again, the intensity is still not enough. The stimulus does, however, disturb the membrane potential locally for as long as 1 millisecond or more after both of these weak stimuli. These local potential changes are called *acute local potentials,* and when they fail to elicit an action potential, they are called *acute subthreshold potentials.*

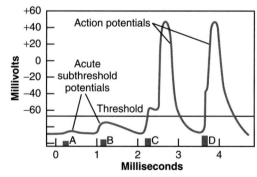

Figure 5-18 Effect of stimuli of increasing voltages to elicit an action potential. Note development of "acute subthreshold potentials" when the stimuli are below the threshold value required for eliciting an action potential.

At point C in Figure 5-18, the stimulus is even stronger. Now the local potential has barely reached the level required to elicit an action potential, called the *threshold level*, but this occurs only after a short "latent period." At point D, the stimulus is still stronger, the acute local potential is also stronger, and the action potential occurs after less of a latent period.

Thus, this figure shows that even a weak stimulus causes a local potential change at the membrane, but the intensity of the local potential must rise to a threshold level before the action potential is set off.

"Refractory Period" After an Action Potential, During Which a New Stimulus Cannot Be Elicited

A new action potential cannot occur in an excitable fiber as long as the membrane is still depolarized from the preceding action potential. The reason for this is that shortly after the action potential is initiated, the sodium channels (or calcium channels, or both) become inactivated and no amount of excitatory signal applied to these channels at this point will open the inactivation gates. The only condition that will allow them to reopen is for the membrane potential to return to or near the original resting membrane potential level. Then, within another small fraction of a second, the inactivation gates of the channels open and a new action potential can be initiated.

The period during which a second action potential cannot be elicited, even with a strong stimulus, is called the *absolute refractory period.* This period for large myelinated nerve fibers is about 1/2500 second. Therefore, one can readily calculate that such a fiber can transmit a maximum of about 2500 impulses per second.

Inhibition of Excitability—"Stabilizers" and Local Anesthetics

In contrast to the factors that increase nerve excitability, still others, called *membrane-stabilizing factors, can decrease excitability.* For instance, *a high extracellular fluid calcium ion concentration* decreases membrane permeability to sodium ions and simultaneously reduces excitability. Therefore, calcium ions are said to be a "stabilizer."

Local Anesthetics. Among the most important stabilizers are the many substances used clinically as local anesthetics, including *procaine* and *tetracaine.* Most of these act directly on the activation gates of the sodium channels, making it much more difficult for these gates to open, thereby reducing membrane excitability. When excitability has been reduced so low that the ratio of *action potential strength to excitability threshold* (called the "safety factor") is reduced below 1.0, nerve impulses fail to pass along the anesthetized nerves.

Recording Membrane Potentials and Action Potentials

Cathode Ray Oscilloscope. Earlier in this chapter, we noted that the membrane potential changes extremely rapidly during the course of an action potential. Indeed, most of the action potential complex of large nerve fibers takes place in less than 1/1000 second. In some figures of this chapter, an electrical meter has been shown recording these potential changes. However, it must be understood that any meter capable of recording most action potentials must be capable

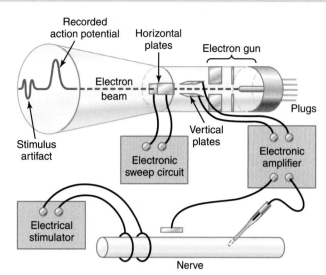

Figure 5-19 Cathode ray oscilloscope for recording transient action potentials.

of responding extremely rapidly. For practical purposes, the only common type of meter that is capable of responding accurately to the rapid membrane potential changes is the cathode ray oscilloscope.

Figure 5-19 shows the basic components of a cathode ray oscilloscope. The cathode ray tube itself is composed basically of an *electron gun* and a *fluorescent screen* against which electrons are fired. Where the electrons hit the screen surface, the fluorescent material glows. If the electron beam is moved across the screen, the spot of glowing light also moves and draws a fluorescent line on the screen.

In addition to the electron gun and fluorescent surface, the cathode ray tube is provided with two sets of electrically charged plates—one set positioned on the two sides of the electron beam, and the other set positioned above and below. Appropriate electronic control circuits change the voltage on these plates so that the electron beam can be bent up or down in response to electrical signals coming from recording electrodes on nerves. The beam of electrons also is swept horizontally across the screen at a constant time rate by an internal electronic circuit of the oscilloscope. This gives the record shown on the face of the cathode ray tube in the figure, giving a time base horizontally and voltage changes from the nerve electrodes shown vertically. Note at the left end of the record a small *stimulus artifact* caused by the electrical stimulus used to elicit the nerve action potential. Then further to the right is the recorded action potential itself.

Bibliography

Alberts B, Johnson A, Lewis J, et al: *Molecular Biology of the Cell*, ed 3, New York, 2008, Garland Science.

Biel M, Wahl-Schott C, Michalakis S, Zong X: Hyperpolarization-activated cation channels: from genes to function, *Physiol Rev* 89:847, 2009.

Blaesse P, Airaksinen MS, Rivera C, Kaila K: Cation-chloride cotransporters and neuronal function, *Neuron* 61:820, 2009.

Dai S, Hall DD, Hell JW: Supramolecular assemblies and localized regulation of voltage-gated ion channels, *Physiol Rev* 89:411, 2009.

Hodgkin AL, Huxley AF: Quantitative description of membrane current and its application to conduction and excitation in nerve, *J Physiol (Lond)* 117:500, 1952.

Kandel ER, Schwartz JH, Jessell TM: *Principles of Neural Science*, ed 4, New York, 2000, McGraw-Hill.

Kleber AG, Rudy Y: Basic mechanisms of cardiac impulse propagation and associated arrhythmias, *Physiol Rev* 84:431, 2004.

Luján R, Maylie J, Adelman JP: New sites of action for GIRK and SK channels, *Nat Rev Neurosci* 10:475, 2009.

Mangoni ME, Nargeot J: Genesis and regulation of the heart automaticity, *Physiol Rev* 88:919, 2008.

Perez-Reyes E: Molecular physiology of low-voltage-activated T-type calcium channels, *Physiol Rev* 83:117, 2003.

Poliak S, Peles E: The local differentiation of myelinated axons at nodes of Ranvier, *Nat Rev Neurosci* 12:968, 2003.

Schafer DP, Rasband MN: Glial regulation of the axonal membrane at nodes of Ranvier, *Curr Opin Neurobiol* 16:508, 2006.

Vacher H, Mohapatra DP, Trimmer JS: Localization and targeting of voltage-dependent ion channels in mammalian central neurons, *Physiol Rev* 88:1407, 2008.

Contraction of Skeletal Muscle

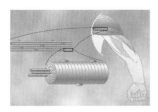 About 40 percent of the body is skeletal muscle, and perhaps another 10 percent is smooth and cardiac muscle. Some of the same basic principles of contraction apply to all three different types of muscle. In this chapter, function of skeletal muscle is considered mainly; the specialized functions of smooth muscle are discussed in Chapter 8, and cardiac muscle is discussed in Chapter 9.

Physiologic Anatomy of Skeletal Muscle

Skeletal Muscle Fiber

Figure 6-1 shows the organization of skeletal muscle, demonstrating that all skeletal muscles are composed of numerous fibers ranging from 10 to 80 micrometers in diameter. Each of these fibers is made up of successively smaller subunits, also shown in Figure 6-1 and described in subsequent paragraphs.

In most skeletal muscles, each fiber extends the entire length of the muscle. Except for about 2 percent of the fibers, each fiber is usually innervated by only one nerve ending, located near the middle of the fiber.

The Sarcolemma Is a Thin Membrane Enclosing a Skeletal Muscle Fiber. The sarcolemma consists of a true cell membrane, called the *plasma membrane,* and an outer coat made up of a thin layer of polysaccharide material that contains numerous thin collagen fibrils. At each end of the muscle fiber, this surface layer of the sarcolemma fuses with a tendon fiber. The tendon fibers in turn collect into bundles to form the muscle tendons that then insert into the bones.

Myofibrils Are Composed of Actin and Myosin Filaments. Each muscle fiber contains several hundred to several thousand *myofibrils,* which are demonstrated by the many small open dots in the cross-sectional view of Figure 6-1*C.* Each myofibril (Figure 6-1*D* and *E*) is composed of about 1500 adjacent *myosin filaments* and

3000 *actin filaments,* which are large polymerized protein molecules that are responsible for the actual muscle contraction. These can be seen in longitudinal view in the electron micrograph of Figure 6-2 and are represented diagrammatically in Figure 6-1, parts *E* through *L.* The thick filaments in the diagrams are *myosin,* and the thin filaments are *actin.*

Note in Figure 6-1*E* that the myosin and actin filaments partially interdigitate and thus cause the myofibrils to have alternate light and dark bands, as illustrated in Figure 6-2. The light bands contain only actin filaments and are called *I bands* because they are *isotropic* to polarized light. The dark bands contain myosin filaments, as well as the ends of the actin filaments where they overlap the myosin, and are called *A bands* because they are *anisotropic* to polarized light. Note also the small projections from the sides of the myosin filaments in Figure 6-1*E* and *L.* These are *cross-bridges.* It is the interaction between these cross-bridges and the actin filaments that causes contraction.

Figure 6-1*E* also shows that the ends of the actin filaments are attached to a so-called *Z disc.* From this disc, these filaments extend in both directions to interdigitate with the myosin filaments. The Z disc, which itself is composed of filamentous proteins different from the actin and myosin filaments, passes crosswise across the myofibril and also crosswise from myofibril to myofibril, attaching the myofibrils to one another all the way across the muscle fiber. Therefore, the entire muscle fiber has light and dark bands, as do the individual myofibrils. These bands give skeletal and cardiac muscle their striated appearance.

The portion of the myofibril (or of the whole muscle fiber) that lies between two successive Z discs is called a *sarcomere.* When the muscle fiber is contracted, as shown at the bottom of Figure 6-5, the length of the sarcomere is about 2 micrometers. At this length, the actin filaments completely overlap the myosin filaments, and the tips of the actin filaments are just beginning to overlap one another. As discussed later, at this length the muscle is capable of generating its greatest force of contraction.

SKELETAL MUSCLE

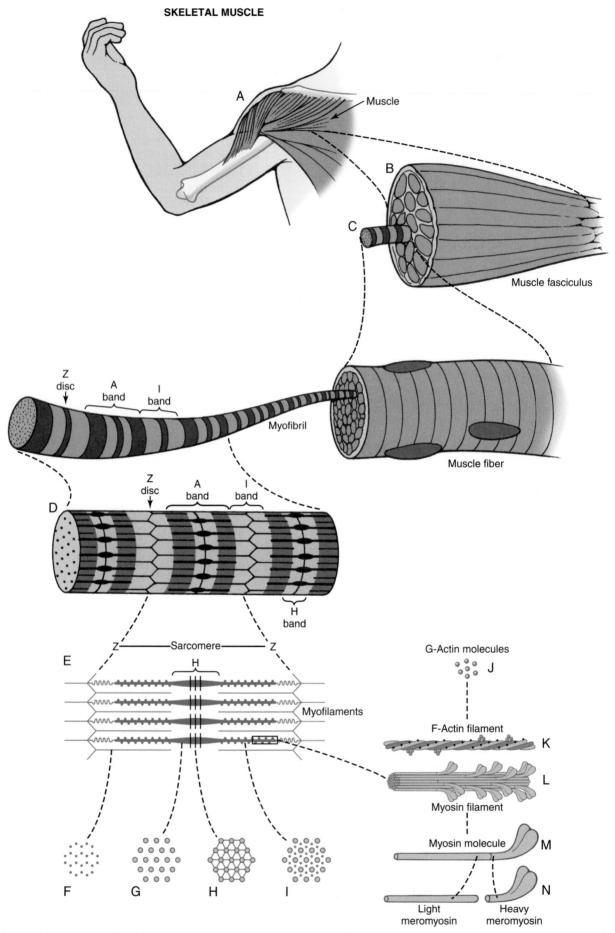

Figure 6-1 Organization of skeletal muscle, from the gross to the molecular level. *F, G, H,* and *I* are cross sections at the levels indicated.

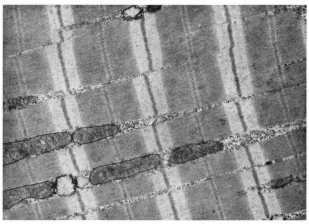

Figure 6-2 Electron micrograph of muscle myofibrils showing the detailed organization of actin and myosin filaments. Note the mitochondria lying between the myofibrils. (From Fawcett DW: The Cell. Philadelphia: WB Saunders, 1981.)

Titin Filamentous Molecules Keep the Myosin and Actin Filaments in Place. The side-by-side relationship between the myosin and actin filaments is difficult to maintain. This is achieved by a large number of filamentous molecules of a protein called *titin* (Figure 6-3). Each titin molecule has a molecular weight of about 3 million, which makes it one of the largest protein molecules in the body. Also, because it is filamentous, it is *very springy.* These springy titin molecules act as a framework that holds the myosin and actin filaments in place so that the contractile machinery of the sarcomere will work. One end of the titin molecule is elastic and is attached to the Z disk, acting as a spring and changing length as the sarcomere contracts and relaxes. The other part of the titin molecule tethers it to the myosin thick filament. The titin molecule itself also appears to act as a template for initial formation of portions of the contractile filaments of the sarcomere, especially the myosin filaments.

Sarcoplasm Is the Intracellular Fluid Between Myofibrils. The many myofibrils of each muscle fiber are suspended side by side in the muscle fiber. The spaces between the myofibrils are filled with intracellular fluid

called *sarcoplasm,* containing large quantities of potassium, magnesium, and phosphate, plus multiple protein enzymes. Also present are tremendous numbers of *mitochondria* that lie parallel to the myofibrils. These supply the contracting myofibrils with large amounts of energy in the form of adenosine triphosphate (ATP) formed by the mitochondria.

Sarcoplasmic Reticulum Is a Specialized Endoplasmic Reticulum of Skeletal Muscle. Also in the sarcoplasm surrounding the myofibrils of each muscle fiber is an extensive reticulum (Figure 6-4), called the *sarcoplasmic reticulum.* This reticulum has a special organization that is extremely important in controlling muscle contraction, as discussed in Chapter 7. The rapidly contracting types of muscle fibers have especially extensive sarcoplasmic reticula.

General Mechanism of Muscle Contraction

The initiation and execution of muscle contraction occur in the following sequential steps.

1. An action potential travels along a motor nerve to its endings on muscle fibers.

2. At each ending, the nerve secretes a small amount of the neurotransmitter substance *acetylcholine.*

3. The acetylcholine acts on a local area of the muscle fiber membrane to open multiple "acetylcholine-gated" cation channels through protein molecules floating in the membrane.

4. Opening of the acetylcholine-gated channels allows large quantities of sodium ions to diffuse to the interior of the muscle fiber membrane. This causes a local depolarization that in turn leads to opening of

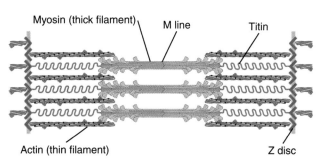

Figure 6-3 Organization of proteins in a sarcomere. Each titin molecule extends from the *Z disc* to the *M line.* Part of the titin molecule is closely associated with the myosin thick filament, whereas the rest of the molecule is springy and changes length as the sarcomere contracts and relaxes.

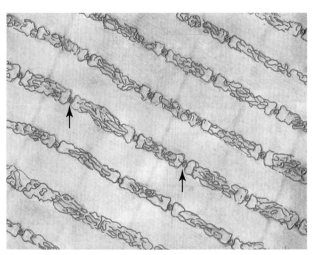

Figure 6-4 Sarcoplasmic reticulum in the extracellular spaces between the myofibrils, showing a longitudinal system paralleling the myofibrils. Also shown in cross section are T tubules (*arrows*) that lead to the exterior of the fiber membrane and are important for conducting the electrical signal into the center of the muscle fiber. (From Fawcett DW: The Cell. Philadelphia: WB Saunders, 1981.)

voltage-gated sodium channels. This initiates an action potential at the membrane.

5. The action potential travels along the muscle fiber membrane in the same way that action potentials travel along nerve fiber membranes.

6. The action potential depolarizes the muscle membrane, and much of the action potential electricity flows through the center of the muscle fiber. Here it causes the sarcoplasmic reticulum to release large quantities of calcium ions that have been stored within this reticulum.

7. The calcium ions initiate attractive forces between the actin and myosin filaments, causing them to slide alongside each other, which is the contractile process.

8. After a fraction of a second, the calcium ions are pumped back into the sarcoplasmic reticulum by a Ca^{++} membrane pump and remain stored in the reticulum until a new muscle action potential comes along; this removal of calcium ions from the myofibrils causes the muscle contraction to cease.

We now describe the molecular machinery of the muscle contractile process.

Molecular Mechanism of Muscle Contraction

Sliding Filament Mechanism of Muscle Contraction. Figure 6-5 demonstrates the basic mechanism of muscle contraction. It shows the relaxed state of a sarcomere (top) and the contracted state (bottom). In the relaxed state, the ends of the actin filaments extending from two successive Z discs barely begin to overlap one another. Conversely, in the contracted state, these actin filaments have been pulled inward among the myosin filaments, so their ends overlap one another to their

maximum extent. Also, the Z discs have been pulled by the actin filaments up to the ends of the myosin filaments. Thus, muscle contraction occurs by a *sliding filament mechanism.*

But what causes the actin filaments to slide inward among the myosin filaments? This is caused by forces generated by interaction of the cross-bridges from the myosin filaments with the actin filaments. Under resting conditions, these forces are inactive. But when an action potential travels along the muscle fiber, this causes the sarcoplasmic reticulum to release large quantities of calcium ions that rapidly surround the myofibrils. The calcium ions in turn activate the forces between the myosin and actin filaments, and contraction begins. But energy is needed for the contractile process to proceed. This energy comes from high-energy bonds in the ATP molecule, which is degraded to adenosine diphosphate (ADP) to liberate the energy. In the next few sections, we describe what is known about the details of these molecular processes of contraction.

Molecular Characteristics of the Contractile Filaments

Myosin Filaments Are Composed of Multiple Myosin Molecules. Each of the myosin molecules, shown in Figure 6-6A, has a molecular weight of about 480,000. Figure 6-6B shows the organization of many molecules to form a myosin filament, as well as interaction of this filament on one side with the ends of two actin filaments.

The *myosin molecule* (see Figure 6-6A) is composed of six polypeptide chains—two *heavy chains,* each with a molecular weight of about 200,000, and four *light chains* with molecular weights of about 20,000 each. The two heavy chains wrap spirally around each other to form a double

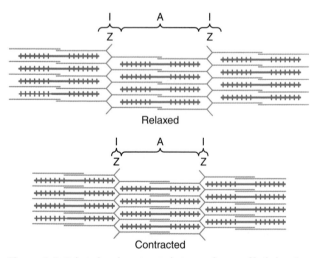

Figure 6-5 Relaxed and contracted states of a myofibril showing (*top*) sliding of the actin filaments (*pink*) into the spaces between the myosin filaments (*red*) and (*bottom*) pulling of the Z membranes toward each other.

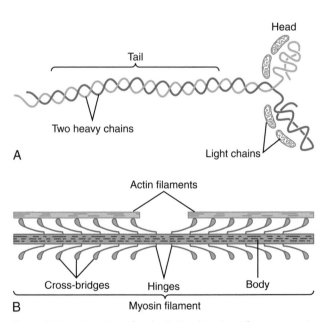

Figure 6-6 *A,* Myosin molecule. *B,* Combination of many myosin molecules to form a myosin filament. Also shown are thousands of myosin *cross-bridges* and interaction between the *heads* of the cross-bridges with adjacent actin filaments.

helix, which is called the *tail* of the myosin molecule. One end of each of these chains is folded bilaterally into a globular polypeptide structure called a myosin *head.* Thus, there are two free heads at one end of the double-helix myosin molecule. The four light chains are also part of the myosin head, two to each head. These light chains help control the function of the head during muscle contraction.

The *myosin filament* is made up of 200 or more individual myosin molecules. The central portion of one of these filaments is shown in Figure 6-6*B*, displaying the tails of the myosin molecules bundled together to form the *body* of the filament, while many heads of the molecules hang outward to the sides of the body. Also, part of the body of each myosin molecule hangs to the side along with the head, thus providing an *arm* that extends the head outward from the body, as shown in the figure. The protruding arms and heads together are called *cross-bridges.* Each cross-bridge is flexible at two points called *hinges*—one where the arm leaves the body of the myosin filament, and the other where the head attaches to the arm. The hinged arms allow the heads to be either extended far outward from the body of the myosin filament or brought close to the body. The hinged heads in turn participate in the actual contraction process, as discussed in the following sections.

The total length of each myosin filament is uniform, almost exactly 1.6 micrometers. Note, however, that there are no cross-bridge heads in the center of the myosin filament for a distance of about 0.2 micrometer because the hinged arms extend away from the center.

Now, to complete the picture, the myosin filament itself is twisted so that each successive pair of cross-bridges is axially displaced from the previous pair by 120 degrees. This ensures that the cross-bridges extend in all directions around the filament.

ATPase Activity of the Myosin Head. Another feature of the myosin head that is essential for muscle contraction is that it functions as an *ATPase enzyme.* As explained later, this property allows the head to cleave ATP and use the energy derived from the ATP's high-energy phosphate bond to energize the contraction process.

Actin Filaments Are Composed of Actin, Tropomyosin, and Troponin. The backbone of the actin filament is a double-stranded *F-actin protein molecule,* represented by the two lighter-colored strands in Figure 6-7. The two strands are wound in a helix in the same manner as the myosin molecule.

Each strand of the double F-actin helix is composed of polymerized *G-actin molecules,* each having a molecular weight of about 42,000. Attached to each one of the G-actin molecules is one molecule of ADP. It is believed that these ADP molecules are the active sites on the actin filaments with which the cross-bridges of the myosin filaments interact to cause muscle contraction. The active sites on the two F-actin strands of the double helix are staggered, giving one active site on the overall actin filament about every 2.7 nanometers.

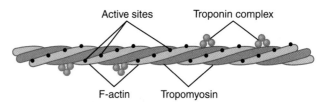

Figure 6-7 Actin filament, composed of two helical strands of *F-actin* molecules and two strands of *tropomyosin* molecules that fit in the grooves between the actin strands. Attached to one end of each tropomyosin molecule is a *troponin* complex that initiates contraction.

Each actin filament is about 1 micrometer long. The bases of the actin filaments are inserted strongly into the Z discs; the ends of the filaments protrude in both directions to lie in the spaces between the myosin molecules, as shown in Figure 6-5.

Tropomyosin Molecules. The actin filament also contains another protein, *tropomyosin.* Each molecule of tropomyosin has a molecular weight of 70,000 and a length of 40 nanometers. These molecules are wrapped spirally around the sides of the F-actin helix. In the resting state, the tropomyosin molecules lie on top of the active sites of the actin strands so that attraction cannot occur between the actin and myosin filaments to cause contraction.

Troponin and Its Role in Muscle Contraction. Attached intermittently along the sides of the tropomyosin molecules are still other protein molecules called *troponin.* These are actually complexes of three loosely bound protein subunits, each of which plays a specific role in controlling muscle contraction. One of the subunits (troponin I) has a strong affinity for actin, another (troponin T) for tropomyosin, and a third (troponin C) for calcium ions. This complex is believed to attach the tropomyosin to the actin. The strong affinity of the troponin for calcium ions is believed to initiate the contraction process, as explained in the next section.

Interaction of One Myosin Filament, Two Actin Filaments, and Calcium Ions to Cause Contraction

Inhibition of the Actin Filament by the Troponin-Tropomyosin Complex; Activation by Calcium Ions. A pure actin filament without the presence of the troponin-tropomyosin complex (but in the presence of magnesium ions and ATP) binds instantly and strongly with the heads of the myosin molecules. Then, if the troponin-tropomyosin complex is added to the actin filament, the binding between myosin and actin does not take place. Therefore, it is believed that the active sites on the normal actin filament of the relaxed muscle are inhibited or physically covered by the troponin-tropomyosin complex. Consequently, the sites cannot attach to the heads of the myosin filaments to cause contraction. Before contraction can take place, the inhibitory effect of the troponin-tropomyosin complex must itself be inhibited.

This brings us to the role of the calcium ions. In the presence of large amounts of calcium ions, the inhibitory effect of the troponin-tropomyosin on the actin filaments is itself inhibited. The mechanism of this is not known, but one suggestion is the following: When calcium ions combine with troponin C, each molecule of which can bind strongly with up to four calcium ions, the troponin complex supposedly undergoes a conformational change that in some way tugs on the tropomyosin molecule and moves it deeper into the groove between the two actin strands. This "uncovers" the active sites of the actin, thus allowing these to attract the myosin cross-bridge heads and cause contraction to proceed. Although this is a hypothetical mechanism, it does emphasize that the normal relation between the troponin-tropomyosin complex and actin is altered by calcium ions, producing a new condition that leads to contraction.

Interaction Between the "Activated" Actin Filament and the Myosin Cross-Bridges—The "Walk-Along" Theory of Contraction. As soon as the actin filament becomes activated by the calcium ions, the heads of the cross-bridges from the myosin filaments become attracted to the active sites of the actin filament, and this, in some way, causes contraction to occur. Although the precise manner by which this interaction between the cross-bridges and the actin causes contraction is still partly theoretical, one hypothesis for which considerable evidence exists is the "walk-along" theory (or *"ratchet" theory*) of contraction.

Figure 6-8 demonstrates this postulated walk-along mechanism for contraction. The figure shows the heads of two cross-bridges attaching to and disengaging from active sites of an actin filament. It is postulated that when a head attaches to an active site, this attachment simultaneously causes profound changes in the intramolecular forces between the head and arm of its cross-bridge. The new alignment of forces causes the head to tilt toward the arm and to drag the actin filament along with it. This tilt of the head is called the *power stroke.* Then, immediately after tilting, the head automatically breaks away from the active site. Next, the head returns to its extended direction. In this position, it combines with a new active site farther down along the actin filament; then the head tilts again to cause a new power stroke, and the actin filament moves another step. Thus, the heads of the cross-bridges bend back and forth and step by step walk along the actin filament, pulling the ends of two successive actin filaments toward the center of the myosin filament.

Each one of the cross-bridges is believed to operate independently of all others, each attaching and pulling in a continuous repeated cycle. Therefore, the greater the number of cross-bridges in contact with the actin filament at any given time, the greater the force of contraction.

ATP as the Source of Energy for Contraction— Chemical Events in the Motion of the Myosin Heads. When a muscle contracts, work is performed and energy is required. Large amounts of ATP are cleaved to form ADP during the contraction process; the greater the

amount of work performed by the muscle, the greater the amount of ATP that is cleaved, which is called the *Fenn effect.* The following sequence of events is believed to be the means by which this occurs:

1. Before contraction begins, the heads of the cross-bridges bind with ATP. The ATPase activity of the myosin head immediately cleaves the ATP but leaves the cleavage products, ADP plus phosphate ion, bound to the head. In this state, the conformation of the head is such that it extends perpendicularly toward the actin filament but is not yet attached to the actin.

2. When the troponin-tropomyosin complex binds with calcium ions, active sites on the actin filament are uncovered and the myosin heads then bind with these, as shown in Figure 6-8.

3. The bond between the head of the cross-bridge and the active site of the actin filament causes a conformational change in the head, prompting the head to tilt toward the arm of the cross-bridge. This provides the *power stroke* for pulling the actin filament. The energy that activates the power stroke is the energy already stored, like a "cocked" spring, by the conformational change that occurred in the head when the ATP molecule was cleaved earlier.

4. Once the head of the cross-bridge tilts, this allows release of the ADP and phosphate ion that were previously attached to the head. At the site of release of the ADP, a new molecule of ATP binds. This binding of new ATP causes detachment of the head from the actin.

5. After the head has detached from the actin, the new molecule of ATP is cleaved to begin the next cycle, leading to a new power stroke. That is, the energy again "cocks" the head back to its perpendicular condition, ready to begin the new power stroke cycle.

6. When the cocked head (with its stored energy derived from the cleaved ATP) binds with a new active site on the actin filament, it becomes uncocked and once again provides a new power stroke.

Thus, the process proceeds again and again until the actin filaments pull the Z membrane up against the ends of the myosin filaments or until the load on the muscle becomes too great for further pulling to occur.

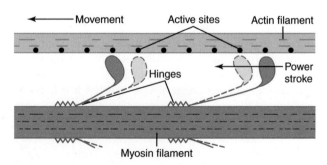

Figure 6-8 "Walk-along" mechanism for contraction of the muscle.

The Amount of Actin and Myosin Filament Overlap Determines Tension Developed by the Contracting Muscle

Figure 6-9 shows the effect of sarcomere length and amount of myosin-actin filament overlap on the active tension developed by a contracting muscle fiber. To the right, shown in black, are different degrees of overlap of the myosin and actin filaments at different sarcomere lengths. At point D on the diagram, the actin filament has pulled all the way out to the end of the myosin filament, with no actin-myosin overlap. At this point, the tension developed by the activated muscle is zero. Then, as the sarcomere shortens and the actin filament begins to overlap the myosin filament, the tension increases progressively until the sarcomere length decreases to about 2.2 micrometers. At this point, the actin filament has already overlapped all the cross-bridges of the myosin filament but has not yet reached the center of the myosin filament. With further shortening, the sarcomere maintains full tension until point B is reached, at a sarcomere length of about 2 micrometers. At this point, the ends of the two actin filaments begin to overlap each other in addition to overlapping the myosin filaments. As the sarcomere length falls from 2 micrometers down to about 1.65 micrometers, at point A, the strength of contraction decreases rapidly. At this point, the two Z discs of the sarcomere abut the ends of the myosin filaments. Then, as contraction proceeds to still shorter sarcomere lengths, the ends of the myosin filaments are crumpled and, as shown in the figure, the strength of contraction approaches zero, but the sarcomere has now contracted to its shortest length.

Effect of Muscle Length on Force of Contraction in the Whole Intact Muscle.
The top curve of Figure 6-10 is similar to that in Figure 6-9, but the curve in Figure 6-10 depicts tension of the intact, whole muscle rather than of a single muscle fiber. The whole muscle has a large

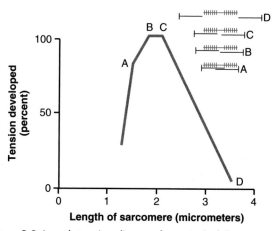

Figure 6-9 Length-tension diagram for a single fully contracted sarcomere, showing maximum strength of contraction when the sarcomere is 2.0 to 2.2 micrometers in length. At the upper right are the relative positions of the actin and myosin filaments at different sarcomere lengths from *point A* to *point D*. (Modified from Gordon AM, Huxley AF, Julian FJ: The length-tension diagram of single vertebrate striated muscle fibers. J Physiol 171:28P, 1964.)

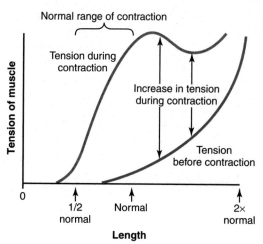

Figure 6-10 Relation of muscle length to tension in the muscle both before and during muscle contraction.

amount of connective tissue in it; also, the sarcomeres in different parts of the muscle do not always contract the same amount. Therefore, the curve has somewhat different dimensions from those shown for the individual muscle fiber, but it exhibits the same general form for the slope *in the normal range of contraction,* as noted in Figure 6-10.

Note in Figure 6-10 that when the muscle is at its normal *resting* length, which is at a sarcomere length of about 2 micrometers, it contracts upon activation with the approximate maximum force of contraction. However, the *increase* in tension that occurs during contraction, called *active tension,* decreases as the muscle is stretched beyond its normal length—that is, to a sarcomere length greater than about 2.2 micrometers. This is demonstrated by the decreased length of the arrow in the figure at greater than normal muscle length.

Relation of Velocity of Contraction to Load
A skeletal muscle contracts rapidly when it contracts against no load—to a state of full contraction in about 0.1 second for the average muscle. When loads are applied, the velocity of contraction becomes progressively less as the load increases, as shown in Figure 6-11. That is, when the

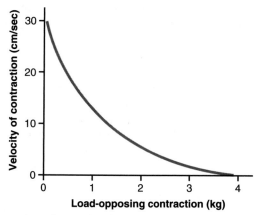

Figure 6-11 Relation of load to velocity of contraction in a skeletal muscle with a cross section of 1 square centimeter and a length of 8 centimeters.

load has been increased to equal the maximum force that the muscle can exert, the velocity of contraction becomes zero and no contraction results, despite activation of the muscle fiber.

This decreasing velocity of contraction with load is caused by the fact that a load on a contracting muscle is a reverse force that opposes the contractile force caused by muscle contraction. Therefore, the net force that is available to cause velocity of shortening is correspondingly reduced.

Energetics of Muscle Contraction

Work Output During Muscle Contraction

When a muscle contracts against a load, it performs *work*. This means that *energy* is transferred from the muscle to the external load to lift an object to a greater height or to overcome resistance to movement.

In mathematical terms, work is defined by the following equation:

$$W = L \times D$$

in which W is the work output, L is the load, and D is the distance of movement against the load. The energy required to perform the work is derived from the chemical reactions in the muscle cells during contraction, as described in the following sections.

Sources of Energy for Muscle Contraction

We have already seen that muscle contraction depends on energy supplied by ATP. Most of this energy is required to actuate the walk-along mechanism by which the cross-bridges pull the actin filaments, but small amounts are required for (1) pumping calcium ions from the sarcoplasm into the sarcoplasmic reticulum after the contraction is over and (2) pumping sodium and potassium ions through the muscle fiber membrane to maintain appropriate ionic environment for propagation of muscle fiber action potentials.

The concentration of ATP in the muscle fiber, about 4 millimolar, is sufficient to maintain full contraction for only 1 to 2 seconds at most. The ATP is split to form ADP, which transfers energy from the ATP molecule to the contracting machinery of the muscle fiber. Then, as described in Chapter 2, the ADP is rephosphorylated to form new ATP within another fraction of a second, which allows the muscle to continue its contraction. There are several sources of the energy for this rephosphorylation.

The first source of energy that is used to reconstitute the ATP is the substance *phosphocreatine,* which carries a high-energy phosphate bond similar to the bonds of ATP. The high-energy phosphate bond of phosphocreatine has a slightly higher amount of free energy than that of each ATP bond, as is discussed more fully in Chapters 67 and 72. Therefore, phosphocreatine is instantly cleaved, and its released energy causes bonding of a new phosphate ion to ADP to reconstitute the ATP. However, the total amount of phosphocreatine in the muscle fiber is also very little—only about five times as great as the ATP. Therefore, the combined energy of both the stored ATP and the phosphocreatine in the muscle is capable of causing maximal muscle contraction for only 5 to 8 seconds.

The second important source of energy, which is used to reconstitute both ATP and phosphocreatine, is "glycolysis" of *glycogen* previously stored in the muscle cells. Rapid enzymatic breakdown of the glycogen to pyruvic acid and lactic acid liberates energy that is used to convert ADP to ATP; the ATP can then be used directly to energize additional muscle contraction and also to re-form the stores of phosphocreatine.

The importance of this glycolysis mechanism is twofold. First, the glycolytic reactions can occur even in the absence of oxygen, so muscle contraction can be sustained for many seconds and sometimes up to more than a minute, even when oxygen delivery from the blood is not available. Second, the rate of formation of ATP by the glycolytic process is about 2.5 times as rapid as ATP formation in response to cellular foodstuffs reacting with oxygen. However, so many end products of glycolysis accumulate in the muscle cells that glycolysis also loses its capability to sustain maximum muscle contraction after about 1 minute.

The third and final source of energy is *oxidative metabolism.* This means combining oxygen with the end products of glycolysis and with various other cellular foodstuffs to liberate ATP. More than 95 percent of all energy used by the muscles for sustained, long-term contraction is derived from this source. The foodstuffs that are consumed are carbohydrates, fats, and protein. For extremely long-term maximal muscle activity—over a period of many hours—by far the greatest proportion of energy comes from fats, but for periods of 2 to 4 hours, as much as one half of the energy can come from stored carbohydrates.

The detailed mechanisms of these energetic processes are discussed in Chapters 67 through 72. In addition, the importance of the different mechanisms of energy release during performance of different sports is discussed in Chapter 84 on sports physiology.

Efficiency of Muscle Contraction. The efficiency of an engine or a motor is calculated as the percentage of energy input that is converted into work instead of heat. The percentage of the input energy to muscle (the chemical energy in nutrients) that can be converted into work, even under the best conditions, is less than 25 percent, with the remainder becoming heat. The reason for this low efficiency is that about one half of the energy in foodstuffs is lost during the formation of ATP, and even then, only 40 to 45 percent of the energy in the ATP itself can later be converted into work.

Maximum efficiency can be realized only when the muscle contracts at a moderate velocity. If the muscle contracts slowly or without any movement, small amounts of *maintenance heat* are released during contraction, even though little or no work is performed, thereby decreasing the conversion efficiency to as little as zero. Conversely, if contraction is too rapid, large proportions of the energy are used to overcome viscous friction within the muscle itself, and this, too, reduces the efficiency of contraction. Ordinarily, maximum efficiency is developed when the velocity of contraction is about 30 percent of maximum.

Characteristics of Whole Muscle Contraction

Many features of muscle contraction can be demonstrated by eliciting single *muscle twitches.* This can be accomplished by instantaneous electrical excitation of the nerve to a muscle or by passing a short electrical stimulus through the muscle itself, giving rise to a single, sudden contraction lasting for a fraction of a second.

Isometric Versus Isotonic Contraction. Muscle contraction is said to be *isometric* when the muscle does not shorten during contraction and *isotonic* when it does shorten but the tension on the muscle remains constant throughout the contraction. Systems for recording the two types of muscle contraction are shown in Figure 6-12.

In the isometric system, the muscle contracts against a force transducer without decreasing the muscle length, as shown on the right in Figure 6-12. In the isotonic system, the muscle shortens against a fixed load; this is illustrated on the left in the figure, showing a muscle lifting a pan of weights. The characteristics of isotonic contraction depend on the load against which the muscle contracts, as well as the inertia of the load. However, the isometric system records strictly changes in force of muscle contraction itself. Therefore, the isometric system is most often used when comparing the functional characteristics of different muscle types.

Characteristics of Isometric Twitches Recorded from Different Muscles. The human body has many sizes of skeletal muscles—from the small stapedius muscle in the middle ear, measuring only a few millimeters long and a millimeter or so in diameter, up to the large quadriceps muscle, a half million times as large as the stapedius. Further, the fibers may be as small as 10 micrometers in diameter or as large as 80 micrometers. Finally, the energetics of muscle contraction vary considerably from one muscle to another. Therefore, it is no wonder that the mechanical characteristics of muscle contraction differ among muscles.

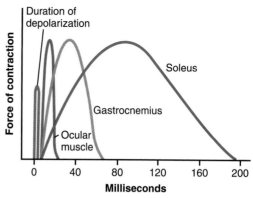

Figure 6-13 Duration of isometric contractions for different types of mammalian skeletal muscles, showing a latent period between the action potential (depolarization) and muscle contraction.

Figure 6-13 shows records of isometric contractions of three types of skeletal muscle: an ocular muscle, which has a duration of *isometric* contraction of less than 1/50 second; the gastrocnemius muscle, which has a duration of contraction of about 1/15 second; and the soleus muscle, which has a duration of contraction of about 1/5 second. It is interesting that these durations of contraction are adapted to the functions of the respective muscles. Ocular movements must be extremely rapid to maintain fixation of the eyes on specific objects to provide accuracy of vision. The gastrocnemius muscle must contract moderately rapidly to provide sufficient velocity of limb movement for running and jumping, and the soleus muscle is concerned principally with slow contraction for continual, long-term support of the body against gravity.

Fast Versus Slow Muscle Fibers. As we discuss more fully in Chapter 84 on sports physiology, every muscle of the body is composed of a mixture of so-called *fast* and *slow* muscle fibers, with still other fibers gradated between these two extremes. Muscles that react rapidly, including anterior tibialis, are composed mainly of "fast" fibers with only small numbers of the slow variety. Conversely, muscles such as soleus that respond slowly but with prolonged contraction are composed mainly of "slow" fibers. The differences between these two types of fibers are as follows.

Slow Fibers (Type 1, Red Muscle). (1) Smaller fibers. (2) Also innervated by smaller nerve fibers. (3) More extensive blood vessel system and capillaries to supply extra amounts of oxygen. (4) Greatly increased numbers of mitochondria, also to support high levels of oxidative metabolism. (5) Fibers contain large amounts of myoglobin, an iron-containing protein similar to hemoglobin in red blood cells. Myoglobin combines with oxygen and stores it until needed; this also greatly speeds oxygen transport to the mitochondria. The myoglobin gives the slow muscle a reddish appearance and the name *red muscle.*

Fast Fibers (Type II, White Muscle). (1) Large fibers for great strength of contraction. (2) Extensive sarcoplasmic reticulum for rapid release of calcium ions to initiate contraction. (3) Large amounts of glycolytic enzymes for rapid release of energy by the glycolytic process. (4) Less extensive blood supply because oxidative metabolism is of secondary importance. (5) Fewer mitochondria, also because oxidative metabolism is secondary. A deficit of red myoglobin in fast muscle gives it the name *white muscle.*

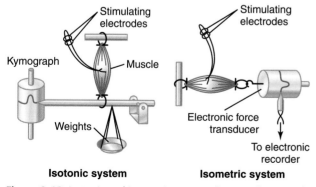

Figure 6-12 Isotonic and isometric systems for recording muscle contractions.

Mechanics of Skeletal Muscle Contraction

Motor Unit—All the Muscle Fibers Innervated by a Single Nerve Fiber. Each motoneuron that leaves the spinal cord innervates multiple muscle fibers, the number depending on the type of muscle. All the muscle fibers innervated by a single nerve fiber are called a *motor unit.* In general, small muscles that react rapidly and whose control must be exact have more nerve fibers for fewer muscle fibers (for instance, as few as two or three muscle fibers per motor unit in some of the laryngeal muscles). Conversely, large muscles that do not require fine control, such as the soleus muscle, may have several hundred muscle fibers in a motor unit. An average figure for all the muscles of the body is questionable, but a good guess would be about 80 to 100 muscle fibers to a motor unit.

The muscle fibers in each motor unit are not all bunched together in the muscle but overlap other motor units in microbundles of 3 to 15 fibers. This interdigitation allows the separate motor units to contract in support of one another rather than entirely as individual segments.

Muscle Contractions of Different Force—Force Summation. *Summation* means the adding together of individual twitch contractions to increase the intensity of overall muscle contraction. Summation occurs in two ways: (1) by increasing the number of motor units contracting simultaneously, which is called *multiple fiber summation,* and (2) by increasing the frequency of contraction, which is called *frequency summation* and can lead to *tetanization.*

Multiple Fiber Summation. When the central nervous system sends a weak signal to contract a muscle, the smaller motor units of the muscle may be stimulated in preference to the larger motor units. Then, as the strength of the signal increases, larger and larger motor units begin to be excited as well, with the largest motor units often having as much as 50 times the contractile force of the smallest units. This is called the *size principle.* It is important because it allows the gradations of muscle force during weak contraction to occur in small steps, whereas the steps become progressively greater when large amounts of force are required. The cause of this size principle is that the smaller motor units are driven by small motor nerve fibers, and the small motoneurons in the spinal cord are more excitable than the larger ones, so naturally they are excited first.

Another important feature of multiple fiber summation is that the different motor units are driven asynchronously by the spinal cord, so contraction alternates among motor units one after the other, thus providing smooth contraction even at low frequencies of nerve signals.

Frequency Summation and Tetanization. Figure 6-14 shows the principles of frequency summation and tetanization. To the left are displayed individual twitch contractions occurring one after another at low frequency of stimulation. Then, as the frequency increases, there comes a point where each new contraction occurs before the preceding one is over. As a result, the second contraction is added partially to the first, so the total strength of contraction rises progressively with increasing frequency. When the frequency reaches a critical level, the successive contractions eventually become so rapid that they fuse together and the whole muscle contraction appears to be completely smooth and continuous, as shown in the figure. This is called *tetanization.* At a slightly higher frequency, the strength of contraction reaches its

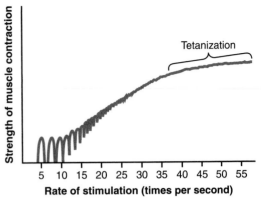

Figure 6-14 Frequency summation and tetanization.

maximum, so any additional increase in frequency beyond that point has no further effect in increasing contractile force. This occurs because enough calcium ions are maintained in the muscle sarcoplasm, even between action potentials, so that full contractile state is sustained without allowing any relaxation between the action potentials.

Maximum Strength of Contraction. The maximum strength of tetanic contraction of a muscle operating at a normal muscle length averages between 3 and 4 kilograms per square centimeter of muscle, or 50 pounds per square inch. Because a quadriceps muscle can have up to 16 square inches of muscle belly, as much as 800 pounds of tension may be applied to the patellar tendon. Thus, one can readily understand how it is possible for muscles to pull their tendons out of their insertions in bone.

Changes in Muscle Strength at the Onset of Contraction— The Staircase Effect (Treppe). When a muscle begins to contract after a long period of rest, its initial strength of contraction may be as little as one-half its strength 10 to 50 muscle twitches later. That is, the strength of contraction increases to a plateau, a phenomenon called the *staircase effect,* or *treppe.*

Although all the possible causes of the staircase effect are not known, it is believed to be caused primarily by increasing calcium ions in the cytosol because of the release of more and more ions from the sarcoplasmic reticulum with each successive muscle action potential and failure of the sarcoplasm to recapture the ions immediately.

Skeletal Muscle Tone. Even when muscles are at rest, a certain amount of tautness usually remains. This is called *muscle tone.* Because normal skeletal muscle fibers do not contract without an action potential to stimulate the fibers, skeletal muscle tone results entirely from a low rate of nerve impulses coming from the spinal cord. These, in turn, are controlled partly by signals transmitted from the brain to the appropriate spinal cord anterior motoneurons and partly by signals that originate in *muscle spindles* located in the muscle itself. Both of these are discussed in relation to muscle spindle and spinal cord function in Chapter 54.

Muscle Fatigue. Prolonged and strong contraction of a muscle leads to the well-known state of muscle fatigue. Studies in athletes have shown that muscle fatigue increases in almost direct proportion to the rate of depletion of muscle glycogen. Therefore, fatigue results mainly from inability of the contractile and metabolic processes of the muscle fibers to continue supplying the same work output. However, experiments have also shown that transmission of the nerve signal through the neuromuscular junction, which is discussed in Chapter 7, can diminish at least a small amount after intense prolonged muscle activity, thus further diminishing muscle contraction. Interruption of blood flow through a contracting muscle leads to almost complete muscle fatigue within 1 or 2 minutes because of the loss of nutrient supply, especially loss of oxygen.

Lever Systems of the Body. Muscles operate by applying tension to their points of insertion into bones, and the bones in turn form various types of lever systems. Figure 6-15 shows the lever system activated by the biceps muscle to lift the forearm. If we assume that a large biceps muscle has a cross-sectional area of 6 square inches, the maximum force of contraction would be about 300 pounds. When the forearm is at right angles with the upper arm, the tendon attachment of the biceps is about 2 inches anterior to the fulcrum at the elbow and the total length of the forearm lever is about 14 inches. Therefore, the amount of lifting power of the biceps at the hand would be only one seventh of the 300 pounds of muscle force, or about 43 pounds. When the arm is fully extended, the attachment of the biceps is much less than 2 inches anterior to the fulcrum and the force with which the hand can be brought forward is also much less than 43 pounds.

In short, an analysis of the lever systems of the body depends on knowledge of (1) the point of muscle insertion, (2) its distance from the fulcrum of the lever, (3) the length of the lever arm, and (4) the position of the lever. Many types of movement are required in the body, some of which need great strength and others of which need large distances of movement. For this reason, there are many different types of muscle; some are long and contract a long distance, and some are short but have large cross-sectional areas and can provide extreme strength of contraction over short distances. The study of different types of muscles, lever systems, and their movements is called *kinesiology* and is an important scientific component of human physioanatomy.

"Positioning" of a Body Part by Contraction of Agonist and Antagonist Muscles on Opposite Sides of a Joint— "Coactivation" of Antagonist Muscles. Virtually all body movements are caused by simultaneous contraction of agonist and antagonist muscles on opposite sides of joints. This is called coactivation of the agonist and antagonist muscles, and it is controlled by the motor control centers of the brain and spinal cord.

The position of each separate part of the body, such as an arm or a leg, is determined by the relative degrees of contraction of the agonist and antagonist sets of muscles. For instance, let us assume that an arm or a leg is to be placed in a midrange position. To achieve this, agonist and antagonist muscles are excited about equally. Remember that an elongated muscle contracts with more force than a shortened muscle, which was demonstrated in Figure 6-10, showing maximum strength of contraction at full functional muscle length and almost no strength of contraction at half-normal length. Therefore, the elongated muscle on one side of a joint can contract with far greater force than the shorter muscle on the opposite side. As an arm or leg moves toward its midposition, the strength of the longer muscle decreases, whereas the strength of the shorter muscle increases until the two strengths equal each other. At this point, movement of the arm or leg stops. Thus, by varying the ratios of the degree of activation of the agonist and antagonist muscles, the nervous system directs the positioning of the arm or leg.

We learn in Chapter 54 that the motor nervous system has additional important mechanisms to compensate for different muscle loads when directing this positioning process.

Remodeling of Muscle to Match Function

All the muscles of the body are continually being remodeled to match the functions that are required of them. Their diameters are altered, their lengths are altered, their strengths are altered, their vascular supplies are altered, and even the types of muscle fibers are altered at least slightly. This remodeling process is often quite rapid, within a few weeks. Indeed, experiments in animals have shown that muscle contractile proteins in some smaller, more active muscles can be replaced in as little as 2 weeks.

Muscle Hypertrophy and Muscle Atrophy. When the total mass of a muscle increases, this is called *muscle hypertrophy.* When it decreases, the process is called *muscle atrophy.*

Virtually all muscle hypertrophy results from an increase in the number of actin and myosin filaments in each muscle fiber, causing enlargement of the individual muscle fibers; this is called simply *fiber hypertrophy.* Hypertrophy occurs to a much greater extent when the muscle is loaded during the contractile process. Only a few strong contractions each day are required to cause significant hypertrophy within 6 to 10 weeks.

The manner in which forceful contraction leads to hypertrophy is not known. It is known, however, that the rate of synthesis of muscle contractile proteins is far greater when hypertrophy is developing, leading also to progressively greater numbers of both actin and myosin filaments in the myofibrils, often increasing as much as 50 percent. In turn, some of the myofibrils themselves have been observed to split within hypertrophying muscle to form new myofibrils, but how important this is in usual muscle hypertrophy is still unknown.

Along with the increasing size of myofibrils, the enzyme systems that provide energy also increase. This is especially true of the enzymes for glycolysis, allowing rapid supply of energy during short-term forceful muscle contraction.

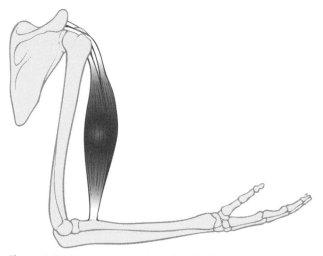

Figure 6-15 Lever system activated by the biceps muscle.

When a muscle remains unused for many weeks, the rate of degradation of the contractile proteins is more rapid than the rate of replacement. Therefore, muscle atrophy occurs. The pathway that appears to account for much of the protein degradation in a muscle undergoing atrophy is the *ATP-dependent ubiquitin-proteasome pathway*. Proteasomes are large protein complexes that degrade damaged or unneeded proteins by *proteolysis*, a chemical reaction that breaks peptide bonds. Ubiquitin is a regulatory protein that basically labels which cells will be targeted for proteasomal degradation.

Adjustment of Muscle Length. Another type of hypertrophy occurs when muscles are stretched to greater than normal length. This causes new sarcomeres to be added at the ends of the muscle fibers, where they attach to the tendons. In fact, new sarcomeres can be added as rapidly as several per minute in newly developing muscle, illustrating the rapidity of this type of hypertrophy.

Conversely, when a muscle continually remains shortened to less than its normal length, sarcomeres at the ends of the muscle fibers can actually disappear. It is by these processes that muscles are continually remodeled to have the appropriate length for proper muscle contraction.

Hyperplasia of Muscle Fibers. Under rare conditions of extreme muscle force generation, the actual number of muscle fibers has been observed to increase (but only by a few percentage points), in addition to the fiber hypertrophy process. This increase in fiber number is called *fiber hyperplasia*. When it does occur, the mechanism is linear splitting of previously enlarged fibers.

Effects of Muscle Denervation. When a muscle loses its nerve supply, it no longer receives the contractile signals that are required to maintain normal muscle size. Therefore, atrophy begins almost immediately. After about 2 months, degenerative changes also begin to appear in the muscle fibers themselves. If the nerve supply to the muscle grows back rapidly, full return of function can occur in as little as 3 months, but from that time onward, the capability of functional return becomes less and less, with no further return of function after 1 to 2 years.

In the final stage of denervation atrophy, most of the muscle fibers are destroyed and replaced by fibrous and fatty tissue. The fibers that do remain are composed of a long cell membrane with a lineup of muscle cell nuclei but with few or no contractile properties and little or no capability of regenerating myofibrils if a nerve does regrow.

The fibrous tissue that replaces the muscle fibers during denervation atrophy also has a tendency to continue shortening for many months, which is called *contracture*. Therefore, one of the most important problems in the practice of physical therapy is to keep atrophying muscles from developing debilitating and disfiguring contractures. This is achieved by daily stretching of the muscles or use of appliances that keep the muscles stretched during the atrophying process.

Recovery of Muscle Contraction in Poliomyelitis: Development of Macromotor Units. When some but not all nerve fibers to a muscle are destroyed, as commonly occurs in poliomyelitis, the remaining nerve fibers branch off to form new axons that then innervate many of the paralyzed muscle fibers. This causes large motor units called *macromotor units*, which can contain as many as five times the normal number of muscle fibers for each motoneuron coming from the spinal cord. This decreases the fineness of control one has over the muscles but does allow the muscles to regain varying degrees of strength.

Rigor Mortis

Several hours after death, all the muscles of the body go into a state of *contracture* called "rigor mortis"; that is, the muscles contract and become rigid, even without action potentials. This rigidity results from loss of all the ATP, which is required to cause separation of the cross-bridges from the actin filaments during the relaxation process. The muscles remain in rigor until the muscle proteins deteriorate about 15 to 25 hours later, which presumably results from autolysis caused by enzymes released from lysosomes. All these events occur more rapidly at higher temperatures.

Bibliography

Allen DG, Lamb GD, Westerblad H: Skeletal muscle fatigue: cellular mechanisms, *Physiol Rev* 88:287, 2008.

Berchtold MW, Brinkmeier H, Muntener M: Calcium ion in skeletal muscle: its crucial role for muscle function, plasticity, and disease, *Physiol Rev* 80:1215, 2000.

Cheng H, Lederer WJ: Calcium sparks, *Physiol Rev* 88:1491, 2008.

Clanton TL, Levine S: Respiratory muscle fiber remodeling in chronic hyperinflation: dysfunction or adaptation? *J Appl Physiol* 107:324, 2009.

Clausen T: Na+-K+ pump regulation and skeletal muscle contractility, *Physiol Rev* 83:1269, 2003.

Dirksen RT: Checking your SOCCs and feet: the molecular mechanisms of Ca2+ entry in skeletal muscle, *J Physiol* 587:3139, 2009.

Fitts RH: The cross-bridge cycle and skeletal muscle fatigue, *J Appl Physiol* 104:551, 2008.

Glass DJ: Signalling pathways that mediate skeletal muscle hypertrophy and atrophy, *Nat Cell Biol* 5:87, 2003.

Gordon AM, Regnier M, Homsher E: Skeletal and cardiac muscle contractile activation: tropomyosin "rocks and rolls", *News Physiol Sci* 16:49, 2001.

Gunning P, O'Neill G, Hardeman E: Tropomyosin-based regulation of the actin cytoskeleton in time and space, *Physiol Rev* 88:1, 2008.

Huxley AF, Gordon AM: Striation patterns in active and passive shortening of muscle, *Nature (Lond)* 193:280, 1962.

Kjær M: Role of extracellular matrix in adaptation of tendon and skeletal muscle to mechanical loading, *Physiol Rev* 84:649, 2004.

Lynch GS, Ryall JG: Role of beta-adrenoceptor signaling in skeletal muscle: implications for muscle wasting and disease, *Physiol Rev* 88:729, 2008.

MacIntosh BR: Role of calcium sensitivity modulation in skeletal muscle performance, *News Physiol Sci* 18:222, 2003.

Phillips SM, Glover EI, Rennie MJ: Alterations of protein turnover underlying disuse atrophy in human skeletal muscle, *J Appl Physiol* 107:645, 2009.

Powers SK, Jackson MJ: Exercise-induced oxidative stress: cellular mechanisms and impact on muscle force production, *Physiol Rev* 88:1243, 2008.

Sandri M: Signaling in muscle atrophy and hypertrophy, *Physiology (Bethesda)* 160, 2008.

Sieck GC, Regnier M: Plasticity and energetic demands of contraction in skeletal and cardiac muscle, *J Appl Physiol* 90:1158, 2001.

Treves S, Vukcevic M, Maj M, et al: Minor sarcoplasmic reticulum membrane components that modulate excitation-contraction coupling in striated muscles, *J Physiol* 587:3071, 2009.

Excitation of Skeletal Muscle: Neuromuscular Transmission and Excitation-Contraction Coupling

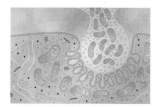

Transmission of Impulses from Nerve Endings to Skeletal Muscle Fibers: The Neuromuscular Junction

The skeletal muscle fibers are innervated by large, myelinated nerve fibers that originate from large motoneurons in the anterior horns of the spinal cord. As pointed out in Chapter 6, each nerve fiber, after entering the muscle belly, normally branches and stimulates from three to several hundred skeletal muscle fibers. Each nerve ending makes a junction, called the *neuromuscular junction*, with the muscle fiber near its midpoint. The action potential initiated in the muscle fiber by the nerve signal travels in both directions toward the muscle fiber ends. With the exception of about 2 percent of the muscle fibers, there is only one such junction per muscle fiber.

Physiologic Anatomy of the Neuromuscular Junction—The Motor End Plate. Figure 7-1*A* and *B* shows the neuromuscular junction from a large, myelinated nerve fiber to a skeletal muscle fiber. The nerve fiber forms a complex of *branching nerve terminals* that invaginate into the surface of the muscle fiber but lie outside the muscle fiber plasma membrane. The entire structure is called the *motor end plate.* It is covered by one or more Schwann cells that insulate it from the surrounding fluids.

Figure 7-1*C* shows an electron micrographic sketch of the junction between a single axon terminal and the muscle fiber membrane. The invaginated membrane is called the *synaptic gutter* or *synaptic trough,* and the space between the terminal and the fiber membrane is called the *synaptic space* or *synaptic cleft.* This space is 20 to 30 nanometers wide. At the bottom of the gutter are numerous smaller *folds* of the muscle membrane called *subneural clefts,* which greatly increase the surface area at which the synaptic transmitter can act.

In the axon terminal are many mitochondria that supply adenosine triphosphate (ATP), the energy source that is used for synthesis of an excitatory transmitter, *acetylcholine.* The acetylcholine in turn excites the muscle fiber membrane. Acetylcholine is synthesized in the cytoplasm of the terminal, but it is absorbed rapidly into many small *synaptic vesicles,* about 300,000 of which are normally in the terminals of a single end plate. In the synaptic space are large quantities of the enzyme *acetylcholinesterase,* which destroys acetylcholine a few milliseconds after it has been released from the synaptic vesicles.

Secretion of Acetylcholine by the Nerve Terminals

When a nerve impulse reaches the neuromuscular junction, about 125 vesicles of acetylcholine are released from the terminals into the synaptic space. Some of the details of this mechanism can be seen in Figure 7-2, which shows an expanded view of a synaptic space with the neural membrane above and the muscle membrane and its subneural clefts below.

On the inside surface of the neural membrane are linear *dense bars,* shown in cross section in Figure 7-2. To each side of each dense bar are protein particles that penetrate the neural membrane; these are *voltage-gated calcium channels.* When an action potential spreads over the terminal, these channels open and allow calcium ions to diffuse from the synaptic space to the interior of the nerve terminal. The calcium ions, in turn, are believed to exert an attractive influence on the acetylcholine vesicles, drawing them to the neural membrane adjacent to the dense bars. The vesicles then fuse with the neural membrane and empty their acetylcholine into the synaptic space by the process of *exocytosis.*

Although some of the aforementioned details are speculative, it is known that the effective stimulus for causing acetylcholine release from the vesicles is entry of calcium ions and that acetylcholine from the vesicles is then emptied through the neural membrane adjacent to the dense bars.

Effect of Acetylcholine on the Postsynaptic Muscle Fiber Membrane to Open Ion Channels. Figure 7-2 also shows many small *acetylcholine receptors* in the muscle fiber membrane; these are *acetylcholine-gated ion channels,* and they are located almost entirely near the mouths of the subneural clefts lying immediately below the dense bar areas, where the acetylcholine is emptied into the synaptic space.

Figure 7-1 Different views of the motor end plate. *A,* Longitudinal section through the end plate. *B,* Surface view of the end plate. *C,* Electron micrographic appearance of the contact point between a single axon terminal and the muscle fiber membrane. (Redrawn from Fawcett DW, as modified from Couteaux R, in Bloom W, Fawcett DW: A Textbook of Histology. Philadelphia: WB Saunders, 1986.)

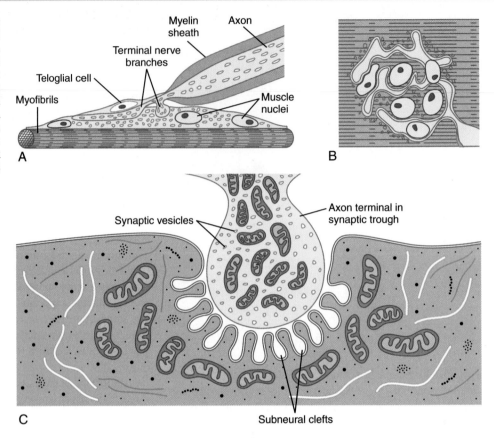

Figure 7-2 Release of acetylcholine from synaptic vesicles at the neural membrane of the neuromuscular junction. Note the proximity of the release sites in the neural membrane to the acetylcholine receptors in the muscle membrane, at the mouths of the subneural clefts.

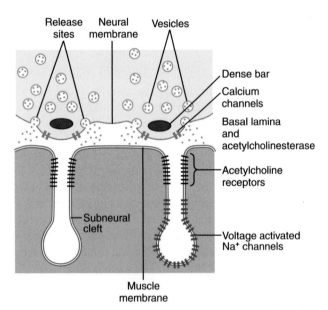

Each receptor is a protein complex that has a total molecular weight of 275,000. The complex is composed of five subunit proteins, two *alpha* proteins and one each of *beta, delta,* and *gamma* proteins. These protein molecules penetrate all the way through the membrane, lying side by side in a circle to form a tubular channel, illus-

trated in Figure 7-3. The channel remains constricted, as shown in section A of the figure, until two acetylcholine molecules attach respectively to the two *alpha* subunit proteins. This causes a conformational change that opens the channel, as shown in section B of the figure.

The acetylcholine-gated channel has a diameter of about 0.65 nanometer, which is large enough to allow the important positive ions—sodium (Na^+), potassium (K^+), and calcium (Ca^{++})—to move easily through the opening. Conversely, negative ions, such as chloride ions, do not pass through because of strong negative charges in the mouth of the channel that repel these negative ions.

In practice, far more sodium ions flow through the acetylcholine-gated channels than any other ions, for two reasons. First, there are only two positive ions in large concentration: sodium ions in the extracellular fluid and potassium ions in the intracellular fluid. Second, the negative potential on the inside of the muscle membrane, −80 to −90 millivolts, pulls the positively charged sodium ions to the inside of the fiber, while simultaneously preventing efflux of the positively charged potassium ions when they attempt to pass outward.

As shown in Figure 7-3B, the principal effect of opening the acetylcholine-gated channels is to allow large numbers of sodium ions to pour to the inside of the fiber, carrying with them large numbers of positive charges. This creates a local positive potential change inside the muscle fiber membrane, called the *end plate potential.* In turn, this end plate potential initiates an action potential that spreads along the muscle membrane and thus causes muscle contraction.

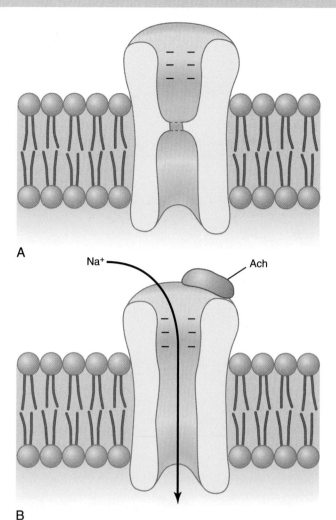

Figure 7-3 Acetylcholine-gated channel. *A,* Closed state. *B,* After acetylcholine (Ach) has become attached and a conformational change has opened the channel, allowing sodium ions to enter the muscle fiber and excite contraction. Note the negative charges at the channel mouth that prevent passage of negative ions such as chloride ions.

Destruction of the Released Acetylcholine by Acetylcholinesterase. The acetylcholine, once released into the synaptic space, continues to activate the acetylcholine receptors as long as the acetylcholine persists in the space. However, it is removed rapidly by two means: (1) Most of the acetylcholine is destroyed by the enzyme *acetylcholinesterase,* which is attached mainly to the spongy layer of fine connective tissue that fills the synaptic space between the presynaptic nerve terminal and the postsynaptic muscle membrane. (2) A small amount of acetylcholine diffuses out of the synaptic space and is then no longer available to act on the muscle fiber membrane.

The short time that the acetylcholine remains in the synaptic space—a few milliseconds at most—normally is sufficient to excite the muscle fiber. Then the rapid removal of the acetylcholine prevents continued muscle re-excitation after the muscle fiber has recovered from its initial action potential.

End Plate Potential and Excitation of the Skeletal Muscle Fiber. The sudden insurgence of sodium ions into the muscle fiber when the acetylcholine-gated channels open causes the electrical potential inside the fiber at the *local area of the end plate* to increase in the positive direction as much as 50 to 75 millivolts, creating a *local potential* called the *end plate potential.* Recall from Chapter 5 that a sudden increase in nerve membrane potential of more than 20 to 30 millivolts is normally sufficient to initiate more and more sodium channel opening, thus initiating an action potential at the muscle fiber membrane.

Figure 7-4 shows the principle of an end plate potential initiating the action potential. This figure shows three separate end plate potentials. End plate potentials A and C are too weak to elicit an action potential, but they do produce weak local end plate voltage changes, as recorded in the figure. By contrast, end plate potential B is much stronger and causes enough sodium channels to open so that the self-regenerative effect of more and more sodium ions flowing to the interior of the fiber initiates an action potential. The weakness of the end plate potential at point A was caused by poisoning of the muscle fiber with *curare,* a drug that blocks the gating action of acetylcholine on the acetylcholine channels by competing for the acetylcholine receptor sites. The weakness of the end plate potential at point C resulted from the effect of *botulinum toxin,* a bacterial poison that decreases the quantity of acetylcholine release by the nerve terminals.

Safety Factor for Transmission at the Neuromuscular Junction; Fatigue of the Junction. Ordinarily, each impulse that arrives at the neuromuscular junction causes about three times as much end plate potential as that required to stimulate the muscle fiber. Therefore, the normal neuromuscular junction is said to have a high *safety factor.* However, stimulation of the nerve fiber at rates greater than 100 times per second for several minutes often diminishes the number of acetylcholine vesicles so much that impulses fail to pass into the muscle

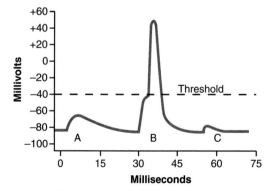

Figure 7-4 End plate potentials (in millivolts). *A,* Weakened end plate potential recorded in a curarized muscle, too weak to elicit an action potential. *B,* Normal end plate potential eliciting a muscle action potential. *C,* Weakened end plate potential caused by botulinum toxin that decreases end plate release of acetylcholine, again too weak to elicit a muscle action potential.

fiber. This is called *fatigue* of the neuromuscular junction, and it is the same effect that causes fatigue of synapses in the central nervous system when the synapses are overexcited. Under normal functioning conditions, measurable fatigue of the neuromuscular junction occurs rarely, and even then only at the most exhausting levels of muscle activity.

Molecular Biology of Acetylcholine Formation and Release

Because the neuromuscular junction is large enough to be studied easily, it is one of the few synapses of the nervous system for which most of the details of chemical transmission have been worked out. The formation and release of acetylcholine at this junction occur in the following stages:

1. Small vesicles, about 40 nanometers in size, are formed by the Golgi apparatus in the cell body of the motoneuron in the spinal cord. These vesicles are then transported by axoplasm that "streams" through the core of the axon from the central cell body in the spinal cord all the way to the neuromuscular junction at the tips of the peripheral nerve fibers. About 300,000 of these small vesicles collect in the nerve terminals of a single skeletal muscle end plate.

2. Acetylcholine is synthesized in the cytosol of the nerve fiber terminal but is immediately transported through the membranes of the vesicles to their interior, where it is stored in highly concentrated form, about 10,000 molecules of acetylcholine in each vesicle.

3. When an action potential arrives at the nerve terminal, it opens many calcium channels in the membrane of the nerve terminal because this terminal has an abundance of voltage-gated calcium channels. As a result, the calcium ion concentration inside the terminal membrane increases about 100-fold, which in turn increases the rate of fusion of the acetylcholine vesicles with the terminal membrane about 10,000-fold. This fusion makes many of the vesicles rupture, allowing *exocytosis* of acetylcholine into the synaptic space. About 125 vesicles usually rupture with each action potential. Then, after a few milliseconds, the acetylcholine is split by acetylcholinesterase into acetate ion and choline and the choline is reabsorbed actively into the neural terminal to be reused to form new acetylcholine. This sequence of events occurs within a period of 5 to 10 milliseconds.

4. The number of vesicles available in the nerve ending is sufficient to allow transmission of only a few thousand nerve-to-muscle impulses. Therefore, for continued function of the neuromuscular junction, new vesicles need to be re-formed rapidly. Within a few seconds after each action potential is over, "coated pits" appear in the terminal nerve membrane, caused by contractile proteins in the nerve ending, especially the protein *clathrin*, which is attached to the membrane in the areas of the original vesicles. Within about 20 seconds, the proteins contract and cause the pits to break away to the interior of the membrane, thus forming new vesicles. Within another few seconds, acetylcholine is transported to the interior of these vesicles, and they are then ready for a new cycle of acetylcholine release.

Drugs That Enhance or Block Transmission at the Neuromuscular Junction

Drugs That Stimulate the Muscle Fiber by Acetylcholine-Like Action. Many compounds, including *methacholine, carbachol,* and *nicotine,* have the same effect on the muscle fiber as does acetylcholine. The difference between these drugs and acetylcholine is that the drugs are not destroyed by cholinesterase or are destroyed so slowly that their action often persists for many minutes to several hours. The drugs work by causing localized areas of depolarization of the muscle fiber membrane at the motor end plate where the acetylcholine receptors are located. Then, every time the muscle fiber recovers from a previous contraction, these depolarized areas, by virtue of leaking ions, initiate a new action potential, thereby causing a state of muscle spasm.

Drugs That Stimulate the Neuromuscular Junction by Inactivating Acetylcholinesterase. Three particularly well-known drugs, *neostigmine, physostigmine,* and *diisopropyl fluorophosphate,* inactivate the acetylcholinesterase in the synapses so that it no longer hydrolyzes acetylcholine. Therefore, with each successive nerve impulse, additional acetylcholine accumulates and stimulates the muscle fiber repetitively. This causes *muscle spasm* when even a few nerve impulses reach the muscle. Unfortunately, it can also cause death due to laryngeal spasm, which smothers the person.

Neostigmine and physostigmine combine with acetylcholinesterase to inactivate the acetylcholinesterase for up to several hours, after which these drugs are displaced from the acetylcholinesterase so that the esterase once again becomes active. Conversely, diisopropyl fluorophosphate, which is a powerful "nerve" gas poison, inactivates acetylcholinesterase for weeks, which makes this a particularly lethal poison.

Drugs That Block Transmission at the Neuromuscular Junction. A group of drugs known as *curariform drugs* can prevent passage of impulses from the nerve ending into the muscle. For instance, D-tubocurarine blocks the action of acetylcholine on the muscle fiber acetylcholine receptors, thus preventing sufficient increase in permeability of the muscle membrane channels to initiate an action potential.

Myasthenia Gravis Causes Muscle Paralysis

Myasthenia gravis, which occurs in about 1 in every 20,000 persons, causes muscle paralysis because of inability of the neuromuscular junctions to transmit enough signals from the nerve fibers to the muscle fibers. Pathologically, antibodies that attack the acetylcholine receptors have been demonstrated in the blood of most patients with myasthenia gravis. Therefore, it is believed that myasthenia gravis is an autoimmune disease in which the patients have developed antibodies that block or destroy their own acetylcholine receptors at the postsynaptic neuromuscular junction.

Regardless of the cause, the end plate potentials that occur in the muscle fibers are mostly too weak to initiate opening of the voltage-gated sodium channels so that muscle fiber depolarization does not occur. If the disease is intense enough, the patient dies of paralysis—in particular, paralysis of the respiratory muscles. The disease can usually be ameliorated for several hours by administering *neostigmine* or some other anticholinesterase drug, which allows larger than normal amounts of acetylcholine to accumulate in the synaptic space. Within minutes, some of these paralyzed people can begin to function almost normally, until a new dose of neostigmine is required a few hours later.

Muscle Action Potential

Almost everything discussed in Chapter 5 regarding initiation and conduction of action potentials in nerve fibers applies equally to skeletal muscle fibers, except for quantitative differences. Some of the quantitative aspects of muscle potentials are the following:

1. Resting membrane potential: about −80 to −90 millivolts in skeletal fibers—the same as in large myelinated nerve fibers.

2. Duration of action potential: 1 to 5 milliseconds in skeletal muscle—about five times as long as in large myelinated nerves.

3. Velocity of conduction: 3 to 5 m/sec—about 1/13 the velocity of conduction in the large myelinated nerve fibers that excite skeletal muscle.

Spread of the Action Potential to the Interior of the Muscle Fiber by Way of "Transverse Tubules"

The skeletal muscle fiber is so large that action potentials spreading along its surface membrane cause almost no current flow deep within the fiber. Yet to cause maximum muscle contraction, current must penetrate deeply into the muscle fiber to the vicinity of the separate myofibrils. This is achieved by transmission of action potentials along *transverse tubules* (T tubules) that penetrate all the way through the muscle fiber from one side of the fiber to the other, as illustrated in Figure 7-5. The T tubule action potentials cause release of calcium ions inside the muscle fiber in the immediate vicinity of the myofibrils, and these calcium ions then cause contraction. This overall process is called *excitation-contraction* coupling.

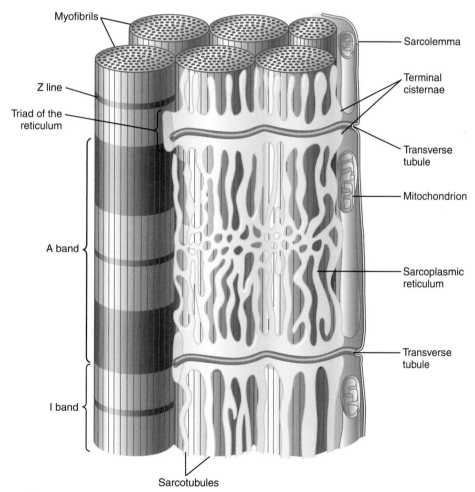

Figure 7-5 Transverse (T) tubule–sarcoplasmic reticulum system. Note that the T tubules communicate with the outside of the cell membrane, and deep in the muscle fiber, each T tubule lies adjacent to the ends of longitudinal sarcoplasmic reticulum tubules that surround all sides of the actual myofibrils that contract. This illustration was drawn from frog muscle, which has one T tubule per sarcomere, located at the Z line. A similar arrangement is found in mammalian heart muscle, but mammalian skeletal muscle has two T tubules per sarcomere, located at the A-I band junctions.

Excitation-Contraction Coupling

Transverse Tubule–Sarcoplasmic Reticulum System

Figure 7-5 shows myofibrils surrounded by the T tubule–sarcoplasmic reticulum system. The T tubules are small and run transverse to the myofibrils. They begin at the cell membrane and penetrate all the way from one side of the muscle fiber to the opposite side. Not shown in the figure is the fact that these tubules branch among themselves and form entire *planes* of T tubules interlacing among all the separate myofibrils. Also, *where the T tubules originate from the cell membrane, they are open to the exterior of the muscle fiber.* Therefore, they communicate with the extracellular fluid surrounding the muscle fiber and they themselves contain extracellular fluid in their lumens. In other words, the T tubules are actually internal extensions of the cell membrane. Therefore, when an action potential spreads over a muscle fiber membrane, a potential change also spreads along the T tubules to the deep interior of the muscle fiber. The electrical currents surrounding these T tubules then elicit the muscle contraction.

Figure 7-5 also shows a *sarcoplasmic reticulum,* in yellow. This is composed of two major parts: (1) large chambers called *terminal cisternae* that abut the T tubules and (2) long longitudinal tubules that surround all surfaces of the actual contracting myofibrils.

Release of Calcium Ions by the Sarcoplasmic Reticulum

One of the special features of the sarcoplasmic reticulum is that within its vesicular tubules is an excess of calcium ions in high concentration, and many of these ions are released from each vesicle when an action potential occurs in the adjacent T tubule.

Figures 7-6 and 7-7 show that the action potential of the T tubule causes current flow into the sarcoplasmic reticular cisternae where they abut the T tubule. As the action potential reaches the T tubule, the voltage change is sensed by *dihydropyridine receptors* that are linked to *calcium release channels,* also called *ryanodine receptor channels,* in the adjacent sarcoplasmic reticular cisternae (see Figure 7-6). Activation of dihydropyridine receptors triggers the opening of the calcium release channels in the cisternae, as well as in their attached longitudinal tubules. These channels remain open for a few milliseconds, releasing calcium ions into the sarcoplasm surrounding the myofibrils and causing contraction, as discussed in Chapter 6.

Calcium Pump for Removing Calcium Ions from the Myofibrillar Fluid After Contraction Occurs. Once the calcium ions have been released from the sarcoplasmic tubules and have diffused among the myofibrils, muscle contraction continues as long as the calcium ions remain in high concentration. However, a continually active calcium pump located in the walls of the sarcoplasmic reticulum pumps calcium ions away from the myofibrils back into the sarcoplasmic tubules (see Figure 7-6). This pump can concentrate the calcium ions about 10,000-fold inside the tubules. In addition, inside the reticulum is a protein called *calsequestrin* that can bind up to 40 times more calcium.

Excitatory "Pulse" of Calcium Ions. The normal resting state concentration ($<10^{-7}$ molar) of calcium ions in the cytosol that bathes the myofibrils is too little to elicit contraction. Therefore, the troponin-tropomyosin complex keeps the actin filaments inhibited and maintains a relaxed state of the muscle.

Conversely, full excitation of the T tubule and sarcoplasmic reticulum system causes enough release of calcium ions to increase the concentration in the

Figure 7-6 Excitation-contraction coupling in skeletal muscle. The *top panel* shows an action potential in the T tubule that causes a conformational change in the voltage-sensing dihydropyridine (DHP) receptors, opening the Ca++ release channels in the terminal cisternae of the sarcoplasmic reticulum and permitting Ca++ to rapidly diffuse into the sarcoplasm and initiate muscle contraction. During repolarization (*bottom panel*) the conformational change in the DHP receptor closes the Ca++ release channels and Ca++ is transported from the sarcoplasm into the sarcoplasmic reticulum by an ATP-dependent calcium pump.

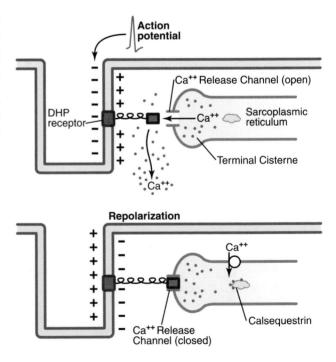

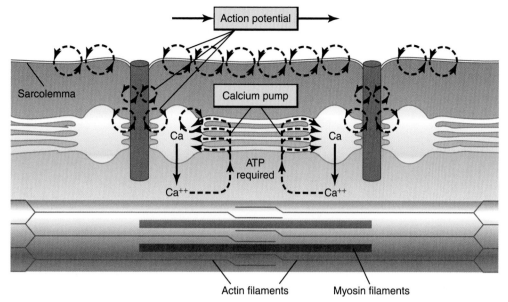

Figure 7-7 Excitation-contraction coupling in the muscle, showing (1) an action potential that causes release of calcium ions from the sarcoplasmic reticulum and then (2) re-uptake of the calcium ions by a calcium pump.

myofibrillar fluid to as high as 2×10^{-4} molar concentration, a 500-fold increase, which is about 10 times the level required to cause maximum muscle contraction. Immediately thereafter, the calcium pump depletes the calcium ions again. The total duration of this calcium "pulse" in the usual *skeletal muscle* fiber lasts about 1/20 of a second, although it may last several times as long in some fibers and several times less in others. (In heart muscle, the calcium pulse lasts about one third of a second because of the long duration of the cardiac action potential.)

During this calcium pulse, muscle contraction occurs. If the contraction is to continue without interruption for long intervals, a series of calcium pulses must be initiated by a continuous series of repetitive action potentials, as discussed in Chapter 6.

Bibliography

Also see references for Chapters 5 and 6.

Brown RH Jr: Dystrophin-associated proteins and the muscular dystrophies, *Annu Rev Med* 48:457, 1997.

Chaudhuri A, Behan PO: Fatigue in neurological disorders, *Lancet* 363:978, 2004.

Cheng H, Lederer WJ: Calcium sparks, *Physiol Rev* 88:1491, 2008.

Engel AG, Ohno K, Shen XM, Sine SM: Congenital myasthenic syndromes: multiple molecular targets at the neuromuscular junction, *Ann N Y Acad Sci* 998:138, 2003.

Fagerlund MJ, Eriksson LI: Current concepts in neuromuscular transmission, *Br J Anaesth* 103:108, 2009.

Haouzi P, Chenuel B, Huszczuk A: Sensing vascular distension in skeletal muscle by slow conducting afferent fibers: neurophysiological basis and implication for respiratory control, *J Appl Physiol* 96:407, 2004.

Hirsch NP: Neuromuscular junction in health and disease, *Br J Anaesth* 99:132, 2007.

Keesey JC: Clinical evaluation and management of myasthenia gravis, *Muscle Nerve* 29:484, 2004.

Korkut C, Budnik V: WNTs tune up the neuromuscular junction, *Nat Rev Neurosci* 10:627, 2009.

Leite JF, Rodrigues-Pinguet N, Lester HA: Insights into channel function via channel dysfunction, *J Clin Invest* 111:436, 2003.

Meriggioli MN, Sanders DB: Autoimmune myasthenia gravis: emerging clinical and biological heterogeneity, *Lancet Neurol* 8:475, 2009.

Rekling JC, Funk GD, Bayliss DA, et al: Synaptic control of motoneuronal excitability, *Physiol Rev* 80:767, 2000.

Rosenberg PB: Calcium entry in skeletal muscle, *J Physiol* 587:3149, 2009.

Toyoshima C, Nomura H, Sugita Y: Structural basis of ion pumping by Ca^{2+}-ATPase of sarcoplasmic reticulum, *FEBS Lett* 555:106, 2003.

Van der Kloot W, Molgo J: Quantal acetylcholine release at the vertebrate neuromuscular junction, *Physiol Rev* 74:899, 1994.

Vincent A: Unraveling the pathogenesis of myasthenia gravis, *Nat Rev Immunol* 10:797, 2002.

Vincent A, McConville J, Farrugia ME, et al: Antibodies in myasthenia gravis and related disorders, *Ann N Y Acad Sci* 998:324, 2003.

Excitation and Contraction of Smooth Muscle

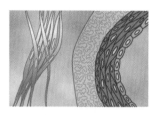

Contraction of Smooth Muscle

In Chapters 6 and 7, the discussion was concerned with skeletal muscle. We now turn to smooth muscle, which is composed of far smaller fibers—usually 1 to 5 micrometers in diameter and only 20 to 500 micrometers in length. In contrast, skeletal muscle fibers are as much as 30 times greater in diameter and hundreds of times as long. Many of the same principles of contraction apply to smooth muscle as to skeletal muscle. Most important, essentially the same attractive forces between myosin and actin filaments cause contraction in smooth muscle as in skeletal muscle, but the internal physical arrangement of smooth muscle fibers is different.

Types of Smooth Muscle

The smooth muscle of each organ is distinctive from that of most other organs in several ways: (1) physical dimensions, (2) organization into bundles or sheets, (3) response to different types of stimuli, (4) characteristics of innervation, and (5) function. Yet for the sake of simplicity, smooth muscle can generally be divided into two major types, which are shown in Figure 8-1: *multi-unit smooth muscle* and *unitary* (or *single-unit*) *smooth muscle.*

Multi-Unit Smooth Muscle. This type of smooth muscle is composed of discrete, separate smooth muscle fibers. Each fiber operates independently of the others and often is innervated by a single nerve ending, as occurs for skeletal muscle fibers. Further, the outer surfaces of these fibers, like those of skeletal muscle fibers, are covered by a thin layer of basement membrane–like substance, a mixture of fine collagen and glycoprotein that helps insulate the separate fibers from one another.

The most important characteristic of multi-unit smooth muscle fibers is that each fiber can contract independently of the others, and their control is exerted mainly by nerve signals. In contrast, a major share of control of unitary smooth muscle is exerted by non-nervous stimuli. Some examples of multi-unit smooth muscle are the ciliary muscle of the eye, the iris muscle of the eye, and the pilo-erector muscles that cause erection of the hairs when stimulated by the sympathetic nervous system.

Unitary Smooth Muscle. This type is also called *syncytial smooth muscle* or *visceral smooth muscle.* The term "unitary" is confusing because it does not mean single muscle fibers. Instead, it means a mass of hundreds to thousands of smooth muscle fibers that contract together as a single unit. The fibers usually are arranged in sheets or bundles, and their cell membranes are adherent to one another at multiple points so that force generated in one muscle fiber can be transmitted to the next. In addition, the cell membranes are joined by many *gap junctions* through which ions can flow freely from one muscle cell to the next so that action potentials or simple ion flow without action potentials can travel from one fiber to the next and cause the muscle fibers to contract together. This type of smooth muscle is also known as *syncytial smooth muscle* because of its syncytial interconnections among fibers. It is also called *visceral smooth muscle* because it is found in the walls of most viscera of the body, including the gastrointestinal tract, bile ducts, ureters, uterus, and many blood vessels.

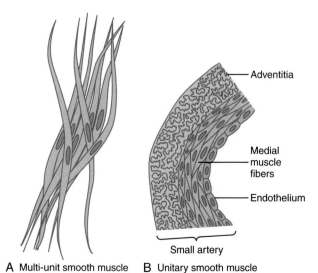

A Multi-unit smooth muscle B Unitary smooth muscle

Figure 8-1 Multi-unit (*A*) and unitary (*B*) smooth muscle.

Contractile Mechanism in Smooth Muscle

Chemical Basis for Smooth Muscle Contraction

Smooth muscle contains both *actin* and *myosin filaments*, having chemical characteristics similar to those of the actin and myosin filaments in skeletal muscle. It does not contain the normal troponin complex that is required in the control of skeletal muscle contraction, so the mechanism for control of contraction is different. This is discussed in detail later in this chapter.

Chemical studies have shown that actin and myosin filaments derived from smooth muscle interact with each other in much the same way that they do in skeletal muscle. Further, the contractile process is activated by calcium ions, and adenosine triphosphate (ATP) is degraded to adenosine diphosphate (ADP) to provide the energy for contraction.

There are, however, major differences between the physical organization of smooth muscle and that of skeletal muscle, as well as differences in excitation-contraction coupling, control of the contractile process by calcium ions, duration of contraction, and amount of energy required for contraction.

Physical Basis for Smooth Muscle Contraction

Smooth muscle does not have the same striated arrangement of actin and myosin filaments as is found in skeletal muscle. Instead, electron micrographic techniques suggest the physical organization exhibited in Figure 8-2. This figure shows large numbers of actin filaments attached to so-called *dense bodies.* Some of these bodies are attached to the cell membrane. Others are dispersed inside the cell. Some of the membrane-dense bodies of adjacent cells are bonded together by intercellular protein bridges. It is mainly through these bonds that the force of contraction is transmitted from one cell to the next.

Interspersed among the actin filaments in the muscle fiber are myosin filaments. These have a diameter more than twice that of the actin filaments. In electron micrographs, one usually finds 5 to 10 times as many actin filaments as myosin filaments.

To the right in Figure 8-2 is a postulated structure of an individual contractile unit within a smooth muscle cell, showing large numbers of actin filaments radiating from two dense bodies; the ends of these filaments overlap a myosin filament located midway between the dense bodies. This contractile unit is similar to the contractile unit of skeletal muscle, but without the regularity of the skeletal muscle structure; in fact, the dense bodies of smooth muscle serve the same role as the Z discs in skeletal muscle.

There is another difference: Most of the myosin filaments have what are called "sidepolar" cross-bridges arranged so that the bridges on one side hinge in one direction and those on the other side hinge in the opposite direction. This allows the myosin to pull an actin filament in one direction on one side while simultaneously pulling another actin filament in the opposite direction on the other side. The value of this organization is that it

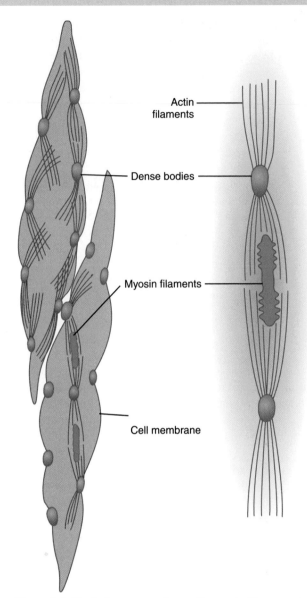

Figure 8-2 Physical structure of smooth muscle. The upper left-hand fiber shows actin filaments radiating from dense bodies. The lower left-hand fiber and the right-hand diagram demonstrate the relation of myosin filaments to actin filaments.

allows smooth muscle cells to contract as much as 80 percent of their length instead of being limited to less than 30 percent, as occurs in skeletal muscle.

Comparison of Smooth Muscle Contraction and Skeletal Muscle Contraction

Although most skeletal muscles contract and relax rapidly, most smooth muscle contraction is prolonged tonic contraction, sometimes lasting hours or even days. Therefore, it is to be expected that both the physical and the chemical characteristics of smooth muscle versus skeletal muscle contraction would differ. Following are some of the differences.

Slow Cycling of the Myosin Cross-Bridges. The rapidity of cycling of the myosin cross-bridges in smooth muscle—that is, their attachment to actin, then release from the actin, and reattachment for the next cycle—is much slower than in skeletal muscle; in fact, the frequency is as little as 1/10 to 1/300 that in skeletal muscle. Yet the *fraction of time* that the cross-bridges remain attached to the actin filaments, which is a major factor that determines the force of contraction, is believed to be greatly increased in smooth muscle. A possible reason for the slow cycling is that the cross-bridge heads have far less ATPase activity than in skeletal muscle, so degradation of the ATP that energizes the movements of the cross-bridge heads is greatly reduced, with corresponding slowing of the rate of cycling.

Low Energy Requirement to Sustain Smooth Muscle Contraction. Only 1/10 to 1/300 as much energy is required to sustain the same tension of contraction in smooth muscle as in skeletal muscle. This, too, is believed to result from the slow attachment and detachment cycling of the cross-bridges and because only one molecule of ATP is required for each cycle, regardless of its duration.

This sparsity of energy utilization by smooth muscle is exceedingly important to the overall energy economy of the body because organs such as the intestines, urinary bladder, gallbladder, and other viscera often maintain tonic muscle contraction almost indefinitely.

Slowness of Onset of Contraction and Relaxation of the Total Smooth Muscle Tissue. A typical smooth muscle tissue begins to contract 50 to 100 milliseconds after it is excited, reaches full contraction about 0.5 second later, and then declines in contractile force in another 1 to 2 seconds, giving a total contraction time of 1 to 3 seconds. This is about 30 times as long as a single contraction of an average skeletal muscle fiber. But because there are so many types of smooth muscle, contraction of some types can be as short as 0.2 second or as long as 30 seconds.

The slow onset of contraction of smooth muscle, as well as its prolonged contraction, is caused by the slowness of attachment and detachment of the cross-bridges with the actin filaments. In addition, the initiation of contraction in response to calcium ions is much slower than in skeletal muscle, as discussed later.

Maximum Force of Contraction Is Often Greater in Smooth Muscle Than in Skeletal Muscle. Despite the relatively few myosin filaments in smooth muscle, and despite the slow cycling time of the cross-bridges, the maximum force of contraction of smooth muscle is often greater than that of skeletal muscle—as great as 4 to 6 kg/cm² cross-sectional area for smooth muscle, in comparison with 3 to 4 kilograms for skeletal muscle. This great force of smooth muscle contraction results from the prolonged period of attachment of the myosin cross-bridges to the actin filaments.

"Latch" Mechanism Facilitates Prolonged Holding of Contractions of Smooth Muscle. Once smooth muscle has developed full contraction, the amount of continuing excitation can usually be reduced to far less than the initial level yet the muscle maintains its full force of contraction. Further, the energy consumed to maintain contraction is often minuscule, sometimes as little as 1/300 the energy required for comparable sustained skeletal muscle contraction. This is called the "latch" mechanism.

The importance of the latch mechanism is that it can maintain prolonged tonic contraction in smooth muscle for hours with little use of energy. Little continued excitatory signal is required from nerve fibers or hormonal sources.

Stress-Relaxation of Smooth Muscle. Another important characteristic of smooth muscle, especially the visceral unitary type of smooth muscle of many hollow organs, is its ability to return to nearly its original *force* of contraction seconds or minutes after it has been elongated or shortened. For example, a sudden increase in fluid volume in the urinary bladder, thus stretching the smooth muscle in the bladder wall, causes an immediate large increase in pressure in the bladder. However, during the next 15 seconds to a minute or so, despite continued stretch of the bladder wall, the pressure returns almost exactly back to the original level. Then, when the volume is increased by another step, the same effect occurs again.

Conversely, when the volume is suddenly decreased, the pressure falls drastically at first but then rises in another few seconds or minutes to or near to the original level. These phenomena are called *stress-relaxation* and *reverse stress-relaxation.* Their importance is that, except for short periods of time, they allow a hollow organ to maintain about the same amount of pressure inside its lumen despite long-term, large changes in volume.

Regulation of Contraction by Calcium Ions

As is true for skeletal muscle, the initiating stimulus for most smooth muscle contraction is an increase in intracellular calcium ions. This increase can be caused in different types of smooth muscle by nerve stimulation of the smooth muscle fiber, hormonal stimulation, stretch of the fiber, or even change in the chemical environment of the fiber.

Yet smooth muscle does not contain troponin, the regulatory protein that is activated by calcium ions to cause skeletal muscle contraction. Instead, smooth muscle contraction is activated by an entirely different mechanism, as follows.

Calcium Ions Combine with Calmodulin to Cause Activation of Myosin Kinase and Phosphorylation of the Myosin Head.
In place of troponin, smooth muscle cells contain a large amount of another regulatory protein called *calmodulin* (Figure 8-3). Although this protein is similar to troponin, it is different in the manner in which it initiates contraction. Calmodulin does this by activating the myosin cross-bridges. This activation and subsequent contraction occur in the following sequence:

1. The calcium ions bind with calmodulin.

2. The calmodulin-calcium complex then joins with and activates *myosin light chain kinase,* a phosphorylating enzyme.

3. One of the light chains of each myosin head, called the *regulatory chain,* becomes phosphorylated in response to this myosin kinase. When this chain is not phosphorylated, the attachment-detachment cycling of the myosin head with the actin filament does not occur.

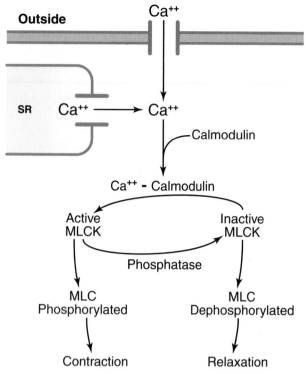

Figure 8-3 Intracellular calcium ion (Ca⁺⁺) concentration increases when Ca⁺⁺ enters the cell through calcium channels in the cell membrane or the sarcoplasmic reticulum (SR). The Ca⁺⁺ binds to calmodulin to form a Ca⁺⁺-calmodulin complex, which then activates myosin light chain kinase (MLCK). The MLCK phosphorylates the myosin light chain (MLC) leading to contraction of the smooth muscle. When Ca⁺⁺ concentration decreases, due to pumping of Ca⁺⁺ out of the cell, the process is reversed and myosin phosphatase removes the phosphate from MLC, leading to relaxation.

But when the regulatory chain is phosphorylated, the head has the capability of binding repetitively with the actin filament and proceeding through the entire cycling process of intermittent "pulls," the same as occurs for skeletal muscle, thus causing muscle contraction.

Myosin Phosphatase Is Important in Cessation of Contraction.

When the calcium ion concentration falls below a critical level, the aforementioned processes automatically reverse, except for the phosphorylation of the myosin head. Reversal of this requires another enzyme, *myosin phosphatase* (see Figure 8-3), located in the cytosol of the smooth muscle cell, which splits the phosphate from the regulatory light chain. Then the cycling stops and contraction ceases. The time required for relaxation of muscle contraction, therefore, is determined to a great extent by the amount of active myosin phosphatase in the cell.

Possible Mechanism for Regulation of the Latch Phenomenon

Because of the importance of the latch phenomenon in smooth muscle, and because this phenomenon allows long-term maintenance of tone in many smooth muscle organs without much expenditure of energy, many attempts have been made to explain it. Among the many mechanisms that have been postulated, one of the simplest is the following.

When the myosin kinase and myosin phosphatase enzymes are both strongly activated, the cycling frequency of the myosin heads and the velocity of contraction are great. Then, as the activation of the enzymes decreases, the cycling frequency decreases, but at the same time, the deactivation of these enzymes allows the myosin heads to remain attached to the actin filament for a longer and longer proportion of the cycling period. Therefore, the number of heads attached to the actin filament at any given time remains large. Because the number of heads attached to the actin determines the static force of contraction, tension is maintained, or "latched"; yet little energy is used by the muscle because ATP is not degraded to ADP except on the rare occasion when a head detaches.

Nervous and Hormonal Control of Smooth Muscle Contraction

Although skeletal muscle fibers are stimulated exclusively by the nervous system, smooth muscle can be stimulated to contract by multiple types of signals: by nervous signals, by hormonal stimulation, by stretch of the muscle, and in several other ways. The principal reason for the difference is that the smooth muscle membrane contains many types of receptor proteins that can initiate the contractile process. Still other receptor proteins inhibit smooth muscle contraction, which is another difference from skeletal muscle. Therefore, in this section, we discuss nervous control of smooth muscle contraction, followed by hormonal control and other means of control.

Neuromuscular Junctions of Smooth Muscle

Physiologic Anatomy of Smooth Muscle Neuromuscular Junctions. Neuromuscular junctions of the highly structured type found on skeletal muscle fibers do not occur in smooth muscle. Instead, the *autonomic nerve fibers* that innervate smooth muscle generally branch diffusely on top of a sheet of muscle fibers, as shown in Figure 8-4. In most instances, these fibers

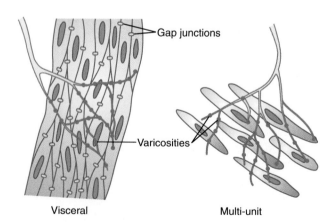

Figure 8-4 Innervation of smooth muscle.

do not make direct contact with the smooth muscle fiber cell membranes but instead form so-called *diffuse junctions* that secrete their transmitter substance into the matrix coating of the smooth muscle often a few nanometers to a few micrometers away from the muscle cells; the transmitter substance then diffuses to the cells. Furthermore, where there are many layers of muscle cells, the nerve fibers often innervate only the outer layer. Muscle excitation travels from this outer layer to the inner layers by action potential conduction in the muscle mass or by additional diffusion of the transmitter substance.

The axons that innervate smooth muscle fibers do not have typical branching end feet of the type in the motor end plate on skeletal muscle fibers. Instead, most of the fine terminal axons have multiple *varicosities* distributed along their axes. At these points the *Schwann cells* that envelop the axons are interrupted so that transmitter substance can be secreted through the walls of the varicosities. In the varicosities are vesicles similar to those in the skeletal muscle end plate that contain transmitter substance. But in contrast to the vesicles of skeletal muscle junctions, which always contain acetylcholine, the vesicles of the autonomic nerve fiber endings contain *acetylcholine* in some fibers and *norepinephrine* in others—and occasionally other substances as well.

In a few instances, particularly in the multi-unit type of smooth muscle, the varicosities are separated from the muscle cell membrane by as little as 20 to 30 nanometers—the same width as the synaptic cleft that occurs in the skeletal muscle junction. These are called *contact junctions,* and they function in much the same way as the skeletal muscle neuromuscular junction; the rapidity of contraction of these smooth muscle fibers is considerably faster than that of fibers stimulated by the diffuse junctions.

Excitatory and Inhibitory Transmitter Substances Secreted at the Smooth Muscle Neuromuscular Junction. The most important transmitter substances secreted by the autonomic nerves innervating smooth muscle are *acetylcholine* and *norepinephrine,* but they are never secreted by the same nerve fibers. Acetylcholine is an excitatory transmitter substance for smooth muscle fibers in some organs but an inhibitory transmitter for smooth muscle in other organs. When acetylcholine excites a muscle fiber, norepinephrine ordinarily inhibits it. Conversely, when acetylcholine inhibits a fiber, norepinephrine usually excites it.

But why are these responses different? The answer is that both acetylcholine and norepinephrine excite or inhibit smooth muscle by first binding with a *receptor protein* on the surface of the muscle cell membrane. Some of the receptor proteins are *excitatory receptors,* whereas others are *inhibitory receptors.* Thus, the type of receptor determines whether the smooth muscle is inhibited or excited and also determines which of the two transmitters, acetylcholine or norepinephrine, is effective in

causing the excitation or inhibition. These receptors are discussed in more detail in Chapter 60 in relation to function of the autonomic nervous system.

Membrane Potentials and Action Potentials in Smooth Muscle

Membrane Potentials in Smooth Muscle. The quantitative voltage of the membrane potential of smooth muscle depends on the momentary condition of the muscle. In the normal resting state, the intracellular potential is usually about −50 to −60 millivolts, which is about 30 millivolts less negative than in skeletal muscle.

Action Potentials in Unitary Smooth Muscle. Action potentials occur in unitary smooth muscle (such as visceral muscle) in the same way that they occur in skeletal muscle. They do not normally occur in most multi-unit types of smooth muscle, as discussed in a subsequent section.

The action potentials of visceral smooth muscle occur in one of two forms: (1) spike potentials or (2) action potentials with plateaus.

Spike Potentials. Typical spike action potentials, such as those seen in skeletal muscle, occur in most types of unitary smooth muscle. The duration of this type of action potential is 10 to 50 milliseconds, as shown in Figure 8-5A. Such action potentials can be elicited in many ways, for example, by electrical stimulation, by the

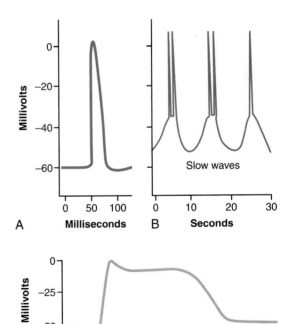

Figure 8-5 *A,* Typical smooth muscle action potential (spike potential) elicited by an external stimulus. *B,* Repetitive spike potentials, elicited by slow rhythmical electrical waves that occur spontaneously in the smooth muscle of the intestinal wall. *C,* Action potential with a plateau, recorded from a smooth muscle fiber of the uterus.

action of hormones on the smooth muscle, by the action of transmitter substances from nerve fibers, by stretch, or as a result of spontaneous generation in the muscle fiber itself, as discussed subsequently.

Action Potentials with Plateaus. Figure 8-5C shows a smooth muscle action potential with a plateau. The onset of this action potential is similar to that of the typical spike potential. However, instead of rapid repolarization of the muscle fiber membrane, the repolarization is delayed for several hundred to as much as 1000 milliseconds (1 second). The importance of the plateau is that it can account for the prolonged contraction that occurs in some types of smooth muscle, such as the ureter, the uterus under some conditions, and certain types of vascular smooth muscle. (Also, this is the type of action potential seen in cardiac muscle fibers that have a prolonged period of contraction, as discussed in Chapters 9 and 10.)

Calcium Channels Are Important in Generating the Smooth Muscle Action Potential. The smooth muscle cell membrane has far more voltage-gated calcium channels than does skeletal muscle but few voltage-gated sodium channels. Therefore, sodium participates little in the generation of the action potential in most smooth muscle. Instead, flow of calcium ions to the interior of the fiber is mainly responsible for the action potential. This occurs in the same self-regenerative way as occurs for the sodium channels in nerve fibers and in skeletal muscle fibers. However, the calcium channels open many times more slowly than do sodium channels, and they also remain open much longer. This accounts in large measure for the prolonged plateau action potentials of some smooth muscle fibers.

Another important feature of calcium ion entry into the cells during the action potential is that the calcium ions act directly on the smooth muscle contractile mechanism to cause contraction. Thus, the calcium performs two tasks at once.

Slow Wave Potentials in Unitary Smooth Muscle Can Lead to Spontaneous Generation of Action Potentials. Some smooth muscle is self-excitatory. That is, action potentials arise within the smooth muscle cells themselves without an extrinsic stimulus. This is often associated with a basic *slow wave rhythm* of the membrane potential. A typical slow wave in a visceral smooth muscle of the gut is shown in Figure 8-5B. The slow wave itself is not the action potential. That is, it is not a self-regenerative process that spreads progressively over the membranes of the muscle fibers. Instead, it is a local property of the smooth muscle fibers that make up the muscle mass.

The cause of the slow wave rhythm is unknown. One suggestion is that the slow waves are caused by waxing and waning of the pumping of positive ions (presumably sodium ions) outward through the muscle fiber membrane; that is, the membrane potential becomes more negative when sodium is pumped rapidly and less negative when the sodium pump becomes less active. Another suggestion is that the conductances of the ion channels increase and decrease rhythmically.

The importance of the slow waves is that, when they are strong enough, they can initiate action potentials. The slow waves themselves cannot cause muscle contraction. However, when the peak of the negative slow wave potential inside the cell membrane rises in the positive direction from −60 to about −35 millivolts (the approximate threshold for eliciting action potentials in most visceral smooth muscle), an action potential develops and spreads over the muscle mass and contraction occurs. Figure 8-5B demonstrates this effect, showing that at each peak of the slow wave, one or more action potentials occur. These repetitive sequences of action potentials elicit rhythmical contraction of the smooth muscle mass. Therefore, the slow waves are called *pacemaker waves*. In Chapter 62, we see that this type of pacemaker activity controls the rhythmical contractions of the gut.

Excitation of Visceral Smooth Muscle by Muscle Stretch. When visceral (unitary) smooth muscle is stretched sufficiently, spontaneous action potentials are usually generated. They result from a combination of (1) the normal slow wave potentials and (2) decrease in overall negativity of the membrane potential caused by the stretch itself. This response to stretch allows the gut wall, when excessively stretched, to contract automatically and rhythmically. For instance, when the gut is overfilled by intestinal contents, local automatic contractions often set up peristaltic waves that move the contents away from the overfilled intestine, usually in the direction of the anus.

Depolarization of Multi-Unit Smooth Muscle Without Action Potentials

The smooth muscle fibers of multi-unit smooth muscle (such as the muscle of the iris of the eye or the piloerector muscle of each hair) normally contract mainly in response to nerve stimuli. The nerve endings secrete acetylcholine in the case of some multi-unit smooth muscles and norepinephrine in the case of others. In both instances, the transmitter substances cause depolarization of the smooth muscle membrane, and this in turn elicits contraction. Action potentials usually do not develop; the reason is that the fibers are too small to generate an action potential. (When action potentials are elicited in *visceral unitary smooth muscle*, 30 to 40 smooth muscle fibers must depolarize simultaneously before a self-propagating action potential ensues.) Yet in small smooth muscle cells, even without an action potential, the local depolarization (called the *junctional potential*) caused by the nerve transmitter substance itself spreads "electrotonically" over the entire fiber and is all that is necessary to cause muscle contraction.

Effect of Local Tissue Factors and Hormones to Cause Smooth Muscle Contraction Without Action Potentials

Probably half of all smooth muscle contraction is initiated by stimulatory factors acting directly on the smooth muscle contractile machinery and without action potentials. Two types of non-nervous and nonaction potential stimulating factors often involved are (1) local tissue chemical factors and (2) various hormones.

Smooth Muscle Contraction in Response to Local Tissue Chemical Factors.
In Chapter 17, we discuss control of contraction of the arterioles, meta-arterioles, and precapillary sphincters. The smallest of these vessels have little or no nervous supply. Yet the smooth muscle is highly contractile, responding rapidly to changes in local chemical conditions in the surrounding interstitial fluid.

In the normal resting state, many of these small blood vessels remain contracted. But when extra blood flow to the tissue is necessary, multiple factors can relax the vessel wall, thus allowing for increased flow. In this way, a powerful local feedback control system controls the blood flow to the local tissue area. Some of the specific control factors are as follows:

1. Lack of oxygen in the local tissues causes smooth muscle relaxation and, therefore, vasodilatation.
2. Excess carbon dioxide causes vasodilatation.
3. Increased hydrogen ion concentration causes vasodilatation.

Adenosine, lactic acid, increased potassium ions, diminished calcium ion concentration, and increased body temperature can all cause local vasodilatation.

Effects of Hormones on Smooth Muscle Contraction.
Many circulating hormones in the blood affect smooth muscle contraction to some degree, and some have profound effects. Among the more important of these are *norepinephrine, epinephrine, acetylcholine, angiotensin, endothelin, vasopressin, oxytocin, serotonin,* and *histamine.*

A hormone causes contraction of a smooth muscle cell when the muscle cell membrane contains *hormone-gated excitatory receptors* for the respective hormone. Conversely, the hormone causes inhibition if the membrane contains *inhibitory receptors* for the hormone rather than excitatory receptors.

Mechanisms of Smooth Muscle Excitation or Inhibition by Hormones or Local Tissue Factors.
Some hormone receptors in the smooth muscle membrane open sodium or calcium ion channels and depolarize the membrane, the same as after nerve stimulation. Sometimes action potentials result, or action potentials that are already occurring may be enhanced. In other cases, depolarization occurs without action potentials and this depolarization allows calcium ion entry into the cell, which promotes the contraction.

Inhibition, in contrast, occurs when the hormone (or other tissue factor) *closes the sodium and calcium channels* to prevent entry of these positive ions; inhibition also occurs if the normally closed *potassium channels are opened,* allowing positive potassium ions to diffuse out of the cell. Both of these actions increase the degree of negativity inside the muscle cell, a state called *hyperpolarization,* which strongly inhibits muscle contraction.

Sometimes smooth muscle contraction or inhibition is initiated by hormones without directly causing any change in the membrane potential. In these instances, the hormone may activate a membrane receptor that does not open any ion channels but instead causes an internal change in the muscle fiber, such as release of calcium ions from the intracellular sarcoplasmic reticulum; the calcium then induces contraction. To inhibit contraction, other receptor mechanisms are known to activate the enzyme *adenylate cyclase* or *guanylate cyclase* in the cell membrane; the portions of the receptors that protrude to the interior of the cells are coupled to these enzymes, causing the formation of *cyclic adenosine monophosphate* (cAMP) or *cyclic guanosine monophosphate* (cGMP), so-called *second messengers.* The cAMP or cGMP has many effects, one of which is to change the degree of phosphorylation of several enzymes that indirectly inhibit contraction. The pump that moves calcium ions from the sarcoplasm into the sarcoplasmic reticulum is activated, as well as the cell membrane pump that moves calcium ions out of the cell itself; these effects reduce the calcium ion concentration in the sarcoplasm, thereby inhibiting contraction.

Smooth muscles have considerable diversity in how they initiate contraction or relaxation in response to different hormones, neurotransmitters, and other substances. In some instances, the same substance may cause either relaxation or contraction of smooth muscles in different locations. For example, norepinephrine inhibits contraction of smooth muscle in the intestine but stimulates contraction of smooth muscle in blood vessels.

Source of Calcium Ions That Cause Contraction Through the Cell Membrane and from the Sarcoplasmic Reticulum

Although the contractile process in smooth muscle, as in skeletal muscle, is activated by calcium ions, the source of the calcium ions differs. An important difference is that the sarcoplasmic reticulum, which provides virtually all the calcium ions for skeletal muscle contraction, is only slightly developed in most smooth muscle. Instead, most of the calcium ions that cause contraction enter the muscle cell from the extracellular fluid at the time of the action potential or other stimulus. That is, the concentration of calcium ions in the extracellular fluid is greater than 10^{-3} molar, in comparison with less than 10^{-7} molar inside the smooth muscle cell; this causes rapid diffusion of the calcium ions into the cell from the extracellular fluid when the calcium channels open. The time required for this diffusion to occur averages 200 to 300 milliseconds and is called the *latent period* before contraction begins. This latent period is about 50 times as great for smooth muscle as for skeletal muscle contraction.

Role of the Smooth Muscle Sarcoplasmic Reticulum.

Figure 8-6 shows a few slightly developed sarcoplasmic tubules that lie near the cell membrane in some larger smooth muscle cells. Small invaginations of the cell membrane, called *caveolae,* abut the surfaces of these tubules. The caveolae suggest a rudimentary analog of the transverse tubule system of skeletal muscle. When an action potential is transmitted into the caveolae, this is believed to excite calcium ion release from the abutting sarcoplasmic tubules in the same way that action potentials in skeletal muscle transverse tubules cause release of calcium ions from the skeletal muscle longitudinal sarcoplasmic tubules. In general, the more extensive the sarcoplasmic reticulum in the smooth muscle fiber, the more rapidly it contracts.

Smooth Muscle Contraction Is Dependent on Extracellular Calcium Ion Concentration.

Although changing the extracellular fluid calcium ion concentration from normal has little effect on the force of contraction of skeletal muscle, this is not true for most smooth muscle. When the extracellular fluid calcium ion concentration falls to about 1/3 to 1/10 normal, smooth muscle contraction usually ceases. Therefore, the force of contraction of smooth muscle is usually highly dependent on extracellular fluid calcium ion concentration.

A Calcium Pump Is Required to Cause Smooth Muscle Relaxation.

To cause relaxation of smooth muscle after it has contracted, the calcium ions must be removed from the intracellular fluids. This removal is achieved by a *calcium pump* that pumps calcium ions out of the smooth muscle fiber back into the extracellular fluid, or into a sarcoplasmic reticulum, if it is present. This pump is slow-acting in comparison with the fast-acting sarcoplasmic reticulum pump in skeletal muscle. Therefore, a single smooth muscle contraction often lasts for seconds rather than hundredths to tenths of a second, as occurs for skeletal muscle.

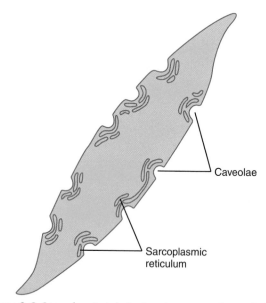

Figure 8-6 Sarcoplasmic tubules in a large smooth muscle fiber showing their relation to invaginations in the cell membrane called *caveolae.*

Caveolae

Sarcoplasmic reticulum

Bibliography

Also see references for Chapters 5 and 6.

Andersson KE, Arner A: Pharmacology of the lower urinary tract: basis for current and future treatments of urinary incontinence, *Physiol Rev* 84:935, 2004.

Berridge MJ: Smooth muscle cell calcium activation mechanisms, *J Physiol* 586:5047, 2008.

Blaustein MP, Lederer WJ: Sodium/calcium exchange: its physiological implications, *Physiol Rev* 79:763, 1999.

Cheng H, Lederer WJ: Calcium sparks, *Physiol Rev* 88:1491, 2008.

Davis MJ, Hill MA: Signaling mechanisms underlying the vascular myogenic response, *Physiol Rev* 79:387, 1999.

Drummond HA, Grifoni SC, Jernigan NLA: New trick for an old dogma: ENaC proteins as mechanotransducers in vascular smooth muscle, *Physiology (Bethesda)* 23:23, 2008.

Harnett KM, Biancani P: Calcium-dependent and calcium-independent contractions in smooth muscles, *Am J Med* 115(Suppl 3A):24S, 2003.

Hilgers RH, Webb RC: Molecular aspects of arterial smooth muscle contraction: focus on Rho, *Exp Biol Med (Maywood)* 230:829, 2005.

House SJ, Potier M, Bisaillon J, Singer HA, Trebak M: The non-excitable smooth muscle: calcium signaling and phenotypic switching during vascular disease, *Pflugers Arch* 456:769, 2008.

Huizinga JD, Lammers WJ: Gut peristalsis is governed by a multitude of cooperating mechanisms, *Am J Physiol Gastrointest Liver Physiol* 296:G1, 2009.

Kuriyama H, Kitamura K, Itoh T, Inoue R: Physiological features of visceral smooth muscle cells, with special reference to receptors and ion channels, *Physiol Rev* 78:811, 1998.

Morgan KG, Gangopadhyay SS: Cross-bridge regulation by thin filament-associated proteins, *J Appl Physiol* 91:953, 2001.

Somlyo AP, Somlyo AV: Ca^{2+} sensitivity of smooth muscle and nonmuscle myosin II: modulated by G proteins, kinases, and myosin phosphatase, *Physiol Rev* 83:1325, 2003.

Stephens NL: Airway smooth muscle, *Lung* 179:333, 2001.

Touyz RM: Transient receptor potential melastatin 6 and 7 channels, magnesium transport, and vascular biology: implications in hypertension, *Am J Physiol Heart Circ Physiol* 294:H1103, 2008.

Walker JS, Wingard CJ, Murphy RA: Energetics of crossbridge phosphorylation and contraction in vascular smooth muscle, *Hypertension* 23:1106, 1994.

Wamhoff BR, Bowles DK, Owens GK: Excitation-transcription coupling in arterial smooth muscle, *Circ Res* 98:868, 2006.

Webb RC: Smooth muscle contraction and relaxation, *Adv Physiol Educ* 27:201, 2003.

III
UNIT

The Heart

9. Cardiac Muscle; The Heart as a Pump and Function of the Heart Valves

10. Rhythmical Excitation of the Heart

11. The Normal Electrocardiogram

12. Electrocardiographic Interpretation of Cardiac Muscle and Coronary Blood Flow Abnormalities: Vectorial Analysis

13. Cardiac Arrhythmias and Their Electrocardiographic Interpretation

Cardiac Muscle; The Heart as a Pump and Function of the Heart Valves

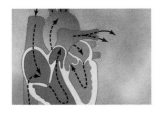

With this chapter we begin discussion of the heart and circulatory system. The heart, shown in Figure 9-1, is actually two separate pumps: a *right heart* that pumps blood through the lungs, and a *left heart* that pumps blood through the peripheral organs. In turn, each of these hearts is a pulsatile two-chamber pump composed of an *atrium* and a *ventricle.* Each atrium is a weak primer pump for the ventricle, helping to move blood into the ventricle. The ventricles then supply the main pumping force that propels the blood either (1) through the pulmonary circulation by the right ventricle or (2) through the peripheral circulation by the left ventricle.

Special mechanisms in the heart cause a continuing succession of heart contractions called *cardiac rhythmicity,* transmitting action potentials throughout the cardiac muscle to cause the heart's rhythmical beat. This rhythmical control system is explained in Chapter 10. In this chapter, we explain how the heart operates as a pump, beginning with the special features of cardiac muscle itself.

again. One also notes immediately from this figure that cardiac muscle is *striated* in the same manner as in skeletal muscle. Further, cardiac muscle has typical myofibrils that contain *actin* and *myosin filaments* almost identical to those found in skeletal muscle; these filaments lie side by side and slide along one another during contraction in the same manner as occurs in skeletal muscle (see Chapter 6). But in other ways, cardiac muscle is quite different from skeletal muscle, as we shall see.

Cardiac Muscle as a Syncytium. The dark areas crossing the cardiac muscle fibers in Figure 9-2 are called *intercalated discs;* they are actually cell membranes that separate individual cardiac muscle cells from one another. That is, cardiac muscle fibers are made up of many individual cells connected in series and in parallel with one another.

At each intercalated disc the cell membranes fuse with one another in such a way that they form permeable "communicating" junctions (gap junctions) that allow rapid diffusion of ions. Therefore, from a functional point of view, ions move with ease in the intracellular fluid along the longitudinal axes of the cardiac muscle fibers so that

Physiology of Cardiac Muscle

The heart is composed of three major types of cardiac muscle: *atrial muscle, ventricular muscle,* and specialized *excitatory* and *conductive muscle* fibers. The atrial and ventricular types of muscle contract in much the same way as skeletal muscle, except that the duration of contraction is much longer. The specialized excitatory and conductive fibers, however, contract only feebly because they contain few contractile fibrils; instead, they exhibit either automatic rhythmical electrical discharge in the form of action potentials or conduction of the action potentials through the heart, providing an excitatory system that controls the rhythmical beating of the heart.

Physiologic Anatomy of Cardiac Muscle

Figure 9-2 shows the histology of cardiac muscle, demonstrating cardiac muscle fibers arranged in a latticework, with the fibers dividing, recombining, and then spreading

HEAD AND UPPER EXTREMITY

Aorta

Pulmonary artery

Superior vena cava

Lungs

Right atrium

Pulmonary valve

Pulmonary veins

Left atrium

Tricuspid valve

Mitral valve

Right ventricle

Aortic valve

Inferior vena cava

Left ventricle

TRUNK AND LOWER EXTREMITY

Figure 9-1 Structure of the heart, and course of blood flow through the heart chambers and heart valves.

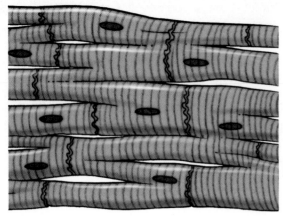

Figure 9-2 "Syncytial," interconnecting nature of cardiac muscle fibers.

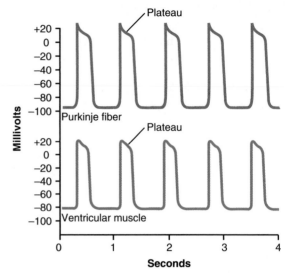

Figure 9-3 Rhythmical action potentials (in millivolts) from a Purkinje fiber and from a ventricular muscle fiber, recorded by means of microelectrodes.

action potentials travel easily from one cardiac muscle cell to the next, past the intercalated discs. Thus, cardiac muscle is a *syncytium* of many heart muscle cells in which the cardiac cells are so interconnected that when one of these cells becomes excited, the action potential spreads to all of them, from cell to cell throughout the latticework interconnections.

The heart actually is composed of two syncytiums: the *atrial syncytium,* which constitutes the walls of the two atria, and the *ventricular syncytium,* which constitutes the walls of the two ventricles. The atria are separated from the ventricles by fibrous tissue that surrounds the atrioventricular (A-V) valvular openings between the atria and ventricles. Normally, potentials are not conducted from the atrial syncytium into the ventricular syncytium directly through this fibrous tissue. Instead, they are conducted only by way of a specialized conductive system called the *A-V bundle,* a bundle of conductive fibers several millimeters in diameter that is discussed in detail in Chapter 10.

This division of the muscle of the heart into two functional syncytiums allows the atria to contract a short time ahead of ventricular contraction, which is important for effectiveness of heart pumping.

Action Potentials in Cardiac Muscle

The *action potential* recorded in a ventricular muscle fiber, shown in Figure 9-3, averages about 105 millivolts, which means that the intracellular potential rises from a very negative value, about –85 millivolts, between beats to a slightly positive value, about +20 millivolts, during each beat. After the initial *spike,* the membrane remains depolarized for about 0.2 second, exhibiting a *plateau* as shown in the figure, followed at the end of the plateau by abrupt repolarization. The presence of this plateau in the action potential causes ventricular contraction to last as much as 15 times as long in cardiac muscle as in skeletal muscle.

What Causes the Long Action Potential and the Plateau? At this point, we address the questions: Why is the action potential of cardiac muscle so long and why does it have a plateau, whereas that of skeletal muscle

does not? The basic biophysical answers to these questions were presented in Chapter 5, but they merit summarizing here as well.

At least two major differences between the membrane properties of cardiac and skeletal muscle account for the prolonged action potential and the plateau in cardiac muscle. First, the *action potential of skeletal muscle* is caused almost entirely by sudden opening of large numbers of so-called *fast sodium channels* that allow tremendous numbers of sodium ions to enter the skeletal muscle fiber from the extracellular fluid. These channels are called "fast" channels because they remain open for only a few thousandths of a second and then abruptly close. At the end of this closure, repolarization occurs, and the action potential is over within another thousandth of a second or so.

In *cardiac muscle, the action potential* is caused by opening of two types of channels: (1) the same *fast sodium channels* as those in skeletal muscle and (2) another entirely different population of *slow calcium channels,* which are also called *calcium-sodium channels.* This second population of channels differs from the fast sodium channels in that they are slower to open and, even more important, remain open for several tenths of a second. During this time, a large quantity of both calcium and sodium ions flows through these channels to the interior of the cardiac muscle fiber, and this maintains a prolonged period of depolarization, *causing the plateau* in the action potential. Further, the calcium ions that enter during this plateau phase activate the muscle contractile process, while the calcium ions that cause skeletal muscle contraction are derived from the intracellular sarcoplasmic reticulum.

The second major functional difference between cardiac muscle and skeletal muscle that helps account for both the prolonged action potential and its plateau is this: Immediately after the onset of the action potential, the permeability of the cardiac muscle membrane for potassium ions *decreases* about fivefold, an effect that does not occur in skeletal muscle. This decreased potassium permeability may result from the excess calcium influx through the calcium channels just noted. Regardless of the cause, the decreased potassium permeability greatly decreases the outflux of positively charged potassium ions during the action potential plateau and thereby prevents early return of the action potential voltage to its resting level. When the slow calcium-sodium channels do close at the end of 0.2 to 0.3 second and the influx of calcium and sodium ions ceases, the membrane permeability for potassium ions also increases rapidly; this rapid loss of potassium from the fiber immediately returns the membrane potential to its resting level, thus ending the action potential.

Velocity of Signal Conduction in Cardiac Muscle. The velocity of conduction of the excitatory action potential signal along both *atrial and ventricular muscle fibers* is about 0.3 to 0.5 m/sec, or about $\frac{1}{250}$ the velocity in very large nerve fibers and about $\frac{1}{10}$ the velocity in skeletal muscle fibers. The velocity of conduction in the specialized heart conductive system—in the *Purkinje fibers*—is as great as 4 m/sec in most parts of the system, which allows reasonably rapid conduction of the excitatory signal to the different parts of the heart, as explained in Chapter 10.

Refractory Period of Cardiac Muscle. Cardiac muscle, like all excitable tissue, is refractory to restimulation during the action potential. Therefore, the refractory period of the heart is the interval of time, as shown to the left in Figure 9-4, during which a normal cardiac impulse cannot re-excite an already excited area of cardiac muscle. The normal refractory period of the ventricle is 0.25 to 0.30 second, which is about the duration of the prolonged plateau action potential. There is an additional *relative refractory period* of about 0.05 second during which the muscle is more difficult than normal to excite but nevertheless can be excited by a very strong excitatory signal, as demonstrated by the early "premature" contraction in the second example of Figure 9-4. The refractory period of atrial muscle is much shorter than that for the ventricles (about 0.15 second for the atria compared with 0.25 to 0.30 second for the ventricles).

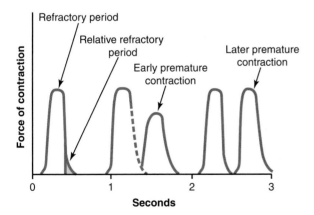

Figure 9-4 Force of ventricular heart muscle contraction, showing also duration of the refractory period and relative refractory period, plus the effect of premature contraction. Note that premature contractions do not cause wave summation, as occurs in skeletal muscle.

Excitation-Contraction Coupling—Function of Calcium Ions and the *Transverse Tubules*

The term "excitation-contraction coupling" refers to the mechanism by which the action potential causes the myofibrils of muscle to contract. This was discussed for skeletal muscle in Chapter 7. Once again, there are differences in this mechanism in cardiac muscle that have important effects on the characteristics of heart muscle contraction.

As is true for skeletal muscle, when an action potential passes over the cardiac muscle membrane, the action potential spreads to the interior of the cardiac muscle fiber along the membranes of the transverse (T) tubules. The T tubule action potentials in turn act on the membranes of the *longitudinal sarcoplasmic tubules* to cause release of calcium ions into the muscle sarcoplasm from the sarcoplasmic reticulum. In another few thousandths of a second, these calcium ions diffuse into the myofibrils and catalyze the chemical reactions that promote sliding of the actin and myosin filaments along one another; this produces the muscle contraction.

Thus far, this mechanism of excitation-contraction coupling is the same as that for skeletal muscle, but there is a second effect that is quite different. In addition to the calcium ions that are released into the sarcoplasm from the cisternae of the sarcoplasmic reticulum, calcium ions also diffuse into the sarcoplasm from the T tubules themselves at the time of the action potential, which opens voltage-dependent calcium channels in the membrane of the T tubule (Figure 9-5). Calcium entering the cell then activates *calcium release channels*, also called *ryanodine receptor channels*, in the sarcoplasmic reticulum membrane, triggering the release of calcium into the sarcoplasm. Calcium ions in the sarcoplasm then interact with troponin to initiate cross-bridge formation and contraction by the same basic mechanism as described for skeletal muscle in Chapter 6.

Without the calcium from the T tubules, the strength of cardiac muscle contraction would be reduced considerably because the sarcoplasmic reticulum of cardiac muscle is less well developed than that of skeletal muscle and does not store enough calcium to provide full contraction. The T tubules of cardiac muscle, however, have a diameter 5 times as great as that of the skeletal muscle tubules, which means a volume 25 times as great. Also, inside the T tubules is a large quantity of mucopolysaccharides that are electronegatively charged and bind an abundant store of calcium ions, keeping these always available for diffusion to the interior of the cardiac muscle fiber when a T tubule action potential appears.

The strength of contraction of cardiac muscle depends to a great extent on the concentration of calcium ions in the extracellular fluids. In fact, a heart placed in a calcium-free solution will quickly stop beating. The reason for this is that the openings of the T tubules pass directly through the cardiac muscle cell membrane into the extracellular spaces surrounding the cells, allowing the same

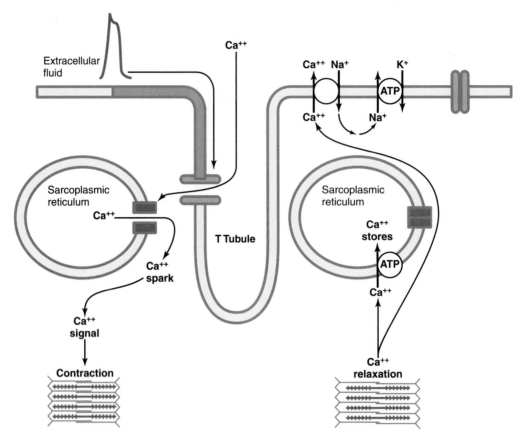

Figure 9-5 Mechanisms of excitation-contraction coupling and relaxation in cardiac muscle.

extracellular fluid that is in the cardiac muscle interstitium to percolate through the T tubules as well. Consequently, the quantity of calcium ions in the T tubule system (i.e., the availability of calcium ions to cause cardiac muscle contraction) depends to a great extent on the extracellular fluid calcium ion concentration.

In contrast, the strength of skeletal muscle contraction is hardly affected by moderate changes in extracellular fluid calcium concentration because skeletal muscle contraction is caused almost entirely by calcium ions released from the sarcoplasmic reticulum *inside* the skeletal muscle fiber.

At the end of the plateau of the cardiac action potential, the influx of calcium ions to the interior of the muscle fiber is suddenly cut off, and the calcium ions in the sarcoplasm are rapidly pumped back out of the muscle fibers into both the sarcoplasmic reticulum and the T tubule–extracellular fluid space. Transport of calcium back into the sarcoplasmic reticulum is achieved with the help of a calcium-ATPase pump (see Figure 9-5). Calcium ions are also removed from the cell by a sodium-calcium exchanger. The sodium that enters the cell during this exchange is then transported out of the cell by the sodium-potassium ATPase pump. As a result, the contraction ceases until a new action potential comes along.

Duration of Contraction. Cardiac muscle begins to contract a few milliseconds after the action potential begins and continues to contract until a few milliseconds after the action potential ends. Therefore, the duration of contraction of cardiac muscle is mainly a function of the duration of the action potential, *including the plateau*—about 0.2 second in atrial muscle and 0.3 second in ventricular muscle.

Cardiac Cycle

The cardiac events that occur from the beginning of one heartbeat to the beginning of the next are called the *cardiac cycle.* Each cycle is initiated by spontaneous generation of an action potential in the *sinus node,* as explained in Chapter 10. This node is located in the superior lateral wall of the right atrium near the opening of the superior vena cava, and the action potential travels from here rapidly through both atria and then through the A-V bundle into the ventricles. Because of this special arrangement of the conducting system from the atria into the ventricles, there is a delay of more than 0.1 second during passage of the cardiac impulse from the atria into the ventricles. This allows the atria to contract ahead of ventricular contraction, thereby pumping blood into the ventricles before the strong ventricular contraction begins. Thus, the atria act as *primer pumps* for the ventricles, and the ventricles in turn provide the major source of power for moving blood through the body's vascular system.

Diastole and Systole

The cardiac cycle consists of a period of relaxation called *diastole*, during which the heart fills with blood, followed by a period of contraction called *systole*.

The total *duration of the cardiac cycle*, including systole and diastole, is the reciprocal of the heart rate. For example, if heart rate is 72 beats/min, the duration of the cardiac cycle is 1/72 beats/min—about 0.0139 minutes per beat, or 0.833 second per beat.

Figure 9-6 shows the different events during the cardiac cycle for the left side of the heart. The top three curves show the pressure changes in the aorta, left ventricle, and left atrium, respectively. The fourth curve depicts the changes in left ventricular volume, the fifth the electrocardiogram, and the sixth a phonocardiogram, which is a recording of the sounds produced by the heart—mainly by the heart valves—as it pumps. It is especially important that the reader study in detail this figure and understand the causes of all the events shown.

Effect of Heart Rate on Duration of Cardiac Cycle. When heart rate increases, the duration of each cardiac cycle decreases, including the contraction and relaxation phases. The duration of the action potential and the period of contraction (systole) also decrease, but not by as great a percentage as does the relaxation phase (diastole). At a normal heart rate of 72 beats/min, systole comprises about 0.4 of the entire cardiac cycle. At three times the normal heart rate, systole is about 0.65 of the entire cardiac cycle. This means that the heart beating at a very fast rate does not remain relaxed long enough to allow complete filling of the cardiac chambers before the next contraction.

Relationship of the Electrocardiogram to the Cardiac Cycle

The electrocardiogram in Figure 9-6 shows the *P, Q, R, S,* and *T waves,* which are discussed in Chapters 11, 12, and 13. They are electrical voltages generated by the heart and recorded by the electrocardiograph from the surface of the body.

The *P wave* is caused by *spread of depolarization* through the atria, and this is followed by atrial contraction, which causes a slight rise in the atrial pressure curve immediately after the electrocardiographic P wave.

About 0.16 second after the onset of the P wave, the *QRS waves* appear as a result of electrical depolarization of the ventricles, which initiates contraction of the ventricles and causes the ventricular pressure to begin rising, as also shown in the figure. Therefore, the QRS complex begins slightly before the onset of ventricular systole.

Finally, one observes the *ventricular T wave* in the electrocardiogram. This represents the stage of repolarization of the ventricles when the ventricular muscle fibers begin to relax. Therefore, the T wave occurs slightly before the end of ventricular contraction.

Function of the Atria as Primer Pumps

Blood normally flows continually from the great veins into the atria; about 80 percent of the blood flows directly through the atria into the ventricles even before the atria contract. Then, atrial contraction usually causes an additional 20 percent filling of the ventricles. Therefore, the atria simply function as primer pumps that increase the ventricular pumping effectiveness as much as 20 percent. However, the heart can continue to operate under most conditions

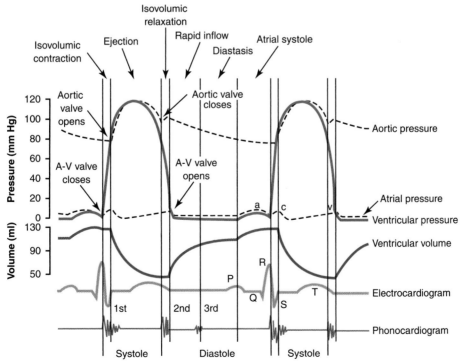

Figure 9-6 Events of the cardiac cycle for left ventricular function, showing changes in left atrial pressure, left ventricular pressure, aortic pressure, ventricular volume, the electrocardiogram, and the phonocardiogram.

even without this extra 20 percent effectiveness because it normally has the capability of pumping 300 to 400 percent more blood than is required by the resting body. Therefore, when the atria fail to function, the difference is unlikely to be noticed unless a person exercises; then acute signs of heart failure occasionally develop, especially shortness of breath.

> **Pressure Changes in the Atria—a, c, and v Waves.** In the atrial pressure curve of Figure 9-6, three minor pressure elevations, called the *a, c,* and *v atrial pressure waves,* are noted.
>
> The *a wave* is caused by atrial contraction. Ordinarily, the *right* atrial pressure increases 4 to 6 mm Hg during atrial contraction, and the *left* atrial pressure increases about 7 to 8 mm Hg.
>
> The *c wave* occurs when the ventricles begin to contract; it is caused partly by slight backflow of blood into the atria at the onset of ventricular contraction but mainly by bulging of the A-V valves backward toward the atria because of increasing pressure in the ventricles.
>
> The *v wave* occurs toward the end of ventricular contraction; it results from slow flow of blood into the atria from the veins while the A-V valves are closed during ventricular contraction. Then, when ventricular contraction is over, the A-V valves open, allowing this stored atrial blood to flow rapidly into the ventricles and causing the v wave to disappear.

Function of the Ventricles as Pumps

Filling of the Ventricles During Diastole. During ventricular systole, large amounts of blood accumulate in the right and left atria because of the closed A-V valves. Therefore, as soon as systole is over and the ventricular pressures fall again to their low diastolic values, the moderately increased pressures that have developed in the atria during ventricular systole immediately push the A-V valves open and allow blood to flow rapidly into the ventricles, as shown by the rise of the left *ventricular volume curve* in Figure 9-6. This is called the *period of rapid filling of the ventricles.*

The period of rapid filling lasts for about the first third of diastole. During the middle third of diastole, only a small amount of blood normally flows into the ventricles; this is blood that continues to empty into the atria from the veins and passes through the atria directly into the ventricles.

During the last third of diastole, the atria contract and give an additional thrust to the inflow of blood into the ventricles; this accounts for about 20 percent of the filling of the ventricles during each heart cycle.

Emptying of the Ventricles During Systole

Period of Isovolumic (Isometric) Contraction. Immediately after ventricular contraction begins, the ventricular pressure rises abruptly, as shown in Figure 9-6, causing the A-V valves to close. Then an additional 0.02 to 0.03 second is required for the ventricle to build up sufficient pressure to push the semilunar (aortic and pulmonary) valves open against the pressures in the aorta and pulmonary artery. Therefore, during this period, contraction is occurring in the ventricles, but there is

no emptying. This is called the period of *isovolumic* or *isometric contraction,* meaning that tension is increasing in the muscle but little or no shortening of the muscle fibers is occurring.

Period of Ejection. When the left ventricular pressure rises slightly above 80 mm Hg (and the right ventricular pressure slightly above 8 mm Hg), the ventricular pressures push the semilunar valves open. Immediately, blood begins to pour out of the ventricles, with about 70 percent of the blood emptying occurring during the first third of the period of ejection and the remaining 30 percent emptying during the next two thirds. Therefore, the first third is called the *period of rapid ejection,* and the last two thirds, the *period of slow ejection.*

Period of Isovolumic (Isometric) Relaxation. At the end of systole, ventricular relaxation begins suddenly, allowing both the right and left *intraventricular pressures* to decrease rapidly. The elevated pressures in the distended large arteries that have just been filled with blood from the contracted ventricles immediately push blood back toward the ventricles, which snaps the aortic and pulmonary valves closed. For another 0.03 to 0.06 second, the ventricular muscle continues to relax, even though the ventricular volume does not change, giving rise to the period of *isovolumic* or *isometric relaxation.* During this period, the intraventricular pressures decrease rapidly back to their low diastolic levels. Then the A-V valves open to begin a new cycle of ventricular pumping.

End-Diastolic Volume, End-Systolic Volume, and Stroke Volume Output. During diastole, normal filling of the ventricles increases the volume of each ventricle to about 110 to 120 ml. This volume is called the *end-diastolic volume.* Then, as the ventricles empty during systole, the volume decreases about 70 ml, which is called the *stroke volume output.* The remaining volume in each ventricle, about 40 to 50 ml, is called the *end-systolic volume.* The fraction of the end-diastolic volume that is ejected is called the *ejection fraction*—usually equal to about 60 percent.

When the heart contracts strongly, the end-systolic volume can be decreased to as little as 10 to 20 ml. Conversely, when large amounts of blood flow into the ventricles during diastole, the ventricular end-diastolic volumes can become as great as 150 to 180 ml in the healthy heart. By both increasing the end-diastolic volume and decreasing the end-systolic volume, the stroke volume output can be increased to more than double normal.

Function of the Valves

Atrioventricular Valves. The *A-V valves* (the *tricuspid* and *mitral* valves) prevent backflow of blood from the ventricles to the atria during systole, and the *semilunar valves* (the *aortic* and *pulmonary artery* valves) prevent backflow from the aorta and pulmonary arteries into the ventricles during diastole. These valves, shown in Figure 9-7 for the left ventricle, close and open *passively.* That is, they close when a backward pressure gradient pushes

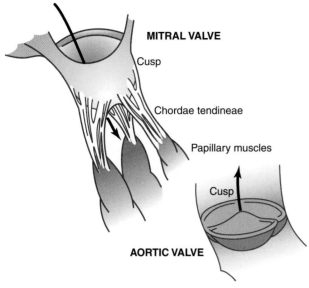

MITRAL VALVE

Cusp

Chordae tendineae

Papillary muscles

Cusp

AORTIC VALVE

Figure 9-7 Mitral and aortic valves (the left ventricular valves).

blood backward, and they open when a forward pressure gradient forces blood in the forward direction. For anatomical reasons, the thin, filmy A-V valves require almost no backflow to cause closure, whereas the much heavier semilunar valves require rather rapid backflow for a few milliseconds.

Function of the Papillary Muscles. Figure 9-7 also shows papillary muscles that attach to the vanes of the A-V valves by the *chordae tendineae.* The papillary muscles contract when the ventricular walls contract, but contrary to what might be expected, they *do not* help the valves to close. Instead, they pull the vanes of the valves inward toward the ventricles to prevent their bulging too far backward toward the atria during ventricular contraction. If a chorda tendinea becomes ruptured or if one of the papillary muscles becomes paralyzed, the valve bulges far backward during ventricular contraction, sometimes so far that it leaks severely and results in severe or even lethal cardiac incapacity.

Aortic and Pulmonary Artery Valves. The aortic and pulmonary artery semilunar valves function quite differently from the A-V valves. First, the high pressures in the arteries at the end of systole cause the semilunar valves to snap to the closed position, in contrast to the much softer closure of the A-V valves. Second, because of smaller openings, the velocity of blood ejection through the aortic and pulmonary valves is far greater than that through the much larger A-V valves. Also, because of the rapid closure and rapid ejection, the edges of the aortic and pulmonary valves are subjected to much greater mechanical abrasion than are the A-V valves. Finally, the A-V valves are supported by the chordae tendineae, which is not true for the semilunar valves. It is obvious from the anatomy of the aortic and pulmonary valves (as shown for the aortic valve at the bottom of Figure 9-7) that they must be constructed with an especially strong yet very pliable fibrous tissue base to withstand the extra physical stresses.

Aortic Pressure Curve

When the left ventricle contracts, the ventricular pressure increases rapidly until the aortic valve opens. Then, after the valve opens, the pressure in the ventricle rises much less rapidly, as shown in Figure 9-6, because blood immediately flows out of the ventricle into the aorta and then into the systemic distribution arteries.

The entry of blood into the arteries causes the walls of these arteries to stretch and the pressure to increase to about 120 mm Hg.

Next, at the end of systole, after the left ventricle stops ejecting blood and the aortic valve closes, the elastic walls of the arteries maintain a high pressure in the arteries, even during diastole.

A so-called *incisura* occurs in the aortic pressure curve when the aortic valve closes. This is caused by a short period of backward flow of blood immediately before closure of the valve, followed by sudden cessation of the backflow.

After the aortic valve has closed, the pressure in the aorta decreases slowly throughout diastole because the blood stored in the distended elastic arteries flows continually through the peripheral vessels back to the veins. Before the ventricle contracts again, the aortic pressure usually has fallen to about 80 mm Hg (diastolic pressure), which is two thirds the maximal pressure of 120 mm Hg (systolic pressure) that occurs in the aorta during ventricular contraction.

The pressure curves in the *right ventricle* and *pulmonary artery* are similar to those in the aorta, except that the pressures are only about one sixth as great, as discussed in Chapter 14.

Relationship of the Heart Sounds to Heart Pumping

When listening to the heart with a stethoscope, one does not hear the opening of the valves because this is a relatively slow process that normally makes no noise. However, when the valves close, the vanes of the valves and the surrounding fluids vibrate under the influence of sudden pressure changes, giving off sound that travels in all directions through the chest.

When the ventricles contract, one first hears a sound caused by closure of the A-V valves. The vibration is low in pitch and relatively long-lasting and is known as the *first heart sound.* When the aortic and pulmonary valves close at the end of systole, one hears a rapid snap because these valves close rapidly, and the surroundings vibrate for a short period. This sound is called the *second heart sound.* The precise causes of the heart sounds are discussed more fully in Chapter 23, in relation to listening to the sounds with the stethoscope.

Work Output of the Heart

The *stroke work output* of the heart is the amount of energy that the heart converts to work during each heartbeat while pumping blood into the arteries. *Minute work output* is the total amount of energy converted to work in 1 minute; this is equal to the stroke work output times the heart rate per minute.

Work output of the heart is in two forms. First, by far the major proportion is used to move the blood from the low-pressure veins to the high-pressure arteries. This is called *volume-pressure work* or *external work*. Second, a minor proportion of the energy is used to accelerate the blood to its velocity of ejection through the aortic and pulmonary valves. This is the *kinetic energy of blood flow* component of the work output.

Right ventricular external work output is normally about one sixth the work output of the left ventricle because of the sixfold difference in systolic pressures that the two ventricles pump. The additional work output of each ventricle required to create kinetic energy of blood flow is proportional to the mass of blood ejected times the square of velocity of ejection.

Ordinarily, the work output of the left ventricle required to create kinetic energy of blood flow is only about 1 percent of the total work output of the ventricle and therefore is ignored in the calculation of the total stroke work output. But in certain abnormal conditions, such as aortic stenosis, in which blood flows with great velocity through the stenosed valve, more than 50 percent of the total work output may be required to create kinetic energy of blood flow.

Graphical Analysis of Ventricular Pumping

Figure 9-8 shows a diagram that is especially useful in explaining the pumping mechanics of the *left* ventricle. The most important components of the diagram are the two curves labeled "diastolic pressure" and "systolic pressure." These curves are volume-pressure curves.

The diastolic pressure curve is determined by filling the heart with progressively greater volumes of blood and then measuring the diastolic pressure immediately before ventricular contraction occurs, which is the *end-diastolic pressure* of the ventricle.

The systolic pressure curve is determined by recording the systolic pressure achieved during ventricular contraction at each volume of filling.

Until the volume of the noncontracting ventricle rises above about 150 ml, the "diastolic" pressure does not increase greatly. Therefore, up to this volume, blood can flow easily into the ventricle from the atrium. Above 150 ml, the ventricular diastolic pressure increases rapidly, partly because of fibrous tissue in the heart that will stretch no more and partly because the pericardium that surrounds the heart becomes filled nearly to its limit.

During ventricular contraction, the "systolic" pressure increases even at low ventricular volumes and reaches a maximum at a ventricular volume of 150 to 170 ml. Then, as the volume increases still further, the systolic pressure actually decreases under some conditions, as demonstrated by the falling systolic pressure curve in Figure 9-8, because at these great volumes, the actin and myosin filaments of the cardiac muscle fibers are pulled apart far enough that the strength of each cardiac fiber contraction becomes less than optimal.

Note especially in the figure that the maximum systolic pressure for the normal *left* ventricle is between 250 and 300 mm Hg, but this varies widely with each person's heart strength and degree of heart stimulation by cardiac nerves. For the normal *right* ventricle, the maximum systolic pressure is between 60 and 80 mm Hg.

"Volume-Pressure Diagram" During the Cardiac Cycle; Cardiac Work Output. The red lines in Figure 9-8 form a loop called the *volume-pressure diagram* of the cardiac cycle for normal function of the *left* ventricle. A more detailed version of this loop is shown in Figure 9-9. It is divided into four phases.

Phase I: Period of filling. This phase in the volume-pressure diagram begins at a ventricular volume of about 50 ml and a diastolic pressure of 2 to 3 mm Hg. The amount of blood that remains in the ventricle after the previous heartbeat, 50 ml, is called the *end-systolic volume*. As venous blood flows into the ventricle from the left atrium, the ventricular volume normally increases to about 120 ml, called the *end-diastolic volume*, an increase of 70 ml. Therefore, the volume-pressure diagram during phase I extends along the line labeled "I," from point A to point B, with the volume increasing to 120 ml and the diastolic pressure rising to about 5 to 7 mm Hg.

Phase II: Period of isovolumic contraction. During isovolumic contraction, the volume of the ventricle does not change because all valves are closed. However, the pressure inside the ventricle increases to equal the pressure in the aorta, at a pressure value of about 80 mm Hg, as depicted by point C.

Phase III: Period of ejection. During ejection, the systolic pressure rises even higher because of still more contraction of the ventricle. At the same time, the volume of the ventricle decreases because the aortic valve has now opened and blood flows out of the ventricle into the aorta. Therefore, the curve labeled "III," or "period of ejection," traces the changes in volume and systolic pressure during this period of ejection.

Phase IV: Period of isovolumic relaxation. At the end of the period of ejection (point D), the aortic valve closes, and the ventricular pressure falls back to the diastolic pressure level. The line labeled "IV" traces this decrease in intraventricular pressure without any change in volume. Thus, the ventricle returns to its starting point, with about 50 ml of blood left in the ventricle and at an atrial pressure of 2 to 3 mm Hg.

Readers well trained in the basic principles of physics will recognize that the area subtended by this functional

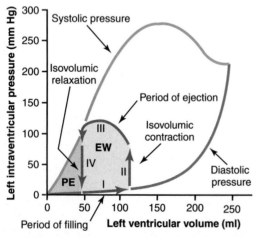

Figure 9-8 Relationship between left ventricular volume and intraventricular pressure during diastole and systole. Also shown by the heavy red lines is the "volume-pressure diagram," demonstrating changes in intraventricular volume and pressure during the normal cardiac cycle. EW, net external work.

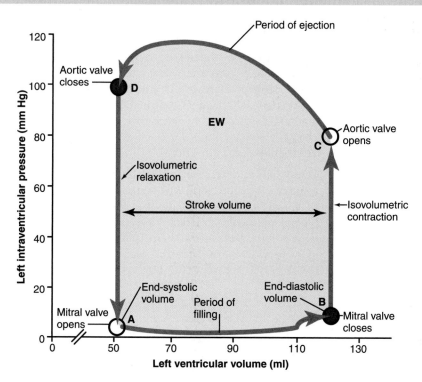

Figure 9-9 The "volume-pressure diagram" demonstrating changes in intraventricular volume and pressure during a single cardiac cycle (*red line*). The tan shaded area represents the net external work (*EW*) output by the left ventricle during the cardiac cycle.

volume-pressure diagram (the tan shaded area, labeled EW) represents the *net external work output* of the ventricle during its contraction cycle. In experimental studies of cardiac contraction, this diagram is used for calculating cardiac work output.

When the heart pumps large quantities of blood, the area of the work diagram becomes much larger. That is, it extends far to the right because the ventricle fills with more blood during diastole, it rises much higher because the ventricle contracts with greater pressure, and it usually extends farther to the left because the ventricle contracts to a smaller volume—especially if the ventricle is stimulated to increased activity by the sympathetic nervous system.

Concepts of Preload and Afterload. In assessing the contractile properties of muscle, it is important to specify the degree of tension on the muscle when it begins to contract, which is called the *preload,* and to specify the load against which the muscle exerts its contractile force, which is called the *afterload.*

For cardiac contraction, the *preload* is usually considered to be the end-diastolic pressure when the ventricle has become filled.

The *afterload* of the ventricle is the pressure in the aorta leading from the ventricle. In Figure 9-8, this corresponds to the systolic pressure described by the phase III curve of the volume-pressure diagram. (Sometimes the afterload is loosely considered to be the resistance in the circulation rather than the pressure.)

The importance of the concepts of preload and afterload is that in many abnormal functional states of the heart or circulation, the pressure during filling of the ventricle (the preload), the arterial pressure against which the ventricle must contract (the afterload), or both are severely altered from normal.

Chemical Energy Required for Cardiac Contraction: Oxygen Utilization by the Heart

Heart muscle, like skeletal muscle, uses chemical energy to provide the work of contraction. Approximately 70 to 90 percent of this energy is normally derived from oxidative metabolism of fatty acids with about 10 to 30 percent coming from other nutrients, especially lactate and glucose. Therefore, the rate of oxygen consumption by the heart is an excellent measure of the chemical energy liberated while the heart performs its work. The different chemical reactions that liberate this energy are discussed in Chapters 67 and 68.

Experimental studies have shown that oxygen consumption of the heart and the chemical energy expended during contraction are directly related to the total shaded area in Figure 9-8. This shaded portion consists of the *external work* (EW) as explained earlier and an additional portion called the *potential energy,* labeled PE. The potential energy represents additional work that could be accomplished by contraction of the ventricle if the ventricle should empty completely all the blood in its chamber with each contraction.

Oxygen consumption has also been shown to be nearly proportional to the *tension* that occurs in the heart muscle during contraction multiplied by the *duration of time* that the contraction persists, called the *tension-time index.* Because tension is high when systolic pressure is high, correspondingly more oxygen is used. Also, much more chemical energy is expended even at normal systolic pressures when the ventricle is abnormally dilated because the heart muscle tension during contraction is proportional to pressure times the diameter of the ventricle. This becomes especially important in heart failure where the heart ventricle is dilated and, paradoxically, the amount of chemical energy required for a given amount of work output is greater than normal even though the heart is already failing.

Efficiency of Cardiac Contraction. During heart muscle contraction, most of the expended chemical energy is converted into *heat* and a much smaller portion into *work output*. The ratio of work output to total chemical energy expenditure is called the *efficiency of cardiac contraction,* or simply *efficiency of the heart.* Maximum efficiency of the normal heart is between 20 and 25 percent. In heart failure, this can decrease to as low as 5 to 10 percent.

Regulation of Heart Pumping

When a person is at rest, the heart pumps only 4 to 6 liters of blood each minute. During severe exercise, the heart may be required to pump four to seven times this amount. The basic means by which the volume pumped by the heart is regulated are (1) intrinsic cardiac regulation of pumping in response to changes in volume of blood flowing into the heart and (2) control of heart rate and strength of heart pumping by the autonomic nervous system.

Intrinsic Regulation of Heart Pumping—The Frank-Starling Mechanism

In Chapter 20, we will learn that under most conditions, the amount of blood pumped by the heart each minute is normally determined almost entirely by the rate of blood flow into the heart from the veins, which is called *venous return.* That is, each peripheral tissue of the body controls its own local blood flow, and all the local tissue flows combine and return by way of the veins to the right atrium. The heart, in turn, automatically pumps this incoming blood into the arteries so that it can flow around the circuit again.

This intrinsic ability of the heart to adapt to increasing volumes of inflowing blood is called the *Frank-Starling mechanism of the heart,* in honor of Otto Frank and Ernest Starling, two great physiologists of a century ago. Basically, the Frank-Starling mechanism means that the greater the heart muscle is stretched during filling, the greater is the force of contraction and the greater the quantity of blood pumped into the aorta. Or, stated another way: *Within physiologic limits, the heart pumps all the blood that returns to it by the way of the veins.*

What Is the Explanation of the Frank-Starling Mechanism? When an extra amount of blood flows into the ventricles, the cardiac muscle itself is stretched to greater length. This in turn causes the muscle to contract with increased force because the actin and myosin filaments are brought to a more nearly optimal degree of overlap for force generation. Therefore, the ventricle, because of its increased pumping, automatically pumps the extra blood into the arteries.

This ability of stretched muscle, up to an optimal length, to contract with increased work output is characteristic of all striated muscle, as explained in Chapter 6, and is not simply a characteristic of cardiac muscle.

In addition to the important effect of lengthening the heart muscle, still another factor increases heart pumping when its volume is increased. Stretch of the right atrial wall directly increases the heart rate by 10 to 20 percent; this, too, helps increase the amount of blood pumped each minute, although its contribution is much less than that of the Frank-Starling mechanism.

Ventricular Function Curves

One of the best ways to express the functional ability of the ventricles to pump blood is by *ventricular function curves,* as shown in Figures 9-10 and 9-11. Figure 9-10 shows a type of ventricular function curve called the *stroke work output curve.* Note that as the atrial pressure for each side of the heart increases, the stroke work output for that side increases until it reaches the limit of the ventricle's pumping ability.

Figure 9-11 shows another type of ventricular function curve called the *ventricular volume output curve.* The two curves of this figure represent function of the two ventricles of the human heart based on data extrapolated from lower animals. As the right and left atrial pressures increase, the respective ventricular volume outputs per minute also increase.

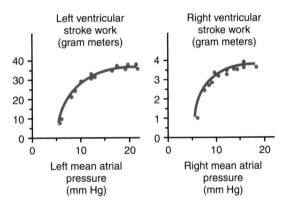

Figure 9-10 Left and right ventricular function curves recorded from dogs, depicting *ventricular stroke work output* as a function of left and right mean atrial pressures. (Curves reconstructed from data in Sarnoff SJ: Myocardial contractility as described by ventricular function curves. Physiol Rev 35:107, 1955.)

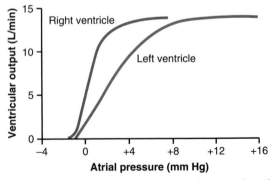

Figure 9-11 Approximate normal right and left *ventricular volume output curves* for the normal resting human heart as extrapolated from data obtained in dogs and data from human beings.

Thus, *ventricular function curves* are another way of expressing the Frank-Starling mechanism of the heart. That is, as the ventricles fill in response to higher atrial pressures, each ventricular volume and strength of cardiac muscle contraction increase, causing the heart to pump increased quantities of blood into the arteries.

Control of the Heart by the Sympathetic and Parasympathetic Nerves

The pumping effectiveness of the heart also is controlled by the *sympathetic* and *parasympathetic (vagus)* nerves, which abundantly supply the heart, as shown in Figure 9-12. For given levels of atrial pressure, the amount of blood pumped each minute *(cardiac output)* often can be increased more than 100 percent by sympathetic stimulation. By contrast, the output can be decreased to as low as zero or almost zero by vagal (parasympathetic) stimulation.

Mechanisms of Excitation of the Heart by the Sympathetic Nerves. Strong sympathetic stimulation can increase the heart rate in young adult humans from the normal rate of 70 beats/min up to 180 to 200 and, rarely, even 250 beats/min. Also, sympathetic stimulation increases the force of heart contraction to as much as double normal, thereby increasing the volume of blood pumped and increasing the ejection pressure. Thus, sympathetic stimulation often can increase the maximum cardiac output as much as twofold to threefold, in addition to the increased output caused by the Frank-Starling mechanism already discussed.

Conversely, *inhibition* of the sympathetic nerves to the heart can decrease cardiac pumping to a moderate extent in the following way: Under normal conditions, the sympathetic nerve fibers to the heart discharge continuously at a slow rate that maintains pumping at about 30 percent above that with no sympathetic stimulation. Therefore, when the activity of the sympathetic nervous system is depressed below normal, this decreases both heart rate and strength of ventricular muscle contraction, thereby decreasing the level of cardiac pumping as much as 30 percent below normal.

Parasympathetic (Vagal) Stimulation of the Heart. Strong stimulation of the parasympathetic nerve fibers in the vagus nerves to the heart can stop the heartbeat for a few seconds, but then the heart usually "escapes" and beats at a rate of 20 to 40 beats/min as long as the parasympathetic stimulation continues. In addition, strong vagal stimulation can decrease the strength of heart muscle contraction by 20 to 30 percent.

The vagal fibers are distributed mainly to the atria and not much to the ventricles, where the power contraction of the heart occurs. This explains the effect of vagal stimulation mainly to decrease heart rate rather than to decrease greatly the strength of heart contraction. Nevertheless, the great decrease in heart rate combined with a slight decrease in heart contraction strength can decrease ventricular pumping 50 percent or more.

Effect of Sympathetic or Parasympathetic Stimulation on the Cardiac Function Curve. Figure 9-13 shows four cardiac function curves. They are similar to the ventricular function curves of Figure 9-11. However, they represent function of the entire heart rather than of a single ventricle; they show the relation between right atrial pressure at the input of the right heart and cardiac output from the left ventricle into the aorta.

The curves of Figure 9-13 demonstrate that at any given right atrial pressure, the cardiac output increases during increased sympathetic stimulation and decreases during increased parasympathetic stimulation. These changes in output caused by autonomic nervous system stimulation result both from *changes in heart rate* and from *changes in contractile strength of the heart* because both change in response to the nerve stimulation.

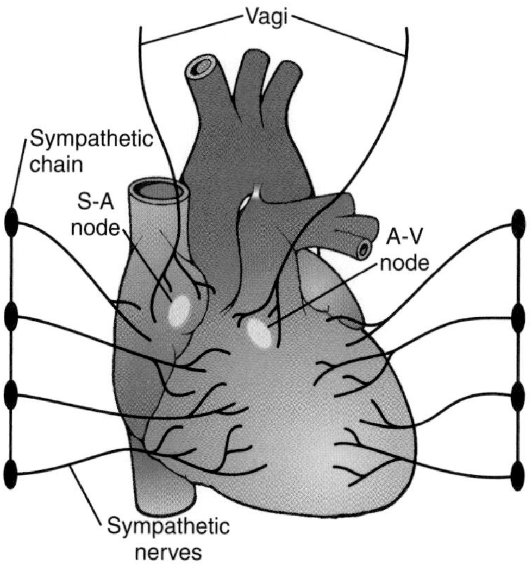

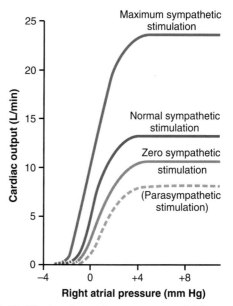

Figure 9-12 Cardiac *sympathetic* and *parasympathetic* nerves. (The vagus nerves to the heart are parasympathetic nerves.)

Figure 9-13 Effect on the cardiac output curve of different degrees of sympathetic or parasympathetic stimulation.

Effect of Potassium and Calcium Ions on Heart Function

In the discussion of membrane potentials in Chapter 5, it was pointed out that potassium ions have a marked effect on membrane potentials, and in Chapter 6 it was noted that calcium ions play an especially important role in activating the muscle contractile process. Therefore, it is to be expected that the concentration of each of these two ions in the extracellular fluids should also have important effects on cardiac pumping.

Effect of Potassium Ions. Excess potassium in the extracellular fluids causes the heart to become dilated and flaccid and also slows the heart rate. Large quantities also can block conduction of the cardiac impulse from the atria to the ventricles through the A-V bundle. Elevation of potassium concentration to only 8 to 12 mEq/L—two to three times the normal value—can cause such weakness of the heart and abnormal rhythm that death occurs.

These effects result partially from the fact that a high potassium concentration in the extracellular fluids decreases the resting membrane potential in the cardiac muscle fibers, as explained in Chapter 5. That is, high extracellular fluid potassium concentration partially depolarizes the cell membrane, causing the membrane potential to be less negative. As the membrane potential decreases, the intensity of the action potential also decreases, which makes contraction of the heart progressively weaker.

Effect of Calcium Ions. An excess of calcium ions causes effects almost exactly opposite to those of potassium ions, causing the heart to go toward spastic contraction. This is caused by a direct effect of calcium ions to initiate the cardiac contractile process, as explained earlier in the chapter.

Conversely, deficiency of calcium ions causes cardiac *flaccidity*, similar to the effect of high potassium. Fortunately, calcium ion levels in the blood normally are regulated within a very narrow range. Therefore, cardiac effects of abnormal calcium concentrations are seldom of clinical concern.

Effect of Temperature on Heart Function

Increased body temperature, as occurs when one has fever, causes a greatly increased heart rate, sometimes to double normal. Decreased temperature causes a greatly decreased heart rate, falling to as low as a few beats per minute when a person is near death from hypothermia in the body temperature range of 60° to 70°F. These effects presumably result from the fact that heat increases the permeability of the cardiac muscle membrane to ions that control heart rate, resulting in acceleration of the self-excitation process.

Contractile strength of the heart often is enhanced temporarily by a moderate increase in temperature, as occurs during body exercise, but prolonged elevation of temperature exhausts the metabolic systems of the heart and eventually causes weakness. Therefore, optimal function of the heart depends greatly on proper control of body

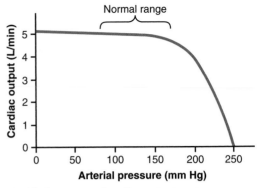

Figure 9-14 Constancy of cardiac output up to a pressure level of 160 mm Hg. Only when the arterial pressure rises above this normal limit does the increasing pressure load cause the cardiac output to fall significantly.

temperature by the temperature control mechanisms explained in Chapter 73.

Increasing the Arterial Pressure Load (up to a Limit) Does Not Decrease the Cardiac Output

Note in Figure 9-14 that increasing the arterial pressure in the aorta does not decrease the cardiac output until the mean arterial pressure rises above about 160 mm Hg. In other words, during normal function of the heart at normal systolic arterial pressures (80 to 140 mm Hg), the cardiac output is determined almost entirely by the ease of blood flow through the body's tissues, which in turn controls *venous return* of blood to the heart. This is the principal subject of Chapter 20.

Bibliography

Bers DM: Altered cardiac myocyte Ca regulation in heart failure, *Physiology (Bethesda)* 21:380, 2006.

Bers DM: Calcium cycling and signaling in cardiac myocytes, *Annu Rev Physiol* 70:23, 2008.

Brette F, Orchard C: T-tubule function in mammalian cardiac myocytes, *Circ Res* 92:1182, 2003.

Chantler PD, Lakatta EG, Najjar SS: Arterial-ventricular coupling: mechanistic insights into cardiovascular performance at rest and during exercise, *J Appl Physiol* 105:1342, 2008.

Cheng H, Lederer WJ: Calcium sparks, *Physiol Rev* 88:1491, 2008.

Clancy CE, Kass RS: Defective cardiac ion channels: from mutations to clinical syndromes, *J Clin Invest* 110:1075, 2002.

Couchonnal LF, Anderson ME: The role of calmodulin kinase II in myocardial physiology and disease, *Physiology (Bethesda)* 23:151, 2008.

Fuchs F, Smith SH: Calcium, cross-bridges, and the Frank-Starling relationship, *News Physiol Sci* 16:5, 2001.

Guyton AC: Determination of cardiac output by equating venous return curves with cardiac response curves, *Physiol Rev* 35:123, 1955.

Guyton AC, Jones CE, Coleman TG: *Circulatory Physiology: Cardiac Output and Its Regulation*, 2nd ed, Philadelphia, 1973, WB Saunders.

Kang M, Chung KY, Walker JW: G-protein coupled receptor signaling in myocardium: not for the faint of heart, *Physiology (Bethesda)* 22:174, 2007.

Knaapen P, Germans T, Knuuti J, et al: Myocardial energetic and efficiency: current status of the noninvasive approach, *Circulation* 115:918, 2007.

Mangoni ME, Nargeot J: Genesis and regulation of the heart automaticity, *Physiol Rev* 88:919, 2008.

Korzick DH: Regulation of cardiac excitation-contraction coupling: a cellular update, *Adv Physiol Educ* 27:192, 2003.

Olson EN: A decade of discoveries in cardiac biology, *Nat Med* 10:467, 2004.

Rudy Y, Ackerman MJ, Bers DM, et al: Systems approach to understanding electromechanical activity in the human heart: a National Heart, Lung, and Blood Institute workshop summary, *Circulation* 118:1202, 2008.

Saks V, Dzeja P, Schlattner U, et al: Cardiac system bioenergetics: metabolic basis of the Frank-Starling law, *J Physiol* 571:253, 2006.

Sarnoff SJ: Myocardial contractility as described by ventricular function curves, *Physiol Rev* 35:107, 1955.

Starling EH: *The Linacre Lecture on the Law of the Heart*, London, 1918, Longmans Green.

CHAPTER 10

Rhythmical Excitation of the Heart

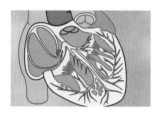

The heart is endowed with a special system for (1) generating rhythmical electrical impulses to cause rhythmical contraction of the heart muscle and (2) conducting these impulses rapidly through the heart. When this system functions normally, the atria contract about one sixth of a second ahead of ventricular contraction, which allows filling of the ventricles before they pump the blood through the lungs and peripheral circulation. Another special importance of the system is that it allows all portions of the ventricles to contract almost simultaneously, which is essential for most effective pressure generation in the ventricular chambers.

This rhythmical and conductive system of the heart is susceptible to damage by heart disease, especially by ischemia of the heart tissues resulting from poor coronary blood flow. The effect is often a bizarre heart rhythm or abnormal sequence of contraction of the heart chambers, and the pumping effectiveness of the heart often is affected severely, even to the extent of causing death.

Specialized Excitatory and Conductive System of the Heart

Figure 10-1 shows the specialized excitatory and conductive system of the heart that controls cardiac contractions. The figure shows the sinus node (also called sinoatrial or S-A node), in which the normal rhythmical impulses are generated; the internodal pathways that conduct impulses from the sinus node to the atrioventricular (A-V) node; the A-V node, in which impulses from the atria are delayed before passing into the ventricles; the A-V bundle, which conducts impulses from the atria into the ventricles; and the left and right bundle branches of Purkinje fibers, which conduct the cardiac impulses to all parts of the ventricles.

Sinus (Sinoatrial) Node

The sinus node (also called *sinoatrial node*) is a small, flattened, ellipsoid strip of specialized cardiac muscle about 3 millimeters wide, 15 millimeters long, and 1 millimeter thick. It is located in the superior posterolateral wall of the right atrium immediately below and slightly lateral to the opening of the superior vena cava. The fibers of this node have almost no contractile muscle filaments and are each only 3 to 5 micrometers in diameter, in contrast to a diameter of 10 to 15 micrometers for the surrounding atrial muscle fibers. However, the sinus nodal fibers connect directly with the atrial muscle fibers so that any action potential that begins in the sinus node spreads immediately into the atrial muscle wall.

Automatic Electrical Rhythmicity of the Sinus Fibers

Some cardiac fibers have the capability of *self-excitation*, a process that can cause automatic rhythmical discharge and contraction. This is especially true of the fibers of the heart's specialized conducting system, including the fibers of the sinus node. For this reason, the sinus node ordinarily controls the rate of beat of the entire heart, as discussed in detail later in this chapter. First, let us describe this automatic rhythmicity.

Mechanism of Sinus Nodal Rhythmicity. Figure 10-2 shows action potentials recorded from inside a sinus nodal fiber for three heartbeats and, by comparison, a single ventricular muscle fiber action potential. Note that the "resting membrane potential" of the sinus nodal fiber between discharges has a negativity of about −55 to −60 millivolts, in comparison with −85 to −90 millivolts for the ventricular muscle fiber. The cause of this lesser negativity is that the cell membranes of the sinus fibers are naturally leaky to sodium and calcium ions, and positive charges of the entering sodium and calcium ions neutralize some of the intracellular negativity.

Before attempting to explain the rhythmicity of the sinus nodal fibers, first recall from the discussions of Chapters 5 and 9 that cardiac muscle has three types of membrane ion channels that play important roles in causing the voltage changes of the action potential. They are (1) *fast sodium channels*, (2) *slow sodium-calcium channels*, and (3) *potassium channels*.

Opening of the fast sodium channels for a few 10,000 ths of a second is responsible for the rapid upstroke spike of the action potential observed in ventricular muscle, because of rapid influx of positive sodium ions to the

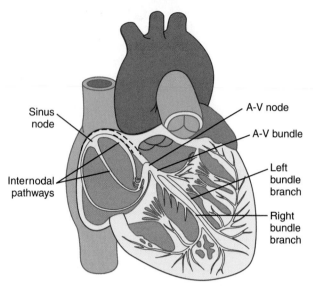

Figure 10-1 Sinus node and the Purkinje system of the heart, showing also the A-V node, atrial internodal pathways, and ventricular bundle branches.

interior of the fiber. Then the "plateau" of the ventricular action potential is caused primarily by slower opening of the slow sodium-calcium channels, which lasts for about 0.3 second. Finally, opening of potassium channels allows diffusion of large amounts of positive potassium ions in the outward direction through the fiber membrane and returns the membrane potential to its resting level.

But there is a difference in the function of these channels in the sinus nodal fiber because the "resting" potential is much less negative—only –55 millivolts in the nodal fiber instead of the –90 millivolts in the ventricular muscle fiber. At this level of –55 millivolts, the fast sodium channels mainly have already become "inactivated," which means that they have become blocked. The cause of this is that any time the membrane potential remains less negative than about –55 millivolts for more than a few milliseconds, the inactivation gates on the inside of the cell membrane that close the fast sodium channels become closed and remain so. Therefore, only the slow sodium-calcium channels can open (i.e., can become "activated")

and thereby cause the action potential. As a result, the atrial nodal action potential is slower to develop than the action potential of the ventricular muscle. Also, after the action potential does occur, return of the potential to its negative state occurs slowly as well, rather than the abrupt return that occurs for the ventricular fiber.

Self-Excitation of Sinus Nodal Fibers. Because of the high sodium ion concentration in the extracellular fluid outside the nodal fiber, as well as a moderate number of already open sodium channels, positive sodium ions from outside the fibers normally tend to leak to the inside. Therefore, between heartbeats, influx of positively charged sodium ions causes a slow rise in the resting membrane potential in the positive direction. Thus, as shown in Figure 10-2, the "resting" potential gradually rises and becomes less negative between each two heartbeats. When the potential reaches a threshold voltage of about –40 millivolts, the sodium-calcium channels become "activated," thus causing the action potential. Therefore, basically, the inherent leakiness of the sinus nodal fibers to sodium and calcium ions causes their self-excitation.

Why does this leakiness to sodium and calcium ions not cause the sinus nodal fibers to remain depolarized all the time? The answer is that two events occur during the course of the action potential to prevent this. First, the sodium-calcium channels become inactivated (i.e., they close) within about 100 to 150 milliseconds after opening, and second, at about the same time, greatly increased numbers of potassium channels open. Therefore, influx of positive calcium and sodium ions through the sodium-calcium channels ceases, while at the same time large quantities of positive potassium ions diffuse out of the fiber. Both of these effects reduce the intracellular potential back to its negative resting level and therefore terminate the action potential. Furthermore, the potassium channels remain open for another few tenths of a second, temporarily continuing movement of positive charges out of the cell, with resultant excess negativity inside the fiber; this is called *hyperpolarization.* The hyperpolarization state initially carries the "resting" membrane potential down to about –55 to –60 millivolts at the termination of the action potential.

Why is this new state of hyperpolarization not maintained forever? The reason is that during the next few tenths of a second after the action potential is over, progressively more and more potassium channels close. The inward-leaking sodium and calcium ions once again overbalance the outward flux of potassium ions, and this causes the "resting" potential to drift upward once more, finally reaching the threshold level for discharge at a potential of about –40 millivolts. Then the entire process begins again: self-excitation to cause the action potential, recovery from the action potential, hyperpolarization after the action potential is over, drift of the "resting" potential to threshold, and finally re-excitation to elicit another cycle. This process continues indefinitely throughout a person's life.

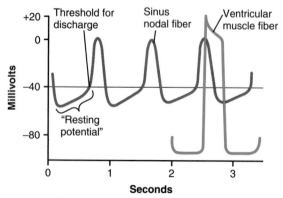

Figure 10-2 Rhythmical discharge of a sinus nodal fiber. Also, the sinus nodal action potential is compared with that of a ventricular muscle fiber.

Internodal Pathways and Transmission of the Cardiac Impulse Through the Atria

The ends of the sinus nodal fibers connect directly with surrounding atrial muscle fibers. Therefore, action potentials originating in the sinus node travel outward into these atrial muscle fibers. In this way, the action potential spreads through the entire atrial muscle mass and, eventually, to the A-V node. The velocity of conduction in most atrial muscle is about 0.3 m/sec, but conduction is more rapid, about 1 m/sec, in several small bands of atrial fibers. One of these, called the *anterior interatrial band,* passes through the anterior walls of the atria to the left atrium. In addition, three other small bands curve through the anterior, lateral, and posterior atrial walls and terminate in the A-V node; shown in Figures 10-1 and 10-3, these are called, respectively, the *anterior, middle, and posterior internodal pathways.* The cause of more rapid velocity of conduction in these bands is the presence of specialized conduction fibers. These fibers are similar to even more rapidly conducting "Purkinje fibers" of the ventricles, which are discussed as follows.

Atrioventricular Node and Delay of Impulse Conduction from the Atria to the Ventricles

The atrial conductive system is organized so that the cardiac impulse does not travel from the atria into the ventricles too rapidly; this delay allows time for the atria to empty their blood into the ventricles before ventricular contraction begins. It is primarily the A-V node and its adjacent conductive fibers that delay this transmission into the ventricles.

The A-V node is located in the posterior wall of the right atrium immediately behind the tricuspid valve, as shown in Figure 10-1. And Figure 10-3 shows diagrammatically the different parts of this node, plus its connections with the entering atrial internodal pathway fibers and the exiting A-V bundle. The figure also shows the approximate intervals of time in fractions of a second between initial onset of the cardiac impulse in the sinus node and its subsequent appearance in the A-V nodal system. Note that the impulse, after traveling through the internodal pathways, reaches the A-V node about 0.03 second after its origin in the sinus node. Then there is a delay of another 0.09 second in the A-V node itself before the impulse enters the penetrating portion of the A-V bundle, where it passes into the ventricles. A final delay of another 0.04 second occurs mainly in this penetrating A-V bundle, which is composed of multiple small fascicles passing through the fibrous tissue separating the atria from the ventricles.

Thus, the total delay in the A-V nodal and A-V bundle system is about 0.13 second. This, in addition to the initial conduction delay of 0.03 second from the sinus node to the A-V node, makes a total delay of 0.16 second before the excitatory signal finally reaches the contracting muscle of the ventricles.

Cause of the Slow Conduction. The slow conduction in the transitional, nodal, and penetrating A-V bundle fibers is caused mainly by diminished numbers of gap junctions between successive cells in the conducting pathways, so there is great resistance to conduction of excitatory ions from one conducting fiber to the next. Therefore, it is easy to see why each succeeding cell is slow to be excited.

Rapid Transmission in the Ventricular Purkinje System

Special Purkinje fibers lead from the A-V node through the A-V bundle into the ventricles. Except for the initial portion of these fibers where they penetrate the A-V fibrous barrier, they have functional characteristics that are quite the opposite of those of the A-V nodal fibers. They are very large fibers, even larger than the normal ventricular muscle fibers, and they transmit action potentials at a velocity of 1.5 to 4.0 m/sec, a velocity about 6 times that in the usual ventricular muscle and 150 times that in some of the A-V nodal fibers. This allows almost instantaneous transmission of the cardiac impulse throughout the entire remainder of the ventricular muscle.

The rapid transmission of action potentials by Purkinje fibers is believed to be caused by a very high level of permeability of the gap junctions at the intercalated discs between the successive cells that make up the Purkinje fibers. Therefore, ions are transmitted easily from one cell to the next, thus enhancing the velocity of transmission. The Purkinje fibers also have very few myofibrils, which means that they contract little or not at all during the course of impulse transmission.

One-Way Conduction Through the A-V Bundle. A special characteristic of the A-V bundle is the inability, except in abnormal states, of action potentials to travel backward from the ventricles to the atria. This prevents re-entry of cardiac impulses by this route from

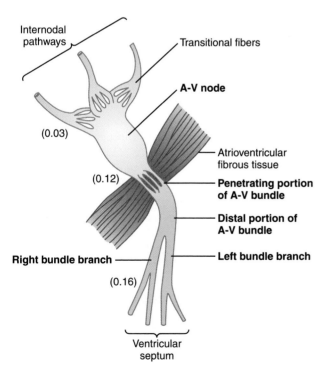

Internodal pathways

Transitional fibers

A-V node

(0.03)

Atrioventricular fibrous tissue

(0.12)

Penetrating portion of A-V bundle

Distal portion of A-V bundle

Right bundle branch

Left bundle branch

(0.16)

Ventricular septum

Figure 10-3 Organization of the A-V node. The numbers represent the interval of time from the origin of the impulse in the sinus node. The values have been extrapolated to human beings.

the ventricles to the atria, allowing only forward conduction from the atria to the ventricles.

Furthermore, it should be recalled that everywhere, except at the A-V bundle, the atrial muscle is separated from the ventricular muscle by a continuous fibrous barrier, a portion of which is shown in Figure 10-3. This barrier normally acts as an insulator to prevent passage of the cardiac impulse between atrial and ventricular muscle through any other route besides forward conduction through the A-V bundle itself. (In rare instances, an abnormal muscle bridge does penetrate the fibrous barrier elsewhere besides at the A-V bundle. Under such conditions, the cardiac impulse can re-enter the atria from the ventricles and cause a serious cardiac arrhythmia.)

Distribution of the Purkinje Fibers in the Ventricles— The Left and Right Bundle Branches. After penetrating the fibrous tissue between the atrial and ventricular muscle, the distal portion of the A-V bundle passes downward in the ventricular septum for 5 to 15 millimeters toward the apex of the heart, as shown in Figures 10-1 and 10-3. Then the bundle divides into left and right bundle branches that lie beneath the endocardium on the two respective sides of the ventricular septum. Each branch spreads downward toward the apex of the ventricle, progressively dividing into smaller branches. These branches in turn course sidewise around each ventricular chamber and back toward the base of the heart. The ends of the Purkinje fibers penetrate about one third of the way into the muscle mass and finally become continuous with the cardiac muscle fibers.

From the time the cardiac impulse enters the bundle branches in the ventricular septum until it reaches the terminations of the Purkinje fibers, the total elapsed time averages only 0.03 second. Therefore, once the cardiac impulse enters the ventricular Purkinje conductive system, it spreads almost immediately to the entire ventricular muscle mass.

Transmission of the Cardiac Impulse in the Ventricular Muscle

Once the impulse reaches the ends of the Purkinje fibers, it is transmitted through the ventricular muscle mass by the ventricular muscle fibers themselves. The velocity of transmission is now only 0.3 to 0.5 m/sec, one sixth that in the Purkinje fibers.

The cardiac muscle wraps around the heart in a double spiral, with fibrous septa between the spiraling layers; therefore, the cardiac impulse does not necessarily travel directly outward toward the surface of the heart but instead angulates toward the surface along the directions of the spirals. Because of this, transmission from the endocardial surface to the epicardial surface of the ventricle requires as much as another 0.03 second, approximately equal to the time required for transmission through the entire ventricular portion of the Purkinje system. Thus, the total time for transmission of the cardiac impulse from the initial bundle branches to the last of the ventricular muscle fibers in the normal heart is about 0.06 second.

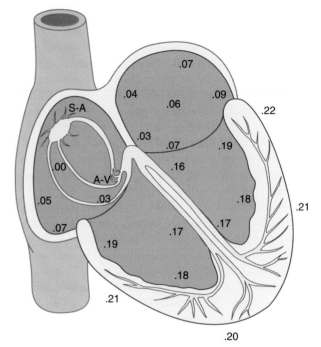

Figure 10-4 Transmission of the cardiac impulse through the heart, showing the time of appearance (in fractions of a second after initial appearance at the sinoatrial node) in different parts of the heart.

Summary of the Spread of the Cardiac Impulse Through the Heart

Figure 10-4 shows in summary form the transmission of the cardiac impulse through the human heart. The numbers on the figure represent the intervals of time, in fractions of a second, that lapse between the origin of the cardiac impulse in the sinus node and its appearance at each respective point in the heart. Note that the impulse spreads at moderate velocity through the atria but is delayed more than 0.1 second in the A-V nodal region before appearing in the ventricular septal A-V bundle. Once it has entered this bundle, it spreads very rapidly through the Purkinje fibers to the entire endocardial surfaces of the ventricles. Then the impulse once again spreads slightly less rapidly through the ventricular muscle to the epicardial surfaces.

It is important that the student learn in detail the course of the cardiac impulse through the heart and the precise times of its appearance in each separate part of the heart, because a thorough quantitative knowledge of this process is essential to the understanding of electrocardiography, which is discussed in Chapters 11 through 13.

Control of Excitation and Conduction in the Heart

Sinus Node as the Pacemaker of the Heart

In the discussion thus far of the genesis and transmission of the cardiac impulse through the heart, we have noted that the impulse normally arises in the sinus node. In some abnormal conditions, this is not the case. Other parts of the heart can also exhibit intrinsic rhythmical excitation in the same way that the sinus nodal fibers do; this is particularly true of the A-V nodal and Purkinje fibers.

The A-V nodal fibers, when not stimulated from some outside source, discharge at an intrinsic rhythmical rate of 40 to 60 times per minute, and the Purkinje fibers discharge at a rate somewhere between 15 and 40 times per minute. These rates are in contrast to the normal rate of the sinus node of 70 to 80 times per minute.

Why then does the sinus node rather than the A-V node or the Purkinje fibers control the heart's rhythmicity? The answer derives from the fact that the discharge rate of the sinus node is considerably faster than the natural self-excitatory discharge rate of either the A-V node or the Purkinje fibers. Each time the sinus node discharges, its impulse is conducted into both the A-V node and the Purkinje fibers, also discharging their excitable membranes. But the sinus node discharges again before either the A-V node or the Purkinje fibers can reach their own thresholds for self-excitation. Therefore, the new impulse from the sinus node discharges both the A-V node and the Purkinje fibers before self-excitation can occur in either of these.

Thus, the sinus node controls the beat of the heart because its rate of rhythmical discharge is faster than that of any other part of the heart. Therefore, the sinus node is virtually always the pacemaker of the normal heart.

Abnormal Pacemakers—"Ectopic" Pacemaker. Occasionally some other part of the heart develops a rhythmical discharge rate that is more rapid than that of the sinus node. For instance, this sometimes occurs in the A-V node or in the Purkinje fibers when one of these becomes abnormal. In either case, the pacemaker of the heart shifts from the sinus node to the A-V node or to the excited Purkinje fibers. Under rarer conditions, a place in the atrial or ventricular muscle develops excessive excitability and becomes the pacemaker.

A pacemaker elsewhere than the sinus node is called an "*ectopic*" *pacemaker.* An ectopic pacemaker causes an abnormal sequence of contraction of the different parts of the heart and can cause significant debility of heart pumping.

Another cause of shift of the pacemaker is blockage of transmission of the cardiac impulse from the sinus node to the other parts of the heart. The new pacemaker then occurs most frequently at the A-V node or in the penetrating portion of the A-V bundle on the way to the ventricles.

When A-V block occurs—that is, when the cardiac impulse fails to pass from the atria into the ventricles through the A-V nodal and bundle system—the atria continue to beat at the normal rate of rhythm of the sinus node, while a new pacemaker usually develops in the Purkinje system of the ventricles and drives the ventricular muscle at a new rate somewhere between 15 and 40 beats per minute. After sudden A-V bundle block, the Purkinje system does not begin to emit its intrinsic

rhythmical impulses until 5 to 20 seconds later because, before the blockage, the Purkinje fibers had been "overdriven" by the rapid sinus impulses and, consequently, are in a suppressed state. During these 5 to 20 seconds, the ventricles fail to pump blood, and the person faints after the first 4 to 5 seconds because of lack of blood flow to the brain. This delayed pickup of the heartbeat is called *Stokes-Adams syndrome.* If the delay period is too long, it can lead to death.

Role of the Purkinje System in Causing Synchronous Contraction of the Ventricular Muscle

It is clear from our description of the Purkinje system that normally the cardiac impulse arrives at almost all portions of the ventricles within a narrow span of time, exciting the first ventricular muscle fiber only 0.03 to 0.06 second ahead of excitation of the last ventricular muscle fiber. This causes all portions of the ventricular muscle in both ventricles to begin contracting at almost the same time and then to continue contracting for about another 0.3 second.

Effective pumping by the two ventricular chambers requires this synchronous type of contraction. If the cardiac impulse should travel through the ventricles slowly, much of the ventricular mass would contract before contraction of the remainder, in which case the overall pumping effect would be greatly depressed. Indeed, in some types of cardiac debilities, several of which are discussed in Chapters 12 and 13, slow transmission does occur, and the pumping effectiveness of the ventricles is decreased as much as 20 to 30 percent.

Control of Heart Rhythmicity and Impulse Conduction by the Cardiac Nerves: Sympathetic and Parasympathetic Nerves

The heart is supplied with both sympathetic and parasympathetic nerves, as shown in Figure 9-10 of Chapter 9. The parasympathetic nerves (the vagi) are distributed mainly to the S-A and A-V nodes, to a lesser extent to the muscle of the two atria, and very little directly to the ventricular muscle. The sympathetic nerves, conversely, are distributed to all parts of the heart, with strong representation to the ventricular muscle, as well as to all the other areas.

Parasympathetic (Vagal) Stimulation Can Slow or Even Block Cardiac Rhythm and Conduction—"Ventricular Escape." Stimulation of the parasympathetic nerves to the heart (the vagi) causes the hormone *acetylcholine* to be released at the vagal endings. This hormone has two major effects on the heart. First, it decreases the rate of rhythm of the sinus node, and second, it decreases the excitability of the A-V junctional fibers between the atrial musculature and the A-V node, thereby slowing transmission of the cardiac impulse into the ventricles.

Weak to moderate vagal stimulation slows the rate of heart pumping, often to as little as one-half normal.

And strong stimulation of the vagi can stop completely the rhythmical excitation by the sinus node or block completely transmission of the cardiac impulse from the atria into the ventricles through the A-V node. In either case, rhythmical excitatory signals are no longer transmitted into the ventricles. The ventricles stop beating for 5 to 20 seconds, but then some small area in the Purkinje fibers, usually in the ventricular septal portion of the A-V bundle, develops a rhythm of its own and causes ventricular contraction at a rate of 15 to 40 beats per minute. This phenomenon is called *ventricular escape.*

Mechanism of the Vagal Effects. The acetylcholine released at the vagal nerve endings greatly increases the permeability of the fiber membranes to potassium ions, which allows rapid leakage of potassium out of the conductive fibers. This causes increased negativity inside the fibers, an effect called *hyperpolarization,* which makes this excitable tissue much less excitable, as explained in Chapter 5.

In the sinus node, the state of hyperpolarization alters the "resting" membrane potential of the sinus nodal fibers to a level considerably more negative than usual, to −65 to −75 millivolts rather than the normal level of −55 to −60 millivolts. Therefore, the initial rise of the sinus nodal membrane potential caused by inward sodium and calcium leakage requires much longer to reach the threshold potential for excitation. This greatly slows the rate of rhythmicity of these nodal fibers. If the vagal stimulation is strong enough, it is possible to stop entirely the rhythmical self-excitation of this node.

In the A-V node, a state of hyperpolarization caused by vagal stimulation makes it difficult for the small atrial fibers entering the node to generate enough electricity to excite the nodal fibers. Therefore, the safety factor for transmission of the cardiac impulse through the transitional fibers into the A-V nodal fibers decreases. A moderate decrease simply delays conduction of the impulse, but a large decrease blocks conduction entirely.

Effect of Sympathetic Stimulation on Cardiac Rhythm and Conduction. Sympathetic stimulation causes essentially the opposite effects on the heart to those caused by vagal stimulation, as follows: First, it increases the rate of sinus nodal discharge. Second, it increases the rate of conduction, as well as the level of excitability in all portions of the heart. Third, it increases greatly the force of contraction of all the cardiac musculature, both atrial and ventricular, as discussed in Chapter 9.

In short, sympathetic stimulation increases the overall activity of the heart. Maximal stimulation can almost triple the frequency of heartbeat and can increase the strength of heart contraction as much as twofold.

Mechanism of the Sympathetic Effect. Stimulation of the sympathetic nerves releases the hormone *norepineph-* *rine* at the sympathetic nerve endings. Norepinephrine in turn stimulates *beta-1 adrenergic receptors,* which mediate the effects on heart rate. The precise mechanism by which beta-1 adrenergic stimulation acts on cardiac muscle fibers is somewhat unclear, but the belief is that it increases the permeability of the fiber membrane to sodium and calcium ions. In the sinus node, an increase of sodium-calcium permeability causes a more positive resting potential and also causes increased rate of upward drift of the diastolic membrane potential toward the threshold level for self-excitation, thus accelerating self-excitation and, therefore, increasing the heart rate.

In the A-V node and A-V bundles, increased sodium-calcium permeability makes it easier for the action potential to excite each succeeding portion of the conducting fiber bundles, thereby decreasing the conduction time from the atria to the ventricles.

The increase in permeability to calcium ions is at least partially responsible for the increase in contractile strength of the cardiac muscle under the influence of sympathetic stimulation, because calcium ions play a powerful role in exciting the contractile process of the myofibrils.

Bibliography

Barbuti A, DiFrancesco D: Control of cardiac rate by "funny" channels in health and disease, *Ann N Y Acad Sci* 1123:213, 2008.

Baruscotti M, Robinson RB: Electrophysiology and pacemaker function of the developing sinoatrial node, *Am J Physiol Heart Circ Physiol* 293:H2613, 2007.

Cheng H, Lederer WJ: Calcium sparks, *Physiol Rev* 88:1491, 2008.

Chien KR, Domian IJ, Parker KK: Cardiogenesis and the complex biology of regenerative cardiovascular medicine, *Science* 322:1494, 2008.

Dobrzynski H, Boyett MR, Anderson RH: New insights into pacemaker activity: promoting understanding of sick sinus syndrome, *Circulation* 115:1921, 2007.

James TN: Structure and function of the sinus node, AV node and His bundle of the human heart: part I—structure, *Prog Cardiovasc Dis* 45:235, 2002.

James TN: Structure and function of the sinus node, AV node and His bundle of the human heart: part II—function, *Prog Cardiovasc Dis* 45:327, 2003.

Kléber AG, Rudy Y: Basic mechanisms of cardiac impulse propagation and associated arrhythmias, *Physiol Rev* 84:431, 2004.

Lakatta EG, Vinogradova TM, Maltsev VA: The missing link in the mystery of normal automaticity of cardiac pacemaker cells, *Ann N Y Acad Sci* 1123:41, 2008.

Leclercq C, Hare JM: Ventricular resynchronization: current state of the art, *Circulation* 109:296, 2004.

Mangoni ME, Nargeot J: Genesis and regulation of the heart automaticity, *Physiol Rev* 88:919, 2008.

Mazgalev TN, Ho SY, Anderson RH: Anatomic-electrophysiological correlations concerning the pathways for atrioventricular conduction, *Circulation* 103:2660, 2001.

Schram G, Pourrier M, Melnyk P, et al: Differential distribution of cardiac ion channel expression as a basis for regional specialization in electrical function, *Circ Res* 90:939, 2002.

Yasuma F, Hayano J: Respiratory sinus arrhythmia: why does the heartbeat synchronize with respiratory rhythm? *Chest* 125:683, 2004.

The Normal Electrocardiogram

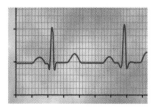

When the cardiac impulse passes through the heart, electrical current also spreads from the heart into the adjacent tissues surrounding the heart. A small portion of the current spreads all the way to the surface of the body. If electrodes are placed on the skin on opposite sides of the heart, electrical potentials generated by the current can be recorded; the recording is known as an electrocardiogram. A normal electrocardiogram for two beats of the heart is shown in Figure 11-1.

Characteristics of the Normal Electrocardiogram

The normal electrocardiogram (see Figure 11-1) is composed of a P wave, a QRS complex, and a T wave. The QRS complex is often, but not always, three separate waves: the Q wave, the R wave, and the S wave.

The P wave is caused by electrical potentials generated when the atria depolarize before atrial contraction begins. The QRS complex is caused by potentials generated when the ventricles depolarize before contraction, that is, as the depolarization wave spreads through the ventricles. Therefore, both the P wave and the components of the QRS complex are *depolarization waves*.

The T wave is caused by potentials generated as the ventricles recover from the state of depolarization. This process normally occurs in ventricular muscle 0.25 to 0.35 second after depolarization, and the T wave is known as a *repolarization wave.*

Thus, the electrocardiogram is composed of both depolarization and repolarization waves. The principles of depolarization and repolarization are discussed in Chapter 5. The distinction between depolarization waves and repolarization waves is so important in electrocardiography that further clarification is necessary.

Depolarization Waves versus Repolarization Waves

Figure 11-2 shows a single cardiac muscle fiber in four stages of depolarization and repolarization, the color red designating depolarization. During depolarization, the normal negative potential inside the fiber reverses and becomes slightly positive inside and negative outside.

In Figure 11-2A, depolarization, demonstrated by red positive charges inside and red negative charges outside, is traveling from left to right. The first half of the fiber has already depolarized, while the remaining half is still polarized. Therefore, the left electrode on the outside of the fiber is in an area of negativity, and the right electrode is in an area of positivity; this causes the meter to record positively. To the right of the muscle fiber is shown a record

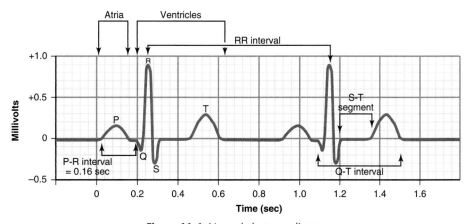

Figure 11-1 Normal electrocardiogram.

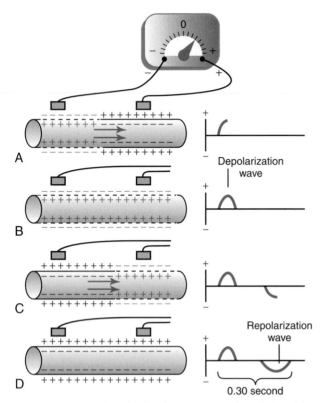

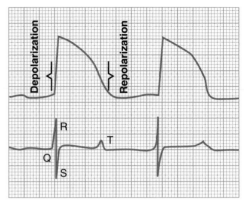

Figure 11-3 *Above,* Monophasic action potential from a ventricular muscle fiber during normal cardiac function, showing rapid depolarization and then repolarization occurring slowly during the plateau stage but rapidly toward the end. *Below,* Electrocardiogram recorded simultaneously.

Figure 11-2 Recording the depolarization wave (*A* and *B*) and the repolarization wave (*C* and *D*) from a cardiac muscle fiber.

of changes in potential between the two electrodes, as recorded by a high-speed recording meter. Note that when depolarization has reached the halfway mark in Figure 11-2*A*, the record has risen to a maximum positive value.

In Figure 11-2*B*, depolarization has extended over the entire muscle fiber, and the recording to the right has returned to the zero baseline because both electrodes are now in areas of equal negativity. The completed wave is a depolarization wave because it results from spread of depolarization along the muscle fiber membrane.

Figure 11-2*C* shows halfway repolarization of the same muscle fiber, with positivity returning to the outside of the fiber. At this point, the left electrode is in an area of positivity, and the right electrode is in an area of negativity. This is opposite to the polarity in Figure 11-2*A*. Consequently, the recording, as shown to the right, becomes negative.

In Figure 11-2*D*, the muscle fiber has completely repolarized, and both electrodes are now in areas of positivity so that no potential difference is recorded between them. Thus, in the recording to the right, the potential returns once more to zero. This completed negative wave is a repolarization wave because it results from spread of repolarization along the muscle fiber membrane.

Relation of the Monophasic Action Potential of Ventricular Muscle to the QRS and T Waves in the Standard Electrocardiogram. The monophasic action potential of ventricular muscle, discussed in Chapter 10, normally lasts between 0.25 and 0.35 second. The top part of Figure 11-3 shows a monophasic action potential

recorded from a microelectrode inserted to the inside of a single ventricular muscle fiber. The upsweep of this action potential is caused by depolarization, and the return of the potential to the baseline is caused by repolarization.

Note in the lower half of the figure a simultaneous recording of the electrocardiogram from this same ventricle, which shows the QRS waves appearing at the beginning of the monophasic action potential and the T wave appearing at the end. Note especially that *no potential is recorded in the electrocardiogram when the ventricular muscle is either completely polarized or completely depolarized.* Only when the muscle is partly polarized and partly depolarized does current flow from one part of the ventricles to another part and therefore current also flows to the surface of the body to produce the electrocardiogram.

Relationship of Atrial and Ventricular Contraction to the Waves of the Electrocardiogram

Before contraction of muscle can occur, depolarization must spread through the muscle to initiate the chemical processes of contraction. Refer again to Figure 11-1; the P wave occurs at the beginning of contraction of the atria, and the QRS complex of waves occurs at the beginning of contraction of the ventricles. The ventricles remain contracted until after repolarization has occurred, that is, until after the end of the T wave.

The atria repolarize about 0.15 to 0.20 second after termination of the P wave. This is also approximately when the QRS complex is being recorded in the electrocardiogram. Therefore, the atrial repolarization wave, known as the *atrial T wave,* is usually obscured by the much larger QRS complex. For this reason, an atrial T wave seldom is observed in the electrocardiogram.

The ventricular repolarization wave is the T wave of the normal electrocardiogram. Ordinarily, ventricular muscle begins to repolarize in some fibers about 0.20 second after the beginning of the depolarization wave (the QRS complex), but in many other fibers, it takes as long as 0.35 second. Thus, the process of ventricular repolarization extends over a long period, about 0.15 second. For this reason, the T wave in the normal electrocardiogram is a prolonged wave, but the voltage of the T wave is considerably less than the voltage of the QRS complex, partly because of its prolonged length.

Voltage and Time Calibration of the Electrocardiogram

All recordings of electrocardiograms are made with appropriate calibration lines on the recording paper. Either these calibration lines are already ruled on the paper, as is the case when a pen recorder is used, or they are recorded on the paper at the same time that the electrocardiogram is recorded, which is the case with the photographic types of electrocardiographs.

As shown in Figure 11-1, the horizontal calibration lines are arranged so that 10 of the small line divisions upward or downward in the standard electrocardiogram represent 1 millivolt, with positivity in the upward direction and negativity in the downward direction.

The vertical lines on the electrocardiogram are time calibration lines. A typical electrocardiogram is run at a paper speed of 25 millimeters per second, although faster speeds are sometimes used. Therefore, each 25 millimeters in the horizontal direction is 1 second, and each 5-millimeter segment, indicated by the dark vertical lines, represents 0.20 second. The 0.20-second intervals are then broken into five smaller intervals by thin lines, each of which represents 0.04 second.

Normal Voltages in the Electrocardiogram. The recorded voltages of the waves in the normal electrocardiogram depend on the manner in which the electrodes are applied to the surface of the body and how close the electrodes are to the heart. When one electrode is placed directly over the ventricles and a second electrode is placed elsewhere on the body remote from the heart, the voltage of the QRS complex may be as great as 3 to 4 millivolts. Even this voltage is small in comparison with the monophasic action potential of 110 millivolts recorded directly at the heart muscle membrane. When electrocardiograms are recorded from electrodes on the two arms or on one arm and one leg, the voltage of the QRS complex usually is 1.0 to 1.5 millivolts from the top of the R wave to the bottom of the S wave; the voltage of the P wave is between 0.1 and 0.3 millivolts; and that of the T wave is between 0.2 and 0.3 millivolts.

P-Q or P-R Interval. The time between the beginning of the P wave and the beginning of the QRS complex is the interval between the beginning of electrical excitation of the atria and the beginning of excitation of the ventricles. This period is called the *P-Q interval*. The normal P-Q interval is about 0.16 second. (Often this interval is called the *P-R interval* because the Q wave is likely to be absent.)

Q-T Interval. Contraction of the ventricle lasts almost from the beginning of the Q wave (or R wave, if the Q wave is absent) to the end of the T wave. This interval is called the *Q-T interval* and ordinarily is about 0.35 second.

Rate of Heartbeat as Determined from the Electrocardiogram. The rate of heartbeat can be determined easily from an electrocardiogram because the heart rate is the reciprocal of the time interval between two successive heartbeats. If the interval between two beats as determined from the time calibration lines is 1 second, the heart rate is 60 beats per minute. The normal interval between two successive QRS complexes in the adult person is about 0.83 second. This is a heart rate of 60/0.83 times per minute, or 72 beats per minute.

Methods for Recording Electrocardiograms

Sometimes the electrical currents generated by the cardiac muscle during each beat of the heart change electrical potentials and polarities on the respective sides of the heart in less than 0.01 second. Therefore, it is essential that any apparatus for recording electrocardiograms be capable of responding rapidly to these changes in potentials.

Recorders for Electrocardiographs

Many modern clinical electrocardiographs use computer-based systems and electronic display, whereas others use a direct pen recorder that writes the electrocardiogram with a pen directly on a moving sheet of paper. Sometimes the pen is a thin tube connected at one end to an inkwell, and its recording end is connected to a powerful electromagnet system that is capable of moving the pen back and forth at high speed. As the paper moves forward, the pen records the electrocardiogram. The movement of the pen is controlled by appropriate electronic amplifiers connected to electrocardiographic electrodes on the patient.

Other pen recording systems use special paper that does not require ink in the recording stylus. One such paper turns black when it is exposed to heat; the stylus itself is made very hot by electrical current flowing through its tip. Another type turns black when electrical current flows from the tip of the stylus through the paper to an electrode at its back. This leaves a black line on the paper where the stylus touches.

Flow of Current Around the Heart during the Cardiac Cycle

Recording Electrical Potentials from a Partially Depolarized Mass of Syncytial Cardiac Muscle

Figure 11-4 shows a syncytial mass of cardiac muscle that has been stimulated at its centralmost point. Before stimulation, all the exteriors of the muscle cells had been positive and the interiors negative. For reasons presented in Chapter 5 in the discussion of membrane potentials, as soon as an area of cardiac syncytium becomes depolarized, negative charges leak to the outsides of the depolarized muscle fibers, making this part of the surface

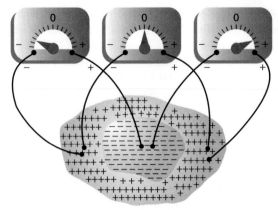

Figure 11-4 Instantaneous potentials develop on the surface of a cardiac muscle mass that has been depolarized in its center.

electronegative, as represented by the negative signs in Figure 11-4. The remaining surface of the heart, which is still polarized, is represented by the positive signs. Therefore, a meter connected with its negative terminal on the area of depolarization and its positive terminal on one of the still-polarized areas, as shown to the right in the figure, records positively.

Two other electrode placements and meter readings are also demonstrated in Figure 11-4. These should be studied carefully, and the reader should be able to explain the causes of the respective meter readings. Because the depolarization spreads in all directions through the heart, the potential differences shown in the figure persist for only a few thousandths of a second, and the actual voltage measurements can be accomplished only with a high-speed recording apparatus.

Flow of Electrical Currents in the Chest Around the Heart

Figure 11-5 shows the ventricular muscle lying within the chest. Even the lungs, although mostly filled with air, conduct electricity to a surprising extent, and fluids in other tissues surrounding the heart conduct electricity even more easily. Therefore, the heart is actually suspended in a conductive medium. When one portion of the ventricles depolarizes and therefore becomes electronegative with respect to the remainder, electrical current flows from the depolarized area to the polarized area in large circuitous routes, as noted in the figure.

It should be recalled from the discussion of the Purkinje system in Chapter 10 that the cardiac impulse first arrives in the ventricles in the septum and shortly thereafter spreads to the inside surfaces of the remainder of the ventricles, as shown by the red areas and the negative signs in Figure 11-5. This provides electronegativity on the insides of the ventricles and electropositivity on the outer walls of the ventricles, with electrical current flowing through the fluids surrounding the ventricles along elliptical paths, as demonstrated by the curving arrows in the figure. If one algebraically averages all the lines of current flow (the elliptical lines), one finds that *the*

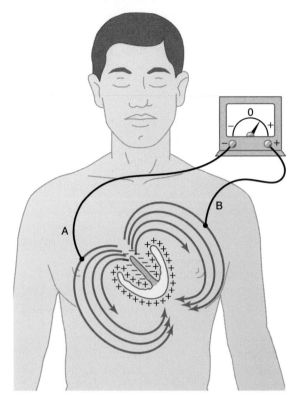

Figure 11-5 Flow of current in the chest around partially depolarized ventricles.

average current flow occurs with negativity toward the base of the heart and with positivity toward the apex.

During most of the remainder of the depolarization process, current also continues to flow in this same direction, while depolarization spreads from the endocardial surface outward through the ventricular muscle mass. Then, immediately before depolarization has completed its course through the ventricles, the average direction of current flow reverses for about 0.01 second, flowing from the ventricular apex toward the base, because the last part of the heart to become depolarized is the outer walls of the ventricles near the base of the heart.

Thus, in normal heart ventricles, current flows from negative to positive primarily in the direction from the base of the heart toward the apex during almost the entire cycle of depolarization, except at the very end. And if a meter is connected to electrodes on the surface of the body as shown in Figure 11-5, the electrode nearer the base will be negative, whereas the electrode nearer the apex will be positive, and the recording meter will show positive recording in the electrocardiogram.

Electrocardiographic Leads

Three Bipolar Limb Leads

Figure 11-6 shows electrical connections between the patient's limbs and the electrocardiograph for recording electrocardiograms from the so-called *standard bipolar*

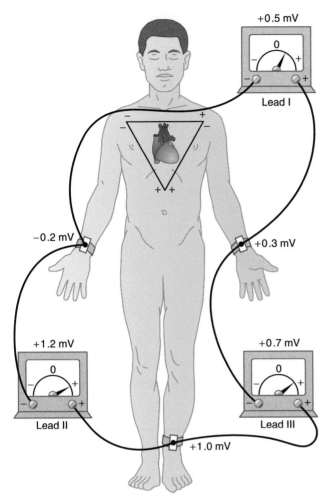

Figure 11-6 Conventional arrangement of electrodes for recording the standard electrocardiographic leads. Einthoven's triangle is superimposed on the chest.

limb leads. The term "bipolar" means that the electrocardiogram is recorded from two electrodes located on different sides of the heart—in this case, on the limbs. Thus, a "lead" is not a single wire connecting from the body but a combination of two wires and their electrodes to make a complete circuit between the body and the electrocardiograph. The electrocardiograph in each instance is represented by an electrical meter in the diagram, although the actual electrocardiograph is a high-speed recording meter with a moving paper.

Lead I. In recording limb lead I, the negative terminal of the electrocardiograph is connected to the right arm and the positive terminal to the left arm. Therefore, when the point where the right arm connects to the chest is electronegative with respect to the point where the left arm connects, the electrocardiograph records positively, that is, above the zero voltage line in the electrocardiogram. When the opposite is true, the electrocardiograph records below the line.

Lead II. To record limb lead II, the negative terminal of the electrocardiograph is connected to the right arm and the positive terminal to the left leg. Therefore, when the right arm is negative with respect to the left leg, the electrocardiograph records positively.

Lead III. To record limb lead III, the negative terminal of the electrocardiograph is connected to the left arm and the positive terminal to the left leg. This means that the electrocardiograph records positively when the left arm is negative with respect to the left leg.

Einthoven's Triangle. In Figure 11-6, the triangle, called *Einthoven's triangle*, is drawn around the area of the heart. This illustrates that the two arms and the left leg form apices of a triangle surrounding the heart. The two apices at the upper part of the triangle represent the points at which the two arms connect electrically with the fluids around the heart, and the lower apex is the point at which the left leg connects with the fluids.

Einthoven's Law. Einthoven's law states that if the electrical potentials of any two of the three bipolar limb electrocardiographic leads are known at any given instant, the third one can be determined mathematically by simply summing the first two. Note, however, that the positive and negative signs of the different leads must be observed when making this summation.

For instance, let us assume that momentarily, as noted in Figure 11-6, the right arm is –0.2 millivolts (negative) with respect to the average potential in the body, the left arm is +0.3 millivolts (positive), and the left leg is +1.0 millivolts (positive). Observing the meters in the figure, one can see that lead I records a positive potential of +0.5 millivolts because this is the difference between the –0.2 millivolts on the right arm and the +0.3 millivolts on the left arm. Similarly, lead III records a positive potential of +0.7 millivolts, and lead II records a positive potential of +1.2 millivolts because these are the instantaneous potential differences between the respective pairs of limbs.

Now, note that the sum of the voltages in leads I and III equals the voltage in lead II; that is, 0.5 plus 0.7 equals 1.2. Mathematically, this principle, called Einthoven's law, holds true at any given instant while the three "standard" bipolar electrocardiograms are being recorded.

Normal Electrocardiograms Recorded from the Three Standard Bipolar Limb Leads. Figure 11-7 shows recordings of the electrocardiograms in leads I, II, and III. It is obvious that the electrocardiograms in these three leads are similar to one another because they all record positive P waves and positive T waves, and the major portion of the QRS complex is also positive in each electrocardiogram.

On analysis of the three electrocardiograms, it can be shown, with careful measurements and proper observance of polarities, that at any given instant the sum of the potentials in leads I and III equals the potential in lead II, thus illustrating the validity of Einthoven's law.

Because the recordings from all the bipolar limb leads are similar to one another, it does not matter greatly which lead is recorded when one wants to diagnose different cardiac arrhythmias, because diagnosis of arrhythmias depends mainly on the time relations between the different waves of the cardiac cycle. But when one wants to diagnose damage in the ventricular or atrial muscle or in the Purkinje conducting system, it matters greatly which

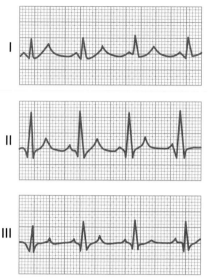

Figure 11-7 Normal electrocardiograms recorded from the three standard electrocardiographic leads.

leads are recorded, because abnormalities of cardiac muscle contraction or cardiac impulse conduction do change the patterns of the electrocardiograms markedly in some leads yet may not affect other leads. Electrocardiographic interpretation of these two types of conditions—cardiac myopathies and cardiac arrhythmias—is discussed separately in Chapters 12 and 13.

Chest Leads (Precordial Leads)

Often electrocardiograms are recorded with one electrode placed on the anterior surface of the chest directly over the heart at one of the points shown in Figure 11-8. This electrode is connected to the positive terminal of the electrocardiograph, and the negative electrode, called the *indifferent electrode*, is connected through equal electrical resistances to the right arm, left arm, and left leg all at the same time, as also shown in the figure. Usually six standard chest leads are recorded, one at a time, from the anterior chest wall, the chest electrode being placed sequentially at the six points shown in the diagram. The different recordings are known as leads V1, V2, V3, V4, V5, and V6.

Figure 11-9 illustrates the electrocardiograms of the healthy heart as recorded from these six standard chest leads. Because the heart surfaces are close to the chest wall, each chest lead records mainly the electrical potential of the cardiac musculature immediately beneath the electrode. Therefore, relatively minute abnormalities in the ventricles, particularly in the anterior ventricular wall, can cause marked changes in the electrocardiograms recorded from individual chest leads.

In leads V1 and V2, the QRS recordings of the normal heart are mainly negative because, as shown in Figure 11-8, the chest electrode in these leads is nearer to the base of the heart than to the apex, and the base of the heart is the direction of electronegativity during most of

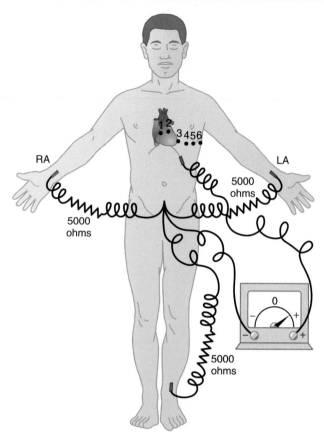

Figure 11-8 Connections of the body with the electrocardiograph for recording chest leads. LA, left arm; RA, right arm.

the ventricular depolarization process. Conversely, the QRS complexes in leads V4, V5, and V6 are mainly positive because the chest electrode in these leads is nearer the heart apex, which is the direction of electropositivity during most of depolarization.

Augmented Unipolar Limb Leads

Another system of leads in wide use is the *augmented unipolar limb lead*. In this type of recording, two of the limbs are connected through electrical resistances to the negative terminal of the electrocardiograph, and the third limb is connected to the positive terminal. When the positive terminal is on the right arm, the lead is known as the aVR lead; when on the left arm, the aVL lead; and when on the left leg, the aVF lead.

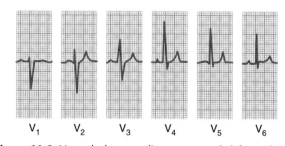

Figure 11-9 Normal electrocardiograms recorded from the six standard chest leads.

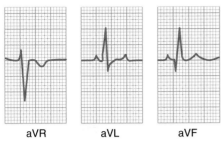

aVR   aVL   aVF

Figure 11-10 Normal electrocardiograms recorded from the three augmented unipolar limb leads.

Normal recordings of the augmented unipolar limb leads are shown in Figure 11-10. They are all similar to the standard limb lead recordings, except that the recording from the aVR lead is inverted. (Why does this inversion occur? Study the polarity connections to the electrocardiograph to determine this.)

Bibliography

See bibliography for Chapter 13.

UNIT III

Electrocardiographic Interpretation of Cardiac Muscle and Coronary Blood Flow Abnormalities: Vectorial Analysis

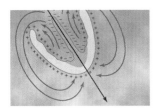

From the discussion in Chapter 10 of impulse transmission through the heart, it is obvious that any change in the pattern of this transmission can cause abnormal electrical potentials around the heart and, consequently, alter the shapes of the waves in the electrocardiogram. For this reason, most serious abnormalities of the heart muscle can be diagnosed by analyzing the contours of the waves in the different electrocardiographic leads.

Principles of Vectorial Analysis of Electrocardiograms

Use of Vectors to Represent Electrical Potentials

Before it is possible to understand how cardiac abnormalities affect the contours of the electrocardiogram, one must first become thoroughly familiar with the concept of *vectors* and *vectorial analysis* as applied to electrical potentials in and around the heart.

Several times in Chapter 11 it was pointed out that heart current flows in a particular direction in the heart at a given instant during the cardiac cycle. A vector is an arrow that points in the direction of the electrical potential generated by the current flow, *with the arrowhead in the positive direction.* Also, by convention, the length of the arrow is drawn *proportional to the voltage of the potential.*

"Resultant" Vector in the Heart at Any Given Instant. Figure 12-1 shows, by the shaded area and the negative signs, depolarization of the ventricular septum and parts of the apical endocardial walls of the two ventricles. At this instant of heart excitation, electrical current flows between the depolarized areas inside the heart and the nondepolarized areas on the outside of the heart, as indicated by the long elliptical arrows. Some current also flows inside the heart chambers directly from the depolarized areas toward the still polarized areas. Overall, considerably more current flows downward from the base of the ventricles toward the apex than in the upward direction. Therefore, the summated vector of the generated potential at this particular instant, called the *instantaneous mean vector,* is represented by the long *black* arrow drawn through the center of the ventricles in a direction from base toward apex. Furthermore, because the summated current is considerable in quantity, the potential is large and the vector is long.

Direction of a Vector Is Denoted in Terms of Degrees

When a vector is exactly horizontal and directed toward the person's left side, the vector is said to extend in the direction of 0 degrees, as shown in Figure 12-2. From this zero reference point, the scale of vectors rotates clockwise: when the vector extends from above and straight downward, it has a direction of +90 degrees; when it extends from the person's left to right, it has a direction of +180 degrees; and when it extends straight upward, it has a direction of −90 (or +270) degrees.

In a normal heart, the average direction of the vector during spread of the depolarization wave through the ventricles, called the *mean QRS vector,* is about +59 degrees, which is shown by vector A drawn through the center of Figure 12-2 in the +59-degree direction. This means that during most of the depolarization wave, the apex of the heart remains positive with respect to the base of the heart, as discussed later in the chapter.

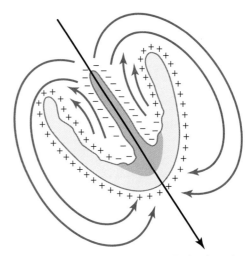

Figure 12-1 Mean vector through the partially depolarized ventricles.

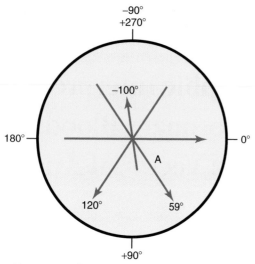

Figure 12-2 Vectors drawn to represent potentials for several different hearts, and the "axis" of the potential (expressed in degrees) for each heart.

Axis for Each Standard Bipolar Lead and Each Unipolar Limb Lead

In Chapter 11, the three standard bipolar and the three unipolar limb leads are described. Each lead is actually a pair of electrodes connected to the body on opposite sides of the heart, and the direction from negative electrode to positive electrode is called the "axis" of the lead. Lead I is recorded from two electrodes placed respectively on the two arms. Because the electrodes lie exactly in the horizontal direction, with the positive electrode to the left, the axis of lead I is 0 degrees.

In recording lead II, electrodes are placed on the right arm and left leg. The right arm connects to the torso in the upper right-hand corner and the left leg connects in the lower left-hand corner. Therefore, the direction of this lead is about +60 degrees.

By similar analysis, it can be seen that lead III has an axis of about +120 degrees; lead aVR, +210 degrees; aVF, +90 degrees; and aVL –30 degrees. The directions of the axes of all these leads are shown in Figure 12-3, which is

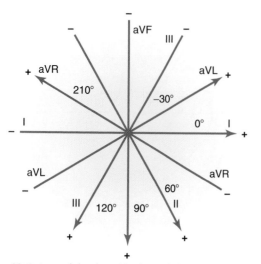

Figure 12-3 Axes of the three bipolar and three unipolar leads.

known as the *hexagonal reference system.* The polarities of the electrodes are shown by the plus and minus signs in the figure. *The reader must learn these axes and their polarities, particularly for the bipolar limb leads I, II, and III, to understand the remainder of this chapter.*

Vectorial Analysis of Potentials Recorded in Different Leads

Now that we have discussed, first, the conventions for representing potentials across the heart by means of vectors and, second, the axes of the leads, it is possible to use these together to determine the instantaneous potential that will be recorded in the electrocardiogram of each lead for a given vector in the heart, as follows.

Figure 12-4 shows a partially depolarized heart; vector *A* represents the instantaneous mean direction of current flow in the ventricles. In this instance, the direction of the vector is +55 degrees, and the voltage of the potential, represented by the length of vector *A,* is 2 mv. In the diagram below the heart, vector *A* is shown again, and a line is drawn to represent the axis of lead I in the 0-degree direction. To determine how much of the voltage in vector *A* will be recorded in lead I, a line perpendicular to the axis of lead I is drawn from the tip of vector *A* to the lead I axis, and a so-called *projected vector (B)* is drawn along the lead I axis. The arrow of this projected vector points toward the positive end of the lead I axis, which means that the record momentarily being recorded in the electrocardiogram of lead I is positive. And the instantaneous recorded voltage will be equal to the length of *B* divided by the length of *A* times 2 millivolts, or about 1 millivolt.

Figure 12-5 shows another example of vectorial analysis. In this example, vector *A* represents the electrical potential and its axis at a given instant during ventricular depolarization in a heart in which the left side of the heart depolarizes more rapidly than the right. In this instance, the instantaneous vector has a direction of 100 degrees, and its voltage is again 2 millivolts. To determine the potential actually recorded in lead I, we draw a perpendicular line from the tip of vector *A* to the lead I axis and find projected vector *B*. Vector *B* is very short and this time in the negative direction, indicating that at this

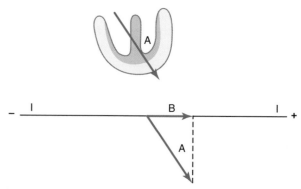

Figure 12-4 Determination of a projected vector B along the axis of lead I when vector A represents the instantaneous potential in the ventricles.

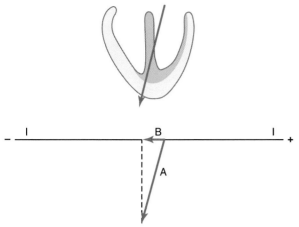

Figure 12-5 Determination of the projected vector B along the axis of lead I when vector A represents the instantaneous potential in the ventricles.

particular instant, the recording in lead I will be negative (below the zero line in the electrocardiogram), and the voltage recorded will be slight, about −0.3 millivolts. This figure demonstrates that *when the vector in the heart is in a direction almost perpendicular to the axis of the lead, the voltage recorded in the electrocardiogram of this lead is very low.* Conversely, *when the heart vector has almost exactly the same axis as the lead axis, essentially the entire voltage of the vector will be recorded.*

Vectorial Analysis of Potentials in the Three Standard Bipolar Limb Leads. In Figure 12-6, vector *A* depicts the instantaneous electrical potential of a partially depolarized heart. To determine the potential recorded at this instant in the electrocardiogram for each one of the three standard bipolar limb leads, perpendicular lines (the dashed lines) are drawn from the tip of vector *A* to the three lines representing the axes of the three different standard leads, as shown in the figure. The projected vector *B* depicts the potential recorded at that instant in lead I, projected vector *C* depicts the potential in lead II, and projected vector *D* depicts the potential in lead III. In each of these, the record in the electrocardiogram is positive—that is,

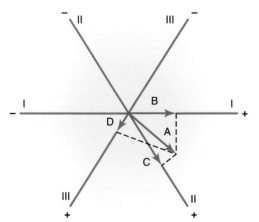

Figure 12-6 Determination of projected vectors in leads I, II, and III when vector A represents the instantaneous potential in the ventricles.

above the zero line—because the projected vectors point in the positive directions along the axes of all the leads. The potential in lead I (vector *B*) is about one-half that of the actual potential in the heart (vector *A*); in lead II (vector *C*), it is almost equal to that in the heart; and in lead III (vector *D*), it is about one-third that in the heart.

An identical analysis can be used to determine potentials recorded in augmented limb leads, except that the respective axes of the augmented leads (see Figure 12-3) are used in place of the standard bipolar limb lead axes used for Figure 12-6.

Vectorial Analysis of the Normal Electrocardiogram

Vectors That Occur at Successive Intervals during Depolarization of the Ventricles—the QRS Complex

When the cardiac impulse enters the ventricles through the atrioventricular bundle, the first part of the ventricles to become depolarized is the left endocardial surface of the septum. Then depolarization spreads rapidly to involve both endocardial surfaces of the septum, as demonstrated by the darker shaded portion of the ventricle in Figure 12-7A. Next, depolarization spreads along the endocardial surfaces of the remainder of the two ventricles, as shown in Figure 12-7B and C. Finally, it spreads through the ventricular muscle to the outside of the heart, as shown progressively in Figure 12-7C, D, and E.

At each stage in Figure 12-7, parts A to E, the instantaneous mean electrical potential of the ventricles is represented by a red vector superimposed on the ventricle in each figure. Each of these vectors is then analyzed by the method described in the preceding section to determine the voltages that will be recorded at each instant in each of the three standard electrocardiographic leads. To the right in each figure is shown progressive development of the electrocardiographic QRS complex. *Keep in mind that a positive vector in a lead will cause recording in the electrocardiogram above the zero line, whereas a negative vector will cause recording below the zero line.*

Before proceeding with further consideration of vectorial analysis, it is essential that this analysis of the successive normal vectors presented in Figure 12-7 be understood. Each of these analyses should be studied in detail by the procedure given here. A short summary of this sequence follows.

In Figure 12-7A, the ventricular muscle has just begun to be depolarized, representing an instant about 0.01 second after the onset of depolarization. At this time, the vector is short because only a small portion of the ventricles—the septum—is depolarized. Therefore, all electrocardiographic voltages are low, as recorded to the right of the ventricular muscle for each of the leads. The voltage in lead II is greater than the voltages in leads I and III because the heart vector extends mainly in the same direction as the axis of lead II.

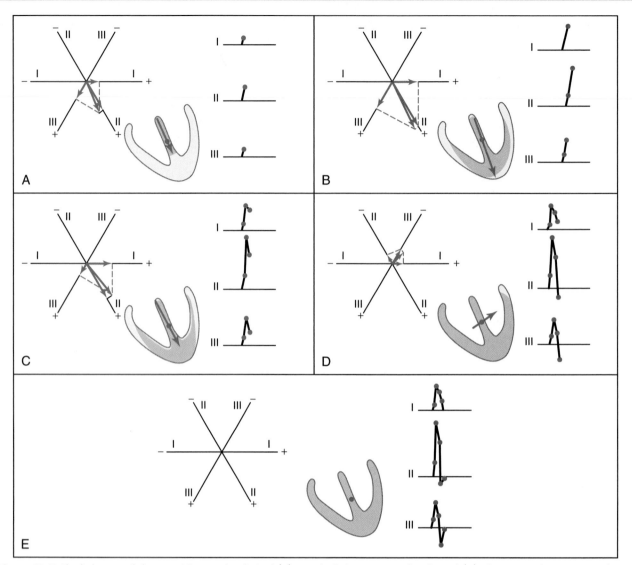

Figure 12-7 Shaded areas of the ventricles are depolarized (−); nonshaded areas are still polarized (+). The ventricular vectors and QRS complexes 0.01 second after onset of ventricular depolarization *(A)*; 0.02 second after onset of depolarization *(B)*; 0.035 second after onset of depolarization *(C)*; 0.05 second after onset of depolarization *(D)*; and after depolarization of the ventricles is complete, 0.06 second after onset *(E)*.

In Figure 12-7*B*, which represents about 0.02 second after onset of depolarization, the heart vector is long because much of the ventricular muscle mass has become depolarized. Therefore, the voltages in all electrocardiographic leads have increased.

In Figure 12-7*C*, about 0.035 second after onset of depolarization, the heart vector is becoming shorter and the recorded electrocardiographic voltages are lower because the outside of the heart apex is now electronegative, neutralizing much of the positivity on the other epicardial surfaces of the heart. Also, the axis of the vector is beginning to shift toward the left side of the chest because the left ventricle is slightly slower to depolarize than the right. Therefore, the ratio of the voltage in lead I to that in lead III is increasing.

In Figure 12-7*D*, about 0.05 second after onset of depolarization, the heart vector points toward the base of the left ventricle, and it is short because only a minute portion of the ventricular muscle is still polarized positive. Because

of the direction of the vector at this time, the voltages recorded in leads II and III are both negative—that is, below the line—whereas the voltage of lead I is still positive.

In Figure 12-7*E*, about 0.06 second after onset of depolarization, the entire ventricular muscle mass is depolarized so that no current flows around the heart and no electrical potential is generated. The vector becomes zero, and the voltages in all leads become zero.

Thus, the QRS complexes are completed in the three standard bipolar limb leads.

Sometimes the QRS complex has a slight negative depression at its beginning in one or more of the leads, which is not shown in Figure 12-7; this depression is the Q wave. When it occurs, it is caused by initial depolarization of the left side of the septum before the right side, which creates a weak vector from left to right for a fraction of a second before the usual base-to-apex vector occurs. The major positive deflection shown in Figure 12-7 is the R wave, and the final negative deflection is the S wave.

Electrocardiogram during Repolarization—the T Wave

After the ventricular muscle has become depolarized, about 0.15 second later, repolarization begins and proceeds until complete at about 0.35 second. This repolarization causes the T wave in the electrocardiogram.

Because the septum and endocardial areas of the ventricular muscle depolarize first, it seems logical that these areas should repolarize first as well. However, this is not the usual case because the septum and other endocardial areas have a longer period of contraction than most of the external surfaces of the heart. Therefore, *the greatest portion of ventricular muscle mass to repolarize first is the entire outer surface of the ventricles, especially near the apex of the heart.* The endocardial areas, conversely, normally repolarize last. This sequence of repolarization is postulated to be caused by the high blood pressure inside the ventricles during contraction, which greatly reduces coronary blood flow to the endocardium, thereby slowing repolarization in the endocardial areas.

Because the outer apical surfaces of the ventricles repolarize before the inner surfaces, the positive end of the overall ventricular vector during repolarization is toward the apex of the heart. As a result, the normal T wave in all three bipolar limb leads is positive, which is also the polarity of most of the normal QRS complex.

In Figure 12-8, five stages of repolarization of the ventricles are denoted by progressive increase of the light tan areas—the repolarized areas. At each stage, the vector extends from the base of the heart toward the apex until it disappears in the last stage. At first, the vector is relatively small because the area of repolarization is small. Later, the vector becomes stronger because of greater degrees of repolarization. Finally, the vector becomes weaker again because the areas of depolarization still persisting become

so slight that the total quantity of current flow decreases. These changes also demonstrate that the vector is greatest when about half the heart is in the polarized state and about half is depolarized.

The changes in the electrocardiograms of the three standard limb leads during repolarization are noted under each of the ventricles, depicting the progressive stages of repolarization. Thus, over about 0.15 second, the period of time required for the whole process to take place, the T wave of the electrocardiogram is generated.

Depolarization of the Atria—the P Wave

Depolarization of the atria begins in the sinus node and spreads in all directions over the atria. Therefore, the point of original electronegativity in the atria is about at the point of entry of the superior vena cava where the sinus node lies, and the direction of initial depolarization is denoted by the black vector in Figure 12-9. Furthermore, the vector remains generally in this direction throughout the process of normal atrial depolarization. Because this direction is generally in the positive directions of the axes of the three standard bipolar limb leads I, II, and III, the electrocardiograms recorded from the atria during depolarization are also usually positive in all three of these leads, as shown in Figure 12-9. This record of atrial depolarization is known as the atrial P wave.

Repolarization of the Atria—the Atrial T Wave. Spread of depolarization through the atrial muscle is *much slower than in the ventricles* because the atria have no Purkinje system for fast conduction of the depolarization signal. Therefore, the musculature around the sinus node becomes depolarized a long time before the musculature in distal parts of the atria. Because of this, *the area in the atria that also becomes repolarized first is the sinus nodal region, the area that had originally become depolarized first.* Thus, when repolarization begins, the region around the sinus node becomes positive with respect to the rest of the atria. Therefore, the atrial repolarization

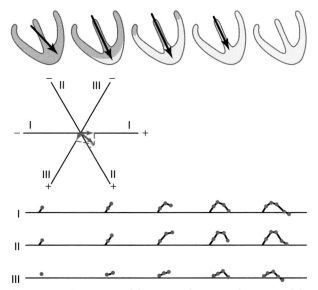

Figure 12-8 Generation of the T wave during repolarization of the ventricles, showing also vectorial analysis of the first stage of repolarization. The total time from the beginning of the T wave to its end is approximately 0.15 second.

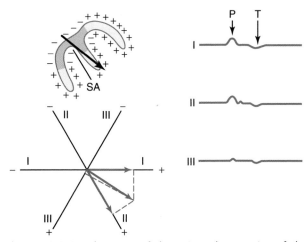

Figure 12-9 Depolarization of the atria and generation of the P wave, showing the maximum vector through the atria and the resultant vectors in the three standard leads. At the right are the atrial P and T waves. SA, sinoatrial node.

vector is *backward to the vector of depolarization.* (Note that this is opposite to the effect that occurs in the ventricles.) Therefore, as shown to the right in Figure 12-9, the so-called atrial T wave follows about 0.15 second after the atrial P wave, but this T wave is on the opposite side of the zero reference line from the P wave; that is, it is normally negative rather than positive in the three standard bipolar limb leads.

In the normal electrocardiogram, the *atrial* T wave appears at about the same time that the QRS complex of the ventricles appears. Therefore, it is almost always totally obscured by the large *ventricular* QRS complex, although in some very abnormal states, it does appear in the recorded electrocardiogram.

Vectorcardiogram

It has been noted in the discussion up to this point that the vector of current flow through the heart changes rapidly as the impulse spreads through the myocardium. It changes in two aspects: First, the vector increases and decreases in length because of increasing and decreasing voltage of the vector. Second, the vector changes direction because of changes in the average direction of the electrical potential from the heart. The so-called *vectorcardiogram* depicts these changes at different times during the cardiac cycle, as shown in Figure 12-10.

In the large vectorcardiogram of Figure 12-10, point 5 is the *zero reference point,* and this point is the negative end of all the successive vectors. While the heart muscle is polarized between heartbeats, the positive end of the vector remains at the zero point because there is no vectorial electrical potential. However, as soon as current begins to flow through the ventricles at the beginning of ventricular depolarization, the positive end of the vector leaves the zero reference point.

When the septum first becomes depolarized, the vector extends downward toward the apex of the ventricles, but it is relatively weak, thus generating the first portion of the ventricular vectorcardiogram, as shown by the positive end of vector 1. As more of the ventricular muscle becomes depolarized, the vector becomes stronger and stronger, usually swinging slightly to one side. Thus, vector 2 of Figure 12-10 represents the state of depolarization of the ventricles about 0.02 second after vector 1. After another 0.02 second, vector 3 represents the potential, and vector 4 occurs in another 0.01 second. Finally, the ventricles become totally depolarized, and the vector becomes zero once again, as shown at point 5.

The elliptical figure generated by the positive ends of the vectors is called the *QRS vectorcardiogram.* Vectorcardiograms can be recorded on an oscilloscope by connecting body surface electrodes from the neck and lower abdomen to the vertical plates of the oscilloscope and connecting chest surface electrodes from each side of the heart to the horizontal plates. When the vector changes, the spot of light on the oscilloscope follows the course of the positive end of the changing vector, thus inscribing the vectorcardiogram on the oscilloscopic screen.

Mean Electrical Axis of the Ventricular QRS—and Its Significance

The vectorcardiogram during ventricular depolarization (the QRS vectorcardiogram) shown in Figure 12-10 is that of a normal heart. Note from this vectorcardiogram that the preponderant direction of the vectors of the ventricles during depolarization is mainly toward the apex of the heart. That is, during most of the cycle of ventricular depolarization, the direction of the electrical potential (negative to positive) is from the base of the ventricles toward the apex. This preponderant direction of the potential during depolarization is called the *mean electrical axis of the ventricles.* The mean electrical axis of the normal ventricles is 59 degrees. In many pathological conditions of the heart, this direction changes markedly, sometimes even to opposite poles of the heart.

Determining the Electrical Axis from Standard Lead Electrocardiograms

Clinically, the electrical axis of the heart is usually estimated from the standard bipolar limb lead electrocardiograms rather than from the vectorcardiogram. Figure 12-11 shows a method for doing this. After recording the standard leads, one determines the net potential and polarity of the recordings in leads I and III. In lead I of Figure 12-11, the recording is positive, and in lead III, the recording is mainly positive but negative during part of the cycle. If any part of a recording is negative, *this negative potential is subtracted from the positive part of the potential* to determine the *net potential* for that lead, as shown by the arrow to the right of the QRS complex for lead III. Then each net potential for leads I and III is plotted on the axes of the respective leads, with the base of the potential at the point of intersection of the axes, as shown in Figure 12-11.

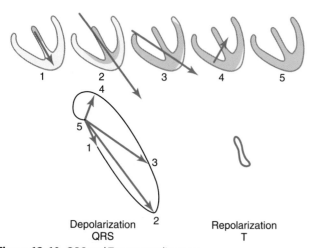

Depolarization   Repolarization
QRS   T

Figure 12-10 QRS and T vectorcardiograms.

Chapter 12 Electrocardiographic Interpretation of Cardiac Muscle and Coronary Blood Flow Abnormalities: Vectorial Analysis

UNIT III

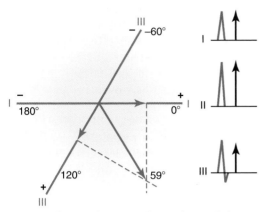

Figure 12-11 Plotting the mean electrical axis of the ventricles from two electrocardiographic leads (leads I and III).

If the net potential of lead I is positive, it is plotted in a positive direction along the line depicting lead I. Conversely, if this potential is negative, it is plotted in a negative direction. Also, for lead III, the net potential is placed with its base at the point of intersection, and, if positive, it is plotted in the positive direction along the line depicting lead III. If it is negative, it is plotted in the negative direction.

To determine the vector of the total QRS ventricular mean electrical potential, one draws perpendicular lines (the dashed lines in the figure) from the apices of leads I and III, respectively. The point of intersection of these two perpendicular lines represents, by vectorial analysis, the apex of the *mean* QRS vector in the ventricles, and the point of intersection of the lead I and lead III axes represents the negative end of the mean vector. Therefore, the *mean QRS vector* is drawn between these two points. The approximate average potential generated by the ventricles during depolarization is represented by the length of this mean QRS vector, and the mean electrical axis is represented by the direction of the mean vector. Thus, the orientation of the mean electrical axis of the normal ventricles, as determined in Figure 12-11, is 59 degrees positive (+59 degrees).

Abnormal Ventricular Conditions That Cause Axis Deviation

Although the mean electrical axis of the ventricles averages about 59 degrees, this axis can swing even in the normal heart from about 20 degrees to about 100 degrees. The causes of the normal variations are mainly anatomical differences in the Purkinje distribution system or in the musculature itself of different hearts. However, a number of abnormal conditions of the heart can cause axis deviation beyond the normal limits, as follows.

Change in the Position of the Heart in the Chest. If the heart itself is angulated to the left, the mean electrical axis of the heart also *shifts to the left*. Such shift occurs (1) at the end of deep expiration, (2) when a person

lies down, because the abdominal contents press upward against the diaphragm, and (3) quite frequently in obese people whose diaphragms normally press upward against the heart all the time due to increased visceral adiposity.

Likewise, angulation of the heart to the right causes the mean electrical axis of the ventricles to *shift to the right*. This occurs (1) at the end of deep inspiration, (2) when a person stands up, and (3) normally in tall, lanky people whose hearts hang downward.

Hypertrophy of One Ventricle. When one ventricle greatly hypertrophies, *the axis of the heart shifts toward the hypertrophied ventricle* for two reasons. First, a far greater quantity of muscle exists on the hypertrophied side of the heart than on the other side, and this allows generation of greater electrical potential on that side. Second, more time is required for the depolarization wave to travel through the hypertrophied ventricle than through the normal ventricle. Consequently, the *normal* ventricle becomes depolarized considerably in advance of the *hypertrophied* ventricle, and this causes a strong vector from the normal side of the heart toward the hypertrophied side, which remains strongly positively charged. Thus, the axis deviates toward the hypertrophied ventricle.

Vectorial Analysis of Left Axis Deviation Resulting from Hypertrophy of the Left Ventricle. Figure 12-12 shows the three standard bipolar limb lead electrocardiograms. Vectorial analysis demonstrates left axis deviation with mean electrical axis pointing in the −15-degree direction. This is a typical electrocardiogram caused by increased muscle mass of the left ventricle. In this instance, the axis deviation was caused by *hypertension* (high arterial blood pressure), which caused the left ventricle to hypertrophy so that it could pump blood against elevated systemic arterial pressure. A similar picture of left axis deviation occurs when the

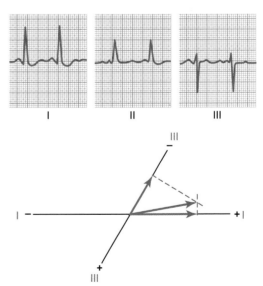

Figure 12-12 Left axis deviation in a *hypertensive heart (hypertrophic left ventricle)*. Note the slightly prolonged QRS complex as well.

left ventricle hypertrophies as a result of *aortic valvular stenosis, aortic valvular regurgitation,* or any number of *congenital heart conditions* in which the left ventricle enlarges while the right ventricle remains relatively normal in size.

Vectorial Analysis of Right Axis Deviation Resulting from Hypertrophy of the Right Ventricle. The electrocardiogram of Figure 12-13 shows intense right axis deviation, to an electrical axis of 170 degrees, which is 111 degrees to the right of the normal 59-degree mean ventricular QRS axis. The right axis deviation demonstrated in this figure was caused by hypertrophy of the right ventricle as a result of *congenital pulmonary valve stenosis.* Right axis deviation also can occur in other congenital heart conditions that cause hypertrophy of the right ventricle, such as *tetralogy of Fallot* and *interventricular septal defect.*

Bundle Branch Block Causes Axis Deviation. Ordinarily, the lateral walls of the two ventricles depolarize at almost the same instant because both the left and the right bundle branches of the Purkinje system transmit the cardiac impulse to the two ventricular walls at almost the same instant. As a result, the potentials generated by the two ventricles (on the two opposite sides of the heart) almost neutralize each other. But if only one of the major bundle branches is blocked, the cardiac impulse spreads through the normal ventricle long before it spreads through the other. Therefore, depolarization of the two ventricles does not occur even nearly simultaneously, and the depolarization potentials do not neutralize each other. As a result, axis deviation occurs as follows.

Vectorial Analysis of Left Axis Deviation in Left Bundle Branch Block. When the left bundle branch is blocked, cardiac depolarization spreads through the right ventricle two to three times as rapidly as through the left ventricle. Consequently, much of the left ventricle remains polarized for as long as 0.1 second after the right ventricle has become totally depolarized. Thus, the right ventricle becomes electronegative, whereas the left ventricle remains electropositive during most of the depolarization process, and a strong vector projects from the right ventricle toward the left ventricle. In other words, there is intense left axis deviation of about −50 degrees because the positive end of the vector points toward the left ventricle. This is demonstrated in Figure 12-14, which shows typical left axis deviation resulting from left bundle branch block.

Because of slowness of impulse conduction when the Purkinje system is blocked, in addition to axis deviation, the duration of the QRS complex is greatly prolonged because of extreme slowness of depolarization in the affected side of the heart. One can see this by observing the excessive widths of the QRS waves in Figure 12-14. This is discussed in greater detail later in the chapter. This extremely prolonged QRS complex differentiates bundle branch block from axis deviation caused by hypertrophy.

Vectorial Analysis of Right Axis Deviation in Right Bundle Branch Block. When the right bundle branch is blocked, the left ventricle depolarizes far more rapidly than the right ventricle, so the left side of the ventricles becomes electronegative as long as 0.1 second before the right. Therefore, a strong vector develops, with its negative end toward the left ventricle and its positive end toward the right ventricle. In other words, intense right axis deviation occurs. Right axis deviation caused by right bundle branch block is demonstrated, and its vector is

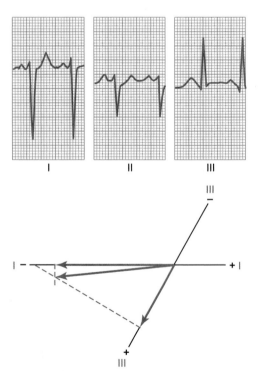

Figure 12-13 High-voltage electrocardiogram in *congenital pulmonary valve stenosis **with right ventricular hypertrophy.*** Intense right axis deviation and a slightly prolonged QRS complex also are seen.

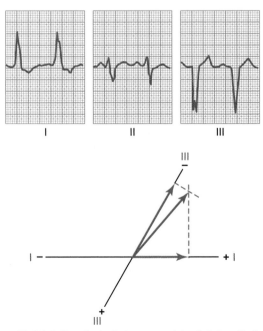

Figure 12-14 Left axis deviation caused by *left bundle branch block.* Note also the greatly prolonged QRS complex.

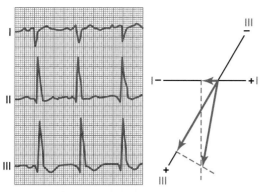

Figure 12-15 Right axis deviation caused by *right bundle branch block*. Note also the greatly prolonged QRS complex.

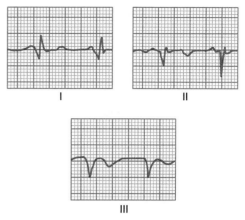

Figure 12-16 Low-voltage electrocardiogram following local damage throughout the ventricles caused by *previous myocardial infarction*.

analyzed, in Figure 12-15, which shows an axis of about 105 degrees instead of the normal 59 degrees and a prolonged QRS complex because of slow conduction.

Conditions That Cause Abnormal Voltages of the QRS Complex

Increased Voltage in the Standard Bipolar Limb Leads

Normally, the voltages in the three standard bipolar limb leads, as measured from the peak of the R wave to the bottom of the S wave, vary between 0.5 and 2.0 millivolts, with lead III usually recording the lowest voltage and lead II the highest. However, these relations are not invariable, even for the normal heart. In general, when the sum of the voltages of all the QRS complexes of the three standard leads is greater than 4 millivolts, the patient is considered to have a high-voltage electrocardiogram.

The cause of high-voltage QRS complexes most often is increased muscle mass of the heart, which ordinarily results from *hypertrophy of the muscle* in response to excessive load on one part of the heart or the other. For example, the right ventricle hypertrophies when it must pump blood through a stenotic pulmonary valve, and the left ventricle hypertrophies when a person has high blood pressure. The increased quantity of muscle causes generation of increased quantities of electricity around the heart. As a result, the electrical potentials recorded in the electrocardiographic leads are considerably greater than normal, as shown in Figures 12-12 and 12-13.

Decreased Voltage of the Electrocardiogram

Decreased Voltage Caused by Cardiac Myopathies. One of the most common causes of decreased voltage of the QRS complex is a series of *old myocardial infarctions* with resultant *diminished muscle mass*. This also causes the depolarization wave to move through the ventricles slowly and prevents major portions of the heart from becoming massively depolarized all at once. Consequently, this condition causes some prolongation of the QRS complex along with the decreased voltage. Figure 12-16 shows

a typical low-voltage electrocardiogram with prolongation of the QRS complex, which is common after multiple small infarctions of the heart have caused local delays of impulse conduction and reduced voltages due to loss of muscle mass throughout the ventricles.

Decreased Voltage Caused by Conditions Surrounding the Heart. One of the most important causes of decreased voltage in electrocardiographic leads is *fluid in the pericardium*. Because extracellular fluid conducts electrical currents with great ease, a large portion of the electricity flowing out of the heart is conducted from one part of the heart to another through the pericardial fluid. Thus, this effusion effectively "short-circuits" the electrical potentials generated by the heart, decreasing the electrocardiographic voltages that reach the outside surfaces of the body. *Pleural effusion,* to a lesser extent, also can "short-circuit" the electricity around the heart so that the voltages at the surface of the body and in the electrocardiograms are decreased.

Pulmonary emphysema can decrease the electrocardiographic potentials, but for a different reason than that of pericardial effusion. In pulmonary emphysema, conduction of electrical current through the lungs is depressed considerably because of excessive quantity of air in the lungs. Also, the chest cavity enlarges, and the lungs tend to envelop the heart to a greater extent than normally. Therefore, the lungs act as an insulator to prevent spread of electrical voltage from the heart to the surface of the body, and this results in decreased electrocardiographic potentials in the various leads.

Prolonged and Bizarre Patterns of the QRS Complex

Prolonged QRS Complex as a Result of Cardiac Hypertrophy or Dilatation

The QRS complex lasts as long as depolarization continues to spread through the ventricles—that is, as long as part of the ventricles is depolarized and part is still polarized.

Therefore, *prolonged conduction* of the impulse through the ventricles always causes a prolonged QRS complex. Such prolongation often occurs when one or both ventricles are hypertrophied or dilated, owing to the longer pathway that the impulse must then travel. The normal QRS complex lasts 0.06 to 0.08 second, whereas in hypertrophy or dilatation of the left or right ventricle, the QRS complex may be prolonged to 0.09 to 0.12 second.

Prolonged QRS Complex Resulting from Purkinje System Blocks

When the Purkinje fibers are blocked, the cardiac impulse must then be conducted by the ventricular muscle instead of by way of the Purkinje system. This decreases the velocity of impulse conduction to about one third of normal. Therefore, if complete block of one of the bundle branches occurs, the duration of the QRS complex is usually increased to 0.14 second or greater.

In general, a QRS complex is considered to be abnormally long when it lasts more than 0.09 second; when it lasts more than 0.12 second, the prolongation is almost certainly caused by pathological block somewhere in the ventricular conduction system, as shown by the electrocardiograms for bundle branch block in Figures 12-14 and 12-15.

Conditions That Cause Bizarre QRS Complexes

Bizarre patterns of the QRS complex most frequently are caused by two conditions: (1) destruction of cardiac muscle in various areas throughout the ventricular system, with replacement of this muscle by scar tissue, and (2) multiple small local blocks in the conduction of impulses at many points in the Purkinje system. As a result, cardiac impulse conduction becomes irregular, causing rapid shifts in voltages and axis deviations. This often causes double or even triple peaks in some of the electrocardiographic leads, such as those shown in Figure 12-14.

Current of Injury

Many different cardiac abnormalities, especially those that damage the heart muscle itself, often cause part of the heart to remain partially or totally *depolarized all the time.* When this occurs, current flows between the pathologically depolarized and the normally polarized areas even between heartbeats. This is called a *current of injury.* Note especially that *the injured part of the heart is negative, because this is the part that is depolarized and emits negative charges into the surrounding fluids, whereas the remainder of the heart is neutral or positive polarity.*

Some abnormalities that can cause current of injury are (1) *mechanical trauma,* which sometimes makes the membranes remain so permeable that full repolarization cannot take place; (2) *infectious processes* that damage the muscle membranes; and (3) *ischemia of local areas of heart muscle caused by local coronary occlusions,* which is by far the most common cause of current of injury in the heart. During ischemia, not enough nutrients from the coronary blood supply are available to the heart muscle to maintain normal membrane polarization.

Effect of Current of Injury on the QRS Complex

In Figure 12-17, a small area in the base of the left ventricle is newly infarcted (loss of coronary blood flow). Therefore, during the T-P interval—that is, when the normal ventricular muscle is totally polarized—abnormal *negative* current still flows from the infarcted area at the base of the left ventricle and spreads toward the rest of the ventricles.

The vector of this "current of injury," as shown in the first heart in Figure 12-17, is in a direction of about 125 degrees, with the base of the vector, the *negative end,* toward the injured muscle. As shown in the lower portions of the figure, even before the QRS complex begins, *this vector causes an initial record in lead I below the zero potential line,* because the projected vector of the current of injury in lead I points toward the negative end of the lead I axis. In lead II, the record is above the line because the projected vector points more toward the positive terminal of the lead. In lead III, the projected vector points in the same direction as the positive terminal of lead III so that the record is positive. Furthermore, because the vector lies almost exactly in the direction of the axis of lead III, the voltage of the current of injury in lead III is much greater than in either lead I or lead II.

As the heart then proceeds through its normal process of depolarization, the septum first becomes depolarized; then the depolarization spreads down to the apex and back toward the bases of the ventricles. The last portion of the ventricles to become totally depolarized is the base of the right ventricle, because the base of the left ventricle is already totally and permanently depolarized. By vectorial analysis, the successive stages of electrocardiogram generation by the depolarization wave traveling through the ventricles can be constructed graphically, as demonstrated in the lower part of Figure 12-17.

When the heart becomes totally depolarized, at the end of the depolarization process (as noted by the next-to-last stage in Figure 12-17), all the ventricular muscle is in a negative state. Therefore, at this instant in the electrocardiogram, no current flows from the ventricles to the electrocardiographic electrodes because now both the injured heart muscle and the contracting muscle are depolarized.

Next, as repolarization takes place, all of the heart finally repolarizes, except the area of permanent depolarization in the injured base of the left ventricle. Thus, repolarization causes a return of the current of injury in each lead, as noted at the far right in Figure 12-17.

The J Point—the Zero Reference Potential for Analyzing Current of Injury

One might think that the electrocardiograph machines for recording electrocardiograms could determine when no current is flowing around the heart. However, many

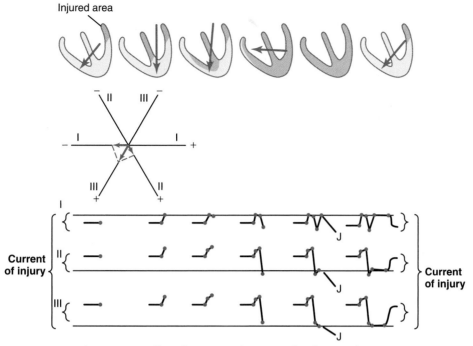

Figure 12-17 Effect of a current of injury on the electrocardiogram.

stray currents exist in the body, such as currents resulting from "skin potentials" and from differences in ionic concentrations in different fluids of the body. Therefore, when two electrodes are connected between the arms or between an arm and a leg, these stray currents make it impossible to predetermine the exact zero reference level in the electrocardiogram.

For these reasons, the following procedure must be used to determine the zero potential level: First, one notes *the exact point at which the wave of depolarization just completes its passage through the heart*, which occurs at the end of the QRS complex. At exactly this point, all parts of the ventricles have become depolarized, including both the damaged parts and the normal parts, so no current is flowing around the heart. Even the current of injury disappears at this point. Therefore, the potential of the electrocardiogram at this instant is at zero voltage. This point is known as the "J" point in the electrocardiogram, as shown in Figure 12-18.

Then, for analysis of the electrical axis of the injury potential caused by a current of injury, a horizontal line is drawn in the electrocardiogram for each lead at the level of the J point. This horizontal line is then the *zero potential level* in the electrocardiogram from which all potentials caused by currents of injury must be measured.

Use of the J Point in Plotting Axis of Injury Potential. Figure 12-18 shows electrocardiograms (leads I and III) from an injured heart. Both records show injury potentials. In other words, the J point of each of these two electrocardiograms is not on the same line as the T-P segment. In the figure, a horizontal line has been drawn through the J point to represent the zero voltage level in each of the two recordings. The injury potential in each

lead is the difference between the voltage of the electrocardiogram immediately before onset of the P wave and the zero voltage level determined from the J point. In lead I, the recorded voltage of the injury potential is above the zero potential level and is, therefore, positive. Conversely, in lead III, the injury potential is below the zero voltage level and, therefore, is negative.

At the bottom in Figure 12-18, the respective injury potentials in leads I and III are plotted on the coordinates of these leads, and the resultant vector of the injury potential for the whole ventricular muscle mass

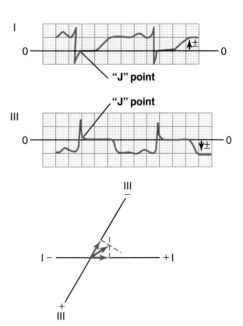

Figure 12-18 J point as the zero reference potential of the electrocardiograms for leads I and III. Also, the method for plotting the axis of the injury potential is shown by the lowermost panel.

is determined by vectorial analysis as described. In this instance, the resultant vector extends from the right side of the ventricles toward the left and slightly upward, with an axis of about −30 degrees. If one places this vector for the injury potential directly over the ventricles, *the negative end of the vector points toward the permanently depolarized, "injured" area of the ventricles.* In the example shown in Figure 12-18, the injured area would be in the lateral wall of the right ventricle.

This analysis is obviously complex. However, it is essential that the student go over it again and again until he or she understands it thoroughly. No other aspect of electrocardiographic analysis is more important.

Coronary Ischemia as a Cause of Injury Potential

Insufficient blood flow to the cardiac muscle depresses the metabolism of the muscle for three reasons: (1) lack of oxygen, (2) excess accumulation of carbon dioxide, and (3) lack of sufficient food nutrients. Consequently, repolarization of the muscle membrane cannot occur in areas of severe myocardial ischemia. Often the heart muscle does not die because the blood flow is sufficient to maintain life of the muscle even though it is not sufficient to cause repolarization of the membranes. As long as this state exists, an injury potential continues to flow during the diastolic portion (the T-P portion) of each heart cycle.

Extreme ischemia of the cardiac muscle occurs after coronary occlusion, and a strong current of injury flows from the infarcted area of the ventricles during the T-P interval between heartbeats, as shown in Figures 12-19 and 12-20. Therefore, one of the most important diagnostic features of electrocardiograms recorded after acute coronary thrombosis is the current of injury.

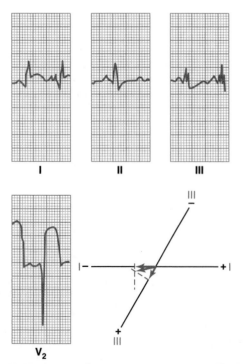

Figure 12-19 Current of injury in *acute anterior wall infarction.* Note the intense injury potential in lead V₂.

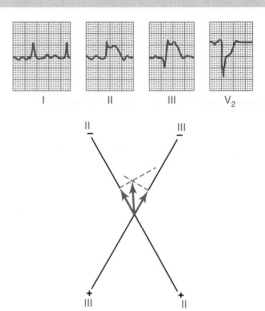

Figure 12-20 Injury potential in *acute posterior wall, apical infarction.*

Acute Anterior Wall Infarction. Figure 12-19 shows the electrocardiogram in the three standard bipolar limb leads and in one chest lead (lead V_2) recorded from a patient with acute anterior wall cardiac infarction. The most important diagnostic feature of this electrocardiogram is the intense injury potential in chest lead V_2. If one draws a zero horizontal potential line through the J point of this electrocardiogram, a strong *negative* injury potential during the T-P interval is found, which means that the chest electrode over the front of the heart is in an area of strongly negative potential. In other words, the negative end of the injury potential vector in this heart is against the anterior chest wall. This means that the current of injury is emanating from the anterior wall of the ventricles, which diagnoses this condition as *anterior wall infarction.*

Analyzing the injury potentials in leads I and III, one finds a negative potential in lead I and a positive potential in lead III. This means that the resultant vector of the injury potential in the heart is about +150 degrees, with the negative end pointing toward the left ventricle and the positive end pointing toward the right ventricle. Thus, in this particular electrocardiogram, the current of injury is coming mainly from the left ventricle, as well as from the anterior wall of the heart. Therefore, one would conclude that this anterior wall infarction almost certainly is caused by thrombosis of the anterior descending branch of the left coronary artery.

Posterior Wall Infarction. Figure 12-20 shows the three standard bipolar limb leads and one chest lead (lead V_2) from a patient with posterior wall infarction. The major diagnostic feature of this electrocardiogram is also in the chest lead. If a zero potential reference line is drawn through the J point of this lead, it is readily apparent that during the T-P interval, the potential of the current of injury is positive. This means that the positive end of the vector is in the direction of the anterior chest wall, and the negative end (injured end of the vector) points away from the chest wall. In other words, the current of injury is coming from the back of the heart opposite to the anterior chest wall, which is the reason this type of electrocardiogram is the basis for diagnosing posterior wall infarction.

If one analyzes the injury potentials from leads II and III of Figure 12-20, it is readily apparent that the injury potential is negative in both leads. By vectorial analysis, as shown in the figure, one finds that the resultant vector of the injury potential is about −95 degrees, with the negative end pointing downward and the positive end pointing upward. Thus, because the infarct, as indicated by the chest lead, is on the posterior wall of the heart and, as indicated by the injury potentials in leads II and III, is in the apical portion of the heart, one would suspect that this infarct is near the apex on the posterior wall of the left ventricle.

Infarction in Other Parts of the Heart. By the same procedures demonstrated in the preceding discussions of anterior and posterior wall infarctions, it is possible to determine the locus of any infarcted area emitting a current of injury, regardless of which part of the heart is involved. In making such vectorial analyses, it must be remembered that *the positive end of the injury potential vector points toward the normal cardiac muscle, and the negative end points toward the injured portion of the heart that is emitting the current of injury.*

Recovery from Acute Coronary Thrombosis. Figure 12-21 shows a V_3 chest lead from a patient with acute posterior wall infarction, demonstrating changes in the electrocardiogram from the day of the attack to 1 week later, 3 weeks later, and finally 1 year later. From this electrocardiogram, one can see that the injury potential is strong immediately after the acute attack (T-P segment displaced positively from the S-T segment). However, after about 1 week, the injury potential has diminished considerably, and after 3 weeks, it is gone. After that, the electrocardiogram does not change greatly during the next year. This is the usual recovery pattern after acute myocardial infarction of moderate degree, showing that the *new collateral coronary blood flow* develops enough to re-establish appropriate nutrition to most of the infarcted area.

Conversely, in some patients with myocardial infarction, the infarcted area never redevelops adequate coronary blood supply. Often, some of the heart muscle

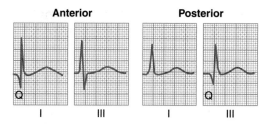

Figure 12-22 Electrocardiograms of anterior and posterior wall infarctions that occurred about 1 year previously, showing a Q wave in lead I in anterior wall infarction and a Q wave in lead III in *posterior wall infarction.*

dies, but if the muscle does not die, it will continue to show an injury potential as long as the ischemia exists, particularly during bouts of exercise when the heart is overloaded.

Old Recovered Myocardial Infarction. Figure 12-22 shows leads I and III after *anterior infarction* and leads I and III after *posterior infarction* about 1 year after the acute heart attack. The records show what might be called the "ideal" configurations of the QRS complex in these types of recovered myocardial infarction. Usually a Q wave has developed at the beginning of the QRS complex in lead I in anterior infarction because of loss of muscle mass in the anterior wall of the left ventricle, but in posterior infarction, a Q wave has developed at the beginning of the QRS complex in lead III because of loss of muscle in the posterior apical part of the ventricle.

These configurations are certainly not found in all cases of old cardiac infarction. Local loss of muscle and local points of cardiac signal conduction block can cause very bizarre QRS patterns (especially prominent Q waves, for instance), decreased voltage, and QRS prolongation.

Current of Injury in Angina Pectoris. "Angina pectoris" means pain from the heart felt in the pectoral regions of the upper chest. This pain usually also radiates into the left neck area and down the left arm. The pain is typically caused by moderate ischemia of the heart. Usually, no pain is felt as long as the person is quiet, but as soon as he or she overworks the heart, the pain appears.

An injury potential sometimes appears in the electrocardiogram during an attack of severe angina pectoris because the coronary insufficiency becomes great enough to prevent adequate repolarization of some areas of the heart during diastole.

Abnormalities in the T Wave

Earlier in the chapter, it was pointed out that the T wave is normally positive in all the standard bipolar limb leads and that this is caused by repolarization of the apex and outer surfaces of the ventricles ahead of the intraventricular surfaces. That is, the T wave becomes abnormal when the normal sequence of repolarization does not occur. Several factors can change this sequence of repolarization.

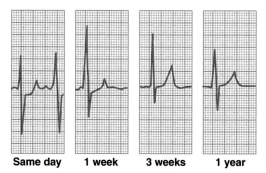

| Same day | 1 week | 3 weeks | 1 year |

Figure 12-21 Recovery of the myocardium after *moderate posterior wall infarction,* demonstrating disappearance of the injury potential that is present on the first day after the infarction and still slightly present at 1 week.

141

Effect of Slow Conduction of the Depolarization Wave on the Characteristics of the T Wave

Referring to Figure 12-14, note that the QRS complex is considerably prolonged. The reason for this prolongation is *delayed conduction in the left ventricle* resulting from left bundle branch block. This causes the left ventricle to become depolarized about 0.08 second after depolarization of the right ventricle, which gives a strong mean QRS vector *to the left.* However, the refractory periods of the right and left ventricular muscle masses are not greatly different from each other. Therefore, the right ventricle begins to repolarize long before the left ventricle; this causes strong positivity in the right ventricle and negativity in the left ventricle at the time that the T wave is developing. In other words, the mean axis of the T wave is now deviated *to the right,* which is opposite the mean electrical axis of the QRS complex in the same electrocardiogram. Thus, when conduction of the depolarization impulse through the ventricles is greatly delayed, the T wave is almost always of opposite polarity to that of the QRS complex.

Shortened Depolarization in Portions of the Ventricular Muscle as a Cause of T Wave Abnormalities

If the base of the ventricles should exhibit an abnormally short period of depolarization, that is, a shortened action potential, repolarization of the ventricles would not begin at the apex as it normally does. Instead, the base of the ventricles would repolarize ahead of the apex, and the vector of repolarization would point from the apex toward the base of the heart, opposite to the standard vector of repolarization. Consequently, the T wave in all three standard leads would be negative rather than the usual positive. Thus, the simple fact that the base of the ventricles has a shortened period of depolarization is sufficient to cause marked changes in the T wave, even to the extent of changing the entire T wave polarity, as shown in Figure 12-23.

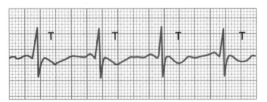

Figure 12-23 Inverted T wave resulting from mild *ischemia at the apex* of the ventricles.

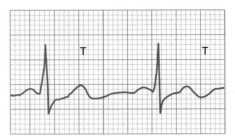

Figure 12-24 Biphasic T wave caused by *digitalis toxicity*.

Mild ischemia is by far the most common cause of shortening of depolarization of cardiac muscle because this increases current flow through the potassium channels. When the ischemia occurs in only one area of the heart, the depolarization period of this area decreases out of proportion to that in other portions. As a result, definite changes in the T wave can take place. The ischemia might result from chronic, progressive coronary occlusion; acute coronary occlusion; or relative coronary insufficiency that occurs during exercise.

One means for detecting mild coronary insufficiency is to have the patient exercise and to record the electrocardiogram, noting whether changes occur in the T waves. The changes in the T waves need not be specific because any change in the T wave in any lead—inversion, for instance, or a biphasic wave—is often evidence enough that some portion of the ventricular muscle has a period of depolarization out of proportion to the rest of the heart, caused by mild to moderate coronary insufficiency.

Effect of Digitalis on the T Wave. As discussed in Chapter 22, digitalis is a drug that can be used during coronary insufficiency to increase the strength of cardiac muscle contraction. But when overdosages of digitalis are given, depolarization duration in one part of the ventricles may be increased out of proportion to that of other parts. As a result, nonspecific changes, such as T wave inversion or biphasic T waves, may occur in one or more of the electrocardiographic leads. A biphasic T wave caused by excessive administration of digitalis is shown in Figure 12-24. Therefore, changes in the T wave during digitalis administration are often the earliest signs of digitalis toxicity.

Bibliography

See bibliography for Chapter 13.

Cardiac Arrhythmias and Their Electrocardiographic Interpretation

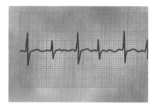

Some of the most distressing types of heart malfunction occur not as a result of abnormal heart muscle but because of abnormal rhythm of the heart. For instance, sometimes the beat of the atria is not coordinated with the beat of the ventricles, so the atria no longer function as primer pumps for the ventricles.

The purpose of this chapter is to discuss the physiology of common cardiac arrhythmias and their effects on heart pumping, as well as their diagnosis by electrocardiography. The causes of the cardiac arrhythmias are usually one or a combination of the following abnormalities in the rhythmicity-conduction system of the heart:

1. Abnormal rhythmicity of the pacemaker.

2. Shift of the pacemaker from the sinus node to another place in the heart.

3. Blocks at different points in the spread of the impulse through the heart.

4. Abnormal pathways of impulse transmission through the heart.

5. Spontaneous generation of spurious impulses in almost any part of the heart.

Abnormal Sinus Rhythms

Tachycardia

The term "tachycardia" means *fast heart rate,* usually defined in an adult person as faster than 100 beats/min. An electrocardiogram recorded from a patient with tachycardia is shown in Figure 13-1. This electrocardiogram is normal except that the heart rate, as determined from the time intervals between QRS complexes, is about 150 per minute instead of the normal 72 per minute.

Some causes of tachycardia include increased body temperature, stimulation of the heart by the sympathetic nerves, or toxic conditions of the heart.

The heart rate increases about 10 beats/min for each degree of Fahrenheit (18 beats per degree Celsius) increase in body temperature, up to a body temperature of about 105°F (40.5°C); beyond this, the heart rate may decrease because of progressive debility of the heart muscle as a result of the fever. Fever causes tachycardia because increased temperature increases the rate of metabolism of the sinus node, which in turn directly increases its excitability and rate of rhythm.

Many factors can cause the sympathetic nervous system to excite the heart, as we discuss at multiple points in this text. For instance, when a patient loses blood and passes into a state of shock or semishock, sympathetic reflex stimulation of the heart often increases the heart rate to 150 to 180 beats/min.

Simple weakening of the myocardium usually increases the heart rate because the weakened heart does not pump blood into the arterial tree to a normal extent, and this elicits sympathetic reflexes to increase the heart rate.

Bradycardia

The term "bradycardia" means a slow heart rate, usually defined as fewer than 60 beats/min. Bradycardia is shown by the electrocardiogram in Figure 13-2.

Bradycardia in Athletes. The athlete's heart is larger and considerably stronger than that of a normal person, which allows the athlete's heart to pump a large stroke

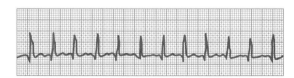

Figure 13-1 Sinus tachycardia (lead I).

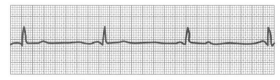

Figure 13-2 Sinus bradycardia (lead III).

volume output per beat even during periods of rest. When the athlete is at rest, excessive quantities of blood pumped into the arterial tree with each beat initiate feedback circulatory reflexes or other effects to cause bradycardia.

Vagal Stimulation as a Cause of Bradycardia. Any circulatory reflex that stimulates the vagus nerves causes release of acetylcholine at the vagal endings in the heart, thus giving a parasympathetic effect. Perhaps the most striking example of this occurs in patients with *carotid sinus syndrome.* In these patients, the pressure receptors (baroreceptors) in the carotid sinus region of the carotid artery walls are excessively sensitive. Therefore, even mild external pressure on the neck elicits a strong baroreceptor reflex, causing intense vagal-acetylcholine effects on the heart, including extreme bradycardia. Indeed, sometimes this reflex is so powerful that it actually stops the heart for 5 to 10 seconds.

Sinus Arrhythmia

Figure 13-3 shows a *cardiotachometer* recording of the heart rate, at first during normal and then (in the second half of the record) during deep respiration. A cardiotachometer is an instrument that records *by the height of successive spikes* the duration of the interval between the successive QRS complexes in the electrocardiogram. Note from this record that the heart rate increased and decreased no more than 5 percent during quiet respiration (left half of the record). Then, *during deep respiration,* the heart rate increased and decreased with each respiratory cycle by as much as 30 percent.

Sinus arrhythmia can result from any one of many circulatory conditions that alter the strengths of the sympathetic and parasympathetic nerve signals to the heart sinus node. In the "respiratory" type of sinus arrhythmia, as shown in Figure 13-3, this results mainly from "spillover" of signals from the medullary respiratory center into the adjacent vasomotor center during inspiratory and expiratory cycles of respiration. The spillover signals cause alternate increase and decrease in the number of impulses transmitted through the sympathetic and vagus nerves to the heart.

Abnormal Rhythms That Result from Block of Heart Signals Within the Intracardiac Conduction Pathways

Sinoatrial Block

In rare instances, the impulse from the sinus node is blocked before it enters the atrial muscle. This phenomenon is demonstrated in Figure 13-4, which shows

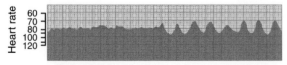

Figure 13-3 Sinus arrhythmia as recorded by a cardiotachometer. To the left is the record when the subject was breathing normally; to the right, when breathing deeply.

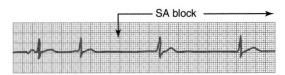

Figure 13-4 Sinoatrial nodal block, with A-V nodal rhythm during the block period (lead III).

sudden cessation of P waves, with resultant standstill of the atria. However, the ventricles pick up a new rhythm, the impulse usually originating spontaneously in the atrioventricular (A-V) node, so the rate of the ventricular QRS-T complex is slowed but not otherwise altered.

Atrioventricular Block

The only means by which impulses ordinarily can pass from the atria into the ventricles is through the *A-V bundle,* also known as the *bundle of His.* Conditions that can either decrease the rate of impulse conduction in this bundle or block the impulse entirely are as follows:

1. *Ischemia of the A-V node or A-V bundle fibers* often delays or blocks conduction from the atria to the ventricles. Coronary insufficiency can cause ischemia of the A-V node and bundle in the same way that it can cause ischemia of the myocardium.

2. *Compression of the A-V bundle* by scar tissue or by calcified portions of the heart can depress or block conduction from the atria to the ventricles.

3. *Inflammation of the A-V node or A-V bundle* can depress conductivity from the atria to the ventricles. Inflammation results frequently from different types of myocarditis, caused, for example, by diphtheria or rheumatic fever.

4. *Extreme stimulation of the heart by the vagus nerves* in rare instances blocks impulse conduction through the A-V node. Such vagal excitation occasionally results from strong stimulation of the baroreceptors in people with *carotid sinus syndrome,* discussed earlier in relation to bradycardia.

Incomplete Atrioventricular Heart Block

Prolonged P-R (or P-Q) Interval—First-Degree Block. The usual lapse of time between *beginning* of the P wave and *beginning* of the QRS complex is about 0.16 second when the heart is beating at a normal rate. This so-called *P-R interval* usually decreases in length with faster heartbeat and increases with slower heartbeat. In general, when the P-R interval increases to greater than 0.20 second, the P-R interval is said to be prolonged and the patient is said to have *first-degree incomplete heart block.*

Figure 13-5 shows an electrocardiogram with prolonged P-R interval; the interval in this instance is about

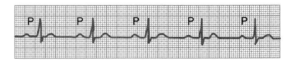

Figure 13-5 Prolonged P-R interval caused by first degree A-V heart block (lead II).

0.30 second instead of the normal 0.20 or less. Thus, first-degree block is defined as a *delay* of conduction from the atria to the ventricles but not actual blockage of conduction. The P-R interval seldom increases above 0.35 to 0.45 second because, by that time, conduction through the A-V bundle is depressed so much that conduction stops entirely. One means for determining the severity of some heart diseases—*acute rheumatic heart disease*, for instance—is to measure the P-R interval.

Second-Degree Block. When conduction through the A-V bundle is slowed enough to increase the P-R interval to 0.25 to 0.45 second, the action potential is sometimes strong enough to pass through the bundle into the ventricles and sometimes not strong enough. In this instance, there will be an atrial P wave but no QRS-T wave, and it is said that there are "dropped beats" of the ventricles. This condition is called *second-degree heart block.*

Figure 13-6 shows P-R intervals of 0.30 second, as well as one dropped ventricular beat as a result of failure of conduction from the atria to the ventricles.

At times, every other beat of the ventricles is dropped, so a "2:1 rhythm" develops, with the atria beating twice for every single beat of the ventricles. At other times, rhythms of 3:2 or 3:1 also develop.

Complete A-V Block (Third-Degree Block). When the condition causing poor conduction in the A-V node or A-V bundle becomes severe, complete block of the impulse from the atria into the ventricles occurs. In this instance, the ventricles spontaneously establish their own signal, usually originating in the A-V node or A-V bundle. Therefore, the P waves become dissociated from the QRS-T complexes, as shown in Figure 13-7. Note that the *rate of rhythm of the atria* in this electrocardiogram is about 100 beats per minute, whereas the *rate of ventricular beat* is less than 40 per minute. Furthermore, there is no relation between the rhythm of the P waves and that of the QRS-T complexes because the ventricles have "escaped" from control by the atria, and they are beating at their own natural rate, controlled most often by rhythmical signals generated in the A-V node or A-V bundle.

Stokes-Adams Syndrome—Ventricular Escape. In some patients with A-V block, the total block comes and goes; that is, impulses are conducted from the atria into the ventricles for a period of time and then suddenly impulses are not conducted. The duration of block may be a few seconds, a few minutes, a few hours, or even weeks or longer before conduction returns. This condition occurs in hearts with borderline ischemia of the conductive system.

Each time A-V conduction ceases, the ventricles often do not start their own beating until after a delay of 5 to 30 seconds. This results from the phenomenon called *overdrive suppression.* This means that ventricular excitability is at first in a suppressed state because the ventricles have been driven by the atria at a rate greater than their natural rate of rhythm. However, after a few seconds, some part of the Purkinje system beyond the block, usually in the distal part of the A-V node beyond the blocked point in the node, or in the A-V bundle, begins discharging rhythmically at a rate of 15 to 40 times per minute and acting as the pacemaker of the ventricles. This is called *ventricular escape.*

Because the brain cannot remain active for more than 4 to 7 seconds without blood supply, most patients faint a few seconds after complete block occurs because the heart does not pump any blood for 5 to 30 seconds, until the ventricles "escape." After escape, however, the slowly beating ventricles usually pump enough blood to allow rapid recovery from the faint and then to sustain the person. These periodic fainting spells are known as the *Stokes-Adams syndrome.*

Occasionally the interval of ventricular standstill at the onset of complete block is so long that it becomes detrimental to the patient's health or even causes death. Consequently, most of these patients are provided with an *artificial pacemaker,* a small battery-operated electrical stimulator planted beneath the skin, with electrodes usually connected to the right ventricle. The pacemaker provides continued rhythmical impulses that take control of the ventricles.

Incomplete Intraventricular Block—Electrical Alternans

Most of the same factors that can cause A-V block can also block impulse conduction in the peripheral ventricular Purkinje system. Figure 13-8 shows the condition known as *electrical alternans,* which results from partial intraventricular block every other heartbeat.

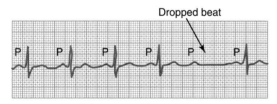

Figure 13-6 Second degree A-V block, showing occasional failure of the ventricles to receive the excitatory signals (lead V_3).

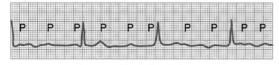

Figure 13-7 Complete A-V block (lead II).

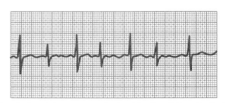

Figure 13-8 Partial intraventricular block—"electrical alternans" (lead III).

This electrocardiogram also shows *tachycardia* (rapid heart rate), which is probably the reason the block has occurred, because when the rate of the heart is rapid, it may be impossible for some portions of the Purkinje system to recover from the previous refractory period quickly enough to respond during every succeeding heartbeat. Also, many conditions that depress the heart, such as ischemia, myocarditis, or digitalis toxicity, can cause incomplete intraventricular block, resulting in electrical alternans.

Premature Contractions

A premature contraction is a contraction of the heart before the time that normal contraction would have been expected. This condition is also called *extrasystole, premature beat,* or *ectopic beat.*

Causes of Premature Contractions. Most premature contractions result from *ectopic foci* in the heart, which emit abnormal impulses at odd times during the cardiac rhythm. Possible causes of ectopic foci are (1) local areas of ischemia; (2) small calcified plaques at different points in the heart, which press against the adjacent cardiac muscle so that some of the fibers are irritated; and (3) toxic irritation of the A-V node, Purkinje system, or myocardium caused by drugs, nicotine, or caffeine. Mechanical initiation of premature contractions is also frequent during cardiac catheterization; large numbers of premature contractions often occur when the catheter enters the right ventricle and presses against the endocardium.

Premature Atrial Contractions

Figure 13-9 shows a single premature atrial contraction. The P wave of this beat occurred too soon in the heart cycle; the P-R interval is shortened, indicating that the ectopic origin of the beat is in the atria near the A-V node. Also, the interval between the premature contraction and the next succeeding contraction is slightly prolonged, which is called a *compensatory pause.* One of the reasons for this is that the premature contraction originated in the atrium some distance from the sinus node, and the impulse had to travel through a considerable amount of atrial muscle before it discharged the sinus node. Consequently, the sinus node discharged late in the premature cycle, and this made the succeeding sinus node discharge also late in appearing.

Premature atrial contractions occur frequently in otherwise healthy people. Indeed, they often occur in athletes whose hearts are in very healthy condition. Mild toxic conditions resulting from such factors as smoking, lack of sleep, ingestion of too much coffee, alcoholism, and use of various drugs can also initiate such contractions.

Pulse Deficit. When the heart contracts ahead of schedule, the ventricles will not have filled with blood normally, and the stroke volume output during that contraction is depressed or almost absent. Therefore, the pulse wave passing to the peripheral arteries after a premature contraction may be so weak that it cannot be felt in the radial artery. Thus, a deficit in the number of radial pulses occurs when compared with the actual number of contractions of the heart.

A-V Nodal or A-V Bundle Premature Contractions

Figure 13-10 shows a premature contraction that originated in the A-V node or in the A-V bundle. The P wave is missing from the electrocardiographic record of the premature contraction. Instead, the P wave is superimposed onto the QRS-T complex because the cardiac impulse traveled backward into the atria at the same time that it traveled forward into the ventricles; this P wave slightly distorts the QRS-T complex, but the P wave itself cannot be discerned as such. In general, A-V nodal premature contractions have the same significance and causes as atrial premature contractions.

Premature Ventricular Contractions

The electrocardiogram of Figure 13-11 shows a series of premature ventricular contractions (PVCs) alternating with normal contractions. PVCs cause specific effects in the electrocardiogram, as follows:

1. The QRS complex is usually considerably prolonged. The reason is that the impulse is conducted mainly through slowly conducting muscle of the ventricles rather than through the Purkinje system.

2. The QRS complex has a high voltage for the following reasons: when the normal impulse passes through the heart, it passes through both ventricles nearly simultaneously; consequently, in the normal heart, the depolarization waves of the two sides of the heart—mainly of opposite polarity to each other—partially neutralize each other in the electrocardiogram. When a PVC

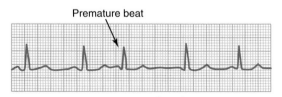

Figure 13-9 Atrial premature beat (lead I).

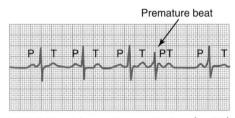

Figure 13-10 A-V nodal premature contraction (lead III).

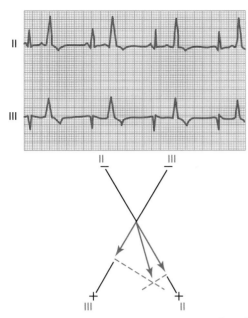

Figure 13-11 Premature ventricular contractions (PVCs) demonstrated by the large abnormal QRS-T complexes (leads II and III). Axis of the premature contractions is plotted in accordance with the principles of vectorial analysis explained in Chapter 12; this shows the origin of the PVC to be near the base of the ventricles.

occurs, the impulse almost always travels in only one direction, so there is no such neutralization effect, and one entire side or end of the ventricles is depolarized ahead of the other; this causes large electrical potentials, as shown for the PVCs in Figure 13-11.

3. After almost all PVCs, the T wave has an electrical potential polarity exactly opposite to that of the QRS complex because the *slow conduction of the impulse* through the cardiac muscle causes the muscle fibers that depolarize first also to repolarize first.

Some PVCs are relatively benign in their effects on overall pumping by the heart; they can result from such factors as cigarettes, excessive intake of coffee, lack of sleep, various mild toxic states, and even emotional irritability. Conversely, many other PVCs result from stray impulses or re-entrant signals that originate around the borders of infarcted or ischemic areas of the heart. The presence of such PVCs is not to be taken lightly. Statistics show that people with significant numbers of PVCs have a much higher than normal chance of developing spontaneous lethal ventricular fibrillation, presumably initiated by one of the PVCs. This is especially true when the PVCs occur during the vulnerable period for causing fibrillation, just at the end of the T wave when the ventricles are coming out of refractoriness, as explained later in the chapter.

Vector Analysis of the Origin of an Ectopic Premature Ventricular Contraction.

In Chapter 12, the principles of vectorial analysis are explained. Applying these principles, one can determine from the electrocar-

diogram in Figure 13-11 the point of origin of the PVC as follows: Note that the potentials of the premature contractions in leads II and III are both strongly positive. Plotting these potentials on the axes of leads II and III and solving by vectorial analysis for the mean QRS vector in the heart, one finds that the vector of this premature contraction has its negative end (origin) at the base of the heart and its positive end toward the apex. Thus, the first portion of the heart to become depolarized during this premature contraction is near the base of the ventricles, which therefore is the locus of the ectopic focus.

Disorders of Cardiac Repolarization—The Long QT Syndromes.

Recall that the Q wave corresponds to ventricular depolarization while the T wave corresponds to ventricular repolarization. The Q-T interval is the time from the Q point to the end of the T wave. Disorders that delay repolarization of ventricular muscle following the action potential cause prolonged ventricular action potentials and therefore excessively long Q-T intervals on the electrocardiogram, a condition called *long QT syndrome* (LQTS).

The major reason that the long QT syndrome is of concern is that delayed repolarization of ventricular muscle increases a person's susceptibility to develop ventricular arrhythmias called *torsades de pointes,* which literally means "twisting of the points." This type of arrhythmia has the features shown in Figure 13-12. The shape of the QRS complex may change over time with the onset of arrhythmia usually following a premature beat, a pause, and then another beat with a long Q-T interval, which may trigger arrhythmias, tachycardia, and in some instances ventricular fibrillation.

Disorders of cardiac repolarization that lead to LQTS may be inherited or acquired. The congenital forms of LQTS are rare disorders caused by mutations of sodium or potassium channel genes. At least 10 different mutations of these genes that can cause variable degrees of Q-T prolongation have been identified.

More common are the acquired forms of LQTS that are associated with plasma electrolyte disturbances, such as hypomagnesemia, hypokalemia, or hypocalcemia, or with administration of excess amounts of antiarrhythmic drugs such as quinidine or some antibiotics such as fluoroquinolones or erythromycin that prolong the Q-T interval.

Although some people with LQTS show no major symptoms (other than the prolonged Q-T interval), others exhibit fainting and ventricular arrhythmias that may be precipitated by physical exercise, intense emotions such as fright or anger, or when startled by a noise. The ventricular arrhythmias associated with LQTS can, in some cases, deteriorate into ventricular fibrillation and sudden death.

Treatment for LQTS may include magnesium sulfate for acute LQTS, and for long-term LQTS antiarrhythmia medications, such as beta-adrenergic blockers, or surgical implantation of a cardiac defibrillator are used.

Premature depolarization

Repetitive premature depolarization

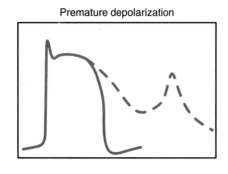
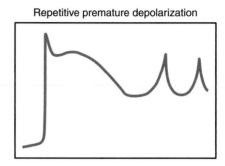

Torsades de pointes

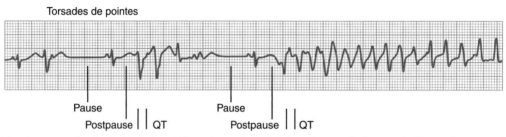

Pause

Postpause | | QT

Pause

Postpause | | QT

Figure 13-12 Development of arrhythmias in long QT syndrome (LQTS). When the ventricular muscle fiber action potential is prolonged as a result of delayed repolarization, a premature depolarization (*dashed line in top left figure*) may occur before complete repolarization. Repetitive premature depolarizations (*right top figure*) may lead to multiple depolarizations under certain conditions. In torsades de pointes (*bottom figure*), premature ventricular beats lead pauses, postpause prolongation of the Q-T interval, and arrhythmias. (Redrawn from Murray KT, Roden DM: Disorders of cardiac repolarization: the long QT syndromes. In: Crawford MG, DiMarco JP [eds]: Cardiology. London: Mosby, 2001.)

Paroxysmal Tachycardia

Some abnormalities in different portions of the heart, including the atria, the Purkinje system, or the ventricles, can occasionally cause rapid rhythmical discharge of impulses that spread in all directions throughout the heart. This is believed to be caused most frequently by re-entrant circus movement feedback pathways that set up local repeated self–re-excitation. Because of the rapid rhythm in the irritable focus, this focus becomes the pacemaker of the heart.

The term "paroxysmal" means that the heart rate becomes rapid in paroxysms, with the paroxysm beginning suddenly and lasting for a few seconds, a few minutes, a few hours, or much longer. Then the paroxysm usually ends as suddenly as it began, with the pacemaker of the heart instantly shifting back to the sinus node.

Paroxysmal tachycardia often can be stopped by eliciting a vagal reflex. A type of vagal reflex sometimes elicited for this purpose is to press on the neck in the regions of the carotid sinuses, which may cause enough of a vagal reflex to stop the paroxysm. Various drugs may also be used. Two drugs frequently used are quinidine and lidocaine, either of which depresses the normal increase in sodium permeability of the cardiac muscle membrane during generation of the action potential, thereby often blocking the rhythmical discharge of the focal point that is causing the paroxysmal attack.

Atrial Paroxysmal Tachycardia

Figure 13-13 demonstrates in the middle of the record a sudden increase in the heart rate from about 95 to about 150 beats per minute. On close study of the

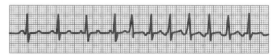

Figure 13-13 Atrial paroxysmal tachycardia—onset in middle of record (lead I).

electrocardiogram during the rapid heartbeat, an inverted P wave is seen before each QRS-T complex, and this P wave is partially superimposed onto the normal T wave of the preceding beat. This indicates that the origin of this paroxysmal tachycardia is in the atrium, but because the P wave is abnormal in shape, the origin is not near the sinus node.

A-V Nodal Paroxysmal Tachycardia. Paroxysmal tachycardia often results from an aberrant rhythm that involves the A-V node. This usually causes almost normal QRS-T complexes but totally missing or obscured P waves.

Atrial or A-V nodal paroxysmal tachycardia, both of which are called *supraventricular tachycardias*, usually occurs in young, otherwise healthy people, and they generally grow out of the predisposition to tachycardia after adolescence. In general, supraventricular tachycardia frightens a person tremendously and may cause weakness during the paroxysm, but only seldom does permanent harm come from the attack.

Ventricular Paroxysmal Tachycardia

Figure 13-14 shows a typical short paroxysm of ventricular tachycardia. The electrocardiogram of ventricular paroxysmal tachycardia has the appearance of a series of

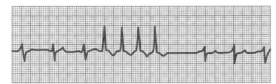

Figure 13-14 Ventricular paroxysmal tachycardia (lead III).

ventricular premature beats occurring one after another without any normal beats interspersed.

Ventricular paroxysmal tachycardia is usually a serious condition for two reasons. First, this type of tachycardia usually does not occur unless considerable ischemic damage is present in the ventricles. Second, *ventricular tachycardia frequently initiates the lethal condition of ventricular fibrillation* because of rapid repeated stimulation of the ventricular muscle, as we discuss in the next section.

Sometimes intoxication from the heart treatment drug *digitalis* causes irritable foci that lead to ventricular tachycardia. Conversely, *quinidine,* which increases the refractory period and threshold for excitation of cardiac muscle, may be used to block irritable foci causing ventricular tachycardia.

Ventricular Fibrillation

The most serious of all cardiac arrhythmias is ventricular fibrillation, which, if not stopped within 1 to 3 minutes, is almost invariably fatal. Ventricular fibrillation results from cardiac impulses that have gone berserk within the ventricular muscle mass, stimulating first one portion of the ventricular muscle, then another portion, then another, and eventually feeding back onto itself to re-excite the same ventricular muscle over and over—never stopping. When this happens, many small portions of the ventricular muscle will be contracting at the same time, while equally as many other portions will be relaxing. Thus, there is never a coordinate contraction of all the ventricular muscle at once, which is required for a pumping cycle of the heart. Despite massive movement of stimulatory signals throughout the ventricles, the ventricular chambers neither enlarge nor contract but remain in an indeterminate stage of partial contraction, pumping either no blood or negligible amounts. Therefore, after fibrillation begins, unconsciousness occurs within 4 to 5 seconds for lack of blood flow to the brain, and irretrievable death of tissues begins to occur throughout the body within a few minutes.

Multiple factors can spark the beginning of ventricular fibrillation—a person may have a normal heartbeat one moment, but 1 second later, the ventricles are in fibrillation. Especially likely to initiate fibrillation are (1) sudden electrical shock of the heart or (2) ischemia of the heart muscle, of its specialized conducting system, or both.

Phenomenon of Re-entry—"Circus Movements" as the Basis for Ventricular Fibrillation

When the *normal* cardiac impulse in the normal heart has traveled through the extent of the ventricles, it has no place to go because all the ventricular muscle is refractory and cannot conduct the impulse farther. Therefore, that impulse dies, and the heart awaits a new action potential to begin in the atrial sinus node.

Under some circumstances, however, this normal sequence of events does not occur. Therefore, let us explain more fully the background conditions that can initiate re-entry and lead to "circus movements," which in turn cause ventricular fibrillation.

Figure 13-15 shows several small cardiac muscle strips cut in the form of circles. If such a strip is stimulated at the 12 o'clock position *so that the impulse travels in only one direction,* the impulse spreads progressively around the circle until it returns to the 12 o'clock position. If the originally stimulated muscle fibers are still in a refractory state, the impulse then dies out because refractory muscle cannot transmit a second impulse. But there are three different conditions that can cause this impulse to continue to travel around the circle, that is, to cause "re-entry" of the impulse into muscle that has already been excited. This is called a "circus movement."

First, if the *pathway around the circle is too long,* by the time the impulse returns to the 12 o'clock position, the originally stimulated muscle will no longer be refractory and the impulse will continue around the circle again and again.

Second, if the length of the pathway remains constant but the *velocity of conduction becomes decreased* enough, an increased interval of time will elapse before the impulse returns to the 12 o'clock position. By this time, the originally stimulated muscle might be out of the refractory state, and the impulse can continue around the circle again and again.

Third, *the refractory period of the muscle might become greatly shortened.* In this case, the impulse could also continue around and around the circle.

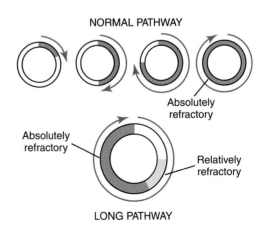

Figure 13-15 Circus movement, showing annihilation of the impulse in the short pathway and continued propagation of the impulse in the long pathway.

All these conditions occur in different pathological states of the human heart, as follows: (1) A long pathway typically occurs in dilated hearts. (2) Decreased rate of conduction frequently results from (a) blockage of the Purkinje system, (b) ischemia of the muscle, (c) high blood potassium levels, or (d) many other factors. (3) A shortened refractory period commonly occurs in response to various drugs, such as epinephrine, or after repetitive electrical stimulation. Thus, in many cardiac disturbances, re-entry can cause abnormal patterns of cardiac contraction or abnormal cardiac rhythms that ignore the pace-setting effects of the sinus node.

Chain Reaction Mechanism of Fibrillation

In ventricular fibrillation, one sees many separate and small contractile waves spreading at the same time in different directions over the cardiac muscle. The re-entrant impulses in fibrillation are not simply a single impulse moving in a circle, as shown in Figure 13-15. Instead, they have degenerated into a series of multiple wave fronts that have the appearance of a "chain reaction." One of the best ways to explain this process in fibrillation is to describe the initiation of fibrillation by electric shock caused by 60-cycle alternating electric current.

Fibrillation Caused by 60-Cycle Alternating Current. At a central point in the ventricles of heart A in Figure 13-16, a 60-cycle electrical stimulus is applied through a stimulating electrode. The first cycle of the electrical stimulus causes a depolarization wave to spread in all directions, leaving all the muscle beneath the electrode in a refractory state. After about 0.25 second, part of this muscle begins to come out of the refractory state. Some portions come out of refractoriness before other portions. This state of events is depicted in heart A by many lighter patches, which represent excitable cardiac muscle, and dark patches, which represent still refractory muscle. Now, continuing 60-cycle stimuli from the electrode can cause impulses to travel only in certain directions through the heart but not in all directions. Thus, in heart A, certain impulses travel for short distances, until they reach refractory areas of the heart, and then are blocked. But other impulses pass between the refractory areas and continue to travel in the excitable areas. Then, several events transpire in rapid succession, all occurring simultaneously and eventuating in a state of fibrillation.

First, block of the impulses in some directions but successful transmission in other directions creates one of the necessary conditions for a re-entrant signal to develop—that is, *transmission of some of the depolarization waves around the heart in only some directions but not other directions.*

Second, the rapid stimulation of the heart causes two changes in the cardiac muscle itself, both of which predispose to circus movement: (1) The *velocity of conduction through the heart muscle decreases,* which allows a longer time interval for the impulses to travel around the heart. (2) The *refractory period of the muscle is shortened,* allowing re-entry of the impulse into previously excited heart muscle within a much shorter time than normally.

Third, one of the most important features of fibrillation is the *division of impulses,* as demonstrated in heart A. When a depolarization wave reaches a refractory area in the heart, it travels to both sides around the refractory area. Thus, a single impulse becomes two impulses. Then, when each of these reaches another refractory area, it, too, divides to form two more impulses. In this way, many new wave fronts are continually being formed in the heart by progressive *chain reactions* until, finally, there are many small depolarization waves traveling in many directions at the same time. Furthermore, this irregular pattern of impulse travel causes *many circuitous routes for the impulses to travel, greatly lengthening the conductive pathway, which is one of the conditions that sustains the fibrillation.* It also results in a continual irregular pattern of patchy refractory areas in the heart.

One can readily see when a vicious circle has been initiated: More and more impulses are formed; these cause more and more patches of refractory muscle, and the refractory patches cause more and more division of the impulses. Therefore, any time a single area of cardiac muscle comes out of refractoriness, an impulse is close at hand to re-enter the area.

Heart B in Figure 13-16 demonstrates the final state that develops in fibrillation. Here one can see many impulses traveling in all directions, some dividing and increasing the number of impulses, whereas others are blocked by refractory areas. In fact, a single electric shock during this vulnerable period frequently can lead to an odd pattern of impulses spreading multidirectionally around refractory areas of muscle, which will lead to fibrillation.

Electrocardiogram in Ventricular Fibrillation

In ventricular fibrillation, the electrocardiogram is bizarre (Figure 13-17) and ordinarily shows no tendency toward a regular rhythm of any type. During the first few seconds

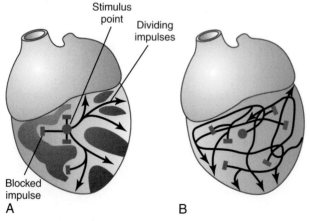

Figure 13-16 A, Initiation of fibrillation in a heart when patches of refractory musculature are present. B, Continued propagation of *fibrillatory impulses* in the fibrillating ventricle.

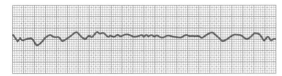

Figure 13-17 Ventricular fibrillation (lead II).

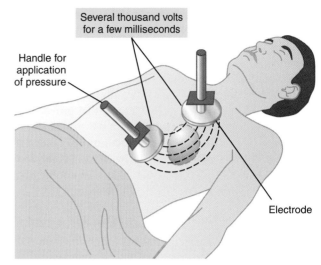

Figure 13-18 Application of electrical current to the chest to stop ventricular fibrillation.

of ventricular fibrillation, relatively large masses of muscle contract simultaneously, and this causes coarse, irregular waves in the electrocardiogram. After another few seconds, the coarse contractions of the ventricles disappear, and the electrocardiogram changes into a new pattern of low-voltage, very irregular waves. Thus, no repetitive electrocardiographic pattern can be ascribed to ventricular fibrillation. Instead, the ventricular muscle contracts at as many as 30 to 50 small patches of muscle at a time, and electrocardiographic potentials change constantly and spasmodically because the electrical currents in the heart flow first in one direction and then in another and seldom repeat any specific cycle.

The voltages of the waves in the electrocardiogram in ventricular fibrillation are usually about 0.5 millivolt when ventricular fibrillation first begins, but they decay rapidly so that after 20 to 30 seconds, they are usually only 0.2 to 0.3 millivolt. Minute voltages of 0.1 millivolt or less may be recorded for 10 minutes or longer after ventricular fibrillation begins. As already pointed out, because no pumping of blood occurs during ventricular fibrillation, this state is lethal unless stopped by some heroic therapy, such as immediate electroshock through the heart, as explained in the next section.

Electroshock Defibrillation of the Ventricles

Although a moderate alternating-current voltage applied directly to the ventricles almost invariably throws the ventricles into fibrillation, a strong high-voltage alternating electrical current passed through the ventricles for a fraction of a second can stop fibrillation by throwing all the ventricular muscle into refractoriness simultaneously. This is accomplished by passing intense current through large electrodes placed on two sides of the heart. The current penetrates most of the fibers of the ventricles at the same time, thus stimulating essentially all parts of the ventricles simultaneously and causing them all to become refractory. All action potentials stop, and the heart remains quiescent for 3 to 5 seconds, after which it begins to beat again, usually with the sinus node or some other part of the heart becoming the pacemaker. However, the same re-entrant focus that had originally thrown the ventricles into fibrillation often is still present, in which case fibrillation may begin again immediately.

When electrodes are applied directly to the two sides of the heart, fibrillation can usually be stopped using 110 volts of 60-cycle alternating current applied for 0.1 second or 1000 volts of direct current applied for a few thousandths of a second. When applied through two electrodes on the chest wall, as shown in Figure 13-18, the usual procedure is to charge a large electrical capacitor up to several thousand volts and then to cause the capacitor to discharge for a few thousandths of a second through the electrodes and through the heart.

Hand Pumping of the Heart (Cardiopulmonary Resuscitation) as an Aid to Defibrillation

Unless defibrillated within 1 minute after fibrillation begins, the heart is usually too weak to be revived by defibrillation because of the lack of nutrition from coronary blood flow. However, it is still possible to revive the heart by preliminarily pumping the heart by hand (intermittent hand squeezing) and then defibrillating the heart later. In this way, small quantities of blood are delivered into the aorta and a renewed coronary blood supply develops. Then, after a few minutes of hand pumping, electrical defibrillation often becomes possible. Indeed, fibrillating hearts have been pumped by hand for as long as 90 minutes followed by successful defibrillation.

A technique for pumping the heart without opening the chest consists of intermittent thrusts of pressure on the chest wall along with artificial respiration. This, plus defibrillation, is called *cardiopulmonary resuscitation*, or CPR.

Lack of blood flow to the brain for more than 5 to 8 minutes usually causes permanent mental impairment or even destruction of brain tissue. Even if the heart is revived, the person may die from the effects of brain damage or may live with permanent mental impairment.

Atrial Fibrillation

Remember that except for the conducting pathway through the A-V bundle, the atrial muscle mass is separated from the ventricular muscle mass by fibrous tissue. Therefore, ventricular fibrillation often occurs without atrial fibrillation. Likewise, fibrillation often occurs in the

151

atria without ventricular fibrillation (shown to the right in Figure 13-20).

The mechanism of atrial fibrillation is identical to that of ventricular fibrillation, except that the process occurs only in the atrial muscle mass instead of the ventricular mass. A frequent cause of atrial fibrillation is atrial enlargement resulting from heart valve lesions that prevent the atria from emptying adequately into the ventricles, or from ventricular failure with excess damming of blood in the atria. The dilated atrial walls provide ideal conditions of a long conductive pathway, as well as slow conduction, both of which predispose to atrial fibrillation.

Pumping Characteristics of the Atria during Atrial Fibrillation.

For the same reasons that the ventricles will not pump blood during ventricular fibrillation, neither do the atria pump blood in atrial fibrillation. Therefore, the atria become useless as primer pumps for the ventricles. Even so, blood flows passively through the atria into the ventricles, and the efficiency of ventricular pumping is decreased only 20 to 30 percent. Therefore, in contrast to the lethality of ventricular fibrillation, a person can live for months or even years with atrial fibrillation, although at reduced efficiency of overall heart pumping.

Electrocardiogram in Atrial Fibrillation.

Figure 13-19 shows the electrocardiogram during atrial fibrillation. Numerous small depolarization waves spread in all directions through the atria during atrial fibrillation. Because the waves are weak and many of them are of opposite polarity at any given time, they usually almost completely electrically neutralize one another. Therefore, in the electrocardiogram, one can see either no P waves from the atria or only a fine, high-frequency, very low voltage wavy record. Conversely, the QRS-T complexes are normal unless there is some pathology of the ventricles, but their timing is irregular, as explained next.

Irregularity of Ventricular Rhythm during Atrial Fibrillation.

When the atria are fibrillating, impulses arrive from the atrial muscle at the A-V node rapidly but also irregularly. Because the A-V node will not pass a second impulse for about 0.35 second after a previous one, at least 0.35 second must elapse between one ventricular contraction and the next. Then an additional but variable interval of 0 to 0.6 second occurs before one of the irregular atrial fibrillatory impulses happens to arrive at the A-V node. Thus, the interval between successive

ventricular contractions varies from a minimum of about 0.35 second to a maximum of about 0.95 second, causing a very irregular heartbeat. In fact, this irregularity, demonstrated by the variable spacing of the heartbeats in the electrocardiogram of Figure 13-19, is one of the clinical findings used to diagnose the condition. Also, because of the rapid rate of the fibrillatory impulses in the atria, the ventricle is driven at a fast heart rate, usually between 125 and 150 beats per minute.

Electroshock Treatment of Atrial Fibrillation.

In the same manner that ventricular fibrillation can be converted back to a normal rhythm by electroshock, so too can atrial fibrillation be converted by electroshock. The procedure is essentially the same as for ventricular fibrillation conversion—passage of a single strong electric shock through the heart, which throws the entire heart into refractoriness for a few seconds; a normal rhythm often follows *if the heart is capable of this.*

Atrial Flutter

Atrial flutter is another condition caused by a circus movement in the atria. It is different from atrial fibrillation, in that the electrical signal travels as a single large wave always in one direction around and around the atrial muscle mass, as shown to the left in Figure 13-20. Atrial flutter causes a rapid rate of contraction of the atria, usually between 200 and 350 beats per minute. However, because one side of the atria is contracting while the other side is relaxing, the amount of blood pumped by the atria is slight. Furthermore, the signals reach the A-V node too rapidly for all of them to be passed into the ventricles, because the refractory periods of the A-V node and A-V bundle are too long to pass more than a fraction of the atrial signals. Therefore, there are usually two to three beats of the atria for every single beat of the ventricles.

Figure 13-21 shows a typical electrocardiogram in atrial flutter. The P waves are strong because of contraction of semicoordinate masses of muscle. However, note

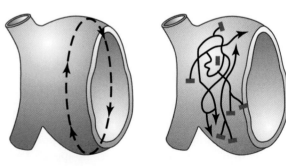

Atrial flutter   Atrial fibrillation

Figure 13-20 Pathways of impulses in atrial flutter and atrial fibrillation.

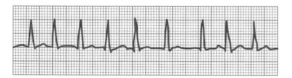

Figure 13-19 Atrial fibrillation (lead I). The waves that can be seen are ventricular QRS and T waves.

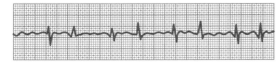

Figure 13-21 Atrial flutter—2:1 and 3:1 atrial to ventricle rhythm (lead I).

in the record that a QRS-T complex follows an atrial P wave only once for every two to three beats of the atria, giving a 2:1 or 3:1 rhythm.

Cardiac Arrest

A final serious abnormality of the cardiac rhythmicity-conduction system is *cardiac arrest.* This results from cessation of all electrical control signals in the heart. That is, no spontaneous rhythm remains.

Cardiac arrest may occur *during deep anesthesia,* when many patients develop severe hypoxia because of inadequate respiration. The hypoxia prevents the muscle fibers and conductive fibers from maintaining normal electrolyte concentration differentials across their membranes, and their excitability may be so affected that the automatic rhythmicity disappears.

In most instances of cardiac arrest from anesthesia, prolonged cardiopulmonary resuscitation (many minutes or even hours) is quite successful in re-establishing a normal heart rhythm. In some patients, severe myocardial disease can cause permanent or semipermanent cardiac arrest, which can cause death. To treat the condition, rhythmical electrical impulses from an *implanted electronic cardiac pacemaker* have been used successfully to keep patients alive for months to years.

Bibliography

Antzelevitch C: Role of spatial dispersion of repolarization in inherited and acquired sudden cardiac death syndromes, *Am J Physiol Heart Circ Physiol* 293:H2024, 2007.

Awad MM, Calkins H, Judge DP: Mechanisms of disease: molecular genetics of arrhythmogenic right ventricular dysplasia/cardiomyopathy, *Nat Clin Pract Cardiovasc Med* 5:258, 2008.

Barbuti A, DiFrancesco D: Control of cardiac rate by "funny" channels in health and disease, *Ann N Y Acad Sci* 1123:213, 2008.

Cheng H, Lederer WJ: Calcium sparks, *Physiol Rev* 88:1491, 2008.

Dobrzynski H, Boyett MR, Anderson RH: New insights into pacemaker activity: promoting understanding of sick sinus syndrome, *Circulation* 115:1921, 2007.

Elizari MV, Acunzo RS, Ferreiro M: Hemiblocks revisited, *Circulation* 115:1154, 2007.

Jalife J: Ventricular fibrillation: mechanisms of initiation and maintenance, *Annu Rev Physiol* 62:25, 2000.

Lubitz SA, Fischer A, Fuster V: Catheter ablation for atrial fibrillation, *BMJ* 336:819, 2008.

Maron BJ: Sudden death in young athletes, *N Engl J Med* 349:1064, 2003.

Morita H, Wu J, Zipes DP: The QT syndromes: long and short, *Lancet* 372:750, 2008.

Murray KT, Roden DM: Disorders of cardiac repolarization: the long QT syndromes. In Crawford MG, DiMarco JP, editors: Cardiology, London, 2001, Mosby.

Myerburg RJ: Implantable cardioverter-defibrillators after myocardial infarction, *N Engl J Med* 359:2245, 2008.

Passman R, Kadish A: Sudden death prevention with implantable devices, *Circulation* 116:561, 2007.

Roden DM: Drug-induced prolongation of the QT interval, *N Engl J Med* 350:1013, 2004.

Sanguinetti MC: Tristani-Firouzi M: hERG potassium channels and cardiac arrhythmia, *Nature* 440:463, 2006.

Swynghedauw B, Baillard C, Milliez P: The long QT interval is not only inherited but is also linked to cardiac hypertrophy, *J Mol Med* 81:336, 2003.

Wang K, Asinger RW, Marriott HJ: ST-segment elevation in conditions other than acute myocardial infarction, *N Engl J Med* 349:2128, 2003.

Zimetbaum PJ, Josephson ME: Use of the electrocardiogram in acute myocardial infarction, *N Engl J Med* 348:933, 2003.

UNIT III

IV

UNIT

The Circulation

14. Overview of the Circulation; Biophysics of Pressure, Flow, and Resistance

15. Vascular Distensibility and Functions of the Arterial and Venous Systems

16. The Microcirculation and Lymphatic System: Capillary Fluid Exchange, Interstitial Fluid, and Lymph Flow

17. Local and Humoral Control of Tissue Blood Flow

18. Nervous Regulation of the Circulation, and Rapid Control of Arterial Pressure

19. Role of the Kidneys in Long-Term Control of Arterial Pressure and in Hypertension; The Integrated System for Arterial Pressure Regulation

20. Cardiac Output, Venous Return, and Their Regulation

21. Muscle Blood Flow and Cardiac Output During Exercise; the Coronary Circulation and Ischemic Heart Disease

22. Cardiac Failure

23. Heart Valves and Heart Sounds; Valvular and Congenital Heart Defects

24. Circulatory Shock and Its Treatment

Overview of the Circulation; Biophysics of Pressure, Flow, and Resistance

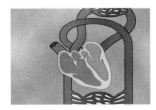

The function of the circulation is to service the needs of the body tissues—to transport nutrients to the body tissues, to transport waste products away, to transport hormones from one part of the body to another, and, in general, to maintain an appropriate environment in all the tissue fluids of the body for optimal survival and function of the cells.

The rate of blood flow through many tissues is controlled mainly in response to tissue need for nutrients. In some organs, such as the kidneys, the circulation serves additional functions. Blood flow to the kidney, for example, is far in excess of its metabolic requirements and is related to its excretory function, which demands that a large volume of blood be filtered each minute.

The heart and blood vessels, in turn, are controlled to provide the necessary cardiac output and arterial pressure to cause the needed tissue blood flow. What are the mechanisms for controlling blood volume and blood flow, and how does this relate to all the other functions of the circulation? These are some of the topics and questions that we discuss in this section on the circulation.

Physical Characteristics of the Circulation

The circulation, shown in Figure 14-1, is divided into the *systemic circulation* and the *pulmonary circulation.* Because the systemic circulation supplies blood flow to all the tissues of the body except the lungs, it is also called the *greater circulation* or *peripheral circulation.*

Functional Parts of the Circulation. Before discussing the details of circulatory function, it is important to understand the role of each part of the circulation.

The function of the *arteries* is to transport blood *under high pressure* to the tissues. For this reason, the arteries have strong vascular walls, and blood flows at a high velocity in the arteries.

The *arterioles* are the last small branches of the arterial system; they act as *control conduits* through which blood is released into the capillaries. Arterioles have strong muscular walls that can close the arterioles completely or can, by relaxing, dilate the vessels severalfold, thus having the capability of vastly altering blood flow in each tissue in response to its needs.

The function of the *capillaries* is to exchange fluid, nutrients, electrolytes, hormones, and other substances between the blood and the interstitial fluid. To serve this role, the capillary walls are very thin and have numerous minute *capillary pores* permeable to water and other small molecular substances.

The *venules* collect blood from the capillaries and gradually coalesce into progressively larger veins.

The *veins* function as conduits for transport of blood from the venules back to the heart; equally important, they serve as a major reservoir of extra blood. Because the pressure in the venous system is very low, the venous walls are thin. Even so, they are muscular enough to contract or expand and thereby act as a controllable reservoir for the extra blood, either a small or a large amount, depending on the needs of the circulation.

Volumes of Blood in the Different Parts of the Circulation. Figure 14-1 gives an overview of the circulation and lists the percentage of the total blood volume in major segments of the circulation. For instance, about 84 percent of the entire blood volume of the body is in the systemic circulation and 16 percent is in the heart and lungs. Of the 84 percent in the systemic circulation, 64 percent is in the veins, 13 percent in the arteries, and 7 percent in the systemic arterioles and capillaries. The heart contains 7 percent of the blood, and the pulmonary vessels, 9 percent.

Most surprising is the low blood volume in the capillaries. It is here, however, that the most important function of the circulation occurs, diffusion of substances back and forth between the blood and the tissues. This function is discussed in detail in Chapter 16.

Cross-Sectional Areas and Velocities of Blood Flow. If all the *systemic vessels* of each type were put side by side, their approximate total cross-sectional areas for the average human being would be as follows:

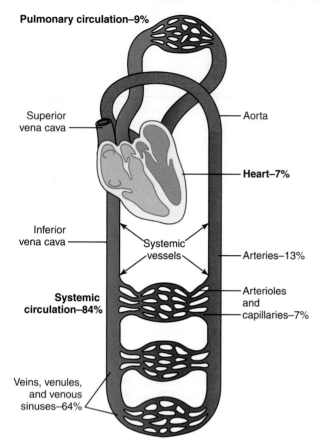

Pulmonary circulation—9%

Superior vena cava

Aorta

Heart—7%

Inferior vena cava

Systemic vessels

Arteries—13%

Systemic circulation—84%

Arterioles and capillaries—7%

Veins, venules, and venous sinuses—64%

Figure 14-1 Distribution of blood (in percentage of total blood) in the different parts of the circulatory system.

Vessel	Cross-Sectional Area (cm²)
Aorta	2.5
Small arteries	20
Arterioles	40
Capillaries	2500
Venules	250
Small veins	80
Venae cavae	8

Note particularly the much larger cross-sectional areas of the veins than of the arteries, averaging about four times those of the corresponding arteries. This explains the large blood storage capacity of the venous system in comparison with the arterial system.

Because the same volume of blood flow (F) must pass through each segment of the circulation each minute, the velocity of blood flow (v) is inversely proportional to vascular cross-sectional area (A):

$$v = F/A$$

Thus, under resting conditions, the velocity averages about 33 cm/sec in the aorta but only 1/1000 as rapidly in the capillaries, about 0.3 mm/sec. However, because the capillaries have a typical length of only 0.3 to 1 millimeter, the blood remains in the capillaries for only 1 to 3 seconds. This short time is surprising because all

diffusion of nutrient food substances and electrolytes that occurs through the capillary walls must do so in this short time.

Pressures in the Various Portions of the Circulation. Because the heart pumps blood continually into the aorta, the mean pressure in the aorta is high, averaging about 100 mm Hg. Also, because heart pumping is pulsatile, the arterial pressure alternates between a *systolic pressure level* of 120 mm Hg and a *diastolic pressure level* of 80 mm Hg, as shown on the left side of Figure 14-2.

As the blood flows through the *systemic circulation,* its mean pressure falls progressively to about 0 mm Hg by the time it reaches the termination of the venae cavae where they empty into the right atrium of the heart.

The pressure in the systemic capillaries varies from as high as 35 mm Hg near the arteriolar ends to as low as 10 mm Hg near the venous ends, but their average "functional" pressure in most vascular beds is about 17 mm Hg, a pressure low enough that little of the plasma leaks through the minute *pores* of the capillary walls, even though nutrients can *diffuse* easily through these same pores to the outlying tissue cells.

Note at the far right side of Figure 14-2 the respective pressures in the different parts of the *pulmonary circulation.* In the pulmonary arteries, the pressure is pulsatile, just as in the aorta, but the pressure is far less: *pulmonary artery systolic pressure* averages about 25 mm Hg and *diastolic pressure* 8 mm Hg, with a mean pulmonary arterial pressure of only 16 mm Hg. The mean pulmonary capillary pressure averages only 7 mm Hg. Yet the total blood flow through the lungs each minute is the same as through the systemic circulation. The low pressures of the pulmonary system are in accord with the needs of the lungs because all that is required is to expose the blood in the pulmonary capillaries to oxygen and other gases in the pulmonary alveoli.

Basic Principles of Circulatory Function

Although the details of circulatory function are complex, there are three basic principles that underlie all functions of the system.

1. **The rate of blood flow to each tissue of the body is almost always precisely controlled in relation to the tissue need.** When tissues are active, they need a greatly increased supply of nutrients and therefore much more blood flow than when at rest—occasionally as much as 20 to 30 times the resting level. Yet the heart normally cannot increase its cardiac output more than four to seven times greater than resting levels. Therefore, it is not possible simply to increase blood flow everywhere in the body when a particular tissue demands increased flow. Instead, the microvessels of each tissue continuously monitor tissue needs, such as the availability of oxygen and other nutrients

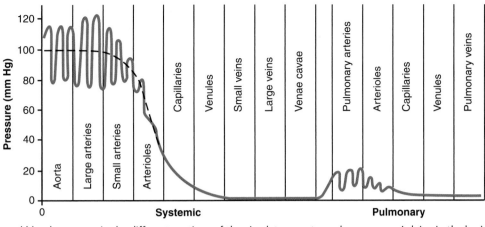

Figure 14-2 Normal blood pressures in the different portions of the circulatory system when a person is lying in the horizontal position.

and the accumulation of carbon dioxide and other tissue waste products, and these in turn act directly on the local blood vessels, dilating or constricting them, to control local blood flow precisely to that level required for the tissue activity. Also, nervous control of the circulation from the central nervous system and hormones provide additional help in controlling tissue blood flow.

2. **The cardiac output is controlled mainly by the sum of all the local tissue flows.** When blood flows through a tissue, it immediately returns by way of the veins to the heart. The heart responds automatically to this increased inflow of blood by pumping it immediately back into the arteries. Thus, the heart acts as an automaton, responding to the demands of the tissues. The heart, however, often needs help in the form of special nerve signals to make it pump the required amounts of blood flow.

3. **Arterial pressure regulation is generally independent of either local blood flow control or cardiac output control.** The circulatory system is provided with an extensive system for controlling the arterial blood pressure. For instance, if at any time the pressure falls significantly below the normal level of about 100 mm Hg, within seconds a barrage of nervous reflexes elicits a series of circulatory changes to raise the pressure back toward normal. The nervous signals especially (a) increase the force of heart pumping, (b) cause contraction of the large venous reservoirs to provide more blood to the heart, and (c) cause generalized constriction of most of the arterioles throughout the body so that more blood accumulates in the large arteries to increase the arterial pressure. Then, over more prolonged periods, hours and days, the kidneys play an additional major role in pressure control both by secreting pressure-controlling hormones and by regulating the blood volume.

Thus, in summary, the needs of the individual tissues are served specifically by the circulation. In the remainder of this chapter, we begin to discuss the basic details of the management of tissue blood flow and control of cardiac output and arterial pressure.

Interrelationships of Pressure, Flow, and Resistance

Blood flow through a blood vessel is determined by two factors: (1) *pressure difference* of the blood between the two ends of the vessel, also sometimes called "pressure gradient" along the vessel, which is the force that pushes the blood through the vessel, and (2) the impediment to blood flow through the vessel, which is called *vascular resistance*. Figure 14-3 demonstrates these relationships, showing a blood vessel segment located anywhere in the circulatory system.

P_1 represents the pressure at the origin of the vessel; at the other end, the pressure is P_2. Resistance occurs as a result of friction between the flowing blood and the intravascular endothelium all along the inside of the vessel. The flow through the vessel can be calculated by the following formula, which is called *Ohm's law*:

$$F = \frac{\Delta P}{R}$$

in which F is blood flow, ΔP is the pressure difference $(P_1 - P_2)$ between the two ends of the vessel, and R is the resistance. This formula states that the blood flow is directly proportional to the pressure difference but inversely proportional to the resistance.

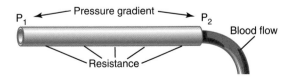

Figure 14-3 Interrelationships of pressure, resistance, and blood flow.

Note that it is the *difference* in pressure between the two ends of the vessel, not the absolute pressure in the vessel, that determines rate of flow. For example, if the pressure at both ends of a vessel is 100 mm Hg and yet no difference exists between the two ends, there will be no flow despite the presence of 100 mm Hg pressure.

Ohm's law, illustrated in Equation 1, expresses the most important of all the relations that the reader needs to understand to comprehend the hemodynamics of the circulation. Because of the extreme importance of this formula, the reader should also become familiar with its other algebraic forms:

$$\Delta P = F \times R$$

$$R = \frac{\Delta P}{F}$$

Blood Flow

Blood flow means the quantity of blood that passes a given point in the circulation in a given period of time. Ordinarily, blood flow is expressed in *milliliters per minute* or *liters per minute,* but it can be expressed in milliliters per second or in any other units of flow and time.

The overall blood flow in the total circulation of an adult person at rest is about 5000 ml/min. This is called the *cardiac output* because it is the amount of blood pumped into the aorta by the heart each minute.

Methods for Measuring Blood Flow. Many mechanical and mechanoelectrical devices can be inserted in series with a blood vessel or, in some instances, applied to the outside of the vessel to measure flow. They are called *flowmeters.*

Electromagnetic Flowmeter. One of the most important devices for measuring blood flow without opening the vessel is the electromagnetic flowmeter, the principles of which are illustrated in Figure 14-4. Figure 14-4*A* shows the generation of electromotive force (electrical voltage) in a wire that is moved rapidly in a cross-wise direction through a magnetic field. This is the well-known principle for production of electricity by the electric generator. Figure 14-4*B* shows that the same principle applies for generation of electromotive force in blood that is moving through a magnetic field. In this case, a blood vessel is placed between the poles of a strong magnet, and electrodes are placed on the two sides of the vessel perpendicular to the magnetic lines of force. When blood flows through the vessel, an electrical voltage proportional to the rate of blood flow is generated between the two electrodes, and this is recorded using an appropriate voltmeter or electronic recording apparatus. Figure 14-4*C* shows an actual "probe" that is placed on a large blood vessel to record its blood flow. The probe contains both the strong magnet and the electrodes.

A special advantage of the electromagnetic flowmeter is that it can record changes in flow in less than 1/100 of a second, allowing accurate recording of pulsatile changes in flow, as well as steady flow.

Ultrasonic Doppler Flowmeter. Another type of flowmeter that can be applied to the outside of the vessel and that has many of the same advantages as the electromagnetic flowmeter is the *ultrasonic Doppler flowmeter,* shown in Figure 14-5. A minute piezoelectric crystal is mounted at one end in the wall of the device. This crystal, when energized with an appropriate electronic apparatus, transmits ultrasound at a frequency of several hundred thousand cycles per second downstream along the flowing

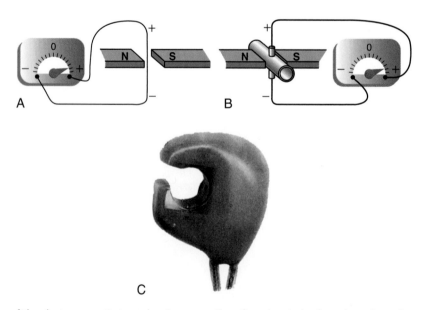

A   B   C

Figure 14-4 Flowmeter of the electromagnetic type, showing generation of an electrical voltage in a wire as it passes through an electromagnetic field (*A*); generation of an electrical voltage in electrodes on a blood vessel when the vessel is placed in a strong magnetic field and blood flows through the vessel (*B*); and a modern electromagnetic flowmeter probe for chronic implantation around blood vessels (*C*).

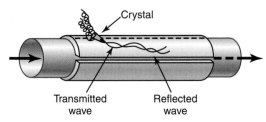

Figure 14-5 Ultrasonic Doppler flowmeter.

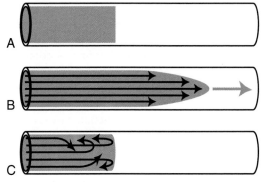

Figure 14-6 *A*, Two fluids (one dyed red, and the other clear) before flow begins; *B*, the same fluids 1 second after flow begins; *C*, turbulent flow, with elements of the fluid moving in a disorderly pattern.

blood. A portion of the sound is reflected by the red blood cells in the flowing blood. The reflected ultrasound waves then travel backward from the blood cells toward the crystal. These reflected waves have a lower frequency than the transmitted wave because the red cells are moving away from the transmitter crystal. This is called the *Doppler effect.* (It is the same effect that one experiences when a train approaches and passes by while blowing its whistle. Once the whistle has passed by the person, the pitch of the sound from the whistle suddenly becomes much lower than when the train is approaching.)

For the flowmeter shown in Figure 14-5, the high-frequency ultrasound wave is intermittently cut off, and the reflected wave is received back onto the crystal and amplified greatly by the electronic apparatus. Another portion of the electronic apparatus determines the frequency difference between the transmitted wave and the reflected wave, thus determining the velocity of blood flow. As long as diameter of a blood vessel does not change, changes in blood flow in the vessel are directly related to changes in flow velocity.

Like the electromagnetic flowmeter, the ultrasonic Doppler flowmeter is capable of recording rapid, pulsatile changes in flow, as well as steady flow.

Laminar Flow of Blood in Vessels. When blood flows at a steady rate through a long, smooth blood vessel, it flows in *streamlines*, with each layer of blood remaining the same distance from the vessel wall. Also, the central-most portion of the blood stays in the center of the vessel. This type of flow is called *laminar flow* or *streamline flow*, and it is the opposite of *turbulent flow*, which is blood flowing in all directions in the vessel and continually mixing within the vessel, as discussed subsequently.

Parabolic Velocity Profile during Laminar Flow. When laminar flow occurs, the velocity of flow in the center of the vessel is far greater than that toward the outer edges. This is demonstrated in Figure 14-6. In Figure 14-6*A*, a vessel contains two fluids, the one at the left colored by a dye and the one at the right a clear fluid, but there is no flow in the vessel. When the fluids are made to flow, a parabolic interface develops between them, as shown 1 second later in Figure 14-6*B*; the portion of fluid adjacent to the vessel wall has hardly moved, the portion slightly away from the wall has moved a small distance, and the portion in the center of the vessel has moved a long distance. This effect is called the "parabolic profile for velocity of blood flow."

The cause of the parabolic profile is the following: The fluid molecules touching the wall move slowly because of adherence to the vessel wall. The next layer of molecules slips over these, the third layer over the second, the fourth layer over the third, and so forth. Therefore, the fluid in the middle of the vessel can move rapidly because many layers of slipping molecules exist between the middle of the vessel and the vessel wall; thus, each layer toward the center flows progressively more rapidly than the outer layers.

Turbulent Flow of Blood under Some Conditions. When the rate of blood flow becomes too great, when it passes by an obstruction in a vessel, when it makes a sharp turn, or when it passes over a rough surface, the flow may then become *turbulent*, or disorderly, rather than streamlined (see Figure 14-6*C*). Turbulent flow means that the blood flows crosswise in the vessel and along the vessel, usually forming whorls in the blood, called *eddy currents*. These are similar to the whirlpools that one frequently sees in a rapidly flowing river at a point of obstruction.

When eddy currents are present, the blood flows with much greater resistance than when the flow is streamlined, because eddies add tremendously to the overall friction of flow in the vessel.

The tendency for turbulent flow increases in direct proportion to the velocity of blood flow, the diameter of the blood vessel, and the density of the blood and is inversely proportional to the viscosity of the blood, in accordance with the following equation:

$$Re = \frac{v \cdot d \cdot \rho}{\eta}$$

where Re is *Reynolds' number* and is the measure of the tendency for turbulence to occur, v is the mean velocity of blood flow (in centimeters/second), d is the vessel diameter (in centimeters), ρ is density, and η is the viscosity (in poise). The viscosity of blood is normally about $\frac{1}{30}$ poise, and the density is only slightly greater than 1. When Reynolds' number rises above 200 to 400, turbulent flow will occur at some branches of vessels but will die out along the smooth portions of the vessels. However, when Reynolds' number rises above approximately 2000, turbulence will usually occur even in a straight, smooth vessel.

Reynolds' number for flow in the vascular system even normally rises to 200 to 400 in large arteries; as a result there is almost always some turbulence of flow at the branches of these vessels. In the proximal portions of the aorta and pulmonary artery, Reynolds' number can rise to several thousand during the rapid phase of ejection by the ventricles; this causes considerable turbulence in the proximal aorta and pulmonary artery where many conditions are appropriate for turbulence: (1) high velocity of blood flow, (2) pulsatile nature of the flow, (3) sudden change in vessel diameter, and (4) large vessel diameter. However, in small vessels, Reynolds' number is almost never high enough to cause turbulence.

Blood Pressure

Standard Units of Pressure. Blood pressure almost always is measured in millimeters of mercury (mm Hg) because the mercury manometer has been used as the standard reference for measuring pressure since its invention in 1846 by Poiseuille. Actually, blood pressure means the *force exerted by the blood against any unit area of the vessel wall*. When one says that the pressure in a vessel is 50 mm Hg, this means that the force exerted is sufficient to push a column of mercury against gravity up to a level 50 millimeters high. If the pressure is 100 mm Hg, it will push the column of mercury up to 100 millimeters.

Occasionally, pressure is measured in *centimeters of water (cm H_2O)*. A pressure of 10 cm H_2O means a pressure sufficient to raise a column of water against gravity to a height of 10 centimeters. *One millimeter of mercury pressure equals 1.36 cm water pressure* because the specific gravity of mercury is 13.6 times that of water, and 1 centimeter is 10 times as great as 1 millimeter.

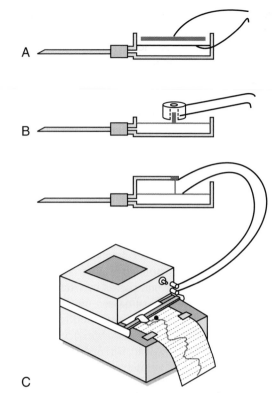

Figure 14-7 Principles of three types of electronic transducers for recording rapidly changing blood pressures (explained in the text).

In Figure 14-7*A*, a simple metal plate is placed a few hundredths of a centimeter above the membrane. When the membrane bulges, the membrane comes closer to the plate, which increases the *electrical capacitance* between these two, and this change in capacitance can be recorded using an appropriate electronic system.

In Figure 14-7*B*, a small iron slug rests on the membrane, and this can be displaced upward into a center space inside an electrical wire coil. Movement of the iron into the coil increases the *inductance* of the coil, and this, too, can be recorded electronically.

Finally, in Figure 14-7*C*, a very thin, stretched resistance wire is connected to the membrane. When this wire is stretched greatly, its resistance increases; when it is stretched less, its resistance decreases. These changes, too, can be recorded by an electronic system.

The electrical signals from the transducer are sent to an amplifier and then to an appropriate recording device. With some of these high-fidelity types of recording systems, pressure cycles up to 500 cycles per second have been recorded accurately. In common use are recorders capable of registering pressure changes that occur as rapidly as 20 to 100 cycles per second, in the manner shown on the recording paper in Figure 14-7*C*.

High-Fidelity Methods for Measuring Blood Pressure. The mercury in a manometer has so much inertia that it cannot rise and fall rapidly. For this reason, the mercury manometer, although excellent for recording steady pressures, cannot respond to pressure changes that occur more rapidly than about one cycle every 2 to 3 seconds. Whenever it is desired to record rapidly changing pressures, some other type of pressure recorder is necessary. Figure 14-7 demonstrates the basic principles of three electronic pressure *transducers* commonly used for converting blood pressure and/or rapid changes in pressure into electrical signals and then recording the electrical signals on a high-speed electrical recorder. Each of these transducers uses a very thin, highly stretched metal membrane that forms one wall of the fluid chamber. The fluid chamber in turn is connected through a needle or catheter inserted into the blood vessel in which the pressure is to be measured. When the pressure is high, the membrane bulges slightly, and when it is low, it returns toward its resting position.

Resistance to Blood Flow

Units of Resistance. Resistance is the impediment to blood flow in a vessel, but it cannot be measured by any direct means. Instead, resistance must be calculated from measurements of blood flow and pressure difference between two points in the vessel. If the pressure difference between two points is 1 mm Hg and the flow is 1 ml/sec, the resistance is said to be 1 *peripheral resistance unit*, usually abbreviated *PRU*.

Expression of Resistance in CGS Units. Occasionally, a basic physical unit called the CGS (centimeters, grams, seconds) unit is used to express resistance. This unit is dyne sec/cm^5. Resistance in these units can be calculated by the following formula:

$$R\left(\text{in }\frac{\text{dyne sec}}{\text{cm}^5}\right) = \frac{1333 \times \text{mm Hg}}{\text{ml/sec}}$$

Total Peripheral Vascular Resistance and Total Pulmonary Vascular Resistance. The rate of blood flow through the entire circulatory system is equal to the rate of blood pumping by the heart—that is, it is equal to the cardiac output. In the adult human being, this is approximately 100 ml/sec. The pressure difference from the systemic arteries to the systemic veins is about 100 mm Hg. Therefore, the resistance of the entire systemic circulation, called the *total peripheral resistance*, is about 100/100, or 1 peripheral resistance unit (PRU).

In conditions in which all the blood vessels throughout the body become strongly constricted, the total peripheral resistance occasionally rises to as high as 4 PRU. Conversely, when the vessels become greatly dilated, the resistance can fall to as little as 0.2 PRU.

In the pulmonary system, the mean pulmonary arterial pressure averages 16 mm Hg and the mean left atrial pressure averages 2 mm Hg, giving a net pressure difference of 14 mm. Therefore, when the cardiac output is normal at about 100 ml/sec, the *total pulmonary vascular resistance* calculates to be about 0.14 PRU (about one seventh that in the systemic circulation).

"Conductance" of Blood in a Vessel and Its Relation to Resistance.

Conductance is a measure of the blood flow through a vessel for a given pressure difference. This is generally expressed in terms of milliliters per second per millimeter of mercury pressure, but it can also be expressed in terms of liters per second per millimeter of mercury or in any other units of blood flow and pressure.

It is evident that conductance is the exact reciprocal of resistance in accord with the following equation:

$$\text{Conductance} = \frac{1}{\text{Resistance}}$$

Very Slight Changes in Diameter of a Vessel Can Change Its Conductance Tremendously!

Slight changes in the diameter of a vessel cause tremendous changes in the vessel's ability to conduct blood when the blood flow is streamlined. This is demonstrated

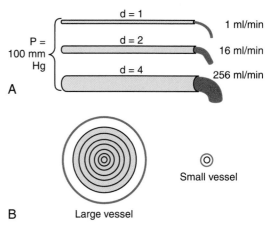

Figure 14-8 *A*, Demonstration of the effect of vessel diameter on blood flow. *B*, Concentric rings of blood flowing at different velocities; the farther away from the vessel wall, the faster the flow.

by the experiment illustrated in Figure 14-8*A*, which shows three vessels with relative diameters of 1, 2, and 4 but with the same pressure difference of 100 mm Hg between the two ends of the vessels. Although the diameters of these vessels increase only fourfold, the respective flows are 1, 16, and 256 ml/min, which is a 256-fold increase in flow. Thus, the conductance of the vessel increases in proportion to the *fourth power of the diameter*, in accordance with the following formula:

$$\text{Conductance} \propto \text{Diameter}^4$$

Poiseuille's Law. The cause of this great increase in conductance when the diameter increases can be explained by referring to Figure 14-8*B*, which shows cross sections of a large and a small vessel. The concentric rings inside the vessels indicate that the velocity of flow in each ring is different from that in the adjacent rings because of *laminar* flow, which was discussed earlier in the chapter. That is, the blood in the ring touching the wall of the vessel is barely flowing because of its adherence to the vascular endothelium. The next ring of blood toward the center of the vessel slips past the first ring and, therefore, flows more rapidly. The third, fourth, fifth, and sixth rings likewise flow at progressively increasing velocities. Thus, the blood that is near the wall of the vessel flows slowly, whereas that in the middle of the vessel flows much more rapidly.

In the small vessel, essentially all the blood is near the wall, so the extremely rapidly flowing central stream of blood simply does not exist. By integrating the velocities of all the concentric rings of flowing blood and multiplying them by the areas of the rings, one can derive the following formula, known as Poiseuille's law:

$$F = \frac{\pi \Delta P r^4}{8\eta l}$$

in which F is the rate of blood flow, ΔP is the pressure difference between the ends of the vessel, r is the radius of the vessel, l is length of the vessel, and η is viscosity of the blood.

UNIT IV

Note particularly in this equation that the rate of blood flow is directly proportional to the *fourth power of the radius* of the vessel, which demonstrates once again that the diameter of a blood vessel (which is equal to twice the radius) plays by far the greatest role of all factors in determining the rate of blood flow through a vessel.

Importance of the Vessel Diameter "Fourth Power Law" in Determining Arteriolar Resistance. In the systemic circulation, about two thirds of the total systemic resistance to blood flow is arteriolar resistance in the small arterioles. The internal diameters of the arterioles range from as little as 4 micrometers to as great as 25 micrometers. However, their strong vascular walls allow the internal diameters to change tremendously, often as much as fourfold. From the fourth power law discussed earlier that relates blood flow to diameter of the vessel, one can see that a fourfold increase in vessel diameter can increase the flow as much as 256-fold. Thus, this fourth power law makes it possible for the arterioles, responding with only small changes in diameter to nervous signals or local tissue chemical signals, either to turn off almost completely the blood flow to the tissue or at the other extreme to cause a vast increase in flow. Indeed, ranges of blood flow of more than 100-fold in separate tissue areas have been recorded between the limits of maximum arteriolar constriction and maximum arteriolar dilatation.

Resistance to Blood Flow in Series and Parallel Vascular Circuits. Blood pumped by the heart flows from the high-pressure part of the systemic circulation (i.e., aorta) to the low-pressure side (i.e., vena cava) through many miles of blood vessels arranged in series and in parallel. The arteries, arterioles, capillaries, venules, and veins are collectively arranged in series. When blood vessels are arranged in series, flow through each blood vessel is the same and the total resistance to blood flow (R_{total}) is equal to the sum of the resistances of each vessel:

$$R_{total} = R_1 + R_2 + R_3 + R_4 \cdots$$

The total peripheral vascular resistance is therefore equal to the sum of resistances of the arteries, arterioles, capillaries, venules, and veins. In the example shown in Figure 14-9A, the total vascular resistance is equal to the sum of R_1 and R_2.

Blood vessels branch extensively to form parallel circuits that supply blood to the many organs and tissues of the body. This parallel arrangement permits each tissue to regulate its own blood flow, to a great extent, independently of flow to other tissues.

For blood vessels arranged in parallel (Figure 14-9B), the total resistance to blood flow is expressed as:

$$\frac{1}{R_{total}} = \frac{1}{R_1} + \frac{1}{R_2} + \frac{1}{R_3} + \frac{1}{R_4} \cdots$$

It is obvious that for a given pressure gradient, far greater amounts of blood will flow through this parallel system than through any of the individual blood vessels. Therefore, the total resistance is far less than the resistance of any single blood vessel. Flow through each of the parallel vessels in Figure 14-9B is determined by the pressure gradient and its own resistance, not the resistance of the other parallel blood vessels. However, increasing the resistance of any of the blood vessels increases the total vascular resistance.

It may seem paradoxical that adding more blood vessels to a circuit reduces the total vascular resistance. Many parallel blood vessels, however, make it easier for blood to flow through the circuit because each parallel vessel provides another pathway, or *conductance*, for blood flow. The total conductance (C_{total}) for blood flow is the sum of the conductance of each parallel pathway:

$$C_{total} = C_1 + C_2 + C_3 + C_4 \cdots$$

For example, brain, kidney, muscle, gastrointestinal, skin, and coronary circulations are arranged in parallel, and each tissue contributes to the overall conductance of the systemic circulation. Blood flow through each tissue is a fraction of the total blood flow (cardiac output) and is determined by the resistance (the reciprocal of conductance) for blood flow in the tissue, as well as the pressure gradient. Therefore, amputation of a limb or surgical removal of a kidney also removes a parallel circuit and reduces the total vascular conductance and total blood flow (i.e., cardiac output) while increasing total peripheral vascular resistance.

Effect of Blood Hematocrit and Blood Viscosity on Vascular Resistance and Blood Flow

Note especially that another of the important factors in Poiseuille's equation is the viscosity of the blood. The greater the viscosity, the less the flow in a vessel if all other factors are constant. Furthermore, *the viscosity of normal blood is about three times as great as the viscosity of water.*

But what makes the blood so viscous? It is mainly the large numbers of suspended red cells in the blood, each of which exerts frictional drag against adjacent cells and against the wall of the blood vessel.

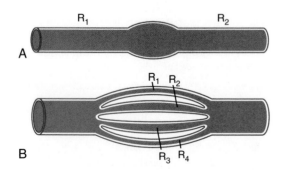

Figure 14-9 Vascular resistances: *A*, in series and *B*, in parallel.

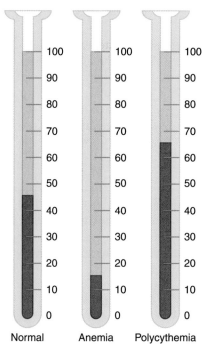

Figure 14-10 Hematocrits in a healthy (normal) person and in patients with anemia and polycythemia.

Hematocrit. The proportion of the blood that is red blood cells is called the *hematocrit*. Thus, if a person has a hematocrit of 40, this means that 40 percent of the blood volume is cells and the remainder is plasma. The hematocrit of adult men averages about 42, while that of women averages about 38. These values vary tremendously, depending on whether the person has anemia, on the degree of bodily activity, and on the altitude at which the person resides. These changes in hematocrit are discussed in relation to the red blood cells and their oxygen transport function in Chapter 32.

Hematocrit is determined by centrifuging blood in a calibrated tube, as shown in Figure 14-10. The calibration allows direct reading of the percentage of cells.

Effect of Hematocrit on Blood Viscosity. The viscosity of blood increases drastically as the hematocrit increases, as shown in Figure 14-11. The viscosity of

whole blood at normal hematocrit is about 3; this means that three times as much pressure is required to force whole blood as to force water through the same blood vessel. When the hematocrit rises to 60 or 70, which it often does in *polycythemia,* the blood viscosity can become as great as 10 times that of water, and its flow through blood vessels is greatly retarded.

Other factors that affect blood viscosity are the plasma protein concentration and types of proteins in the plasma, but these effects are so much less than the effect of hematocrit that they are not significant considerations in most hemodynamic studies. The viscosity of blood plasma is about 1.5 times that of water.

Effects of Pressure on Vascular Resistance and Tissue Blood Flow

"Autoregulation" Attenuates the Effect of Arterial Pressure on Tissue Blood Flow. From the discussion thus far, one might expect an increase in arterial pressure to cause a proportionate increase in blood flow through the various tissues of the body. However, the effect of arterial pressure on blood flow in many tissues is usually far less than one would expect, as shown in Figure 14-12. The reason for this is that an increase in arterial pressure not only increases the force that pushes blood through the vessels but it also initiates compensatory increases in vascular resistance within a few seconds through activation of the local control mechanisms discussed in Chapter 17. Conversely, with reductions in arterial pressure most vascular resistance is promptly reduced in most tissues and blood flow is maintained relatively constant. The ability of each tissue to adjust its vascular resistance and to maintain normal blood flow during changes in arterial pressure between approximately 70 and 175 mm Hg is called *blood flow autoregulation.*

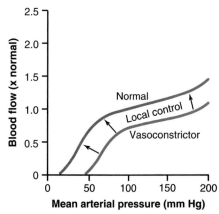

Figure 14-12 Effect of changes in arterial pressure over a period of several minutes on blood flow in a tissue such as skeletal muscle. Note that between pressure of 70 and 175 mm Hg blood flow is "autoregulated." The *blue line* shows the effect of sympathetic nerve stimulation or vasoconstriction by hormones such as norepinephrine, angiotensin II, vasopressin, or endothelin on this relationship. Reduced tissue blood flow is rarely maintained for more than a few hours due to activation of local autoregulatory mechanisms that eventually return blood flow toward normal.

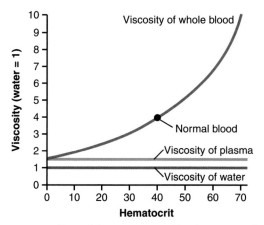

Figure 14-11 Effect of hematocrit on blood viscosity. (Water viscosity = 1.)

Note in Figure 14-12 that changes in blood flow can be caused by strong sympathetic stimulation, which *constricts* the blood vessels. Likewise, hormonal vasoconstrictors, such as *norepinephrine, angiotensin II, vasopressin,* or *endothelin,* can also reduce blood flow, at least transiently.

Changes in tissue blood flow rarely last for more than a few hours even when increases in arterial pressure or increased levels of vasoconstrictors are sustained. The reason for the relative constancy of blood flow is that each tissue's local autoregulatory mechanisms eventually override most of the effects of vasoconstrictors in order to provide a blood flow that is appropriate for the needs of the tissue.

Pressure-Flow Relationship in Passive Vascular Beds. In isolated blood vessels or in tissues that do not exhibit autoregulation, changes in arterial pressure may have important effects on blood flow. In fact, the effect of pressure on blood flow may be greater than predicted by Poiseuille's equation, as shown by the upward curving lines in Figure 14-13. The reason for this is that increased arterial pressure not only increases the force that pushes blood through the vessels but it also distends the elastic vessels, actually *decreasing* vascular resistance. Conversely, decreased arterial pressure in passive blood vessels increases resistance as the elastic vessels gradually collapse due to reduced distending pressure. When pressure falls below a critical level, called the *critical closing pressure,* flow ceases as the blood vessels are completely collapsed.

Sympathetic stimulation and other vasoconstrictors can alter the passive pressure-flow relationship shown in Figure 14-13. Thus, *inhibition of* sympathetic activity

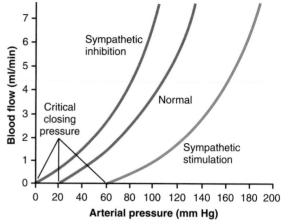

Figure 14-13 Effect of arterial pressure on blood flow through a *passive* blood vessel at different degrees of vascular tone caused by increased or decreased sympathetic stimulation of the vessel.

greatly dilates the vessels and can increase the blood flow twofold or more. Conversely, very strong sympathetic stimulation *can constrict* the vessels so much that blood flow occasionally decreases to as low as zero for a few seconds despite high arterial pressure.

In reality, there are few physiological conditions in which tissues display the passive pressure-flow relationship shown in Figure 14-13. Even in tissues that do not effectively autoregulate blood flow during acute changes in arterial pressure, blood flow is regulated according to the needs of the tissue when the pressure changes are sustained, as discussed in Chapter 17.

Bibliography

See bibliography for Chapter 15.

Vascular Distensibility and Functions of the Arterial and Venous Systems

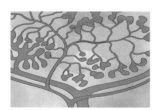

Vascular Distensibility

A valuable characteristic of the vascular system is that all blood vessels are *distensible.* The distensible nature of the arteries allows them to accommodate the pulsatile output of the heart and to average out the pressure pulsations. This provides smooth, continuous flow of blood through the very small blood vessels of the tissues.

The most distensible by far of all the vessels are the veins. Even slight increases in venous pressure cause the veins to store 0.5 to 1.0 liter of extra blood. Therefore, the veins provide a *reservoir function* for storing large quantities of extra blood that can be called into use whenever required elsewhere in the circulation.

Units of Vascular Distensibility. Vascular distensibility normally is expressed as the fractional increase in volume for each millimeter of mercury rise in pressure, in accordance with the following formula:

$$\text{Vascular distensibility} = \frac{\text{Increase in volume}}{\text{Increase in pressure} \times \text{Original volume}}$$

That is, if 1 mm Hg causes a vessel that originally contained 10 millimeters of blood to increase its volume by 1 milliliter, the distensibility would be 0.1 per mm Hg, or 10 percent per mm Hg.

Difference in Distensibility of the Arteries and the Veins. Anatomically, the walls of the arteries are far stronger than those of the veins. Consequently, the veins, on average, are about eight times more distensible than the arteries. That is, a given increase in pressure causes about eight times as much increase in blood in a vein as in an artery of comparable size.

In the pulmonary circulation, the pulmonary vein distensibilities are similar to those of the systemic circulation. But the pulmonary arteries normally operate under pressures about one sixth of those in the systemic arterial system, and

their distensibilities are correspondingly greater, about six times the distensibility of systemic arteries.

Vascular Compliance (or Vascular Capacitance)

In hemodynamic studies, it usually is much more important to know the *total quantity of blood* that can be stored in a given portion of the circulation for each mm Hg pressure rise than to know the distensibilities of the individual vessels. This value is called the *compliance* or *capacitance* of the respective vascular bed; that is,

$$\text{Vascular compliance} = \frac{\text{Increase in volume}}{\text{Increase in pressure}}$$

Compliance and distensibility are quite different. A highly distensible vessel that has a slight volume may have far less compliance than a much less distensible vessel that has a large volume because *compliance is equal to distensibility times volume.*

The compliance of a systemic vein is about 24 times that of its corresponding artery because it is about 8 times as distensible and it has a volume about 3 times as great ($8 \times 3 = 24$).

Volume-Pressure Curves of the Arterial and Venous Circulations

A convenient method for expressing the relation of pressure to volume in a vessel or in any portion of the circulation is to use the so-called *volume-pressure curve.* The red and blue solid curves in Figure 15-1 represent, respectively, the volume-pressure curves of the normal systemic arterial system and venous system, showing that when the arterial system of the average adult person (including all the large arteries, small arteries, and arterioles) is filled with about 700 milliliters of blood, the mean arterial pressure is 100 mm Hg, but when it is filled with only 400 milliliters of blood, the pressure falls to zero.

In the entire systemic venous system, the volume normally ranges from 2000 to 3500 milliliters, and a change of several hundred millimeters in this volume is required to change the venous pressure only 3 to 5 mm Hg. This mainly explains why as much as one half liter of blood can be

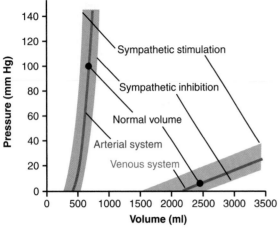

Figure 15-1 "Volume-pressure curves" of the systemic arterial and venous systems, showing the effects of stimulation or inhibition of the sympathetic nerves to the circulatory system.

transfused into a healthy person in only a few minutes without greatly altering function of the circulation.

Effect of Sympathetic Stimulation or Sympathetic Inhibition on the Volume-Pressure Relations of the Arterial and Venous Systems.

Also shown in Figure 15-1 are the effects of exciting or inhibiting the vascular sympathetic nerves on the volume-pressure curves. It is evident that increase in vascular smooth muscle tone caused by sympathetic stimulation increases the pressure at each volume of the arteries or veins, whereas sympathetic inhibition decreases the pressure at each volume. Control of the vessels in this manner by the sympathetics is a valuable means for diminishing the dimensions of one segment of the circulation, thus transferring blood to other segments. For instance, an increase in vascular tone throughout the systemic circulation often causes large volumes of blood to shift into the heart, which is one of the principal methods that the body uses to increase heart pumping.

Sympathetic control of vascular capacitance is also highly important during hemorrhage. Enhancement of sympathetic tone, especially to the veins, reduces the vessel sizes enough that the circulation continues to operate almost normally even when as much as 25 percent of the total blood volume has been lost.

Delayed Compliance (Stress-Relaxation) of Vessels

The term "delayed compliance" means that a vessel exposed to increased volume at first exhibits a large increase in pressure, but progressive delayed stretching of smooth muscle in the vessel wall allows the pressure to return back toward normal over a period of minutes to hours. This effect is shown in Figure 15-2. In this figure, the pressure is recorded in a small segment of a vein that is occluded at both ends. An extra volume of blood is suddenly injected until the pressure rises from 5 to 12 mm Hg. Even though none of the blood is removed after it is injected, the pressure begins to decrease immediately and approaches about 9 mm Hg after several minutes. In other words, the volume of blood injected causes immediate

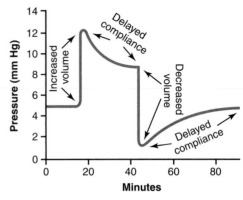

Figure 15-2 Effect on the intravascular pressure of injecting a volume of blood into a venous segment and later removing the excess blood, demonstrating the principle of delayed compliance.

elastic distention of the vein, but then the smooth muscle fibers of the vein begin to "creep" to longer lengths, and their tensions correspondingly decrease. This effect is a characteristic of all smooth muscle tissue and is called *stress-relaxation*, which was explained in Chapter 8.

Delayed compliance is a valuable mechanism by which the circulation can accommodate extra blood when necessary, such as after too large a transfusion. Delayed compliance in the reverse direction is one of the ways in which the circulation automatically adjusts itself over a period of minutes or hours to diminished blood volume after serious hemorrhage.

Arterial Pressure Pulsations

With each beat of the heart a new surge of blood fills the arteries. Were it not for distensibility of the arterial system, all of this new blood would have to flow through the peripheral blood vessels almost instantaneously, only during cardiac systole, and no flow would occur during diastole. However, the compliance of the arterial tree normally reduces the pressure pulsations to almost no pulsations by the time the blood reaches the capillaries; therefore, tissue blood flow is mainly continuous with very little pulsation.

A typical record of the *pressure pulsations* at the root of the aorta is shown in Figure 15-3. In the healthy young adult, the pressure at the top of each pulse, called the *systolic pressure*, is about 120 mm Hg. At the lowest point of each pulse, called the *diastolic pressure*, it is about 80 mm Hg. The difference between these two pressures, about 40 mm Hg, is called the *pulse pressure*.

Two major factors affect the pulse pressure: (1) the *stroke volume output* of the heart and (2) the *compliance (total distensibility)* of the arterial tree. A third, less important factor, is the character of ejection from the heart during systole.

In general, the greater the stroke volume output, the greater the amount of blood that must be accommodated in the arterial tree with each heartbeat, and, therefore, the greater the pressure rise and fall during systole and diastole, thus causing a greater pulse pressure. Conversely, the less the compliance of the arterial system, the greater the

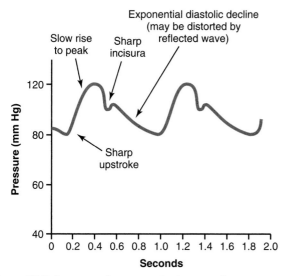

Figure 15-3 Pressure pulse contour in the ascending aorta.

rise in pressure for a given stroke volume of blood pumped into the arteries. For instance, as demonstrated by the middle top curves in Figure 15-4, the pulse pressure in old age sometimes rises to as much as twice normal, because the arteries have become hardened with *arteriosclerosis* and therefore are relatively noncompliant.

In effect, pulse pressure is determined approximately by the *ratio of stroke volume output to compliance of the arterial tree.* Any condition of the circulation that affects either of these two factors also affects the pulse pressure:

Pulse Pressure ≈ stroke volume/arterial compliance

Abnormal Pressure Pulse Contours

Some conditions of the circulation also cause *abnormal contours of the pressure pulse wave* in addition to altering the pulse pressure. Especially distinctive among these are aortic stenosis, patent ductus arteriosus, and aortic regurgitation, each of which is shown in Figure 15-4.

In *aortic valve stenosis,* the diameter of the aortic valve opening is reduced significantly, and the aortic pressure pulse is decreased significantly because of diminished blood flow outward through the stenotic valve.

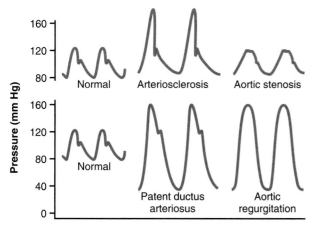

Figure 15-4 Aortic pressure pulse contours in arteriosclerosis, aortic stenosis, patent ductus arteriosus, and aortic regurgitation.

In *patent ductus arteriosus,* one half or more of the blood pumped into the aorta by the left ventricle flows immediately backward through the wide-open ductus into the pulmonary artery and lung blood vessels, thus allowing the diastolic pressure to fall very low before the next heartbeat.

In *aortic regurgitation,* the aortic valve is absent or will not close completely. Therefore, after each heartbeat, the blood that has just been pumped into the aorta flows immediately backward into the left ventricle. As a result, the aortic pressure can fall all the way to zero between heartbeats. Also, there is no incisura in the aortic pulse contour because there is no aortic valve to close.

Transmission of Pressure Pulses to the Peripheral Arteries

When the heart ejects blood into the aorta during systole, at first only the proximal portion of the aorta becomes distended because the inertia of the blood prevents sudden blood movement all the way to the periphery. However, the rising pressure in the proximal aorta rapidly overcomes this inertia, and the wave front of distention spreads farther and farther along the aorta, as shown in Figure 15-5. This is called *transmission of the pressure pulse* in the arteries.

The velocity of pressure pulse transmission in the normal aorta is 3 to 5 m/sec; in the large arterial branches, 7 to 10 m/sec; and in the small arteries, 15 to 35 m/sec. In general, the greater the compliance of each vascular segment, the slower the velocity, which explains the slow transmission in the aorta and the much faster transmission in the much less compliant small distal arteries. In the aorta, the velocity of transmission of the pressure pulse is 15 or more times the velocity of blood flow because the

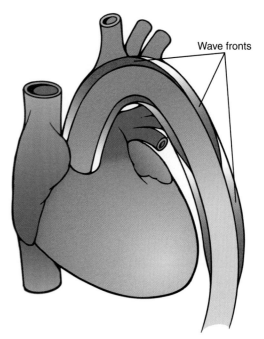

Figure 15-5 Progressive stages in transmission of the pressure pulse along the aorta.

pressure pulse is simply a moving wave of *pressure* that involves little forward total movement of blood volume.

Damping of the Pressure Pulses in the Smaller Arteries, Arterioles, and Capillaries.

Figure 15-6 shows typical changes in the contours of the pressure pulse as the pulse travels into the peripheral vessels. Note especially in the three lower curves that the intensity of pulsation becomes progressively less in the smaller arteries, the arterioles, and, especially, the capillaries. In fact, only when the aortic pulsations are extremely large or the arterioles are greatly dilated can pulsations be observed in the capillaries.

This progressive diminution of the pulsations in the periphery is called *damping* of the pressure pulses. The cause of this is twofold: (1) resistance to blood movement in the vessels and (2) compliance of the vessels. The resistance damps the pulsations because a small amount of blood must flow forward at the pulse wave front to distend the next segment of the vessel; the greater the resistance, the more difficult it is for this to occur. The compliance damps the pulsations because the more compliant a vessel, the greater the quantity of blood required at the pulse wave front to cause an increase in pressure. Therefore, *the degree of damping is almost directly proportional to the product of resistance times compliance.*

Clinical Methods for Measuring Systolic and Diastolic Pressures

It is not reasonable to use pressure recorders that require needle insertion into an artery for making routine arterial pressure measurements in human patients, although these are used on occasion when special studies are necessary. Instead, the clinician determines systolic and diastolic pressures by indirect means, usually by the *auscultatory method*.

Auscultatory Method.

Figure 15-7 shows the auscultatory method for determining systolic and diastolic arterial pressures. A stethoscope is placed over the antecubital artery and a blood pressure cuff is inflated around the upper arm. As long as the cuff continues to compress the arm with too little pressure to close the brachial artery, no sounds are heard from the antecubital artery with the stethoscope. However, when the cuff pressure is great enough to close the artery during part of the arterial pressure cycle, a sound then is heard with each pulsation. These sounds are called *Korotkoff sounds,*

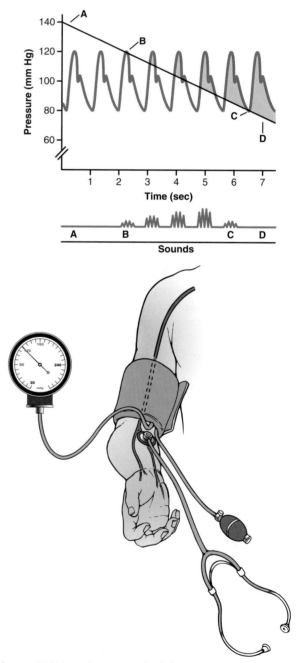

Figure 15-7 Auscultatory method for measuring systolic and diastolic arterial pressures.

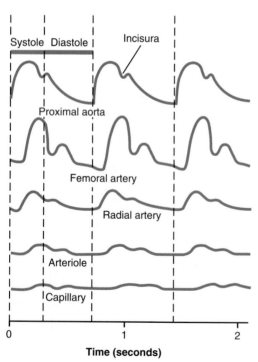

Figure 15-6 Changes in the pulse pressure contour as the pulse wave travels toward the smaller vessels.

named after *Nikolai Korotkoff*, a Russian physician who described them in 1905.

The Korotkoff sounds are believed to be caused mainly by blood jetting through the partly occluded vessel and by vibrations of the vessel wall. The jet causes turbulence in the vessel beyond the cuff, and this sets up the vibrations heard through the stethoscope.

In determining blood pressure by the auscultatory method, the pressure in the cuff is first elevated well above arterial systolic pressure. As long as this cuff pressure is higher than systolic pressure, the brachial artery remains collapsed so that no blood jets into the lower artery during any part of the pressure cycle. Therefore, no Korotkoff sounds are heard in the lower artery. But then the cuff pressure gradually is reduced. Just as soon as the pressure in the cuff falls below systolic pressure (point B, Figure 15-7), blood begins to slip through the artery beneath the cuff during the peak of systolic pressure, and one begins to hear *tapping* sounds from the antecubital artery in synchrony with the heartbeat. As soon as these sounds begin to be heard, the pressure level indicated by the manometer connected to the cuff is about equal to the systolic pressure.

As the pressure in the cuff is lowered still more, the Korotkoff sounds change in quality, having less of the tapping quality and more of a rhythmical and harsher quality. Then, finally, when the pressure in the cuff falls near diastolic pressure, the sounds suddenly change to a muffled quality (point C, Figure 15-7). One notes the manometer pressure when the Korotkoff sounds change to the muffled quality and this pressure is about equal to the diastolic pressure, although it slightly overestimates the diastolic pressure determined by direct intra-arterial catheter. As the cuff pressure falls a few mm Hg further, the artery no longer closes during diastole, which means that the basic factor causing the sounds (the jetting of blood through a squeezed artery) is no longer present. Therefore, the sounds disappear entirely. Many clinicians believe that the pressure at which the Korotkoff sounds completely disappear should be used as the diastolic pressure, except in situations in which the disappearance of sounds cannot reliably be determined because sounds are audible even after complete deflation of the cuff. For example, in patients with arteriovenous fistulas for hemodialysis or with aortic insufficiency, Korotkoff sounds may be heard after complete deflation of the cuff.

The auscultatory method for determining systolic and diastolic pressures is not entirely accurate, but it usually gives values within 10 percent of those determined by direct catheter measurement from inside the arteries.

Normal Arterial Pressures as Measured by the Auscultatory Method. Figure 15-8 shows the approximate normal systolic and diastolic arterial pressures at different ages. The progressive increase in pressure with age results from the effects of aging on the blood pressure control mechanisms. We shall see in Chapter 19 that the kidneys are primarily responsible for this long-term regulation of arterial pressure; and it is well known that

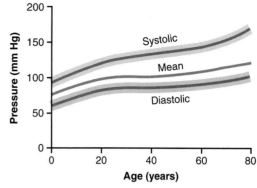

Figure 15-8 Changes in systolic, diastolic, and mean arterial pressures with age. The shaded areas show the approximate normal ranges.

the kidneys exhibit definitive changes with age, especially after the age of 50 years.

A slight extra increase in *systolic* pressure usually occurs beyond the age of 60 years. This results from decreasing distensibility, or "hardening," of the arteries, which is often a result of *atherosclerosis*. The final effect is a higher systolic pressure with considerable increase in pulse pressure, as previously explained.

Mean Arterial Pressure. The mean arterial pressure is the average of the arterial pressures measured millisecond by millisecond over a period of time. It is not equal to the average of systolic and diastolic pressure because at normal heart rates, a greater fraction of the cardiac cycle is spent in diastole than is systole; thus, the arterial pressure remains nearer to diastolic pressure than to systolic pressure during the greater part of the cardiac cycle. The mean arterial pressure is therefore determined about 60 percent by the diastolic pressure and 40 percent by the systolic pressure. Note in Figure 15-8 that the mean pressure (solid green line) at all ages is nearer to the diastolic pressure than to the systolic pressure. However, at very high heart rates diastole comprises a smaller fraction of the cardiac cycle and the mean arterial pressure is more closely approximated as the average of systolic and diastolic pressures.

Veins and Their Functions

For years, the veins were considered to be nothing more than passageways for flow of blood to the heart, but it is now apparent that they perform other special functions that are necessary for operation of the circulation. Especially important, they are capable of constricting and enlarging and thereby storing either small or large quantities of blood and making this blood available when it is required by the remainder of the circulation. The peripheral veins can also propel blood forward by means of a so-called *venous pump*, and they even help to regulate cardiac output, an exceedingly important function that is described in detail in Chapter 20.

Venous Pressures—Right Atrial Pressure (Central Venous Pressure) and Peripheral Venous Pressures

To understand the various functions of the veins, it is first necessary to know something about pressure in the veins and what determines the pressure.

Blood from all the systemic veins flows into the right atrium of the heart; therefore, the pressure in the right atrium is called the *central venous pressure.*

Right atrial pressure is regulated by a balance between (1) the ability of the heart to pump blood out of the right atrium and ventricle into the lungs and *(2) the tendency for blood to flow from the peripheral veins into the right atrium.* If the right heart is pumping strongly, the right atrial pressure decreases. Conversely, weakness of the heart elevates the right atrial pressure. Also, any effect that causes rapid inflow of blood into the right atrium from the peripheral veins elevates the right atrial pressure. Some of the factors that can increase this venous return (and thereby increase the right atrial pressure) are (1) increased blood volume, (2) increased large vessel tone throughout the body with resultant increased peripheral venous pressures, and (3) dilatation of the arterioles, which decreases the peripheral resistance and allows rapid flow of blood from the arteries into the veins.

The same factors that regulate right atrial pressure also contribute to regulation of cardiac output because the amount of blood pumped by the heart depends on both the ability of the heart to pump and the tendency for blood to flow into the heart from the peripheral vessels. Therefore, we will discuss regulation of right atrial pressure in much more depth in Chapter 20 in connection with regulation of cardiac output.

The *normal right atrial pressure* is about 0 mm Hg, which is equal to the atmospheric pressure around the body. It can increase to 20 to 30 mm Hg under very abnormal conditions, such as (1) serious heart failure or (2) after massive transfusion of blood, which greatly increases the total blood volume and causes excessive quantities of blood to attempt to flow into the heart from the peripheral vessels.

The lower limit to the right atrial pressure is usually about −3 to −5 mm Hg below atmospheric pressure. This is also the pressure in the chest cavity that surrounds the heart. The right atrial pressure approaches these low values when the heart pumps with exceptional vigor or when blood flow into the heart from the peripheral vessels is greatly depressed, such as after severe hemorrhage.

Venous Resistance and Peripheral Venous Pressure

Large veins have so little resistance to blood flow *when they are distended* that the resistance then is almost zero and is of almost no importance. However, as shown in Figure 15-9, most of the large veins that enter the thorax are compressed at many points by the surrounding tissues so that blood flow is impeded at these points. For instance, the veins from the arms are compressed by their sharp angulations over the first rib. Also, the pressure in the neck veins often falls so low that the atmospheric pressure on the outside of the neck causes these veins to

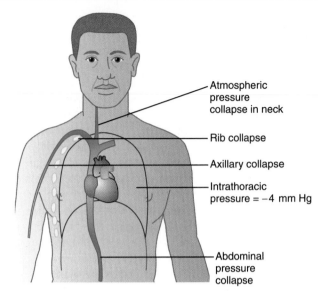

Figure 15-9 Compression points that tend to collapse the veins entering the thorax.

collapse. Finally, veins coursing through the abdomen are often compressed by different organs and by the intra-abdominal pressure, so they usually are at least partially collapsed to an ovoid or slitlike state. For these reasons, the *large veins do usually offer some resistance to blood flow,* and because of this, the pressure in the more peripheral small veins in a person lying down is usually +4 to +6 mm Hg greater than the right atrial pressure.

Effect of High Right Atrial Pressure on Peripheral Venous Pressure. When the right atrial pressure rises above its normal value of 0 mm Hg, blood begins to back up in the large veins. This enlarges the veins, and even the collapse points in the veins open up when the right atrial pressure rises above +4 to +6 mm Hg. Then, as the right atrial pressure rises still further, the additional increase causes a corresponding rise in peripheral venous pressure in the limbs and elsewhere. Because the heart must be weakened to cause a rise in right atrial pressure as high as +4 to +6 mm Hg, one often finds that the peripheral venous pressure is not noticeably elevated even in the early stages of heart failure.

Effect of Intra-abdominal Pressure on Venous Pressures of the Leg. The pressure in the abdominal cavity of a recumbent person normally averages about +6 mm Hg, but it can rise to +15 to +30 mm Hg as a result of pregnancy, large tumors, abdominal obesity, or excessive fluid (called "ascites") in the abdominal cavity. When the intra-abdominal pressure does rise, the pressure in the veins of the legs must rise *above* the abdominal pressure before the abdominal veins will open and allow the blood to flow from the legs to the heart. Thus, if the intra-abdominal pressure is +20 mm Hg, the lowest possible pressure in the femoral veins is also about +20 mm Hg.

Effect of Gravitational Pressure on Venous Pressure

In any body of water that is exposed to air, the pressure at the surface of the water is equal to atmospheric pressure, but the pressure rises 1 mm Hg for each 13.6 millimeters of distance below the surface. This pressure results from the weight of the water and therefore is called *gravitational pressure* or *hydrostatic pressure.*

Gravitational pressure also occurs in the vascular system of the human being because of weight of the blood in the vessels, as shown in Figure 15-10. When a person is standing, the pressure in the right atrium remains about 0 mm Hg because the heart pumps into the arteries any excess blood that attempts to accumulate at this point. However, in an adult *who is standing absolutely still,* the pressure in the veins of the feet is about +90 mm Hg simply because of the gravitational weight of the blood in the veins between the heart and the feet. The venous pressures at other levels of the body are proportionately between 0 and 90 mm Hg.

In the arm veins, the pressure at the level of the top rib is usually about +6 mm Hg because of compression of the subclavian vein as it passes over this rib. The gravitational pressure down the length of the arm then is determined by the distance below the level of this rib. Thus, if the gravitational difference between the level of the rib and the hand is +29 mm Hg, this gravitational pressure is added to the +6 mm Hg pressure caused by compression of the vein as it crosses the rib, making a total of +35 mm Hg pressure in the veins of the hand.

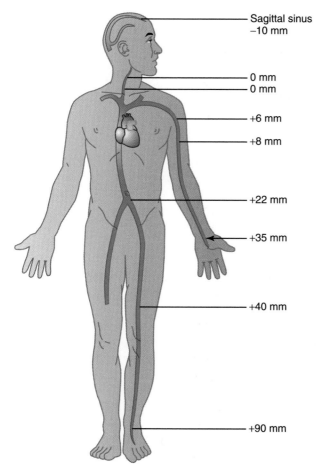

Sagittal sinus
−10 mm

0 mm
0 mm

+6 mm

+8 mm

+22 mm

+35 mm

+40 mm

+90 mm

Figure 15-10 Effect of gravitational pressure on the venous pressures throughout the body in the standing person.

The neck veins of a person standing upright collapse almost completely all the way to the skull because of atmospheric pressure on the outside of the neck. This collapse causes the pressure in these veins to remain at zero along their entire extent. The reason for this is that any tendency for the pressure to rise above this level opens the veins and allows the pressure to fall back to zero because of flow of the blood. Conversely, any tendency for the neck vein pressure to fall below zero collapses the veins still more, which further increases their resistance and again returns the pressure back to zero.

The veins inside the skull, on the other hand, are in a noncollapsible chamber (the skull cavity) so that they cannot collapse. Consequently, *negative pressure can exist in the dural sinuses of the head;* in the standing position, the venous pressure in the sagittal sinus at the top of the brain is about −10 mm Hg because of the hydrostatic "suction" between the top of the skull and the base of the skull. Therefore, if the sagittal sinus is opened during surgery, air can be sucked immediately into the venous system; the air may even pass downward to cause air embolism in the heart, and death can ensue.

Effect of the Gravitational Factor on Arterial and Other Pressures. The gravitational factor also affects pressures in the peripheral arteries and capillaries, in addition to its effects in the veins. For instance, a standing person who has a mean arterial pressure of 100 mm Hg at the level of the heart has an arterial pressure in the feet of about 190 mm Hg. Therefore, when one states that the arterial pressure is 100 mm Hg, this generally means that this is the pressure at the gravitational level of the heart but not necessarily elsewhere in the arterial vessels.

Venous Valves and the "Venous Pump": Their Effects on Venous Pressure

Were it not for valves in the veins, the gravitational pressure effect would cause the venous pressure in the feet always to be about +90 mm Hg in a standing adult. However, every time one moves the legs, one tightens the muscles and compresses the veins in or adjacent to the muscles, and this squeezes the blood out of the veins. But the valves in the veins, shown in Figure 15-11, are arranged so that the direction of venous blood flow can be only toward the heart. Consequently, every time a person moves the legs or even tenses the leg muscles, a certain amount of venous blood is propelled toward the heart. This pumping system is known as the "venous pump" or "muscle pump," and it is efficient enough that under ordinary circumstances, the venous pressure in the feet of a walking adult remains less than +20 mm Hg.

If a person stands perfectly still, the venous pump does not work, and the venous pressures in the lower legs increase to the full gravitational value of 90 mm Hg in about 30 seconds. The pressures in the capillaries also increase greatly, causing fluid to leak from the circulatory system into the tissue spaces. As a result, the legs swell and the blood volume diminishes. Indeed, 10 to 20 percent of the blood volume can be lost from the circulatory

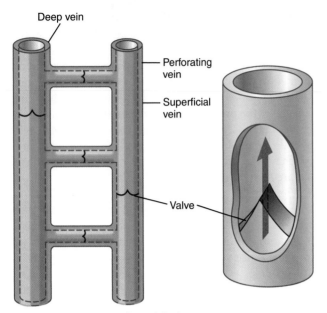

Figure 15-11 Venous valves of the leg.

system within the 15 to 30 minutes of standing absolutely still, as often occurs when a soldier is made to stand at rigid attention.

Venous Valve Incompetence Causes "Varicose" Veins. The valves of the venous system frequently become "incompetent" or sometimes even are destroyed. This is especially true when the veins have been overstretched by excess venous pressure lasting weeks or months, as occurs in pregnancy or when one stands most of the time. Stretching the veins increases their cross-sectional areas, but the leaflets of the valves do not increase in size. Therefore, the leaflets of the valves no longer close completely. When this develops, the pressure in the veins of the legs increases greatly because of failure of the venous pump; this further increases the sizes of the veins and finally destroys the function of the valves entirely. Thus, the person develops "varicose veins," which are characterized by large, bulbous protrusions of the veins beneath the skin of the entire leg, particularly the lower leg.

Whenever people with varicose veins stand for more than a few minutes, the venous and capillary pressures become very high and leakage of fluid from the capillaries causes constant edema in the legs. The edema in turn prevents adequate diffusion of nutritional materials from the capillaries to the muscle and skin cells, so the muscles become painful and weak and the skin frequently becomes gangrenous and ulcerates. The best treatment for such a condition is continual elevation of the legs to a level at least as high as the heart. Tight binders on the legs also can be of considerable assistance in preventing the edema and its sequelae.

Clinical Estimation of Venous Pressure. The venous pressure often can be estimated by simply observing the degree of distention of the peripheral veins—especially of the neck veins. For instance, in the sitting position, the neck veins are never distended in the normal quietly resting person. However, when the right atrial pressure becomes increased to as much as +10 mm Hg, the lower veins of the neck begin to protrude; and at +15 mm Hg atrial pressure essentially all the veins in the neck become distended.

Direct Measurement of Venous Pressure and Right Atrial Pressure

Venous pressure can also be measured with ease by inserting a needle directly into a vein and connecting it to a pressure recorder. The only means by which *right atrial pressure* can be measured accurately is by inserting a catheter through the peripheral veins and into the right atrium. Pressures measured through such *central venous catheters* are used almost routinely in some types of hospitalized cardiac patients to provide constant assessment of heart pumping ability.

Pressure Reference Level for Measuring Venous and Other Circulatory Pressures

In discussions up to this point, we often have spoken of right atrial pressure as being 0 mm Hg and arterial pressure as being 100 mm Hg, but we have not stated the gravitational level in the circulatory system to which this pressure is referred. There is one point in the circulatory system at which gravitational pressure factors caused by changes in body position of a healthy person usually do not affect the pressure measurement by more than 1 to 2 mm Hg. This is at or near the level of the tricuspid valve, as shown by the crossed axes in Figure 15-12. Therefore, all circulatory pressure measurements discussed in this text are referred to this level, which is called the *reference level for pressure measurement.*

The reason for lack of gravitational effects at the tricuspid valve is that the heart automatically prevents significant gravitational changes in pressure at this point in the following way:

If the pressure at the tricuspid valve rises slightly above normal, the right ventricle fills to a greater extent than usual, causing the heart to pump blood more rapidly and therefore to decrease the pressure at the tricuspid valve back toward the normal mean value. Conversely, if the pressure falls, the right ventricle fails to fill adequately, its pumping decreases, and blood dams up in the venous system until

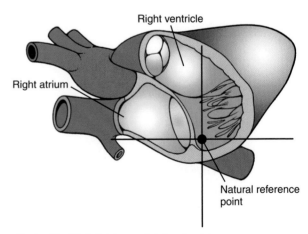

Figure 15-12 Reference point for circulatory pressure measurement (located near the tricuspid valve).

the pressure at the tricuspid level again rises to the normal value. In other words, *the heart acts as a feedback regulator of pressure* at the tricuspid valve.

When a person is lying on his or her back, the tricuspid valve is located at almost exactly 60 percent of the chest thickness in front of the back. This is the *zero pressure reference level* for a person lying down.

Blood Reservoir Function of the Veins

As pointed out in Chapter 14, more than 60 percent of all the blood in the circulatory system is usually in the veins. For this reason and also because the veins are so compliant, it is said that the venous system serves as a *blood reservoir* for the circulation.

When blood is lost from the body and the arterial pressure begins to fall, nervous signals are elicited from the carotid sinuses and other pressure-sensitive areas of the circulation, as discussed in Chapter 18. These in turn elicit nerve signals from the brain and spinal cord mainly through sympathetic nerves to the veins, causing them to constrict. This takes up much of the slack in the circulatory system caused by the lost blood. Indeed, even after as much as 20 percent of the total blood volume has been lost, the circulatory system often functions almost normally because of this variable reservoir function of the veins.

Specific Blood Reservoirs. Certain portions of the circulatory system are so extensive and/or so compliant that they are called "specific blood reservoirs." These include (1) the *spleen,* which sometimes can decrease in size sufficiently to release as much as 100 milliliters of blood into other areas of the circulation; (2) the *liver,* the sinuses of which can release several hundred milliliters of blood into the remainder of the circulation; (3) the *large abdominal veins,* which can contribute as much as 300 milliliters; and (4) the *venous plexus beneath the skin,* which also can contribute several hundred milliliters. The *heart* and the *lungs,* although not parts of the systemic venous reservoir system, must also be considered blood reservoirs. The heart, for instance, shrinks during sympathetic stimulation and in this way can contribute some 50 to 100 milliliters of blood; the lungs can contribute another 100 to 200 milliliters when the pulmonary pressures decrease to low values.

The Spleen as a Reservoir for Storing Red Blood Cells. Figure 15-13 shows that the spleen has two separate areas for storing blood: the *venous sinuses* and the *pulp.* The sinuses can swell the same as any other part of the venous system and store whole blood.

In the splenic pulp, the capillaries are so permeable that whole blood, including the red blood cells, oozes through the capillary walls into a trabecular mesh, forming the *red pulp.* The red cells are trapped by the trabeculae, while the plasma flows on into the venous sinuses and then into the general circulation. As a consequence, the red pulp of

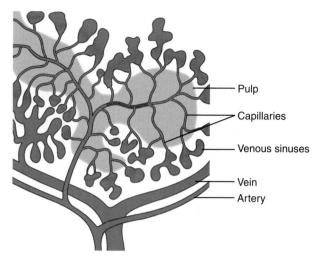

Figure 15-13 Functional structures of the spleen. (Courtesy Dr. Don W. Fawcett, Montana.)

the spleen is a *special reservoir that contains large quantities of concentrated red blood cells.* These can then be expelled into the general circulation whenever the sympathetic nervous system becomes excited and causes the spleen and its vessels to contract. As much as 50 milliliters of concentrated red blood cells can be released into the circulation, raising the hematocrit 1 to 2 percent.

In other areas of the splenic pulp are islands of white blood cells, which collectively are called the *white pulp.* Here lymphoid cells are manufactured similar to those manufactured in the lymph nodes. They are part of the body's immune system, described in Chapter 34.

Blood-Cleansing Function of the Spleen—Removal of Old Cells

Blood cells passing through the splenic pulp before entering the sinuses undergo thorough squeezing. Therefore, it is to be expected that fragile red blood cells would not withstand the trauma. For this reason, many of the red blood cells destroyed in the body have their final demise in the spleen. After the cells rupture, the released hemoglobin and the cell stroma are digested by the reticuloendothelial cells of the spleen, and the products of digestion are mainly reused by the body as nutrients, often for making new blood cells.

Reticuloendothelial Cells of the Spleen

The pulp of the spleen contains many large phagocytic reticuloendothelial cells, and the venous sinuses are lined with similar cells. These cells function as part of a cleansing system for the blood, acting in concert with a similar system of reticuloendothelial cells in the venous sinuses of the liver. When the blood is invaded by infectious agents, the reticuloendothelial cells of the spleen rapidly remove debris, bacteria, parasites, and so forth. Also, in many chronic infectious processes, the spleen enlarges in the same manner that lymph nodes enlarge and then performs its cleansing function even more avidly.

Bibliography

Badeer HS: Hemodynamics for medical students, *Am J Physiol (Adv Physiol Educ)* 25:44, 2001.

Guyton AC: *Arterial pressure and hypertension*, Philadelphia, 1980, WB Saunders.

Guyton AC, Jones CE: Central venous pressure: physiological significance and clinical implications, *Am Heart J* 86:431, 1973.

Guyton AC, Jones CE, Coleman TG: *Circulatory physiology: cardiac output and its regulation*, Philadelphia, 1973, WB Saunders.

Hall JE: Integration and regulation of cardiovascular function, *Am J Physiol (Adv Physiol Educ)* 22:S174, 1999.

Hicks JW, Badeer HS: Gravity and the circulation: "open" vs. "closed" systems, *Am J Physiol* 262:R725–R732, 1992.

Jones DW, Appel LJ, Sheps SG, et al: Measuring blood pressure accurately: New and persistent challenges, *JAMA* 289:1027, 2003.

Kass DA: Ventricular arterial stiffening: integrating the pathophysiology, *Hypertension* 46:185, 2005.

Kurtz TW, Griffin KA, Bidani AK, et al: Recommendations for blood pressure measurement in humans and experimental animals. Part 2: Blood pressure measurement in experimental animals: a statement for professionals from the Subcommittee of Professional and Public Education of the American Heart Association Council on High Blood Pressure Research, *Hypertension* 45:299, 2005.

O'Rourke MF, Nichols WW: Aortic diameter, aortic stiffness, and wave reflection increase with age and isolated systolic hypertension, *Hypertension* 45:652, 2005.

Laurent S, Boutouyrie P, Lacolley P: Structural and genetic bases of arterial stiffness, *Hypertension* 45:1050, 2005.

Pickering TG, Hall JE, Appel LJ, et al: Recommendations for blood pressure measurement in humans and experimental animals: Part 1: blood pressure measurement in humans: a statement for professionals from the Subcommittee of Professional and Public Education of the American Heart Association Council on High Blood Pressure Research, *Hypertension* 45:142, 2005.

Wilkinson IB, Franklin SS, Cockcroft JR: Nitric oxide and the regulation of large artery stiffness: from physiology to pharmacology, *Hypertension* 44:112, 2004.

The Microcirculation and Lymphatic System: Capillary Fluid Exchange, Interstitial Fluid, and Lymph Flow

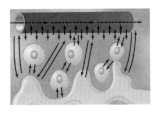

The most purposeful function of the circulation occurs in the microcirculation: This is *transport of nutrients to the tissues and removal of cell excreta*. The small arterioles control blood flow to each tissue, and local conditions in the tissues in turn control the diameters of the arterioles. Thus, each tissue, in most instances, controls its own blood flow in relation to its individual needs, a subject that is discussed in Chapter 17.

The walls of the capillaries are extremely thin, constructed of single-layer, highly permeable endothelial cells. Therefore, water, cell nutrients, and cell excreta can all interchange quickly and easily between the tissues and the circulating blood.

The peripheral circulation of the whole body has about 10 billion capillaries with a total surface area estimated to be 500 to 700 square meters (about one-eighth the surface area of a football field). Indeed, it is rare that any single functional cell of the body is more than 20 to 30 micrometers away from a capillary.

Structure of the Microcirculation and Capillary System

The microcirculation of each organ is organized specifically to serve that organ's needs. In general, each nutrient artery entering an organ branches six to eight times before the arteries become small enough to be called *arterioles*, which generally have internal diameters of only 10 to 15 micrometers. Then the arterioles themselves branch two to five times, reaching diameters of 5 to 9 micrometers at their ends where they supply blood to the capillaries.

The arterioles are highly muscular, and their diameters can change manyfold. The metarterioles (the terminal arterioles) do not have a continuous muscular coat, but smooth muscle fibers encircle the vessel at intermittent points, as shown in Figure 16-1 by the black dots on the sides of the metarteriole.

At the point where each true capillary originates from a metarteriole, a smooth muscle fiber usually encircles

the capillary. This is called the *precapillary sphincter.* This sphincter can open and close the entrance to the capillary.

The venules are larger than the arterioles and have a much weaker muscular coat. Yet the pressure in the venules is much less than that in the arterioles, so the venules can still contract considerably despite the weak muscle.

This typical arrangement of the capillary bed is not found in all parts of the body, although a similar arrangement may serve the same purposes. Most important, the metarterioles and the precapillary sphincters are in close contact with the tissues they serve. Therefore, the local conditions of the tissues—the concentrations of nutrients, end products of metabolism, hydrogen ions, and so forth—can cause direct effects on the vessels to control local blood flow in each small tissue area.

Structure of the Capillary Wall. Figure 16-2 shows the ultramicroscopic structure of typical endothelial cells in the capillary wall as found in most organs of the body, especially in muscles and connective tissue. Note that the wall is composed of a unicellular layer of endothelial cells and is surrounded by a thin basement membrane on the outside of the capillary. The total thickness of the capillary wall is only about 0.5 micrometer. The internal diameter of the capillary is 4 to 9 micrometers, barely large enough for red blood cells and other blood cells to squeeze through.

"Pores" in the Capillary Membrane. Figure 16-2 shows two small passageways connecting the interior of the capillary with the exterior. One of these is an *intercellular cleft*, which is the thin-slit, curving channel that lies at the bottom of the figure between adjacent endothelial cells. Each cleft is interrupted periodically by short ridges of protein attachments that hold the endothelial cells together, but between these ridges fluid can percolate freely through the cleft. The cleft normally has a uniform spacing with a width of about 6 to 7 nanometers (60 to 70 angstroms), slightly smaller than the diameter of an albumin protein molecule.

Because the intercellular clefts are located only at the edges of the endothelial cells, they usually represent no more than 1/1000 of the total surface area of the capillary wall. Nevertheless, the rate of thermal motion of water

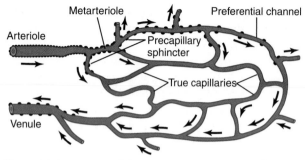

Figure 16-1 Structure of the mesenteric capillary bed. (Redrawn from Zweifach BW: Factors Regulating Blood Pressure. New York: Josiah Macy, Jr., Foundation, 1950.)

molecules, as well as most water-soluble ions and small solutes, is so rapid that all of these diffuse with ease between the interior and exterior of the capillaries through these "slit-pores," the intercellular clefts.

Present in the endothelial cells are many minute *plasmalemmal vesicles*, also called *caveolae (small caves)*. These form from oligomers of proteins called *caveolins* that are associated with molecules of *cholesterol* and *sphingolipids*. Although the precise functions of caveolae are still unclear, they are believed to play a role in *endocytosis* (the process by which the cell engulfs material from outside the cell) and *transcytosis* of macromolecules across endothelial cells. The caveolae at the surface of the

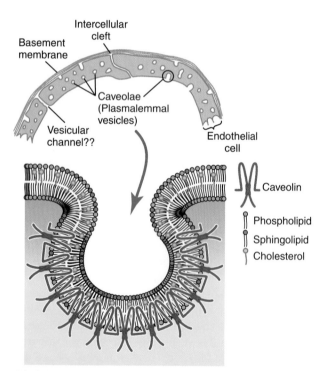

Figure 16-2 Structure of the capillary wall. Note especially the *intercellular cleft* at the junction between adjacent endothelial cells; it is believed that most water-soluble substances diffuse through the capillary membrane along the clefts. Small membrane invaginations, called *caveolae*, are believed to play a role in transporting macromolecules across the cell membrane. Caveolae contain caveolins, proteins which interact with cholesterol and polymerize to form the caveolae.

cell appear to imbibe small packets of plasma or extracellular fluid that contain plasma proteins. These vesicles can then move slowly through the endothelial cell. Some of these vesicles may coalesce to form *vesicular channels* all the way through the endothelial cell, which is demonstrated in Figure 16-2.

Special Types of "Pores" Occur in the Capillaries of Certain Organs. The "pores" in the capillaries of some organs have special characteristics to meet the peculiar needs of the organs. Some of these characteristics are as follows:

1. In the *brain*, the junctions between the capillary endothelial cells are mainly "tight" junctions that allow only extremely small molecules such as water, oxygen, and carbon dioxide to pass into or out of the brain tissues.

2. In the *liver*, the opposite is true. The clefts between the capillary endothelial cells are wide open so that almost all dissolved substances of the plasma, including the plasma proteins, can pass from the blood into the liver tissues.

3. The pores of the *gastrointestinal capillary membranes* are midway between those of the muscles and those of the liver.

4. In the *glomerular capillaries of the kidney*, numerous small oval windows called *fenestrae* penetrate all the way through the middle of the endothelial cells so that tremendous amounts of very small molecular and ionic substances (but not the large molecules of the plasma proteins) can filter through the glomeruli without having to pass through the clefts between the endothelial cells.

Flow of Blood in the Capillaries—Vasomotion

Blood usually does not flow continuously through the capillaries. Instead, it flows intermittently, turning on and off every few seconds or minutes. The cause of this intermittency is the phenomenon called *vasomotion*, which means intermittent contraction of the metarterioles and precapillary sphincters (and sometimes even the very small arterioles as well).

Regulation of Vasomotion. The most important factor found thus far to affect the degree of opening and closing of the metarterioles and precapillary sphincters is the concentration of *oxygen* in the tissues. When the rate of oxygen usage by the tissue is great so that tissue oxygen concentration decreases below normal, the intermittent periods of capillary blood flow occur more often, and the duration of each period of flow lasts longer, thereby allowing the capillary blood to carry increased quantities of oxygen (as well as other nutrients) to the tissues.

This effect, along with multiple other factors that control local tissue blood flow, is discussed in Chapter 17.

Average Function of the Capillary System

Despite the fact that blood flow through each capillary is intermittent, so many capillaries are present in the tissues that their overall function becomes averaged. That is, there is an *average rate of blood flow* through each tissue capillary bed, an *average capillary pressure* within the capillaries, and an *average rate of transfer of substances* between the blood of the capillaries and the surrounding interstitial fluid. In the remainder of this chapter, we are concerned with these averages, although one must remember that the average functions are, in reality, the functions of literally billions of individual capillaries, each operating intermittently in response to local conditions in the tissues.

Exchange of Water, Nutrients, and Other Substances Between the Blood and Interstitial Fluid

Diffusion Through the Capillary Membrane

By far the most important means by which substances are transferred between the plasma and the interstitial fluid is *diffusion*. Figure 16-3 demonstrates this process, showing that as the blood flows along the lumen of the capillary, tremendous numbers of water molecules and dissolved particles diffuse back and forth through the capillary wall, providing continual mixing between the interstitial fluid and the plasma. *Diffusion results from thermal motion of the water molecules and dissolved substances in the fluid,* the different molecules and ions moving first in one direction and then another, bouncing randomly in every direction.

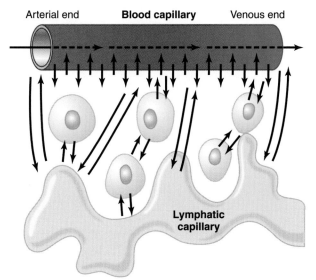

Figure 16-3 Diffusion of fluid molecules and dissolved substances between the capillary and interstitial fluid spaces.

Lipid-Soluble Substances Can Diffuse Directly Through the Cell Membranes of the Capillary Endothelium. If a substance is lipid soluble, it can diffuse directly through the cell membranes of the capillary without having to go through the pores. Such substances include *oxygen* and *carbon dioxide.* Because these substances can permeate all areas of the capillary membrane, their rates of transport through the capillary membrane are many times faster than the rates for lipid-insoluble substances, such as sodium ions and glucose that can go only through the pores.

Water-Soluble, Non-Lipid-Soluble Substances Diffuse Through Intercellular "Pores" in the Capillary Membrane. Many substances needed by the tissues are soluble in water but cannot pass through the lipid membranes of the endothelial cells; such substances include *water molecules* themselves, *sodium ions, chloride ions,* and *glucose.* Despite the fact that not more than 1/1000 of the surface area of the capillaries is represented by the intercellular clefts between the endothelial cells, the velocity of thermal molecular motion in the clefts is so great that even this small area is sufficient to allow tremendous diffusion of water and water-soluble substances through these cleft-pores. To give one an idea of the rapidity with which these substances diffuse, *the rate at which water molecules diffuse through the capillary membrane is about 80 times as great as the rate at which plasma itself flows linearly along the capillary.* That is, the water of the plasma is exchanged with the water of the interstitial fluid 80 times before the plasma can flow the entire distance through the capillary.

Effect of Molecular Size on Passage Through the Pores. The width of the capillary intercellular cleft-pores, 6 to 7 nanometers, is about 20 times the diameter of the water molecule, which is the smallest molecule that normally passes through the capillary pores. Conversely, the diameters of plasma protein molecules are slightly greater than the width of the pores. Other substances, such as sodium ions, chloride ions, glucose, and urea, have intermediate diameters. Therefore, the permeability of the capillary pores for different substances varies according to their molecular diameters.

Table 16-1 gives the relative permeabilities of the capillary pores in skeletal muscle for substances commonly encountered, demonstrating, for instance, that the permeability for glucose molecules is 0.6 times that for water molecules, whereas the permeability for albumin molecules is very, very slight, only 1/1000 that for water molecules.

A word of caution must be issued at this point. The capillaries in various tissues have extreme differences in their permeabilities. For instance, the membranes of the liver capillary sinusoids are so permeable that even plasma proteins pass freely through these walls, almost as easily as water and other substances. Also, the permeability of the renal glomerular membrane for water

UNIT IV

Table 16-1 Relative Permeability of Skeletal Muscle Capillary Pores to Different-Sized Molecules

Substance	Molecular Weight	Permeability
Water	18	1.00
NaCl	58.5	0.96
Urea	60	0.8
Glucose	180	0.6
Sucrose	342	0.4
Inulin	5,000	0.2
Myoglobin	17,600	0.03
Hemoglobin	68,000	0.01
Albumin	69,000	0.001

Data from Pappenheimer JR: Passage of molecules through capillary walls. Physiol Rev 33:387, 1953.

and electrolytes is about 500 times the permeability of the muscle capillaries, but this is not true for the plasma proteins; for these, the capillary permeabilities are very slight, as in other tissues and organs. When we study these different organs later in this text, it should become clear why some tissues—the liver, for instance—require greater degrees of capillary permeability than others to transfer tremendous amounts of nutrients between the blood and liver parenchymal cells, and the kidneys to allow filtration of large quantities of fluid for formation of urine.

Effect of Concentration Difference on Net Rate of Diffusion Through the Capillary Membrane. The "net" rate of diffusion of a substance through any membrane is proportional to the *concentration difference of the substance* between the two sides of the membrane. That is, the greater the difference between the concentrations of any given substance on the two sides of the capillary membrane, the greater the net movement of the substance in one direction through the membrane. For instance, the concentration of oxygen in capillary blood is normally greater than in the interstitial fluid. Therefore, large quantities of oxygen normally move from the blood toward the tissues. Conversely, the concentration of carbon dioxide is greater in the tissues than in the blood, which causes excess carbon dioxide to move into the blood and to be carried away from the tissues.

The rates of diffusion through the capillary membranes of most nutritionally important substances are so great that only slight concentration differences suffice to cause more than adequate transport between the plasma and interstitial fluid. For instance, the concentration of oxygen in the interstitial fluid immediately outside the capillary is no more than a few percent less than its concentration in the plasma of the blood, yet this slight difference causes enough oxygen to move from the blood into the interstitial

spaces to provide all the oxygen required for tissue metabolism, often as much as several liters of oxygen per minute during very active states of the body.

Interstitium and Interstitial Fluid

About one sixth of the total volume of the body consists of spaces between cells, which collectively are called the *interstitium.* The fluid in these spaces is the *interstitial fluid.*

The structure of the interstitium is shown in Figure 16-4. It contains two major types of solid structures: (1) *collagen fiber bundles* and (2) *proteoglycan filaments.* The collagen fiber bundles extend long distances in the interstitium. They are extremely strong and therefore provide most of the tensional strength of the tissues. The proteoglycan filaments, however, are extremely thin coiled or twisted molecules composed of about 98 percent *hyaluronic acid* and 2 percent protein. These molecules are so thin that they cannot be seen with a light microscope and are difficult to demonstrate even with the electron microscope. Nevertheless, they form a mat of very fine reticular filaments aptly described as a "brush pile."

"Gel" in the Interstitium. The fluid in the interstitium is derived by filtration and diffusion from the capillaries. It contains almost the same constituents as plasma except for much lower concentrations of proteins because proteins do not easily pass outward through the pores of the capillaries. The interstitial fluid is entrapped mainly in the minute spaces among the proteoglycan filaments. This combination of proteoglycan filaments and fluid entrapped within them has the characteristics of a *gel* and therefore is called *tissue gel.*

Because of the large number of proteoglycan filaments, it is *difficult for fluid to flow* easily through the tissue gel.

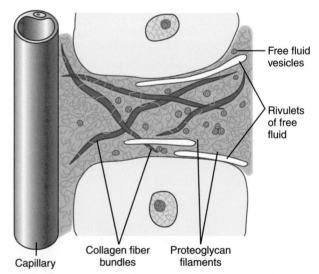

Figure 16-4 Structure of the interstitium. Proteoglycan filaments are everywhere in the spaces between the collagen fiber bundles. Free fluid vesicles and small amounts of free fluid in the form of rivulets occasionally also occur.

Instead, *fluid mainly diffuses* through the gel; that is, it moves molecule by molecule from one place to another by kinetic, thermal motion rather than by large numbers of molecules moving together.

Diffusion through the gel occurs about 95 to 99 percent as rapidly as it does through free fluid. For the short distances between the capillaries and the tissue cells, this diffusion allows rapid transport through the interstitium not only of water molecules but also of electrolytes, small molecular weight nutrients, cellular excreta, oxygen, carbon dioxide, and so forth.

"Free" Fluid in the Interstitium. Although almost all the fluid in the interstitium normally is entrapped within the tissue gel, occasionally small *rivulets of "free" fluid* and *small free fluid vesicles* are also present, which means fluid that is free of the proteoglycan molecules and therefore can flow freely. When a dye is injected into the circulating blood, it often can be seen to flow through the interstitium in the small rivulets, usually coursing along the surfaces of collagen fibers or surfaces of cells.

The amount of "free" fluid present in *normal* tissues is slight, usually less than 1 percent. Conversely, when the tissues develop *edema, these small pockets and rivulets of free fluid expand tremendously* until one half or more of the edema fluid becomes freely flowing fluid independent of the proteoglycan filaments.

Fluid Filtration Across Capillaries Is Determined by Hydrostatic and Colloid Osmotic Pressures, as Well as Capillary Filtration Coefficient

The hydrostatic pressure in the capillaries tends to force fluid and its dissolved substances through the capillary pores into the interstitial spaces. Conversely, osmotic pressure caused by the plasma proteins (called *colloid osmotic pressure*) tends to cause fluid movement by osmosis from the interstitial spaces into the blood. This osmotic pressure exerted by the plasma proteins normally prevents significant loss of fluid volume from the blood into the interstitial spaces.

Also important is the *lymphatic system,* which returns to the circulation the small amounts of excess protein and fluid that leak from the blood into the interstitial spaces. In the remainder of this chapter, we discuss the mechanisms that control capillary filtration and lymph flow function together to regulate the respective volumes of the plasma and the interstitial fluid.

Hydrostatic and Colloid Osmotic Forces Determine Fluid Movement Through the Capillary Membrane. Figure 16-5 shows the four primary forces that determine whether fluid will move out of the blood into the interstitial fluid or in the opposite direction. These forces, called "Starling forces" in honor of the physiologist who first demonstrated their importance, are:

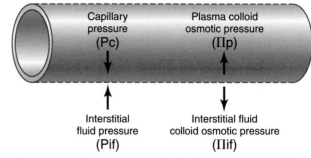

Figure 16-5 Fluid pressure and colloid osmotic pressure forces operate at the capillary membrane, tending to move fluid either outward or inward through the membrane pores.

1. The *capillary pressure* (Pc), which tends to force fluid *outward* through the capillary membrane.
2. The *interstitial fluid pressure* (Pif), which tends to force fluid *inward* through the capillary membrane when Pif is positive but outward when Pif is negative.
3. The capillary *plasma colloid osmotic pressure* (Πp), which tends to cause osmosis of fluid *inward* through the capillary membrane.
4. The *interstitial fluid colloid osmotic pressure* (Πif), which tends to cause osmosis of fluid *outward* through the capillary membrane.

If the sum of these forces—the *net filtration pressure*—is positive, there will be a net *fluid filtration* across the capillaries. If the sum of the Starling forces is negative, there will be a net *fluid absorption* from the interstitial spaces into the capillaries. The net filtration pressure (NFP) is calculated as:

$$NFP = Pc - Pif - \Pi p + \Pi if$$

As discussed later, the NFP is slightly positive under normal conditions, resulting in a net filtration of fluid across the capillaries into the interstitial space in most organs. The rate of fluid filtration in a tissue is also determined by the number and size of the pores in each capillary, as well as the number of capillaries in which blood is flowing. These factors are usually expressed together as the *capillary filtration coefficient* (K_f). The K_f is therefore a measure of the capacity of the capillary membranes to filter water for a given NFP and is usually expressed as ml/min per mm Hg net filtration pressure.

The rate of capillary fluid filtration is therefore determined as:

$$Filtration = K_f \times NFP$$

In the following sections we discuss each of the forces that determine the rate of capillary fluid filtration.

Capillary Hydrostatic Pressure

Various methods have been used to estimate the capillary hydrostatic pressure: (1) *direct micropipette cannulation of the capillaries,* which has given an average mean capillary pressure of about 25 mm Hg in some tissues such as the skeletal muscle and the gut, and (2) *indirect functional measurement of the capillary pressure,* which has given a capillary pressure averaging about 17 mm Hg in these tissues.

Micropipette Method for Measuring Capillary Pressure.

To measure pressure in a capillary by cannulation, a microscopic glass pipette is thrust directly into the capillary, and the pressure is measured by an appropriate micromanometer system. Using this method, capillary pressures have been measured in capillaries of exposed tissues of animals and in large capillary loops of the eponychium at the base of the fingernail in humans. These measurements have given pressures of 30 to 40 mm Hg in the arterial ends of the capillaries, 10 to 15 mm Hg in the venous ends, and about 25 mm Hg in the middle.

In some capillaries, such as the *glomerular capillaries* of the kidneys, the pressures measured by the micropipette method are much higher, averaging about 60 mm Hg. The *peritubular capillaries* of the kidneys, in contrast, have hydrostatic pressure that average only about 13 mm Hg. Thus, the capillary hydrostatic pressures in different tissues are highly variable, depending on the particular tissue and the physiological condition.

Isogravimetric Method for Indirectly Measuring "Functional" Capillary Pressure.

Figure 16-6 demonstrates an *isogravimetric* method for indirectly estimating capillary pressure. This figure shows a section of gut held up by one arm of a gravimetric balance. Blood is perfused through the blood vessels of the gut wall. When the arterial pressure is decreased, the resulting decrease in capillary pressure allows the osmotic pressure of the plasma proteins to cause absorption of fluid out of the gut wall and makes the weight of the gut decrease. This immediately causes displacement of the balance arm. To prevent this weight decrease, the venous pressure is increased an amount sufficient to overcome the effect of decreasing the arterial pressure. In other words, the capillary pressure is kept constant while simultaneously (1) decreasing the arterial pressure and (2) increasing the venous pressure.

In the graph in the lower part of the figure, the changes in arterial and venous pressures that exactly nullify all weight changes are shown. The arterial and venous lines meet each other at a value of 17 mm Hg. Therefore, the capillary pressure must have remained at this same level of 17 mm Hg throughout these maneuvers; otherwise, either filtration or absorption of fluid through the capillary walls would have occurred. Thus, in a roundabout way, the "functional" capillary pressure in this tissue is measured to be about 17 mm Hg.

It is clear that the isogravimetric method, which determines the capillary pressure that exactly balances all the forces tending to move fluid into or out of the capillaries, gives a lower value compared with the capillary pressure measured directly with a micropipette. A major reason for this is that capillary fluid filtration is not exactly balanced

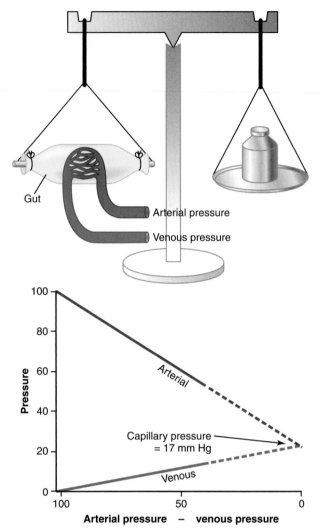

Figure 16-6 Isogravimetric method for measuring capillary pressure.

with fluid reabsorption in most tissues. The fluid that is filtered in excess of what is reabsorbed is carried away by lymph vessels in most tissues. In the glomerular capillaries of the kidneys, a very large amount of fluid, approximately 125 ml/min, is continuously filtered.

Interstitial Fluid Hydrostatic Pressure

There are several methods for measuring interstitial fluid hydrostatic pressure and each of these gives slightly different values, depending on the method used and the tissue in which the pressure is measured. In loose subcutaneous tissue, interstitial fluid pressure measured by the different methods is usually a few millimeters of mercury less than atmospheric pressure; that is, the values are called *negative interstitial fluid pressure.* In other tissues that are surrounded by capsules, such as the kidneys, the interstitial pressure is generally *positive* (greater than atmospheric pressure). The methods most widely used have been (1) direct cannulation of the tissues with a micropipette, (2) measurement of the pressure from implanted perforated capsules, and (3) measurement of the pressure from a cotton wick inserted into the tissue.

Measurement of Interstitial Fluid Pressure Using the Micropipette. The same type of micropipette used for measuring capillary pressure can also be used in some tissues for measuring interstitial fluid pressure. The tip of the micropipette is about 1 micrometer in diameter, but even this is 20 or more times larger than the sizes of the spaces between the proteoglycan filaments of the interstitium. Therefore, the pressure that is measured is probably the pressure in a free fluid pocket.

The first pressures measured using the micropipette method ranged from −1 to +2 mm Hg but were usually slightly positive. With experience and improved equipment for making such measurements, more recent pressures have averaged about −2 mm Hg, giving average pressure values in *loose* tissues, such as skin, that are slightly less than atmospheric pressure.

Measurement of Interstitial Free Fluid Pressure in Implanted Perforated Hollow Capsules. Interstitial free fluid pressure measured by this method when using 2-centimeter diameter capsules in normal *loose* subcutaneous tissue averages about −6 mm Hg, but with smaller capsules, the values are not greatly different from the −2 mm Hg measured by the micropipette.

Interstitial Fluid Pressures in Tightly Encased Tissues

Some tissues of the body are surrounded by tight encasements, such as the cranial vault around the brain, the strong fibrous capsule around the kidney, the fibrous sheaths around the muscles, and the sclera around the eye. In most of these, regardless of the method used for measurement, the interstitial fluid pressures are positive. However, these interstitial fluid pressures almost invariably are still less than the pressures exerted on the outsides of the tissues by their encasements. For instance, the cerebrospinal fluid pressure surrounding the brain of an animal lying on its side averages about +10 mm Hg, whereas the *brain interstitial fluid pressure* averages about +4 to +6 mm Hg. In the kidneys, the capsular pressure surrounding the kidney averages about +13 mm Hg, whereas the reported *renal interstitial fluid pressures* have averaged about +6 mm Hg. Thus, if one remembers that the pressure exerted on the skin is atmospheric pressure, which is considered to be zero pressure, one might formulate a general rule that the normal interstitial fluid pressure is usually several millimeters of mercury negative with respect to the pressure that surrounds each tissue.

Is the True Interstitial Fluid Pressure in Loose Subcutaneous Tissue Subatmospheric?

The concept that the interstitial fluid pressure is subatmospheric in some tissues of the body began with clinical observations that could not be explained by the previously held concept that interstitial fluid pressure was always positive. Some of the pertinent observations are the following:

1. When a skin graft is placed on a concave surface of the body, such as in an eye socket after removal of the eye, before the skin becomes attached to the sublying socket, fluid tends to collect underneath the graft. Also, the skin attempts to shorten, with the result that it tends to pull it away from the concavity. Nevertheless, some negative force underneath the skin causes absorption of the fluid and usually literally pulls the skin back into the concavity.

2. Less than 1 mm Hg of positive pressure is required to inject large volumes of fluid into loose subcutaneous tissues, such as beneath the lower eyelid, in the axillary space, and in the scrotum. Amounts of fluid calculated to be more than 100 times the amount of fluid normally in the interstitial space, when injected into these areas, cause no more than about 2 mm Hg of positive pressure. The importance of these observations is that they show that such tissues do not have strong fibers that can prevent the accumulation of fluid. Therefore, some other mechanism, such as a low compliance system, must be available to prevent such fluid accumulation.

3. In most natural cavities of the body where there is free fluid in dynamic equilibrium with the surrounding interstitial fluids, the pressures that have been measured have been negative. Some of these are the following:

   Intrapleural space: −8 mm Hg
   Joint synovial spaces: −4 to −6 mm Hg
   Epidural space: −4 to −6 mm Hg

4. The implanted capsule for measuring the interstitial fluid pressure can be used to record dynamic changes in this pressure. The changes are approximately those that one would calculate to occur (1) when the arterial pressure is increased or decreased, (2) when fluid is injected into the surrounding tissue space, or (3) when a highly concentrated colloid osmotic agent is injected into the blood to absorb fluid from the tissue spaces. It is not likely that these dynamic changes could be recorded this accurately unless the capsule pressure closely approximated the true interstitial pressure.

Summary—An Average Value for Negative Interstitial Fluid Pressure in Loose Subcutaneous Tissue. Although the aforementioned different methods give slightly different values for interstitial fluid pressure, there currently is a general belief among most physiologists that the true interstitial fluid pressure in *loose* subcutaneous tissue is slightly less subatmospheric, averaging about −3 mm Hg.

Pumping by the Lymphatic System Is the Basic Cause of the Negative Interstitial Fluid Pressure

The lymphatic system is discussed later in the chapter, but we need to understand here the basic role that this system plays in determining interstitial fluid pressure. The lymphatic system is a "scavenger" system that removes excess fluid, excess protein molecules, debris, and other matter from the tissue spaces. Normally, when fluid enters the terminal lymphatic capillaries, the lymph vessel walls automatically contract for a few seconds and pump the fluid into the blood circulation. This overall process creates the slight negative pressure that has been measured for fluid in the interstitial spaces.

Plasma Colloid Osmotic Pressure

Proteins in the Plasma Cause Colloid Osmotic Pressure. In the basic discussion of osmotic pressure in Chapter 4, it was pointed out that only those molecules or ions that fail to pass through the pores of a semipermeable membrane exert osmotic pressure. Because the proteins are the only dissolved constituents in the plasma and interstitial fluids that do not readily pass through the capillary pores, it is the proteins of the plasma and interstitial fluids that are responsible for the osmotic pressures on the two sides of the capillary membrane. To distinguish this osmotic pressure from that which occurs at the cell membrane, it is called either *colloid osmotic pressure* or *oncotic pressure*. The term "colloid" osmotic pressure is derived from the fact that a protein solution resembles a colloidal solution despite the fact that it is actually a true molecular solution.

Normal Values for Plasma Colloid Osmotic Pressure. The colloid osmotic pressure of normal human plasma averages about 28 mm Hg; 19 mm of this is caused by molecular effects of the dissolved protein and 9 mm by the *Donnan effect*—that is, extra osmotic pressure caused by sodium, potassium, and the other cations held in the plasma by the proteins.

Effect of the Different Plasma Proteins on Colloid Osmotic Pressure. The plasma proteins are a mixture that contains albumin, with an average molecular weight of 69,000; globulins, 140,000; and fibrinogen, 400,000. Thus, 1 gram of globulin contains only half as many molecules as 1 gram of albumin, and 1 gram of fibrinogen contains only one sixth as many molecules as 1 gram of albumin. It should be recalled from the discussion of osmotic pressure in Chapter 4 that osmotic pressure is determined by the *number of molecules* dissolved in a fluid rather than by the mass of these molecules. Therefore, when corrected for number of molecules rather than mass, the following chart gives both the relative mass concentrations (g/dl) of the different types of proteins in normal plasma and their respective contributions to the total plasma colloid osmotic pressure (Πp).

	g/dl	Πp (mm Hg)
Albumin	4.5	21.8
Globulins	2.5	6.0
Fibrinogen	0.3	0.2
Total	7.3	28.0

Thus, about 80 percent of the total colloid osmotic pressure of the plasma results from the albumin fraction, 20 percent from the globulins, and almost none from the fibrinogen. Therefore, from the point of view of capillary and tissue fluid dynamics, it is mainly albumin that is important.

Interstitial Fluid Colloid Osmotic Pressure

Although the size of the usual capillary pore is smaller than the molecular sizes of the plasma proteins, this is not true of all the pores. Therefore, small amounts of plasma proteins do leak through the pores into the interstitial spaces through pores and by transcytosis in small vesicles.

The total quantity of protein in the entire 12 liters of interstitial fluid of the body is slightly greater than the total quantity of protein in the plasma itself, but because this volume is four times the volume of plasma, the average protein *concentration* of the interstitial fluid is usually only 40 percent of that in plasma, or about 3 g/dl. Quantitatively, one finds that the average interstitial fluid colloid osmotic pressure for this concentration of proteins is about 8 mm Hg.

Exchange of Fluid Volume Through the Capillary Membrane

Now that the different factors affecting fluid movement through the capillary membrane have been discussed, it is possible to put all these together to see how the capillary system maintains normal fluid volume distribution between the plasma and the interstitial fluid.

The average capillary pressure at the arterial ends of the capillaries is 15 to 25 mmHg greater than at the venous ends. Because of this difference, fluid "filters" out of the capillaries at their arterial ends, but at their venous ends fluid is reabsorbed back into the capillaries. Thus, a small amount of fluid actually "flows" through the tissues from the arterial ends of the capillaries to the venous ends. The dynamics of this flow are as follows.

Analysis of the Forces Causing Filtration at the Arterial End of the Capillary. The approximate average forces operative at the *arterial end* of the capillary that cause movement through the capillary membrane are shown as follows:

	mm Hg
Forces tending to move fluid outward:	
Capillary pressure (arterial end of capillary)	30
Negative interstitial free fluid pressure	3
Interstitial fluid colloid osmotic pressure	8
TOTAL OUTWARD FORCE	41
Forces tending to move fluid inward:	
Plasma colloid osmotic pressure	28
TOTAL INWARD FORCE	28
Summation of forces:	
Outward	41
Inward	28
NET OUTWARD FORCE (AT ARTERIAL END)	13

Thus, the summation of forces at the arterial end of the capillary shows a net *filtration pressure* of 13 mm Hg, tending to move fluid outward through the capillary pores.

This 13 mm Hg filtration pressure causes, on average, about 1/200 of the plasma in the flowing blood to filter out of the arterial ends of the capillaries into the interstitial spaces each time the blood passes through the capillaries.

Analysis of Reabsorption at the Venous End of the Capillary.

The low blood pressure at the venous end of the capillary changes the balance of forces in favor of absorption as follows:

	mm Hg
Forces tending to move fluid inward:	
Plasma colloid osmotic pressure	28
TOTAL INWARD FORCE	28
Forces tending to move fluid outward:	
Capillary pressure (venous end of capillary)	10
Negative interstitial free fluid pressure	3
Interstitial fluid colloid osmotic pressure	8
TOTAL OUTWARD FORCE	21
Summation of forces:	
Inward	28
Outward	21
NET INWARD FORCE	7

Thus, the force that causes fluid to move into the capillary, 28 mm Hg, is greater than that opposing reabsorption, 21 mm Hg. The difference, 7 mm Hg, is the *net reabsorption pressure* at the venous ends of the capillaries. This reabsorption pressure is considerably less than the filtration pressure at the capillary arterial ends, but remember that the venous capillaries are more numerous and more permeable than the arterial capillaries, so that less reabsorption pressure is required to cause inward movement of fluid.

The reabsorption pressure causes about nine tenths of the fluid that has filtered out of the arterial ends of the capillaries to be reabsorbed at the venous ends. The remaining one tenth flows into the lymph vessels and returns to the circulating blood.

Starling Equilibrium for Capillary Exchange

Ernest H. Starling pointed out more than a century ago that under normal conditions, a state of near-equilibrium exists in most capillaries. That is, the amount of fluid filtering outward from the arterial ends of capillaries equals almost exactly the fluid returned to the circulation by absorption. The slight disequilibrium that does occur accounts for the fluid that is eventually returned to the circulation by way of the lymphatics.

The following chart shows the principles of the Starling equilibrium. For this chart, the pressures in the arterial and venous capillaries are averaged to calculate mean *functional* capillary pressure for the entire length of the capillary. This calculates to be 17.3 mm Hg.

	mm Hg
Mean forces tending to move fluid outward:	
Mean capillary pressure	17.3
Negative interstitial free fluid pressure	3.0
Interstitial fluid colloid osmotic pressure	8.0
TOTAL OUTWARD FORCE	28.3
Mean force tending to move fluid inward:	
Plasma colloid osmotic pressure	28.0
TOTAL INWARD FORCE	28.0
Summation of mean forces:	
Outward	28.3
Inward	28.0
NET OUTWARD FORCE	0.3

Thus, for the total capillary circulation, we find a near-equilibrium between the total outward forces, 28.3 mm Hg, and the total inward force, 28.0 mm Hg. This slight imbalance of forces, 0.3 mm Hg, causes slightly more filtration of fluid into the interstitial spaces than reabsorption. This slight excess of filtration is called *net filtration*, and it is the fluid that must be returned to the circulation through the lymphatics. The normal rate of net filtration *in the entire body*, not including the kidneys, is only about 2 ml/min.

Filtration Coefficient. In the previous example, an average net imbalance of forces at the capillary membranes of 0.3 mm Hg causes net fluid filtration in the entire body of 2 ml/min. Expressing this for each millimeter of mercury imbalance, one finds a net filtration rate of 6.67 ml/min of fluid per mm Hg for the entire body. This is called the whole body capillary *filtration coefficient*.

The filtration coefficient can also be expressed for separate parts of the body in terms of rate of filtration per minute per mm Hg per 100 grams of tissue. On this basis, the filtration coefficient of the average tissue is about 0.01 ml/min/mm Hg/100 g of tissue. But, because of extreme differences in permeabilities of the capillary systems in different tissues, this coefficient varies more than 100-fold among the different tissues. It is very small in brain and muscle, moderately large in subcutaneous tissue, large in the intestine, and extreme in the liver and glomerulus of the kidney where the pores are either numerous or wide open. By the same token, the permeation of proteins through the capillary membranes varies greatly as well. The concentration of protein in the interstitial fluid of muscles is about 1.5 g/dl; in subcutaneous tissue, 2 g/dl; in intestine, 4 g/dl; and in liver, 6 g/dl.

Effect of Abnormal Imbalance of Forces at the Capillary Membrane

If the mean capillary pressure rises above 17 mm Hg, the net force tending to cause filtration of fluid into the tissue spaces rises. Thus, a 20 mm Hg rise in mean capillary pressure causes an increase in net filtration pressure from 0.3 mm Hg to 20.3 mm Hg, which results in 68 times as much net filtration of fluid into the interstitial spaces as normally occurs. To prevent accumulation of excess fluid in these spaces would require 68 times the normal flow of fluid into the lymphatic system, an amount that is 2 to 5 times too much for the lymphatics to carry away. As a result, fluid will begin to accumulate in the interstitial spaces and edema will result.

Conversely, if the capillary pressure falls very low, net reabsorption of fluid into the capillaries will occur instead of net filtration and the blood volume will increase at the expense of the interstitial fluid volume. These effects of imbalance at the capillary membrane in relation to the development of different kinds of edema are discussed in Chapter 25.

Lymphatic System

The lymphatic system represents an accessory route through which fluid can flow from the interstitial spaces into the blood. Most important, the lymphatics can carry proteins and large particulate matter away from the tissue spaces, neither of which can be removed by absorption directly into the blood capillaries. This return of proteins to the blood from the interstitial spaces is an essential function without which we would die within about 24 hours.

Lymph Channels of the Body

Almost all tissues of the body have special lymph channels that drain excess fluid directly from the interstitial spaces. The exceptions include the superficial portions of the skin, the central nervous system, the endomysium of muscles, and the bones. But, even these tissues have minute interstitial channels called *prelymphatics* through which interstitial fluid can flow; this fluid eventually empties either into lymphatic vessels or, in the case of the brain, into the cerebrospinal fluid and then directly back into the blood.

Essentially all the lymph vessels from the lower part of the body eventually empty into the *thoracic duct*, which in turn empties into the blood venous system at the juncture of the *left* internal jugular vein and left subclavian vein, as shown in Figure 16-7.

Lymph from the left side of the head, the left arm, and parts of the chest region also enters the thoracic duct before it empties into the veins.

Lymph from the right side of the neck and head, the right arm, and parts of the right thorax enters the *right lymph duct* (much smaller than the thoracic duct), which empties into the blood venous system at the juncture of the *right* subclavian vein and internal jugular vein.

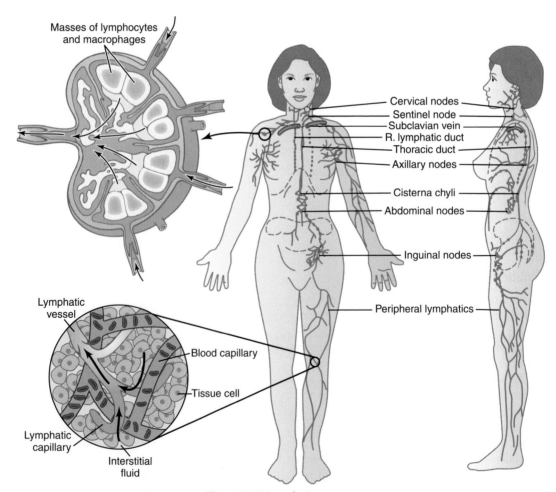

Figure 16-7 Lymphatic system.

Terminal Lymphatic Capillaries and Their Permeability. Most of the fluid filtering from the *arterial ends* of *blood capillaries* flows among the cells and finally is reabsorbed back into the *venous ends* of the *blood capillaries;* but on the average, about one tenth of the fluid instead enters the *lymphatic capillaries* and returns to the blood through the lymphatic system rather than through the venous capillaries. The total quantity of all this lymph is normally only 2 to 3 liters each day.

The fluid that returns to the circulation by way of the lymphatics is extremely important because substances of high molecular weight, such as proteins, cannot be absorbed from the tissues in any other way, although they can enter the lymphatic capillaries almost unimpeded. The reason for this is a special structure of the lymphatic capillaries, demonstrated in Figure 16-8. This figure shows the endothelial cells of the lymphatic capillary attached by *anchoring filaments* to the surrounding connective tissue. At the junctions of adjacent endothelial cells, the edge of one endothelial cell overlaps the edge of the adjacent cell in such a way that the overlapping edge is free to flap inward, thus forming a minute valve that opens to the interior of the lymphatic capillary. Interstitial fluid, along with its suspended particles, can push the valve open and flow directly into the lymphatic capillary. But this fluid has difficulty leaving the capillary once it has entered because any backflow closes the flap valve. Thus, the lymphatics have valves at the very tips of the terminal lymphatic capillaries, as well as valves along their larger vessels up to the point where they empty into the blood circulation.

Formation of Lymph

Lymph is derived from interstitial fluid that flows into the lymphatics. Therefore, lymph as it first enters the terminal lymphatics has almost the same composition as the interstitial fluid.

The protein concentration in the interstitial fluid of most tissues averages about 2 g/dl, and the protein concentration of lymph flowing from these tissues is near this value. In the liver, lymph formed has a protein concentration as high as 6 g/dl, and lymph formed in the intestines has a protein concentration as high as 3 to 4 g/dl. Because about two thirds of all lymph normally is derived from the liver and intestines, the thoracic duct lymph, which is a mixture of lymph from all areas of the body, usually has a protein concentration of 3 to 5 g/dl.

The lymphatic system is also one of the major routes for absorption of nutrients from the gastrointestinal tract, especially for absorption of virtually all fats in food, as discussed in Chapter 65. Indeed, after a fatty meal, thoracic duct lymph sometimes contains as much as 1 to 2 percent fat.

Finally, even large particles, such as bacteria, can push their way between the endothelial cells of the lymphatic capillaries and in this way enter the lymph. As the lymph passes through the lymph nodes, these particles are almost entirely removed and destroyed, as discussed in Chapter 33.

Rate of Lymph Flow

About 100 milliliters per hour of lymph flows through the *thoracic duct* of a resting human, and approximately another 20 milliliters flows into the circulation each hour through other channels, making a total estimated lymph flow of about 120 ml/hr or 2 to 3 liters per day.

Effect of Interstitial Fluid Pressure on Lymph Flow. Figure 16-9 shows the effect of different levels of interstitial fluid pressure on lymph flow as measured in dog legs. Note that normal lymph flow is very little at interstitial fluid pressures more negative than the normal value of −6 mm Hg. Then, as the pressure rises to 0 mm Hg (atmospheric pressure), flow increases more than 20-fold. Therefore, any factor that increases interstitial fluid

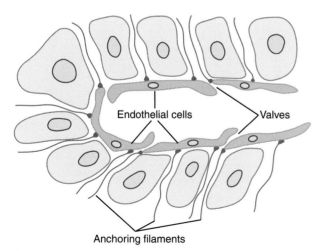

Figure 16-8 Special structure of the lymphatic capillaries that permits passage of substances of high molecular weight into the lymph.

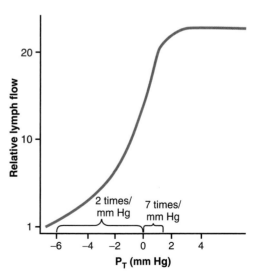

Figure 16-9 Relation between interstitial fluid pressure and lymph flow in the leg of a dog. Note that lymph flow reaches a maximum when the interstitial pressure, P_T, rises slightly above atmospheric pressure (0 mm Hg). (Courtesy Drs. Harry Gibson and Aubrey Taylor.)

pressure also increases lymph flow if the lymph vessels are functioning normally. Such factors include the following:

- Elevated capillary hydrostatic pressure
- Decreased plasma colloid osmotic pressure
- Increased interstitial fluid colloid osmotic pressure
- Increased permeability of the capillaries

All of these cause a balance of fluid exchange at the blood capillary membrane to favor fluid movement into the interstitium, thus increasing interstitial fluid volume, interstitial fluid pressure, and lymph flow all at the same time.

However, note in Figure 16-9 that when the interstitial fluid pressure becomes 1 or 2 mm Hg greater than atmospheric pressure (>0 mm Hg), lymph flow fails to rise any further at still higher pressures. This results from the fact that the increasing tissue pressure not only increases entry of fluid into the lymphatic capillaries but also compresses the outside surfaces of the larger lymphatics, thus impeding lymph flow. At the higher pressures, these two factors balance each other almost exactly, so lymph flow reaches what is called the "maximum lymph flow rate." This is illustrated by the upper level plateau in Figure 16-9.

Lymphatic Pump Increases Lymph Flow. Valves exist in all lymph channels; typical valves are shown in Figure 16-10 in collecting lymphatics into which the lymphatic capillaries empty.

Motion pictures of exposed lymph vessels in animals and in human beings show that when a collecting lymphatic or larger lymph vessel becomes stretched with fluid, the smooth muscle in the wall of the vessel automatically contracts. Furthermore, each segment of the lymph vessel between successive valves functions as a separate automatic pump. That is, even slight filling of a segment causes it to contract and the fluid is pumped through the next valve into the next lymphatic segment. This fills the subsequent segment, and a few seconds later it, too, contracts, the process continuing all along the lymph vessel until the fluid is finally emptied into the blood circulation. In a very large lymph vessel such as the thoracic duct, this lymphatic pump can generate pressures as great as 50 to 100 mm Hg.

Pumping Caused by External Intermittent Compression of the Lymphatics. In addition to the pumping caused by intrinsic intermittent contraction of the lymph vessel walls, any external factor that intermittently compresses the lymph vessel also can cause pumping. In order of their importance, such factors are as follows:

- Contraction of surrounding skeletal muscles
- Movement of the parts of the body
- Pulsations of arteries adjacent to the lymphatics
- Compression of the tissues by objects outside the body

The lymphatic pump becomes very active during exercise, often increasing lymph flow 10- to 30-fold. Conversely, during periods of rest, lymph flow is sluggish, almost zero.

Lymphatic Capillary Pump. The terminal lymphatic capillary is also capable of pumping lymph, in addition to the pumping by the larger lymph vessels. As explained earlier in the chapter, the walls of the lymphatic capillaries are tightly adherent to the surrounding tissue cells by means of their anchoring filaments. Therefore, each time excess fluid enters the tissue and causes the tissue to swell, the anchoring filaments pull on the wall of the lymphatic capillary and fluid flows into the terminal lymphatic capillary through the junctions between the endothelial cells. Then, when the tissue is compressed, the pressure inside the capillary increases and causes the overlapping edges of the endothelial cells to close like valves. Therefore, the pressure pushes the lymph forward into the collecting lymphatic instead of backward through the cell junctions.

The lymphatic capillary endothelial cells also contain a few contractile actomyosin filaments. In some animal tissues (e.g., the bat's wing) these filaments have been observed to cause rhythmical contraction of the lymphatic capillaries in the same way that many of the small blood and larger lymphatic vessels also contract rhythmically. Therefore, it is probable that at least part of lymph

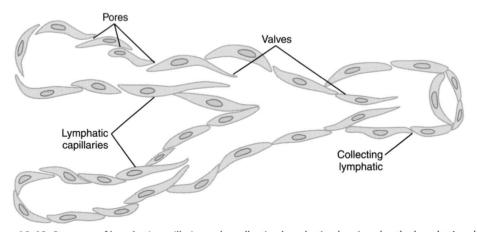

Figure 16-10 Structure of lymphatic capillaries and a collecting lymphatic, showing also the lymphatic valves.

pumping results from lymph capillary endothelial cell contraction in addition to contraction of the larger muscular lymphatics.

Summary of Factors That Determine Lymph Flow. From the previous discussion, one can see that the two primary factors that determine lymph flow are (1) the interstitial fluid pressure and (2) the activity of the lymphatic pump. Therefore, one can state that, roughly, *the rate of lymph flow is determined by the product of interstitial fluid pressure times the activity of the lymphatic pump.*

Role of the Lymphatic System in Controlling Interstitial Fluid Protein Concentration, Interstitial Fluid Volume, and Interstitial Fluid Pressure

It is already clear that the lymphatic system functions as an "overflow mechanism" to return to the circulation excess proteins and excess fluid volume from the tissue spaces. Therefore, the lymphatic system also plays a central role in controlling (1) the concentration of proteins in the interstitial fluids, (2) the volume of interstitial fluid, and (3) the interstitial fluid pressure. Let us explain how these factors interact.

First, remember that small amounts of proteins leak continuously out of the blood capillaries into the interstitium. Only minute amounts, if any, of the leaked proteins return to the circulation by way of the venous ends of the blood capillaries. Therefore, these proteins tend to accumulate in the interstitial fluid, and this in turn increases the colloid osmotic pressure of the interstitial fluids.

Second, the increasing colloid osmotic pressure in the interstitial fluid shifts the balance of forces at the blood capillary membranes in favor of fluid filtration into the interstitium. Therefore, in effect, fluid is translocated osmotically outward through the capillary wall by the proteins and into the interstitium, thus increasing both interstitial fluid volume and interstitial fluid pressure.

Third, the increasing interstitial fluid pressure greatly increases the rate of lymph flow, as explained previously. This in turn carries away the excess interstitial fluid volume and excess protein that has accumulated in the spaces.

Thus, once the interstitial fluid protein concentration reaches a certain level and causes a comparable increase in interstitial fluid volume and interstitial fluid pressure, the return of protein and fluid by way of the lymphatic system becomes great enough to balance exactly the rate of leakage of these into the interstitium from the blood capillaries. Therefore, the quantitative values of all these factors reach a steady state; they will remain balanced at these steady state levels until something changes the rate of leakage of proteins and fluid from the blood capillaries.

Significance of Negative Interstitial Fluid Pressure as a Means for Holding the Body Tissues Together

Traditionally, it has been assumed that the different tissues of the body are held together entirely by connective tissue fibers. However, at many places in the body, connective tissue fibers are very weak or even absent. This occurs particularly at points where tissues slide over one another, such as the skin sliding over the back of the hand or over the face. Yet even at these places, the tissues are held together by the negative interstitial fluid pressure, which is actually a partial vacuum. When the tissues lose their negative pressure, fluid accumulates in the spaces and the condition known as *edema* occurs. This is discussed in Chapter 25.

Bibliography

Dejana E: Endothelial cell-cell junctions: happy together, *Nat Rev Mol Cell Biol* 5:261, 2004.

Gashev AA: Physiologic aspects of lymphatic contractile function: current perspectives, *Ann N Y Acad Sci* 979:178, 2002.

Gratton JP, Bernatchez P, Sessa WC: Caveolae and caveolins in the cardiovascular system, *Circ Res* 94:1408, 2004.

Guyton AC: Concept of negative interstitial pressure based on pressures in implanted perforated capsules, *Circ Res* 12:399, 1963.

Guyton AC: Interstitial fluid pressure: II. Pressure-volume curves of interstitial space, *Circ Res* 16:452, 1965.

Guyton AC, Granger HJ, Taylor AE: Interstitial fluid pressure, *Physiol Rev* 51:527, 1971.

Michel CC, Curry FE: Microvascular permeability, *Physiol Rev* 79:703, 1999.

Mehta D, Malik AB: Signaling mechanisms regulating endothelial permeability, *Physiol Rev* 86:279, 2006.

Miyasaka M, Tanaka T: Lymphocyte trafficking across high endothelial venules: dogmas and enigmas, *Nat Rev Immunol* 4:360, 2004.

Parker JC: Hydraulic conductance of lung endothelial phenotypes and Starling safety factors against edema, *Am J Physiol Lung Cell Mol Physiol* 292:L378, 2007.

Parker JC, Townsley MI: Physiological determinants of the pulmonary filtration coefficient, *Am J Physiol Lung Cell Mol Physiol* 295:L235, 2008.

Predescu SA, Predescu DN, Malik AB: Molecular determinants of endothelial transcytosis and their role in endothelial permeability, *Am J Physiol Lung Cell Mol Physiol* 293:L823, 2007.

Oliver G: Lymphatic vasculature development, *Nat Rev Immunol* 4:35, 2004.

Taylor AE, Granger DN: Exchange of macromolecules across the microcirculation. In Renkin EM, Michel CC, editors: *Handbook of Physiology*, Sec 2, vol IV, Bethesda, MD, 1984, American Physiological Society, pp 467.

Local and Humoral Control of Tissue Blood Flow

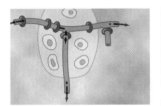

Local Control of Blood Flow in Response to Tissue Needs

One of the most fundamental principles of circulatory function is the ability of each tissue to control its own local blood flow in proportion to its metabolic needs.

What are some of the specific needs of the tissues for blood flow? The answer to this is manyfold, including the following:

1. Delivery of oxygen to the tissues.

2. Delivery of other nutrients, such as glucose, amino acids, and fatty acids.

3. Removal of carbon dioxide from the tissues.

4. Removal of hydrogen ions from the tissues.

5. Maintenance of proper concentrations of other ions in the tissues.

6. Transport of various hormones and other substances to the different tissues.

Certain organs have special requirements. For instance, blood flow to the skin determines heat loss from the body and in this way helps to control body temperature. Also, delivery of adequate quantities of blood plasma to the kidneys allows the kidneys to excrete the waste products of the body and to regulate body fluid volumes and electrolytes.

We shall see that these factors exert extreme degrees of local blood flow control and that different tissues place different levels of importance on these factors in controlling blood flow.

Variations in Blood Flow in Different Tissues and Organs. Note in Table 17-1 the very large blood flows in some organs—for example, several hundred ml/min per 100 g of thyroid or adrenal gland tissue and a total blood flow of 1350 ml/min in the liver, which is 95 ml/min/100 g of liver tissue.

Also note the extremely large blood flow through the kidneys—1100 ml/min. This extreme amount of flow is required for the kidneys to perform their function of cleansing the blood of waste products.

Conversely, most surprising is the low blood flow to all the *inactive* muscles of the body, only a total of 750 ml/min, even though the muscles constitute between 30 and 40 percent of the total body mass. In the resting state, the metabolic activity of the muscles is very low, and so also is the blood flow, only 4 ml/min/100 g. Yet, during heavy exercise, muscle metabolic activity can increase more than 60-fold and the blood flow as much as 20-fold, increasing to as high as 16,000 ml/min in the body's total muscle vascular bed (or 80 ml/min/100 g of muscle).

Importance of Blood Flow Control by the Local Tissues. One might ask the simple question: Why not simply allow a very large blood flow all the time through every tissue of the body, always enough to supply the tissue's needs whether the activity of the tissue is little or great? The answer is equally simple: To do this would require many times more blood flow than the heart can pump.

Experiments have shown that the blood flow to each tissue usually is regulated at the minimal level that will supply the tissue's requirements—no more, no less. For instance, in tissues for which the most important requirement is delivery of oxygen, the blood flow is always controlled at a level only slightly more than required to maintain full tissue oxygenation but no more than this. By controlling local blood flow in such an exact way, the tissues almost never suffer from oxygen nutritional deficiency and the workload on the heart is kept at a minimum.

Mechanisms of Blood Flow Control

Local blood flow control can be divided into two phases: (1) acute control and (2) long-term control.

Acute control is achieved by rapid changes in local vasodilation or vasoconstriction of the arterioles, metarterioles, and precapillary sphincters, occurring within seconds to minutes to provide very rapid maintenance of appropriate local tissue blood flow.

Long-term control, however, means slow, controlled changes in flow over a period of days, weeks, or even

Table 17-1 Blood Flow to Different Organs and Tissues Under Basal Conditions

	Percent of Cardiac Output	ml/min	ml/min/100 g of Tissue Weight
Brain	14	700	50
Heart	4	200	70
Bronchi	2	100	25
Kidneys	22	1100	360
Liver	27	1350	95
Portal	(21)	(1050)	
Arterial	(6)	(300)	
Muscle (inactive state)	15	750	4
Bone	5	250	3
Skin (cool weather)	6	300	3
Thyroid gland	1	50	160
Adrenal glands	0.5	25	300
Other tissues	3.5	175	1.3
Total	100.0	5000	

months. In general, these long-term changes provide even better control of the flow in proportion to the needs of the tissues. These changes come about as a result of an increase or decrease in the physical sizes and numbers of actual blood vessels supplying the tissues.

Acute Control of Local Blood Flow

Effect of Tissue Metabolism on Local Blood Flow. Figure 17-1 shows the approximate acute effect on blood flow of increasing the rate of metabolism in a local tissue, such as in a skeletal muscle. Note that an increase in metabolism up to eight times normal increases the blood flow acutely about fourfold.

Acute Local Blood Flow Regulation When Oxygen Availability Changes. One of the most necessary of the metabolic nutrients is oxygen. Whenever the availability of oxygen to the tissues decreases, such as (1) at high altitude at the top of a high mountain, (2) in pneumonia, (3) in carbon monoxide poisoning (which poisons the ability of hemoglobin to transport oxygen), or (4) in cyanide poisoning (which poisons the ability of the tissues to use oxygen), the blood flow through the tissues increases markedly. Figure 17-2 shows that as the arterial oxygen saturation decreases to about 25 percent of normal, the blood flow through an isolated leg increases about threefold; that is, the blood flow increases almost enough, but not quite enough, to make up for the decreased amount of oxygen in the blood, thus almost maintaining a relatively constant supply of oxygen to the tissues.

Total cyanide poisoning of oxygen usage by a local tissue area can cause local blood flow to increase as much as sevenfold, thus demonstrating the extreme effect of oxygen deficiency to increase blood flow.

There are two basic theories for the regulation of local blood flow when either the rate of tissue metabolism changes or the availability of oxygen changes. They are (1) the *vasodilator theory* and (2) the *oxygen lack theory*.

Vasodilator Theory for Acute Local Blood Flow Regulation—Possible Special Role of Adenosine. According to this theory, the greater the rate of metabolism or the less the availability of oxygen or some other nutrients to a tissue, the greater the rate of formation of *vasodilator substances* in the tissue cells. The vasodilator substances then are believed to diffuse through the tissues to the precapillary sphincters, metarterioles, and arterioles to cause dilation. Some of the different vasodilator substances that have been suggested are *adenosine,*

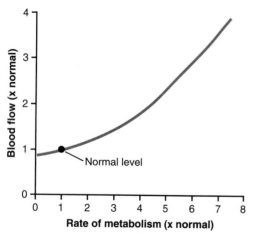

Figure 17-1 Effect of increasing rate of metabolism on tissue blood flow.

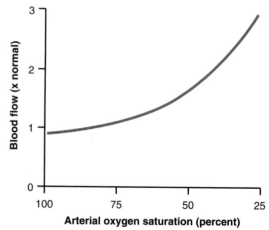

Figure 17-2 Effect of decreasing arterial oxygen saturation on blood flow through an isolated dog leg.

carbon dioxide, adenosine phosphate compounds, histamine, potassium ions, and *hydrogen ions.*

Vasodilator substances may be released from the tissue in response to oxygen deficiency. For instance, experiments have shown that decreased availability of oxygen can cause both adenosine and lactic acid (containing hydrogen ions) to be released into the spaces between the tissue cells; these substances then cause intense acute vasodilation and therefore are responsible, or partially responsible, for the local blood flow regulation. Vasodilator substances, such as carbon dioxide, lactic acid, and potassium ions, tend to increase in the tissues when blood flow is reduced and cell metabolism continues at the same rate, or when cell metabolism is suddenly increased. As the concentration of vasodilator metabolites increases, this causes vasodilation of the arterioles, increasing the tissue blood flow and returning the tissue concentration of the metabolites toward normal.

Many physiologists believe that *adenosine* is an important local vasodilator for controlling local blood flow. For example, minute quantities of adenosine are released from heart muscle cells when coronary blood flow becomes too little, and this causes enough local vasodilation in the heart to return coronary blood flow back to normal. Also, whenever the heart becomes more active than normal and the heart's metabolism increases an extra amount, this, too, causes increased utilization of oxygen, followed by (1) decreased oxygen concentration in the heart muscle cells with (2) consequent degradation of adenosine triphosphate (ATP), which (3) increases the release of adenosine. It is believed that much of this adenosine leaks out of the heart muscle cells to cause coronary vasodilation, providing increased coronary blood flow to supply the increased nutrient demands of the active heart.

Although research evidence is less clear, many physiologists also have suggested that the same adenosine mechanism is an important controller of blood flow in skeletal muscle and many other tissues, as well as in the heart. It has been difficult, however, to prove that sufficient quantities of any single vasodilator substance, including adenosine, are indeed formed in the tissues to cause all the measured increase in blood flow. It is likely that a combination of several different vasodilators released by the tissues contributes to blood flow regulation.

Oxygen Lack Theory for Local Blood Flow Control. Although the vasodilator theory is widely accepted, several critical facts have made other physiologists favor still another theory, which can be called either the *oxygen lack theory* or, more accurately, the *nutrient lack theory* (because other nutrients besides oxygen are involved). Oxygen (and other nutrients as well) is required as one of the metabolic nutrients to cause vascular muscle contraction. Therefore, in the absence of adequate oxygen, it is reasonable to believe that the blood vessels simply would relax and therefore naturally dilate. Also, increased utilization of oxygen in the tissues as a result of increased metabolism theoretically could

decrease the availability of oxygen to the smooth muscle fibers in the local blood vessels, and this, too, would cause local vasodilation.

A mechanism by which the oxygen lack theory could operate is shown in Figure 17-3. This figure shows a tissue unit, consisting of a metarteriole with a single sidearm capillary and its surrounding tissue. At the origin of the capillary is a *precapillary sphincter,* and around the metarteriole are several other smooth muscle fibers. Observing such a tissue under a microscope—for example, in a bat's wing—one sees that the precapillary sphincters are normally either completely open or completely closed. The number of precapillary sphincters that are open at any given time is roughly proportional to the requirements of the tissue for nutrition. The precapillary sphincters and metarterioles open and close cyclically several times per minute, with the duration of the open phases being proportional to the metabolic needs of the tissues for oxygen. The cyclical opening and closing is called *vasomotion.*

Let us explain how oxygen concentration in the local tissue could regulate blood flow through the area. Because smooth muscle requires oxygen to remain contracted, one might assume that the strength of contraction of the sphincters would increase with an increase in oxygen concentration. Consequently, when the oxygen concentration in the tissue rises above a certain level, the precapillary and metarteriole sphincters presumably would close until the tissue cells consume the excess oxygen. But when the excess oxygen is gone and the oxygen concentration falls low enough, the sphincters would open once more to begin the cycle again.

Thus, on the basis of available data, either a *vasodilator substance theory* or an *oxygen lack theory* could explain acute local blood flow regulation in response to the metabolic needs of the tissues. Probably the truth lies in a combination of the two mechanisms.

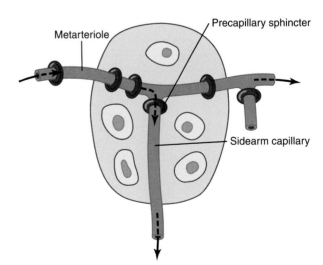

Figure 17-3 Diagram of a tissue unit area for explanation of acute local feedback control of blood flow, showing a *metarteriole* passing through the tissue and a *sidearm capillary* with its *precapillary sphincter* for controlling capillary blood flow.

Possible Role of Other Nutrients Besides Oxygen in Control of Local Blood Flow. Under special conditions, it has been shown that lack of glucose in the perfusing blood can cause local tissue vasodilation. Also, it is possible that this same effect occurs when other nutrients, such as amino acids or fatty acids, are deficient, although this has not been studied adequately. In addition, vasodilation occurs in the vitamin deficiency disease *beriberi,* in which the patient has deficiencies of the vitamin B substances *thiamine, niacin,* and *riboflavin.* In this disease, the peripheral vascular blood flow almost everywhere in the body often increases twofold to threefold. Because all these vitamins are necessary for oxygen-induced phosphorylation, which is required to produce ATP in the tissue cells, one can well understand how deficiency of these vitamins might lead to diminished smooth muscle contractile ability and therefore also local vasodilation.

Special Examples of Acute "Metabolic" Control of Local Blood Flow

The mechanisms that we have described thus far for local blood flow control are called "metabolic mechanisms" because all of them function in response to the metabolic needs of the tissues. Two additional special examples of metabolic control of local blood flow are *reactive hyperemia* and *active hyperemia.*

Reactive Hyperemia. When the blood supply to a tissue is blocked for a few seconds to as long as an hour or more and then is unblocked, blood flow through the tissue usually increases immediately to four to seven times normal; this increased flow will continue for a few seconds if the block has lasted only a few seconds but sometimes continues for as long as many hours if the blood flow has been stopped for an hour or more. This phenomenon is called *reactive hyperemia.*

Reactive hyperemia is another manifestation of the local "metabolic" blood flow regulation mechanism; that is, lack of flow sets into motion all of those factors that cause vasodilation. After short periods of vascular occlusion, the extra blood flow during the reactive hyperemia phase lasts long enough to repay almost exactly the tissue oxygen deficit that has accrued during the period of occlusion. This mechanism emphasizes the close connection between local blood flow regulation and delivery of oxygen and other nutrients to the tissues.

Active Hyperemia. When any tissue becomes highly active, such as an exercising muscle, a gastrointestinal gland during a hypersecretory period, or even the brain during rapid mental activity, the rate of blood flow through the tissue increases. Here again, by simply applying the basic principles of local blood flow control, one can easily understand this *active hyperemia.* The increase in local metabolism causes the cells to devour tissue fluid nutrients rapidly and also to release large quantities of vasodilator substances. The result is to dilate the local blood vessels and, therefore, to increase local blood flow. In this way, the active tissue receives the additional nutrients required to sustain its new level of function. As pointed out earlier, active hyperemia in skeletal muscle can increase local muscle blood flow as much as 20-fold during intense exercise.

"Autoregulation" of Blood Flow When the Arterial Pressure Changes from Normal—"Metabolic" and "Myogenic" Mechanisms

In any tissue of the body, a rapid increase in arterial pressure causes an immediate rise in blood flow. But, within less than a minute, the blood flow in most tissues returns almost to the normal level, even though the arterial pressure is kept elevated. This return of flow toward normal is called "*autoregulation*" of blood flow. After autoregulation has occurred, the local blood flow in most body tissues will be related to arterial pressure approximately in accord with the solid "acute" curve in Figure 17-4. Note that between arterial pressures of about 70 mm Hg and 175 mm Hg the blood flow increases only 20 to 30 percent even though the arterial pressure increases 150 percent.

For almost a century, two views have been proposed to explain this acute autoregulation mechanism. They have been called (1) the metabolic theory and (2) the myogenic theory.

The *metabolic theory* can be understood easily by applying the basic principles of local blood flow regulation discussed in previous sections. Thus, when the arterial pressure becomes too great, the excess flow provides too much oxygen and too many other nutrients to the tissues and "washes out" the vasodilators released by the tissues. These nutrients (especially oxygen) and decreased tissue levels of vasodilators then cause the blood vessels to constrict and the flow to return nearly to normal despite the increased pressure.

The *myogenic theory,* however, suggests that still another mechanism not related to tissue metabolism explains the phenomenon of autoregulation. This theory is based on the observation that sudden stretch of small blood vessels causes the smooth muscle of the vessel wall

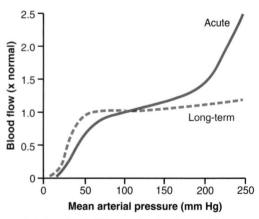

Figure 17-4 Effect of different levels of arterial pressure on blood flow through a muscle. The *solid red curve* shows the effect if the arterial pressure is raised over a period of a few minutes. The *dashed green curve* shows the effect if the arterial pressure is raised slowly over a period of many weeks.

to contract. Therefore, it has been proposed that when high arterial pressure stretches the vessel, this in turn causes reactive vascular constriction that reduces blood flow nearly back to normal. Conversely, at low pressures, the degree of stretch of the vessel is less, so that the smooth muscle relaxes, reducing vascular resistance and helping to return flow toward normal.

The myogenic response is inherent to vascular smooth muscle and can occur in the absence of neural or hormonal influences. It is most pronounced in arterioles but can also be observed in arteries, venules, veins, and even lymphatic vessels. Myogenic contraction is initiated by stretch-induced vascular depolarization, which then rapidly increases calcium ion entry from the extracellular fluid into the cells, causing them to contract. Changes in vascular pressure may also open or close other ion channels that influence vascular contraction. The precise mechanisms by which changes in pressure cause opening or closing of vascular ion channels are still uncertain but likely involve mechanical effects of pressure on extracellular proteins that are tethered to cytoskeleton elements of the vascular wall or to the ion channels themselves.

The myogenic mechanism appears to be important in preventing excessive stretch of blood vessel when blood pressure is increased. However, the role of the myogenic mechanism in blood flow regulation is unclear because this pressure-sensing mechanism cannot directly detect changes in blood flow in the tissue. Indeed, metabolic factors appear to override the myogenic mechanism in circumstances where the metabolic demands of the tissues are significantly increased, such as during vigorous muscle exercise, which can cause dramatic increases in skeletal muscle blood flow.

Special Mechanisms for Acute Blood Flow Control in Specific Tissues

Although the general mechanisms for local blood flow control discussed thus far are present in almost all tissues of the body, distinctly different mechanisms operate in a few special areas. All mechanisms are discussed throughout this text in relation to specific organs, but two notable ones are as follows:

1. In the *kidneys*, blood flow control is vested to a great extent in a mechanism called *tubuloglomerular feedback*, in which the composition of the fluid in the early distal tubule is detected by an epithelial structure of the distal tubule itself called the *macula densa*. This is located where the distal tubule lies adjacent to the afferent and efferent arterioles at the nephron *juxtaglomerular apparatus*. When too much fluid filters from the blood through the glomerulus into the tubular system, feedback signals from the macula densa cause constriction of the afferent arterioles, in this way reducing both renal blood flow and glomerular filtration rate back to or near to normal. The details of this mechanism are discussed in Chapter 26.

2. In the *brain*, in addition to control of blood flow by tissue oxygen concentration, the concentrations of carbon dioxide and hydrogen ions play prominent roles. An increase of either or both of these dilates the cerebral vessels and allows rapid washout of the excess carbon dioxide or hydrogen ions from the brain tissues. This is important because the *level of excitability of the brain itself is highly dependent on exact control of both carbon dioxide concentration and hydrogen ion concentration*. This special mechanism for cerebral blood flow control is presented in Chapter 61.

3. In the *skin*, blood flow control is closely linked to regulation of body temperature. Cutaneous and subcutaneous flow regulates heat loss from the body by metering the flow of heat from the core to the surface of the body, where heat is lost to the environment. Skin blood flow is controlled largely by the central nervous system through the sympathetic nerves, as discussed in Chapter 73. Although skin blood flow is only about 3 ml/min/100 g of tissue in cool weather, large changes from that value can occur as needed. When humans are exposed to body heating, skin blood flow may increase manyfold, to as high as *7 to 8 L/min* for the entire body. When body temperature is reduced, skin blood flow decreases, falling to barely above zero at very low temperatures. Even with severe vasoconstriction, skin blood flow is usually great enough to meet the basic metabolic demands of the skin.

Control of Tissue Blood Flow by Endothelial-Derived Relaxing or Constricting Factors

The endothelial cells lining the blood vessels synthesize several substances that, when released, can affect the degree of relaxation or contraction of the arterial wall. For many of these endothelial-derived relaxing or constrictor factors, the physiological roles are just beginning to be understood and clinical applications have, in most cases, not yet been developed.

Nitric Oxide—A Vasodilator Released from Healthy Endothelial Cells. The most important of the endothelial-derived relaxing factors is *nitric oxide (NO)*, a lipophilic gas that is released from endothelial cells in response to a variety of chemical and physical stimuli. *Nitric oxide synthase (NOS) enzymes* in endothelial cells synthesize NO from *arginine* and oxygen and by reduction of inorganic nitrate. After diffusing out of the endothelial cell, NO has a half-life in the blood of only about 6 seconds and acts mainly in the local tissues where it is released. NO activates *soluble guanylate cyclases* in vascular smooth muscle cells (Figure 17-5), resulting in conversion of cyclic guanosine triphosphate (cGTP) to cyclic guanosine monophosphate (cGMP) and activation of *cGMP-dependent protein kinase (PKG)*, which has several actions that cause the blood vessels to relax.

When blood flows through the arteries and arterioles, this causes *shear stress* on the endothelial cells because of viscous drag of the blood against the vascular walls.

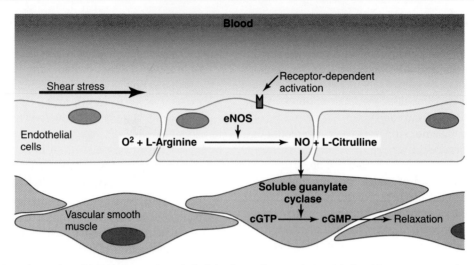

Figure 17-5 Nitric oxide synthase (eNOS) enzyme in endothelial cells synthesizes nitric oxide (NO) from arginine and oxygen. NO activates soluble guanylate cyclases in vascular smooth muscle cells, resulting in conversion of cyclic guanosine triphosphate (cGTP) to cyclic guanosine monophosphate (cGMP) which ultimately causes the blood vessels to relax.

This stress contorts the endothelial cells in the direction of flow and causes significant increase in the release of NO. The NO then relaxes the blood vessels. This is fortunate because the local metabolic mechanisms for controlling tissue blood flow dilate mainly the very small arteries and arterioles in each tissue. Yet, when blood flow through a microvascular portion of the circulation increases, this secondarily stimulates the release of NO from larger vessels due to increased flow and shear stress in these vessels. The released NO increases the diameters of the larger upstream blood vessels whenever microvascular blood flow increases downstream. Without such a response, the effectiveness of local blood flow control would be decreased because a significant part of the resistance to blood flow is in the upstream small arteries.

NO synthesis and release from endothelial cells are also stimulated by some vasoconstrictors, such as *angiotensin II*, which bind to specific receptors on endothelial cells. The increased NO release protects against excessive vasoconstriction.

When endothelial cells are damaged by chronic hypertension or atherosclerosis, impaired NO synthesis may contribute to excessive vasoconstriction and worsening of the hypertension and endothelial damage, which, if untreated, may eventually cause vascular injury and damage to vulnerable tissues such as the heart, kidneys, and brain.

Even before NO was discovered, clinicians used nitroglycerin, amyl nitrates, and other nitrate derivatives to treat patients suffering from *angina pectoris,* severe chest pain caused by ischemia of the heart muscle. These drugs, when broken down chemically, release NO and evoke dilation of blood vessels throughout the body, including the coronary blood vessels.

Other important applications of NO physiology and pharmacology are the development and clinical use of drugs (e.g., sildenafil) that inhibit *cGMP specific phosphodiesterase-5 (PDE-5),* an enzyme that degrades cGMP. By preventing the degradation of cGMP the PDE-5 inhibi-

tors effectively prolong the actions of NO to cause vasodilation. The primary clinical use of the PDE-5 inhibitors is to treat erectile dysfunction. Penile erection is caused by parasympathetic nerve impulses through the pelvic nerves to the penis, where the neurotransmitters acetylcholine and NO are released. By preventing the degradation of NO, the PDE-5 inhibitors enhance the dilation of the blood vessels in the penis and aid in erection, as discussed in Chapter 80.

Endothelin—A Powerful Vasoconstrictor Released from Damaged Endothelium. Endothelial cells also release vasoconstrictor substances. The most important of these is *endothelin,* a large 21 amino acid peptide that requires only nanogram quantities to cause powerful vasoconstriction. This substance is present in the endothelial cells of all or most blood vessels but greatly increases when the vessels are injured. The usual stimulus for release is damage to the endothelium, such as that caused by crushing the tissues or injecting a traumatizing chemical into the blood vessel. After severe blood vessel damage, release of local endothelin and subsequent vasoconstriction helps to prevent extensive bleeding from arteries as large as 5 millimeters in diameter that might have been torn open by crushing injury.

Increased endothelin release is also believed to contribute to vasoconstriction when the endothelium is damaged by hypertension. Drugs that block endothelin receptors have been used to treat *pulmonary hypertension* but have not generally been used for lowering blood pressure in patients with systemic arterial hypertension.

Long-Term Blood Flow Regulation

Thus far, most of the mechanisms for local blood flow regulation that we have discussed act within a few seconds to a few minutes after the local tissue conditions have changed. Yet, even after full activation of these acute mechanisms, the blood flow usually is adjusted only about three quarters of the way to the exact additional requirements of the tissues. For instance, when the arterial pressure suddenly increases from 100 to 150 mm Hg, the blood flow increases almost instantaneously about 100 percent. Then, within 30 seconds to 2 minutes, the flow decreases back to about 10 to 15 percent above the original control value. This illustrates the rapidity of the acute mechanisms for local blood flow regulation, but at the same time, it demonstrates that the regulation is still incomplete because there remains a 10 to 15 percent excess blood flow.

However, over a period of hours, days, and weeks, a long-term type of local blood flow regulation develops in addition to the acute control. This long-term regulation gives far more complete control of blood flow. For instance, in the aforementioned example, if the arterial pressure remains at 150 mm Hg indefinitely, within a few weeks the blood flow through the tissues gradually approaches almost exactly the normal flow level. Figure 17-4 shows by the dashed green curve the extreme effectiveness of this long-term local blood flow regulation. Note that once the long-term regulation has had time to occur, long-term changes in arterial pressure between 50 and 250 mm Hg have little effect on the rate of local blood flow.

Long-term regulation of blood flow is especially important when the metabolic demands of a tissue change. Thus, if a tissue becomes chronically overactive and therefore requires increased quantities of oxygen and other nutrients, the arterioles and capillary vessels usually increase both in number and size within a few weeks to match the needs of the tissue—unless the circulatory system has become pathological or too old to respond.

Mechanism of Long-Term Regulation—Change in "Tissue Vascularity"

The mechanism of long-term local blood flow regulation is principally to change the amount of vascularity of the tissues. For instance, if the metabolism in a tissue is increased for a prolonged period, vascularity increases, a process generally called *angiogenesis;* if the metabolism is decreased, vascularity decreases. Figure 17-6 shows the large increase in the number of capillaries in a rat anterior tibialis muscle that was stimulated electrically to contract for short periods of time each day for 30 days, compared with the unstimulated muscle in the other leg of the animal.

Thus, there is actual physical reconstruction of the tissue vasculature to meet the needs of the tissues. This reconstruction occurs rapidly (within days) in young animals. It also occurs rapidly in new growth tissue, such as in scar tissue and cancerous tissue; however, it occurs much slower in old, well-established tissues. Therefore, the time required for long-term regulation to take place may be only a few days in the neonate or as long as months in the elderly person. Furthermore, the final degree of response is much better in younger tissues than in older, so that in the neonate, the vascularity will adjust to match almost exactly the needs of the tissue for blood flow, whereas in

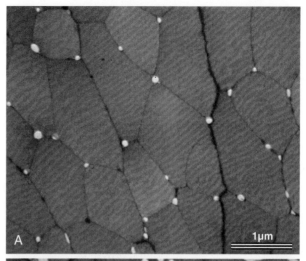

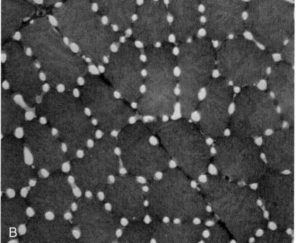

Figure 17-6 Large increase in the number of capillaries (*white dots*) in a rat anterior tibialis muscle that was stimulated electrically to contract for short periods of time each day for 30 days (*B*), compared with the unstimulated muscle (*A*). The 30 days of intermittent electrical stimulation converted the predominantly fast twitch, glycolytic anterior tibialis muscle to a predominantly slow twitch, oxidative muscle with increased numbers of capillaries and decreased fiber diameter as shown. (Photo courtesy Dr. Thomas Adair.)

older tissues, vascularity frequently lags far behind the needs of the tissues.

Role of Oxygen in Long-Term Regulation. Oxygen is important not only for acute control of local blood flow but also for long-term control. One example of this is increased vascularity in tissues of animals that live at high altitudes, where the atmospheric oxygen is low. A second example is that fetal chicks hatched in low oxygen have up to twice as much tissue blood vessel conductivity as is normally true. This same effect is also dramatically demonstrated in premature human babies put into oxygen tents for therapeutic purposes. The excess oxygen causes almost immediate cessation of new vascular growth in the retina of the premature baby's eyes and even causes degeneration of some of the small vessels that already have formed. Then when the infant is taken out of the oxygen tent, there is explosive overgrowth of new vessels to make up for the sudden decrease in available oxygen; indeed, there is often so much overgrowth that the retinal vessels grow out from the retina into the eye's vitreous humor and eventually cause blindness. (This condition is called *retrolental fibroplasia*.)

Importance of Vascular Endothelial Growth Factor in Formation of New Blood Vessels

A dozen or more factors that increase growth of new blood vessels have been found, almost all of which are small peptides. Three of those that have been best characterized are *vascular endothelial growth factor (VEGF), fibroblast growth factor,* and *angiogenin,* each of which has been isolated from tissues that have inadequate blood supply. Presumably, it is deficiency of tissue oxygen or other nutrients, or both, that leads to formation of the vascular growth factors (also called "angiogenic factors").

Essentially all the angiogenic factors promote new vessel growth in the same way. They cause new vessels to sprout from other small vessels. The first step is dissolution of the basement membrane of the endothelial cells at the point of sprouting. This is followed by rapid reproduction of new endothelial cells that stream outward through the vessel wall in extended cords directed toward the source of the angiogenic factor. The cells in each cord continue to divide and rapidly fold over into a tube. Next, the tube connects with another tube budding from another donor vessel (another arteriole or venule) and forms a capillary loop through which blood begins to flow. If the flow is great enough, smooth muscle cells eventually invade the wall, so some of the new vessels eventually grow to be new arterioles or venules or perhaps even larger vessels. Thus, angiogenesis explains the manner in which metabolic factors in local tissues can cause growth of new vessels.

Certain other substances, such as some steroid hormones, have exactly the opposite effect on small blood vessels, occasionally even causing dissolution of vascular cells and disappearance of vessels. Therefore, blood vessels can also be made to disappear when not needed. Peptides produced in the tissues can also block the growth of new blood vessels. For example, *angiostatin,* a fragment of the protein plasminogen, is a naturally occurring inhibitor of angiogenesis. *Endostatin* is another antiangiogenic peptide that is derived from the breakdown of collagen type XVII. Although the precise physiological functions of these antiangiogenic substances are still unknown, there is great interest in their potential use in arresting blood vessel growth in cancerous tumors and therefore preventing the large increases in blood flow needed to sustain the nutrient supply of rapidly growing tumors.

Vascularity Is Determined by Maximum Blood Flow Need, Not by Average Need. An especially valuable characteristic of long-term vascular control is that vascularity is determined mainly by the *maximum* level of blood flow need rather than by average need. For instance, during heavy exercise the need for whole body blood flow often increases to six to eight times the resting blood flow. This great excess of flow may not be required for more than a few minutes each day. Nevertheless, even this short need can cause enough VEGF to be formed by the muscles to increase their vascularity as required. Were it not for this capability, every time that a person attempted heavy exercise, the muscles would fail to receive the required nutrients, especially the required oxygen, so that the muscles simply would fail to contract.

However, after extra vascularity does develop, the extra blood vessels normally remain mainly vasoconstricted, opening to allow extra flow only when appropriate local stimuli such as oxygen lack, nerve vasodilatory stimuli, or other stimuli call forth the required extra flow.

Development of Collateral Circulation— a Phenomenon of Long-Term Local Blood Flow Regulation

When an artery or a vein is blocked in virtually any tissue of the body, a new vascular channel usually develops around the blockage and allows at least partial resupply of blood to the affected tissue. The first stage in this process is dilation of small vascular loops that already connect the vessel above the blockage to the vessel below. This dilation occurs within the first minute or two, indicating that the dilation is likely mediated by metabolic factors that relax the muscle fibers of the small vessels involved. After this initial opening of collateral vessels, the blood flow often is still less than one quarter that is needed to supply all the tissue needs. However, further opening occurs within the ensuing hours, so within 1 day as much as half the tissue needs may be met, and within a few days the blood flow is usually sufficient to meet the tissue needs.

The collateral vessels continue to grow for many months thereafter, almost always forming multiple small collateral channels rather than one single large vessel. Under resting conditions, the blood flow usually returns very near to normal, but the new channels seldom become large enough to supply the blood flow needed during strenuous tissue activity. Thus, the development of collateral vessels follows the usual principles of both acute and long-term local blood flow control, the acute control being rapid metabolic dilation, followed chronically by growth and enlargement of new vessels over a period of weeks and months.

The most important example of the development of collateral blood vessels occurs after thrombosis of one of the coronary arteries. Almost all people by the age of 60 years have had at least one of the smaller branch coronary vessels closed, or at least partially occluded. Yet most people do not know that this has happened because collaterals have developed rapidly enough to prevent myocardial damage. It is in those other instances in which coronary insufficiency occurs too rapidly or too severely for collaterals to develop that serious heart attacks occur.

Humoral Control of the Circulation

Humoral control of the circulation means control by substances secreted or absorbed into the body fluids—such as hormones and locally produced factors. Some of these substances are formed by special glands and transported in the blood throughout the entire body. Others are formed in local tissue areas and cause only local circulatory effects. Among the most important of the humoral factors that affect circulatory function are the following.

Vasoconstrictor Agents

Norepinephrine and Epinephrine. *Norepinephrine* is an especially powerful vasoconstrictor hormone; *epinephrine* is less so and in some tissues even causes mild vasodilation. (A special example of vasodilation caused by epinephrine occurs to dilate the coronary arteries during increased heart activity.)

When the sympathetic nervous system is stimulated in most or all parts of the body during stress or exercise, the sympathetic nerve endings in the individual tissues release norepinephrine, which excites the heart and contracts the veins and arterioles. In addition, the sympathetic nerves to the adrenal medullae cause these glands to secrete both norepinephrine and epinephrine into the blood. These hormones then circulate to all areas of the body and cause almost the same effects on the circulation as direct sympathetic stimulation, thus providing a dual system of control: (1) direct nerve stimulation and (2) indirect effects of norepinephrine and/or epinephrine in the circulating blood.

Angiotensin II. Angiotensin II is another powerful vasoconstrictor substance. As little as *one millionth* of a gram can increase the arterial pressure of a human being 50 mm Hg or more.

The effect of angiotensin II is to constrict powerfully the small arterioles. If this occurs in an isolated tissue area, the blood flow to that area can be severely depressed. However, the real importance of angiotensin II is that it normally acts on many of the arterioles of the body at the same time to increase the *total peripheral resistance,* thereby increasing the arterial pressure. Thus, this hormone plays an integral role in the regulation of arterial pressure, as is discussed in detail in Chapter 19.

Vasopressin. *Vasopressin,* also called *antidiuretic hormone,* is even more powerful than angiotensin II as a vasoconstrictor, thus making it one of the body's most potent vascular constrictor substances. It is formed in nerve cells in the hypothalamus of the brain (see Chapters 28 and 75) but is then transported downward by nerve axons to the posterior pituitary gland, where it is finally secreted into the blood.

It is clear that vasopressin could have enormous effects on circulatory function. Yet normally, only minute amounts of vasopressin are secreted, so most physiologists have thought that vasopressin plays little role in vascular control. However, experiments have shown that the concentration of circulating blood vasopressin after severe hemorrhage can increase enough to raise the arterial pressure as much as 60 mm Hg. In many instances, this can, by itself, bring the arterial pressure almost back up to normal.

Vasopressin has a major function to increase greatly water reabsorption from the renal tubules back into the blood (discussed in Chapter 28), and therefore to help control body fluid volume. That is why this hormone is also called *antidiuretic hormone.*

Vasodilator Agents

Bradykinin. Several substances called *kinins* cause powerful vasodilation when formed in the blood and tissue fluids of some organs.

The kinins are small polypeptides that are split away by proteolytic enzymes from alpha2-globulins in the plasma or tissue fluids. A proteolytic enzyme of particular importance for this purpose is *kallikrein,* which is present in the blood and tissue fluids in an inactive form. This inactive kallikrein is activated by maceration of the blood, by tissue inflammation, or by other similar chemical or physical effects on the blood or tissues. As kallikrein becomes activated, it acts immediately on alpha2-globulin to release a kinin called *kallidin* that is then converted by tissue enzymes into *bradykinin.* Once formed, bradykinin persists for only a few minutes because it is inactivated by the enzyme *carboxypeptidase* or by *converting enzyme,* the same enzyme that also plays an essential role in activating angiotensin, as discussed in Chapter 19. The activated kallikrein enzyme is destroyed by a *kallikrein inhibitor* also present in the body fluids.

Bradykinin causes both powerful *arteriolar dilation* and *increased capillary permeability.* For instance, injection of *1 microgram* of bradykinin into the brachial artery of a person increases blood flow through the arm as much as sixfold, and even smaller amounts injected locally into tissues can cause marked local edema resulting from increase in capillary pore size.

There is reason to believe that kinins play special roles in regulating blood flow and capillary leakage of fluids in inflamed tissues. It also is believed that bradykinin plays a normal role to help regulate blood flow in the skin, as well as in the salivary and gastrointestinal glands.

Histamine. Histamine is released in essentially every tissue of the body if the tissue becomes damaged or inflamed or is the subject of an allergic reaction. Most of the histamine is derived from *mast cells* in the damaged tissues and from *basophils* in the blood.

Histamine has a powerful vasodilator effect on the arterioles and, like bradykinin, has the ability to increase greatly capillary porosity, allowing leakage of both fluid and plasma protein into the tissues. In many pathological conditions, the intense arteriolar dilation and increased capillary porosity produced by histamine cause tremendous quantities of fluid to leak out of the circulation into the tissues, inducing edema. The local vasodilatory and edema-producing effects of histamine are especially prominent during allergic reactions and are discussed in Chapter 34.

Vascular Control by Ions and Other Chemical Factors

Many different ions and other chemical factors can either dilate or constrict local blood vessels. Most of them have little function in *overall regulation* of the circulation, but some specific effects are:

1. An increase in *calcium ion* concentration causes *vasoconstriction.* This results from the general effect of calcium to stimulate smooth muscle contraction, as discussed in Chapter 8.

2. An increase in *potassium ion* concentration, within the physiological range, causes *vasodilation.* This results from the ability of potassium ions to inhibit smooth muscle contraction.

3. An increase in *magnesium* ion concentration causes *powerful vasodilation* because magnesium ions inhibit smooth muscle contraction.

4. An *increase in hydrogen ion* concentration (decrease in pH) causes dilation of the arterioles. Conversely, *slight decrease in hydrogen ion* concentration causes arteriolar constriction.

5. *Anions* that have significant effects on blood vessels are *acetate* and *citrate,* both of which cause mild degrees of vasodilation.

6. An *increase in carbon dioxide concentration* causes moderate vasodilation in most tissues but marked vasodilation in the brain. Also, carbon dioxide in the blood, acting on the brain vasomotor center, has an extremely powerful indirect effect, transmitted through the sympathetic nervous vasoconstrictor system, to cause widespread vasoconstriction throughout the body.

Most Vasodilators or Vasoconstrictors Have Little Effect on Long-Term Blood Flow Unless They Alter Metabolic Rate of the Tissues. In most cases, tissue blood flow and cardiac output (the sum of flow to all of the body's tissues) are not substantially altered, except for a day or two, in experimental studies when one chronically infuses large amounts of powerful vasoconstrictors such as angiotensin II or vasodilators such as bradykinin. Why is blood flow not significantly altered in most tissues even in the presence of very large amounts of these vasoactive agents?

To answer this question we must return to one of the fundamental principles of circulatory function that we previously discussed—the ability of each tissue to *autoregulate* its own blood flow according to the metabolic needs and other functions of the tissue. Administration of a powerful vasoconstrictor, such as angiotensin II, may cause transient decreases in tissue blood flow and cardiac output but usually has little long-term effect if it does not alter metabolic rate of the tissues. Likewise, most vasodilators cause only short-term changes in tissue blood flow and cardiac output if they do not alter tissue metabolism. Therefore, blood flow is generally regulated according to the specific needs of the tissues as long as the arterial pressure is adequate to perfuse the tissues.

Bibliography

Adair TH: Growth regulation of the vascular system: an emerging role for adenosine, Am J Physiol Regul Integr Comp Physiol 289:R283, 2005.
Campbell WB, Falck JR: Arachidonic acid metabolites as endothelium-derived hyperpolarizing factors, Hypertension 49:590, 2007.
Drummond HA, Grifoni SC, Jernigan NL: A new trick for an old dogma: ENaC proteins as mechanotransducers in vascular smooth muscle, Physiology (Bethesda) 23:23, 2008.
Dhaun N, Goddard J, Kohan DE, et al: Role of endothelin-1 in clinical hypertension: 20 years on, Hypertension 52:452, 2008.
Ferrara N, Gerber HP, LeCouter J: The biology of VEGF and its receptors, Nat Med 9:669, 2003.
Folkman J: Angiogenesis, Annu Rev Med 57:1, 2006.
Folkman J: Angiogenesis: an organizing principle for drug discovery? Nat Rev Drug Discov 6:273, 2007.
Guyton AC, Coleman TG, Granger HJ: Circulation: overall regulation, Annu Rev Physiol 34:13, 1972.
Hall JE, Brands MW, Henegar JR: Angiotensin II and long-term arterial pressure regulation: the overriding dominance of the kidney, J Am Soc Nephrol 10(Suppl 12):S258, 1999.
Heerkens EH, Izzard AS, Heagerty AM: Integrins, vascular remodeling, and hypertension, Hypertension 49:1, 2007.
Hester RL, Hammer LW: Venular-arteriolar communication in the regulation of blood flow, Am J Physiol Regul Integr Comp Physiol 282:R1280, 2002.
Hodnett BL, Hester RL: Regulation of muscle blood flow in obesity, Microcirculation 14:273, 2007.
Horowitz A, Simons M: Branching morphogenesis, Circ Res 103:784, 2008.
Humphrey JD: Mechanisms of arterial remodeling in hypertension: coupled roles of wall shear and intramural stress, Hypertension 52:195, 2008.
Jain RK, di Tomaso E, Duda DG, et al: Angiogenesis in brain tumours, Nat Rev Neurosci 8:610, 2007.
Keeley EC, Mehrad B, Strieter RM: Chemokines as mediators of neovascularization, Arterioscler Thromb Vasc Biol 28:1928, 2008.
Renkin EM: Control of microcirculation and blood-tissue exchange. In Renkin EM, Michel CC (eds.): Handbook of Physiology, Sec 2, vol IV, Bethesda, 1984, American Physiological Society, pp 627.
Roman RJ: P-450 metabolites of arachidonic acid in the control of cardiovascular function, Physiol Rev 82:131, 2002.

Nervous Regulation of the Circulation, and Rapid Control of Arterial Pressure

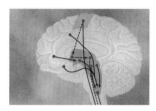

Nervous Regulation of the Circulation

As discussed in Chapter 17, adjustment of blood flow in the tissues and organs of the body is mainly the function of local tissue control mechanisms. In this chapter we discuss how nervous control of the circulation has more global functions, such as redistributing blood flow to different areas of the body, increasing or decreasing pumping activity by the heart, and providing very rapid control of systemic arterial pressure.

The nervous system controls the circulation almost entirely through the *autonomic nervous system.* The total function of this system is presented in Chapter 60, and this subject was also introduced in Chapter 17. For our present discussion, we will consider additional specific anatomical and functional characteristics, as follows.

Autonomic Nervous System

By far the most important part of the autonomic nervous system for regulating the circulation is the *sympathetic nervous system.* The *parasympathetic nervous system,* however, contributes importantly to regulation of heart function, as described later in the chapter.

Sympathetic Nervous System. Figure 18-1 shows the anatomy of sympathetic nervous control of the circulation. Sympathetic vasomotor nerve fibers leave the spinal cord through all the thoracic spinal nerves and through the first one or two lumbar spinal nerves. They then pass immediately into a *sympathetic chain,* one of which lies on each side of the vertebral column. Next, they pass by two routes to the circulation: (1) through specific *sympathetic nerves* that innervate mainly the vasculature of the internal viscera and the heart, as shown on the right side of Figure 18-1, and (2) almost immediately into peripheral portions of the *spinal nerves* distributed to the vasculature of the peripheral areas. The precise pathways of these fibers in the spinal cord and in the sympathetic chains are discussed in Chapter 60.

Sympathetic Innervation of the Blood Vessels. Figure 18-2 shows distribution of sympathetic nerve fibers to the blood vessels, demonstrating that in most tissues all the vessels *except* the capillaries are innervated. Precapillary sphincters and metarterioles are innervated in some tissues, such as the mesenteric blood vessels, although their sympathetic innervation is usually not as dense as in the small arteries, arterioles, and veins.

The innervation of the *small arteries* and *arterioles* allows sympathetic stimulation to increase *resistance* to blood flow and thereby to *decrease* rate of blood flow through the tissues.

The innervation of the large vessels, particularly of the *veins,* makes it possible for sympathetic stimulation to *decrease* the volume of these vessels. This can push blood into the heart and thereby play a major role in regulation of heart pumping, as we explain later in this and subsequent chapters.

Sympathetic Nerve Fibers to the Heart. Sympathetic fibers also go directly to the heart, as shown in Figure 18-1 and as discussed in Chapter 9. It should be recalled that sympathetic stimulation markedly increases the activity of the heart, both increasing the heart rate and enhancing its strength and volume of pumping.

Parasympathetic Control of Heart Function, Especially Heart Rate. Although the parasympathetic nervous system is exceedingly important for many other autonomic functions of the body, such as control of multiple gastrointestinal actions, it plays only a minor role in regulation of vascular function in most tissues. Its most important circulatory effect is to control heart rate by way of *parasympathetic nerve fibers* to the heart in the *vagus nerves,* shown in Figure 18-1 by the dashed red line from the brain medulla directly to the heart.

The effects of parasympathetic stimulation on heart function were discussed in detail in Chapter 9. Principally, parasympathetic stimulation causes a marked *decrease* in heart rate and a slight decrease in heart muscle contractility.

Sympathetic Vasoconstrictor System and Its Control by the Central Nervous System

The sympathetic nerves carry tremendous numbers of *vasoconstrictor nerve fibers* and only a few vasodilator fibers. The vasoconstrictor fibers are distributed to essentially all

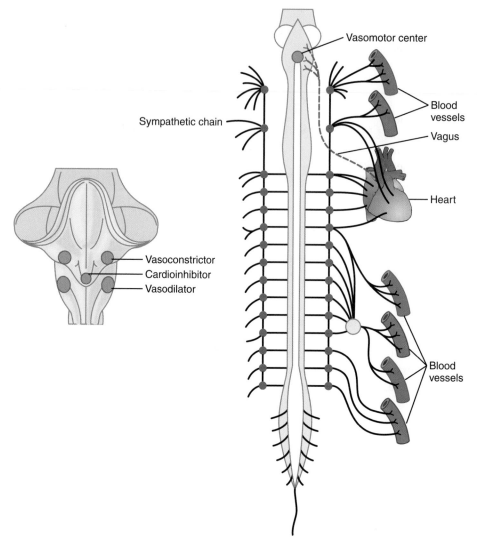

Figure 18-1 Anatomy of *sympathetic nervous control* of the circulation. Also shown by the dashed red line, a vagus nerve that carries *parasympathetic signals* to the heart.

segments of the circulation, but more to some tissues than others. This sympathetic vasoconstrictor effect is especially powerful in the kidneys, intestines, spleen, and skin but much less potent in skeletal muscle and the brain.

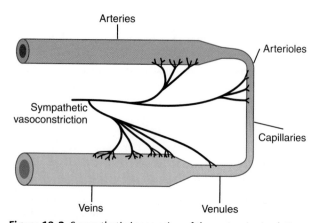

Figure 18-2 Sympathetic innervation of the systemic circulation.

Vasomotor Center in the Brain and Its Control of the Vasoconstrictor System. Located bilaterally mainly in the reticular substance of the medulla and of the lower third of the pons is an area called the *vasomotor center,* shown in Figures 18-1 and 18-3. This center transmits parasympathetic impulses through the vagus nerves to the heart and transmits sympathetic impulses through the spinal cord and peripheral sympathetic nerves to virtually all arteries, arterioles, and veins of the body.

Although the total organization of the vasomotor center is still unclear, experiments have made it possible to identify certain important areas in this center, as follows:

1. A *vasoconstrictor area* located bilaterally in the anterolateral portions of the upper medulla. The neurons originating in this area distribute their fibers to all levels of the spinal cord, where they excite preganglionic vasoconstrictor neurons of the sympathetic nervous system.

2. A *vasodilator area* located bilaterally in the anterolateral portions of the lower half of the medulla. The fibers from these neurons project upward to the vasoconstrictor area just described; they inhibit the vasoconstrictor activity of this area, thus causing vasodilation.

3. A *sensory area* located bilaterally in the *tractus solitarius* in the posterolateral portions of the medulla and lower pons. The neurons of this area receive sensory nerve signals from the circulatory system mainly through the *vagus* and *glossopharyngeal nerves*, and output signals from this sensory area then help to control activities of both the vasoconstrictor and vasodilator areas of the vasomotor center, thus providing "reflex" control of many circulatory functions. An example is the baroreceptor reflex for controlling arterial pressure, which we describe later in this chapter.

Continuous Partial Constriction of the Blood Vessels Is Normally Caused by Sympathetic Vasoconstrictor Tone.

Under normal conditions, the vasoconstrictor area of the vasomotor center transmits signals continuously to the sympathetic vasoconstrictor nerve fibers over the entire body, causing slow firing of these fibers at a rate of about one half to two impulses per second. This continual firing is called *sympathetic vasoconstrictor tone*. These impulses normally maintain a partial state of contraction in the blood vessels, called *vasomotor tone*.

Figure 18-4 demonstrates the significance of vasoconstrictor tone. In the experiment of this figure, total spinal anesthesia was administered to an animal. This blocked all transmission of sympathetic nerve impulses from the spinal cord to the periphery. As a result, the arterial pressure fell from 100 to 50 mm Hg, demonstrating the effect of losing vasoconstrictor tone throughout the body. A few minutes later, a small amount of the hormone norepinephrine was injected into the blood (norepinephrine is the principal vasoconstrictor hormonal substance secreted at the endings of the sympathetic vasoconstrictor nerve fibers throughout the body). As this injected hormone was transported in the blood to blood vessels, the vessels once again became constricted and the arterial pressure rose to a level even greater than normal for 1 to 3 minutes, until the norepinephrine was destroyed.

Control of Heart Activity by the Vasomotor Center.

At the same time that the vasomotor center regulates the amount of vascular constriction, it also controls heart activity. The *lateral* portions of the vasomotor center transmit excitatory impulses through the sympathetic nerve fibers to the heart when there is need to increase heart rate and contractility. Conversely, when there is need to decrease heart pumping, the *medial* portion of the vasomotor center sends signals to the adjacent *dorsal motor nuclei of the vagus nerves*, which then transmit parasympathetic impulses through the vagus nerves to the heart to decrease heart rate and heart contractility. Therefore,

the vasomotor center can either increase or decrease heart activity. Heart rate and strength of heart contraction ordinarily increase when vasoconstriction occurs and ordinarily decrease when vasoconstriction is inhibited.

Control of the Vasomotor Center by Higher Nervous Centers.

Large numbers of small neurons located throughout the *reticular substance* of the *pons, mesencephalon,* and *diencephalon* can either excite or inhibit the vasomotor center. This reticular substance is shown in Figure 18-3 by the rose-colored area. In general, the neurons in the more lateral and superior portions of the reticular substance cause excitation, whereas the more medial and inferior portions cause inhibition.

The *hypothalamus* plays a special role in controlling the vasoconstrictor system because it can exert either powerful excitatory or inhibitory effects on the vasomotor center. The *posterolateral portions* of the hypothalamus cause mainly excitation, whereas the *anterior portion* can cause either mild excitation or inhibition, depending on the precise part of the anterior hypothalamus stimulated.

Many parts of the *cerebral cortex* can also excite or inhibit the vasomotor center. Stimulation of the *motor cortex,* for instance, excites the vasomotor center because of impulses transmitted downward into the hypothalamus and then to the vasomotor center. Also, stimulation of the *anterior temporal lobe,* the *orbital areas of the frontal cortex,* the *anterior part of the cingulate gyrus,* the *amygdala,* the *septum,* and the *hippocampus* can all either excite or inhibit the vasomotor center, depending on the precise portions of these areas that are stimulated and on the intensity of stimulus. Thus, widespread basal areas of the brain can have profound effects on cardiovascular function.

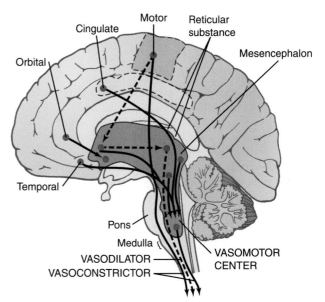

Figure 18-3 Areas of the brain that play important roles in the nervous regulation of the circulation. The *dashed lines* represent inhibitory pathways.

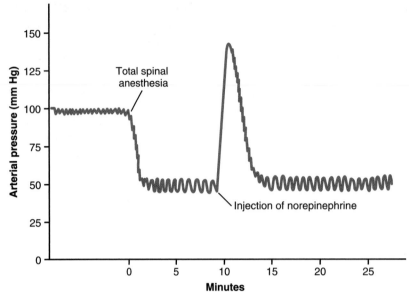

Figure 18-4 Effect of total spinal anesthesia on the arterial pressure, showing marked decrease in pressure resulting from loss of "vasomotor tone."

Norepinephrine—The Sympathetic Vasoconstrictor Transmitter Substance. The substance secreted at the endings of the vasoconstrictor nerves is almost entirely norepinephrine, which acts directly on the *alpha adrenergic receptors* of the vascular smooth muscle to cause vasoconstriction, as discussed in Chapter 60.

Adrenal Medullae and Their Relation to the Sympathetic Vasoconstrictor System. Sympathetic impulses are transmitted to the adrenal medullae at the same time that they are transmitted to the blood vessels. They cause the medullae to *secrete both epinephrine and norepinephrine into the circulating blood.* These two hormones are carried in the blood stream to all parts of the body, where they act directly on all blood vessels, usually to cause vasoconstriction. In a few tissues epinephrine causes vasodilation because it also has a "beta" adrenergic receptor stimulatory effect, which dilates rather than constricts certain vessels, as discussed in Chapter 60.

Sympathetic *Vasodilator* System and Its Control by the Central Nervous System. The sympathetic nerves to skeletal muscles carry sympathetic *vasodilator* fibers, as well as constrictor fibers. In some animals such as the cat, these dilator fibers release *acetylcholine,* not norepinephrine, at their endings, although in primates, the vasodilator effect is believed to be caused by epinephrine exciting specific beta-adrenergic receptors in the muscle vasculature.

The pathway for central nervous system control of the vasodilator system is shown by the dashed lines in Figure 18-3. The principal area of the brain controlling this system is the *anterior hypothalamus.*

Possible Unimportance of the Sympathetic Vasodilator System. It is doubtful that the sympathetic vasodilator system plays a major role in the control of the circulation in the human being because complete block of the sympathetic nerves to the muscles hardly affects the ability of these muscles to control their own blood flow in response to their needs. Yet some experiments suggest that at the onset of exercise, the sympathetic vasodilator system might cause initial vasodilation in skeletal muscles to allow *anticipatory increase in blood flow* even before the muscles require increased nutrients.

Emotional Fainting—Vasovagal Syncope. A particularly interesting vasodilatory reaction occurs in people who experience intense emotional disturbances that cause fainting. In this case, the muscle vasodilator system becomes activated, and at the same time, the vagal cardioinhibitory center transmits strong signals to the heart to slow the heart rate markedly. The arterial pressure falls rapidly, which reduces blood flow to the brain and causes the person to lose consciousness. This overall effect is called *vasovagal syncope.* Emotional fainting begins with disturbing thoughts in the cerebral cortex. The pathway probably then goes to the vasodilatory center of the anterior hypothalamus next to the vagal centers of the medulla, to the heart through the vagus nerves, and also through the spinal cord to the *sympathetic vasodilator* nerves of the muscles.

Role of the Nervous System in Rapid Control of Arterial Pressure

One of the most important functions of nervous control of the circulation is its capability to cause rapid increases in arterial pressure. For this purpose, the entire vasoconstrictor and cardioaccelerator functions of the sympathetic nervous system are stimulated together. At the same time, there is reciprocal inhibition of parasympathetic vagal inhibitory signals to the heart. Thus, three major changes occur simultaneously, each of which helps to increase arterial pressure. They are as follows:

1. *Most arterioles of the systemic circulation are constricted.* This greatly increases the total peripheral resistance, thereby increasing the arterial pressure.

2. *The veins especially (but the other large vessels of the circulation as well) are strongly constricted.* This displaces blood out of the large peripheral blood vessels toward the heart, thus increasing the volume of blood in the heart chambers. The stretch of the heart then causes the heart to beat with far greater force and therefore to pump increased quantities of blood. This, too, increases the arterial pressure.

3. Finally, *the heart itself is directly stimulated by the autonomic nervous system, further enhancing cardiac pumping.* Much of this is caused by an increase in the heart rate, the rate sometimes increasing to as great as three times normal. In addition, sympathetic nervous signals have a significant direct effect to increase contractile force of the heart muscle, this, too, increasing the capability of the heart to pump larger volumes of blood. During strong sympathetic stimulation, the heart can pump about two times as much blood as under normal conditions. This contributes still more to the acute rise in arterial pressure.

Rapidity of Nervous Control of Arterial Pressure.

An especially important characteristic of nervous control of arterial pressure is its rapidity of response, beginning within seconds and often increasing the pressure to two times normal within 5 to 10 seconds. Conversely, sudden inhibition of nervous cardiovascular stimulation can decrease the arterial pressure to as little as one-half normal within 10 to 40 seconds. Therefore, nervous control of arterial pressure is by far the most rapid of all our mechanisms for pressure control.

Increase in Arterial Pressure During Muscle Exercise and Other Types of Stress

An important example of the ability of the nervous system to increase the arterial pressure is the increase in pressure that occurs during muscle exercise. During heavy exercise, the muscles require greatly increased blood flow. Part of this increase results from local vasodilation of the muscle vasculature caused by increased metabolism of the muscle cells, as explained in Chapter 17. Additional increase results from simultaneous elevation of arterial pressure caused by sympathetic stimulation of the overall circulation during exercise. In most heavy exercise, the arterial pressure rises about 30 to 40 percent, which increases blood flow almost an additional twofold.

The increase in arterial pressure during exercise results mainly from the following effect: At the same time that the motor areas of the brain become activated to cause exercise, most of the reticular activating system of the brain stem is also activated, which includes greatly increased stimulation of the vasoconstrictor and cardioacceleratory areas of the vasomotor center. These increase the arterial

pressure instantaneously to keep pace with the increase in muscle activity.

In many other types of stress besides muscle exercise, a similar rise in pressure can also occur. For instance, during extreme fright, the arterial pressure sometimes rises by as much as 75 to 100 mm Hg within a few seconds. This is called the *alarm reaction,* and it provides an excess of arterial pressure that can immediately supply blood to the muscles of the body that might need to respond instantly to cause flight from danger.

Reflex Mechanisms for Maintaining Normal Arterial Pressure

Aside from the exercise and stress functions of the autonomic nervous system to increase arterial pressure, there are multiple subconscious special nervous control mechanisms that operate all the time to maintain the arterial pressure at or near normal. Almost all of these are *negative feedback reflex mechanisms,* which we explain in the following sections.

Baroreceptor Arterial Pressure Control System— Baroreceptor Reflexes

By far the best known of the nervous mechanisms for arterial pressure control is the *baroreceptor reflex.* Basically, this reflex is initiated by stretch receptors, called either *baroreceptors* or *pressoreceptors,* located at specific points in the walls of several large systemic arteries. A rise in arterial pressure stretches the baroreceptors and causes them to transmit signals into the central nervous system. "Feedback" signals are then sent back through the autonomic nervous system to the circulation to reduce arterial pressure downward toward the normal level.

Physiologic Anatomy of the Baroreceptors and Their Innervation.

Baroreceptors are spray-type nerve endings that lie in the walls of the arteries; they are stimulated when stretched. A few baroreceptors are located in the wall of almost every large artery of the thoracic and neck regions; but, as shown in Figure 18-5, baroreceptors are extremely abundant in (1) the wall of each internal carotid artery slightly above the carotid bifurcation, an area known as the *carotid sinus,* and (2) the wall of the aortic arch.

Figure 18-5 shows that signals from the "carotid baroreceptors" are transmitted through small *Hering's nerves* to the *glossopharyngeal nerves* in the high neck, and then to the *tractus solitarius* in the medullary area of the brain stem. Signals from the "aortic baroreceptors" in the arch of the aorta are transmitted through the *vagus nerves* also to the same tractus solitarius of the medulla.

Response of the Baroreceptors to Arterial Pressure.

Figure 18-6 shows the effect of different arterial pressure levels on the rate of impulse transmission in a Hering's carotid sinus nerve. Note that the carotid sinus baroreceptors are not stimulated at all by pressures between 0 and 50 to 60 mm Hg, but above these levels, they respond progressively more rapidly and reach a

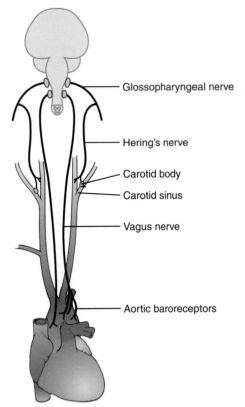

Figure 18-5 The baroreceptor system for controlling arterial pressure.

maximum at about 180 mm Hg. The responses of the aortic baroreceptors are similar to those of the carotid receptors except that they operate, in general, at arterial pressure levels about 30 mm Hg higher.

Note especially that in the normal operating range of arterial pressure, around 100 mm Hg, even a slight change in pressure causes a strong change in the baroreflex signal to readjust arterial pressure back toward normal. Thus, the baroreceptor feedback mechanism functions most effectively in the pressure range where it is most needed.

The baroreceptors respond rapidly to changes in arterial pressure; in fact, the rate of impulse firing increases in the fraction of a second during each systole and decreases again during diastole. Furthermore, the baroreceptors *respond much more to a rapidly changing pressure* than to a stationary pressure. That is, if the mean arterial pressure is 150 mm Hg but at that moment is rising rapidly, the rate of impulse transmission may be as much as twice that when the pressure is stationary at 150 mm Hg.

Circulatory Reflex Initiated by the Baroreceptors. After the baroreceptor signals have entered the tractus solitarius of the medulla, secondary signals *inhibit the vasoconstrictor center* of the medulla and *excite the vagal parasympathetic center.* The net effects are (1) *vasodilation* of the veins and arterioles throughout the peripheral circulatory system and (2) *decreased heart rate* and *strength of heart contraction.* Therefore, excitation of the baroreceptors by high pressure in the arteries reflexly *causes the arterial pressure to decrease* because of both a decrease in peripheral resistance and a decrease in cardiac output. Conversely, low pressure has opposite effects, reflexly causing the pressure to rise back toward normal.

Figure 18-7 shows a typical reflex change in arterial pressure caused by occluding the two common carotid arteries. This reduces the carotid sinus pressure; as a result, signals from the baroreceptors decrease and cause less inhibitory effect on the vasomotor center. The vasomotor center then becomes much more active than usual, causing the aortic arterial pressure to rise and remain elevated during the 10 minutes that the carotids are occluded. Removal of the occlusion allows the pressure in the carotid sinuses to rise, and the carotid sinus reflex now causes the aortic pressure to fall immediately to slightly below normal as a momentary overcompensation and then return to normal in another minute.

Function of the Baroreceptors During Changes in Body Posture. The ability of the baroreceptors to maintain relatively constant arterial pressure in the upper body

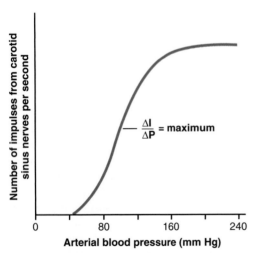

Figure 18-6 Activation of the baroreceptors at different levels of arterial pressure. ΔI, change in carotid sinus nerve impulses per second; ΔP, change in arterial blood pressure in mm Hg.

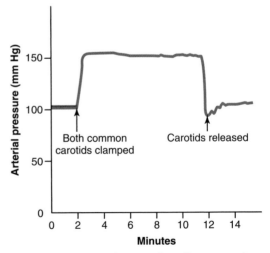

Figure 18-7 Typical carotid sinus reflex effect on aortic arterial pressure caused by clamping both common carotids (after the two vagus nerves have been cut).

is important when a person stands up after having been lying down. Immediately on standing, the arterial pressure in the head and upper part of the body tends to fall, and marked reduction of this pressure could cause loss of consciousness. However, the falling pressure at the baroreceptors elicits an immediate reflex, resulting in strong sympathetic discharge throughout the body. This minimizes the decrease in pressure in the head and upper body.

Pressure "Buffer" Function of the Baroreceptor Control System. Because the baroreceptor system opposes either increases or decreases in arterial pressure, it is called a *pressure buffer system* and the nerves from the baroreceptors are called *buffer nerves.*

Figure 18-8 shows the importance of this buffer function of the baroreceptors. The upper record in this figure shows an arterial pressure recording for 2 hours from a normal dog, and the lower record shows an arterial pressure recording from a dog whose baroreceptor nerves from both the carotid sinuses and the aorta had been removed. Note the extreme variability of pressure in the denervated dog caused by simple events of the day, such as lying down, standing, excitement, eating, defecation, and noises.

Figure 18-9 shows the frequency distributions of the mean arterial pressures recorded for a 24-hour day in both the normal dog and the denervated dog. Note that when the baroreceptors were functioning normally the mean

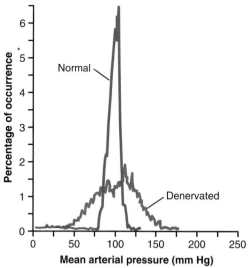

Figure 18-9 Frequency distribution curves of the arterial pressure for a 24-hour period in a normal dog and in the same dog several weeks after the baroreceptors had been denervated. (Redrawn from Cowley AW Jr, Liard JP, Guyton AC: Role of baroreceptor reflex in daily control of arterial blood pressure and other variables in dogs. Circ Res 32:564, 1973. By permission of the American Heart Association, Inc.)

arterial pressure remained throughout the day within a narrow range between 85 and 115 mm Hg—indeed, during most of the day at almost exactly 100 mm Hg. Conversely, after denervation of the baroreceptors, the frequency distribution curve became the broad, low curve of the figure, showing that the pressure range increased 2.5-fold, frequently falling to as low as 50 mm Hg or rising to over 160 mm Hg. Thus, one can see the extreme variability of pressure in the absence of the arterial baroreceptor system.

In summary, a primary purpose of the arterial baroreceptor system is to reduce the minute-by-minute variation in arterial pressure to about one-third that which would occur if the baroreceptor system was not present.

Are the Baroreceptors Important in Long-Term Regulation of Arterial Pressure? Although the arterial baroreceptors provide powerful moment-to-moment control of arterial pressure, their importance in long-term blood pressure regulation has been controversial. One reason that the baroreceptors have been considered by some physiologists to be relatively unimportant in chronic regulation of arterial pressure chronically is that they tend to *reset* in 1 to 2 days to the pressure level to which they are exposed. That is, if the arterial pressure rises from the normal value of 100 mm Hg to 160 mm Hg, a very high rate of baroreceptor impulses are at first transmitted. During the next few minutes, the rate of firing diminishes considerably; then it diminishes much more slowly during the next 1 to 2 days, at the end of which time the rate of firing will have returned to nearly normal despite the fact that the mean arterial pressure still remains at 160 mm Hg. Conversely, when the arterial pressure falls to a very low level, the baroreceptors at first transmit no impulses,

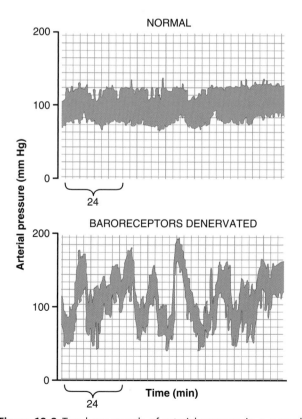

Figure 18-8 Two-hour records of arterial pressure in a normal dog (*above*) and in the same dog (*below*) several weeks after the baroreceptors had been denervated. (Redrawn from Cowley AW Jr, Liard JF, Guyton AC: Role of baroreceptor reflex in daily control of arterial blood pressure and other variables in dogs. Circ Res 32:564, 1973. By permission of the American Heart Association, Inc.)

but gradually, over 1 to 2 days, the rate of baroreceptor firing returns toward the control level.

This "resetting" of the baroreceptors may attenuate their potency as a control system for correcting disturbances that tend to change arterial pressure for longer than a few days at a time. Experimental studies, however, have suggested that the baroreceptors do not completely reset and may therefore contribute to long-term blood pressure regulation, especially by influencing sympathetic nerve activity of the kidneys. For example, with prolonged increases in arterial pressure, the baroreceptor reflexes may mediate decreases in renal sympathetic nerve activity that promote increased excretion of sodium and water by the kidneys. This, in turn, causes a gradual decrease in blood volume, which helps to restore arterial pressure toward normal. Thus, long-term regulation of mean arterial pressure by the baroreceptors requires interaction with additional systems, principally the renal–body fluid–pressure control system (along with its associated nervous and hormonal mechanisms), discussed in Chapters 19 and 29.

Control of Arterial Pressure by the Carotid and Aortic Chemoreceptors—Effect of Oxygen Lack on Arterial Pressure.

Closely associated with the baroreceptor pressure control system is a *chemoreceptor reflex* that operates in much the same way as the baroreceptor reflex except that *chemoreceptors*, instead of stretch receptors, initiate the response.

The chemoreceptors are chemosensitive cells sensitive to oxygen lack, carbon dioxide excess, and hydrogen ion excess. They are located in several small *chemoreceptor organs* about 2 millimeters in size (two *carotid bodies*, one of which lies in the bifurcation of each common carotid artery, and usually one to three *aortic bodies* adjacent to the aorta). The chemoreceptors excite nerve fibers that, along with the baroreceptor fibers, pass through Hering's nerves and the vagus nerves into the vasomotor center of the brain stem.

Each carotid or aortic body is supplied with an abundant blood flow through a small nutrient artery, so the chemoreceptors are always in close contact with arterial blood. Whenever the arterial pressure falls below a critical level, the chemoreceptors become stimulated because diminished blood flow causes decreased oxygen, as well as excess buildup of carbon dioxide and hydrogen ions that are not removed by the slowly flowing blood.

The signals transmitted from the chemoreceptors *excite* the vasomotor center, and this elevates the arterial pressure back toward normal. However, this chemoreceptor reflex is not a powerful arterial pressure controller until the arterial pressure falls below 80 mm Hg. Therefore, it is at the lower pressures that this reflex becomes important to help prevent further decreases in arterial pressure.

The chemoreceptors are discussed in much more detail in Chapter 41 in relation to *respiratory control*, in which they play a far more important role than in blood pressure control.

Atrial and Pulmonary Artery Reflexes Regulate Arterial Pressure.

Both the atria and the pulmonary arteries have in their walls stretch receptors called *low-pressure receptors*. They are similar to the baroreceptor stretch receptors of the large systemic arteries. These low-pressure receptors play an important role, especially in minimizing arterial pressure changes in response to changes in blood volume. For example, if 300 milliliters of blood suddenly are infused into a dog with all receptors intact, the arterial pressure rises only about 15 mm Hg. With the *arterial baroreceptors* denervated, the pressure rises about 40 mm Hg. If the *low-pressure receptors* also are denervated, the arterial pressure rises about 100 mm Hg.

Thus, one can see that even though the low-pressure receptors in the pulmonary artery and in the atria cannot detect the systemic arterial pressure, they do detect simultaneous increases in pressure in the low-pressure areas of the circulation caused by increase in volume, and they elicit reflexes parallel to the baroreceptor reflexes to make the total reflex system more potent for control of arterial pressure.

Atrial Reflexes That Activate the Kidneys—The "Volume Reflex."

Stretch of the atria also causes significant reflex dilation of the afferent arterioles in the kidneys. Signals are also transmitted simultaneously from the atria to the hypothalamus to decrease secretion of antidiuretic hormone (ADH). The decreased afferent arteriolar resistance in the kidneys causes the glomerular capillary pressure to rise, with resultant increase in filtration of fluid into the kidney tubules. The diminution of ADH diminishes the reabsorption of water from the tubules. Combination of these two effects—increase in glomerular filtration and decrease in reabsorption of the fluid—increases fluid loss by the kidneys and reduces an increased blood volume back toward normal. (We will also see in Chapter 19 that atrial stretch caused by increased blood volume also elicits a hormonal effect on the kidneys—release of *atrial natriuretic peptide*—that adds still further to the excretion of fluid in the urine and return of blood volume toward normal.)

All these mechanisms that tend to return the blood volume back toward normal after a volume overload act indirectly as pressure controllers, as well as blood volume controllers, because excess volume drives the heart to greater cardiac output and leads, therefore, to greater arterial pressure. This volume reflex mechanism is discussed again in Chapter 29, along with other mechanisms of blood volume control.

Atrial Reflex Control of Heart Rate (the Bainbridge Reflex).

An increase in atrial pressure also causes an increase in heart rate, sometimes increasing the heart rate as much as 75 percent. A small part of this increase is caused by a direct effect of the increased atrial volume to stretch the sinus node; it was pointed out in Chapter 10 that such direct stretch can increase the heart rate as much as 15 percent. An additional 40 to 60 percent increase in rate is caused by a nervous reflex called the *Bainbridge reflex*. The stretch receptors of the atria that elicit the Bainbridge reflex transmit their afferent signals through the vagus nerves to the medulla of the brain. Then efferent signals are transmitted back through vagal and sympathetic nerves to increase heart rate and strength of heart contraction. Thus, this reflex helps prevent damming of blood in the veins, atria, and pulmonary circulation.

Central Nervous System Ischemic Response—Control of Arterial Pressure by the Brain's Vasomotor Center in Response to Diminished Brain Blood Flow

Most nervous control of blood pressure is achieved by reflexes that originate in the baroreceptors, the chemoreceptors, and the low-pressure receptors, all of which are located in the peripheral circulation outside the brain. However, when blood flow to the vasomotor center in the lower brain stem becomes decreased severely enough to cause nutritional deficiency—that is, to cause *cerebral ischemia*—the vasoconstrictor and cardioaccelerator neurons in the vasomotor center respond directly to the ischemia and become strongly excited. When this occurs, the systemic arterial pressure often rises to a level as high as the heart can possibly pump. This effect is believed to be caused by failure of the slowly flowing blood to carry carbon dioxide away from the brain stem vasomotor center: At low levels of blood flow to the vasomotor center, the local concentration of carbon dioxide increases greatly and has an extremely potent effect in stimulating the sympathetic vasomotor nervous control areas in the brain's medulla.

It is possible that other factors, such as buildup of lactic acid and other acidic substances in the vasomotor center, also contribute to the marked stimulation and elevation in arterial pressure. This arterial pressure elevation in response to cerebral ischemia is known as the *central nervous system (CNS) ischemic response.*

The ischemic effect on vasomotor activity can elevate the mean arterial pressure dramatically, sometimes to as high as 250 mm Hg for as long as 10 minutes. *The degree of sympathetic vasoconstriction caused by intense cerebral ischemia is often so great that some of the peripheral vessels become totally or almost totally occluded.* The kidneys, for instance, often entirely cease their production of urine because of renal arteriolar constriction in response to the sympathetic discharge. Therefore, *the CNS ischemic response is one of the most powerful of all the activators of the sympathetic vasoconstrictor system.*

Importance of the CNS Ischemic Response as a Regulator of Arterial Pressure. Despite the powerful nature of the CNS ischemic response, it does not become significant until the arterial pressure falls far below normal, down to 60 mm Hg and below, reaching its greatest degree of stimulation at a pressure of 15 to 20 mm Hg. Therefore, it is not one of the normal mechanisms for regulating arterial pressure. Instead, it operates principally as an *emergency pressure control system that acts rapidly and very powerfully to prevent further

decrease in arterial pressure whenever blood flow to the brain decreases dangerously close to the lethal level.* It is sometimes called the "last ditch stand" pressure control mechanism.

Cushing Reaction to Increased Pressure Around the Brain. The so-called *Cushing reaction* is a special type of CNS ischemic response that results from increased pressure of the cerebrospinal fluid around the brain in the cranial vault. For instance, when the cerebrospinal fluid pressure rises to equal the arterial pressure, it compresses the whole brain, as well as the arteries in the brain, and cuts off the blood supply to the brain. This initiates a CNS ischemic response that causes the arterial pressure to rise. When the arterial pressure has risen to a level higher than the cerebrospinal fluid pressure, blood will flow once again into the vessels of the brain to relieve the brain ischemia. Ordinarily, the blood pressure comes to a new equilibrium level slightly higher than the cerebrospinal fluid pressure, thus allowing blood to begin again to flow through the brain. The Cushing reaction helps protect the vital centers of the brain from loss of nutrition if ever the cerebrospinal fluid pressure rises high enough to compress the cerebral arteries.

Special Features of Nervous Control of Arterial Pressure

Role of the Skeletal Nerves and Skeletal Muscles in Increasing Cardiac Output and Arterial Pressure

Although most rapidly acting nervous control of the circulation is effected through the autonomic nervous system, at least two conditions in which the skeletal nerves and muscles also play major roles in circulatory responses are the following.

Abdominal Compression Reflex. When a baroreceptor or chemoreceptor reflex is elicited, nerve signals are transmitted simultaneously through skeletal nerves to skeletal muscles of the body, particularly to the abdominal muscles. This compresses all the venous reservoirs of the abdomen, helping to translocate blood out of the abdominal vascular reservoirs toward the heart. As a result, increased quantities of blood are made available for the heart to pump. This overall response is called the *abdominal compression reflex.* The resulting effect on the circulation is the same as that caused by sympathetic vasoconstrictor impulses when they constrict the veins: an increase in both cardiac output and arterial pressure. The abdominal compression reflex is probably much more important than has been realized in the past because it is well known that people whose skeletal muscles have been paralyzed are considerably more prone to hypotensive episodes than are people with normal skeletal muscles.

Increased Cardiac Output and Arterial Pressure Caused by Skeletal Muscle Contraction During Exercise. When the skeletal muscles contract during exercise, they compress blood vessels throughout the body. Even anticipation of exercise tightens the muscles, thereby compressing the vessels in the muscles and in the abdomen. The resulting effect is to translocate blood from the peripheral vessels into the heart and lungs and, therefore, to increase the cardiac output. This is an essential effect in helping to cause the fivefold to sevenfold increase in cardiac output that sometimes occurs in heavy exercise. The increase in cardiac output in turn is an essential ingredient in increasing the arterial pressure during exercise, an increase usually from a normal mean of 100 mm Hg up to 130 to 160 mm Hg.

Respiratory Waves in the Arterial Pressure

With each cycle of respiration, the arterial pressure usually rises and falls 4 to 6 mm Hg in a wavelike manner, causing *respiratory waves* in the arterial pressure. The waves result from several different effects, some of which are reflex in nature, as follows:

1. Many of the "breathing signals" that arise in the respiratory center of the medulla "spill over" into the vasomotor center with each respiratory cycle.

2. Every time a person inspires, the pressure in the thoracic cavity becomes more negative than usual, causing the blood vessels in the chest to expand. This reduces the quantity of blood returning to the left side of the heart and thereby momentarily decreases the cardiac output and arterial pressure.

3. The pressure changes caused in the thoracic vessels by respiration can excite vascular and atrial stretch receptors.

Although it is difficult to analyze the exact relations of all these factors in causing the respiratory pressure waves, the net result during normal respiration is usually an increase in arterial pressure during the early part of expiration and a decrease in pressure during the remainder of the respiratory cycle. During deep respiration, the blood pressure can rise and fall as much as 20 mm Hg with each respiratory cycle.

Arterial Pressure "Vasomotor" Waves—Oscillation of Pressure Reflex Control Systems

Often while recording arterial pressure from an animal, in addition to the small pressure waves caused by respiration, some much larger waves are also noted—as great as 10 to 40 mm Hg at times—that rise and fall more slowly than the respiratory waves. The duration of each cycle varies from 26 seconds in the anesthetized dog to 7 to 10 seconds in the unanesthetized human. These waves are called *vasomotor waves* or *"Mayer waves."* Such records are demonstrated in Figure 18-10, showing the cyclical rise and fall in arterial pressure.

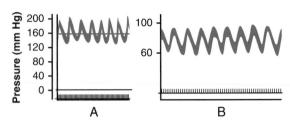

Figure 18-10 *A,* Vasomotor waves caused by oscillation of the CNS ischemic response. *B,* Vasomotor waves caused by baroreceptor reflex oscillation.

The cause of vasomotor waves is "reflex oscillation" of one or more nervous pressure control mechanisms, some of which are the following.

Oscillation of the Baroreceptor and Chemoreceptor Reflexes. The vasomotor waves of Figure 18-10B are often seen in experimental pressure recordings, although usually much less intense than shown in the figure. They are caused mainly by oscillation of the *baroreceptor reflex.* That is, a high pressure excites the baroreceptors; this then inhibits the sympathetic nervous system and lowers the pressure a few seconds later. The decreased pressure in turn reduces the baroreceptor stimulation and allows the vasomotor center to become active once again, elevating the pressure to a high value. The response is not instantaneous, and it is delayed until a few seconds later. This high pressure then initiates another cycle, and the oscillation continues on and on.

The *chemoreceptor reflex* can also oscillate to give the same type of waves. This reflex usually oscillates simultaneously with the baroreceptor reflex. It probably plays the major role in causing vasomotor waves when the arterial pressure is in the range of 40 to 80 mm Hg because in this low range, chemoreceptor control of the circulation becomes powerful, whereas baroreceptor control becomes weaker.

Oscillation of the CNS Ischemic Response. The record in Figure 18-10A resulted from oscillation of the CNS ischemic pressure control mechanism. In this experiment, the cerebrospinal fluid pressure was raised to 160 mm Hg, which compressed the cerebral vessels and initiated a CNS ischemic pressure response up to 200 mm Hg. When the arterial pressure rose to such a high value, the brain ischemia was relieved and the sympathetic nervous system became inactive. As a result, the arterial pressure fell rapidly back to a much lower value, causing brain ischemia once again. The ischemia then initiated another rise in pressure. Again the ischemia was relieved and again the pressure fell. This repeated itself cyclically as long as the cerebrospinal fluid pressure remained elevated.

Thus, any reflex pressure control mechanism can oscillate if the intensity of "feedback" is strong enough and if there is a delay between excitation of the pressure receptor and the subsequent pressure response. The vasomotor waves are of considerable theoretical importance because they show that the nervous reflexes that control arterial pressure obey the same principles as those applicable to mechanical and electrical control systems. For instance, if the feedback "gain" is too great in the guiding mechanism of an automatic pilot for an airplane and there is also delay in response time of the guiding mechanism, the plane will oscillate from side to side instead of following a straight course.

Bibliography

Cao WH, Fan W, Morrison SF: Medullary pathways mediating specific sympathetic responses to activation of dorsomedial hypothalamus, *Neuroscience* 126:229, 2004.

Cowley AW Jr: Long-term control of arterial blood pressure, *Physiol Rev* 72:231, 1992.

DiBona GF: Physiology in perspective: the wisdom of the body. Neural control of the kidney, *Am J Physiol Regul Integr Comp Physiol* 289:R633, 2005.

Esler M, Lambert G, Brunner-La Rocca HP, et al: Sympathetic nerve activity and neurotransmitter release in humans: translation from pathophysiology into clinical practice, *Acta Physiol Scand* 177:275, 2003.

Freeman R: Clinical practice. Neurogenic orthostatic hypotension, *N Engl J Med* 358:615, 2008.

Goldstein DS, Robertson D, Esler M, et al: Dysautonomias: clinical disorders of the autonomic nervous system, *Ann Intern Med* 137:753, 2002.

Guyton AC: *Arterial pressure and hypertension*, Philadelphia, 1980, WB Saunders.

Guyenet PG: The sympathetic control of blood pressure, *Nat Rev Neurosci* 7:335, 2006.

Joyner MJ: Baroreceptor function during exercise: resetting the record, *Exp Physiol* 91:27, 2006.

Lohmeier TE, Dwyer TM, Irwin ED, et al: Prolonged activation of the baroreflex abolishes obesity-induced hypertension, *Hypertension* 49:1307, 2007.

Lohmeier TE, Hildebrandt DA, Warren S, et al: Recent insights into the interactions between the baroreflex and the kidneys in hypertension, *Am J Physiol Regul Integr Comp Physiol* 288:R828, 2005.

Ketch T, Biaggioni I, Robertson R, Robertson D: Four faces of baroreflex failure: hypertensive crisis, volatile hypertension, orthostatic tachycardia, and malignant vagotonia, *Circulation* 105:2518, 2002.

Mifflin SW: What does the brain know about blood pressure? *News Physiol Sci* 16:266, 2001.

Olshansky B, Sabbah HN, Hauptman PJ, et al: Parasympathetic nervous system and heart failure: pathophysiology and potential implications for therapy, *Circulation* 118:863, 2008.

Schultz HD, Li YL, Ding Y: Arterial chemoreceptors and sympathetic nerve activity: implications for hypertension and heart failure, *Hypertension* 50:6, 2007.

Zucker IH: Novel mechanisms of sympathetic regulation in chronic heart failure, *Hypertension* 48:1005, 2006.

Role of the Kidneys in Long-Term Control of Arterial Pressure and in Hypertension: The Integrated System for Arterial Pressure Regulation

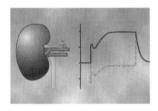

Short-term control of arterial pressure by the sympathetic nervous system, as discussed in Chapter 18, occurs primarily through the effects of the nervous system on total peripheral vascular resistance and capacitance, as well as on cardiac pumping ability.

The body, however, also has powerful mechanisms for regulating arterial pressure week after week and month after month. This long-term control of arterial pressure is closely intertwined with homeostasis of body fluid volume, which is determined by the balance between the fluid intake and output. For long-term survival, fluid intake and output must be precisely balanced, a task that is performed by multiple nervous and hormonal controls, and by local control systems within the kidneys that regulate their excretion of salt and water. In this chapter we discuss these renal–body fluid systems that play a dominant role in long-term blood pressure regulation.

Renal–Body Fluid System for Arterial Pressure Control

The renal–body fluid system for arterial pressure control acts slowly but powerfully as follows: If blood volume increases and vascular capacitance is not altered, arterial pressure will also increase. The rising pressure in turn causes the kidneys to excrete the excess volume, thus returning the pressure back toward normal.

In the phylogenetic history of animal development, this renal–body fluid system for pressure control is a primitive one. It is fully operative in one of the lowest of vertebrates, the hagfish. This animal has a low arterial pressure, only 8 to 14 mm Hg, and this pressure increases almost directly in proportion to its blood volume. The hagfish continually drinks sea water, which is absorbed into its blood, increasing the blood volume and blood pressure. However, when the pressure rises too high, the kidney simply excretes the excess volume into the urine and relieves the pressure. At low pressure, the kidney excretes less fluid than

is ingested. Therefore, because the hagfish continues to drink, extracellular fluid volume, blood volume, and pressure all build up again to the higher levels.

Throughout the ages, this primitive mechanism of pressure control has survived almost as it functions in the hagfish; in the humans, kidney output of water and salt is just as sensitive to pressure changes as in the hagfish, if not more so. Indeed, an increase in arterial pressure in the human of only a few mm Hg can double renal output of water, which is called *pressure diuresis*, as well as double the output of salt, which is called *pressure natriuresis*.

In the human being, the renal–body fluid system for arterial pressure control, just as in the hagfish, is a fundamental mechanism for long-term arterial pressure control. However, through the stages of evolution, multiple refinements have been added to make this system much more exact in its control in the human being. An especially important refinement, as discussed later, has been the addition of the renin-angiotensin mechanism.

Quantitation of Pressure Diuresis as a Basis for Arterial Pressure Control

Figure 19-1 shows the approximate average effect of different arterial pressure levels on urinary volume output by an isolated kidney, demonstrating markedly increased urine volume output as the pressure rises. This increased urinary output is the phenomenon of *pressure diuresis*. The curve in this figure is called a *renal urinary output curve* or a *renal function curve*. In the human being, at an arterial pressure of 50 mm Hg, the urine output is essentially zero. At 100 mm Hg it is normal, and at 200 mm Hg it is about six to eight times normal. Furthermore, not only does increasing the arterial pressure increase urine volume output, but it causes approximately equal increase in sodium output, which is the phenomenon of *pressure natriuresis*.

An Experiment Demonstrating the Renal–Body Fluid System for Arterial Pressure Control. Figure 19-2 shows the results of an experiment in dogs in which all the nervous reflex mechanisms for blood pressure control were first blocked. Then the arterial pressure was suddenly elevated by infusing about 400 ml of blood intravenously. Note the rapid increase in cardiac output

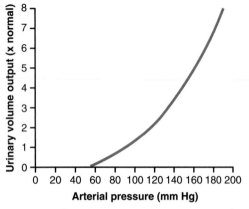

Figure 19-1 Typical renal urinary output curve measured in a perfused isolated kidney, showing pressure diuresis when the arterial pressure rises above normal.

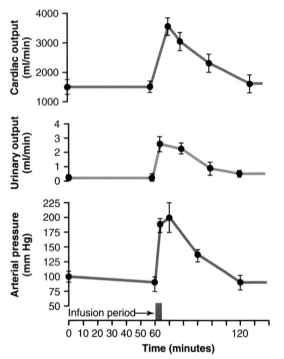

Figure 19-2 Increases in cardiac output, urinary output, and arterial pressure caused by increased blood volume in dogs whose nervous pressure control mechanisms had been blocked. This figure shows return of arterial pressure to normal after about an hour of fluid loss into the urine. (Courtesy Dr. William Dobbs.)

to about double normal and increase in mean arterial pressure to 205 mm Hg, 115 mm Hg above its resting level. Shown by the middle curve is the effect of this increased arterial pressure on urine output, which increased 12-fold. Along with this tremendous loss of fluid in the urine, both the cardiac output and the arterial pressure returned to normal during the subsequent hour. Thus, one sees an extreme capability of the kidneys to eliminate fluid volume from the body in response to high arterial pressure and in so doing to return the arterial pressure back to normal.

Arterial Pressure Control by the Renal–Body Fluid Mechanism—"Near Infinite Feedback Gain" Feature. Figure 19-3 shows a graphical method that

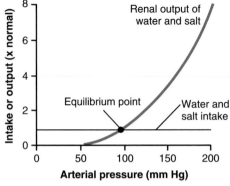

Figure 19-3 Analysis of arterial pressure regulation by equating the "renal output curve" with the "salt and water intake curve." The equilibrium point describes the level to which the arterial pressure will be regulated. (That small portion of the salt and water intake that is lost from the body through nonrenal routes is ignored in this and similar figures in this chapter.)

can be used for analyzing arterial pressure control by the renal–body fluid system. This analysis is based on two separate curves that intersect each other: (1) the renal output curve for water and salt in response to rising arterial pressure, which is the same renal output curve as that shown in Figure 19-1, and (2) the line that represents the net water and salt intake.

Over a long period, the water and salt output must equal the intake. Furthermore, the only place on the graph in Figure 19-3 at which output equals intake is where the two curves intersect, which is called the *equilibrium point*. Now, let us see what happens if the arterial pressure increases above, or decreases below, the equilibrium point.

First, assume that the arterial pressure rises to 150 mm Hg. At this level, the renal output of water and salt is about three times as great as the intake. Therefore, the body loses fluid, the blood volume decreases, and the arterial pressure decreases. Furthermore, this "negative balance" of fluid will not cease until the pressure falls *all the way* back exactly to the equilibrium level. Indeed, even when the arterial pressure is only 1 mm Hg greater than the equilibrium level, there still is slightly more loss of water and salt than intake, so the pressure continues to fall that last 1 mm Hg *until the pressure eventually returns exactly to the equilibrium point.*

If the arterial pressure falls below the equilibrium point, the intake of water and salt is greater than the output. Therefore, body fluid volume increases, blood volume increases, and the arterial pressure rises until once again it returns *exactly* to the equilibrium point. This return of the arterial pressure *always back to the equilibrium point* is the *near infinite feedback gain principle* for control of arterial pressure by the renal–body fluid mechanism.

Two Determinants of the Long-Term Arterial Pressure Level. In Figure 19-3, one can also see that two basic long-term factors determine the long-term arterial pressure level. This can be explained as follows.

As long as the two curves representing (1) renal output of salt and water and (2) intake of salt and water remain exactly as they are shown in Figure 19-3, the mean arterial pressure level will eventually readjust to 100 mm Hg, which is the pressure level depicted by the equilibrium point of this figure. Furthermore, there are only two ways in which the pressure of this equilibrium point can be changed from the 100 mm Hg level. One of these is by shifting the pressure level of the renal output curve for salt and water, and the other is by changing the level of the water and salt intake line. Therefore, expressed simply, the two primary determinants of the long-term arterial pressure level are as follows:

1. The degree of pressure shift of the renal output curve for water and salt

2. The level of the water and salt intake

Operation of these two determinants in the control of arterial pressure is demonstrated in Figure 19-4. In Figure 19-4A, some abnormality of the kidneys has caused the renal output curve to shift 50 mm Hg in the high-pressure direction (to the right). Note that the equilibrium point has also shifted to 50 mm Hg higher than normal. Therefore, one can state that if the renal output curve shifts to a new pressure level, the arterial pressure will follow to this new pressure level within a few days.

Figure 19-4B shows how a change in the level of salt and water intake also can change the arterial pressure. In this case, the intake level has increased fourfold and the equilibrium point has shifted to a pressure level of 160 mm Hg,

60 mm Hg above the normal level. Conversely, a decrease in the intake level would reduce the arterial pressure.

Thus, it is *impossible to change the long-term mean arterial pressure level* to a new value without changing one or both of the two basic determinants of long-term arterial pressure—either (1) the level of salt and water intake or (2) the degree of shift of the renal function curve along the pressure axis. However, if either of these is changed, one finds the arterial pressure thereafter to be regulated at a new pressure level, the arterial pressure at which the two new curves intersect.

The Chronic Renal Output Curve Is Much Steeper than the Acute Curve. An important characteristic of pressure natriuresis (and pressure diuresis) is that chronic changes in arterial pressure, lasting for days or months, have much greater effect on renal output of salt and water than observed during acute changes in pressure (Figure 19-5). Thus, when the kidneys are functioning normally, the *chronic renal output curve* is much steeper than the acute curve.

The powerful effects of chronic increases in arterial pressure on urine output are because increased pressure not only has direct hemodynamic effects on the kidney to increase excretion, but also indirect effects mediated by nervous and hormonal changes that occur when blood pressure is increased. For example, increased arterial pressure decreases activity of the sympathetic nervous system and various hormones such as angiotensin II and aldosterone that tend to reduce salt and water excretion by the kidneys. Reduced activity of these *antinatriuretic* systems therefore amplifies the effectiveness of pressure natriuresis and diuresis in raising salt and water excretion during chronic increases in arterial pressure (see Chapters 27 and 29 for further discussion).

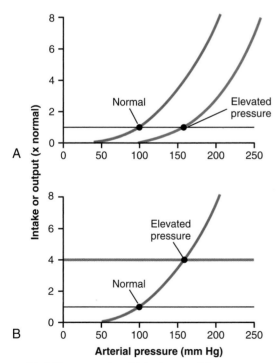

A

B

Figure 19-4 Two ways in which the arterial pressure can be increased: *A,* by shifting the renal output curve in the right-hand direction toward a higher pressure level or *B,* by increasing the intake level of salt and water.

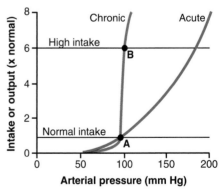

Figure 19-5 Acute and chronic renal output curves. Under steady-state conditions renal output of salt and water is equal to intake of salt and water. *A* and *B* represent the equilibrium points for long-term regulation of arterial pressure when salt intake is normal or six times normal, respectively. Because of the steepness of the chronic renal output curve, increased salt intake causes only small changes in arterial pressure. In persons with impaired kidney function, the steepness of the renal output curve may be reduced, similar to the acute curve, resulting in increased sensitivity of arterial pressure to changes in salt intake.

Conversely, when blood pressure is reduced, the sympathetic nervous system is activated and formation of antinatriuretic hormones is increased, adding to the direct effects of reduced pressure to decrease renal output of salt and water. This combination of direct effects of pressure on the kidneys and indirect effects of pressure on the sympathetic nervous system and various hormone systems make pressure natriuresis and diuresis extremely powerful for long-term control of arterial pressure and body fluid volumes.

The importance of neural and hormonal influences on pressure natriuresis is especially evident during chronic changes in sodium intake. If the kidneys and the nervous and hormonal mechanisms are functioning normally, chronic increases in intakes of salt and water to as high as six times normal are usually associated with only small increases in arterial pressure. Note that the blood pressure equilibrium point B on the curve is nearly the same as point A, the equilibrium point at normal salt intake. Conversely, decreases in salt and water intake to as low as one-sixth normal typically have little effect on arterial pressure. Thus, many persons are said to be *salt insensitive* because large variations in salt intake do not change blood pressure more than a few mm Hg.

Individuals with kidney injury or excessive secretion of antinatriuretic hormones such as angiotensin II or aldosterone, however, may be *salt sensitive* with an attenuated renal output curve similar to the acute curve shown in Figure 19-5. In these cases, even moderate increases in salt intake may cause significant increases in arterial pressure.

Some of the factors include loss of functional nephrons due to kidney injury, or excessive formation of antinatriuretic hormones such as angiotensin II or aldosterone. For example, surgical reduction of kidney mass or injury to the kidney due to hypertension, diabetes, and various kidney diseases all cause blood pressure to be more sensitive to changes in salt intake. In these instances, greater than normal increases in arterial pressure are required to raise renal output sufficiently to maintain a balance between the intake and output of salt and water.

There is some evidence that long-term high salt intake, lasting for several years, may actually damage the kidneys and eventually make blood pressure more salt sensitive. We will discuss salt sensitivity of blood pressure in patients with hypertension later in this chapter.

Failure of Increased Total Peripheral Resistance to Elevate the Long-Term Level of Arterial Pressure if Fluid Intake and Renal Function Do Not Change

Now is the chance for the reader to see whether he or she really understands the renal–body fluid mechanism for arterial pressure control. Recalling the basic equation for arterial pressure—*arterial pressure* equals *cardiac output* times *total peripheral resistance*—it is clear that an increase in total peripheral resistance should elevate the arterial pressure. Indeed, *when the total peripheral resistance is acutely increased,* the arterial pressure does rise

immediately. Yet if the kidneys continue to function normally, the acute rise in arterial pressure usually is not maintained. Instead, the arterial pressure returns all the way to normal within a day or so. Why?

The answer to this is the following: Increasing resistance in the blood vessels everywhere else in the body *besides in the kidneys* does not change the equilibrium point for blood pressure control as dictated by the kidneys (see again Figures 19-3 and 19-4). Instead, the kidneys immediately begin to respond to the high arterial pressure, causing pressure diuresis and pressure natriuresis. Within hours, large amounts of salt and water are lost from the body, and this continues until the arterial pressure returns to the pressure level of the equilibrium point. At this point blood pressure is normalized and extracellular fluid volume and blood volume are decreased to levels below normal.

As proof of this principle that changes in total peripheral resistance do not affect the long-term level of arterial pressure if function of the kidneys is still normal, carefully study Figure 19-6. This figure shows the approximate cardiac outputs and the arterial pressures in different clinical conditions in which the *long-term total peripheral resistance* is either much less than or much greater than normal, but kidney excretion of salt and water is normal. Note in all these different clinical conditions that the arterial pressure is also exactly normal.

A word of caution is necessary at this point in our discussion. Many times when the total peripheral resistance increases, *this also increases the intrarenal vascular resistance at the same time,* which alters the function of the kidney and can cause hypertension by shifting the renal

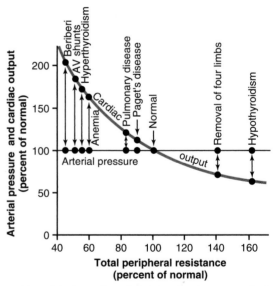

Figure 19-6 Relations of total peripheral resistance to the long-term levels of arterial pressure and cardiac output in different clinical abnormalities. In these conditions, the kidneys were functioning normally. Note that changing the whole-body total peripheral resistance caused equal and opposite changes in cardiac output but in all cases had no effect on arterial pressure. (Redrawn from Guyton AC: Arterial Pressure and Hypertension. Philadelphia: WB Saunders, 1980.)

function curve to a higher pressure level, in the manner shown in Figure 19-4*A*. We see an example of this later in this chapter when we discuss hypertension caused by vasoconstrictor mechanisms. But *it is the increase in renal resistance* that is the culprit, *not the increased total peripheral resistance*—an important distinction.

Increased Fluid Volume Can Elevate Arterial Pressure by Increasing Cardiac Output or Total Peripheral Resistance

The overall mechanism by which increased extracellular fluid volume may elevate arterial pressure, if vascular capacity is not simultaneously increased, is shown in Figure 19-7. The sequential events are (1) increased extracellular fluid volume (2) increases the blood volume, which (3) increases the mean circulatory filling pressure, which (4) increases venous return of blood to the heart, which (5) increases cardiac output, which (6) increases arterial pressure. The increased arterial pressure, in turn, increases real excretion of salt and water and may return extracellular fluid volume to nearly normal if kidney function is normal.

Note especially in this schema the two ways in which an increase in cardiac output can increase the arterial pressure. One of these is the direct effect of increased cardiac output to increase the pressure, and the other is an indirect effect to raise total peripheral vascular resistance

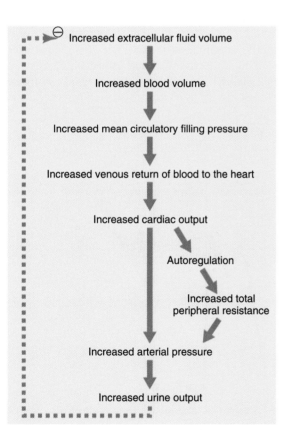

Figure 19-7 Sequential steps by which increased extracellular fluid volume increases the arterial pressure. Note especially that increased cardiac output has both a *direct effect* to increase arterial pressure and an *indirect effect* by first increasing the total peripheral resistance.

through *autoregulation* of blood flow. The second effect can be explained as follows.

Referring to Chapter 17, let us recall that whenever an excess amount of blood flows through a tissue, the local tissue vasculature constricts and decreases the blood flow back toward normal. This phenomenon is called "autoregulation," which means simply regulation of blood flow by the tissue itself. When increased blood volume increases the cardiac output, the blood flow increases in all tissues of the body, so this autoregulation mechanism constricts blood vessels all over the body. This in turn increases the total peripheral resistance.

Finally, because arterial pressure is equal to *cardiac output* times *total peripheral resistance*, the secondary increase in total peripheral resistance that results from the autoregulation mechanism helps greatly in increasing the arterial pressure. For instance, only a 5 to 10 percent increase in cardiac output can increase the arterial pressure from the normal mean arterial pressure of 100 mm Hg up to 150 mm Hg. In fact, the slight increase in cardiac output is often not measurable.

Importance of Salt (NaCl) in the Renal–Body Fluid Schema for Arterial Pressure Regulation

Although the discussions thus far have emphasized the importance of volume in regulation of arterial pressure, experimental studies have shown that an increase in salt intake is far more likely to elevate the arterial pressure than is an increase in water intake. The reason for this is that pure water is normally excreted by the kidneys almost as rapidly as it is ingested, but salt is not excreted so easily. As salt accumulates in the body, it also indirectly increases the extracellular fluid volume for two basic reasons:

1. When there is excess salt in the extracellular fluid, the osmolality of the fluid increases, and this in turn stimulates the thirst center in the brain, making the person drink extra amounts of water to return the extracellular salt concentration to normal. This increases the extracellular fluid volume.

2. The increase in osmolality caused by the excess salt in the extracellular fluid also stimulates the hypothalamic-posterior pituitary gland secretory mechanism to secrete increased quantities of *antidiuretic hormone.* (This is discussed in Chapter 28.) The antidiuretic hormone then causes the kidneys to reabsorb greatly increased quantities of water from the renal tubular fluid, thereby diminishing the excreted volume of urine but increasing the extracellular fluid volume.

Thus, for these important reasons, the amount of salt that accumulates in the body is the main determinant of the extracellular fluid volume. Because only small increases in extracellular fluid and blood volume can often increase the arterial pressure greatly if the vascular capacity is not simultaneously increased, accumulation of even a small amount of extra salt in the body can lead to considerable elevation of arterial pressure.

As discussed previously, raising salt intake in the absence of impaired kidney function or excessive formation of antinatriuretic hormones usually does not increase arterial pressure much because the kidneys rapidly eliminate the excess salt and blood volume is hardly altered.

Chronic Hypertension (High Blood Pressure) Is Caused by Impaired Renal Fluid Excretion

When a person is said to have chronic *hypertension* (or "high blood pressure"), it is meant that his or her *mean arterial pressure* is greater than the upper range of the accepted normal measure. A *mean* arterial pressure greater than 110 mm Hg (normal is about 90 mm Hg) is considered to be hypertensive. (This level of *mean* pressure occurs when the *diastolic* blood pressure is greater than about 90 mm Hg and the *systolic* pressure is greater than about 135 mm Hg.) In severe hypertension, the *mean* arterial pressure can rise to 150 to 170 mm Hg, with *diastolic* pressure as high as 130 mm Hg and *systolic* pressure occasionally as high as 250 mm Hg.

Even moderate elevation of arterial pressure leads to shortened life expectancy. At severely high pressures—mean arterial pressures 50 percent or more above normal—a person can expect to live no more than a few more years unless appropriately treated. The lethal effects of hypertension are caused mainly in three ways:

1. Excess workload on the heart leads to early heart failure and coronary heart disease, often causing death as a result of a heart attack.

2. The high pressure frequently damages a major blood vessel in the brain, followed by death of major portions of the brain; this is a *cerebral infarct.* Clinically it is called a "stroke." Depending on which part of the brain is involved, a stroke can cause paralysis, dementia, blindness, or multiple other serious brain disorders.

3. High pressure almost always causes injury in the kidneys, producing many areas of renal destruction and, eventually, kidney failure, uremia, and death.

Lessons learned from the type of hypertension called "volume-loading hypertension" have been crucial in understanding the role of the renal–body fluid volume mechanism for arterial pressure regulation. Volume-loading hypertension means hypertension caused by excess accumulation of extracellular fluid in the body, some examples of which follow.

Experimental Volume-Loading Hypertension Caused by Reduced Renal Mass Along with Simultaneous Increase in Salt Intake. Figure 19-8 shows a typical experiment demonstrating volume-loading hypertension in a group of dogs with 70 percent of their kidney mass removed. At the first circled point on the curve, the two poles of one of the kidneys were removed, and at the second circled point, the entire opposite kidney was removed, leaving the animals with only 30 percent of normal renal mass. Note that removal of this amount of kidney mass increased the arterial pressure an average of only 6 mm Hg. Then, the dogs were given salt solution to drink instead of water. Because *salt* solution fails to quench the thirst, the dogs drank two to four times the normal amounts of volume, and within a few days, their average arterial pressure rose to about 40 mm Hg above normal. After 2 weeks, the dogs were given tap water again instead of salt solution; the pressure returned to normal within 2 days. Finally, at the end of the experiment, the dogs were given salt solution again, and this time the pressure

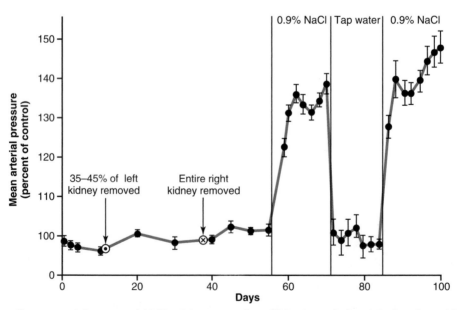

Figure 19-8 Average effect on arterial pressure of drinking 0.9 percent saline solution instead of water in four dogs with 70 percent of their renal tissue removed. (Redrawn from Langston JB, Guyton AC, Douglas BH, et al: Effect of changes in salt intake on arterial pressure and renal function in partially nephrectomized dogs. Circ Res 12:508, 1963. By permission of the American Heart Association, Inc.)

rose much more rapidly to an even higher level because the dogs had already learned to tolerate the salt solution and therefore drank much more. Thus, this experiment demonstrates volume-loading hypertension.

If the reader considers again the basic determinants of long-term arterial pressure regulation, he or she can immediately understand why hypertension occurred in the volume-loading experiment of Figure 19-8. First, reduction of the kidney mass to 30 percent of normal greatly reduced the ability of the kidneys to excrete salt and water. Therefore, salt and water accumulated in the body and in a few days raised the arterial pressure high enough to excrete the excess salt and water intake.

Sequential Changes in Circulatory Function During the Development of Volume-Loading Hypertension. It is especially instructive to study the sequential changes in circulatory function during progressive development of volume-loading hypertension. Figure 19-9 shows these sequential changes. A week or so before the point labeled "0" days, the kidney mass had already been decreased to only 30 percent of normal. Then, at this point, the intake of salt and water was increased to about six times normal and kept at this high intake thereafter. The acute effect was to increase extracellular fluid volume, blood volume, and cardiac output to 20 to 40 percent above normal. Simultaneously, the arterial pressure began to rise but not nearly so much at first as did the fluid volumes and cardiac output. The reason for this slower rise in pressure can be discerned by studying the total peripheral resistance curve, which shows an initial *decrease* in total peripheral resistance. This decrease was caused by the baroreceptor mechanism discussed in Chapter 18, which tried to prevent the rise in pressure. However, after 2 to 4 days, the baroreceptors adapted (reset) and were no longer able to prevent the rise in pressure. At this time, the arterial pressure had risen almost to its full height because of the increase in cardiac output, even though the total peripheral resistance was still almost at the normal level.

After these early acute changes in the circulatory variables had occurred, more prolonged secondary changes occurred during the next few weeks. Especially important was a *progressive increase in total peripheral resistance*, while at the same time *the cardiac output decreased almost all the way back to normal*, mainly as a result of *the long-term blood flow autoregulation* mechanism that is discussed in detail in Chapter 17 and earlier in this chapter. That is, after the cardiac output had risen to a high level and had initiated the hypertension, the excess blood flow through the tissues then caused progressive constriction of the local arterioles, thus returning the local blood flows in all the body tissues and also the cardiac output almost all the way back to normal, while simultaneously causing a *secondary increase in total peripheral resistance*.

Note, too, that the extracellular fluid volume and blood volume returned almost all the way back to normal along with the decrease in cardiac output. This resulted from

two factors: First, the increase in arteriolar resistance decreased the capillary pressure, which allowed the fluid in the tissue spaces to be absorbed back into the blood. Second, the elevated arterial pressure now caused the kidneys to excrete the excess volume of fluid that had initially accumulated in the body.

Last, let us take stock of the final state of the circulation several weeks after the initial onset of volume loading. We find the following effects:

1. Hypertension
2. Marked increase in total peripheral resistance
3. Almost complete return of the extracellular fluid volume, blood volume, and cardiac output back to normal

Therefore, we can divide volume-loading hypertension into two separate sequential stages: The first stage results from increased fluid volume causing increased cardiac output. This increase in cardiac output mediates the hypertension. The second stage in volume-loading hypertension is characterized by high blood pressure and high total peripheral resistance but return of the cardiac output so near to normal that the usual measuring techniques frequently cannot detect an abnormally elevated cardiac output.

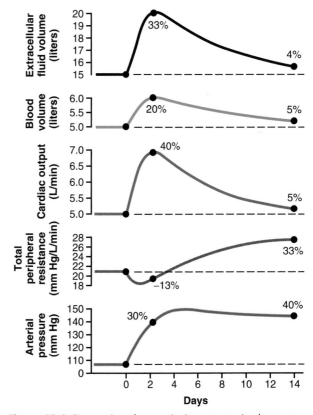

Figure 19-9 Progressive changes in important circulatory system variables during the first few weeks of *volume-loading hypertension.* Note especially the initial increase in cardiac output as the basic cause of the hypertension. Subsequently, the autoregulation mechanism returns the cardiac output almost to normal while simultaneously causing a *secondary increase in total peripheral resistance.* (Modified from Guyton AC: Arterial Pressure and Hypertension. Philadelphia: WB Saunders, 1980.)

Thus, the increased total peripheral resistance in volume-loading hypertension occurs after the hypertension has developed and, therefore, is secondary to the hypertension rather than being the cause of the hypertension.

Volume-Loading Hypertension in Patients Who Have No Kidneys but Are Being Maintained on an Artificial Kidney

When a patient is maintained on an artificial kidney, it is especially important to keep the patient's body fluid volume at a normal level—that is, it is important to remove an appropriate amount of water and salt each time the patient is dialyzed. If this is not done and extracellular fluid volume is allowed to increase, hypertension almost invariably develops in exactly the same way as shown in Figure 19-9. That is, the cardiac output increases at first and causes hypertension. Then the autoregulation mechanism returns the cardiac output back toward normal while causing a secondary increase in total peripheral resistance. Therefore, in the end, the hypertension is a high peripheral resistance type of hypertension.

Hypertension Caused by Primary Aldosteronism

Another type of volume-loading hypertension is caused by excess aldosterone in the body or, occasionally, by excesses of other types of steroids. A small tumor in one of the adrenal glands occasionally secretes large quantities of aldosterone, which is the condition called "primary aldosteronism." As discussed in Chapters 27 and 29, aldosterone increases the rate of reabsorption of salt and water by the tubules of the kidneys, thereby reducing the loss of these in the urine while at the same time causing an increase in blood volume and extracellular fluid volume. Consequently, hypertension occurs. And, if salt intake is increased at the same time, the hypertension becomes even greater. Furthermore, if the condition persists for months or years, the excess arterial pressure often causes pathological changes in the kidneys that make the kidneys retain even more salt and water in addition to that caused directly by the aldosterone. Therefore, the hypertension often finally becomes lethally severe.

Here again, in the early stages of this type of hypertension, the cardiac output is increased, but in later stages, the cardiac output generally returns almost to normal while the total peripheral resistance becomes secondarily elevated, as explained earlier in the chapter for primary volume-loading hypertension.

The Renin-Angiotensin System: Its Role in Arterial Pressure Control

Aside from the capability of the kidneys to control arterial pressure through changes in extracellular fluid volume, the kidneys also have another powerful mechanism for controlling pressure. It is the renin-angiotensin system.

Renin is a protein enzyme released by the kidneys when the arterial pressure falls too low. In turn, it raises the arterial pressure in several ways, thus helping to correct the initial fall in pressure.

Components of the Renin-Angiotensin System

Figure 19-10 shows the functional steps by which the renin-angiotensin system helps to regulate arterial pressure.

Renin is synthesized and stored in an inactive form called *prorenin* in the *juxtaglomerular cells* (JG cells) of the kidneys. The JG cells are modified smooth muscle cells located *in the walls of the afferent arterioles immediately proximal to the glomeruli.* When the arterial pressure falls, intrinsic reactions in the kidneys themselves cause many of the prorenin molecules in the JG cells to split and release renin. Most of the renin enters the renal blood and then passes out of the kidneys to circulate throughout the entire body. However, small amounts of the renin do remain in the local fluids of the kidney and initiate several intrarenal functions.

Renin itself is an enzyme, not a vasoactive substance. As shown in the schema of Figure 19-10, renin acts enzymatically on another plasma protein, a globulin called *renin substrate* (or *angiotensinogen*), to release a 10-amino acid peptide, *angiotensin I.* Angiotensin I has mild vasoconstrictor properties but not enough to cause significant changes in circulatory function. The renin persists in the blood for 30 minutes to 1 hour and continues to cause formation of still more angiotensin I during this entire time.

Within a few seconds to minutes after formation of angiotensin I, two additional amino acids are split from

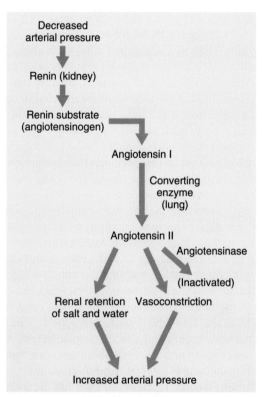

Figure 19-10 Renin-angiotensin vasoconstrictor mechanism for arterial pressure control.

the angiotensin I to form the 8-amino acid peptide *angiotensin II*. This conversion occurs to a great extent in the lungs while the blood flows through the small vessels of the lungs, catalyzed by an enzyme called *angiotensin converting enzyme* that is present in the endothelium of the lung vessels. Other tissues such as the kidneys and blood vessels also contain converting enzyme and therefore form angiotensin II locally.

Angiotensin II is an extremely powerful vasoconstrictor, and it also affects circulatory function in other ways as well. However, it persists in the blood only for 1 or 2 minutes because it is rapidly inactivated by multiple blood and tissue enzymes collectively called *angiotensinases*.

During its persistence in the blood, angiotensin II has two principal effects that can elevate arterial pressure. The first of these, *vasoconstriction in many areas of the body*, occurs rapidly. Vasoconstriction occurs intensely in the arterioles and much less so in the veins. Constriction of the arterioles increases the total peripheral resistance, thereby raising the arterial pressure, as demonstrated at the bottom of the schema in Figure 19-10. Also, the mild constriction of the veins promotes increased venous return of blood to the heart, thereby helping the heart pump against the increasing pressure.

The second principal means by which angiotensin II increases the arterial pressure is to *decrease excretion of both salt and water* by the kidneys. This slowly increases the extracellular fluid volume, which then increases the arterial pressure during subsequent hours and days. This long-term effect, acting through the extracellular fluid volume mechanism, is even more powerful than the acute vasoconstrictor mechanism in eventually raising the arterial pressure.

Rapidity and Intensity of the Vasoconstrictor Pressure Response to the Renin-Angiotensin System

Figure 19-11 shows a typical experiment demonstrating the effect of hemorrhage on the arterial pressure under two separate conditions: (1) with the renin-angiotensin system functioning and (2) without the system functioning (the system was interrupted by a renin-blocking antibody). Note that after hemorrhage—enough to cause

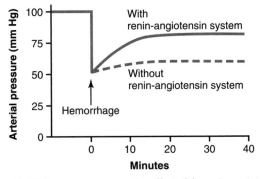

Figure 19-11 Pressure-compensating effect of the renin-angiotensin vasoconstrictor system after severe hemorrhage. (Drawn from experiments by Dr. Royce Brough.)

acute decrease of the arterial pressure to 50 mm Hg—the arterial pressure rose back to 83 mm Hg when the renin-angiotensin system was functional. Conversely, it rose to only 60 mm Hg when the renin-angiotensin system was blocked. This shows that the renin-angiotensin system is powerful enough to return the arterial pressure at least halfway back to normal within a few minutes after severe hemorrhage. Therefore, sometimes it can be of lifesaving service to the body, especially in circulatory shock.

Note also that the renin-angiotensin vasoconstrictor system requires about 20 minutes to become fully active. Therefore, it is somewhat slower to act for blood pressure control than are the nervous reflexes and the sympathetic norepinephrine-epinephrine system.

Effect of Angiotensin II in the Kidneys to Cause Renal Retention of Salt and Water—An Important Means for Long-Term Control of Arterial Pressure

Angiotensin II causes the kidneys to retain both salt and water in two major ways:

1. Angiotensin II acts directly on the kidneys to cause salt and water retention.

2. Angiotensin II causes the adrenal glands to secrete aldosterone, and the aldosterone in turn increases salt and water reabsorption by the kidney tubules.

Thus, whenever excess amounts of angiotensin II circulate in the blood, the entire long-term renal–body fluid mechanism for arterial pressure control automatically becomes set to a higher arterial pressure level than normal.

Mechanisms of the Direct Renal Effects of Angiotensin II to Cause Renal Retention of Salt and Water. Angiotensin has several direct renal effects that make the kidneys retain salt and water. One major effect is to constrict the renal arterioles, thereby diminishing blood flow through the kidneys. The slow flow of blood reduces the pressure in the peritubular capillaries, which causes rapid reabsorption of fluid from the tubules. Angiotensin II also has important direct actions on the tubular cells themselves to increase tubular reabsorption of sodium and water. The total result of all these effects is significant, sometimes decreasing urine output to less than one fifth of normal.

Stimulation of Aldosterone Secretion by Angiotensin II, and the Effect of Aldosterone to Increase Salt and Water Retention by the Kidneys. Angiotensin II is also one of the most powerful stimulators of aldosterone secretion by the adrenal glands, as we shall discuss in relation to body fluid regulation in Chapter 29 and in relation to adrenal gland function in Chapter 77. Therefore, when the renin-angiotensin system becomes activated, the rate of aldosterone secretion usually also increases; and an important subsequent function of aldosterone is to cause marked increase in sodium reabsorption by the kidney tubules, thus increasing the total body extracellular fluid sodium. This increased sodium then causes water retention, as already explained, increasing the extracellular fluid volume and leading secondarily to still more long-term elevation of the arterial pressure.

Thus both the direct effect of angiotensin on the kidney and its effect acting through aldosterone are important in long-term arterial pressure control. However, research in our laboratory has suggested that the direct effect of angiotensin on the kidneys is perhaps three or more times as potent as the indirect effect acting through aldosterone—even though the indirect effect is the one most widely known.

Quantitative Analysis of Arterial Pressure Changes Caused by Angiotensin II. Figure 19-12 shows a quantitative analysis of the effect of angiotensin in arterial pressure control. This figure shows two renal output curves, as well as a line depicting a normal level of sodium intake. The left-hand renal output curve is that measured in dogs whose renin-angiotensin system had been blocked by an angiotensin-converting enzyme inhibitor drug that blocks the conversion of angiotensin I to angiotensin II. The right-hand curve was measured in dogs infused continuously with angiotensin II at a level about 2.5 times the normal rate of angiotensin formation in the blood. Note the shift of the renal output curve toward higher pressure levels under the influence of angiotensin II. This shift is caused by both the direct effects of angiotensin II on the kidney and the indirect effect acting through aldosterone secretion, as explained earlier.

Finally, note the two equilibrium points, one for zero angiotensin showing an arterial pressure level of 75 mm Hg, and one for elevated angiotensin showing a pressure level of 115 mm Hg. Therefore, the effect of angiotensin to cause renal retention of salt and water can have a powerful effect in promoting chronic elevation of the arterial pressure.

Role of the Renin-Angiotensin System in Maintaining a Normal Arterial Pressure Despite Large Variations in Salt Intake

One of the most important functions of the renin-angiotensin system is to allow a person to eat either very small or very large amounts of salt without causing great changes in either extracellular fluid volume or arterial pressure. This function is explained by the schema in Figure 19-13, which shows that the initial effect of increased salt intake is to elevate the extracellular fluid volume, in turn elevating the arterial pressure. Then, the increased arterial pressure causes increased blood flow through the kidneys, as well as other effects, which reduce the rate of secretion of renin to a much lower level and lead sequentially to decreased renal retention of salt and water, return of the extracellular fluid volume almost to normal, and, finally, return of the arterial pressure also almost to normal. Thus, the renin-angiotensin system is an automatic feedback mechanism that helps maintain the arterial pressure at or near the normal level even when salt intake is increased. Or, when salt intake is decreased below normal, exactly opposite effects take place.

To emphasize the efficacy of the renin-angiotensin system in controlling arterial pressure, when the system functions normally, the pressure rises no more than 4 to 6 mm Hg in response to as much as a 50-fold increase in salt intake. Conversely, when the renin-angiotensin system is blocked, the same increase in salt intake sometimes causes the pressure to rise 10 times the normal increase, often as much as 50 to 60 mm Hg.

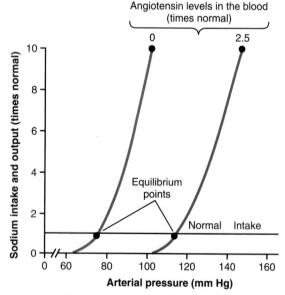

Figure 19-12 Effect of two angiotensin II levels in the blood on the renal output curve, showing regulation of the arterial pressure at an equilibrium point of 75 mm Hg when the angiotensin II level is low and at 115 mm Hg when the angiotensin II level is high.

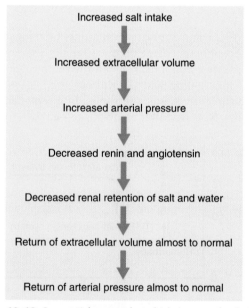

Figure 19-13 Sequential events by which increased salt intake increases the arterial pressure, but feedback decrease in activity of the renin angiotensin system returns the arterial pressure almost to the normal level.

Types of Hypertension in Which Angiotensin Is Involved: Hypertension Caused by a Renin-Secreting Tumor or by Infusion of Angiotensin II

Occasionally a tumor of the renin-secreting juxtaglomerular cells *(the JG cells)* occurs and secretes tremendous quantities of renin; in turn, equally large quantities of angiotensin II are formed. In all patients in whom this has occurred, severe hypertension has developed. Also, when large amounts of angiotensin II are infused continuously for days or weeks into animals, similar severe long-term hypertension develops.

We have already noted that angiotensin II can increase the arterial pressure in two ways:

1. By constricting the arterioles throughout the entire body, thereby increasing the total peripheral resistance and arterial pressure; this effect occurs within seconds after one begins to infuse angiotensin.

2. By causing the kidneys to retain salt and water; over a period of days, this, too, causes hypertension and is the principal cause of the long-term continuation of the elevated pressure.

"One-Kidney" Goldblatt Hypertension. When one kidney is removed and a constrictor is placed on the renal artery of the remaining kidney, as shown in Figure 19-14, the immediate effect is greatly reduced pressure in the renal artery beyond the constrictor, as demonstrated by the dashed curve in the figure. Then, within seconds or minutes, the systemic arterial pressure begins to rise and continues to rise for several days. The pressure usually rises rapidly for the first hour or so, and this is followed by a slower additional rise during the next several days. When the *systemic* arterial pressure reaches its new stable pressure level, the *renal* arterial pressure (the dashed curve in the figure) will have returned almost all the way back to normal. The hypertension produced in this way is called *"one-kidney" Goldblatt hypertension* in honor of Dr. Harry Goldblatt, who first studied the important quantitative features of hypertension caused by renal artery constriction.

The early rise in arterial pressure in Goldblatt hypertension is caused by the renin-angiotensin vasoconstrictor mechanism. That is, because of poor blood flow through the kidney after acute constriction of the renal artery, large quantities of renin are secreted by the kidney, as demonstrated by the lowermost curve in Figure 19-14, and this increases angiotensin II and aldosterone in the blood. The angiotensin in turn raises the arterial pressure acutely. The secretion of renin rises to a peak in an hour or so but returns nearly to normal in 5 to 7 days because the *renal* arterial pressure by that time has also risen back to normal, so the kidney is no longer ischemic.

The second rise in arterial pressure is caused by retention of salt and water by the constricted kidney (that is also stimulated by angiotensin II and aldosterone). In 5 to 7 days, the body fluid volume will have increased enough

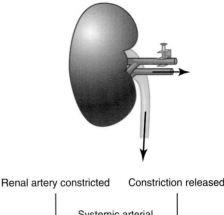

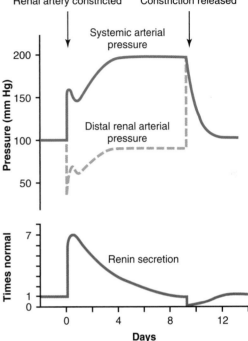

Figure 19-14 Effect of placing a constricting clamp on the renal artery of one kidney after the other kidney has been removed. Note the changes in systemic arterial pressure, renal artery pressure distal to the clamp, and rate of renin secretion. The resulting hypertension is called "one-kidney" Goldblatt hypertension.

to raise the arterial pressure to its new sustained level. The quantitative value of this sustained pressure level is determined by the degree of constriction of the renal artery. That is, the aortic pressure must rise high enough so that renal arterial pressure distal to the constrictor is enough to cause normal urine output.

A similar scenario occurs in patients with stenosis of the renal artery of a single remaining kidney, as sometimes occurs after a person receives a kidney transplant. Also, functional or pathological increases in resistance of the renal arterioles, due to atherosclerosis or excessive levels of vasoconstrictors, can cause hypertension through the same mechanisms as constriction of the main renal artery.

"Two-Kidney" Goldblatt Hypertension. Hypertension also can result when the artery to only one kidney is constricted while the artery to the other kidney

223

is normal. This hypertension results from the following mechanism: The constricted kidney secretes renin and also retains salt and water because of decreased renal arterial pressure in this kidney. Then the "normal" opposite kidney retains salt and water because of the renin produced by the ischemic kidney. This renin causes formation of angiotension II and aldosterone, both of which circulate to the opposite kidney and cause it also to retain salt and water. Thus, both kidneys, but for different reasons, become salt and water retainers. Consequently, hypertension develops.

The clinical counterpart of "two-kidney Goldblatt" hypertension occurs when there is stenosis of a single renal artery, for example caused by atherosclerosis, in a person who has two kidneys.

Hypertension Caused by Diseased Kidneys That Secrete Renin Chronically. Often, patchy areas of one or both kidneys are diseased and become ischemic because of local vascular constrictions, whereas other areas of the kidneys are normal. When this occurs, almost identical effects occur as in the two-kidney type of Goldblatt hypertension. That is, the patchy ischemic kidney tissue secretes renin, and this in turn, acting through the formation of angiotensin II, causes the remaining kidney mass also to retain salt and water. Indeed, one of the most common causes of renal hypertension, especially in older persons, is such patchy ischemic kidney disease.

Other Types of Hypertension Caused by Combinations of Volume Loading and Vasoconstriction

Hypertension in the Upper Part of the Body Caused by Coarctation of the Aorta. One out of every few thousand babies is born with pathological constriction or blockage of the aorta at a point beyond the aortic arterial branches to the head and arms but proximal to the renal arteries, a condition called coarctation of the aorta. When this occurs, blood flow to the lower body is carried by multiple, small collateral arteries in the body wall, with much vascular resistance between the upper aorta and the lower aorta. As a consequence, the arterial pressure in the upper part of the body may be 40 to 50 percent higher than that in the lower body.

The mechanism of this upper-body hypertension is almost identical to that of one-kidney Goldblatt hypertension. That is, when a constrictor is placed on the aorta above the renal arteries, the blood pressure in both kidneys at first falls, renin is secreted, angiotensin and aldosterone are formed, and hypertension occurs in the upper body. The arterial pressure in the lower body at the level of the kidneys rises approximately to normal, but high pressure persists in the upper body. The kidneys are no longer ischemic, so secretion of renin and formation of angiotensin and aldosterone return to normal. Likewise, in coarctation of the aorta, the arterial pressure in the lower body is usually almost normal, whereas the pressure in the upper body is far higher than normal.

Role of Autoregulation in the Hypertension Caused by Aortic Coarctation. A significant feature of hypertension caused by aortic coarctation is that blood flow in the arms, where the pressure may be 40 to 60 percent above normal, is almost exactly normal. Also, blood flow in the legs, where the pressure is not elevated, is almost exactly normal. How could this be, with the pressure in the upper body 40 to 60 percent greater than in the lower body? The answer is not that there are differences in vasoconstrictor substances in the blood of the upper and lower body, because the same blood flows to both areas. Likewise, the nervous system innervates both areas of the circulation similarly, so there is no reason to believe that there is a difference in nervous control of the blood vessels. The only reasonable answer is that *long-term autoregulation develops so nearly completely* that the local blood flow control mechanisms have compensated almost 100 percent for the differences in pressure. The result is that, in both the high-pressure area and the low-pressure area, the local blood flow is controlled almost exactly in accord with the needs of the tissue and not in accord with the level of the pressure. One of the reasons these observations are so important is that they demonstrate how nearly complete the long-term autoregulation process can be.

Hypertension in Preeclampsia (Toxemia of Pregnancy). Approximately 5 to 10 percent of expectant mothers develop a syndrome called *preeclampsia* (also called *toxemia of pregnancy*). One of the manifestations of preeclampsia is hypertension that usually subsides after delivery of the baby. Although the precise causes of preeclampsia are not completely understood, ischemia of the placenta and subsequent release by the placenta of toxic factors are believed to play a role in causing many of the manifestations of this disorder, including hypertension in the mother. Substances released by the ischemic placenta, in turn, cause dysfunction of vascular endothelial cells throughout the body, including the blood vessels of the kidneys. This *endothelial dysfunction decreases release of nitric oxide* and other vasodilator substances, causing vasoconstriction, decreased rate of fluid filtration from the glomeruli into the renal tubules, impaired renal-pressure natriuresis, and development of hypertension.

Another pathological abnormality that may contribute to hypertension in preeclampsia is thickening of the kidney glomerular membranes (perhaps caused by an autoimmune process), which also reduces the rate of glomerular fluid filtration. For obvious reasons, the arterial pressure level required to cause normal formation of urine becomes elevated, and the long-term level of arterial pressure becomes correspondingly elevated. These patients are especially prone to extra degrees of hypertension when they have excess salt intake.

Neurogenic Hypertension. *Acute neurogenic hypertension* can be caused by strong *stimulation of the sympathetic nervous system.* For instance, when a person becomes excited for any reason or at times during states of anxiety, the sympathetic system becomes excessively stimulated, peripheral vasoconstriction occurs everywhere in the body, and *acute* hypertension ensues.

Acute Neurogenic Hypertension Caused by Sectioning the Baroreceptor Nerves. Another type of *acute* neurogenic hypertension occurs when the nerves leading from the baroreceptors are cut or when the tractus solitarius is destroyed in each side of the medulla oblongata (these are the areas where the nerves from the carotid and aortic baroreceptors connect in the brain stem). The sudden cessation of normal nerve signals from the baroreceptors has the same effect on the nervous pressure control mechanisms as a sudden reduction of the arterial pressure in the aorta and carotid arteries. That is, loss of the normal inhibitory effect on the vasomotor center caused by normal baroreceptor nervous signals allows the vasomotor center suddenly to become extremely active and the mean arterial pressure to increase from 100 mm Hg to as high as 160 mm Hg. The pressure returns to nearly normal within about 2 days because the response of the vasomotor center to the absent baroreceptor signal fades away, which is called central "resetting" of the baroreceptor pressure control mechanism. Therefore, the neurogenic hypertension caused by sectioning the baroreceptor nerves is mainly an acute type of hypertension, not a chronic type.

Genetic Causes of Hypertension. Spontaneous hereditary hypertension has been observed in several strains of animals, including different strains of rats, rabbits, and at least one strain of dogs. In the strain of rats that has been studied to the greatest extent, the Okamoto spontaneously hypertensive rat strain, there is evidence that in early development of the hypertension, the sympathetic nervous system is considerably more active than in normal rats. In the later stages of this type of hypertension, structural changes have been observed in the nephrons of the kidneys: (1) increased preglomerular renal arterial resistance and (2) decreased permeability of the glomerular membranes. These structural changes could also contribute to the long-term continuance of the hypertension. In other strains of hypertensive rats, impaired renal function also has been observed.

In humans, several different gene mutations have been identified that can cause hypertension. These forms of hypertension are called *monogenic hypertension* because they are caused by mutation of a single gene. An interesting feature of these genetic disorders is that they all cause excessive salt and water reabsorption by the renal tubules. In some cases the increased reabsorption is due to gene mutations that directly increase transport of sodium or chloride in the renal tubular epithelial cells. In other instances, the gene mutations cause increased synthesis or activity of hormones that stimulate renal tubular salt and water reabsorption. Thus, in all monogenic hypertensive disorders discovered thus far, the final common pathway to hypertension appears to be increased salt reabsorption and expansion of extracellular fluid volume. Monogenic hypertension, however, is rare and all of the known forms together account for less than 1% of human hypertension.

"Primary (Essential) Hypertension"

About 90 to 95 percent of all people who have hypertension are said to have "primary hypertension," also widely known as "essential hypertension" by many clinicians. These terms mean simply that *the hypertension is of unknown origin,* in contrast to those forms of hypertension that are *secondary* to known causes, such as renal artery stenosis or monogenic forms of hypertension.

In most patients, *excess weight gain* and *sedentary lifestyle* appear to play a major role in causing hypertension. The majority of patients with hypertension are overweight, and studies of different populations suggest that excess weight gain and obesity may account for as much as 65 to 75 percent of the risk for developing primary hypertension. Clinical studies have clearly shown the value of weight loss for reducing blood pressure in most patients with hypertension. In fact, clinical guidelines for treating hypertension recommend increased physical activity and weight loss as a first step in treating most patients with hypertension.

Some of the characteristics of primary hypertension caused by excess weight gain and obesity include:

1. *Cardiac output is increased* due, in part, to the additional blood flow required for the extra adipose tissue. However, blood flow in the heart, kidneys, gastrointestinal tract, and skeletal muscle also increases with weight gain due to increased metabolic rate and growth of the organs and tissues in response to their increased metabolic demands. As the hypertension is sustained for many months and years, total peripheral vascular resistance may be increased.

2. *Sympathetic nerve activity, especially in the kidneys, is increased in overweight patients.* The causes of increased sympathetic activity in obesity are not fully understood, but recent studies suggest that hormones, such as *leptin,* released from fat cells may directly stimulate multiple regions of the hypothalamus, which, in turn, have an excitatory influence on the vasomotor centers of the brain medulla.

3. *Angiotensin II and aldosterone levels are increased two-fold to threefold in many obese patients.* This may be caused partly by increased sympathetic nerve stimulation, which increases renin release by the kidneys and therefore formation of angiotensin II, which, in turn, stimulates the adrenal gland to secrete aldosterone.

4. *The renal-pressure natriuresis mechanism is impaired, and the kidneys will not excrete adequate amounts of salt and water unless the arterial pressure is high or unless kidney function is somehow improved.* In other words, if the mean arterial pressure in the essential hypertensive person is 150 mm Hg, acute reduction of the mean arterial pressure artificially to the normal value of 100 mm Hg (but without otherwise altering renal function except for the decreased pressure) will cause almost total anuria, and the person will retain salt and water until the pressure rises back to the elevated value of 150 mm Hg. Chronic reductions in arterial pressure with effective antihypertensive therapies, however, usually do not cause marked salt and water retention by the kidneys because these therapies also improve renal-pressure natriuresis, as discussed later.

Experimental studies in obese animals and obese patients suggest that impaired renal-pressure natriuresis in obesity

225

hypertension is caused mainly by increased renal tubular reabsorption of salt and water due to increased sympathetic nerve activity and increased levels of angiotensin II and aldosterone. However, if hypertension is not effectively treated, there may also be vascular damage in the kidneys that can reduce the glomerular filtration rate and increase the severity of the hypertension. Eventually uncontrolled hypertension associated with obesity can lead to severe vascular injury and complete loss of kidney function.

Graphical Analysis of Arterial Pressure Control in Essential Hypertension.

Figure 19-15 is a graphical analysis of essential hypertension. The curves of this figure are called *sodium-loading renal function curves* because the arterial pressure in each instance is increased very slowly, over many days or weeks, by gradually increasing the level of sodium intake. The sodium-loading type of curve can be determined by increasing the level of sodium intake to a new level every few days, then waiting for the renal output of sodium to come into balance with the intake, and at the same time recording the changes in arterial pressure.

When this procedure is used in essential hypertensive patients, two types of curves, shown to the right in Figure 19-15, can be recorded in essential hypertensive patients, one called (1) *salt-insensitive* hypertension and the other (2) *salt-sensitive* hypertension. Note in both instances that the curves are shifted to the right, to a higher pressure level than for normal people. Now, let us plot on this same graph (1) a normal level of salt intake and (2) a high level of salt intake representing 3.5 times the normal intake. In the case of the person with salt-insensitive essential hypertension, the arterial pressure does not increase significantly when changing from normal salt intake to high salt intake. Conversely, in those patients who have

salt-sensitive essential hypertension, the high salt intake significantly exacerbates the hypertension.

Two additional points should be emphasized: (1) Salt sensitivity of blood pressure is not an all-or-none characteristic—it is a quantitative characteristic, with some individuals being more salt sensitive than others. (2) Salt sensitivity of blood pressure is not a fixed characteristic; instead, blood pressure usually becomes more salt sensitive as a person ages, especially after 50 or 60 years of age.

The reason for the difference between salt-insensitive essential hypertension and salt-sensitive hypertension is presumably related to structural or functional differences in the kidneys of these two types of hypertensive patients. For example, salt-sensitive hypertension may occur with different types of chronic renal disease due to gradual loss of the functional units of the kidneys (the *nephrons*) or to normal aging as discussed in Chapter 31. Abnormal function of the renin-angiotensin system can also cause blood pressure to become salt sensitive, as discussed previously in this chapter.

Treatment of Essential Hypertension.

Current guidelines for treating hypertension recommend, as a first step, lifestyle modifications that are aimed at increasing physical activity and weight loss in most patients. Unfortunately, many patients are unable to lose weight, and pharmacological treatment with antihypertensive drugs must be initiated.

Two general classes of drugs are used to treat hypertension: (1) *vasodilator drugs* that increase renal blood flow and (2) *natriuretic or diuretic drugs* that decrease tubular reabsorption of salt and water.

Vasodilator drugs usually cause vasodilation in many other tissues of the body, as well as in the kidneys. Different ones act in one of the following ways: (1) by inhibiting sympathetic nervous signals to the kidneys or by blocking the action of the sympathetic transmitter substance on the renal vasculature and renal tubules, (2) by directly relaxing the smooth muscle of the renal vasculature, or (3) by blocking the action of the renin-angiotensin system on the renal vasculature or renal tubules.

Those drugs that reduce reabsorption of salt and water by the renal tubules include especially drugs that block active transport of sodium through the tubular wall; this blockage in turn also prevents the reabsorption of water, as explained earlier in the chapter. These natriuretic or diuretic drugs are discussed in greater detail in Chapter 31.

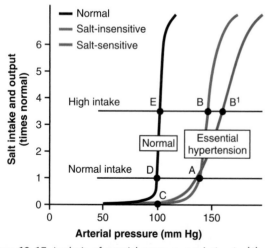

Figure 19-15 Analysis of arterial pressure regulation in (1) non-salt-sensitive essential hypertension and (2) salt-sensitive essential hypertension. (Redrawn from Guyton AC, Coleman TG, Young DB, et al: Salt balance and long-term blood pressure control. Annu Rev Med 31:15, 1980. With permission, from the *Annual Review of Medicine,* © 1980, by Annual Reviews http://www.AnnualReviews.org.)

Summary of the Integrated, Multifaceted System for Arterial Pressure Regulation

By now, it is clear that arterial pressure is regulated not by a single pressure controlling system but instead by several interrelated systems, each of which performs a specific function. For instance, when a person bleeds severely so that the pressure falls suddenly, two problems confront the pressure control system. The first is survival, that is, to return the arterial pressure immediately to a high enough level that the person can live through the acute episode. The second is to return the blood volume and arterial eventually to their normal levels so that the circulatory system can reestablish full normality, not merely back to the levels required for survival.

In Chapter 18, we saw that the first line of defense against acute changes in arterial pressure is the nervous control system. In this chapter, we have emphasized a second line of defense achieved mainly by kidney mechanisms for long-term control of arterial pressure. However, there are other pieces to the puzzle. Figure 19-16 helps to put these together.

Figure 19-16 shows the approximate immediate (seconds and minutes) and long-term (hours and days) control responses, expressed as feedback gain, of eight arterial pressure control mechanisms. These mechanisms can be divided into three groups: (1) those that react rapidly, within seconds or minutes; (2) those that respond over an intermediate time period, minutes or hours; and (3) those that provide long-term arterial pressure regulation, days, months, and years. Let us see how they fit together as a total, integrated system for pressure control.

Rapidly Acting Pressure Control Mechanisms, Acting Within Seconds or Minutes. The rapidly acting pressure control mechanisms are almost entirely acute nervous reflexes or other nervous responses. Note in Figure 19-16 the three mechanisms that show responses within seconds. They are (1) the baroreceptor feedback mechanism, (2) the central nervous system ischemic

mechanism, and (3) the chemoreceptor mechanism. Not only do these mechanisms begin to react within seconds, but they are also powerful. After any acute fall in pressure, as might be caused by severe hemorrhage, the nervous mechanisms combine (1) to cause constriction of the veins and transfer of blood into the heart, (2) to cause increased heart rate and contractility of the heart to provide greater pumping capacity by the heart, and (3) to cause constriction of most peripheral arterioles to impede flow of blood out of the arteries; all these effects occur almost instantly to raise the arterial pressure back into a survival range.

When the pressure suddenly rises too high, as might occur in response to rapid transfusion of excess blood, the same control mechanisms operate in the reverse direction, again returning the pressure back toward normal.

Pressure Control Mechanisms That Act After Many Minutes. Several pressure control mechanisms exhibit significant responses only after a few minutes following acute arterial pressure change. Three of these, shown in Figure 19-16, are (1) the renin-angiotensin vasoconstrictor mechanism, (2) stress-relaxation of the vasculature, and (3) shift of fluid through the tissue capillary walls in and out of the circulation to readjust the blood volume as needed.

We have already described at length the role of the renin-angiotensin vasoconstrictor system to provide a semiacute means for increasing the arterial pressure when this is necessary. The *stress-relaxation mechanism* is demonstrated by the following example: When the pressure in the blood vessels becomes too high, they become stretched and keep on stretching more and more for minutes or hours; as a result, the pressure in the vessels falls toward normal. This continuing stretch of the vessels, called *stress-relaxation,* can serve as an intermediate-term pressure "buffer."

The *capillary fluid shift mechanism* means simply that any time capillary pressure falls too low, fluid is absorbed from the tissues through the capillary membranes and into the circulation, thus building up the blood volume and increasing the pressure in the circulation. Conversely, when the capillary pressure rises too high, fluid is lost out of the circulation into the tissues, thus reducing the blood volume, as well as virtually all the pressures throughout the circulation.

These three intermediate mechanisms become mostly activated within 30 minutes to several hours. During this time, the nervous mechanisms usually become less and less effective, which explains the importance of these nonnervous, intermediate time pressure control measures.

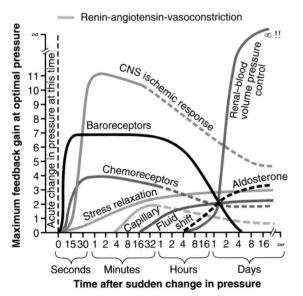

Figure 19-16 Approximate potency of various arterial pressure control mechanisms at different time intervals after onset of a disturbance to the arterial pressure. Note especially the infinite gain (∞) of the renal body fluid pressure control mechanism that occurs after a few weeks' time. (Redrawn from Guyton AC: Arterial Pressure and Hypertension. Philadelphia: WB Saunders, 1980.)

Long-Term Mechanisms for Arterial Pressure Regulation. The goal of this chapter has been to explain the role of the kidneys in long-term control of arterial pressure. To the far right in Figure 19-16 is shown the renal–blood volume pressure control mechanism (which is the same as the renal–body fluid pressure control mechanism), demonstrating that it takes a few hours to begin showing significant response. Yet it eventually develops a feedback gain for control of arterial pressure nearly equal to infinity. This means that this mechanism can eventually return the arterial pressure nearly *all the way* back, not merely partway back, to that pressure level that provides normal output of salt and water by the kidneys. By now, the reader should be familiar with this concept, which has been the major point of this chapter.

Many factors can affect the pressure-regulating level of the renal–body fluid mechanism. One of these, shown in Figure 19-16, is aldosterone. A decrease in arterial pressure leads within minutes to an increase in aldosterone secretion, and over the next hour or days, this plays an important role in modifying the pressure control characteristics of the renal–body fluid mechanism.

Especially important is interaction of the renin-angiotensin system with the aldosterone and renal fluid mechanisms. For instance, a person's salt intake varies tremendously from one day to another. We have seen in this chapter that the salt intake can decrease to as little as one-tenth normal or can increase to 10 to 15 times normal and yet the regulated level of the mean arterial pressure will change only a few mm Hg if the renin-angiotensin-aldosterone system is fully operative. But, without a functional renin-angiotensin-aldosterone system, blood pressure becomes very sensitive to changes in salt intake.

Thus, arterial pressure control begins with the life-saving measures of the nervous pressure controls, then continues with the sustaining characteristics of the intermediate pressure controls, and, finally, is stabilized at the long-term pressure level by the renal–body fluid mechanism. This long-term mechanism in turn has multiple interactions with the renin-angiotensin-aldosterone system, the nervous system, and several other factors that provide special blood pressure control capabilities for special purposes.

Bibliography

Chobanian AV, Bakris GL, Black HR, et al: Joint National Committee on Prevention, Detection, Evaluation, and Treatment of High Blood Pressure. National High Blood Pressure Education Program Coordinating Committee. Seventh Report of the Joint National Committee on prevention, detection, evaluation, and treatment of high blood pressure, *Hypertension* 42:1206, 2003.

Coffman TM, Crowley SD: Kidney in hypertension: Guyton redux, *Hypertension* 51:811, 2008.

Cowley AW Jr: Long-term control of arterial blood pressure, *Physiol Rev* 72:231, 1992.

Guyton AC: *Arterial pressure and hypertension*, Philadelphia, 1980, WB Saunders.

Guyton AC: Blood pressure control—special role of the kidneys and body fluids, *Science* 252:1813, 1991.

Hall JE: The kidney, hypertension, and obesity, *Hypertension* 41:625, 2003.

Hall JE, Brands MW, Henegar JR: Angiotensin II and long-term arterial pressure regulation: the overriding dominance of the kidney, *J Am Soc Nephrol* 10(Suppl 12):S258, 1999.

Hall JE, Granger JP, Hall ME, et al: Pathophysiology of hypertension. In Fuster V, O'Rourke RA, Walsh RA, et al, eds.: *Hurst's The Heart*, ed 12, New York, 2008, McGraw-Hill Medical, pp 1570.

Hall JE, da Silva AA, Brandon E, et al: Pathophysiology of obesity hypertension and target organ injury. In Lip GYP, Hall JE, eds.: *Comprehensive Hypertension*, New York, 2007, Elsevier, pp 447.

LaMarca BD, Gilbert J, Granger JP: Recent progress toward the understanding of the pathophysiology of hypertension during preeclampsia, *Hypertension* 51:982, 2008.

Lohmeier TE, Hildebrandt DA, Warren S, et al: Recent insights into the interactions between the baroreflex and the kidneys in hypertension, *Am J Physiol Regul Integr Comp Physiol* 288:R828, 2005.

Oparil S, Zaman MA, Calhoun DA: Pathogenesis of hypertension, *Ann Intern Med* 139:761, 2003.

Reckelhoff JF, Fortepiani LA: Novel mechanisms responsible for postmenopausal hypertension, *Hypertension* 43:918, 2004.

Rossier BC, Schild L: Epithelial sodium channel: mendelian versus essential hypertension, *Hypertension* 52:595, 2008.

Cardiac Output, Venous Return, and Their Regulation

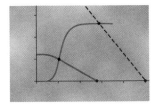

Cardiac output is the quantity of blood pumped into the aorta each minute by the heart. This is also the quantity of blood that flows through the circulation. Cardiac output is one of the most important factors that we have to consider in relation to the circulation because it is the sum of the blood flows to all of the tissues of the body.

Venous return is the quantity of blood flowing from the veins into the right atrium each minute. The venous return and the cardiac output must equal each other except for a few heartbeats at a time when blood is temporarily stored in or removed from the heart and lungs.

Normal Values for Cardiac Output at Rest and During Activity

Cardiac output varies widely with the level of activity of the body. The following factors, among others, directly affect cardiac output: (1) the basic level of body metabolism, (2) whether the person is exercising, (3) the person's age, and (4) size of the body.

For *young, healthy men,* resting cardiac output averages about 5.6 L/min. For *women,* this value is about 4.9 L/min. When one considers the factor of age as well—because with increasing age, body activity and mass of some tissues (e.g., skeletal muscle) diminish—the average cardiac output for the resting adult, in round numbers, is often stated to be about 5 L/min.

Cardiac Index

Experiments have shown that the cardiac output increases approximately in proportion to the surface area of the body. Therefore, cardiac output is frequently stated in terms of the *cardiac index,* which is the *cardiac output per square meter of body surface area.* The normal human being weighing 70 kilograms has a body surface area of about 1.7 square meters, which means that the normal average cardiac index for adults is about 3 L/min/m^2 of body surface area.

Effect of Age on Cardiac Output. Figure 20-1 shows the cardiac output, expressed as cardiac index, at different ages. Rising rapidly to a level greater than 4 L/min/m^2 at age 10 years, the cardiac index declines to about 2.4 L/min/m^2 at age 80 years. We explain later in the chapter that the cardiac output is regulated throughout life almost directly in proportion to the overall bodily metabolic activity. Therefore, the declining cardiac index is indicative of declining activity or declining muscle mass with age.

Control of Cardiac Output by Venous Return—Role of the Frank-Starling Mechanism of the Heart

When one states that cardiac output is controlled by venous return, this means that it is not the heart itself that is normally the primary controller of cardiac output. Instead, it is the various factors of the peripheral circulation that affect flow of blood into the heart from the veins, called *venous return,* that are the primary controllers.

The main reason peripheral factors are usually more important than the heart itself in controlling cardiac output is that the heart has a built-in mechanism that normally allows it to pump automatically whatever amount of blood that flows into the right atrium from the veins. This mechanism, called the *Frank-Starling law of the heart,* was discussed in Chapter 9. Basically, this law states that when increased quantities of blood flow into the heart, the increased blood stretches the walls of the heart chambers. As a result of the stretch, the cardiac muscle contracts with increased force, and this empties the extra blood that has entered from the systemic circulation. Therefore, the blood that flows into the heart is automatically pumped without delay into the aorta and flows again through the circulation.

Another important factor, discussed in Chapter 10, is that stretching the heart causes the heart to pump faster—at an increased heart rate. That is, stretch of the *sinus node* in the wall of the right atrium has a direct effect on the rhythmicity of the node itself to increase heart rate as much as 10 to 15 percent. In addition, the

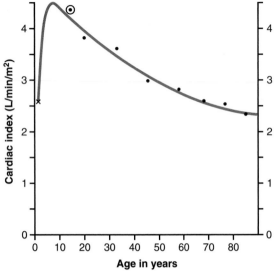

Figure 20-1 *Cardiac index* for the human being (cardiac output per square meter of surface area) at different ages. (Redrawn from Guyton AC, Jones CE, Coleman TB: Circulatory Physiology: Cardiac Output and Its Regulation, 2nd ed. Philadelphia: WB Saunders, 1973.)

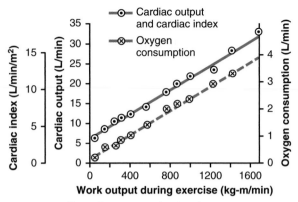

Figure 20-2 Effect of increasing levels of exercise to increase cardiac output (*red solid line*) and oxygen consumption (*blue dashed line*). (Redrawn from Guyton AC, Jones CE, Coleman TB: Circulatory Physiology: Cardiac Output and Its Regulation, 2nd ed. Philadelphia: WB Saunders, 1973.)

stretched right atrium initiates a nervous reflex called the *Bainbridge reflex,* passing first to the vasomotor center of the brain and then back to the heart by way of the sympathetic nerves and vagi, also to increase the heart rate.

Under most normal unstressful conditions, the cardiac output is controlled almost entirely by peripheral factors that determine venous return. However, we discuss later in the chapter that if the returning blood does become more than the heart can pump, then the heart becomes the limiting factor that determines cardiac output.

Cardiac Output Regulation Is the Sum of Blood Flow Regulation in All the Local Tissues of the Body—Tissue Metabolism Regulates Most Local Blood Flow

The venous return to the heart is the sum of all the local blood flows through all the individual tissue segments of the peripheral circulation. Therefore, it follows that cardiac output regulation is the sum of all the local blood flow regulations.

The mechanisms of local blood flow regulation were discussed in Chapter 17. In most tissues, blood flow increases mainly in proportion to each tissue's metabolism. For instance, local blood flow almost always increases when tissue oxygen consumption increases; this effect is demonstrated in Figure 20-2 for different levels of exercise. Note that at each increasing level of work output during exercise, the oxygen consumption and the cardiac output increase in parallel to each other.

To summarize, cardiac output is determined by the sum of all the various factors throughout the body that control local blood flow. All the local blood flows summate

to form the venous return, and the heart automatically pumps this returning blood back into the arteries to flow around the system again.

Effect of Total Peripheral Resistance on the Long-Term Cardiac Output Level. Figure 20-3 is the same as Figure 19-6. It is repeated here to illustrate an extremely important principle in cardiac output control: Under many conditions, the long-term cardiac output level varies reciprocally with changes in total peripheral resistance, as long as the arterial pressure is unchanged. Note in Figure 20-3 that when the total peripheral resistance is exactly normal (at the 100 percent mark in the figure), the cardiac output is also normal. Then, when

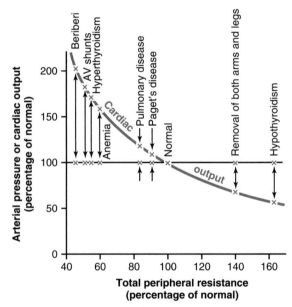

Figure 20-3 Chronic effect of different levels of total peripheral resistance on cardiac output, showing a reciprocal relationship between total peripheral resistance and cardiac output. (Redrawn from Guyton AC: Arterial Pressure and Hypertension. Philadelphia: WB Saunders, 1980.)

the total peripheral resistance increases above normal, the cardiac output falls; conversely, when the total peripheral resistance decreases, the cardiac output increases. One can easily understand this by reconsidering one of the forms of Ohm's law, as expressed in Chapter 14:

$$\text{Cardiac Output} = \frac{\text{Arterial Pressure}}{\text{Total Peripheral Resistance}}$$

The meaning of this formula, and of Figure 20-3, is simply the following: Any time the long-term level of total peripheral resistance changes (but no other functions of the circulation change), the cardiac output changes quantitatively in exactly the opposite direction.

The Heart Has Limits for the Cardiac Output That It Can Achieve

There are definite limits to the amount of blood that the heart can pump, which can be expressed quantitatively in the form of *cardiac output curves.*

Figure 20-4 demonstrates the *normal cardiac output curve,* showing the cardiac output per minute at each level of right atrial pressure. This is one type of *cardiac function curve,* which was discussed in Chapter 9. Note that the plateau level of this normal cardiac output curve is about 13 L/min, 2.5 times the normal cardiac output of about 5 L/min. This means that the normal human heart, functioning without any special stimulation, can pump an amount of venous return up to about 2.5 times the normal venous return before the heart becomes a limiting factor in the control of cardiac output.

Shown in Figure 20-4 are several other cardiac output curves for hearts that are not pumping normally. The uppermost curves are for *hypereffective hearts* that are pumping better than normal. The lowermost curves are for *hypoeffective hearts* that are pumping at levels below normal.

Factors That Cause a Hypereffective Heart

Two types of factors can make the heart a better pump than normal: (1) nervous stimulation and (2) hypertrophy of the heart muscle.

Effect of Nervous Excitation to Increase Heart Pumping. In Chapter 9, we saw that a combination of (1) sympathetic *stimulation* and (2) parasympathetic *inhibition* does two things to increase the pumping effectiveness of the heart: (1) It greatly increases the heart rate—sometimes, in young people, from the normal level of 72 beats/min up to 180 to 200 beats/min—and (2) it increases the strength of heart contraction (which is called increased "contractility") to twice its normal strength. Combining these two effects, maximal nervous excitation of the heart can raise the plateau level of the cardiac output curve to almost twice the plateau of the normal curve, as shown by the 25-L/min level of the uppermost curve in Figure 20-4.

Increased Pumping Effectiveness Caused by Heart Hypertrophy. A long-term increased workload, but not so much excess load that it damages the heart, causes the heart muscle to increase in mass and contractile strength in the same way that heavy exercise causes skeletal muscles to hypertrophy. For instance, it is common for the hearts of marathon runners to be increased in mass by 50 to 75 percent. This increases the plateau level of the cardiac output curve, sometimes 60 to 100 percent, and therefore allows the heart to pump much greater than usual amounts of cardiac output.

When one combines nervous excitation of the heart and hypertrophy, as occurs in marathon runners, the total effect can allow the heart to pump as much 30 to 40 L/min, about 2½ times the level that can be achieved in the average person; this increased level of pumping is one of the most important factors in determining the runner's running time.

Factors That Cause a Hypoeffective Heart

Any factor that decreases the heart's ability to pump blood causes hypoeffectivity. Some of the factors that can do this are the following:

- Increased arterial pressure against which the heart must pump, such as in hypertension
- Inhibition of nervous excitation of the heart
- Pathological factors that cause abnormal heart rhythm or rate of heartbeat
- Coronary artery blockage, causing a "heart attack"
- Valvular heart disease
- Congenital heart disease
- Myocarditis, an inflammation of the heart muscle
- Cardiac hypoxia

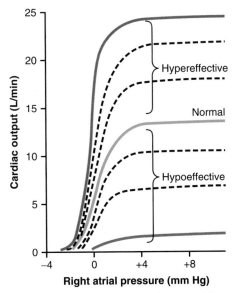

Figure 20-4 Cardiac output curves for the normal heart and for hypoeffective and hypereffective hearts. (Redrawn from Guyton AC, Jones CE, Coleman TB: Circulatory Physiology: Cardiac Output and Its Regulation, 2nd ed. Philadelphia: WB Saunders, 1973.)

Role of the Nervous System in Controlling Cardiac Output

Importance of the Nervous System in Maintaining Arterial Pressure When Peripheral Blood Vessels Are Dilated and Venous Return and Cardiac Output Increase

Figure 20-5 shows an important difference in cardiac output control with and without a functioning autonomic nervous system. The solid curves demonstrate the effect in the normal dog of intense dilation of the peripheral blood vessels caused by administering the drug dinitrophenol, which increased the metabolism of virtually all tissues of the body about fourfold. Note that with nervous control to keep the arterial pressure from falling, dilating all the peripheral blood vessels caused almost no change in arterial pressure but increased the cardiac output almost fourfold. However, after autonomic control of the nervous system had been blocked, none of the normal circulatory reflexes for maintaining the arterial pressure could function. Vasodilation of the vessels with dinitrophenol (dashed curves) then caused a profound fall in arterial pressure to about one-half normal, and the cardiac output rose only 1.6-fold instead of 4-fold.

Thus, maintenance of a normal arterial pressure by the nervous reflexes, by mechanisms explained in Chapter 18, is essential to achieve high cardiac outputs when the peripheral tissues dilate their vessels to increase the venous return.

Effect of the Nervous System to *Increase* the Arterial Pressure During Exercise. During exercise, intense increase in metabolism in active skeletal muscles acts directly on the muscle arterioles to relax them and to allow adequate oxygen and other nutrients needed to sustain muscle contraction. Obviously, this greatly decreases the total peripheral resistance, which normally would decrease the arterial pressure as well. However, the nervous system immediately compensates. The same brain activity that sends motor signals to the muscles sends simultaneous signals into the autonomic nervous centers of the brain to excite circulatory activity, causing large vein constriction, increased heart rate, and increased contractility of the heart. All these changes acting together increase the arterial pressure above normal, which in turn forces still more blood flow through the active muscles.

In summary, when local tissue blood vessels dilate and thereby increase venous return and cardiac output above normal, the nervous system plays an exceedingly important role in preventing the arterial pressure from falling to disastrously low levels. In fact, during exercise, the nervous system goes even further, providing additional signals to raise the arterial pressure even above normal, which serves to increase the cardiac output an extra 30 to 100 percent.

Pathologically High or Low Cardiac Outputs

In healthy humans, the average cardiac outputs are surprisingly constant from one person to another. However, multiple clinical abnormalities can cause either high or low cardiac outputs. Some of the more important of these are shown in Figure 20-6.

High Cardiac Output Caused by Reduced Total Peripheral Resistance

The left side of Figure 20-6 identifies conditions that commonly cause cardiac outputs higher than normal. One of the distinguishing features of these conditions is that *they all result from chronically reduced total peripheral resistance*. None of them result from excessive excitation of the heart itself, which we will explain subsequently. For the present, let us look at some of the conditions that can decrease the peripheral resistance and at the same time increase the cardiac output to above normal.

1. *Beriberi.* This disease is caused by insufficient quantity of the vitamin *thiamine (vitamin B₁)* in the diet. Lack of this vitamin causes diminished ability of the tissues to use some cellular nutrients, and the local tissue blood flow mechanisms in turn cause marked compensatory peripheral vasodilation. Sometimes the total peripheral resistance decreases to as little as one-half normal. Consequently, the long-term levels of venous return and cardiac output also often increase to twice normal.

2. *Arteriovenous fistula (shunt).* Earlier, we pointed out that whenever a fistula (also called an *AV shunt*) occurs between a major artery and a major vein, tremendous amounts of blood flow directly from the artery into the vein. This, too, greatly decreases the total peripheral resistance and, likewise, increases the venous return and cardiac output.

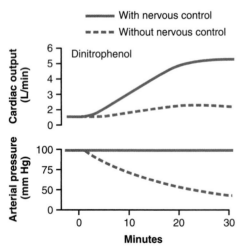

Figure 20-5 Experiment in a dog to demonstrate the importance of nervous maintenance of the arterial pressure as a prerequisite for cardiac output control. Note that with pressure control, the metabolic stimulant *dinitrophenol* increases cardiac output greatly; without pressure control, the arterial pressure falls and the cardiac output rises very little. (Drawn from experiments by Dr. M. Banet.)

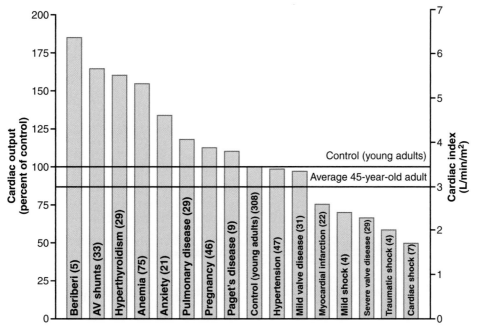

Figure 20-6 Cardiac output in different pathological conditions. The numbers in parentheses indicate number of patients studied in each condition. (Redrawn from Guyton AC, Jones CE, Coleman TB: Circulatory Physiology: Cardiac Output and Its Regulation, 2nd ed. Philadelphia: WB Saunders, 1973.)

3. *Hyperthyroidism.* In hyperthyroidism, the metabolism of most tissues of the body becomes greatly increased. Oxygen usage increases, and vasodilator products are released from the tissues. Therefore, the total peripheral resistance decreases markedly because of the local tissue blood flow control reactions throughout the body; consequently, the venous return and cardiac output often increase to 40 to 80 percent above normal.

4. *Anemia.* In anemia, two peripheral effects greatly decrease the total peripheral resistance. One of these is reduced viscosity of the blood, resulting from the decreased concentration of red blood cells. The other is diminished delivery of oxygen to the tissues, which causes local vasodilation. As a consequence, the cardiac output increases greatly.

Any other factor that decreases the total peripheral resistance chronically also increases the cardiac output if arterial pressure does not decrease too much.

Low Cardiac Output

Figure 20-6 shows at the far right several conditions that cause abnormally low cardiac output. These conditions fall into two categories: (1) those abnormalities that cause the pumping effectiveness of the heart to fall too low and (2) those that cause venous return to fall too low.

Decreased Cardiac Output Caused by Cardiac Factors. Whenever the heart becomes severely damaged, regardless of the cause, its limited level of pumping may fall below that needed for adequate blood flow to the tissues. Some examples of this include (1) *severe coronary blood vessel blockage and consequent myocardial infarction,* (2) *severe valvular heart disease,* (3) *myocarditis,* (4) *cardiac tamponade,* and (5) *cardiac metabolic*

derangements. The effects of several of these are shown on the right in Figure 20-6, demonstrating the low cardiac outputs that result.

When the cardiac output falls so low that the tissues throughout the body begin to suffer nutritional deficiency, the condition is called *cardiac shock.* This is discussed fully in Chapter 22 in relation to cardiac failure.

Decrease in Cardiac Output Caused by Noncardiac Peripheral Factors—Decreased Venous Return. Anything that interferes with venous return also can lead to decreased cardiac output. Some of these factors are the following:

1. *Decreased blood volume.* By far, the most common noncardiac peripheral factor that leads to decreased cardiac output is decreased blood volume, resulting most often from hemorrhage. It is clear why this condition decreases the cardiac output: Loss of blood decreases the filling of the vascular system to such a low level that there is not enough blood in the peripheral vessels to create peripheral vascular pressures high enough to push the blood back to the heart.

2. *Acute venous dilation.* On some occasions, the peripheral veins become acutely vasodilated. This results most often when the sympathetic nervous system suddenly becomes inactive. For instance, fainting often results from sudden loss of sympathetic nervous system activity, which causes the peripheral capacitative vessels, especially the veins, to dilate markedly. This decreases the filling pressure of the vascular system because the blood volume can no longer create adequate pressure in the now flaccid peripheral blood vessels. As a result, the blood "pools" in the vessels and does not return to the heart.

233

3. *Obstruction of the large veins.* On rare occasions, the large veins leading into the heart become obstructed, so the blood in the peripheral vessels cannot flow back into the heart. Consequently, the cardiac output falls markedly.

4. *Decreased tissue mass, especially decreased skeletal muscle mass.* With normal aging or with prolonged periods of physical inactivity, there is usually a reduction in the size of the skeletal muscles. This, in turn, decreases the total oxygen consumption and blood flow needs of the muscles, resulting in decreases in skeletal muscle blood flow and cardiac output.

5. *Decreased metabolic rate of the tissues.* If tissue metabolic rate is reduced, such as occurs in skeletal muscle during prolonged bed rest, the oxygen consumption and nutrition needs of the tissues will also be lower. This decreases blood flow to the tissues, resulting in reduced cardiac output. Other conditions, such as *hypothyroidism,* may also reduce metabolic rate and therefore tissue blood flow and cardiac output.

Regardless of the cause of low cardiac output, whether it be a peripheral factor or a cardiac factor, if ever the cardiac output falls below that level required for adequate nutrition of the tissues, the person is said to suffer *circulatory shock.* This condition can be lethal within a few minutes to a few hours. Circulatory shock is such an important clinical problem that it is discussed in detail in Chapter 24.

A More Quantitative Analysis of Cardiac Output Regulation

Our discussion of cardiac output regulation thus far is adequate for understanding the factors that control cardiac output in most simple conditions. However, to understand cardiac output regulation in especially stressful situations, such as the extremes of exercise, cardiac failure, and circulatory shock, a more complex quantitative analysis is presented in the following sections.

To perform the more quantitative analysis, it is necessary to distinguish separately the two primary factors concerned with cardiac output regulation: (1) the pumping ability of the heart, as represented by *cardiac output curves,* and (2) the peripheral factors that affect flow of blood from the veins into the heart, as represented by *venous return curves.* Then one can put these curves together in a quantitative way to show how they interact with each other to determine cardiac output, venous return, and right atrial pressure at the same time.

Cardiac Output Curves Used in the Quantitative Analysis

Some of the cardiac output curves used to depict quantitative heart pumping effectiveness have already been shown in Figure 20-4. However, an additional set of curves is required to show the effect on cardiac output caused by changing external pressures on the outside of the heart, as explained in the next section.

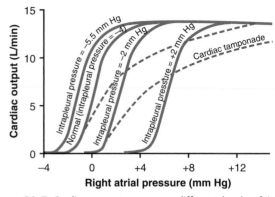

Figure 20-7 Cardiac output curves at different levels of intrapleural pressure and at different degrees of cardiac tamponade. (Redrawn from Guyton AC, Jones CE, Coleman TB: Circulatory Physiology: Cardiac Output and Its Regulation, 2nd ed. Philadelphia: WB Saunders, 1973.)

Effect of External Pressure Outside the Heart on Cardiac Output Curves. Figure 20-7 shows the effect of changes in external cardiac pressure on the cardiac output curve. The normal external pressure is equal to the normal intrapleural pressure (the pressure in the chest cavity), which is −4 mm Hg. Note in the figure that a rise in intrapleural pressure, to −2 mm Hg, shifts the entire cardiac output curve to the right by the same amount. This shift occurs because to fill the cardiac chambers with blood requires an extra 2 mm Hg right atrial pressure to overcome the increased pressure on the outside of the heart. Likewise, an increase in intrapleural pressure to +2 mm Hg requires a 6 mm Hg increase in right atrial pressure from the normal −4 mm Hg, which shifts the entire cardiac output curve 6 mm Hg to the right.

Some of the factors that can alter the external pressure on the heart and thereby shift the cardiac output curve are the following:

1. *Cyclical changes of intrapleural pressure during respiration,* which are about ±2 mm Hg during normal breathing but can be as much as ±50 mm Hg during strenuous breathing.

2. *Breathing against a negative pressure,* which shifts the curve to a more negative right atrial pressure (to the left).

3. *Positive pressure breathing,* which shifts the curve to the right.

4. *Opening the thoracic cage,* which increases the intrapleural pressure to 0 mm Hg and shifts the cardiac output curve to the right 4 mm Hg.

5. *Cardiac tamponade,* which means accumulation of a large quantity of fluid in the pericardial cavity around the heart with resultant increase in external cardiac pressure and shifting of the curve to the right. Note in Figure 20-7 that cardiac tamponade shifts the upper parts of the curves farther to the right than the lower parts because the external "tamponade" pressure rises to higher values as the chambers of the heart fill to increased volumes during high cardiac output.

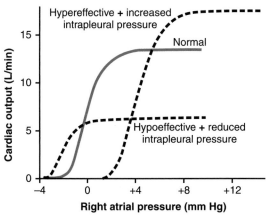

Figure 20-8 Combinations of two major patterns of cardiac output curves showing the effect of alterations in both extracardiac pressure and effectiveness of the heart as a pump. (Redrawn from Guyton AC, Jones CE, Coleman TB: Circulatory Physiology: Cardiac Output and Its Regulation, 2nd ed. Philadelphia: WB Saunders, 1973.)

Combinations of Different Patterns of Cardiac Output Curves. Figure 20-8 shows that the final cardiac output curve can change as a result of simultaneous changes in (a) external cardiac pressure and (b) effectiveness of the heart as a pump. For example, the combination of a hypereffective heart and increased intrapleural pressure would lead to increased maximum level of cardiac output due to the increased pumping capability of the heart but the cardiac output curve would be shifted to the right (to higher atrial pressures) due to the increased intrapleural pressure. Thus, by knowing what is happening to the external pressure, as well as to the capability of the heart as a pump, one can express the momentary ability of the heart to pump blood by a single cardiac output curve.

Venous Return Curves

There remains the entire systemic circulation that must be considered before total analysis of cardiac regulation can be achieved. To analyze the function of the systemic circulation, we first remove the heart and lungs from the circulation of an animal and replace them with a pump and artificial oxygenator system. Then, different factors, such as blood volume, vascular resistances, and central venous pressure in the right atrium, are altered to determine how the systemic circulation operates in different circulatory states. In these studies, one finds three principal factors that affect venous return to the heart from the systemic circulation. They are as follows:

1. *Right atrial pressure,* which exerts a backward force on the veins to impede flow of blood from the veins into the right atrium.

2. Degree of filling of the systemic circulation (measured by the *mean systemic filling pressure*), which forces the systemic blood toward the heart (this is the pressure measured everywhere in the systemic circulation when all flow of blood is stopped and is discussed in detail later).

3. *Resistance to blood flow* between the peripheral vessels and the right atrium.

These factors can all be expressed quantitatively by the *venous return curve,* as we explain in the next sections.

Normal Venous Return Curve

In the same way that the cardiac output curve relates pumping of blood by the heart to right atrial pressure, the *venous return curve relates venous return also to right atrial pressure*—that is, the venous flow of blood into the heart from the systemic circulation at different levels of right atrial pressure.

The curve in Figure 20-9 is the *normal* venous return curve. This curve shows that when heart pumping capability becomes diminished and causes the right atrial pressure to rise, the backward force of the rising atrial pressure on the veins of the systemic circulation decreases venous return of blood to the heart. *If all nervous circulatory reflexes are prevented from acting,* venous return decreases to zero when the right atrial pressure rises to about +7 mm Hg. Such a slight rise in right atrial pressure causes a drastic decrease in venous return because the systemic circulation is a distensible bag, so any increase in back pressure causes blood to dam up in this bag instead of returning to the heart.

At the same time that the right atrial pressure is rising and causing venous stasis, pumping by the heart also approaches zero because of decreasing venous return. Both the arterial and the venous pressures come to equilibrium when all flow in the systemic circulation ceases at a pressure of 7 mm Hg, which, by definition, is the *mean systemic filling pressure (Psf).*

Plateau in the Venous Return Curve at Negative Atrial Pressures Caused by Collapse of the Large Veins. When the right atrial pressure falls *below* zero—that is, below atmospheric pressure—further increase in venous return almost ceases. And by the time the right atrial pressure has fallen to about –2 mm Hg, the venous return will have reached a plateau. It remains at this plateau level even though the right atrial pressure falls to –20 mm Hg, –50 mm Hg, or even further. This plateau is caused by *collapse of the veins* entering the chest. Negative pressure

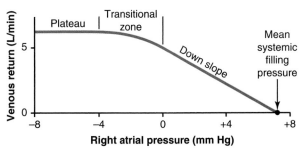

Figure 20-9 Normal *venous return curve.* The plateau is caused by *collapse* of the large veins entering the chest when the right atrial pressure falls below atmospheric pressure. Note also that venous return becomes zero when the right atrial pressure rises to equal the mean systemic filling pressure.

in the right atrium sucks the walls of the veins together where they enter the chest, which prevents any additional flow of blood from the peripheral veins. Consequently, even very negative pressures in the right atrium cannot increase venous return significantly above that which exists at a normal atrial pressure of 0 mm Hg.

Mean Circulatory Filling Pressure and Mean Systemic Filling Pressure, and Their Effect on Venous Return

When heart pumping is stopped by shocking the heart with electricity to cause ventricular fibrillation or is stopped in any other way, flow of blood everywhere in the circulation ceases a few seconds later. Without blood flow, the pressures everywhere in the circulation become equal. This equilibrated pressure level is called the *mean circulatory filling pressure.*

Effect of Blood Volume on Mean Circulatory Filling Pressure. The greater the volume of blood in the circulation, the greater is the mean circulatory filling pressure because extra blood volume stretches the walls of the vasculature. The *red curve* in Figure 20-10 shows the approximate normal effect of different levels of blood volume on the mean circulatory filling pressure. Note that at a blood volume of about 4000 milliliters, the mean circulatory filling pressure is close to zero because this is the "unstressed volume" of the circulation, but at a volume of 5000 milliliters, the filling pressure is the normal value of 7 mm Hg. Similarly, at still higher volumes, the mean circulatory filling pressure increases almost linearly.

Effect of Sympathetic Nervous Stimulation of the Circulation on Mean Circulatory Filling Pressure. The *green curve* and *blue curve* in Figure 20-10 show the effects, respectively, of high and low levels of sympathetic nervous activity on the mean circulatory filling pressure.

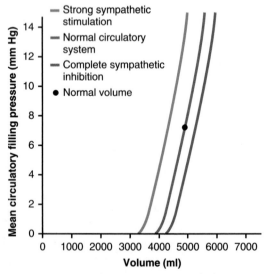

Figure 20-10 Effect of changes in total blood volume on the *mean circulatory filling pressure* (i.e., "volume-pressure curves" for the entire circulatory system). These curves also show the effects of strong sympathetic stimulation and complete sympathetic inhibition.

Strong sympathetic stimulation constricts all the systemic blood vessels, as well as the larger pulmonary blood vessels and even the chambers of the heart. Therefore, the capacity of the system decreases so that at each level of blood volume, the mean circulatory filling pressure is increased. At normal blood volume, maximal sympathetic stimulation increases the mean circulatory filling pressure from 7 mm Hg to about 2.5 times that value, or about 17 mm Hg.

Conversely, complete inhibition of the sympathetic nervous system relaxes both the blood vessels and the heart, decreasing the mean circulatory filling pressure from the normal value of 7 mm Hg down to about 4 mm Hg. Before leaving Figure 20-10, note specifically how steep the curves are. This means that even slight changes in blood volume or slight changes in the capacity of the system caused by various levels of sympathetic activity can have large effects on the mean circulatory filling pressure.

Mean Systemic Filling Pressure and Its Relation to Mean Circulatory Filling Pressure. The *mean systemic filling pressure,* Psf, is slightly different from the mean circulatory filling pressure. It is the pressure measured everywhere *in the systemic circulation* after blood flow has been stopped by clamping the large blood vessels at the heart, so the pressures in the systemic circulation can be measured independently from those in the pulmonary circulation. The mean systemic pressure, although almost impossible to measure in the living animal, is the important pressure for determining venous return. *The mean systemic filling pressure, however, is almost always nearly equal to the mean circulatory filling pressure* because the pulmonary circulation has less than one eighth as much capacitance as the systemic circulation and only about one tenth as much blood volume.

Effect on the Venous Return Curve of Changes in Mean Systemic Filling Pressure. Figure 20-11 shows the effects on the venous return curve caused by increasing or decreasing the mean systemic filling pressure (Psf). Note in Figure 20-11 that the normal mean systemic filling pressure is 7 mm Hg. Then, for the uppermost curve

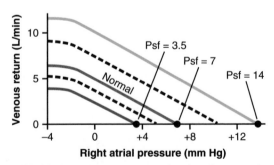

Figure 20-11 Venous return curves showing the normal curve when the mean systemic filling pressure (Psf) is 7 mm Hg and the effect of altering the Psf to either 3.5 or 14 mm Hg. (Redrawn from Guyton AC, Jones CE, Coleman TB: Circulatory Physiology: Cardiac Output and Its Regulation, 2nd ed. Philadelphia: WB Saunders, 1973.)

in the figure, the mean systemic filling pressure has been increased to 14 mm Hg, and for the lowermost curve, has been decreased to 3.5 mm Hg. These curves demonstrate that the greater the mean systemic filling pressure (which also means the greater the "tightness" with which the circulatory system is filled with blood), the more the venous return curve shifts *upward* and *to the right*. Conversely, the lower the mean systemic filling pressure, the more the curve shifts *downward* and *to the left*.

To express this another way, the greater the system is filled, the easier it is for blood to flow into the heart. The less the filling, the more difficult it is for blood to flow into the heart.

"Pressure Gradient for Venous Return"—When This Is Zero, There Is No Venous Return. When the right atrial pressure rises to equal the mean systemic filling pressure, there is no longer any pressure difference between the peripheral vessels and the right atrium. Consequently, there can no longer be any blood flow from any peripheral vessels back to the right atrium. However, when the right atrial pressure falls progressively lower than the mean systemic filling pressure, the flow to the heart increases proportionately, as one can see by studying any of the venous return curves in Figure 20-11. That is, *the greater the difference between the mean systemic filling pressure and the right atrial pressure, the greater becomes the venous return*. Therefore, the difference between these two pressures is called the *pressure gradient for venous return*.

Resistance to Venous Return

In the same way that mean systemic filling pressure represents a pressure pushing venous blood from the periphery toward the heart, there is also resistance to this venous flow of blood. It is called the *resistance to venous return*. Most of the resistance to venous return occurs in the veins, although some occurs in the arterioles and small arteries as well.

Why is venous resistance so important in determining the resistance to venous return? The answer is that when the resistance in the veins increases, blood begins to be dammed up, mainly in the veins themselves. But the venous pressure rises very little because the veins are highly distensible. Therefore, this rise in venous pressure is not very effective in overcoming the resistance, and blood flow into the right atrium decreases drastically. Conversely, when arteriolar and small artery resistances increase, blood accumulates in the arteries, which have a capacitance only one thirtieth as great as that of the veins. Therefore, even slight accumulation of blood in the arteries raises the pressure greatly—30 times as much as in the veins—and this high pressure does overcome much of the increased resistance. Mathematically, it turns out that about two thirds of the so-called "resistance to venous return" is determined by venous resistance, and about one third by the arteriolar and small artery resistance.

Venous return can be calculated by the following formula:

$$VR = \frac{Psf - PRA}{RVR}$$

in which *VR* is venous return, *Psf* is mean systemic filling pressure, *PRA* is right atrial pressure, and *RVR* is resistance to venous return. In the healthy human adult, the values for these are as follows: venous return equals 5 L/min, mean systemic filling pressure equals 7 mm Hg, right atrial pressure equals 0 mm Hg, and resistance to venous return equals 1.4 mm Hg per L/min of blood flow.

Effect of Resistance to Venous Return on the Venous Return Curve. Figure 20-12 demonstrates the effect of different levels of resistance to venous return on the venous return curve, showing that a *decrease* in this resistance to one-half normal allows twice as much flow of blood and, therefore, *rotates the curve upward* to twice as great a slope. Conversely, an *increase* in resistance to twice normal *rotates the curve downward* to one half as great a slope.

Note also that when the right atrial pressure rises to equal the mean systemic filling pressure, venous return becomes zero at all levels of resistance to venous return because when there is no pressure gradient to cause flow of blood, it makes no difference what the resistance is in the circulation; the flow is still zero. Therefore, *the highest level to which the right atrial pressure can rise*, regardless of how much the heart might fail, is equal to the mean systemic filling pressure.

Combinations of Venous Return Curve Patterns. Figure 20-13 shows effects on the venous return curve caused by simultaneous changes in mean systemic pressure (Psf) and resistance to venous return, demonstrating that both these factors can operate simultaneously.

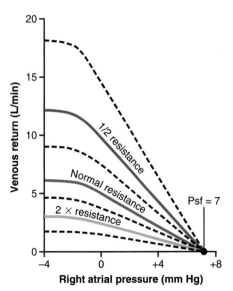

Figure 20-12 Venous return curves depicting the effect of altering the "resistance to venous return." Psf, mean systemic filling pressure. (Redrawn from Guyton AC, Jones CE, Coleman TB: Circulatory Physiology: Cardiac Output and Its Regulation, 2nd ed. Philadelphia: WB Saunders, 1973.)

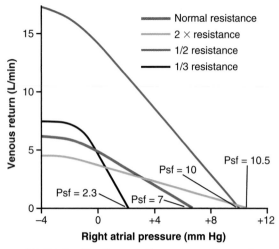

Figure 20-13 Combinations of the major patterns of venous return curves, showing the effects of simultaneous changes in mean systemic filling pressure (Psf) and in "resistance to venous return." (Redrawn from Guyton AC, Jones CE, Coleman TB: Circulatory Physiology: Cardiac Output and Its Regulation, 2nd ed. Philadelphia: WB Saunders, 1973.)

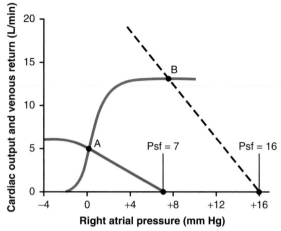

Figure 20-14 The two *solid curves* demonstrate an analysis of cardiac output and right atrial pressure when the cardiac output (*red line*) and venous return (*blue line*) curves are normal. Transfusion of blood equal to 20 percent of the blood volume causes the venous return curve to become the *dashed curve;* as a result, the cardiac output and right atrial pressure shift from point *A* to point *B*. Psf, mean systemic filling pressure.

Analysis of Cardiac Output and Right Atrial Pressure Using Simultaneous Cardiac Output and Venous Return Curves

In the complete circulation, the heart and the systemic circulation must operate together. This means that (1) the venous return from the systemic circulation must equal the cardiac output from the heart and (2) the right atrial pressure is the same for both the heart and the systemic circulation.

Therefore, one can predict the cardiac output and right atrial pressure in the following way: (1) Determine the momentary pumping ability of the heart and depict this in the form of a cardiac output curve; (2) determine the momentary state of flow from the systemic circulation into the heart and depict this in the form of a venous return curve; and (3) "equate" these curves against each other, as shown in Figure 20-14.

Two curves in the figure depict the *normal cardiac output curve* (red line) and the *normal venous return curve* (blue line). There is only one point on the graph, point A, at which the venous return equals the cardiac output and at which the right atrial pressure is the same for both the heart and the systemic circulation. Therefore, in the normal circulation, the right atrial pressure, cardiac output, and venous return are all depicted by point A, called the *equilibrium point,* giving a normal value for cardiac output of 5 L/min and a right atrial pressure of 0 mm Hg.

Effect of Increased Blood Volume on Cardiac Output. A sudden increase in blood volume of about 20 percent increases the cardiac output to about 2.5 to 3 times normal. An analysis of this effect is shown in Figure 20-14. Immediately on infusing the large quantity of extra blood, the increased filling of the system causes the mean systemic filling pressure (Psf) to increase to 16 mm Hg, which shifts the venous return curve to the right. At the same time, the increased blood volume distends the blood vessels, thus reducing their resistance and thereby reducing the resistance to venous return, which rotates the curve upward. As a result of these two effects, the venous return curve of Figure 20-14 is shifted to the right. This new curve equates with the cardiac output curve at point B, showing that the cardiac output and venous return increase 2.5 to 3 times, and that the right atrial pressure rises to about +8 mm Hg.

Further Compensatory Effects Initiated in Response to Increased Blood Volume. The greatly increased cardiac output caused by increased blood volume lasts for only a few minutes because several compensatory effects immediately begin to occur: (1) The increased cardiac output *increases the capillary pressure* so that fluid begins to transude out of the capillaries into the tissues, thereby returning the blood volume toward normal. (2) The increased pressure in the veins causes the veins to continue distending gradually by the mechanism called *stress-relaxation,* especially causing the venous blood reservoirs, such as the liver and spleen, to distend, thus *reducing the mean systemic pressure.* (3) The excess blood flow through the peripheral tissues causes autoregulatory increase in the peripheral vascular resistance, thus increasing the *resistance to venous return.* These factors cause the mean systemic filling pressure to return back toward normal and the resistance vessels of the systemic circulation to constrict. Therefore, gradually, over a period of 10 to 40 minutes, the cardiac output returns almost to normal.

Effect of Sympathetic Stimulation on Cardiac Output. Sympathetic stimulation affects both the heart and the systemic circulation: (1) It *makes the heart a stronger pump.* (2) In the systemic circulation, it *increases*

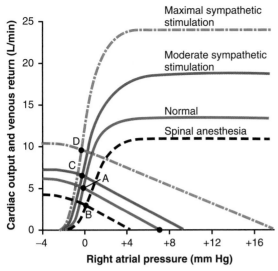

Figure 20-15 Analysis of the effect on cardiac output of (1) moderate sympathetic stimulation (from point *A* to point *C*), (2) maximal sympathetic stimulation (point *D*), and (3) sympathetic inhibition caused by total spinal anesthesia (point *B*). (Redrawn from Guyton AC, Jones CE, Coleman TB: Circulatory Physiology: Cardiac Output and Its Regulation, 2nd ed. Philadelphia: WB Saunders, 1973.)

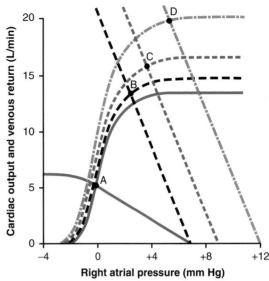

Figure 20-16 Analysis of successive changes in cardiac output and right atrial pressure in a human being after a large arteriovenous (AV) fistula is suddenly opened. The stages of the analysis, as shown by the equilibrium points, are *A*, normal conditions; *B*, immediately after opening the AV fistula; *C*, 1 minute or so after the sympathetic reflexes have become active; and *D*, several weeks after the blood volume has increased and the heart has begun to hypertrophy. (Redrawn from Guyton AC, Jones CE, Coleman TB: Circulatory Physiology: Cardiac Output and Its Regulation, 2nd ed. Philadelphia: WB Saunders, 1973.)

the mean systemic filling pressure because of contraction of the peripheral vessels, especially the veins, and it *increases the resistance to venous return.*

In Figure 20-15, the *normal* cardiac output and venous return curves are depicted; these equate with each other at point A, which represents a normal venous return and cardiac output of 5 L/min and a right atrial pressure of 0 mm Hg. Note in the figure that maximal sympathetic stimulation (green curves) increases the mean systemic filling pressure to 17 mm Hg (depicted by the point at which the venous return curve reaches the zero venous return level). And the sympathetic stimulation also increases pumping effectiveness of the heart by nearly 100 percent. As a result, the cardiac output rises from the normal value at equilibrium point A to about double normal at equilibrium point D—and yet *the right atrial pressure hardly changes.* Thus, different degrees of sympathetic stimulation can increase the cardiac output progressively to about twice normal *for short periods of time*, until other compensatory effects occur within seconds or minutes.

Effect of Sympathetic Inhibition on Cardiac Output.
The sympathetic nervous system can be blocked by inducing *total spinal anesthesia* or by using some drug, such as *hexamethonium*, that blocks transmission of nerve signals through the autonomic ganglia. The lowermost curves in Figure 20-15 show the effect of sympathetic inhibition caused by total spinal anesthesia, demonstrating that (1) the *mean systemic filling pressure falls to about 4 mm Hg* and (2) the *effectiveness of the heart as a pump decreases to about 80 percent of normal.* The cardiac output falls from point A to point B, which is a decrease to about 60 percent of normal.

Effect of Opening a Large Arteriovenous Fistula.
Figure 20-16 shows various stages of circulatory changes that occur after opening a large arteriovenous fistula, that is, after making an opening directly between a large artery and a large vein.

1. The two red curves crossing at point A show the normal condition.

2. The curves crossing at point B show the circulatory condition *immediately after opening the large fistula.* The principal effects are (1) a sudden and precipitous rotation of the venous return curve upward caused by the *large decrease in resistance to venous return* when blood is allowed to flow with almost no impediment directly from the large arteries into the venous system, bypassing most of the resistance elements of the peripheral circulation, and (2) a *slight increase in the level of the cardiac output curve* because opening the fistula decreases the peripheral resistance and allows an acute fall in arterial pressure against which the heart can pump more easily. The net result, depicted by point B, is an *increase in cardiac output from 5 L/min up to 13 L/min and an increase in right atrial pressure to about +3 mm Hg.*

3. Point C represents the effects about 1 minute later, after the sympathetic nerve reflexes have restored the arterial pressure almost to normal and caused two other effects: (1) an increase in the mean systemic filling pressure (because of constriction of all veins and arteries) from 7 to 9 mm Hg, thus shifting the venous return

curve 2 mm Hg to the right, and (2) further elevation of the cardiac output curve because of sympathetic nervous excitation of the heart. The cardiac output now rises to almost 16 L/min, and the right atrial pressure to about 4 mm Hg.

4. Point D shows the effect after several more weeks. By this time, the blood volume has increased because the slight reduction in arterial pressure and the sympathetic stimulation have both reduced kidney output of urine. The mean systemic filling pressure has now risen to +12 mm Hg, shifting the venous return curve another 3 mm Hg to the right. Also, the prolonged increased workload on the heart has caused the heart muscle to hypertrophy slightly, raising the level of the cardiac output curve still further. Therefore, point D shows a cardiac output now of almost 20 L/min and a right atrial pressure of about 6 mm Hg.

Other Analyses of Cardiac Output Regulation. In Chapter 21, analysis of cardiac output regulation during exercise is presented, and in Chapter 22, analyses of cardiac output regulation at various stages of congestive heart failure are shown.

Methods for Measuring Cardiac Output

In animal experiments, one can cannulate the aorta, pulmonary artery, or great veins entering the heart and measure the cardiac output using any type of flowmeter. An electromagnetic or ultrasonic flowmeter can also be placed on the aorta or pulmonary artery to measure cardiac output.

In the human, except in rare instances, cardiac output is measured by indirect methods that do not require surgery. Two of the methods that have been used for experimental studies are the *oxygen Fick method* and the *indicator dilution method.*

Cardiac output can also be estimated by *echocardiography,* a method that uses ultrasound waves from a transducer placed on the chest wall or passed into the patient's esophagus to measure the size of the heart's chambers, as well as the velocity of blood flowing from the left ventricle into the aorta. Stroke volume is calculated from the velocity of blood flowing into the aorta and the aorta cross-sectional area determined from the aorta diameter that is measured by ultrasound imaging. Cardiac output is then calculated from the product of the stroke volume and the heart rate.

Pulsatile Output of the Heart as Measured by an Electromagnetic or Ultrasonic Flowmeter

Figure 20-17 shows a recording in a dog of blood flow in the root of the aorta made using an electromagnetic flowmeter. It demonstrates that the blood flow rises rapidly to a peak during systole, and then at the end of systole reverses for a fraction of a second. This reverse flow causes the aortic valve to close and the flow to return to zero.

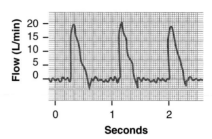

Figure 20-17 Pulsatile blood flow in the root of the aorta recorded using an electromagnetic flowmeter.

Measurement of Cardiac Output Using the Oxygen Fick Principle

The Fick principle is explained by Figure 20-18. This figure shows that 200 milliliters of oxygen are being absorbed from the lungs into the pulmonary blood each minute. It also shows that the blood entering the right heart has an oxygen concentration of 160 milliliters per liter of blood, whereas that leaving the left heart has an oxygen concentration of 200 milliliters per liter of blood. From these data, one can calculate that each liter of blood passing through the lungs absorbs 40 milliliters of oxygen.

Because the total quantity of oxygen absorbed into the blood from the lungs each minute is 200 milliliters, dividing 200 by 40 calculates a total of five 1-liter portions of blood that must pass through the pulmonary circulation each minute to absorb this amount of oxygen. Therefore, the quantity of blood flowing through the lungs each minute is 5 liters, which is also a measure of the cardiac output. Thus, the cardiac output can be calculated by the following formula:

Cardiac output (L/min)

$$= \frac{\textbf{O}_2 \textbf{ absorbed per minute by the lungs (ml/min)}}{\textbf{Arteriovenous O}_2 \textbf{ difference (ml/L of blood)}}$$

In applying this Fick procedure for measuring cardiac output in the human being, *mixed venous blood* is usually obtained through a catheter inserted up the brachial vein of the forearm, through the subclavian vein, down to the right atrium, and, finally, into the right ventricle or

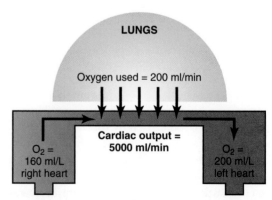

Figure 20-18 Fick principle for determining cardiac output.

pulmonary artery. And *systemic arterial blood* can then be obtained from any systemic artery in the body. The *rate of oxygen absorption* by the lungs is measured by the rate of disappearance of oxygen from the respired air, using any type of oxygen meter.

Indicator Dilution Method for Measuring Cardiac Output

To measure cardiac output by the so-called "indicator dilution method," a small amount of *indicator,* such as a dye, is injected into a large systemic vein or, preferably, into the right atrium. This passes rapidly through the right side of the heart, then through the blood vessels of the lungs, through the left side of the heart, and, finally, into the systemic arterial system. The concentration of the dye is recorded as the dye passes through one of the peripheral arteries, giving a curve as shown in Figure 20-19. In each of these instances, 5 milligrams of Cardio-Green dye was injected at zero time. In the top recording, none of the dye passed into the arterial tree until about 3 seconds after the injection, but then the arterial concentration of the dye rose rapidly to a maximum in about 6 to 7 seconds. After that, the concentration fell rapidly, but before the concentration reached zero, some of the dye had already circulated all the way through some of the peripheral systemic vessels and returned through the heart for a second time. Consequently, the dye concentration in the artery began to rise again. For the purpose of calculation, it is necessary to *extrapolate* the early down-slope of the curve to the zero point, as shown by the dashed portion of each curve. In this way, the *extrapolated time-concentration curve* of the dye in the systemic artery without recirculation can be measured in its first portion and estimated reasonably accurately in its latter portion.

Once the extrapolated time-concentration curve has been determined, one then calculates the mean concentration of dye in the arterial blood for the duration of the curve. For instance, in the top example of Figure 20-19, this was done by measuring the area under the entire initial and extrapolated curve and then averaging the concentration of dye for the duration of the curve; one can see from the shaded rectangle straddling the curve in the upper figure that the average concentration of dye was 0.25 mg/dl of blood and that the duration of this average value was 12 seconds. A total of 5 milligrams of dye had been injected at the beginning of the experiment. For blood carrying only 0.25 milligram of dye in each 100 milliliters to carry the entire 5 milligrams of dye through the heart and lungs in 12 seconds, a total of 20 portions each with 100 milliliters of blood would have passed through the heart during the 12 seconds, which would be the same as a cardiac output of 2 L/12 sec, or 10 L/min. We leave it to the reader to calculate the cardiac output from the bottom *extrapolated* curve of Figure 20-19. To summarize, the cardiac output can be determined using the following formula:

$$\text{Cardiac output (ml/min)} =$$

$$\frac{\text{Milligrams of dye injected} \times 60}{\left(\begin{array}{c}\text{Average concentration of dye}\\\text{in each milliliter of blood}\\\text{for the duration of the curve}\end{array}\right) \times \left(\begin{array}{c}\text{Duration of}\\\text{the curve}\\\text{in seconds}\end{array}\right)}$$

Bibliography

Gaasch WH, Zile MR: Left ventricular diastolic dysfunction and diastolic heart failure, *Annu Rev Med* 55:373, 2004.

Guyton AC: Venous return. In Hamilton WF, editor: *Handbook of Physiology,* Sec 2, vol 2, Baltimore, 1963, Williams & Wilkins, p 1099.

Guyton AC: Determination of cardiac output by equating venous return curves with cardiac response curves, *Physiol Rev* 35:123, 1955.

Guyton AC, Jones CE, Coleman TG: *Circulatory physiology: cardiac output and its regulation,* Philadelphia, 1973, WB Saunders.

Guyton AC, Lindsey AW, Kaufmann BN: Effect of mean circulatory filling pressure and other peripheral circulatory factors on cardiac output, *Am J Physiol* 180:463–468, 1955.

Hall JE: Integration and regulation of cardiovascular function, *Am J Physiol* 277:S174, 1999.

Hall JE: The pioneering use of systems analysis to study cardiac output regulation, *Am J Physiol Regul Integr Comp Physiol* 287:R1009, 2004.

Klein I, Danzi S: Thyroid disease and the heart, *Circulation* 116:1725, 2007.

Koch WJ, Lefkowitz RJ, Rockman HA: Functional consequences of altering myocardial adrenergic receptor signaling, *Annu Rev Physiol* 62:237, 2000.

Mathews L, Singh RK: Cardiac output monitoring, *Ann Card Anaesth* 11:56, 2008.

Rothe CF: Mean circulatory filling pressure: its meaning and measurement, *J Appl Physiol* 74:499, 1993.

Rothe CF: Reflex control of veins and vascular capacitance, *Physiol Rev* 63:1281, 1983.

Sarnoff SJ, Berglund E: Ventricular function. 1. Starling's law of the heart, studied by means of simultaneous right and left ventricular function curves in the dog, *Circulation* 9:706–718, 1953.

Uemura K, Sugimachi M, Kawada T, et al: A novel framework of circulatory equilibrium, *Am J Physiol Heart Circ Physiol* 286:H2376, 2004.

Vatner SF, Braunwald E: Cardiovascular control mechanisms in the conscious state, *N Engl J Med* 293:970, 1975.

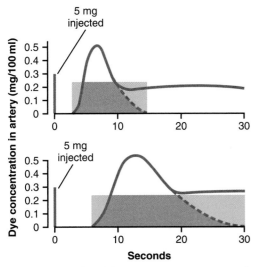

Figure 20-19 *Extrapolated dye concentration curves* used to calculate two separate cardiac outputs by the dilution method. (The rectangular areas are the calculated average concentrations of dye in the arterial blood for the durations of the respective extrapolated curves.)

Muscle Blood Flow and Cardiac Output During Exercise; the Coronary Circulation and Ischemic Heart Disease

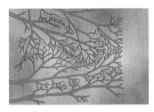

In this chapter we consider (1) blood flow to the skeletal muscles and (2) coronary artery blood flow to the heart. Regulation of each of these is achieved mainly by local control of vascular resistance in response to muscle tissue metabolic needs.

We also discuss the physiology of related subjects such as (1) cardiac output control during exercise, (2) characteristics of heart attacks, and (3) the pain of angina pectoris.

Blood Flow Regulation in Skeletal Muscle at Rest and During Exercise

Very strenuous exercise is one of the most stressful conditions that the normal circulatory system faces. This is true because there is such a large mass of skeletal muscle in the body, all of it requiring large amounts of blood flow. Also, the cardiac output often must increase in the nonathlete to four to five times normal, or in the well-trained athlete to six to seven times normal, to satisfy the metabolic needs of the exercising muscles.

Rate of Blood Flow Through the Muscles

During rest, blood flow through skeletal muscle averages 3 to 4 ml/min/100 g of muscle. During extreme exercise in the well-conditioned athlete, this can increase 25- to 50-fold, rising to 100 to 200 ml/min/100 g of muscle. Peak blood flows as high as 400 ml/min/100 g of muscle have been reported in thigh muscles of endurance-trained athletes.

Blood Flow During Muscle Contractions. Figure 21-1 shows a record of blood flow changes in a calf muscle of a human leg during strong rhythmical muscular exercise. Note that the flow increases and decreases with each muscle contraction. At the end of the contractions, the blood flow remains very high for a few seconds but then returns toward normal during the next few minutes.

The cause of the lower flow during the muscle contraction phase of exercise is compression of the blood vessels by the contracted muscle. During strong tetanic contraction, which causes sustained compression of the blood vessels, the blood flow can be almost stopped, but this also causes rapid weakening of the contraction.

Increased Blood Flow in Muscle Capillaries During Exercise. During rest, some muscle capillaries have little or no flowing blood. But during strenuous exercise, all the capillaries open. This opening of dormant capillaries diminishes the distance that oxygen and other nutrients must diffuse from the capillaries to the contracting muscle fibers and sometimes contributes a twofold to threefold increased capillary surface area through which oxygen and nutrients can diffuse from the blood to the tissues.

Control of Blood Flow in Skeletal Muscles

Local Regulation—Decreased Oxygen in Muscle Greatly Enhances Flow. The tremendous increase in muscle blood flow that occurs during skeletal muscle activity is caused mainly by chemicals acting directly on the muscle arterioles to cause dilation. One of the most important chemical effects is reduction of oxygen in the muscle tissues. When muscles are active they use oxygen rapidly, thereby decreasing the oxygen concentration in the tissue fluids. This in turn causes local arteriolar vasodilation because the arteriolar walls cannot maintain contraction in the absence of oxygen and because oxygen deficiency causes release of vasodilator substances. Adenosine may be an important vasodilator substance, but experiments have shown that even large amounts of adenosine infused directly into a muscle artery cannot increase blood flow to the same extent as during intense exercise and cannot sustain vasodilation in skeletal muscle for more than about 2 hours.

Fortunately, even after the muscle blood vessels have become insensitive to the vasodilator effects of adenosine, still other vasodilator factors continue to maintain increased capillary blood flow as long as the exercise continues. These factors include (1) potassium ions, (2) adenosine triphosphate (ATP), (3) lactic acid, and (4) carbon dioxide. We still do not know quantitatively how great a role each of these plays in increasing muscle

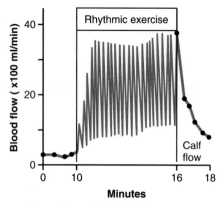

Figure 21-1 Effects of muscle exercise on blood flow in the calf of a leg during strong rhythmical contraction. The blood flow was much less during contractions than between contractions. (Adapted from Barcroft H, Dornhorst AC: The blood flow through the human calf during rhythmic exercise. J Physiol 109:402, 1949.)

blood flow during muscle activity; this subject was discussed in additional detail in Chapter 17.

Nervous Control of Muscle Blood Flow. In addition to local tissue vasodilator mechanisms, skeletal muscles are provided with sympathetic vasoconstrictor nerves and (in some species of animals) sympathetic vasodilator nerves as well.

Sympathetic Vasoconstrictor Nerves. The sympathetic vasoconstrictor nerve fibers secrete norepinephrine at their nerve endings. When maximally activated, this can decrease blood flow through resting muscles to as little as one-half to one-third normal. This vasoconstriction is of physiologic importance in circulatory shock and during other periods of stress when it is necessary to maintain a normal or even high arterial pressure.

In addition to the norepinephrine secreted at the sympathetic vasoconstrictor nerve endings, the medullae of the two adrenal glands also secrete large amounts of norepinephrine plus even more epinephrine into the circulating blood during strenuous exercise. The circulating norepinephrine acts on the muscle vessels to cause a vasoconstrictor effect similar to that caused by direct sympathetic nerve stimulation. The epinephrine, however, often has a slight vasodilator effect because epinephrine excites more of the beta-adrenergic receptors of the vessels, which are vasodilator receptors, in contrast to the alpha vasoconstrictor receptors excited especially by norepinephrine. These receptors are discussed in Chapter 60.

Total Body Circulatory Readjustments During Exercise

Three major effects occur during exercise that are essential for the circulatory system to supply the tremendous blood flow required by the muscles. They are (1) mass discharge of the sympathetic nervous system throughout the body with consequent stimulatory effects on the entire circulation, (2) increase in arterial pressure, and (3) increase in cardiac output.

Effects of Mass Sympathetic Discharge

At the onset of exercise, signals are transmitted not only from the brain to the muscles to cause muscle contraction but also into the vasomotor center to initiate sympathetic discharge throughout the body. Simultaneously, the parasympathetic signals to the heart are attenuated. Therefore, three major circulatory effects result.

First, the heart is stimulated to greatly increased heart rate and increased pumping strength as a result of the sympathetic drive to the heart plus release of the heart from normal parasympathetic inhibition.

Second, most of the arterioles of the peripheral circulation are strongly contracted, except for the arterioles in the active muscles, which are strongly vasodilated by the local vasodilator effects in the muscles, as noted earlier. Thus, the heart is stimulated to supply the increased blood flow required by the muscles, while at the same time blood flow through most nonmuscular areas of the body is temporarily reduced, thereby "lending" blood supply to the muscles. This accounts for as much as 2 L/min of extra blood flow to the muscles, which is exceedingly important when one thinks of a person running for his life—even a fractional increase in running speed may make the difference between life and death. Two of the peripheral circulatory systems, the coronary and cerebral systems, are spared this vasoconstrictor effect because both these circulatory areas have poor vasoconstrictor innervation—fortunately so because both the heart and the brain are as essential to exercise as are the skeletal muscles.

Third, the muscle walls of the veins and other capacitative areas of the circulation are contracted powerfully, which greatly increases the mean systemic filling pressure. As we learned in Chapter 20, this is one of the most important factors in promoting increase in venous return of blood to the heart and, therefore, in increasing the cardiac output.

Increase in Arterial Pressure During Exercise Due to Sympathetic Stimulation

An important effect of increased sympathetic stimulation in exercise is to increase the arterial pressure. This results from multiple stimulatory effects, including (1) vasoconstriction of the arterioles and small arteries in most tissues of the body except the active muscles, (2) increased pumping activity by the heart, and (3) a great increase in mean systemic filling pressure caused mainly by venous contraction. These effects, working together, almost always increase the arterial pressure during exercise. This increase can be as little as 20 mm Hg or as great as 80 mm Hg, depending on the conditions under which the exercise is performed. When a person performs exercise under tense conditions but uses only a few muscles, the sympathetic nervous response still occurs everywhere in the body. In the few active muscles, vasodilation occurs, but everywhere else in the body the effect is mainly vasoconstriction, often increasing the mean arterial pressure to as high as 170 mm Hg. Such a condition might occur in a person standing on a ladder and nailing with a hammer on the ceiling above. The tenseness of the situation is obvious.

Conversely, when a person performs massive whole-body exercise, such as running or swimming, the increase in arterial pressure is often only 20 to 40 mm Hg. This lack of a large increase in pressure results from the extreme vasodilation that occurs simultaneously in large masses of active muscle.

Why Is the Arterial Pressure Increase During Exercise Important? When muscles are stimulated maximally in a laboratory experiment but without allowing the arterial pressure to rise, muscle blood flow seldom rises more than about eightfold. Yet, we know from studies of marathon runners that muscle blood flow can increase from as little as 1 L/min for the whole body during rest to more than 20 L/min during maximal activity. Therefore, it is clear that muscle blood flow can increase much more than occurs in the aforementioned simple laboratory experiment. What is the difference? Mainly, the arterial pressure rises during normal exercise. Let us assume, for instance, that the arterial pressure rises 30 percent, a common increase during heavy exercise. This 30 percent increase causes 30 percent more force to push blood through the muscle tissue vessels. But this is not the only important effect; the extra pressure also stretches the walls of the vessels, and this effect, along with the locally released vasodilators and higher blood pressure, may increase muscle total flow to more than 20 times normal.

Importance of the Increase in Cardiac Output During Exercise

Many different physiologic effects occur at the same time during exercise to increase cardiac output approximately in proportion to the degree of exercise. In fact, the ability of the circulatory system to provide increased cardiac output for delivery of oxygen and other nutrients to the muscles during exercise is equally as important as the strength of the muscles themselves in setting the limit for continued muscle work. For instance, marathon runners who can increase their cardiac outputs the most are generally the same persons who have record-breaking running times.

Graphical Analysis of the Changes in Cardiac Output During Heavy Exercise. Figure 21-2 shows a graphical analysis of the large increase in cardiac output that occurs during heavy exercise. The cardiac output and venous return curves crossing at point A give the analysis for the normal circulation, and the curves crossing at point B analyze heavy exercise. Note that the great increase in cardiac output requires significant changes in both the cardiac output curve and the venous return curve, as follows.

The increased level of the cardiac output curve is easy to understand. It results almost entirely from sympathetic stimulation of the heart that causes (1) increased heart rate, often up to rates as high as 170 to 190 beats/min, and (2) increased strength of contraction of the heart, often to as much as twice normal. Without this increased level

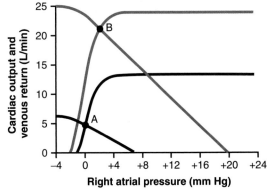

Figure 21-2 Graphical analysis of change in cardiac output and right atrial pressure with onset of strenuous exercise. *Black curves,* normal circulation. *Red curves,* heavy exercise.

of cardiac function, the increase in cardiac output would be limited to the plateau level of the normal heart, which would be a maximum increase of cardiac output of only about 2.5-fold rather than the 4-fold that can commonly be achieved by the untrained runner and the 7-fold that can be achieved in some marathon runners.

Now study the venous return curves. If no change occurred from the normal venous return curve, the cardiac output could hardly rise at all in exercise because the upper plateau level of the normal venous return curve is only 6 L/min. Yet two important changes do occur:

1. The mean systemic filling pressure rises tremendously at the onset of heavy exercise. This results partly from the sympathetic stimulation that contracts the veins and other capacitative parts of the circulation. In addition, tensing of the abdominal and other skeletal muscles of the body compresses many of the internal vessels, thus providing more compression of the entire capacitative vascular system, causing a still greater increase in mean systemic filling pressure. During maximal exercise, these two effects together can increase the mean systemic filling pressure from a normal level of 7 mm Hg to as high as 30 mm Hg.

2. The slope of the venous return curve rotates upward. This is caused by decreased resistance in virtually all the blood vessels in active muscle tissue, which also causes resistance to venous return to decrease, thus increasing the upward slope of the venous return curve.

Therefore, the combination of increased mean systemic filling pressure and decreased resistance to venous return raises the entire level of the venous return curve.

In response to the changes in both the venous return curve and the cardiac output curve, the new equilibrium point in Figure 21-2 for cardiac output and right atrial pressure is now point B, in contrast to the normal level at point A. Note especially that the right atrial pressure has hardly changed, having risen only 1.5 mm Hg. In fact, in a person with a strong heart, the right atrial pressure often falls below normal in very heavy exercise because of the greatly increased sympathetic stimulation of the heart during exercise.

Coronary Circulation

About one third of all deaths in industrialized countries of the Western world result from coronary artery disease, and almost all elderly people have at least some impairment of the coronary artery circulation. For this reason, understanding normal and pathological physiology of the coronary circulation is one of the most important subjects in medicine.

Physiologic Anatomy of the Coronary Blood Supply

Figure 21-3 shows the heart and its coronary blood supply. Note that the main coronary arteries lie on the surface of the heart and smaller arteries then penetrate from the surface into the cardiac muscle mass. It is almost entirely through these arteries that the heart receives its nutritive blood supply. Only the inner 1/10 millimeter of the endocardial surface can obtain significant nutrition directly from the blood inside the cardiac chambers, so this source of muscle nutrition is minuscule.

The *left coronary artery* supplies mainly the anterior and left lateral portions of the left ventricle, whereas the *right coronary artery* supplies most of the right ventricle, as well as the posterior part of the left ventricle in 80 to 90 percent of people.

Most of the coronary venous blood flow from the left ventricular muscle returns to the right atrium of the heart by way of the *coronary sinus*, which is about 75 percent of the total coronary blood flow. And most of the coronary venous blood from the right ventricular muscle returns through small anterior cardiac veins that flow directly into the right atrium, not by way of the coronary sinus. A very small amount of coronary venous blood also flows back into the heart through very minute *thebesian veins*, which empty directly into all chambers of the heart.

Normal Coronary Blood Flow—About 5 Percent of Cardiac Output

The resting coronary blood flow in the resting human being averages 70 ml/min/100 g heart weight, or about 225 ml/min, which is about 4 to 5 percent of the total cardiac output.

During strenuous exercise, the heart in the young adult increases its cardiac output fourfold to sevenfold, and it pumps this blood against a higher than normal arterial pressure. Consequently, the work output of the heart under severe conditions may increase sixfold to ninefold. At the same time, the coronary blood flow increases threefold to fourfold to supply the extra nutrients needed by the heart. This increase is not as much as the increase in workload, which means that the ratio of energy expenditure by the heart to coronary blood flow increases. Thus, the "efficiency" of cardiac utilization of energy increases to make up for the relative deficiency of coronary blood supply.

Phasic Changes in Coronary Blood Flow During Systole and Diastole—Effect of Cardiac Muscle Compression. Figure 21-4 shows the changes in blood flow through the nutrient capillaries of the left ventricular coronary system in ml/min in the human heart during systole and diastole, as extrapolated from studies in experimental animals. Note from this diagram that the coronary capillary blood flow in the left ventricle muscle falls to a low value during systole, which is opposite to flow in vascular beds elsewhere in the body. The reason for this is strong compression of the left ventricular muscle around the intramuscular vessels during systolic contraction.

During diastole, the cardiac muscle relaxes and no longer obstructs blood flow through the left ventricular muscle capillaries, so blood flows rapidly during all of diastole.

Blood flow through the coronary capillaries of the right ventricle also undergoes phasic changes during the cardiac cycle, but because the force of contraction of the right ventricular muscle is far less than that of the left ventricular muscle, the inverse phasic changes are only partial, in contrast to those in the left ventricular muscle.

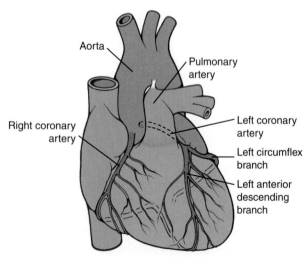

Figure 21-3 The coronary arteries.

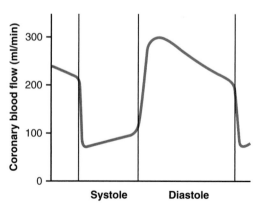

Figure 21-4 Phasic flow of blood through the coronary capillaries of the human left ventricle during cardiac systole and diastole (as extrapolated from measured flows in dogs).

Epicardial Versus Subendocardial Coronary Blood Flow—Effect of Intramyocardial Pressure. Figure 21-5 demonstrates the special arrangement of the coronary vessels at different depths in the heart muscle, showing on the outer surface *epicardial coronary arteries* that supply most of the muscle. Smaller, intramuscular arteries derived from the epicardial arteries penetrate the muscle, supplying the needed nutrients. Lying immediately beneath the endocardium is a plexus of *subendocardial arteries*. During systole, blood flow through the subendocardial plexus of the left ventricle, where the intramuscular coronary vessels are compressed greatly by ventricular muscle contraction, tends to be reduced. But the extra vessels of the subendocardial plexus normally compensate for this. Later in the chapter, we explain how this peculiar difference between blood flow in the epicardial and subendocardial arteries plays an important role in certain types of coronary ischemia.

Control of Coronary Blood Flow

Local Muscle Metabolism Is the Primary Controller of Coronary Flow

Blood flow through the coronary system is regulated mostly by local arteriolar vasodilation in response to the nutritional needs of cardiac muscle. That is, whenever the vigor of cardiac contraction is increased, the rate of coronary blood flow also increases. Conversely, decreased heart activity is accompanied by decreased coronary flow. This local regulation of coronary blood flow is almost identical to that occurring in many other tissues of the body, especially in the skeletal muscles.

Oxygen Demand as a Major Factor in Local Coronary Blood Flow Regulation. Blood flow in the coronary arteries usually is regulated almost exactly in proportion to the need of the cardiac musculature for oxygen. Normally, about 70 percent of the oxygen in the coronary arterial blood is removed as the blood flows through the heart muscle. Because not much oxygen is left, very little additional oxygen can be supplied to the heart musculature unless the coronary blood flow increases. Fortunately, the coronary blood flow does increase almost in direct proportion to any additional metabolic consumption of oxygen by the heart.

However, the exact means by which increased oxygen consumption causes coronary dilation has not been determined. It is speculated by many research workers that a decrease in the oxygen concentration in the heart

causes vasodilator substances to be released from the muscle cells and that these dilate the arterioles. A substance with great vasodilator propensity is adenosine. In the presence of very low concentrations of oxygen in the muscle cells, a large proportion of the cell's ATP degrades to adenosine monophosphate; then small portions of this are further degraded and release adenosine into the tissue fluids of the heart muscle, with resultant increase in local coronary blood flow. After the adenosine causes vasodilation, much of it is reabsorbed into the cardiac cells to be reused.

Adenosine is not the only vasodilator product that has been identified. Others include adenosine phosphate compounds, potassium ions, hydrogen ions, carbon dioxide, prostaglandins, and nitric oxide. Yet the mechanisms of coronary vasodilation during increased cardiac activity have not been fully explained by adenosine. Pharmacologic agents that block or partially block the vasodilator effect of adenosine do not prevent coronary vasodilation caused by increased heart muscle activity. Studies in skeletal muscle have also shown that continued infusion of adenosine maintains vascular dilation for only 1 to 3 hours, and yet muscle activity still dilates the local blood vessels even when the adenosine can no longer dilate them. Therefore, the other vasodilator mechanisms listed earlier should be remembered.

Nervous Control of Coronary Blood Flow

Stimulation of the autonomic nerves to the heart can affect coronary blood flow both directly and indirectly. The direct effects result from action of the nervous transmitter substances acetylcholine from the vagus nerves and norepinephrine and epinephrine from the sympathetic nerves on the coronary vessels themselves. The indirect effects result from secondary changes in coronary blood flow caused by increased or decreased activity of the heart.

The indirect effects, which are mostly opposite to the direct effects, play a far more important role in normal control of coronary blood flow. Thus, sympathetic stimulation, which releases norepinephrine and epinephrine, increases both heart rate and heart contractility and increases the rate of metabolism of the heart. In turn, the increased metabolism of the heart sets off local blood flow regulatory mechanisms for dilating the coronary vessels, and the blood flow increases approximately in proportion to the metabolic needs of the heart muscle. In contrast, vagal stimulation, with its release of acetylcholine, slows the heart and has a slight depressive effect on heart contractility. These effects in turn decrease cardiac oxygen consumption and, therefore, indirectly constrict the coronary arteries.

Direct Effects of Nervous Stimuli on the Coronary Vasculature. The distribution of parasympathetic (vagal) nerve fibers to the ventricular coronary system is not very great. However, the acetylcholine released by parasympathetic stimulation has a direct effect to dilate the coronary arteries.

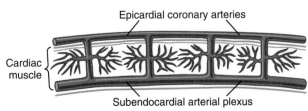

Epicardial coronary arteries

Cardiac muscle

Subendocardial arterial plexus

Figure 21-5 Diagram of the epicardial, intramuscular, and subendocardial coronary vasculature.

247

There is much more extensive sympathetic innervation of the coronary vessels. In Chapter 60, we see that the sympathetic transmitter substances norepinephrine and epinephrine can have either vascular constrictor or vascular dilator effects, depending on the presence or absence of constrictor or dilator receptors in the blood vessel walls. The constrictor receptors are called *alpha receptors* and the dilator receptors are called *beta receptors.* Both alpha and beta receptors exist in the coronary vessels. In general, the epicardial coronary vessels have a preponderance of alpha receptors, whereas the intramuscular arteries may have a preponderance of beta receptors. Therefore, sympathetic stimulation can, at least theoretically, cause slight overall coronary constriction or dilation, but usually constriction. In some people, the alpha vasoconstrictor effects seem to be disproportionately severe, and these people can have vasospastic myocardial ischemia during periods of excess sympathetic drive, often with resultant anginal pain.

Metabolic factors, especially myocardial oxygen consumption, are the major controllers of myocardial blood flow. Whenever the direct effects of nervous stimulation alter the coronary blood flow in the wrong direction, the metabolic control of coronary flow usually overrides the direct coronary nervous effects within seconds.

Special Features of Cardiac Muscle Metabolism

The basic principles of cellular metabolism, discussed in Chapters 67 through 72, apply to cardiac muscle the same as for other tissues, but there are some quantitative differences. Most important, under resting conditions, cardiac muscle normally consumes fatty acids to supply most of its energy instead of carbohydrates (about 70 percent of the energy is derived from fatty acids). However, as is also true of other tissues, under anaerobic or ischemic conditions, cardiac metabolism must call on anaerobic glycolysis mechanisms for energy. Unfortunately, glycolysis consumes tremendous quantities of the blood glucose and at the same time forms large amounts of lactic acid in the cardiac tissue, which is probably one of the causes of cardiac pain in cardiac ischemic conditions, as discussed later in this chapter.

As is true in other tissues, more than 95 percent of the metabolic energy liberated from foods is used to form ATP in the mitochondria. This ATP in turn acts as the conveyer of energy for cardiac muscular contraction and other cellular functions. In severe coronary ischemia, the ATP degrades first to adenosine diphosphate, then to adenosine monophosphate and adenosine. Because the cardiac muscle cell membrane is slightly permeable to adenosine, much of this can diffuse from the muscle cells into the circulating blood.

The released adenosine is believed to be one of the substances that causes dilation of the coronary arterioles during coronary hypoxia, as discussed earlier. However, loss of adenosine also has a serious cellular consequence. Within as little as 30 minutes of severe coronary ischemia, as occurs after a myocardial infarct, about one half of the adenine base can be lost from the affected cardiac muscle cells. Furthermore, this loss can be replaced by new synthesis of adenine at a rate of only 2 percent per hour. Therefore, once a serious bout of coronary ischemia has persisted for 30 or more minutes, relief of the ischemia may be too late to prevent injury and death of the cardiac cells. This almost certainly is one of the major causes of cardiac cellular death during myocardial ischemia.

Ischemic Heart Disease

The most common cause of death in Western culture is ischemic heart disease, which results from insufficient coronary blood flow. About 35 percent of people in the United States die of this cause. Some deaths occur suddenly as a result of acute coronary occlusion or fibrillation of the heart, whereas other deaths occur slowly over a period of weeks to years as a result of progressive weakening of the heart pumping process. In this chapter, we discuss acute coronary ischemia caused by acute coronary occlusion and myocardial infarction. In Chapter 22, we discuss congestive heart failure, the most frequent cause of which is slowly increasing coronary ischemia and weakening of the cardiac muscle.

Atherosclerosis as a Cause of Ischemic Heart Disease. The most frequent cause of diminished coronary blood flow is atherosclerosis. The atherosclerotic process is discussed in connection with lipid metabolism in Chapter 68. Briefly, this process is the following.

In people who have genetic predisposition to atherosclerosis, who are overweight or obese and have a sedentary lifestyle, or who have high blood pressure and damage to the endothelial cells of the coronary blood vessels, large quantities of cholesterol gradually become deposited beneath the endothelium at many points in arteries throughout the body. Gradually, these areas of deposit are invaded by fibrous tissue and frequently become calcified. The net result is the development of atherosclerotic plaques that actually protrude into the vessel lumens and either block or partially block blood flow. A common site for development of atherosclerotic plaques is the first few centimeters of the major coronary arteries.

Acute Coronary Occlusion

Acute occlusion of a coronary artery most frequently occurs in a person who already has underlying atherosclerotic coronary heart disease but almost never in a person with a normal coronary circulation. Acute occlusion can result from any one of several effects, two of which are the following:

1. The atherosclerotic plaque can cause a local blood clot called a *thrombus,* which in turn occludes the artery. The thrombus usually occurs where the arteriosclerotic plaque has broken through the endothelium, thus coming in direct contact with the flowing blood. Because the plaque presents an unsmooth surface, blood platelets adhere to it, fibrin is deposited, and red

Chapter 21   Muscle Blood Flow and Cardiac Output During Exercise; the Coronary Circulation and Ischemic Heart Disease

UNIT IV

blood cells become entrapped to form a blood clot that grows until it occludes the vessel. Or, occasionally, the clot breaks away from its attachment on the atherosclerotic plaque and flows to a more peripheral branch of the coronary arterial tree, where it blocks the artery at that point. A thrombus that flows along the artery in this way and occludes the vessel more distally is called a *coronary embolus.*

2. Many clinicians believe that local muscular spasm of a coronary artery also can occur. The spasm might result from direct irritation of the smooth muscle of the arterial wall by the edges of an arteriosclerotic plaque, or it might result from local nervous reflexes that cause excess coronary vascular wall contraction. The spasm may then lead to *secondary thrombosis* of the vessel.

Lifesaving Value of Collateral Circulation in the Heart. The degree of damage to the heart muscle caused either by slowly developing atherosclerotic constriction of the coronary arteries or by sudden coronary occlusion is determined to a great extent by the degree of collateral circulation that has already developed or that can open within minutes after the occlusion.

In a normal heart, almost no large communications exist among the larger coronary arteries. But many anastomoses do exist among the smaller arteries sized 20 to 250 micrometers in diameter, as shown in Figure 21-6.

When a sudden occlusion occurs in one of the larger coronary arteries, the small anastomoses begin to dilate within seconds. But the blood flow through these minute collaterals is usually less than one-half that needed to keep alive most of the cardiac muscle that they now supply; the diameters of the collateral vessels do not enlarge much more for the next 8 to 24 hours. But then collateral flow does begin to increase, doubling by the second or third

day and often reaching normal or almost normal coronary flow within about 1 month. Because of these developing collateral channels, many patients recover almost completely from various degrees of coronary occlusion when the area of muscle involved is not too great.

When atherosclerosis constricts the coronary arteries slowly over a period of many years rather than suddenly, collateral vessels can develop at the same time while the atherosclerosis becomes more and more severe. Therefore, the person may never experience an acute episode of cardiac dysfunction. But, eventually, the sclerotic process develops beyond the limits of even the collateral blood supply to provide the needed blood flow, and sometimes the collateral blood vessels themselves develop atherosclerosis. When this occurs, the heart muscle becomes severely limited in its work output, often so much so that the heart cannot pump even normally required amounts of blood flow. This is one of the most common causes of the cardiac failure that occurs in vast numbers of older people.

Myocardial Infarction

Immediately after an acute coronary occlusion, blood flow ceases in the coronary vessels beyond the occlusion except for small amounts of collateral flow from surrounding vessels. The area of muscle that has either zero flow or so little flow that it cannot sustain cardiac muscle function is said to be *infarcted.* The overall process is called a *myocardial infarction.*

Soon after the onset of the infarction, small amounts of collateral blood begin to seep into the infarcted area, and this, combined with progressive dilation of local blood vessels, causes the area to become overfilled with stagnant blood. Simultaneously the muscle fibers use the last vestiges of the oxygen in the blood, causing the hemoglobin to become totally deoxygenated. Therefore, the infarcted area takes on a bluish-brown hue, and the blood vessels of the area appear to be engorged despite lack of blood flow. In later stages, the vessel walls become highly permeable and leak fluid; the local muscle tissue becomes edematous, and the cardiac muscle cells begin to swell because of diminished cellular metabolism. Within a few hours of almost no blood supply, the cardiac muscle cells die.

Cardiac muscle requires about 1.3 ml of oxygen per 100 grams of muscle tissue per minute just to remain alive. This is in comparison with about 8 ml of oxygen per 100 grams delivered to the normal resting left ventricle each minute. Therefore, if there is even 15 to 30 percent of normal resting coronary blood flow, the muscle will not die. In the central portion of a large infarct, however, where there is almost no collateral blood flow, the muscle does die.

Subendocardial Infarction. The subendocardial muscle frequently becomes infarcted even when there is no evidence of infarction in the outer surface portions of the heart. The reason for this is that the subendocardial muscle has extra difficulty obtaining adequate blood flow because the blood vessels in the subendocardium

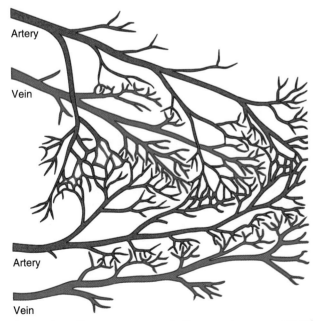

Figure 21-6 Minute anastomoses in the normal coronary arterial system.

Artery

Vein

Artery

Vein

are intensely compressed by systolic contraction of the heart, as explained earlier. Therefore, any condition that compromises blood flow to any area of the heart usually causes damage first in the subendocardial regions, and the damage then spreads outward toward the epicardium.

Causes of Death After Acute Coronary Occlusion

The most common causes of death after acute myocardial infarction are (1) decreased cardiac output; (2) damming of blood in the pulmonary blood vessels and then death resulting from pulmonary edema; (3) fibrillation of the heart; and, occasionally, (4) rupture of the heart.

Decreased Cardiac Output—Systolic Stretch and Cardiac Shock.

When some of the cardiac muscle fibers are not functioning and others are too weak to contract with great force, the overall pumping ability of the affected ventricle is proportionately depressed. Indeed, the overall pumping strength of the infarcted heart is often decreased more than one might expect because of a phenomenon called *systolic stretch*, shown in Figure 21-7. That is, when the normal portions of the ventricular muscle contract, the ischemic portion of the muscle, whether it is dead or simply nonfunctional, instead of contracting is forced outward by the pressure that develops inside the ventricle. Therefore, much of the pumping force of the ventricle is dissipated by bulging of the area of nonfunctional cardiac muscle.

When the heart becomes incapable of contracting with sufficient force to pump enough blood into the peripheral arterial tree, cardiac failure and death of peripheral tissues ensue as a result of peripheral ischemia. This condition is called *coronary shock, cardiogenic shock, cardiac shock,* or

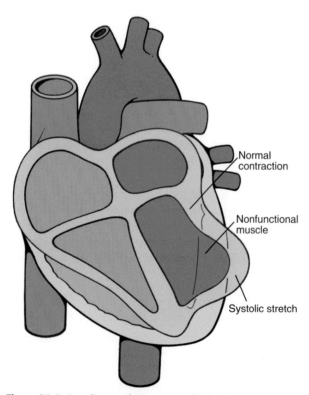

Figure 21-7 Systolic stretch in an area of ischemic cardiac muscle.

Normal contraction

Nonfunctional muscle

Systolic stretch

low cardiac output failure. It is discussed more fully in the next chapter. Cardiac shock almost always occurs when more than 40 percent of the left ventricle is infarcted. And death occurs in over 70 percent of patients once they develop cardiac shock.

Damming of Blood in the Body's Venous System.

When the heart is not pumping blood forward, it must be damming blood in the atria and in the blood vessels of the lungs or in the systemic circulation. This leads to increased capillary pressures, particularly in the lungs.

This damming of blood in the veins often causes little difficulty during the first few hours after myocardial infarction. Instead, symptoms develop a few days later for the following reason: The acutely diminished cardiac output leads to diminished blood flow to the kidneys. Then, for reasons that are discussed in Chapter 22, the kidneys fail to excrete enough urine. This adds progressively to the total blood volume and, therefore, leads to congestive symptoms. Consequently, many patients who seemingly are getting along well during the first few days after onset of heart failure will suddenly develop acute pulmonary edema and often will die within a few hours after appearance of the initial pulmonary symptoms.

Fibrillation of the Ventricles After Myocardial Infarction.

Many people who die of coronary occlusion die because of sudden ventricular fibrillation. The tendency to develop fibrillation is especially great after a large infarction, but fibrillation can sometimes occur after small occlusions as well. Indeed, some patients with chronic coronary insufficiency die suddenly from fibrillation without any acute infarction.

There are two especially dangerous periods after coronary infarction during which fibrillation is most likely to occur. The first is during the first 10 minutes after the infarction occurs. Then there is a short period of relative safety, followed by a second period of cardiac irritability beginning 1 hour or so later and lasting for another few hours. Fibrillation can also occur many days after the infarct but less likely so.

At least four factors enter into the tendency for the heart to fibrillate:

1. Acute loss of blood supply to the cardiac muscle causes rapid depletion of potassium from the ischemic musculature. This also increases the potassium concentration in the extracellular fluids surrounding the cardiac muscle fibers. Experiments in which potassium has been injected into the coronary system have demonstrated that an elevated extracellular potassium concentration increases the irritability of the cardiac musculature and, therefore, its likelihood of fibrillating.

2. Ischemia of the muscle causes an "injury current," which is described in Chapter 12 in relation to electrocardiograms in patients with acute myocardial infarction.

That is, the ischemic musculature often cannot completely repolarize its membranes after a heartbeat, so the external surface of this muscle remains negative with respect to normal cardiac muscle membrane potential elsewhere in the heart. Therefore, electric current flows from this ischemic area of the heart to the normal area and can elicit abnormal impulses that can cause fibrillation.

3. Powerful sympathetic reflexes often develop after massive infarction, principally because the heart does not pump an adequate volume of blood into the arterial tree, which leads to reduced blood pressure. The sympathetic stimulation also increases irritability of the cardiac muscle and thereby predisposes to fibrillation.

4. Cardiac muscle weakness caused by the myocardial infarction often causes the ventricle to dilate excessively. This increases the pathway length for impulse conduction in the heart and frequently causes abnormal conduction pathways all the way around the infarcted area of the cardiac muscle. Both of these effects predispose to development of circus movements because, as discussed in Chapter 13, excess prolongation of conduction pathways in the ventricles allows impulses to re-enter muscle that is already recovering from refractoriness, thereby initiating a "circus movement" cycle of new excitation and causing the process to continue on and on.

Rupture of the Infarcted Area. During the first day or so after an acute infarct, there is little danger of rupture of the ischemic portion of the heart, but a few days later, the dead muscle fibers begin to degenerate, and the heart wall becomes stretched very thin. When this happens, the dead muscle bulges outward severely with each heart contraction, and this systolic stretch becomes greater and greater until finally the heart ruptures. In fact, one of the means used in assessing progress of severe myocardial infarction is to record by cardiac imaging (i.e., x-rays) whether the degree of systolic stretch is worsening.

When a ventricle does rupture, loss of blood into the pericardial space causes rapid development of *cardiac tamponade*—that is, compression of the heart from the outside by blood collecting in the pericardial cavity. Because of this compression of the heart, blood cannot flow into the right atrium, and the patient dies of suddenly decreased cardiac output.

Stages of Recovery from Acute Myocardial Infarction

The upper left part of Figure 21-8 shows the effects of acute coronary occlusion in a patient with a small area of muscle ischemia; to the right is shown a heart with a large area of ischemia. When the area of ischemia is small, little or no death of the muscle cells may occur, but part of the muscle often does become temporarily nonfunctional because of inadequate nutrition to support muscle contraction.

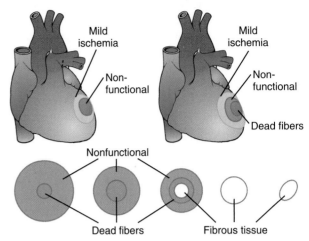

Figure 21-8 *Top,* Small and large areas of coronary ischemia. *Bottom,* Stages of recovery from myocardial infarction.

When the area of ischemia is large, some of the muscle fibers in the center of the area die rapidly, within 1 to 3 hours where there is total cessation of coronary blood supply. Immediately around the dead area is a nonfunctional area, with failure of contraction and usually failure of impulse conduction. Then, extending circumferentially around the nonfunctional area is an area that is still contracting but weakly so because of mild ischemia.

Replacement of Dead Muscle by Scar Tissue. In the lower part of Figure 21-8, the various stages of recovery after a large myocardial infarction are shown. Shortly after the occlusion, the muscle fibers in the center of the ischemic area die. Then, during the ensuing days, this area of dead fibers becomes bigger because many of the marginal fibers finally succumb to the prolonged ischemia. At the same time, because of enlargement of collateral arterial channels supplying the outer rim of the infarcted area, much of the nonfunctional muscle recovers. After a few days to 3 weeks, most of the nonfunctional muscle becomes functional again or dies—one or the other. In the meantime, fibrous tissue begins developing among the dead fibers because ischemia can stimulate growth of fibroblasts and promote development of greater than normal quantities of fibrous tissue. Therefore, the dead muscle tissue is gradually replaced by fibrous tissue. Then, because it is a general property of fibrous tissue to undergo progressive contraction and dissolution, the fibrous scar may grow smaller over a period of several months to a year.

Finally, the normal areas of the heart gradually hypertrophy to compensate at least partially for the lost dead cardiac musculature. By these means, the heart recovers either partially or almost completely within a few months.

Value of Rest in Treating Myocardial Infarction. The degree of cardiac cellular death is determined by the degree of ischemia and the workload on the heart muscle.

When the workload is greatly increased, such as during exercise, in severe emotional strain, or as a result of fatigue, the heart needs increased oxygen and other nutrients for sustaining its life. Furthermore, anastomotic blood vessels that supply blood to ischemic areas of the heart must also still supply the areas of the heart that they normally supply. When the heart becomes excessively active, the vessels of the normal musculature become greatly dilated. This allows most of the blood flowing into the coronary vessels to flow through the normal muscle tissue, thus leaving little blood to flow through the small anastomotic channels into the ischemic area so that the ischemic condition worsens. This condition is called the *"coronary steal" syndrome.* Consequently, one of the most important factors in the treatment of a patient with myocardial infarction is observance of absolute body rest during the recovery process.

Function of the Heart After Recovery from Myocardial Infarction

Occasionally, a heart that has recovered from a large myocardial infarction returns almost to full functional capability, but more frequently its pumping capability is permanently decreased below that of a healthy heart. This does not mean that the person is necessarily a cardiac invalid or that the resting cardiac output is depressed below normal, because the normal heart is capable of pumping 300 to 400 percent more blood per minute than the body requires during rest—that is, a normal person has a "cardiac reserve" of 300 to 400 percent. Even when the cardiac reserve is reduced to as little as 100 percent, the person can still perform most normal daily activities but not strenuous exercise that would overload the heart.

Pain in Coronary Heart Disease

Normally, a person cannot "feel" his or her heart, but ischemic cardiac muscle often does cause pain sensation, sometimes severe. Exactly what causes this pain is not known, but it is believed that ischemia causes the muscle to release acidic substances, such as lactic acid, or other pain-promoting products, such as histamine, kinins, or cellular proteolytic enzymes, that are not removed rapidly enough by the slowly moving coronary blood flow. The high concentrations of these abnormal products then stimulate pain nerve endings in the cardiac muscle, sending pain impulses through sensory afferent nerve fibers into the central nervous system.

Angina Pectoris

In most people who develop progressive constriction of their coronary arteries, cardiac pain, called *angina pectoris,* begins to appear whenever the load on the heart becomes too great in relation to the available coronary blood flow. This pain is usually felt beneath the upper sternum over the heart, and in addition it is often referred to distant surface areas of the body, most commonly to the left arm and left shoulder but also frequently to the neck and even to the side of the face. The reason for this distribution of pain is that the heart originates during embryonic life in the neck, as do the arms. Therefore, both the heart and these surface areas of the body receive pain nerve fibers from the same spinal cord segments.

Most people who have chronic angina pectoris feel pain when they exercise or when they experience emotions that increase metabolism of the heart or temporarily constrict the coronary vessels because of sympathetic vasoconstrictor nerve signals. Anginal pain is also exacerbated by cold temperatures or by having a full stomach, both of which increase the workload of the heart. The pain usually lasts for only a few minutes. However, some patients have such severe and lasting ischemia that the pain is present all the time. The pain is frequently described as hot, pressing, and constricting; it is of such quality that it usually makes the patient stop all unnecessary body activity and come to a complete state of rest.

Treatment with Drugs. Several vasodilator drugs, when administered during an acute anginal attack, can often give immediate relief from the pain. Commonly used short-acting vasodilators are *nitroglycerin* and other *nitrate drugs.* Other vasodilators, such as angiotensin converting enzyme inhibitors, angiotensin receptor blockers, calcium channel blockers, and ranolazine, may be beneficial in treating chronic stable angina pectoris.

Another class of drugs used for prolonged treatment of angina pectoris is the *beta blockers,* such as propranolol. These drugs block sympathetic beta-adrenergic receptors, which prevents sympathetic enhancement of heart rate and cardiac metabolism during exercise or emotional episodes. Therefore, therapy with a beta blocker decreases the need of the heart for extra metabolic oxygen during stressful conditions. For obvious reasons, this can also reduce the number of anginal attacks, as well as their severity.

Surgical Treatment of Coronary Artery Disease

Aortic-Coronary Bypass Surgery. In many patients with coronary ischemia, the constricted areas of the coronary arteries are located at only a few discrete points blocked by atherosclerotic disease and the coronary vessels elsewhere are normal or almost normal. A surgical procedure was developed in the 1960s, called *aortic-coronary bypass,* for removing a section of a subcutaneous vein from an arm or leg and then grafting this vein from the root of the aorta to the side of a peripheral coronary artery beyond the atherosclerotic blockage point. One to five such grafts are usually performed, each of which supplies a peripheral coronary artery beyond a block.

Anginal pain is relieved in most patients. Also, in patients whose hearts have not become too severely damaged before the operation, the coronary bypass procedure may provide the patient with normal survival expectation. If the heart has already been severely damaged, however, the bypass procedure is likely to be of little value.

Coronary Angioplasty. Since the 1980s, a procedure has been used to open partially blocked coronary vessels before they become totally occluded. This procedure, called *coronary artery angioplasty,* is the following: A small balloon-tipped catheter, about 1 millimeter in diameter, is passed under radiographic guidance into the coronary system and pushed through the partially occluded artery until the balloon portion of the catheter straddles the partially occluded point. Then the balloon is inflated with high pressure, which markedly stretches the diseased artery. After this procedure is performed, the blood flow through the vessel often increases threefold to fourfold, and more than 75 percent of the patients who undergo the procedure are relieved of the coronary ischemic symptoms for at least several years, although many of the patients still eventually require coronary bypass surgery.

Small stainless steel mesh tubes called "stents" are sometimes placed inside a coronary artery dilated by angioplasty to hold the artery open, thus preventing its restenosis. Within a few weeks after the stent is placed in the coronary artery, the endothelium usually grows over the metal surface of the stent, allowing blood to flow smoothly through the stent. However, reclosure (restenosis) of the blocked coronary artery occurs in about 25 to 40 percent of patients treated with angioplasty, often within 6 months of the initial procedure. This is usually due to excessive formation of scar tissue that develops underneath the healthy new endothelium that has grown over the stent. Stents that slowly release drugs (drug-eluting stents) may help to prevent the excessive growth of scar tissue.

Newer procedures for opening atherosclerotic coronary arteries are constantly in experimental development. One of these employs a laser beam from the tip of a coronary artery catheter aimed at the atherosclerotic lesion. The laser literally dissolves the lesion without substantially damaging the rest of the arterial wall.

Bibliography

Cohn PF, Fox KM, Daly C: Silent myocardial ischemia, *Circulation* 108:1263, 2003.

Dalal H, Evans PH, Campbell JL: Recent developments in secondary prevention and cardiac rehabilitation after acute myocardial infarction, *BMJ* 328:693, 2004.

Duncker DJ, Bache RJ: Regulation of coronary blood flow during exercise, *Physiol Rev* 88:1009, 2008.

Freedman SB, Isner JM: Therapeutic angiogenesis for coronary artery disease, *Ann Intern Med* 136:54, 2002.

Gehlbach BK, Geppert E: The pulmonary manifestations of left heart failure, *Chest* 125:669, 2004.

González-Alonso J, Crandall CG, Johnson JM: The cardiovascular challenge of exercising in the heat, *J Physiol* 586:45, 2008.

Guyton AC, Jones CE, Coleman TG: *Circulatory pathology: Cardiac output and its regulation*, Philadelphia, 1973, WB Saunders.

Hester RL, Hammer LW: Venular-arteriolar communication in the regulation of blood flow, *Am J Physiol* 282:R1280, 2002.

Joyner MJ, Wilkins BW: Exercise hyperaemia: is anything obligatory but the hyperaemia? *J Physiol* 583:855, 2007.

Koerselman J, van der Graaf Y, de Jaegere PP, et al: Coronary collaterals: an important and underexposed aspect of coronary artery disease, *Circulation* 107:2507, 2003.

Levine BD: VO2max: what do we know, and what do we still need to know? *J Physiol* 586:25, 2008.

Reynolds HR, Hochman J: Cardiogenic shock: current concepts and improving outcomes, *Circulation* 117:686, 2008.

Richardson RS: Oxygen transport and utilization: an integration of the muscle systems, *Adv Physiol Educ* 27:183, 2003.

Renault MA, Losordo DW: Therapeutic myocardial angiogenesis, *Microvasc Res* 74:159, 2007.

Saltin B: Exercise hyperaemia: magnitude and aspects on regulation in humans, *J Physiol* 583:819, 2007.

Tsai AG, Johnson PC, Intaglietta M: Oxygen gradients in the microcirculation, *Physiol Rev* 83:933, 2003.

Yellon DM, Downey JM: Preconditioning the myocardium: from cellular physiology to clinical cardiology, *Physiol Rev* 83:1113, 2003.

Cardiac Failure

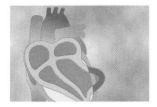

One of the most important ailments that must be treated by the physician is cardiac failure ("heart failure"). This can result from any heart condition that reduces the ability of the heart to pump blood. The cause is usually decreased contractility of the myocardium resulting from diminished coronary blood flow. However, failure can also be caused by damaged heart valves, external pressure around the heart, vitamin B deficiency, primary cardiac muscle disease, or any other abnormality that makes the heart a hypoeffective pump.

In this chapter, we discuss mainly cardiac failure caused by ischemic heart disease resulting from partial blockage of the coronary blood vessels, the most common cause of heart failure. In Chapter 23, we discuss valvular and congenital heart disease.

Definition of Cardiac Failure. The term "cardiac failure" means simply failure of the heart to pump enough blood to satisfy the needs of the body.

Circulatory Dynamics in Cardiac Failure

Acute Effects of Moderate Cardiac Failure

If a heart suddenly becomes severely damaged, such as by myocardial infarction, the pumping ability of the heart is immediately depressed. As a result, two main effects occur: (1) reduced cardiac output and (2) damming of blood in the veins, resulting in increased venous pressure.

The progressive changes in heart pumping effectiveness at different times after an acute myocardial infarction are shown graphically in Figure 22-1. The top curve of this figure shows a normal cardiac output curve. Point A on this curve is the normal operating point, showing a normal cardiac output under resting conditions of 5 L/min and a right atrial pressure of 0 mm Hg.

Immediately after the heart becomes damaged, the cardiac output curve becomes greatly lowered, falling to the lowest curve at the bottom of the graph. Within a few seconds, a new circulatory state is established at point B, illustrating that the cardiac output has fallen to 2 L/min, about two-fifths normal, whereas the right atrial pressure has risen to +4 mm Hg because venous blood returning to the heart from the body is dammed up in the right atrium. This low cardiac output is still sufficient to sustain life for perhaps a few hours, but it is likely to be associated with fainting. Fortunately, this acute stage usually lasts for only a few seconds because sympathetic nervous reflexes occur almost immediately and compensate, to a great extent, for the damaged heart, as follows.

Compensation for Acute Cardiac Failure by Sympathetic Nervous Reflexes. When the cardiac output falls precariously low, many of the circulatory reflexes discussed in Chapter 18 are rapidly activated. The best known of these is the *baroreceptor reflex,* which is activated by diminished arterial pressure. The *chemoreceptor reflex,* the *central nervous system ischemic response,* and even *reflexes that originate in the damaged heart* also likely contribute to activating the sympathetic nervous system. The sympathetics therefore become strongly stimulated within a few seconds, and the parasympathetic nervous signals to the heart become reciprocally inhibited at the same time.

Strong sympathetic stimulation has major effects on the heart itself and on the peripheral vasculature. If all the ventricular musculature is diffusely damaged but is still functional, sympathetic stimulation strengthens this damaged musculature. If part of the muscle is nonfunctional and part of it is still normal, the normal muscle is strongly stimulated by sympathetic stimulation, in this way partially compensating for the nonfunctional muscle. Thus, *the heart becomes a stronger pump* as a result of sympathetic stimulation. This effect is illustrated in Figure 22-1, showing after sympathetic compensation about twofold elevation of the very low cardiac output curve.

Sympathetic stimulation also increases venous return because it increases the tone of most of the blood vessels of the circulation, especially the veins, *raising the mean systemic filling* pressure to 12 to 14 mm Hg, almost 100 percent above normal. As discussed in Chapter 20, this increased filling pressure greatly increases the tendency for blood to flow from the veins back into the heart.

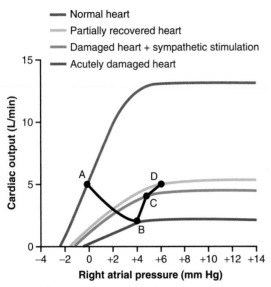

Figure 22-1 Progressive changes in the cardiac output curve after acute myocardial infarction. Both the cardiac output and right atrial pressure change progressively from point A to point D (illustrated by the black line) over a period of seconds, minutes, days, and weeks.

Therefore, the damaged heart becomes primed with more inflowing blood than usual, and the right atrial pressure rises still further, which helps the heart to pump still larger quantities of blood. Thus, in Figure 22-1, the new circulatory state is depicted by point C, showing a cardiac output of 4.2 L/min and a right atrial pressure of 5 mm Hg.

The sympathetic reflexes become maximally developed in about 30 seconds. Therefore, a person who has a sudden, moderate heart attack might experience nothing more than cardiac pain and a few seconds of fainting. Shortly thereafter, with the aid of the sympathetic reflex compensations, the cardiac output may return to a level adequate to sustain the person if he or she remains quiet, although the pain might persist.

Chronic Stage of Failure—Fluid Retention and Compensated Cardiac Output

After the first few minutes of an acute heart attack, a prolonged semichronic state begins, characterized mainly by two events: (1) retention of fluid by the kidneys and (2) varying degrees of recovery of the heart itself over a period of weeks to months, as illustrated by the light green curve in Figure 22-1; this was also discussed in Chapter 21.

Renal Retention of Fluid and Increase in Blood Volume Occur for Hours to Days

A low cardiac output has a profound effect on renal function, sometimes causing anuria when the cardiac output falls to 50 to 60 percent of normal. In general, the urine output remains below normal as long as the cardiac output and arterial pressure remain significantly less than normal; urine output usually does not return all the way to normal after an acute heart attack until the cardiac output and arterial pressure rise almost to normal levels.

Moderate Fluid Retention in Cardiac Failure Can Be Beneficial. Many cardiologists have considered fluid retention always to have a detrimental effect in cardiac failure. But it is now known that a moderate increase in body fluid and blood volume is an important factor in helping to compensate for the diminished pumping ability of the heart by increasing the venous return. The increased blood volume increases venous return in two ways: First, it increases the mean systemic filling pressure, which *increases the pressure gradient for causing venous flow of blood toward the heart*. Second, it distends the veins, which *reduces the venous resistance* and allows even more ease of flow of blood to the heart.

If the heart is not too greatly damaged, this increased venous return can often fully compensate for the heart's diminished pumping ability—enough that even when the heart's pumping ability is reduced to as low as 40 to 50 percent of normal, the increased venous return can often cause entirely nearly normal cardiac output as long as the person remains in a quiet resting state.

When the heart's pumping capability is reduced further, blood flow to the kidneys finally becomes too low for the kidneys to excrete enough salt and water to equal salt and water intake. Therefore, fluid retention begins and continues indefinitely, unless major therapeutic procedures are used to prevent this. Furthermore, because the heart is already pumping at its maximum pumping capacity, *this excess fluid no longer has a beneficial effect* on the circulation. Instead, the fluid retention increases the workload on the already damaged heart and severe edema develops throughout the body, which can be very detrimental in itself and can lead to death.

Detrimental Effects of Excess Fluid Retention in Severe Cardiac Failure. In contrast to the beneficial effects of moderate fluid retention in cardiac failure, in severe failure extreme excesses of fluid can have serious physiological consequences. They include (1) increasing the workload on the damaged heart, (2) overstretching of the heart, thus weakening the heart still more; (3) filtration of fluid into the lungs, causing pulmonary edema and consequent deoxygenation of the blood; and (4) development of extensive edema in most parts of the body. These detrimental effects of excessive fluid are discussed in later sections of this chapter.

Recovery of the Myocardium After Myocardial Infarction

After a heart becomes suddenly damaged as a result of myocardial infarction, the natural reparative processes of the body begin to help restore normal cardiac function. For instance, a new collateral blood supply begins to penetrate the peripheral portions of the infarcted area of the heart, often causing much of the heart muscle in the fringe areas to become functional again. Also, the undamaged portion of the heart musculature hypertrophies, in this way offsetting much of the cardiac damage.

The degree of recovery depends on the type of cardiac damage, and it varies from no recovery to almost complete recovery. After acute myocardial infarction, the heart ordinarily recovers rapidly during the first few days and weeks and achieves most of its final state of recovery within 5 to 7 weeks, although mild degrees of additional recovery can continue for months.

Cardiac Output Curve After Partial Recovery. Figure 22-1 shows function of the partially recovered heart a week or so after acute myocardial infarction. By this time, considerable fluid has been retained in the body and the tendency for venous return has increased markedly as well; therefore, the right atrial pressure has risen even more. As a result, the state of the circulation is now changed from point C to point D, which shows a normal cardiac output of 5 L/min but right atrial pressure increased to 6 mm Hg.

Because the cardiac output has returned to normal, renal output of fluid also returns to normal and no further fluid retention occurs, except that *the retention of fluid that has already occurred continues to maintain moderate excesses of fluid*. Therefore, except for the high right atrial pressure represented by point D in this figure, the person now has essentially normal cardiovascular dynamics *as long as he or she remains at rest*.

If the heart recovers to a significant extent and if adequate fluid volume has been retained, the sympathetic stimulation gradually abates toward normal for the following reasons: The partial recovery of the heart can elevate the cardiac output curve the same as sympathetic stimulation can. Therefore, as the heart recovers even slightly, the fast pulse rate, cold skin, and pallor resulting from sympathetic stimulation in the acute stage of cardiac failure gradually disappear.

Summary of the Changes That Occur After Acute Cardiac Failure—"Compensated Heart Failure"

To summarize the events discussed in the past few sections describing the dynamics of circulatory changes after an acute, moderate heart attack, we can divide the stages into (1) the instantaneous effect of the cardiac damage; (2) compensation by the sympathetic nervous system, which occurs mainly within the first 30 seconds to 1 minute; and (3) chronic compensations resulting from partial heart recovery and renal retention of fluid. All these changes are shown graphically by the black line in Figure 22-1. The progression of this line shows the normal state of the circulation (point A), the state a few seconds after the heart attack but before sympathetic reflexes have occurred (point B), the rise in cardiac output toward normal caused by sympathetic stimulation (point C), and final return of the cardiac output to almost normal after several days to several weeks of partial cardiac recovery and fluid retention (point D). This final state is called *compensated heart failure*.

Compensated Heart Failure. Note especially in Figure 22-1 that the maximum pumping ability of the partly recovered heart, as depicted by the plateau level of the light green curve, is still depressed to less than one-half normal. This demonstrates that an increase in right atrial pressure can maintain the cardiac output at a normal level despite continued weakness of the heart. Thus, many people, especially older people, have normal resting cardiac outputs but mildly to moderately elevated right atrial pressures because of various degrees of "compensated heart failure." These persons may not know that they have cardiac damage because the damage often has occurred a little at a time, and the compensation has occurred concurrently with the progressive stages of damage.

When a person is in compensated heart failure, any attempt to perform heavy exercise usually causes immediate return of the symptoms of acute failure because the heart is not able to increase its pumping capacity to the levels required for the exercise. Therefore, it is said that the *cardiac reserve* is reduced in compensated heart failure. This concept of cardiac reserve is discussed more fully later in the chapter.

Dynamics of Severe Cardiac Failure— Decompensated Heart Failure

If the heart becomes severely damaged, no amount of compensation, either by sympathetic nervous reflexes or by fluid retention, can make the excessively weakened heart pump a normal cardiac output. As a consequence, the cardiac output cannot rise high enough to make the kidneys excrete normal quantities of fluid. Therefore, fluid continues to be retained, the person develops more and more edema, and this state of events eventually leads to death. This is called *decompensated heart failure*. Thus, the main cause of decompensated heart failure is failure of the heart to pump sufficient blood to make the kidneys excrete daily the necessary amounts of fluid.

Graphical Analysis of Decompensated Heart Failure. Figure 22-2 shows greatly depressed cardiac output at different times (points A to F) after the heart has become severely weakened. Point A on this curve represents the approximate state of the circulation before any compensation has occurred, and point B, the state a few minutes later after sympathetic stimulation has

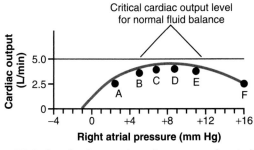

Figure 22-2 Greatly depressed cardiac output that indicates decompensated heart disease. Progressive fluid retention raises the right atrial pressure over a period of days, and the cardiac output progresses from point A to point F, until death occurs.

compensated as much as it can but before fluid retention has begun. At this time, the cardiac output has risen to 4 L/min and the right atrial pressure has risen to 5 mm Hg. The person appears to be in reasonably good condition, but this state will not remain stable because the cardiac output has not risen high enough to cause adequate kidney excretion of fluid; therefore, fluid retention continues and can eventually be the cause of death. These events can be explained quantitatively in the following way.

Note the straight line in Figure 22-2, at a cardiac output level of 5 L/min. This is approximately the critical cardiac output level that is required in the normal adult person to make the kidneys re-establish normal fluid balance—that is, for the output of salt and water to be as great as the intake of these. At any cardiac output below this level, all the fluid-retaining mechanisms discussed in the earlier section remain in play and the body fluid volume increases progressively. And because of this progressive increase in fluid volume, the mean systemic filling pressure of the circulation continues to rise; this forces progressively increasing quantities of blood from the person's peripheral veins into the right atrium, thus increasing the right atrial pressure. After 1 day or so, the state of the circulation changes in Figure 22-2 from point B to point C—the right atrial pressure rising to 7 mm Hg and the cardiac output to 4.2 L/min. Note again that the cardiac output is still not high enough to cause normal renal output of fluid; therefore, fluid continues to be retained. After another day or so, the right atrial pressure rises to 9 mm Hg, and the circulatory state becomes that depicted by point D. Still, the cardiac output is not enough to establish normal fluid balance.

After another few days of fluid retention, the right atrial pressure has risen still further, but by now, cardiac function is beginning to decline toward a lower level. This decline is caused by overstretch of the heart, edema of the heart muscle, and other factors that diminish the heart's pumping performance. It is now clear that further retention of fluid will be more detrimental than beneficial to the circulation. Yet the cardiac output still is not high enough to bring about normal renal function, so fluid retention not only continues but accelerates because of the falling cardiac output (and falling arterial pressure that also occurs). Consequently, within a few days, the state of the circulation has reached point F on the curve, with the cardiac output now less than 2.5 L/min and the right atrial pressure 16 mm Hg. This state has approached or reached incompatibility with life, and the patient dies unless this chain of events can be reversed. This state of heart failure in which the failure continues to worsen is called *decompensated heart failure.*

Thus, one can see from this analysis that failure of the cardiac output (and arterial pressure) to rise to the critical level required for normal renal function results in (1) progressive retention of more and more fluid, which causes (2) progressive elevation of the mean systemic filling pressure, and (3) progressive elevation of the right atrial pressure until finally the heart is so overstretched or so edematous that it cannot pump even moderate quantities of blood and, therefore, fails completely. Clinically, one detects this serious condition of decompensation principally by the progressing edema, especially edema of the lungs, which leads to bubbling *rales* (a crackling sound) in the lungs and to *dyspnea* (air hunger). Lack of appropriate therapy when this state of events occurs rapidly leads to death.

Treatment of Decompensation. The decompensation process can often be stopped by (1) *strengthening the heart* in any one of several ways, especially by administration of a cardiotonic drug, such as *digitalis,* so that the heart becomes strong enough to pump adequate quantities of blood required to make the kidneys function normally again, or (2) *administering diuretic drugs to increase kidney excretion* while at the same time reducing water and salt intake, which brings about a balance between fluid intake and output despite low cardiac output.

Both methods stop the decompensation process by re-establishing normal fluid balance so that at least as much fluid leaves the body as enters it.

Mechanism of Action of the Cardiotonic Drugs Such as Digitalis. Cardiotonic drugs, such as digitalis, when administered to a person with a healthy heart, have little effect on increasing the contractile strength of the cardiac muscle. However, when administered to a person with a chronically failing heart, the same drugs can sometimes increase the strength of the failing myocardium as much as 50 to 100 percent. Therefore, they are one of the mainstays of therapy in chronic heart failure.

Digitalis and other cardiotonic glycosides are believed to strengthen heart contractions by increasing the quantity of calcium ions in muscle fibers. This effect is likely due to inhibition of sodium-potassium ATPase in cardiac cell membranes. Inhibition of the sodium-potassium pump increases intracellular sodium concentration and slows the sodium-calcium exchange pump, which extrudes calcium from the cell in exchange for sodium. Because the sodium-calcium exchange pump relies on a high sodium gradient across the cell membrane, accumulation of sodium inside the cell reduces its activity.

In the failing heart muscle, the sarcoplasmic reticulum fails to accumulate normal quantities of calcium and, therefore, cannot release enough calcium ions into the free-fluid compartment of the muscle fibers to cause full contraction of the muscle. The effect of digitalis to depress the sodium-calcium exchange pump and raise calcium ion concentration in cardiac muscle provides the extra calcium needed to increase the muscle contractile force. Therefore, it is usually beneficial to depress the calcium pumping mechanism a moderate amount using digitalis, allowing the muscle fiber intracellular calcium level to rise slightly.

Unilateral Left Heart Failure

In the discussions thus far in this chapter, we have considered failure of the heart as a whole. Yet, in a large number of patients, especially those with early acute failure, left-sided failure predominates over right-sided failure, and, in rare instances, the right side fails without significant failure of the left side. Therefore, we need to discuss the special features of unilateral heart failure.

When the left side of the heart fails without concomitant failure of the right side, blood continues to be pumped into the lungs with usual right heart vigor, whereas it is not pumped adequately out of the lungs by the left heart into the systemic circulation. As a result, the *mean pulmonary filling pressure* rises because of shift of large volumes of blood from the systemic circulation into the pulmonary circulation.

As the volume of blood in the lungs increases, the pulmonary capillary pressure increases, and if this rises above a value approximately equal to the colloid osmotic pressure of the plasma, about 28 mm Hg, fluid begins to filter out of the capillaries into the lung interstitial spaces and alveoli, resulting in pulmonary edema.

Thus, among the most important problems of left heart failure are *pulmonary vascular congestion* and *pulmonary edema.* In severe, acute left heart failure, pulmonary edema occasionally occurs so rapidly that it can cause death by suffocation in 20 to 30 minutes, which we discuss later in the chapter.

Low-Output Cardiac Failure—Cardiogenic Shock

In many instances after acute heart attacks and often after prolonged periods of slow progressive cardiac deterioration, the heart becomes incapable of pumping even the minimal amount of blood flow required to keep the body alive. Consequently, the body tissues begin to suffer and even to deteriorate, often leading to death within a few hours to a few days. The picture then is one of circulatory shock, as explained in Chapter 24. Even the cardiovascular system suffers from lack of nutrition, and it, too (along with the remainder of the body), deteriorates, thus hastening death. This circulatory shock syndrome caused by inadequate cardiac pumping is called *cardiogenic shock* or simply *cardiac shock.* Once a person develops cardiogenic shock, the survival rate is often less than 30 percent even with appropriate medical care.

Vicious Circle of Cardiac Deterioration in Cardiogenic Shock.

The discussion of circulatory shock in Chapter 24 emphasizes the tendency for the heart to become progressively more damaged when its coronary blood supply is reduced during the course of the shock. That is, the low arterial pressure that occurs during shock reduces the coronary blood supply even more. This makes the heart still weaker, which makes the arterial pressure fall still more, which makes the shock progressively worse, the process eventually becoming a vicious circle of cardiac deterioration. In cardiogenic shock caused by myocardial infarction, this problem is greatly compounded by already existing coronary vessel blockage. For instance, in a healthy heart, the arterial pressure usually must be reduced below about 45 mm Hg before cardiac deterioration sets in. However, in a heart that already has a blocked major coronary vessel, deterioration begins when the coronary arterial pressure falls below 80 to 90 mm Hg. In other words, even a small decrease in arterial pressure can now set off a vicious circle of cardiac deterioration. For this reason, in treating myocardial infarction, it is extremely important to prevent even short periods of hypotension.

Physiology of Treatment.

Often a patient dies of cardiogenic shock before the various compensatory processes can return the cardiac output (and arterial pressure) to a life-sustaining level. Therefore, treatment of this condition is one of the most important problems in the management of acute heart attacks.

Immediate administration of digitalis is often used for strengthening the heart if the ventricular muscle shows signs of deterioration. Also, infusion of whole blood, plasma, or a blood pressure–raising drug is used to sustain the arterial pressure. If the arterial pressure can be elevated high enough, the coronary blood flow often will increase enough to prevent the vicious circle of deterioration. And this allows enough time for appropriate compensatory mechanisms in circulatory system to correct the shock.

Some success has also been achieved in saving the lives of patients in cardiogenic shock by using one of the following procedures: (1) surgically removing the clot in the coronary artery, often in combination with coronary bypass graft, or (2) catheterizing the blocked coronary artery and infusing either *streptokinase* or *tissue-type plasminogen activator* enzymes that cause dissolution of the clot. The results are occasionally astounding when one of these procedures is instituted within the first hour of cardiogenic shock but of little, if any, benefit after 3 hours.

Edema in Patients with Cardiac Failure

Inability of Acute Cardiac Failure to Cause *Peripheral* Edema.

Acute *left* heart failure can cause rapid congestion of the lungs, with development of *pulmonary edema* and even death within minutes to hours.

However, either left or right heart failure is very slow to cause *peripheral edema.* This can best be explained by referring to Figure 22-3. When a previously healthy heart acutely fails as a pump, the aortic pressure falls and the right atrial pressure rises. As the cardiac output approaches zero, these two pressures approach each other at an equilibrium value of about 13 mm Hg.

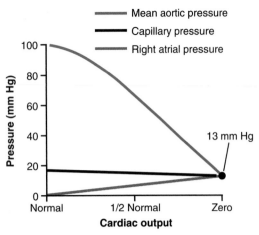

Figure 22-3 Progressive changes in mean aortic pressure, peripheral tissue capillary pressure, and right atrial pressure as the cardiac output falls from normal to zero.

Capillary pressure also falls from its normal value of 17 mm Hg to the new equilibrium pressure of 13 mm Hg. Thus, *severe acute cardiac failure often causes a fall in peripheral capillary pressure rather than a rise.* Therefore, animal experiments, as well as experience in humans, show that acute cardiac failure almost never causes immediate development of peripheral edema.

Long-Term Fluid Retention by the Kidneys—the Cause of Peripheral Edema in Persisting Heart Failure

After the first day or so of overall heart failure or of right-ventricular heart failure, peripheral edema does begin to occur principally *because of fluid retention by the kidneys*. The retention of fluid increases the mean systemic filling pressure, resulting in increased tendency for blood to return to the heart. This elevates the right atrial pressure to a still higher value and returns the arterial pressure back toward normal. Therefore, *the capillary pressure now also rises markedly*, thus causing loss of fluid into the tissues and development of severe edema.

There are several known causes of the reduced renal output of urine during cardiac failure.

1. **Decreased glomerular filtration rate.** A decrease in cardiac output has a tendency to reduce the glomerular pressure in the kidneys because of (1) *reduced arterial pressure* and (2) *intense sympathetic constriction of the afferent arterioles of the kidney.* As a consequence, except in the mildest degrees of heart failure, the glomerular filtration rate becomes less than normal. It is clear from the discussion of kidney function in Chapters 26 through 29 that *even a slight decrease in glomerular filtration often markedly decreases urine output.* When the cardiac output falls to about one-half normal, this can result in almost complete anuria.

2. **Activation of the renin-angiotensin system and increased reabsorption of water and salt by the renal tubules.** The reduced blood flow to the kidneys causes marked increase in *renin secretion* by the kidneys, and this in turn increases the *formation of angiotensin II,* as described in Chapter 19. The angiotensin in turn has a direct effect on the arterioles of the kidneys to decrease further the blood flow through the kidneys, which reduces the pressure in the peritubular capillaries surrounding the renal tubules, promoting greatly increased reabsorption of both water and salt from the tubules. Angiotensin also acts directly on the renal tubular epithelial cells to stimulate reabsorption of salt and water. Therefore, loss of water and salt into the urine decreases greatly, and large quantities of salt and water accumulate in the blood and interstitial fluids everywhere in the body.

3. **Increased aldosterone secretion.** In the chronic stage of heart failure, large quantities of aldosterone are secreted by the adrenal cortex. This results mainly from the effect of angiotensin to stimulate aldosterone secretion by the adrenal cortex. But some of the increase in aldosterone secretion often results from increased plasma potassium. Excess potassium is one of the most powerful stimuli known for aldosterone secretion, and the potassium concentration rises in response to reduced renal function in cardiac failure.

   The elevated aldosterone level further increases the reabsorption of sodium from the renal tubules. This in turn leads to a secondary increase in water reabsorption for two reasons: First, as the sodium is reabsorbed, it reduces the osmotic pressure in the tubules but increases the osmotic pressure in the renal interstitial fluids; these changes promote osmosis of water into the blood. Second, the absorbed sodium and anions that go with the sodium, mainly chloride ions, increase the osmotic concentration of the extracellular fluid everywhere in the body. This elicits *antidiuretic hormone* secretion by the hypothalamic-posterior pituitary gland system (discussed in Chapter 29). The antidiuretic hormone in turn promotes still greater increase in tubular reabsorption of water.

4. **Activation of the sympathetic nervous system.** As discussed previously, heart failure causes marked activation of the sympathetic nervous system, which in turn has several effects that lead to salt and water retention by the kidneys: (1) constriction of renal afferent arterioles, which reduces glomerular filtration rate; (2) stimulation of renal tubular reabsorption of salt and water by activation of alpha-adrenergic receptors on tubular epithelial cells; (3) stimulation of renin release and angiotensin II formation, which increases renal tubular reabsorption; and (4) stimulation of antidiuretic hormone release from the posterior pituitary, which then increases water reabsorption by the renal tubules. These effects of sympathetic stimulation are discussed in more detail in Chapters 26 and 27.

Role of Atrial Natriuretic Peptide to Delay Onset of Cardiac Decompensation. *Atrial natriuretic peptide*

(ANP) is a hormone released by the atrial walls of the heart when they become stretched. Because heart failure almost always increases both the right and left atrial pressures that stretch the atrial walls, the circulating levels of ANP in the blood may increase 5- to 10-fold in severe heart failure. The ANP in turn has a direct effect on the kidneys to increase greatly their excretion of salt and water. Therefore, ANP plays a natural role to help prevent extreme congestive symptoms during cardiac failure. The renal effects of ANP are discussed in Chapter 29.

Acute Pulmonary Edema in Late-Stage Heart Failure—Another Lethal Vicious Circle

A frequent cause of death in heart failure is *acute pulmonary edema* occurring in patients who have already had chronic heart failure for a long time. When this occurs in a person without new cardiac damage, it usually is set off by some temporary overload of the heart, such as might result from a bout of heavy exercise, some emotional experience, or even a severe cold. The acute pulmonary edema is believed to result from the following vicious circle:

1. A temporarily increased load on the already weak left ventricle initiates the vicious circle. Because of limited pumping capacity of the left heart, blood begins to dam up in the lungs.

2. The increased blood in the lungs elevates the pulmonary capillary pressure, and a small amount of fluid begins to transude into the lung tissues and alveoli.

3. The increased fluid in the lungs diminishes the degree of oxygenation of the blood.

4. The decreased oxygen in the blood further weakens the heart and also weakens the arterioles everywhere in the body, thus causing peripheral vasodilation.

5. The peripheral vasodilation increases venous return of blood from the peripheral circulation still more.

6. The increased venous return further increases the damming of the blood in the lungs, leading to still more transudation of fluid, more arterial oxygen desaturation, more venous return, and so forth. Thus, a vicious circle has been established.

Once this vicious circle has proceeded beyond a certain critical point, it will continue until death of the patient unless heroic therapeutic measures are used within minutes. The types of heroic therapeutic measures that can reverse the process and save the patient's life include the following:

1. Putting tourniquets on both arms and legs to sequester much of the blood in the veins and, therefore, decrease the workload on the left side of the heart

2. Giving a rapidly acting diuretic, such as furosemide, to cause rapid loss of fluid from the body

3. Giving the patient pure oxygen to breathe to reverse the blood oxygen desaturation, the heart deterioration, and the peripheral vasodilation

4. Giving the patient a rapidly acting cardiotonic drug, such as digitalis, to strengthen the heart

This vicious circle of acute pulmonary edema can proceed so rapidly that death can occur in 20 minutes to 1 hour. Therefore, any procedure that is to be successful must be instituted immediately.

Cardiac Reserve

The maximum percentage that the cardiac output can increase above normal is called the *cardiac reserve*. Thus, in the healthy young adult, the cardiac reserve is 300 to 400 percent. In athletically trained persons, it is 500 to 600 percent or more. But in heart failure, there is no cardiac reserve. As an example of normal reserve, during severe exercise the cardiac output of a healthy young adult can rise to about five times normal; this is an increase above normal of 400 percent—that is, *a cardiac reserve of 400 percent*.

Any factor that prevents the heart from pumping blood satisfactorily will decrease the cardiac reserve. This can result from ischemic heart disease, primary myocardial disease, vitamin deficiency that affects cardiac muscle, physical damage to the myocardium, valvular heart disease, and many other factors, some of which are shown in Figure 22-4.

Diagnosis of Low Cardiac Reserve—Exercise Test. As long as persons with low cardiac reserve remain in a state of rest, they usually will not experience major symptoms of heart disease. However, a diagnosis of low cardiac reserve usually can be easily made by requiring the person to exercise either on a treadmill or by walking up and down steps, either of which requires greatly increased cardiac output. The increased load on the heart rapidly uses up the small amount of reserve that is available, and the cardiac output soon fails to rise high enough to sustain the body's new level of activity. The acute effects are as follows:

1. Immediate and sometimes extreme shortness of breath (dyspnea) resulting from failure of the heart to pump

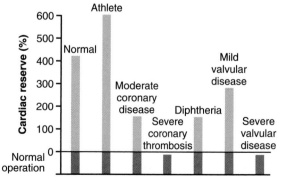

Figure 22-4 Cardiac reserve in different conditions, showing less than zero reserve for two of the conditions.

sufficient blood to the tissues, thereby causing tissue ischemia and creating a sensation of air hunger

2. Extreme muscle fatigue resulting from muscle ischemia, thus limiting the person's ability to continue with the exercise

3. Excessive increase in heart rate because the nervous reflexes to the heart overreact in an attempt to overcome the inadequate cardiac output

Exercise tests are part of the armamentarium of the cardiologist. These tests take the place of cardiac output measurements that cannot be made with ease in most clinical settings.

Quantitative Graphical Method for Analysis of Cardiac Failure

Although it is possible to understand most general principles of cardiac failure using mainly qualitative logic, as we have done thus far in this chapter, one can grasp the importance of the different factors in cardiac failure with far greater depth by using more quantitative approaches. One such approach is the graphical method for analysis of cardiac output regulation introduced in Chapter 20. In the remaining sections of this chapter, we analyze several aspects of cardiac failure, using this graphical technique.

Graphical Analysis of Acute Heart Failure and Chronic Compensation

Figure 22-5 shows *cardiac output* and *venous return curves* for different states of the heart and peripheral circulation. The two curves passing through Point A are (1) the *normal cardiac output curve* and (2) the *normal venous return curve*. As pointed out in Chapter 20, there is only one point on each of these two curves at which the circulatory system can operate—point A where the two curves cross. Therefore, the normal state of the circulation is a cardiac output and venous return of 5 L/min and a right atrial pressure of 0 mm Hg.

Effect of Acute Heart Attack. During the first few seconds after a moderately severe heart attack, the cardiac output curve falls to the *lowermost curve*. During these few seconds, the venous return curve still has not changed because the peripheral circulatory system is still operating normally. Therefore, the new state of the circulation is depicted by point B, where the new cardiac output curve crosses the normal venous return curve. Thus, the right atrial pressure rises immediately to 4 mm Hg, whereas the cardiac output falls to 2 L/min.

Effect of Sympathetic Reflexes. Within the next 30 seconds, the sympathetic reflexes become very active. They raise both the cardiac output and the venous return curves. Sympathetic stimulation can increase the plateau level of the cardiac output curve as much as 30 to 100 percent. It can also increase the mean systemic filling pressure (depicted by the point where the venous return curve crosses the zero venous return axis) by several millimeters of mercury—in this figure, from a normal value of 7 mm Hg up to 10 mm Hg. This increase in mean systemic filling pressure shifts the entire venous return curve to the right and upward. The new cardiac output and venous return curves now equilibrate at point C, that is, at a right atrial pressure of +5 mm Hg and a cardiac output of 4 L/min.

Compensation During the Next Few Days. During the ensuing week, the cardiac output and venous return curves rise further because of (1) some recovery of the heart and (2) renal retention of salt and water, which raises the mean systemic filling pressure still further—this time up to +12 mm Hg. The two new curves now equilibrate at point D. Thus, the cardiac output has now returned to normal. The right atrial pressure, however, has risen still further to +6 mm Hg. Because the cardiac output is now normal, renal output is also normal, so a new state of equilibrated fluid balance has been achieved. The circulatory system will continue to function at point D and remain stable, with a normal cardiac output and an elevated right atrial pressure, until some additional extrinsic factor changes either the cardiac output curve or the venous return curve.

Using this technique for analysis, one can see especially the importance of moderate fluid retention and how it eventually leads to a new stable state of the circulation in mild to moderate heart failure. And one can also see the interrelation between mean systemic filling pressure and cardiac pumping at various degrees of heart failure.

Note that the events described in Figure 22-5 are the same as those presented in Figure 22-1, but in Figure 22-5, they are presented in a more quantitative manner.

Graphical Analysis of "Decompensated" Cardiac Failure

The black cardiac output curve in Figure 22-6 is the same as the curve shown in Figure 22-2, a greatly depressed curve that has already reached a degree of recovery as great as this heart can achieve. In this figure, we have added venous return curves that occur during successive days after the acute fall of the cardiac output curve to this low level. At point A, the curve at time zero equates with the normal venous return curve to give a cardiac output of about 3 L/min. However, stimulation of the sympathetic nervous system, caused by this low cardiac output, increases the mean systemic filling pressure within 30 seconds from 7 to 10.5 mm Hg. This shifts the venous

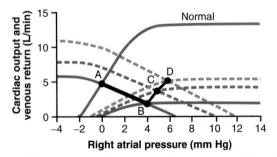

Figure 22-5 Progressive changes in cardiac output and right atrial pressure during different stages of cardiac failure.

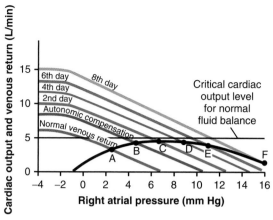

Figure 22-6 Graphical analysis of decompensated heart disease showing progressive shift of the venous return curve to the right as a result of continued fluid retention.

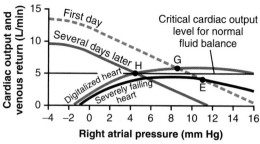

Figure 22-7 Treatment of decompensated heart disease showing the effect of digitalis in elevating the cardiac output curve, this in turn causing increased urine output and progressive shift of the venous return curve to the left.

return curve upward and to the right to produce the curve labeled "autonomic compensation." Thus, the new venous return curve equates with the cardiac output curve at point B. The cardiac output has been improved to a level of 4 L/min but at the expense of an additional rise in right atrial pressure to 5 mm Hg.

The cardiac output of 4 L/min is still too low to cause the kidneys to function normally. Therefore, fluid continues to be retained, and the mean systemic filling pressure rises from 10.5 to almost 13 mm Hg. Now the venous return curve becomes that labeled "2nd day" and equilibrates with the cardiac output curve at point C. The cardiac output rises to 4.2 L/min and the right atrial pressure to 7 mm Hg.

During the succeeding days, the cardiac output never rises quite high enough to re-establish normal renal function. Fluid continues to be retained, the mean systemic filling pressure continues to rise, the venous return curve continues to shift to the right, and the equilibrium point between the venous return curve and the cardiac output curve also shifts progressively to point D, to point E, and, finally, to point F. The equilibration process is now on the down slope of the cardiac output curve, so further retention of fluid causes even more severe cardiac edema and a detrimental effect on cardiac output. The condition accelerates downhill until death occurs.

Thus, "decompensation" results from the fact that the cardiac output curve never rises to the critical level of 5 L/min needed to re-establish normal kidney excretion of fluid that would be required to cause balance between fluid input and output.

Treatment of Decompensated Heart Disease with Digitalis. Let us assume that the stage of decompensation has already reached point E in Figure 22-6, and let us proceed to the same point E in Figure 22-7. At this time, digitalis is given to strengthen the heart. This raises the cardiac output curve to the level shown in Figure 22-7, but there is not an immediate change in the venous return curve. Therefore, the new cardiac output curve equates

with the venous return curve at point G. The cardiac output is now 5.7 L/min, a value greater than the critical level of 5 liters required to make the kidneys excrete normal amounts of urine. Therefore, the kidneys eliminate much more fluid than normally, causing *diuresis*, a well-known therapeutic effect of digitalis.

The progressive loss of fluid over a period of several days reduces the mean systemic filling pressure back down to 11.5 mm Hg, and the new venous return curve becomes the curve labeled "Several days later." This curve equates with the cardiac output curve of the digitalized heart at point H, at an output of 5 L/min and a right atrial pressure of 4.6 mm Hg. This cardiac output is precisely that required for normal fluid balance. Therefore, no additional fluid will be lost and none will be gained. Consequently, the circulatory system has now stabilized, or in other words, the decompensation of the heart failure has been "compensated." And to state this another way, the final steady-state condition of the circulation is defined by the crossing point of three curves: the cardiac output curve, the venous return curve, and the critical level for normal fluid balance. The compensatory mechanisms automatically stabilize the circulation when all three curves cross at the same point.

Graphical Analysis of High-Output Cardiac Failure

Figure 22-8 gives an analysis of two types of high-output cardiac failure. One of these is caused by an *arteriovenous fistula* that overloads the heart because of excessive venous return, even though the pumping capability of the heart is not depressed. The other is caused by *beriberi*, in which the venous return is greatly increased because of diminished systemic vascular resistance, but at the same time, the pumping capability of the heart is depressed.

Arteriovenous Fistula. The "normal" curves of Figure 22-8 depict the normal cardiac output and normal venous return curves. These equate with each other at point A, which depicts a normal cardiac output of 5 L/min and a normal right atrial pressure of 0 mm Hg.

Now let us assume that the systemic vascular resistance (the *total peripheral vascular resistance*) becomes greatly decreased because of opening a large arteriovenous fistula (a direct opening between a large artery and a large vein). The venous return curve rotates upward to give the curve

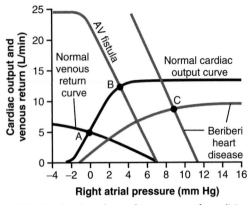

Figure 22-8 Graphical analysis of two types of conditions that can cause high-output cardiac failure: (1) arteriovenous (AV) fistula and (2) beriberi heart disease.

The two blue curves (cardiac output curve and venous return curve) intersect with each other at point C, which describes the circulatory condition in beriberi, with a right atrial pressure in this instance of 9 mm Hg and a cardiac output about 65 percent above normal; this high cardiac output occurs despite the weak heart, as demonstrated by the depressed plateau level of the cardiac output curve.

labeled "AV fistula." This venous return curve equates with the normal cardiac output curve at point B, with a cardiac output of 12.5 L/min and a right atrial pressure of 3 mm Hg. Thus, the cardiac output has become greatly elevated, the right atrial pressure is slightly elevated, and there are mild signs of peripheral congestion. If the person attempts to exercise, he or she will have little cardiac reserve because the heart is already at near-maximum capacity to pump the extra blood through the arteriovenous fistula. This condition resembles a failure condition and is called "high-output failure," but in reality, the heart is overloaded by excess venous return.

Beriberi. Figure 22-8 shows the approximate changes in the cardiac output and venous return curves caused by *beriberi.* The decreased level of the cardiac output curve is caused by weakening of the heart because of the avitaminosis (mainly lack of thiamine) that causes the beriberi syndrome. The weakening of the heart has decreased the blood flow to the kidneys. Therefore, the kidneys have retained a large amount of extra body fluid, which in turn has increased the mean systemic filling pressure (represented by the point where the venous return curve now intersects the zero cardiac output level) from the normal value of 7 mm Hg up to 11 mm Hg. This has shifted the venous return curve to the right. Finally, the venous return curve has rotated upward from the normal curve because the avitaminosis has dilated the peripheral blood vessels, as explained in Chapter 17.

Bibliography

Abraham WT, Greenberg BH, Yancy CW: Pharmacologic therapies across the continuum of left ventricular dysfunction, *Am J Cardiol* 102:21G–28G, 2008.

Andrew P: Diastolic heart failure demystified, *Chest* 124:744, 2003.

Bers DM: Altered cardiac myocyte Ca regulation in heart failure, *Physiology (Bethesda)* 21:380, 2006.

Braunwald E: Biomarkers in heart failure, *N Engl J Med* 358:2148, 2008.

Dorn GW 2nd, Molkentin JD: Manipulating cardiac contractility in heart failure: data from mice and men, *Circulation* 109:150, 2004.

Floras JS: Sympathetic activation in human heart failure: diverse mechanisms, therapeutic opportunities, *Acta Physiol Scand* 177:391, 2003.

Guyton AC, Jones CE, Coleman TG: *Circulatory physiology: cardiac output and its regulation*, Philadelphia, 1973, WB Saunders.

Haddad F, Doyle R, Murphy DJ, et al: Right ventricular function in cardiovascular disease, part II: pathophysiology, clinical importance, and management of right ventricular failure, *Circulation* 117:1717, 2008.

Ikeda Y, Hoshijima M, Chien KR: Toward biologically targeted therapy of calcium cycling defects in heart failure, *Physiology (Bethesda)* 23:6, 2008.

Lohmeier TE: Neurohumoral regulation of arterial pressure in hemorrhage and heart failure, *Am J Physiol Regul Integr Comp Physiol* 283:R810, 2002.

Mehra MR, Gheorghiade M, Bonow RO: Mitral regurgitation in chronic heart failure: more questions than answers? *Curr Cardiol Rep* 6:96, 2004.

McMurray J, Pfeffer MA: New therapeutic options in congestive heart failure: Part I, *Circulation* 105:2099, 2002.

McMurray J, Pfeffer MA: New therapeutic options in congestive heart failure: Part II, *Circulation* 105:2223, 2002.

Morita H, Seidman J, Seidman CE: Genetic causes of human heart failure, *J Clin Invest* 115:518, 2005.

Pfisterer M: Right ventricular involvement in myocardial infarction and cardiogenic shock, *Lancet* 362:392, 2003.

Pitt B: Aldosterone blockade in patients with chronic heart failure, *Cardiol Clin* 26:15, 2008.

Reynolds HR, Hochman JS: Cardiogenic shock: Current concepts and improving outcomes, *Circulation* 117:686, 2008.

Spodick DH: Acute cardiac tamponade, *N Engl J Med* 349:684, 2003.

Zile MR, Brutsaert DL: New concepts in diastolic dysfunction and diastolic heart failure: Part I: diagnosis, prognosis, and measurements of diastolic function, *Circulation* 105:1387, 2002.

Zucker IH: Novel mechanisms of sympathetic regulation in chronic heart failure, *Hypertension* 48:1005, 2006.

Heart Valves and Heart Sounds; Valvular and Congenital Heart Defects

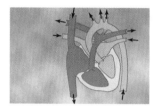

Function of the heart valves was discussed in Chapter 9, where it was pointed out that *closing* of the valves causes audible sounds. Ordinarily, no audible sounds occur when the valves open. In this chapter, we first discuss the factors that cause the sounds in the heart under normal and abnormal conditions. Then we discuss the overall circulatory changes that occur when valvular or congenital heart defects are present.

Heart Sounds

Normal Heart Sounds

Listening with a stethoscope to a normal heart, one hears a sound usually described as "lub, dub, lub, dub." The "lub" is associated with closure of the atrioventricular (A-V) valves at the beginning of systole, and the "dub" is associated with closure of the semilunar (aortic and pulmonary) valves at the end of systole. The "lub" sound is called the *first heart sound*, and the "dub" is called the *second heart sound*, because the normal pumping cycle of the heart is considered to start when the A-V valves close at the onset of ventricular systole.

Causes of the First and Second Heart Sounds. The earliest explanation for the cause of the heart sounds was that the "slapping" together of the valve leaflets sets up vibrations. However, this has been shown to cause little, if any, of the sound, because the blood between the leaflets cushions the slapping effect and prevents significant sound. Instead, the cause is *vibration of the taut valves immediately after closure*, along with *vibration of the adjacent walls of the heart and major vessels around the heart.* That is, in generating the first heart sound, contraction of the ventricles first causes sudden backflow of blood against the A-V valves (the tricuspid and mitral valves), causing them to close and bulge toward the atria until the chordae tendineae abruptly stop the back bulging. The elastic tautness of the chordae tendineae and of

the valves then causes the back-surging blood to bounce forward again into each respective ventricle. This causes the blood and the ventricular walls, as well as the taut valves, to vibrate and causes vibrating turbulence in the blood. The vibrations travel through the adjacent tissues to the chest wall, where they can be heard as sound by using the stethoscope.

The second heart sound results from sudden closure of the semilunar valves at the end of systole. When the semilunar valves close, they bulge backward toward the ventricles and their elastic stretch recoils the blood back into the arteries, which causes a short period of reverberation of blood back and forth between the walls of the arteries and the semilunar valves, as well as between these valves and the ventricular walls. The vibrations occurring in the arterial walls are then transmitted mainly along the arteries. When the vibrations of the vessels or ventricles come into contact with a "sounding board," such as the chest wall, they create sound that can be heard.

Duration and Pitch of the First and Second Heart Sounds. The duration of each of the heart sounds is slightly more than 0.10 second—the first sound about 0.14 second, and the second about 0.11 second. The reason for the shorter second sound is that the semilunar valves are more taut than the A-V valves, so they vibrate for a shorter time than do the A-V valves.

The audible range of frequency (pitch) in the first and second heart sounds, as shown in Figure 23-1, begins at the lowest frequency the ear can detect, about 40 cycles/sec, and goes up above 500 cycles/sec. When special electronic apparatus is used to record these sounds, by far a larger proportion of the recorded sound is at frequencies and sound levels below the audible range, going down to 3 to 4 cycles/sec and peaking at about 20 cycles/sec, as illustrated by the lower shaded area in Figure 23-1. For this reason, major portions of the heart sounds can be recorded electronically in phonocardiograms even though they cannot be heard with a stethoscope.

The second heart sound normally has a higher frequency than the first heart sound for two reasons: (1) the tautness of the semilunar valves in comparison with the much less taut A-V valves, and (2) the greater elas-

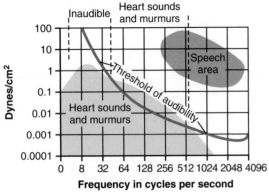

Figure 23-1 Amplitude of different-frequency vibrations in the heart sounds and heart murmurs in relation to the threshold of audibility, showing that the range of sounds that can be heard is between 40 and 520 cycles/sec. (Modified from Butterworth JS, Chassin JL, McGrath JJ: Cardiac Auscultation, 2nd ed, New York: Grune & Stratton, 1960.)

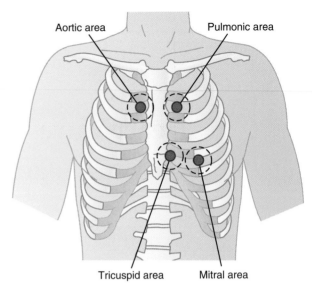

Figure 23-2 Chest areas from which sound from each valve is best heard.

tic coefficient of the taut arterial walls that provide the principal vibrating chambers for the second sound, in comparison with the much looser, less elastic ventricular chambers that provide the vibrating system for the first heart sound. The clinician uses these differences to distinguish special characteristics of the two respective sounds.

Third Heart Sound. Occasionally a weak, rumbling third heart sound is heard at the beginning of the *middle third of diastole.* A logical but unproved explanation of this sound is oscillation of blood back and forth between the walls of the ventricles initiated by inrushing blood from the atria. This is analogous to running water from a faucet into a paper sack, the inrushing water reverberating back and forth between the walls of the sack to cause vibrations in its walls. The reason the third heart sound does not occur until the middle third of diastole is believed to be that in the early part of diastole, the ventricles are not filled sufficiently to create even the small amount of elastic tension necessary for reverberation. The frequency of this sound is usually so low that the ear cannot hear it, yet it can often be recorded in the phonocardiogram.

Atrial Heart Sound (Fourth Heart Sound). An atrial heart sound can sometimes be recorded in the phonocardiogram, but it can almost never be heard with a stethoscope because of its weakness and very low frequency—usually 20 cycles/sec or less. This sound occurs when the atria contract, and presumably, it is caused by the inrush of blood into the ventricles, which initiates vibrations similar to those of the third heart sound.

Chest Surface Areas for Auscultation of Normal Heart Sounds

Listening to the sounds of the body, usually with the aid of a stethoscope, is called *auscultation.* Figure 23-2 shows the areas of the chest wall from which the different heart valvular sounds can best be distinguished. Although the

sounds from all the valves can be heard from all these areas, the cardiologist distinguishes the sounds from the different valves by a process of elimination. That is, he or she moves the stethoscope from one area to another, noting the loudness of the sounds in different areas and gradually picking out the sound components from each valve.

The areas for listening to the different heart sounds are not directly over the valves themselves. The aortic area is upward along the aorta because of sound transmission up the aorta, and the pulmonic area is upward along the pulmonary artery. The tricuspid area is over the right ventricle, and the mitral area is over the apex of the left ventricle, which is the portion of the heart nearest the surface of the chest; the heart is rotated so that the remainder of the left ventricle lies more posteriorly.

Phonocardiogram

If a microphone specially designed to detect low-frequency sound is placed on the chest, the heart sounds can be amplified and recorded by a high-speed recording apparatus. The recording is called a *phonocardiogram,* and the heart sounds appear as waves, as shown schematically in Figure 23-3. Recording A is an example of normal heart sounds, showing the vibrations of the first, second, and third heart sounds and even the very weak atrial sound. Note specifically that the third and atrial heart sounds are each a very low rumble. The third heart sound can be recorded in only one third to one half of all people, and the atrial heart sound can be recorded in perhaps one fourth of all people.

Valvular Lesions

Rheumatic Valvular Lesions

By far the greatest number of valvular lesions results from *rheumatic fever.* Rheumatic fever is an autoimmune disease in which the heart valves are likely to be damaged or

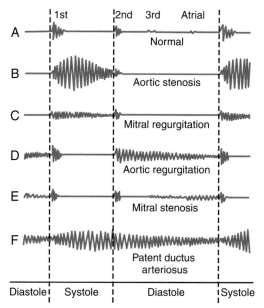

Figure 23-3 Phonocardiograms from normal and abnormal hearts.

destroyed. It is usually initiated by streptococcal toxin in the following manner.

The sequence of events almost always begins with a preliminary streptococcal infection caused specifically by group A hemolytic streptococci. These bacteria initially cause a sore throat, scarlet fever, or middle ear infection. But the streptococci also release several different proteins against which the person's reticuloendothelial system produces *antibodies.* The antibodies react not only with the streptococcal protein but also with other protein tissues of the body, often causing severe immunologic damage. These reactions continue to take place as long as the antibodies persist in the blood—1 year or more.

Rheumatic fever causes damage especially in certain susceptible areas, such as the heart valves. The degree of heart valve damage is directly correlated with the concentration and persistence of the antibodies. The principles of immunity that relate to this type of reaction are discussed in Chapter 34, and it is noted in Chapter 31 that acute glomerular nephritis of the kidneys has a similar immunologic basis.

In rheumatic fever, large hemorrhagic, fibrinous, bulbous lesions grow along the inflamed edges of the heart valves. Because the mitral valve receives more trauma during valvular action than any of the other valves, it is the one most often seriously damaged, and the aortic valve is the second most frequently damaged. The right heart valves, the tricuspid and pulmonary valves, are usually affected much less severely, probably because the low-pressure stresses that act on these valves are slight compared with the high-pressure stresses that act on the left heart valves.

Scarring of the Valves. The lesions of acute rheumatic fever frequently occur on adjacent valve leaflets simultaneously, so the edges of the leaflets become stuck together. Then, weeks, months, or years later, the lesions become scar tissue, permanently fusing portions of adjacent valve

leaflets. Also, the free edges of the leaflets, which are normally filmy and free-flapping, often become solid, scarred masses.

A valve in which the leaflets adhere to one another so extensively that blood cannot flow through it normally is said to be *stenosed.* Conversely, when the valve edges are so destroyed by scar tissue that they cannot close as the ventricles contract, *regurgitation* (backflow) of blood occurs when the valve should be closed. Stenosis usually does not occur without the coexistence of at least some degree of regurgitation, and vice versa.

Other Causes of Valvular Lesions. Stenosis or lack of one or more leaflets of a valve also occurs occasionally as a *congenital defect.* Complete lack of leaflets is rare; *congenital stenosis* is more common, as is discussed later in this chapter.

Heart Murmurs Caused by Valvular Lesions

As shown by the phonocardiograms in Figure 23-3, many abnormal heart sounds, known as "heart murmurs," occur when there are abnormalities of the valves, as follows.

Systolic Murmur of Aortic Stenosis. In aortic stenosis, blood is ejected from the left ventricle through only a small fibrous opening of the aortic valve. Because of the resistance to ejection, sometimes the blood pressure in the left ventricle rises as high as 300 mm Hg, while the pressure in the aorta is still normal. Thus, a nozzle effect is created *during systole,* with blood jetting at tremendous velocity through the small opening of the valve. This causes *severe turbulence* of the blood in the root of the aorta. The turbulent blood impinging against the aortic walls causes intense vibration, and a loud murmur (see recording B, Figure 23-3) occurs during systole and is transmitted throughout the superior thoracic aorta and even into the large arteries of the neck. This sound is harsh and in severe stenosis may be so loud that it can be heard several feet away from the patient. Also, the sound vibrations can often be felt with the hand on the upper chest and lower neck, a phenomenon known as a *"thrill."*

Diastolic Murmur of Aortic Regurgitation. In aortic regurgitation, no abnormal sound is heard during systole, but *during diastole,* blood flows backward from the high-pressure aorta into the left ventricle, causing a "blowing" murmur of relatively high pitch with a swishing quality heard maximally over the left ventricle (see recording D, Figure 23-3). This murmur results from *turbulence* of blood jetting backward into the blood already in the low-pressure diastolic left ventricle.

Systolic Murmur of Mitral Regurgitation. In mitral regurgitation, blood flows backward through the mitral valve into the left atrium *during systole.* This also causes a high-frequency "blowing," swishing sound (see recording C, Figure 23-3) similar to that of aortic regurgitation but occurring during systole rather than diastole. It is transmitted most strongly into the left atrium. However, the left atrium is so deep within the chest that it is difficult to hear this sound directly over the atrium. As a result, the sound of mitral regurgitation is transmitted to the chest wall mainly through the left ventricle to the apex of the heart.

Diastolic Murmur of Mitral Stenosis. In mitral stenosis, blood passes with difficulty through the stenosed mitral valve from the left atrium into the left ventricle, and because the pressure in the left atrium seldom rises above 30 mm Hg, a large pressure differential forcing blood from the left atrium into the left ventricle does not develop. Consequently, the abnormal sounds heard in mitral stenosis (see recording E, Figure 23-3) are usually weak and of very low frequency, so most of the sound spectrum is below the low-frequency end of human hearing.

During the early part of diastole, a left ventricle with a stenotic mitral valve has so little blood in it and its walls are so flabby that blood does not reverberate back and forth between the walls of the ventricle. For this reason, even in severe mitral stenosis, no murmur may be heard during the first third of diastole. Then, after partial filling, the ventricle has stretched enough for blood to reverberate and a low rumbling murmur begins.

Phonocardiograms of Valvular Murmurs. Phonocardiograms B, C, D, and E of Figure 23-3 show, respectively, idealized records obtained from patients with aortic stenosis, mitral regurgitation, aortic regurgitation, and mitral stenosis. It is obvious from these phonocardiograms that the aortic stenotic lesion causes the loudest murmur, and the mitral stenotic lesion causes the weakest. The phonocardiograms show how the intensity of the murmurs varies during different portions of systole and diastole, and the relative timing of each murmur is also evident. Note especially that the murmurs of aortic stenosis and mitral regurgitation occur only during systole, whereas the murmurs of aortic regurgitation and mitral stenosis occur only during diastole. If the reader does not understand this timing, extra review should be undertaken until it is understood.

Abnormal Circulatory Dynamics in Valvular Heart Disease

Dynamics of the Circulation in Aortic Stenosis and Aortic Regurgitation

In *aortic stenosis,* the contracting left ventricle fails to empty adequately, whereas in *aortic regurgitation,* blood flows backward into the ventricle from the aorta after the ventricle has just pumped the blood into the aorta. Therefore, in either case, the *net stroke volume output* of the heart is reduced.

Several important compensations take place that can ameliorate the severity of the circulatory defects. Some of these compensations are the following.

Hypertrophy of the Left Ventricle. In both aortic stenosis and aortic regurgitation, the left ventricular musculature hypertrophies because of the increased ventricular workload.

In *regurgitation,* the left ventricular chamber also enlarges to hold all the regurgitant blood from the aorta. Sometimes the left ventricular muscle mass increases fourfold to fivefold, creating a tremendously large left side of the heart.

When the aortic valve is seriously *stenosed,* the hypertrophied muscle allows the left ventricle to develop as much as 400 mm Hg intraventricular pressure at systolic peak.

In severe aortic regurgitation, sometimes the hypertrophied muscle allows the left ventricle to pump a stroke volume output as great as 250 ml, although as much as three fourths of this blood returns to the ventricle during diastole, and only one fourth flows through the aorta to the body.

Increase in Blood Volume. Another effect that helps compensate for the diminished net pumping by the left ventricle is increased blood volume. This results from (1) an initial slight decrease in arterial pressure, plus (2) peripheral circulatory reflexes that the decrease in pressure induces. These together diminish renal output of urine, causing the blood volume to increase and the mean arterial pressure to return to normal. Also, red cell mass eventually increases because of a slight degree of tissue hypoxia.

The increase in blood volume tends to increase venous return to the heart. This, in turn, causes the left ventricle to pump with the extra power required to overcome the abnormal pumping dynamics.

Eventual Failure of the Left Ventricle and Development of Pulmonary Edema

In the early stages of aortic stenosis or aortic regurgitation, the intrinsic ability of the left ventricle to adapt to increasing loads prevents significant abnormalities in circulatory function in the person during rest, other than increased work output required of the left ventricle. Therefore, considerable degrees of aortic stenosis or aortic regurgitation often occur before the person knows that he or she has serious heart disease (such as a resting left ventricular systolic pressure as high as 200 mm Hg in aortic stenosis or a left ventricular stroke volume output as high as double normal in aortic regurgitation).

Beyond a critical stage in these aortic valve lesions, the left ventricle finally cannot keep up with the work demand. As a consequence, the left ventricle dilates and cardiac output begins to fall; blood simultaneously dams up in the left atrium and in the lungs behind the failing left ventricle. The left atrial pressure rises progressively, and at mean left atrial pressures above 25 to 40 mm Hg, serious edema appears in the lungs, as discussed in detail in Chapter 38.

Dynamics of Mitral Stenosis and Mitral Regurgitation

In mitral stenosis, blood flow from the left atrium into the left ventricle is impeded, and in mitral regurgitation, much of the blood that has flowed into the left ventricle during diastole leaks back into the left atrium during systole rather than being pumped into the aorta. Therefore, either of these conditions reduces net movement of blood from the left atrium into the left ventricle.

Pulmonary Edema in Mitral Valvular Disease. The buildup of blood in the left atrium causes progressive increase in left atrial pressure, and this eventually results in development of serious pulmonary edema. Ordinarily, lethal edema does not occur until the mean left atrial pressure rises above 25 mm Hg and sometimes as high as 40 mm Hg, because the lung lymphatic vessels enlarge manyfold and can rapidly carry fluid away from the lung tissues.

Enlarged Left Atrium and Atrial Fibrillation. The high left atrial pressure in mitral valvular disease also causes progressive enlargement of the left atrium, which increases the distance that the cardiac electrical excitatory impulse must travel in the atrial wall. This pathway may eventually become so long that it predisposes to development of excitatory signal *circus movements,* as discussed in Chapter 13. Therefore, in late stages of mitral valvular disease, especially in mitral stenosis, atrial fibrillation usually occurs. This further reduces the pumping effectiveness of the heart and causes further cardiac debility.

Compensation in Early Mitral Valvular Disease. As also occurs in aortic valvular disease and in many types of congenital heart disease, the blood volume increases in mitral valvular disease principally because of diminished excretion of water and salt by the kidneys. This increased blood volume increases venous return to the heart, thereby helping to overcome the effect of the cardiac debility. Therefore, after compensation, cardiac output may fall only minimally until the late stages of mitral valvular disease, even though the left atrial pressure is rising.

As the left atrial pressure rises, blood begins to dam up in the lungs, eventually all the way back to the pulmonary artery. In addition, incipient edema of the lungs causes pulmonary arteriolar constriction. These two effects together increase systolic pulmonary arterial pressure and also right ventricular pressure, sometimes to as high as 60 mm Hg, which is more than double normal. This, in turn, causes hypertrophy of the right side of the heart, which partially compensates for its increased workload.

Circulatory Dynamics During Exercise in Patients with Valvular Lesions

During exercise, large quantities of venous blood are returned to the heart from the peripheral circulation. Therefore, all the dynamic abnormalities that occur in the different types of valvular heart disease become tremendously exacerbated. Even in mild valvular heart disease, in which the symptoms may be unrecognizable at rest, severe symptoms often develop during heavy exercise. For instance, in patients with aortic valvular lesions, exercise can cause acute left ventricular failure followed by *acute pulmonary edema.* Also, in patients with mitral disease, exercise can cause so much damming of blood in the lungs that serious or even lethal pulmonary edema may ensue in as little as 10 minutes.

Even in mild to moderate cases of valvular disease, the patient's *cardiac reserve* diminishes in proportion to the severity of the valvular dysfunction. That is, the cardiac output does not increase as much as it should during exercise. Therefore, the muscles of the body fatigue rapidly because of too little increase in muscle blood flow.

Abnormal Circulatory Dynamics in Congenital Heart Defects

Occasionally, the heart or its associated blood vessels are malformed during fetal life; the defect is called a *congenital anomaly.* There are three major types of congenital anomalies of the heart and its associated vessels: (1) *stenosis* of the channel of blood flow at some point in the heart or in a closely allied major blood vessel; (2) an anomaly that allows blood to flow backward from the left side of the heart or aorta to the right side of the heart or pulmonary artery, thus failing to flow through the systemic circulation-called a *left-to-right shunt;* and (3) an anomaly that allows blood to flow directly from the right side of the heart into the left side of the heart, thus failing to flow through the lungs—called a *right-to-left shunt.*

The effects of the different stenotic lesions are easily understood. For instance, *congenital aortic valve stenosis* results in the same dynamic effects as aortic valve stenosis caused by other valvular lesions, namely, a tendency to develop serious pulmonary edema and a reduced cardiac output.

Another type of congenital stenosis is *coarctation of the aorta,* often occurring near the level of the diaphragm. This causes the arterial pressure in the upper part of the body (above the level of the coarctation) to be much greater than the pressure in the lower body because of the great resistance to blood flow through the coarctation to the lower body; part of the blood must go around the coarctation through small collateral arteries, as discussed in Chapter 19.

Patent Ductus Arteriosus—a Left-to-Right Shunt

During fetal life, the lungs are collapsed, and the elastic compression of the lungs that keeps the alveoli collapsed keeps most of the lung blood vessels collapsed as well. Therefore, resistance to blood flow through the lungs is so great that the pulmonary arterial pressure is high in the fetus. Also, because of low resistance to blood flow from the aorta through the large vessels of the placenta, the pressure in the aorta of the fetus is lower than normal—in fact, lower than in the pulmonary artery. This causes almost all the pulmonary arterial blood to flow through a special artery present in the fetus that connects the pulmonary artery with the aorta (Figure 23-4), called the *ductus arteriosus*, thus bypassing the lungs. This allows immediate recirculation of the blood through the systemic arteries of the fetus without the blood going through the lungs. This lack of blood flow through the lungs is not detrimental to the fetus because the blood is oxygenated by the placenta.

Closure of the Ductus Arteriosus After Birth.

As soon as a baby is born and begins to breathe, the lungs inflate; not only do the alveoli fill with air, but also the resistance to blood flow through the pulmonary vascular tree decreases tremendously, allowing the pulmonary arterial pressure to fall. Simultaneously, the aortic pressure rises because of sudden cessation of blood flow from the aorta through the placenta. Thus, the pressure in the pulmonary artery falls, while that in the aorta rises. As a result, forward blood flow through the ductus arteriosus ceases suddenly at birth, and in fact, blood begins to flow backward through the ductus from the aorta into the pulmonary artery. This new state of backward blood flow causes the ductus arteriosus to become occluded within a few hours to a few days in most babies, so blood flow through the ductus does not persist. The ductus is believed to close because the oxygen concentration of the aortic blood now flowing through it is about twice as high as that of the blood flowing from the pulmonary artery into the ductus during fetal life. The oxygen presumably constricts the muscle in the ductus wall. This is discussed further in Chapter 83.

Unfortunately, in about 1 of every 5500 babies, the ductus does not close, causing the condition known as *patent ductus arteriosus*, which is shown in Figure 23-4.

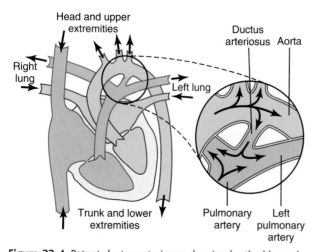

Figure 23-4 Patent ductus arteriosus, showing by the blue color that venous blood changes into oxygenated blood at different points in the circulation. The right-hand diagram shows backflow of blood from the aorta into the pulmonary artery and then through the lungs for a second time.

Dynamics of the Circulation with a Persistent Patent Ductus.

During the early months of an infant's life, a patent ductus usually does not cause severely abnormal function. But as the child grows older, the differential between the high pressure in the aorta and the lower pressure in the pulmonary artery progressively increases, with corresponding increase in backward flow of blood from the aorta into the pulmonary artery. Also, the high aortic blood pressure usually causes the diameter of the partially open ductus to increase with time, making the condition even worse.

Recirculation Through the Lungs. In an older child with a patent ductus, one half to two thirds of the aortic blood flows backward through the ductus into the pulmonary artery, then through the lungs, and finally back into the left ventricle and aorta, passing through the lungs and left side of the heart two or more times for every one time that it passes through the systemic circulation. These people *do not show cyanosis until later in life, when the heart fails or the lungs become congested.* Indeed, early in life, the arterial blood is often better oxygenated than normal because of the extra times it passes through the lungs.

Diminished Cardiac and Respiratory Reserve. The major effects of patent ductus arteriosus on the patient are decreased cardiac and respiratory reserve. The left ventricle is pumping about two or more times the normal cardiac output, and the maximum that it can pump after hypertrophy of the heart has occurred is about four to seven times normal. Therefore, during exercise, the net blood flow through the remainder of the body can never increase to the levels required for strenuous activity. With even moderately strenuous exercise, the person is likely to become weak and may even faint from momentary heart failure.

The high pressures in the pulmonary vessels caused by excess flow through the lungs often lead to pulmonary congestion and pulmonary edema. As a result of the excessive load on the heart, and especially because the pulmonary congestion becomes progressively more severe with age, most patients with uncorrected patent ductus die from heart disease between ages 20 and 40 years.

Heart Sounds: Machinery Murmur.

In a newborn infant with patent ductus arteriosus, occasionally no abnormal heart sounds are heard because the quantity of reverse blood flow through the ductus may be insufficient to cause a heart murmur. But as the baby grows older, reaching age 1 to 3 years, a harsh, blowing murmur begins to be heard in the pulmonary artery area of the chest, as shown in recording F, Figure 23-3. This sound is much more intense during systole when the aortic pressure is high and much less intense during diastole when the aortic pressure falls low, so that the murmur waxes and wanes with each beat of the heart, creating the so-called *machinery murmur*.

Surgical Treatment. Surgical treatment of patent ductus arteriosus is extremely simple; one need only ligate the patent ductus or divide it and then close the two ends. In fact, this was one of the first successful heart surgeries ever performed.

Tetralogy of Fallot—a Right-to-Left Shunt

Tetralogy of Fallot is shown in Figure 23-5; it is the most common cause of "blue baby." Most of the blood bypasses the lungs, so the aortic blood is mainly unoxygenated venous blood. In this condition, four abnormalities of the heart occur simultaneously:

1. The aorta originates from the right ventricle rather than the left, or it overrides a hole in the septum, as shown in Figure 23-5, receiving blood from both ventricles.

2. The pulmonary artery is stenosed, so much lower than normal amounts of blood pass from the right ventricle into the lungs; instead, most of the blood passes directly into the aorta, thus bypassing the lungs.

3. Blood from the left ventricle flows either through a ventricular septal hole into the right ventricle and then into the aorta or directly into the aorta that overrides this hole.

4. Because the right side of the heart must pump large quantities of blood against the high pressure in the aorta, its musculature is highly developed, causing an enlarged right ventricle.

Abnormal Circulatory Dynamics. It is readily apparent that the major physiological difficulty caused by

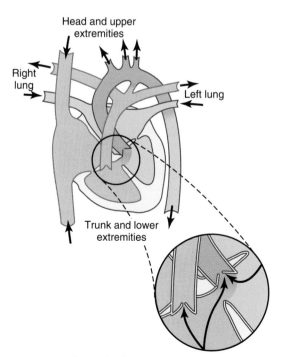

Figure 23-5 Tetralogy of Fallot, showing by the blue color that most of the venous blood is shunted from the right ventricle into the aorta without passing through the lungs.

tetralogy of Fallot is the shunting of blood past the lungs without its becoming oxygenated. As much as 75 percent of the venous blood returning to the heart passes directly from the right ventricle into the aorta without becoming oxygenated.

A diagnosis of tetralogy of Fallot is usually based on (1) the fact that the baby's skin is *cyanotic* (blue); (2) measurement of high systolic pressure in the right ventricle, recorded through a catheter; (3) characteristic changes in the radiological silhouette of the heart, showing an enlarged right ventricle; and (4) angiograms (x-ray pictures) showing abnormal blood flow through the interventricular septal hole and into the overriding aorta, but much less flow through the stenosed pulmonary artery.

Surgical Treatment. Tetralogy of Fallot can usually be treated successfully by surgery. The usual operation is to open the pulmonary stenosis, close the septal defect, and reconstruct the flow pathway into the aorta. When surgery is successful, the average life expectancy increases from only 3 to 4 years to 50 or more years.

Causes of Congenital Anomalies

Congenital heart disease is not uncommon, occurring in about 8 of every 1000 live births. One of the most common causes of congenital heart defects is a viral infection in the mother during the first trimester of pregnancy when the fetal heart is being formed. Defects are particularly prone to develop when the expectant mother contracts German measles; thus, obstetricians may advise termination of pregnancy if German measles occurs in the first trimester.

Some congenital defects of the heart are hereditary because the same defect has been known to occur in identical twins, as well as in succeeding generations. Children of patients surgically treated for congenital heart disease have about a 10 times greater chance of having congenital heart disease than other children do. Congenital defects of the heart are also frequently associated with other congenital defects of the baby's body.

Use of Extracorporeal Circulation During Cardiac Surgery

It is almost impossible to repair intracardiac defects surgically while the heart is still pumping. Therefore, many types of artificial *heart-lung machines* have been developed to take the place of the heart and lungs during the course of operation. Such a system is called *extracorporeal circulation.* The system consists principally of a pump and an oxygenating device. Almost any type of pump that does not cause hemolysis of the blood seems to be suitable.

Methods used for oxygenating blood include (1) bubbling oxygen through the blood and removing the bubbles from the blood before passing it back into the patient,

(2) dripping the blood downward over the surfaces of plastic sheets in the presence of oxygen, (3) passing the blood over surfaces of rotating discs, or (4) passing the blood between thin membranes or through thin tubes that are permeable to oxygen and carbon dioxide.

The different systems have all been fraught with difficulties, including hemolysis of the blood, development of small clots in the blood, likelihood of small bubbles of oxygen or small emboli of antifoam agent passing into the arteries of the patient, necessity for large quantities of blood to prime the entire system, failure to exchange adequate quantities of oxygen, and necessity to use heparin to prevent blood coagulation in the extracorporeal system. Heparin also interferes with adequate hemostasis during the surgical procedure. Yet despite these difficulties, in the hands of experts, patients can be kept alive on artificial heart-lung machines for many hours while operations are performed on the inside of the heart.

Hypertrophy of the Heart in Valvular and Congenital Heart Disease

Hypertrophy of cardiac muscle is one of the most important mechanisms by which the heart adapts to increased workloads, whether these loads are caused by increased pressure against which the heart muscle must contract or by increased cardiac output that must be pumped. Some physicians believe that the increased strength of contraction of the heart muscle causes the hypertrophy; others believe that the increased metabolic rate of the muscle is the primary stimulus. Regardless of which of these is correct, one can calculate approximately how much hypertrophy will occur in each chamber of the heart by multiplying ventricular output by the pressure against which the ventricle must work, with emphasis on pressure. Thus, hypertrophy occurs in most types of valvular and congenital disease, sometimes causing heart weights as great as 800 grams instead of the normal 300 grams.

Detrimental Effects of Late Stages of Cardiac Hypertrophy. Although the most common cause of cardiac hypertrophy is hypertension, almost all forms of cardiac diseases including valvular and congenital disease can stimulate enlargement of the heart.

"Physiological" cardiac hypertrophy is generally considered to be a compensatory response of the heart to increased workload and is usually beneficial for maintaining cardiac output in the face of abnormalities that impair the heart's effectiveness as a pump. However, extreme degrees of hypertrophy can lead to heart failure. One of the reasons for this is that the coronary vasculature typically does not increase to the same extent as the mass of cardiac muscle increases. The second reason is that fibrosis often develops in the muscle, especially in the subendocardial muscle where the coronary blood flow is poor, with fibrous tissue replacing degenerating muscle fibers. Because of the disproportionate increase in muscle mass relative to coronary blood flow, relative ischemia may develop as the cardiac muscle hypertrophies and coronary blood flow insufficiency may ensue. Anginal pain is therefore a frequent accompaniment of cardiac hypertrophy associated with valvular and congenital heart diseases. Enlargement of the heart is also associated with greater risk for developing arrhythmias, which in turn can lead to further impairment of cardiac function and sudden death because of fibrillation.

Bibliography

Braunwald E, Seidman CE, Sigwart U: Contemporary evaluation and management of hypertrophic cardiomyopathy, *Circulation* 106:1312, 2002.

Carabello BA: The current therapy for mitral regurgitation, *J Am Coll Cardiol* 52:319, 2008.

Dal-Bianco JP, Khandheria BK, Mookadam F, et al: Management of asymptomatic severe aortic stenosis, *J Am Coll Cardiol* 52:1279, 2008.

Dorn GW 2nd: The fuzzy logic of physiological cardiac hypertrophy, *Hypertension* 49:962, 2007.

Hoffman JI, Kaplan S: The incidence of congenital heart disease, *J Am Coll Cardiol* 39:1890, 2002.

Jenkins KJ, Correa A, Feinstein JA, et al: Noninherited risk factors and congenital cardiovascular defects: current knowledge: a scientific statement from the American Heart Association Council on Cardiovascular Disease in the Young: endorsed by the American Academy of Pediatrics, *Circulation* 115:2995, 2007.

Maron BJ: Hypertrophic cardiomyopathy: a systematic review, *JAMA* 287:1308, 2002.

McDonald M, Currie BJ, Carapetis JR: Acute rheumatic fever: a chink in the chain that links the heart to the throat? *Lancet Infect Dis* 4:240, 2004.

Nishimura RA, Holmes DR Jr: Clinical practice: hypertrophic obstructive cardiomyopathy, *N Engl J Med* 350:1320, 2004.

Reimold SC, Rutherford JD: Clinical practice: valvular heart disease in pregnancy, *N Engl J Med* 349:52, 2003.

Rhodes JF, Hijazi ZM, Sommer RJ: Pathophysiology of congenital heart disease in the adult, part II. Simple obstructive lesions, *Circulation* 117:1228, 2008.

Schoen FJ: Evolving concepts of cardiac valve dynamics: the continuum of development, functional structure, pathobiology, and tissue engineering, *Circulation* 118:1864, 2008.

Sommer RJ, Hijazi ZM, Rhodes JF Jr: Pathophysiology of congenital heart disease in the adult: part I: shunt lesions, *Circulation* 117:1090, 2008.

Sommer RJ, Hijazi ZM, Rhodes JF: Pathophysiology of congenital heart disease in the adult: part III: complex congenital heart disease, *Circulation* 117:1340, 2008.

Circulatory Shock and Its Treatment

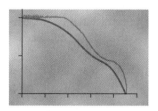 *Circulatory shock* means generalized inadequate blood flow through the body, to the extent that the body tissues are damaged, especially because of too little oxygen and other nutrients delivered to the tissue cells. Even the cardiovascular system itself—the heart musculature, walls of the blood vessels, vasomotor system, and other circulatory parts—begins to deteriorate, so the shock, once begun, is prone to become progressively worse.

Physiologic Causes of Shock

Circulatory Shock Caused by Decreased Cardiac Output

Shock usually results from inadequate cardiac output. Therefore, any condition that reduces the cardiac output far below normal will likely lead to circulatory shock. Two types of factors can severely reduce cardiac output:

1. *Cardiac abnormalities that decrease the ability of the heart to pump blood.* These include especially myocardial infarction but also toxic states of the heart, severe heart valve dysfunction, heart arrhythmias, and other conditions. The circulatory shock that results from diminished cardiac pumping ability is called *cardiogenic shock.* This is discussed in detail in Chapter 22 where it is pointed out that as many as 70 percent of people who develop cardiogenic shock do not survive.

2. *Factors that decrease venous return* also decrease cardiac output because the heart cannot pump blood that does not flow into it. The most common cause of decreased venous return is *diminished blood volume,* but venous return can also be reduced as a result of *decreased vascular tone,* especially of the venous blood reservoirs, or *obstruction to blood flow* at some point in the circulation, especially in the venous return pathway to the heart.

Circulatory Shock That Occurs Without Diminished Cardiac Output

Occasionally, cardiac output is normal or even greater than normal, yet the person is in circulatory shock. This can result from (1) *excessive metabolic rate, so even a normal cardiac output is inadequate,* or (2) *abnormal tissue perfusion patterns, so most of the cardiac output is passing through blood vessels besides those that supply the local tissues with nutrition.*

The specific causes of shock are discussed later in the chapter. For the present, it is important to note that all of them lead to *inadequate delivery of nutrients to critical tissues and critical organs and also cause inadequate removal of cellular waste products from the tissues.*

What Happens to the Arterial Pressure in Circulatory Shock?

In the minds of many physicians, the arterial pressure level is the principal measure of adequacy of circulatory function. However, the arterial pressure can often be seriously misleading. At times, a person may be in severe shock and still have an almost normal arterial pressure because of powerful nervous reflexes that keep the pressure from falling. At other times, the arterial pressure can fall to half of normal, but the person still has normal tissue perfusion and is not in shock.

In most types of shock, especially shock caused by severe blood loss, the arterial blood pressure decreases at the same time the cardiac output decreases, although usually not as much.

Tissue Deterioration Is the End Result of Circulatory Shock

Once circulatory shock reaches a critical state of severity, regardless of its initiating cause, *the shock itself leads to more shock.* That is, the inadequate blood flow causes the body tissues to begin deteriorating, including the heart and circulatory system itself. This causes an even greater decrease in cardiac output, and a vicious circle ensues, with progressively increasing circulatory shock, less adequate tissue perfusion, more shock, and so forth until death. It is with this late stage of circulatory shock that we are especially concerned, because appropriate physiologic treatment can often reverse the rapid slide to death.

Stages of Shock

Because the characteristics of circulatory shock change with different degrees of severity, shock is divided into the following three major stages:

1. A *nonprogressive stage* (sometimes called the *compensated stage*), in which the normal circulatory compensatory mechanisms eventually cause full recovery without help from outside therapy.

2. A *progressive stage*, in which, without therapy, the shock becomes steadily worse until death.

3. An *irreversible stage*, in which the shock has progressed to such an extent that all forms of known therapy are inadequate to save the person's life, even though, for the moment, the person is still alive.

Now, let us discuss the stages of circulatory shock caused by decreased blood volume, which illustrate the basic principles. Then we will consider special characteristics of shock initiated by other causes.

Shock Caused by Hypovolemia— Hemorrhagic Shock

Hypovolemia means diminished blood volume. Hemorrhage is the most common cause of hypovolemic shock. Hemorrhage *decreases the filling pressure of the circulation* and, as a consequence, decreases venous return. As a result, the cardiac output falls below normal and shock may ensue.

Relationship of Bleeding Volume to Cardiac Output and Arterial Pressure

Figure 24-1 shows the approximate effects on both cardiac output and arterial pressure of removing blood from the circulatory system over a period of about 30 minutes. About 10 percent of the total blood volume can be removed with almost no effect on either arterial pressure or cardiac output, but greater blood loss usually dimin-

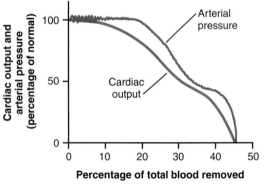

Figure 24-1 Effect of hemorrhage on cardiac output and arterial pressure.

ishes the cardiac output first and later the arterial pressure, both of which fall to zero when about 40 to 45 percent of the total blood volume has been removed.

Sympathetic Reflex Compensations in Shock— Their Special Value to Maintain Arterial Pressure. The decrease in arterial pressure after hemorrhage, as well as decreases in pressures in the pulmonary arteries and veins in the thorax, causes powerful sympathetic reflexes (initiated mainly by the arterial baroreceptors and other vascular stretch receptors, as explained in Chapter 18). These reflexes stimulate the sympathetic vasoconstrictor system in most tissues of the body, resulting in three important effects: (1) The arterioles constrict in most parts of the systemic circulation, thereby increasing the total peripheral resistance. (2) The veins and venous reservoirs constrict, thereby helping to maintain adequate venous return despite diminished blood volume. (3) Heart activity increases markedly, sometimes increasing the heart rate from the normal value of 72 beats/min to as high as 160 to 180 beats/min.

Value of the Sympathetic Nervous Reflexes. In the absence of the sympathetic reflexes, only 15 to 20 percent of the blood volume can be removed over a period of 30 minutes before a person dies; this is in contrast to a 30 to 40 percent loss of blood volume that a person can sustain when the reflexes are intact. Therefore, the reflexes extend the amount of blood loss that can occur without causing death to about twice that which is possible in their absence.

Greater Effect of the Sympathetic Nervous Reflexes in Maintaining Arterial Pressure than in Maintaining Cardiac Output. Referring again to Figure 24-1, note that the arterial pressure is maintained at or near normal levels in the hemorrhaging person longer than is the cardiac output. The reason for this is that the sympathetic reflexes are geared more for maintaining arterial pressure than for maintaining cardiac output. They increase the arterial pressure mainly by increasing the total peripheral resistance, which has no beneficial effect on cardiac output; however, the *sympathetic constriction of the veins is important to keep venous return and cardiac output from falling too much*, in addition to their role in maintaining arterial pressure.

Especially interesting is the second plateau occurring at about 50 mm Hg in the arterial pressure curve of Figure 24-1. This results from activation of the central nervous system ischemic response, which causes extreme stimulation of the sympathetic nervous system when the brain begins to suffer from lack of oxygen or from excess buildup of carbon dioxide, as discussed in Chapter 18. This effect of the central nervous system ischemic response can be called the "last-ditch stand" of the sympathetic reflexes in their attempt to keep the arterial pressure from falling too low.

Protection of Coronary and Cerebral Blood Flow by the Reflexes. A special value of the maintenance of normal arterial pressure even in the presence of decreasing cardiac output is protection of blood flow through the coronary and cerebral circulatory systems. The sympathetic stimulation does not cause significant constriction of either the cerebral or the cardiac vessels. In addition, in both vascular beds, local blood flow autoregulation is excellent, which prevents moderate decreases in arterial pressure from significantly decreasing their blood flows. Therefore, blood flow through the heart and brain is maintained essentially at normal levels as long as the arterial pressure does not fall below about 70 mm Hg, despite the fact that blood flow in some other areas of the body might be decreased to as little as one third to one quarter normal by this time because of vasoconstriction.

Progressive and Nonprogressive Hemorrhagic Shock

Figure 24-2 shows an experiment that demonstrates the effects of different degrees of sudden acute hemorrhage on the subsequent course of arterial pressure. The animals were anesthetized and bled rapidly until their arterial pressures fell to different levels. Those animals whose pressures fell immediately to no lower than 45 mm Hg (groups I, II, and III) all eventually recovered; the recovery occurred rapidly if the pressure fell only slightly (group I) but occurred slowly if it fell almost to the 45 mm Hg level (group III). When the arterial pressure fell below 45 mm Hg (groups IV, V, and VI), all the animals died, although many of them hovered between life and death for hours before the circulatory system deteriorated to the stage of death.

This experiment demonstrates that the circulatory system can recover as long as the degree of hemorrhage is no greater than a certain critical amount. Crossing this critical threshold by even a few milliliters of blood loss makes the eventual difference between life and death. Thus, hemorrhage beyond a certain critical level causes shock to become *progressive*. That is, *the shock itself causes still more shock*, and the condition becomes a vicious circle that eventually leads to deterioration of the circulation and to death.

Nonprogressive Shock—Compensated Shock

If shock is not severe enough to cause its own progression, the person eventually recovers. Therefore, shock of this lesser degree is called *nonprogressive shock*, or *compensated shock*, meaning that the sympathetic reflexes and other factors compensate enough to prevent further deterioration of the circulation.

The factors that cause a person to recover from moderate degrees of shock are all the negative feedback control mechanisms of the circulation that attempt to return cardiac output and arterial pressure back to normal levels. They include the following:

1. *Baroreceptor reflexes*, which elicit powerful sympathetic stimulation of the circulation.

2. *Central nervous system ischemic response*, which elicits even more powerful sympathetic stimulation throughout the body but is not activated significantly until the arterial pressure falls below 50 mm Hg.

3. *Reverse stress-relaxation of the circulatory system*, which causes the blood vessels to contract around the diminished blood volume so that the blood volume that is available more adequately fills the circulation.

4. *Increased secretion of renin by the kidneys and formation of angiotensin II*, which constricts the peripheral arteries and also causes decreased output of water and salt by the kidneys, both of which help prevent progression of shock.

5. *Increased secretion by the posterior pituitary gland of vasopressin (antidiuretic hormone)*, which constricts the peripheral arteries and veins and greatly increases water retention by the kidneys.

6. *Increased secretion by the adrenal medullae of epinephrine and norepinephrine*, which constricts the peripheral arteries and veins and increases the heart rate.

7. *Compensatory mechanisms that return the blood volume back toward normal*, including absorption of large quantities of fluid from the intestinal tract, absorption of fluid into the blood capillaries from the interstitial spaces of the body, conservation of water and salt by the kidneys, and increased thirst and increased appetite for salt, which make the person drink water and eat salty foods if able.

The sympathetic reflexes and increased secretion of catecholamines by the adrenal medullae provide rapid help toward bringing about recovery because they become maximally activated within 30 seconds to a few minutes after hemorrhage.

The angiotensin and vasopressin mechanisms, as well as the reverse stress-relaxation that causes contraction of the blood vessels and venous reservoirs, all require 10 minutes to 1 hour to respond completely, but they aid greatly in increasing the arterial pressure or increasing the circulatory filling pressure and thereby increasing the return of blood to the heart.

Finally, readjustment of blood volume by absorption of fluid from the interstitial spaces and intestinal tract, as well as oral ingestion and absorption of additional quantities of water and salt, may require from 1 to 48 hours,

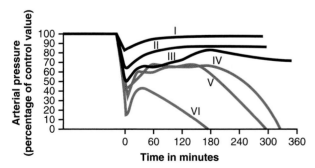

Figure 24-2 Time course of arterial pressure in dogs after different degrees of acute hemorrhage. Each curve represents average results from six dogs.

but recovery eventually takes place, provided the shock does not become severe enough to enter the progressive stage.

"Progressive Shock" Is Caused by a Vicious Circle of Cardiovascular Deterioration

Figure 24-3 shows some of the positive feedbacks that further depress cardiac output in shock, thus causing the shock to become progressive. Some of the more important feedbacks are the following.

Cardiac Depression. When the arterial pressure falls low enough, *coronary blood flow decreases below that required for adequate nutrition of the myocardium.* This weakens the heart muscle and thereby decreases the cardiac output more. Thus, a positive feedback cycle has developed, whereby the shock becomes more and more severe.

Figure 24-4 shows cardiac output curves extrapolated to the human heart from studies in experimental animals, demonstrating progressive deterioration of the heart at different times after the onset of shock. An anesthetized dog was bled until the arterial pressure fell to 30 mm Hg, and the pressure was held at this level by further bleeding or retransfusion of blood as required. Note from the second curve in the figure that there was little deterioration of the heart during the first 2 hours, but by 4 hours, the heart had deteriorated about 40 percent; then, rapidly, during the last hour of the experiment (after 4 hours of low coronary blood pressure), the heart deteriorated completely.

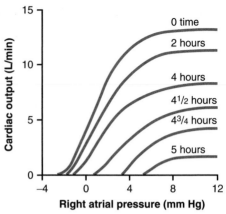

Figure 24-4 Cardiac output curves of the heart at different times after hemorrhagic shock begins. (These curves are extrapolated to the human heart from data obtained in dog experiments by Dr. J. W. Crowell.)

Thus, one of the important features of progressive shock, whether it is hemorrhagic in origin or caused in another way, is eventual progressive deterioration of the heart. In the early stages of shock, this plays very little role in the condition of the person, partly because deterioration of the heart is not severe during the first hour or so of shock, but mainly because the heart has tremendous reserve capability that normally allows it to pump 300 to 400 percent more blood than is required by the body for adequate tissue nutrition. In the latest stages of shock, however, deterioration of the heart is probably the

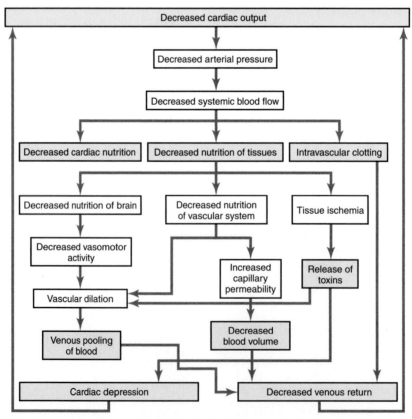

Figure 24-3 Different types of "positive feedback" that can lead to progression of shock.

most important factor in the final lethal progression of the shock.

Vasomotor Failure. In the early stages of shock, various circulatory reflexes cause intense activity of the sympathetic nervous system. This, as discussed earlier, helps delay depression of the cardiac output and especially helps prevent decreased arterial pressure. However, there comes a point when diminished blood flow to the brain's vasomotor center depresses the center so much that it, too, becomes progressively less active and finally totally inactive. For instance, *complete circulatory arrest to the brain* causes, during the first 4 to 8 minutes, the most intense of all sympathetic discharges, but by the end of 10 to 15 minutes, the vasomotor center becomes so depressed that no further evidence of sympathetic discharge can be demonstrated. Fortunately, the vasomotor center usually does not fail in the early stages of shock if the arterial pressure remains above 30 mm Hg.

Blockage of Very Small Vessels—"Sludged Blood." In time, blockage occurs in many of the very small blood vessels in the circulatory system and this also causes the shock to progress. The initiating cause of this blockage is sluggish blood flow in the microvessels. Because tissue metabolism continues despite the low flow, large amounts of acid, both carbonic acid and lactic acid, continue to empty into the local blood vessels and greatly increase the local acidity of the blood. This acid, plus other deterioration products from the ischemic tissues, causes local blood agglutination, resulting in minute blood clots, leading to very small plugs in the small vessels. Even if the vessels do not become plugged, an increased tendency for the blood cells to stick to one another makes it more difficult for blood to flow through the microvasculature, giving rise to the term *sludged blood.*

Increased Capillary Permeability. After many hours of capillary hypoxia and lack of other nutrients, the permeability of the capillaries gradually increases, and large quantities of fluid begin to transude into the tissues. This decreases the blood volume even more, with a resultant further decrease in cardiac output, making the shock still more severe. Capillary hypoxia does not cause increased capillary permeability until the late stages of prolonged shock.

Release of Toxins by Ischemic Tissue. Throughout the history of research in the field of shock, it has been suggested that shock causes tissues to release toxic substances, such as histamine, serotonin, and tissue enzymes, that cause further deterioration of the circulatory system. Experimental studies have proved the significance of at least one toxin, *endotoxin,* in some types of shock.

Cardiac Depression Caused by Endotoxin. *Endotoxin* is released from the bodies of dead gram-negative bacteria in the intestines. Diminished blood flow to the intestines often causes enhanced formation and absorption of this toxic substance. The circulating toxin then causes increased cellular metabolism despite inadequate nutrition of the cells; this has a specific effect on the heart muscle, causing *cardiac depression.* Endotoxin can play a major role in some types of shock, especially "septic shock," discussed later in the chapter.

Generalized Cellular Deterioration. As shock becomes severe, many signs of generalized cellular deterioration occur throughout the body. One organ especially affected is the *liver,* as illustrated in Figure 24-5. This occurs mainly because of lack of enough nutrients to support the normally high rate of metabolism in liver cells, but also partly because of the exposure of the liver cells to any vascular toxin or other abnormal metabolic factor occurring in shock.

Among the damaging cellular effects that are known to occur in most body tissues are the following:

1. Active transport of sodium and potassium through the cell membrane is greatly diminished. As a result, sodium and chloride accumulate in the cells and potassium is lost from the cells. In addition, the cells begin to swell.

2. Mitochondrial activity in the liver cells, as well as in many other tissues of the body, becomes severely depressed.

3. Lysosomes in the cells in widespread tissue areas begin to break open, with intracellular release of *hydrolases* that cause further intracellular deterioration.

4. Cellular metabolism of nutrients, such as glucose, eventually becomes greatly depressed in the last stages of shock. The actions of some hormones are depressed as well, including almost 100 percent depression of the action of insulin.

All these effects contribute to further deterioration of many organs of the body, including especially (1) the *liver,* with depression of its many metabolic and detoxification functions; (2) the *lungs,* with eventual development of pulmonary edema and poor ability to oxygenate the blood; and (3) the *heart,* thereby further depressing its contractility.

Tissue Necrosis in Severe Shock—Patchy Areas of Necrosis Occur Because of Patchy Blood Flows in Different Organs. Not all cells of the body are equally damaged by shock because some tissues have better blood supplies than others. For instance, the cells adjacent to the arterial ends of capillaries receive better nutrition than cells adjacent to the venous ends of the same capillaries. Therefore, more nutritive deficiency occurs around the venous ends of capillaries than elsewhere. For instance, Figure 24-5 shows necrosis in the center of a liver lobule, the portion of the lobule that is last to be exposed to the blood as it passes through the liver sinusoids.

Similar punctate lesions occur in heart muscle, although here a definite repetitive pattern, such as occurs in the liver, cannot be demonstrated. Nevertheless, the cardiac lesions play an important role in leading to the final irreversible stage of shock. Deteriorative lesions also occur in the kidneys, especially in the epithelium of the kidney tubules, leading to kidney failure and occasionally uremic death several days later. Deterioration of the lungs

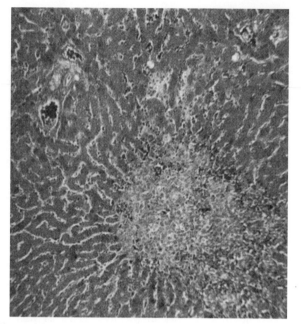

Figure 24-5 Necrosis of the central portion of a liver lobule in severe circulatory shock. (Courtesy Dr. J. W. Crowell.)

also often leads to respiratory distress and death several days later—called the *shock lung syndrome.*

Acidosis in Shock. Most metabolic derangements that occur in shocked tissue can lead to acidosis all through the body. This results from poor delivery of oxygen to the tissues, which greatly diminishes oxidative metabolism of the foodstuffs. When this occurs, the cells obtain most of their energy by the anaerobic process of glycolysis, which leads to tremendous quantities of *excess lactic acid* in the blood. In addition, poor blood flow through tissues prevents normal removal of carbon dioxide. The carbon dioxide reacts locally in the cells with water to form high concentrations of intracellular carbonic acid; this, in turn, reacts with various tissue chemicals to form still other intracellular acidic substances. Thus, another deteriorative effect of shock is both generalized and local tissue acidosis, leading to further progression of the shock itself.

Positive Feedback Deterioration of Tissues in Shock and the Vicious Circle of Progressive Shock

All the factors just discussed that can lead to further progression of shock are types of *positive feedback*. That is, each increase in the degree of shock causes a further increase in the shock.

However, positive feedback does not necessarily lead to a vicious circle. Whether a vicious circle develops depends on the intensity of the positive feedback. In mild degrees of shock, the negative feedback mechanisms of the circulation—sympathetic reflexes, reverse stress-relaxation mechanism of the blood reservoirs, absorption of fluid into the blood from the interstitial spaces, and others—can easily overcome the positive feedback influences and, therefore, cause recovery. But in severe degrees of shock, the deteriorative feedback mechanisms become more and more powerful, leading to such rapid deterioration of the

circulation that all the normal negative feedback systems of circulatory control acting together cannot return the cardiac output to normal.

Considering once again the principles of positive feedback and vicious circle discussed in Chapter 1, one can readily understand why there is a critical cardiac output level above which a person in shock recovers and below which a person enters a vicious circle of circulatory deterioration that proceeds until death.

Irreversible Shock

After shock has progressed to a certain stage, transfusion or any other type of therapy becomes incapable of saving the person's life. The person is then said to be in the *irreversible stage of shock.* Ironically, even in this irreversible stage, therapy can, on rare occasions, return the arterial pressure and even the cardiac output to normal or near normal for short periods, but the circulatory system nevertheless continues to deteriorate, and death ensues in another few minutes to few hours.

Figure 24-6 demonstrates this effect, showing that transfusion during the irreversible stage can sometimes cause the cardiac output (as well as the arterial pressure) to return to nearly normal. However, the cardiac output soon begins to fall again, and subsequent transfusions have less and less effect. By this time, multiple deteriorative changes have occurred in the muscle cells of the heart that may not necessarily affect the heart's *immediate* ability to pump blood but, over a long period, depress heart pumping enough to cause death. Beyond a certain point, so much tissue damage has occurred, so many destructive enzymes have been released into the body fluids, so much acidosis has developed, and so many other destructive factors are now in progress that even a normal cardiac output for a few minutes cannot reverse the continuing deterioration. Therefore, in severe shock, a stage is eventually reached at which the person will die even though vigorous therapy might still return the cardiac output to normal for short periods.

Depletion of Cellular High-Energy Phosphate Reserves in Irreversible Shock. The high-energy phosphate reserves in the tissues of the body, especially in the liver and the heart, are greatly diminished in severe degrees

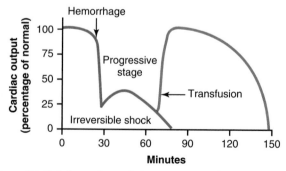

Figure 24-6 Failure of transfusion to prevent death in irreversible shock.

of shock. Essentially all the *creatine phosphate* has been degraded, and almost all the *adenosine triphosphate* has downgraded to *adenosine diphosphate, adenosine monophosphate,* and, eventually, *adenosine.* Then much of this adenosine diffuses out of the cells into the circulating blood and is converted into uric acid, a substance that cannot re-enter the cells to reconstitute the adenosine phosphate system. New adenosine can be synthesized at a rate of only about 2 percent of the normal cellular amount an hour, meaning that once the high-energy phosphate stores of the cells are depleted, they are difficult to replenish.

Thus, one of the most devastating end results of deterioration in shock, and the one that is perhaps most significant for development of the final state of irreversibility, is this cellular depletion of these high-energy compounds.

Hypovolemic Shock Caused by Plasma Loss

Loss of plasma from the circulatory system, even without loss of red blood cells, can sometimes be severe enough to reduce the total blood volume markedly, causing typical hypovolemic shock similar in almost all details to that caused by hemorrhage. Severe plasma loss occurs in the following conditions:

1. *Intestinal obstruction* may cause severely reduced plasma volume. Distention of the intestine in intestinal obstruction partly blocks venous blood flow in the intestinal walls, which increases intestinal capillary pressure. This in turn causes fluid to leak from the capillaries into the intestinal walls and also into the intestinal lumen. Because the lost fluid has high protein content, the result is reduced total blood plasma protein, as well as reduced plasma volume.

2. In almost all patients who have *severe burns* or other denuding conditions of the skin, so much plasma is lost through the denuded skin areas that the plasma volume becomes markedly reduced.

The hypovolemic shock that results from plasma loss has almost the same characteristics as the shock caused by hemorrhage, except for one additional complicating factor: the blood viscosity increases greatly as a result of increased red blood cell concentration in the remaining blood, and this exacerbates the sluggishness of blood flow.

Loss of fluid from all fluid compartments of the body is called *dehydration;* this, too, can reduce the blood volume and cause hypovolemic shock similar to that resulting from hemorrhage. Some of the causes of this type of shock are (1) excessive sweating, (2) fluid loss in severe diarrhea or vomiting, (3) excess loss of fluid by the kidneys, (4) inadequate intake of fluid and electrolytes, or (5) destruction of the adrenal cortices, with loss of aldosterone secretion and consequent failure of the kidneys to reabsorb sodium, chloride, and water, which occurs in the absence of the adrenocortical hormone aldosterone.

Hypovolemic Shock Caused by Trauma

One of the most common causes of circulatory shock is trauma to the body. Often the shock results simply from hemorrhage caused by the trauma, but it can also occur even without hemorrhage, because extensive contusion of the body can damage the capillaries sufficiently to allow excessive loss of plasma into the tissues. This results in greatly reduced plasma volume, with resultant hypovolemic shock.

Various attempts have been made to implicate toxic factors released by the traumatized tissues as one of the causes of shock after trauma. However, cross-transfusion experiments into normal animals have failed to show significant toxic elements.

In summary, traumatic shock seems to result mainly from hypovolemia, although there might also be a moderate degree of concomitant neurogenic shock caused by loss of vasomotor tone, as discussed next.

Neurogenic Shock—Increased Vascular Capacity

Shock occasionally results without any loss of blood volume. Instead, the *vascular capacity* increases so much that even the normal amount of blood becomes incapable of filling the circulatory system adequately. One of the major causes of this is *sudden loss of vasomotor tone* throughout the body, resulting especially in massive dilation of the veins. The resulting condition is known as *neurogenic shock.*

The role of vascular capacity in helping to regulate circulatory function was discussed in Chapter 15, where it was pointed out that either an increase in vascular capacity or a decrease in blood volume *reduces the mean systemic filling pressure,* which reduces venous return to the heart. Diminished venous return caused by vascular dilation is called *venous pooling* of blood.

Causes of Neurogenic Shock. Some neurogenic factors that can cause loss of vasomotor tone include the following:

1. *Deep general anesthesia* often depresses the vasomotor center enough to cause vasomotor paralysis, with resulting neurogenic shock.

2. *Spinal anesthesia,* especially when this extends all the way up the spinal cord, blocks the sympathetic nervous outflow from the nervous system and can be a potent cause of neurogenic shock.

3. *Brain damage* is often a cause of vasomotor paralysis. Many patients who have had brain concussion or contusion of the basal regions of the brain develop profound neurogenic shock. Also, even though brain ischemia for a few minutes almost always causes extreme vasomotor stimulation, prolonged ischemia (lasting longer than 5 to 10 minutes) can cause the opposite effect—

total inactivation of the vasomotor neurons in the brain stem, with consequent development of severe neurogenic shock.

Anaphylactic Shock and Histamine Shock

Anaphylaxis is an allergic condition in which the cardiac output and arterial pressure often decrease drastically. This is discussed in Chapter 34. It results primarily from an antigen-antibody reaction that rapidly occurs after an antigen to which the person is sensitive enters the circulation. One of the principal effects is to cause the *basophils* in the blood and *mast* cells in the pericapillary tissues to release *histamine* or a *histamine-like substance.* The histamine causes (1) an increase in vascular capacity because of venous dilation, thus causing a marked decrease in venous return; (2) dilation of the arterioles, resulting in greatly reduced arterial pressure; and (3) greatly increased capillary permeability, with rapid loss of fluid and protein into the tissue spaces. The net effect is a great reduction in venous return and sometimes such serious shock that the person dies within minutes.

Intravenous injection of large amounts of histamine causes "histamine shock," which has characteristics almost identical to those of anaphylactic shock.

Septic Shock

A condition that was formerly known by the popular name "blood poisoning" is now called *septic shock* by most clinicians. This refers to a bacterial infection widely disseminated to many areas of the body, with the infection being borne through the blood from one tissue to another and causing extensive damage. There are many varieties of septic shock because of the many types of bacterial infections that can cause it and because infection in different parts of the body produces different effects.

Septic shock is extremely important to the clinician because other than cardiogenic shock, septic shock is the most frequent cause of shock-related death in the modern hospital.

Some of the typical causes of septic shock include the following:

1. Peritonitis caused by spread of infection from the uterus and fallopian tubes, sometimes resulting from instrumental abortion performed under unsterile conditions.
2. Peritonitis resulting from rupture of the gastrointestinal system, sometimes caused by intestinal disease and sometimes by wounds.
3. Generalized bodily infection resulting from spread of a skin infection such as streptococcal or staphylococcal infection.
4. Generalized gangrenous infection resulting specifically from gas gangrene bacilli, spreading first through

peripheral tissues and finally by way of the blood to the internal organs, especially the liver.

5. Infection spreading into the blood from the kidney or urinary tract, often caused by colon bacilli.

Special Features of Septic Shock. Because of the multiple types of septic shock, it is difficult to categorize this condition. Some features often observed are:

1. High fever.
2. Often marked vasodilation throughout the body, especially in the infected tissues.
3. High cardiac output in perhaps half of patients, caused by arteriolar dilation in the infected tissues and by high metabolic rate and vasodilation elsewhere in the body, resulting from bacterial toxin stimulation of cellular metabolism and from high body temperature.
4. Sludging of the blood, caused by red cell agglutination in response to degenerating tissues.
5. Development of micro-blood clots in widespread areas of the body, a condition called *disseminated intravascular coagulation.* Also, this causes the blood clotting factors to be used up, so hemorrhaging occurs in many tissues, especially in the gut wall of the intestinal tract.

In early stages of septic shock, the patient usually does not have signs of circulatory collapse but only signs of the bacterial infection. As the infection becomes more severe, the circulatory system usually becomes involved either because of direct extension of the infection or secondarily as a result of toxins from the bacteria, with resultant loss of plasma into the infected tissues through deteriorating blood capillary walls. There finally comes a point at which deterioration of the circulation becomes progressive in the same way that progression occurs in all other types of shock. The end stages of septic shock are not greatly different from the end stages of hemorrhagic shock, even though the initiating factors are markedly different in the two conditions.

Physiology of Treatment in Shock

Replacement Therapy

Blood and Plasma Transfusion. If a person is in shock caused by hemorrhage, the best possible therapy is usually transfusion of whole blood. If the shock is caused by plasma loss, the best therapy is administration of plasma; when dehydration is the cause, administration of an appropriate electrolyte solution can correct the shock.

Whole blood is not always available, such as under battlefield conditions. Plasma can usually substitute adequately for whole blood because it increases the blood volume and restores normal hemodynamics. Plasma cannot restore a normal hematocrit, but the human body can usually stand a decrease in hematocrit to about half of normal before serious consequences result, if cardiac output is adequate. Therefore, in emergency conditions, it is reasonable to use plasma in place of whole blood for treatment of hemorrhagic or most other types of hypovolemic shock.

Sometimes plasma is unavailable. In these instances, various *plasma substitutes* have been developed that perform almost exactly the same hemodynamic functions as plasma. One of these is dextran solution.

Dextran Solution as a Plasma Substitute. The principal requirement of a truly effective plasma substitute is that it remain in the circulatory system—that is, does not filter through the capillary pores into the tissue spaces. In addition, the solution must be nontoxic and must contain appropriate electrolytes to prevent derangement of the body's extracellular fluid electrolytes on administration.

To remain in the circulation, the plasma substitute must contain some substance that has a large enough molecular size to exert colloid osmotic pressure. One substance developed for this purpose is *dextran,* a large polysaccharide polymer of glucose. Certain bacteria secrete dextran as a by-product of their growth, and commercial dextran can be manufactured using a bacterial culture procedure. By varying the growth conditions of the bacteria, the molecular weight of the dextran can be controlled to the desired value. Dextrans of appropriate molecular size do not pass through the capillary pores and, therefore, can replace plasma proteins as colloid osmotic agents.

Few toxic reactions have been observed when using purified dextran to provide colloid osmotic pressure; therefore, solutions containing this substance have proved to be a satisfactory substitute for plasma in most fluid replacement therapy.

Treatment of Shock with Sympathomimetic Drugs—Sometimes Useful, Sometimes Not

A *sympathomimetic drug* is a drug that mimics sympathetic stimulation. These drugs include *norepinephrine, epinephrine,* and a large number of long-acting drugs that have the same effect as epinephrine and norepinephrine.

In two types of shock, sympathomimetic drugs have proved to be especially beneficial. The first of these is *neurogenic shock,* in which the sympathetic nervous system is severely depressed. Administering a sympathomimetic drug takes the place of the diminished sympathetic actions and can often restore full circulatory function.

The second type of shock in which sympathomimetic drugs are valuable is *anaphylactic shock,* in which excess histamine plays a prominent role. The sympathomimetic drugs have a vasoconstrictor effect that opposes the vasodilating effect of histamine. Therefore, epinephrine, norepinephrine, or other sympathomimetic drugs are often lifesaving.

Sympathomimetic drugs have not proved to be very valuable in hemorrhagic shock. The reason is that in this type of shock, the sympathetic nervous system is almost always maximally activated by the circulatory reflexes already; so much norepinephrine and epinephrine are already circulating in the blood that sympathomimetic drugs have essentially no additional beneficial effect.

Other Therapy

Treatment by the Head-Down Position. When the pressure falls too low in most types of shock, especially in hemorrhagic and neurogenic shock, placing the patient with the head at least 12 inches lower than the feet helps in promoting venous return, thereby also increasing cardiac output. This head-down position is the first essential step in the treatment of many types of shock.

Oxygen Therapy. Because the major deleterious effect of most types of shock is too little delivery of oxygen to the tissues, giving the patient oxygen to breathe can be of benefit in some instances. However, this frequently is far less beneficial than one might expect, because the problem in most types of shock is not inadequate oxygenation of the blood by the lungs but inadequate transport of the blood after it is oxygenated.

Treatment with Glucocorticoids (Adrenal Cortex Hormones That Control Glucose Metabolism). Glucocorticoids are frequently given to patients in severe shock for several reasons: (1) experiments have shown empirically that glucocorticoids frequently increase the strength of the heart in the late stages of shock; (2) glucocorticoids stabilize lysosomes in tissue cells and thereby prevent release of lysosomal enzymes into the cytoplasm of the cells, thus preventing deterioration from this source; and (3) glucocorticoids might aid in the metabolism of glucose by the severely damaged cells.

Circulatory Arrest

A condition closely allied to circulatory shock is circulatory arrest, in which all blood flow stops. This occurs frequently on the surgical operating table as a result of *cardiac arrest* or *ventricular fibrillation.*

Ventricular fibrillation can usually be stopped by strong electroshock of the heart, the basic principles of which are described in Chapter 13.

Cardiac arrest may result from too little oxygen in the anesthetic gaseous mixture or from a depressant effect of the anesthesia itself. A normal cardiac rhythm can usually be restored by removing the anesthetic and immediately applying cardiopulmonary resuscitation procedures, while at the same time supplying the patient's lungs with adequate quantities of ventilatory oxygen.

Effect of Circulatory Arrest on the Brain

A special problem in circulatory arrest is to prevent detrimental effects in the brain as a result of the arrest. In general, more than 5 to 8 minutes of total circulatory arrest can cause at least some degree of permanent brain damage in more than half of patients. Circulatory arrest for as long as 10 to 15 minutes almost always permanently destroys significant amounts of mental power.

For many years, it was taught that this detrimental effect on the brain was caused by the acute cerebral hypoxia that occurs during circulatory arrest. However, experiments have shown that if blood clots are prevented from occurring in the blood vessels of the brain, this will also prevent much of the early deterioration of the brain during circulatory arrest. For instance, in animal experiments, all the blood was removed from the animal's blood vessels at the beginning of circulatory arrest and then replaced at the end of circulatory arrest so that no intravascular blood clotting could occur. In this experiment, the brain was usually able to withstand up to 30 minutes of circulatory arrest without permanent brain damage. Also, administration of heparin or streptokinase (to prevent blood coagulation) before cardiac arrest was shown to increase the survivability of the brain up to two to four times longer than usual.

It is likely that the severe brain damage that occurs from circulatory arrest is caused mainly by permanent blockage of many small blood vessels by blood clots, thus leading to prolonged ischemia and eventual death of the neurons.

Bibliography

Annane D, Sebille V, Charpentier C, et al: Effect of treatment with low doses of hydrocortisone and fludrocortisone on mortality in patients with septic shock, *JAMA* 288:862, 2002.

Burry LD, Wax RS: Role of corticosteroids in septic shock, *Ann Pharmacother* 38:464, 2004.

Crowell JW, Smith EE: Oxygen deficit and irreversible hemorrhagic shock, *Am J Physiol* 206:313, 1964.

Flierl MA, Rittirsch D, Huber-Lang MS, et al: Molecular events in the cardiomyopathy of sepsis, *Mol Med* 14:327, 2008.

Galli SJ, Tsai M, Piliponsky AM: The development of allergic inflammation, *Nature* 454:445, 2008.

Goodnough LT, Shander A: Evolution in alternatives to blood transfusion, *Hematol J* 4:87, 2003.

Guyton AC, Jones CE, Coleman TG: *Circulatory physiology: cardiac output and its regulation*, Philadelphia, 1973, WB Saunders.

Kemp SF, Lockey RF, Simons FE: Epinephrine: the drug of choice for anaphylaxis. A statement of the World Allergy Organization, *Allergy* 63:1061, 2008.

Martin GS, Mannino DM, Eaton S, et al: The epidemiology of sepsis in the United States from 1979 through 2000, *N Engl J Med* 348:1546, 2003.

Reynolds HR, Hochman J: Cardiogenic shock: current concepts and improving outcomes, *Circulation* 117:686, 2008.

Rushing GD, Britt LD: Reperfusion injury after hemorrhage: a collective review, *Ann Surg* 247:929, 2008.

Toh CH, Dennis M: Disseminated intravascular coagulation: old disease, new hope, *BMJ* 327:974, 2003.

Wheeler AP: Recent developments in the diagnosis and management of severe sepsis, *Chest* 132:1967, 2007.

Wilson M, Davis DP, Coimbra R: Diagnosis and monitoring of hemorrhagic shock during the initial resuscitation of multiple trauma patients: a review, *J Emerg Med* 24:413, 2003.

V

UNIT

The Body Fluids and Kidneys

25. The Body Fluid Compartments: Extracellular and Intracellular Fluids; Edema

26. Urine Formation by the Kidneys: I. Glomerular Filtration, Renal Blood Flow, and Their Control

27. Urine Formation by the Kidneys: II. Tubular Reabsorption and Secretion

28. Urine Concentration and Dilution; Regulation of Extracellular Fluid Osmolarity and Sodium Concentration

29. Renal Regulation of Potassium, Calcium, Phosphate, and Magnesium; Integration of Renal Mechanisms for Control of Blood Volume and Extracellular Fluid Volume

30. Acid-Base Regulation

31. Diuretics, Kidney Diseases

The Body Fluid Compartments: Extracellular and Intracellular Fluids; Edema

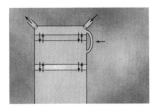

The maintenance of a relatively constant volume and a stable composition of the body fluids is essential for homeostasis, as discussed in Chapter 1. Some of the most common and important problems in clinical medicine arise because of abnormalities in the control systems that maintain this constancy of the body fluids. In this chapter and in the following chapters on the kidneys, we discuss the overall regulation of body fluid volume, constituents of the extracellular fluid, acid-base balance, and control of fluid exchange between extracellular and intracellular compartments.

Fluid Intake and Output Are Balanced During Steady-State Conditions

The relative constancy of the body fluids is remarkable because there is continuous exchange of fluid and solutes with the external environment, as well as within the different compartments of the body. For example, there is a highly variable fluid intake that must be carefully matched by equal output of water from the body to prevent body fluid volumes from increasing or decreasing.

Daily Intake of Water

Water is added to the body by two major sources: (1) It is ingested in the form of liquids or water in the food, which together normally add about 2100 ml/day to the body fluids, and (2) it is synthesized in the body as a result of oxidation of carbohydrates, adding about 200 ml/day. This provides a total water intake of about 2300 ml/day (Table 25-1). Intake of water, however, is highly variable among different people and even within the same person on different days, depending on climate, habits, and level of physical activity.

Daily Loss of Body Water

Insensible Water Loss. Some of the water losses cannot be precisely regulated. For example, there is a continuous loss of water by evaporation from the respiratory tract and diffusion through the skin, which together account for about 700 ml/day of water loss under normal conditions. This is termed *insensible water loss* because we are not consciously aware of it, even though it occurs continually in all living humans.

The insensible water loss through the skin occurs independently of sweating and is present even in people who are born without sweat glands; the average water loss by diffusion through the skin is about 300 to 400 ml/day. This loss is minimized by the cholesterol-filled cornified layer of the skin, which provides a barrier against excessive loss by diffusion. When the cornified layer becomes denuded, as occurs with extensive burns, the rate of evaporation can increase as much as 10-fold, to 3 to 5 L/day. For this reason, burn victims must be given large amounts of fluid, usually intravenously, to balance fluid loss.

Insensible water loss through the respiratory tract averages about 300 to 400 ml/day. As air enters the respiratory tract, it becomes saturated with moisture, to a vapor pressure of about 47 mm Hg, before it is expelled. Because the vapor pressure of the inspired air is usually less than 47 mm Hg, water is continuously lost through the lungs with respiration. In cold weather, the atmospheric vapor pressure decreases to nearly 0, causing an even greater loss of water from the lungs as the temperature decreases. This explains the dry feeling in the respiratory passages in cold weather.

Fluid Loss in Sweat. The amount of water lost by sweating is highly variable, depending on physical activity and environmental temperature. The volume of sweat normally is about 100 ml/day, but in very hot weather or during heavy exercise water loss in sweat occasionally increases to 1 to 2 L/hour. This would rapidly deplete the body fluids if intake were not also increased by activating the thirst mechanism discussed in Chapter 29.

Water Loss in Feces. Only a small amount of water (100 ml/day) normally is lost in the feces. This can increase to several liters a day in people with severe diarrhea. For this reason, severe diarrhea can be life threatening if not corrected within a few days.

Table 25-1 Daily Intake and Output of Water (ml/day)

	Normal	Prolonged, Heavy Exercise
Intake		
Fluids ingested	2100	?
From metabolism	200	200
Total intake	2300	?
Output		
Insensible—skin	350	350
Insensible—lungs	350	650
Sweat	100	5000
Feces	100	100
Urine	1400	500
Total output	2300	6600

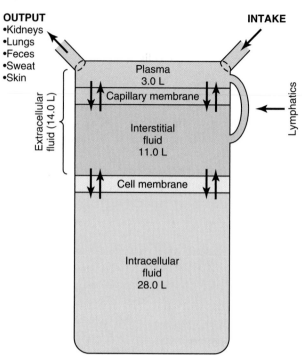

Figure 25-1 Summary of body fluid regulation, including the major body fluid compartments and the membranes that separate these compartments. The values shown are for an average 70-kilogram person.

Water Loss by the Kidneys. The remaining water loss from the body occurs in the urine excreted by the kidneys. There are multiple mechanisms that control the rate of urine excretion. In fact, the most important means by which the body maintains a balance between water intake and output, as well as a balance between intake and output of most electrolytes in the body, is by controlling the rates at which the kidneys excrete these substances. For example, urine volume can be as low as 0.5 L/day in a dehydrated person or as high as 20 L/day in a person who has been drinking tremendous amounts of water.

This variability of intake is also true for most of the electrolytes of the body, such as sodium, chloride, and potassium. In some people, sodium intake may be as low as 20 mEq/day, whereas in others, sodium intake may be as high as 300 to 500 mEq/day. The kidneys are faced with the task of adjusting the excretion rate of water and electrolytes to match precisely the intake of these substances, as well as compensating for excessive losses of fluids and electrolytes that occur in certain disease states. In Chapters 26 through 30, we discuss the mechanisms that allow the kidneys to perform these remarkable tasks.

Body Fluid Compartments

The total body fluid is distributed mainly between two compartments: the *extracellular fluid* and the *intracellular fluid* (Figure 25-1). The extracellular fluid is divided into the *interstitial fluid* and the blood *plasma.*

There is another small compartment of fluid that is referred to as *transcellular fluid.* This compartment includes fluid in the synovial, peritoneal, pericardial, and intraocular spaces, as well as the cerebrospinal fluid; it is usually considered to be a specialized type of extracellular fluid, although in some cases its composition may differ

markedly from that of the plasma or interstitial fluid. All the transcellular fluids together constitute about 1 to 2 liters.

In the average 70-kilogram adult man, the total body water is about 60 percent of the body weight, or about 42 liters. This percentage can change, depending on age, gender, and degree of obesity. As a person grows older, the percentage of total body weight that is fluid gradually decreases. This is due in part to the fact that aging is usually associated with an increased percentage of the body weight being fat, which decreases the percentage of water in the body.

Because women normally have more body fat than men, their total body water averages about 50 percent of the body weight. In premature and newborn babies, the total body water ranges from 70 to 75 percent of body weight. Therefore, when discussing the "average" body fluid compartments, we should realize that variations exist, depending on age, gender, and percentage of body fat.

Intracellular Fluid Compartment

About 28 of the 42 liters of fluid in the body are inside the 100 trillion cells and are collectively called the *intracellular fluid.* Thus, the intracellular fluid constitutes about 40 percent of the total body weight in an "average" person.

The fluid of each cell contains its individual mixture of different constituents, but the concentrations of these substances are similar from one cell to another. In fact, the composition of cell fluids is remarkably similar even in different animals, ranging from the most primitive microorganisms to humans. For this reason, the intracellular fluid of all the different cells together is considered to be one large fluid compartment.

Extracellular Fluid Compartment

All the fluids outside the cells are collectively called the *extracellular fluid.* Together these fluids account for about 20 percent of the body weight, or about 14 liters in a normal 70-kilogram man. The two largest compartments of the extracellular fluid are the *interstitial fluid,* which makes up more than three fourths (11 liters) of the extracellular fluid, and the *plasma,* which makes up almost one fourth of the extracellular fluid, or about 3 liters. The plasma is the noncellular part of the blood; it exchanges substances continuously with the interstitial fluid through the pores of the capillary membranes. These pores are highly permeable to almost all solutes in the extracellular fluid except the proteins. Therefore, the extracellular fluids are constantly mixing, so the plasma and interstitial fluids have about the same composition except for proteins, which have a higher concentration in the plasma.

Blood Volume

Blood contains both extracellular fluid (the fluid in plasma) and intracellular fluid (the fluid in the red blood cells). However, blood is considered to be a separate fluid compartment because it is contained in a chamber of its own, the circulatory system. The blood volume is especially important in the control of cardiovascular dynamics.

The average blood volume of adults is about 7 percent of body weight, or about 5 liters. About 60 percent of the blood is plasma and 40 percent is red blood cells, but these percentages can vary considerably in different people, depending on gender, weight, and other factors.

Hematocrit (Packed Red Cell Volume). The hematocrit is the fraction of the blood composed of red blood cells, as determined by centrifuging blood in a "hematocrit tube" until the cells become tightly packed in the bottom of the tube. It is impossible to completely pack the red cells together; therefore, about 3 to 4 percent of the plasma remains entrapped among the cells, and the true hematocrit is only about 96 percent of the measured hematocrit.

In men, the measured hematocrit is normally about 0.40, and in women, it is about 0.36. In severe *anemia,* the hematocrit may fall as low as 0.10, a value that is barely sufficient to sustain life. Conversely, there are some conditions in which there is excessive production of red blood cells, resulting in *polycythemia.* In these conditions, the hematocrit can rise to 0.65.

Constituents of Extracellular and Intracellular Fluids

Comparisons of the composition of the extracellular fluid, including the plasma and interstitial fluid, and the intracellular fluid are shown in Figures 25-2 and 25-3 and in Table 25-2.

Ionic Composition of Plasma and Interstitial Fluid Is Similar

Because the plasma and interstitial fluid are separated only by highly permeable capillary membranes, their ionic composition is similar. The most important difference between these two compartments is the higher concentration of protein in the plasma; because the capillaries have a low permeability to the plasma proteins, only small amounts of proteins are leaked into the interstitial spaces in most tissues.

Because of the *Donnan effect,* the concentration of positively charged ions (cations) is slightly greater ($\approx$2 percent) in the plasma than in the interstitial fluid. The plasma proteins have a net negative charge and, therefore, tend to bind cations, such as sodium and potassium ions, thus holding extra amounts of these cations in the plasma along with the plasma proteins. Conversely, negatively charged ions (anions) tend to have a slightly higher concentration in the interstitial fluid compared with the plasma, because the negative charges of the plasma proteins repel the negatively charged anions. For practical purposes, however, the concentration of ions in the interstitial fluid and in the plasma is considered to be about equal.

Referring again to Figure 25-2, one can see that the extracellular fluid, including the plasma and the interstitial fluid, contains large amounts of sodium and chloride ions, reasonably large amounts of bicarbonate ions, but only small quantities of potassium, calcium, magnesium, phosphate, and organic acid ions.

The composition of extracellular fluid is carefully regulated by various mechanisms, but especially by the kidneys, as discussed later. This allows the cells to remain continually bathed in a fluid that contains the proper concentration of electrolytes and nutrients for optimal cell function.

Intracellular Fluid Constituents

The intracellular fluid is separated from the extracellular fluid by a cell membrane that is highly permeable to water but not to most of the electrolytes in the body.

In contrast to the extracellular fluid, the intracellular fluid contains only small quantities of sodium and chloride ions and almost no calcium ions. Instead, it contains large amounts of potassium and phosphate ions plus moderate quantities of magnesium and sulfate ions, all of which have low concentrations in the extracellular fluid. Also, cells contain large amounts of protein, almost four times as much as in the plasma.

Measurement of Fluid Volumes in the Different Body Fluid Compartments—the Indicator-Dilution Principle

The volume of a fluid compartment in the body can be measured by placing an indicator substance in the compartment, allowing it to disperse evenly throughout the compartment's fluid, and then analyzing the extent to which the

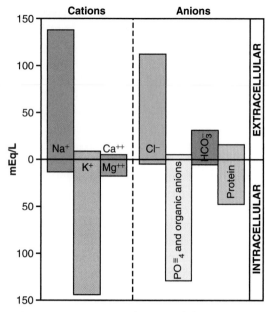

Figure 25-2 Major cations and anions of the intracellular and extracellular fluids. The concentrations of Ca⁺⁺ and Mg⁺⁺ represent the sum of these two ions. The concentrations shown represent the total of free ions and complexed ions.

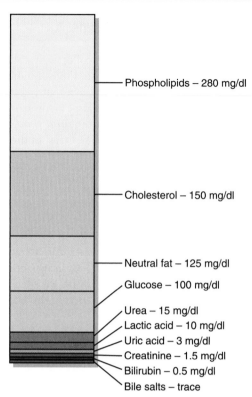

Phospholipids – 280 mg/dl

Cholesterol – 150 mg/dl

Neutral fat – 125 mg/dl
Glucose – 100 mg/dl
Urea – 15 mg/dl
Lactic acid – 10 mg/dl
Uric acid – 3 mg/dl
Creatinine – 1.5 mg/dl
Bilirubin – 0.5 mg/dl
Bile salts – trace

Figure 25-3 Nonelectrolytes of the plasma.

Table 25-2 Osmolar Substances in Extracellular and Intracellular Fluids

	Plasma (mOsm/L H₂O)	Interstitial (mOsm/L H₂O)	Intracellular (mOsm/L H₂O)
Na⁺	142	139	14
K⁺	4.2	4.0	140
Ca⁺⁺	1.3	1.2	0
Mg⁺⁺	0.8	0.7	20
Cl⁻	108	108	4
HCO₃⁻	24	28.3	10
HPO₄⁼, H₂PO₄⁻	2	2	11
SO₄⁼	0.5	0.5	1
Phosphocreatine			45
Carnosine			14
Amino acids	2	2	8
Creatine	0.2	0.2	9
Lactate	1.2	1.2	1.5
Adenosine triphosphate			5
Hexose monophosphate			3.7
Glucose	5.6	5.6	
Protein	1.2	0.2	4
Urea	4	4	4
Others	4.8	3.9	10
Total mOsm/L	301.8	300.8	301.2
Corrected osmolar activity (mOsm/L)	282.0	281.0	281.0
Total osmotic pressure at 37°C (mm Hg)	5443	5423	5423

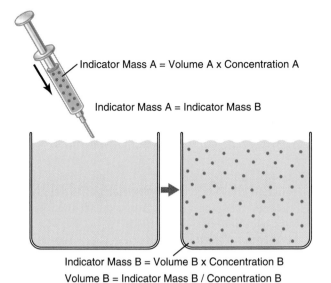

Indicator Mass A = Volume A x Concentration A

Indicator Mass A = Indicator Mass B

Indicator Mass B = Volume B x Concentration B
Volume B = Indicator Mass B / Concentration B

Figure 25-4 Indicator-dilution method for measuring fluid volumes.

substance becomes diluted. Figure 25-4 shows this "indicator-dilution" method of measuring the volume of a fluid compartment. This method is based on the conservation of mass principle, which means that the total mass of a substance after dispersion in the fluid compartment will be the same as the total mass injected into the compartment.

In the example shown in Figure 25-4, a small amount of dye or other substance contained in the syringe is injected into a chamber and the substance is allowed to disperse throughout the chamber until it becomes mixed in equal concentrations in all areas. Then a sample of fluid containing the dispersed substance is removed and the concentration is analyzed chemically, photoelectrically, or by other means. If none of the substance leaks out of the compartment, the total mass of substance in the compartment (Volume B × Concentration B) will equal the total mass of the substance injected (Volume A × Concentration A). By simple rearrangement of the equation, one can calculate the unknown volume of chamber B as

$$\text{Volume B} = \frac{\text{Volume A} \times \text{Concentration A}}{\text{Concentration B}}$$

Note that all one needs to know for this calculation is (1) the total amount of substance injected into the chamber (the numerator of the equation) and (2) the concentration of the fluid in the chamber after the substance has been dispersed (the denominator).

For example, if 1 milliliter of a solution containing 10 mg/ml of dye is dispersed into chamber B and the final concentration in the chamber is 0.01 milligram for each milliliter of fluid, the unknown volume of the chamber can be calculated as follows:

$$\text{Volume B} = \frac{1 \text{ ml} \times 10 \text{ mg/ml}}{0.01 \text{ mg/ml}} = 1000 \text{ ml}$$

This method can be used to measure the volume of virtually any compartment in the body as long as (1) the indicator disperses evenly throughout the compartment, (2) the indicator disperses only in the compartment that is being measured, and (3) the indicator is not metabolized or excreted. Several substances can be used to measure the volume of each of the different body fluids.

Determination of Volumes of Specific Body Fluid Compartments

Measurement of Total Body Water. Radioactive water (tritium, ^3H_2O) or heavy water (deuterium, ^2H_2O) can be used to measure total body water. These forms of water mix with the total body water within a few hours after being injected into the blood, and the dilution principle can be used to calculate total body water (Table 25-3). Another substance that has been used to measure total body water is *antipyrine*, which is very lipid soluble and can rapidly penetrate cell membranes and distribute itself uniformly throughout the intracellular and extracellular compartments.

Measurement of Extracellular Fluid Volume. The volume of extracellular fluid can be estimated using any of several substances that disperse in the plasma and interstitial fluid but do not readily permeate the cell membrane. They include radioactive sodium, radioactive chloride, radioactive iothalamate, thiosulfate ion, and inulin. When any one of these substances is injected into the blood, it usually disperses almost completely throughout the extracellular fluid within 30 to 60 minutes. Some of these substances, however, such as radioactive sodium, may diffuse into the cells in small amounts. Therefore, one frequently speaks of the *sodium space* or the *inulin space,* instead of calling the measurement the true extracellular fluid volume.

Table 25-3 Measurement of Body Fluid Volumes

Volume	Indicators
Total body water	^3H_2O, ^2H_2O, antipyrine
Extracellular fluid	^{22}Na, ^{125}I-iothalamate, thiosulfate, inulin
Intracellular fluid	(Calculated as total body water – Extracellular fluid volume)
Plasma volume	^{125}I-albumin, Evans blue dye (T-1824)
Blood volume	^{51}Cr-labeled red blood cells, or calculated as blood volume = Plasma volume/(1 – Hematocrit)
Interstitial fluid	(Calculated as extracellular fluid volume – Plasma volume)

Calculation of Intracellular Volume. The intracellular volume cannot be measured directly. However, it can be calculated as

Intracellular volume = Total body water – Extracellular volume

Measurement of Plasma Volume. To measure plasma volume, a substance must be used that does not readily penetrate capillary membranes but remains in the vascular system after injection. One of the most commonly used substances for measuring plasma volume is serum albumin labeled with radioactive iodine (^{125}I-albumin). Also, dyes that avidly bind to the plasma proteins, such as *Evans blue dye* (also called *T-1824*), can be used to measure plasma volume.

Calculation of Interstitial Fluid Volume. Interstitial fluid volume cannot be measured directly, but it can be calculated as

**Interstitial fluid volume =
Extracellular fluid volume – Plasma volume**

Measurement of Blood Volume. If one measures plasma volume using the methods described earlier, blood volume can also be calculated if one knows the *hematocrit* (the fraction of the total blood volume composed of cells), using the following equation:

$$\text{Total blood volume} = \frac{\text{Plasma volume}}{1 - \text{Hematocrit}}$$

For example, if plasma volume is 3 liters and hematocrit is 0.40, total blood volume would be calculated as

$$\frac{3 \text{ liters}}{1 - 0.4} = 5 \text{ liters}$$

Another way to measure blood volume is to inject into the circulation red blood cells that have been labeled with radioactive material. After these mix in the circulation, the radioactivity of a mixed blood sample can be measured and the total blood volume can be calculated using the indicator-dilution principle. A substance frequently used to label the red blood cells is radioactive chromium (^{51}Cr), which binds tightly with the red blood cells.

Regulation of Fluid Exchange and Osmotic Equilibrium Between Intracellular and Extracellular Fluid

A frequent problem in treating seriously ill patients is maintaining adequate fluids in one or both of the intracellular and extracellular compartments. As discussed in Chapter 16 and later in this chapter, the relative amounts of extracellular fluid distributed between the plasma and interstitial spaces are determined mainly by the balance of hydrostatic and colloid osmotic forces across the capillary membranes.

The distribution of fluid between intracellular and extracellular compartments, in contrast, is determined mainly by the osmotic effect of the smaller solutes—especially sodium, chloride, and other electrolytes—acting across the cell membrane. The reason for this is that the cell membranes are highly permeable to water but relatively impermeable to even small ions such as sodium and chloride. Therefore, water moves across the cell membrane rapidly and the intracellular fluid remains isotonic with the extracellular fluid.

In the next section, we discuss the interrelations between intracellular and extracellular fluid volumes and the osmotic factors that can cause shifts of fluid between these two compartments.

Basic Principles of Osmosis and Osmotic Pressure

The basic principles of osmosis and osmotic pressure were presented in Chapter 4. Therefore, we review here only the most important aspects of these principles as they apply to volume regulation.

Osmosis is the net diffusion of water across a selectively permeable membrane from a region of high water concentration to one that has a lower water concentration. When a solute is added to pure water, this reduces the concentration of water in the mixture. Thus, the higher the solute concentration in a solution, the lower the water concentration. Further, water diffuses from a region of low solute concentration (high water concentration) to one with a high solute concentration (low water concentration).

Because cell membranes are relatively impermeable to most solutes but highly permeable to water (i.e., selectively permeable), whenever there is a higher concentration of solute on one side of the cell membrane, water diffuses across the membrane toward the region of higher solute concentration. Thus, if a solute such as sodium chloride is added to the extracellular fluid, water rapidly diffuses from the cells through the cell membranes into the extracellular fluid until the water concentration on both sides of the membrane becomes equal. Conversely, if a solute such as sodium chloride is removed from the extracellular fluid, water diffuses from the extracellular fluid through the cell membranes and into the cells. The rate of diffusion of water is called the *rate of osmosis*.

Relation Between Moles and Osmoles. Because the water concentration of a solution depends on the number of solute particles in the solution, a concentration term is necessary to describe the total concentration of solute particles, regardless of their exact composition. The total number of particles in a solution is measured in *osmoles*. One osmole (osm) is equal to 1 mole (mol) (6.02×10^{23})

of solute particles. Therefore, a solution containing 1 mole of glucose in each liter has a concentration of 1 osm/L. If a molecule dissociates into two ions (giving two particles), such as sodium chloride ionizing to give chloride and sodium ions, then a solution containing 1 mol/L will have an osmolar concentration of 2 osm/L. Likewise, a solution that contains 1 mole of a molecule that dissociates into three ions, such as sodium sulfate (Na_2SO_4), will contain 3 osm/L. Thus, the term *osmole* refers to the number of osmotically active particles in a solution rather than to the molar concentration.

In general, the osmole is too large a unit for expressing osmotic activity of solutes in the body fluids.

The term *milliosmole* (mOsm), which equals 1/1000 osmole, is commonly used.

Osmolality and Osmolarity. The osmolal concentration of a solution is called *osmolality* when the concentration is expressed as *osmoles per kilogram of water;* it is called *osmolarity* when it is expressed as *osmoles per liter of solution.* In dilute solutions such as the body fluids, these two terms can be used almost synonymously because the differences are small. In most cases, it is easier to express body fluid quantities in liters of fluid rather than in kilograms of water. Therefore, most of the calculations used clinically and the calculations expressed in the next several chapters are based on osmolarities rather than osmolalities.

Calculation of the Osmolarity and Osmotic Pressure of a Solution. Using van't Hoff's law, one can calculate the potential osmotic pressure of a solution, assuming that the cell membrane is impermeable to the solute.

For example, the osmotic pressure of a 0.9 percent sodium chloride solution is calculated as follows: A 0.9 percent solution means that there is 0.9 gram of sodium chloride per 100 milliliters of solution, or 9 g/L. Because the molecular weight of sodium chloride is 58.5 g/mol, the molarity of the solution is 9 g/L divided by 58.5 g/mol, or about 0.154 mol/L. Because each molecule of sodium chloride is equal to 2 osmoles, the osmolarity of the solution is 0.154 × 2, or 0.308 osm/L. Therefore, the osmolarity of this solution is 308 mOsm/L. The potential osmotic pressure of this solution would therefore be 308 mOsm/L × 19.3 mm Hg/mOsm/L, or 5944 mm Hg.

This calculation is only an approximation because sodium and chloride ions do not behave entirely independently in solution because of interionic attraction between them. One can correct for these deviations from the predictions of van't Hoff's law by using a correction factor called the *osmotic coefficient.* For sodium chloride, the osmotic coefficient is about 0.93. Therefore, the actual osmolarity of a 0.9 percent sodium chloride solution is 308 × 0.93, or about 286 mOsm/L. For practical reasons, the osmotic coefficients of different solutes are sometimes neglected in determining the osmolarity and osmotic pressures of physiologic solutions.

Osmolarity of the Body Fluids. Turning back to Table 25-2, note the approximate osmolarity of the various osmotically active substances in plasma, interstitial fluid, and intracellular fluid. Note that about 80 percent of the total osmolarity of the interstitial fluid and plasma is due to sodium and chloride ions, whereas for intracellular fluid, almost half the osmolarity is due to potassium ions and the remainder is divided among many other intracellular substances.

As shown in Table 25-2, the total osmolarity of each of the three compartments is about 300 mOsm/L, with the plasma being about 1 mOsm/L greater than that of the interstitial and intracellular fluids. The slight difference between plasma and interstitial fluid is caused by the osmotic effects of the plasma proteins, which maintain about 20 mm Hg greater pressure in the capillaries than in the surrounding interstitial spaces, as discussed in Chapter 16.

Corrected Osmolar Activity of the Body Fluids. At the bottom of Table 25-2 are shown *corrected osmolar activities* of plasma, interstitial fluid, and intracellular fluid. The reason for these corrections is that cations and anions exert interionic attraction, which can cause a slight decrease in the osmotic "activity" of the dissolved substance.

Osmotic Equilibrium Is Maintained Between Intracellular and Extracellular Fluids

Large osmotic pressures can develop across the cell membrane with relatively small changes in the concentrations of solutes in the extracellular fluid. As discussed earlier, for each milliosmole concentration gradient of an *impermeant solute* (one that will not permeate the cell membrane), about 19.3 mm Hg osmotic pressure is exerted across the cell membrane. If the cell membrane is exposed to pure water and the osmolarity of intracellular fluid is 282 mOsm/L, the potential osmotic pressure that can develop across the cell membrane is more than 5400 mm Hg. This demonstrates the large force that can move water across the cell membrane when the intracellular and extracellular fluids are not in osmotic equilibrium. As a result of these forces, relatively small changes in the concentration of impermeant solutes in the extracellular fluid can cause large changes in cell volume.

Isotonic, Hypotonic, and Hypertonic Fluids. The effects of different concentrations of impermeant solutes in the extracellular fluid on cell volume are shown in Figure 25-5. If a cell is placed in a solution of impermeant solutes having an osmolarity of 282 mOsm/L, the cells

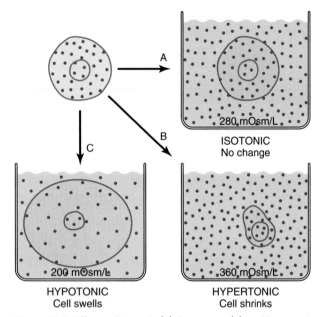

Figure 25-5 Effects of isotonic (*A*), hypertonic (*B*), and hypotonic (*C*) solutions on cell volume.

will not shrink or swell because the water concentration in the intracellular and extracellular fluids is equal and the solutes cannot enter or leave the cell. Such a solution is said to be *isotonic* because it neither shrinks nor swells the cells. Examples of isotonic solutions include a 0.9 percent solution of sodium chloride or a 5 percent glucose solution. These solutions are important in clinical medicine because they can be infused into the blood without the danger of upsetting osmotic equilibrium between the intracellular and extracellular fluids.

If a cell is placed into a *hypotonic* solution that has a lower concentration of impermeant solutes (<282 mOsm/L), water will diffuse into the cell, causing it to swell; water will continue to diffuse into the cell, diluting the intracellular fluid while also concentrating the extracellular fluid until both solutions have about the same osmolarity. Solutions of sodium chloride with a concentration of less than 0.9 percent are hypotonic and cause cells to swell.

If a cell is placed in a *hypertonic* solution having a higher concentration of impermeant solutes, water will flow out of the cell into the extracellular fluid, concentrating the intracellular fluid and diluting the extracellular fluid. In this case, the cell will shrink until the two concentrations become equal. Sodium chloride solutions of greater than 0.9 percent are hypertonic.

Isosmotic, Hyperosmotic, and Hypo-osmotic Fluids. The terms *isotonic, hypotonic,* and *hypertonic* refer to whether solutions will cause a change in cell volume. The tonicity of solutions depends on the concentration of impermeant solutes. Some solutes, however, can permeate the cell membrane. Solutions with an osmolarity the same as the cell are called *isosmotic,* regardless of whether the solute can penetrate the cell membrane.

The terms *hyperosmotic* and *hypo-osmotic* refer to solutions that have a higher or lower osmolarity, respectively, compared with the normal extracellular fluid, without regard for whether the solute permeates the cell membrane. Highly permeating substances, such as urea, can cause transient shifts in fluid volume between the intracellular and extracellular fluids, but given enough time, the concentrations of these substances eventually become equal in the two compartments and have little effect on intracellular volume under steady-state conditions.

Osmotic Equilibrium Between Intracellular and Extracellular Fluids Is Rapidly Attained. The transfer of fluid across the cell membrane occurs so rapidly that any differences in osmolarities between these two compartments are usually corrected within seconds or, at the most, minutes. This rapid movement of water across the cell membrane does not mean that complete equilibrium occurs between the intracellular and extracellular compartments throughout the whole body within the same short period. The reason for this is that fluid usually enters the body through the gut and must be transported by the blood to all tissues before complete osmotic equilibrium can occur. It usually takes about 30 minutes to achieve osmotic equilibrium everywhere in the body after drinking water.

Volume and Osmolality of Extracellular and Intracellular Fluids in Abnormal States

Some of the different factors that can cause extracellular and intracellular volumes to change markedly are ingestion of water, dehydration, intravenous infusion of different types of solutions, loss of large amounts of fluid from the gastrointestinal tract, and loss of abnormal amounts of fluid by sweating or through the kidneys.

One can calculate both the changes in intracellular and extracellular fluid volumes and the types of therapy that should be instituted if the following basic principles are kept in mind:

1. *Water moves rapidly across cell membranes;* therefore, the osmolarities of intracellular and extracellular fluids remain almost exactly equal to each other except for a few minutes after a change in one of the compartments.

2. *Cell membranes are almost completely impermeable to many solutes;* therefore, the number of osmoles in the extracellular or intracellular fluid generally remains constant unless solutes are added to or lost from the extracellular compartment.

With these basic principles in mind, we can analyze the effects of different abnormal fluid conditions on extracellular and intracellular fluid volumes and osmolarities.

Effect of Adding Saline Solution to the Extracellular Fluid

If an *isotonic* saline solution is added to the extracellular fluid compartment, the osmolarity of the extracellular fluid does not change; therefore, no osmosis occurs through the cell membranes. The only effect is an increase in extracellular fluid volume (Figure 25-6*A*). The sodium and chloride largely remain in the extracellular fluid because the cell membrane behaves as though it were virtually impermeable to the sodium chloride.

If a *hypertonic* solution is added to the extracellular fluid, the extracellular osmolarity increases and causes osmosis of water out of the cells into the extracellular compartment (see Figure 25-6*B*). Again, almost all the added sodium chloride remains in the extracellular compartment and fluid diffuses from the cells into the extracellular space to achieve osmotic equilibrium. The net effect is an increase in extracellular volume (greater than the volume of fluid added), a decrease in intracellular volume, and a rise in osmolarity in both compartments.

If a *hypotonic* solution is added to the extracellular fluid, the osmolarity of the extracellular fluid decreases and some of the extracellular water diffuses into the cells until the intracellular and extracellular compartments have the same osmolarity (see Figure 25-6*C*). Both the intracellular and the extracellular volumes are increased by the addition of hypotonic fluid, although the intracellular volume increases to a greater extent.

Calculation of Fluid Shifts and Osmolarities After Infusion of Hypertonic Saline. We can calculate the sequential effects of infusing different solutions on extracellular and intracellular fluid volumes and

osmolarities. For example, if 2 liters of a hypertonic 3.0 percent sodium chloride solution are infused into the extracellular fluid compartment of a 70-kilogram patient whose initial plasma osmolarity is 280 mOsm/L, what would be the intracellular and extracellular fluid volumes and osmolarities after osmotic equilibrium?

The first step is to calculate the initial conditions, including the volume, concentration, and total milliosmoles in each compartment. Assuming that extracellular fluid volume is 20 percent of body weight and intracellular fluid volume is 40 percent of body weight, the following volumes and concentrations can be calculated.

Step 1. Initial Conditions

	Volume (Liters)	Concentration (mOsm/L)	Total (mOsm)
Extracellular fluid	14	280	3,920
Intracellular fluid	28	280	7,840
Total body fluid	42	280	11,760

Next, we calculate the total milliosmoles added to the extracellular fluid in 2 liters of 3.0 percent sodium chloride. A 3.0 percent solution means that there are 3.0 g/100 ml, or 30 grams of sodium chloride per liter. Because the molecular weight of sodium chloride is about 58.5 g/mol, this means that there is about 0.513 mole of sodium chloride per liter of solution. For 2 liters of solution, this would be 1.026 mole of sodium chloride. Because 1 mole of sodium chloride is about equal to 2 osmoles (sodium chloride has two osmotically active particles per

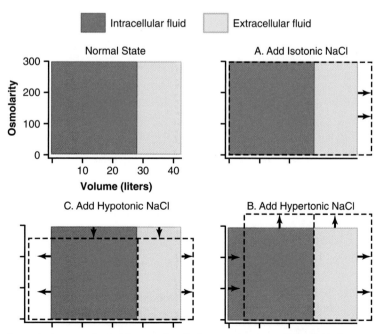

Figure 25-6 Effect of adding isotonic, hypertonic, and hypotonic solutions to the extracellular fluid after osmotic equilibrium. The normal state is indicated by the solid lines, and the shifts from normal are shown by the shaded areas. The volumes of intracellular and extracellular fluid compartments are shown in the abscissa of each diagram, and the osmolarities of these compartments are shown on the ordinates.

mole), the net effect of adding 2 liters of this solution is to add 2052 milliosmoles of sodium chloride to the extracellular fluid.

In Step 2, we calculate the instantaneous effect of adding 2052 milliosmoles of sodium chloride to the extracellular fluid along with 2 liters of volume. There would be no change in the *intracellular fluid* concentration or volume, and there would be no osmotic equilibrium. In the *extracellular fluid,* however, there would be an additional 2051 milliosmoles of total solute, yielding a total of 5971 milliosmoles. Because the extracellular compartment now has 16 liters of volume, the concentration can be calculated by dividing 5971 milliosmoles by 16 liters to yield a concentration of 373 mOsm/L. Thus, the following values would occur instantly after adding the solution.

Step 2. Instantaneous Effect of Adding 2 Liters of 3.0 Percent Sodium Chloride

	Volume (Liters)	Concentration (mOsm/L)	Total (mOsm)
Extracellular fluid	16	373	5,972
Intracellular fluid	28	280	7,840
Total body fluid	44	No equilibrium	13,812

In the third step, we calculate the volumes and concentrations that would occur within a few minutes after osmotic equilibrium develops. In this case, the concentrations in the intracellular and extracellular fluid compartments would be equal and can be calculated by dividing the total milliosmoles in the body, 13,812, by the total volume, which is now 44 liters. This yields a concentration of 313.9 mOsm/L. Therefore, all the body fluid compartments will have this same concentration after osmotic equilibrium. Assuming that no solute or water has been lost from the body and that there is no movement of sodium chloride into or out of the cells, we then calculate the volumes of the intracellular and extracellular compartments. The intracellular fluid volume is calculated by dividing the total milliosmoles in the intracellular fluid (7840) by the concentration (313.9 mOsm/L), to yield a volume of 24.98 liters. Extracellular fluid volume is calculated by dividing the total milliosmoles in extracellular fluid (5972) by the concentration (313.9 mOsm/L), to yield a volume of 19.02 liters. Again, these calculations are based on the assumption that the sodium chloride added to the extracellular fluid remains there and does not move into the cells.

Step 3. Effect of Adding 2 Liters of 3.0 Percent Sodium Chloride After Osmotic Equilibrium

	Volume (Liters)	Concentration (mOsm/L)	Total (mOsm)
Extracellular fluid	19.02	313.9	5,972
Intracellular fluid	24.98	313.9	7,840
Total body fluid	44.0	313.9	13,812

Thus, one can see from this example that adding 2 liters of a hypertonic sodium chloride solution causes more than a 5-liter increase in extracellular fluid volume while decreasing intracellular fluid volume by almost 3 liters.

This method of calculating changes in intracellular and extracellular fluid volumes and osmolarities can be applied to virtually any clinical problem of fluid volume regulation. The reader should be familiar with such calculations because an understanding of the mathematical aspects of osmotic equilibrium between intracellular and extracellular fluid compartments is essential for understanding almost all fluid abnormalities of the body and their treatment.

Glucose and Other Solutions Administered for Nutritive Purposes

Many types of solutions are administered intravenously to provide nutrition to people who cannot otherwise take adequate amounts of nutrition. Glucose solutions are widely used, and amino acid and homogenized fat solutions are used to a lesser extent. When these solutions are administered, their concentrations of osmotically active substances are usually adjusted nearly to isotonicity, or they are given slowly enough that they do not upset the osmotic equilibrium of the body fluids. After the glucose or other nutrients are metabolized, an excess of water often remains, especially if additional fluid is ingested. Ordinarily, the kidneys excrete this in the form of a very dilute urine. The net result, therefore, is the addition of only nutrients to the body.

Clinical Abnormalities of Fluid Volume Regulation: Hyponatremia and Hypernatremia

The primary measurement that is readily available to the clinician for evaluating a patient's fluid status is the plasma sodium concentration. Plasma osmolarity is not routinely measured, but because sodium and its associated anions (mainly chloride) account for more than 90 percent of the solute in the extracellular fluid, plasma sodium concentration is a reasonable indicator of plasma osmolarity under many conditions. When plasma sodium concentration is reduced more than a few milliequivalents below normal (about 142 mEq/L), a person is said to have *hyponatremia.* When plasma sodium concentration is elevated above normal, a person is said to have *hypernatremia.*

Causes of Hyponatremia: Excess Water or Loss of Sodium

Decreased plasma sodium concentration can result from loss of sodium chloride from the extracellular fluid or addition of excess water to the extracellular fluid (Table 25-4).

Table 25-4 Abnormalities of Body Fluid Volume Regulation: Hyponatremia and Hypernatremia

Abnormality	Cause	Plasma Na+ Concentration	Extracellular Fluid Volume	Intracellular Fluid Volume
Hyponatremia—dehydration	Adrenal insufficiency; overuse of diuretics	↓	↓	↑
Hyponatremia—overhydration	Excess ADH (SIADH); bronchogenic tumors	↓	↑	↑
Hypernatremia—dehydration	Diabetes insipidus; excessive sweating	↑	↓	↓
Hypernatremia—overhydration	Cushing's disease; primary aldosteronism	↑	↑	↓

ADH, antidiuretic hormone; SIADH, syndrome of inappropriate ADH.

A primary loss of sodium chloride usually results in *hyponatremia—dehydration* and is associated with decreased extracellular fluid volume. Conditions that can cause hyponatremia owing to loss of sodium chloride include *diarrhea* and *vomiting. Overuse of diuretics* that inhibit the ability of the kidneys to conserve sodium and certain types of sodium-wasting kidney diseases can also cause modest degrees of hyponatremia. Finally, *Addison's disease,* which results from decreased secretion of the hormone aldosterone, impairs the ability of the kidneys to reabsorb sodium and can cause a modest degree of hyponatremia.

Hyponatremia can also be associated with excess water retention, which dilutes the sodium in the extracellular fluid, a condition that is referred to as *hyponatremia—overhydration.* For example, *excessive secretion of antidiuretic hormone,* which causes the kidney tubules to reabsorb more water, can lead to hyponatremia and overhydration.

Consequences of Hyponatremia: Cell Swelling

Rapid changes in cell volume as a result of hyponatremia can have profound effects on tissue and organ function, especially the brain. A rapid reduction in plasma sodium concentration, for example, can cause brain cell edema and neurological symptoms, including headache, nausea, lethargy, and disorientation. If plasma sodium concentration rapidly falls below 115 to 120 mmol/L, brain swelling may lead to seizures, coma, permanent brain damage, and death. Because the skull is rigid, the brain cannot increase its volume by more than about 10 percent without it being forced down the neck *(herniation),* which can lead to permanent brain injury and death.

When hyponatremia evolves more slowly over several days, the brain and other tissues respond by transporting sodium, chloride, potassium, and organic solutes, such as glutamate, from the cells into the extracellular compartment. This attenuates osmotic flow of water into the cells and swelling of the tissues (Figure 25-7).

Transport of solutes from the cells during slowly developing hyponatremia, however, can make the brain vulnerable to injury if the hyponatremia is corrected too rapidly. When hypertonic solutions are added too rapidly to correct hyponatremia, this can outpace the brain's ability to recapture the solutes lost from the cells and may lead to osmotic injury of the neurons that is associated with *demyelination,* a loss of the myelin sheath from nerves. This osmotic-mediated demyelination of neurons can be avoided by limiting the correction of chronic hyponatremia to less than 10 to 12 mmol/L in 24 hours and to less than 18 mmol/L in 48 hours. This slow rate of correction permits the brain to recover the lost osmoles that have occurred as a result of adaptation to chronic hyponatremia.

Hyponatremia is the most common electrolyte disorder encountered in clinical practice and may occur in up to 15% to 25% of hospitalized patients.

Causes of Hypernatremia: Water Loss or Excess Sodium

Increased plasma sodium concentration, which also causes increased osmolarity, can be due to either loss of water from the extracellular fluid, which concentrates the sodium ions, or excess sodium in the extracellular fluid. When there is primary loss of water from the extracellular fluid, this results in *hypernatremia—dehydration.* This condition can occur from an inability to secrete antidiuretic hormone, which is needed for the kidneys to conserve water. As a result of lack of antidiuretic hormone, the kidneys excrete large amounts of dilute urine (a disorder referred to as *diabetes insipidus*), causing dehydration and increased concentration of sodium chloride in the extracellular fluid. In certain types of renal diseases, the kidneys cannot respond to antidiuretic hormone, also causing a type of *nephrogenic diabetes insipidus.* A more common cause of hypernatremia associated with decreased extracellular fluid volume is *dehydration* caused by water intake that is less than water loss, as can occur with sweating during prolonged, heavy exercise.

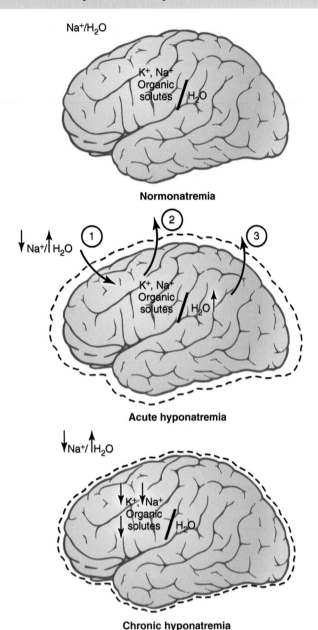

Figure 25-7 Brain cell volume regulation during hyponatremia. During acute hyponatremia, caused by loss of Na$^+$ or excess H$_2$O, there is diffusion of H$_2$O into the cells (*1*) and swelling of the brain tissue. This stimulates transport of Na$^+$, K$^+$, and organic solutes out of the cells (*2*), which then cause water diffusion out of the cells (*3*). With chronic hyponatremia, the brain swelling is attenuated by the transport of solutes from the cells.

Hypernatremia can also occur as a result of excessive sodium chloride added to the extracellular fluid. This often results in *hypernatremia—overhydration* because excess extracellular sodium chloride is usually associated with at least some degree of water retention by the kidneys as well. For example, *excessive secretion of the sodium-retaining hormone aldosterone* can cause a mild degree of hypernatremia and overhydration. The reason that the hypernatremia is not more severe is that increased aldosterone secretion causes the kidneys to reabsorb greater amounts of water, as well as sodium.

Thus, in analyzing abnormalities of plasma sodium concentration and deciding on proper therapy, one should first determine whether the abnormality is caused by a primary loss or gain of sodium or a primary loss or gain of water.

Consequences of Hypernatremia: Cell Shrinkage

Hypernatremia is much less common than hyponatremia and severe symptoms usually occur only with rapid and large increases in plasma sodium concentration above 158 to 160 mmol/L. One reason for this is that hypernatremia promotes intense thirst that protects against a large increase in plasma and extracellular fluid sodium, as discussed in Chapter 28. However, severe hypernatremia can occur in patients with hypothalamic lesions that impair their sense of thirst, in infants who may not have ready access to water, or elderly patients with altered mental status.

Correction of hypernatremia can be achieved by administering hypo-osmotic sodium chloride or dextrose solutions. However, it is prudent to correct the hypernatremia slowly in patients who have had chronic increases in plasma sodium concentration. The reason for this is that hypernatremia also activates defense mechanisms that protect the cell from changes in volume. These defense mechanisms are opposite to those that occur for hyponatremia and consist of mechanisms that increase the intracellular concentration of sodium and other solutes.

Edema: Excess Fluid in the Tissues

Edema refers to the presence of excess fluid in the body tissues. In most instances, edema occurs mainly in the extracellular fluid compartment, but it can involve intracellular fluid as well.

Intracellular Edema

Three conditions are especially prone to cause intracellular swelling: (1) hyponatremia, as discussed earlier; (2) depression of the metabolic systems of the tissues; and (3) lack of adequate nutrition to the cells. For example, when blood flow to a tissue is decreased, the delivery of oxygen and nutrients is reduced. If the blood flow becomes too low to maintain normal tissue metabolism, the cell membrane ionic pumps become depressed. When this occurs, sodium ions that normally leak into the interior of the cell can no longer be pumped out of the cells and the excess intracellular sodium ions cause osmosis of water into the cells. Sometimes this can increase intracellular volume of a tissue area—even of an entire ischemic leg, for example—to two to three times normal. When this occurs, it is usually a prelude to death of the tissue.

Intracellular edema can also occur in inflamed tissues. Inflammation usually increases cell membrane permeability, allowing sodium and other ions to diffuse into the interior of the cell, with subsequent osmosis of water into the cells.

Extracellular Edema

Extracellular fluid edema occurs when there is excess fluid accumulation in the extracellular spaces. There are two general causes of extracellular edema: (1) abnormal leakage of fluid from the plasma to the interstitial spaces across the capillaries, and (2) failure of the lymphatics to return fluid from the interstitium back into the blood, often called *lymphedema*. The most common clinical cause of interstitial fluid accumulation is excessive capillary fluid filtration.

Factors That Can Increase Capillary Filtration

To understand the causes of excessive capillary filtration, it is useful to review the determinants of capillary filtration discussed in Chapter 16. Mathematically, capillary filtration rate can be expressed as

$$\text{Filtration} = K_f \times (P_c - P_{if} - \pi_c + \pi_{if}),$$

where K_f is the capillary filtration coefficient (the product of the permeability and surface area of the capillaries), P_c is the capillary hydrostatic pressure, P_{if} is the interstitial fluid hydrostatic pressure, π_c is the capillary plasma colloid osmotic pressure, and π_{if} is the interstitial fluid colloid osmotic pressure. From this equation, one can see *that any one of the following changes can increase the capillary filtration rate:*

- Increased capillary filtration coefficient.
- Increased capillary hydrostatic pressure.
- Decreased plasma colloid osmotic pressure.

Lymphedema—Failure of the Lymph Vessels to Return Fluid and Protein to the Blood

When lymph vessel function is greatly impaired, due to blockage or loss of the lymph vessels, edema can become especially severe because plasma proteins that leak into the interstitium have no other way to be removed. The rise in protein concentration raises the colloid osmotic pressure of the interstitial fluid, which draws even more fluid out of the capillaries.

Blockage of lymph flow can be especially severe with infections of the lymph nodes, such as occurs with infection by *filaria nematodes (Wuchereria bancrofti),* which are microscopic, threadlike worms. The adult worms live in the human lymph system and are spread from person to person by mosquitoes. People with filarial infections can suffer from severe lymphedema and *elephantiasis* and in men, swelling of the scrotum, called *hydrocele.* Lymphatic filariasis affects over 120 million people in 80 countries throughout the tropics and subtropics of Asia, Africa, the Western Pacific, and parts of the Caribbean and South America.

Lymphedema can also occur in certain types of cancer or after surgery in which lymph vessels are removed or obstructed. For example, large numbers of lymph vessels are removed during radical mastectomy, impairing removal of fluid from the breast and arm areas and causing edema and swelling of the tissue spaces. A few lymph vessels eventually regrow after this type of surgery, so the interstitial edema is usually temporary.

Summary of Causes of Extracellular Edema

A large number of conditions can cause fluid accumulation in the interstitial spaces by abnormal leaking of fluid from the capillaries or by preventing the lymphatics from returning fluid from the interstitium back to the circulation. The following is a partial list of conditions that can cause extracellular edema by these two types of abnormalities:

I. Increased capillary pressure
   A. Excessive kidney retention of salt and water
      1. Acute or chronic kidney failure
      2. Mineralocorticoid excess
   B. High venous pressure and venous constriction
      1. Heart failure
      2. Venous obstruction
      3. Failure of venous pumps
         (a) Paralysis of muscles
         (b) Immobilization of parts of the body
         (c) Failure of venous valves
   C. Decreased arteriolar resistance
      1. Excessive body heat
      2. Insufficiency of sympathetic nervous system
      3. Vasodilator drugs
II. Decreased plasma proteins
   A. Loss of proteins in urine (nephrotic syndrome)
   B. Loss of protein from denuded skin areas
      1. Burns
      2. Wounds
   C. Failure to produce proteins
      1. Liver disease (e.g., cirrhosis)
      2. Serious protein or caloric malnutrition
III. Increased capillary permeability
   A. Immune reactions that cause release of histamine and other immune products
   B. Toxins
   C. Bacterial infections
   D. Vitamin deficiency, especially vitamin C
   E. Prolonged ischemia
   F. Burns
IV. Blockage of lymph return
   A. Cancer
   B. Infections (e.g., filaria nematodes)
   C. Surgery
   D. Congenital absence or abnormality of lymphatic vessels

Edema Caused by Heart Failure. One of the most serious and most common causes of edema is heart failure. In heart failure, the heart fails to pump blood normally from the veins into the arteries; this raises venous pressure and capillary pressure, causing increased capillary filtration. In addition, the arterial pressure tends to fall, causing decreased excretion of salt and water by the kidneys, which increases blood volume and further raises capillary hydrostatic pressure to cause still more edema. Also, blood flow to the kidneys is reduced in heart failure and this stimulates secretion of renin, causing increased formation of angiotensin II and increased secretion of aldosterone, both of which cause additional salt and water retention by the kidneys. Thus, in untreated heart failure, all these factors acting together cause serious generalized extracellular edema.

In patients with left-sided heart failure but without significant failure of the right side of the heart, blood is pumped into the lungs normally by the right side of the heart but cannot escape easily from the pulmonary veins to the left side of the heart because this part of the heart has been greatly weakened. Consequently, all the pulmonary vascular pressures, including pulmonary capillary pressure, rise far above normal, causing serious and life-threatening pulmonary edema. When untreated, fluid accumulation in the lungs can rapidly progress, causing death within a few hours.

Edema Caused by Decreased Kidney Excretion of Salt and Water. As discussed earlier, most sodium chloride added to the blood remains in the extracellular compartment, and only small amounts enter the cells. Therefore, in kidney diseases that compromise urinary excretion of salt and water, large amounts of sodium chloride and water are added to the extracellular fluid. Most of this salt and water leaks from the blood into the interstitial spaces, but some remains in the blood. The main effects of this are to cause (1) widespread increases in interstitial fluid volume (extracellular edema) and (2) hypertension because of the increase in blood volume, as explained in Chapter 19. As an example, children who develop acute glomerulonephritis, in which the renal glomeruli are injured by inflammation and therefore fail to filter adequate amounts of fluid, also develop serious extracellular fluid edema in the entire body; along with the edema, these children usually develop severe hypertension.

Edema Caused by Decreased Plasma Proteins. A reduction in plasma concentration of proteins because of either failure to produce normal amounts of proteins or leakage of proteins from the plasma causes the plasma colloid osmotic pressure to fall. This leads to increased capillary filtration throughout the body and extracellular edema.

One of the most important causes of decreased plasma protein concentration is loss of proteins in the urine in certain kidney diseases, a condition referred to as *nephrotic syndrome.* Multiple types of renal diseases can damage the membranes of the renal glomeruli, causing the mem-

branes to become leaky to the plasma proteins and often allowing large quantities of these proteins to pass into the urine. When this loss exceeds the ability of the body to synthesize proteins, a reduction in plasma protein concentration occurs. Serious generalized edema occurs when the plasma protein concentration falls below 2.5 g/100 ml.

Cirrhosis of the liver is another condition that causes a reduction in plasma protein concentration. Cirrhosis means development of large amounts of fibrous tissue among the liver parenchymal cells. One result is failure of these cells to produce sufficient plasma proteins, leading to decreased plasma colloid osmotic pressure and the generalized edema that goes with this condition.

Another way liver cirrhosis causes edema is that the liver fibrosis sometimes compresses the abdominal portal venous drainage vessels as they pass through the liver before emptying back into the general circulation. Blockage of this portal venous outflow raises capillary hydrostatic pressure throughout the gastrointestinal area and further increases filtration of fluid out of the plasma into the intra-abdominal areas. When this occurs, the combined effects of decreased plasma protein concentration and high portal capillary pressures cause transudation of large amounts of fluid and protein into the abdominal cavity, a condition referred to as *ascites.*

Safety Factors That Normally Prevent Edema

Even though many disturbances can cause edema, usually the abnormality must be severe before serious edema develops. The reason for this is that three major safety factors prevent excessive fluid accumulation in the interstitial spaces: (1) low compliance of the interstitium when interstitial fluid pressure is in the negative pressure range, (2) the ability of lymph flow to increase 10- to 50-fold, and (3) washdown of interstitial fluid protein concentration, which reduces interstitial fluid colloid osmotic pressure as capillary filtration increases.

Safety Factor Caused by Low Compliance of the Interstitium in the Negative Pressure Range

In Chapter 16, we noted that interstitial fluid hydrostatic pressure in most loose subcutaneous tissues of the body is slightly less than atmospheric pressure, averaging about −3 mm Hg. This slight suction in the tissues helps hold the tissues together. Figure 25-8 shows the approximate relations between different levels of interstitial fluid pressure and interstitial fluid volume, as extrapolated to the human being from animal studies. Note in Figure 25-8 that as long as the interstitial fluid pressure is in the negative range, small changes in interstitial fluid volume are associated with relatively large changes in interstitial fluid hydrostatic pressure. Therefore, in the negative pressure range, the *compliance* of the tissues, defined as the change in volume per millimeter of mercury pressure change, is low.

How does the low compliance of the tissues in the negative pressure range act as a safety factor against edema? To answer this question, recall the determinants of capillary

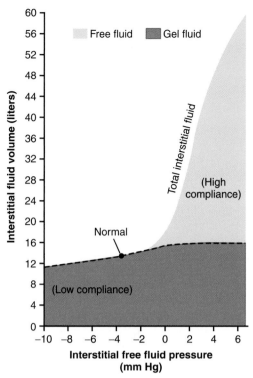

Figure 25-8 Relation between interstitial fluid hydrostatic pressure and interstitial fluid volumes, including total volume, free fluid volume, and gel fluid volume, for loose tissues such as skin. Note that significant amounts of free fluid occur only when the interstitial fluid pressure becomes positive. (Modified from Guyton AC, Granger HJ, Taylor AE: Interstitial fluid pressure. Physiol Rev 51:527, 1971.)

filtration discussed previously. When interstitial fluid hydrostatic pressure increases, this increased pressure tends to oppose further capillary filtration. Therefore, as long as the interstitial fluid hydrostatic pressure is in the negative pressure range, small increases in interstitial fluid volume cause relatively large increases in interstitial fluid hydrostatic pressure, opposing further filtration of fluid into the tissues.

Because the normal interstitial fluid hydrostatic pressure is –3 mm Hg, the interstitial fluid hydrostatic pressure must increase by about 3 mm Hg before large amounts of fluid will begin to accumulate in the tissues. Therefore, the safety factor against edema is a change of interstitial fluid pressure of about 3 mm Hg.

Once interstitial fluid pressure rises above 0 mm Hg, the compliance of the tissues increases markedly, allowing large amounts of fluid to accumulate in the tissues with relatively small additional increases in interstitial fluid hydrostatic pressure. Thus, in the positive tissue pressure range, this safety factor against edema is lost because of the large increase in compliance of the tissues.

Importance of Interstitial Gel in Preventing Fluid Accumulation in the Interstitium. Note in Figure 25-8 that in normal tissues with negative interstitial fluid pressure, virtually all the fluid in the interstitium is in gel form. That is, the fluid is bound in a proteoglycan meshwork so that there are virtually no "free" fluid spaces larger than a few hundredths of a micrometer in diameter. The importance of the gel is that it prevents fluid from *flowing* eas-

ily through the tissues because of impediment from the "brush pile" of trillions of proteoglycan filaments. Also, when the interstitial fluid pressure falls to very negative values, the gel does not contract greatly because the meshwork of proteoglycan filaments offers an elastic resistance to compression. In the negative fluid pressure range, the interstitial fluid volume does not change greatly, regardless of whether the degree of suction is only a few millimeters of mercury negative pressure or 10 to 20 mm Hg negative pressure. In other words, the compliance of the tissues is very low in the negative pressure range.

By contrast, when interstitial fluid pressure rises to the positive pressure range, there is a tremendous accumulation of *free fluid* in the tissues. In this pressure range, the tissues are compliant, allowing large amounts of fluid to accumulate with relatively small additional increases in interstitial fluid hydrostatic pressure. Most of the extra fluid that accumulates is "free fluid" because it pushes the brush pile of proteoglycan filaments apart. Therefore, the fluid can flow freely through the tissue spaces because it is not in gel form. When this occurs, the edema is said to be *pitting edema* because one can press the thumb against the tissue area and push the fluid out of the area. When the thumb is removed, a pit is left in the skin for a few seconds until the fluid flows back from the surrounding tissues. This type of edema is distinguished from *nonpitting edema,* which occurs when the tissue cells swell instead of the interstitium or when the fluid in the interstitium becomes clotted with fibrinogen so that it cannot move freely within the tissue spaces.

Importance of the Proteoglycan Filaments as a "Spacer" for the Cells and in Preventing Rapid Flow of Fluid in the Tissues. The proteoglycan filaments, along with much larger collagen fibrils in the interstitial spaces, act as a "spacer" between the cells. Nutrients and ions do not diffuse readily through cell membranes; therefore, without adequate spacing between the cells, these nutrients, electrolytes, and cell waste products could not be rapidly exchanged between the blood capillaries and cells located at a distance from one another.

The proteoglycan filaments also prevent fluid from flowing too easily through the tissue spaces. If it were not for the proteoglycan filaments, the simple act of a person standing up would cause large amounts of interstitial fluid to flow from the upper body to the lower body. When too much fluid accumulates in the interstitium, as occurs in edema, this extra fluid creates large channels that allow the fluid to flow readily through the interstitium. Therefore, when severe edema occurs in the legs, the edema fluid often can be decreased by simply elevating the legs.

Even though fluid does not *flow* easily through the tissues in the presence of the compacted proteoglycan filaments, different substances within the fluid can *diffuse* through the tissues at least 95 percent as easily as they normally diffuse. Therefore, the usual diffusion of nutrients to the cells and the removal of waste products from the cells are not compromised by the proteoglycan filaments of the interstitium.

Increased Lymph Flow as a Safety Factor Against Edema

A major function of the lymphatic system is to return to the circulation the fluid and proteins filtered from the capillaries into the interstitium. Without this continuous return of the filtered proteins and fluid to the blood, the plasma volume would be rapidly depleted, and interstitial edema would occur.

The lymphatics act as a safety factor against edema because lymph flow can increase 10- to 50-fold when fluid begins to accumulate in the tissues. This allows the lymphatics to carry away large amounts of fluid and proteins in response to increased capillary filtration, preventing the interstitial pressure from rising into the positive pressure range. The safety factor caused by increased lymph flow has been calculated to be about 7 mm Hg.

"Washdown" of the Interstitial Fluid Protein as a Safety Factor Against Edema

As increased amounts of fluid are filtered into the interstitium, the interstitial fluid pressure increases, causing increased lymph flow. In most tissues the protein concentration of the interstitium decreases as lymph flow is increased, because larger amounts of protein are carried away than can be filtered out of the capillaries; the reason for this is that the capillaries are relatively impermeable to proteins, compared with the lymph vessels. Therefore, the proteins are "washed out" of the interstitial fluid as lymph flow increases.

Because the interstitial fluid colloid osmotic pressure caused by the proteins tends to draw fluid out of the capillaries, decreasing the interstitial fluid proteins lowers the net filtration force across the capillaries and tends to prevent further accumulation of fluid. The safety factor from this effect has been calculated to be about 7 mm Hg.

Summary of Safety Factors That Prevent Edema

Putting together all the safety factors against edema, we find the following:

1. The safety factor caused by low tissue compliance in the negative pressure range is about 3 mm Hg.
2. The safety factor caused by increased lymph flow is about 7 mm Hg.
3. The safety factor caused by washdown of proteins from the interstitial spaces is about 7 mm Hg.

Therefore, the total safety factor against edema is about 17 mm Hg. This means that the capillary pressure in a peripheral tissue could theoretically rise by 17 mm Hg, or approximately double the normal value, before marked edema would occur.

Fluids in the "Potential Spaces" of the Body

Some examples of "potential spaces" are pleural cavity, pericardial cavity, peritoneal cavity, and synovial cavities, including both the joint cavities and the bursae.

Virtually all these potential spaces have surfaces that almost touch each other, with only a thin layer of fluid in between, and the surfaces slide over each other. To facilitate the sliding, a viscous proteinaceous fluid lubricates the surfaces.

Fluid Is Exchanged Between the Capillaries and the Potential Spaces. The surface membrane of a potential space usually does not offer significant resistance to the passage of fluids, electrolytes, or even proteins, which all move back and forth between the space and the interstitial fluid in the surrounding tissue with relative ease. Therefore, each potential space is in reality a large tissue space. Consequently, fluid in the capillaries adjacent to the potential space diffuses not only into the interstitial fluid but also into the potential space.

Lymphatic Vessels Drain Protein from the Potential Spaces. Proteins collect in the potential spaces because of leakage out of the capillaries, similar to the collection of protein in the interstitial spaces throughout the body. The protein must be removed through lymphatics or other channels and returned to the circulation. Each potential space is either directly or indirectly connected with lymph vessels. In some cases, such as the pleural cavity and peritoneal cavity, large lymph vessels arise directly from the cavity itself.

Edema Fluid in the Potential Spaces Is Called "Effusion." When edema occurs in the subcutaneous tissues adjacent to the potential space, edema fluid usually collects in the potential space as well and this fluid is called *effusion.* Thus, lymph blockage or any of the multiple abnormalities that can cause excessive capillary filtration can cause effusion in the same way that interstitial edema is caused. The abdominal cavity is especially prone to collect effusion fluid, and in this instance, the effusion is called *ascites.* In serious cases, 20 liters or more of ascitic fluid can accumulate.

The other potential spaces, such as the pleural cavity, pericardial cavity, and joint spaces, can become seriously swollen when there is generalized edema. Also, injury or local infection in any one of the cavities often blocks the lymph drainage, causing isolated swelling in the cavity.

The dynamics of fluid exchange in the pleural cavity are discussed in detail in Chapter 38. These dynamics are mainly representative of all the other potential spaces as well. It is especially interesting that the normal fluid pressure in most or all of the potential spaces in the nonedematous state is *negative* in the same way that this pressure is negative (subatmospheric) in loose subcutaneous tissue. For instance, the interstitial fluid hydrostatic pressure is normally about −7 to −8 mm Hg in the pleural cavity, −3 to −5 mm Hg in the joint spaces, and −5 to −6 mm Hg in the pericardial cavity.

Bibliography

Amiry-Moghaddam M, Ottersen OP: The molecular basis of water transport in the brain, *Nat Rev Neurosci* 4:991, 2003.

Aukland K: Why don't our feet swell in the upright position? *News Physiol Sci* 9:214, 1994.

Gashev AA: Physiologic aspects of lymphatic contractile function: current perspectives, *Ann N Y Acad Sci* 979:178, 2002.

Guyton AC, Granger HJ, Taylor AE: Interstitial fluid pressure, *Physiol Rev* 51:527, 1971.

Halperin ML, Bohn D: Clinical approach to disorders of salt and water balance: emphasis on integrative physiology, *Crit Care Clin* 18:249, 2002.

Hull RP, Goldsmith DJ: Nephrotic syndrome in adults, *British Med J* 336:1185, 2008.

Jussila L, Alitalo K: Vascular growth factors and lymphangiogenesis, *Physiol Rev* 82:673, 2002.

Lymphatic Filariasis. Centers for Disease Control and Prevention: 2008 http://www.cdc.gov/ncidod/dpd/parasites/lymphaticfilariasis/index.htm.

Loh JA, Verbalis JG: Disorders of water and salt metabolism associated with pituitary disease, *Endocrinol Metab Clin North Am* 37:213, 2008.

Oliver G, Srinivasan RS: Lymphatic vasculature development: current concepts, *Ann N Y Acad Sci* 1131:75, 2008.

Parker JC: Hydraulic conductance of lung endothelial phenotypes and Starling safety factors against edema, *Am J Physiol Lung Cell Mol Physiol* 292:L378, 2007.

Parker JC, Townsley MI: Physiological determinants of the pulmonary filtration coefficient, *Am J Physiol Lung Cell Mol Physiol* 295:L235, 2008.

Reynolds RM, Padfield PL, Seckl JR: Disorders of sodium balance, *Br Med J* 332:702, 2006.

Saaristo A, Karkkainen MJ, Alitalo K: Insights into the molecular pathogenesis and targeted treatment of lymphedema, *Ann N Y Acad Sci* 979:94, 2002.

Verbalis JG, Goldsmith SR, Greenberg A, et al: Hyponatremia treatment guidelines 2007: expert panel recommendations, *Am J Med* 120 (11 Suppl 1):S1, 2007.

UNIT V

Urine Formation by the Kidneys: I. Glomerular Filtration, Renal Blood Flow, and Their Control

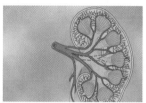

Multiple Functions of the Kidneys

Most people are familiar with one important function of the kidneys—to rid the body of waste materials that are either ingested or produced by metabolism. A second function that is especially critical is to control the volume and composition of the body fluids. For water and virtually all electrolytes in the body, the balance between intake (due to ingestion or metabolic production) and output (due to excretion or metabolic consumption) is maintained largely by the kidneys. This regulatory function of the kidneys maintains the stable internal environment necessary for the cells to perform their various activities.

The kidneys perform their most important functions by filtering the plasma and removing substances from the filtrate at variable rates, depending on the needs of the body. Ultimately, the kidneys "clear" unwanted substances from the filtrate (and therefore from the blood) by excreting them in the urine while returning substances that are needed back to the blood.

Although this chapter and the next few chapters focus mainly on the control of renal excretion of water, electrolytes, and metabolic waste products, the kidneys serve many important homeostatic functions, including the following:

- Excretion of metabolic waste products and foreign chemicals
- Regulation of water and electrolyte balances
- Regulation of body fluid osmolality and electrolyte concentrations
- Regulation of arterial pressure
- Regulation of acid-base balance
- Secretion, metabolism, and excretion of hormones
- Gluconeogenesis

Excretion of Metabolic Waste Products, Foreign Chemicals, Drugs, and Hormone Metabolites. The kidneys are the primary means for eliminating waste products of metabolism that are no longer needed by the body. These products include *urea* (from the metabolism of amino acids), *creatinine* (from muscle creatine), *uric acid* (from nucleic acids), *end products of hemoglobin breakdown* (such as bilirubin), and *metabolites of various hormones.* These waste products must be eliminated from the body as rapidly as they are produced. The kidneys also eliminate most toxins and other foreign substances that are either produced by the body or ingested, such as pesticides, drugs, and food additives.

Regulation of Water and Electrolyte Balances. For maintenance of homeostasis, excretion of water and electrolytes must precisely match intake. If intake exceeds excretion, the amount of that substance in the body will increase. If intake is less than excretion, the amount of that substance in the body will decrease.

Intake of water and many electrolytes is governed mainly by a person's eating and drinking habits, requiring the kidneys to adjust their excretion rates to match the intakes of various substances. Figure 26-1 shows the response of the kidneys to a sudden 10-fold increase in sodium intake from a low level of 30 mEq/day to a high level of 300 mEq/day. Within 2 to 3 days after raising the sodium intake, renal excretion also increases to about 300 mEq/day so that a balance between intake and output is re-established. However, during the 2 to 3 days of renal adaptation to the high sodium intake, there is a modest accumulation of sodium that raises extracellular fluid volume slightly and triggers hormonal changes and other compensatory responses that signal the kidneys to increase their sodium excretion.

The capacity of the kidneys to alter sodium excretion in response to changes in sodium intake is enormous. Experimental studies have shown that in many people, sodium intake can be increased to 1500 mEq/day (more than 10 times normal) or decreased to 10 mEq/day (less than one-tenth normal) with relatively small changes in extracellular fluid volume or plasma sodium concentration. This is also true for water and for most other electrolytes, such as chloride, potassium, calcium, hydrogen, magnesium, and phosphate ions. In the next few chapters, we discuss the specific mechanisms that permit the kidneys to perform these amazing feats of homeostasis.

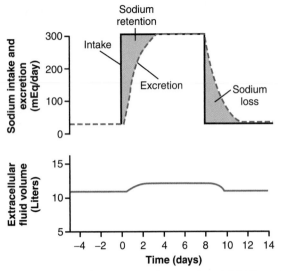

Figure 26-1 Effect of increasing sodium intake 10-fold (from 30 to 300 mEq/day) on urinary sodium excretion and extracellular fluid volume. The shaded areas represent the net sodium retention or the net sodium loss, determined from the difference between sodium intake and sodium excretion.

Regulation of Arterial Pressure. As discussed in Chapter 19, the kidneys play a dominant role in long-term regulation of arterial pressure by excreting variable amounts of sodium and water. The kidneys also contribute to short-term arterial pressure regulation by secreting hormones and vasoactive factors or substances (e.g., *renin*) that lead to the formation of vasoactive products (e.g., angiotensin II).

Regulation of Acid-Base Balance. The kidneys contribute to acid-base regulation, along with the lungs and body fluid buffers, by excreting acids and by regulating the body fluid buffer stores. The kidneys are the only means of eliminating from the body certain types of acids, such as sulfuric acid and phosphoric acid, generated by the metabolism of proteins.

Regulation of Erythrocyte Production. The kidneys secrete *erythropoietin,* which stimulates the production of red blood cells by *hematopoietic stem cells* in the bone marrow, as discussed in Chapter 32. One important stimulus for erythropoietin secretion by the kidneys is *hypoxia*. The kidneys normally account for almost all the erythropoietin secreted into the circulation. In people with severe kidney disease or who have had their kidneys removed and have been placed on hemodialysis, severe anemia develops as a result of decreased erythropoietin production.

Regulation of 1,25-Dihydroxyvitamin D$_3$ Production. The kidneys produce the active form of vitamin D, 1,25-dihydroxyvitamin D$_3$ (*calcitriol*), by hydroxylating this vitamin at the "number 1" position. Calcitriol is essential for normal calcium deposition in bone and calcium reabsorption by the gastrointestinal tract. As

discussed in Chapter 79, calcitriol plays an important role in calcium and phosphate regulation.

Glucose Synthesis. The kidneys synthesize glucose from amino acids and other precursors during prolonged fasting, a process referred to as *gluconeogenesis*. The kidneys' capacity to add glucose to the blood during prolonged periods of fasting rivals that of the liver.

With chronic kidney disease or acute failure of the kidneys, these homeostatic functions are disrupted and severe abnormalities of body fluid volumes and composition rapidly occur. With complete renal failure, enough potassium, acids, fluid, and other substances accumulate in the body to cause death within a few days, unless clinical interventions such as hemodialysis are initiated to restore, at least partially, the body fluid and electrolyte balances.

Physiologic Anatomy of the Kidneys

General Organization of the Kidneys and Urinary Tract

The two kidneys lie on the posterior wall of the abdomen, outside the peritoneal cavity (Figure 26-2). Each kidney of the adult human weighs about 150 grams and is about the size of a clenched fist. The medial side of each kidney contains an indented region called the *hilum* through which pass the renal artery and vein, lymphatics, nerve supply, and ureter, which carries the final urine from the kidney to the bladder, where it is stored until emptied. The kidney is surrounded by a tough, fibrous *capsule* that protects its delicate inner structures.

If the kidney is bisected from top to bottom, the two major regions that can be visualized are the outer *cortex* and the inner *medulla* regions. The medulla is divided into 8 to 10 cone-shaped masses of tissue called *renal pyramids*. The base of each pyramid originates at the border between the cortex and medulla and terminates in the *papilla*, which projects into the space of the *renal pelvis*, a funnel-shaped continuation of the upper end of the ureter. The outer border of the pelvis is divided into open-ended pouches called *major calyces* that extend downward and divide into *minor calyces*, which collect urine from the tubules of each papilla. The walls of the calyces, pelvis, and ureter contain contractile elements that propel the urine toward the *bladder*, where urine is stored until it is emptied by *micturition,* discussed later in this chapter.

Renal Blood Supply

Blood flow to the two kidneys is normally about 22 percent of the cardiac output, or 1100 ml/min. The renal artery enters the kidney through the hilum and then branches progressively to form the *interlobar arteries, arcuate arteries, interlobular arteries* (also called *radial arteries*) and *afferent arterioles,* which lead to the *glomerular capillaries,* where large amounts of fluid and solutes (except the plasma proteins) are filtered to begin urine

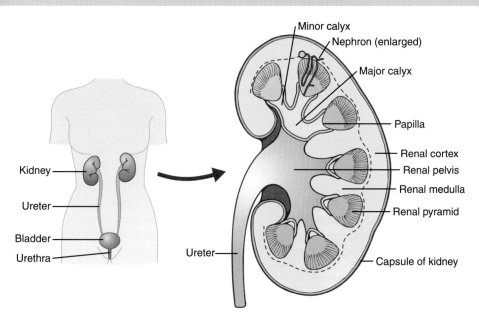

Minor calyx
Nephron (enlarged)
Major calyx
Papilla
Renal cortex
Renal pelvis
Renal medulla
Renal pyramid
Capsule of kidney
Kidney
Ureter
Bladder
Urethra
Ureter

Figure 26-2 General organization of the kidneys and the urinary system.

formation (Figure 26-3). The distal ends of the capillaries of each glomerulus coalesce to form the *efferent arteriole,* which leads to a second capillary network, the *peritubular capillaries,* that surrounds the renal tubules.

The renal circulation is unique in having two capillary beds, the glomerular and peritubular capillaries, which are arranged in series and separated by the efferent arterioles, which help regulate the hydrostatic pressure in both sets of capillaries. High hydrostatic pressure in the glo-

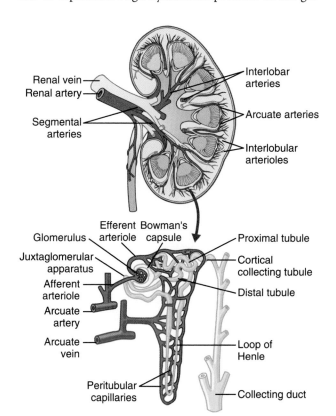

Renal vein
Renal artery
Segmental arteries
Glomerulus
Juxtaglomerular apparatus
Afferent arteriole
Arcuate artery
Arcuate vein
Peritubular capillaries
Efferent arteriole
Bowman's capsule
Interlobar arteries
Arcuate arteries
Interlobular arterioles
Proximal tubule
Cortical collecting tubule
Distal tubule
Loop of Henle
Collecting duct

Figure 26-3 Section of the human kidney showing the major vessels that supply the blood flow to the kidney and schematic of the microcirculation of each nephron.

merular capillaries (about 60 mm Hg) causes rapid fluid filtration, whereas a much lower hydrostatic pressure in the peritubular capillaries (about 13 mm Hg) permits rapid fluid reabsorption. By adjusting the resistance of the afferent and efferent arterioles, the kidneys can regulate the hydrostatic pressure in both the glomerular and the peritubular capillaries, thereby changing the rate of glomerular filtration, tubular reabsorption, or both in response to body homeostatic demands.

The peritubular capillaries empty into the vessels of the venous system, which run parallel to the arteriolar vessels. The blood vessels of the venous system progressively form the *interlobular vein, arcuate vein, interlobar vein,* and *renal vein,* which leaves the kidney beside the renal artery and ureter.

The Nephron Is the Functional Unit of the Kidney

Each kidney in the human contains about 800,000 to 1,000,000 *nephrons,* each capable of forming urine. The kidney cannot regenerate new nephrons. Therefore, with renal injury, disease, or normal aging, there is a gradual decrease in nephron number. After age 40, the number of functioning nephrons usually decreases about 10 percent every 10 years; thus, at age 80, many people have 40 percent fewer functioning nephrons than they did at age 40. This loss is not life threatening because adaptive changes in the remaining nephrons allow them to excrete the proper amounts of water, electrolytes, and waste products, as discussed in Chapter 31.

Each nephron contains (1) a tuft of glomerular capillaries called the *glomerulus,* through which large amounts of fluid are filtered from the blood, and (2) a long *tubule* in which the filtered fluid is converted into urine on its way to the pelvis of the kidney (see Figure 26-3).

The glomerulus contains a network of branching and anastomosing glomerular capillaries that, compared with other capillaries, have high hydrostatic pressure (about

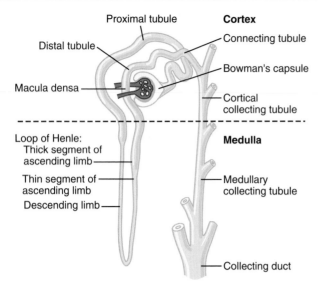

Figure 26-4 Basic tubular segments of the nephron. The relative lengths of the different tubular segments are not drawn to scale.

60 mm Hg). The glomerular capillaries are covered by epithelial cells, and the total glomerulus is encased in *Bowman's capsule.*

Fluid filtered from the glomerular capillaries flows into Bowman's capsule and then into the *proximal tubule,* which lies in the cortex of the kidney (Figure 26-4). From the proximal tubule, fluid flows into the *loop of Henle,* which dips into the renal medulla. Each loop consists of a *descending* and an *ascending limb.* The walls of the descending limb and the lower end of the ascending limb are very thin and therefore are called the *thin segment of the loop of Henle.* After the ascending limb of the loop returns partway back to the cortex, its wall becomes much thicker, and it is referred to as the *thick segment of the ascending limb.*

At the end of the thick ascending limb is a short segment that has in its wall a plaque of specialized epithelial cells, known as the *macula densa.* As discussed later, the macula densa plays an important role in controlling nephron function. Beyond the macula densa, fluid enters the *distal tubule,* which, like the proximal tubule, lies in the renal cortex. This is followed by the *connecting tubule* and the *cortical collecting tubule,* which lead to the *cortical collecting duct.* The initial parts of 8 to 10 cortical collecting ducts join to form a single larger collecting duct that runs downward into the medulla and becomes the *medullary collecting duct.* The collecting ducts merge to form progressively larger ducts that eventually empty into the renal pelvis through the tips of the *renal papillae.* In each kidney, there are about 250 of the very large collecting ducts, each of which collects urine from about 4000 nephrons.

Regional Differences in Nephron Structure: Cortical and Juxtamedullary Nephrons. Although each nephron has all the components described earlier, there are some differences, depending on how deep the nephron lies within the kidney mass. Those nephrons that have glomeruli located in the outer cortex are called *cortical nephrons;* they have short loops of Henle that penetrate only a short distance into the medulla (Figure 26-5).

Figure 26-5 Schematic of relations between blood vessels and tubular structures and differences between cortical and juxtamedullary nephrons.

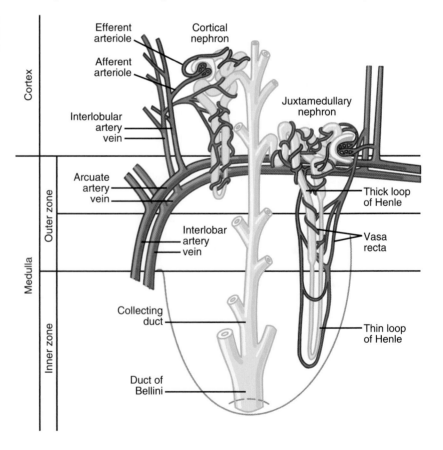

About 20 to 30 percent of the nephrons have glomeruli that lie deep in the renal cortex near the medulla and are called *juxtamedullary nephrons.* These nephrons have long loops of Henle that dip deeply into the medulla, in some cases all the way to the tips of the renal papillae.

The vascular structures supplying the juxtamedullary nephrons also differ from those supplying the cortical nephrons. For the cortical nephrons, the entire tubular system is surrounded by an extensive network of peritubular capillaries. For the juxtamedullary nephrons, long efferent arterioles extend from the glomeruli down into the outer medulla and then divide into specialized peritubular capillaries called *vasa recta* that extend downward into the medulla, lying side by side with the loops of Henle. Like the loops of Henle, the vasa recta return toward the cortex and empty into the cortical veins. This specialized network of capillaries in the medulla plays an essential role in the formation of a concentrated urine and is discussed in Chapter 28.

Micturition

Micturition is the process by which the urinary bladder empties when it becomes filled. This involves two main steps: First, the bladder fills progressively until the tension in its walls rises above a threshold level; this elicits the second step, which is a nervous reflex called the *micturition reflex* that empties the bladder or, if this fails, at least causes a conscious desire to urinate. Although the micturition reflex is an autonomic spinal cord reflex, it can also be inhibited or facilitated by centers in the cerebral cortex or brain stem.

Physiologic Anatomy of the Bladder

The urinary bladder, shown in Figure 26-6, is a smooth muscle chamber composed of two main parts: (1) the *body,* which is the major part of the bladder in which urine collects, and (2) the *neck,* which is a funnel-shaped extension of the body, passing inferiorly and anteriorly into the urogenital triangle and connecting with the urethra. The lower part of the bladder neck is also called the *posterior urethra* because of its relation to the urethra.

The smooth muscle of the bladder is called the *detrusor muscle.* Its muscle fibers extend in all directions and, when contracted, can increase the pressure in the bladder to 40 to 60 mm Hg. Thus, *contraction of the detrusor muscle is a major step in emptying the bladder.* Smooth muscle cells of the detrusor muscle fuse with one another so that low-resistance electrical pathways exist from one muscle

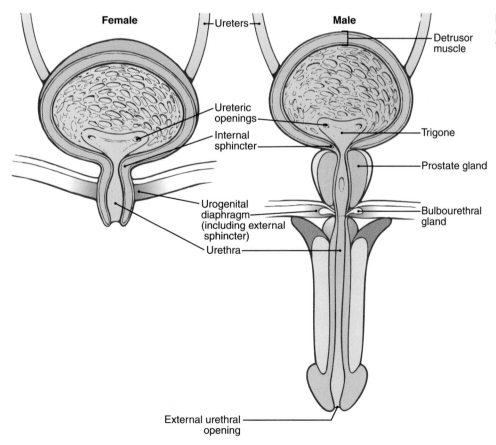

Figure 26-6 Anatomy of the urinary bladder in males and females.

Female

Ureters

Ureteric openings

Internal sphincter

Urogenital diaphragm (including external sphincter)

Urethra

External urethral opening

Male

Detrusor muscle

Trigone

Prostate gland

Bulbourethral gland

Figure 26-7 Innervation of the urinary bladder.

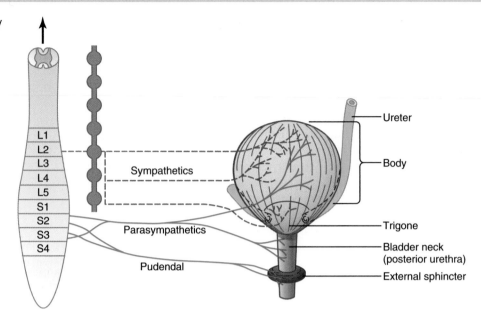

cell to the other. Therefore, an action potential can spread throughout the detrusor muscle, from one muscle cell to the next, to cause contraction of the entire bladder at once.

On the posterior wall of the bladder, lying immediately above the bladder neck, is a small triangular area called the *trigone.* At the lowermost apex of the trigone, the bladder neck opens into the *posterior urethra* and the two ureters enter the bladder at the uppermost angles of the trigone. The trigone can be identified by the fact that its *mucosa,* the inner lining of the bladder, is smooth, in contrast to the remaining bladder mucosa, which is folded to form *rugae.*

Each ureter, as it enters the bladder, courses obliquely through the detrusor muscle and then passes another 1 to 2 centimeters beneath the bladder mucosa before emptying into the bladder.

The bladder neck (posterior urethra) is 2 to 3 centimeters long, and its wall is composed of detrusor muscle interlaced with a large amount of elastic tissue. The muscle in this area is called the *internal sphincter.* Its natural tone normally keeps the bladder neck and posterior urethra empty of urine and, therefore, prevents emptying of the bladder until the pressure in the main part of the bladder rises above a critical threshold.

Beyond the posterior urethra, the urethra passes through the *urogenital diaphragm,* which contains a layer of muscle called the *external sphincter* of the bladder. This muscle is a voluntary skeletal muscle, in contrast to the muscle of the bladder body and bladder neck, which is entirely smooth muscle. The external sphincter muscle is under voluntary control of the nervous system and can be used to consciously prevent urination even when involuntary controls are attempting to empty the bladder.

Innervation of the Bladder

The principal nerve supply of the bladder is by way of the *pelvic nerves,* which connect with the spinal cord through the *sacral plexus,* mainly connecting with cord segments S2 and S3 (Figure 26-7). Coursing through the pelvic nerves are both *sensory nerve fibers* and *motor nerve fibers.* The sensory fibers detect the degree of stretch in the bladder wall. Stretch signals from the posterior urethra are especially strong and are mainly responsible for initiating the reflexes that cause bladder emptying.

The motor nerves transmitted in the pelvic nerves are *parasympathetic fibers.* These terminate on ganglion cells located in the wall of the bladder. Short postganglionic nerves then innervate the detrusor muscle.

In addition to the pelvic nerves, two other types of innervation are important in bladder function. Most important are the *skeletal motor fibers* transmitted through the *pudendal nerve* to the external bladder sphincter. These are *somatic nerve fibers* that innervate and control the voluntary skeletal muscle of the sphincter. Also, the bladder receives *sympathetic innervation* from the sympathetic chain through the *hypogastric nerves,* connecting mainly with the L2 segment of the spinal cord. These sympathetic fibers stimulate mainly the blood vessels and have little to do with bladder contraction. Some sensory nerve fibers also pass by way of the sympathetic nerves and may be important in the sensation of fullness and, in some instances, pain.

Transport of Urine from the Kidney Through the Ureters and into the Bladder

Urine that is expelled from the bladder has essentially the same composition as fluid flowing out of the collecting ducts; there are no significant changes in the composition of urine as it flows through the renal calyces and ureters to the bladder.

Urine flowing from the collecting ducts into the renal calyces stretches the calyces and increases their inherent pacemaker activity, which in turn initiates peristaltic contractions that spread to the renal pelvis and then downward along the length of the ureter, thereby forcing urine from the renal pelvis toward the bladder. In adults, the ureters are normally 25 to 35 centimeters (10 to 14 inches) long.

The walls of the ureters contain smooth muscle and are innervated by both sympathetic and parasympathetic nerves, as well as by an intramural plexus of neurons and nerve fibers that extends along the entire length of the ureters. As with other visceral smooth muscle, *peristaltic contractions in the ureter are enhanced by parasympathetic stimulation and inhibited by sympathetic stimulation.*

The ureters enter the bladder through the *detrusor muscle* in the trigone region of the bladder, as shown in Figure 26-6. Normally, the ureters course obliquely for several centimeters through the bladder wall. The normal tone of the detrusor muscle in the bladder wall tends to compress the ureter, thereby preventing backflow (reflux) of urine from the bladder when pressure builds up in the bladder during micturition or bladder compression. Each peristaltic wave along the ureter increases the pressure within the ureter so that the region passing through the bladder wall opens and allows urine to flow into the bladder.

In some people, the distance that the ureter courses through the bladder wall is less than normal, so contraction of the bladder during micturition does not always lead to complete occlusion of the ureter. As a result, some of the urine in the bladder is propelled backward into the ureter, a condition called *vesicoureteral reflux.* Such reflux can lead to enlargement of the ureters and, if severe, can increase the pressure in the renal calyces and structures of the renal medulla, causing damage to these regions.

Pain Sensation in the Ureters, and the Ureterorenal Reflex. The ureters are well supplied with pain nerve fibers. When a ureter becomes blocked (e.g., by a ureteral stone), intense reflex constriction occurs, associated with severe pain. Also, the pain impulses cause a sympathetic reflex back to the kidney to constrict the renal arterioles, thereby decreasing urine output from the kidney. This effect is called the *ureterorenal reflex* and is important for preventing excessive flow of fluid into the pelvis of a kidney with a blocked ureter.

Filling of the Bladder and Bladder Wall Tone; the Cystometrogram

Figure 26-8 shows the approximate changes in intravesicular pressure as the bladder fills with urine. When there is no urine in the bladder, the intravesicular pressure is about 0, but by the time 30 to 50 milliliters of urine have collected, the pressure rises to 5 to 10 centimeters of water. Additional urine—200 to 300 milliliters—can collect with only a small additional rise in pressure; this constant level of pressure is caused by intrinsic tone of the bladder wall itself. Beyond 300 to 400 milliliters, collection of more urine in the bladder causes the pressure to rise rapidly.

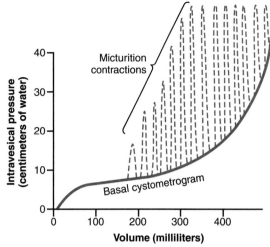

Figure 26-8 Normal cystometrogram, showing also acute pressure waves (*dashed spikes*) caused by micturition reflexes.

Superimposed on the tonic pressure changes during filling of the bladder are periodic acute increases in pressure that last from a few seconds to more than a minute. The pressure peaks may rise only a few centimeters of water or may rise to more than 100 centimeters of water. These pressure peaks are called *micturition waves* in the cystometrogram and are caused by the micturition reflex.

Micturition Reflex

Referring again to Figure 26-8, one can see that as the bladder fills, many superimposed *micturition contractions* begin to appear, as shown by the dashed spikes. They are the result of a stretch reflex initiated by *sensory stretch receptors* in the bladder wall, especially by the receptors in the posterior urethra when this area begins to fill with urine at the higher bladder pressures. Sensory signals from the bladder stretch receptors are conducted to the sacral segments of the cord through the *pelvic nerves* and then reflexively back again to the bladder through the *parasympathetic nerve fibers* by way of these same nerves.

When the bladder is only partially filled, these micturition contractions usually relax spontaneously after a fraction of a minute, the detrusor muscles stop contracting, and pressure falls back to the baseline. As the bladder continues to fill, the micturition reflexes become more frequent and cause greater contractions of the detrusor muscle.

Once a micturition reflex begins, it is "self-regenerative." That is, initial contraction of the bladder activates the stretch receptors to cause a greater increase in sensory impulses from the bladder and posterior urethra, which causes a further increase in reflex contraction of the bladder; thus, the cycle is repeated again and again until the bladder has reached a strong degree of contraction. Then, after a few seconds to more than a minute, the self-regenerative reflex begins to fatigue and the regenerative cycle of the micturition reflex ceases, permitting the bladder to relax.

Thus, the micturition reflex is a single complete cycle of (1) progressive and rapid increase of pressure, (2) a period of sustained pressure, and (3) return of the pressure to the basal tone of the bladder. Once a micturition reflex has occurred but has not succeeded in emptying the bladder, the nervous elements of this reflex usually remain in an inhibited state for a few minutes to 1 hour or more before another micturition reflex occurs. As the bladder becomes more and more filled, micturition reflexes occur more and more often and more and more powerfully.

Once the micturition reflex becomes powerful enough, it causes another reflex, which passes through the *pudendal nerves* to the *external sphincter* to inhibit it. If this inhibition is more potent in the brain than the voluntary constrictor signals to the external sphincter, urination will occur. If not, urination will not occur until the bladder fills still further and the micturition reflex becomes more powerful.

Facilitation or Inhibition of Micturition by the Brain

The micturition reflex is an autonomic spinal cord reflex, but it can be inhibited or facilitated by centers in the brain. These centers include (1) strong *facilitative* and *inhibitory centers in the brain stem, located mainly in the pons,* and (2) several *centers located in the cerebral cortex* that are mainly inhibitory but can become excitatory.

The micturition reflex is the basic cause of micturition, but the higher centers normally exert final control of micturition as follows:

1. The higher centers keep the micturition reflex partially inhibited, except when micturition is desired.

2. The higher centers can prevent micturition, even if the micturition reflex occurs, by tonic contraction of the external bladder sphincter until a convenient time presents itself.

3. When it is time to urinate, the cortical centers can facilitate the sacral micturition centers to help initiate a micturition reflex and at the same time inhibit the external urinary sphincter so that urination can occur.

Voluntary urination is usually initiated in the following way: First, a person voluntarily contracts his or her abdominal muscles, which increases the pressure in the bladder and allows extra urine to enter the bladder neck and posterior urethra under pressure, thus stretching their walls. This stimulates the stretch receptors, which excites the micturition reflex and simultaneously inhibits the external urethral sphincter. Ordinarily, all the urine will be emptied, with rarely more than 5 to 10 milliliters left in the bladder.

Abnormalities of Micturition

Atonic Bladder and Incontinence Caused by Destruction of Sensory Nerve Fibers. Micturition reflex contraction cannot occur if the sensory nerve fibers from the bladder to the spinal cord are destroyed, thereby preventing transmission of stretch signals from the bladder. When this happens, a person loses bladder control, despite intact

efferent fibers from the cord to the bladder and despite intact neurogenic connections within the brain. Instead of emptying periodically, the bladder fills to capacity and overflows a few drops at a time through the urethra. This is called *overflow incontinence.*

A common cause of atonic bladder is crush injury to the sacral region of the spinal cord. Certain diseases can also cause damage to the dorsal root nerve fibers that enter the spinal cord. For example, syphilis can cause constrictive fibrosis around the dorsal root nerve fibers, destroying them. This condition is called *tabes dorsalis,* and the resulting bladder condition is called *tabetic bladder.*

Automatic Bladder Caused by Spinal Cord Damage Above the Sacral Region.   If the spinal cord is damaged above the sacral region but the sacral cord segments are still intact, typical micturition reflexes can still occur. However, they are no longer controlled by the brain. During the first few days to several weeks after the damage to the cord has occurred, the micturition reflexes are suppressed because of the state of "spinal shock" caused by the sudden loss of facilitative impulses from the brain stem and cerebrum. However, if the bladder is emptied periodically by catheterization to prevent bladder injury caused by overstretching of the bladder, the excitability of the micturition reflex gradually increases until typical micturition reflexes return; then, periodic (but unannounced) bladder emptying occurs.

Some patients can still control urination in this condition by stimulating the skin (scratching or tickling) in the genital region, which sometimes elicits a micturition reflex.

Uninhibited Neurogenic Bladder Caused by Lack of Inhibitory Signals from the Brain.   Another abnormality of micturition is the so-called uninhibited neurogenic bladder, which results in frequent and relatively uncontrolled micturition. This condition derives from partial damage in the spinal cord or the brain stem that interrupts most of the inhibitory signals. Therefore, facilitative impulses passing continually down the cord keep the sacral centers so excitable that even a small quantity of urine elicits an uncontrollable micturition reflex, thereby promoting frequent urination.

Urine Formation Results from Glomerular Filtration, Tubular Reabsorption, and Tubular Secretion

The rates at which different substances are excreted in the urine represent the sum of three renal processes, shown in Figure 26-9: (1) glomerular filtration, (2) reabsorption of substances from the renal tubules into the blood, and (3) secretion of substances from the blood into the renal tubules. Expressed mathematically,

Urinary excretion rate =
Filtration rate − Reabsorption rate + Secretion rate

Urine formation begins when a large amount of fluid that is virtually free of protein is filtered from the glomerular capillaries into Bowman's capsule. Most substances in the plasma, except for proteins, are freely filtered, so their concentration in the glomerular filtrate in Bowman's capsule is almost the same as in the plasma. As filtered fluid leaves Bowman's capsule and passes through

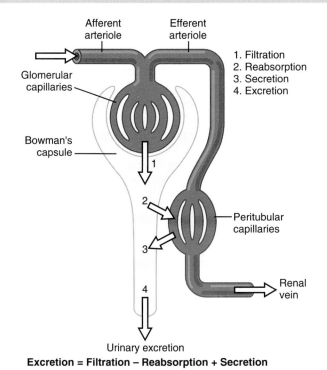

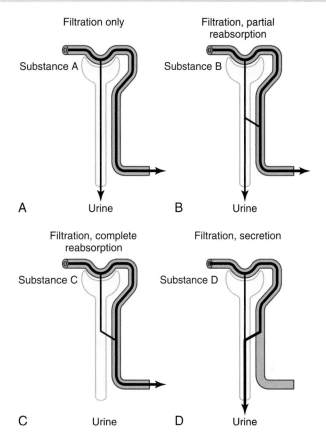

Excretion = Filtration − Reabsorption + Secretion

Figure 26-9 Basic kidney processes that determine the composition of the urine. Urinary excretion rate of a substance is equal to the rate at which the substance is filtered minus its reabsorption rate plus the rate at which it is secreted from the peritubular capillary blood into the tubules.

Figure 26-10 Renal handling of four hypothetical substances. *A*, The substance is freely filtered but not reabsorbed. *B*, The substance is freely filtered, but part of the filtered load is reabsorbed back in the blood. *C*, The substance is freely filtered but is not excreted in the urine because all the filtered substance is reabsorbed from the tubules into the blood. *D*, The substance is freely filtered and is not reabsorbed but is secreted from the peritubular capillary blood into the renal tubules.

the tubules, it is modified by reabsorption of water and specific solutes back into the blood or by secretion of other substances from the peritubular capillaries into the tubules.

Figure 26-10 shows the renal handling of four hypothetical substances. The substance shown in panel A is freely filtered by the glomerular capillaries but is neither reabsorbed nor secreted. Therefore, its excretion rate is equal to the rate at which it was filtered. Certain waste products in the body, such as creatinine, are handled by the kidneys in this manner, allowing excretion of essentially all that is filtered.

In panel B, the substance is freely filtered but is also partly reabsorbed from the tubules back into the blood. Therefore, the rate of urinary excretion is less than the rate of filtration at the glomerular capillaries. In this case, the excretion rate is calculated as the filtration rate minus the reabsorption rate. This is typical for many of the electrolytes of the body such as sodium and chloride ions.

In panel C, the substance is freely filtered at the glomerular capillaries but is not excreted into the urine because all the filtered substance is reabsorbed from the tubules back into the blood. This pattern occurs for some of the nutritional substances in the blood, such as amino acids and glucose, allowing them to be conserved in the body fluids.

The substance in panel D is freely filtered at the glomerular capillaries and is not reabsorbed, but additional quantities of this substance are secreted from the peritubular capillary blood into the renal tubules. This pattern often occurs for organic acids and bases, permitting them

to be rapidly cleared from the blood and excreted in large amounts in the urine. The excretion rate in this case is calculated as filtration rate plus tubular secretion rate.

For each substance in the plasma, a particular combination of filtration, reabsorption, and secretion occurs. The rate at which the substance is excreted in the urine depends on the relative rates of these three basic renal processes.

Filtration, Reabsorption, and Secretion of Different Substances

In general, tubular reabsorption is quantitatively more important than tubular secretion in the formation of urine, but secretion plays an important role in determining the amounts of potassium and hydrogen ions and a few other substances that are excreted in the urine. Most substances that must be cleared from the blood, especially the end products of metabolism such as urea, creatinine, uric acid, and urates, are poorly reabsorbed and are therefore excreted in large amounts in the urine. Certain foreign substances and drugs are also poorly reabsorbed but, in addition, are secreted from the blood into the tubules, so their excretion rates are high.

Conversely, electrolytes, such as sodium ions, chloride ions, and bicarbonate ions, are highly reabsorbed, so only small amounts appear in the urine. Certain nutritional substances, such as amino acids and glucose, are completely reabsorbed from the tubules and do not appear in the urine even though large amounts are filtered by the glomerular capillaries.

Each of the processes—glomerular filtration, tubular reabsorption, and tubular secretion—is regulated according to the needs of the body. For example, when there is excess sodium in the body, the rate at which sodium is filtered increases and a smaller fraction of the filtered sodium is reabsorbed, causing increased urinary excretion of sodium.

For most substances, the rates of filtration and reabsorption are extremely large relative to the rates of excretion. Therefore, subtle adjustments of filtration or reabsorption can lead to relatively large changes in renal excretion. For example, an increase in glomerular filtration rate (GFR) of only 10 percent (from 180 to 198 L/day) would raise urine volume 13-fold (from 1.5 to 19.5 L/day) if tubular reabsorption remained constant. In reality, changes in glomerular filtration and tubular reabsorption usually act in a coordinated manner to produce the necessary changes in renal excretion.

Why Are Large Amounts of Solutes Filtered and Then Reabsorbed by the Kidneys? One might question the wisdom of filtering such large amounts of water and solutes and then reabsorbing most of these substances. One advantage of a high GFR is that it allows the kidneys to rapidly remove waste products from the body that depend mainly on glomerular filtration for their excretion. Most waste products are poorly reabsorbed by the tubules and, therefore, depend on a high GFR for effective removal from the body.

A second advantage of a high GFR is that it allows all the body fluids to be filtered and processed by the kidneys many times each day. Because the entire plasma volume is only about 3 liters, whereas the GFR is about 180 L/day, the entire plasma can be filtered and processed about 60 times each day. This high GFR allows the kidneys to precisely and rapidly control the volume and composition of the body fluids.

Glomerular Filtration—the First Step in Urine Formation

Composition of the Glomerular Filtrate

Urine formation begins with filtration of large amounts of fluid through the glomerular capillaries into Bowman's capsule. Like most capillaries, the glomerular capillaries are relatively impermeable to proteins, so the filtered fluid (called the *glomerular filtrate*) is essentially protein free and devoid of cellular elements, including red blood cells.

The concentrations of other constituents of the glomerular filtrate, including most salts and organic molecules, are similar to the concentrations in the plasma. Exceptions to this generalization include a few low-molecular-weight substances, such as calcium and fatty acids, that are not freely filtered because they are partially bound to the plasma proteins. For example, almost one half of the plasma calcium and most of the plasma fatty acids are bound to proteins and these bound portions are not filtered through the glomerular capillaries.

GFR Is About 20 Percent of the Renal Plasma Flow

As in other capillaries, the GFR is determined by (1) the balance of hydrostatic and colloid osmotic forces acting across the capillary membrane and (2) the capillary filtration coefficient (K_f), the product of the permeability and filtering surface area of the capillaries. The glomerular capillaries have a much higher rate of filtration than most other capillaries because of a high glomerular hydrostatic pressure and a large K_f. In the average adult human, the GFR is about 125 ml/min, or 180 L/day. The fraction of the renal plasma flow that is filtered (the filtration fraction) averages about 0.2; this means that about 20 percent of the plasma flowing through the kidney is filtered through the glomerular capillaries. The filtration fraction is calculated as follows:

$$\text{Filtration fraction} = \text{GFR/Renal plasma flow}$$

Glomerular Capillary Membrane

The glomerular capillary membrane is similar to that of other capillaries, except that it has three (instead of the usual two) major layers: (1) the *endothelium* of the capillary, (2) a *basement membrane*, and (3) a layer of *epithelial cells (podocytes)* surrounding the outer surface of the capillary basement membrane (Figure 26-11). Together, these layers make up the filtration barrier, which, despite the three layers, filters several hundred times as much water and solutes as the usual capillary membrane. Even with this high rate of filtration, the glomerular capillary membrane normally prevents filtration of plasma proteins.

The high filtration rate across the glomerular capillary membrane is due partly to its special characteristics. The capillary *endothelium* is perforated by thousands of small holes called *fenestrae*, similar to the fenestrated capillaries found in the liver. Although the fenestrations are relatively large, endothelial cells are richly endowed with fixed negative charges that hinder the passage of plasma proteins.

Surrounding the endothelium is the *basement membrane*, which consists of a meshwork of collagen and proteoglycan fibrillae that have large spaces through which large amounts of water and small solutes can filter. The basement membrane effectively prevents filtration of plasma proteins, in part because of strong negative electrical charges associated with the proteoglycans.

The final part of the glomerular membrane is a layer of epithelial cells that line the outer surface of the glomerulus. These cells are not continuous but have long footlike processes (podocytes) that encircle the outer surface

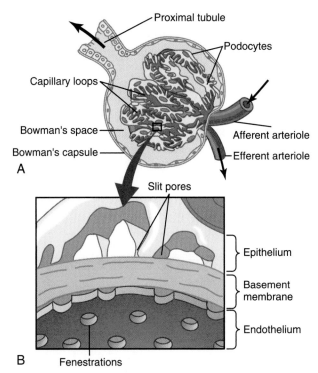

Figure 26-11 *A*, Basic ultrastructure of the glomerular capillaries. *B*, Cross section of the glomerular capillary membrane and its major components: capillary endothelium, basement membrane, and epithelium (podocytes).

Table 26-1 Filterability of Substances by Glomerular Capillaries Based on Molecular Weight

Substance	Molecular Weight	Filterability
Water	18	1.0
Sodium	23	1.0
Glucose	180	1.0
Inulin	5,500	1.0
Myoglobin	17,000	0.75
Albumin	69,000	0.005

of the capillaries (see Figure 26-11). The foot processes are separated by gaps called *slit pores* through which the glomerular filtrate moves. The epithelial cells, which also have negative charges, provide additional restriction to filtration of plasma proteins. Thus, all layers of the glomerular capillary wall provide a barrier to filtration of plasma proteins.

Filterability of Solutes Is Inversely Related to Their Size. The glomerular capillary membrane is thicker than most other capillaries, but it is also much more porous and therefore filters fluid at a high rate. Despite the high filtration rate, the glomerular filtration barrier is selective in determining which molecules will filter, based on their size and electrical charge.

Table 26-1 lists the effect of molecular size on filterability of different molecules. A filterability of 1.0 means that the substance is filtered as freely as water; a filterability of 0.75 means that the substance is filtered only 75 percent as rapidly as water. Note that electrolytes such as sodium and small organic compounds such as glucose are freely filtered. As the molecular weight of the molecule approaches that of albumin, the filterability rapidly decreases, approaching zero.

Negatively Charged Large Molecules Are Filtered Less Easily Than Positively Charged Molecules of Equal Molecular Size. The molecular diameter of the plasma protein albumin is only about 6 nanometers, whereas the pores of the glomerular membrane are thought to be about

8 nanometers (80 angstroms). Albumin is restricted from filtration, however, because of its negative charge and the electrostatic repulsion exerted by negative charges of the glomerular capillary wall proteoglycans.

Figure 26-12 shows how electrical charge affects the filtration of different molecular weight dextrans by the glomerulus. Dextrans are polysaccharides that can be manufactured as neutral molecules or with negative or positive charges. Note that for any given molecular radius, positively charged molecules are filtered much more readily than negatively charged molecules. Neutral dextrans are also filtered more readily than negatively charged dextrans of equal molecular weight. The reason for these differences in filterability is that the negative charges of the basement membrane and the podocytes provide an important means for restricting large negatively charged molecules, including the plasma proteins.

In certain kidney diseases, the negative charges on the basement membrane are lost even before there are noticeable changes in kidney histology, a condition referred to as *minimal change nephropathy*. As a result of this loss of negative charges on the basement membranes, some

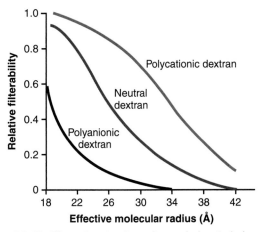

Figure 26-12 Effect of molecular radius and electrical charge of dextran on its filterability by the glomerular capillaries. A value of 1.0 indicates that the substance is filtered as freely as water, whereas a value of 0 indicates that it is not filtered. Dextrans are polysaccharides that can be manufactured as neutral molecules or with negative or positive charges and with varying molecular weights.

of the lower-molecular-weight proteins, especially albumin, are filtered and appear in the urine, a condition known as *proteinuria* or *albuminuria*.

Determinants of the GFR

The GFR is determined by (1) the sum of the hydrostatic and colloid osmotic forces across the glomerular membrane, which gives the *net filtration pressure,* and (2) the glomerular capillary filtration coefficient, K_f. Expressed mathematically, the GFR equals the product of K_f and the net filtration pressure:

$$GFR = K_f \times \text{Net filtration pressure}$$

The net filtration pressure represents the sum of the hydrostatic and colloid osmotic forces that either favor or oppose filtration across the glomerular capillaries (Figure 26-13). These forces include (1) hydrostatic pressure inside the glomerular capillaries (glomerular hydrostatic pressure, P_G), which promotes filtration; (2) the hydrostatic pressure in Bowman's capsule (P_B) outside the capillaries, which opposes filtration; (3) the colloid osmotic pressure of the glomerular capillary plasma proteins (π_G), which opposes filtration; and (4) the colloid osmotic pressure of the proteins in Bowman's capsule (π_B), which promotes filtration. (Under normal conditions, the concentration of protein in the glomerular filtrate is so low that the colloid osmotic pressure of the Bowman's capsule fluid is considered to be zero.)

The GFR can therefore be expressed as

$$GFR = K_f \times (P_G - P_B - \pi_G + \pi_B)$$

Although the normal values for the determinants of GFR have not been measured directly in humans, they have been estimated in animals such as dogs and rats. Based on the results in animals, the approximate normal forces favoring and opposing glomerular filtration in humans are believed to be as follows (see Figure 26-13):

Forces Favoring Filtration (mm Hg)

Glomerular hydrostatic pressure	60
Bowman's capsule colloid osmotic pressure	0

Forces Opposing Filtration (mm Hg)

Bowman's capsule hydrostatic pressure	18
Glomerular capillary colloid osmotic pressure	32

Net filtration pressure = 60 − 18 − 32 = +10 mm Hg

Some of these values can change markedly under different physiologic conditions, whereas others are altered mainly in disease states, as discussed later.

Increased Glomerular Capillary Filtration Coefficient Increases GFR

The K_f is a measure of the product of the hydraulic conductivity and surface area of the glomerular capillaries. The K_f cannot be measured directly, but it is estimated experimentally by dividing the rate of glomerular filtration by net filtration pressure:

$$K_f = GFR/\text{Net filtration pressure}$$

Because total GFR for both kidneys is about 125 ml/min and the net filtration pressure is 10 mm Hg, the normal K_f is calculated to be about 12.5 ml/min/mm Hg of filtration pressure. When K_f is expressed per 100 grams of kidney weight, it averages about 4.2 ml/min/mm Hg, a value about 400 times as high as the K_f of most other capillary systems of the body; the average K_f of many other tissues in the body is only about 0.01 ml/min/mm Hg per 100 grams. This high K_f for the glomerular capillaries contributes tremendously to their rapid rate of fluid filtration.

Although increased K_f raises GFR and decreased K_f reduces GFR, changes in K_f probably do not provide a primary mechanism for the normal day-to-day regulation of GFR. Some diseases, however, lower K_f by reducing the number of functional glomerular capillaries (thereby reducing the surface area for filtration) or by increasing the thickness of the glomerular capillary membrane and reducing its hydraulic conductivity. For example, chronic, uncontrolled hypertension and diabetes mellitus gradually reduce K_f by increasing the thickness of the glomerular capillary basement membrane and, eventually, by damaging the capillaries so severely that there is loss of capillary function.

Increased Bowman's Capsule Hydrostatic Pressure Decreases GFR

Direct measurements, using micropipettes, of hydrostatic pressure in Bowman's capsule and at different points in the proximal tubule in experimental animals suggest that a reasonable estimate for Bowman's capsule pressure in humans is about 18 mm Hg under normal conditions. Increasing the hydrostatic pressure in Bowman's capsule

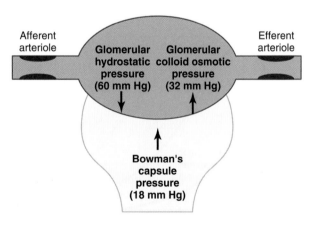

Figure 26-13 Summary of forces causing filtration by the glomerular capillaries. The values shown are estimates for healthy humans.

reduces GFR, whereas decreasing this pressure raises GFR. However, changes in Bowman's capsule pressure normally do not serve as a primary means for regulating GFR.

In certain pathological states associated with obstruction of the urinary tract, Bowman's capsule pressure can increase markedly, causing serious reduction of GFR. For example, precipitation of calcium or of uric acid may lead to "stones" that lodge in the urinary tract, often in the ureter, thereby obstructing outflow of the urinary tract and raising Bowman's capsule pressure. This reduces GFR and eventually can cause *hydronephrosis* (distention and dilation of the renal pelvis and calyces) and can damage or even destroy the kidney unless the obstruction is relieved.

Increased Glomerular Capillary Colloid Osmotic Pressure Decreases GFR

As blood passes from the afferent arteriole through the glomerular capillaries to the efferent arterioles, the plasma protein concentration increases about 25 percent (Figure 26-14). The reason for this is that about one fifth of the fluid in the capillaries filters into Bowman's capsule, thereby concentrating the glomerular plasma proteins that are not filtered. Assuming that the normal colloid osmotic pressure of plasma entering the glomerular capillaries is 28 mm Hg, this value usually rises to about 36 mm Hg by the time the blood reaches the efferent end of the capillaries. Therefore, the average colloid osmotic pressure of the glomerular capillary plasma proteins is midway between 28 and 36 mm Hg, or about 32 mm Hg.

Thus, two factors that influence the glomerular capillary colloid osmotic pressure are (1) the arterial plasma colloid osmotic pressure and (2) the fraction of plasma filtered by the glomerular capillaries (filtration fraction). Increasing the arterial plasma colloid osmotic pressure raises the glomerular capillary colloid osmotic pressure, which in turn decreases GFR.

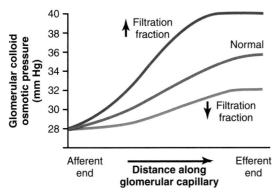

Figure 26-14 Increase in colloid osmotic pressure in plasma flowing through the glomerular capillary. Normally, about one fifth of the fluid in the glomerular capillaries filters into Bowman's capsule, thereby concentrating the plasma proteins that are not filtered. Increases in the filtration fraction (glomerular filtration rate/renal plasma flow) increase the rate at which the plasma colloid osmotic pressure rises along the glomerular capillary; decreases in the filtration fraction have the opposite effect.

Increasing the filtration fraction also concentrates the plasma proteins and raises the glomerular colloid osmotic pressure (see Figure 26-14). Because the filtration fraction is defined as GFR/renal plasma flow, the filtration fraction can be increased either by raising GFR or by reducing renal plasma flow. For example, a reduction in renal plasma flow with no initial change in GFR would tend to increase the filtration fraction, which would raise the glomerular capillary colloid osmotic pressure and tend to reduce GFR. For this reason, changes in renal blood flow can influence GFR independently of changes in glomerular hydrostatic pressure.

With increasing renal blood flow, a lower fraction of the plasma is initially filtered out of the glomerular capillaries, causing a slower rise in the glomerular capillary colloid osmotic pressure and less inhibitory effect on GFR. *Consequently, even with a constant glomerular hydrostatic pressure, a greater rate of blood flow into the glomerulus tends to increase GFR and a lower rate of blood flow into the glomerulus tends to decrease GFR.*

Increased Glomerular Capillary Hydrostatic Pressure Increases GFR

The glomerular capillary hydrostatic pressure has been estimated to be about 60 mm Hg under normal conditions. Changes in glomerular hydrostatic pressure serve as the primary means for physiologic regulation of GFR. Increases in glomerular hydrostatic pressure raise GFR, whereas decreases in glomerular hydrostatic pressure reduce GFR.

Glomerular hydrostatic pressure is determined by three variables, each of which is under physiologic control: (1) *arterial pressure*, (2) *afferent arteriolar resistance*, and (3) *efferent arteriolar resistance*.

Increased arterial pressure tends to raise glomerular hydrostatic pressure and, therefore, to increase GFR. (However, as discussed later, this effect is buffered by autoregulatory mechanisms that maintain a relatively constant glomerular pressure as blood pressure fluctuates.)

Increased resistance of afferent arterioles reduces glomerular hydrostatic pressure and decreases GFR. Conversely, dilation of the afferent arterioles increases both glomerular hydrostatic pressure and GFR (Figure 26-15).

Constriction of the efferent arterioles increases the resistance to outflow from the glomerular capillaries. This raises the glomerular hydrostatic pressure, and as long as the increase in efferent resistance does not reduce renal blood flow too much, GFR increases slightly (see Figure 26-15). However, because efferent arteriolar constriction also reduces renal blood flow, the filtration fraction and glomerular colloid osmotic pressure increase as efferent arteriolar resistance increases. Therefore, if the constriction of efferent arterioles is severe (more than about a threefold increase in efferent arteriolar resistance), the rise in colloid osmotic pressure exceeds the increase in glomerular capillary hydrostatic pressure caused by efferent arteriolar constriction. When this occurs, the *net force* for filtration actually decreases, causing a reduction in GFR.

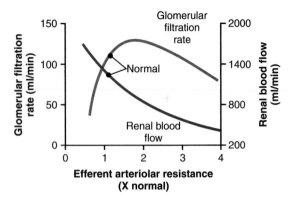

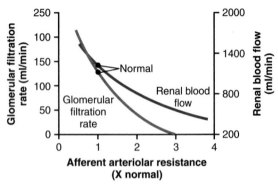

Figure 26-15 Effect of change in afferent arteriolar resistance or efferent arteriolar resistance on glomerular filtration rate and renal blood flow.

Table 26-2 Factors That Can Decrease the Glomerular Filtration Rate (GFR)

Physical Determinants*	Physiologic/Pathophysiologic Causes
$\downarrow K_f \rightarrow \downarrow$ GFR	Renal disease, diabetes mellitus, hypertension
$\uparrow P_B \rightarrow \downarrow$ GFR	Urinary tract obstruction (e.g., kidney stones)
$\uparrow \pi_G \rightarrow \downarrow$ GFR	$\downarrow$ Renal blood flow, increased plasma proteins
$\downarrow P_G \rightarrow \downarrow$ GFR	
$\downarrow A_P \rightarrow \downarrow P_G$	$\downarrow$ Arterial pressure (has only small effect due to autoregulation)
$\downarrow R_E \rightarrow \downarrow P_G$	$\downarrow$ Angiotensin II (drugs that block angiotensin II formation)
$\uparrow R_A \rightarrow \downarrow P_G$	$\uparrow$ Sympathetic activity, vasoconstrictor hormones (e.g., norepinephrine, endothelin)

*Opposite changes in the determinants usually increase GFR.
K_f, glomerular filtration coefficient; P_B, Bowman's capsule hydrostatic pressure; π_G, glomerular capillary colloid osmotic pressure; P_G, glomerular capillary hydrostatic pressure; A_P, systemic arterial pressure; R_E, efferent arteriolar resistance; R_A, afferent arteriolar resistance.

Thus, efferent arteriolar constriction has a biphasic effect on GFR. At moderate levels of constriction, there is a slight increase in GFR, but with severe constriction, there is a decrease in GFR. The primary cause of the eventual decrease in GFR is as follows: As efferent constriction becomes severe and as plasma protein concentration increases, there is a rapid, nonlinear increase in colloid osmotic pressure caused by the Donnan effect; the higher the protein concentration, the more rapidly the colloid osmotic pressure rises because of the interaction of ions bound to the plasma proteins, which also exert an osmotic effect, as discussed in Chapter 16.

To summarize, constriction of afferent arterioles reduces GFR. However, the effect of efferent arteriolar constriction depends on the severity of the constriction; modest efferent constriction raises GFR, but severe efferent constriction (more than a threefold increase in resistance) tends to reduce GFR.

Table 26-2 summarizes the factors that can decrease GFR.

Renal Blood Flow

In an average 70-kilogram man, the combined blood flow through both kidneys is about 1100 ml/min, or about 22 percent of the cardiac output. Considering that the two kidneys constitute only about 0.4 percent of the total body weight, one can readily see that they receive an extremely high blood flow compared with other organs.

As with other tissues, blood flow supplies the kidneys with nutrients and removes waste products. However, the high flow to the kidneys greatly exceeds this need. The purpose of this additional flow is to supply enough plasma for the high rates of glomerular filtration that are necessary for precise regulation of body fluid volumes and solute concentrations. As might be expected, the mechanisms that regulate renal blood flow are closely linked to the control of GFR and the excretory functions of the kidneys.

Renal Blood Flow and Oxygen Consumption

On a per-gram-weight basis, the kidneys normally consume oxygen at twice the rate of the brain but have almost seven times the blood flow of the brain. Thus, the oxygen delivered to the kidneys far exceeds their metabolic needs, and the arterial-venous extraction of oxygen is relatively low compared with that of most other tissues.

A large fraction of the oxygen consumed by the kidneys is related to the high rate of active sodium reabsorption by the renal tubules. If renal blood flow and GFR are reduced and less sodium is filtered, less sodium is reabsorbed and less oxygen is consumed. Therefore, renal oxygen consumption varies in proportion to renal tubular sodium reabsorption, which in turn is closely related to GFR and the rate of sodium filtered (Figure 26-16). If glomerular filtration completely ceases, renal sodium reabsorption also ceases and oxygen consumption decreases to about one-fourth normal. This residual oxygen consumption reflects the basic metabolic needs of the renal cells.

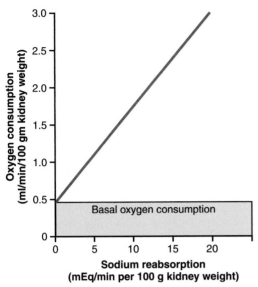

Figure 26-16 Relationship between oxygen consumption and sodium reabsorption in dog kidneys. (Kramer K, Deetjen P: Relation of renal oxygen consumption to blood supply and glomerular filtration during variations of blood pressure. Pflugers Arch Physiol 271:782, 1960.)

Table 26-3 Approximate Pressures and Vascular Resistances in the Circulation of a Normal Kidney

Vessel	Pressure in Vessel (mm Hg)		Percent of Total Renal Vascular Resistance
	Beginning	*End*	
Renal artery	100	100	≈0
Interlobar, arcuate, and interlobular arteries	≈100	85	≈16
Afferent arteriole	85	60	≈26
Glomerular capillaries	60	59	≈1
Efferent arteriole	59	18	≈43
Peritubular capillaries	18	8	≈10
Interlobar, interlobular, and arcuate veins	8	4	≈4
Renal vein	4	≈4	≈0

Determinants of Renal Blood Flow

Renal blood flow is determined by the pressure gradient across the renal vasculature (the difference between renal artery and renal vein hydrostatic pressures), divided by the total renal vascular resistance:

$$\frac{\text{(Renal artery pressure–Renal vein pressure)}}{\text{Total renal vascular resistance}}$$

Renal artery pressure is about equal to systemic arterial pressure, and renal vein pressure averages about 3 to 4 mm Hg under most conditions. As in other vascular beds, the total vascular resistance through the kidneys is determined by the sum of the resistances in the individual vasculature segments, including the arteries, arterioles, capillaries, and veins (Table 26-3).

Most of the renal vascular resistance resides in three major segments: interlobular arteries, afferent arterioles, and efferent arterioles. Resistance of these vessels is controlled by the sympathetic nervous system, various hormones, and local internal renal control mechanisms, as discussed later. An increase in the resistance of any of the vascular segments of the kidneys tends to reduce the renal blood flow, whereas a decrease in vascular resistance increases renal blood flow if renal artery and renal vein pressures remain constant.

Although changes in arterial pressure have some influence on renal blood flow, the kidneys have effective mechanisms for maintaining renal blood flow and GFR relatively constant over an arterial pressure range between 80 and 170 mm Hg, a process called *autoregulation*. This capacity for autoregulation occurs through mechanisms that are completely intrinsic to the kidneys, as discussed later in this chapter.

Blood Flow in the Vasa Recta of the Renal Medulla Is Very Low Compared with Flow in the Renal Cortex

The outer part of the kidney, the renal cortex, receives most of the kidney's blood flow. Blood flow in the renal medulla accounts for only 1 to 2 percent of the total renal blood flow. Flow to the renal medulla is supplied by a specialized portion of the peritubular capillary system called the *vasa recta*. These vessels descend into the medulla in parallel with the loops of Henle and then loop back along with the loops of Henle and return to the cortex before emptying into the venous system. As discussed in Chapter 28, the vasa recta play an important role in allowing the kidneys to form concentrated urine.

Physiologic Control of Glomerular Filtration and Renal Blood Flow

The determinants of GFR that are most variable and subject to physiologic control include the glomerular hydrostatic pressure and the glomerular capillary colloid osmotic pressure. These variables, in turn, are influenced by the sympathetic nervous system, hormones and autacoids (vasoactive substances that are released in the kidneys and act locally), and other feedback controls that are intrinsic to the kidneys.

Sympathetic Nervous System Activation Decreases GFR

Essentially all the blood vessels of the kidneys, including the afferent and the efferent arterioles, are richly innervated by sympathetic nerve fibers. Strong activation of the renal sympathetic nerves can constrict the renal arterioles and decrease renal blood flow and GFR. Moderate or mild sympathetic stimulation has little influence on renal blood flow and GFR. For example, reflex activation of the sympathetic nervous system resulting from moderate decreases in pressure at the carotid sinus baroreceptors or cardiopulmonary receptors has little influence on renal blood flow or GFR.

The renal sympathetic nerves seem to be most important in reducing GFR during severe, acute disturbances lasting for a few minutes to a few hours, such as those elicited by the defense reaction, brain ischemia, or severe hemorrhage. In the healthy resting person, sympathetic tone appears to have little influence on renal blood flow.

Hormonal and Autacoid Control of Renal Circulation

Several hormones and autacoids can influence GFR and renal blood flow, as summarized in Table 26-4.

Norepinephrine, Epinephrine, and Endothelin Constrict Renal Blood Vessels and Decrease GFR.
Hormones that constrict afferent and efferent arterioles, causing reductions in GFR and renal blood flow, include *norepinephrine* and *epinephrine* released from the adrenal medulla. In general, blood levels of these hormones parallel the activity of the sympathetic nervous system; thus, norepinephrine and epinephrine have little influence on renal hemodynamics except under extreme conditions, such as severe hemorrhage.

Another vasoconstrictor, *endothelin*, is a peptide that can be released by damaged vascular endothelial cells of the kidneys, as well as by other tissues. The physiologic role of this autacoid is not completely understood. However, endothelin may contribute to hemostasis (minimizing blood loss) when a blood vessel is severed, which damages the endothelium and releases this powerful vasoconstrictor. Plasma endothelin levels are also increased in certain disease states associated with vascular injury, such as toxemia of pregnancy, acute renal failure, and chronic uremia, and may contribute to renal vasoconstriction and decreased GFR in some of these pathophysiologic conditions.

Table 26-4 Hormones and Autacoids That Influence Glomerular Filtration Rate (GFR)

Hormone or Autacoid	Effect on GFR
Norepinephrine	↓
Epinephrine	↓
Endothelin	↓
Angiotensin II	↔ (prevents ↓)
Endothelial-derived nitric oxide	↑
Prostaglandins	↑

Angiotensin II Preferentially Constricts Efferent Arterioles in Most Physiologic Conditions.
A powerful renal vasoconstrictor, *angiotensin II*, can be considered a circulating hormone, as well as a locally produced autacoid because it is formed in the kidneys and in the systemic circulation. Receptors for angiotensin II are present in virtually all blood vessels of the kidneys. However, the preglomerular blood vessels, especially the afferent arterioles, appear to be relatively protected from angiotensin II–mediated constriction in most physiologic conditions associated with activation of the renin-angiotensin system such as during a low-sodium diet or reduced renal perfusion pressure due to renal artery stenosis. This protection is due to release of vasodilators, especially *nitric oxide* and *prostaglandins*, which counteract the vasoconstrictor effects of angiotensin II in these blood vessels.

The efferent arterioles, however, are highly sensitive to angiotensin II. Because angiotensin II preferentially constricts efferent arterioles in most physiologic conditions, increased angiotensin II levels raise glomerular hydrostatic pressure while reducing renal blood flow. It should be kept in mind that increased angiotensin II formation usually occurs in circumstances associated with decreased arterial pressure or volume depletion, which tend to decrease GFR. In these circumstances, the increased level of angiotensin II, by constricting efferent arterioles, helps *prevent* decreases in glomerular hydrostatic pressure and GFR; at the same time, though, the reduction in renal blood flow caused by efferent arteriolar constriction contributes to decreased flow through the peritubular capillaries, which in turn increases reabsorption of sodium and water, as discussed in Chapter 27.

Thus, increased angiotensin II levels that occur with a low-sodium diet or volume depletion help maintain GFR and normal excretion of metabolic waste products such as urea and creatinine that depend on glomerular filtration for their excretion; at the same time, the angiotensin II-induced constriction of efferent arterioles increases tubular reabsorption of sodium and water, which helps restore blood volume and blood pressure. This effect of angiotensin II in helping to "autoregulate" GFR is discussed in more detail later in this chapter.

Endothelial-Derived Nitric Oxide Decreases Renal Vascular Resistance and Increases GFR.
An autacoid that decreases renal vascular resistance and is released by the vascular endothelium throughout the body is *endothelial-derived nitric oxide*. A basal level of nitric oxide production appears to be important for maintaining vasodilation of the kidneys. This allows the kidneys to excrete normal amounts of sodium and water. Therefore, administration of drugs that inhibit formation of nitric oxide increases renal vascular resistance and decreases GFR and urinary sodium excretion, eventually causing high blood pressure. In some hypertensive patients or in patients with atherosclerosis, damage of the vascular endothelium and impaired nitric oxide production may contribute to increased renal vasoconstriction and elevated blood pressure.

Prostaglandins and Bradykinin Tend to Increase GFR.

Hormones and autacoids that cause vasodilation and increased renal blood flow and GFR include the prostaglandins (PGE_2 and PGI_2) and bradykinin. These substances are discussed in Chapter 17. Although these vasodilators do not appear to be of major importance in regulating renal blood flow or GFR in normal conditions, they may dampen the renal vasoconstrictor effects of the sympathetic nerves or angiotensin II, especially their effects to constrict the afferent arterioles.

By opposing vasoconstriction of afferent arterioles, the prostaglandins may help prevent excessive reductions in GFR and renal blood flow. Under stressful conditions, such as volume depletion or after surgery, the administration of nonsteroidal anti-inflammatory agents, such as aspirin, that inhibit prostaglandin synthesis may cause significant reductions in GFR.

Autoregulation of GFR and Renal Blood Flow

Feedback mechanisms intrinsic to the kidneys normally keep the renal blood flow and GFR relatively constant, despite marked changes in arterial blood pressure. These mechanisms still function in blood-perfused kidneys that have been removed from the body, independent of systemic influences. This relative constancy of GFR and renal blood flow is referred to as *autoregulation* (Figure 26-17).

The primary function of blood flow autoregulation in most tissues other than the kidneys is to maintain the delivery of oxygen and nutrients at a normal level and to remove the waste products of metabolism, despite changes in the arterial pressure. In the kidneys, the normal blood flow is much higher than that required for these functions. The major function of autoregulation in the kidneys is to maintain a relatively constant GFR and to allow precise control of renal excretion of water and solutes.

The GFR normally remains autoregulated (that is, remains relatively constant), despite considerable arterial pressure fluctuations that occur during a person's usual activities. For instance, a decrease in arterial pressure to as low as 75 mm Hg or an increase to as high as 160 mm Hg usually changes GFR less than 10 percent. In general, renal blood flow is autoregulated in parallel with GFR, but GFR is more efficiently autoregulated under certain conditions.

Importance of GFR Autoregulation in Preventing Extreme Changes in Renal Excretion

Although the renal autoregulatory mechanisms are not perfect, they do prevent potentially large changes in GFR and renal excretion of water and solutes that would otherwise occur with changes in blood pressure. One can understand the quantitative importance of autoregulation by considering the relative magnitudes of glomerular filtration, tubular reabsorption, and renal excretion and the changes in renal excretion that would occur without autoregulatory mechanisms.

Normally, GFR is about 180 L/day and tubular reabsorption is 178.5 L/day, leaving 1.5 L/day of fluid to be excreted in the urine. In the absence of autoregulation, a relatively small increase in blood pressure (from 100 to 125 mm Hg) would cause a similar 25 percent increase in GFR (from about 180 to 225 L/day). If tubular reabsorption remained constant at 178.5 L/day, this would increase the urine flow to 46.5 L/day (the difference between GFR and tubular reabsorption)—a total increase in urine of more than 30-fold. Because the total plasma volume is only about 3 liters, such a change would quickly deplete the blood volume.

In reality, changes in arterial pressure usually exert much less of an effect on urine volume for two reasons: (1) renal autoregulation prevents large changes in GFR that would otherwise occur, and (2) there are additional adaptive mechanisms in the renal tubules that cause them to increase their reabsorption rate when GFR rises, a phenomenon referred to as *glomerulotubular balance* (discussed in Chapter 27). Even with these special control mechanisms, changes in arterial pressure still have significant effects on renal excretion of water and sodium; this is referred to as *pressure diuresis* or *pressure natriuresis,* and it is crucial in the regulation of body fluid volumes and arterial pressure, as discussed in Chapters 19 and 29.

Tubuloglomerular Feedback and Autoregulation of GFR

To perform the function of autoregulation, the kidneys have a feedback mechanism that links changes in sodium chloride concentration at the macula densa with the control of renal arteriolar resistance. This feedback helps ensure a relatively constant delivery of sodium chloride to the distal tubule and helps prevent spurious fluctuations in renal excretion that would otherwise occur. In many circumstances, this feedback autoregulates renal blood

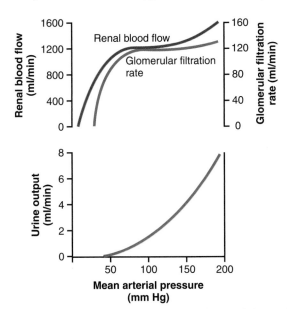

Figure 26-17 Autoregulation of renal blood flow and glomerular filtration rate but lack of autoregulation of urine flow during changes in renal arterial pressure.

flow and GFR in parallel. However, because this mechanism is specifically directed toward stabilizing sodium chloride delivery to the distal tubule, there are instances when GFR is autoregulated at the expense of changes in renal blood flow, as discussed later.

The tubuloglomerular feedback mechanism has two components that act together to control GFR: (1) an afferent arteriolar feedback mechanism and (2) an efferent arteriolar feedback mechanism. These feedback mechanisms depend on special anatomical arrangements of the *juxtaglomerular complex* (Figure 26-18).

The juxtaglomerular complex consists of *macula densa cells* in the initial portion of the distal tubule and *juxtaglomerular cells* in the walls of the afferent and efferent arterioles. The macula densa is a specialized group of epithelial cells in the distal tubules that comes in close contact with the afferent and efferent arterioles. The macula densa cells contain Golgi apparatus, which are intracellular secretory organelles directed toward the arterioles, suggesting that these cells may be secreting a substance toward the arterioles.

Decreased Macula Densa Sodium Chloride Causes Dilation of Afferent Arterioles and Increased Renin Release.

The macula densa cells sense changes in volume delivery to the distal tubule by way of signals that are not completely understood. Experimental studies suggest that decreased GFR slows the flow rate in the loop of Henle, causing increased reabsorption of sodium and chloride ions in the ascending loop of Henle, thereby reducing the

concentration of sodium chloride at the macula densa cells. This decrease in sodium chloride concentration initiates a signal from the macula densa that has two effects (Figure 26-19): (1) It decreases resistance to blood flow in the afferent arterioles, which raises glomerular hydrostatic pressure and helps return GFR toward normal, and (2) it increases renin release from the juxtaglomerular cells of the afferent and efferent arterioles, which are the major storage sites for renin. Renin released from these cells then functions as an enzyme to increase the formation of angiotensin I, which is converted to angiotensin II. Finally, the angiotensin II constricts the efferent arterioles, thereby increasing glomerular hydrostatic pressure and helping to return GFR toward normal.

These two components of the tubuloglomerular feedback mechanism, operating together by way of the special anatomical structure of the juxtaglomerular apparatus, provide feedback signals to both the afferent and the efferent arterioles for efficient autoregulation of GFR during changes in arterial pressure. When both of these mechanisms are functioning together, the GFR changes only a few percentage points, even with large fluctuations in arterial pressure between the limits of 75 and 160 mm Hg.

Blockade of Angiotensin II Formation Further Reduces GFR During Renal Hypoperfusion. As discussed earlier, a preferential constrictor action of angiotensin II on efferent arterioles helps prevent serious reductions in glomerular hydrostatic pressure and GFR when renal perfusion pressure falls below normal. The administration of drugs that block

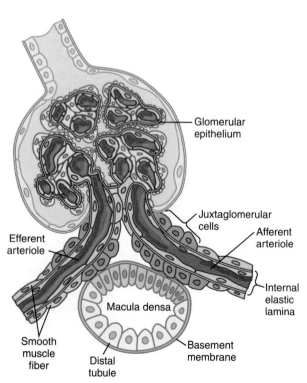

Figure 26-18 Structure of the juxtaglomerular apparatus, demonstrating its possible feedback role in the control of nephron function.

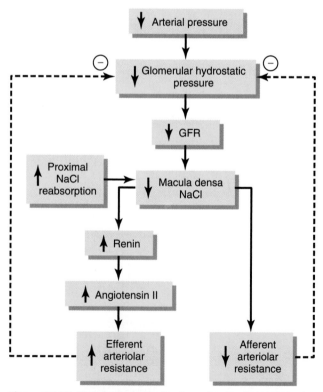

Figure 26-19 Macula densa feedback mechanism for autoregulation of glomerular hydrostatic pressure and glomerular filtration rate (GFR) during decreased renal arterial pressure.

the formation of angiotensin II (angiotensin-converting enzyme inhibitors) or that block the action of angiotensin II (angiotensin II receptor antagonists) causes greater reductions in GFR than usual when the renal arterial pressure falls below normal. Therefore, an important complication of using these drugs to treat patients who have hypertension because of renal artery stenosis (partial blockage of the renal artery) is a severe decrease in GFR that can, in some cases, cause acute renal failure. Nevertheless, angiotensin II–blocking drugs can be useful therapeutic agents in many patients with hypertension, congestive heart failure, and other conditions, as long as they are monitored to ensure that severe decreases in GFR do not occur.

Myogenic Autoregulation of Renal Blood Flow and GFR

Another mechanism that contributes to the maintenance of a relatively constant renal blood flow and GFR is the ability of individual blood vessels to resist stretching during increased arterial pressure, a phenomenon referred to as the *myogenic mechanism.* Studies of individual blood vessels (especially small arterioles) throughout the body have shown that they respond to increased wall tension or wall stretch by contraction of the vascular smooth muscle. Stretch of the vascular wall allows increased movement of calcium ions from the extracellular fluid into the cells, causing them to contract through the mechanisms discussed in Chapter 8. This contraction prevents excessive stretch of the vessel and at the same time, by raising vascular resistance, helps prevent excessive increases in renal blood flow and GFR when arterial pressure increases.

Although the myogenic mechanism probably operates in most arterioles throughout the body, its importance in renal blood flow and GFR autoregulation has been questioned by some physiologists because this pressure-sensitive mechanism has no means of directly detecting changes in renal blood flow or GFR per se. On the other hand, this mechanism may be more important in protecting the kidney from hypertension-induced injury. In response to sudden increases in blood pressure, the myogenic constrictor response in afferent arterioles occurs within seconds and therefore attenuates transmission of increased arterial pressure to the glomerular capillaries.

Other Factors That Increase Renal Blood Flow and GFR: High Protein Intake and Increased Blood Glucose

Although renal blood flow and GFR are relatively stable under most conditions, there are circumstances in which these variables change significantly. For example, *a high protein intake is known to increase both renal blood flow and GFR.* With a chronic high-protein diet, such as one that contains large amounts of meat, the increases in GFR and renal blood flow are due partly to growth of the kidneys. However, GFR and renal blood flow increase 20 to 30 percent within 1 or 2 hours after a person eats a high-protein meal.

One likely explanation for the increased GFR is the following: A high-protein meal increases the release of amino acids into the blood, which are reabsorbed in the proximal tubule. Because amino acids and sodium are reabsorbed together by the proximal tubules, increased amino acid reabsorption also stimulates

sodium reabsorption in the proximal tubules. This decreases sodium delivery to the macula densa (see Figure 26-19), which elicits a tubuloglomerular feedback–mediated decrease in resistance of the afferent arterioles, as discussed earlier. The decreased afferent arteriolar resistance then raises renal blood flow and GFR. This increased GFR allows sodium excretion to be maintained at a nearly normal level while increasing the excretion of the waste products of protein metabolism, such as urea.

A similar mechanism may also explain the marked increases in renal blood flow and GFR that occur with large increases in blood glucose levels in uncontrolled diabetes mellitus. Because glucose, like some of the amino acids, is also reabsorbed along with sodium in the proximal tubule, increased glucose delivery to the tubules causes them to reabsorb excess sodium along with glucose. This, in turn, decreases delivery of sodium chloride to the macula densa, activating a tubuloglomerular feedback-mediated dilation of the afferent arterioles and subsequent increases in renal blood flow and GFR.

These examples demonstrate that renal blood flow and GFR per se are not the primary variables controlled by the tubuloglomerular feedback mechanism. The main purpose of this feedback is to ensure a constant delivery of sodium chloride to the distal tubule, where final processing of the urine takes place. Thus, disturbances that tend to increase reabsorption of sodium chloride at tubular sites before the macula densa tend to elicit increased renal blood flow and GFR, which helps return distal sodium chloride delivery toward normal so that normal rates of sodium and water excretion can be maintained (see Figure 26-19).

An opposite sequence of events occurs when proximal tubular reabsorption is reduced. For example, when the proximal tubules are damaged (which can occur as a result of poisoning by heavy metals, such as mercury, or large doses of drugs, such as tetracyclines), their ability to reabsorb sodium chloride is decreased. As a consequence, large amounts of sodium chloride are delivered to the distal tubule and, without appropriate compensations, would quickly cause excessive volume depletion. One of the important compensatory responses appears to be a tubuloglomerular feedback–mediated renal vasoconstriction that occurs in response to the increased sodium chloride delivery to the macula densa in these circumstances. These examples again demonstrate the importance of this feedback mechanism in ensuring that the distal tubule receives the proper rate of delivery of sodium chloride, other tubular fluid solutes, and tubular fluid volume so that appropriate amounts of these substances are excreted in the urine.

Bibliography

Beeuwkes R III: The vascular organization of the kidney, *Annu Rev Physiol* 42:531, 1980.

Bell PD, Lapointe JY, Peti-Peterdi J: Macula densa cell signaling, *Annu Rev Physiol* 65:481, 2003.

Cowley AW Jr, Mori T, Mattson D, et al: Role of renal NO production in the regulation of medullary blood flow, *Am J Physiol Regul Integr Comp Physiol* 284:R1355, 2003.

Cupples WA, Braam B: Assessment of renal autoregulation, *Am J Physiol Renal Physiol* 292:F1105, 2007.

Deen WN: What determines glomerular capillary permeability? *J Clin Invest* 114:1412, 2004.

DiBona GF: Physiology in perspective: The Wisdom of the Body. Neural control of the kidney, *Am J Physiol Regul Integr Comp Physiol* 289:R633, 2005.

Drummond HA, Grifoni SC, Jernigan NL: A new trick for an old dogma: ENaC proteins as mechanotransducers in vascular smooth muscle, *Physiology (Bethesda)* 23:23, 2008.

UNIT V

Fowler CJ, Griffiths D, de Groat WC: The neural control of micturition, *Nat Rev Neurosci* 9:453, 2008.

Hall JE: Angiotensin II and long-term arterial pressure regulation: the overriding dominance of the kidney, *J Am Soc Nephrol* 10:(Suppl 12):s258, 1999.

Hall JE, Brands MW: The renin-angiotensin-aldosterone system: renal mechanisms and circulatory homeostasis. In Seldin DW, Giebisch G, eds: *The Kidney—Physiology and Pathophysiology*, ed 3, New York, 2000, Raven Press, pp 1009–1046.

Hall JE, Henegar JR, Dwyer TM, et al: Is obesity a major cause of chronic kidney disease? *Adv Ren Replace Ther* 11:41, 2004.

Haraldsson B, Sörensson J: Why do we not all have proteinuria? An update of our current understanding of the glomerular barrier, *News Physiol Sci* 19:7, 2004.

Kriz W, Kaissling B: Structural organization of the mammalian kidney. In Seldin DW, Giebisch G, eds: *The Kidney—Physiology and Pathophysiology*, ed 3, New York, 2000, Raven Press, pp 587–654.

Loutzenhiser R, Griffin K, Williamson G, et al: Renal autoregulation: new perspectives regarding the protective and regulatory roles of the underlying mechanisms, *Am J Physiol Regul Integr Comp Physiol* 290:R1153, 2006.

Pallone TL, Zhang Z, Rhinehart K: Physiology of the renal medullary microcirculation, *Am J Physiol Renal Physiol* 284:F253, 2003.

Roman RJ: P-450 metabolites of arachidonic acid in the control of cardiovascular function, *Physiol Rev* 82:131, 2002.

Schnermann J, Levine DZ: Paracrine factors in tubuloglomerular feedback: adenosine, ATP, and nitric oxide, *Annu Rev Physiol* 65:501, 2003.

CHAPTER 27

Urine Formation by the Kidneys: II. Tubular Reabsorption and Secretion

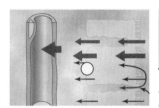

Renal Tubular Reabsorption and Secretion

As the glomerular filtrate enters the renal tubules, it flows sequentially through the successive parts of the tubule—the *proximal tubule,* the *loop of Henle,* the *distal tubule,* the *collecting tubule,* and, finally, the *collecting duct*—before it is excreted as urine. Along this course, some substances are selectively reabsorbed from the tubules back into the blood, whereas others are secreted from the blood into the tubular lumen. Eventually, the urine that is formed and all the substances in the urine represent the sum of three basic renal processes—glomerular filtration, tubular reabsorption, and tubular secretion:

Urinary excretion = Glomerular filtration – Tubular reabsorption + Tubular secretion

For many substances, tubular reabsorption plays a much more important role than secretion in determining the final urinary excretion rate. However, tubular secretion accounts for significant amounts of potassium ions, hydrogen ions, and a few other substances that appear in the urine.

Tubular Reabsorption Is Quantitatively Large and Highly Selective

Table 27-1 shows the renal handling of several substances that are all freely filtered in the kidneys and reabsorbed at variable rates. The rate at which each of these substances is filtered is calculated as

Filtration = Glomerular filtration rate × Plasma concentration

This calculation assumes that the substance is freely filtered and not bound to plasma proteins. For example, if plasma glucose concentration is 1 g/L, the amount of glucose filtered each day is about 180 L/day × 1 g/L, or 180 g/day. Because virtually none of the filtered glucose is normally excreted, the rate of glucose reabsorption is also 180 g/day.

From Table 27-1, two things are immediately apparent. First, the processes of glomerular filtration and tubular reabsorption are quantitatively large relative to urinary excretion for many substances. This means that a small change in glomerular filtration or tubular reabsorption can potentially cause a relatively large change in urinary excretion. For example, a 10 percent decrease in tubular reabsorption, from 178.5 to 160.7 L/day, would increase urine volume from 1.5 to 19.3 L/day (almost a 13-fold increase) if the glomerular filtration rate (GFR) remained constant. In reality, however, changes in tubular reabsorption and glomerular filtration are closely coordinated so that large fluctuations in urinary excretion are avoided.

Second, unlike glomerular filtration, which is relatively nonselective (essentially all solutes in the plasma are filtered except the plasma proteins or substances bound to them), *tubular reabsorption is highly selective.* Some substances, such as glucose and amino acids, are almost completely reabsorbed from the tubules, so the urinary excretion rate is essentially zero. Many of the ions in the plasma, such as sodium, chloride, and bicarbonate, are also highly reabsorbed, but their rates of reabsorption and urinary excretion are variable, depending on the needs of the body. Waste products, such as urea and creatinine, conversely, are poorly reabsorbed from the tubules and excreted in relatively large amounts.

Therefore, by controlling the rate at which they reabsorb different substances, the kidneys regulate the excretion of solutes independently of one another, a capability that is essential for precise control of the body fluid composition. In this chapter, we discuss the mechanisms that allow the kidneys to selectively reabsorb or secrete different substances at variable rates.

Tubular Reabsorption Includes Passive and Active Mechanisms

For a substance to be reabsorbed, it must first be transported (1) across the tubular epithelial membranes into the renal interstitial fluid and then (2) through the peritubular capillary membrane back into the blood (Figure 27-1).

Table 27-1 Filtration, Reabsorption, and Excretion Rates of Different Substances by the Kidneys

	Amount Filtered	Amount Reabsorbed	Amount Excreted	% of Filtered Load Reabsorbed
Glucose (g/day)	180	180	0	100
Bicarbonate (mEq/day)	4,320	4,318	2	>99.9
Sodium (mEq/day)	25,560	25,410	150	99.4
Chloride (mEq/day)	19,440	19,260	180	99.1
Potassium (mEq/day)	756	664	92	87.8
Urea (g/day)	46.8	23.4	23.4	50
Creatinine (g/day)	1.8	0	1.8	0

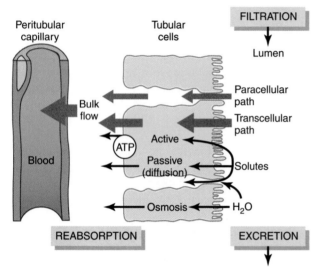

Figure 27-1 Reabsorption of filtered water and solutes from the tubular lumen across the tubular epithelial cells, through the renal interstitium, and back into the blood. Solutes are transported through the cells (*transcellular path*) by passive diffusion or active transport, or between the cells (*paracellular path*) by diffusion. Water is transported through the cells and between the tubular cells by osmosis. Transport of water and solutes from the interstitial fluid into the peritubular capillaries occurs by ultrafiltration (*bulk flow*).

Thus, reabsorption of water and solutes includes a series of transport steps. Reabsorption across the tubular epithelium into the interstitial fluid includes active or passive transport by the same basic mechanisms discussed in Chapter 4 for transport across other membranes of the body. For instance, water and solutes can be transported through the cell membranes themselves *(transcellular route)* or through the spaces between the cell junctions *(paracellular route)*. Then, after absorption across the tubular epithelial cells into the interstitial fluid, water and solutes are transported through the peritubular capillary walls into the blood by *ultrafiltration (bulk flow)* that is mediated by hydrostatic and colloid osmotic forces. The peritubular capillaries behave like the venous ends of most other capillaries because there is a net reabsorptive force that moves the fluid and solutes from the interstitium into the blood.

Active Transport

Active transport can move a solute against an electrochemical gradient and requires energy derived from metabolism. Transport that is coupled directly to an energy source, such as the hydrolysis of adenosine triphosphate (ATP), is termed *primary active transport.* A good example of this is the sodium-potassium ATPase pump that functions throughout most parts of the renal tubule. Transport that is coupled *indirectly* to an energy source, such as that due to an ion gradient, is referred to as *secondary active transport.* Reabsorption of glucose by the renal tubule is an example of secondary active transport. Although solutes can be reabsorbed by active and/ or passive mechanisms by the tubule, water is always reabsorbed by a passive (nonactive) physical mechanism called *osmosis,* which means water diffusion from a region of low solute concentration (high water concentration) to one of high solute concentration (low water concentration).

Solutes Can Be Transported Through Epithelial Cells or Between Cells. Renal tubular cells, like other epithelial cells, are held together by *tight junctions.* Lateral intercellular spaces lie behind the tight junctions and separate the epithelial cells of the tubule. Solutes can be reabsorbed or secreted across the cells through the *transcellular pathway* or between the cells by moving across the tight junctions and intercellular spaces by way of the *paracellular pathway.* Sodium is a substance that moves through both routes, although most of the sodium is transported through the transcellular pathway. In some nephron segments, especially the proximal tubule, water is also reabsorbed across the paracellular pathway, and substances dissolved in the water, especially potassium, magnesium, and chloride ions, are carried with the reabsorbed fluid between the cells.

Primary Active Transport Through the Tubular Membrane Is Linked to Hydrolysis of ATP. *The special importance of primary active transport is that it can move solutes against an electrochemical gradient.* The energy for this active transport comes from the hydrolysis of ATP by way of membrane-bound ATPase; the ATPase is also

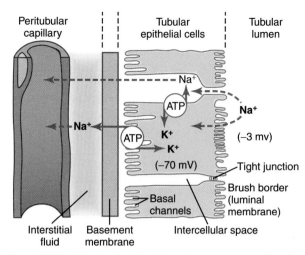

Figure 27-2 Basic mechanism for active transport of sodium through the tubular epithelial cell. The sodium-potassium pump transports sodium from the interior of the cell across the basolateral membrane, creating a low intracellular sodium concentration and a negative intracellular electrical potential. The low intracellular sodium concentration and the negative electrical potential cause sodium ions to diffuse from the tubular lumen into the cell through the brush border.

a component of the carrier mechanism that binds and moves solutes across the cell membranes. The primary active transporters in the kidneys that are known include *sodium-potassium ATPase, hydrogen ATPase, hydrogen-potassium ATPase,* and *calcium ATPase.*

A good example of a primary active transport system is the reabsorption of sodium ions across the proximal tubular membrane, as shown in Figure 27-2. On the basolateral sides of the tubular epithelial cell, the cell membrane has an extensive sodium-potassium ATPase system that hydrolyzes ATP and uses the released energy to transport sodium ions out of the cell into the interstitium. At the same time, potassium is transported from the interstitium to the inside of the cell. The operation of this ion pump maintains low intracellular sodium and high intracellular potassium concentrations and creates a net negative charge of about −70 millivolts within the cell. This active pumping of sodium out of the cell across the *basolateral* membrane of the cell favors passive diffusion of sodium across the *luminal* membrane of the cell, from the tubular lumen into the cell, for two reasons: (1) There is a concentration gradient favoring sodium diffusion into the cell because intracellular sodium concentration is low (12 mEq/L) and tubular fluid sodium concentration is high (140 mEq/L) and (2) the negative, −70-millivolt, intracellular potential attracts the positive sodium ions from the tubular lumen into the cell.

Active reabsorption of sodium by sodium-potassium ATPase occurs in most parts of the tubule. In certain parts of the nephron, there are also additional provisions for moving large amounts of sodium into the cell. In the proximal tubule, there is an extensive brush border on the luminal side of the membrane (the side that faces the tubular lumen) that multiplies the surface area

about 20-fold. There are also carrier proteins that bind sodium ions on the luminal surface of the membrane and release them inside the cell, providing *facilitated diffusion* of sodium through the membrane into the cell. These sodium carrier proteins are also important for secondary active transport of other substances, such as glucose and amino acids, as discussed later.

Thus, the net reabsorption of sodium ions from the tubular lumen back into the blood involves at least three steps:

1. Sodium diffuses across the luminal membrane (also called the *apical membrane*) into the cell down an electrochemical gradient established by the sodium-potassium ATPase pump on the basolateral side of the membrane.

2. Sodium is transported across the basolateral membrane against an electrochemical gradient by the sodium-potassium ATPase pump.

3. Sodium, water, and other substances are reabsorbed from the interstitial fluid into the peritubular capillaries by ultrafiltration, a passive process driven by the hydrostatic and colloid osmotic pressure gradients.

Secondary Active Reabsorption Through the Tubular Membrane. In secondary active transport, two or more substances interact with a specific membrane protein (a carrier molecule) and are transported together across the membrane. As one of the substances (for instance, sodium) diffuses down its electrochemical gradient, the energy released is used to drive another substance (for instance, glucose) against its electrochemical gradient. Thus, secondary active transport does not require energy directly from ATP or from other high-energy phosphate sources. Rather, the direct source of the energy is that liberated by the simultaneous facilitated diffusion of another transported substance down its own electrochemical gradient.

Figure 27-3 shows secondary active transport of glucose and amino acids in the proximal tubule. In both instances, specific carrier proteins in the brush border combine with a sodium ion and an amino acid or a glucose molecule at the same time. These transport mechanisms are so efficient that they remove virtually all the glucose and amino acids from the tubular lumen. After entry into the cell, glucose and amino acids exit across the basolateral membranes by diffusion, driven by the high glucose and amino acid concentrations in the cell facilitated by specific transport proteins.

Sodium glucose co-transporters (SGLT2 and SGLT1) are located on the brush border of proximal tubular cells and carry glucose into the cell cytoplasm against a concentration gradient, as described previously. Approximately 90 percent of the filtered glucose is reabsorbed by SGLT2 in the early part of the proximal tubule (S1 segment) and the residual 10 percent is transported by SGLT1 in the latter segments of the proximal tubule. On the basolateral

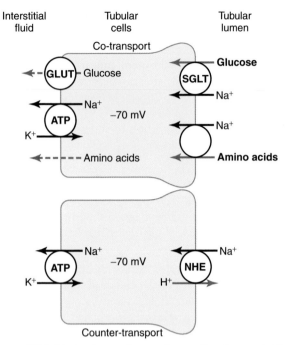

Interstitial fluid **Tubular cells** **Tubular lumen**

Co-transport

GLUT — Glucose

Glucose

SGLT

Na⁺

−70 mV

ATP

K⁺

Na⁺

Amino acids

Na⁺

Amino acids

Counter-transport

Na⁺

−70 mV

ATP

K⁺

NHE

Na⁺

H⁺

Figure 27-3 Mechanisms of secondary active transport. The upper cell shows the *co-transport* of glucose and amino acids along with sodium ions through the apical side of the tubular epithelial cells, followed by facilitated diffusion through the basolateral membranes. The lower cell shows the *counter-transport* of hydrogen ions from the interior of the cell across the apical membrane and into the tubular lumen; movement of sodium ions into the cell, down an electrochemical gradient established by the sodium-potassium pump on the basolateral membrane, provides the energy for transport of the hydrogen ions from inside the cell into the tubular lumen. GLUT, glucose transporter; NHE, sodium-hydrogen exchanger; SGLT, sodium-glucose co-transporter.

side of the membrane, glucose diffuses out of the cell into the interstitial spaces with the help of *glucose transporters* -*GLUT2*, in the S1 segment and *GLUT1* in the latter part (S3 segment) of the proximal tubule.

Although transport of glucose against a chemical gradient does not directly use ATP, the reabsorption of glucose depends on energy expended by the primary active sodium-potassium ATPase pump in the basolateral membrane. Because of the activity of this pump, an electrochemical gradient for facilitated diffusion of sodium across the luminal membrane is maintained, and it is this downhill diffusion of sodium to the interior of the cell that provides the energy for the simultaneous uphill transport of glucose across the luminal membrane. Thus, this reabsorption of glucose is referred to as "secondary active transport" because glucose itself is reabsorbed uphill against a chemical gradient, but it is "secondary" to primary active transport of sodium.

Another important point is that a substance is said to undergo "active" transport when at least one of the steps in the reabsorption involves primary or secondary active transport, even though other steps in the reabsorption process may be passive. For glucose reabsorption, secondary active transport occurs at the luminal membrane, but passive facilitated diffusion occurs at the basolateral membrane, and passive uptake by bulk flow occurs at the peritubular capillaries.

Secondary Active Secretion into the Tubules. Some substances are secreted into the tubules by secondary active transport. This often involves *counter-transport* of the substance with sodium ions. In counter-transport, the energy liberated from the downhill movement of one of the substances (e.g., sodium ions) enables uphill movement of a second substance in the opposite direction.

One example of counter-transport, shown in Figure 27-3, is the active secretion of hydrogen ions coupled to sodium reabsorption in the luminal membrane of the proximal tubule. In this case, sodium entry into the cell is coupled with hydrogen extrusion from the cell by sodium-hydrogen counter-transport. This transport is mediated by a specific protein (*sodium-hydrogen exchanger*) in the brush border of the luminal membrane. As sodium is carried to the interior of the cell, hydrogen ions are forced outward in the opposite direction into the tubular lumen. The basic principles of primary and secondary active transport are discussed in additional detail in Chapter 4.

Pinocytosis—An Active Transport Mechanism for Reabsorption of Proteins. Some parts of the tubule, especially the proximal tubule, reabsorb large molecules such as proteins by *pinocytosis.* In this process the protein attaches to the brush border of the luminal membrane, and this portion of the membrane then invaginates to the interior of the cell until it is completely pinched off and a vesicle is formed containing the protein. Once inside the cell, the protein is digested into its constituent amino acids, which are reabsorbed through the basolateral membrane into the interstitial fluid. Because pinocytosis requires energy, it is considered a form of active transport.

Transport Maximum for Substances That Are Actively Reabsorbed. For most substances that are actively reabsorbed or secreted, there is a limit to the rate at which the solute can be transported, often referred to as the *transport maximum*. This limit is due to saturation of the specific transport systems involved when the amount of solute delivered to the tubule (referred to as *tubular load*) exceeds the capacity of the carrier proteins and specific enzymes involved in the transport process.

The glucose transport system in the proximal tubule is a good example. Normally, measurable glucose does not appear in the urine because essentially all the filtered glucose is reabsorbed in the proximal tubule. However, when the filtered load exceeds the capability of the tubules to reabsorb glucose, urinary excretion of glucose does occur.

In the adult human, the transport maximum for glucose averages about 375 mg/min, whereas the filtered load of glucose is only about 125 mg/min (GFR × plasma glucose = 125 ml/min × 1 mg/ml). With large increases in GFR and/or plasma glucose concentration that increase the

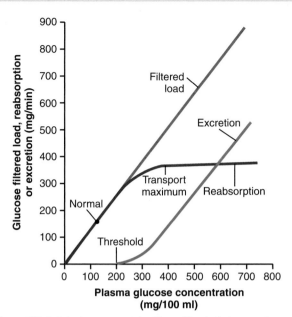

Figure 27-4 Relations among the filtered load of glucose, the rate of glucose reabsorption by the renal tubules, and the rate of glucose excretion in the urine. The *transport maximum* is the maximum rate at which glucose can be reabsorbed from the tubules. The *threshold* for glucose refers to the filtered load of glucose at which glucose first begins to be excreted in the urine.

filtered load of glucose above 375 mg/min, the excess glucose filtered is not reabsorbed and passes into the urine.

Figure 27-4 shows the relation between plasma concentration of glucose, filtered load of glucose, tubular transport maximum for glucose, and rate of glucose loss in the urine. Note that when the plasma glucose concentration is 100 mg/100 ml and the filtered load is at its normal level, 125 mg/min, there is no loss of glucose in the urine. However, when the plasma concentration of glucose rises above about 200 mg/100 ml, increasing the filtered load to about 250 mg/min, a small amount of glucose begins to appear in the urine. This point is termed the *threshold* for glucose. *Note that this appearance of glucose in the urine (at the threshold) occurs before the transport maximum is reached.* One reason for the difference between threshold and transport maximum is that not all nephrons have the same transport maximum for glucose, and some of the nephrons therefore begin to excrete glucose before others have reached their transport maximum. *The overall transport maximum for the kidneys, which is normally about 375 mg/min, is reached when all nephrons have reached their maximal capacity to reabsorb glucose.*

The plasma glucose of a healthy person almost never becomes high enough to cause glucose excretion in the urine, even after eating a meal. However, in uncontrolled *diabetes mellitus*, plasma glucose may rise to high levels, causing the filtered load of glucose to exceed the transport maximum and resulting in urinary glucose excretion. Some of the important transport maximums for substances *actively reabsorbed* by the tubules are as follows:

Substance	Transport Maximum
Glucose	375 mg/min
Phosphate	0.10 mM/min
Sulfate	0.06 mM/min
Amino acids	1.5 mM/min
Urate	15 mg/min
Lactate	75 mg/min
Plasma protein	30 mg/min

Transport Maximums for Substances That Are Actively Secreted. Substances that are *actively secreted* also exhibit transport maximums as follows:

Substance	Transport Maximum
Creatinine	16 mg/min
Para-aminohippuric acid	80 mg/min

Substances That Are Actively Transported but Do Not Exhibit a Transport Maximum. The reason that actively transported solutes often exhibit a transport maximum is that the transport carrier system becomes saturated as the tubular load increases. *Some substances that are passively reabsorbed do not demonstrate a transport maximum* because their rate of transport is determined by other factors, such as (1) the electrochemical gradient for diffusion of the substance across the membrane, (2) the permeability of the membrane for the substance, and (3) the time that the fluid containing the substance remains within the tubule. Transport of this type is referred to as *gradient-time transport* because the rate of transport depends on the electrochemical gradient and the time that the substance is in the tubule, which in turn depends on the tubular flow rate.

Some actively transported substances also have characteristics of gradient-time transport. An example is sodium reabsorption in the proximal tubule. The main reason that sodium transport in the proximal tubule does not exhibit a transport maximum is that other factors limit the reabsorption rate besides the maximum rate of active transport. For example, in the proximal tubules, the maximum transport capacity of the basolateral sodium-potassium ATPase pump is usually far greater than the actual rate of net sodium reabsorption. One of the reasons for this is that a significant amount of sodium transported out of the cell leaks back into the tubular lumen through the epithelial tight junctions. The rate at which this backleak occurs depends on several factors, including (1) the permeability of the tight junctions and (2) the interstitial physical forces, which determine the rate of bulk flow reabsorption from the interstitial fluid into the peritubular capillaries. Therefore, sodium transport in the proximal tubules obeys mainly gradient-time transport principles rather than tubular maximum transport characteristics. This means that the greater the concentration of sodium in the proximal tubules, the greater its reabsorption rate.

327

Also, the slower the flow rate of tubular fluid, the greater the percentage of sodium that can be reabsorbed from the proximal tubules.

In the more distal parts of the nephron, the epithelial cells have much tighter junctions and transport much smaller amounts of sodium. In these segments, sodium reabsorption exhibits a transport maximum similar to that for other actively transported substances. Furthermore, this transport maximum can be increased by certain hormones, such as *aldosterone.*

Passive Water Reabsorption by Osmosis Is Coupled Mainly to Sodium Reabsorption

When solutes are transported out of the tubule by either primary or secondary active transport, their concentrations tend to decrease inside the tubule while increasing in the renal interstitium. This creates a concentration difference that causes osmosis of water in the same direction that the solutes are transported, from the tubular lumen to the renal interstitium. Some parts of the renal tubule, especially the proximal tubule, are highly permeable to water, and water reabsorption occurs so rapidly that there is only a small concentration gradient for solutes across the tubular membrane.

A large part of the osmotic flow of water in the proximal tubules occurs through the so-called *tight junctions* between the epithelial cells, as well as through the cells themselves. The reason for this, as already discussed, is that the junctions between the cells are not as tight as their name would imply and permit significant diffusion of water and small ions. This is especially true in the proximal tubules, which have a high permeability for water and a smaller but significant permeability to most ions, such as sodium, chloride, potassium, calcium, and magnesium.

As water moves across the tight junctions by osmosis, it can also carry with it some of the solutes, a process referred to as *solvent drag.* And because the reabsorption of water, organic solutes, and ions is coupled to sodium reabsorption, changes in sodium reabsorption significantly influence the reabsorption of water and many other solutes.

In the more distal parts of the nephron, beginning in the loop of Henle and extending through the collecting tubule, the tight junctions become far less permeable to water and solutes and the epithelial cells also have a greatly decreased membrane surface area. Therefore, water cannot move easily across the tight junctions of the tubular membrane by osmosis. However, antidiuretic hormone (ADH) greatly increases the water permeability in the distal and collecting tubules, as discussed later.

Thus, water movement across the tubular epithelium can occur only if the membrane is permeable to water, no matter how large the osmotic gradient. In the proximal tubule, the water permeability is always high and water is reabsorbed as rapidly as the solutes. In the ascending loop of Henle, water permeability is always low, so almost no water is reabsorbed despite a large osmotic gradient.

Water permeability in the last parts of the tubules—the distal tubules, collecting tubules, and collecting ducts—can be high or low, depending on the presence or absence of ADH.

Reabsorption of Chloride, Urea, and Other Solutes by Passive Diffusion

When sodium is reabsorbed through the tubular epithelial cell, negative ions such as chloride are transported along with sodium because of electrical potentials. That is, transport of positively charged sodium ions out of the lumen leaves the inside of the lumen negatively charged, compared with the interstitial fluid. This causes chloride ions to diffuse *passively* through the *paracellular pathway.* Additional reabsorption of chloride ions occurs because of a chloride concentration gradient that develops when water is reabsorbed from the tubule by osmosis, thereby concentrating the chloride ions in the tubular lumen (Figure 27-5). Thus, the active reabsorption of sodium is closely coupled to the passive reabsorption of chloride by way of an electrical potential and a chloride concentration gradient.

Chloride ions can also be reabsorbed by secondary active transport. The most important of the secondary active transport processes for chloride reabsorption involves co-transport of chloride with sodium across the luminal membrane.

Urea is also passively reabsorbed from the tubule, but to a much lesser extent than chloride ions. As water is reabsorbed from the tubules (by osmosis coupled to sodium reabsorption), urea concentration in the tubular lumen increases (see Figure 27-5). This creates a concentration gradient favoring the reabsorption of urea. However, urea does not permeate the tubule as readily as water. In some parts of the nephron, especially the inner medullary collecting duct, passive urea reabsorption is facilitated by specific *urea transporters.* Yet, only about one half of the urea that is filtered by the glomerular capillaries is reabsorbed from the tubules. The remainder of the urea passes into the urine, allowing the kidneys to excrete large

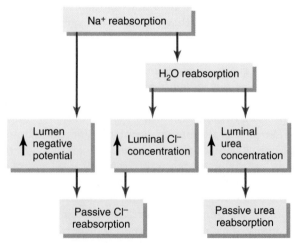

Figure 27-5 Mechanisms by which water, chloride, and urea reabsorption are coupled with sodium reabsorption.

amounts of this waste product of metabolism. In mammals, greater than 90 percent of waste nitrogen, mainly generated in the liver as a product of protein metabolism, is normally excreted by the kidneys as urea.

Another waste product of metabolism, creatinine, is an even larger molecule than urea and is essentially impermeant to the tubular membrane. Therefore, almost none of the creatinine that is filtered is reabsorbed, so that virtually all the creatinine filtered by the glomerulus is excreted in the urine.

Reabsorption and Secretion Along Different Parts of the Nephron

In the previous sections, we discussed the basic principles by which water and solutes are transported across the tubular membrane. With these generalizations in mind, we can now discuss the different characteristics of the individual tubular segments that enable them to perform their specific functions. Only the tubular transport functions that are quantitatively most important are discussed, especially as they relate to the reabsorption of sodium, chloride, and water. In subsequent chapters, we discuss the reabsorption and secretion of other specific substances in different parts of the tubular system.

Proximal Tubular Reabsorption

Normally, about 65 percent of the filtered load of sodium and water and a slightly lower percentage of filtered chloride are reabsorbed by the proximal tubule before the filtrate reaches the loops of Henle. These percentages can be increased or decreased in different physiologic conditions, as discussed later.

Proximal Tubules Have a High Capacity for Active and Passive Reabsorption. The high capacity of the proximal tubule for reabsorption results from its special cellular characteristics, as shown in Figure 27-6. The proximal tubule epithelial cells are highly metabolic and have large numbers of mitochondria to support powerful active transport processes. In addition, the proximal tubular cells have an extensive brush border on the luminal (apical) side of the membrane, as well as an extensive labyrinth of intercellular and basal channels, all of which together provide an extensive membrane surface area on the luminal and basolateral sides of the epithelium for rapid transport of sodium ions and other substances.

The extensive membrane surface of the epithelial brush border is also loaded with protein carrier molecules that transport a large fraction of the sodium ions across the luminal membrane linked by way of the *co-transport* mechanism with multiple organic nutrients such as amino acids and glucose. Additional sodium is transported from the tubular lumen into the cell by *counter-transport* mechanisms that reabsorb sodium while secreting other substances into the tubular lumen, especially hydrogen

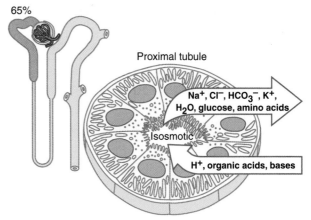

Figure 27-6 Cellular ultrastructure and primary transport characteristics of the proximal tubule. The proximal tubules reabsorb about 65 percent of the filtered sodium, chloride, bicarbonate, and potassium and essentially all the filtered glucose and amino acids. The proximal tubules also secrete organic acids, bases, and hydrogen ions into the tubular lumen.

ions. As discussed in Chapter 30, the secretion of hydrogen ions into the tubular lumen is an important step in the removal of bicarbonate ions from the tubule (by combining H^+ with the HCO_3^- to form H_2CO_3, which then dissociates into H_2O and CO_2).

Although the sodium-potassium ATPase pump provides the major force for reabsorption of sodium, chloride, and water throughout the proximal tubule, there are some differences in the mechanisms by which sodium and chloride are transported through the luminal side of the early and late portions of the proximal tubular membrane.

In the first half of the proximal tubule, sodium is reabsorbed by co-transport along with glucose, amino acids, and other solutes. But in the second half of the proximal tubule, little glucose and amino acids remain to be reabsorbed. Instead, sodium is now reabsorbed mainly with chloride ions. The second half of the proximal tubule has a relatively high concentration of chloride (around 140 mEq/L) compared with the early proximal tubule (about 105 mEq/L) because when sodium is reabsorbed, it preferentially carries with it glucose, bicarbonate, and organic ions in the early proximal tubule, leaving behind a solution that has a higher concentration of chloride. In the second half of the proximal tubule, the higher chloride concentration favors the diffusion of this ion from the tubule lumen through the intercellular junctions into the renal interstitial fluid. Smaller amounts of chloride may also be reabsorbed through specific chloride channels in the proximal tubular cell membrane.

Concentrations of Solutes Along the Proximal Tubule. Figure 27-7 summarizes the changes in concentrations of various solutes along the proximal tubule. Although the *amount* of sodium in the tubular fluid decreases markedly along the proximal tubule, the *concentration* of sodium (and the total osmolarity) remains relatively constant because water permeability of the

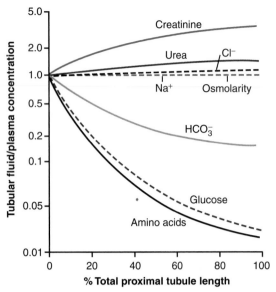

Figure 27-7 Changes in concentrations of different substances in tubular fluid along the proximal convoluted tubule relative to the concentrations of these substances in the plasma and in the glomerular filtrate. A value of 1.0 indicates that the concentration of the substance in the tubular fluid is the same as the concentration in the plasma. Values below 1.0 indicate that the substance is reabsorbed more avidly than water, whereas values above 1.0 indicate that the substance is reabsorbed to a lesser extent than water or is secreted into the tubules.

proximal tubules is so great that water reabsorption keeps pace with sodium reabsorption. Certain organic solutes, such as glucose, amino acids, and bicarbonate, are much more avidly reabsorbed than water, so their concentrations decrease markedly along the length of the proximal tubule. Other organic solutes that are less permeant and not actively reabsorbed, such as creatinine, increase their concentration along the proximal tubule. The total solute concentration, as reflected by osmolarity, remains essentially the same all along the proximal tubule because of the extremely high permeability of this part of the nephron to water.

Secretion of Organic Acids and Bases by the Proximal Tubule. The proximal tubule is also an important site for secretion of organic acids and bases such as *bile salts, oxalate, urate,* and *catecholamines.* Many of these substances are the end products of metabolism and must be rapidly removed from the body. The *secretion* of these substances into the proximal tubule plus *filtration* into the proximal tubule by the glomerular capillaries and the almost total lack of reabsorption by the tubules, all combined, contribute to rapid excretion in the urine.

In addition to the waste products of metabolism, the kidneys secrete many potentially harmful drugs or toxins directly through the tubular cells into the tubules and rapidly clear these substances from the blood. In the case of certain drugs, such as penicillin and salicylates, the rapid clearance by the kidneys creates a problem in maintaining a therapeutically effective drug concentration.

Another compound that is rapidly secreted by the proximal tubule is para-aminohippuric acid (PAH). PAH is secreted so rapidly that the average person can clear about 90 percent of the PAH from the plasma flowing through the kidneys and excrete it in the urine. For this reason, the rate of PAH clearance can be used to estimate the renal plasma flow, as discussed later.

Solute and Water Transport in the Loop of Henle

The loop of Henle consists of three functionally distinct segments: the *thin descending segment,* the *thin ascending segment,* and the *thick ascending segment.* The thin descending and thin ascending segments, as their names imply, have thin epithelial membranes with no brush borders, few mitochondria, and minimal levels of metabolic activity (Figure 27-8).

The descending part of the thin segment is highly permeable to water and moderately permeable to most solutes, including urea and sodium. The function of this nephron segment is mainly to allow simple diffusion of substances through its walls. About 20 percent of the filtered water is reabsorbed in the loop of Henle, and almost

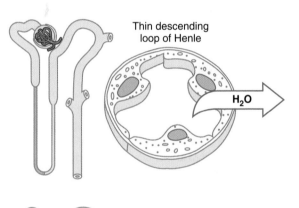

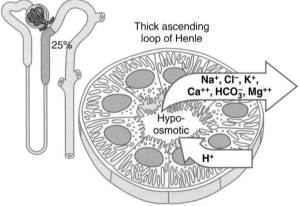

Figure 27-8 Cellular ultrastructure and transport characteristics of the thin descending loop of Henle (*top*) and the thick ascending segment of the loop of Henle (*bottom*). The descending part of the thin segment of the loop of Henle is highly permeable to water and moderately permeable to most solutes but has few mitochondria and little or no active reabsorption. The thick ascending limb of the loop of Henle reabsorbs about 25 percent of the filtered loads of sodium, chloride, and potassium, as well as large amounts of calcium, bicarbonate, and magnesium. This segment also secretes hydrogen ions into the tubular lumen.

all of this occurs in the thin descending limb. The ascending limb, including both the thin and the thick portions, is virtually impermeable to water, a characteristic that is important for concentrating the urine.

The thick segment of the loop of Henle, which begins about halfway up the ascending limb, has thick epithelial cells that have high metabolic activity and are capable of active reabsorption of sodium, chloride, and potassium (see Figure 27-8). About 25 percent of the filtered loads of sodium, chloride, and potassium are reabsorbed in the loop of Henle, mostly in the thick ascending limb. Considerable amounts of other ions, such as calcium, bicarbonate, and magnesium, are also reabsorbed in the thick ascending loop of Henle. The thin segment of the ascending limb has a much lower reabsorptive capacity than the thick segment, and the thin descending limb does not reabsorb significant amounts of any of these solutes.

An important component of solute reabsorption in the thick ascending limb is the sodium-potassium ATPase pump in the epithelial cell basolateral membranes. As in the proximal tubule, the reabsorption of other solutes in the thick segment of the ascending loop of Henle is closely linked to the reabsorptive capability of the sodium-potassium ATPase pump, which maintains a low intracellular sodium concentration. The low intracellular sodium concentration in turn provides a favorable gradient for movement of sodium from the tubular fluid into the cell. *In the thick ascending loop, movement of sodium across the luminal membrane is mediated primarily by a 1-sodium, 2-chloride, 1-potassium co-transporter* (Figure 27-9). This co-transport protein carrier in the luminal membrane uses the potential energy released by downhill diffusion of sodium into the cell to drive the reabsorption of potassium into the cell against a concentration gradient.

The thick ascending limb of the loop of Henle is the site of action of the powerful *"loop" diuretics furosemide, ethacrynic acid,* and *bumetanide,* all of which inhibit the action of the sodium, 2-chloride, potassium co-transporter. These diuretics are discussed in Chapter 31.

The thick ascending limb also has a sodium-hydrogen counter-transport mechanism in its luminal cell membrane that mediates sodium reabsorption and hydrogen secretion in this segment (see Figure 27-9).

There is also significant paracellular reabsorption of cations, such as Mg^{++}, Ca^{++}, Na^+, and K^+, in the thick ascending limb owing to the slight positive charge of the tubular lumen relative to the interstitial fluid. Although the 1-sodium, 2-chloride, 1-potassium co-transporter moves equal amounts of cations and anions into the cell, there is a slight backleak of potassium ions into the lumen, creating a positive charge of about +8 millivolts in the tubular lumen. This positive charge forces cations such as Mg^{++} and Ca^{++} to diffuse from the tubular lumen through the paracellular space and into the interstitial fluid.

The thick segment of the ascending loop of Henle is virtually impermeable to water. Therefore, most of the water delivered to this segment remains in the tubule despite reabsorption of large amounts of solute. The tubular fluid

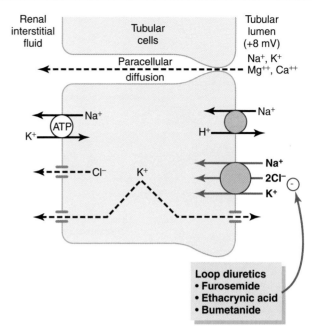

Figure 27-9 Mechanisms of sodium, chloride, and potassium transport in the thick ascending loop of Henle. The sodium-potassium ATPase pump in the basolateral cell membrane maintains a low intracellular sodium concentration and a negative electrical potential in the cell. The 1-sodium, 2-chloride, 1-potassium co-transporter in the luminal membrane transports these three ions from the tubular lumen into the cells, using the potential energy released by diffusion of sodium down an electrochemical gradient into the cells. Sodium is also transported into the tubular cell by sodium-hydrogen counter-transport. The positive charge (+8 mV) of the tubular lumen relative to the interstitial fluid forces cations such as Mg^{++} and Ca^{++} to diffuse from the lumen to the interstitial fluid via the paracellular pathway.

in the ascending limb becomes very dilute as it flows toward the distal tubule, a feature that is important in allowing the kidneys to dilute or concentrate the urine under different conditions, as we discuss much more fully in Chapter 28.

Distal Tubule

The thick segment of the ascending limb of the loop of Henle empties into the *distal tubule.* The first portion of the distal tubule forms the *macula densa,* a group of closely packed epithelial cells that is part of the *juxtaglomerular complex* and provides feedback control of GFR and blood flow in this same nephron.

The next part of the distal tubule is highly convoluted and has many of the same reabsorptive characteristics of the thick segment of the ascending limb of the loop of Henle. That is, it avidly reabsorbs most of the ions, including sodium, potassium, and chloride, but is virtually impermeable to water and urea. For this reason, it is referred to as the *diluting segment* because it also dilutes the tubular fluid.

Approximately 5 percent of the filtered load of sodium chloride is reabsorbed in the early distal tubule. The *sodium-chloride co-transporter* moves sodium chloride from the tubular lumen into the cell, and the

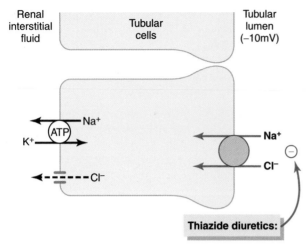

Figure 27-10 Mechanism of sodium chloride transport in the early distal tubule. Sodium and chloride are transported from the tubular lumen into the cell by a co-transporter that is inhibited by thiazide diuretics. Sodium is pumped out of the cell by sodium-potassium ATPase and chloride diffuses into the interstitial fluid via chloride channels.

sodium-potassium ATPase pump transports sodium out of the cell across the basolateral membrane (Figure 27-10). Chloride diffuses out of the cell into the renal interstitial fluid through chloride channels in the basolateral membrane.

The *thiazide diuretics,* which are widely used to treat disorders such as hypertension and heart failure, inhibit the sodium-chloride co-transporter.

Late Distal Tubule and Cortical Collecting Tubule

The second half of the distal tubule and the subsequent cortical collecting tubule have similar functional characteristics. Anatomically, they are composed of two distinct cell types, the *principal cells* and *intercalated cells* (Figure 27-11). The principal cells reabsorb sodium and water from the lumen and secrete potassium ions into the lumen. The intercalated cells reabsorb potassium ions and secrete hydrogen ions into the tubular lumen.

Principal Cells Reabsorb Sodium and Secrete Potassium. Sodium *reabsorption* and potassium *secretion* by the principal cells depend on the activity of a sodium-potassium ATPase pump in each cell's basolateral membrane (Figure 27-12). This pump maintains a low sodium concentration inside the cell and, therefore, favors sodium diffusion into the cell through special channels. The secretion of potassium by these cells from the blood into the tubular lumen involves two steps: (1) Potassium enters the cell because of the sodium-potassium ATPase pump, which maintains a high intracellular potassium concentration, and then (2) once in the cell, potassium diffuses down its concentration gradient across the luminal membrane into the tubular fluid.

The principal cells are the primary sites of action of the *potassium-sparing diuretics,* including spironolactone, eplerenone, amiloride, and triamterene. *Spironolactone*

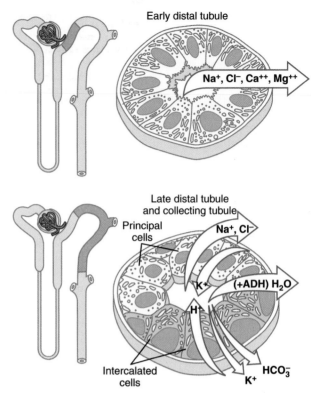

Figure 27-11 Cellular ultrastructure and transport characteristics of the early distal tubule and the late distal tubule and collecting tubule. The early distal tubule has many of the same characteristics as the thick ascending loop of Henle and reabsorbs sodium, chloride, calcium, and magnesium but is virtually impermeable to water and urea. The late distal tubules and cortical collecting tubules are composed of two distinct cell types, the *principal cells* and the *intercalated cells.* The principal cells reabsorb sodium from the lumen and secrete potassium ions into the lumen. The intercalated cells reabsorb potassium and bicarbonate ions from the lumen and secrete hydrogen ions into the lumen. The reabsorption of water from this tubular segment is controlled by the concentration of *antidiuretic hormone.*

and *eplerenone* are mineralocorticoid receptor antagonists that compete with aldosterone for receptor sites in the principal cells and therefore inhibit the stimulatory effects of aldosterone on sodium reabsorption and potassium secretion. *Amiloride* and *triamterene* are sodium channel blockers that directly inhibit the entry of sodium into the sodium channels of the luminal membranes and therefore reduce the amount of sodium that can be transported across the basolateral membranes by the sodium-potassium ATPase pump. This, in turn, decreases transport of potassium into the cells and ultimately reduces potassium secretion into the tubular fluid. For this reason the sodium channel blockers, as well as the aldosterone antagonists, decrease urinary excretion of potassium and act as potassium-sparing diuretics.

Intercalated Cells Secrete Hydrogen and Reabsorb Bicarbonate and Potassium Ions. Hydrogen ion secretion by the intercalated cells is mediated by a hydrogen-ATPase transporter. Hydrogen is generated in this cell by the action of carbonic anhydrase on water and carbon

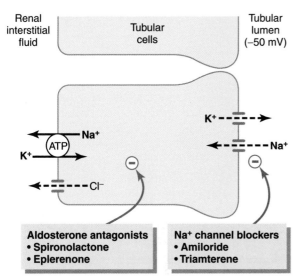

Figure 27-12 Mechanism of sodium chloride reabsorption and potassium secretion in the late distal tubules and cortical collecting tubules. Sodium enters the cell through special channels and is transported out of the cell by the sodium-potassium ATPase pump. Aldosterone antagonists compete with aldosterone for binding sites in the cell and therefore inhibit the effects of aldosterone to stimulate sodium reabsorption and potassium secretion. Sodium channel blockers directly inhibit the entry of sodium into the sodium channels.

dioxide to form carbonic acid, which then dissociates into hydrogen ions and bicarbonate ions. The hydrogen ions are then secreted into the tubular lumen, and for each hydrogen ion secreted, a bicarbonate ion becomes available for reabsorption across the basolateral membrane. A more detailed discussion of this mechanism is presented in Chapter 30. The intercalated cells can also reabsorb potassium ions.

The functional characteristics of the *late distal tubule* and *cortical collecting tubule* can be summarized as follows:

1. The tubular membranes of both segments are almost completely impermeable to urea, similar to the diluting segment of the early distal tubule; thus, almost all the urea that enters these segments passes on through and into the collecting duct to be excreted in the urine, although some reabsorption of urea occurs in the medullary collecting ducts.

2. Both the late distal tubule and the cortical collecting tubule segments reabsorb sodium ions, and the rate of reabsorption is controlled by hormones, especially aldosterone. At the same time, these segments secrete potassium ions from the peritubular capillary blood into the tubular lumen, a process that is also controlled by aldosterone and by other factors such as the concentration of potassium ions in the body fluids.

3. The *intercalated cells* of these nephron segments avidly secrete hydrogen ions by an active *hydrogen-ATPase* mechanism. This process is different from the secondary active secretion of hydrogen ions by the proximal tubule because it is capable of secreting hydrogen ions

against a large concentration gradient, as much as 1000 to 1. This is in contrast to the relatively small gradient (4- to 10-fold) for hydrogen ions that can be achieved by secondary active secretion in the proximal tubule. Thus, the intercalated cells play a key role in acid-base regulation of the body fluids.

4. The permeability of the late distal tubule and cortical collecting duct to water is controlled by the concentration of *ADH*, which is also called *vasopressin*. With high levels of ADH, these tubular segments are permeable to water, but in the absence of ADH, they are virtually impermeable to water. This special characteristic provides an important mechanism for controlling the degree of dilution or concentration of the urine.

Medullary Collecting Duct

Although the medullary collecting ducts reabsorb less than 10 percent of the filtered water and sodium, they are the final site for processing the urine and, therefore, play an extremely important role in determining the final urine output of water and solutes.

The epithelial cells of the collecting ducts are nearly cuboidal in shape with smooth surfaces and relatively few mitochondria (Figure 27-13). Special characteristics of this tubular segment are as follows:

1. The permeability of the medullary collecting duct to water is controlled by the level of ADH. With high levels of ADH, water is avidly reabsorbed into the medullary interstitium, thereby reducing the urine volume and concentrating most of the solutes in the urine.

2. Unlike the cortical collecting tubule, the medullary collecting duct is permeable to urea and there are special *urea transporters* that facilitate urea diffusion across the luminal and basolateral membranes. Therefore, some of the tubular urea is reabsorbed into the medullary interstitium, helping to raise the osmolality in this

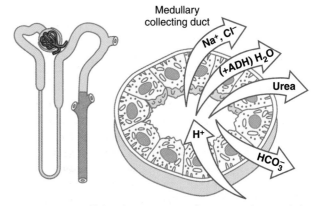

Figure 27-13 Cellular ultrastructure and transport characteristics of the medullary collecting duct. The medullary collecting ducts actively reabsorb sodium and secrete hydrogen ions and are permeable to urea, which is reabsorbed in these tubular segments. The reabsorption of water in medullary collecting ducts is controlled by the concentration of antidiuretic hormone.

region of the kidneys and contributing to the kidneys' overall ability to form concentrated urine. This is discussed in Chapter 28.

3. The medullary collecting duct is capable of secreting hydrogen ions against a large concentration gradient, as also occurs in the cortical collecting tubule. Thus, the medullary collecting duct also plays a key role in regulating acid-base balance.

Summary of Concentrations of Different Solutes in the Different Tubular Segments

Whether a solute will become concentrated in the tubular fluid is determined by the relative degree of reabsorption of that solute versus the reabsorption of water. If a greater percentage of water is reabsorbed, the substance becomes more concentrated. If a greater percentage of the solute is reabsorbed, the substance becomes more diluted.

Figure 27-14 shows the degree of concentration of several substances in the different tubular segments. All the values in this figure represent the tubular fluid concentration divided by the plasma concentration of a substance. If plasma concentration of the substance is assumed to be constant, any change in the ratio of tubular fluid/plasma concentration rate reflects changes in tubular fluid concentration.

As the filtrate moves along the tubular system, the concentration rises to progressively greater than 1.0 if more water is reabsorbed than solute, or if there has been a net secretion of the solute into the tubular fluid. If the concentration ratio becomes progressively less than 1.0, this means that relatively more solute has been reabsorbed than water.

The substances represented at the top of Figure 27-14, such as creatinine, become highly concentrated in the urine. In general, these substances are not needed by the body, and the kidneys have become adapted to reabsorb them only slightly or not at all, or even to secrete them into the tubules, thereby excreting especially great quantities into the urine. Conversely, the substances represented toward the bottom of the figure, such as glucose and amino acids, are all strongly reabsorbed; these are all substances that the body needs to conserve, and almost none of them are lost in the urine.

Tubular Fluid/Plasma Inulin Concentration Ratio Can Be Used to Measure Water Reabsorption by the Renal Tubules. Inulin, a polysaccharide used to measure GFR, is not reabsorbed or secreted by the renal tubules. Changes in inulin concentration at different points along the renal tubule, therefore, reflect changes in the amount of water present in the tubular fluid.

For example, the tubular fluid/plasma concentration ratio for inulin rises to about 3.0 at the end of the proximal tubules, indicating that inulin concentration in the tubular fluid is three times greater than in the plasma and in the glomerular filtrate. Because inulin is not secreted or reabsorbed from the tubules, a tubular fluid/plasma concentration ratio of 3.0 means that only one third of the water that was filtered remains in the renal tubule and that two thirds of the filtered water has been reabsorbed as the fluid passes through the proximal tubule. At the end of the collecting ducts, the tubular fluid/plasma inulin concentration ratio rises to about 125 (see Figure 27-14), indicating that only 1/125 of the filtered water remains in the tubule and that more than 99% has been reabsorbed.

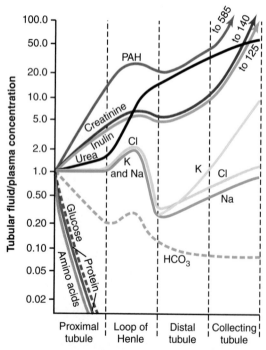

Figure 27-14 Changes in average concentrations of different substances at different points in the tubular system relative to the concentration of that substance in the plasma and in the glomerular filtrate. A value of 1.0 indicates that the concentration of the substance in the tubular fluid is the same as the concentration of that substance in the plasma. Values below 1.0 indicate that the substance is reabsorbed more avidly than water, whereas values above 1.0 indicate that the substance is reabsorbed to a lesser extent than water or is secreted into the tubules.

Regulation of Tubular Reabsorption

Because it is essential to maintain a precise balance between tubular reabsorption and glomerular filtration, there are multiple nervous, hormonal, and local control mechanisms that regulate tubular reabsorption, just as there are for control of glomerular filtration. An important feature of tubular reabsorption is that reabsorption of some solutes can be regulated independently of others, especially through hormonal control mechanisms.

Glomerulotubular Balance—The Ability of the Tubules to Increase Reabsorption Rate in Response to Increased Tubular Load

One of the most basic mechanisms for controlling tubular reabsorption is the intrinsic ability of the tubules to increase their reabsorption rate in response to increased tubular load (increased tubular inflow). This phenomenon is referred to as *glomerulotubular balance.* For example, if GFR is increased from 125 ml/min to 150 ml/min, the absolute rate of proximal tubular reabsorption also increases from about 81 ml/min (65 percent of GFR) to about 97.5 ml/min (65 percent of GFR). Thus, glomerulotubular balance refers to the fact that the total rate of reabsorption increases as the filtered load increases, even though the percentage of GFR reabsorbed in the proximal tubule remains relatively constant at about 65 percent.

Some degree of glomerulotubular balance also occurs in other tubular segments, especially the loop of Henle. The precise mechanisms responsible for this are not fully understood but may be due partly to changes in physical forces in the tubule and surrounding renal interstitium, as discussed later. It is clear that the mechanisms for glomerulotubular balance can occur independently of hormones and can be demonstrated in completely isolated kidneys or even in completely isolated proximal tubular segments.

Glomerulotubular balance helps to prevent overloading of the distal tubular segments when GFR increases. Glomerulotubular balance acts as a second line of defense to buffer the effects of spontaneous changes in GFR on urine output. (The first line of defense, discussed earlier, includes the renal autoregulatory mechanisms, especially tubuloglomerular feedback, which help prevent changes in GFR.) Working together, the autoregulatory and glomerulotubular balance mechanisms prevent large changes in fluid flow in the distal tubules when the arterial pressure changes or when there are other disturbances that would otherwise upset sodium and volume homeostasis.

Peritubular Capillary and Renal Interstitial Fluid Physical Forces

Hydrostatic and colloid osmotic forces govern the rate of reabsorption across the peritubular capillaries, just as they control filtration in the glomerular capillaries. Changes in peritubular capillary reabsorption can in turn influence the hydrostatic and colloid osmotic pressures of the renal interstitium and, ultimately, reabsorption of water and solutes from the renal tubules.

Normal Values for Physical Forces and Reabsorption Rate.
As the glomerular filtrate passes through the renal tubules, more than 99 percent of the water and most of the solutes are normally reabsorbed. Fluid and electrolytes are reabsorbed from the tubules into the renal interstitium and from there into the peritubular capillaries. The normal rate of peritubular capillary reabsorption is about 124 ml/min.

Reabsorption across the peritubular capillaries can be calculated as

$$\text{Reabsorption} = K_f \times \text{Net reabsorptive force}$$

The net reabsorptive force represents the sum of the hydrostatic and colloid osmotic forces that either favor or oppose reabsorption across the peritubular capillaries. These forces include (1) hydrostatic pressure inside the peritubular capillaries (peritubular hydrostatic pressure [P_c]), which opposes reabsorption; (2) hydrostatic pressure in the renal interstitium (P_{if}) outside the capillaries, which favors reabsorption; (3) colloid osmotic pressure of the peritubular capillary plasma proteins (π_c), which favors reabsorption; and (4) colloid osmotic pressure of the proteins in the renal interstitium (π_{if}), which opposes reabsorption.

Figure 27-15 shows the approximate normal forces that favor and oppose peritubular reabsorption. Because the normal peritubular capillary pressure averages about 13 mm Hg and renal interstitial fluid hydrostatic pressure averages 6 mm Hg, there is a positive hydrostatic pressure gradient from the peritubular capillary to the interstitial fluid of about 7 mm Hg, which opposes fluid reabsorption. This is more than counterbalanced by the colloid osmotic pressures that favor reabsorption. The plasma colloid osmotic pressure, which favors reabsorption, is about 32 mm Hg, and the colloid osmotic pressure of the interstitium, which opposes reabsorption, is 15 mm Hg, causing a net colloid osmotic force of about 17 mm Hg, favoring reabsorption. Therefore, subtracting the net hydrostatic forces that oppose reabsorption (7 mm Hg) from the net colloid osmotic forces that favor reabsorption (17 mm Hg) gives a net reabsorptive force of about 10 mm Hg. This is a high value, similar to that found in the glomerular capillaries, but in the opposite direction.

The other factor that contributes to the high rate of fluid reabsorption in the peritubular capillaries is a large filtration coefficient (K_f) because of the high hydraulic conductivity and large surface area of the capillaries. Because the reabsorption rate is normally about 124 ml/min and net reabsorption pressure is 10 mm Hg, K_f normally is about 12.4 ml/min/mm Hg.

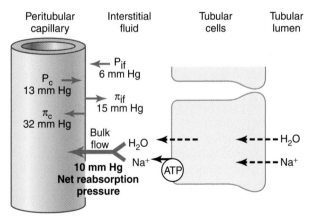

Figure 27-15 Summary of the hydrostatic and colloid osmotic forces that determine fluid reabsorption by the peritubular capillaries. The numerical values shown are estimates of the normal values for humans. The net reabsorptive pressure is normally about 10 mm Hg, causing fluid and solutes to be reabsorbed into the peritubular capillaries as they are transported across the renal tubular cells. ATP, adenosine triphosphate; P_c, peritubular capillary hydrostatic pressure; P_{if}, interstitial fluid hydrostatic pressure; π_c, peritubular capillary colloid osmotic pressure; π_{if}, interstitial fluid colloid osmotic pressure.

Regulation of Peritubular Capillary Physical Forces. The two determinants of peritubular capillary reabsorption that are directly influenced by renal hemodynamic changes are the hydrostatic and colloid osmotic pressures of the peritubular capillaries. The *peritubular capillary hydrostatic pressure* is influenced by the *arterial pressure* and *resistances of the afferent and efferent arterioles.* (1) Increases in arterial pressure tend to raise peritubular capillary hydrostatic pressure and decrease reabsorption rate. This effect is buffered to some extent by autoregulatory mechanisms that maintain relatively constant renal blood flow, as well as relatively constant hydrostatic pressures in the renal blood vessels. (2) Increase in resistance of either the afferent or the efferent arterioles reduces peritubular capillary hydrostatic pressure and tends to increase reabsorption rate. Although constriction of the efferent arterioles increases glomerular capillary hydrostatic pressure, it lowers peritubular capillary hydrostatic pressure.

The second major determinant of peritubular capillary reabsorption is the *colloid osmotic pressure* of the plasma in these capillaries; raising the colloid osmotic pressure increases peritubular capillary reabsorption. *The colloid osmotic pressure of peritubular capillaries is determined by* (1) the *systemic plasma colloid osmotic pressure;* increasing the plasma protein concentration of systemic blood tends to raise peritubular capillary colloid osmotic pressure, thereby increasing reabsorption; and (2) the *filtration fraction;* the higher the filtration fraction, the greater the fraction of plasma filtered through the glomerulus and, consequently, the more concentrated the protein becomes in the plasma that remains behind. Thus, increasing the filtration fraction also tends to increase the peritubular capillary reabsorption rate. Because filtration fraction is defined as the ratio of GFR/renal plasma flow, increased filtration fraction can occur as a result of increased GFR or decreased renal plasma flow. Some renal vasoconstrictors, such as angiotensin II, increase peritubular capillary reabsorption by decreasing renal plasma flow and increasing filtration fraction, as discussed later.

Changes in the peritubular capillary K_f can also influence the reabsorption rate because K_f is a measure of the permeability and surface area of the capillaries. Increases in K_f raise reabsorption, whereas decreases in K_f lower peritubular capillary reabsorption. K_f remains relatively constant in most physiologic conditions. Table 27-2 summarizes the factors that can influence the peritubular capillary reabsorption rate.

Renal Interstitial Hydrostatic and Colloid Osmotic Pressures.

Ultimately, changes in peritubular capillary physical forces influence tubular reabsorption by changing the physical forces in the renal interstitium surrounding the tubules. For example, a decrease in the reabsorptive force across the peritubular capillary membranes, caused by either increased peritubular capillary hydrostatic pressure or decreased peritubular capillary colloid osmotic pressure, reduces the uptake of fluid and

Table 27-2 Factors That Can Influence Peritubular Capillary Reabsorption

$\uparrow P_c \rightarrow \downarrow$ Reabsorption
  • $\downarrow R_A \rightarrow \uparrow P_c$
  • $\downarrow R_E \rightarrow \uparrow P_c$
  • $\uparrow$ Arterial Pressure $\rightarrow \uparrow P_c$
$\uparrow \pi_c \rightarrow \uparrow$ Reabsorption
  • $\uparrow \pi_A \rightarrow \uparrow \pi_c$
  • $\uparrow FF \rightarrow \uparrow \pi_c$
$\uparrow K_f \rightarrow \uparrow$ Reabsorption

P_c, peritubular capillary hydrostatic pressure; R_A and R_E, afferent and efferent arteriolar resistances, respectively; π_c, peritubular capillary colloid osmotic pressure; π_A, arterial plasma colloid osmotic pressure; FF, filtration fraction; K_f, peritubular capillary filtration coefficient.

solutes from the interstitium into the peritubular capillaries. This in turn raises renal interstitial fluid hydrostatic pressure and decreases interstitial fluid colloid osmotic pressure because of dilution of the proteins in the renal interstitium. These changes then decrease the net reabsorption of fluid from the renal tubules into the interstitium, especially in the proximal tubules.

The mechanisms by which changes in interstitial fluid hydrostatic and colloid osmotic pressures influence tubular reabsorption can be understood by examining the pathways through which solute and water are reabsorbed (Figure 27-16). Once the solutes enter the intercellular channels or renal interstitium by active transport or passive diffusion, water is drawn from the tubular lumen into the interstitium by osmosis. And once the water and solutes are in the interstitial spaces, they can either be swept up into the peritubular capillaries or diffuse back through the epithelial junctions into the tubular lumen. The so-called tight junctions between the epithelial cells of the proximal tubule are actually leaky, so considerable amounts of sodium can diffuse in both directions through these junctions. With the normal high rate of peritubular capillary reabsorption, the net movement of water and solutes is into the peritubular capillaries with little backleak into the lumen of the tubule. However, when peritubular capillary reabsorption is reduced, there is increased interstitial fluid hydrostatic pressure and a tendency for greater amounts of solute and water to backleak into the tubular lumen, thereby reducing the rate of net reabsorption (refer again to Figure 27-16).

The opposite is true when there is increased peritubular capillary reabsorption above the normal level. An initial increase in reabsorption by the peritubular capillaries tends to reduce interstitial fluid hydrostatic pressure and raise interstitial fluid colloid osmotic pressure. Both of these forces favor movement of fluid and solutes out of the tubular lumen and into the interstitium; therefore, backleak of water and solutes into the tubular lumen is reduced, and net tubular reabsorption increases.

Thus, through changes in the hydrostatic and colloid osmotic pressures of the renal interstitium, the uptake of water and solutes by the peritubular capillaries is closely

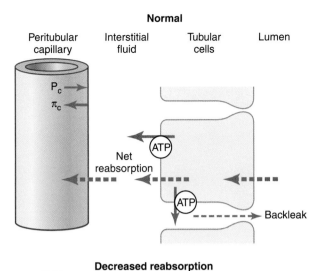

Normal

Peritubular capillary   Interstitial fluid   Tubular cells   Lumen

Net reabsorption

Backleak

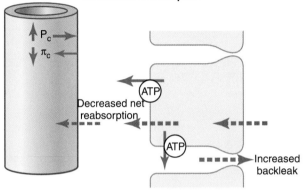

Decreased reabsorption

Decreased net reabsorption

Increased backleak

Figure 27-16 Proximal tubular and peritubular capillary reabsorption under normal conditions (*top*) and during decreased peritubular capillary reabsorption (*bottom*) caused by either increasing peritubular capillary hydrostatic pressure (P_c) or decreasing peritubular capillary colloid osmotic pressure (π_c). Reduced peritubular capillary reabsorption, in turn, decreases the net reabsorption of solutes and water by increasing the amounts of solutes and water that leak back into the tubular lumen through the tight junctions of the tubular epithelial cells, especially in the proximal tubule.

matched to the net reabsorption of water and solutes from the tubular lumen into the interstitium. Therefore, in general, *forces that increase peritubular capillary reabsorption also increase reabsorption from the renal tubules. Conversely, hemodynamic changes that inhibit peritubular capillary reabsorption also inhibit tubular reabsorption of water and solutes.*

Effect of Arterial Pressure on Urine Output— Pressure Natriuresis and Pressure Diuresis

Even small increases in arterial pressure can cause marked increases in urinary excretion of sodium and water, phenomena that are referred to as *pressure natriuresis* and *pressure diuresis.* Because of the autoregulatory mechanisms described in Chapter 26, increasing the arterial pressure between the limits of 75 and 160 mm Hg usually has only a small effect on renal blood flow and GFR. The slight increase in GFR that does occur contributes in part to the effect of increased arterial pressure on urine output. When GFR autoregulation is impaired, as often occurs in

kidney disease, increases in arterial pressure cause much larger increases in GFR.

A second effect of increased renal arterial pressure that raises urine output is that it decreases the percentage of the filtered load of sodium and water that is reabsorbed by the tubules. The mechanisms responsible for this effect include a slight increase in peritubular capillary hydrostatic pressure, especially in the vasa recta of the renal medulla, and a subsequent increase in the renal interstitial fluid hydrostatic pressure. As discussed earlier, an increase in the renal interstitial fluid hydrostatic pressure enhances backleak of sodium into the tubular lumen, thereby reducing the net reabsorption of sodium and water and further increasing the rate of urine output when renal arterial pressure rises.

A third factor that contributes to the pressure natriuresis and pressure diuresis mechanisms is reduced angiotensin II formation. Angiotensin II itself increases sodium reabsorption by the tubules; it also stimulates aldosterone secretion, which further increases sodium reabsorption. Therefore, decreased angiotensin II formation contributes to the decreased tubular sodium reabsorption that occurs when arterial pressure is increased.

Hormonal Control of Tubular Reabsorption

Precise regulation of body fluid volumes and solute concentrations requires the kidneys to excrete different solutes and water at variable rates, sometimes independently of one another. For example, when potassium intake is increased, the kidneys must excrete more potassium while maintaining normal excretion of sodium and other electrolytes. Likewise, when sodium intake is changed, the kidneys must appropriately adjust urinary sodium excretion without major changes in excretion of other electrolytes. Several hormones in the body provide this specificity of tubular reabsorption for different electrolytes and water. Table 27-3 summarizes some of the most important hormones for regulating tubular reabsorption, their principal sites of action on the renal tubule, and their effects on solute and water excretion. Some of these hormones are discussed in more detail in Chapters 28 and 29, but we briefly review their renal tubular actions in the next few paragraphs.

Aldosterone Increases Sodium Reabsorption and Stimulates Potassium Secretion. Aldosterone, secreted by the zona glomerulosa cells of the adrenal cortex, is an important regulator of sodium reabsorption and potassium secretion by the renal tubules. *A major renal tubular site of aldosterone action is on the principal cells of the cortical collecting tubule.* The mechanism by which aldosterone increases sodium reabsorption while at the same time increasing potassium secretion is by stimulating the sodium-potassium ATPase pump on the basolateral side of the cortical collecting tubule membrane. Aldosterone also increases the sodium permeability of the luminal side of the membrane. The cellular mechanisms of aldosterone action are discussed in Chapter 77.

Table 27-3 Hormones That Regulate Tubular Reabsorption

Hormone	Site of Action	Effects
Aldosterone	Collecting tubule and duct	↑ NaCl, H_2O reabsorption, ↑ K^+ secretion
Angiotensin II	Proximal tubule, thick ascending loop of Henle/distal tubule, collecting tubule	↑ NaCl, H_2O reabsorption, ↑ H^+ secretion
Antidiuretic hormone	Distal tubule/collecting tubule and duct	↑ H_2O reabsorption
Atrial natriuretic peptide	Distal tubule/collecting tubule and duct	↓ NaCl reabsorption
Parathyroid hormone	Proximal tubule, thick ascending loop of Henle/distal tubule	↓ $PO_4^{\equiv}$ reabsorption, ↑ Ca^{++} reabsorption

The most important stimuli for aldosterone are (1) increased extracellular potassium concentration and (2) increased angiotensin II levels, which typically occur in conditions associated with sodium and volume depletion or low blood pressure. The increased secretion of aldosterone associated with these conditions causes renal sodium and water retention, helping to increase extracellular fluid volume and restore blood pressure toward normal.

In the absence of aldosterone, as occurs with adrenal destruction or malfunction *(Addison's disease),* there is marked loss of sodium from the body and accumulation of potassium. Conversely, excess aldosterone secretion, as occurs in patients with adrenal tumors *(Conn's syndrome),* is associated with sodium retention and decreased plasma potassium concentration due, in part, to excessive potassium secretion by the kidneys. Although day-to-day regulation of sodium balance can be maintained as long as minimal levels of aldosterone are present, the inability to appropriately adjust aldosterone secretion greatly impairs the regulation of renal potassium excretion and potassium concentration of the body fluids. Thus, aldosterone is even more important as a regulator of potassium concentration than it is for sodium concentration.

Angiotensin II Increases Sodium and Water Reabsorption. Angiotensin II is perhaps the body's most powerful sodium-retaining hormone. As discussed in Chapter 19, angiotensin II formation increases in circumstances associated with low blood pressure and/or low extracellular fluid volume, such as during hemorrhage or loss of salt and water from the body fluids by excessive sweating or severe diarrhea. The increased formation of angiotensin II helps to return blood pressure and extracellular volume toward normal by increasing sodium and water reabsorption from the renal tubules through three main effects:

1. *Angiotensin II stimulates aldosterone secretion,* which in turn increases sodium reabsorption.

2. *Angiotensin II constricts the efferent arterioles,* which has two effects on peritubular capillary dynamics that increase sodium and water reabsorption. First, efferent arteriolar constriction reduces peritubular capillary hydrostatic pressure, which increases net tubular reabsorption, especially from the proximal tubules. Second, efferent arteriolar constriction, by reducing renal blood flow, raises filtration fraction in the glomerulus and increases the concentration of proteins and the colloid osmotic pressure in the peritubular capillaries; this increases the reabsorptive force at the peritubular capillaries and raises tubular reabsorption of sodium and water.

3. *Angiotensin II directly stimulates sodium reabsorption in the proximal tubules, the loops of Henle, the distal tubules, and the collecting tubules.* One of the direct effects of angiotensin II is to stimulate the sodium-potassium ATPase pump on the tubular epithelial cell basolateral membrane. A second effect is to stimulate sodium-hydrogen exchange in the luminal membrane, especially in the proximal tubule. A third effect of angiotensin II is to stimulate sodium-bicarbonate co-transport in the basolateral membrane (Figure 27-17).

Thus, angiotensin II stimulates sodium transport across both the luminal and the basolateral surfaces of the epithelial cell membrane in most renal tubular segments. These multiple actions of angiotensin II cause marked sodium and water retention by the kidneys when angiotensin II levels are increased and play a critical role in

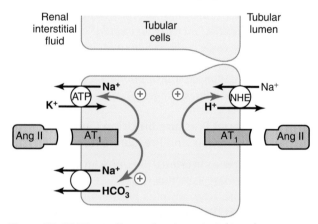

Figure 27-17 Direct effects of angiotensin II (*Ang II*) to increase proximal tubular sodium reabsorption. Ang II stimulates sodium sodium-hydrogen exchange (*NHE*) on the luminal membrane and the sodium-potassium ATPase transporter as well as sodium-bicarbonate co-transport on the basolateral membrane. These same effects of Ang II likely occur in several other parts of the renal tubule, including the loop of Henle, distal tubule, and collecting tubule.

permitting the body to adapt to wide variations in sodium intake without large changes in extracellular fluid volume and blood pressure, as discussed in Chapter 29.

At the same time that angiotensin II increases renal tubular sodium reabsorption, its vasoconstrictor effect on efferent arterioles also aids in the maintenance of normal excretion of metabolic waste products such as urea and creatinine that depend mainly on adequate GFR for their excretion. Thus, increased formation of angiotensin II permits the kidneys to retain sodium and water without causing retention of metabolic waste products.

ADH Increases Water Reabsorption. The most important renal action of ADH is to increase the water permeability of the distal tubule, collecting tubule, and collecting duct epithelia. This effect helps the body to conserve water in circumstances such as dehydration. In the absence of ADH, the permeability of the distal tubules and collecting ducts to water is low, causing the kidneys to excrete large amounts of dilute urine. Thus, the actions of ADH play a key role in controlling the degree of dilution or concentration of the urine, as discussed further in Chapters 28 and 75.

ADH binds to specific V_2 receptors in the late distal tubules, collecting tubules, and collecting ducts, increasing the formation of cyclic AMP and activating protein kinases (Figure 27-18). This, in turn, stimulates the movement of an intracellular protein, called *aquaporin-2 (AQP-2)*, to the luminal side of the cell membranes. The molecules of AQP-2 cluster together and fuse with the cell membrane by exocytosis to form *water channels* that permit rapid diffusion of water through the cells. There are other aquaporins, AQP-3 and AQP-4, in the basolateral side of the cell membrane that provide a path for water to rapidly exit the cells, although these are not believed to be regulated by ADH. Chronic increases in ADH levels also increase the formation of AQP-2 protein in the renal tubular cells by stimulating AQP-2 gene transcription. When the concentration of ADH decreases, the molecules of AQP-2 are shuttled back to the cell cytoplasm, thereby removing the water channels from the luminal membrane and reducing water permeability. These cellular actions of ADH are discussed further in Chapter 75.

Atrial Natriuretic Peptide Decreases Sodium and Water Reabsorption. Specific cells of the cardiac atria, when distended because of plasma volume expansion, secrete a peptide called *atrial natriuretic peptide (ANP)*. Increased levels of this peptide in turn directly inhibit the reabsorption of sodium and water by the renal tubules, especially in the collecting ducts. ANP also inhibits renin secretion and therefore angiotensin II formation, which in turn reduces renal tubular reabsorption. This decreased sodium and water reabsorption increases urinary excretion, which helps to return blood volume back toward normal.

ANP levels are greatly elevated in congestive heart failure when the cardiac atria are stretched because of impaired pumping of the ventricles. The increased ANP helps to attenuate sodium and water retention in heart failure.

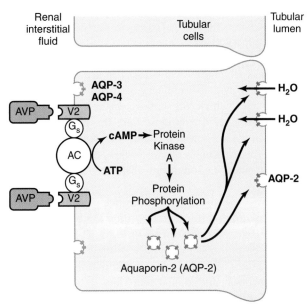

Figure 27-18 Mechanism of action of arginine vasopressin (*AVP*) on the epithelial cells of the late distal tubules, collecting tubules and collecting ducts. AVP binds to its V_2 receptors, which are coupled with stimulatory G proteins (G_s) that activate adenylate cyclase (*AC*) and stimulate formation of cyclic adenosine monophosphate (*cAMP*). This, in turn, activates protein kinase A and phosphorylation of intracellular proteins, causing movement of aquaporin-2 (*AQP-2*) to the luminal side of the cell membrane. The molecules of AQP-2 fuse together to form water channels. On the basolateral side of the cell membrane are other aquaporins, *AQP-3* and *AQP-4*, that permit water to flow out of the cell, although these aquaporins do not appear to be regulated by AVP.

Parathyroid Hormone Increases Calcium Reabsorption. Parathyroid hormone is one of the most important calcium-regulating hormones in the body. Its principal action in the kidneys is to increase tubular reabsorption of calcium, especially in the distal tubules and perhaps also in the loops of Henle. Parathyroid hormone also has other actions, including inhibition of phosphate reabsorption by the proximal tubule and stimulation of magnesium reabsorption by the loop of Henle, as discussed in Chapter 29.

Sympathetic Nervous System Activation Increases Sodium Reabsorption

Activation of the sympathetic nervous system, if severe, can decrease sodium and water excretion by constricting the renal arterioles, thereby reducing GFR. Even low levels of sympathetic activation, however, decrease sodium and water excretion by increasing sodium reabsorption in the proximal tubule, the thick ascending limb of the loop of Henle, and perhaps in more distal parts of the renal tubule. This occurs by activation of α-adrenergic receptors on the renal tubular epithelial cells.

Sympathetic nervous system stimulation also increases renin release and angiotensin II formation, which adds to the overall effect to increase tubular reabsorption and decrease renal excretion of sodium.

Use of Clearance Methods to Quantify Kidney Function

The rates at which different substances are "cleared" from the plasma provide a useful way of quantitating the effectiveness with which the kidneys excrete various substances (Table 27-4). By definition, the *renal clearance of a substance is the volume of plasma that is completely cleared of the substance by the kidneys per unit time.*

This concept is somewhat abstract because there is no single volume of plasma that is *completely* cleared of a substance. However, renal clearance provides a useful way of quantifying the excretory function of the kidneys and, as discussed later, can be used to quantify the rate at which blood flows through the kidneys, as well as the basic functions of the kidneys: glomerular filtration, tubular reabsorption, and tubular secretion.

To illustrate the clearance principle, consider the following example: If the plasma passing through the kidneys contains 1 milligram of a substance in each milliliter and if 1 milligram of this substance is also excreted into the urine each minute, then 1 ml/min of the plasma is "cleared" of the substance. Thus, clearance refers to the volume of plasma that would be necessary to supply the amount of substance excreted in the urine per unit time. Stated mathematically,

$$C_s \times P_s = U_s \times V,$$

where C_s is the clearance rate of a substance s, P_s is the plasma concentration of the substance, U_s is the urine concentration of that substance, and V is the urine flow rate. Rearranging this equation, clearance can be expressed as

$$C_s = \frac{U_s \times V}{P_s}$$

Thus, renal clearance of a substance is calculated from the urinary excretion rate ($U_s \times V$) of that substance divided by its plasma concentration.

Inulin Clearance Can Be Used to Estimate GFR

If a substance is freely filtered (filtered as freely as water) and is not reabsorbed or secreted by the renal tubules, then the rate at which that substance is excreted in the urine ($U_s \times V$) is equal to the filtration rate of the substance by the kidneys (GFR $\times P_s$). Thus,

$$GFR \times P_s = U_s \times V$$

The GFR, therefore, can be calculated as the clearance of the substance as follows:

$$GFR = \frac{U_s \times V}{P_s} = C_s$$

A substance that fits these criteria is *inulin*, a polysaccharide molecule with a molecular weight of about 5200. Inulin, which is not produced in the body, is found in the roots of certain plants and must be administered intravenously to a patient to measure GFR.

Figure 27-19 shows the renal handling of inulin. In this example, the plasma concentration is 1 mg/ml, urine concentration is 125 mg/ml, and urine flow rate is 1 ml/min. Therefore, 125 mg/min of inulin passes into the urine. Then, inulin clearance is calculated as the urine excretion rate of inulin divided by the plasma concentration, which yields a

Table 27-4 Use of Clearance to Quantify Kidney Function

Term	Equation	Units
Clearance rate (C_s)	$C_s = \dfrac{U_s \times \dot{V}}{P_s}$	ml/min
Glomerular filtration rate (GFR)	$GFR = \dfrac{U_{inulin} \times \dot{V}}{P_{inulin}}$	
Clearance ratio	$Clearance\ ratio = \dfrac{C_s}{C_{inulin}}$	None
Effective renal plasma flow (ERPF)	$ERPF = C_{PAH} = \dfrac{U_{PAH} \times \dot{V}}{P_{PAH}}$	ml/min
Renal plasma flow (RPF)	$RPF = \dfrac{C_{PAH}}{E_{PAH}} = \dfrac{(U_{PAH} \times \dot{V}/P_{PAH})}{(P_{PAH} - V_{PAH})/P_{PAH}}$ $= \dfrac{U_{PAH} \times \dot{V}}{P_{PAH} - V_{PAH}}$	ml/min
Renal blood flow (RBF)	$RBF = \dfrac{RPF}{1 - Hematocrit}$	ml/min
Excretion rate	$Excretion\ rate = U_s \times \dot{V}$	mg/min, mmol/min, or mEq/min
Reabsorption rate	$Reabsorption\ rate = Filtered\ load - Excretion\ rate$ $= (GFR \times P_s) - (U_s \times \dot{V})$	mg/min, mmol/min, or mEq/min
Secretion rate	$Secretion\ rate = Excretion\ rate - Filtered\ load$	mg/min, mmol/min, or mEq/min

S, a substance; U, urine concentration; $\dot{V}$, urine flow rate; P, plasma concentration; PAH, para-aminohippuric acid; P_{PAH}, renal arterial PAH concentration; E_{PAH}, PAH extraction ratio; V_{PAH}, renal venous PAH concentration.

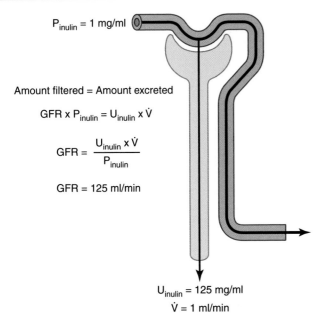

$P_{inulin} = 1 \text{ mg/ml}$

Amount filtered = Amount excreted

$$GFR \times P_{inulin} = U_{inulin} \times \dot{V}$$

$$GFR = \frac{U_{inulin} \times \dot{V}}{P_{inulin}}$$

$$GFR = 125 \text{ ml/min}$$

$$U_{inulin} = 125 \text{ mg/ml}$$
$$\dot{V} = 1 \text{ ml/min}$$

Figure 27-19 Measurement of glomerular filtration rate (*GFR*) from the renal clearance of inulin. Inulin is freely filtered by the glomerular capillaries but is not reabsorbed by the renal tubules. P_{inulin}, plasma inulin concentration; U_{inulin}, urine inulin concentration; $\dot{V}$, urine flow rate.

value of 125 ml/min. Thus, 125 milliliters of plasma flowing through the kidneys must be filtered to deliver the inulin that appears in the urine.

Inulin is not the only substance that can be used for determining GFR. Other substances that have been used clinically to estimate GFR include *radioactive iothalamate* and *creatinine*.

Creatinine Clearance and Plasma Creatinine Concentration Can Be Used to Estimate GFR

Creatinine is a by-product of muscle metabolism and is cleared from the body fluids almost entirely by glomerular filtration. Therefore, the clearance of creatinine can also be used to assess GFR. Because measurement of creatinine clearance does not require intravenous infusion into the patient, this method is much more widely used than inulin clearance for estimating GFR clinically. However, creatinine clearance is not a perfect marker of GFR because a small amount of it is secreted by the tubules, so the amount of creatinine excreted slightly exceeds the amount filtered. There is normally a slight error in measuring plasma creatinine that leads to an overestimate of the plasma creatinine concentration, and fortuitously, these two errors tend to cancel each other. Therefore, creatinine clearance provides a reasonable estimate of GFR.

In some cases, it may not be practical to collect urine in a patient for measuring creatinine clearance (C_{Cr}). An approximation of *changes* in GFR, however, can be obtained by simply measuring plasma creatinine concentration (P_{Cr}), which is inversely proportional to GFR:

$$GFR \approx C_{Cr} = \frac{U_{Cr} \times \dot{V}}{P_{Cr}}$$

If GFR suddenly decreases by 50%, the kidneys will transiently filter and excrete only half as much creatinine, causing

accumulation of creatinine in the body fluids and raising plasma concentration. Plasma concentration of creatinine will continue to rise until the filtered load of creatinine ($P_{Cr} \times GFR$) and creatinine excretion ($U_{Cr} \times \dot{V}$) return to normal and a balance between creatinine production and creatinine excretion is re-established. This will occur when plasma creatinine increases to approximately twice normal, as shown in Figure 27-20.

If GFR falls to one-fourth normal, plasma creatinine would increase to about four times normal and a decrease of GFR to one-eighth normal would raise plasma creatinine to eight times normal. Thus, under steady-state conditions, the creatinine excretion rate equals the rate of creatinine production, despite reductions in GFR. However, this normal rate of creatinine excretion occurs at the expense of elevated plasma creatinine concentration, as shown in Figure 27-21.

PAH Clearance Can Be Used to Estimate Renal Plasma Flow

Theoretically, if a substance is *completely* cleared from the plasma, the clearance rate of that substance is equal to the total renal plasma flow. In other words, the amount of the substance delivered to the kidneys in the blood (renal plasma flow $\times P_s$) would be equal to the amount excreted in the urine ($U_s \times \dot{V}$). Thus, renal plasma flow (RPF) could be calculated as

$$RPF = \frac{U_s \times \dot{V}}{P_s} = C_s$$

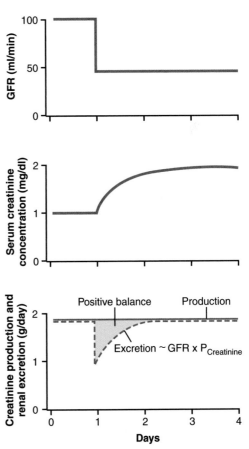

Figure 27-20 Effect of reducing glomerular filtration rate (*GFR*) by 50 percent on serum creatinine concentration and on creatinine excretion rate when the production rate of creatinine remains constant. $P_{Creatinine}$, plasma creatinine concentration.

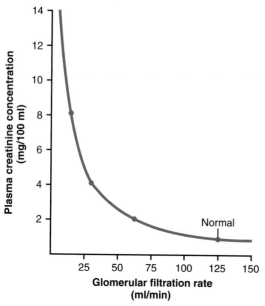

Figure 27-21 Approximate relationship between glomerular filtration rate (GFR) and plasma creatinine concentration under steady-state conditions. Decreasing GFR by 50 percent will increase plasma creatinine to twice normal if creatinine production by the body remains constant.

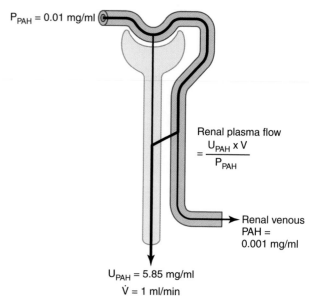

$P_{PAH} = 0.01$ mg/ml

Renal plasma flow
$$= \frac{U_{PAH} \times V}{P_{PAH}}$$

Renal venous
PAH =
0.001 mg/ml

$U_{PAH} = 5.85$ mg/ml
$\dot{V} = 1$ ml/min

Figure 27-22 Measurement of renal plasma flow from the renal clearance of para-aminohippuric acid (*PAH*). PAH is freely filtered by the glomerular capillaries and is also secreted from the peritubular capillary blood into the tubular lumen. The amount of PAH in the plasma of the renal artery is about equal to the amount of PAH excreted in the urine. Therefore, the renal plasma flow can be calculated from the clearance of PAH (C_{PAH}). To be more accurate, one can correct for the percentage of PAH that is still in the blood when it leaves the kidneys. P_{PAH}, arterial plasma PAH concentration; U_{PAH}, urine PAH concentration; $\dot{V}$, urine flow rate.

Because the GFR is only about 20 percent of the total plasma flow, a substance that is completely cleared from the plasma must be excreted by tubular secretion, as well as glomerular filtration (Figure 27-22). There is no known substance that is *completely* cleared by the kidneys. One substance, however, PAH, is about 90 percent cleared from the plasma. Therefore, the clearance of PAH can be used as an approximation of renal plasma flow. To be more accurate, one can correct for the percentage of PAH that is still in the blood when it leaves the kidneys. The percentage of PAH removed from the blood is known as the *extraction ratio of PAH* and averages about 90 percent in normal kidneys. In diseased kidneys, this extraction ratio may be reduced because of inability of damaged tubules to secrete PAH into the tubular fluid.

The calculation of RPF can be demonstrated by the following example: Assume that the plasma concentration of PAH is 0.01 mg/ml, urine concentration is 5.85 mg/ml, and urine flow rate is 1 ml/min. PAH clearance can be calculated from the rate of urinary PAH excretion (5.85 mg/ml × 1 ml/min) divided by the plasma PAH concentration (0.01 mg/ml). Thus, clearance of PAH calculates to be 585 ml/min.

If the extraction ratio for PAH is 90 percent, the actual renal plasma flow can be calculated by dividing 585 ml/min by 0.9, yielding a value of 650 ml/min. Thus, total renal plasma flow can be calculated as

$$\text{Total renal plasma flow} = \frac{\text{PAH clearance}}{\text{PAH extraction ratio}}$$

The extraction ratio (E_{PAH}) is calculated as the difference between the renal arterial PAH (P_{PAH}) and renal venous PAH (V_{PAH}) concentrations, divided by the renal arterial PAH concentration:

$$E_{PAH} = \frac{P_{PAH} - V_{PAH}}{P_{PAH}}$$

One can calculate the total blood flow through the kidneys from the total renal plasma flow and hematocrit (the percentage of red blood cells in the blood). If the hematocrit is 0.45 and the total renal plasma flow is 650 ml/min, the total blood flow through both kidneys is 650/(1 to 0.45), or 1182 ml/min.

Filtration Fraction Is Calculated from GFR Divided by Renal Plasma Flow

To calculate the filtration fraction, which is the fraction of plasma that filters through the glomerular membrane, one must first know the renal plasma flow (PAH clearance) and the GFR (inulin clearance). If renal plasma flow is 650 ml/min and GFR is 125 ml/min, the filtration fraction (FF) is calculated as

$$\text{FF} = \text{GFR/RPF} = 125/650 = 0.19$$

Calculation of Tubular Reabsorption or Secretion from Renal Clearances

If the rates of glomerular filtration and renal excretion of a substance are known, one can calculate whether there is a net reabsorption or a net secretion of that substance by the renal tubules. For example, if the rate of excretion of the substance ($U_s \times \dot{V}$) is less than the filtered load of the substance ($\text{GFR} \times P_s$), then some of the substance must have been reabsorbed from the renal tubules.

Conversely, if the excretion rate of the substance is greater than its filtered load, then the rate at which it appears in the urine represents the sum of the rate of glomerular filtration plus tubular secretion.

The following example demonstrates the calculation of tubular reabsorption. Assume the following laboratory values for a patient were obtained:

Urine flow rate = 1 ml/min

Urine concentration of sodium (U_{Na}) = 70 mEq/L = 70 µEq/ml

Plasma sodium concentration = 140 mEq/L = 140 µEq/ml

GFR (inulin clearance) = 100 ml/min

In this example, the filtered sodium load is GFR × P_{Na}, or 100 ml/min × 140 µEq/ml = 14,000 µEq/min. Urinary sodium excretion (U_{Na} × urine flow rate) is 70 µEq/min. Therefore, tubular reabsorption of sodium is the difference between the filtered load and urinary excretion, or 14,000 µEq/min − 70 µEq/min = 13,930 µEq/min.

Comparisons of Inulin Clearance with Clearances of Different Solutes. The following generalizations can be made by comparing the clearance of a substance with the clearance of inulin, a measure of GFR: (1) If the clearance rate of the substance equals that of inulin, the substance is only filtered and not reabsorbed or secreted; (2) if the clearance rate of a substance is less than inulin clearance, the substance must have been reabsorbed by the nephron tubules; and (3) if the clearance rate of a substance is greater than that of inulin, the substance must be secreted by the nephron tubules. Listed below are the approximate clearance rates for some of the substances normally handled by the kidneys:

Substance	Clearance Rate (ml/min)
Glucose	0
Sodium	0.9
Chloride	1.3
Potassium	12.0
Phosphate	25.0
Inulin	125.0
Creatinine	140.0

Bibliography

Aronson PS: Ion exchangers mediating NaCl transport in the renal proximal tubule, *Cell Biochem Biophys* 36:147, 2002.

Benos DJ, Fuller CM, Shlyonsky VG, et al: Amiloride-sensitive Na⁺ channels: insights and outlooks, *News Physiol Sci* 12:55, 1997.

Bröer S: Amino acid transport across mammalian intestinal and renal epithelia, *Physiol Rev* 88:249, 2008.

Féraille E, Doucet A: Sodium-potassium-adenosine-triphosphatase–dependent sodium transport in the kidney: hormonal control, *Physiol Rev* 81:345, 2001.

Granger JP, Alexander BT, Llinas M: Mechanisms of pressure natriuresis, *Curr Hypertens Rep* 4:152, 2002.

Hall JE, Brands MW: The renin-angiotensin-aldosterone system: renal mechanisms and circulatory homeostasis. In Seldin DW, Giebisch G, eds: *The Kidney—Physiology and Pathophysiology*, ed 3, New York, 2000, Raven Press.

Hall JE, Granger JP: Regulation of fluid and electrolyte balance in hypertension- role of hormones and peptides. In Battegay EJ, Lip GYH, Bakris GL, eds: *Hypertension-Principles and Practice*, Boca Raton, 2005, Taylor and Francis Group, LLC, pp 121–142.

Humphreys MH, Valentin J-P: Natriuretic hormonal agents. In Seldin DW, Giebisch G, eds: *The Kidney—Physiology and Pathophysiology*, ed 3, New York, 2000, Raven Press.

Kellenberger S, Schild L: Epithelial sodium channel/degenerin family of ion channels: A variety of functions for a shared structure, *Physiol Rev* 82:735, 2002.

Nielsen S, Frøkiær J, Marples D, et al: Aquaporins in the kidney: from molecules to medicine, *Physiol Rev* 82:205, 2002.

Palmer LG, Frindt G: Aldosterone and potassium secretion by the cortical collecting duct, *Kidney Int* 57:1324, 2000.

Rahn KH, Heidenreich S, Bruckner D: How to assess glomerular function and damage in humans, *J Hypertens* 17:309, 1999.

Reeves WB, Andreoli TE: Sodium chloride transport in the loop of Henle, distal convoluted tubule and collecting duct. In Seldin DW, Giebisch G, eds: *The Kidney—Physiology and Pathophysiology*, ed 3, New York, 2000, Raven Press.

Reilly RF, Ellison DH: Mammalian distal tubule: physiology, pathophysiology, and molecular anatomy, *Physiol Rev* 80:277, 2000.

Rossier BC, Praderv S, Schild L, et al: Epithelial sodium channel and the control of sodium balance: interaction between genetic and environmental factors, *Annu Rev Physiol* 64:877, 2002.

Russell JM: Sodium-potassium-chloride cotransport, *Physiol Rev* 80:211, 2000.

Schafer JA: Abnormal regulation of ENaC: syndromes of salt retention and salt wasting by the collecting duct, *Am J Physiol Renal Physiol* 283:F221, 2002.

Thomson SC, Blantz RC: Glomerulotubular Balance, Tubuloglomerular Feedback, and Salt Homeostasis, *J Am Soc Nephrol* 19:2272, 2008.

Verrey F, Ristic Z, Romeo E, et al: Novel renal amino acid transporters, *Annu Rev Physiol* 67:557, 2005.

Weinstein AM: Mathematical models of renal fluid and electrolyte transport: acknowledging our uncertainty, *Am J Physiol Renal Physiol* 284:F871, 2003.

Wright EM: Renal Na(+)-glucose cotransporters, *Am J Physiol Renal Physiol* 280:F10, 2001.

UNIT V

Urine Concentration and Dilution; Regulation of Extracellular Fluid Osmolarity and Sodium Concentration

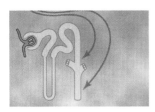

For the cells of the body to function properly, they must be bathed in extracellular fluid with a relatively constant concentration of electrolytes and other solutes. The total concentration of solutes in the extracellular fluid—and therefore the osmolarity—is determined by the amount of solute divided by the volume of the extracellular fluid. Thus, to a large extent, extracellular fluid sodium concentration and osmolarity are regulated by the amount of extracellular water. The total body water is controlled by (1) fluid intake, which is regulated by factors that determine thirst, and (2) renal excretion of water, which is controlled by multiple factors that influence glomerular filtration and tubular reabsorption.

In this chapter, we discuss (1) the mechanisms that cause the kidneys to eliminate excess water by excreting a dilute urine; (2) the mechanisms that cause the kidneys to conserve water by excreting a concentrated urine; (3) the renal feedback mechanisms that control the extracellular fluid sodium concentration and osmolarity; and (4) the thirst and salt appetite mechanisms that determine the intakes of water and salt, which also help to control extracellular fluid volume, osmolarity, and sodium concentration.

Kidneys Excrete Excess Water by Forming Dilute Urine

Normal kidneys have tremendous capability to vary the relative proportions of solutes and water in the urine in response to various challenges. When there is excess water in the body and body fluid osmolarity is reduced, the kidney can excrete urine with an osmolarity as low as 50 mOsm/L, a concentration that is only about one-sixth the osmolarity of normal extracellular fluid. Conversely, when there is a deficit of water and extracellular fluid osmolarity is high, the kidney can excrete urine with a concentration of 1200 to 1400 mOsm/L. Equally important, the kidney can excrete a large volume of dilute urine or a small volume of concentrated urine without major changes in rates of excretion of solutes such as sodium

and potassium. This ability to regulate water excretion independently of solute excretion is necessary for survival, especially when fluid intake is limited.

Antidiuretic Hormone Controls Urine Concentration

There is a powerful feedback system for regulating plasma osmolarity and sodium concentration that operates by altering renal excretion of water independently of the rate of solute excretion. A primary effector of this feedback is *antidiuretic hormone (ADH)*, also called *vasopressin*.

When osmolarity of the body fluids increases above normal (i.e., the solutes in the body fluids become too concentrated), the posterior pituitary gland secretes more ADH, which increases the permeability of the distal tubules and collecting ducts to water, as discussed in Chapter 27. This permits large amounts of water to be reabsorbed and decreases urine volume but does not markedly alter the rate of renal excretion of the solutes.

When there is excess water in the body and extracellular fluid osmolarity is reduced, the secretion of ADH by the posterior pituitary decreases, thereby reducing the permeability of the distal tubule and collecting ducts to water, which causes large amounts of dilute urine to be excreted. Thus, the rate of ADH secretion determines, to a large extent, whether the kidney excretes dilute or concentrated urine.

Renal Mechanisms for Excreting Dilute Urine

When there is a large excess of water in the body, the kidney can excrete as much as 20 L/day of dilute urine, with a concentration as low as 50 mOsm/L. The kidney performs this impressive feat by continuing to reabsorb solutes while failing to reabsorb large amounts of water in the distal parts of the nephron, including the late distal tubule and the collecting ducts.

Figure 28-1 shows the approximate renal responses in a human after ingestion of 1 liter of water. Note that urine volume increases to about six times normal within 45 minutes after the water has been drunk. However, the total amount of solute excreted remains relatively constant because the urine formed becomes very dilute and urine osmolarity decreases from 600 to about 100 mOsm/L.

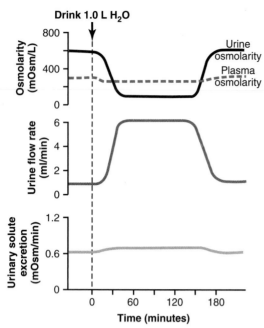

Figure 28-1 Water diuresis in a human after ingestion of 1 liter of water. Note that after water ingestion, urine volume increases and urine osmolarity decreases, causing the excretion of a large volume of dilute urine; however, the total amount of solute excreted by the kidneys remains relatively constant. These responses of the kidneys prevent plasma osmolarity from decreasing markedly during excess water ingestion.

Thus, after ingestion of excess water, the kidney rids the body of the excess water but does not excrete excess amounts of solutes.

When the glomerular filtrate is initially formed, its osmolarity is about the same as that of plasma (300 mOsm/L). To excrete excess water, it is necessary to dilute the filtrate as it passes along the tubule. This is achieved by reabsorbing solutes to a greater extent than water, as shown in Figure 28-2, but this occurs only in certain segments of the tubular system as follows.

Tubular Fluid Remains Isosmotic in the Proximal Tubule. As fluid flows through the proximal tubule, solutes and water are reabsorbed in equal proportions, so little change in osmolarity occurs; thus, the proximal tubule fluid remains isosmotic to the plasma, with an osmolarity of about 300 mOsm/L. As fluid passes down the descending loop of Henle, water is reabsorbed by osmosis and the tubular fluid reaches equilibrium with the surrounding interstitial fluid of the renal medulla, which is very hypertonic—about two to four times the osmolarity of the original glomerular filtrate. Therefore, the tubular fluid becomes more concentrated as it flows into the inner medulla.

Tubular Fluid Is Diluted in the Ascending Loop of Henle. In the ascending limb of the loop of Henle, especially in the thick segment, sodium, potassium, and chloride are avidly reabsorbed. However, this portion of the tubular segment is impermeable to water, even in the presence of large amounts of ADH. Therefore, the tubular fluid becomes more dilute as it flows up the ascending loop of Henle into

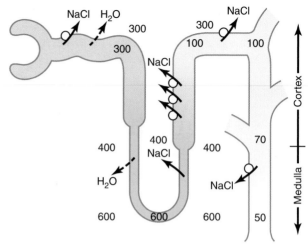

Figure 28-2 Formation of dilute urine when antidiuretic hormone (ADH) levels are very low. Note that in the ascending loop of Henle, the tubular fluid becomes very dilute. In the distal tubules and collecting tubules, the tubular fluid is further diluted by the reabsorption of sodium chloride and the failure to reabsorb water when ADH levels are very low. The failure to reabsorb water and continued reabsorption of solutes lead to a large volume of dilute urine. (Numerical values are in milliosmoles per liter.)

the early distal tubule, with the osmolarity decreasing progressively to about 100 mOsm/L by the time the fluid enters the early distal tubular segment. *Thus, regardless of whether ADH is present or absent, fluid leaving the early distal tubular segment is hypo-osmotic, with an osmolarity of only about one-third the osmolarity of plasma.*

Tubular Fluid in Distal and Collecting Tubules Is Further Diluted in the Absence of ADH. As the dilute fluid in the early distal tubule passes into the late distal convoluted tubule, cortical collecting duct, and collecting duct, there is additional reabsorption of sodium chloride. In the absence of ADH, this portion of the tubule is also impermeable to water and the additional reabsorption of solutes causes the tubular fluid to become even more dilute, decreasing its osmolarity to as low as 50 mOsm/L. The failure to reabsorb water and the continued reabsorption of solutes lead to a large volume of dilute urine.

To summarize, the mechanism for forming dilute urine is to continue reabsorbing solutes from the distal segments of the tubular system while failing to reabsorb water. In healthy kidneys, fluid leaving the ascending loop of Henle and early distal tubule is always dilute, regardless of the level of ADH. In the absence of ADH, the urine is further diluted in the late distal tubule and collecting ducts and a large volume of dilute urine is excreted.

Kidneys Conserve Water by Excreting Concentrated Urine

The ability of the kidney to form urine that is more concentrated than plasma is essential for survival of mammals that live on land, including humans. Water is continuously lost from the body through various routes, including the lungs by evaporation into the expired air, the gastrointestinal tract by way of the feces, the skin through evaporation and perspiration, and the kidneys through the excretion of urine. Fluid intake is required to match this loss, but the ability of the kidney to form a small volume of concentrated urine minimizes the intake of fluid required to maintain homeostasis, a function that is especially important when water is in short supply.

When there is a water deficit in the body, the kidney forms concentrated urine by continuing to excrete solutes while increasing water reabsorption and decreasing the volume of urine formed. The human kidney can produce a maximal urine concentration of 1200 to 1400 mOsm/L, four to five times the osmolarity of plasma.

Some desert animals, such as the Australian hopping mouse, can concentrate urine to as high as 10,000 mOsm/L. This allows the mouse to survive in the desert without drinking water; sufficient water can be obtained through the food ingested and water produced in the body by metabolism of the food. Animals adapted to fresh water environments usually have minimal urine concentrating ability. Beavers, for example, can concentrate the urine only to about 500 mOsm/L.

Obligatory Urine Volume

The maximal concentrating ability of the kidney dictates how much urine volume must be excreted each day to rid the body of waste products of metabolism and ions that are ingested. A normal 70-kilogram human must excrete about 600 milliosmoles of solute each day. If maximal urine concentrating ability is 1200 mOsm/L, the *minimal* volume of urine that must be excreted, called the *obligatory urine volume*, can be calculated as

$$\frac{600 \text{ mOsm/day}}{1200 \text{ mOsm/L}} = 0.5 \text{L/day}$$

This minimal loss of volume in the urine contributes to dehydration, along with water loss from the skin, respiratory tract, and gastrointestinal tract, when water is not available to drink.

The limited ability of the human kidney to concentrate the urine to a maximal concentration of 1200 mOsm/L explains why severe dehydration occurs if one attempts to drink seawater. Sodium chloride concentration in the oceans averages about 3.0 to 3.5 percent, with an osmolarity between about 1000 and 1200 mOsm/L. Drinking 1 liter of seawater with a concentration of 1200 mOsm/L would provide a total sodium chloride intake of 1200 milliosmoles. If maximal urine concentrating ability is 1200 mOsm/L, the amount of urine volume needed to excrete 1200 milliosmoles would be 1200 milliosmoles divided by 1200 mOsm/L, or 1.0 liter. Why then does drinking seawater cause dehydration? The answer is that the kidney must also excrete other solutes, especially urea, which contribute about 600 mOsm/L when the urine is maximally concentrated. Therefore, the maximum concentration of sodium chloride that can be excreted by the kidneys is about 600 mOsm/L. Thus, for every liter of seawater drunk, 1.5 liters of urine volume would be required to rid the body of 1200 milliosmoles of sodium chloride ingested in addition to 600 milliosmoles of other solutes such as urea.

This would result in a net fluid loss of 0.5 liter for every liter of seawater drunk, explaining the rapid dehydration that occurs in shipwreck victims who drink seawater. However, a shipwreck victim's pet Australian hopping mouse could drink with impunity all the seawater it wanted.

Urine Specific Gravity

Urine *specific gravity* is often used in clinical settings to provide a rapid estimate of urine solute concentration. The more concentrated the urine, the higher the urine specific gravity. In most cases, urine specific gravity increases linearly with increasing urine osmolarity (Figure 28-3). Urine specific gravity, however, is a measure of the weight of solutes in a given volume of urine and is therefore determined by the number and size of the solute molecules. This contrasts with osmolarity, which is determined only by the number of solute molecules in a given volume.

Urine specific gravity is generally expressed in grams/ml and, in humans, normally ranges from 1.002 to 1.028 g/ml, rising by .001 for every 35 to 40 mOsmol/L increase in urine osmolarity. This relationship between specific gravity and osmolarity is altered when there are significant amounts of large molecules in the urine, such as glucose, radiocontrast media used for diagnostic purposes, or some antibiotics. In these cases, urine specific gravity measurements may falsely suggest a very concentrated urine, despite a normal urine osmolality.

Dipsticks are available that measure approximate urine specific gravity, but most laboratories measure specific gravity with a refractometer.

Requirements for Excreting a Concentrated Urine—High ADH Levels and Hyperosmotic Renal Medulla

The basic requirements for forming a concentrated urine are (1) a *high level of ADH,* which increases the permeability of the distal tubules and collecting ducts to water,

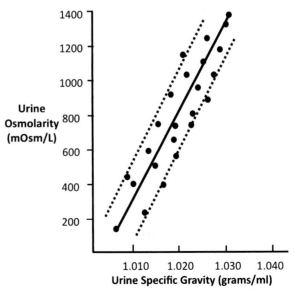

Figure 28-3 Relationship between specific gravity (grams/ml) and osmolarity of the urine.

thereby allowing these tubular segments to avidly reabsorb water, and (2) *a high osmolarity of the renal medullary interstitial fluid*, which provides the osmotic gradient necessary for water reabsorption to occur in the presence of high levels of ADH.

The renal medullary interstitium surrounding the collecting ducts is normally hyperosmotic, so when ADH levels are high, water moves through the tubular membrane by osmosis into the renal interstitium; from there it is carried away by the vasa recta back into the blood. Thus, the urine concentrating ability is limited by the level of ADH and by the degree of hyperosmolarity of the renal medulla. We discuss the factors that control ADH secretion later, but for now, what is the process by which renal medullary interstitial fluid becomes hyperosmotic? This process involves the operation of the *countercurrent mechanism.*

The countercurrent mechanism depends on the special anatomical arrangement of the loops of Henle and the vasa recta, the specialized peritubular capillaries of the renal medulla. In the human, about 25 percent of the nephrons are *juxtamedullary nephrons*, with loops of Henle and vasa recta that go deeply into the medulla before returning to the cortex. Some of the loops of Henle dip all the way to the tips of the renal papillae that project from the medulla into the renal pelvis. Paralleling the long loops of Henle are the vasa recta, which also loop down into the medulla before returning to the renal cortex. And finally, the collecting ducts, which carry urine through the hyperosmotic renal medulla before it is excreted, also play a critical role in the countercurrent mechanism.

Countercurrent Mechanism Produces a Hyperosmotic Renal Medullary Interstitium

The osmolarity of interstitial fluid in almost all parts of the body is about 300 mOsm/L, which is similar to the plasma osmolarity. (As discussed in Chapter 25, the *corrected osmolar activity*, which accounts for intermolecular attraction, is about 282 mOsm/L.) The osmolarity of the interstitial fluid in the medulla of the kidney is much higher and may increase progressively to about 1200 to 1400 mOsm/L in the pelvic tip of the medulla. This means that the renal medullary interstitium has accumulated solutes in great excess of water. Once the high solute concentration in the medulla is achieved, it is maintained by a balanced inflow and outflow of solutes and water in the medulla.

The major factors that contribute to the buildup of solute concentration into the renal medulla are as follows:

1. Active transport of sodium ions and co-transport of potassium, chloride, and other ions out of the thick portion of the ascending limb of the loop of Henle into the medullary interstitium

2. Active transport of ions from the collecting ducts into the medullary interstitium

3. Facilitated diffusion of urea from the inner medullary collecting ducts into the medullary interstitium

4. Diffusion of only small amounts of water from the medullary tubules into the medullary interstitium, far less than the reabsorption of solutes into the medullary interstitium

Special Characteristics of Loop of Henle That Cause Solutes to Be Trapped in the Renal Medulla. The transport characteristics of the loops of Henle are summarized in Table 28-1, along with the properties of the proximal tubules, distal tubules, cortical collecting tubules, and inner medullary collecting ducts.

The most important cause of the high medullary osmolarity is active transport of sodium and co-transport of potassium, chloride, and other ions from the thick ascending loop of Henle into the interstitium. This pump is capable of establishing about a 200-milliosmole concentration gradient between the tubular lumen and the interstitial fluid. Because the thick ascending limb is virtually impermeable to water, the solutes pumped out are

Table 28-1 Summary of Tubule Characteristics—Urine Concentration

		Permeability		
	Active NaCl Transport	**H₂O**	**NaCl**	**Urea**
Proximal tubule	++	++	+	+
Thin descending limb	0	++	+	+
Thin ascending limb	0	0	+	+
Thick ascending limb	++	0	0	0
Distal tubule	+	+ADH	0	0
Cortical collecting tubule	+	+ADH	0	0
Inner medullary collecting duct	+	+ADH	0	++ADH

0, minimal level of active transport or permeability; +, moderate level of active transport or permeability; ++, high level of active transport or permeability; +ADH, permeability to water or urea is increased by ADH.

not followed by osmotic flow of water into the interstitium. Thus, the active transport of sodium and other ions out of the thick ascending loop adds solutes in excess of water to the renal medullary interstitium. There is some passive reabsorption of sodium chloride from the thin ascending limb of Henle's loop, which is also impermeable to water, adding further to the high solute concentration of the renal medullary interstitium.

The descending limb of Henle's loop, in contrast to the ascending limb, is very permeable to water, and the tubular fluid osmolarity quickly becomes equal to the renal medullary osmolarity. Therefore, water diffuses out of the descending limb of Henle's loop into the interstitium and the tubular fluid osmolarity gradually rises as it flows toward the tip of the loop of Henle.

Steps Involved in Causing Hyperosmotic Renal Medullary Interstitium.
Keeping in mind these characteristics of the loop of Henle, let us now discuss how the renal medulla becomes hyperosmotic. First, assume that the loop of Henle is filled with fluid with a concentration of 300 mOsm/L, the same as that leaving the proximal tubule (Figure 28-4, step 1). Next, the active ion pump of the *thick ascending limb* on the loop of Henle reduces the concentration inside the tubule and raises the interstitial concentration; this pump establishes a 200-mOsm/L concentration gradient between the tubular fluid and the interstitial fluid (step 2). The limit to the gradient is about 200 mOsm/L because paracellular diffusion of ions back into the tubule eventually counterbalances transport of ions out of the lumen when the 200-mOsm/L concentration gradient is achieved.

Step 3 is that the tubular fluid in the *descending limb of the loop of Henle* and the interstitial fluid quickly reach osmotic equilibrium because of osmosis of water out of the descending limb. The interstitial osmolarity is maintained at 400 mOsm/L because of continued transport of ions out of the thick ascending loop of Henle. Thus, by itself, the active transport of sodium chloride out of the thick ascending limb is capable of establishing only a 200-mOsm/L concentration gradient, much less than that achieved by the countercurrent system.

Step 4 is additional flow of fluid into the loop of Henle from the proximal tubule, which causes the hyperosmotic fluid previously formed in the descending limb to flow into the ascending limb. Once this fluid is in the ascending limb, additional ions are pumped into the interstitium, with water remaining in the tubular fluid, until a 200-mOsm/L osmotic gradient is established, with the interstitial fluid osmolarity rising to 500 mOsm/L (step 5). Then, once again, the fluid in the descending limb reaches equilibrium with the hyperosmotic medullary interstitial fluid (step 6), and as the hyperosmotic tubular fluid from the descending limb of the loop of Henle flows into the ascending limb, still more solute is continuously pumped out of the tubules and deposited into the medullary interstitium.

These steps are repeated over and over, with the net effect of adding more and more solute to the medulla in excess of water; with sufficient time, *this process gradually traps solutes in the medulla and multiplies the concentration gradient established by the active pumping of ions out of the thick ascending loop of Henle, eventually raising the interstitial fluid osmolarity to 1200 to 1400 mOsm/L as shown in step 7.*

Thus, the repetitive reabsorption of sodium chloride by the thick ascending loop of Henle and continued inflow of new sodium chloride from the proximal tubule into the loop of Henle is called the *countercurrent multiplier*. The sodium chloride reabsorbed from the ascending loop of Henle keeps adding to the newly arrived sodium chloride, thus "multiplying" its concentration in the medullary interstitium.

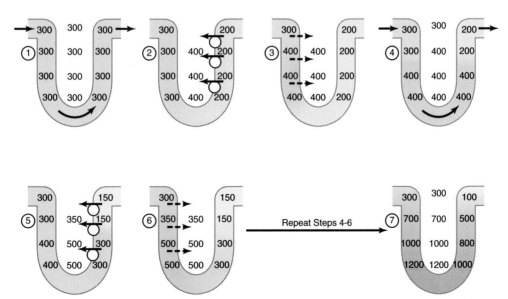

Figure 28-4 Countercurrent multiplier system in the loop of Henle for producing a hyperosmotic renal medulla. (Numerical values are in milliosmoles per liter.)

Role of Distal Tubule and Collecting Ducts in Excreting Concentrated Urine

When the tubular fluid leaves the loop of Henle and flows into the distal convoluted tubule in the renal cortex, the fluid is dilute, with an osmolarity of only about 100 mOsm/L (Figure 28-5). The early distal tubule further dilutes the tubular fluid because this segment, like the ascending loop of Henle, actively transports sodium chloride out of the tubule but is relatively impermeable to water.

As fluid flows into the cortical collecting tubule, the amount of water reabsorbed is critically dependent on the plasma concentration of ADH. In the absence of ADH, this segment is almost impermeable to water and fails to reabsorb water but continues to reabsorb solutes and further dilutes the urine. When there is a high concentration of ADH, the cortical collecting tubule becomes highly permeable to water, so large amounts of water are now reabsorbed from the tubule into the cortex interstitium, where it is swept away by the rapidly flowing peritubular capillaries. *The fact that these large amounts of water are reabsorbed into the cortex, rather than into the renal medulla, helps to preserve the high medullary interstitial fluid osmolarity.*

As the tubular fluid flows along the medullary collecting ducts, there is further water reabsorption from the tubular fluid into the interstitium, but the total amount of water is relatively small compared with that added to the cortex interstitium. The reabsorbed water is quickly carried away by the vasa recta into the venous blood. When high levels of ADH are present, the collecting ducts become permeable to water, so the fluid at the end of the collecting ducts has essentially the same osmolarity as the interstitial fluid of the renal medulla—about

1200 mOsm/L (see Figure 28-4). Thus, by reabsorbing as much water as possible, the kidneys form highly concentrated urine, excreting normal amounts of solutes in the urine while adding water back to the extracellular fluid and compensating for deficits of body water.

Urea Contributes to Hyperosmotic Renal Medullary Interstitium and Formation of Concentrated Urine

Thus far, we have considered only the contribution of sodium chloride to the hyperosmotic renal medullary interstitium. However, urea contributes about 40 to 50 percent of the osmolarity (500 to 600 mOsm/L) of the renal medullary interstitium when the kidney is forming a maximally concentrated urine. Unlike sodium chloride, urea is passively reabsorbed from the tubule. When there is water deficit and blood concentration of ADH is high, large amounts of urea are passively reabsorbed from the inner medullary collecting ducts into the interstitium.

The mechanism for reabsorption of urea into the renal medulla is as follows: As water flows up the ascending loop of Henle and into the distal and cortical collecting tubules, little urea is reabsorbed because these segments are impermeable to urea (see Table 28-1). In the presence of high concentrations of ADH, water is reabsorbed rapidly from the cortical collecting tubule and the urea concentration increases rapidly because urea is not very permeant in this part of the tubule.

As the tubular fluid flows into the inner medullary collecting ducts, still more water reabsorption takes place, causing an even higher concentration of urea in the fluid. This high concentration of urea in the tubular fluid of the inner medullary collecting duct causes urea to diffuse out of the tubule into the renal interstitial fluid. This diffusion is greatly facilitated by specific *urea transporters, UT-A1 and UT-A3*. One of these urea transporters, UT-A3, is activated by ADH, increasing transport of urea out of the inner medullary collecting duct even more when ADH levels are elevated. The simultaneous movement of water and urea out of the inner medullary collecting ducts maintains a high concentration of urea in the tubular fluid and, eventually, in the urine, even though urea is being reabsorbed.

The fundamental role of urea in contributing to urine concentrating ability is evidenced by the fact that people who ingest a high-protein diet, yielding large amounts of urea as a nitrogenous "waste" product, can concentrate their urine much better than people whose protein intake and urea production are low. Malnutrition is associated with a low urea concentration in the medullary interstitium and considerable impairment of urine concentrating ability.

Recirculation of Urea from Collecting Duct to Loop of Henle Contributes to Hyperosmotic Renal Medulla. A healthy person usually excretes about 20 to 50 percent of the filtered load of urea. In general, the rate of urea excretion is determined mainly by two factors: (1) the concentration of urea in the plasma and

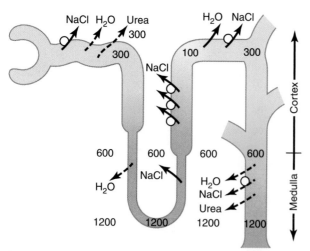

Figure 28-5 Formation of a concentrated urine when antidiuretic hormone (ADH) levels are high. Note that the fluid leaving the loop of Henle is dilute but becomes concentrated as water is absorbed from the distal tubules and collecting tubules. With high ADH levels, the osmolarity of the urine is about the same as the osmolarity of the renal medullary interstitial fluid in the papilla, which is about 1200 mOsm/L. (Numerical values are in milliosmoles per liter.)

(2) the glomerular filtration rate (GFR). In patients with renal disease who have large reductions of GFR, the plasma urea concentration increases markedly, returning the filtered urea load and urea excretion rate to the normal level (equal to the rate of urea production), despite the reduced GFR.

In the proximal tubule, 40 to 50 percent of the filtered urea is reabsorbed, but even so, the tubular fluid urea concentration increases because urea is not nearly as permeant as water. The concentration of urea continues to rise as the tubular fluid flows into the thin segments of the loop of Henle, partly because of water reabsorption out of the descending loop of Henle but also because of some *secretion* of urea into the thin loop of Henle from the medullary interstitium (Figure 28-6). The passive secretion of urea into the thin loops of Henle is facilitated by the urea transporter *UT-A2*.

The thick limb of the loop of Henle, the distal tubule, and the cortical collecting tubule are all relatively impermeable to urea, and very little urea reabsorption occurs in these tubular segments. When the kidney is forming concentrated urine and high levels of ADH are present, reabsorption of water from the distal tubule and cortical collecting tubule further raises the tubular fluid concentration of urea. As this urea flows into the inner medullary collecting duct, the high tubular fluid concentration of urea and specific urea transporters cause urea to diffuse into the medullary interstitium. A moderate share of the urea that moves into the medullary interstitium

eventually diffuses into the thin loop of Henle and then passes upward through the ascending loop of Henle, the distal tubule, the cortical collecting tubule, and back down into the medullary collecting duct again. In this way, urea can recirculate through these terminal parts of the tubular system several times before it is excreted. Each time around the circuit contributes to a higher concentration of urea.

This urea recirculation provides an additional mechanism for forming a hyperosmotic renal medulla. Because urea is one of the most abundant waste products that must be excreted by the kidneys, this mechanism for concentrating urea before it is excreted is essential to the economy of the body fluid when water is in short supply.

When there is excess water in the body, urine flow rate is usually increased and therefore the concentration of urea in the inner medullary collecting ducts is reduced, causing less diffusion of urea into the renal medullary interstitium. ADH levels are also reduced when there is excess body water and this, in turn, decreases the permeability of the inner medullary collecting ducts to both water and urea, and more urea is excreted in the urine.

Countercurrent Exchange in the Vasa Recta Preserves Hyperosmolarity of the Renal Medulla

Blood flow must be provided to the renal medulla to supply the metabolic needs of the cells in this part of the kidney. Without a special medullary blood flow system, the solutes pumped into the renal medulla by the countercurrent multiplier system would be rapidly dissipated.

There are two special features of the renal medullary blood flow that contribute to the preservation of the high solute concentrations:

1. *The medullary blood flow is low,* accounting for less than 5 percent of the total renal blood flow. This sluggish blood flow is sufficient to supply the metabolic needs of the tissues but helps to minimize solute loss from the medullary interstitium.

2. *The vasa recta serve as countercurrent exchangers,* minimizing washout of solutes from the medullary interstitium.

The countercurrent exchange mechanism operates as follows (Figure 28-7): Blood enters and leaves the medulla by way of the vasa recta at the boundary of the cortex and renal medulla. The vasa recta, like other capillaries, are highly permeable to solutes in the blood, except for the plasma proteins. As blood descends into the medulla toward the papillae, it becomes progressively more concentrated, partly by solute entry from the interstitium and partly by loss of water into the interstitium. By the time the blood reaches the tips of the vasa recta, it has a concentration of about 1200 mOsm/L, the same as that of the medullary interstitium. As blood ascends back toward the cortex, it becomes progressively less concentrated as solutes diffuse back out into the medullary interstitium and as water moves into the vasa recta.

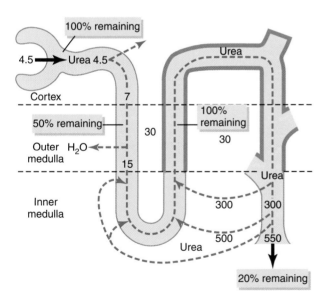

Figure 28-6 Recirculation of urea absorbed from the medullary collecting duct into the interstitial fluid. This urea diffuses into the thin loop of Henle and then passes through the distal tubules, and it finally passes back into the collecting duct. The recirculation of urea helps to trap urea in the renal medulla and contributes to the hyperosmolarity of the renal medulla. The *heavy tan lines,* from the thick ascending loop of Henle to the medullary collecting ducts, indicate that these segments are not very permeable to urea. (Numerical values are in milliosmoles per liter of urea during antidiuresis, when large amounts of antidiuretic hormone are present. Percentages of the filtered load of urea that remain in the tubules are indicated in the blue boxes.)

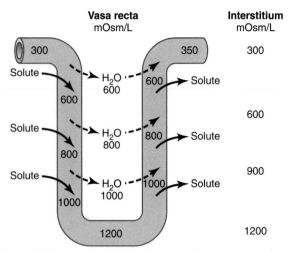

Vasa recta
mOsm/L

Interstitium
mOsm/L

Figure 28-7 Countercurrent exchange in the vasa recta. Plasma flowing down the descending limb of the vasa recta becomes more hyperosmotic because of diffusion of water out of the blood and diffusion of solutes from the renal interstitial fluid into the blood. In the ascending limb of the vasa recta, solutes diffuse back into the interstitial fluid and water diffuses back into the vasa recta. Large amounts of solutes would be lost from the renal medulla without the U shape of the vasa recta capillaries. (Numerical values are in milliosmoles per liter.)

Although there are large amounts of fluid and solute exchange across the vasa recta, there is little net dilution of the concentration of the interstitial fluid at each level of the renal medulla because of the U shape of the vasa recta capillaries, which act as countercurrent exchangers. *Thus, the vasa recta do not create the medullary hyperosmolarity, but they do prevent it from being dissipated.*

The U-shaped structure of the vessels minimizes loss of solute from the interstitium but does not prevent the bulk flow of fluid and solutes into the blood through the usual colloid osmotic and hydrostatic pressures that favor reabsorption in these capillaries. Under steady-state conditions, the vasa recta carry away only as much solute and

water as is absorbed from the medullary tubules and the high concentration of solutes established by the countercurrent mechanism is preserved.

Increased Medullary Blood Flow Reduces Urine Concentrating Ability. Certain vasodilators can markedly increase renal medullary blood flow, thereby "washing out" some of the solutes from the renal medulla and reducing maximum urine concentrating ability. Large increases in arterial pressure can also increase the blood flow of the renal medulla to a greater extent than in other regions of the kidney and tend to wash out the hyperosmotic interstitium, thereby reducing urine concentrating ability. As discussed earlier, maximum concentrating ability of the kidney is determined not only by the level of ADH but also by the osmolarity of the renal medulla interstitial fluid. Even with maximal levels of ADH, urine concentrating ability will be reduced if medullary blood flow increases enough to reduce the hyperosmolarity in the renal medulla.

Summary of Urine Concentrating Mechanism and Changes in Osmolarity in Different Segments of the Tubules

The changes in osmolarity and volume of the tubular fluid as it passes through the different parts of the nephron are shown in Figure 28-8.

Proximal Tubule. About 65 percent of the filtered electrolytes is reabsorbed in the proximal tubule. However, the proximal tubular membranes are highly permeable to water, so that whenever solutes are reabsorbed, water also diffuses through the tubular membrane by osmosis. Therefore, the osmolarity of the fluid remains about the same as the glomerular filtrate, 300 mOsm/L.

Descending Loop of Henle. As fluid flows down the descending loop of Henle, water is absorbed into

Figure 28-8 Changes in osmolarity of the tubular fluid as it passes through the different tubular segments in the presence of high levels of antidiuretic hormone (ADH) and in the absence of ADH. (Numerical values indicate the approximate volumes in milliliters per minute or in osmolarities in milliosmoles per liter of fluid flowing along the different tubular segments.)

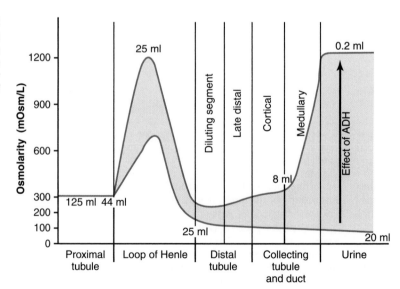

the medulla. The descending limb is highly permeable to water but much less permeable to sodium chloride and urea. Therefore, the osmolarity of the fluid flowing through the descending loop gradually increases until it is nearly equal to that of the surrounding interstitial fluid, which is about 1200 mOsm/L when the blood concentration of ADH is high.

When dilute urine is being formed, owing to low ADH concentrations, the medullary interstitial osmolarity is less than 1200 mOsm/L; consequently, the descending loop tubular fluid osmolarity also becomes less concentrated. This is due partly to the fact that less urea is absorbed into the medullary interstitium from the collecting ducts when ADH levels are low and the kidney is forming a large volume of dilute urine.

Thin Ascending Loop of Henle. The thin ascending limb is essentially impermeable to water but reabsorbs some sodium chloride. Because of the high concentration of sodium chloride in the tubular fluid, owing to water removal from the descending loop of Henle, there is some passive diffusion of sodium chloride from the thin ascending limb into the medullary interstitium. Thus, the tubular fluid becomes more dilute as the sodium chloride diffuses out of the tubule and water remains in the tubule.

Some of the urea absorbed into the medullary interstitium from the collecting ducts also diffuses into the ascending limb, thereby returning the urea to the tubular system and helping to prevent its washout from the renal medulla. This *urea recycling* is an additional mechanism that contributes to the hyperosmotic renal medulla.

Thick Ascending Loop of Henle. The thick part of the ascending loop of Henle is also virtually impermeable to water, but large amounts of sodium, chloride, potassium, and other ions are actively transported from the tubule into the medullary interstitium. Therefore, fluid in the thick ascending limb of the loop of Henle becomes very dilute, falling to a concentration of about 100 mOsm/L.

Early Distal Tubule. The early distal tubule has properties similar to those of the thick ascending loop of Henle, so further dilution of the tubular fluid to about 50 mOsm/L occurs as solutes are reabsorbed while water remains in the tubule.

Late Distal Tubule and Cortical Collecting Tubules. In the late distal tubule and cortical collecting tubules, the osmolarity of the fluid depends on the level of ADH. With high levels of ADH, these tubules are highly permeable to water and significant amounts of water are reabsorbed. Urea, however, is not very permeant in this part of the nephron, resulting in increased urea concentration as water is reabsorbed. This allows most of the urea delivered to the distal tubule and collecting tubule to pass into the inner medullary collecting ducts, from which it is eventually reabsorbed or excreted in the urine. In the absence of ADH, little water is reabsorbed in the late distal tubule and cortical collecting tubule; therefore, osmolarity decreases even further because of continued active reabsorption of ions from these segments.

Inner Medullary Collecting Ducts. The concentration of fluid in the inner medullary collecting ducts also depends on (1) ADH and (2) the surrounding medullary interstitium osmolarity established by the countercurrent mechanism. In the presence of large amounts of ADH, these ducts are highly permeable to water, and water diffuses from the tubule into the interstitial fluid until osmotic equilibrium is reached, with the tubular fluid having about the same concentration as the renal medullary interstitium (1200 to 1400 mOsm/L). Thus, a small volume of concentrated urine is produced when ADH levels are high. Because water reabsorption increases urea concentration in the tubular fluid and because the inner medullary collecting ducts have specific urea transporters that greatly facilitate diffusion, much of the highly concentrated urea in the ducts diffuses out of the tubular lumen into the medullary interstitium. This absorption of the urea into the renal medulla contributes to the high osmolarity of the medullary interstitium and the high concentrating ability of the kidney.

Several important points to consider may not be obvious from this discussion. First, although sodium chloride is one of the principal solutes that contribute to the hyperosmolarity of the medullary interstitium, *the kidney can, when needed, excrete a highly concentrated urine that contains little sodium chloride.* The hyperosmolarity of the urine in these circumstances is due to high concentrations of other solutes, especially of waste products such as urea. One condition in which this occurs is dehydration accompanied by low sodium intake. As discussed in Chapter 29, low sodium intake stimulates formation of the hormones angiotensin II and aldosterone, which together cause avid sodium reabsorption from the tubules while leaving the urea and other solutes to maintain the highly concentrated urine.

Second, *large quantities of dilute urine can be excreted without increasing the excretion of sodium.* This is accomplished by decreasing ADH secretion, which reduces water reabsorption in the more distal tubular segments without significantly altering sodium reabsorption.

And finally, there is an *obligatory urine volume* that is dictated by the maximum concentrating ability of the kidney and the amount of solute that must be excreted. Therefore, if large amounts of solute must be excreted, they must be accompanied by the minimal amount of water necessary to excrete them. For example, if 600 milliosmoles of solute must be excreted each day, this requires *at least* 0.5 liter of urine if maximal urine concentrating ability is 1200 mOsm/L.

Quantifying Renal Urine Concentration and Dilution: "Free Water" and Osmolar Clearances

The process of concentrating or diluting the urine requires the kidneys to excrete water and solutes somewhat independently. When the urine is dilute, water is excreted in excess of solutes. Conversely, when the urine is concentrated, solutes are excreted in excess of water.

The total clearance of solutes from the blood can be expressed as the *osmolar clearance* (C_{osm}); this is the volume of plasma cleared of solutes each minute, in the same way that clearance of a single substance is calculated:

$$C_{osm} = \frac{U_{osm} \times \dot{V}}{P_{osm}}$$

where U_{osm} is the urine osmolarity, $\dot{V}$ is the urine flow rate, and P_{osm} is the plasma osmolarity. For example, if plasma osmolarity is 300 mOsm/L, urine osmolarity is 600 mOsm/L, and urine flow rate is 1 ml/min (0.001 L/min), the rate of osmolar excretion is 0.6 mOsm/min (600 mOsm/L × 0.001 L/min) and osmolar clearance is 0.6 mOsm/min divided by 300 mOsm/L, or 0.002 L/min (2.0 ml/min). This means that 2 milliliters of plasma are being cleared of solute each minute.

Relative Rates at Which Solutes and Water Are Excreted Can Be Assessed Using the Concept of "Free-Water Clearance."

Free-water clearance (C_{H2O}) is calculated as the difference between water excretion (urine flow rate) and osmolar clearance:

$$C_{H_2O} = \dot{V} - C_{osm} = \dot{V} - \frac{(U_{osm} \times \dot{V})}{(P_{osm})}$$

Thus, the rate of free-water clearance represents the rate at which solute-free water is excreted by the kidneys. When free-water clearance is positive, excess water is being excreted by the kidneys; when free-water clearance is negative, excess solutes are being removed from the blood by the kidneys and water is being conserved.

Using the example discussed earlier, if urine flow rate is 1 ml/min and osmolar clearance is 2 ml/min, free-water clearance would be –1 ml/min. This means that instead of water being cleared from the kidneys in excess of solutes, the kidneys are actually returning water back to the systemic circulation, as occurs during water deficits. *Thus, whenever urine osmolarity is greater than plasma osmolarity, free-water clearance is negative, indicating water conservation.*

When the kidneys are forming a dilute urine (i.e., urine osmolarity is less than plasma osmolarity), free-water clearance will be a positive value, denoting that water is being removed from the plasma by the kidneys in excess of solutes. Thus, water free of solutes, called "free water," is being lost from the body and the plasma is being concentrated when free-water clearance is positive.

Disorders of Urinary Concentrating Ability

Impairment in the ability of the kidneys to concentrate or dilute the urine appropriately can occur with one or more of the following abnormalities:

1. *Inappropriate secretion of ADH.* Either too much or too little ADH secretion results in abnormal fluid handling by the kidneys.

2. *Impairment of the countercurrent mechanism.* A hyperosmotic medullary interstitium is required for maximal urine concentrating ability. No matter how much ADH is present, maximal urine concentration is limited by the degree of hyperosmolarity of the medullary interstitium.

3. *Inability of the distal tubule, collecting tubule, and collecting ducts to respond to ADH.*

Failure to Produce ADH: "Central" Diabetes Insipidus. An inability to produce or release ADH from the posterior pituitary can be caused by head injuries or infections, or it can be congenital. Because the distal tubular segments cannot reabsorb water in the absence of ADH, this condition, called *"central" diabetes insipidus,* results in the formation of a large volume of dilute urine with urine volumes that can exceed 15 L/day. The thirst mechanisms, discussed later in this chapter, are activated when excessive water is lost from the body; therefore, as long as the person drinks enough water, large decreases in body fluid water do not occur. The primary abnormality observed clinically in people with this condition is the large volume of dilute urine. However, if water intake is restricted, as can occur in a hospital setting when fluid intake is restricted or the patient is unconscious (e.g., because of a head injury), severe dehydration can rapidly occur.

The treatment for central diabetes insipidus is administration of a synthetic analog of ADH, *desmopressin,* which acts selectively on V_2 receptors to increase water permeability in the late distal and collecting tubules. Desmopressin can be given by injection, as a nasal spray, or orally, and it rapidly restores urine output toward normal.

Inability of the Kidneys to Respond to ADH: "Nephrogenic" Diabetes Insipidus. In some circumstances normal or elevated levels of ADH are present but the renal tubular segments cannot respond appropriately. This condition is referred to as *"nephrogenic" diabetes insipidus* because the abnormality resides in the kidneys. This abnormality can be due to either failure of the countercurrent mechanism to form a hyperosmotic renal medullary interstitium or failure of the distal and collecting tubules and collecting ducts to respond to ADH. In either case, large volumes of dilute urine are formed, which tends to cause dehydration unless fluid intake is increased by the same amount as urine volume is increased.

Many types of renal diseases can impair the concentrating mechanism, especially those that damage the renal medulla (see Chapter 31 for further discussion). Also, impairment of the function of the loop of Henle, as occurs with diuretics that inhibit electrolyte reabsorption by this segment, such as furosemide, can compromise urine concentrating ability. And certain drugs, such as lithium (used to treat manic-depressive disorders) and tetracyclines (used as antibiotics), can impair the ability of the distal nephron segments to respond to ADH.

Nephrogenic diabetes insipidus can be distinguished from central diabetes insipidus by administration of desmopressin, the synthetic analog of ADH. Lack of a prompt decrease in urine volume and an increase in urine osmolarity within

2 hours after injection of desmopressin is strongly suggestive of nephrogenic diabetes insipidus. The treatment for nephrogenic diabetes insipidus is to correct, if possible, the underlying renal disorder. The hypernatremia can also be attenuated by a low-sodium diet and administration of a diuretic that enhances renal sodium excretion, such as a thiazide diuretic.

Control of Extracellular Fluid Osmolarity and Sodium Concentration

Regulation of extracellular fluid osmolarity and sodium concentration are closely linked because sodium is the most abundant ion in the extracellular compartment. Plasma sodium concentration is normally regulated within close limits of 140 to 145 mEq/L, with an average concentration of about 142 mEq/L. Osmolarity averages about 300 mOsm/L (about 282 mOsm/L when corrected for interionic attraction) and seldom changes more than ±2 to 3 percent. As discussed in Chapter 25, these variables must be precisely controlled because they determine the distribution of fluid between the intracellular and extracellular compartments.

Estimating Plasma Osmolarity from Plasma Sodium Concentration

In most clinical laboratories, plasma osmolarity is not routinely measured. However, because sodium and its associated anions account for about 94 percent of the solute in the extracellular compartment, plasma osmolarity (P_{osm}) can be roughly approximated as

$$P_{osm} = 2.1 \times \text{Plasma sodium concentration}$$

For instance, with a plasma sodium concentration of 142 mEq/L, the plasma osmolarity would be estimated from this formula to be about 298 mOsm/L. To be more exact, especially in conditions associated with renal disease, the contribution of two other solutes, glucose and urea, should be included. Such estimates of plasma osmolarity are usually accurate within a few percentage points of those measured directly.

Normally, sodium ions and associated anions (primarily bicarbonate and chloride) represent about 94 percent of the extracellular osmoles, with glucose and urea contributing about 3 to 5 percent of the total osmoles. However, because urea easily permeates most cell membranes, it exerts little *effective* osmotic pressure under steady-state conditions. Therefore, the sodium ions in the extracellular fluid and associated anions are the principal determinants of fluid movement across the cell membrane. Consequently, we can discuss the control of osmolarity and control of sodium ion concentration at the same time.

Although multiple mechanisms control the amount of sodium and water excretion by the kidneys, two primary systems are especially involved in regulating the concentration of sodium and osmolarity of extracellular

fluid: (1) the osmoreceptor-ADH system and (2) the thirst mechanism.

Osmoreceptor-ADH Feedback System

Figure 28-9 shows the basic components of the osmoreceptor-ADH feedback system for control of extracellular fluid sodium concentration and osmolarity. When osmolarity (plasma sodium concentration) increases above normal because of water deficit, for example, this feedback system operates as follows:

1. An increase in extracellular fluid osmolarity (which in practical terms means an increase in plasma sodium concentration) causes the special nerve cells called *osmoreceptor cells*, located in the *anterior hypothalamus* near the supraoptic nuclei, to shrink.

2. Shrinkage of the osmoreceptor cells causes them to fire, sending nerve signals to additional nerve cells in the supraoptic nuclei, which then relay these signals down the stalk of the pituitary gland to the posterior pituitary.

3. These action potentials conducted to the posterior pituitary stimulate the release of ADH, which is stored in secretory granules (or vesicles) in the nerve endings.

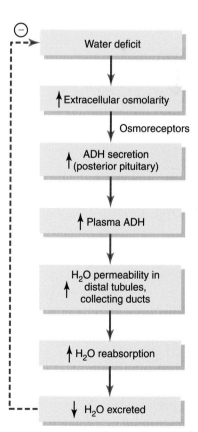

Figure 28-9 Osmoreceptor-antidiuretic hormone (ADH) feedback mechanism for regulating extracellular fluid osmolarity in response to a water deficit.

4. ADH enters the blood stream and is transported to the kidneys, where it increases the water permeability of the late distal tubules, cortical collecting tubules, and medullary collecting ducts.

5. The increased water permeability in the distal nephron segments causes increased water reabsorption and excretion of a small volume of concentrated urine.

Thus, water is conserved in the body while sodium and other solutes continue to be excreted in the urine. This causes dilution of the solutes in the extracellular fluid, thereby correcting the initial excessively concentrated extracellular fluid.

The opposite sequence of events occurs when the extracellular fluid becomes too dilute (hypo-osmotic). For example, with excess water ingestion and a decrease in extracellular fluid osmolarity, less ADH is formed, the renal tubules decrease their permeability for water, less water is reabsorbed, and a large volume of dilute urine is formed. This in turn concentrates the body fluids and returns plasma osmolarity toward normal.

ADH Synthesis in Supraoptic and Paraventricular Nuclei of the Hypothalamus and ADH Release from the Posterior Pituitary

Figure 28-10 shows the neuroanatomy of the hypothalamus and the pituitary gland, where ADH is synthesized and released. The hypothalamus contains two types of *magnocellular (large) neurons that synthesize ADH in the supraoptic and paraventricular nuclei of the hypothalamus,* about five sixths in the supraoptic nuclei and about one sixth in the paraventricular nuclei. Both of these nuclei have axonal extensions to the posterior pituitary. Once ADH is synthesized, it is transported down the axons of the neurons to their tips, terminating in the posterior pituitary gland. When the supraoptic and paraventricular nuclei are stimulated by increased osmolarity or other factors, nerve impulses pass down these nerve endings, changing their membrane permeability and increasing calcium entry. ADH stored in the secretory granules (also called vesicles) of the nerve endings is released in response to increased calcium entry. The released ADH is then carried away in the capillary blood of the posterior pituitary into the systemic circulation.

Secretion of ADH in response to an osmotic stimulus is rapid, so plasma ADH levels can increase severalfold within minutes, thereby providing a rapid means for altering renal excretion of water.

A second neuronal area important in controlling osmolarity and ADH secretion is located along the *anteroventral region of the third ventricle,* called the *AV3V region.* At the upper part of this region is a structure called the *subfornical organ,* and at the inferior part is another structure called the *organum vasculosum* of the *lamina terminalis.* Between these two organs is the *median preoptic nucleus,* which has multiple nerve connections with the two organs, as well as with the supraoptic nuclei and

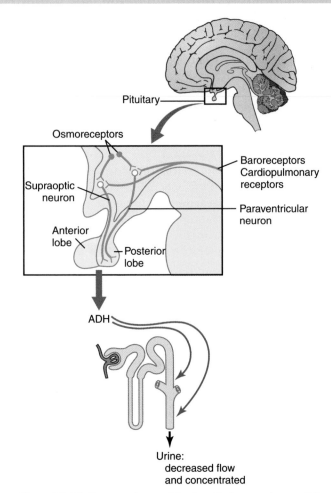

Figure 28-10 Neuroanatomy of the hypothalamus, where antidiuretic hormone (ADH) is synthesized, and the posterior pituitary gland, where ADH is released.

the blood pressure control centers in the medulla of the brain. Lesions of the AV3V region cause multiple deficits in the control of ADH secretion, thirst, sodium appetite, and blood pressure. Electrical stimulation of this region or stimulation by angiotensin II can increase ADH secretion, thirst, and sodium appetite.

In the vicinity of the AV3V region and the supraoptic nuclei are neuronal cells that are excited by small increases in extracellular fluid osmolarity; hence, the term *osmoreceptors* has been used to describe these neurons. These cells send nerve signals to the supraoptic nuclei to control their firing and secretion of ADH. It is also likely that they induce thirst in response to increased extracellular fluid osmolarity.

Both the subfornical organ and the organum vasculosum of the lamina terminalis have vascular supplies that lack the typical blood-brain barrier that impedes the diffusion of most ions from the blood into the brain tissue. This makes it possible for ions and other solutes to cross between the blood and the local interstitial fluid in this region. As a result, the osmoreceptors rapidly respond to changes in osmolarity of the extracellular fluid, exerting powerful control over the secretion of ADH and over thirst, as discussed later.

Stimulation of ADH Release by Decreased Arterial Pressure and/or Decreased Blood Volume

ADH release is also controlled by cardiovascular reflexes that respond to decreases in blood pressure and/or blood volume, including (1) the *arterial baroreceptor reflexes* and (2) *the cardiopulmonary reflexes,* both of which are discussed in Chapter 18. These reflex pathways originate in high-pressure regions of the circulation, such as the aortic arch and carotid sinus, and in the low-pressure regions, especially in the cardiac atria. Afferent stimuli are carried by the vagus and glossopharyngeal nerves with synapses in the nuclei of the tractus solitarius. Projections from these nuclei relay signals to the hypothalamic nuclei that control ADH synthesis and secretion.

Thus, in addition to increased osmolarity, two other stimuli increase ADH secretion: (1) decreased arterial pressure and (2) decreased blood volume. Whenever blood pressure and blood volume are reduced, such as occurs during hemorrhage, increased ADH secretion causes increased fluid reabsorption by the kidneys, helping to restore blood pressure and blood volume toward normal.

Quantitative Importance of Osmolarity and Cardiovascular Reflexes in Stimulating ADH Secretion

As shown in Figure 28-11, either a decrease in effective blood volume or an increase in extracellular fluid osmolarity stimulates ADH secretion. However, ADH is considerably more sensitive to small changes in osmolarity than to similar percentage changes in blood volume. For example, a change in plasma osmolarity of only 1 percent is sufficient to increase ADH levels. By contrast, after blood loss, plasma ADH levels do not change appreciably until blood volume is reduced by about 10 percent. With further decreases in blood volume, ADH levels rapidly increase. Thus, with severe decreases in blood volume, the cardiovascular reflexes play a major role in stimulating ADH secretion. The usual day-to-day regulation of ADH secretion during simple dehydration is effected mainly by changes in plasma osmolarity. Decreased blood volume, however, greatly enhances the ADH response to increased osmolarity.

Other Stimuli for ADH Secretion

ADH secretion can also be increased or decreased by other stimuli to the central nervous system, as well as by various drugs and hormones, as shown in Table 28-2. For example, *nausea* is a potent stimulus for ADH release, which may increase to as much as 100 times normal after vomiting. Also, drugs such as *nicotine* and *morphine* stimulate ADH release, whereas some drugs, such as *alcohol,* inhibit ADH release. The marked diuresis that occurs after ingestion of alcohol is due in part to inhibition of ADH release.

Importance of Thirst in Controlling Extracellular Fluid Osmolarity and Sodium Concentration

The kidneys minimize fluid loss during water deficits through the osmoreceptor-ADH feedback system. Adequate fluid intake, however, is necessary to counterbalance whatever fluid loss does occur through sweating and breathing and through the gastrointestinal tract. Fluid intake is regulated by the thirst mechanism, which, together with the osmoreceptor-ADH mechanism, maintains precise control of extracellular fluid osmolarity and sodium concentration.

Many of the same factors that stimulate ADH secretion also increase thirst, which is defined as the conscious desire for water.

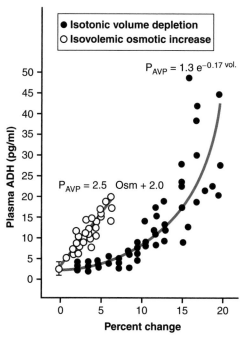

Figure 28-11 The effect of increased plasma osmolarity or decreased blood volume on the level of plasma (P) antidiuretic hormone (ADH), also called *arginine vasopressin* (AVP). (Redrawn from Dunn FL, Brennan TJ, Nelson AE, et al: The role of blood osmolality and volume in regulating vasopressin secretion in the rat. J Clin Invest 52(12):3212, 1973. By copyright permission of the American Society of Clinical Investigation.)

In the figure:
- ● Isotonic volume depletion
- ○ Isovolemic osmotic increase

$$P_{AVP} = 1.3\, e^{-0.17\, vol.}$$

$$P_{AVP} = 2.5\ Osm + 2.0$$

Y-axis: Plasma ADH (pg/ml), values 0, 5, 10, 15, 20, 25, 30, 35, 40, 45, 50
X-axis: Percent change, values 0, 5, 10, 15, 20

Table 28-2 Regulation of ADH Secretion

Increase ADH	Decrease ADH
↑ Plasma osmolarity	↓ Plasma osmolarity
↓ Blood volume	↑ Blood volume
↓ Blood pressure	↑ Blood pressure
Nausea	
Hypoxia	
Drugs:	Drugs:
Morphine	Alcohol
Nicotine	Clonidine (antihypertensive drug)
Cyclophosphamide	Haloperidol (dopamine blocker)

UNIT V

Central Nervous System Centers for Thirst

Referring again to Figure 28-10, the same area along the anteroventral wall of the third ventricle that promotes ADH release also stimulates thirst. Located anterolaterally in the preoptic nucleus is another small area that, when stimulated electrically, causes immediate drinking that continues as long as the stimulation lasts. All these areas together are called the *thirst center.*

The neurons of the thirst center respond to injections of hypertonic salt solutions by stimulating drinking behavior. These cells almost certainly function as osmoreceptors to activate the thirst mechanism, in the same way that the osmoreceptors stimulate ADH release.

Increased osmolarity of the cerebrospinal fluid in the third ventricle has essentially the same effect to promote drinking. It is likely that the *organum vasculosum of the lamina terminalis,* which lies immediately beneath the ventricular surface at the inferior end of the AV3V region, is intimately involved in mediating this response.

Stimuli for Thirst

Table 28-3 summarizes some of the known stimuli for thirst. One of the most important is *increased extracellular fluid osmolarity, which causes intracellular dehydration in the thirst centers,* thereby stimulating the sensation of thirst. The value of this response is obvious: it helps to dilute extracellular fluids and returns osmolarity toward normal.

Decreases in extracellular fluid volume and arterial pressure also stimulate thirst by a pathway that is independent of the one stimulated by increased plasma osmolarity. Thus, blood volume loss by hemorrhage stimulates thirst even though there might be no change in plasma osmolarity. This probably occurs because of neural input from cardiopulmonary and systemic arterial baroreceptors in the circulation.

A third important stimulus for thirst is angiotensin II. Studies in animals have shown that angiotensin II acts on the subfornical organ and on the organum vasculosum of the lamina terminalis. These regions are outside the blood-brain barrier, and peptides such as angiotensin II diffuse into the tissues. Because angiotensin II is also stimulated by factors associated with hypovolemia and low blood pressure, its effect on thirst helps to restore blood volume and blood pressure toward normal, along

with the other actions of angiotensin II on the kidneys to decrease fluid excretion.

Dryness of the mouth and mucous membranes of the esophagus can elicit the sensation of thirst. As a result, a thirsty person may receive relief from thirst almost immediately after drinking water, even though the water has not been absorbed from the gastrointestinal tract and has not yet had an effect on extracellular fluid osmolarity.

Gastrointestinal and pharyngeal stimuli influence thirst. In animals that have an esophageal opening to the exterior so that water is never absorbed into the blood, partial relief of thirst occurs after drinking, although the relief is only temporary. Also, gastrointestinal distention may partially alleviate thirst; for instance, simple inflation of a balloon in the stomach can relieve thirst. However, relief of thirst sensations through gastrointestinal or pharyngeal mechanisms is short-lived; the desire to drink is completely satisfied only when plasma osmolarity and/or blood volume returns to normal.

The ability of animals and humans to "meter" fluid intake is important because it prevents overhydration. After a person drinks water, 30 to 60 minutes may be required for the water to be reabsorbed and distributed throughout the body. If the thirst sensation were not temporarily relieved after drinking water, the person would continue to drink more and more, eventually leading to overhydration and excess dilution of the body fluids. Experimental studies have repeatedly shown that animals drink almost exactly the amount necessary to return plasma osmolarity and volume to normal.

Threshold for Osmolar Stimulus of Drinking

The kidneys must continually excrete an obligatory amount of water even in a dehydrated person, to rid the body of excess solutes that are ingested or produced by metabolism. Water is also lost by evaporation from the lungs and the gastrointestinal tract and by evaporation and sweating from the skin. Therefore, there is always a tendency for dehydration, with resultant increased extracellular fluid sodium concentration and osmolarity.

When the sodium concentration increases only about 2 mEq/L above normal, the thirst mechanism is activated, causing a desire to drink water. This is called the *threshold for drinking.* Thus, even small increases in plasma osmolarity are normally followed by water intake, which restores extracellular fluid osmolarity and volume toward normal. In this way, the extracellular fluid osmolarity and sodium concentration are precisely controlled.

Integrated Responses of Osmoreceptor-ADH and Thirst Mechanisms in Controlling Extracellular Fluid Osmolarity and Sodium Concentration

In a healthy person, the osmoreceptor-ADH and thirst mechanisms work in parallel to precisely regulate extracellular fluid osmolarity and sodium concentration, despite the constant challenges of dehydration. Even with additional challenges, such as high salt intake, these feedback

Table 28-3 Control of Thirst

Increase Thirst	Decrease Thirst
↑ Plasma osmolarity	↓ Plasma osmolarity
↓ Blood volume	↑ Blood volume
↓ Blood pressure	↑ Blood pressure
↑ Angiotensin II	↓ Angiotensin II
Dryness of mouth	Gastric distention

systems are able to keep plasma osmolarity reasonably constant. Figure 28-12 shows that an increase in sodium intake to as high as six times normal has only a small effect on plasma sodium concentration as long as the ADH and thirst mechanisms are both functioning normally.

When either the ADH or the thirst mechanism fails, the other ordinarily can still control extracellular osmolarity and sodium concentration with reasonable effectiveness, as long as there is enough fluid intake to balance the daily obligatory urine volume and water losses caused by respiration, sweating, or gastrointestinal losses. However, if both the ADH and thirst mechanisms fail simultaneously, plasma sodium concentration and osmolarity are poorly controlled; thus, when sodium intake is increased after blocking the total ADH-thirst system, relatively large changes in plasma sodium concentration occur. In the absence of the ADH-thirst mechanisms, no other feedback mechanism is capable of adequately regulating plasma sodium concentration and osmolarity.

Role of Angiotensin II and Aldosterone in Controlling Extracellular Fluid Osmolarity and Sodium Concentration

As discussed in Chapter 27, both angiotensin II and aldosterone play an important role in regulating sodium reabsorption by the renal tubules. When sodium intake is low, increased levels of these hormones stimulate sodium reabsorption by the kidneys and, therefore, prevent large sodium losses, even though sodium intake may be reduced to as low as 10 percent of normal. Conversely, with high sodium intake, decreased formation of these hormones permits the kidneys to excrete large amounts of sodium.

Because of the importance of angiotensin II and aldosterone in regulating sodium excretion by the kidneys, one might mistakenly infer that they also play an important role in regulating extracellular fluid sodium concentration. Although these hormones increase the *amount* of sodium in the extracellular fluid, they also increase the extracellular fluid volume by increasing reabsorption of water along with the sodium. Therefore, *angiotensin II and aldosterone have little effect on sodium **concentration**, except under extreme conditions.*

This relative unimportance of aldosterone in regulating extracellular fluid sodium concentration is shown by the experiment of Figure 28-13. This figure shows the effect on plasma sodium concentration of changing sodium intake more than sixfold under two conditions: (1) under normal conditions and (2) after the aldosterone feedback system was blocked by removing the adrenal glands and infusing the animals with aldosterone at a constant rate so that plasma levels could not change upward or downward. Note that when sodium intake was increased sixfold, plasma concentration changed only about 1 to 2 percent in either case. This indicates that even without a functional aldosterone feedback system, plasma sodium concentration can be well regulated. The same type of experiment has been conducted after blocking angiotensin II formation, with the same result.

There are two primary reasons why changes in angiotensin II and aldosterone do not have a major effect on plasma sodium concentration. First, as discussed earlier, angiotensin II and aldosterone increase both sodium and water reabsorption by the renal tubules, leading to increases in extracellular fluid volume and sodium *quantity* but little change in sodium *concentration*. Second, as long as the ADH-thirst mechanism is functional, any tendency toward increased plasma sodium concentration is compensated for by increased water intake or increased plasma ADH secretion, which tends to dilute the extracellular fluid back toward normal. The ADH-thirst system far overshadows the angiotensin II and aldosterone systems for regulating sodium concentration under normal conditions. Even in patients with *primary aldosteronism*, who have extremely high levels of aldosterone, the plasma sodium concentration usually increases only about 3 to 5 mEq/L above normal.

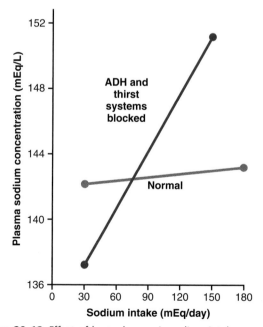

Figure 28-12 Effect of large changes in sodium intake on extracellular fluid sodium concentration in dogs under normal conditions (*red line*) and after the antidiuretic hormone (ADH) and thirst feedback systems had been blocked (*blue line*). Note that control of extracellular fluid sodium concentration is poor in the absence of these feedback systems. (Courtesy Dr. David B. Young.)

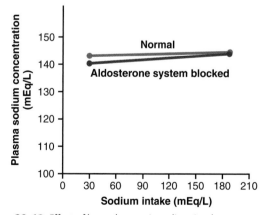

Figure 28-13 Effect of large changes in sodium intake on extracellular fluid sodium concentration in dogs under normal conditions (*red line*) and after the aldosterone feedback system had been blocked (*blue line*). Note that sodium concentration is maintained relatively constant over this wide range of sodium intakes, with or without aldosterone feedback control. (Courtesy Dr. David B. Young.)

Under extreme conditions, caused by complete loss of aldosterone secretion because of adrenalectomy or in patients with Addison's disease (severely impaired secretion or total lack of aldosterone), there is tremendous loss of sodium by the kidneys, which can lead to reductions in plasma sodium concentration. One of the reasons for this is that large losses of sodium eventually cause severe volume depletion and decreased blood pressure, which can activate the thirst mechanism through the cardiovascular reflexes. This leads to a further dilution of the plasma sodium concentration, even though the increased water intake helps to minimize the decrease in body fluid volumes under these conditions.

Thus, there are extreme situations in which plasma sodium concentration may change significantly, even with a functional ADH-thirst mechanism. Even so, the ADH-thirst mechanism is by far the most powerful feedback system in the body for controlling extracellular fluid osmolarity and sodium concentration.

Salt-Appetite Mechanism for Controlling Extracellular Fluid Sodium Concentration and Volume

Maintenance of normal extracellular fluid volume and sodium concentration requires a balance between sodium excretion and sodium intake. In modern civilizations, sodium intake is almost always greater than necessary for homeostasis. In fact, the average sodium intake for individuals in industrialized cultures eating processed foods usually ranges between 100 and 200 mEq/day, even though humans can survive and function normally on 10 to 20 mEq/day. Thus, most people eat far more sodium than is necessary for homeostasis, and there is evidence that our usual high sodium intake may contribute to cardiovascular disorders such as hypertension.

Salt appetite is due in part to the fact that animals and humans like salt and eat it regardless of whether they are salt deficient. There is also a regulatory component to salt appetite in which there is a behavioral drive to obtain salt when there is sodium deficiency in the body. This is particularly important in herbivores, which naturally eat a low-sodium diet, but salt craving may also be important in humans who have extreme deficiency of sodium, such as occurs in Addison's disease. In this instance, there is deficiency of aldosterone secretion, which causes excessive loss of sodium in the urine and leads to decreased extracellular fluid volume and decreased sodium concentration; both of these changes elicit the desire for salt.

In general, the primary stimuli that increase salt appetite are those associated with sodium deficits and decreased blood volume or decreased blood pressure, associated with circulatory insufficiency.

The neuronal mechanism for salt appetite is analogous to that of the thirst mechanism. Some of the same neuronal centers in the AV3V region of the brain seem to be involved because lesions in this region frequently affect both thirst and salt appetite simultaneously in animals. Also, circulatory reflexes elicited by low blood pressure or decreased blood volume affect both thirst and salt appetite at the same time.

Bibliography

Antunes-Rodrigues J, de Castro M, Elias LL, et al: Neuroendocrine control of body fluid metabolism, *Physiol Rev* 84:169, 2004.

Bourque CW: Central mechanisms of osmosensation and systemic osmoregulation, *Nat Rev Neurosci* 9:519–531, 2008.

Cowley AW Jr, Mori T, Mattson D, et al: Role of renal NO production in the regulation of medullary blood flow, *Am J Physiol Regul Integr Comp Physiol* 284:R1355, 2003.

Dwyer TM, Schmidt-Nielsen B: The renal pelvis: machinery that concentrates urine in the papilla, *News Physiol Sci* 18:1, 2003.

Fenton RA, Knepper MA: Mouse models and the urinary concentrating mechanism in the new millennium, *Physiol Rev* 87:1083, 2007.

Finley JJ 4th, Konstam MA, Udelson JE: Arginine vasopressin antagonists for the treatment of heart failure and hyponatremia, *Circulation* 118:410, 2008.

Geerling JC, Loewy AD: Central regulation of sodium appetite, *Exp Physiol* 93:177, 2008.

Kozono D, Yasui M, King LS, et al: Aquaporin water channels: atomic structure molecular dynamics meet clinical medicine, *J Clin Invest* 109:1395, 2002.

Loh JA, Verbalis JG: Disorders of water and salt metabolism associated with pituitary disease, *Endocrinol Metab Clin North Am* 37:213, 2008.

McKinley MJ, Johnson AK: The physiological regulation of thirst and fluid intake, *News Physiol Sci* 19:1, 2004.

Pallone TL, Zhang Z, Rhinehart K: Physiology of the renal medullary microcirculation, *Am J Physiol Renal Physiol* 284:F253, 2003.

Sands JM, Bichet DG: Nephrogenic diabetes insipidus, *Ann Intern Med* 144:186, 2006.

Schrier RW: Body water homeostasis: clinical disorders of urinary dilution and concentration, *J Am Soc Nephrol* 17:1820, 2006.

Sharif-Naeini R, Ciura S, Zhang Z, et al: Contribution of TRPV channels to osmosensory transduction, thirst, and vasopressin release, *Kidney Int* 73:811, 2008.

Renal Regulation of Potassium, Calcium, Phosphate, and Magnesium; Integration of Renal Mechanisms for Control of Blood Volume and Extracellular Fluid Volume

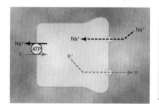

Regulation of Extracellular Fluid Potassium Concentration and Potassium Excretion

Extracellular fluid potassium concentration normally is regulated precisely at about 4.2 mEq/L, seldom rising or falling more than ±0.3 mEq/L. This precise control is necessary because many cell functions are very sensitive to changes in extracellular fluid potassium concentration. For instance, an increase in plasma potassium concentration of only 3 to 4 mEq/L can cause cardiac arrhythmias, and higher concentrations can lead to cardiac arrest or fibrillation.

A special difficulty in regulating extracellular potassium concentration is the fact that more than 98 percent of the total body potassium is contained in the cells and only 2 percent in the extracellular fluid (Figure 29-1). For a 70-kilogram adult, who has about 28 liters of intracellular fluid (40 percent of body weight) and 14 liters of extracellular fluid (20 percent of body weight), about 3920 mEq of potassium are inside the cells and only about 59 mEq are in the extracellular fluid. Also, the potassium contained in a single meal is often as high as 50 mEq, and the daily intake usually ranges between 50 and 200 mEq/day; therefore, failure to rapidly rid the extracellular fluid of the ingested potassium could cause life-threatening *hyperkalemia* (increased plasma potassium concentration). Likewise, a small loss of potassium from the extracellular fluid could cause severe *hypokalemia* (low plasma potassium concentration) in the absence of rapid and appropriate compensatory responses.

Maintenance of balance between intake and output of potassium depends primarily on excretion by the kidneys because the amount excreted in the feces is only about 5 to 10 percent of the potassium intake. Thus, the maintenance of normal potassium balance requires the kidneys to adjust their potassium excretion rapidly and precisely in response to wide variations in intake, as is also true for most other electrolytes.

Control of potassium distribution between the extracellular and intracellular compartments also plays an important role in potassium homeostasis. Because more than 98 percent of the total body potassium is contained in the cells, they can serve as an overflow site for excess extracellular fluid potassium during hyperkalemia or as a source of potassium during hypokalemia. Thus, redistribution of potassium between the intracellular and extracellular fluid compartments provides a first line of defense against changes in extracellular fluid potassium concentration.

Regulation of Internal Potassium Distribution

After ingestion of a normal meal, extracellular fluid potassium concentration would rise to a lethal level if the ingested potassium did not rapidly move into the cells. For example, absorption of 40 mEq of potassium (the amount contained in a meal rich in vegetables and fruit) into an extracellular fluid volume of 14 liters would raise plasma potassium concentration by about 2.9 mEq/L if all the potassium remained in the extracellular compartment. Fortunately, most of the ingested potassium rapidly moves into the cells until the kidneys can eliminate the excess. Table 29-1 summarizes some of the factors that can influence the distribution of potassium between the intracellular and extracellular compartments.

Insulin Stimulates Potassium Uptake into Cells. Insulin is important for increasing cell potassium uptake after a meal. In people who have insulin deficiency owing to diabetes mellitus, the rise in plasma potassium concentration after eating a meal is much greater than normal. Injections of insulin, however, can help to correct the hyperkalemia.

Aldosterone Increases Potassium Uptake into Cells. Increased potassium intake also stimulates secretion of aldosterone, which increases cell potassium uptake. Excess aldosterone secretion (Conn's syndrome) is almost invariably associated with hypokalemia, due in part to movement of extracellular potassium into the cells. Conversely, patients with deficient aldosterone production (Addison's disease) often have clinically significant hyperkalemia due to accumulation of potassium in the extracellular space, as well as to renal retention of potassium.

β-Adrenergic Stimulation Increases Cellular Uptake of Potassium. Increased secretion of catecholamines,

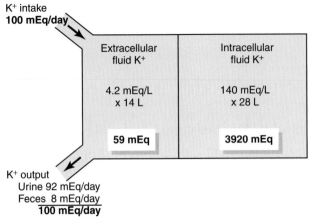

K⁺ intake
100 mEq/day

Extracellular fluid K⁺	Intracellular fluid K⁺
4.2 mEq/L × 14 L	140 mEq/L × 28 L
59 mEq	**3920 mEq**

K⁺ output
Urine 92 mEq/day
Feces 8 mEq/day
100 mEq/day

Figure 29-1 Normal potassium intake, distribution of potassium in the body fluids, and potassium output from the body.

Table 29-1 Factors That Can Alter Potassium Distribution Between the Intracellular and Extracellular Fluid

Factors That Shift K⁺ into Cells (Decrease Extracellular [K⁺])	Factors That Shift K⁺ Out of Cells (Increase Extracellular [K⁺])
• Insulin • Aldosterone • β-adrenergic stimulation • Alkalosis	• Insulin deficiency (diabetes mellitus) • Aldosterone deficiency (Addison's disease) • β-adrenergic blockade • Acidosis • Cell lysis • Strenuous exercise • Increased extracellular fluid osmolarity

especially epinephrine, can cause movement of potassium from the extracellular to the intracellular fluid, mainly by activation of β_2-adrenergic receptors. Conversely, treatment of hypertension with β-adrenergic receptor blockers, such as propranolol, causes potassium to move out of the cells and creates a tendency toward hyperkalemia.

Acid-Base Abnormalities Can Cause Changes in Potassium Distribution. Metabolic acidosis increases extracellular potassium concentration, in part by causing loss of potassium from the cells, whereas metabolic alkalosis decreases extracellular fluid potassium concentration. Although the mechanisms responsible for the effect of hydrogen ion concentration on potassium internal distribution are not completely understood, one effect of increased hydrogen ion concentration is to reduce the activity of the sodium-potassium adenosine triphosphatase (ATPase) pump. This in turn decreases cellular uptake of potassium and raises extracellular potassium concentration.

Cell Lysis Causes Increased Extracellular Potassium Concentration. As cells are destroyed, the large amounts of potassium contained in the cells are released into the

extracellular compartment. This can cause significant hyperkalemia if large amounts of tissue are destroyed, as occurs with severe muscle injury or with red blood cell lysis.

Strenuous Exercise Can Cause Hyperkalemia by Releasing Potassium from Skeletal Muscle. During prolonged exercise, potassium is released from skeletal muscle into the extracellular fluid. Usually the hyperkalemia is mild, but it may be clinically significant after heavy exercise, especially in patients treated with β-adrenergic blockers or in individuals with insulin deficiency. In rare instances, hyperkalemia after exercise may be severe enough to cause cardiac arrhythmias and sudden death.

Increased Extracellular Fluid Osmolarity Causes Redistribution of Potassium from the Cells to Extracellular Fluid. Increased extracellular fluid osmolarity causes osmotic flow of water out of the cells. The cellular dehydration increases intracellular potassium concentration, thereby promoting diffusion of potassium out of the cells and increasing extracellular fluid potassium concentration. Decreased extracellular fluid osmolarity has the opposite effect.

Overview of Renal Potassium Excretion

Renal potassium excretion is determined by the sum of three processes: (1) the rate of potassium filtration (GFR multiplied by the plasma potassium concentration), (2) the rate of potassium reabsorption by the tubules, and (3) the rate of potassium secretion by the tubules. The normal rate of potassium filtration by the glomerular capillaries is about 756 mEq/day (GFR, 180 L/day multiplied by plasma potassium, 4.2 mEq/L); this rate of filtration is relatively constant in healthy persons because of the autoregulatory mechanisms for GFR discussed previously and the precision with which plasma potassium concentration is regulated. Severe decreases in GFR in certain renal diseases, however, can cause serious potassium accumulation and hyperkalemia.

Figure 29-2 summarizes the tubular handling of potassium under normal conditions. About 65 percent of the filtered potassium is reabsorbed in the proximal tubule. Another 25 to 30 percent of the filtered potassium is reabsorbed in the loop of Henle, especially in the thick ascending part where potassium is actively co-transported along with sodium and chloride. In both the proximal tubule and the loop of Henle, a relatively constant fraction of the filtered potassium load is reabsorbed. Changes in potassium reabsorption in these segments can influence potassium excretion, but most of the day-to-day variation of potassium excretion is not due to changes in reabsorption in the proximal tubule or loop of Henle.

Daily Variations in Potassium Excretion Are Caused Mainly by Changes in Potassium Secretion in Distal and Collecting Tubules. The most important sites for regulating potassium excretion are the principal cells

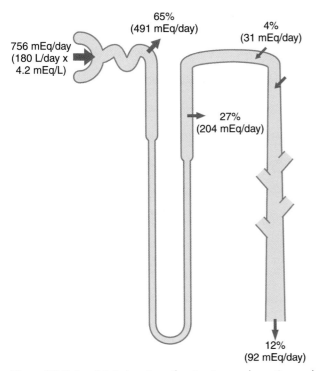

65%
(491 mEq/day)

4%
(31 mEq/day)

756 mEq/day
(180 L/day x
4.2 mEq/L)

27%
(204 mEq/day)

12%
(92 mEq/day)

Figure 29-2 Renal tubular sites of potassium reabsorption and secretion. Potassium is reabsorbed in the proximal tubule and in the ascending loop of Henle, so only about 8 percent of the filtered load is delivered to the distal tubule. Secretion of potassium into the late distal tubules and collecting ducts adds to the amount delivered; therefore, the daily excretion is about 12 percent of the potassium filtered at the glomerular capillaries. The percentages indicate how much of the filtered load is reabsorbed or secreted into the different tubular segments.

of the late distal tubules and cortical collecting tubules. In these tubular segments, potassium can at times be reabsorbed or at other times be secreted, depending on the needs of the body. With a normal potassium intake of 100 mEq/day, the kidneys must excrete about 92 mEq/day (the remaining 8 mEq are lost in the feces). About 31 mEq/day of potassium are secreted into the distal and collecting tubules, accounting for about one third of the excreted potassium.

With high potassium intakes, the required extra excretion of potassium is achieved almost entirely by increasing the secretion of potassium into the distal and collecting tubules. In fact, with extremely high potassium diets, the rate of potassium excretion can exceed the amount of potassium in the glomerular filtrate, indicating a powerful mechanism for secreting potassium.

When potassium intake is low, the secretion rate of potassium in the distal and collecting tubules decreases, causing a reduction in urinary potassium secretion. With extreme reductions in potassium intake, there is net reabsorption of potassium in the distal segments of the nephron, and potassium excretion can fall to 1 percent of the potassium in the glomerular filtrate (to <10 mEq/day). With potassium intakes below this level, severe hypokalemia can develop.

Thus, most of the day-to-day regulation of potassium excretion occurs in the late distal and cortical collecting tubules, where potassium can be either reabsorbed or secreted, depending on the needs of the body. In the next section, we consider the basic mechanisms of potassium secretion and the factors that regulate this process.

Potassium Secretion by Principal Cells of Late Distal and Cortical Collecting Tubules

The cells in the late distal and cortical collecting tubules that secrete potassium are called *principal cells* and make up about 90 percent of the epithelial cells in these regions. Figure 29-3 shows the basic cellular mechanisms of potassium secretion by the principal cells.

Secretion of potassium from the blood into the tubular lumen is a two-step process, beginning with uptake from the interstitium into the cell by the sodium-potassium ATPase pump in the basolateral cell membrane; this pump moves sodium out of the cell into the interstitium and at the same time moves potassium to the interior of the cell.

The second step of the process is passive diffusion of potassium from the interior of the cell into the tubular fluid. The sodium-potassium ATPase pump creates a high intracellular potassium concentration, which provides the driving force for passive diffusion of potassium from the cell into the tubular lumen. The luminal membrane of the principal cells is highly permeable to potassium. One reason for this high permeability is that special channels are specifically permeable to potassium ions, thus allowing these ions to rapidly diffuse across the membrane.

Control of Potassium Secretion by Principal Cells. The primary factors that control potassium secretion by the principal cells of the late distal and cortical collecting tubules are (1) the activity of the sodium-potassium ATPase pump, (2) the electrochemical gradient for potassium secretion from the blood to the tubular lumen,

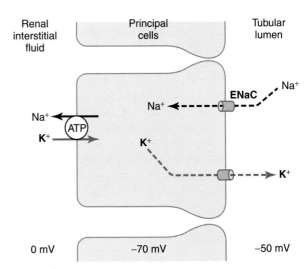

Renal interstitial fluid

Principal cells

Tubular lumen

ENaC

Na+

Na+

Na+

ATP

K+

K+

K+

0 mV

−70 mV

−50 mV

Figure 29-3 Mechanisms of potassium secretion and sodium reabsorption by the principal cells of the late distal and collecting tubules.

and (3) the permeability of the luminal membrane for potassium. These three determinants of potassium secretion are in turn regulated by the factors discussed later.

Intercalated Cells Can Reabsorb Potassium During Potassium Depletion.

In circumstances associated with severe potassium depletion, there is a cessation of potassium secretion and actually a net reabsorption of potassium in the late distal and collecting tubules. This reabsorption occurs through the *intercalated cells;* although this reabsorptive process is not completely understood, one mechanism believed to contribute is a *hydrogen-potassium ATPase* transport mechanism located in the luminal membrane. This transporter reabsorbs potassium in exchange for hydrogen ions secreted into the tubular lumen, and the potassium then diffuses through the basolateral membrane of the cell into the blood. This transporter is necessary to allow potassium reabsorption during extracellular fluid potassium depletion, but under normal conditions it plays only a small role in controlling potassium excretion.

Summary of Factors That Regulate Potassium Secretion: Plasma Potassium Concentration, Aldosterone, Tubular Flow Rate, and Hydrogen Ion Concentration

Because normal regulation of potassium excretion occurs mainly as a result of changes in potassium secretion by the principal cells of the late distal and collecting tubules, in this chapter we discuss the primary factors that influence secretion by these cells. The most important factors that *stimulate* potassium secretion by the principal cells include (1) increased extracellular fluid potassium concentration, (2) increased aldosterone, and (3) increased tubular flow rate.

One factor that *decreases* potassium secretion is increased hydrogen ion concentration (acidosis).

Increased Extracellular Fluid Potassium Concentration Stimulates Potassium Secretion.

The rate of potassium secretion in the late distal and cortical collecting tubules is directly stimulated by increased extracellular fluid potassium concentration, leading to increases in potassium excretion, as shown in Figure 29-4. This effect is especially pronounced when extracellular fluid potassium concentration rises above about 4.1 mEq/L, slightly less than the normal concentration. Increased plasma potassium concentration, therefore, serves as one of the most important mechanisms for increasing potassium secretion and regulating extracellular fluid potassium ion concentration.

Increased extracellular fluid potassium concentration raises potassium secretion by three mechanisms: (1) Increased extracellular fluid potassium concentration stimulates the sodium-potassium ATPase pump, thereby increasing potassium uptake across the basolateral membrane. This in turn increases intracellular potassium ion

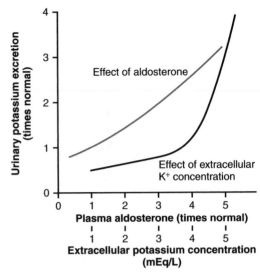

Figure 29-4 Effect of plasma aldosterone concentration (*red line*) and extracellular potassium ion concentration (*black line*) on the rate of urinary potassium excretion. These factors stimulate potassium secretion by the principal cells of the cortical collecting tubules. (Drawn from data in Young DB, Paulsen AW: Interrelated effects of aldosterone and plasma potassium on potassium excretion. Am J Physiol 244:F28, 1983.)

concentration, causing potassium to diffuse across the luminal membrane into the tubule. (2) Increased extracellular potassium concentration increases the potassium gradient from the renal interstitial fluid to the interior of the epithelial cell; this reduces back leakage of potassium ions from inside the cells through the basolateral membrane. (3) Increased potassium concentration stimulates aldosterone secretion by the adrenal cortex, which further stimulates potassium secretion, as discussed next.

Aldosterone Stimulates Potassium Secretion.

Aldosterone stimulates active reabsorption of sodium ions by the principal cells of the late distal tubules and collecting ducts (see Chapter 27). This effect is mediated through a sodium-potassium ATPase pump that transports sodium outward through the basolateral membrane of the cell and into the blood at the same time that it pumps potassium into the cell. Thus, aldosterone also has a powerful effect to control the rate at which the principal cells secrete potassium.

A second effect of aldosterone is to increase the permeability of the luminal membrane for potassium, further adding to the effectiveness of aldosterone in stimulating potassium secretion. Therefore, aldosterone has a powerful effect to increase potassium excretion, as shown in Figure 29-4.

Increased Extracellular Potassium Ion Concentration Stimulates Aldosterone Secretion.

In negative feedback control systems, the factor that is controlled usually has a feedback effect on the controller. In the case of the aldosterone-potassium control system, the rate of aldosterone secretion by the adrenal gland is controlled

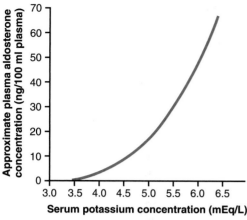

Figure 29-5 Effect of extracellular fluid potassium ion concentration on plasma aldosterone concentration. Note that small changes in potassium concentration cause large changes in aldosterone concentration.

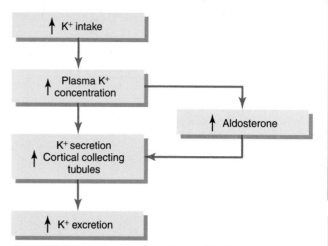

Figure 29-7 Primary mechanisms by which high potassium intake raises potassium excretion. Note that increased plasma potassium concentration directly raises potassium secretion by the cortical collecting tubules and indirectly increases potassium secretion by raising plasma aldosterone concentration.

strongly by extracellular fluid potassium ion concentration. Figure 29-5 shows that an increase in plasma potassium concentration of about 3 mEq/L can increase plasma aldosterone concentration from nearly 0 to as high as 60 ng/100 ml, a concentration almost 10 times normal.

The effect of potassium ion concentration to stimulate aldosterone secretion is part of a powerful feedback system for regulating potassium excretion, as shown in Figure 29-6. In this feedback system, an increase in plasma potassium concentration stimulates aldosterone secretion and, therefore, increases the blood level of aldosterone (block 1). The increase in blood aldosterone then causes a marked increase in potassium excretion by the kidneys (block 2). The increased potassium excretion then reduces the extracellular fluid potassium concentration back toward normal (blocks 3 and 4). Thus, this feedback mechanism acts synergistically with the direct effect of increased extracellular potassium concentration to elevate potassium excretion when potassium intake is raised (Figure 29-7).

Blockade of Aldosterone Feedback System Greatly Impairs Control of Potassium Concentration. In the absence of aldosterone secretion, as occurs in patients with Addison's disease, renal secretion of potassium is impaired, thus causing extracellular fluid potassium concentration to rise to dangerously high levels. Conversely, with excess aldosterone secretion (primary aldosteronism), potassium secretion becomes greatly increased, causing potassium loss by the kidneys and thus leading to hypokalemia.

In addition to its stimulatory effect on renal secretion of potassium, aldosterone also increases cellular uptake of potassium, which contributes to the powerful aldosterone-potassium feedback system, as discussed previously.

The special quantitative importance of the aldosterone feedback system in controlling potassium concentration is shown in Figure 29-8. In this experiment, potassium intake was increased almost sevenfold in dogs under two conditions: (1) under normal conditions and (2) after the aldosterone feedback system had been blocked by removing the adrenal glands and placing the animals on a fixed rate of aldosterone infusion so that plasma aldosterone concentration could neither increase nor decrease.

Note that in the normal animals, a sevenfold increase in potassium intake caused only a slight increase in potassium concentration, from 4.2 to 4.3 mEq/L. Thus, when the aldosterone feedback system is functioning normally, potassium concentration is precisely controlled, despite large changes in potassium intake.

When the aldosterone feedback system was blocked, the same increases in potassium intake caused a much larger increase in potassium concentration, from 3.8 to almost 4.7 mEq/L. Thus, control of potassium concentration is greatly impaired when the aldosterone feedback system is blocked. A similar impairment of potassium regulation is observed in humans with poorly functioning aldosterone feedback systems, such as occurs in patients

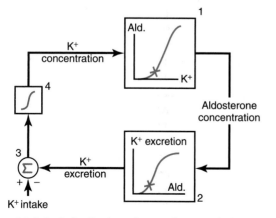

Figure 29-6 Basic feedback mechanism for control of extracellular fluid potassium concentration by aldosterone (*Ald.*).

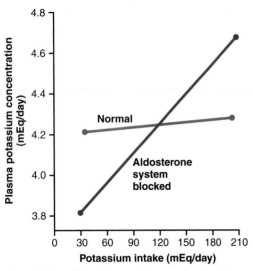

Figure 29-8 Effect of large changes in potassium intake on extracellular fluid potassium concentration under normal conditions (*red line*) and after the aldosterone feedback had been blocked (*blue line*). Note that after blockade of the aldosterone system, regulation of potassium concentration was greatly impaired. (Courtesy Dr. David B. Young.)

with either primary aldosteronism (too much aldosterone) or Addison's disease (too little aldosterone).

Increased Distal Tubular Flow Rate Stimulates Potassium Secretion. A rise in distal tubular flow rate, as occurs with volume expansion, high sodium intake, or treatment with some diuretics, stimulates potassium secretion (Figure 29-9). Conversely, a decrease in distal tubular flow rate, as caused by sodium depletion, reduces potassium secretion.

The effect of tubular flow rate on potassium secretion in the distal and collecting tubules is strongly influenced by potassium intake. When potassium intake is high, increased tubular flow rate has a much greater effect to stimulate potassium secretion than when potassium intake is low (see Figure 29-9).

The mechanism for the effect of high-volume flow rate is as follows: When potassium is secreted into the tubular fluid, the luminal concentration of potassium increases, thereby reducing the driving force for potassium diffusion across the luminal membrane. With increased tubular flow rate, the secreted potassium is continuously flushed down the tubule, so the rise in tubular potassium concentration becomes minimized. Therefore, net potassium secretion is stimulated by increased tubular flow rate.

The effect of increased tubular flow rate is especially important in helping to preserve normal potassium excretion during changes in sodium intake. For example, with a high sodium intake, there is decreased aldosterone secretion, which by itself would tend to decrease the rate of potassium secretion and, therefore, reduce urinary excretion of potassium. However, the high distal tubular flow rate that occurs with a high sodium intake tends to increase potassium secretion (Figure 29-10), as discussed in the previous paragraph. Therefore, the two effects of high sodium intake, decreased aldosterone secretion and

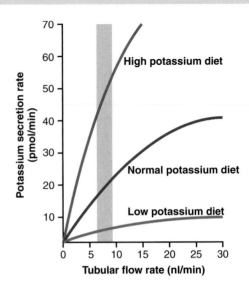

Figure 29-9 Relationship between flow rate in the cortical collecting tubules and potassium secretion and the effect of changes in potassium intake. Note that a high dietary potassium intake greatly enhances the effect of increased tubular flow rate to increase potassium secretion. The *shaded bar* shows the approximate normal tubular flow rate under most physiological conditions. (Data from Malnic G, Berliner RW, Giebisch G. *Am J Physiol* 256:F932, 1989.)

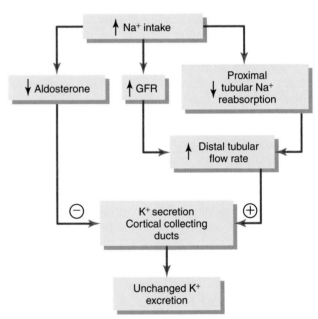

Figure 29-10 Effect of high sodium intake on renal excretion of potassium. Note that a high-sodium diet decreases plasma aldosterone, which tends to decrease potassium secretion by the cortical collecting tubules. However, the high-sodium diet simultaneously increases fluid delivery to the cortical collecting duct, which tends to increase potassium secretion. The opposing effects of a high-sodium diet counterbalance each other, so there is little change in potassium excretion.

the high tubular flow rate, counterbalance each other, so there is little change in potassium excretion. Likewise, with a low sodium intake, there is little change in potassium excretion because of the counterbalancing effects of increased aldosterone secretion and decreased tubular flow rate on potassium secretion.

Acute Acidosis Decreases Potassium Secretion.

Acute increases in hydrogen ion concentration of the extracellular fluid (acidosis) reduce potassium secretion, whereas decreased hydrogen ion concentration (alkalosis) increases potassium secretion. The primary mechanism by which increased hydrogen ion concentration inhibits potassium secretion is by reducing the activity of the sodium-potassium ATPase pump. This in turn decreases intracellular potassium concentration and subsequent passive diffusion of potassium across the luminal membrane into the tubule.

With more prolonged acidosis, lasting over a period of several days, there is an increase in urinary potassium excretion. The mechanism for this effect is due in part to an effect of chronic acidosis to inhibit proximal tubular sodium chloride and water reabsorption, which increases distal volume delivery, thereby stimulating the secretion of potassium. This effect overrides the inhibitory effect of hydrogen ions on the sodium-potassium ATPase pump. *Thus, chronic acidosis leads to a loss of potassium, whereas acute acidosis leads to decreased potassium excretion.*

Beneficial Effects of a Diet High in Potassium and Low in Sodium Content.

For most of human history, the typical diet has been one that is low in sodium and high in potassium content, compared with the typical modern diet. In isolated populations that have not experienced industrialization, such as the Yanomamo tribe living in the Amazon of Northern Brazil, sodium intake may be as low as 10 to 20 mmol/day while potassium intake may be as high as 200 mmol/day. This is due to their consumption of a diet containing large amounts of fruits and vegetables and no processed foods. Populations consuming this type of diet typically do not experience age-related increases in blood pressure and cardiovascular diseases.

With industrialization and increased consumption of processed foods, which often have high sodium and low potassium content, there have been dramatic increases in sodium intake and decreases in potassium intake. In most industrialized countries potassium consumption averages only 30 to 70 mmol/day while sodium intake averages 140 to 180 mmol/day.

Experimental and clinical studies have shown that the combination of high sodium and low potassium intake increases the risk for hypertension and associated cardiovascular and kidney diseases. A diet rich in potassium, however, seems to protect against the adverse effects of a high-sodium diet, reducing blood pressure and the risk for stroke, coronary artery disease, and kidney disease. The beneficial effects of increasing potassium intake are especially apparent when combined with a low-sodium diet.

Dietary guidelines published by U.S. National Academy of Sciences, the American Heart Association, and other organizations recommend reducing dietary intake sodium chloride to around 65 mmol/day (corresponding to 1.5 g/day of sodium or 3.8 g/day sodium chloride), while increasing potassium intake to 120 mmol/day (4.7 g/day) for healthy adults.

Control of Renal Calcium Excretion and Extracellular Calcium Ion Concentration

The mechanisms for regulating calcium ion concentration are discussed in detail in Chapter 79, along with the endocrinology of the calcium-regulating hormones, parathyroid hormone (PTH), and calcitonin. Therefore, calcium ion regulation is discussed only briefly in this chapter.

Extracellular fluid calcium ion concentration normally remains tightly controlled within a few percentage points of its normal level, 2.4 mEq/L. When calcium ion concentration falls to low levels *(hypocalcemia)*, the excitability of nerve and muscle cells increases markedly and can in extreme cases result in *hypocalcemic tetany*. This is characterized by spastic skeletal muscle contractions. *Hypercalcemia* (increased calcium concentration) depresses neuromuscular excitability and can lead to cardiac arrhythmias.

About 50 percent of the total calcium in the plasma (5 mEq/L) exists in the ionized form, which is the form that has biological activity at cell membranes. The remainder is either bound to the plasma proteins (about 40 percent) or complexed in the non-ionized form with anions such as phosphate and citrate (about 10 percent).

Changes in plasma hydrogen ion concentration can influence the degree of calcium binding to plasma proteins. With acidosis, less calcium is bound to the plasma proteins. Conversely, in alkalosis, a greater amount of calcium is bound to the plasma proteins. Therefore, *patients with alkalosis are more susceptible to hypocalcemic tetany.*

As with other substances in the body, the intake of calcium must be balanced with the net loss of calcium over the long term. Unlike ions such as sodium and chloride, however, a large share of calcium excretion occurs in the feces. The usual rate of dietary calcium intake is about 1000 mg/day, with about 900 mg/day of calcium excreted in the feces. Under certain conditions, fecal calcium excretion can exceed calcium ingestion because calcium can also be secreted into the intestinal lumen. Therefore, the gastrointestinal tract and the regulatory mechanisms that influence intestinal calcium absorption and secretion play a major role in calcium homeostasis, as discussed in Chapter 79.

Almost all the calcium in the body (99 percent) is stored in the bone, with only about 0.1 percent in the extracellular fluid and 1.0 percent in the intracellular fluid and cell organelles. The bone, therefore, acts as a large reservoir for storing calcium and as a source of calcium when extracellular fluid calcium concentration tends to decrease.

One of the most important regulators of bone uptake and release of calcium is PTH. When extracellular fluid calcium concentration falls below normal, the parathyroid glands are directly stimulated by the low calcium levels to promote increased secretion of PTH. This hormone then acts directly on the bones to increase the resorption of bone salts (release of salts from the bones) and to release large amounts of calcium into the extracellular fluid, thereby returning calcium levels back toward normal. When calcium ion concentration is elevated, PTH secretion decreases, so almost no bone resorption occurs; instead, excess calcium is deposited in the bones. Thus, the day-to-day regulation of calcium ion concentration is mediated in large part by the effect of PTH on bone resorption.

The bones, however, do not have an inexhaustible supply of calcium. Therefore, over the long term, the intake of calcium must be balanced with calcium excretion by the gastrointestinal tract and the kidneys. The most important regulator of calcium reabsorption at both of these sites is PTH. *Thus, PTH regulates plasma calcium concentration through three main effects: (1) by stimulating bone resorption; (2) by stimulating activation of vitamin D, which then increases intestinal reabsorption of calcium; and (3) by directly increasing renal tubular calcium reabsorption* (Figure 29-11). The control of gastrointestinal calcium reabsorption and calcium exchange in the bones is discussed elsewhere, and the remainder of this section focuses on the mechanisms that control renal calcium excretion.

Control of Calcium Excretion by the Kidneys

Calcium is both filtered and reabsorbed in the kidneys but not secreted. Therefore, the rate of renal calcium excretion is calculated as

Renal calcium excretion =
Calcium filtered – Calcium reabsorbed

Only about 50 percent of the plasma calcium is ionized, with the remainder being bound to the plasma proteins or complexed with anions such as phosphate. Therefore, only about 50 percent of the plasma calcium can be filtered at the glomerulus. Normally, about 99 percent of the filtered calcium is reabsorbed by the tubules, with only about 1 percent of the filtered calcium being excreted. About 65 percent of the filtered calcium is reabsorbed in the proximal tubule, 25 to 30 percent is reabsorbed in the loop of Henle, and 4 to 9 percent is reabsorbed in the distal and collecting tubules. This pattern of reabsorption is similar to that for sodium.

As is true with the other ions, calcium excretion is adjusted to meet the body's needs. With an increase in calcium intake, there is also increased renal calcium excretion, although much of the increase of calcium intake is eliminated in the feces. With calcium depletion, calcium excretion by the kidneys decreases as a result of enhanced tubular reabsorption.

Proximal Tubular Calcium Reabsorption. Most of the calcium reabsorption in the proximal tubule occurs through the paracellular pathway, dissolved in water and carried with the reabsorbed fluid as it flows between the cells. Only about 20% of proximal tubular calcium reabsorption occurs through the transcellular pathway in two steps: (1) calcium diffuses from the tubular lumen into the cell down an electrochemical gradient due to the much higher concentration of calcium in the tubular lumen, compared with the epithelial cell cytoplasm, and because the cell interior has a negative relative to the tubular lumen; (2) calcium exits the cell across the basolateral membrane by a calcium-ATPase pump and by sodium-calcium counter-transporter (Figure 29-12).

Loop of Henle and Distal Tubule Calcium Reabsorption. In the loop of Henle, calcium reabsorption is restricted to the thick ascending limb. Approximately 50% of calcium reabsorption in the thick ascending limb occurs through the paracellular route by passive diffusion due to the slight positive charge of the tubular lumen relative to the interstitial fluid. The remaining 50% of calcium reabsorption in the thick ascending limb occurs through the transcellular pathway, a process that is stimulated by PTH.

In the distal tubule, calcium reabsorption occurs almost entirely by active transport through the cell membrane. The mechanism for this active transport is similar to that in the proximal tubule and thick ascending limb and involves diffusion across the luminal membrane through calcium channels and exit across the basolateral membrane by a calcium-ATPase pump, as well as a

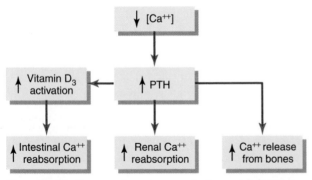

Figure 29-11 Compensatory responses to decreased plasma ionized calcium concentration mediated by parathyroid hormone (PTH) and vitamin D.

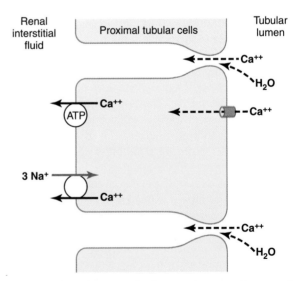

Figure 29-12 Mechanisms of calcium reabsorption by paracellular and transcellular pathways in the proximal tubular cells.

sodium-calcium counter transport mechanism. In this segment, as well as in the loops of Henle, PTH stimulates calcium reabsorption. Vitamin D (Calcitrol) and calcitonin also stimulate calcium reabsorption in the thick ascending limb of Henle's loop and in the distal tubule, although these hormones are not as important quantitatively as PTH in reducing renal calcium excretion.

Factors that Regulate Tubular Calcium Reabsorption. One of the primary controllers of renal tubular calcium reabsorption is PTH. Increased levels of PTH stimulate calcium reabsorption in the thick ascending loops of Henle and distal tubules, which reduces urinary excretion of calcium. Conversely, reduction of PTH promotes calcium excretion by decreasing reabsorption in the loops of Henle and distal tubules.

In the proximal tubule, calcium reabsorption usually parallels sodium and water reabsorption and is independent of PTH. Therefore, in instances of extracellular volume expansion or increased arterial pressure—both of which decrease proximal sodium and water reabsorption—there is also reduction in calcium reabsorption and, consequently, increased urinary excretion of calcium. Conversely, with extracellular volume contraction or decreased blood pressure, calcium excretion decreases primarily because of increased proximal tubular reabsorption.

Another factor that influences calcium reabsorption is the plasma concentration of phosphate. Increased plasma phosphate stimulates PTH, which increases calcium reabsorption by the renal tubules, thereby reducing calcium excretion. The opposite occurs with reduction in plasma phosphate concentration.

Calcium reabsorption is also stimulated by metabolic alkalosis and inhibited by metabolic acidosis. Most of the effect of hydrogen ion concentration on calcium excretion results from changes in calcium reabsorption in the distal tubule.

A summary of the factors that are known to influence calcium excretion by the renal tubules is shown in Table 29-2.

Regulation of Renal Phosphate Excretion

Phosphate excretion by the kidneys is controlled primarily by an overflow mechanism that can be explained as follows: The renal tubules have a normal transport maximum for reabsorbing phosphate of about 0.1 mM/min. When less than this amount of phosphate is present in the glomerular filtrate, essentially *all* the filtered phosphate is reabsorbed. When more than this is present, the *excess* is excreted. Therefore, phosphate normally begins to spill into the urine when its concentration in the extracellular fluid rises above a threshold of about 0.8 mM/L, which gives a tubular load of phosphate of about 0.1 mM/min, assuming a GFR of 125 ml/min. Because most people ingest large quantities of phosphate in milk products and meat, the concentration of phosphate is usually maintained above 1 mM/L, a level at which there is continual excretion of phosphate into the urine.

The proximal tubule normally reabsorbs 75 to 80 percent of the filtered phosphate. The distal tubule reabsorbs about 10 percent of the filtered load, and only very small amounts are reabsorbed in the loop of Henle, collecting tubules, and collecting ducts. Approximately 10 percent of the filtered phosphate is excreted in the urine.

In the proximal tubule, phosphate reabsorption occurs mainly through the transcellular pathway. Phosphate enters the cell from the lumen by a sodium-phosphate co-transporter and exits the cell across the basolateral membrane by a process that is not well understood but may involve a counter transport mechanism in which phosphate is exchanged for an anion.

Changes in tubular phosphate reabsorptive capacity can also occur in different conditions and influence phosphate excretion. For instance, a diet low in phosphate can, over time, increase the reabsorptive transport maximum for phosphate, thereby reducing the tendency for phosphate to spill over into the urine.

PTH can play a significant role in regulating phosphate concentration through two effects: (1) PTH promotes bone resorption, thereby dumping large amounts of phosphate ions into the extracellular fluid from the bone salts, and (2) PTH decreases the transport maximum for phosphate by the renal tubules, so a greater proportion of the tubular phosphate is lost in the urine. *Thus, whenever plasma PTH is increased, tubular phosphate reabsorption is decreased and more phosphate is excreted.* These interrelations among phosphate, PTH, and calcium are discussed in more detail in Chapter 79.

Control of Renal Magnesium Excretion and Extracellular Magnesium Ion Concentration

More than one half of the body's magnesium is stored in the bones. Most of the rest resides within the cells, with less than 1 percent located in the extracellular fluid. Although the total plasma magnesium concentration is about 1.8 mEq/L, more than one half of this is bound to plasma proteins. Therefore, the free ionized concentration of magnesium is only about 0.8 mEq/L.

The normal daily intake of magnesium is about 250 to 300 mg/day, but only about one half of this intake is absorbed by the gastrointestinal tract. To maintain

Table 29-2 Factors That Alter Renal Calcium Excretion

↓ Calcium Excretion	↑ Calcium Excretion
↑Parathyroid hormone (PTH)	↓ PTH
↓ Extracellular fluid volume	↑ Extracellular fluid volume
↓ Blood pressure	↑ Blood pressure
↑ Plasma phosphate	↓ Plasma phosphate
Metabolic alkalosis	Metabolic acidosis
Vitamin D$_3$	

magnesium balance, the kidneys must excrete this absorbed magnesium, about one half the daily intake of magnesium, or 125 to 150 mg/day. The kidneys normally excrete about 10 to 15 percent of the magnesium in the glomerular filtrate.

Renal excretion of magnesium can increase markedly during magnesium excess or decrease to almost nil during magnesium depletion. Because magnesium is involved in many biochemical processes in the body, including activation of many enzymes, its concentration must be closely regulated.

Regulation of magnesium excretion is achieved mainly by changing tubular reabsorption. The proximal tubule usually reabsorbs only about 25 percent of the filtered magnesium. The primary site of reabsorption is the loop of Henle, where about 65 percent of the filtered load of magnesium is reabsorbed. Only a small amount (usually <5 percent) of the filtered magnesium is reabsorbed in the distal and collecting tubules.

The mechanisms that regulate magnesium excretion are not well understood, but the following disturbances lead to increased magnesium excretion: (1) increased extracellular fluid magnesium concentration, (2) extracellular volume expansion, and (3) increased extracellular fluid calcium concentration.

Integration of Renal Mechanisms for Control of Extracellular Fluid

Extracellular fluid volume is determined mainly by the balance between intake and output of water and salt. In many instances, salt and fluid intakes are dictated by a person's habits rather than by physiologic control mechanisms. Therefore, the burden of extracellular volume regulation is usually placed on the kidneys, which must adapt their excretion of salt and water to match intake of salt and water under steady-state conditions.

In discussing the regulation of extracellular fluid volume, we consider the factors that regulate the amount of sodium chloride in the extracellular fluid because changes in extracellular fluid sodium chloride content usually cause parallel changes in extracellular fluid volume, provided the antidiuretic hormone (ADH)-thirst mechanisms are operative. When the ADH-thirst mechanisms are functioning normally, a change in the amount of sodium chloride in the extracellular fluid is matched by a similar change in the amount of extracellular water, so osmolality and sodium concentration are maintained relatively constant.

Sodium Intake and Excretion Are Precisely Matched Under Steady-State Conditions

An important consideration in overall control of sodium excretion—or excretion of most electrolytes, for that matter—is that under steady-state conditions, excretion by the kidneys is determined by intake. To maintain life, a person must, over the long term, excrete almost precisely the amount of sodium ingested. Therefore, even with disturbances that cause major changes in kidney function, balance between intake and output of sodium usually is restored within a few days.

If disturbances of kidney function are not too severe, sodium balance may be achieved mainly by intrarenal adjustments with minimal changes in extracellular fluid volume or other systemic adjustments. But when perturbations to the kidneys are severe and intrarenal compensations are exhausted, systemic adjustments must be invoked, such as changes in blood pressure, changes in circulating hormones, and alterations of sympathetic nervous system activity.

These adjustments can be costly in terms of overall homeostasis because they cause other changes throughout the body that may, in the long run, be damaging. For example, impaired kidney function may lead to increased blood pressure that, in turn, helps to maintain normal sodium excretion. Over the long term the high blood pressure may cause injury to the blood vessels, heart, and other organs. These compensations, however, are necessary because a sustained imbalance between fluid and electrolyte intake and excretion would quickly lead to accumulation or loss of electrolytes and fluid, causing cardiovascular collapse within a few days. Thus, one can view the systemic adjustments that occur in response to abnormalities of kidney function as a necessary trade-off that brings electrolyte and fluid excretion back in balance with intake.

Sodium Excretion Is Controlled by Altering Glomerular Filtration or Tubular Sodium Reabsorption Rates

The two variables that influence sodium and water excretion are the rates of glomerular filtration and tubular reabsorption:

Excretion = Glomerular filtration − Tubular reabsorption

GFR normally is about 180 L/day, tubular reabsorption is 178.5 L/day, and urine excretion is 1.5 L/day. Thus, small changes in GFR or tubular reabsorption potentially can cause large changes in renal excretion. For example, a 5 percent increase in GFR (to 189 L/day) would cause a 9 L/day increase in urine volume, if tubular compensations did not occur; this would quickly cause catastrophic changes in body fluid volumes. Similarly, small changes in tubular reabsorption, in the absence of compensatory adjustments of GFR, would also lead to dramatic changes in urine volume and sodium excretion. Tubular reabsorption and GFR usually are regulated precisely, so excretion by the kidneys can be exactly matched to intake of water and electrolytes.

Even with disturbances that alter GFR or tubular reabsorption, changes in urinary excretion are minimized by various buffering mechanisms. For example, if the kidneys become greatly vasodilated and GFR increases (as can occur with certain drugs or high fever), this raises sodium chloride delivery to the tubules, which in turn leads to at least two intrarenal compensations: (1) increased tubular reabsorption of much of the extra sodium chloride filtered, called *glomerulotubular balance,* and (2) *macula densa feedback,* in which increased sodium chloride delivery to the distal tubule causes afferent arteriolar constriction and return of GFR toward normal. Likewise, abnormalities of tubular reabsorption in the proximal tubule or loop of Henle are partially compensated for by these same intrarenal feedbacks.

Because neither of these two mechanisms operates perfectly to restore distal sodium chloride delivery all the way back to normal, changes in either GFR or tubular reabsorption can lead to significant changes in urine sodium and water excretion. When this happens, other feedback mechanisms come into play, such as changes in blood pressure and changes in various hormones, and eventually return sodium excretion to equal sodium intake. In the next few sections, we review how these mechanisms operate together to control sodium and water balance and in so doing act also to control extracellular fluid volume. All these feedback mechanisms control renal excretion of sodium and water by altering either GFR or tubular reabsorption.

Importance of Pressure Natriuresis and Pressure Diuresis in Maintaining Body Sodium and Fluid Balance

One of the most basic and powerful mechanisms for the maintenance of sodium and fluid balance, as well as for controlling blood volume and extracellular fluid volume, is the effect of blood pressure on sodium and water excretion—called the *pressure natriuresis* and *pressure diuresis* mechanisms, respectively. As discussed in Chapter 19, this feedback between the kidneys and the circulatory system also plays a dominant role in long-term blood pressure regulation.

Pressure diuresis refers to the effect of increased blood pressure to raise urinary volume excretion, whereas pressure natriuresis refers to the rise in sodium excretion that occurs with elevated blood pressure. Because pressure diuresis and natriuresis usually occur in parallel, we refer to these mechanisms simply as "pressure natriuresis" in the following discussion.

Figure 29-13 shows the effect of arterial pressure on urinary sodium output. Note that acute increases in blood pressure of 30 to 50 mm Hg cause a twofold to threefold increase in urinary sodium output. This effect is independent of changes in activity of the sympathetic nervous system or of various hormones, such as angiotensin II, ADH, or aldosterone, because pressure natriuresis can be demonstrated in an isolated kidney that has been removed from the influence of these factors. With chronic increases in blood pressure, the effectiveness of pressure natriuresis is greatly enhanced because the increased blood pressure also, after a short time delay, suppresses renin release and, therefore, decreases formation of angiotensin II and aldosterone. As discussed previously, decreased levels of

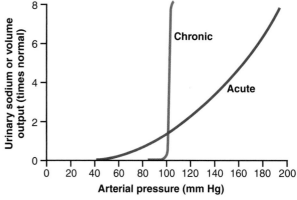

Figure 29-13 Acute and chronic effects of arterial pressure on sodium output by the kidneys (pressure natriuresis). Note that chronic increases in arterial pressure cause much greater increases in sodium output than those measured during acute increases in arterial pressure.

angiotensin II and aldosterone inhibit renal tubular reabsorption of sodium, thereby amplifying the direct effects of increased blood pressure to raise sodium and water excretion.

Pressure Natriuresis and Diuresis Are Key Components of a Renal-Body Fluid Feedback for Regulating Body Fluid Volumes and Arterial Pressure

The effect of increased blood pressure to raise urine output is part of a powerful feedback system that operates to maintain balance between fluid intake and output, as shown in Figure 29-14. This is the same mechanism that is discussed in Chapter 19 for arterial pressure control. The extracellular fluid volume, blood volume, cardiac output, arterial pressure, and urine output are all controlled at the same time as separate parts of this basic feedback mechanism.

During changes in sodium and fluid intake, this feedback mechanism helps to maintain fluid balance and to minimize changes in blood volume, extracellular fluid volume, and arterial pressure as follows:

1. An increase in fluid intake (assuming that sodium accompanies the fluid intake) above the level of urine output causes a temporary accumulation of fluid in the body.

2. As long as fluid intake exceeds urine output, fluid accumulates in the blood and interstitial spaces, causing parallel increases in blood volume and extracellular fluid volume. As discussed later, the actual increases in these variables are usually small because of the effectiveness of this feedback.

3. An increase in blood volume raises mean circulatory filling pressure.

4. An increase in mean circulatory filling pressure raises the pressure gradient for venous return.

5. An increased pressure gradient for venous return elevates cardiac output.

6. An increased cardiac output raises arterial pressure.

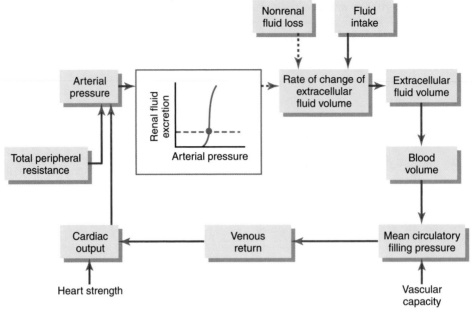

Figure 29-14 Basic renal-body fluid feedback mechanism for control of blood volume, extracellular fluid volume, and arterial pressure. *Solid lines* indicate positive effects, and *dashed lines* indicate negative effects.

7. An increased arterial pressure increases urine output by way of pressure diuresis. The steepness of the normal pressure natriuresis relation indicates that only a slight increase in blood pressure is required to raise urinary excretion severalfold.

8. The increased fluid excretion balances the increased intake, and further accumulation of fluid is prevented.

Thus, the renal-body fluid feedback mechanism operates to prevent continuous accumulation of salt and water in the body during increased salt and water intake. As long as kidney function is normal and the pressure diuresis mechanism is operating effectively, large changes in salt and water intake can be accommodated with only slight changes in blood volume, extracellular fluid volume, cardiac output, and arterial pressure.

The opposite sequence of events occurs when fluid intake falls below normal. In this case, there is a tendency toward decreased blood volume and extracellular fluid volume, as well as reduced arterial pressure. Even a small decrease in blood pressure causes a large decrease in urine output, thereby allowing fluid balance to be maintained with minimal changes in blood pressure, blood volume, or extracellular fluid volume. The effectiveness of this mechanism in preventing large changes in blood volume is demonstrated in Figure 29-15, which shows that changes in blood volume are almost imperceptible despite large variations in daily intake of water and electrolytes, except when intake becomes so low that it is not sufficient to make up for fluid losses caused by evaporation or other inescapable losses.

As discussed later, there are nervous and hormonal systems, in addition to intrarenal mechanisms, that can raise sodium excretion to match increased sodium intake even without measureable increases in arterial pressure

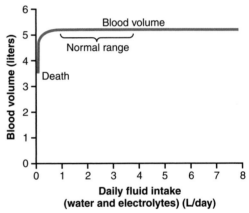

Figure 29-15 Approximate effect of changes in daily fluid intake on blood volume. Note that blood volume remains relatively constant in the normal range of daily fluid intakes.

in many persons. Other individuals who are more "salt sensitive" have significant increases in arterial pressure with even moderate increases in sodium intake. With prolonged high-sodium intake, lasting over several years, high blood pressure may occur even in those persons who are not initially salt sensitive. When blood pressure does rise, pressure natriuresis provides a critical means of maintaining balance between sodium intake and urinary sodium excretion.

Precision of Blood Volume and Extracellular Fluid Volume Regulation

By studying Figure 29-14, one can see why the blood volume remains almost exactly constant despite extreme changes in daily fluid intake. The reason for this is the following: (1) A slight change in blood volume causes a marked change in cardiac output, (2) a slight change in cardiac output causes a large change in blood pressure, and (3) a slight change in blood pressure causes a large change in urine output. These factors work together to provide effective feedback control of blood volume.

The same control mechanisms operate whenever there is a blood loss because of hemorrhage. In this case, a fall in blood pressure along with nervous and hormonal factors discussed later cause fluid retention by the kidneys. Other parallel processes occur to reconstitute the red blood cells and plasma proteins in the blood. If abnormalities of red blood cell volume remain, such as occurs when there is deficiency of erythropoietin or other factors needed to stimulate red blood cell production, the plasma volume will simply make up the difference, and the overall blood volume will return essentially to normal despite the low red blood cell mass.

Distribution of Extracellular Fluid Between the Interstitial Spaces and Vascular System

From Figure 29-14 it is apparent that blood volume and extracellular fluid volume are usually controlled in parallel with each other. Ingested fluid initially goes into the blood, but it rapidly becomes distributed between the interstitial spaces and the plasma. Therefore, blood volume and extracellular fluid volume usually are controlled simultaneously.

There are circumstances, however, in which the distribution of extracellular fluid between the interstitial spaces and blood can vary greatly. As discussed in Chapter 25, *the principal factors that can cause accumulation of fluid in the interstitial spaces include (1) increased capillary hydrostatic pressure, (2) decreased plasma colloid osmotic pressure, (3) increased permeability of the capillaries, and (4) obstruction of lymphatic vessels.* In all these conditions, an unusually high proportion of the extracellular fluid becomes distributed to the interstitial spaces.

Figure 29-16 shows the normal distribution of fluid between the interstitial spaces and the vascular system and the distribution that occurs in edema states. When small amounts of fluid accumulate in the blood as a result of either too much fluid intake or a decrease in renal output of fluid, about 20 to 30 percent of it stays in the blood and increases the blood volume. The remainder is distributed to the interstitial spaces. When the extracellular fluid volume rises more than 30 to 50 percent above normal, almost all the additional fluid goes into the interstitial spaces and little remains in the blood. This occurs because once the interstitial fluid pressure rises from its normally negative value to become positive, the tissue interstitial spaces become compliant and large amounts of fluid then pour into the tissues without interstitial fluid pressure rising much more. In other words, the safety factor against edema, owing to a rising interstitial fluid pressure that counteracts fluid accumulation in the tissues, is lost once the tissues become highly compliant.

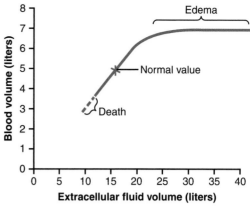

Figure 29-16 Approximate relation between extracellular fluid volume and blood volume, showing a nearly linear relation in the normal range but also showing the failure of blood volume to continue rising when the extracellular fluid volume becomes excessive. When this occurs, the additional extracellular fluid volume resides in the interstitial spaces and edema results.

Thus, under normal conditions, the interstitial spaces act as an "overflow" reservoir for excess fluid, sometimes increasing in volume 10 to 30 liters. This causes edema, as explained in Chapter 25, but it also acts as an important overflow release valve for the circulation, protecting the cardiovascular system against dangerous overload that could lead to pulmonary edema and cardiac failure.

To summarize, extracellular fluid volume and blood volume are controlled simultaneously, but the quantitative amounts of fluid distribution between the interstitium and the blood depend on the physical properties of the circulation and the interstitial spaces, as well as on the dynamics of fluid exchange through the capillary membranes.

Nervous and Hormonal Factors Increase the Effectiveness of Renal-Body Fluid Feedback Control

In Chapter 27, we discuss the nervous and hormonal factors that influence GFR and tubular reabsorption and, therefore, renal excretion of salt and water. These nervous and hormonal mechanisms usually act in concert with the pressure natriuresis and pressure diuresis mechanisms, making them more effective in minimizing the changes in blood volume, extracellular fluid volume, and arterial pressure that occur in response to day-to-day challenges. However, abnormalities of kidney function or of the various nervous and hormonal factors that influence the kidneys can lead to serious changes in blood pressure and body fluid volumes, as discussed later.

Sympathetic Nervous System Control of Renal Excretion: Arterial Baroreceptor and Low-Pressure Stretch Receptor Reflexes

Because the kidneys receive extensive sympathetic innervation, changes in sympathetic activity can alter renal sodium and water excretion, as well as regulation of extracellular fluid volume under some conditions. For example, when blood volume is reduced by hemorrhage, pressures in the pulmonary blood vessels and other low-pressure regions of the thorax decrease, causing reflex activation of the sympathetic nervous system. This in turn increases renal sympathetic nerve activity, which has several effects to decrease sodium and water excretion: (1) constriction of the renal arterioles, with resultant decreased GFR of the sympathetic activation if severe; (2) increased tubular reabsorption of salt and water; and (3) stimulation of renin release and increased angiotensin II and aldosterone formation, both of which further increase tubular reabsorption. And if the reduction in blood volume is great enough to lower systemic arterial pressure, further activation of the sympathetic nervous system occurs because of decreased stretch of the arterial barore-ceptors located in the carotid sinus and aortic arch. All these reflexes together play an important role in the rapid restitution of blood volume that occurs in acute conditions such as hemorrhage. Also, reflex inhibition of renal sympathetic activity may contribute to the rapid elimination of excess fluid in the circulation that occurs after eating a meal that contains large amounts of salt and water.

Role of Angiotensin II in Controlling Renal Excretion

One of the body's most powerful controllers of sodium excretion is angiotensin II. Changes in sodium and fluid intake are associated with reciprocal changes in angiotensin II formation, and this in turn contributes greatly to the maintenance of body sodium and fluid balances. That is, when sodium intake is elevated above normal, renin secretion is decreased, causing decreased angiotensin II formation. Because angiotensin II has several important effects in increasing tubular reabsorption of sodium, as explained in Chapter 27, a reduced level of angiotensin II decreases tubular reabsorption of sodium and water, thus increasing the kidneys' excretion of sodium and water. The net result is to minimize the rise in extracellular fluid volume and arterial pressure that would otherwise occur when sodium intake increases.

Conversely, when sodium intake is reduced below normal, increased levels of angiotensin II cause sodium and water retention and oppose reductions in arterial blood pressure that would otherwise occur. Thus, changes in activity of the renin-angiotensin system act as a powerful amplifier of the pressure natriuresis mechanism for maintaining stable blood pressures and body fluid volumes.

Importance of Changes in Angiotensin II in Altering Pressure Natriuresis. The importance of angiotensin II in making the pressure natriuresis mechanism more effective is shown in Figure 29-17. Note that when the angiotensin control of natriuresis is fully functional, the pressure natriuresis curve is steep (normal curve), indicating that only minor changes in blood pressure are necessary to increase sodium excretion when sodium intake is raised.

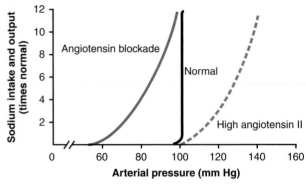

Figure 29-17 Effects of excessive angiotensin II formation and blocking angiotensin II formation on the renal-pressure natriuresis curve. Note that high levels of angiotensin II formation decrease the slope of pressure natriuresis, making blood pressure very sensitive to changes in sodium intake. Blockade of angiotensin II formation shifts pressure natriuresis to lower blood pressures.

In contrast, when angiotensin levels cannot be decreased in response to increased sodium intake (high angiotensin II curve), as occurs in some hypertensive patients who have impaired ability to decrease renin secretion, the pressure natriuresis curve is not nearly as steep. Therefore, when sodium intake is raised, much greater increases in arterial pressure are necessary to increase sodium excretion and maintain sodium balance. For example, in most people, a 10-fold increase in sodium intake causes an increase of only a few millimeters of mercury in arterial pressure, whereas in subjects who cannot suppress angiotensin II formation appropriately in response to excess sodium, the same rise in sodium intake causes blood pressure to rise as much as 50 mm Hg. Thus, the inability to suppress angiotensin II formation when there is excess sodium reduces the slope of pressure natriuresis and makes arterial pressure very salt sensitive, as discussed in Chapter 19.

The use of drugs to block the effects of angiotensin II has proved to be important clinically for improving the kidneys' ability to excrete salt and water. When angiotensin II formation is blocked with an angiotensin-converting enzyme inhibitor (see Figure 29-17) or an angiotensin II receptor antagonist, the renal-pressure natriuresis curve is shifted to lower pressures; this indicates an enhanced ability of the kidneys to excrete sodium because normal levels of sodium excretion can now be maintained at reduced arterial pressures. This shift of pressure natriuresis provides the basis for the chronic blood pressure–lowering effects in hypertensive patients of the angiotensin-converting enzyme inhibitors and angiotensin II receptor antagonists.

Excessive Angiotensin II Does Not Usually Cause Large Increases in Extracellular Fluid Volume Because Increased Arterial Pressure Counterbalances Angiotensin-Mediated Sodium Retention. Although angiotensin II is one of the most powerful sodium- and water-retaining hormones in the body, neither a decrease nor an increase in circulating angiotensin II has a large effect on extracellular fluid volume or blood volume as long as heart failure or kidney failure does not occur. The reason for this is that with large increases in angiotensin II levels, as occurs with a renin-secreting tumor of the kidney, the high angiotensin II levels initially cause sodium and water retention by the kidneys and a small increase in extracellular fluid volume. This also initiates a rise in arterial pressure that quickly increases kidney output of sodium and water, thereby overcoming the sodium- and water-retaining effects of the angiotensin II and re-establishing a balance between intake and output of sodium at a higher blood pressure. Conversely, after blockade of angiotensin II formation, as occurs when an angiotensin-converting enzyme inhibitor is administered, there is initial loss of sodium and water, but the fall in blood pressure offsets this effect and sodium excretion is once again restored to normal.

If the heart is weakened or there is underlying heart disease, cardiac pumping ability may not be great enough to raise arterial pressure enough to overcome the sodium retaining effects of high levels of angiotensin II; in these instances angiotensin II may cause large amounts of sodium and water retention that may progress to *congestive heart failure.* Blockade of angiotensin II formation may, in these cases, relieve some of the sodium and water retention and attenuate the large expansion of extracellular fluid volume associated with heart failure.

Role of Aldosterone in Controlling Renal Excretion

Aldosterone increases sodium reabsorption, especially in the cortical collecting tubules. The increased sodium reabsorption is also associated with increased water reabsorption and potassium secretion. Therefore, the net effect of aldosterone is to make the kidneys retain sodium and water but also to increase potassium excretion in the urine.

The function of aldosterone in regulating sodium balance is closely related to that described for angiotensin II. That is, with reduction in sodium intake, the increased angiotensin II levels that occur stimulate aldosterone secretion, which in turn contributes to the reduction in urinary sodium excretion and, therefore, to the maintenance of sodium balance. Conversely, with high sodium intake, suppression of aldosterone formation decreases tubular reabsorption, allowing the kidneys to excrete larger amounts of sodium. Thus, changes in aldosterone formation also aid the pressure natriuresis mechanism in maintaining sodium balance during variations in salt intake.

During Chronic Oversecretion of Aldosterone, the Kidneys "Escape" from Sodium Retention as Arterial Pressure Rises.
Although aldosterone has powerful effects on sodium reabsorption, when there is excessive infusion of aldosterone or excessive formation of aldosterone, as occurs in patients with tumors of the adrenal gland (Conn's syndrome), the increased sodium reabsorption and decreased sodium excretion by the kidneys are transient. After 1 to 3 days of sodium and water retention, the extracellular fluid volume rises by about 10 to 15 percent and there is a simultaneous increase in arterial blood pressure. When the arterial pressure rises sufficiently, the kidneys "escape" from the

sodium and water retention and thereafter excrete amounts of sodium equal to the daily intake, despite continued presence of high levels of aldosterone. The primary reason for the escape is the pressure natriuresis and diuresis that occur when the arterial pressure rises.

In patients with adrenal insufficiency who do not secrete enough aldosterone (Addison's disease), there is increased excretion of sodium and water, reduction in extracellular fluid volume, and a tendency toward low blood pressure. In the complete absence of aldosterone, the volume depletion may be severe unless the person is allowed to eat large amounts of salt and drink large amounts of water to balance the increased urine output of salt and water.

Role of ADH in Controlling Renal Water Excretion

As discussed in Chapter 28, ADH plays an important role in allowing the kidneys to form a small volume of concentrated urine while excreting normal amounts of salt. This effect is especially important during water deprivation, which strongly elevates plasma levels of ADH that in turn increase water reabsorption by the kidneys and help to minimize the decreases in extracellular fluid volume and arterial pressure that would otherwise occur. Water deprivation for 24 to 48 hours normally causes only a small decrease in extracellular fluid volume and arterial pressure. However, if the effects of ADH are blocked with a drug that antagonizes the action of ADH to promote water reabsorption in the distal and collecting tubules, the same period of water deprivation causes a substantial fall in both extracellular fluid volume and arterial pressure. Conversely, when there is excess extracellular volume, *decreased* ADH levels reduce reabsorption of water by the kidneys, thus helping to rid the body of the excess volume.

Excess ADH Secretion Usually Causes Only Small Increases in Extracellular Fluid Volume but Large Decreases in Sodium Concentration.
Although ADH is important in regulating extracellular fluid volume, excessive levels of ADH seldom cause large increases in arterial pressure or extracellular fluid volume. Infusion of large amounts of ADH into animals initially causes renal retention of water and a 10 to 15 percent increase in extracellular fluid volume. As the arterial pressure rises in response to this increased volume, much of the excess volume is excreted because of the pressure diuresis mechanism. Also, the rise in blood pressure causes pressure natriuresis and loss of sodium from the extracellular fluid. After several days of ADH infusion, the blood volume and extracellular fluid volume are elevated no more than 5 to 10 percent and the arterial pressure is also elevated by less than 10 mm Hg. The same is true for patients with *inappropriate ADH syndrome,* in which ADH levels may be elevated severalfold.

Thus, high levels of ADH do not cause major increases of either body fluid volume or arterial pressure, although *high ADH levels can cause severe reductions in extracellular sodium ion concentration.* The reason for this is that increased water reabsorption by the kidneys dilutes the extracellular sodium, and at the same time, the small increase in blood pressure that does occur causes loss of sodium from the extracellular fluid in the urine through pressure natriuresis.

In patients who have lost their ability to secrete ADH because of destruction of the supraoptic nuclei, the urine volume may become 5 to 10 times normal. This is almost always compensated for by ingestion of enough water to maintain fluid balance. If free access to water is prevented, the inability to secrete ADH may lead to marked reductions in blood volume and arterial pressure.

Role of Atrial Natriuretic Peptide in Controlling Renal Excretion

Thus far, we have discussed mainly the role of sodium- and water-retaining hormones in controlling extracellular fluid volume. However, several different natriuretic hormones may also contribute to volume regulation. One of the most important of the natriuretic hormones is a peptide referred to as *atrial natriuretic peptide (ANP),* released by the cardiac atrial muscle fibers. The stimulus for release of this peptide appears to be increased stretch of the atria, which can result from excess blood volume. Once released by the cardiac atria, ANP enters the circulation and acts on the kidneys to cause small increases in GFR and decreases in sodium reabsorption by the collecting ducts. These combined actions of ANP lead to increased excretion of salt and water, which helps to compensate for the excess blood volume.

Changes in ANP levels probably help to minimize changes in blood volume during various disturbances, such as increased salt and water intake. However, excessive production of ANP or even complete lack of ANP does not cause major changes in blood volume because these effects can easily be overcome by small changes in blood pressure, acting through pressure natriuresis. For example, infusions of large amounts of ANP initially raise urine output of salt and water and cause slight decreases in blood volume. In less than 24 hours, this effect is overcome by a slight decrease in blood pressure that returns urine output toward normal, despite continued excess of ANP.

Integrated Responses to Changes in Sodium Intake

The integration of the different control systems that regulate sodium and fluid excretion under normal conditions can be summarized by examining the homeostatic responses to progressive increases in dietary sodium intake. As discussed previously, the kidneys have an amazing capability to match their excretion of salt and water to intakes that can range from as low as one tenth of normal to as high as 10 times normal.

High Sodium Intake Suppresses Antinatriuretic Systems and Activates Natriuretic Systems. As sodium intake is increased, sodium output initially lags slightly behind intake. The time delay results in a small increase in the cumulative sodium balance, which causes a slight increase in extracellular fluid volume. It is mainly this small increase in extracellular fluid volume that triggers various mechanisms in the body to increase sodium excretion. These mechanisms include the following:

1. *Activation of low-pressure receptor reflexes* that originate from the stretch receptors of the right atrium and the pulmonary blood vessels. Signals from the stretch receptors go to the brain stem and there inhibit sympathetic nerve activity to the kidneys to decrease tubular sodium reabsorption. This mechanism is most important in the first few hours—or perhaps the first day—after a large increase in salt and water intake.

2. *Suppression of angiotensin II formation,* caused by increased arterial pressure and extracellular fluid volume expansion, decreases tubular sodium reabsorption by eliminating the normal effect of angiotensin II to increase sodium reabsorption. Also, reduced angiotensin II decreases aldosterone secretion, thus further reducing tubular sodium reabsorption.

3. *Stimulation of natriuretic systems,* especially ANP, contributes further to increased sodium excretion. Thus, the combined activation of natriuretic systems and suppression of sodium- and water-retaining systems leads to an increase in sodium excretion when sodium intake is increased. The opposite changes take place when sodium intake is reduced below normal levels.

4. *Small increases in arterial pressure,* caused by volume expansion, may occur with large increases in sodium intake; this raises sodium excretion through pressure natriuresis. As discussed previously, if the nervous, hormonal, and intrarenal mechanisms are operating effectively, measurable increases in blood pressure may not occur even with large increases in sodium intake over several days. However, when high sodium intake is sustained for months or years, the kidneys may become damaged and less effective in excreting sodium, necessitating increased blood pressure to maintain sodium balance through the pressure natriuresis mechanism.

Conditions That Cause Large Increases in Blood Volume and Extracellular Fluid Volume

Despite the powerful regulatory mechanisms that maintain blood volume and extracellular fluid volume reasonably constant, there are abnormal conditions that can cause large increases in both of these variables. Almost all of these conditions result from circulatory abnormalities.

Increased Blood Volume and Extracellular Fluid Volume Caused by Heart Diseases

In congestive heart failure, blood volume may increase 15 to 20 percent and extracellular fluid volume sometimes increases by 200 percent or more. The reason for this can be understood by re-examination of Figure 29-14. Initially, heart failure reduces cardiac output and, consequently, decreases arterial pressure. This in turn activates multiple sodium-retaining systems, especially the renin-angiotensin, aldosterone, and sympathetic nervous systems. In addition, the low blood pressure itself causes the kidneys to retain salt and water. Therefore, the kidneys retain volume in an attempt to return the arterial pressure and cardiac output toward normal.

If the heart failure is not too severe, the rise in blood volume can often return cardiac output and arterial pressure virtually all the way to normal and sodium excretion will eventually increase back to normal, although there will remain increased extracellular fluid volume and blood volume to keep the weakened heart pumping adequately. However, if the heart is greatly weakened, arterial pressure may not be able to increase enough to restore urine output to normal. When this occurs, the kidneys continue to retain volume until the person develops severe circulatory congestion and may eventually die of pulmonary edema.

In myocardial failure, heart valvular disease, and congenital abnormalities of the heart, increased blood volume serves as an important circulatory compensation, which helps to return cardiac output and blood pressure toward normal. This allows even the weakened heart to maintain a life-sustaining level of cardiac output.

Increased Blood Volume Caused by Increased Capacity of Circulation

Any condition that increases vascular capacity will also cause the blood volume to increase to fill this extra capacity. An increase in vascular capacity initially reduces mean circulatory filling pressure (see Figure 29-14), which leads to decreased cardiac output and decreased arterial pressure. The fall in pressure causes salt and water retention by the kidneys until the blood volume increases sufficiently to fill the extra capacity.

In pregnancy the increased vascular capacity of the uterus, placenta, and other enlarged organs of the woman's body regularly increases the blood volume 15 to 25 percent. Similarly, in patients who have large varicose veins of the legs, which in rare instances may hold up to an extra liter of blood, the blood volume simply increases to fill the extra vascular capacity. In these cases, salt and water are retained by the kidneys until the total vascular bed is filled enough to raise blood pressure to the level required to balance renal output of fluid with daily intake of fluid.

Conditions That Cause Large Increases in Extracellular Fluid Volume but with Normal Blood Volume

In several conditions extracellular fluid volume becomes markedly increased but blood volume remains normal or even slightly reduced. These conditions are usually initiated by leakage of fluid and protein into the interstitium, which tends to decrease the blood volume. The kidneys' response to these conditions is similar to the response after hemorrhage. That is, the kidneys retain salt and water in an attempt to restore blood volume toward normal. Much of the extra fluid, however, leaks into the interstitium, causing further edema.

Nephrotic Syndrome—Loss of Plasma Proteins in Urine and Sodium Retention by the Kidneys

The general mechanisms that lead to extracellular edema are reviewed in Chapter 25. One of the most important clinical causes of edema is the so-called *nephrotic syndrome.* In nephrotic syndrome, the glomerular capillaries leak large amounts of protein into the filtrate and the urine because of increased glomerular capillary permeability. Thirty to 50 grams of plasma protein can be lost in the urine each day, sometimes causing the plasma protein concentration to fall to less than one-third normal. As a consequence of the decreased plasma protein concentration, the plasma colloid osmotic pressure falls to low levels. This causes the capillaries all over the body to filter large amounts of fluid into the various tissues, which in turn causes edema and decreases the plasma volume.

Renal sodium retention in nephrotic syndrome occurs through multiple mechanisms activated by leakage of protein and fluid from the plasma into the interstitial fluid, including stimulation of various sodium-retaining systems such as the renin-angiotensin system, aldosterone, and the sympathetic nervous system. The kidneys continue to retain sodium and water until plasma volume is restored nearly to normal. However, because of the large amount of sodium and water retention, the plasma protein concentration becomes further diluted, causing still more fluid to leak into the tissues of the body. The net result is massive fluid retention by the kidneys until tremendous extracellular edema occurs unless treatment is instituted to restore the plasma proteins.

Liver Cirrhosis—Decreased Synthesis of Plasma Proteins by the Liver and Sodium Retention by the Kidneys

A similar sequence of events occurs in cirrhosis of the liver as in nephrotic syndrome, except that in liver cirrhosis, the reduction in plasma protein concentration results from destruction of liver cells, thus reducing the ability of the liver to synthesize enough plasma proteins. Cirrhosis is also associated with large amounts of fibrous tissue in the liver structure, which greatly impedes the flow of portal blood through the liver. This in turn raises capillary pressure throughout the portal vascular bed, which also contributes to the leakage of fluid and proteins into the peritoneal cavity, a condition called *ascites.*

Once fluid and protein are lost from the circulation, the renal responses are similar to those observed in other conditions associated with decreased plasma volume. That is, the kidneys continue to retain salt and water until plasma volume and arterial pressure are restored to normal. In some cases, plasma volume may actually increase above normal because of increased vascular capacity in cirrhosis; the high pressures in the portal circulation can greatly distend veins and therefore increase vascular capacity.

Bibliography

Appel LJ, Brands MW, Daniels SR, et al: Dietary approaches to prevent and treat hypertension: a scientific statement from the American Heart Association, *Hypertension* 47:296, 2006.

Antunes-Rodrigues J, de Castro M, Elias LL, et al: Neuroendocrine control of body fluid metabolism, *Physiol Rev* 84:169, 2004.

Cowley AW Jr: Long-term control of arterial pressure, *Physiol Rev* 72:231, 1992.

Giebisch G, Hebert SC, Wang WH: New aspects of renal potassium transport, *Pflugers Arch* 446:289, 2003.

Guyton AC: Blood pressure control—special role of the kidneys and body fluids, *Science* 252:1813, 1991.

Granger JP, Hall JE: Role of the kidney in hypertension. In Lip GYH, Hall JE, eds: *Comprehensive Hypertension*, Philadelphia, 2008, Mosby-Elsevier, pp 241–264.

Hall JE, Granger JP, Hall ME, et al: Pathophysiology of hypertension. In *Hurst's The Heart*, ed 12, New York, 2008, McGraw-Hill Medical, pp 1570–1609.

Hall JE, Brands MW: The renin-angiotensin-aldosterone system: renal mechanisms and circulatory homeostasis. In Seldin DW, Giebisch G, eds: *The Kidney—Physiology and Pathophysiology*, ed 3, New York, 2000, Raven Press, pp 1009–1046.

Hall JE: Angiotensin II and long-term arterial pressure regulation: the overriding dominance of the kidney, *J Am Soc Nephrol* 10(Suppl 12):s258, 1999.

Hebert SC, Desir G, Giebisch G, et al: Molecular diversity and regulation of renal potassium channels, *Physiol Rev* 85:319, 2005.

Hoenderop JG, Bindels RJ: Epithelial Ca2+ and Mg2+ channels in health and disease, *J Am Soc Nephrol* 16:15, 2005.

Huang CL, Kuo E: Mechanism of hypokalemia in magnesium deficiency, *J Am Soc Nephrol* 18:2649, 2007.

Murer H, Hernando N, Forster I, et al: Regulation of Na/Pi transporter in the proximal tubule, *Annu Rev Physiol* 65:531, 2003.

Schrier RW: Decreased effective blood volume in edematous disorders: what does this mean? *J Am Soc Nephrol* 18:2028, 2007.

Suki WN, Lederer ED, Rouse D: Renal transport of calcium magnesium and phosphate. In: Brenner BM, ed: *The Kidney*, ed 6, Philadelphia, 2000, WB Saunders, pp 520–574.

Suzuki Y, Landowski CP, Hediger MA: Mechanisms and regulation of epithelial Ca2+ absorption in health and disease, *Annu Rev Physiol* 70:257, 2008.

Wall SM: Recent advances in our understanding of intercalated cells, *Curr Opin Nephrol Hypertens* 14:480, 2005.

Warnock DG: Renal genetic disorders related to K+ and Mg2+, *Annu Rev Physiol* 64:845, 2002.

Worcester EM, Coe FL: New insights into the pathogenesis of idiopathic hypercalciuria, *Semin Nephrol* 28:120, 2008.

Young DB: Quantitative analysis of aldosterone's role in potassium regulation, *Am J Physiol* 255:F811, 1988.

Young DB: Analysis of long-term potassium regulation, *Endocr Rev* 6:24, 1985.

Acid-Base Regulation

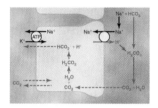

Regulation of hydrogen ion (H⁺) balance is similar in some ways to the regulation of other ions in the body. For instance, there must be a balance between the intake or production of H⁺ and the net removal of H⁺ from the body to achieve homeostasis. And, as is true for other ions, the kidneys play a key role in regulating H⁺ removal from the body. However, precise control of extracellular fluid H⁺ concentration involves much more than simple elimination of H⁺ by the kidneys. There are also multiple acid-base buffering mechanisms involving the blood, cells, and lungs that are essential in maintaining normal H⁺ concentrations in both the extracellular and intracellular fluid.

In this chapter, the various mechanisms that contribute to the regulation of H⁺ concentration are discussed, with special emphasis on the control of renal H⁺ secretion and renal reabsorption, production, and excretion of bicarbonate ions (HCO_3^-), one of the key components of acid-base control systems in the body fluids.

H⁺ Concentration Is Precisely Regulated

Precise H⁺ regulation is essential because the activities of almost all enzyme systems in the body are influenced by H⁺ concentration. Therefore, changes in H⁺ concentration alter virtually all cell and body functions.

Compared with other ions, the H⁺ concentration of the body fluids normally is kept at a low level. For example, the concentration of sodium in extracellular fluid (142 mEq/L) is about 3.5 million times as great as the normal concentration of H⁺, which averages only 0.00004 mEq/L. Equally important, the normal variation in H⁺ concentration in extracellular fluid is only about one millionth as great as the normal variation in sodium ion (Na⁺) concentration. Thus, the precision with which H⁺ is regulated emphasizes its importance to the various cell functions.

Acids and Bases—Their Definitions and Meanings

A hydrogen ion is a single free proton released from a hydrogen atom. Molecules containing hydrogen atoms that can release hydrogen ions in solutions are referred to as *acids*. An example is hydrochloric acid (HCl), which ionizes in water to form hydrogen ions (H⁺) and chloride ions (Cl⁻). Likewise, carbonic acid (H_2CO_3) ionizes in water to form H⁺ and bicarbonate ions (HCO_3^-).

A *base* is an ion or a molecule that can accept an H⁺. For example, HCO_3^- is a base because it can combine with H⁺ to form H_2CO_3. Likewise, $HPO_4^=$ is a base because it can accept an H⁺ to form $H_2PO_4^-$. The proteins in the body also function as bases because some of the amino acids that make up proteins have net negative charges that readily accept H⁺. The protein hemoglobin in the red blood cells and proteins in the other cells of the body are among the most important of the body's bases.

The terms *base* and *alkali* are often used synonymously. An *alkali* is a molecule formed by the combination of one or more of the alkaline metals—sodium, potassium, lithium, and so forth—with a highly basic ion such as a hydroxyl ion (OH⁻). The base portion of these molecules reacts quickly with H⁺ to remove it from solution; they are, therefore, typical bases. For similar reasons, the term *alkalosis* refers to excess removal of H⁺ from the body fluids, in contrast to the excess addition of H⁺, which is referred to as *acidosis*.

Strong and Weak Acids and Bases. A strong acid is one that rapidly dissociates and releases especially large amounts of H⁺ in solution. An example is HCl. Weak acids are less likely to dissociate their ions and, therefore, release H⁺ with less vigor. An example is H_2CO_3. A strong base is one that reacts rapidly and strongly with H⁺ and, therefore, quickly removes these from a solution. A typical example is OH⁻, which reacts with H⁺ to form water (H_2O). A typical weak base is HCO_3^- because it binds with H⁺ much more weakly than does OH⁻. Most acids and bases in the extracellular fluid that are involved in normal acid-base regulation are weak acids and bases. The most important ones that we discuss in detail are H_2CO_3 and HCO_3^- base.

Normal H$^+$ Concentration and pH of Body Fluids and Changes That Occur in Acidosis and Alkalosis.

As discussed earlier, the blood H$^+$ concentration is normally maintained within tight limits around a normal value of about 0.00004 mEq/L (40 nEq/L). Normal variations are only about 3 to 5 nEq/L, but under extreme conditions, the H$^+$ concentration can vary from as low as 10 nEq/L to as high as 160 nEq/L without causing death.

Because H$^+$ concentration normally is low, and because these small numbers are cumbersome, it is customary to express H$^+$ concentration on a logarithm scale, using pH units. pH is related to the actual H$^+$ concentration by the following formula (H$^+$ concentration [H$^+$] is expressed in *equivalents* per liter):

$$pH = \log \frac{1}{[H^+]} = -\log[H^+]$$

For example, the normal [H$^+$] is 40 nEq/L (0.00000004 Eq/L). Therefore, the normal pH is

$$pH = -\log[0.00000004]$$
$$pH = 7.4$$

From this formula, one can see that pH is inversely related to the H$^+$ concentration; therefore, a low pH corresponds to a high H$^+$ concentration and a high pH corresponds to a low H$^+$ concentration.

The normal pH of arterial blood is 7.4, whereas the pH of venous blood and interstitial fluids is about 7.35 because of the extra amounts of carbon dioxide (CO_2) released from the tissues to form H_2CO_3 in these fluids (Table 30-1). Because the normal pH of arterial blood is 7.4, a person is considered to have *acidosis* when the pH falls below this value and to have *alkalosis* when the pH rises above 7.4. The lower limit of pH at which a person can live more than a few hours is about 6.8, and the upper limit is about 8.0.

Intracellular pH usually is slightly lower than plasma pH because the metabolism of the cells produces acid, especially H_2CO_3. Depending on the type of cells, the pH of intracellular fluid has been estimated to range between 6.0 and 7.4. Hypoxia of the tissues and poor blood flow to the tissues can cause acid accumulation and decreased intracellular pH.

The pH of urine can range from 4.5 to 8.0, depending on the acid-base status of the extracellular fluid. As discussed later, the kidneys play a major role in correcting abnormalities of extracellular fluid H$^+$ concentration by excreting acids or bases at variable rates.

An extreme example of an acidic body fluid is the HCl secreted into the stomach by the oxyntic (parietal) cells of the stomach mucosa, as discussed in Chapter 64. The H$^+$ concentration in these cells is about 4 million times greater than the hydrogen concentration in blood, with a pH of 0.8. In the remainder of this chapter, we discuss the regulation of extracellular fluid H$^+$ concentration.

Defending Against Changes in H$^+$ Concentration: Buffers, Lungs, and Kidneys

Three primary systems regulate the H$^+$ concentration in the body fluids to prevent acidosis or alkalosis: (1) the *chemical acid-base buffer systems of the body fluids*, which immediately combine with acid or base to prevent excessive changes in H$^+$ concentration; (2) the *respiratory center*, which regulates the removal of CO_2 (and, therefore, H_2CO_3) from the extracellular fluid; and (3) the *kidneys*, which can excrete either acid or alkaline urine, thereby readjusting the extracellular fluid H$^+$ concentration toward normal during acidosis or alkalosis.

When there is a change in H$^+$ concentration, the *buffer systems* of the body fluids react within seconds to minimize these changes. Buffer systems do not eliminate H$^+$ from or add them to the body but only keep them tied up until balance can be re-established.

The second line of defense, the *respiratory system*, acts within a few minutes to eliminate CO_2 and, therefore, H_2CO_3 from the body.

These first two lines of defense keep the H$^+$ concentration from changing too much until the more slowly responding third line of defense, the *kidneys*, can eliminate the excess acid or base from the body. Although the kidneys are relatively slow to respond compared with the other defenses, over a period of hours to several days, they are by far the most powerful of the acid-base regulatory systems.

Table 30-1 pH and H$^+$ Concentration of Body Fluids

	H$^+$ Concentration (mEq/L)	pH
Extracellular fluid		
Arterial blood	4.0×10^{-5}	7.40
Venous blood	4.5×10^{-5}	7.35
Interstitial fluid	4.5×10^{-5}	7.35
Intracellular fluid	1×10^{-3} to 4×10^{-5}	6.0-7.4
Urine	3×10^{-2} to 1×10^{-5}	4.5-8.0
Gastric HCl	160	0.8

Buffering of H$^+$ in the Body Fluids

A buffer is any substance that can reversibly bind H$^+$. The general form of the buffering reaction is

$$\textbf{Buffer} + \textbf{H}^+ \rightleftharpoons \textbf{H Buffer}$$

In this example, a free H$^+$ combines with the buffer to form a weak acid (H buffer) that can either remain as an unassociated molecule or dissociate back to buffer and H$^+$. When the H$^+$ concentration increases, the reaction is forced to the right and more H$^+$ binds to the buffer, as long as buffer is available. Conversely, when the H⁺ concentration decreases, the reaction shifts toward the left and H⁺ is released from the buffer. In this way, changes in H⁺ concentration are minimized.

The importance of the body fluid buffers can be quickly realized if one considers the low concentration of H⁺ in the body fluids and the relatively large amounts of acids produced by the body each day. For example, about 80 milliequivalents of H⁺ is either ingested or produced each day by metabolism, whereas the H⁺ concentration of the body fluids normally is only about 0.00004 mEq/L. Without buffering, the daily production and ingestion of acids would cause huge changes in body fluid H⁺ concentration.

The action of acid-base buffers can perhaps best be explained by considering the buffer system that is quantitatively the most important in the extracellular fluid—the bicarbonate buffer system.

Bicarbonate Buffer System

The bicarbonate buffer system consists of a water solution that contains two ingredients: (1) a weak acid, H_2CO_3, and (2) a bicarbonate salt, such as $NaHCO_3$.

H_2CO_3 is formed in the body by the reaction of CO_2 with H_2O.

$$CO_2 + H_2O \underset{\text{carbonic anhydrase}}{\overset{}{\rightleftharpoons}} H_2CO_3$$

This reaction is slow, and exceedingly small amounts of H_2CO_3 are formed unless the enzyme *carbonic anhydrase* is present. This enzyme is especially abundant in the walls of the lung alveoli, where CO_2 is released; carbonic anhydrase is also present in the epithelial cells of the renal tubules, where CO_2 reacts with H_2O to form H_2CO_3.

H_2CO_3 ionizes weakly to form small amounts of H⁺ and HCO_3^-.

$$H_2CO_3 \rightleftharpoons H^+ + HCO_3^-$$

The second component of the system, bicarbonate salt, occurs predominantly as sodium bicarbonate ($NaHCO_3$) in the extracellular fluid. $NaHCO_3$ ionizes almost completely to form HCO_3^- and Na⁺, as follows:

$$NaHCO_3 \rightleftharpoons Na^+ + HCO_3^-$$

Now, putting the entire system together, we have the following:

$$CO_2 + H_2O \rightleftharpoons H_2CO_3 \rightleftharpoons H^+ + \underbrace{HCO_3^-}_{+ Na^+}$$

Because of the weak dissociation of H_2CO_3, the H⁺ concentration is extremely small.

When a strong acid such as HCl is added to the bicarbonate buffer solution, the increased H⁺ released from the acid (HCl → H⁺ + Cl⁻) is buffered by HCO_3^-.

$$\uparrow H^+ + HCO_3^- \rightarrow H_2CO_3 \rightarrow CO_2 + H_2O$$

As a result, more H_2CO_3 is formed, causing increased CO_2 and H_2O production. From these reactions, one can see that H⁺ from the strong acid HCl reacts with HCO_3^- to form the very weak acid H_2CO_3, which in turn forms CO_2 and H_2O. The excess CO_2 greatly stimulates respiration, which eliminates the CO_2 from the extracellular fluid.

The opposite reactions take place when a strong base, such as sodium hydroxide (NaOH), is added to the bicarbonate buffer solution.

$$NaOH + H_2CO_3 \rightarrow NaHCO_3 + H_2O$$

In this case, the OH⁻ from the NaOH combines with H_2CO_3 to form additional HCO_3^-. Thus, the weak base $NaHCO_3$ replaces the strong base NaOH. At the same time, the concentration of H_2CO_3 decreases (because it reacts with NaOH), causing more CO_2 to combine with H_2O to replace the H_2CO_3.

$$CO_2 + H_2O \longrightarrow H_2CO_3 \longrightarrow \uparrow HCO_3^- + H^+$$
$$+ \qquad\qquad\qquad +$$
$$NaOH \qquad\qquad\qquad Na$$

The net result, therefore, is a tendency for the CO_2 levels in the blood to decrease, but the decreased CO_2 in the blood inhibits respiration and decreases the rate of CO_2 expiration. The rise in blood HCO_3^- that occurs is compensated for by increased renal excretion of HCO_3^-.

Quantitative Dynamics of the Bicarbonate Buffer System
All acids, including H_2CO_3, are ionized to some extent. From mass balance considerations, the concentrations of H⁺ and HCO_3^- are proportional to the concentration of H_2CO_3.

$$H_2CO_3 \rightleftharpoons H^+ + HCO_3^-$$

For any acid, the concentration of the acid relative to its dissociated ions is defined by the *dissociation constant K'*.

$$K' = \frac{H^+ \times HCO_3^-}{H_2CO_3} \tag{1}$$

This equation indicates that in an H_2CO_3 solution, the amount of free H⁺ is equal to

$$H^+ = K' \times \frac{H_2CO_3}{HCO_3^-} \tag{2}$$

The concentration of undissociated H_2CO_3 cannot be measured in solution because it rapidly dissociates into CO_2 and H_2O or to H⁺ and HCO_3^-. However, the CO_2 dissolved in the blood is directly proportional to the amount of undissociated H_2CO_3. Therefore, equation 2 can be rewritten as

$$H^+ = K \times \frac{CO_2}{HCO_3^-} \tag{3}$$

The dissociation constant (K) for equation 3 is only about $1/400$ of the dissociation constant (K') of equation 2 because the proportionality ratio between H_2CO_3 and CO_2 is 1:400.

Equation 3 is written in terms of the total amount of CO_2 dissolved in solution. However, most clinical laboratories measure the blood CO_2 tension (PCO_2) rather than the actual amount of CO_2. Fortunately, the amount of CO_2 in the blood is a linear function of P_{CO_2} multiplied by the solubility coefficient for CO_2; under physiologic conditions, the solubility coefficient for CO_2 is 0.03 mmol/mm Hg at body temperature. This means that 0.03 millimole of H_2CO_3 is present in the blood for each mm Hg P_{CO_2} measured. Therefore, equation 3 can be rewritten as

$$H^+ = K \times \frac{(0.03 \times P_{CO_2})}{HCO_3^-} \qquad (4)$$

Henderson-Hasselbalch Equation. As discussed earlier, it is customary to express H^+ concentration in pH units rather than in actual concentrations. Recall that pH is defined as $pH = -\log H^+$.

The dissociation constant can be expressed in a similar manner.

$$pK = -\log K$$

Therefore, we can express the H^+ concentration in equation 4 in pH units by taking the negative logarithm of that equation, which yields

$$-\log H^+ = -\log K - \log \frac{(0.03 \times P_{CO_2})}{HCO_3^-} \qquad (5)$$

Therefore,

$$pH = pK - \log \frac{(0.03 \times P_{CO_2})}{HCO_3^-} \qquad (6)$$

Rather than work with a negative logarithm, we can change the sign of the logarithm and invert the numerator and denominator in the last term, using the law of logarithms to yield

$$pH = pK + \log \frac{HCO_3^-}{(0.03 \times P_{CO_2})} \qquad (7)$$

For the bicarbonate buffer system, the pK is 6.1, and equation 7 can be written as

$$pH = 6.1 + \log \frac{HCO_3^-}{0.03 \times P_{CO_2}} \qquad (8)$$

Equation 8 is the Henderson-Hasselbalch equation, and with it, one can calculate the pH of a solution if the molar concentration of HCO_3^- and the P_{CO_2} are known.

From the Henderson-Hasselbalch equation, it is apparent that an increase in HCO_3^- concentration causes the pH to rise, shifting the acid-base balance toward alkalosis. An increase in P_{CO_2} causes the pH to decrease, shifting the acid-base balance toward acidosis.

The Henderson-Hasselbalch equation, in addition to defining the determinants of normal pH regulation and acid-base balance in the extracellular fluid, provides insight into the physiologic control of acid and base composition of the extracellular fluid. As discussed later, *the HCO_3^- concentration is regulated mainly by the kidneys, whereas the P_{CO_2} in extracellular fluid is controlled by the rate of respiration.* By increasing the rate of respiration, the lungs remove CO_2 from the plasma, and by decreasing respiration, the lungs elevate P_{CO_2}. Normal physiologic acid-base homeostasis results from the coordinated efforts of both of these organs, the lungs and the kidneys, and acid-base disorders occur when one or both of these control mechanisms are impaired, thus altering either the HCO_3^- concentration or the P_{CO_2} of extracellular fluid.

When disturbances of acid-base balance result from a primary change in extracellular fluid HCO_3^- concentration, they are referred to as *metabolic* acid-base disorders. Therefore, acidosis caused by a primary decrease in HCO_3^- concentration is termed *metabolic acidosis*, whereas alkalosis caused by a primary increase in HCO_3^- concentration is called *metabolic alkalosis*. Acidosis caused by an increase in P_{CO_2} is called *respiratory acidosis*, whereas alkalosis caused by a decrease in P_{CO_2} is termed *respiratory alkalosis*.

Bicarbonate Buffer System Titration Curve. Figure 30-1 shows the changes in pH of the extracellular fluid when the ratio of HCO_3^- to CO_2 in extracellular fluid is altered. When the concentrations of these two components are equal, the right-hand portion of equation 8 becomes the log of 1, which is equal to 0. Therefore, when the two components of the buffer system are equal, the pH of the solution is the same as the pK (6.1) of the bicarbonate buffer system. When base is added to the system, part of the dissolved CO_2 is converted into HCO_3^- causing an increase in the ratio of HCO_3^- to CO_2 and increasing the pH, as is evident from the Henderson-Hasselbalch equation. When acid is added, it is buffered by HCO_3^-, which is then converted into dissolved CO_2, decreasing the ratio of HCO_3^- to CO_2 and decreasing the pH of the extracellular fluid.

"Buffer Power" Is Determined by the Amount and Relative Concentrations of the Buffer Components. From the titration curve in Figure 30-1, several points are apparent. First, the pH of the system is the same as the pK when each of the components (HCO_3^- and CO_2) constitutes 50 percent of the total concentration of the buffer system. Second, the buffer system is most effective in the central part of the curve, where the pH is near the pK of the system. This means that the change in pH for any given amount of acid or base added to the system is least when the pH is near the pK of the system. The buffer system is still reasonably effective for 1.0 pH unit on either side of the pK, which for the bicarbonate buffer system extends from a pH of about 5.1 to 7.1 units. Beyond these limits, the buffering power rapidly diminishes. And when all the CO_2 has been converted into HCO_3^- or when all the HCO_3^- has been converted into CO_2, the system has no more buffering power.

The absolute concentration of the buffers is also an important factor in determining the buffer power of a system. With low concentrations of the buffers, only a small amount of acid or base added to the solution changes the pH considerably.

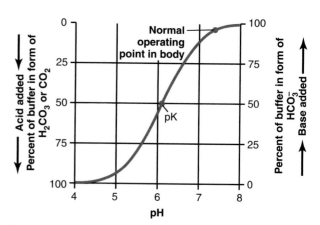

Figure 30-1 Titration curve for bicarbonate buffer system showing the pH of extracellular fluid when the percentages of buffer in the form of HCO_3^- and CO_2 (or H_2CO_3) are altered.

Bicarbonate Buffer System Is the Most Important Extracellular Buffer. From the titration curve shown in Figure 30-1, one would not expect the bicarbonate buffer system to be powerful, for two reasons: First, the pH of the extracellular fluid is about 7.4, whereas the pK of the bicarbonate buffer system is 6.1. This means that there is about 20 times as much of the bicarbonate buffer system in the form of HCO_3^- as in the form of dissolved CO_2. For this reason, this system operates on the portion of the buffering curve where the slope is low and the buffering power is poor. Second, the concentrations of the two elements of the bicarbonate system, CO_2 and HCO_3^-, are not great.

Despite these characteristics, the bicarbonate buffer system is the most powerful extracellular buffer in the body. This apparent paradox is due mainly to the fact that the two elements of the buffer system, HCO_3^- and CO_2, are regulated, respectively, by the kidneys and the lungs, as discussed later. As a result of this regulation, the pH of the extracellular fluid can be precisely controlled by the relative rate of removal and addition of HCO_3^- by the kidneys and the rate of removal of CO_2 by the lungs.

Phosphate Buffer System

Although the phosphate buffer system is not important as an extracellular fluid buffer, it plays a major role in buffering renal tubular fluid and intracellular fluids.

The main elements of the phosphate buffer system are $H_2PO_4^-$ and $HPO_4^=$. When a strong acid such as HCl is added to a mixture of these two substances, the hydrogen is accepted by the base $HPO_4^=$ and converted to $H_2PO_4^-$.

$$HCl + Na_2HPO_4 \rightarrow NaH_2PO_4 + NaCl$$

The result of this reaction is that the strong acid, HCl, is replaced by an additional amount of a weak acid, NaH_2PO_4, and the decrease in pH is minimized.

When a strong base, such as NaOH, is added to the buffer system, the OH^- is buffered by the $H_2PO_4^-$ to form additional amounts of $HPO_4^= + H_2O$.

$$NaOH + NaH_2PO_4 \rightarrow Na_2HPO_4 + H_2O$$

In this case, a strong base, NaOH, is traded for a weak base, Na_2HPO_4, causing only a slight increase in pH.

The phosphate buffer system has a pK of 6.8, which is not far from the normal pH of 7.4 in the body fluids; this allows the system to operate near its maximum buffering power. However, its concentration in the extracellular fluid is low, only about 8 percent of the concentration of the bicarbonate buffer. Therefore, the total buffering power of the phosphate system in the extracellular fluid is much less than that of the bicarbonate buffering system.

In contrast to its rather insignificant role as an extracellular buffer, *the phosphate buffer is especially important in the tubular fluids of the kidneys,* for two reasons: (1) phosphate usually becomes greatly concentrated in the tubules, thereby increasing the buffering power of the phosphate system, and (2) the tubular fluid usually has a considerably lower pH than the extracellular fluid does, bringing the operating range of the buffer closer to the pK (6.8) of the system.

The phosphate buffer system is also important in buffering intracellular fluid because the concentration of phosphate in this fluid is many times that in the extracellular fluid. Also, the pH of intracellular fluid is lower than that of extracellular fluid and therefore is usually closer to the pK of the phosphate buffer system compared with the extracellular fluid.

Proteins Are Important Intracellular Buffers

Proteins are among the most plentiful buffers in the body because of their high concentrations, especially within the cells.

The pH of the cells, although slightly lower than in the extracellular fluid, nevertheless changes approximately in proportion to extracellular fluid pH changes. There is a slight diffusion of H^+ and HCO_3^- through the cell membrane, although these ions require several hours to come to equilibrium with the extracellular fluid, except for rapid equilibrium that occurs in the red blood cells. CO_2, however, can rapidly diffuse through all the cell membranes. *This diffusion of the elements of the bicarbonate buffer system causes the pH in intracellular fluid to change when there are changes in extracellular pH.* For this reason, the buffer systems within the cells help prevent changes in the pH of extracellular fluid but may take several hours to become maximally effective.

In the red blood cell, hemoglobin (Hb) is an important buffer, as follows:

$$H^+ + Hb \rightleftharpoons HHb$$

Approximately 60 to 70 percent of the total chemical buffering of the body fluids is inside the cells, and most of this results from the intracellular proteins. However, except for the red blood cells, the slowness with which H^+ and HCO_3^- move through the cell membranes often delays for several hours the maximum ability of the intracellular proteins to buffer extracellular acid-base abnormalities.

In addition to the high concentration of proteins in the cells, another factor that contributes to their buffering power is the fact that the pKs of many of these protein systems are fairly close to intracellular pH.

Isohydric Principle: All Buffers in a Common Solution Are in Equilibrium with the Same H⁺ Concentration
We have been discussing buffer systems as though they operated individually in the body fluids. However, they all work together because H^+ is common to the reactions of all these systems. Therefore, whenever there is a change in H^+ concentration in the extracellular fluid, the balance of all the buffer systems changes at the same time. This phenomenon

is called the *isohydric principle* and is illustrated by the following formula:

$$H^+ = K_1 \times \frac{HA_1}{A_1} = K_2 \times \frac{HA_2}{A_2} = K_3 \times \frac{HA_3}{A_3}$$

K_1, K_2, K_3 are the dissociation constants of three respective acids, HA_1, HA_2, HA_3, and A_1, A_2, A_3 are the concentrations of the free negative ions that constitute the bases of the three buffer systems.

The implication of this principle is that any condition that changes the balance of one of the buffer systems also changes the balance of all the others because the buffer systems actually buffer one another by shifting H^+ back and forth between them.

Respiratory Regulation of Acid-Base Balance

The second line of defense against acid-base disturbances is control of extracellular fluid CO_2 concentration by the lungs. An increase in ventilation eliminates CO_2 from extracellular fluid, which, by mass action, reduces the H^+ concentration. Conversely, decreased ventilation increases CO_2, thus also increasing H^+ concentration in the extracellular fluid.

Pulmonary Expiration of CO_2 Balances Metabolic Formation of CO_2

CO_2 is formed continually in the body by intracellular metabolic processes. After it is formed, it diffuses from the cells into the interstitial fluids and blood and the flowing blood transports it to the lungs, where it diffuses into the alveoli and then is transferred to the atmosphere by pulmonary ventilation. About 1.2 mol/L of dissolved CO_2 normally is in the extracellular fluid, corresponding to a Pco_2 of 40 mm Hg.

If the rate of metabolic formation of CO_2 increases, the Pco_2 of the extracellular fluid is likewise increased. Conversely, a decreased metabolic rate lowers the Pco_2. If the rate of pulmonary ventilation is increased, CO_2 is blown off from the lungs and the Pco_2 in the extracellular fluid decreases. Therefore, changes in either pulmonary ventilation or the rate of CO_2 formation by the tissues can change the extracellular fluid Pco_2.

Increasing Alveolar Ventilation Decreases Extracellular Fluid H^+ Concentration and Raises pH

If the metabolic formation of CO_2 remains constant, the only other factor that affects Pco_2 in extracellular fluid is the rate of alveolar ventilation. The higher the alveolar ventilation, the lower the Pco_2; conversely, the lower the alveolar ventilation rate, the higher the Pco_2. As discussed previously, when CO_2 concentration increases, the H_2CO_3 concentration and H^+ concentration also increase, thereby lowering extracellular fluid pH.

Figure 30-2 shows the approximate changes in blood pH that are caused by increasing or decreasing the rate of alveolar ventilation. Note that increasing alveolar

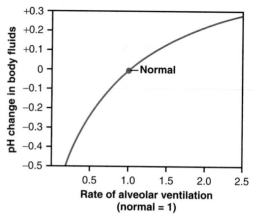

Figure 30-2 Change in extracellular fluid pH caused by increased or decreased rate of alveolar ventilation, expressed as times normal.

ventilation to about twice normal raises the pH of the extracellular fluid by about 0.23. If the pH of the body fluids is 7.40 with normal alveolar ventilation, doubling the ventilation rate raises the pH to about 7.63. Conversely, a decrease in alveolar ventilation to one fourth normal reduces the pH by 0.45. That is, if the pH is 7.4 at a normal alveolar ventilation, reducing the ventilation to one fourth normal reduces the pH to 6.95. Because the alveolar ventilation rate can change markedly, from as low as 0 to as high as 15 times normal, one can easily understand how much the pH of the body fluids can be changed by the respiratory system.

Increased H^+ Concentration Stimulates Alveolar Ventilation

Not only does the alveolar ventilation rate influence H^+ concentration by changing the Pco_2 of the body fluids, but the H^+ concentration affects the rate of alveolar ventilation. Thus, Figure 30-3 shows that the alveolar ventilation rate increases four to five times normal as the pH decreases from the normal value of 7.4 to the strongly acidic value of 7.0. Conversely, when plasma pH rises above 7.4, this causes a decrease in the ventilation rate. As one can see from the graph, the change in ventilation rate per unit pH change is much greater at reduced levels

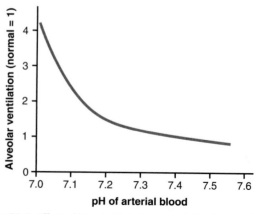

Figure 30-3 Effect of blood pH on the rate of alveolar ventilation.

of pH (corresponding to elevated H⁺ concentration) compared with increased levels of pH. The reason for this is that as the alveolar ventilation rate decreases, owing to an increase in pH (decreased H⁺ concentration), the amount of oxygen added to the blood decreases and the partial pressure of oxygen (P_{O_2}) in the blood also decreases, which stimulates the ventilation rate. Therefore, the respiratory compensation for an increase in pH is not nearly as effective as the response to a marked reduction in pH.

Feedback Control of H⁺ Concentration by the Respiratory System.

Because increased H⁺ concentration stimulates respiration, and because increased alveolar ventilation decreases the H⁺ concentration, the respiratory system acts as a typical negative feedback controller of H⁺ concentration.

$$\uparrow[H^+] \rightarrow \uparrow \text{Alveolar ventilation}$$
$$\ominus \cdots\cdots\cdots\cdots \downarrow P_{CO_2}$$

That is, whenever the H⁺ concentration increases above normal, the respiratory system is stimulated and alveolar ventilation increases. This decreases the P_{CO_2} in extracellular fluid and reduces H⁺ concentration back toward normal. Conversely, if H⁺ concentration falls below normal, the respiratory center becomes depressed, alveolar ventilation decreases, and H⁺ concentration increases back toward normal.

Efficiency of Respiratory Control of H⁺ Concentration.

Respiratory control cannot return the H⁺ concentration all the way back to normal when a disturbance outside the respiratory system has altered pH. Ordinarily, the respiratory mechanism for controlling H⁺ concentration has an effectiveness between 50 and 75 percent, corresponding to a *feedback gain* of 1 to 3. That is, if the pH is suddenly decreased by adding acid to the extracellular fluid and pH falls from 7.4 to 7.0, the respiratory system can return the pH to a value of about 7.2 to 7.3. This response occurs within 3 to 12 minutes.

Buffering Power of the Respiratory System.

Respiratory regulation of acid-base balance is a physiologic type of buffer system because it acts rapidly and keeps the H⁺ concentration from changing too much until the slowly responding kidneys can eliminate the imbalance. In general, the overall buffering power of the respiratory system is one to two times as great as the buffering power of all other chemical buffers in the extracellular fluid combined. That is, one to two times as much acid or base can normally be buffered by this mechanism as by the chemical buffers.

Impairment of Lung Function Can Cause Respiratory Acidosis.

We have discussed thus far the role of the *normal* respiratory mechanism as a means of buffering changes in H⁺ concentration. However, *abnormalities of respiration* can also cause changes in H⁺ concentration. For example, an impairment of lung function, such as severe emphysema, decreases the ability of the lungs to eliminate CO_2; this causes a buildup of CO_2 in the extracellular fluid and a tendency toward *respiratory acidosis*. Also, the ability to respond to metabolic acidosis is impaired because the compensatory reductions in P_{CO_2} that would normally occur by means of increased ventilation are blunted. In these circumstances, the kidneys represent the sole remaining physiologic mechanism for returning pH toward normal after the initial chemical buffering in the extracellular fluid has occurred.

Renal Control of Acid-Base Balance

The kidneys control acid-base balance by excreting either acidic or basic urine. Excreting acidic urine reduces the amount of acid in extracellular fluid, whereas excreting basic urine removes base from the extracellular fluid.

The overall mechanism by which the kidneys excrete acidic or basic urine is as follows: Large numbers of HCO_3^- are filtered continuously into the tubules, and if they are excreted into the urine this removes base from the blood. Large numbers of H⁺ are also secreted into the tubular lumen by the tubular epithelial cells, thus removing acid from the blood. If more H⁺ is secreted than HCO_3^- is filtered, there will be a net loss of acid from the extracellular fluid. Conversely, if more HCO_3^- is filtered than H⁺ is secreted, there will be a net loss of base.

As discussed previously, each day the body produces about 80 mEq of nonvolatile acids, mainly from the metabolism of proteins. These acids are called *nonvolatile* because they are not H_2CO_3 and, therefore, cannot be excreted by the lungs. The primary mechanism for removal of these acids from the body is renal excretion. The kidneys must also prevent the loss of bicarbonate in the urine, a task that is quantitatively more important than the excretion of nonvolatile acids. Each day the kidneys filter about 4320 mEq of bicarbonate (180 L/day × 24 mEq/L); under normal conditions, almost all this is reabsorbed from the tubules, thereby conserving the primary buffer system of the extracellular fluid.

As discussed later, both the reabsorption of bicarbonate and the excretion of H⁺ are accomplished through the process of H⁺ secretion by the tubules. Because the HCO_3^- must react with a secreted H⁺ to form H_2CO_3 before it can be reabsorbed, 4320 mEq of H⁺ must be secreted each day just to reabsorb the filtered bicarbonate. Then an additional 80 mEq of H⁺ must be secreted to rid the body of the nonvolatile acids produced each day, for a total of 4400 mEq of H⁺ secreted into the tubular fluid each day.

When there is a reduction in the extracellular fluid H⁺ concentration (alkalosis), the kidneys fail to reabsorb all the filtered HCO_3^-, thereby increasing the excretion of HCO_3^-. Because HCO_3^- normally buffers H⁺ in the extracellular fluid, this loss of HCO_3^- is the same as adding an H⁺ to the extracellular fluid. Therefore, in alkalosis, the removal of HCO_3^- raises the extracellular fluid H⁺ concentration back toward normal.

In acidosis, the kidneys do not excrete HCO_3^- into the urine but reabsorb all the filtered HCO_3^- and produce new HCO_3^-, which is added back to the extracellular fluid. This reduces the extracellular fluid H^+ concentration back toward normal.

Thus, the kidneys regulate extracellular fluid H^+ concentration through three fundamental mechanisms: (1) secretion of H^+, (2) reabsorption of filtered HCO_3^-, and (3) production of new HCO_3^-. All these processes are accomplished through the same basic mechanism, as discussed in the next few sections.

Secretion of H^+ and Reabsorption of HCO_3^- by the Renal Tubules

Hydrogen ion secretion and HCO_3^- reabsorption occur in virtually all parts of the tubules except the descending and ascending thin limbs of the loop of Henle. Figure 30-4 summarizes HCO_3^- reabsorption along the tubule. Keep in mind that for each HCO_3^- reabsorbed, a H^+ must be secreted.

About 80 to 90 percent of the bicarbonate reabsorption (and H^+ secretion) occurs in the proximal tubule, so only a small amount of HCO_3^- flows into the distal tubules and collecting ducts. In the thick ascending loop of Henle, another 10 percent of the filtered HCO_3^- is reabsorbed, and the remainder of the reabsorption takes place in the distal tubule and collecting duct. As discussed previously, the mechanism by which HCO_3^- is reabsorbed also involves tubular secretion of H^+, but different tubular segments accomplish this task differently.

H^+ is Secreted by Secondary Active Transport in the Early Tubular Segments

The epithelial cells of the proximal tubule, the thick segment of the ascending loop of Henle, and the early distal tubule all secrete H^+ into the tubular fluid by sodium-hydrogen counter-transport, as shown in Figure 30-5. This secondary active secretion of H^+ is coupled with the transport of Na^+ into the cell at the luminal membrane by the *sodium-hydrogen exchanger* protein, and the energy for H^+ secretion against a concentration gradient is derived from the sodium gradient favoring Na^+ movement into the cell. This gradient is established by the sodium-potassium adenosine triphosphatase (ATPase) pump in the basolateral membrane. About 95 percent of the bicarbonate is reabsorbed in this manner, requiring about 4000 mEq of H^+ to be secreted each day by the tubules. This mechanism, however, does not establish a very high H^+ concentration in the tubular fluid; the tubular fluid becomes very acidic only in the collecting tubules and collecting ducts.

Figure 30-5 shows how the process of H^+ secretion achieves HCO_3^- reabsorption. The secretory process begins when CO_2 either diffuses into the tubular cells or is formed by metabolism in the tubular epithelial cells. CO_2, under the influence of the enzyme *carbonic anhydrase*, combines with H_2O to form H_2CO_3, which dissociates into HCO_3^- and H^+. The H^+ is secreted from the cell into the tubular lumen by sodium-hydrogen counter-transport. That is, when Na^+ moves from the lumen of the tubule to the interior of the cell, it first combines with a carrier protein in the luminal border of the cell membrane; at the same time, an H^+ in the interior of the cells combines with the carrier protein. The Na^+ moves into the cell down a concentration gradient that has been established by the sodium-potassium ATPase pump in the basolateral membrane. The gradient for Na^+ movement into the cell then

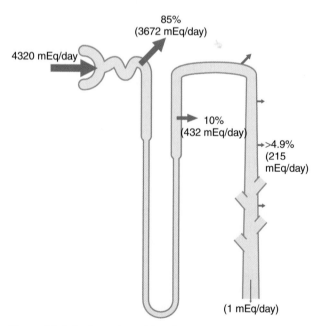

85%
(3672 mEq/day)

4320 mEq/day

10%
(432 mEq/day)

>4.9%
(215 mEq/day)

(1 mEq/day)

Figure 30-4 Reabsorption of bicarbonate in different segments of the renal tubule. The percentages of the filtered load of HCO_3^- absorbed by the various tubular segments are shown, as well as the number of milliequivalents reabsorbed per day under normal conditions.

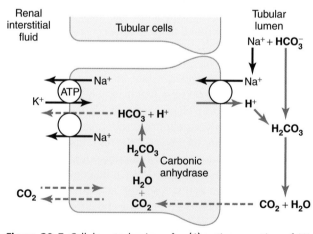

Figure 30-5 Cellular mechanisms for (1) active secretion of H^+ into the renal tubule; (2) tubular reabsorption of HCO_3^- by combination with H^+ to form carbonic acid, which dissociates to form carbon dioxide and water; and (3) sodium ion reabsorption in exchange for H^+ secreted. This pattern of H^+ secretion occurs in the proximal tubule, the thick ascending segment of the loop of Henle, and the early distal tubule.

provides the energy for moving H$^+$ in the opposite direction from the interior of the cell to the tubular lumen.

The HCO$_3^-$ generated in the cell (when H$^+$ dissociates from H$_2$CO$_3$) then moves downhill across the basolateral membrane into the renal interstitial fluid and the peritubular capillary blood. The net result is that for every H$^+$ secreted into the tubular lumen, an HCO$_3^-$ enters the blood.

Filtered HCO$_3^-$ is Reabsorbed by Interaction with H$^+$ in the Tubules

Bicarbonate ions do not readily permeate the luminal membranes of the renal tubular cells; therefore, HCO$_3^-$ that is filtered by the glomerulus cannot be directly reabsorbed. Instead, HCO$_3^-$ is reabsorbed by a special process in which it first combines with H$^+$ to form H$_2$CO$_3$, which eventually becomes CO$_2$ and H$_2$O, as shown in Figure 30-5.

This reabsorption of HCO$_3^-$ is initiated by a reaction in the tubules between HCO$_3^-$ filtered at the glomerulus and H$^+$ secreted by the tubular cells. The H$_2$CO$_3$ formed then dissociates into CO$_2$ and H$_2$O. The CO$_2$ can move easily across the tubular membrane; therefore, it instantly diffuses into the tubular cell, where it recombines with H$_2$O, under the influence of carbonic anhydrase, to generate a new H$_2$CO$_3$ molecule. This H$_2$CO$_3$ in turn dissociates to form HCO$_3^-$ and H$^+$; the HCO$_3^-$ then diffuses through the basolateral membrane into the interstitial fluid and is taken up into the peritubular capillary blood. The transport of HCO$_3$ across the basolateral membrane is facilitated by two mechanisms: (1) Na$^+$-HCO$_3^-$ co-transport in the proximal tubules and (2) Cl$^-$-HCO$_3^-$ exchange in the late segments of the proximal tubule, the thick ascending loop of Henle, and in the collecting tubules and ducts.

Thus, each time an H$^+$ is formed in the tubular epithelial cells, an HCO$_3^-$ is also formed and released back into the blood. The net effect of these reactions is "reabsorption" of HCO$_3^-$ from the tubules, although the HCO$_3^-$ that actually enters the extracellular fluid is not the same as that filtered into the tubules. The reabsorption of filtered HCO$_3^-$ does not result in net secretion of H$^+$ because the secreted H$^+$ combines with the filtered HCO$_3^-$ and is therefore not excreted.

HCO$_3^-$ is "Titrated" Against H$^+$ in the Tubules. Under normal conditions, the rate of tubular H$^+$ secretion is about 4400 mEq/day, and the rate of filtration by HCO$_3^-$ is about 4320 mEq/day. Thus, the quantities of these two ions entering the tubules are almost equal, and they combine with each other to form CO$_2$ and H$_2$O. Therefore, it is said that HCO$_3^-$ and H$^+$ normally "titrate" each other in the tubules.

The titration process is not quite exact because there is usually a slight excess of H$^+$ in the tubules to be excreted in the urine. This excess H$^+$ (about 80 mEq/day) rids the body of nonvolatile acids produced by metabolism. As discussed later, most of this H$^+$ is not excreted as free H$^+$ but rather in combination with other urinary buffers, especially phosphate and ammonia.

When there is an excess of HCO$_3^-$ over H$^+$ in the urine, as occurs in metabolic alkalosis, the excess HCO$_3^-$ cannot be reabsorbed; therefore, the excess HCO$_3^-$ is left in the tubules and eventually excreted into the urine, which helps correct the metabolic alkalosis.

In acidosis, there is excess H$^+$ relative to HCO$_3^-$ causing complete reabsorption of the HCO$_3^-$; the excess H$^+$ passes into the urine. The excess H$^+$ is buffered in the tubules by phosphate and ammonia and eventually excreted as salts. Thus, the basic mechanism by which the kidneys correct either acidosis or alkalosis is incomplete titration of H$^+$ against HCO$_3^-$, leaving one or the other to pass into the urine and be removed from the extracellular fluid.

Primary Active Secretion of H$^+$ in the Intercalated Cells of Late Distal and Collecting Tubules

Beginning in the late distal tubules and continuing through the remainder of the tubular system, the tubular epithelium secretes H$^+$ by *primary active transport*. The characteristics of this transport are different from those discussed for the proximal tubule, loop of Henle, and early distal tubule.

The mechanism for primary active H$^+$ secretion is shown in Figure 30-6. It occurs at the luminal membrane of the tubular cell, where H$^+$ is transported directly by a specific protein, a *hydrogen-transporting ATPase*. The energy required for pumping the H$^+$ is derived from the breakdown of ATP to adenosine diphosphate.

Primary active secretion of H$^+$ occurs in special types of cells called the *intercalated cells* of the late distal tubule and in the collecting tubules. Hydrogen ion secretion in these cells is accomplished in two steps: (1) the dissolved CO$_2$ in this cell combines with H$_2$O to form H$_2$CO$_3$, and (2) the H$_2$CO$_3$ then dissociates into HCO$_3^-$, which is reabsorbed into the blood, plus H$^+$, which is secreted into the tubule by means of the hydrogen-ATPase mechanism. For each H$^+$ secreted, an HCO$_3^-$ is reabsorbed, similar to the process in the proximal tubules. The main difference is

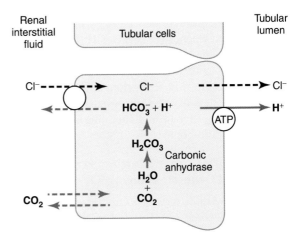

Figure 30-6 Primary active secretion of H$^+$ through the luminal membrane of the intercalated epithelial cells of the late distal and collecting tubules. Note that one HCO$_3^-$ is absorbed for each H$^+$ secreted, and a chloride ion is passively secreted along with the H$^+$.

that H⁺ moves across the luminal membrane by an active H⁺ pump instead of by counter-transport, as occurs in the early parts of the nephron.

Although the secretion of H⁺ in the late distal tubule and collecting tubules accounts for only about 5 percent of the total H⁺ secreted, this mechanism is important in forming maximally acidic urine. In the proximal tubules, H⁺ concentration can be increased only about threefold to fourfold and the tubular fluid pH can be reduced to only about 6.7, although large *amounts* of H⁺ are secreted by this nephron segment. However, H⁺ concentration can be increased as much as 900-fold in the collecting tubules. This decreases the pH of the tubular fluid to about 4.5, which is the lower limit of pH that can be achieved in normal kidneys.

Combination of Excess H⁺ with Phosphate and Ammonia Buffers in the Tubule Generates "New" HCO_3^-

When H⁺ is secreted in excess of the HCO_3^- filtered into the tubular fluid, only a small part of the excess H⁺ can be excreted in the ionic form (H⁺) in the urine. The reason for this is that the minimal urine pH is about 4.5, corresponding to an H⁺ concentration of $10^{-4.5}$ mEq/L, or 0.03 mEq/L. Thus, for each liter of urine formed, a maximum of only about 0.03 mEq of free H⁺ can be excreted. To excrete the 80 mEq of nonvolatile acid formed by metabolism each day, about 2667 liters of urine would have to be excreted if the H⁺ remained free in solution.

The excretion of large amounts of H⁺ (on occasion as much as 500 mEq/day) in the urine is accomplished primarily by combining the H⁺ with buffers in the tubular fluid. The most important buffers are phosphate buffer and ammonia buffer. Other weak buffer systems, such as urate and citrate, are much less important.

When H⁺ is titrated in the tubular fluid with HCO_3^-, this leads to reabsorption of one HCO_3^- for each H⁺ secreted, as discussed earlier. But when there is excess H⁺ in the urine, it combines with buffers other than HCO_3^-, and this leads to generation of new HCO_3^- that can also enter the blood. Thus, when there is excess H⁺ in the extracellular fluid, the kidneys not only reabsorb all the filtered HCO_3^- but also generate new HCO_3^-, thereby helping to replenish the HCO_3^- lost from the extracellular fluid in acidosis. In the next two sections, we discuss the mechanisms by which phosphate and ammonia buffers contribute to the generation of new HCO_3^-.

Phosphate Buffer System Carries Excess H⁺ into the Urine and Generates New HCO_3^-

The phosphate buffer system is composed of $HPO_4^=$ and $H_2PO_4^-$. Both become concentrated in the tubular fluid because water is normally reabsorbed to a greater extent than phosphate by the renal tubules. Therefore, although phosphate is not an important extracellular fluid buffer, it is much more effective as a buffer in the tubular fluid.

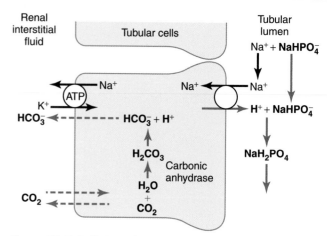

Figure 30-7 Buffering of secreted H⁺ by filtered phosphate ($NaHPO_4^-$). Note that a new HCO_3^- is returned to the blood for each $NaHPO_4^-$ that reacts with a secreted H⁺.

Another factor that makes phosphate important as a tubular buffer is the fact that the pK of this system is about 6.8. Under normal conditions, the urine is slightly acidic, and the urine pH is near the pK of the phosphate buffer system. Therefore, in the tubules, the phosphate buffer system normally functions near its most effective range of pH.

Figure 30-7 shows the sequence of events by which H⁺ is excreted in combination with phosphate buffer and the mechanism by which new HCO_3^- is added to the blood. The process of H⁺ secretion into the tubules is the same as described earlier. As long as there is excess HCO_3^- in the tubular fluid, most of the secreted H⁺ combines with HCO_3^-. However, once all the HCO_3^- has been reabsorbed and is no longer available to combine with H⁺, any excess H⁺ can combine with $HPO_4^=$ and other tubular buffers. After the H⁺ combines with $HPO_4^=$ to form $H_2PO_4^-$, it can be excreted as a sodium salt (NaH_2PO_4), carrying with it the excess H⁺.

There is one important difference in this sequence of H⁺ excretion from that discussed previously. In this case, the HCO_3^- that is generated in the tubular cell and enters the peritubular blood represents a net gain of HCO_3^- by the blood, rather than merely a replacement of filtered HCO_3^-. *Therefore, whenever an H⁺ secreted into the tubular lumen combines with a buffer other than HCO_3^-, the net effect is addition of a new HCO_3^- to the blood.* This demonstrates one of the mechanisms by which the kidneys are able to replenish the extracellular fluid stores of HCO_3^-.

Under normal conditions, much of the filtered phosphate is reabsorbed, and only about 30 to 40 mEq/day are available for buffering H⁺. Therefore, much of the buffering of excess H⁺ in the tubular fluid in acidosis occurs through the ammonia buffer system.

Excretion of Excess H⁺ and Generation of New HCO_3^- by the Ammonia Buffer System

A second buffer system in the tubular fluid that is even more important quantitatively than the phosphate buffer system is composed of ammonia (NH_3) and the ammonium ion (NH_4^+). Ammonium ion is synthesized

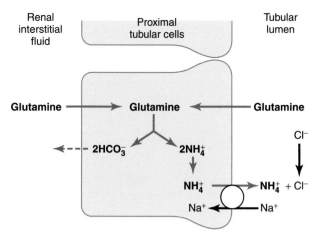

Figure 30-8 Production and secretion of ammonium ion (NH_4^+) by proximal tubular cells. Glutamine is metabolized in the cell, yielding NH_4^+ and bicarbonate. The NH_4^+ is secreted into the lumen by a sodium-NH_4^+ exchanger. For each glutamine molecule metabolized, two NH_4^+ are produced and secreted and two HCO_3^- are returned to the blood.

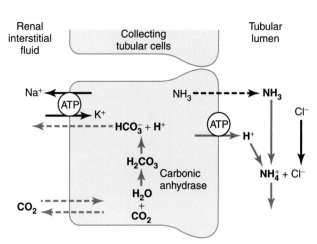

Figure 30-9 Buffering of hydrogen ion secretion by ammonia (NH_3) in the collecting tubules. Ammonia diffuses into the tubular lumen, where it reacts with secreted H^+ to form NH_4^+, which is then excreted. For each NH_4^+ excreted, a new HCO_3^- is formed in the tubular cells and returned to the blood.

from glutamine, which comes mainly from the metabolism of amino acids in the liver. The glutamine delivered to the kidneys is transported into the epithelial cells of the proximal tubules, thick ascending limb of the loop of Henle, and distal tubules (Figure 30-8). Once inside the cell, each molecule of glutamine is metabolized in a series of reactions to ultimately form two NH_4^+ and two HCO_3^-. The NH_4^+ is secreted into the tubular lumen by a counter-transport mechanism in exchange for sodium, which is reabsorbed. The HCO_3^- is transported across the basolateral membrane, along with the reabsorbed Na^+, into the interstitial fluid and is taken up by the peritubular capillaries. Thus, for each molecule of glutamine metabolized in the proximal tubules, two NH_4^+ are secreted into the urine and two HCO_3^- are reabsorbed into the blood. *The HCO_3^- generated by this process constitutes new bicarbonate.*

In the collecting tubules, the addition of NH_4^+ to the tubular fluids occurs through a different mechanism (Figure 30-9). Here, H^+ is secreted by the tubular membrane into the lumen, where it combines with NH_3 to form NH_4^+, which is then excreted. The collecting ducts are permeable to NH_3, which can easily diffuse into the tubular lumen. However, the luminal membrane of this part of the tubules is much less permeable to NH_4^+; therefore, once the H^+ has reacted with NH_3 to form NH_4^+, the NH_4^+ is trapped in the tubular lumen and eliminated in the urine. *For each NH_4^+ excreted, a new HCO_3^- is generated and added to the blood.*

Chronic Acidosis Increases NH_4^+ Excretion. One of the most important features of the renal ammonium-ammonia buffer system is that it is subject to physiologic control. An increase in extracellular fluid H^+ concentration stimulates renal glutamine metabolism and, therefore, increases the formation of NH_4^+ and new HCO_3^- to be used in H^+ buffering; a decrease in H^+ concentration has the opposite effect.

Under *normal conditions,* the amount of H^+ eliminated by the ammonia buffer system accounts for about 50 percent of the acid excreted and 50 percent of the new HCO_3^- generated by the kidneys. However, with *chronic acidosis,* the rate of NH_4^+ excretion can increase to as much as 500 mEq/day. *Therefore, with chronic acidosis, the dominant mechanism by which acid is eliminated is excretion of NH_4^+.* This also provides the most important mechanism for generating new bicarbonate during chronic acidosis.

Quantifying Renal Acid-Base Excretion

Based on the principles discussed earlier, we can quantify the kidneys' net excretion of acid or net addition or elimination of HCO_3^- from the blood as follows.

Bicarbonate excretion is calculated as the urine flow rate multiplied by urinary HCO_3^- concentration. This number indicates how rapidly the kidneys are removing HCO_3^- from the blood (which is the same as adding an H^+ to the blood). In alkalosis, the loss of HCO_3^- helps return the plasma pH toward normal.

The amount of new HCO_3^- contributed to the blood at any given time is equal to the amount of H^+ secreted that ends up in the tubular lumen with nonbicarbonate urinary buffers. As discussed previously, the primary sources of nonbicarbonate urinary buffers are NH_4^+ and phosphate. Therefore, the amount of HCO_3^- added to the blood (and H^+ excreted by NH_4^+) is calculated by measuring NH_4^+ excretion (urine flow rate multiplied by urinary NH_4^+ concentration).

The rest of the nonbicarbonate, non-NH_4^+ buffer excreted in the urine is measured by determining a value known as *titratable acid.* The amount of titratable acid in the urine is measured by titrating the urine with a strong base, such as NaOH, to a pH of 7.4, the pH of normal plasma, and the pH of the glomerular filtrate. This titration reverses the events that occurred in the tubular lumen when the tubular fluid was titrated by secreted H^+. Therefore, the number of milliequivalents of NaOH required to return the urinary pH to 7.4 equals the number of milliequivalents of H^+ added to the tubular fluid that combined with phosphate and other organic buffers. The titratable acid measurement does not include H^+ in association with NH_4^+ because the pK of the ammonia-ammonium reaction is 9.2, and titration with NaOH to a pH of 7.4 does not remove the H^+ from NH_4^+.

Thus, the *net acid excretion* by the kidneys can be assessed as

Net acid excretion = NH_4^+ excretion + Urinary titratable acid $- HCO_3^-$ excretion

The reason we subtract HCO_3^- excretion is that the loss of HCO_3^- is the same as the addition of H^+ to the blood. To maintain acid-base balance, the net acid excretion must equal the nonvolatile acid production in the body. In acidosis, the net acid excretion increases markedly, especially because of increased NH_4^+ excretion, thereby removing acid from the blood. The net acid excretion also equals the rate of net HCO_3^- addition to the blood. *Therefore, in acidosis, there is a net addition of HCO_3^- back to the blood as more NH_4^+ and urinary titratable acid are excreted.*

In alkalosis, titratable acid and NH_4^+ excretion drop to 0, whereas HCO_3^- excretion increases. *Therefore, in alkalosis, there is a negative net acid secretion.* This means that there is a net loss of HCO_3^- from the blood (which is the same as adding H^+ to the blood) and that no new HCO_3^- is generated by the kidneys.

Regulation of Renal Tubular H+ Secretion

As discussed earlier, H^+ secretion by the tubular epithelium is necessary for both HCO_3^- reabsorption and generation of new HCO_3^- associated with titratable acid formation. Therefore, the rate of H^+ secretion must be carefully regulated if the kidneys are to effectively perform their functions in acid-base homeostasis. Under normal conditions, the kidney tubules must secrete at least enough H^+ to reabsorb almost all the HCO_3^- that is filtered, and there must be enough H^+ left over to be excreted as titratable acid or NH_4^+ to rid the body of the nonvolatile acids produced each day from metabolism.

In alkalosis, tubular secretion of H^+ is reduced to a level that is too low to achieve complete HCO_3^- reabsorption, enabling the kidneys to increase HCO_3^- excretion. In this condition, titratable acid and ammonia are not excreted because there is no excess H^+ available to combine with nonbicarbonate buffers; therefore, there is no new HCO_3^- added to the urine in alkalosis. During acidosis, the tubular H^+ secretion is increased sufficiently to reabsorb all the filtered HCO_3^- with enough H^+ left over to excrete large amounts of NH_4^+ and titratable acid, thereby contributing large amounts of new HCO_3^- to the total body extracellular fluid. *The most important stimuli for increasing H^+ secretion by the tubules in acidosis are (1) an increase in Pco_2 of the extracellular fluid in respiratory acidosis*

and (2) an increase in H^+ concentration of the extracellular fluid (decreased pH) respiratory or metabolic acidosis.

The tubular cells respond directly to an increase in Pco_2 of the blood, as occurs in respiratory acidosis, with an increase in the rate of H^+ secretion as follows: The increased Pco_2 raises the Pco_2 of the tubular cells, causing increased formation of H^+ in the tubular cells, which in turn stimulates the secretion of H^+. The second factor that stimulates H^+ secretion is an increase in extracellular fluid H^+ concentration (decreased pH).

A special factor that can increase H^+ secretion under some pathophysiologic conditions is excessive aldosterone secretion. Aldosterone stimulates the secretion of H^+ by the intercalated cells of the collecting duct. Therefore, excessive secretion of aldosterone, as occurs in Conn's syndrome, can increase secretion of H^+ into the tubular fluid and, consequently, increase the amount of HCO_3^- added back to the blood. This usually causes alkalosis in patients with excessive aldosterone secretion.

The tubular cells usually respond to a decrease in H^+ concentration (alkalosis) by reducing H^+ secretion. The decreased H^+ secretion results from decreased extracellular Pco_2, as occurs in respiratory alkalosis, or from a decrease in H^+ concentration per se, as occurs in both respiratory and metabolic alkalosis.

Table 30-2 summarizes the major factors that influence H^+ secretion and HCO_3^- reabsorption. Some of these are not directly related to the regulation of acid-base balance. For example, H^+ secretion is coupled to Na^+ reabsorption by the Na^+-H^+ exchanger in the proximal tubule and thick ascending loop of Henle. Therefore, factors that stimulate Na^+ reabsorption, such as decreased extracellular fluid volume, may also secondarily increase H^+ secretion.

Extracellular fluid volume depletion stimulates sodium reabsorption by the renal tubules and increases H^+ secretion and HCO_3^- reabsorption through multiple mechanisms, including (1) increased angiotensin II levels, which directly stimulate the activity of the Na^+-H^+ exchanger in the renal tubules, and (2) increased aldosterone levels, which stimulate H^+ secretion by the intercalated cells of the cortical collecting tubules. Therefore, extracellular fluid volume depletion tends to cause alkalosis due to excess H^+ secretion and HCO_3^- reabsorption.

Table 30-2 Factors That Increase or Decrease H^+ Secretion and HCO_3^- Reabsorption by the Renal Tubules

Increase H+ Secretion and HCO_3^- Reabsorption	Decrease H+ Secretion and HCO_3^- Reabsorption
↑Pco_2	↓ Pco_2
↑ H^+, ↓ HCO_3^-	↓ H^+, ↑ HCO_3^-
↓ Extracellular fluid volume	↑ Extracellular fluid volume
↑ Angiotensin II	↓ Angiotensin II
↑ Aldosterone	↓ Aldosterone
Hypokalemia	Hyperkalemia

Changes in plasma potassium concentration can also influence H$^+$ secretion, with hypokalemia stimulating and hyperkalemia inhibiting H$^+$ secretion in the proximal tubule. A decreased plasma potassium concentration tends to increase the H$^+$ concentration in the renal tubular cells. This, in turn, stimulates H$^+$ secretion and HCO$_3^-$ reabsorption and leads to alkalosis. Hyperkalemia decreases H$^+$ secretion and HCO$_3^-$ reabsorption and tends to cause acidosis.

Renal Correction of Acidosis—Increased Excretion of H$^+$ and Addition of HCO$_3^-$ to the Extracellular Fluid

Now that we have described the mechanisms by which the kidneys secrete H$^+$ and reabsorb HCO$_3^-$, we can explain how the kidneys readjust the pH of the extracellular fluid when it becomes abnormal.

Referring to equation 8, the Henderson-Hasselbalch equation, we can see that acidosis occurs when the ratio of HCO$_3^-$ to CO$_2$ in the extracellular fluid decreases, thereby decreasing pH. If this ratio decreases because of a fall in HCO$_3^-$, the acidosis is referred to as *metabolic acidosis.* If the pH falls because of an increase in Pco$_2$, the acidosis is referred to as *respiratory acidosis.*

Acidosis Decreases the Ratio of HCO$_3^-$/H$^+$ in Renal Tubular Fluid

Both respiratory and metabolic acidosis cause a decrease in the ratio of HCO$_3^-$ to H$^+$ in the renal tubular fluid. As a result, there is excess H$^+$ in the renal tubules, causing complete reabsorption of HCO$_3^-$ and still leaving additional H$^+$ available to combine with the urinary buffers NH$_4^+$ and HPO$_4^=$. Thus, in acidosis, the kidneys reabsorb all the filtered HCO$_3^-$ and contribute new HCO$_3^-$ through the formation of NH$_4^+$ and titratable acid.

In metabolic acidosis, an excess of H$^+$ over HCO$_3^-$ occurs in the tubular fluid primarily because of decreased filtration of HCO$_3^-$. This decreased filtration of HCO$_3^-$ is caused mainly by a decrease in the extracellular fluid concentration of HCO$_3^-$.

In respiratory acidosis, the excess H$^+$ in the tubular fluid is due mainly to the rise in extracellular fluid Pco$_2$, which stimulates H$^+$ secretion.

As discussed previously, with chronic acidosis, regardless of whether it is respiratory or metabolic, there is an increase in the production of NH$_4^+$, which further contributes to the excretion of H$^+$ and the addition of new HCO$_3^-$ to the extracellular fluid. With severe chronic acidosis, as much as 500 mEq/day of H$^+$ can be excreted in the urine, mainly in the form of NH$_4^+$; this, in turn, contributes up to 500 mEq/day of new HCO$_3^-$ that is added to the blood.

Thus, with chronic acidosis, the increased secretion of H$^+$ by the tubules helps eliminate excess H$^+$ from the body and increases the quantity of HCO$_3^-$ in the extracellular fluid. This increases the HCO$_3^-$ part of the bicarbonate buffer system, which, in accordance with the Henderson-Hasselbalch equation, helps raise the extracellular pH and corrects the acidosis. If the acidosis is metabolically mediated, additional compensation by the lungs causes a reduction in Pco$_2$, also helping to correct the acidosis.

Table 30-3 summarizes the characteristics associated with respiratory and metabolic acidosis, as well as respiratory and metabolic alkalosis, which are discussed in the next section. Note that in *respiratory acidosis,* there is a reduction in pH, an increase in extracellular fluid H$^+$ concentration, and an increase in Pco$_2$, which is the initial cause of the acidosis. *The compensatory response is an increase in plasma HCO$_3^-$, caused by the addition of new HCO$_3^-$ to the extracellular fluid by the kidneys.* The rise in HCO$_3^-$ helps offset the increase in Pco$_2$, thereby returning the plasma pH toward normal.

In *metabolic acidosis,* there is also a decrease in pH and a rise in extracellular fluid H$^+$ concentration. However, in this case, the primary abnormality is a decrease in plasma HCO$_3^-$. *The primary compensations include increased ventilation rate, which reduces Pco$_2$, and renal compensation, which, by adding new HCO$_3^-$ to the extracellular fluid, helps minimize the initial fall in extracellular HCO$_3^-$ concentration.*

Renal Correction of Alkalosis—Decreased Tubular Secretion of H$^+$ and Increased Excretion of HCO$_3^-$

The compensatory responses to alkalosis are basically opposite to those that occur in acidosis. In alkalosis, the ratio of HCO$_3^-$ to CO$_2$ in the extracellular fluid increases,

Table 30-3 Characteristics of Primary Acid-Base Disturbances

	pH	H$^+$	Pco$_2$	HCO$_3^-$
Normal	7.4	40 mEq/L	40 mm Hg	24 mEq/L
Respiratory acidosis	↓	↑	↑↑	↑
Respiratory alkalosis	↑	↓	↓↓	↓
Metabolic acidosis	↓	↑	↓	↓↓
Metabolic alkalosis	↑	↓	↑	↑↑

The primary event is indicated by the double arrows (↑↑ or ↓↓). Note that respiratory acid-base disorders are initiated by an increase or decrease in Pco$_2$, whereas metabolic disorders are initiated by an increase or decrease in HCO$_3^-$.

causing a rise in pH (a decrease in H⁺ concentration), as is evident from the Henderson-Hasselbalch equation.

Alkalosis Increases the Ratio of HCO_3^-/H^+ in Renal Tubular Fluid

Regardless of whether the alkalosis is caused by metabolic or respiratory abnormalities, there is still an increase in the ratio of HCO_3^- to H⁺ in the renal tubular fluid. The net effect of this is an excess of HCO_3^- that cannot be reabsorbed from the tubules and is, therefore, excreted in the urine. Thus, in alkalosis, HCO_3^- is removed from the extracellular fluid by renal excretion, which has the same effect as adding an H⁺ to the extracellular fluid. This helps return the H⁺ concentration and pH back toward normal.

Table 30-3 shows the overall characteristics of respiratory and metabolic alkalosis. In *respiratory alkalosis,* there is an increase in extracellular fluid pH and a decrease in H⁺ concentration. *The cause of the alkalosis is a decrease in plasma Pco_2, caused by hyperventilation.* The reduction in Pco_2 then leads to a decrease in the rate of H⁺ secretion by the renal tubules. The decrease in H⁺ secretion reduces the amount of H⁺ in the renal tubular fluid. Consequently, there is not enough H⁺ to react with all the HCO_3^- that is filtered. Therefore, the HCO_3^- that cannot react with H⁺ is not reabsorbed and is excreted in the urine. This results in a decrease in plasma HCO_3^- concentration and correction of the alkalosis. *Therefore, the compensatory response to a primary reduction in Pco_2 in respiratory alkalosis is a reduction in plasma HCO_3^- concentration, caused by increased renal excretion of HCO_3^-.*

In *metabolic alkalosis,* there is also an increase in plasma pH and a decrease in H⁺ concentration. *The cause of metabolic alkalosis, however, is a rise in the extracellular fluid HCO_3^- concentration.* This is partly compensated for by a reduction in the respiration rate, which increases Pco_2 and helps return the extracellular fluid pH toward normal. In addition, the increase in HCO_3^- concentration in the extracellular fluid leads to an increase in the filtered load of HCO_3^-, which in turn causes an excess of HCO_3^- over H⁺ secreted in the renal tubular fluid. The excess HCO_3^- in the tubular fluid fails to be reabsorbed because there is no H⁺ to react with, and it is excreted in the urine. *In metabolic alkalosis, the primary compensations are decreased ventilation, which raises Pco_2, and increased renal HCO_3^- excretion, which helps compensate for the initial rise in extracellular fluid HCO_3^- concentration.*

Clinical Causes of Acid-Base Disorders

Respiratory Acidosis Results from Decreased Ventilation and Increased Pco₂

From the previous discussion, it is obvious that any factor that decreases the rate of pulmonary ventilation also increases the Pco_2 of extracellular fluid. This causes an increase in H_2CO_3

and H⁺ concentration, thus resulting in acidosis. Because the acidosis is caused by an abnormality in respiration, it is called *respiratory acidosis.*

Respiratory acidosis can occur from pathological conditions that damage the respiratory centers or that decrease the ability of the lungs to eliminate CO_2. For example, damage to the respiratory center in the medulla oblongata can lead to respiratory acidosis. Also, obstruction of the passageways of the respiratory tract, pneumonia, emphysema, or decreased pulmonary membrane surface area, as well as any factor that interferes with the exchange of gases between the blood and the alveolar air, can cause respiratory acidosis.

In respiratory acidosis, the compensatory responses available are (1) the buffers of the body fluids and (2) the kidneys, which require several days to compensate for the disorder.

Respiratory Alkalosis Results from Increased Ventilation and Decreased Pco₂

Respiratory alkalosis is caused by excessive ventilation by the lungs. Rarely does this occur because of physical pathological conditions. However, a psychoneurosis can occasionally increase breathing to the extent that a person becomes alkalotic.

A physiologic type of respiratory alkalosis occurs when a person ascends to high altitude. The low oxygen content of the air stimulates respiration, which causes loss of CO_2 and development of mild respiratory alkalosis. Again, the major means for compensation are the chemical buffers of the body fluids and the ability of the kidneys to increase HCO_3^- excretion.

Metabolic Acidosis Results from Decreased Extracellular Fluid HCO_3^- Concentration

The term *metabolic acidosis* refers to all other types of acidosis besides those caused by excess CO_2 in the body fluids. Metabolic acidosis can result from several general causes: (1) failure of the kidneys to excrete metabolic acids normally formed in the body, (2) formation of excess quantities of metabolic acids in the body, (3) addition of metabolic acids to the body by ingestion or infusion of acids, and (4) loss of base from the body fluids, which has the same effect as adding an acid to the body fluids. Some specific conditions that cause metabolic acidosis are the following.

Renal Tubular Acidosis. This type of acidosis results from a defect in renal secretion of H⁺ or in reabsorption of HCO_3^-, or both. These disorders are generally of two types: (1) impairment of renal tubular HCO_3^- reabsorption, causing loss of HCO_3^- in the urine, or (2) inability of the renal tubular H⁺ secretory mechanism to establish normal acidic urine, causing the excretion of alkaline urine. In these cases, inadequate amounts of titratable acid and NH_4^+ are excreted, so there is net accumulation of acid in the body fluids. Some causes of renal tubular acidosis include chronic renal failure, insufficient aldosterone secretion (Addison's disease), and several hereditary and acquired disorders that impair tubular function, such as Fanconi's syndrome (see Chapter 31).

Diarrhea. Severe diarrhea is probably the most frequent cause of metabolic acidosis. *The cause of this acidosis is the loss of large amounts of sodium bicarbonate into the feces.* The gastrointestinal secretions normally contain large amounts of bicarbonate, and diarrhea results in the loss of HCO_3^- from the body, which has the same effect as losing large amounts of bicarbonate in the urine. This form of metabolic acidosis can be particularly serious and can cause death, especially in young children.

Vomiting of Intestinal Contents. Vomiting of gastric contents alone would cause loss of acid and a tendency toward alkalosis because the stomach secretions are highly acidic. However, vomiting large amounts from deeper in the gastrointestinal tract, which sometimes occurs, causes loss of bicarbonate and results in metabolic acidosis in the same way that diarrhea causes acidosis.

Diabetes Mellitus. Diabetes mellitus is caused by lack of insulin secretion by the pancreas (type I diabetes) or by insufficient insulin secretion to compensate for decreased sensitivity to the effects of insulin (type II diabetes). In the absence of sufficient insulin, the normal use of glucose for metabolism is prevented. Instead, some of the fats are split into acetoacetic acid, and this is metabolized by the tissues for energy in place of glucose. With severe diabetes mellitus, blood acetoacetic acid levels can rise very high, causing severe metabolic acidosis. In an attempt to compensate for this acidosis, large amounts of acid are excreted in the urine, sometimes as much as 500 mmol/day.

Ingestion of Acids. Rarely are large amounts of acids ingested in normal foods. However, severe metabolic acidosis occasionally results from the ingestion of certain acidic poisons. Some of these include acetylsalicylics (aspirin) and methyl alcohol (which forms formic acid when it is metabolized).

Chronic Renal Failure. When kidney function declines markedly, there is a buildup of the anions of weak acids in the body fluids that are not being excreted by the kidneys. In addition, the decreased glomerular filtration rate reduces the excretion of phosphates and NH_4^+, which reduces the amount of HCO_3^- added back to the body fluids. Thus, chronic renal failure can be associated with severe metabolic acidosis.

Metabolic Alkalosis Results from Increased Extracellular Fluid HCO_3^- Concentration

When there is excess retention of HCO_3^- or loss of H^+ from the body, this causes metabolic alkalosis. Metabolic alkalosis is not nearly as common as metabolic acidosis, but some of the causes of metabolic alkalosis are as follows.

Administration of Diuretics (Except the Carbonic Anhydrase Inhibitors). All diuretics cause increased flow of fluid along the tubules, usually increasing flow in the distal and collecting tubules. This leads to increased reabsorption of Na^+ from these parts of the nephrons. Because the sodium reabsorption here is coupled with H^+ secretion, the enhanced sodium reabsorption also leads to an increase in H^+ secretion and an increase in bicarbonate reabsorption. These changes lead to the development of alkalosis, characterized by increased extracellular fluid bicarbonate concentration.

Excess Aldosterone. When large amounts of aldosterone are secreted by the adrenal glands, a mild metabolic alkalosis develops. As discussed previously, aldosterone promotes extensive reabsorption of Na^+ from the distal and collecting tubules and at the same time stimulates the secretion of H^+ by the intercalated cells of the collecting tubules. This increased secretion of H^+ leads to its increased excretion by the kidneys and, therefore, metabolic alkalosis.

Vomiting of Gastric Contents. Vomiting of the gastric contents alone, without vomiting of the lower gastrointestinal contents, causes loss of the HCl secreted by the stomach mucosa. The net result is a loss of acid from the extracellular fluid and development of metabolic alkalosis. This type of alkalosis occurs especially in neonates who have pyloric obstruction caused by hypertrophied pyloric sphincter muscles.

Ingestion of Alkaline Drugs. A common cause of metabolic alkalosis is ingestion of alkaline drugs, such as sodium bicarbonate, for the treatment of gastritis or peptic ulcer.

Treatment of Acidosis or Alkalosis

The best treatment for acidosis or alkalosis is to correct the condition that caused the abnormality. This is often difficult, especially in chronic diseases that cause impaired lung function or kidney failure. In these circumstances, various agents can be used to neutralize the excess acid or base in the extracellular fluid.

To neutralize excess acid, large amounts of *sodium bicarbonate* can be ingested by mouth. The sodium bicarbonate is absorbed from the gastrointestinal tract into the blood and increases the HCO_3^- portion of the bicarbonate buffer system, thereby increasing pH toward normal. Sodium bicarbonate can also be infused intravenously, but because of the potentially dangerous physiologic effects of such treatment, other substances are often used instead, such as *sodium lactate* and *sodium gluconate.* The lactate and gluconate portions of the molecules are metabolized in the body, leaving the sodium in the extracellular fluid in the form of sodium bicarbonate and thereby increasing the pH of the fluid toward normal.

For the treatment of alkalosis, *ammonium chloride* can be administered by mouth. When the ammonium chloride is absorbed into the blood, the ammonia portion is converted by the liver into urea. This reaction liberates HCl, which immediately reacts with the buffers of the body fluids to shift the H^+ concentration in the acidic direction. Ammonium chloride occasionally is infused intravenously, but NH_4^+ is highly toxic and this procedure can be dangerous. Another substance used occasionally is *lysine monohydrochloride.*

Clinical Measurements and Analysis of Acid-Base Disorders

Appropriate therapy of acid-base disorders requires proper diagnosis. The simple acid-base disorders described previously can be diagnosed by analyzing three measurements from an arterial blood sample: pH, plasma HCO_3^- concentration, and P_{CO_2}.

The diagnosis of simple acid-base disorders involves several steps, as shown in Figure 30-10. By examining the pH, one can determine whether the disorder is acidosis or alkalosis. A pH less than 7.4 indicates acidosis, whereas a pH greater than 7.4 indicates alkalosis.

The second step is to examine the plasma P_{CO_2} and HCO_3^- concentration. The normal value for P_{CO_2} is about 40 mm Hg, and for HCO_3^-, it is 24 mEq/L. If the disorder has been characterized as acidosis and the plasma P_{CO_2} is increased, there must be a respiratory component to the acidosis. After renal compensation, the plasma HCO_3^- concentration in respiratory acidosis would tend to increase above normal. *Therefore, the expected values for a simple respiratory acidosis would be reduced plasma pH, increased P_{CO_2},*

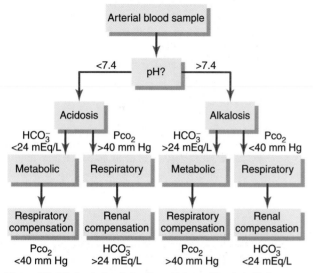

Figure 30-10 Analysis of simple acid-base disorders. If the compensatory responses are markedly different from those shown at the bottom of the figure, one should suspect a mixed acid-base disorder.

and increased plasma HCO$_3^-$ concentration after partial renal compensation.

For metabolic acidosis, there would also be a decrease in plasma pH. However, with metabolic acidosis, the primary abnormality is a decrease in plasma HCO$_3^-$ concentration. Therefore, if a low pH is associated with a low HCO$_3^-$ concentration, there must be a metabolic component to the acidosis. In simple metabolic acidosis, the Pco$_2$ is reduced because of partial respiratory compensation, in contrast to respiratory acidosis, in which Pco$_2$ is increased. *Therefore, in simple metabolic acidosis, one would expect to find a low pH,*

a low plasma HCO$_3^-$ concentration, and a reduction in Pco$_2$ after partial respiratory compensation.

The procedures for categorizing the types of alkalosis involve the same basic steps. First, alkalosis implies that there is an increase in plasma pH. If the increase in pH is associated with decreased Pco$_2$, there must be a respiratory component to the alkalosis. If the rise in pH is associated with increased HCO$_3^-$, there must be a metabolic component to the alkalosis. *Therefore, in simple respiratory alkalosis, one would expect to find increased pH, decreased Pco$_2$, and decreased HCO$_3^-$ concentration in the plasma. In simple metabolic alkalosis, one would expect to find increased pH, increased plasma HCO$_3^-$, and increased Pco$_2$.*

Complex Acid-Base Disorders and Use of the Acid-Base Nomogram for Diagnosis

In some instances, acid-base disorders are not accompanied by appropriate compensatory responses. When this occurs, the abnormality is referred to as a *mixed acid-base disorder.* This means that there are two or more underlying causes for the acid-base disturbance. For example, a patient with low pH would be categorized as acidotic. If the disorder was metabolically mediated, this would also be accompanied by a low plasma HCO$_3^-$ concentration and, after appropriate respiratory compensation, a low Pco$_2$. However, if the low plasma pH and low HCO$_3^-$ concentration are associated with elevated Pco$_2$, one would suspect a respiratory component to the acidosis, as well as a metabolic component. Therefore, this disorder would be categorized as a mixed acidosis. This could occur, for example, in a patient with acute HCO$_3^-$ loss from the gastrointestinal tract because of diarrhea (metabolic acidosis) who also has emphysema (respiratory acidosis).

A convenient way to diagnose acid-base disorders is to use an acid-base nomogram, as shown in Figure 30-11. This

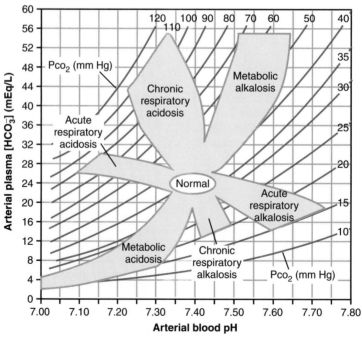

Figure 30-11 Acid-base nomogram showing arterial blood pH, arterial plasma HCO$_3^-$, and Pco$_2$ values. The central open circle shows the approximate limits for acid-base status in normal people. The shaded areas in the nomogram show the approximate limits for the normal compensations caused by simple metabolic and respiratory disorders. For values lying outside the shaded areas, one should suspect a mixed acid-base disorder. (Adapted from Cogan MG, Rector FC Jr: Acid-Base Disorders in the Kidney, 3rd ed. Philadelphia: WB Saunders, 1986.)

diagram can be used to determine the type of acidosis or alkalosis, as well as its severity. In this acid-base diagram, pH, HCO_3^- concentration, and P_{CO_2} values intersect according to the Henderson-Hasselbalch equation. The central open circle shows normal values and the deviations that can still be considered within the normal range. The shaded areas of the diagram show the 95 percent confidence limits for the normal compensations to simple metabolic and respiratory disorders.

When using this diagram, one must assume that sufficient time has elapsed for a full compensatory response, which is 6 to 12 hours for the ventilatory compensations in primary metabolic disorders and 3 to 5 days for the metabolic compensations in primary respiratory disorders. If a value is within the shaded area, this suggests that there is a simple acid-base disturbance. Conversely, if the values for pH, bicarbonate, or P_{CO_2} lie outside the shaded area, this suggests that there may be a mixed acid-base disorder.

It is important to recognize that an acid-base value within the shaded area does not *always* mean that there is a simple acid-base disorder. With this reservation in mind, the acid-base diagrams can be used as a quick means of determining the specific type and severity of an acid-base disorder.

For example, assume that the arterial plasma from a patient yields the following values: pH 7.30, plasma HCO_3^- concentration 12.0 mEq/L, and plasma P_{CO_2} 25 mm Hg. With these values, one can look at the diagram and find that this represents a simple metabolic acidosis, with appropriate respiratory compensation that reduces the P_{CO_2} from its normal value of 40 mm Hg to 25 mm Hg.

A second example would be a patient with the following values: pH 7.15, plasma HCO_3^- concentration 7 mEq/L, and plasma P_{CO_2} 50 mm Hg. In this example, the patient is acidotic, and there appears to be a metabolic component because the plasma HCO_3^- concentration is lower than the normal value of 24 mEq/L. However, the respiratory compensation that would normally reduce P_{CO_2} is absent and P_{CO_2} is slightly increased above the normal value of 40 mm Hg. This is consistent with a mixed acid-base disturbance consisting of metabolic acidosis, as well as a respiratory component.

The acid-base diagram serves as a quick way to assess the type and severity of disorders that may be contributing to abnormal pH, P_{CO_2}, and plasma bicarbonate concentrations. In a clinical setting, the patient's history and other physical findings also provide important clues concerning causes and treatment of the acid-base disorders.

Use of Anion Gap to Diagnose Acid-Base Disorders

The concentrations of anions and cations in plasma must be equal to maintain electrical neutrality. Therefore, there is no real "anion gap" in the plasma. However, only certain cations and anions are routinely measured in the clinical laboratory. The cation normally measured is Na^+, and the anions are usually Cl^- and HCO_3^-. The "anion gap" (which is only a diagnostic concept) is the difference between unmeasured anions and unmeasured cations and is estimated as

$$\text{Plasma anion gap} = [Na^+] - [HCO_3^-] - [Cl^-]$$
$$= 144 - 24 - 108 = 12 \text{ mEq/L}$$

The anion gap will increase if unmeasured anions rise or if unmeasured cations fall. The most important unmeasured cations include calcium, magnesium, and potassium, and the

Table 30-4 Metabolic Acidosis Associated with Normal or Increased Plasma Anion Gap

Increased Anion Gap (Normochloremia)	Normal Anion Gap (Hyperchloremia)
Diabetes mellitus (ketoacidosis)	Diarrhea
Lactic acidosis	Renal tubular acidosis
Chronic renal failure	Carbonic anhydrase inhibitors
Aspirin (acetylsalicylic acid) poisoning	Addison's disease
Methanol poisoning	
Ethylene glycol poisoning	
Starvation	

major unmeasured anions are albumin, phosphate, sulfate, and other organic anions. Usually the unmeasured anions exceed the unmeasured cations, and the anion gap ranges between 8 and 16 mEq/L.

The plasma anion gap is used mainly in diagnosing different causes of metabolic acidosis. In metabolic acidosis, the plasma HCO_3^- is reduced. If the plasma sodium concentration is unchanged, the concentration of anions (either Cl^- or an unmeasured anion) must increase to maintain electroneutrality. If plasma Cl^- increases in proportion to the fall in plasma HCO_3^-, the anion gap will remain normal. This is often referred to as *hyperchloremic metabolic acidosis*.

If the decrease in plasma HCO_3^- is not accompanied by increased Cl^-, there must be increased levels of unmeasured anions and therefore an increase in the calculated anion gap. Metabolic acidosis caused by excess nonvolatile acids (besides HCl), such as lactic acid or ketoacids, is associated with an increased plasma anion gap because the fall in HCO_3^- is not matched by an equal increase in Cl^-. Some examples of metabolic acidosis associated with a normal or increased anion gap are shown in Table 30-4. By calculating the anion gap, one can narrow some of the potential causes of metabolic acidosis.

Bibliography

Attmane-Elakeb A, Amlal H, Bichara M: Ammonium carriers in medullary thick ascending limb, *Am J Physiol Renal Physiol* 280:F1, 2001.

Alpern RJ: Renal acidification mechanisms. In Brenner BM, ed: *The Kidney*, ed 6, Philadelphia, 2000, WB Saunders, pp 455–519.

Breton S, Brown D: New insights into the regulation of V-ATPase-dependent proton secretion, *Am J Physiol Renal Physiol* 292:F1, 2007.

Decoursey TE: Voltage-gated proton channels and other proton transfer pathways, *Physiol Rev* 83:475, 2003.

Fry AC, Karet FE: Inherited renal acidoses, *Physiology (Bethesda)* 22:202, 2007.

Gennari FJ, Maddox DA: Renal regulation of acid-base homeostasis. In Seldin DW, Giebisch G, eds: *The Kidney—Physiology and Pathophysiology*, ed 3, New York, 2000, Raven Press, pp 2015–2054.

Good DW: Ammonium transport by the thick ascending limb of Henle's loop, *Ann Rev Physiol* 56:623, 1994.

Igarashi I, Sekine T, Inatomi J, et al: Unraveling the molecular pathogenesis of isolated proximal renal tubular acidosis, *J Am Soc Nephrol* 13:2171, 2002.

Karet FE: Inherited distal renal tubular acidosis, *J Am Soc Nephrol* 13:2178, 2002.

Kraut JA, Madias NE: Serum anion gap: its uses and limitations in clinical medicine, *Clin J Am Soc Nephrol* 2:162, 2007.

Laffey JG, Kavanagh BP: Hypocapnia, *N Engl J Med* 347:43, 2002.

Lemann J Jr, Bushinsky DA, Hamm LL: Bone buffering of acid and base in humans, *Am J Physiol Renal Physiol* 285:F811, 2003.

Madias NE, Adrogue HJ: Cross-talk between two organs: how the kidney responds to disruption of acid-base balance by the lung, *Nephron Physiol* 93:61, 2003.

Purkerson JM, Schwartz GJ: The role of carbonic anhydrases in renal physiology, *Kidney Int* 71:103, 2007.

Wagner CA, Finberg KE, Breton S, et al: Renal vacuolar H+-ATPase, *Physiol Rev* 84:1263, 2004.

Wesson DE, Alpern RJ, Seldin DW: Clinical syndromes of metabolic alkalosis. In Seldin DW, Giebisch G, eds: *The Kidney—Physiology and Pathophysiology*, ed 3, New York, 2000, Raven Press, pp 2055–2072.

White NH: Management of diabetic ketoacidosis, *Rev Endocr Metab Disord* 4:343, 2003.

Diuretics, Kidney Diseases

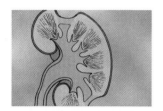

Diuretics and Their Mechanisms of Action

A diuretic is a substance that increases the rate of urine volume output, as the name implies. Most diuretics also increase urinary excretion of solutes, especially sodium and chloride. In fact, most diuretics that are used clinically act by decreasing the rate of sodium reabsorption from the tubules, which causes natriuresis (increased sodium output), which in turn causes diuresis (increased water output). That is, in most cases, increased water output occurs secondary to inhibition of tubular sodium reabsorption because sodium remaining in the tubules acts osmotically to decrease water reabsorption. Because the renal tubular reabsorption of many solutes, such as potassium, chloride, magnesium, and calcium, is also influenced secondarily by sodium reabsorption, many diuretics raise renal output of these solutes as well.

The most common clinical use of diuretics is to reduce extracellular fluid volume, especially in diseases associated with edema and hypertension. As discussed in Chapter 25, loss of sodium from the body mainly decreases extracellular fluid volume; therefore, diuretics are most often administered in clinical conditions in which extracellular fluid volume is expanded.

Some diuretics can increase urine output more than 20-fold within a few minutes after they are administered. However, the effect of most diuretics on renal output of salt and water subsides within a few days (Figure 31-1). This is due to activation of other compensatory mechanisms initiated by decreased extracellular fluid volume. For example, a decrease in extracellular fluid volume may reduce arterial pressure and glomerular filtration rate (GFR) and increase renin secretion and angiotensin II formation; all these responses, together, eventually override the chronic effects of the diuretic on urine output. Thus, in the steady state, urine output becomes equal to intake, but only after reductions in arterial pressure and extracellular fluid volume have occurred, relieving the hypertension or edema that prompted the use of diuretics in the first place.

The many diuretics available for clinical use have different mechanisms of action and, therefore, inhibit tubular reabsorption at different sites along the renal nephron. The general classes of diuretics and their mechanisms of action are shown in Table 31-1.

Osmotic Diuretics Decrease Water Reabsorption by Increasing Osmotic Pressure of Tubular Fluid

Injection into the blood stream of substances that are not easily reabsorbed by the renal tubules, such as urea, mannitol, and sucrose, causes a marked increase in the concentration of osmotically active molecules in the tubules. The osmotic pressure of these solutes then reduces water reabsorption, flushing large amounts of tubular fluid into the urine.

Large volumes of urine are also formed in certain diseases associated with excess solutes that fail to be reabsorbed from the tubular fluid. For example, when the blood glucose concentration rises to high levels in diabetes mellitus, the increased filtered load of glucose into the tubules exceeds their capacity to reabsorb glucose (i.e., exceeds their *transport maximum* for glucose). Above a plasma glucose concentration of about 250 mg/dl, little of the extra glucose is reabsorbed by the tubules; instead, the excess glucose remains in the tubules, acts as an osmotic diuretic, and causes rapid loss of fluid into the urine. In patients with diabetes mellitus, the high urine output is balanced by a high level of fluid intake owing to activation of the thirst mechanism.

"Loop" Diuretics Decrease Active Sodium-Chloride-Potassium Reabsorption in the Thick Ascending Loop of Henle

Furosemide, ethacrynic acid, and *bumetanide* are powerful diuretics that decrease active reabsorption in the thick ascending limb of the loop of Henle by blocking the 1-sodium, 2-chloride, 1-potassium co-transporter located in the luminal membrane of the epithelial cells. These "loop" diuretics are among the most powerful of the clinically used diuretics.

By blocking active sodium-chloride-potassium co-transport in the luminal membrane of the loop of Henle, the loop diuretics raise urine output of sodium, chloride,

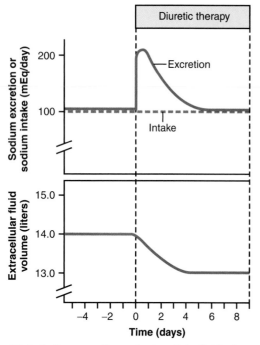

Figure 31-1 Sodium excretion and extracellular fluid volume during diuretic administration. The immediate increase in sodium excretion is accompanied by a decrease in extracellular fluid volume. If sodium intake is held constant, compensatory mechanisms will eventually return sodium excretion to equal sodium intake, thus re-establishing sodium balance.

potassium, and other electrolytes, as well as water, for two reasons: (1) they greatly increase the quantities of solutes delivered to the distal parts of the nephrons, and these act as osmotic agents to prevent water reabsorption as well; and (2) they disrupt the countercurrent multiplier system by decreasing absorption of ions from the loop of Henle into the medullary interstitium, thereby decreasing the osmolarity of the medullary interstitial fluid. Because of this effect, loop diuretics impair the ability of the kidneys to either concentrate or dilute the urine. Urinary dilution is impaired because the inhibition of sodium and chloride

reabsorption in the loop of Henle causes more of these ions to be excreted along with increased water excretion. Urinary concentration is impaired because the renal medullary interstitial fluid concentration of these ions, and therefore renal medullary osmolarity, is reduced. Consequently, reabsorption of fluid from the collecting ducts is decreased, so the maximal concentrating ability of the kidneys is also greatly reduced. In addition, decreased renal medullary interstitial fluid osmolarity reduces absorption of water from the descending loop of Henle. Because of these multiple effects, 20 to 30 percent of the glomerular filtrate may be delivered into the urine, causing, under acute conditions, urine output to be as great as 25 times normal for at least a few minutes.

Thiazide Diuretics Inhibit Sodium-Chloride Reabsorption in the Early Distal Tubule

The thiazide derivatives, such as chlorothiazide, act mainly on the early distal tubules to block the sodium-chloride co-transporter in the luminal membrane of the tubular cells. Under favorable conditions, these agents may cause a maximum of 5 to 10 percent of the glomerular filtrate to pass into the urine. This is about the same amount of sodium normally reabsorbed by the distal tubules.

Carbonic Anhydrase Inhibitors Block Sodium Bicarbonate Reabsorption in the Proximal Tubules

Acetazolamide inhibits the enzyme *carbonic anhydrase*, which is critical for the reabsorption of bicarbonate in the proximal tubule, as discussed in Chapter 30. Carbonic anhydrase is abundant in the proximal tubule, the primary site of action of carbonic anhydrase inhibitors. Some carbonic anhydrase is also present in other tubular cells, such as in the intercalated cells of the collecting tubule.

Because H^+ secretion and HCO_3^- reabsorption in the proximal tubules are coupled to sodium reabsorption through the sodium-hydrogen ion counter-transport mechanism in the luminal membrane, decreasing HCO_3^-

Table 31-1 Classes of Diuretics, Their Mechanisms of Action, and Tubular Sites of Action

Class of Diuretic	Mechanism of Action	Tubular Site of Action
Osmotic diuretics (mannitol)	Inhibit water and solute reabsorption by increasing osmolarity of tubular fluid	Mainly proximal tubules
Loop diuretics (furosemide, bumetanide)	Inhibit Na^+-K^+-Cl^- co-transport in luminal membrane	Thick ascending loop of Henle
Thiazide diuretics (hydrochlorothiazide, chlorthalidone)	Inhibit Na^+-Cl^- co-transport in luminal membrane	Early distal tubules
Carbonic anhydrase inhibitors (acetazolamide)	Inhibit H^+ secretion and HCO_3^- reabsorption, which reduces Na^+ reabsorption	Proximal tubules
Aldosterone antagonists (spironolactone, eplerenone)	Inhibit action of aldosterone on tubular receptor, decrease Na^+ reabsorption, and decrease K^+ secretion	Collecting tubules
Sodium channel blockers (triamterene, amiloride)	Block entry of Na^+ into Na^+ channels of luminal membrane, decrease Na^+ reabsorption, and decrease K^+ secretion	Collecting tubules

reabsorption also reduces sodium reabsorption. The blockage of sodium and HCO_3^- reabsorption from the tubular fluid causes these ions to remain in the tubules and act as an osmotic diuretic. Predictably, a disadvantage of the carbonic anhydrase inhibitors is that they cause some degree of acidosis because of the excessive loss of HCO_3^- in the urine.

Competitive Inhibitors of Aldosterone Decrease Sodium Reabsorption from and Potassium Secretion into the Cortical Collecting Tubule

Spironolactone and *eplerenone* are mineralocorticoid receptor antagonists that compete with aldosterone for receptor binding sites in the cortical collecting tubule epithelial cells and, therefore, can decrease the reabsorption of sodium and secretion of potassium in this tubular segment. As a consequence, sodium remains in the tubules and acts as an osmotic diuretic, causing increased excretion of water, as well as sodium. Because these drugs also block the effect of aldosterone to promote potassium secretion in the tubules, they decrease the excretion of potassium. Mineralocorticoid receptor antagonists also cause movement of potassium from the cells to the extracellular fluid. In some instances, this causes extracellular fluid potassium concentration to increase excessively. For this reason, spironolactone and other mineralocorticoid receptor antagonists are referred to as *potassium-sparing diuretics.* Many of the other diuretics cause loss of potassium in the urine, in contrast to the mineralocorticoid receptor antagonists, which "spare" the loss of potassium.

Diuretics That Block Sodium Channels in the Collecting Tubules Decrease Sodium Reabsorption

Amiloride and *triamterene* also inhibit sodium reabsorption and potassium secretion in the collecting tubules, similar to the effects of spironolactone. However, at the cellular level, these drugs act directly to block the entry of sodium into the sodium channels of the luminal membrane of the collecting tubule epithelial cells. Because of this decreased sodium entry into the epithelial cells, there is also decreased sodium transport across the cells' basolateral membranes and, therefore, decreased activity of the sodium-potassium-adenosine triphosphatase pump. This decreased activity reduces the transport of potassium into the cells and ultimately decreases the secretion of potassium into the tubular fluid. For this reason, the sodium channel blockers are also potassium-sparing diuretics and decrease the urinary excretion rate of potassium.

Kidney Diseases

Diseases of the kidneys are among the most important causes of death and disability in many countries throughout the world. For example, in 2009, more than 26 million adults in the United States were estimated to have chronic kidney disease, and many more millions of people have acute renal failure or less severe forms of kidney dysfunction.

Severe kidney diseases can be divided into two main categories: (1) *acute renal failure,* in which the kidneys abruptly stop working entirely or almost entirely but may eventually recover nearly normal function, and (2) *chronic renal failure,* in which there is progressive loss of function of more and more nephrons that gradually decreases overall kidney function. Within these two general categories, there are many specific kidney diseases that can affect the kidney blood vessels, glomeruli, tubules, renal interstitium, and parts of the urinary tract outside the kidney, including the ureters and bladder. In this chapter, we discuss specific physiologic abnormalities that occur in a few of the more important types of kidney diseases.

Acute Renal Failure

The causes of acute renal failure can be divided into three main categories:

1. Acute renal failure resulting from decreased blood supply to the kidneys; this condition is often referred to as *prerenal acute renal failure* to reflect the fact that the abnormality occurs as a result of an abnormality originating outside the kidneys. For example, prerenal acute renal failure can be a consequence of heart failure with reduced cardiac output and low blood pressure or conditions associated with diminished blood volume and low blood pressure, such as severe hemorrhage.

2. *Intrarenal acute renal failure* resulting from abnormalities within the kidney itself, including those that affect the blood vessels, glomeruli, or tubules.

3. *Postrenal acute renal failure,* resulting from obstruction of the urinary collecting system anywhere from the calyces to the outflow from the bladder. The most common causes of obstruction of the urinary tract outside the kidney are kidney stones, caused by precipitation of calcium, urate, or cystine.

Prerenal Acute Renal Failure Caused by Decreased Blood Flow to the Kidney

The kidneys normally receive an abundant blood supply of about 1100 ml/min, or about 20 to 25 percent of the cardiac output. The main purpose of this high blood flow to the kidneys is to provide enough plasma for the high rates of glomerular filtration needed for effective regulation of body fluid volumes and solute concentrations. Therefore, decreased renal blood flow is usually accompanied by decreased GFR and decreased urine output of water and solutes. Consequently, conditions that acutely diminish blood flow to the kidneys usually cause *oliguria,* which refers to diminished urine output below the level of intake of water and solutes. This causes accumulation of water and solutes in the body fluids. If renal blood flow is markedly reduced, total cessation of urine output can occur, a condition referred to as *anuria.*

Table 31-2 Some Causes of Prerenal Acute Renal Failure

Intravascular Volume Depletion
Hemorrhage (trauma, surgery, postpartum, gastrointestinal)
Diarrhea or vomiting
Burns
Cardiac Failure
Myocardial infarction
Valvular damage
Peripheral Vasodilation and Resultant Hypotension
Anaphylactic shock
Anesthesia
Sepsis, severe infections
Primary renal hemodynamic abnormalities
Renal artery stenosis, embolism, or thrombosis of renal artery or vein

Table 31-3 Some Causes of Intrarenal Acute Renal Failure

Small Vessel and /or Glomerular Injury
Vasculitis (polyarteritis nodosa)
Cholesterol emboli
Malignant hypertension
Acute glomerulonephritis
Tubular Epithelial Injury (Tubular Necrosis)
Acute tubular necrosis due to ischemia
Acute tubular necrosis due to toxins (heavy metals, ethylene glycol, insecticides, poison mushrooms, carbon tetrachloride)
Renal Interstitial Inury
Acute pyelonephritis
Acute allergic interstitial nephritis

As long as renal blood flow does not fall below about 20 to 25 percent of normal, acute renal failure can usually be reversed if the cause of the ischemia is corrected before damage to the renal cells has occurred. Unlike some tissues, the kidney can endure a relatively large reduction in blood flow before actual damage to the renal cells occurs. The reason for this is that as renal blood flow is reduced, the GFR and the amount of sodium chloride filtered by the glomeruli (as well as the filtration rate of water and other electrolytes) are reduced. This decreases the amount of sodium chloride that must be reabsorbed by the tubules, which use most of the energy and oxygen consumed by the normal kidney. Therefore, as renal blood flow and GFR fall, the requirement for renal oxygen consumption is also reduced. As the GFR approaches zero, oxygen consumption of the kidney approaches the rate that is required to keep the renal tubular cells alive even when they are not reabsorbing sodium. When blood flow is reduced below this basal requirement, which is usually less than 20 to 25 percent of the normal renal blood flow, the renal cells start to become hypoxic, and further decreases in renal blood flow, if prolonged, will cause damage or even death of the renal cells, especially the tubular epithelial cells.

If the cause of prerenal acute renal failure is not corrected and ischemia of the kidney persists longer than a few hours, this type of renal failure can evolve into intrarenal acute renal failure, as discussed later. Acute reduction of renal blood flow is a common cause of acute renal failure in hospitalized patients, especially those who have suffered severe injuries. Table 31-2 shows some of the common causes of decreased renal blood flow and prerenal acute renal failure.

Intrarenal Acute Renal Failure Caused by Abnormalities Within the Kidney

Abnormalities that originate within the kidney and that abruptly diminish urine output fall into the general category of *intrarenal acute renal failure*. This category of acute renal failure can be further divided into (1) conditions that injure the glomerular capillaries or other small renal vessels, (2) conditions that damage the renal tubular epithelium, and (3) conditions that cause damage to the renal interstitium. This type of classification refers to the primary site of injury, but because the renal vasculature and tubular system are functionally interdependent, damage to the renal blood vessels can lead to tubular damage, and primary tubular damage can lead to damage of the renal blood vessels. Some causes of intrarenal acute renal failure are listed in Table 31-3.

Acute Renal Failure Caused by Glomerulonephritis

Acute glomerulonephritis is a type of *intrarenal* acute renal failure usually caused by an abnormal immune reaction that damages the glomeruli. In about 95 percent of the patients with this disease, damage to the glomeruli occurs 1 to 3 weeks after an infection elsewhere in the body, usually caused by certain types of group A beta streptococci. The infection may have been a streptococcal sore throat, streptococcal tonsillitis, or even streptococcal infection of the skin. It is not the infection itself that damages the kidneys. Instead, over a few weeks, as antibodies develop against the streptococcal antigen, the antibodies and antigen react with each other to form an insoluble immune complex that becomes entrapped in the glomeruli, especially in the basement membrane portion of the glomeruli.

Once the immune complex has deposited in the glomeruli, many of the cells of the glomeruli begin to proliferate, but mainly the mesangial cells that lie between the endothelium and the epithelium. In addition, large numbers of white blood cells become entrapped in the glomeruli. Many of the glomeruli become blocked by this inflammatory reaction, and those that are not blocked usually become excessively permeable, allowing both protein and red blood cells to leak from the blood of the glomerular capillaries into the glomerular filtrate. In severe cases, either total or almost complete renal shutdown occurs.

The acute inflammation of the glomeruli usually subsides in about 2 weeks and, in most patients, the kidneys return to almost normal function within the next few weeks to few months. Sometimes, however, many of the glomeruli are destroyed beyond repair, and in a small percentage of patients, progressive renal deterioration continues indefinitely, leading to *chronic renal failure*, as described in a subsequent section of this chapter.

Tubular Necrosis as a Cause of Acute Renal Failure

Another cause of intrarenal acute renal failure is *tubular necrosis,* which means destruction of epithelial cells in the tubules. Some common causes of tubular necrosis are (1) severe ischemia and inadequate supply of oxygen and nutrients to the tubular epithelial cells and (2) poisons, toxins, or medications that destroy the tubular epithelial cells.

Acute Tubular Necrosis Caused by Severe Renal Ischemia

Severe ischemia of the kidney can result from circulatory shock or any other disturbance that severely impairs the blood supply to the kidney. If the ischemia is severe enough to seriously impair the delivery of nutrients and oxygen to the renal tubular epithelial cells, and if the insult is prolonged, damage or eventual destruction of the epithelial cells can occur. When this happens, tubular cells "slough off" and plug many of the nephrons, so that there is no urine output from the blocked nephrons; the affected nephrons often fail to excrete urine even when renal blood flow is restored to normal, as long as the tubules remain plugged. The most common causes of ischemic damage to the tubular epithelium are the prerenal causes of acute renal failure associated with circulatory shock, as discussed earlier in this chapter.

Acute Tubular Necrosis Caused by Toxins or Medications

There is a long list of renal poisons and medications that can damage the tubular epithelium and cause acute renal failure. Some of these are *carbon tetrachloride, heavy metals* (such as mercury and lead), *ethylene glycol* (which is a major component in antifreeze), various *insecticides,* some *medications* (such as tetracyclines) used as antibiotics, and *cis-platinum,* which is used in treating certain cancers. Each of these substances has a specific toxic action on the renal tubular epithelial cells, causing death of many of them. As a result, the epithelial cells slough away from the basement membrane and plug the tubules. In some instances, the basement membrane also is destroyed. If the basement membrane remains intact, new tubular epithelial cells can grow along the surface of the membrane, so the tubule may repair itself within 10 to 20 days.

Postrenal Acute Renal Failure Caused by Abnormalities of the Lower Urinary Tract

Multiple abnormalities in the lower urinary tract can block or partially block urine flow and therefore lead to acute renal failure even when the kidneys' blood supply and other functions are initially normal. If the urine output of only one kidney is diminished, no major change in body fluid composition will occur because the contralateral kidney can increase its urine output sufficiently to maintain relatively normal levels of extracellular electrolytes and solutes, as well as normal extracellular fluid volume. With this type of renal failure, normal kidney function can be restored if the basic cause of the problem is corrected within a few hours. But chronic obstruction of the urinary tract, lasting for several days or weeks, can lead to irreversible kidney damage. Some of the causes of postrenal acute failure include (1) bilateral obstruction of the ureters or renal pelvises caused by large stones or blood clots, (2) bladder obstruction, and (3) obstruction of the urethra.

Physiologic Effects of Acute Renal Failure

A major physiologic effect of acute renal failure is retention in the blood and extracellular fluid of water, waste products of metabolism, and electrolytes. This can lead to water and salt overload, which, in turn, can lead to edema and hypertension. Excessive retention of potassium, however, is often a more serious threat to patients with acute renal failure because increases in plasma potassium concentration (hyperkalemia) above 8 mEq/L (only twice normal) can be fatal. Because the kidneys are also unable to excrete sufficient hydrogen ions, patients with acute renal failure develop metabolic acidosis, which in itself can be lethal or can aggravate the hyperkalemia.

In the most severe cases of acute renal failure, complete anuria occurs. The patient will die in 8 to 14 days unless kidney function is restored or unless an artificial kidney is used to rid the body of the excessive retained water, electrolytes, and waste products of metabolism. Other effects of diminished urine output, as well as treatment with an artificial kidney, are discussed in the next section in relation to chronic renal failure.

Chronic Renal Failure: An Irreversible Decrease in the Number of Functional Nephrons

Chronic renal failure results from progressive and irreversible loss of large numbers of functioning nephrons. Serious clinical symptoms often do not occur until the number of functional nephrons falls to at least 70 to 75 percent below normal. In fact, relatively normal blood concentrations of most electrolytes and normal body fluid volumes can still be maintained until the number of functioning nephrons decreases below 20 to 25 percent of normal.

Table 31-4 Some Causes of Chronic Renal Failure

Metablolic Disorders
Diabetes mellitus
Obesity
Amyloidosis
Hypertension
Renal Vascular Disorders
Atherosclerosis
Nephrosclerosis-hypertension
Immunologic Disorders
Glomerulonephritis
Polyarteritis nodosa
Lupus erythematosus
Infections
Pyelonephritis
Tuberculosis
Primary Tubular Disorders
Nephrotoxins (analgesics, heavy metals)
Urinary Tract Obstruction
Renal calculi
Hypertrophy of prostate
Urethral constriction
Congenital Disorders
Polycystic disease
Congenital absence of kidney tissue (renal hypoplasia)

Table 31-4 gives some of the most important causes of chronic renal failure. In general, chronic renal failure, like acute renal failure, can occur because of disorders of the blood vessels, glomeruli, tubules, renal interstitium, and lower urinary tract. Despite the wide variety of diseases that can lead to chronic renal failure, the end result is essentially the same—a decrease in the number of functional nephrons.

Vicious Cycle of Chronic Renal Failure Leading to End-Stage Renal Disease

In many cases, an initial insult to the kidney leads to progressive deterioration of kidney function and further loss of nephrons to the point where the person must be placed on dialysis treatment or transplanted with a functional kidney to survive. This condition is referred to as *end-stage renal disease (ESRD)*.

Studies in laboratory animals have shown that surgical removal of large portions of the kidney initially causes adaptive changes in the remaining nephrons that lead to increased blood flow, increased GFR, and increased urine output in the surviving nephrons. The exact mechanisms responsible for these changes are not well understood but involve hypertrophy (growth of the various structures of the surviving nephrons), as well as functional changes that decrease vascular resistance and tubular reabsorption in the surviving nephrons. These adaptive changes permit a person to excrete normal amounts of water and solutes even when kidney mass is reduced to 20 to 25 percent of normal. Over a period of several years, however, these renal adaptive changes may lead to further injury of the remaining nephrons, particularly to the glomeruli of these nephrons.

The cause of this additional injury is not known, but some investigators believe that it may be related in part to increased pressure or stretch of the remaining glomeruli, which occurs as a result of functional vasodilation or increased blood pressure; the chronic increase in pressure and stretch of the small arterioles and glomeruli are believed to cause injury and sclerosis of these vessels (replacement of normal tissue with connective tissue). These sclerotic lesions can eventually obliterate the glomerulus, leading to further reduction in kidney function, further adaptive changes in the remaining nephrons, and a slowly progressing vicious cycle that eventually terminates in ESRD (Figure 31-2). The only proven method of slowing down this progressive loss of kidney function is to lower arterial pressure and glomerular hydrostatic pressure, especially by using drugs such as angiotensin-converting enzyme inhibitors or angiotensin II receptor antagonists.

Table 31-5 gives the most common causes of ESRD. In the early 1980s, *glomerulonephritis* in all its various forms was believed to be the most common initiating cause of

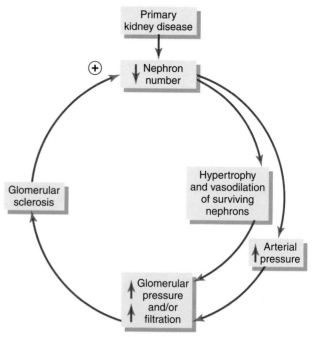

Figure 31-2 Vicious circle that can occur with primary kidney disease. Loss of nephrons because of disease may increase pressure and flow in the surviving glomerular capillaries, which in turn may eventually injure these "normal" capillaries as well, thus causing progressive sclerosis and eventual loss of these glomeruli.

Table 31-5 Most Common Causes of End-Stage Renal Disease (ESRD)

Cause	Percentage of Total ESRD Patients
Diabetes mellitus	45
Hypertension	27
Glomerulonephritis	8
Polycystic kidney disease	2
Other/unknown	18

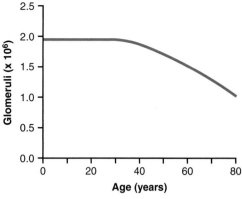

Figure 31-3 Effect of aging on the number of functional glomeruli.

ESRD. In recent years, *diabetes mellitus* and *hypertension* have become recognized as the leading causes of ESRD, together accounting for more than 70 percent of all chronic renal failure.

Excessive weight gain (obesity) appears to be the most important risk factor for the two main causes of ESRD—diabetes and hypertension. As discussed in Chapter 78, type II diabetes, which is closely linked to obesity, accounts for more than 90 percent of all diabetes mellitus. Excess weight gain is also a major cause of essential hypertension, accounting for as much as 65 to 75 percent of the risk for developing hypertension in adults. In addition to causing renal injury through diabetes and hypertension, obesity may have additive or synergistic effects to worsen renal function in patients with preexisting kidney disease.

Injury to the Renal Vasculature as a Cause of Chronic Renal Failure

Many types of vascular lesions can lead to renal ischemia and death of kidney tissue. The most common of these are (1) *atherosclerosis* of the larger renal arteries, with progressive sclerotic constriction of the vessels; (2) *fibromuscular hyperplasia* of one or more of the large arteries, which also causes occlusion of the vessels; and (3) *nephrosclerosis,* caused by sclerotic lesions of the smaller arteries, arterioles, and glomeruli.

Atherosclerotic or hyperplastic lesions of the large arteries frequently affect one kidney more than the other and, therefore, cause unilaterally diminished kidney function. As discussed in Chapter 19, hypertension often occurs when the artery of one kidney is constricted while the artery of the other kidney is still normal, a condition analogous to "two-kidney" Goldblatt hypertension.

Benign nephrosclerosis, the most common form of kidney disease, is seen to at least some extent in about 70 percent of postmortem examinations in people who die after the age of 60. This type of vascular lesion occurs in the smaller interlobular arteries and in the afferent arterioles of the kidney. It is believed to begin with leakage of plasma through the intimal membrane of these vessels. This causes fibrinoid deposits to develop in the medial layers of these vessels, followed by progressive thickening of the vessel wall that eventually constricts the vessels and, in some cases, occludes them. Because there is essentially no collateral circulation among the smaller renal arteries, occlusion of one or more of them causes destruction of a comparable number of nephrons. Therefore, much of the kidney tissue becomes replaced by small amounts of fibrous

tissue. When sclerosis occurs in the glomeruli, the injury is referred to as *glomerulosclerosis.*

Nephrosclerosis and glomerulosclerosis occur to some extent in most people after the fourth decade of life, causing about a 10 percent decrease in the number of functional nephrons each 10 years after age 40 (Figure 31-3). This loss of glomeruli and overall nephron function is reflected by a progressive decrease in both renal blood flow and GFR. Even in "normal" people, kidney plasma flow and GFR decrease by 40 to 50 percent by age 80.

The frequency and severity of nephrosclerosis and glomerulosclerosis are greatly increased by concurrent *hypertension* or *diabetes mellitus.* In fact, diabetes mellitus and hypertension are the two most important causes of ESRD, as discussed previously. Thus, benign nephrosclerosis in association with severe hypertension can lead to a rapidly progressing *malignant nephrosclerosis.* The characteristic histological features of malignant nephrosclerosis include large amounts of fibrinoid deposits in the arterioles and progressive thickening of the vessels, with severe ischemia occurring in the affected nephrons. For unknown reasons, the incidence of malignant nephrosclerosis and severe glomerulosclerosis is significantly higher in blacks than in whites of similar ages who have similar degrees of severity of hypertension or diabetes.

Injury to the Glomeruli as a Cause of Chronic Renal Failure—Glomerulonephritis

Chronic glomerulonephritis can be caused by several diseases that cause inflammation and damage to the capillary loops in the glomeruli of the kidneys. In contrast to the acute form of this disease, chronic glomerulonephritis is a slowly progressive disease that often leads to irreversible renal failure. It may be a primary kidney disease, following acute glomerulonephritis, or it may be secondary to systemic diseases, such as *lupus erythematosus.*

In most cases, chronic glomerulonephritis begins with accumulation of precipitated antigen-antibody complexes in the glomerular membrane. In contrast to acute glomerulonephritis, streptococcal infections account for only a small percentage of patients with the chronic form of glomerulonephritis. Accumulation of antigen-antibody complex in the glomerular membranes causes inflammation, progressive thickening of the membranes, and eventual invasion of the glomeruli by fibrous tissue. In the later stages of the disease, the glomerular capillary filtration coefficient becomes greatly reduced because of decreased numbers of filtering capillaries in the glomerular tufts and because of thickened glomerular membranes. In the final stages of the disease, many glomeruli are replaced by fibrous tissue and are, therefore, unable to filter fluid.

Injury to the Renal Interstitium as a Cause of Chronic Renal Failure—Interstitial Nephritis

Primary or secondary disease of the renal interstitium is referred to as *interstitial nephritis*. In general, this can result from vascular, glomerular, or tubular damage that destroys individual nephrons, or it can involve primary damage to the renal interstitium by poisons, drugs, and bacterial infections.

Renal interstitial injury caused by bacterial infection is called *pyelonephritis*. The infection can result from different types of bacteria but especially from *Escherichia coli* that originate from fecal contamination of the urinary tract. These bacteria reach the kidneys either by way of the blood stream or, more commonly, by ascension from the lower urinary tract by way of the ureters to the kidneys.

Although the normal bladder is able to clear bacteria readily, there are two general clinical conditions that may interfere with the normal flushing of bacteria from the bladder: (1) the inability of the bladder to empty completely, leaving residual urine in the bladder, and (2) the existence of obstruction of urine outflow. With impaired ability to flush bacteria from the bladder, the bacteria multiply and the bladder becomes inflamed, a condition termed *cystitis*. Once cystitis has occurred, it may remain localized without ascending to the kidney, or in some people, bacteria may reach the renal pelvis because of a pathological condition in which urine is propelled up one or both of the ureters during micturition. This condition is called *vesicoureteral reflux* and is due to the failure of the bladder wall to occlude the ureter during micturition; as a result, some of the urine is propelled upward toward the kidney, carrying with it bacteria that can reach the renal pelvis and renal medulla, where they can initiate the infection and inflammation associated with pyelonephritis.

Pyelonephritis begins in the renal medulla and therefore usually affects the function of the medulla more than it affects the cortex, at least in the initial stages. Because one of the primary functions of the medulla is to provide the countercurrent mechanism for concentrating urine, patients with pyelonephritis frequently have markedly impaired ability to concentrate the urine.

With long-standing pyelonephritis, invasion of the kidneys by bacteria not only causes damage to the renal medulla interstitium but also results in progressive damage of renal tubules, glomeruli, and other structures throughout the kidney. Consequently, large parts of functional renal tissue are lost and chronic renal failure can develop.

Nephrotic Syndrome—Excretion of Protein in the Urine Because of Increased Glomerular Permeability

Many patients with kidney disease develop the *nephrotic syndrome*, which is characterized by loss of large quantities of plasma proteins into the urine. In some instances, this occurs without evidence of other major abnormalities of kidney function, but more often it is associated with some degree of renal failure.

The cause of the protein loss in the urine is increased permeability of the glomerular membrane. Therefore, any disease that increases the permeability of this membrane can cause the nephrotic syndrome. Such diseases include (1) *chronic glomerulonephritis*, which affects primarily the glomeruli and often causes greatly increased permeability of the glomerular membrane; (2) *amyloidosis*, which results from deposition of an abnormal proteinoid substance in the walls of the blood vessels and seriously damages the basement membrane of the glomeruli; and (3) *minimal change nephrotic syndrome*, which is associated with no major abnormality in the glomerular capillary membrane that can be detected with light microscopy. As discussed in Chapter 26, minimal change nephropathy has been found to be associated with loss of the negative charges that are normally present in the glomerular capillary basement membrane. Immunologic studies have also shown abnormal immune reactions in some cases, suggesting that the loss of the negative charges may have resulted from antibody attack on the membrane. Loss of normal negative charges in the basement membrane of the glomerular capillaries allows proteins, especially albumin, to pass through the glomerular membrane with ease because the negative charges in the basement membrane normally repel the negatively charged plasma proteins.

Minimal-change nephropathy can occur in adults, but more frequently it occurs in children between the ages of 2 and 6 years. Increased permeability of the glomerular capillary membrane occasionally allows as much as 40 grams of plasma protein loss into the urine each day, which is an extreme amount for a young child. Therefore, the child's plasma protein concentration often falls below 2 g/dl and the colloid osmotic pressure falls from a normal value of 28 to less than 10 mm Hg. As a consequence of this low colloid osmotic pressure in the plasma, large amounts of fluid leak from the capillaries all over the body into most of the tissues, causing severe edema, as discussed in Chapter 25.

Nephron Function in Chronic Renal Failure

Loss of Functional Nephrons Requires the Surviving Nephrons to Excrete More Water and Solutes. It would be reasonable to suspect that decreasing the number of functional nephrons, which reduces the GFR, would also cause major decreases in renal excretion of water and solutes. Yet patients who have lost up to 75 to 80 percent of their nephrons are able to excrete normal amounts of water and electrolytes without serious accumulation of any of these in the body fluids. Further reduction in the number of nephrons, however, leads to electrolyte and fluid retention, and death usually ensues when the number of nephrons falls below 5 to 10 percent of normal.

In contrast to the electrolytes, many of the waste products of metabolism, such as urea and creatinine, accumulate almost in proportion to the number of nephrons that have been destroyed. The reason for this is that substances such as creatinine and urea depend largely on glomerular filtration for their excretion, and they are not reabsorbed as avidly as the electrolytes. Creatinine, for example, is not reabsorbed at all, and the excretion rate is approximately equal to the rate at which it is filtered.

Creatinine filtration rate = GFR × Plasma creatinine concentration
= Creatinine excretion rate

Therefore, if GFR decreases, the creatinine excretion rate also transiently decreases, causing accumulation of creatinine in the body fluids and raising plasma concentration until the excretion rate of creatinine returns to normal—the same rate at which creatinine is produced in the body (Figure 31-4). Thus, under steady-state conditions the creatinine excretion rate equals the rate of creatinine production, despite reductions in GFR; however, this normal rate of creatinine excretion occurs at the expense of elevated plasma creatinine concentration, as shown in curve A of Figure 31-5.

Some solutes, such as phosphate, urate, and hydrogen ions, are often maintained near the normal range until GFR falls below 20 to 30 percent of normal. Thereafter, the plasma concentrations of these substances rise, but not in proportion to the fall in GFR, as shown in curve B of Figure 31-5. Maintenance of relatively constant plasma concentrations of these solutes as GFR declines is accomplished by excreting progressively larger fractions of the amounts of these solutes that are filtered at the glomerular capillaries; this occurs by decreasing the rate of tubular reabsorption or, in some instances, by increasing tubular secretion rates.

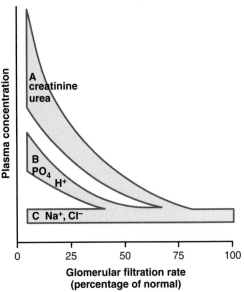

Figure 31-5 Representative patterns of adaptation for different types of solutes in chronic renal failure. Curve A shows the approximate changes in the plasma concentrations of solutes such as creatinine and urea that are filtered and poorly reabsorbed. Curve B shows the approximate concentrations for solutes such as phosphate, urate, and hydrogen ion. Curve C shows the approximate concentrations for solutes such as sodium and chloride.

In the case of sodium and chloride ions, their plasma concentrations are maintained virtually constant even with severe decreases in GFR (see curve C of Figure 31-5). This is accomplished by greatly decreasing tubular reabsorption of these electrolytes.

For example, with a 75 percent loss of functional nephrons, each surviving nephron must excrete four times as much sodium and four times as much volume as under normal conditions (Table 31-6).

Part of this adaptation occurs because of increased blood flow and increased GFR in each of the surviving nephrons, owing to hypertrophy of the blood vessels and glomeruli, as well as functional changes that cause the blood vessels to dilate. Even with large decreases in the total GFR, normal rates of renal excretion can still be maintained by decreasing the rate at which the tubules reabsorb water and solutes.

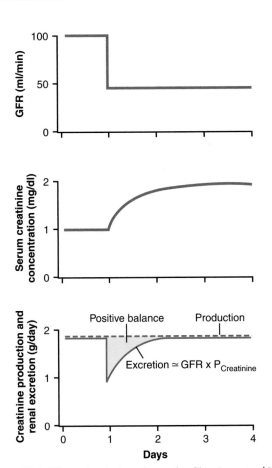

Figure 31-4 Effect of reducing glomerular filtration rate (GFR) by 50 percent on serum creatinine concentration and on creatinine excretion rate when the production rate of creatinine remains constant.

Table 31-6 Total Kidney Excretion and Excretion per Nephron in Renal Failure

	Normal	75% Loss of Nephrons
Number of nephrons	2,000,000	500,000
Total GFR (ml/min)	125	40
Single nephron GFR (nl/min)	62.5	80
Volume excreted for all nephrons (ml/min)	1.5	1.5
Volume excreted per nephron (nl/min)	0.75	3.0

GFR, glomerular filtration rate.

Isosthenuria—Inability of the Kidney to Concentrate or Dilute the Urine. One important effect of the rapid rate of tubular flow that occurs in the remaining nephrons of diseased kidneys is that the renal tubules lose their ability to fully concentrate or dilute the urine. The concentrating ability of the kidney is impaired mainly because (1) the rapid flow of tubular fluid through the collecting ducts prevents adequate water reabsorption, and (2) the rapid flow through both the loop of Henle and the collecting ducts prevents the countercurrent mechanism from operating effectively to concentrate the medullary interstitial fluid solutes. Therefore, as progressively more nephrons are destroyed, the maximum concentrating ability of the kidney declines and urine osmolarity and specific gravity (a measure of the total solute concentration) approach the osmolarity and specific gravity of the glomerular filtrate, as shown in Figure 31-6.

The diluting mechanism in the kidney is also impaired when the number of nephrons decreases because the rapid flushing of fluid through the loops of Henle and the high load of solutes such as urea cause a relatively high solute concentration in the tubular fluid of this part of the nephron. As a consequence, the diluting capacity of the kidney is impaired and the minimal urine osmolality and specific gravity approach those of the glomerular filtrate. Because the concentrating mechanism becomes impaired to a greater extent than does the diluting mechanism in chronic renal failure, an important clinical test of renal function is to determine how well the kidneys can concentrate urine when a person's water intake is restricted for 12 or more hours.

Effects of Renal Failure on the Body Fluids—Uremia

The effect of renal failure on the body fluids depends on (1) water and food intake and (2) the degree of impairment of renal function. Assuming that a person with complete renal failure continues to ingest the same amounts of water and food, the concentrations of different substances in the extracellular fluid are approximately those shown in Figure 31-7. Important effects include (1) *generalized edema* resulting from water and salt retention; (2) *acidosis* resulting from failure of the kidneys to rid the body of normal acidic products; (3) *high concentration of the nonprotein*

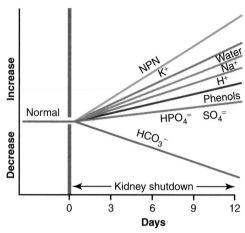

Figure 31-7 Effect of kidney failure on extracellular fluid constituents. NPN, nonprotein nitrogens.

nitrogens—especially urea, creatinine, and uric acid—resulting from failure of the body to excrete the metabolic end products of proteins; and (4) *high concentrations of other substances* excreted by the kidney, including *phenols, sulfates, phosphates, potassium,* and *guanidine bases.* This total condition is called *uremia* because of the high concentration of urea in the body fluids.

Water Retention and Development of Edema in Renal Failure. If water intake is restricted immediately after acute renal failure begins, the total body fluid content may become only slightly increased. If fluid intake is not limited and the patient drinks in response to the normal thirst mechanisms, the body fluids begin to increase immediately and rapidly.

With chronic partial kidney failure, accumulation of fluid may not be severe, as long as salt and fluid intake are not excessive, until kidney function falls to 25 percent of normal or lower. The reason for this, as discussed previously, is that the surviving nephrons excrete larger amounts of salt and water. Even the small fluid retention that does occur, along with increased secretion of renin and angiotensin II that usually occurs in ischemic kidney disease, often causes severe hypertension in chronic renal failure. Almost all patients with kidney function so reduced as to require dialysis to preserve life develop hypertension. In many of these patients, severe reduction of salt intake or removal of extracellular fluid by dialysis can control the hypertension. The remaining patients continue to have hypertension even after excess sodium has been removed by dialysis. In this group, removal of the ischemic kidneys usually corrects the hypertension (as long as fluid retention is prevented by dialysis) because it removes the source of excessive renin secretion and subsequent increased angiotensin II formation.

Uremia—Increase in Urea and Other Nonprotein Nitrogens (Azotemia). The nonprotein nitrogens include urea, uric acid, creatinine, and a few less important compounds. These, in general, are the end products of protein metabolism and must be removed from the body to ensure continued normal protein metabolism in the cells. The concentrations of these, particularly of urea, can rise to as high as 10 times normal during 1 to 2 weeks of total renal failure. With chronic renal failure, the concentrations rise approximately in proportion to the degree of reduction in functional nephrons. For this reason, measuring the concentrations of

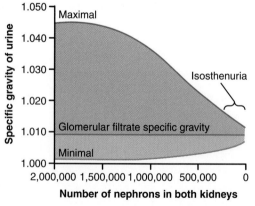

Figure 31-6 Development of isosthenuria in a patient with decreased numbers of functional nephrons.

these substances, especially of urea and creatinine, provides an important means for assessing the degree of renal failure.

Acidosis in Renal Failure. Each day the body normally produces about 50 to 80 millimoles more metabolic acid than metabolic alkali. Therefore, when the kidneys fail to function, acid accumulates in the body fluids. The buffers of the body fluids normally can buffer 500 to 1000 millimoles of acid without lethal increases in extracellular fluid H$^+$ concentration, and the phosphate compounds in the bones can buffer an additional few thousand millimoles of H$^+$. However, when this buffering power is used up, the blood pH falls drastically and the patient will become comatose and die if the pH falls below about 6.8.

Anemia in Chronic Renal Failure Caused by Decreased Erythropoietin Secretion. Patients with severe chronic renal failure almost always develop *anemia*. The most important cause of this is decreased renal secretion of *erythropoietin,* which stimulates the bone marrow to produce red blood cells. If the kidneys are seriously damaged, they are unable to form adequate quantities of erythropoietin, which leads to diminished red blood cell production and consequent anemia.

The availability since 1989 of recombinant erythropoietin, however, has provided a means of treating anemia in patients with chronic renal failure.

Osteomalacia in Chronic Renal Failure Caused by Decreased Production of Active Vitamin D and by Phosphate Retention by the Kidneys. Prolonged renal failure also causes *osteomalacia,* a condition in which the bones are partially absorbed and, therefore, become greatly weakened. An important cause of this condition is the following: Vitamin D must be converted by a two-stage process, first in the liver and then in the kidneys, into 1,25-dihydroxycholecalciferol before it is able to promote calcium absorption from the intestine. Therefore, serious damage to the kidney greatly reduces the blood concentration of *active* vitamin D, which in turn decreases intestinal absorption of calcium and the availability of calcium to the bones.

Another important cause of demineralization of the skeleton in chronic renal failure is the rise in serum phosphate concentration that occurs as a result of decreased GFR. This rise in serum phosphate increases binding of phosphate with calcium in the plasma, thus decreasing the plasma serum *ionized* calcium concentration, which, in turn, stimulates *parathyroid hormone* secretion. This secondary hyperparathyroidism then stimulates the release of calcium from bones, causing further demineralization of the bones.

Hypertension and Kidney Disease

As discussed earlier in this chapter, hypertension can exacerbate injury to the glomeruli and blood vessels of the kidneys and is a major cause of end-stage renal disease. Abnormalities of kidney function can also cause hypertension, as discussed in detail in Chapter 19. Thus, the relation between hypertension and kidney disease can, in some instances, propagate a vicious cycle: primary kidney damage leads to increased blood pressure, which causes further damage to the kidneys, further increases in blood pressure, and so forth, until end-stage renal disease develops.

Not all types of kidney disease cause hypertension because damage to certain portions of the kidney causes uremia without hypertension. Nevertheless, some types of renal damage are particularly prone to cause hypertension. A classification of kidney disease relative to hypertensive or nonhypertensive effects is the following.

Renal Lesions That Reduce the Ability of the Kidneys to Excrete Sodium and Water Promote Hypertension. Renal lesions that decrease the ability of the kidneys to excrete sodium and water almost invariably cause hypertension. Therefore, lesions that either *decrease GFR* or *increase tubular reabsorption* usually lead to hypertension of varying degrees. Some specific types of renal abnormalities that can cause hypertension are as follows:

1. *Increased renal vascular resistance,* which reduces renal blood flow and GFR. An example is hypertension caused by renal artery stenosis.
2. *Decreased glomerular capillary filtration coefficient, which reduces GFR.* An example of this is chronic glomerulonephritis, which causes inflammation and thickening of the glomerular capillary membranes, thereby reducing the glomerular capillary filtration coefficient.
3. *Excessive tubular sodium reabsorption.* An example is hypertension caused by excessive aldosterone secretion, which increases sodium reabsorption mainly in the cortical collecting tubules.

Once hypertension has developed, renal excretion of sodium and water returns to normal because the high arterial pressure causes pressure natriuresis and pressure diuresis, so intake and output of sodium and water become balanced once again. Even when there are large increases in renal vascular resistance or decreases in the glomerular capillary coefficient, the GFR may still return to nearly normal levels after the arterial blood pressure rises. Likewise, when tubular reabsorption is increased, as occurs with excessive aldosterone secretion, the urinary excretion rate is initially reduced but then returns to normal as arterial pressure rises. Thus, after hypertension develops, there may be no obvious sign of impaired excretion of sodium and water other than the hypertension. As explained in Chapter 19, normal excretion of sodium and water at an elevated arterial pressure means that pressure natriuresis and pressure diuresis have been reset to a higher arterial pressure.

Hypertension Caused by Patchy Renal Damage and Increased Renal Secretion of Renin. If one part of the kidney is ischemic and the remainder is not ischemic, such as occurs when one renal artery is severely constricted, the ischemic renal tissue secretes large quantities of renin. This secretion leads to increased formation of angiotensin II, which can cause hypertension. The most likely sequence of events in causing this hypertension, as discussed in Chapter 19, is (1) the ischemic kidney tissue itself excretes less than normal amounts of water and salt; (2) the renin secreted by the ischemic kidney, as well as the subsequent increased angiotensin II formation, affects the nonischemic kidney tissue, causing it also to retain salt and water; and (3) excess salt and water cause hypertension in the usual manner.

A similar type of hypertension can result when patchy areas of one or both kidneys become ischemic as a result of arteriosclerosis or vascular injury in specific portions of the kidneys. When this occurs, the ischemic nephrons excrete less salt and water but secrete greater amounts of renin, which causes increased angiotensin II formation. The high levels of angiotensin II then impair the ability of the surrounding otherwise normal nephrons to excrete sodium and water. As a result, hypertension develops, which restores the overall excretion of sodium and water by the kidney, so balance between intake and output of salt and water is maintained, but at the expense of high blood pressure.

Kidney Diseases That Cause Loss of Entire Nephrons Lead to Renal Failure but May Not Cause Hypertension. Loss of large numbers of whole nephrons, such as occurs with the loss of one kidney and part of another kidney, almost always leads to renal failure if the amount of kidney tissue lost is great enough. If the remaining nephrons are normal and the salt intake is not excessive, this condition might not cause clinically significant hypertension because even a slight rise in blood pressure will raise the GFR and decrease tubular sodium reabsorption sufficiently to promote enough water and salt excretion in the urine, even with the few nephrons that remain intact. However, a patient with this type of abnormality may become severely hypertensive if additional stresses are imposed, such as eating a large amount of salt. In this case, the kidneys simply cannot clear adequate quantities of salt at a normal blood pressure with the small number of functioning nephrons that remain. Increased blood pressure restores excretion of salt and water to match intake of salt and water under steady-state conditions.

Effective treatment of hypertension requires that the kidneys' capability to excrete salt and water is increased, either by increasing GFR or by decreasing tubular reabsorption, so that balance between intake and renal excretion of salt and water excretion can be maintained at lower blood pressures. This can be achieved by drugs that block the effects of nervous and hormonal signals that cause the kidneys to retain salt and water (e.g., with β-adrenergic blockers, angiotensin receptor antagonists, or angiotensin-converting enzyme inhibitors) or with diuretic drugs that directly inhibit renal tubular reabsorption of salt and water.

Specific Tubular Disorders

In Chapter 27, we point out that several mechanisms are responsible for transporting different individual substances across the tubular epithelial membranes. In Chapter 3, we also point out that each cellular enzyme and each carrier protein is formed in response to a respective gene in the nucleus. If any required gene happens to be absent or abnormal, the tubules may be deficient in one of the appropriate carrier proteins or one of the enzymes needed for solute transport by the renal tubular epithelial cells. In other instances, too much of the enzyme or carrier protein is produced. Thus, many hereditary tubular disorders occur because of abnormal transport of individual substances or groups of substances through the tubular membrane. In addition, damage to the tubular epithelial membrane by toxins or ischemia can cause important renal tubular disorders.

Renal Glycosuria—Failure of the Kidneys to Reabsorb Glucose. In this condition the blood glucose concentration may be normal, but the transport mechanism for tubular reabsorption of glucose is greatly limited or absent. Consequently, despite a normal blood glucose level, large amounts of glucose pass into the urine each day. Because diabetes mellitus is also associated with the presence of glucose in the urine, renal glycosuria, which is a relatively benign condition, must be ruled out before making the diagnosis of diabetes mellitus.

Aminoaciduria—Failure of the Kidneys to Reabsorb Amino Acids. Some amino acids share mutual transport systems for reabsorption, whereas other amino acids have their own distinct transport systems. Rarely, a condition called *generalized aminoaciduria* results from deficient reabsorption of all amino acids; more frequently, deficiencies of specific carrier systems may result in (1) *essential cystinuria,* in which large amounts of cystine fail to be reabsorbed and often crystallize in the urine to form renal stones; (2) *simple glycinuria,* in which glycine fails to be reabsorbed; or (3) *beta-aminoisobutyricaciduria,* which occurs in about 5 percent of all people but apparently has no major clinical significance.

Renal Hypophosphatemia—Failure of the Kidneys to Reabsorb Phosphate. In renal hypophosphatemia, the renal tubules fail to reabsorb large enough quantities of phosphate ions when the phosphate concentration of the body fluids falls very low. This condition usually does not cause serious immediate abnormalities because the phosphate concentration of the extracellular fluid can vary widely without causing major cellular dysfunction. Over a long period, a low phosphate level causes diminished calcification of the bones, causing the person to develop rickets. This type of rickets is refractory to vitamin D therapy, in contrast to the rapid response of the usual type of rickets, as discussed in Chapter 79.

Renal Tubular Acidosis—Failure of the Tubules to Secrete Hydrogen Ions. In this condition, the renal tubules are unable to secrete adequate amounts of hydrogen ions. As a result, large amounts of sodium bicarbonate are continually lost in the urine. This causes a continued state of metabolic acidosis, as discussed in Chapter 30. This type of renal abnormality can be caused by hereditary disorders, or it can occur as a result of widespread injury to the renal tubules.

Nephrogenic Diabetes Insipidus—Failure of the Kidneys to Respond to Antidiuretic Hormone. Occasionally, the renal tubules do not respond to antidiuretic hormone, causing large quantities of dilute urine to be excreted. As long as the person is supplied with plenty of water, this condition seldom causes severe difficulty. However, when adequate quantities of water are not available, the person rapidly becomes dehydrated.

Fanconi's Syndrome—A Generalized Reabsorptive Defect of the Renal Tubules. Fanconi's syndrome is usually associated with increased urinary excretion of virtually all amino acids, glucose, and phosphate. In severe cases, other manifestations are also observed, such as (1) failure to reabsorb sodium bicarbonate, which results in metabolic acidosis; (2) increased excretion of potassium and sometimes calcium; and (3) nephrogenic diabetes insipidus.

There are multiple causes of Fanconi's syndrome, which results from a generalized inability of the renal tubular cells to transport various substances. Some of these causes include (1) hereditary defects in cell transport mechanisms, (2) toxins or drugs that injure the renal tubular epithelial cells, and (3) injury to the renal tubular cells as a result of ischemia. The proximal tubular cells are especially affected in Fanconi's syndrome caused by tubular injury because these cells reabsorb and secrete many of the drugs and toxins that can cause damage.

Bartter's Syndrome—Decreased Sodium, Chloride, and Potassium Reabsorption in the Loops of Henle. *Bartter's syndrome* is an autosomal recessive disorder caused by impaired function of the 1-sodium, 2-chloride, 1-potassium co-transporter, or by defects in potassium channels in the luminal membrane or chloride channels in the basolateral membrane of the thick ascending loop of Henle. These disorders result in increased excretion of water, sodium, chloride, potassium, and calcium by the kidneys. The salt and water loss leads to mild volume depletion, resulting in activation of the renin-angiotensin-aldosterone system. The increased aldosterone and high distal tubular flow, due to impaired loop of Henle reabsorption, stimulate potassium and hydrogen secretion in the collecting tubules, leading to hypokalemia and metabolic alkalosis.

Gitelman's Syndrome—Decreased Sodium Chloride Reabsorption in the Distal Tubules. *Gitelman's syndrome* is an autosomal recessive disorder of the thiazide-sensitive sodium-chloride co-transporter in the distal tubules. Patients with Gitelman's syndrome have some of the same characteristics as patients with Bartter's syndrome—salt and water loss, mild water volume depletion, and activation of the renin-angiotensin-aldosterone system—although these abnormalities are usually less severe in Gitelman's syndrome.

Because the tubular defects in Bartter's or Gitelman's syndrome cannot be corrected, treatment is usually focused on replacing the losses of sodium chloride and potassium. Some studies suggest that blockade of prostaglandin synthesis with nonsteroidal anti-inflammatory drugs and administration of aldosterone antagonists, such as spironolactone, may be useful in correcting the hypokalemia.

Liddle's Syndrome—Increased Sodium Reabsorption. *Liddle's syndrome* is a rare autosomal dominant disorder resulting from various mutations in the amiloride-sensitive epithelial sodium channel (ENaC) in the distal and collecting tubules. These mutations cause excessive activity of ENaC, resulting in increased reabsorption of sodium and water, hypertension, and metabolic alkalosis similar to the changes that occur with oversecretion of aldosterone (primary aldosteronism).

Patients with Liddle's syndrome, however, have decreased levels of aldosterone due to sodium retention and compensatory decreases in renin secretion and angiotensin II levels, which, in turn, decrease adrenal secretion of aldosterone. Fortunately, Liddle's syndrome can be treated with the diuretic amiloride, which blocks the excessive ENaC activity.

Treatment of Renal Failure by Transplantation or by Dialysis with an Artificial Kidney

Severe loss of kidney function, either acutely or chronically, is a threat to life and requires removal of toxic waste products and restoration of body fluid volume and composition toward normal. This can be accomplished by kidney transplantation or by dialysis with an artificial kidney. More than 500,000 patients in the United States are currently receiving some form of ESRD therapy.

Successful transplantation of a single donor kidney to a patient with ESRD can restore kidney function to a level that is sufficient to maintain essentially normal homeostasis of body fluids and electrolytes. Approximately 16,000 kidney transplants are performed each year in the United States. Patients who receive kidney transplants typically live longer and have fewer health problems than those who are maintained on dialysis. Maintenance of immunosuppressive therapy is required for almost all patients to help prevent acute

rejection and loss of the transplanted kidney. The side effects of drugs that suppress the immune system include increased risk for infections and for some cancers, although the amount of immunosuppressive therapy can usually be reduced over time to greatly reduce these risks.

More than 350,000 people in the United States with irreversible renal failure or total kidney removal are being maintained chronically by dialysis with artificial kidneys. Dialysis is also used in certain types of acute renal failure to tide the patient over until the kidneys resume their function. If the loss of kidney function is irreversible, it is necessary to perform dialysis chronically to maintain life. Because dialysis cannot maintain completely normal body fluid composition and cannot replace all the multiple functions performed by the kidneys, the health of patients maintained on artificial kidneys usually remains significantly impaired.

Basic Principles of Dialysis. The basic principle of the artificial kidney is to pass blood through minute blood channels bounded by a thin membrane. On the other side of the membrane is a *dialyzing fluid* into which unwanted substances in the blood pass by diffusion.

Figure 31-8 shows the components of one type of artificial kidney in which blood flows continually between two thin membranes of cellophane; outside the membrane is a dialyzing fluid. The cellophane is porous enough to allow the constituents of the plasma, except the plasma proteins, to diffuse in both directions—from plasma into the dialyzing fluid or from the dialyzing fluid back into the plasma.

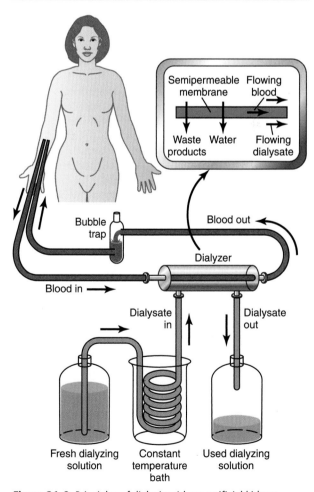

Figure 31-8 Principles of dialysis with an artificial kidney.

If the concentration of a substance is greater in the plasma than in the dialyzing fluid, there will be a net transfer of the substance from the plasma into the dialyzing fluid.

The rate of movement of solute across the dialyzing membrane depends on (1) the concentration gradient of the solute between the two solutions, (2) the permeability of the membrane to the solute, (3) the surface area of the membrane, and (4) the length of time that the blood and fluid remain in contact with the membrane.

Thus, the maximum rate of solute transfer occurs initially when the concentration gradient is greatest (when dialysis is begun) and slows down as the concentration gradient is dissipated. In a flowing system, as is the case with "hemodialysis," in which blood and dialysate fluid flow through the artificial kidney, the dissipation of the concentration gradient can be reduced and diffusion of solute across the membrane can be optimized by increasing the flow rate of the blood, the dialyzing fluid, or both.

In normal operation of the artificial kidney, blood flows continually or intermittently back into the vein. The total amount of blood in the artificial kidney at any one time is usually less than 500 milliliters, the rate of flow may be several hundred milliliters per minute, and the total diffusion surface area is between 0.6 and 2.5 square meters. To prevent coagulation of the blood in the artificial kidney, a small amount of heparin is infused into the blood as it enters the artificial kidney. In addition to diffusion of solutes, mass transfer of solutes and water can be produced by applying a hydrostatic pressure to force the fluid and solutes across the membranes of the dialyzer; such filtration is called *bulk flow*.

Dialyzing Fluid. Table 31-7 compares the constituents in a typical dialyzing fluid with those in normal plasma and uremic plasma. Note that the concentrations of ions and other substances in dialyzing fluid are not the same as the concentrations in normal plasma or in uremic plasma. Instead, they are adjusted to levels that are needed to cause appropriate movement of water and solutes through the membrane during dialysis.

Note that there is no phosphate, urea, urate, sulfate, or creatinine in the dialyzing fluid; however, these are present in high concentrations in the uremic blood. Therefore, when a uremic patient is dialyzed, these substances are lost in large quantities into the dialyzing fluid.

The effectiveness of the artificial kidney can be expressed in terms of the amount of plasma that is cleared of different substances each minute, which, as discussed in Chapter 27, is the primary means for expressing the functional effectiveness of the kidneys themselves to rid the body of unwanted substances. Most artificial kidneys can clear urea from the plasma at a rate of 100 to 225 ml/min, which shows that at least for the excretion of urea, the artificial kidney can function about twice as rapidly as two normal kidneys together, whose urea clearance is only 70 ml/min. Yet the artificial kidney is used for only 4 to 6 hours per day, three times a week. Therefore, the overall plasma clearance is still considerably limited when the artificial kidney replaces the normal kidneys. Also, it is important to keep in mind that the artificial kidney cannot replace some of the other functions of the kidneys, such as secretion of erythropoietin, which is necessary for red blood cell production.

Table 31-7 Comparison of Dialyzing Fluid with Normal and Uremic Plasma

Constituent	Normal Plasma	Dialyzing Fluid	Uremic Plasma
Electrolytes (mEq/L)			
Na^+	142	133	142
K^+	5	1.0	7
Ca^{++}	3	3.0	2
Mg^{++}	1.5	1.5	1.5
Cl^-	107	105	107
HCO_3^-	24	35.7	14
$Lactate^-$	1.2	1.2	1.2
$HPO_4^=$	3	0	9
$Urate^-$	0.3	0	2
$Sulfate^=$	0.5	0	3
Nonelectrolytes			
Glucose	100	125	100
Urea	26	0	200
Creatinine	1	0	6

Bibliography

Andreoli TE, ed: *Cecil's Essentials of Medicine*, ed 6, Philadelphia, 2004, WB Saunders.

Calhoun DA, Jones D, Textor S, et al: Resistant hypertension: diagnosis, evaluation, and treatment: a scientific statement from the American Heart Association Professional Education Committee of the Council for High Blood Pressure Research, *Hypertension* 51:1403, 2008.

Devarajan P: Update on mechanisms of ischemic acute kidney injury, *J Am Soc Nephrol* 17:1503, 2006.

Grantham JJ: Clinical practice, Autosomal dominant polycystic kidney disease, *N Engl J Med* 359:1477, 2008.

Griffin KA, Kramer H, Bidani AK: Adverse renal consequences of obesity, *Am J Physiol Renal Physiol* 294:F685, 2008.

Hall JE: The kidney, hypertension, and obesity, *Hypertension* 41:625, 2003.

Hall JE, da Silva AA, Brandon E, et al: Pathophysiology of obesity hypertension and target organ injury. In Lip GYP, Hall JE, editors: *Comprehensive Hypertension*, New York, 2007, Elsevier, pp 447–468.

Hall JE, Henegar JR, Dwyer TM, et al: Is obesity a major cause of chronic renal disease?, *Adv Ren Replace Ther* 11:41, 2004.

Mitch WE: Acute renal failure. In Goldman F, Bennett JC, editors: *Cecil Textbook of Medicine*, ed 21, Philadelphia, 2000, WB Saunders, pp 567–570.

Molitoris BA: Transitioning to therapy in ischemic acute renal failure, *J Am Soc Nephrol* 14:265, 2003.

Rodriguez-Iturbe B, Musser JM: The current state of poststreptococcal glomerulonephritis, *J Am Soc Nephrol* 19:1855, 2008.

Rossier BC, Schild L: Epithelial sodium channel: Mendelian versus essential hypertension, *Hypertension* 52:595, 2008.

Sarnak MJ, Levey AS, Schoolwerth AC, et al: Kidney disease as a risk factor for development of cardiovascular disease, *Hypertension* 42:1050, 2003.

Singri N, Ahya SN, Levin ML: Acute renal failure, *JAMA* 289:747, 2003.

United States Renal Data System. http://www.usrds.org/.

Wilcox CS: New insights into diuretic use in patients with chronic renal disease, *J Am Soc Nephrol* 13:798, 2002.

Blood Cells, Immunity, and Blood Coagulation

32. Red Blood Cells, Anemia, and Polycythemia

33. Resistance of the Body to Infection: I. Leukocytes, Granulocytes, the Monocyte-Macrophage System, and Inflammation

34. Resistance of the Body to Infection: II. Immunity and Allergy Innate Immunity

35. Blood Types; Transfusion; Tissue and Organ Transplantation

36. Hemostasis and Blood Coagulation

CHAPTER 32

Red Blood Cells, Anemia, and Polycythemia

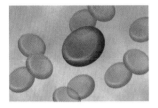

With this chapter we begin discussing the *blood cells* and cells of the *macrophage system* and *lymphatic system*. We first present the functions of red blood cells, which are the most abundant cells of the blood and are necessary for the delivery of oxygen to the tissues.

Red Blood Cells (Erythrocytes)

A major function of red blood cells, also known as *erythrocytes*, is to transport *hemoglobin*, which in turn carries oxygen from the lungs to the tissues. In some lower animals, hemoglobin circulates as free protein in the plasma, not enclosed in red blood cells. When it is free in the plasma of the human being, about 3 percent of it leaks through the capillary membrane into the tissue spaces or through the glomerular membrane of the kidney into the glomerular filtrate each time the blood passes through the capillaries. Therefore, hemoglobin must remain inside red blood cells to effectively perform its functions in humans.

The red blood cells have other functions besides transport of hemoglobin. For instance, they contain a large quantity of *carbonic anhydrase*, an enzyme that catalyzes the reversible reaction between carbon dioxide (CO_2) and water to form carbonic acid (H_2CO_3), increasing the rate of this reaction several thousandfold. The rapidity of this reaction makes it possible for the water of the blood to transport enormous quantities of CO_2 in the form of bicarbonate ion (HCO_3^-) from the tissues to the lungs, where it is reconverted to CO_2 and expelled into the atmosphere as a body waste product. The hemoglobin in the cells is an excellent *acid-base buffer* (as is true of most proteins), so the red blood cells are responsible for most of the acid-base buffering power of whole blood.

Shape and Size of Red Blood Cells. Normal red blood cells, shown in Figure 32-3, are biconcave discs having a mean diameter of about 7.8 micrometers and a thickness of 2.5 micrometers at the thickest point and 1 micrometer or less in the center. The average volume of the red blood cell is 90 to 95 cubic micrometers.

The shapes of red blood cells can change remarkably as the cells squeeze through capillaries. Actually, the red blood cell is a "bag" that can be deformed into almost any shape. Furthermore, because the normal cell has a great excess of cell membrane for the quantity of material inside, deformation does not stretch the membrane greatly and, consequently, does not rupture the cell, as would be the case with many other cells.

Concentration of Red Blood Cells in the Blood. In healthy men, the average number of red blood cells per cubic millimeter is 5,200,000 (±300,000); in women, it is 4,700,000 (±300,000). Persons living at high altitudes have greater numbers of red blood cells, as discussed later.

Quantity of Hemoglobin in the Cells. Red blood cells have the ability to concentrate hemoglobin in the cell fluid up to about 34 grams in each 100 milliliters of cells. The concentration does not rise above this value because this is the metabolic limit of the cell's hemoglobin-forming mechanism. Furthermore, in normal people, the percentage of hemoglobin is almost always near the maximum in each cell. However, when hemoglobin formation is deficient, the percentage of hemoglobin in the cells may fall considerably below this value and the volume of the red cell may also decrease because of diminished hemoglobin to fill the cell.

When the hematocrit (the percentage of blood that is in cells—normally, 40 to 45 percent) and the quantity of hemoglobin in each respective cell are normal, the whole blood of men contains an average of 15 grams of hemoglobin per 100 milliliters of cells; for women, it contains an average of 14 grams per 100 milliliters.

As discussed in connection with blood transport of oxygen in Chapter 40, each gram of pure hemoglobin combines with 1.34 ml of oxygen. Therefore, in a normal man a maximum of about 20 milliliters of oxygen can be carried in combination with hemoglobin in each 100 milliliters of blood, and in a normal woman 19 milliliters of oxygen can be carried.

Production of Red Blood Cells

Areas of the Body That Produce Red Blood Cells.
In the early weeks of embryonic life, primitive, nucleated red blood cells are produced in the *yolk sac.* During the middle trimester of gestation, the *liver* is the main organ for production of red blood cells but reasonable numbers are also produced in the *spleen* and *lymph nodes.* Then, during the last month or so of gestation and after birth, red blood cells are produced exclusively in the *bone marrow.*

As demonstrated in Figure 32-1, the bone marrow of essentially all bones produces red blood cells until a person is 5 years old. The marrow of the long bones,

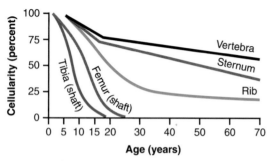

Figure 32-1 Relative rates of red blood cell production in the bone marrow of different bones at different ages.

except for the proximal portions of the humeri and tibiae, becomes quite fatty and produces no more red blood cells after about age 20 years. Beyond this age, most red cells continue to be produced in the marrow of the membranous bones, such as the vertebrae, sternum, ribs, and ilia. Even in these bones, the marrow becomes less productive as age increases.

Genesis of Blood Cells

Pluripotential Hematopoietic Stem Cells, Growth Inducers, and Differentiation Inducers. The blood cells begin their lives in the bone marrow from a single type of cell called the *pluripotential hematopoietic stem cell,* from which all the cells of the circulating blood are eventually derived. Figure 32-2 shows the successive divisions of the pluripotential cells to form the different circulating blood cells. As these cells reproduce, a small portion of them remains exactly like the original pluripotential cells and is retained in the bone marrow to maintain a supply of these, although their numbers diminish with age. Most of the reproduced cells, however, differentiate to form the other cell types shown to the right in Figure 32-2. The intermediate-stage cells are very much like the pluripotential stem cells, even though they have already become committed to a particular line of cells and are called *committed stem cells.*

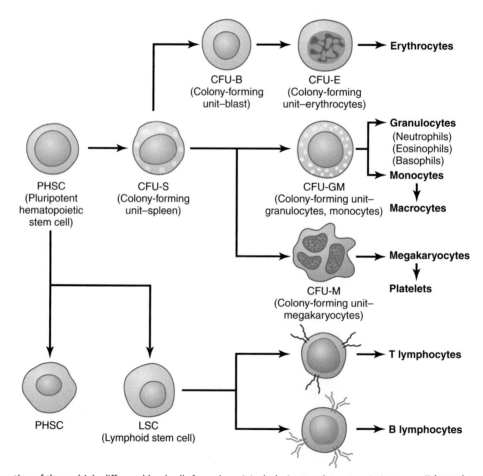

Figure 32-2 Formation of the multiple different blood cells from the original *pluripotent hematopoietic stem cell (PHSC)* in the bone marrow.

The different committed stem cells, when grown in culture, will produce colonies of specific types of blood cells. A committed stem cell that produces erythrocytes is called a *colony-forming unit-erythrocyte,* and the abbreviation CFU-E is used to designate this type of stem cell. Likewise, colony-forming units that form granulocytes and monocytes have the designation CFU-GM and so forth.

Growth and reproduction of the different stem cells are controlled by multiple proteins called *growth inducers.* Four major growth inducers have been described, each having different characteristics. One of these, *interleukin-3,* promotes growth and reproduction of virtually all the different types of committed stem cells, whereas the others induce growth of only specific types of cells.

The growth inducers promote growth but not differentiation of the cells. This is the function of another set of proteins called *differentiation inducers.* Each of these causes one type of committed stem cell to differentiate one or more steps toward a final adult blood cell.

Formation of the growth inducers and differentiation inducers is itself controlled by factors outside the bone marrow. For instance, in the case of erythrocytes (red blood cells), exposure of the blood to low oxygen for a long time causes growth induction, differentiation, and production of greatly increased numbers of erythrocytes, as discussed later in the chapter. In the case of some of the white blood cells, infectious diseases cause growth, differentiation, and eventual formation of specific types of white blood cells that are needed to combat each infection.

Stages of Differentiation of Red Blood Cells

The first cell that can be identified as belonging to the red blood cell series is the *proerythroblast,* shown at the starting point in Figure 32-3. Under appropriate stimulation, large numbers of these cells are formed from the CFU-E stem cells.

Once the proerythroblast has been formed, it divides multiple times, eventually forming many mature red blood cells. The first-generation cells are called *basophil erythroblasts* because they stain with basic dyes; the cell at this time has accumulated very little hemoglobin. In the succeeding generations, as shown in Figure 32-3, the cells become filled with hemoglobin to a concentration of about 34 percent, the nucleus condenses to a small size, and its final remnant is absorbed or extruded from the cell. At the same time, the endoplasmic reticulum is also reabsorbed. The cell at this stage is called a *reticulocyte* because it still contains a small amount of basophilic material, consisting of remnants of the Golgi apparatus, mitochondria, and a few other cytoplasmic organelles. During this reticulocyte stage, the cells pass from the bone marrow into the blood capillaries by *diapedesis* (squeezing through the pores of the capillary membrane).

The remaining basophilic material in the reticulocyte normally disappears within 1 to 2 days, and the cell is then a *mature erythrocyte.* Because of the short life of the reticulocytes, their concentration among all the red cells of the blood is normally slightly less than 1 percent.

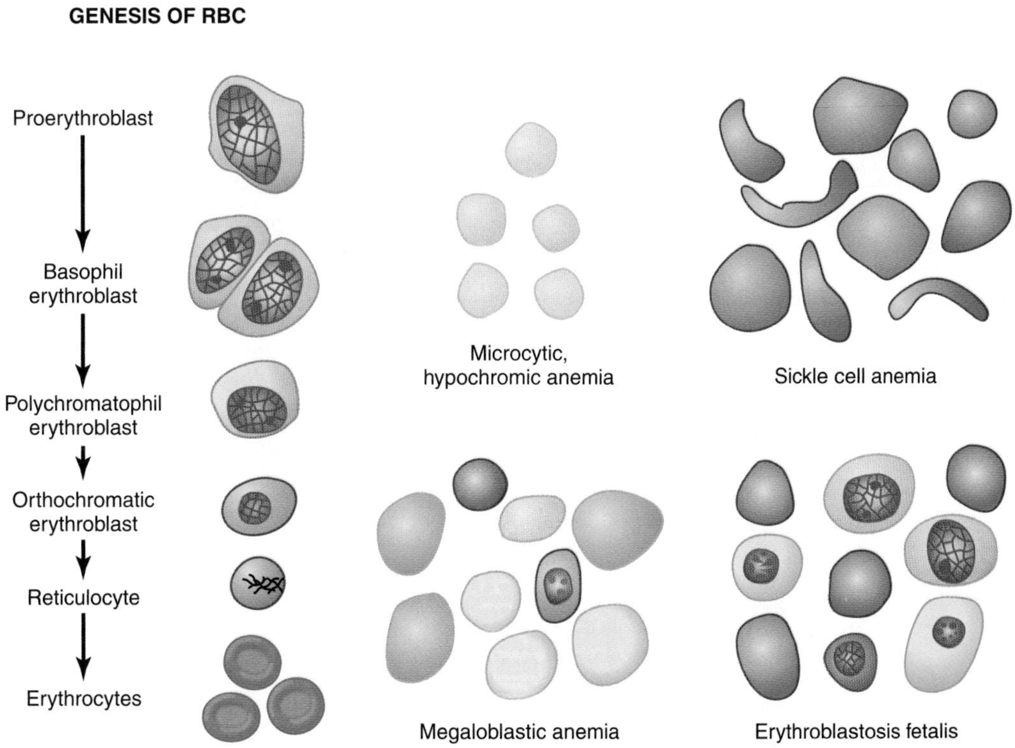

GENESIS OF RBC

Figure 32-3 Genesis of normal red blood cells (RBCs) and characteristics of RBCs in different types of anemias.

Regulation of Red Blood Cell Production—Role of Erythropoietin

The total mass of red blood cells in the circulatory system is regulated within narrow limits, so (1) adequate red cells are always available to provide sufficient transport of oxygen from the lungs to the tissues, yet (2) the cells do not become so numerous that they impede blood flow. This control mechanism is diagrammed in Figure 32-4 and is as follows.

Tissue Oxygenation Is the Most Essential Regulator of Red Blood Cell Production. Any condition that causes the quantity of oxygen transported to the tissues to decrease ordinarily increases the rate of red blood cell production. Thus, when a person becomes extremely *anemic* as a result of hemorrhage or any other condition, the bone marrow begins to produce large quantities of red blood cells. Also, destruction of major portions of the bone marrow by any means, especially by x-ray therapy, causes hyperplasia of the remaining bone marrow, thereby attempting to supply the demand for red blood cells in the body.

At very *high altitudes,* where the quantity of oxygen in the air is greatly decreased, insufficient oxygen is transported to the tissues and red cell production is greatly increased. In this case, it is not the concentration of red blood cells in the blood that controls red cell production but the amount of oxygen transported to the tissues in relation to tissue demand for oxygen.

Various diseases of the circulation that cause decreased tissue blood flow, and particularly those that cause failure of oxygen absorption by the blood as it passes through the lungs, can also increase the rate of red cell production. This is especially apparent in prolonged *cardiac failure* and in many *lung diseases* because the tissue hypoxia resulting from these conditions increases red cell production, with a resultant increase in hematocrit and usually total blood volume as well.

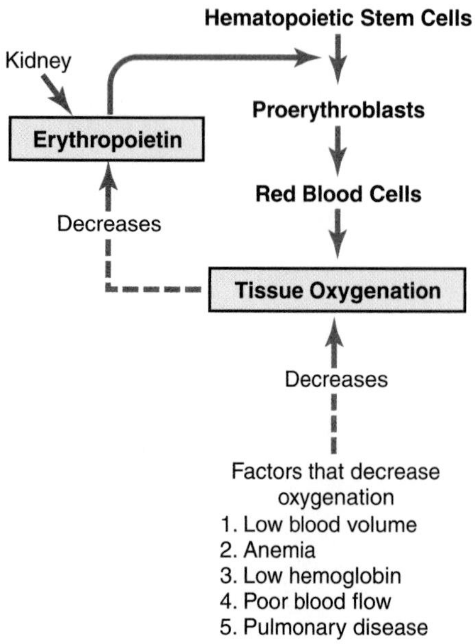

Erythropoietin Stimulates Red Cell Production, and Its Formation Increases in Response to Hypoxia. The principal stimulus for red blood cell production in low oxygen states is a circulating hormone called *erythropoietin,* a glycoprotein with a molecular weight of about 34,000. In the absence of erythropoietin, hypoxia has little or no effect to stimulate red blood cell production. But when the erythropoietin system is functional, hypoxia causes a marked increase in erythropoietin production and the erythropoietin in turn enhances red blood cell production until the hypoxia is relieved.

Role of the Kidneys in Formation of Erythropoietin. Normally, about 90 percent of all erythropoietin is formed in the kidneys; the remainder is formed mainly in the liver. It is not known exactly where in the kidneys the erythropoietin is formed. Some studies suggest that erythropoietin is secreted mainly by fibroblast-like interstitial cells surrounding the tubules in the cortex and outer medulla secrete, where much of the kidney's oxygen consumption occurs. It is likely that other cells, including the renal epithelial cells themselves, also secrete the erythropoietin in response to hypoxia.

Renal tissue hypoxia leads to increased tissue levels of *hypoxia-inducible factor-1* (HIF-1), which serves as a transcription factor for a large number of hypoxia-inducible genes, including the erythropoietin gene. HIF-1 binds to a *hypoxia response element* residing in the erythropoietin gene, inducing transcription of mRNA and, ultimately, increased erythropoietin synthesis.

At times, hypoxia in other parts of the body, but not in the kidneys, stimulates kidney erythropoietin secretion, which suggests that there might be some nonrenal sensor that sends an additional signal to the kidneys to produce this hormone. In particular, both norepinephrine and epinephrine and several of the prostaglandins stimulate erythropoietin production.

When both kidneys are removed from a person or when the kidneys are destroyed by renal disease, the person invariably becomes very anemic because the 10 percent of the normal erythropoietin formed in other tissues (mainly in the liver) is sufficient to cause only one third to one half the red blood cell formation needed by the body.

Effect of Erythropoietin in Erythrogenesis. When an animal or a person is placed in an atmosphere of low oxygen, erythropoietin begins to be formed within minutes to hours, and it reaches maximum production within 24 hours. Yet almost no new red blood cells appear in the circulating blood until about 5 days later. From this fact, as well as from other studies, it has been determined that the important effect of erythropoietin is to stimulate the production of proerythroblasts from hematopoietic stem cells in the bone marrow. In addition, once the proerythroblasts are formed, the erythropoietin causes these cells to pass more rapidly through the different erythroblastic stages than they normally do, further speeding up the production of new red blood cells. The rapid production of

Figure 32-4 Function of the erythropoietin mechanism to increase production of red blood cells when tissue oxygenation decreases.

cells continues as long as the person remains in a low oxygen state or until enough red blood cells have been produced to carry adequate amounts of oxygen to the tissues despite the low oxygen; at this time, the rate of erythropoietin production decreases to a level that will maintain the required number of red cells but not an excess.

In the absence of erythropoietin, few red blood cells are formed by the bone marrow. At the other extreme, when large quantities of erythropoietin are formed and if there is plenty of iron and other required nutrients available, the rate of red blood cell production can rise to perhaps 10 or more times normal. Therefore, the erythropoietin mechanism for controlling red blood cell production is a powerful one.

Maturation of Red Blood Cells—Requirement for Vitamin B$_{12}$ (Cyanocobalamin) and Folic Acid

Because of the continuing need to replenish red blood cells, the erythropoietic cells of the bone marrow are among the most rapidly growing and reproducing cells in the entire body. Therefore, as would be expected, their maturation and rate of production are affected greatly by a person's nutritional status.

Especially important for final maturation of the red blood cells are two vitamins, *vitamin B$_{12}$* and *folic acid.* Both of these are essential for the synthesis of DNA because each, in a different way, is required for the formation of thymidine triphosphate, one of the essential building blocks of DNA. Therefore, lack of either vitamin B$_{12}$ or folic acid causes abnormal and diminished DNA and, consequently, failure of nuclear maturation and cell division. Furthermore, the erythroblastic cells of the bone marrow, in addition to failing to proliferate rapidly, produce mainly larger than normal red cells called *macrocytes* and the cell itself has a flimsy membrane and is often irregular, large, and oval instead of the usual biconcave disc. These poorly formed cells, after entering the circulating blood, are capable of carrying oxygen normally, but their fragility causes them to have a short life, one-half to one-third normal. Therefore, it is said that deficiency of either vitamin B$_{12}$ or folic acid causes *maturation failure* in the process of erythropoiesis.

Maturation Failure Caused by Poor Absorption of Vitamin B$_{12}$ from the Gastrointestinal Tract—Pernicious Anemia. A common cause of red blood cell maturation failure is failure to absorb vitamin B$_{12}$ from the gastrointestinal tract. This often occurs in the disease *pernicious anemia,* in which the basic abnormality is an *atrophic gastric mucosa* that fails to produce normal gastric secretions. The parietal cells of the gastric glands secrete a glycoprotein called *intrinsic factor,* which combines with vitamin B$_{12}$ in food and makes the B$_{12}$ available for absorption by the gut. It does this in the following way: (1) Intrinsic factor binds tightly with the vitamin B$_{12}$. In this bound state, the B$_{12}$ is protected from digestion by the gastrointestinal secretions. (2) Still in the bound state, intrinsic factor binds to specific receptor sites on the brush border

membranes of the mucosal cells in the ileum. (3) Then, vitamin B$_{12}$ is transported into the blood during the next few hours by the process of pinocytosis, carrying intrinsic factor and the vitamin together through the membrane. Lack of intrinsic factor, therefore, decreases availability of vitamin B$_{12}$ because of faulty absorption of the vitamin.

Once vitamin B$_{12}$ has been absorbed from the gastrointestinal tract, it is first stored in large quantities in the liver and then released slowly as needed by the bone marrow. The minimum amount of vitamin B$_{12}$ required each day to maintain normal red cell maturation is only 1 to 3 micrograms, and the normal storage in the liver and other body tissues is about 1000 times this amount. Therefore, 3 to 4 years of defective B$_{12}$ absorption are usually required to cause maturation failure anemia.

Failure of Maturation Caused by Deficiency of Folic Acid (Pteroylglutamic Acid). Folic acid is a normal constituent of green vegetables, some fruits, and meats (especially liver). However, it is easily destroyed during cooking. Also, people with gastrointestinal absorption abnormalities, such as the frequently occurring small intestinal disease called *sprue,* often have serious difficulty absorbing both folic acid and vitamin B$_{12}$. Therefore, in many instances of maturation failure, the cause is deficiency of intestinal absorption of both folic acid and vitamin B$_{12}$.

Formation of Hemoglobin

Synthesis of hemoglobin begins in the proerythroblasts and continues even into the reticulocyte stage of the red blood cells. Therefore, when reticulocytes leave the bone marrow and pass into the blood stream, they continue to form minute quantities of hemoglobin for another day or so until they become mature erythrocytes.

Figure 32-5 shows the basic chemical steps in the formation of hemoglobin. First, succinyl-CoA, formed in the Krebs metabolic cycle (as explained in Chapter 67), binds with glycine to form a pyrrole molecule. In turn, four pyrroles combine to form protoporphyrin IX, which then combines with iron to form the *heme* molecule. Finally, each heme molecule combines with a long polypeptide chain, a *globin* synthesized by ribosomes, forming a subunit of hemoglobin called a *hemoglobin chain* (Figure 32-6). Each chain has a molecular weight of about 16,000; four of these in turn bind together loosely to form the whole hemoglobin molecule.

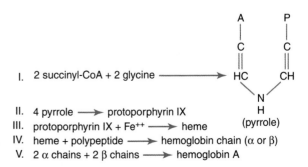

Figure 32-5 Formation of hemoglobin.

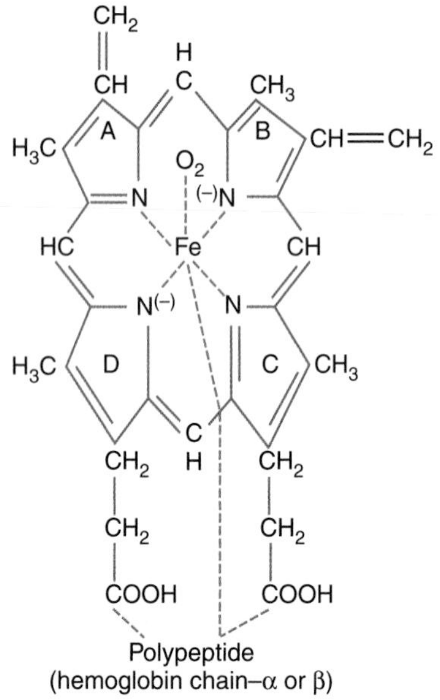

Figure 32-6 Basic structure of the hemoglobin molecule, showing one of the four heme chains that bind together to form the hemoglobin molecule.

There are several slight variations in the different subunit hemoglobin chains, depending on the amino acid composition of the polypeptide portion. The different types of chains are designated *alpha chains, beta chains, gamma chains,* and *delta chains.* The most common form of hemoglobin in the adult human being, *hemoglobin A,* is a combination of *two alpha chains* and *two beta chains.* Hemoglobin A has a molecular weight of 64,458.

Because each hemoglobin chain has a heme prosthetic group containing an atom of iron, and because there are four hemoglobin chains in each hemoglobin molecule, one finds four iron atoms in each hemoglobin molecule; each of these can bind loosely with one molecule of oxygen, making a total of four molecules of oxygen (or eight oxygen atoms) that can be transported by each hemoglobin molecule.

The types of hemoglobin chains in the hemoglobin molecule determine the binding affinity of the hemoglobin for oxygen. Abnormalities of the chains can alter the physical characteristics of the hemoglobin molecule as well. For instance, in *sickle cell anemia,* the amino acid *valine* is substituted for *glutamic acid* at one point in each of the two beta chains. When this type of hemoglobin is exposed to low oxygen, it forms elongated crystals inside the red blood cells that are sometimes 15 micrometers in length. These make it almost impossible for the cells to pass through many small capillaries, and the spiked ends of the crystals are likely to rupture the cell membranes, leading to sickle cell anemia.

Combination of Hemoglobin with Oxygen. The most important feature of the hemoglobin molecule is its ability to combine loosely and reversibly with oxygen. This ability is discussed in detail in Chapter 40 in relation to respiration because the primary function of hemoglobin

in the body is to combine with oxygen in the lungs and then to release this oxygen readily in the peripheral tissue capillaries, where the gaseous tension of oxygen is much lower than in the lungs.

Oxygen *does not* combine with the two positive bonds of the iron in the hemoglobin molecule. Instead, it binds loosely with one of the so-called coordination bonds of the iron atom. This is an extremely loose bond, so the combination is easily reversible. Furthermore, the oxygen does not become ionic oxygen but is carried as molecular oxygen (composed of two oxygen atoms) to the tissues, where, because of the loose, readily reversible combination, it is released into the tissue fluids still in the form of molecular oxygen rather than ionic oxygen.

Iron Metabolism

Because iron is important for the formation not only of hemoglobin but also of other essential elements in the body (e.g., *myoglobin, cytochromes, cytochrome oxidase, peroxidase, catalase*), it is important to understand the means by which iron is utilized in the body. The total quantity of iron in the body averages 4 to 5 grams, about 65 percent of which is in the form of hemoglobin. About 4 percent is in the form of myoglobin, 1 percent is in the form of the various heme compounds that promote intracellular oxidation, 0.1 percent is combined with the protein transferrin in the blood plasma, and 15 to 30 percent is stored for later use, mainly in the reticuloendothelial system and liver parenchymal cells, principally in the form of ferritin.

Transport and Storage of Iron. Transport, storage, and metabolism of iron in the body are diagrammed in Figure 32-7 and can be explained as follows: When iron is absorbed from the small intestine, it immediately combines in the blood plasma with a beta globulin, *apotransferrin,* to form *transferrin,* which is then transported in the plasma. The iron is loosely bound in the transferrin and, consequently, can be released to any tissue cell at any point in the body. Excess iron in the blood is deposited especially in the liver hepatocytes and less in the reticuloendothelial cells of the bone marrow.

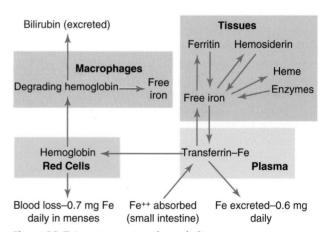

Figure 32-7 Iron transport and metabolism.

In the cell cytoplasm, iron combines mainly with a protein, *apoferritin*, to form *ferritin*. Apoferritin has a molecular weight of about 460,000, and varying quantities of iron can combine in clusters of iron radicals with this large molecule; therefore, ferritin may contain only a small amount of iron or a large amount. This iron stored as ferritin is called *storage iron.*

Smaller quantities of the iron in the storage pool are in an extremely insoluble form called *hemosiderin.* This is especially true when the total quantity of iron in the body is more than the apoferritin storage pool can accommodate. Hemosiderin collects in cells in the form of large clusters that can be observed microscopically as large particles. In contrast, ferritin particles are so small and dispersed that they usually can be seen in the cell cytoplasm only with the electron microscope.

When the quantity of iron in the plasma falls low, some of the iron in the ferritin storage pool is removed easily and transported in the form of transferrin in the plasma to the areas of the body where it is needed. A unique characteristic of the transferrin molecule is that it binds strongly with receptors in the cell membranes of erythroblasts in the bone marrow. Then, along with its bound iron, it is ingested into the erythroblasts by endocytosis. There the transferrin delivers the iron directly to the mitochondria, where heme is synthesized. In people who do not have adequate quantities of transferrin in their blood, failure to transport iron to the erythroblasts in this manner can cause severe *hypochromic anemia* (i.e., red cells that contain much less hemoglobin than normal).

When red blood cells have lived their life span of about 120 days and are destroyed, the hemoglobin released from the cells is ingested by monocyte-macrophage cells. There, iron is liberated and is stored mainly in the ferritin pool to be used as needed for the formation of new hemoglobin.

Daily Loss of Iron. A man excretes about 0.6 mg of iron each day, mainly into the feces. Additional quantities of iron are lost when bleeding occurs. For a woman, additional menstrual loss of blood brings long-term iron loss to an average of about 1.3 mg/day.

Absorption of Iron from the Intestinal Tract

Iron is absorbed from all parts of the small intestine, mostly by the following mechanism. The liver secretes moderate amounts of *apotransferrin* into the bile, which flows through the bile duct into the duodenum. Here, the apotransferrin binds with free iron and also with certain iron compounds, such as hemoglobin and myoglobin from meat, two of the most important sources of iron in the diet. This combination is called *transferrin.* It, in turn, is attracted to and binds with receptors in the membranes of the intestinal epithelial cells. Then, by pinocytosis, the transferrin molecule, carrying its iron store, is absorbed into the epithelial cells and later released into the blood capillaries beneath these cells in the form of *plasma transferrin.*

Iron absorption from the intestines is extremely slow, at a maximum rate of only a few milligrams per day. This means that even when tremendous quantities of iron are present in the food, only small proportions can be absorbed.

Regulation of Total Body Iron by Controlling Rate of Absorption. When the body has become saturated with iron so that essentially all apoferritin in the iron storage areas is already combined with iron, the rate of additional iron absorption from the intestinal tract becomes greatly decreased. Conversely, when the iron stores have become depleted, the rate of absorption can accelerate probably five or more times normal. Thus, total body iron is regulated mainly by altering the rate of absorption.

Life Span of Red Blood Cells is About 120 Days

When red blood cells are delivered from the bone marrow into the circulatory system, they normally circulate an average of 120 days before being destroyed. Even though mature red cells do not have a nucleus, mitochondria, or endoplasmic reticulum, they do have cytoplasmic enzymes that are capable of metabolizing glucose and forming small amounts of ATP. These enzymes also (1) maintain pliability of the cell membrane, (2) maintain membrane transport of ions, (3) keep the iron of the cells' hemoglobin in the ferrous form rather than ferric form, and (4) prevent oxidation of the proteins in the red cells. Even so, the metabolic systems of old red cells become progressively less active and the cells become more and more fragile, presumably because their life processes wear out.

Once the red cell membrane becomes fragile, the cell ruptures during passage through some tight spot of the circulation. Many of the red cells self-destruct in the spleen, where they squeeze through the red pulp of the spleen. There, the spaces between the structural trabeculae of the red pulp, through which most of the cells must pass, are only 3 micrometers wide, in comparison with the 8-micrometer diameter of the red cell. When the spleen is removed, the number of old abnormal red cells circulating in the blood increases considerably.

Destruction of Hemoglobin. When red blood cells burst and release their hemoglobin, the hemoglobin is phagocytized almost immediately by macrophages in many parts of the body, but especially by the Kupffer cells of the liver and macrophages of the spleen and bone marrow. During the next few hours to days, the macrophages release iron from the hemoglobin and pass it back into the blood, to be carried by transferrin either to the bone marrow for the production of new red blood cells or to the liver and other tissues for storage in the form of ferritin. The porphyrin portion of the hemoglobin molecule is converted by the macrophages, through a series of stages, into the bile pigment *bilirubin*, which is released into

419

the blood and later removed from the body by secretion through the liver into the bile; this is discussed in relation to liver function in Chapter 70.

Anemias

Anemia means deficiency of hemoglobin in the blood, which can be caused by either too few red blood cells or too little hemoglobin in the cells. Some types of anemia and their physiologic causes are the following.

Blood Loss Anemia. After rapid hemorrhage the body replaces the fluid portion of the plasma in 1 to 3 days, but this leaves a low concentration of red blood cells. If a second hemorrhage does not occur, the red blood cell concentration usually returns to normal within 3 to 6 weeks.

In chronic blood loss a person frequently cannot absorb enough iron from the intestines to form hemoglobin as rapidly as it is lost. Red cells that are much smaller than normal and have too little hemoglobin inside them are then produced, giving rise to *microcytic, hypochromic anemia*, which is shown in Figure 32-3.

Aplastic Anemia. *Bone marrow aplasia* means lack of functioning bone marrow. For instance, a person exposed to high-dose radiation or chemotherapy for cancer treatment can damage stem cells of the bone marrow, followed in a few weeks by anemia. Likewise, high doses of certain toxic chemicals, such as insecticides or benzene in gasoline, may cause the same effect. In autoimmune disorders, such as lupus erythematosus, the immune system begins attacking healthy cells such as bone marrow stem cells, which may lead to aplastic anemia. In about half of aplastic anemia cases the cause is unknown, a condition called *idiopathic aplastic anemia*.

People with severe aplastic anemia usually die unless treated with blood transfusions, which can temporarily increase the numbers of red blood cells, or by bone marrow transplantation.

Megaloblastic Anemia. Based on the earlier discussions of vitamin B_{12}, folic acid, and intrinsic factor from the stomach mucosa, one can readily understand that loss of any one of these can lead to slow reproduction of erythroblasts in the bone marrow. As a result, the red cells grow too large, with odd shapes, and are called *megaloblasts.* Thus, atrophy of the stomach mucosa, as occurs in *pernicious anemia,* or loss of the entire stomach after surgical total gastrectomy can lead to megaloblastic anemia. Also, patients who have intestinal sprue, in which folic acid, vitamin B_{12}, and other vitamin B compounds are poorly absorbed, often develop megaloblastic anemia. Because in these states the erythroblasts cannot proliferate rapidly enough to form normal numbers of red blood cells, those red cells that are formed are mostly oversized, have bizarre shapes, and have fragile membranes. These

cells rupture easily, leaving the person in dire need of an adequate number of red cells.

Hemolytic Anemia. Different abnormalities of the red blood cells, many of which are hereditarily acquired, make the cells fragile, so they rupture easily as they go through the capillaries, especially through the spleen. Even though the number of red blood cells formed may be normal, or even much greater than normal in some hemolytic diseases, the life span of the fragile red cell is so short that the cells are destroyed faster than they can be formed and serious anemia results.

In *hereditary spherocytosis,* the red cells are very small and *spherical* rather than being biconcave discs. These cells cannot withstand compression forces because they do not have the normal loose, baglike cell membrane structure of the biconcave discs. On passing through the splenic pulp and some other tight vascular beds, they are easily ruptured by even slight compression.

In *sickle cell anemia,* which is present in 0.3 to 1.0 percent of West African and American blacks, the cells have an abnormal type of hemoglobin called *hemoglobin S,* containing faulty beta chains in the hemoglobin molecule, as explained earlier in the chapter. When this hemoglobin is exposed to low concentrations of oxygen, it precipitates into long crystals inside the red blood cell. These crystals elongate the cell and give it the appearance of a sickle rather than a biconcave disc. The precipitated hemoglobin also damages the cell membrane, so the cells become highly fragile, leading to serious anemia. Such patients frequently experience a vicious circle of events called a sickle cell disease "crisis," in which low oxygen tension in the tissues causes sickling, which leads to ruptured red cells, which causes a further decrease in oxygen tension and still more sickling and red cell destruction. Once the process starts, it progresses rapidly, eventuating in a serious decrease in red blood cells within a few hours and, in some cases, death.

In *erythroblastosis fetalis,* Rh-positive red blood cells in the fetus are attacked by antibodies from an Rh-negative mother. These antibodies make the Rh-positive cells fragile, leading to rapid rupture and causing the child to be born with serious anemia. This is discussed in Chapter 35 in relation to the Rh factor of blood. The extremely rapid formation of new red cells to make up for the destroyed cells in erythroblastosis fetalis causes a large number of early *blast* forms of red cells to be released from the bone marrow into the blood.

Effects of Anemia on Function of the Circulatory System

The viscosity of the blood, which was discussed in Chapter 14, depends largely on the blood concentration of red blood cells. In severe anemia, the blood viscosity may fall to as low as 1.5 times that of water rather than the normal value of about 3. This decreases the resistance to blood flow in the peripheral blood vessels, so far greater than normal quantities of blood flow through the tissues and return to the heart, thereby greatly increasing cardiac output. Moreover, hypoxia resulting from diminished transport of oxygen by the blood causes the peripheral tissue blood vessels to dilate, allowing a further increase in the return of blood to the heart and increasing the cardiac output to a still higher level—sometimes three to four times normal. Thus, one of the major effects of anemia is greatly *increased cardiac output,* as well as *increased pumping workload on the heart.*

The increased cardiac output in anemia partially offsets the reduced oxygen-carrying effect of the anemia because even though each unit quantity of blood carries only small quantities of oxygen, the rate of blood flow may be increased enough that almost normal quantities of oxygen are actually delivered to the tissues. However, when a person with anemia begins to exercise, the heart is not capable of pumping much greater quantities of blood than it is already pumping. Consequently, during exercise, which greatly increases tissue demand for oxygen, extreme tissue hypoxia results and *acute cardiac failure* may ensue.

Polycythemia

Secondary Polycythemia. Whenever the tissues become hypoxic because of too little oxygen in the breathed air, such as at high altitudes, or because of failure of oxygen delivery to the tissues, such as in cardiac failure, the blood-forming organs automatically produce large quantities of extra red blood cells. This condition is called *secondary polycythemia,* and the red cell count commonly rises to 6 to 7 million/mm³, about 30 percent above normal.

A common type of secondary polycythemia, called *physiologic polycythemia,* occurs in natives who live at altitudes of 14,000 to 17,000 feet, where the atmospheric oxygen is very low. The blood count is generally 6 to 7 million/mm³; this allows these people to perform reasonably high levels of continuous work even in a rarefied atmosphere.

Polycythemia Vera (Erythremia). In addition to those people who have physiologic polycythemia, others have a pathological condition known as *polycythemia vera,* in which the red blood cell count may be 7 to 8 million/mm³ and the hematocrit may be 60 to 70 percent instead of the normal 40 to 45 percent. Polycythemia vera is caused by a genetic aberration in the hemocytoblastic cells that produce the blood cells. The blast cells no longer stop producing red cells when too many cells are already present. This causes excess production of red blood cells in the same manner that a breast tumor causes excess production of a specific type of breast cell. It usually causes excess production of white blood cells and platelets as well.

In polycythemia vera, not only does the hematocrit increase, but the total blood volume also increases, on some occasions to almost twice normal. As a result, the entire vascular system becomes intensely engorged. Also, many blood capillaries become plugged by the viscous blood; the viscosity of the blood in polycythemia vera sometimes increases from the normal of 3 times the viscosity of water to 10 times that of water.

Effect of Polycythemia on Function of the Circulatory System

Because of the greatly increased viscosity of the blood in polycythemia, blood flow through the peripheral blood vessels is often very sluggish. In accordance with the factors that regulate return of blood to the heart, as discussed in Chapter 20, increasing blood viscosity *decreases* the rate of venous return to the heart. Conversely, the blood volume is greatly increased in polycythemia, which tends to *increase* venous return. Actually, the cardiac output in polycythemia is not far from normal because these two factors more or less neutralize each other.

The arterial pressure is also normal in most people with polycythemia, although in about one third of them, the arterial pressure is elevated. This means that the blood pressure–regulating mechanisms can usually offset the tendency for increased blood viscosity to increase peripheral resistance and, thereby, increase arterial pressure. Beyond certain limits, however, these regulations fail and hypertension develops.

The color of the skin depends to a great extent on the quantity of blood in the skin subpapillary venous plexus. In polycythemia vera, the quantity of blood in this plexus is greatly increased. Further, because the blood passes sluggishly through the skin capillaries before entering the venous plexus, a larger than normal quantity of hemoglobin is deoxygenated. The blue color of all this deoxygenated hemoglobin masks the red color of the oxygenated hemoglobin. Therefore, a person with polycythemia vera ordinarily has a ruddy complexion with a bluish (cyanotic) tint to the skin.

Bibliography

Alayash AI: Oxygen therapeutics: can we tame haemoglobin? *Nat Rev Drug Discov* 3:152, 2004.

Alleyne M, Horne MK, Miller JL: Individualized treatment for iron-deficiency anemia in adults, *Am J Med* 121:943, 2008.

Claster S, Vichinsky EP: Managing sickle cell disease, *BMJ* 327:1151, 2003.

de Montalembert M: Management of sickle cell disease, *BMJ.* 337:a1397, 2008.

Elliott S, Pham E, Macdougall IC: Erythropoietins: a common mechanism of action, *Exp Hematol* 36:1573, 2008.

Fandrey J: Oxygen-dependent and tissue-specific regulation of erythropoietin gene expression, *Am J Physiol Regul Integr Comp Physiol* 286:R977, 2004.

Hentze MW, Muckenthaler MU, Andrews NC: Balancing acts: molecular control of mammalian iron metabolism, *Cell* 117:285, 2004.

Kato GJ, Gladwin MT: Evolution of novel small-molecule therapeutics targeting sickle cell vasculopathy, *JAMA* 300:2638, 2008.

Lappin T: The cellular biology of erythropoietin receptors, *Oncologist* 8(Suppl 1):15, 2003.

Maxwell P: HIF-1: an oxygen response system with special relevance to the kidney, *J Am Soc Nephrol* 14:2712, 2003.

Metcalf D: Hematopoietic cytokines, *Blood* 111:485, 2008.

Nangaku M, Eckardt KU: Hypoxia and the HIF system in kidney disease, *J Mol Med* 85:1325, 2007.

Percy MJ, Rumi E: Genetic origins and clinical phenotype of familial and acquired erythrocytosis and thrombocytosis, *Am J Hematol* 84:46, 2009.

Pietrangelo A: Hereditary hemochromatosis—a new look at an old disease, *N Engl J Med* 350:2383, 2004.

Platt OS: Hydroxyurea for the treatment of sickle cell anemia, *N Engl J Med* 27;358:1362, 2008.

Resistance of the Body to Infection: I. Leukocytes, Granulocytes, the Monocyte-Macrophage System, and Inflammation

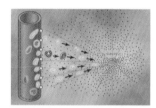

Our bodies are exposed continually to bacteria, viruses, fungi, and parasites, all of which occur normally and to varying degrees in the skin, the mouth, the respiratory passageways, the intestinal tract, the lining membranes of the eyes, and even the urinary tract. Many of these infectious agents are capable of causing serious abnormal physiologic function or even death if they invade the deeper tissues. In addition, we are exposed intermittently to other highly infectious bacteria and viruses besides those that are normally present, and these can cause acute lethal diseases such as pneumonia, streptococcal infection, and typhoid fever.

Our bodies have a special system for combating the different infectious and toxic agents. This system is composed of blood leukocytes (white blood cells) and tissue cells derived from leukocytes. These cells work together in two ways to prevent disease: (1) by actually destroying invading bacteria or viruses by *phagocytosis* and (2) by forming *antibodies* and *sensitized lymphocytes*, which may destroy or inactivate the invader. This chapter is concerned with the first of these methods, and Chapter 34 with the second.

Leukocytes (White Blood Cells)

The leukocytes, also called *white blood cells*, are the *mobile units* of the body's protective system. They are formed partially in the bone marrow (*granulocytes* and *monocytes* and a few *lymphocytes*) and partially in the lymph tissue (*lymphocytes* and *plasma cells*). After formation, they are transported in the blood to different parts of the body where they are needed.

The real value of the white blood cells is that most of them are specifically transported to areas of serious infection and inflammation, thereby providing a rapid and potent defense against infectious agents. As we see later, the granulocytes and monocytes have a special ability to "seek out and destroy" a foreign invader.

General Characteristics of Leukocytes

Types of White Blood Cells. Six types of white blood cells are normally present in the blood. They are *polymorphonuclear neutrophils, polymorphonuclear eosinophils, polymorphonuclear basophils, monocytes, lymphocytes,* and, occasionally, *plasma cells.* In addition, there are large numbers of *platelets,* which are fragments of another type of cell similar to the white blood cells found in the bone marrow, the *megakaryocyte.* The first three types of cells, the polymorphonuclear cells, all have a granular appearance, as shown in cell numbers 7, 10, and 12 in Figure 33-1, and for this reason are called *granulocytes,* or, in clinical terminology, "polys," because of the multiple nuclei.

The granulocytes and monocytes protect the body against invading organisms mainly by ingesting them (i.e., by *phagocytosis*). The lymphocytes and plasma cells function mainly in connection with the immune system; this is discussed in Chapter 34. Finally, the function of platelets is specifically to activate the blood clotting mechanism, which is discussed in Chapter 36.

Concentrations of the Different White Blood Cells in the Blood. The adult human being has about 7000 white blood cells per *microliter* of blood (in comparison with 5 million red blood cells). Of the total white blood cells, the normal percentages of the different types are approximately the following:

Polymorphonuclear neutrophils	62.0%
Polymorphonuclear eosinophils	2.3%
Polymorphonuclear basophils	0.4%
Monocytes	5.3%
Lymphocytes	30.0%

The number of platelets, which are only cell fragments, in each microliter of blood is normally about 300,000.

Genesis of the White Blood Cells

Early differentiation of the pluripotential hematopoietic stem cell into the different types of committed stem cells is shown in Figure 32-2 in the previous chapter. Aside from those cells committed to form red blood cells, two major

Genesis of Myelocytes　　　　**Genesis of Lymphocytes**

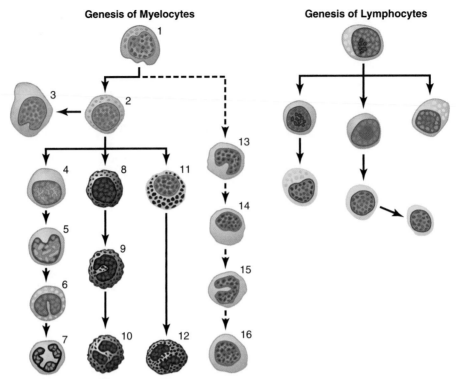

Figure 33-1 Genesis of white blood cells. The different cells of the myelocyte series are *1*, myeloblast; *2*, promyelocyte; *3*, megakaryocyte; *4*, neutrophil myelocyte; *5*, young neutrophil metamyelocyte; *6*, "band" neutrophil metamyelocyte; *7*, polymorphonuclear neutrophil; *8*, eosinophil myelocyte; *9*, eosinophil metamyelocyte; *10*, polymorphonuclear eosinophil; *11*, basophil myelocyte; *12*, polymorphonuclear basophil; *13-16*, stages of monocyte formation.

lineages of *white blood cells* are formed, the myelocytic and the lymphocytic lineages. The left side of Figure 33-1 shows the *myelocytic lineage*, beginning with the *myeloblast*; the right shows the *lymphocytic lineage*, beginning with the *lymphoblast*.

The granulocytes and monocytes are formed only in the bone marrow. Lymphocytes and plasma cells are produced mainly in the various lymphogenous tissues—especially the lymph glands, spleen, thymus, tonsils, and various pockets of lymphoid tissue elsewhere in the body, such as in the bone marrow and in so-called Peyer's patches underneath the epithelium in the gut wall.

The white blood cells formed in the bone marrow are stored within the marrow until they are needed in the circulatory system. Then, when the need arises, various factors cause them to be released (these factors are discussed later). Normally, about three times as many white blood cells are stored in the marrow as circulate in the entire blood. This represents about a 6-day supply of these cells.

The lymphocytes are mostly stored in the various lymphoid tissues, except for a small number that are temporarily being transported in the blood.

As shown in Figure 33-1, megakaryocytes (cell 3) are also formed in the bone marrow. These megakaryocytes fragment in the bone marrow; the small fragments, known as *platelets* (or *thrombocytes*), then pass into the blood. They are very important in the initiation of blood clotting.

Life Span of the White Blood Cells

The life of the granulocytes after being released from the bone marrow is normally 4 to 8 hours circulating in the blood and another 4 to 5 days in tissues where they are needed. In times of serious tissue infection, this total life span is often shortened to only a few hours because the granulocytes proceed even more rapidly to the infected area, perform their functions, and, in the process, are themselves destroyed.

The monocytes also have a short transit time, 10 to 20 hours in the blood, before wandering through the capillary membranes into the tissues. Once in the tissues, they swell to much larger sizes to become *tissue macrophages,* and, in this form, can live for months unless destroyed while performing phagocytic functions. These tissue macrophages are the basis of the *tissue macrophage system,* discussed in greater detail later, which provides continuing defense against infection.

Lymphocytes enter the circulatory system continually, along with drainage of lymph from the lymph nodes and other lymphoid tissue. After a few hours, they pass out of the blood back into the tissues by diapedesis. Then they re-enter the lymph and return to the blood again and again; thus, there is continual circulation of lymphocytes through the body. The lymphocytes have life spans of weeks or months, depending on the body's need for these cells.

The platelets in the blood are replaced about once every 10 days; in other words, about 30,000 platelets are formed each day for each microliter of blood.

Neutrophils and Macrophages Defend Against Infections

It is mainly the neutrophils and tissue macrophages that attack and destroy invading bacteria, viruses, and other injurious agents. The neutrophils are mature cells that can attack and destroy bacteria even in the circulating blood. Conversely, the tissue macrophages begin life as blood monocytes, which are immature cells while still in the blood and have little ability to fight infectious agents at that time. However, once they enter the tissues, they begin to swell—sometimes increasing their diameters as much as fivefold—to as great as 60 to 80 micrometers, a size that can barely be seen with the naked eye. These cells are now called *macrophages,* and they are extremely capable of combating disease agents in the tissues.

White Blood Cells Enter the Tissue Spaces by Diapedesis.
Neutrophils and monocytes can squeeze through the pores of the blood capillaries by *diapedesis.* That is, even though a pore is much smaller than a cell, a small portion of the cell slides through the pore at a time; the portion sliding through is momentarily constricted to the size of the pore, as shown in Figure 33-2 and 33-6.

White Blood Cells Move Through Tissue Spaces by Ameboid Motion.
Both neutrophils and macrophages can move through the tissues by ameboid motion, described in Chapter 2. Some cells move at velocities as great as 40 μm/min, a distance as great as their own length each minute.

White Blood Cells Are Attracted to Inflamed Tissue Areas by Chemotaxis.
Many different chemical substances in the tissues cause both neutrophils and macrophages to move toward the source of the chemical. This phenomenon, shown in Figure 33-2, is known as *chemotaxis.*

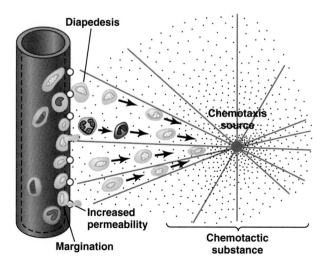

Figure 33-2 Movement of neutrophils by *diapedesis* through capillary pores and by *chemotaxis* toward an area of tissue damage.

When a tissue becomes inflamed, at least a dozen different products that can cause chemotaxis toward the inflamed area are formed. They include (1) some of the bacterial or viral toxins, (2) degenerative products of the inflamed tissues themselves, (3) several reaction products of the "complement complex" (discussed in Chapter 34) activated in inflamed tissues, and (4) several reaction products caused by plasma clotting in the inflamed area, as well as other substances.

As shown in Figure 33-2, chemotaxis depends on the concentration gradient of the chemotactic substance. The concentration is greatest near the source, which directs the unidirectional movement of the white cells. Chemotaxis is effective up to 100 micrometers away from an inflamed tissue. Therefore, because almost no tissue area is more than 50 micrometers away from a capillary, the chemotactic signal can easily move hordes of white cells from the capillaries into the inflamed area.

Phagocytosis

The most important function of the neutrophils and macrophages is *phagocytosis,* which means cellular ingestion of the offending agent. Phagocytes must be selective of the material that is phagocytized; otherwise, normal cells and structures of the body might be ingested. Whether phagocytosis will occur depends especially on three selective procedures.

First, most natural structures in the tissues have smooth surfaces, which resist phagocytosis. But if the surface is rough, the likelihood of phagocytosis is increased.

Second, most natural substances of the body have protective protein coats that repel the phagocytes. Conversely, most dead tissues and foreign particles have no protective coats, which makes them subject to phagocytosis.

Third, the immune system of the body (described in detail in Chapter 34) develops *antibodies* against infectious agents such as bacteria. The antibodies then adhere to the bacterial membranes and thereby make the bacteria especially susceptible to phagocytosis. To do this, the antibody molecule also combines with the C3 product of the *complement cascade,* which is an additional part of the immune system discussed in the next chapter. The C3 molecules, in turn, attach to receptors on the phagocyte membrane, thus initiating phagocytosis. This selection and phagocytosis process is called *opsonization.*

Phagocytosis by Neutrophils.
The neutrophils entering the tissues are already mature cells that can immediately begin phagocytosis. On approaching a particle to be phagocytized, the neutrophil first attaches itself to the particle and then projects pseudopodia in all directions around the particle. The pseudopodia meet one another on the opposite side and fuse. This creates an enclosed chamber that contains the phagocytized particle. Then the chamber invaginates to the inside of the cytoplasmic cavity and breaks away from the outer cell membrane to

UNIT VI

form a free-floating *phagocytic vesicle* (also called a *phagosome*) inside the cytoplasm. A single neutrophil can usually phagocytize 3 to 20 bacteria before the neutrophil itself becomes inactivated and dies.

Phagocytosis by Macrophages. Macrophages are the end-stage product of monocytes that enter the tissues from the blood. When activated by the immune system, as described in Chapter 34, they are much more powerful phagocytes than neutrophils, often capable of phagocytizing as many as 100 bacteria. They also have the ability to engulf much larger particles, even whole red blood cells or, occasionally, malarial parasites, whereas neutrophils are not capable of phagocytizing particles much larger than bacteria. Also, after digesting particles, macrophages can extrude the residual products and often survive and function for many more months.

Once Phagocytized, Most Particles Are Digested by Intracellular Enzymes. Once a foreign particle has been phagocytized, lysosomes and other cytoplasmic granules in the neutrophil or macrophage immediately come in contact with the phagocytic vesicle, and their membranes fuse, thereby dumping many digestive enzymes and bactericidal agents into the vesicle. Thus, the phagocytic vesicle now becomes a *digestive vesicle,* and digestion of the phagocytized particle begins immediately.

Both neutrophils and macrophages contain an abundance of lysosomes filled with *proteolytic enzymes* especially geared for digesting bacteria and other foreign protein matter. The lysosomes of macrophages (but not of neutrophils) also contain large amounts of *lipases,* which digest the thick lipid membranes possessed by some bacteria such as the tuberculosis bacillus.

Both Neutrophils and Macrophages Can Kill Bacteria. In addition to the digestion of ingested bacteria in phagosomes, neutrophils and macrophages contain *bactericidal agents* that kill most bacteria even when the lysosomal enzymes fail to digest them. This is especially important because some bacteria have protective coats or other factors that prevent their destruction by digestive enzymes. Much of the killing effect results from several powerful *oxidizing agents* formed by enzymes in the membrane of the phagosome or by a special organelle called the *peroxisome.* These oxidizing agents include large quantities of *superoxide* (O_2^-), *hydrogen peroxide* (H_2O_2), and *hydroxyl ions* (OH^-), all of which are lethal to most bacteria, even in small quantities. Also, one of the lysosomal enzymes, myeloperoxidase, catalyzes the reaction between H_2O_2 and chloride ions to form hypochlorite, which is exceedingly bactericidal.

Some bacteria, notably the tuberculosis bacillus, have coats that are resistant to lysosomal digestion and also secrete substances that partially resist the killing effects of the neutrophils and macrophages. These bacteria are responsible for many of the chronic diseases, an example of which is tuberculosis.

Monocyte-Macrophage Cell System (Reticuloendothelial System)

In the preceding paragraphs, we described the macrophages mainly as mobile cells that are capable of wandering through the tissues. However, after entering the tissues and becoming macrophages, another large portion of monocytes becomes attached to the tissues and remains attached for months or even years until they are called on to perform specific local protective functions. They have the same capabilities as the mobile macrophages to phagocytize large quantities of bacteria, viruses, necrotic tissue, or other foreign particles in the tissue. And, when appropriately stimulated, they can break away from their attachments and once again become mobile macrophages that respond to chemotaxis and all the other stimuli related to the inflammatory process. Thus, the body has a widespread "monocyte-macrophage system" in virtually all tissue areas.

The total combination of monocytes, mobile macrophages, fixed tissue macrophages, and a few specialized endothelial cells in the bone marrow, spleen, and lymph nodes is called the *reticuloendothelial system.* However, all or almost all these cells originate from monocytic stem cells; therefore, the reticuloendothelial system is almost synonymous with the monocyte-macrophage system. Because the term *reticuloendothelial system* is much better known in medical literature than the term *monocyte-macrophage system,* it should be remembered as a generalized phagocytic system located in all tissues, especially in those tissue areas where large quantities of particles, toxins, and other unwanted substances must be destroyed.

Tissue Macrophages in the Skin and Subcutaneous Tissues (Histiocytes). Although the skin is mainly impregnable to infectious agents, this is no longer true when the skin is broken. When infection begins in a subcutaneous tissue and local inflammation ensues, local tissue macrophages can divide in situ and form still more macrophages. Then they perform the usual functions of attacking and destroying the infectious agents, as described earlier.

Macrophages in the Lymph Nodes. Essentially no particulate matter that enters the tissues, such as bacteria, can be absorbed directly through the capillary membranes into the blood. Instead, if the particles are not destroyed locally in the tissues, they enter the lymph and flow to the lymph nodes located intermittently along the course of the lymph flow. The foreign particles are then trapped in these nodes in a meshwork of sinuses lined by *tissue macrophages.*

Figure 33-3 illustrates the general organization of the lymph node, showing lymph entering through the lymph node capsule by way of *afferent lymphatics,* then flowing through the *nodal medullary sinuses,* and finally passing

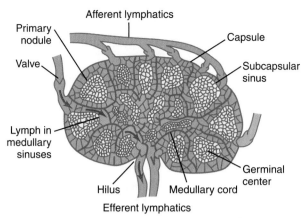

Figure 33-3 Functional diagram of a lymph node. (Redrawn from Ham AW: Histology, 6th ed. Philadelphia: JB Lippincott, 1969.) (Modified from Gartner LP, Hiatt JL: Color Textbook of Histology, 2nd ed. Philadelphia: WB Saunders, 2001.)

out the *hilus* into *efferent lymphatics* that eventually empty into the venous blood.

Large numbers of macrophages line the lymph sinuses, and if any particles enter the sinuses by way of the lymph, the macrophages phagocytize them and prevent general dissemination throughout the body.

Alveolar Macrophages in the Lungs. Another route by which invading organisms frequently enter the body is through the lungs. Large numbers of tissue macrophages are present as integral components of the alveolar walls. They can phagocytize particles that become entrapped in the alveoli. If the particles are digestible, the macrophages can also digest them and release the digestive products into the lymph. If the particle is not digestible, the macrophages often form a "giant cell" capsule around the particle until such time—if ever—that it can be slowly dissolved. Such capsules are frequently formed around tuberculosis bacilli, silica dust particles, and even carbon particles.

Macrophages (Kupffer Cells) in the Liver Sinusoids. Still another route by which bacteria invade the body is through the gastrointestinal tract. Large numbers of bacteria from ingested food constantly pass through the gastrointestinal mucosa into the portal blood. Before this blood enters the general circulation, it passes through the liver sinusoids, which are lined with tissue macrophages called *Kupffer cells*, shown in Figure 33-4. These cells form such an effective particulate filtration system that almost none of the bacteria from the gastrointestinal tract passes from the portal blood into the general systemic circulation. Indeed, motion pictures of phagocytosis by Kupffer cells have demonstrated phagocytosis of a single bacterium in less than $1/100$ of a second.

Macrophages of the Spleen and Bone Marrow. If an invading organism succeeds in entering the general circulation, there are other lines of defense by the tissue macrophage system, especially by macrophages of

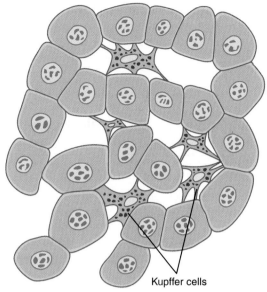

Figure 33-4 Kupffer cells lining the liver sinusoids, showing phagocytosis of India ink particles into the cytoplasm of the Kupffer cells. (Redrawn from Copenhaver WM et al: Bailey's Textbook of Histology, 10th ed. Baltimore: Williams & Wilkins, 1971.)

the spleen and bone marrow. In both these tissues, macrophages become entrapped by the reticular meshwork of the two organs and when foreign particles come in contact with these macrophages, they are phagocytized.

The spleen is similar to the lymph nodes, except that blood, instead of lymph, flows through the tissue spaces of the spleen. Figure 33-5 shows a small peripheral segment of spleen tissue. Note that a small artery penetrates from the splenic capsule into the *splenic pulp* and terminates in small capillaries. The capillaries are highly porous, allowing whole blood to pass out of the capillaries into *cords of red pulp*. The blood then gradually *squeezes* through the trabecular meshwork of these cords and eventually returns to the circulation through the endothelial walls of the *venous sinuses*. The trabeculae of the red pulp are lined with vast numbers of macrophages, and the venous

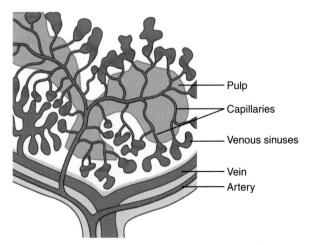

Figure 33-5 Functional structures of the spleen. (Modified from Bloom W, Fawcett DW: A Textbook of Histology, 10th ed. Philadelphia: WB Saunders, 1975.)

sinuses are also lined with macrophages. This peculiar passage of blood through the cords of the red pulp provides an exceptional means of phagocytizing unwanted debris in the blood, including especially old and abnormal red blood cells.

Inflammation: Role of Neutrophils and Macrophages

Inflammation

When tissue injury occurs, whether caused by bacteria, trauma, chemicals, heat, or any other phenomenon, multiple substances are released by the injured tissues and cause dramatic secondary changes in the surrounding uninjured tissues. This entire complex of tissue changes is called *inflammation.*

Inflammation is characterized by (1) vasodilation of the local blood vessels, with consequent excess local blood flow; (2) increased permeability of the capillaries, allowing leakage of large quantities of fluid into the interstitial spaces; (3) often clotting of the fluid in the interstitial spaces because of increased amounts of fibrinogen and other proteins leaking from the capillaries; (4) migration of large numbers of granulocytes and monocytes into the tissue; and (5) swelling of the tissue cells. Some of the many tissue products that cause these reactions are *histamine, bradykinin, serotonin, prostaglandins,* several different *reaction products of the complement system* (described in Chapter 34), *reaction products of the blood clotting system,* and multiple substances called *lymphokines* that are released by sensitized T cells (part of the immune system; also discussed in Chapter 34). Several of these substances strongly activate the macrophage system, and within a few hours, the macrophages begin to devour the destroyed tissues. But at times, the macrophages also further injure the still-living tissue cells.

"Walling-Off" Effect of Inflammation. One of the first results of inflammation is to "wall off" the area of injury from the remaining tissues. The tissue spaces and the lymphatics in the inflamed area are blocked by fibrinogen clots so that after a while, fluid barely flows through the spaces. This walling-off process delays the spread of bacteria or toxic products.

The intensity of the inflammatory process is usually proportional to the degree of tissue injury. For instance, when *staphylococci* invade tissues, they release extremely lethal cellular toxins. As a result, inflammation develops rapidly—indeed, much more rapidly than the staphylococci themselves can multiply and spread. Therefore, local staphylococcal infection is characteristically walled off rapidly and prevented from spreading through the body. Streptococci, in contrast, do not cause such intense local tissue destruction. Therefore, the walling-off process develops slowly over many hours, while many streptococci reproduce and migrate. As a result, streptococci

often have a far greater tendency to spread through the body and cause death than do staphylococci, even though staphylococci are far more destructive to the tissues.

Macrophage and Neutrophil Responses During Inflammation

Tissue Macrophage Is a First Line of Defense Against Infection. Within minutes after inflammation begins, the macrophages already present in the tissues, whether histiocytes in the subcutaneous tissues, alveolar macrophages in the lungs, microglia in the brain, or others, immediately begin their phagocytic actions. When activated by the products of infection and inflammation, the first effect is rapid enlargement of each of these cells. Next, many of the previously sessile macrophages break loose from their attachments and become mobile, forming the first line of defense against infection during the first hour or so. The numbers of these early mobilized macrophages often are not great, but they are lifesaving.

Neutrophil Invasion of the Inflamed Area Is a Second Line of Defense. Within the first hour or so after inflammation begins, large numbers of neutrophils begin to invade the inflamed area from the blood. This is caused by inflammatory cytokines (e.g., TNF, IL-1) and other biochemical products produced by the inflamed tissues that initiate the following reactions:

1. They cause increased expression of *adhesion molecules, such as selectins and intracellular adhesion molecule-1 (ICAM-1)* on the surface of endothelial cells in the capillaries and venules. These adhesion molecules, reacting with complementary *integrin* molecules on the neutrophils, cause the neutrophils to stick to the capillary and venule walls in the inflamed area. This effect is called *margination* and is shown in Figure 33-2 and in more detail in Figure 33-6.

2. They also cause the intercellular attachments between the endothelial cells of the capillaries and small venules to loosen, allowing openings large enough for neutrophils to crawl through by *diapedesis,* directly from the blood into the tissue spaces.

3. They then cause *chemotaxis* of the neutrophils toward the injured tissues, as explained earlier.

Thus, within several hours after tissue damage begins, the area becomes well supplied with neutrophils. Because the blood neutrophils are already mature cells, they are ready to immediately begin their scavenger functions for killing bacteria and removing foreign matter.

Acute Increase in Number of Neutrophils in the Blood—"Neutrophilia." Also within a few hours after the onset of acute, severe inflammation, the number of neutrophils in the blood sometimes increases fourfold to fivefold—from a normal of 4000 to 5000 to 15,000 to 25,000 neutrophils per microliter. This is called *neutrophilia,* which means an increase in the number of neutrophils in the blood. Neutrophilia is caused by products of inflammation that enter the blood stream, are transported to the bone marrow, and there act on the stored neutrophils of the marrow to mobilize these into the circulating blood. This makes even more neutrophils available to the inflamed tissue area.

Second Macrophage Invasion into the Inflamed Tissue Is a Third Line of Defense. Along with the invasion of neutrophils, monocytes from the blood enter the inflamed tissue and enlarge to become macrophages. However, the number of monocytes in the circulating blood is low: Also, the storage pool of monocytes in the bone marrow is much less than that of neutrophils. Therefore, the buildup of macrophages in the inflamed tissue area is much slower than that of neutrophils, requiring several days to become effective. Furthermore, even after invading the inflamed tissue, monocytes are still immature cells, requiring 8 hours or more to swell to much larger sizes and develop tremendous quantities of lysosomes; only then do they acquire the full capacity of *tissue macrophages* for phagocytosis. Yet, after several days to several weeks, the macrophages finally come

to dominate the phagocytic cells of the inflamed area because of greatly increased bone marrow production of new monocytes, as explained later.

As already pointed out, macrophages can phagocytize far more bacteria (about five times as many) and far larger particles, including even neutrophils themselves and large quantities of necrotic tissue, than can neutrophils. Also, the macrophages play an important role in initiating the development of antibodies, as we discuss in Chapter 34.

Increased Production of Granulocytes and Monocytes by the Bone Marrow Is a Fourth Line of Defense. The fourth line of defense is greatly increased production of both granulocytes and monocytes by the bone marrow. This results from stimulation of the granulocytic and monocytic progenitor cells of the marrow. However, it takes 3 to 4 days before newly formed granulocytes and monocytes reach the stage of leaving the bone marrow. If the stimulus from the inflamed tissue continues, the bone marrow can continue to produce these cells in tremendous quantities for months and even years, sometimes at a rate 20 to 50 times normal.

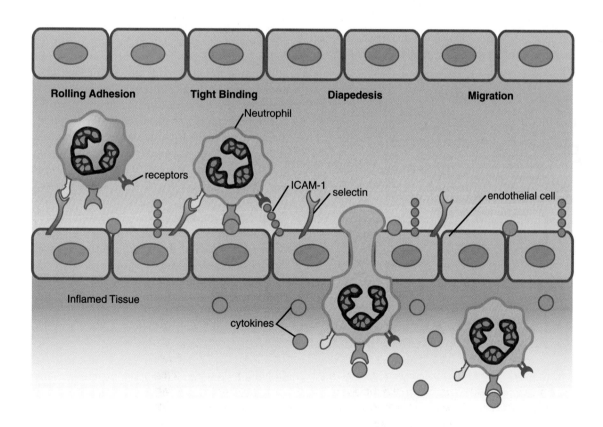

Figure 33-6 Migration of neutrophil from the blood into inflamed tissue. Cytokines and other biochemical products of the inflamed tissue cause increased expression of selectins and intracellular adhesion molecule-1 (ICAM-1) in the surface of endothelial cells. These adhesion molecules bind to complementary molecules/receptors on the neutrophil, causing it to adhere to the wall of the capillary or venule. The neutrophil then migrates through the vessel wall by diapedesis toward the site of tissue injury.

Feedback Control of the Macrophage and Neutrophil Responses

Although more than two dozen factors have been implicated in control of the macrophage response to inflammation, five of these are believed to play dominant roles. They are shown in Figure 33-7 and consist of (1) *tumor necrosis factor* (TNF), (2) *interleukin-1* (IL-1), (3) *granulocyte-monocyte colony-stimulating factor* (GM-CSF), (4) *granulocyte colony-stimulating factor* (G-CSF), and (5) *monocyte colony-stimulating factor* (M-CSF). These factors are formed by activated macrophage cells in the inflamed tissues and in smaller quantities by other inflamed tissue cells.

The cause of the increased production of granulocytes and monocytes by the bone marrow is mainly the three colony-stimulating factors, one of which, GM-CSF, stimulates both granulocyte and monocyte production; the other two, G-CSF and M-CSF, stimulate granulocyte and monocyte production, respectively. This combination of TNF, IL-1, and colony-stimulating factors provides a powerful feedback mechanism that begins with tissue inflammation and proceeds to formation of large numbers of defensive white blood cells that help remove the cause of the inflammation.

Formation of Pus

When neutrophils and macrophages engulf large numbers of bacteria and necrotic tissue, essentially all the neutrophils and many, if not most, of the macrophages eventually die. After several days, a cavity is often excavated in the inflamed tissues. It contains varying portions of necrotic tissue, dead neutrophils, dead macrophages, and tissue fluid. This mixture is commonly known as *pus*. After the infection has been suppressed, the dead cells and necrotic tissue in the pus gradually autolyze over a period of days, and the end products are eventually absorbed into the surrounding tissues and lymph until most of the evidence of tissue damage is gone.

Eosinophils

The eosinophils normally constitute about 2 percent of all the blood leukocytes. Eosinophils are weak phagocytes, and they exhibit chemotaxis, but in comparison with the neutrophils, it is doubtful that the eosinophils are significant in protecting against the usual types of infection.

Eosinophils, however, are often produced in large numbers in people with parasitic infections, and they migrate in large numbers into tissues diseased by parasites. Although most parasites are too large to be phagocytized by eosinophils or any other phagocytic cells, eosinophils attach themselves to the parasites by way of special surface molecules and release substances that kill many of the parasites. For instance, one of the most widespread infections is *schistosomiasis*, a parasitic infection found in as many as one third of the population of some developing countries in Asia, Africa, and South America; the parasite can invade any part of the body. Eosinophils attach themselves to the juvenile forms of the parasite and kill many of them. They do so in several ways: (1) by releasing hydrolytic enzymes from their granules, which are modified lysosomes; (2) probably by also releasing highly reactive forms of oxygen that are especially lethal to parasites; and (3) by releasing from the granules a highly larvacidal polypeptide called *major basic protein*.

In a few areas of the world, another parasitic disease that causes eosinophilia is *trichinosis*. This results from invasion of the body's muscles by the *Trichinella* parasite ("pork worm") after a person eats undercooked infested pork.

Eosinophils also have a special propensity to collect in tissues in which allergic reactions occur, such as in the peribronchial tissues of the lungs in people with asthma and in the skin after allergic skin reactions. This is caused at least partly by the fact that many mast cells and basophils participate in allergic reactions, as we discuss in the next paragraph. The mast cells and basophils release an *eosinophil chemotactic factor* that causes eosinophils to migrate toward the inflamed allergic tissue. The eosinophils are believed to detoxify some of the inflammation-inducing substances released by the mast cells and basophils and probably also to phagocytize and destroy allergen-antibody complexes, thus preventing excess spread of the local inflammatory process.

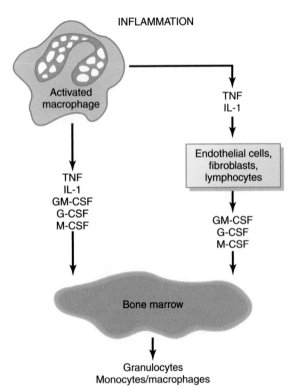

Figure 33-7 Control of bone marrow production of granulocytes and monocyte-macrophages in response to multiple growth factors released from activated macrophages in an inflamed tissue. G-CSF, granulocyte colony-stimulating factor; GM-CSF, granulocyte-monocyte colony-stimulating factor; IL-1, interleukin-1; M-CSF, monocyte colony-stimulating factor; TNF, tumor necrosis factor.

Basophils

The basophils in the circulating blood are similar to the large tissue *mast cells* located immediately outside many of the capillaries in the body. Both mast cells and basophils liberate *heparin* into the blood, a substance that can prevent blood coagulation.

The mast cells and basophils also release *histamine*, as well as smaller quantities of *bradykinin* and *serotonin*. Indeed, it is mainly the mast cells in inflamed tissues that release these substances during inflammation.

The mast cells and basophils play an important role in some types of allergic reactions because the type of antibody that causes allergic reactions, the immunoglobulin E (IgE) type, has a special propensity to become attached to mast cells and basophils. Then, when the specific antigen for the specific IgE antibody subsequently reacts with the antibody, the resulting attachment of antigen to antibody causes the mast cell or basophil to rupture and release large quantities of *histamine, bradykinin, serotonin, heparin, slow-reacting substance of anaphylaxis,* and a number of *lysosomal enzymes.* These cause local vascular and tissue reactions that cause many, if not most, of the allergic manifestations. These reactions are discussed in greater detail in Chapter 34.

Leukopenia

A clinical condition known as *leukopenia,* in which the bone marrow produces very few white blood cells, occasionally occurs. This leaves the body unprotected against many bacteria and other agents that might invade the tissues.

Normally, the human body lives in symbiosis with many bacteria because all the mucous membranes of the body are constantly exposed to large numbers of bacteria. The mouth almost always contains various spirochetal, pneumococcal, and streptococcal bacteria, and these same bacteria are present to a lesser extent in the entire respiratory tract. The distal gastrointestinal tract is especially loaded with colon bacilli. Furthermore, one can always find bacteria on the surfaces of the eyes, urethra, and vagina. Any decrease in the number of white blood cells immediately allows invasion of adjacent tissues by bacteria that are already present.

Within 2 days after the bone marrow stops producing white blood cells, ulcers may appear in the mouth and colon, or the person might develop some form of severe respiratory infection. Bacteria from the ulcers rapidly invade surrounding tissues and the blood. Without treatment, death often ensues in less than a week after acute total leukopenia begins.

Irradiation of the body by x-rays or gamma rays, or exposure to drugs and chemicals that contain benzene or anthracene nuclei, is likely to cause aplasia of the bone marrow. Indeed, some common drugs, such as chloramphenicol (an antibiotic), thiouracil (used to treat thyrotoxicosis), and even various barbiturate hypnotics, on very rare occasions cause leukopenia, thus setting off the entire infectious sequence of this malady.

After moderate irradiation injury to the bone marrow, some stem cells, myeloblasts, and hemocytoblasts may remain undestroyed in the marrow and are capable of regenerating the bone marrow, provided sufficient time is available. A patient properly treated with transfusions, plus antibiotics and other drugs to ward off infection, usually develops enough new bone marrow within weeks to months for blood cell concentrations to return to normal.

Leukemias

Uncontrolled production of white blood cells can be caused by cancerous mutation of a myelogenous or lymphogenous cell. This causes *leukemia,* which is usually characterized by greatly increased numbers of abnormal white blood cells in the circulating blood.

Types of Leukemia. Leukemias are divided into two general types: *lymphocytic leukemias* and *myelogenous leukemias.* The lymphocytic leukemias are caused by cancerous production of lymphoid cells, usually beginning in a lymph node or other lymphocytic tissue and spreading to other areas of the body. The second type of leukemia, myelogenous leukemia, begins by cancerous production of young myelogenous cells in the bone marrow and then spreads throughout the body so that white blood cells are produced in many extramedullary tissues—especially in the lymph nodes, spleen, and liver.

In myelogenous leukemia, the cancerous process occasionally produces partially differentiated cells, resulting in what might be called *neutrophilic leukemia, eosinophilic leukemia, basophilic leukemia,* or *monocytic leukemia.* More frequently, however, the leukemia cells are bizarre and undifferentiated and not identical to any of the normal white blood cells. Usually, the more undifferentiated the cell, the more *acute* is the leukemia, often leading to death within a few months if untreated. With some of the more differentiated cells, the process can be *chronic,* sometimes developing slowly over 10 to 20 years. Leukemic cells, especially the very undifferentiated cells, are usually nonfunctional for providing the normal protection against infection.

Effects of Leukemia on the Body

The first effect of leukemia is metastatic growth of leukemic cells in abnormal areas of the body. Leukemic cells from the bone marrow may reproduce so greatly that they invade the surrounding bone, causing pain and, eventually, a tendency for bones to fracture easily.

Almost all leukemias eventually spread to the spleen, lymph nodes, liver, and other vascular regions, regardless of whether the origin of the leukemia is in the bone marrow or the lymph nodes. Common effects in leukemia are the development of infection, severe anemia, and a bleeding tendency caused by thrombocytopenia (lack of platelets). These effects result mainly from displacement of the normal bone marrow and lymphoid cells by the nonfunctional leukemic cells.

Finally, an important effect of leukemia on the body is excessive use of metabolic substrates by the growing cancerous cells. The leukemic tissues reproduce new cells so rapidly that tremendous demands are made on the body reserves for foodstuffs, specific amino acids, and vitamins. Consequently, the energy of the patient is greatly depleted, and excessive utilization of amino acids by the leukemic cells causes especially rapid deterioration of the normal protein tissues of the body. Thus, while the leukemic tissues grow, other tissues become debilitated. After metabolic starvation has continued long enough, this alone is sufficient to cause death.

Bibliography

Alexander JS, Granger DN: Lymphocyte trafficking mediated by vascular adhesion protein-1: implications for immune targeting and cardiovascular disease, *Circ Res* 86:1190, 2000.

Blander JM, Medzhitov R: Regulation of phagosome maturation by signals from toll-like receptors, *Science* 304:1014, 2004.

Bromley SK, Mempel TR, Luster AD: Orchestrating the orchestrators: chemokines in control of T cell traffic, *Nat Immunol* 9:970, 2008.

Ferrajoli A, O'Brien SM: Treatment of chronic lymphocytic leukemia, *Semin Oncol* 31(Suppl 4):60, 2004.

Huynh KK, Kay JG, Stow JL, et al: Fusion, fission, and secretion during phagocytosis, *Physiology (Bethesda)* 22:366, 2007.

Johnson LA, Jackson DG: Cell traffic and the lymphatic endothelium, *Ann N Y Acad Sci* 1131:119, 2008.

Kinchen JM, Ravichandran KS: Phagosome maturation: going through the acid test, *Nat Rev Mol Cell Biol* 9:781, 2008.

Kunkel EJ, Butcher EC: Plasma-cell homing, *Nat Rev Immunol* 3:822, 2003.

Kvietys PR, Sandig M: Neutrophil diapedesis: paracellular or transcellular? *News Physiol Sci* 16:15, 2001.

Medzhitov R: Origin and physiological roles of inflammation, *Nature* 24:454, 428, 2008.

Ossovskaya VS, Bunnett NW: Protease-activated receptors: contribution to physiology and disease, *Physiol Rev* 84:579, 2004.

Pui CH, Relling MV, Downing JR: Acute lymphoblastic leukemia, *N Engl J Med* 350:1535, 2004.

Ricardo SD, van Goor H, Eddy AA: Macrophage diversity in renal injury and repair, *J Clin Invest* 118:3522, 2008.

Sigmundsdottir H, Butcher EC: Environmental cues, dendritic cells and the programming of tissue-selective lymphocyte trafficking, *Nat Immunol* 9:981, 2008.

Smith KA, Griffin JD: Following the cytokine signaling pathway to leukemogenesis: a chronology, *J Clin Invest* 118:3564, 2008.

Viola A, Luster AD: Chemokines and their receptors: drug targets in immunity and inflammation, *Annu Rev Pharmacol Toxicol* 48:171, 2008.

Werner S, Grose R: Regulation of wound healing by growth factors and cytokines, *Physiol Rev* 83:835, 2003.

Zullig S, Hengartner MO: Cell biology: tickling macrophages, a serious business, *Science* 304:1123, 2004.

Resistance of the Body to Infection: II. Immunity and Allergy

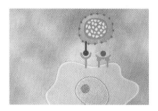 The human body has the ability to resist almost all types of organisms or toxins that tend to damage the tissues and organs. This capability is called *immunity*. Much of immunity is *acquired immunity* that does not develop until after the body is first attacked by a bacterium, virus, or toxin, often requiring weeks or months to develop the immunity. An additional portion of immunity results from general processes, rather than from processes directed at specific disease organisms. This is called *innate immunity*. It includes the following:

1. Phagocytosis of bacteria and other invaders by white blood cells and cells of the tissue macrophage system, as described in Chapter 33.

2. Destruction of swallowed organisms by the acid secretions of the stomach and the digestive enzymes.

3. Resistance of the skin to invasion by organisms.

4. Presence in the blood of certain chemical compounds that attach to foreign organisms or toxins and destroy them. Some of these compounds are (1) *lysozyme,* a mucolytic polysaccharide that attacks bacteria and causes them to dissolute; (2) *basic polypeptides,* which react with and inactivate certain types of gram-positive bacteria; (3) *the complement complex* that is described later, a system of about 20 proteins that can be activated in various ways to destroy bacteria; and (4) *natural killer lymphocytes* that can recognize and destroy foreign cells, tumor cells, and even some infected cells.

This innate immunity makes the human body resistant to such diseases as some paralytic viral infections of animals, hog cholera, cattle plague, and distemper—a viral disease that kills a large percentage of dogs that become afflicted with it. Conversely, many lower animals are resistant or even immune to many human diseases, such as poliomyelitis, mumps, human cholera, measles, and syphilis, which are very damaging or even lethal to human beings.

Acquired (Adaptive) Immunity

In addition to its generalized innate immunity, the human body has the ability to develop extremely powerful specific immunity against individual invading agents such as lethal bacteria, viruses, toxins, and even foreign tissues from other animals. This is called *acquired* or *adaptive immunity.* Acquired immunity is caused by a special immune system that forms antibodies and/or activated lymphocytes that attack and destroy the specific invading organism or toxin. It is with this acquired immunity mechanism and some of its associated reactions, especially the allergies, that this chapter is concerned.

Acquired immunity can often bestow extreme protection. For instance, certain toxins, such as the paralytic botulinum toxin or the tetanizing toxin of tetanus, can be protected against in doses as high as 100,000 times the amount that would be lethal without immunity. This is the reason the treatment process known as *immunization* is so important in protecting human beings against disease and against toxins, as explained in the course of this chapter.

Basic Types of Acquired Immunity—Humoral and Cell-Mediated

Two basic but closely allied types of acquired immunity occur in the body. In one of these the body develops circulating antibodies, which are globulin molecules in the blood plasma that are capable of attacking the invading agent. This type of immunity is called *humoral immunity* or *B-cell immunity* (because B lymphocytes produce the antibodies). The second type of acquired immunity is achieved through the formation of large numbers of activated *T lymphocytes* that are specifically crafted in the lymph nodes to destroy the foreign agent. This type of immunity is called *cell-mediated immunity* or *T-cell immunity* (because the activated lymphocytes are T lymphocytes). We shall see shortly that both the antibodies and the activated lymphocytes are formed in the lymphoid tissues of the body. Let us discuss the initiation of the immune process by *antigens.*

Both Types of Acquired Immunity Are Initiated by Antigens

Because acquired immunity does not develop until after invasion by a foreign organism or toxin, it is clear that the body must have some mechanism for recognizing this invasion. Each toxin or each type of organism almost always contains one or more specific chemical compounds in its makeup that are different from all other compounds. In general, these are proteins or large polysaccharides, and it is they that initiate the acquired immunity. These substances are called *antigens* (*anti*body *gen*erations).

For a substance to be antigenic, it usually must have a high molecular weight, 8000 or greater. Furthermore, the process of antigenicity usually depends on regularly recurring molecular groups, called *epitopes*, on the surface of the large molecule. This also explains why proteins and large polysaccharides are almost always antigenic, because both of these have this stereochemical characteristic.

Lymphocytes Are Responsible for Acquired Immunity

Acquired immunity is the product of the body's lymphocytes. In people who have a genetic lack of lymphocytes or whose lymphocytes have been destroyed by radiation or chemicals, no acquired immunity can develop. And within days after birth, such a person dies of fulminating bacterial infection unless treated by heroic measures. Therefore, it is clear that the lymphocytes are essential to survival of the human being.

The lymphocytes are located most extensively in the lymph nodes, but they are also found in special lymphoid tissues such as the spleen, submucosal areas of the gastrointestinal tract, thymus, and bone marrow. The lymphoid tissue is distributed advantageously in the body to intercept invading organisms or toxins before they can spread too widely.

In most instances, the invading agent first enters the tissue fluids and then is carried by lymph vessels to the lymph node or other lymphoid tissue. For instance, the lymphoid tissue of the gastrointestinal walls is exposed immediately to antigens invading from the gut. The lymphoid tissue of the throat and pharynx (the tonsils and adenoids) is well located to intercept antigens that enter by way of the upper respiratory tract. The lymphoid tissue in the lymph nodes is exposed to antigens that invade the peripheral tissues of the body. And, finally, the lymphoid tissue of the spleen, thymus, and bone marrow plays the specific role of intercepting antigenic agents that have succeeded in reaching the circulating blood.

Two Types of Lymphocytes Promote "Cell-Mediated" Immunity or "Humoral" Immunity—the T and B Lymphocytes. Although most lymphocytes in normal lymphoid tissue look alike when studied under a microscope, these cells are distinctly divided into two major populations. One of the populations, the T lymphocytes, is responsible for forming the activated lymphocytes that provide "cell-mediated" immunity, and the other population, the B lymphocytes, is responsible for forming antibodies that provide "humoral" immunity.

Both types of lymphocytes are derived originally in the embryo from *pluripotent hematopoietic stem cells* that form *common lymphoid progenitor cells* as one of their most important offspring as they differentiate. Almost all of the lymphocytes that are formed eventually end up in the lymphoid tissue, but before doing so, they are further differentiated or "preprocessed" in the following ways.

The lymphoid progenitor cells that are destined to eventually form activated T lymphocytes first migrate to and are preprocessed in the thymus gland, and thus they are called "T" lymphocytes to designate the role of the thymus. They are responsible for cell-mediated immunity.

The other population of lymphocytes—the B lymphocytes that are destined to form antibodies—are preprocessed in the liver during mid–fetal life and in the bone marrow in late fetal life and after birth. This population of cells was first discovered in birds, which have a special preprocessing organ called the *bursa of Fabricius*. For this reason, these lymphocytes are called "B" lymphocytes to designate the role of the bursa, and they are responsible for humoral immunity. Figure 34-1 shows the two lymphocyte systems for the formation, respectively, of (1) the activated T lymphocytes and (2) the antibodies.

Preprocessing of the T and B Lymphocytes

Although all lymphocytes in the body originate from *lymphocyte-committed stem cells* of the embryo, these stem cells themselves are incapable of forming directly either activated T lymphocytes or antibodies. Before they can do so, they must be further differentiated in appropriate processing areas as follows.

Thymus Gland Preprocesses the T Lymphocytes. The T lymphocytes, after origination in the bone marrow, first migrate to the thymus gland. Here they divide rapidly and at the same time develop extreme diversity for reacting against different specific antigens. That is, one thymic lymphocyte develops specific reactivity against one antigen. Then the next lymphocyte develops specificity against another antigen. This continues until there are thousands of different types of thymic lymphocytes with specific reactivities against many thousands of different antigens. These different types of preprocessed T lymphocytes now leave the thymus and spread by way of the blood throughout the body to lodge in lymphoid tissue everywhere.

The thymus also makes certain that any T lymphocytes leaving the thymus will not react against proteins or other antigens that are present in the body's own tissues; otherwise, the T lymphocytes would be lethal to the person's own body in only a few days. The thymus selects which T lymphocytes will be released by first mixing them with virtually all the specific "self-antigens" from the body's own tissues. If a T lymphocyte reacts, it is destroyed and phagocytized instead of being released. This happens to

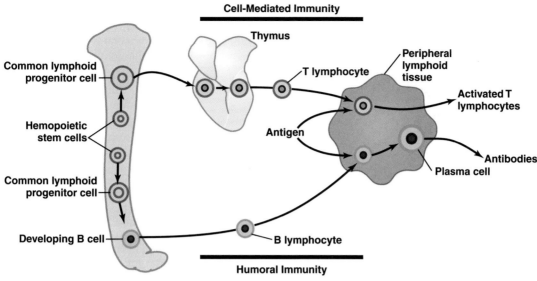

Figure 34-1 Formation of antibodies and sensitized lymphocytes by a lymph node in response to antigens. This figure also shows the origin of thymic (*T*) and bursal (*B*) lymphocytes that respectively are responsible for the cell-mediated and humoral immune processes.

up to 90 percent of the cells. Thus, the only cells that are finally released are those that are nonreactive against the body's own antigens—they react only against antigens from an outside source, such as from a bacterium, a toxin, or even transplanted tissue from another person.

Most of the preprocessing of T lymphocytes in the thymus occurs shortly before birth of a baby and for a few months after birth. Beyond this period, removal of the thymus gland diminishes (but does not eliminate) the T-lymphocytic immune system. However, removal of the thymus several months before birth can prevent development of all cell-mediated immunity. Because this cellular type of immunity is mainly responsible for rejection of transplanted organs, such as hearts and kidneys, one can transplant organs with much less likelihood of rejection if the thymus is removed from an animal a reasonable time before its birth.

Liver and Bone Marrow Preprocess the B Lymphocytes. Much less is known about the details for preprocessing B lymphocytes than for preprocessing T lymphocytes. In the human being, B lymphocytes are known to be preprocessed in the liver during mid–fetal life and in the bone marrow during late fetal life and after birth.

B lymphocytes are different from T lymphocytes in two ways: First, instead of the whole cell developing reactivity against the antigen, as occurs for the T lymphocytes, the B lymphocytes actively secrete *antibodies* that are the reactive agents. These agents are large protein molecules that are capable of combining with and destroying the antigenic substance, which is explained elsewhere in this chapter and in Chapter 33. Second, the B lymphocytes have even greater diversity than the T lymphocytes, thus forming many millions of types of B-lymphocyte antibodies with different specific reactivities. After preprocessing, the B lymphocytes, like the T lymphocytes, migrate

to lymphoid tissue throughout the body, where they lodge near but slightly removed from the T-lymphocyte areas.

T Lymphocytes and B-Lymphocyte Antibodies React Highly Specifically Against Specific Antigens—Role of Lymphocyte Clones

When specific antigens come in contact with T and B lymphocytes in the lymphoid tissue, certain of the T lymphocytes become activated to form activated T cells, and certain of the B lymphocytes become activated to form antibodies. The activated T cells and antibodies in turn react highly specifically against the particular types of antigens that initiated their development. The mechanism of this specificity is the following.

Millions of Specific Types of Lymphocytes Are Stored in the Lymphoid Tissue. Millions of different types of preformed B lymphocytes and preformed T lymphocytes that are capable of forming highly specific types of antibodies or T cells have been stored in the lymph tissue, as explained earlier. Each of these preformed lymphocytes is capable of forming only one type of antibody or one type of T cell with a single type of specificity. And only the specific type of antigen with which it can react can activate it. Once the specific lymphocyte is activated by its antigen, it reproduces wildly, forming tremendous numbers of duplicate lymphocytes (Figure 34-2). If it is a B lymphocyte, its progeny will eventually secrete the specific type of antibody that then circulates throughout the body. If it is a T lymphocyte, its progeny are specific sensitized T cells that are released into the lymph and then carried to the blood and circulated through all the tissue fluids and back into the lymph, sometimes circulating around and around in this circuit for months or years.

All the different lymphocytes that are capable of forming one specific antibody or T cell are called a *clone of lymphocytes*. That is, the lymphocytes in each clone are

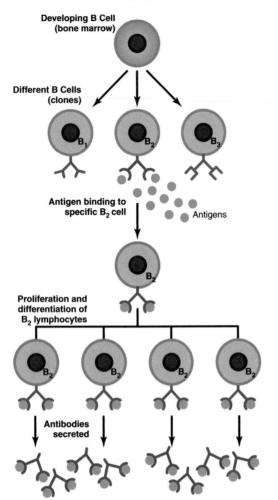

Figure 34-2 An antigen activates only the lymphocytes that have cell surface receptors that are complementary and recognize a specific antigen. Millions of different clones of lymphocytes exist (shown as *B1, B2,* and *B3*). When the lymphocyte clone (*B2* in this example) is activated by its antigen, it reproduces to form large numbers of duplicate lymphocytes, which then secrete antibodies.

alike and are derived originally from one or a few early lymphocytes of its specific type.

Origin of the Many Clones of Lymphocytes

Only several hundred to a few thousand genes code for the millions of different types of antibodies and T lymphocytes. At first, it was a mystery how it was possible for so few genes to code for the millions of different specificities of antibody molecules or T cells that can be produced by the lymphoid tissue, especially when one considers that a single gene is usually necessary for the formation of each different type of protein. This mystery has now been solved.

The whole gene for forming each type of T cell or B cell is never present in the original stem cells from which the functional immune cells are formed. Instead, there are only "gene segments"—actually, hundreds of such segments—but not whole genes. During preprocessing of the respective T- and B-cell lymphocytes, these gene

segments become mixed with one another in random combinations, in this way finally forming whole genes.

Because there are several hundred types of gene segments, as well as millions of different combinations in which the segments can be arranged in single cells, one can understand the millions of different cell gene types that can occur. For each functional T or B lymphocyte that is finally formed, the gene structure codes for only a single antigen specificity. These mature cells then become the highly specific T and B cells that spread to and populate the lymphoid tissue.

Mechanism for Activating a Clone of Lymphocytes

Each clone of lymphocytes is responsive to only a single type of antigen (or to several similar antigens that have almost exactly the same stereochemical characteristics). The reason for this is the following: In the case of the B lymphocytes, each of these has on the surface of its cell membrane about 100,000 antibody molecules that will react highly specifically with only one specific type of antigen. Therefore, when the appropriate antigen comes along, it immediately attaches to the antibody in the cell membrane; this leads to the activation process, which we describe in more detail subsequently. In the case of the T lymphocytes, molecules similar to antibodies, called *surface receptor proteins* (or *T-cell markers*), are on the surface of the T-cell membrane, and these are also highly specific for one specified activating antigen. An antigen therefore stimulates only those cells that have complementary receptors for the antigen and are already committed to respond to it.

Role of Macrophages in the Activation Process. Aside from the lymphocytes in lymphoid tissue, literally millions of macrophages are also present in the same tissue. These line the sinusoids of the lymph nodes, spleen, and other lymphoid tissue, and they lie in apposition to many of the lymph node lymphocytes. Most invading organisms are first phagocytized and partially digested by the macrophages, and the antigenic products are liberated into the macrophage cytosol. The macrophages then pass these antigens by cell-to-cell contact directly to the lymphocytes, thus leading to activation of the specified lymphocytic clones. The macrophages, in addition, secrete a special activating substance, *interleukin-1*, that promotes still further growth and reproduction of the specific lymphocytes.

Role of the T Cells in Activation of the B Lymphocytes. Most antigens activate both T lymphocytes and B lymphocytes at the same time. Some of the T cells that are formed, called *helper cells,* secrete specific substances (collectively called *lymphokines*) that activate the specific B lymphocytes. Indeed, without the aid of these helper T cells, the quantity of antibodies formed by the B lymphocytes is usually slight. We discuss this cooperative relationship between helper T cells and B cells after we describe the mechanisms of the T-cell system of immunity.

Specific Attributes of the B-Lymphocyte System— Humoral Immunity and the Antibodies

Formation of Antibodies by Plasma Cells. Before exposure to a specific antigen, the clones of B lymphocytes remain dormant in the lymphoid tissue. On entry of a foreign antigen, macrophages in the lymphoid tissue phagocytize the antigen and then present it to adjacent B lymphocytes. In addition, the antigen is presented to T cells at the same time, and activated helper T cells are formed. These helper cells also contribute to extreme activation of the B lymphocytes, as we discuss more fully later.

Those B lymphocytes specific for the antigen immediately enlarge and take on the appearance of *lymphoblasts*. Some of the lymphoblasts further differentiate to form plasmablasts, which are precursors of plasma cells. In the *plasmablasts*, the cytoplasm expands and the rough endoplasmic reticulum vastly proliferates. The plasmablasts then begin to divide at a rate of about once every 10 hours for about nine divisions, giving in 4 days a total population of about 500 cells for each original plasmablast. The mature plasma cell then produces gamma globulin antibodies at an extremely rapid rate—about 2000 molecules per second for each plasma cell. In turn, the antibodies are secreted into the lymph and carried to the circulating blood. This process continues for several days or weeks until finally exhaustion and death of the plasma cells occur.

Formation of "Memory" Cells—Difference Between Primary Response and Secondary Response.

A few of the lymphoblasts formed by activation of a clone of B lymphocytes do not go on to form plasma cells but instead form moderate numbers of new B lymphocytes similar to those of the original clone. In other words, the B-cell population of the specifically activated clone becomes greatly enhanced, and the new B lymphocytes are added to the original lymphocytes of the same clone. They also circulate throughout the body to populate all the lymphoid tissue; immunologically, however, they remain dormant until activated once again by a new quantity of the same antigen. These lymphocytes are called *memory cells*. Subsequent exposure to the same antigen will cause a much more rapid and much more potent antibody response this second time around, because there are many more memory cells than there were original B lymphocytes of the specific clone.

Figure 34-3 shows the differences between the primary response for forming antibodies that occurs on first exposure to a specific antigen and the secondary response that occurs after second exposure to the same antigen. Note the 1-week delay in the appearance of the primary response, its weak potency, and its short life. The secondary response, by contrast, begins rapidly after exposure to the antigen (often within hours), is far more potent, and forms antibodies for many months rather than for only a few weeks. The increased potency and duration of the secondary response explain why immunization is usually accomplished by injecting antigen in multiple doses

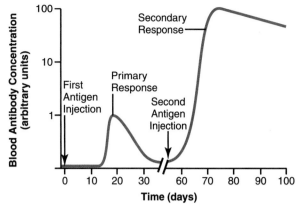

Figure 34-3 Time course of the antibody response in the circulating blood to a primary injection of antigen and to a secondary injection several weeks later.

with periods of several weeks or several months between injections.

Nature of the Antibodies

The antibodies are gamma globulins called *immunoglobulins* (abbreviated as *Ig*), and they have molecular weights between 160,000 and 970,000. They usually constitute about 20 percent of all the plasma proteins.

All the immunoglobulins are composed of combinations of *light* and *heavy polypeptide chains*. Most are a combination of two light and two heavy chains, as shown in Figure 34-4. However, some of the immunoglobulins have combinations of as many as 10 heavy and 10 light chains, which give rise to high-molecular-weight immunoglobulins. Yet, in all immunoglobulins, each heavy chain is paralleled by a light chain at one of its ends, thus forming a heavy-light pair, and there are always at least 2 and as many as 10 such pairs in each immunoglobulin molecule.

Figure 34-4 shows a designated end of each light and heavy chain, called the *variable portion*; the remainder of

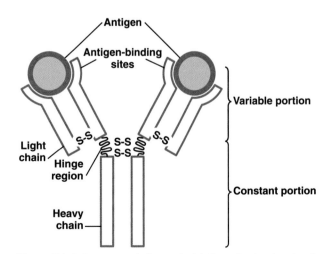

Figure 34-4 Structure of the typical IgG antibody, showing it to be composed of two heavy polypeptide chains and two light polypeptide chains. The antigen binds at two different sites on the variable portions of the chains.

each chain is called the *constant portion.* The variable portion is different for each specificity of antibody, and it is this portion that attaches specifically to a particular type of antigen. The constant portion of the antibody determines other properties of the antibody, establishing such factors as diffusivity of the antibody in the tissues, adherence of the antibody to specific structures within the tissues, attachment to the complement complex, the ease with which the antibodies pass through membranes, and other biological properties of the antibody. A combination of noncovalent and covalent bonds (disulfide) holds the light and heavy chains together.

Specificity of Antibodies. Each antibody is specific for a particular antigen; this is caused by its unique structural organization of amino acids in the variable portions of both the light and heavy chains. The amino acid organization has a different steric shape for each antigen specificity, so when an antigen comes in contact with it, multiple prosthetic groups of the antigen fit as a mirror image with those of the antibody, thus allowing rapid and tight bonding between the antibody and the antigen. When the antibody is highly specific, there are so many bonding sites that the antibody-antigen coupling is exceedingly strong, held together by (1) hydrophobic bonding, (2) hydrogen bonding, (3) ionic attractions, and (4) van der Waals forces. It also obeys the thermodynamic mass action law.

$$K_a = \frac{\text{Concentration of bound antibody-antigen}}{\begin{array}{c}\text{Concentration of antibody} \\ \times \text{ Concentration of antigen}\end{array}}$$

Ka is called the *affinity constant* and is a measure of how tightly the antibody binds with the antigen.

Note, especially, in Figure 34-4 that there are two variable sites on the illustrated antibody for attachment of antigens, making this type of antibody bivalent. A small proportion of the antibodies, which consist of combinations of up to 10 light and 10 heavy chains, have as many as 10 binding sites.

Classes of Antibodies. There are five general classes of antibodies, respectively named *IgM, IgG, IgA, IgD,* and *IgE.* Ig stands for immunoglobulin, and the other five respective letters designate the respective classes.

For the purpose of our present limited discussion, two of these classes of antibodies are of particular importance: IgG, which is a bivalent antibody and constitutes about 75 percent of the antibodies of the normal person, and IgE, which constitutes only a small percentage of the antibodies but is especially involved in allergy. The IgM class is also interesting because a large share of the antibodies formed during the primary response are of this type. These antibodies have 10 binding sites that make them exceedingly effective in protecting the body against invaders, even though there are not many IgM antibodies.

Mechanisms of Action of Antibodies

Antibodies act mainly in two ways to protect the body against invading agents: (1) by direct attack on the invader

and (2) by activation of the "complement system" that then has multiple means of its own for destroying the invader.

Direct Action of Antibodies on Invading Agents. Figure 34-5 shows antibodies (designated by the red Y-shaped bars) reacting with antigens (designated by the shaded objects). Because of the bivalent nature of the antibodies and the multiple antigen sites on most invading agents, the antibodies can inactivate the invading agent in one of several ways, as follows:

1. *Agglutination,* in which multiple large particles with antigens on their surfaces, such as bacteria or red cells, are bound together into a clump
2. *Precipitation,* in which the molecular complex of soluble antigen (such as tetanus toxin) and antibody becomes so large that it is rendered insoluble and precipitates
3. *Neutralization,* in which the antibodies cover the toxic sites of the antigenic agent
4. *Lysis,* in which some potent antibodies are occasionally capable of directly attacking membranes of cellular agents and thereby cause rupture of the agent

These direct actions of antibodies attacking the antigenic invaders often are not strong enough to play a major role in protecting the body against the invader. Most of the protection comes through the amplifying effects of the complement system described next.

Complement System for Antibody Action

"Complement" is a collective term that describes a system of about 20 proteins, many of which are enzyme precursors. The principal actors in this system are 11 proteins designated C1 through C9, B, and D, shown in Figure 34-6. All these are present normally among the plasma proteins in the blood, as well as among the proteins that leak out of the capillaries into the tissue spaces. The enzyme precursors are normally inactive, but they can be activated mainly by the so-called *classic pathway.*

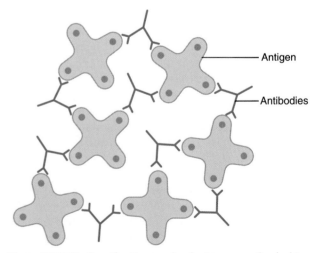

Figure 34-5 Binding of antigen molecules to one another by bivalent antibodies.

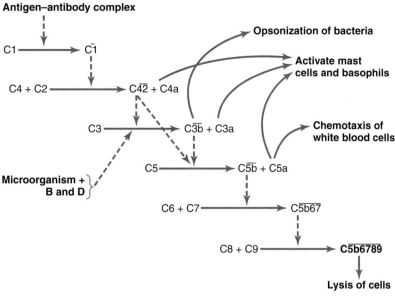

Figure 34-6 Cascade of reactions during activation of the classic pathway of complement. (Modified from Alexander JW, Good RA: Fundamentals of Clinical Immunology. Philadelphia: WB Saunders, 1977.)

Classic Pathway. The classic pathway is initiated by an antigen-antibody reaction. That is, when an antibody binds with an antigen, a specific reactive site on the "constant" portion of the antibody becomes uncovered, or "activated," and this in turn binds directly with the C1 molecule of the complement system, setting into motion a "cascade" of sequential reactions, shown in Figure 34-6, beginning with activation of the proenzyme C1 itself. The C1 enzymes that are formed then activate successively increasing quantities of enzymes in the later stages of the system so that from a small beginning, an extremely large "amplified" reaction occurs. Multiple end products are formed, as shown to the right in the figure, and several of these cause important effects that help to prevent damage to the body's tissues caused by the invading organism or toxin. Among the more important effects are the following:

1. *Opsonization and phagocytosis.* One of the products of the complement cascade, C3b, strongly activates phagocytosis by both neutrophils and macrophages, causing these cells to engulf the bacteria to which the antigen-antibody complexes are attached. This process is called *opsonization.* It often enhances the number of bacteria that can be destroyed by many hundredfold.

2. *Lysis.* One of the most important of all the products of the complement cascade is the lytic complex, which is a combination of multiple complement factors and designated C5b6789. This has a direct effect of rupturing the cell membranes of bacteria or other invading organisms.

3. *Agglutination.* The complement products also change the surfaces of the invading organisms, causing them to adhere to one another, thus promoting agglutination.

4. *Neutralization of viruses.* The complement enzymes and other complement products can attack the structures of some viruses and thereby render them nonvirulent.

5. *Chemotaxis.* Fragment C5a initiates chemotaxis of neutrophils and macrophages, thus causing large numbers of these phagocytes to migrate into the tissue area adjacent to the antigenic agent.

6. *Activation of mast cells and basophils.* Fragments C3a, C4a, and C5a activate mast cells and basophils, causing them to release histamine, heparin, and several other substances into the local fluids. These substances in turn cause increased local blood flow, increased leakage of fluid and plasma protein into the tissue, and other local tissue reactions that help inactivate or immobilize the antigenic agent. The same factors play a major role in inflammation (which was discussed in Chapter 33) and in allergy, as we discuss later.

7. *Inflammatory effects.* In addition to inflammatory effects caused by activation of the mast cells and basophils, several other complement products contribute to local inflammation. These products cause (1) the already increased blood flow to increase still further, (2) the capillary leakage of proteins to be increased, and (3) the interstitial fluid proteins to coagulate in the tissue spaces, thus preventing movement of the invading organism through the tissues.

Special Attributes of the T-Lymphocyte System— Activated T Cells and Cell-Mediated Immunity

Release of Activated T Cells from Lymphoid Tissue and Formation of Memory Cells. On exposure to the proper antigen, as presented by adjacent macrophages, the T lymphocytes of a specific lymphocyte clone proliferate and release large numbers of activated, specifically reacting T cells in ways that parallel antibody release by activated B cells. The principal difference is that instead of releasing antibodies, whole activated T cells are formed and released into the lymph. These then pass into the circulation and are distributed throughout the body, passing through the capillary walls into the tissue spaces, back into the lymph and blood once again, and circulating again and again throughout the body, sometimes lasting for months or even years.

Also, *T-lymphocyte memory cells* are formed in the same way that B memory cells are formed in the antibody system. That is, when a clone of T lymphocytes is activated by an antigen, many of the newly formed lymphocytes are preserved in the lymphoid tissue to become additional T lymphocytes of that specific clone; in fact, these memory cells even spread throughout the lymphoid tissue of the entire body. Therefore, on subsequent exposure to the same antigen anywhere in the body, release of activated T cells occurs far more rapidly and much more powerfully than had occurred during first exposure.

Antigen-Presenting Cells, MHC Proteins, and Antigen Receptors on the T Lymphocytes. T-cell responses are extremely antigen specific, like the antibody responses of B cells, and are at least as important as antibodies in defending against infection. In fact, acquired immune responses usually require assistance from T cells to begin the process, and T cells play a major role in actually helping to eliminate invading pathogens.

Although B lymphocytes recognize intact antigens, T lymphocytes respond to antigens only when they are bound to specific molecules called *MHC proteins* on the surface of *antigen-presenting cells* in the lymphoid tissues (Figure 34-7). The three major types of antigen-presenting cells are *macrophages*, *B lymphocytes*, and *dendritic cells*. The dendritic cells, the most potent of the antigen-presenting cells, are located throughout the body, and their only known function is to present antigens to T cells. Interaction of cell adhesion proteins is critical in

permitting the T cells to bind to antigen-presenting cells long enough to become activated.

The MHC proteins are encoded by a large group of genes called the *major histocompatibility complex (MHC)*. The MHC proteins bind peptide fragments of antigen proteins that are degraded inside antigen-presenting cells and then transport them to the cell surface. There are two types of MHC proteins: (1) *MHC I proteins*, which present antigens to *cytotoxic T cells*, and (2) *MHC II proteins*, which present antigens to *T helper cells*. The specific functions of cytotoxic and helper T cells are discussed later.

The antigens on the surface of antigen-presenting cells bind with receptor molecules on the surfaces of T cells in the same way that they bind with plasma protein antibodies. These receptor molecules are composed of a variable unit similar to the variable portion of the humoral antibody, but its stem section is firmly bound to the cell membrane of the T lymphocyte. There are as many as 100,000 receptor sites on a single T cell.

Several Types of T Cells and Their Different Functions

It has become clear that there are multiple types of T cells. They are classified into three major groups: (1) *helper T cells*, (2) *cytotoxic T cells*, and (3) *suppressor T cells*. The functions of each of these are distinct.

Helper T Cells—Their Role in Overall Regulation of Immunity

The helper T cells are by far the most numerous of the T cells, usually constituting more than three quarters of all of them. As their name implies, they help in the functions of the immune system, and they do so in many ways. In fact, they serve as the major regulator of virtually all immune functions, as shown in Figure 34-8. They do this by forming a series of protein mediators, called *lymphokines*, that act on other cells of the immune system, as well as on bone marrow cells. Among the important lymphokines secreted by the helper T cells are the following:

Interleukin-2

Interleukin-3

Interleukin-4

Interleukin-5

Interleukin-6

Granulocyte-monocyte colony-stimulating factor

Interferon-γ

Specific Regulatory Functions of the Lymphokines. In the absence of the lymphokines from the helper T cells, the remainder of the immune system is almost paralyzed. In fact, it is the helper T cells that are inactivated or destroyed by the *acquired immunodeficiency syndrome (AIDS) virus*, which leaves the body almost totally unprotected against infectious disease, therefore leading

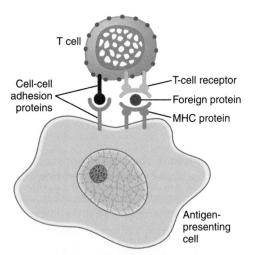

Figure 34-7 Activation of T cells requires interaction of T-cell receptors with an antigen (foreign protein) that is transported to the surface of the antigen-presenting cell by a major histocompatibility complex (MHC) protein. Cell-to-cell adhesion proteins enable the T cell to bind to the antigen-presenting cell long enough to become activated.

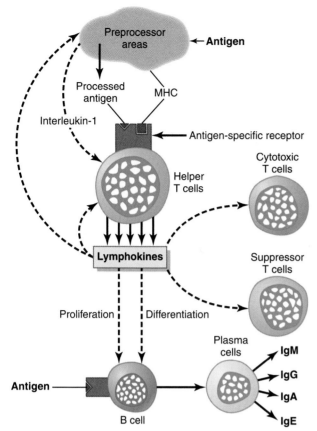

Figure 34-8 Regulation of the immune system, emphasizing a pivotal role of the helper T cells. MHC, major histocompatibility complex.

to the now well-known debilitating and lethal effects of AIDS. Some of the specific regulatory functions are the following.

Stimulation of Growth and Proliferation of Cytotoxic T Cells and Suppressor T Cells. In the absence of helper T cells, the clones for producing cytotoxic T cells and suppressor T cells are activated only slightly by most antigens. The lymphokine interleukin-2 has an especially strong stimulatory effect in causing growth and proliferation of both cytotoxic and suppressor T cells. In addition, several of the other lymphokines have less potent effects.

Stimulation of B-Cell Growth and Differentiation to Form Plasma Cells and Antibodies. The direct actions of antigen to cause B-cell growth, proliferation, formation of plasma cells, and secretion of antibodies are also slight without the "help" of the helper T cells. Almost all the interleukins participate in the B-cell response, but especially interleukins 4, 5, and 6. In fact, these three interleukins have such potent effects on the B cells that they have been called B-cell stimulating factors or B-cell growth factors.

Activation of the Macrophage System. The lymphokines also affect the macrophages. First, they slow or stop the migration of the macrophages after they have been chemotactically attracted into the inflamed tissue area, thus causing great accumulation of macrophages. Second, they activate the macrophages to cause far more efficient phagocytosis, allowing them to attack and destroy increasing numbers of invading bacteria or other tissue-destroying agents.

Feedback Stimulatory Effect on the Helper Cells Themselves. Some of the lymphokines, especially interleukin-2, have a direct positive feedback effect in stimulating activation of the helper T cells themselves. This acts as an amplifier by further enhancing the helper cell response, as well as the entire immune response to an invading antigen.

Cytotoxic T Cells Are "Killer" Cells

The cytotoxic T cell is a direct-attack cell that is capable of killing microorganisms and, at times, even some of the body's own cells. For this reason, these cells are called *killer cells.* The receptor proteins on the surfaces of the cytotoxic cells cause them to bind tightly to those organisms or cells that contain the appropriate binding-specific antigen. Then, they kill the attacked cell in the manner shown in Figure 34-9. After binding, the cytotoxic T cell secretes hole-forming proteins, called *perforins,* that literally punch round holes in the membrane of the attacked cell. Then fluid flows rapidly into the cell from the interstitial space. In addition, the cytotoxic T cell releases cytotoxic substances directly into the attacked cell. Almost immediately, the attacked cell becomes greatly swollen, and it usually dissolves shortly thereafter.

Especially important, these cytotoxic killer cells can pull away from the victim cells after they have punched holes and delivered cytotoxic substances and then move on to kill more cells. Indeed, some of these cells persist for months in the tissues.

Some of the cytotoxic T cells are especially lethal to tissue cells that have been invaded by viruses because many virus particles become entrapped in the membranes of the tissue cells and attract T cells in response to the viral antigenicity. The cytotoxic cells also play an important role in destroying cancer cells, heart transplant cells, or other types of cells that are foreign to the person's own body.

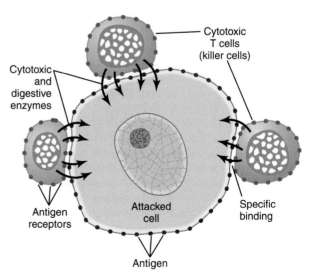

Figure 34-9 Direct destruction of an invading cell by sensitized lymphocytes (cytotoxic T cells).

Suppressor T Cells

Much less is known about the suppressor T cells than about the others, but they are capable of suppressing the functions of both cytotoxic and helper T cells. It is believed that these suppressor functions serve the purpose of preventing the cytotoxic cells from causing excessive immune reactions that might be damaging to the body's own tissues. For this reason, the suppressor cells are classified, along with the helper T cells, as *regulatory T cells*. It is probable that the suppressor T-cell system plays an important role in limiting the ability of the immune system to attack a person's own body tissues, called *immune tolerance*, as we discuss in the next section.

Tolerance of the Acquired Immunity System to One's Own Tissues—Role of Preprocessing in the Thymus and Bone Marrow

If a person should become immune to his or her own tissues, the process of acquired immunity would destroy the individual's own body. The immune mechanism normally "recognizes" a person's own tissues as being distinctive from bacteria or viruses, and the person's immunity system forms few antibodies or activated T cells against his or her own antigens.

Most Tolerance Results from Clone Selection During Preprocessing. It is believed that most tolerance develops during preprocessing of T lymphocytes in the thymus and of B lymphocytes in the bone marrow. The reason for this belief is that injecting a strong antigen into a fetus while the lymphocytes are being preprocessed in these two areas prevents development of clones of lymphocytes in the lymphoid tissue that are specific for the injected antigen. Experiments have shown that specific immature lymphocytes in the thymus, when exposed to a strong antigen, become lymphoblastic, proliferate considerably, and then combine with the stimulating antigen—an effect that is believed to cause the cells themselves to be destroyed by the thymic epithelial cells before they can migrate to and colonize the total body lymphoid tissue.

It is believed that during the preprocessing of lymphocytes in the thymus and bone marrow, all or most of those clones of lymphocytes that are specific to damage the body's own tissues are self-destroyed because of their continual exposure to the body's antigens.

Failure of the Tolerance Mechanism Causes Autoimmune Diseases. Sometimes people lose their immune tolerance of their own tissues. This occurs to a greater extent the older a person becomes. It usually occurs after destruction of some of the body's own tissues, which releases considerable quantities of "self-antigens" that circulate in the body and presumably cause acquired immunity in the form of either activated T cells or antibodies.

Several specific diseases that result from autoimmunity include (1) *rheumatic fever*, in which the body becomes immunized against tissues in the joints and heart, especially the heart valves, after exposure to a specific type of streptococcal toxin that has an epitope in its molecular structure similar to the structure of some of the body's own self-antigens; (2) one type of *glomerulonephritis*, in which the person becomes immunized against the basement membranes of glomeruli; (3) *myasthenia gravis*, in which immunity develops against the acetylcholine receptor proteins of the neuromuscular junction, causing paralysis; and (4) *lupus erythematosus*, in which the person becomes immunized against many different body tissues at the same time, a disease that causes extensive damage and often rapid death.

Immunization by Injection of Antigens

Immunization has been used for many years to produce acquired immunity against specific diseases. A person can be immunized by injecting dead organisms that are no longer capable of causing disease but that still have some of their chemical antigens. This type of immunization is used to protect against typhoid fever, whooping cough, diphtheria, and many other types of bacterial diseases.

Immunity can be achieved against toxins that have been treated with chemicals so that their toxic nature has been destroyed even though their antigens for causing immunity are still intact. This procedure is used in immunizing against tetanus, botulism, and other similar toxic diseases.

And, finally, a person can be immunized by being infected with live organisms that have been "attenuated." That is, these organisms either have been grown in special culture media or have been passed through a series of animals until they have mutated enough that they will not cause disease but do still carry specific antigens required for immunization. This procedure is used to protect against smallpox, yellow fever, poliomyelitis, measles, and many other viral diseases.

Passive Immunity

Thus far, all the acquired immunity we have discussed has been *active immunity*. That is, the person's own body develops either antibodies or activated T cells in response to invasion of the body by a foreign antigen. However, temporary immunity can be achieved in a person without injecting any antigen. This is done by infusing antibodies, activated T cells, or both obtained from the blood of someone else or from some other animal that has been actively immunized against the antigen.

Antibodies last in the body of the recipient for 2 to 3 weeks, and during that time, the person is protected against the invading disease. Activated T cells last for a few weeks if transfused from another person but only for a few hours to a few days if transfused from an animal. Such transfusion of antibodies or T lymphocytes to confer immunity is called *passive immunity*.

Allergy and Hypersensitivity

An important undesirable side effect of immunity is the development, under some conditions, of allergy or other types of immune hypersensitivity. There are several types of allergy and other hypersensitivities, some of which occur only in people who have a specific allergic tendency.

Allergy Caused by Activated T Cells: Delayed-Reaction Allergy

Delayed-reaction allergy is caused by activated T cells and not by antibodies. In the case of poison ivy, the toxin of poison ivy in itself does not cause much harm to the tissues. However, on repeated exposure, it does cause the formation of activated helper and cytotoxic T cells. Then, after subsequent exposure to the poison ivy toxin, within a day or so, the activated T cells diffuse from the circulating blood in large numbers into the skin to respond to the poison ivy toxin. And, at the same time, these T cells elicit a cell-mediated type of immune reaction. Remembering that this type of immunity can cause release of many toxic substances from the activated T cells, as well as extensive invasion of the tissues by macrophages along with their subsequent effects, one can well understand that the eventual result of some delayed-reaction allergies can be serious tissue damage. The damage normally occurs in the tissue area where the instigating antigen is present, such as in the skin in the case of poison ivy, or in the lungs to cause lung edema or asthmatic attacks in the case of some airborne antigens.

Allergies in the "Allergic" Person Who Has Excess IgE Antibodies

Some people have an "allergic" tendency. Their allergies are called *atopic allergies* because they are caused by a nonordinary response of the immune system. The allergic tendency is genetically passed from parent to child and is characterized by the presence of large quantities of IgE antibodies in the blood. These antibodies are called *reagins* or *sensitizing antibodies* to distinguish them from the more common IgG antibodies. When an *allergen* (defined as an antigen that reacts specifically with a specific type of IgE reagin antibody) enters the body, an allergen-reagin reaction takes place and a subsequent allergic reaction occurs.

A special characteristic of the IgE antibodies (the reagins) is a strong propensity to attach to mast cells and basophils. Indeed, a single mast cell or basophil can bind as many as half a million molecules of IgE antibodies. Then, when an antigen (an allergen) that has multiple binding sites binds with several IgE antibodies that are already attached to a mast cell or basophil, this causes immediate change in the membrane of the mast cell or basophil, perhaps resulting from a physical effect of the antibody molecules to contort the cell membrane. At any

rate, many of the mast cells and basophils rupture; others release special agents immediately or shortly thereafter, including *histamine, protease, slow-reacting substance of anaphylaxis* (which is a mixture of toxic leukotrienes), *eosinophil chemotactic substance, neutrophil chemotactic substance, heparin,* and *platelet activating factors*. These substances cause such effects as dilation of the local blood vessels; attraction of eosinophils and neutrophils to the reactive site; increased permeability of the capillaries with loss of fluid into the tissues; and contraction of local smooth muscle cells. Therefore, several different tissue responses can occur, depending on the type of tissue in which the allergen-reagin reaction occurs. Among the different types of allergic reactions caused in this manner are the following.

Anaphylaxis. When a specific allergen is injected directly into the circulation, the allergen can react with basophils of the blood and mast cells in the tissues located immediately outside the small blood vessels if the basophils and mast cells have been sensitized by attachment of IgE reagins. Therefore, a widespread allergic reaction occurs throughout the vascular system and closely associated tissues. This is called *anaphylaxis*. Histamine is released into the circulation and causes body-wide vasodilation, as well as increased permeability of the capillaries with resultant marked loss of plasma from the circulation. Occasionally, a person who experiences this reaction dies of circulatory shock within a few minutes unless treated with epinephrine to oppose the effects of the histamine.

Also released from the activated basophils and mast cells is a mixture of leukotrienes called *slow-reacting substance of anaphylaxis*. These leukotrienes can cause spasm of the smooth muscle of the bronchioles, eliciting an asthma-like attack, sometimes causing death by suffocation.

Urticaria. Urticaria results from antigen entering specific skin areas and causing localized anaphylactoid reactions. Histamine released locally causes (1) vasodilation that induces an immediate red flare and (2) increased local permeability of the capillaries that leads to local circumscribed areas of swelling of the skin within another few minutes. The swellings are commonly called *hives*. Administration of antihistamine drugs to a person before exposure will prevent the hives.

Hay Fever. In hay fever, the allergen-reagin reaction occurs in the nose. Histamine released in response to the reaction causes local intranasal vascular dilation, with resultant increased capillary pressure and increased capillary permeability. Both these effects cause rapid fluid leakage into the nasal cavities and into associated deeper tissues of the nose; and the nasal linings become swollen and secretory. Here again, use of antihistamine drugs can prevent this swelling reaction. But other products of the allergen-reagin reaction can still cause irritation of the nose, eliciting the typical sneezing syndrome.

Asthma. Asthma often occurs in the "allergic" type of person. In such a person, the allergen-reagin reaction occurs in the bronchioles of the lungs. Here, an important product released from the mast cells is believed to be the *slow-reacting substance of anaphylaxis*, which causes spasm of the bronchiolar smooth muscle. Consequently, the person has difficulty breathing until the reactive products of the allergic reaction have been removed. Administration of antihistamine medication has less effect on the course of asthma because histamine does not appear to be the major factor eliciting the asthmatic reaction.

Bibliography

Alberts B, Johnson A, Lewis J, et al: *Molecular Biology of the Cell*, ed 5, New York, 2008, Garland Science.

Anderson GP: Endotyping asthma: new insights into key pathogenic mechanisms in a complex, heterogeneous disease, *Lancet* 372:1107, 2008.

Barton GM: A calculated response: control of inflammation by the innate immune system, *J Clin Invest* 118:413, 2008.

Cossart P, Sansonetti PJ: Bacterial invasion: the paradigms of enteroinvasive pathogens, *Science* 304:242, 2004.

Dorshkind K, Montecino-Rodriguez E, Signer RA: The ageing immune system: is it ever too old to become young again? *Nat Rev Immunol* 9:57, 2009.

Eisenbarth GS, Gottlieb PA: Autoimmune polyendocrine syndromes, *N Engl J Med* 350:2068, 2004.

Fanta CH: Asthma, *N Engl J Med* 360:1002, 2009.

Figdor CG, de Vries IJ, Lesterhuis WJ, et al: Dendritic cell immunotherapy: mapping the way, *Nat Med* 10:475, 2004.

Grossman Z, Min B, Meier-Schellersheim M, et al: Concomitant regulation of T-cell activation and homeostasis, *Nat Rev Immunol* 4:387, 2004.

Kupper TS, Fuhlbrigge RC: Immune surveillance in the skin: mechanisms and clinical consequences, *Nat Rev Immunol* 4:211, 2004.

Linton PJ, Dorshkind K: Age-related changes in lymphocyte development and function, *Nat Immunol* 5:133, 2004.

Mackay IR: Autoimmunity since the 1957 clonal selection theory: a little acorn to a large oak, *Immunol Cell Biol* 86:67, 2008.

Medzhitov R: Recognition of microorganisms and activation of the immune response, *Nature* 449:819, 2007.

Mizushima N, Levine B, Cuervo AM, et al: Autophagy fights disease through cellular self-digestion, *Nature* 45:1069, 2008.

Petrie HT: Cell migration and the control of post-natal T-cell lymphopoiesis in the thymus, *Nat Rev Immunol* 3:859, 2003.

Rahman A, Isenberg DA: Systemic lupus erythematosus, *N Engl J Med* 358:929, 2008.

Vivier E, Anfossi N: Inhibitory NK-cell receptors on T cells: witness of the past, actors of the future, *Nat Rev Immunol* 4:190, 2004.

Welner RS, Pelayo R, Kincade PW: Evolving views on the genealogy of B cells, *Nat Rev Immunol* 8:95, 2008.

Blood Types; Transfusion; Tissue and Organ Transplantation

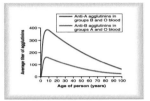

Antigenicity Causes Immune Reactions of Blood

When blood transfusions from one person to another were first attempted, immediate or delayed agglutination and hemolysis of the red blood cells often occurred, resulting in typical transfusion reactions that frequently led to death. Soon it was discovered that the bloods of different people have different antigenic and immune properties so that antibodies in the plasma of one blood will react with antigens on the surfaces of the red cells of another blood type. If proper precautions are taken, one can determine ahead of time whether the antibodies and antigens present in the donor and recipient bloods will cause a transfusion reaction.

Multiplicity of Antigens in the Blood Cells. At least 30 commonly occurring antigens and hundreds of other rare antigens, each of which can at times cause antigen-antibody reactions, have been found on the surfaces of the cell membranes of human blood cells. Most of the antigens are weak and therefore are of importance principally for studying the inheritance of genes to establish parentage.

Two particular types of antigens are much more likely than the others to cause blood transfusion reactions. They are the *O-A-B* system of antigens and the *Rh* system.

O-A-B Blood Types

A and B Antigens—Agglutinogens

Two antigens—type A and type B—occur on the surfaces of the red blood cells in a large proportion of human beings. It is these antigens (also called *agglutinogens* because they often cause blood cell agglutination) that cause most blood transfusion reactions. Because of the way these agglutinogens are inherited, people may have neither of them on their cells, they may have one, or they may have both simultaneously.

Major O-A-B Blood Types. In transfusing blood from one person to another, the bloods of donors and recipients are normally classified into four major O-A-B blood types, as shown in Table 35-1, depending on the presence or absence of the two agglutinogens, the A and B agglutinogens. When neither A nor B agglutinogen is present, the blood is *type O*. When only type A agglutinogen is present, the blood is *type A*. When only type B agglutinogen is present, the blood is *type B*. When both A and B agglutinogens are present, the blood is *type AB*.

Genetic Determination of the Agglutinogens. Two genes, one on each of two paired chromosomes, determine the O-A-B blood type. These genes can be any one of three types but only one type on each of the two chromosomes: type O, type A, or type B. The type O gene is either functionless or almost functionless, so it causes no significant type O agglutinogen on the cells. Conversely, the type A and type B genes do cause strong agglutinogens on the cells.

The six possible combinations of genes, as shown in Table 35-1, are OO, OA, OB, AA, BB, and AB. These combinations of genes are known as the *genotypes*, and each person is one of the six genotypes.

One can also observe from Table 35-1 that a person with genotype OO produces no agglutinogens, and therefore the blood type is O. A person with genotype OA or AA produces type A agglutinogens and therefore has blood type A. Genotypes OB and BB give type B blood, and genotype AB gives type AB blood.

Relative Frequencies of the Different Blood Types. The prevalence of the different blood types among one group of persons studied was approximately:

O	47%
A	41%
B	9%
AB	3%

It is obvious from these percentages that the O and A genes occur frequently, whereas the B gene is infrequent.

Table 35-1 Blood Types with Their Genotypes and Their Constituent Agglutinogens and Agglutinins

Genotypes	Blood Types	Agglutinogens	Agglutinins
OO	O	–	Anti-A and Anti-B
OA or AA	A	A	Anti-B
OB or BB	B	B	Anti-A
AB	AB	A and B	–

Agglutinins

When type A agglutinogen *is not present* in a person's red blood cells, antibodies known as *anti-A agglutinins* develop in the plasma. Also, when type B agglutinogen *is not present* in the red blood cells, antibodies known as *anti-B agglutinins* develop in the plasma.

Thus, referring once again to Table 35-1, note that type O blood, although containing no agglutinogens, does contain both *anti-A* and *anti-B agglutinins*; type A blood contains type A agglutinogens and *anti-B agglutinins*; type B blood contains type B agglutinogens and anti-A agglutinins. Finally, type AB blood contains both A and B agglutinogens but no agglutinins.

Titer of the Agglutinins at Different Ages. Immediately after birth, the quantity of agglutinins in the plasma is almost zero. Two to 8 months after birth, an infant begins to produce agglutinins—anti-A agglutinins when type A agglutinogens are not present in the cells, and anti-B agglutinins when type B agglutinogens are not in the cells. Figure 35-1 shows the changing titers of the anti-A and anti-B agglutinins at different ages. A maximum titer is usually reached at 8 to 10 years of age, and this gradually declines throughout the remaining years of life.

Origin of Agglutinins in the Plasma. The agglutinins are gamma globulins, as are almost all antibodies, and they are produced by the same bone marrow and lymph gland cells that produce antibodies to any other antigens. Most of them are IgM and IgG immunoglobulin molecules.

But why are these agglutinins produced in people who do not have the respective agglutinogens in their red blood cells? The answer to this is that small amounts of type A and B antigens enter the body in food, in bacteria, and in other ways, and these substances initiate the development of the anti-A and anti-B agglutinins.

For instance, infusion of group A antigen into a recipient having a non-A blood type causes a typical immune response with formation of greater quantities of anti-A agglutinins than ever. Also, the neonate has few, if any, agglutinins, showing that agglutinin formation occurs almost entirely after birth.

Agglutination Process in Transfusion Reactions

When bloods are mismatched so that anti-A or anti-B plasma agglutinins are mixed with red blood cells that contain A or B agglutinogens, respectively, the red cells agglutinate as a result of the agglutinins' attaching themselves to the red blood cells. Because the agglutinins have 2 binding sites (IgG type) or 10 binding sites (IgM type), a single agglutinin can attach to two or more red blood cells at the same time, thereby causing the cells to be bound together by the agglutinin. This causes the cells to clump, which is the process of "agglutination." Then these clumps plug small blood vessels throughout the circulatory system. During ensuing hours to days, either physical distortion of the cells or attack by phagocytic white blood cells destroys the membranes of the agglutinated cells, releasing hemoglobin into the plasma, which is called "*hemolysis*" of the red blood cells.

Acute Hemolysis Occurs in Some Transfusion Reactions. Sometimes, when recipient and donor bloods are mismatched, immediate hemolysis of red cells occurs in the circulating blood. In this case, the antibodies cause lysis of the red blood cells by activating the complement system, which releases proteolytic enzymes (the *lytic complex*) that rupture the cell membranes, as described in Chapter 34. *Immediate* intravascular hemolysis is far less common than agglutination followed by *delayed* hemolysis, because not only does there have to be a high titer of antibodies for lysis to occur, but also a different type of antibody seems to be required, mainly the IgM antibodies; these antibodies are called *hemolysins*.

Blood Typing

Before giving a transfusion to a person, it is necessary to determine the blood type of the recipient's blood and the blood type of the donor blood so that the bloods can be appropriately matched. This is called *blood typing* and *blood matching*, and these are performed in the following way: The red blood cells are first separated from the plasma and diluted with saline. One portion is then mixed with anti-A agglutinin and another portion with anti-B agglutinin. After several minutes, the mixtures are

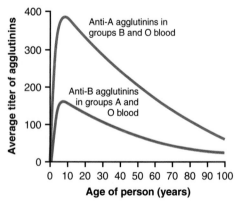

Figure 35-1 Average titers of anti-A and anti-B agglutinins in the plasmas of people with different blood types.

Table 35-2 Blood Typing, Showing Agglutination of Cells of the Different Blood Types with Anti-A or Anti-B Agglutinins in the Sera

Red Blood Cell Types	Sera	
	Anti-A	*Anti-B*
O	–	–
A	+	–
B	–	+
AB	+	+

observed under a microscope. If the red blood cells have become clumped—that is, "agglutinated"—one knows that an antibody-antigen reaction has resulted.

Table 35-2 lists the presence (+) or absence (–) of agglutination of the four types of red blood cells. Type O red blood cells have no agglutinogens and therefore do not react with either the anti-A or the anti-B agglutinins. Type A blood has A agglutinogens and therefore agglutinates with anti-A agglutinins. Type B blood has B agglutinogens and agglutinates with anti-B agglutinins. Type AB blood has both A and B agglutinogens and agglutinates with both types of agglutinins.

Rh Blood Types

Along with the O-A-B blood type system, the Rh blood type system is also important when transfusing blood. The major difference between the O-A-B system and the Rh system is the following: In the O-A-B system, the plasma agglutinins responsible for causing transfusion reactions develop spontaneously, whereas in the Rh system, spontaneous agglutinins almost never occur. Instead, the person must first be massively exposed to an Rh antigen, such as by transfusion of blood containing the Rh antigen, before enough agglutinins to cause a significant transfusion reaction will develop.

Rh Antigens—"Rh-Positive" and "Rh-Negative" People. There are six common types of Rh antigens, each of which is called an *Rh factor*. These types are designated C, D, E, c, d, and e. A person who has a C antigen does not have the c antigen, but the person missing the C antigen always has the c antigen. The same is true for the D-d and E-e antigens. Also, because of the manner of inheritance of these factors, each person has one of each of the three pairs of antigens.

The type D antigen is widely prevalent in the population and considerably more antigenic than the other Rh antigens. Anyone who has this type of antigen is said to be *Rh positive*, whereas a person who does not have type D antigen is said to be *Rh negative*. However, it must be noted that even in Rh-negative people, some of the other Rh antigens can still cause transfusion reactions, although the reactions are usually much milder.

About 85 percent of all white people are Rh positive and 15 percent, Rh negative. In American blacks, the percentage of Rh-positives is about 95 percent, whereas in African blacks, it is virtually 100 percent.

Rh Immune Response

Formation of Anti-Rh Agglutinins. When red blood cells containing Rh factor are injected into a person whose blood does not contain the Rh factor—that is, into an Rh-negative person—anti-Rh agglutinins develop slowly, reaching maximum concentration of agglutinins about 2 to 4 months later. This immune response occurs to a much greater extent in some people than in others. With multiple exposures to the Rh factor, an Rh-negative person eventually becomes strongly "sensitized" to Rh factor.

Characteristics of Rh Transfusion Reactions. If an Rh-negative person has never before been exposed to Rh-positive blood, transfusion of Rh-positive blood into that person will likely cause no immediate reaction. However, anti-Rh antibodies can develop in sufficient quantities during the next 2 to 4 weeks to cause agglutination of those transfused cells that are still circulating in the blood. These cells are then hemolyzed by the tissue macrophage system. Thus, a *delayed* transfusion reaction occurs, although it is usually mild. On subsequent transfusion of Rh-positive blood into the same person, who is now already immunized against the Rh factor, the transfusion reaction is greatly enhanced and can be immediate and as severe as a transfusion reaction caused by mismatched type A or B blood.

Erythroblastosis Fetalis ("Hemolytic Disease of the Newborn")

Erythroblastosis fetalis is a disease of the fetus and newborn child characterized by agglutination and phagocytosis of the fetus's red blood cells. In most instances of erythroblastosis fetalis, the mother is Rh negative and the father Rh positive. The baby has inherited the Rh-positive antigen from the father, and the mother develops anti-Rh agglutinins from exposure to the fetus's Rh antigen. In turn, the mother's agglutinins diffuse through the placenta into the fetus and cause red blood cell agglutination.

Incidence of the Disease. An Rh-negative mother having her first Rh-positive child usually does not develop sufficient anti-Rh agglutinins to cause any harm. However, about 3 percent of second Rh-positive babies exhibit some signs of erythroblastosis fetalis; about 10 percent of third babies exhibit the disease; and the incidence rises progressively with subsequent pregnancies.

Effect of the Mother's Antibodies on the Fetus. After anti-Rh antibodies have formed in the mother, they diffuse slowly through the placental membrane into the fetus's blood. There they cause agglutination of the fetus's blood. The agglutinated red blood cells subsequently hemolyze, releasing hemoglobin into the blood. The fetus's macrophages then convert the hemoglobin into bilirubin, which causes the baby's skin to become yellow (jaundiced). The antibodies can also attack and damage other cells of the body.

Clinical Picture of Erythroblastosis. The jaundiced, erythroblastotic newborn baby is usually anemic at birth, and the anti-Rh agglutinins from the mother usually circulate in the infant's blood for another 1 to 2 months after birth, destroying more and more red blood cells.

The hematopoietic tissues of the infant attempt to replace the hemolyzed red blood cells. The liver and spleen become greatly enlarged and produce red blood cells in the same manner that they normally do during the middle of gestation. Because of the rapid production of red cells, many early forms of red blood cells, including many *nucleated blastic forms,* are passed from the baby's bone marrow into the circulatory system, and it is because of the presence of these nucleated blastic red blood cells that the disease is called *erythroblastosis fetalis.*

Although the severe anemia of erythroblastosis fetalis is usually the cause of death, many children who barely survive the anemia exhibit permanent mental impairment or damage to motor areas of the brain because of precipitation of bilirubin in the neuronal cells, causing destruction of many, a condition called *kernicterus.*

Treatment of the Erythroblastotic Neonate. One treatment for erythroblastosis fetalis is to replace the neonate's blood with Rh-negative blood. About 400 milliliters of Rh-negative blood is infused over a period of 1.5 or more hours while the neonate's own Rh-positive blood is being removed. This procedure may be repeated several times during the first few weeks of life, mainly to keep the bilirubin level low and thereby prevent kernicterus. By the time these transfused Rh-negative cells are replaced with the infant's own Rh-positive cells, a process that requires 6 or more weeks, the anti-Rh agglutinins that had come from the mother will have been destroyed.

Prevention of Erythroblastosis Fetalis. The D antigen of the Rh blood group system is the primary culprit in causing immunization of an Rh-negative mother to an Rh-positive fetus. In the 1970s, a dramatic reduction in the incidence of erythroblastosis fetalis was achieved with the development of *Rh immunoglobulin globin, an anti-D antibody* that is administered to the expectant mother starting at 28 to 30 weeks of gestation. The anti-D antibody is also administered to Rh-negative women who deliver Rh-positive babies to prevent sensitization of the mothers to the D antigen. This greatly reduces the risk of developing large amounts of D antibodies during the second pregnancy.

The mechanism by which Rh immunoglobulin globin prevents sensitization of the D antigen is not completely understood, but one effect of the anti-D antibody is to inhibit antigen-induced B lymphocyte antibody production in the expectant mother. The administered anti-D antibody also attaches to D-antigen sites on Rh-positive fetal red blood cells that may cross the placenta and enter the circulation of the expectant mother, thereby interfering with the immune response to the D antigen.

Transfusion Reactions Resulting from Mismatched Blood Types

If donor blood of one blood type is transfused into a recipient who has another blood type, a transfusion reaction is likely to occur in which the red blood cells *of the donor blood* are agglutinated. It is rare that the transfused blood causes agglutination *of the recipient's cells,* for the following reason: The plasma portion of the donor blood immediately becomes diluted by all the plasma of the recipient, thereby decreasing the titer of the infused agglutinins to a level usually too low to cause agglutination. Conversely, the small amount of infused blood does not significantly dilute the agglutinins in the recipient's plasma. Therefore, the recipient's agglutinins can still agglutinate the mismatched donor cells.

As explained earlier, all transfusion reactions eventually cause either immediate hemolysis resulting from hemolysins or later hemolysis resulting from phagocytosis of agglutinated cells. The hemoglobin released from the red cells is then converted by the phagocytes into bilirubin and later excreted in the bile by the liver, as discussed in Chapter 70. The concentration of bilirubin in the body fluids often rises high enough to cause *jaundice*—that is, the person's internal tissues and skin become *colored with yellow bile pigment.* But if liver function is normal, the bile pigment will be excreted into the intestines by way of the liver bile, so jaundice usually does not appear in an adult person unless more than 400 milliliters of blood is hemolyzed in less than a day.

Acute Kidney Shutdown After Transfusion Reactions. One of the most lethal effects of transfusion reactions is *kidney failure,* which can begin within a few minutes to few hours and continue until the person dies of renal failure.

The kidney shutdown seems to result from three causes: First, the antigen-antibody reaction of the transfusion reaction releases toxic substances from the hemolyzing blood that cause powerful renal vasoconstriction. Second, loss of circulating red cells in the recipient, along with production of toxic substances from the hemolyzed cells and from the immune reaction, often causes circulatory shock. The arterial blood pressure falls very low, and renal blood flow and urine output decrease. Third, if the total amount of free hemoglobin released into the circulating blood is greater than the quantity that can bind with *"haptoglobin"* (a plasma protein that binds small amounts of hemoglobin), much of the excess leaks through the glomerular membranes into the kidney tubules. If this amount is still slight, it can be reabsorbed through the tubular epithelium into the blood and will cause no harm; if it is great, then only a small percentage is reabsorbed. Yet water continues to be reabsorbed, causing the tubular hemoglobin concentration to rise so high that the hemoglobin precipitates and blocks many of the kidney tubules. Thus, renal vasoconstriction, circulatory shock, and renal tubular blockage together cause acute renal shutdown.

If the shutdown is complete and fails to resolve, the patient dies within a week to 12 days, as explained in Chapter 31, unless treated with an artificial kidney.

Transplantation of Tissues and Organs

Most of the different antigens of red blood cells that cause transfusion reactions are also widely present in other cells of the body, and each bodily tissue has its own additional complement of antigens. Consequently, foreign cells transplanted anywhere into the body of a recipient can produce immune reactions. In other words, most recipients are just as able to resist invasion by foreign tissue cells as to resist invasion by foreign bacteria or red cells.

Autografts, Isografts, Allografts, and Xenografts. A transplant of a tissue or whole organ from one part of the same animal to another part is called an *autograft;* from one identical twin to another, an *isograft;* from one human being to another or from any animal to another animal of the same species, an *allograft;* and from a lower animal to a human being or from an animal of one species to one of another species, a *xenograft.*

Transplantation of Cellular Tissues. In the case of *autografts* and *isografts,* cells in the transplant contain virtually the same types of antigens as in the tissues of the recipient and will almost always continue to live normally and indefinitely if an adequate blood supply is provided.

At the other extreme, in the case of *xenografts,* immune reactions almost always occur, causing death of the cells in the graft within 1 day to 5 weeks after transplantation unless some specific therapy is used to prevent the immune reactions.

Some of the different cellular tissues and organs that have been transplanted as allografts, either experimentally or for therapeutic purposes, from one person to another are skin, kidney, heart, liver, glandular tissue, bone marrow, and lung. With proper "matching" of tissues between persons, many kidney allografts have been successful for at least 5 to 15 years, and allograft liver and heart transplants for 1 to 15 years.

Attempts to Overcome Immune Reactions in Transplanted Tissue

Because of the extreme potential importance of transplanting certain tissues and organs, serious attempts have been made to prevent antigen-antibody reactions associated with transplantation. The following specific procedures have met with some degrees of clinical or experimental success.

Tissue Typing—the Human Leukocyte Antigen (HLA) Complex of Antigens

The most important antigens for causing graft rejection are a complex called the *HLA antigens.* Six of these antigens are present on the tissue cell membranes of each person, but there are about 150 different HLA antigens to choose from. Therefore, this represents more than a trillion possible combinations. Consequently, it is virtually impossible for two persons, except in the case of identical twins, to have the same six HLA antigens. Development of significant immunity against any one of these antigens can cause graft rejection.

The HLA antigens occur on the white blood cells, as well as on the tissue cells. Therefore, tissue typing for these antigens is done on the membranes of lymphocytes that have been separated from the person's blood. The lymphocytes are mixed with appropriate antisera and complement; after incubation, the cells are tested for membrane damage, usually by testing the rate of trans-membrane uptake by the lymphocytic cells of a special dye.

Some of the HLA antigens are not severely antigenic, for which reason a precise match of some antigens between donor and recipient is not always essential to allow allograft acceptance. Therefore, by obtaining the best possible match between donor and recipient, the grafting procedure has become far less hazardous. The best success has been with tissue-type matches between siblings and between parent and child. The match in identical twins is exact, so transplants between identical twins are almost never rejected because of immune reactions.

Prevention of Graft Rejection by Suppressing the Immune System

If the immune system were completely suppressed, graft rejection would not occur. In fact, in a person who has serious depression of the immune system, grafts can be successful without the use of significant therapy to prevent rejection. But in the normal person, even with the best possible tissue typing, allografts seldom resist rejection for more than a few days or weeks without use of specific therapy to suppress the immune system. Furthermore, because the T cells are mainly the portion of the immune system important for killing grafted cells, their suppression is much more important than suppression of plasma antibodies. Some of the therapeutic agents that have been used for this purpose include the following:

1. *Glucocorticoid hormones isolated from adrenal cortex glands (or drugs with glucocorticoid-like activity),* which suppress the growth of all lymphoid tissue and, therefore, decrease formation of antibodies and T cells.

2. *Various drugs that have a toxic effect on the lymphoid system* and, therefore, block formation of antibodies and T cells, especially the drug *azathioprine.*

3. *Cyclosporine,* which has a specific inhibitory effect on the formation of helper T cells and, therefore, is especially efficacious in blocking the T-cell rejection reaction. This has proved to be one of the most valuable of all the drugs because it does not depress some other portions of the immune system.

Use of these agents often leaves the person unprotected from infectious disease; therefore, sometimes bacterial and viral infections become rampant. In addition, the incidence of cancer is several times as great in an immunosuppressed person, presumably because the immune system is important in destroying many early cancer cells before they can begin to proliferate.

Transplantation of living tissues in human beings has had important success mainly because of the development of drugs that suppress the responses of the immune system. With the introduction of improved immunosuppressive agents, successful organ transplantation has become much more common. The current approach to immunosuppressive therapy attempts to balance acceptable rates of rejection with moderation in the adverse effects of immunosuppressive drugs.

Bibliography

Avent ND, Reid ME: The Rh blood group system: a review, *Blood* 95:375, 2000.

An X, Mohandas N: Disorders of red cell membrane, *Br J Haematol* 141:367, 2008.

Bowman J: Thirty-five years of Rh prophylaxis, *Transfusion* 43:1661, 2003.

Burton NM, Anstee DJ: Structure, function and significance of Rh proteins in red cells, *Curr Opin Hematol* 15:625, 2008.

Gonzalez-Rey E, Chorny A, Delgado M: Regulation of immune tolerance by anti-inflammatory neuropeptides, *Nat Rev Immunol* 7:52, 2007.

Horn KD: The classification, recognition and significance of polyagglutination in transfusion medicine, *Blood Rev* 13:36, 1999.

Hunt SA, Haddad F: The changing face of heart transplantation, *J Am Coll Cardiol* 52:587, 2008.

Miller J, Mathew JM, Esquenazi V: Toward tolerance to human organ transplants: a few additional corollaries and questions, *Transplantation* 77:940, 2004.

Olsson ML, Clausen H: Modifying the red cell surface: towards an ABO-universal blood supply, *Br J Haematol* 140:3, 2008.

Shimizu K, Mitchell RN: The role of chemokines in transplant graft arterial disease, *Arterioscler Thromb Vasc Biol* 28:1937, 2008.

Spahn DR, Pasch T: Physiological properties of blood substitutes, *News Physiol Sci* 16:38, 2001.

Stroncek DF, Rebulla P: Platelet transfusions, *Lancet* 370:427, 2007.

Sumpter TL, Wilkes DS: Role of autoimmunity in organ allograft rejection: a focus on immunity to type V collagen in the pathogenesis of lung transplant rejection, *Am J Physiol Lung Cell Mol Physiol* 286:L1129, 2004.

Westhoff CM: The structure and function of the Rh antigen complex, *Semin Hematol* 44:42, 2007.

Yazer MH, Hosseini-Maaf B, Olsson ML: Blood grouping discrepancies between ABO genotype and phenotype caused by O alleles, *Curr Opin Hematol* 15:618, 2008.

CHAPTER 36

Hemostasis and Blood Coagulation

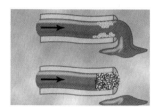

Events in Hemostasis

The term *hemostasis* means prevention of blood loss. Whenever a vessel is severed or ruptured, hemostasis is achieved by several mechanisms: (1) vascular constriction, (2) formation of a platelet plug, (3) formation of a blood clot as a result of blood coagulation, and (4) eventual growth of fibrous tissue into the blood clot to close the hole in the vessel permanently.

Vascular Constriction

Immediately after a blood vessel has been cut or ruptured, the trauma to the vessel wall causes the smooth muscle in the wall to contract; this instantaneously reduces the flow of blood from the ruptured vessel. The contraction results from (1) local myogenic spasm, (2) local autacoid factors from the traumatized tissues and blood platelets, and (3) nervous reflexes. The nervous reflexes are initiated by pain nerve impulses or other sensory impulses that originate from the traumatized vessel or nearby tissues. However, even more vasoconstriction probably results from local *myogenic contraction* of the blood vessels initiated by direct damage to the vascular wall. And, for the smaller vessels, the platelets are responsible for much of the vasoconstriction by releasing a vasoconstrictor substance, *thromboxane A₂*.

The more severely a vessel is traumatized, the greater the degree of vascular spasm. The spasm can last for many minutes or even hours, during which time the processes of platelet plugging and blood coagulation can take place.

Formation of the Platelet Plug

If the cut in the blood vessel is very small—indeed, many very small vascular holes do develop throughout the body each day—the cut is often sealed by a *platelet plug*, rather than by a blood clot. To understand this, it is important that we first discuss the nature of platelets themselves.

Physical and Chemical Characteristics of Platelets

Platelets (also called *thrombocytes*) are minute discs 1 to 4 micrometers in diameter. They are formed in the bone marrow from *megakaryocytes*, which are extremely large cells of the hematopoietic series in the marrow; the megakaryocytes fragment into the minute platelets either in the bone marrow or soon after entering the blood, especially as they squeeze through capillaries. The normal concentration of platelets in the blood is between 150,000 and 300,000 per microliter.

Platelets have many functional characteristics of whole cells, even though they do not have nuclei and cannot reproduce. In their cytoplasm are such active factors as (1) *actin* and *myosin molecules,* which are contractile proteins similar to those found in muscle cells, and still another contractile protein, *thrombosthenin,* that can cause the platelets to contract; (2) residuals of both the *endoplasmic reticulum* and the *Golgi apparatus* that synthesize various enzymes and especially store large quantities of calcium ions; (3) mitochondria and enzyme systems that are capable of forming *adenosine triphosphate* (ATP) and *adenosine diphosphate* (ADP); (4) enzyme systems that synthesize *prostaglandins,* which are local hormones that cause many vascular and other local tissue reactions; (5) an important protein called *fibrin-stabilizing factor,* which we discuss later in relation to blood coagulation; and (6) a *growth factor* that causes vascular endothelial cells, vascular smooth muscle cells, and fibroblasts to multiply and grow, thus causing cellular growth that eventually helps repair damaged vascular walls.

The cell membrane of the platelets is also important. On its surface is a coat of *glycoproteins* that repulses adherence to normal endothelium and yet causes adherence to *injured* areas of the vessel wall, especially to injured endothelial cells and even more so to any exposed collagen from deep within the vessel wall. In addition, the platelet membrane contains large amounts of *phospholipids* that activate multiple stages in the blood-clotting process, as we discuss later.

Thus, the platelet is an active structure. It has a half-life in the blood of 8 to 12 days, so over several weeks its functional processes run out. Then it is eliminated from the circulation mainly by the tissue macrophage system. More than one half of the platelets are removed by macrophages in the spleen, where the blood passes through a latticework of tight trabeculae.

Mechanism of the Platelet Plug

Platelet repair of vascular openings is based on several important functions of the platelet. When platelets come in contact with a damaged vascular surface, especially with collagen fibers in the vascular wall, the platelets immediately change their own characteristics drastically. They begin to swell; they assume irregular forms with numerous irradiating pseudopods protruding from their surfaces; their contractile proteins contract forcefully and cause the release of granules that contain multiple active factors; they become sticky so that they adhere to collagen in the tissues and to a protein called *von Willebrand factor* that leaks into the traumatized tissue from the plasma; they secrete large quantities of ADP; and their enzymes form *thromboxane A₂*. The ADP and thromboxane in turn act on nearby platelets to activate them as well, and the stickiness of these additional platelets causes them to adhere to the original activated platelets.

Therefore, at the site of any opening in a blood vessel wall, the damaged vascular wall activates successively increasing numbers of platelets that themselves attract more and more additional platelets, thus forming a *platelet plug.* This is at first a loose plug, but it is usually successful in blocking blood loss if the vascular opening is small. Then, during the subsequent process of blood coagulation, *fibrin threads* form. These attach tightly to the platelets, thus constructing an unyielding plug.

Importance of the Platelet Mechanism for Closing Vascular Holes. The platelet-plugging mechanism is extremely important for closing minute ruptures in very small blood vessels that occur many thousands of times daily. Indeed, multiple small holes through the endothelial cells themselves are often closed by platelets actually fusing with the endothelial cells to form additional endothelial cell membrane. A person who has few blood platelets develops each day literally thousands of small hemorrhagic areas under the skin and throughout the internal tissues, but this does not occur in the normal person.

Blood Coagulation in the Ruptured Vessel

The third mechanism for hemostasis is formation of the blood clot. The clot begins to develop in 15 to 20 seconds if the trauma to the vascular wall has been severe, and in 1 to 2 minutes if the trauma has been minor. Activator substances from the traumatized vascular wall, from platelets, and from blood proteins adhering to the traumatized vascular wall initiate the clotting process. The physical events of this process are shown in Figure 36-1, and Table 36-1 lists the most important of the clotting factors.

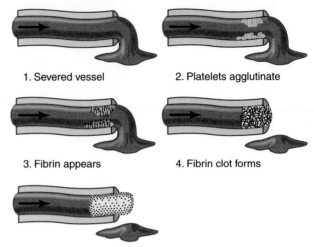

1. Severed vessel   2. Platelets agglutinate

3. Fibrin appears   4. Fibrin clot forms

5. Clot retraction occurs

Figure 36-1 Clotting process in a traumatized blood vessel. (Modified from Seegers WH: Hemostatic Agents, 1948. Courtesy of Charles C Thomas, Publisher, Ltd., Springfield, Ill.)

Within 3 to 6 minutes after rupture of a vessel, if the vessel opening is not too large, the entire opening or broken end of the vessel is filled with clot. After 20 minutes to an hour, the clot retracts; this closes the vessel still further. Platelets also play an important role in this clot retraction, as is discussed later.

Table 36-1 Clotting Factors in Blood and Their Synonyms

Clotting Factor	Synonyms
Fibrinogen	Factor I
Prothrombin	Factor II
Tissue factor	Factor III; tissue thromboplastin
Calcium	Factor IV
Factor V	Proaccelerin; labile factor; Ac-globulin (Ac-G)
Factor VII	Serum prothrombin conversion accelerator (SPCA); proconvertin; stable factor
Factor VIII	Antihemophilic factor (AHF); antihemophilic globulin (AHG); antihemophilic factor A
Factor IX	Plasma thromboplastin component (PTC); Christmas factor; antihemophilic factor B
Factor X	Stuart factor; Stuart-Prower factor
Factor XI	Plasma thromboplastin antecedent (PTA); antihemophilic factor C
Factor XII	Hageman factor
Factor XIII	Fibrin-stabilizing factor
Prekallikrein	Fletcher factor
High-molecular-weight kininogen	Fitzgerald factor; HMWK (high-molecular-weight kininogen)
Platelets	

Fibrous Organization or Dissolution of the Blood Clot

Once a blood clot has formed, it can follow one of two courses: (1) It can become invaded by *fibroblasts,* which subsequently form connective tissue all through the clot, or (2) it can dissolve. The usual course for a clot that forms in a small hole of a vessel wall is invasion by fibroblasts, beginning within a few hours after the clot is formed (which is promoted at least partially by *growth factor* secreted by platelets). This continues to complete organization of the clot into fibrous tissue within about 1 to 2 weeks.

Conversely, when excess blood has leaked into the tissues and tissue clots have occurred where they are not needed, special substances within the clot itself usually become activated. These function as enzymes to dissolve the clot, as discussed later in the chapter.

Mechanism of Blood Coagulation

Basic Theory. More than 50 important substances that cause or affect blood coagulation have been found in the blood and in the tissues—some that promote coagulation, called *procoagulants,* and others that inhibit coagulation, called *anticoagulants.* Whether blood will coagulate depends on the balance between these two groups of substances. In the blood stream, the anticoagulants normally predominate, so the blood does not coagulate while it is circulating in the blood vessels. But when a vessel is ruptured, procoagulants from the area of tissue damage become "activated" and override the anticoagulants, and then a clot does develop.

General Mechanism. Clotting takes place in three essential steps: (1) In response to rupture of the vessel or damage to the blood itself, a complex cascade of chemical reactions occurs in the blood involving more than a dozen blood coagulation factors. The net result is formation of a complex of activated substances collectively called *prothrombin activator.* (2) The prothrombin activator catalyzes conversion of *prothrombin* into *thrombin.* (3) The thrombin acts as an enzyme to convert *fibrinogen* into *fibrin fibers* that enmesh platelets, blood cells, and plasma to form the clot.

Let us discuss first the mechanism by which the blood clot itself is formed, beginning with conversion of prothrombin to thrombin; then we will come back to the initiating stages in the clotting process by which prothrombin activator is formed.

Conversion of Prothrombin to Thrombin

First, prothrombin activator is formed as a result of rupture of a blood vessel or as a result of damage to special substances in the blood. Second, the prothrombin activator, in the presence of sufficient amounts of ionic Ca^{++}, causes conversion of prothrombin to thrombin (Figure 36-2). Third,

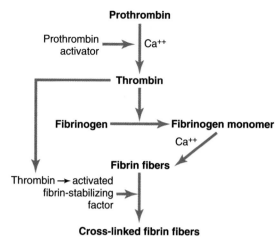

Figure 36-2 Schema for conversion of prothrombin to thrombin and polymerization of fibrinogen to form fibrin fibers.

the thrombin causes polymerization of fibrinogen molecules into fibrin fibers within another 10 to 15 seconds. Thus, the rate-limiting factor in causing blood coagulation is usually the formation of prothrombin activator and not the subsequent reactions beyond that point, because these terminal steps normally occur rapidly to form the clot.

Platelets also play an important role in the conversion of prothrombin to thrombin because much of the prothrombin first attaches to prothrombin receptors on the platelets already bound to the damaged tissue.

Prothrombin and Thrombin. Prothrombin is a plasma protein, an alpha2-globulin, having a molecular weight of 68,700. It is present in normal plasma in a concentration of about 15 mg/dl. It is an unstable protein that can split easily into smaller compounds, one of which is *thrombin,* which has a molecular weight of 33,700, almost exactly one half that of prothrombin.

Prothrombin is formed continually by the liver, and it is continually being used throughout the body for blood clotting. If the liver fails to produce prothrombin, in a day or so prothrombin concentration in the plasma falls too low to provide normal blood coagulation.

Vitamin K is required by the liver for normal activation of prothrombin, as well as a few other clotting factors. Therefore, either lack of vitamin K or the presence of liver disease that prevents normal prothrombin formation can decrease the prothrombin level so low that a bleeding tendency results.

Conversion of Fibrinogen to Fibrin—Formation of the Clot

Fibrinogen. Fibrinogen is a high-molecular-weight protein (MW = 340,000) that occurs in the plasma in quantities of 100 to 700 mg/dl. Fibrinogen is formed in the liver, and liver disease can decrease the concentration of circulating fibrinogen, as it does the concentration of prothrombin, pointed out earlier.

Because of its large molecular size, little fibrinogen normally leaks from the blood vessels into the interstitial fluids, and because fibrinogen is one of the essential factors in the coagulation process, interstitial fluids ordinarily do not coagulate. Yet, when the permeability of the capillaries becomes pathologically increased, fibrinogen does then leak into the tissue fluids in sufficient quantities to allow clotting of these fluids in much the same way that plasma and whole blood can clot.

Action of Thrombin on Fibrinogen to Form Fibrin. Thrombin is a protein *enzyme* with weak proteolytic capabilities. It acts on fibrinogen to remove four low-molecular-weight peptides from each molecule of fibrinogen, forming one molecule of *fibrin monomer* that has the automatic capability to polymerize with other fibrin monomer molecules to form fibrin fibers. Therefore, many fibrin monomer molecules polymerize within seconds into *long fibrin fibers* that constitute the *reticulum* of the blood clot.

In the early stages of polymerization, the fibrin monomer molecules are held together by weak noncovalent hydrogen bonding, and the newly forming fibers are not cross-linked with one another; therefore, the resultant clot is weak and can be broken apart with ease. But another process occurs during the next few minutes that greatly strengthens the fibrin reticulum. This involves a substance called *fibrin-stabilizing factor* that is present in small amounts in normal plasma globulins but is also released from platelets entrapped in the clot. Before fibrin-stabilizing factor can have an effect on the fibrin fibers, it must itself be activated. The same thrombin that causes fibrin formation also activates the fibrin-stabilizing factor. Then this activated substance operates as an enzyme to cause *covalent bonds* between more and more of the fibrin monomer molecules, as well as multiple cross-linkages between adjacent fibrin fibers, thus adding tremendously to the three-dimensional strength of the fibrin meshwork.

Blood Clot. The clot is composed of a meshwork of fibrin fibers running in all directions and entrapping blood cells, platelets, and plasma. The fibrin fibers also adhere to damaged surfaces of blood vessels; therefore, the blood clot becomes adherent to any vascular opening and thereby prevents further blood loss.

Clot Retraction—Serum. Within a few minutes after a clot is formed, it begins to contract and usually expresses most of the fluid from the clot within 20 to 60 minutes. The fluid expressed is called *serum* because all its fibrinogen and most of the other clotting factors have been removed; in this way, serum differs from plasma. Serum cannot clot because it lacks these factors.

Platelets are necessary for clot retraction to occur. Therefore, failure of clot retraction is an indication that the number of platelets in the circulating blood might be low. Electron micrographs of platelets in blood clots show that they become attached to the fibrin fibers in such a way that they actually bond different fibers together. Furthermore,

platelets entrapped in the clot continue to release procoagulant substances, one of the most important of which is *fibrin-stabilizing factor*, which causes more and more cross-linking bonds between adjacent fibrin fibers. In addition, the platelets themselves contribute directly to clot contraction by activating platelet thrombosthenin, actin, and myosin molecules, which are all contractile proteins in the platelets and cause strong contraction of the platelet spicules attached to the fibrin. This also helps compress the fibrin meshwork into a smaller mass. The contraction is activated and accelerated by thrombin, as well as by calcium ions released from calcium stores in the mitochondria, endoplasmic reticulum, and Golgi apparatus of the platelets.

As the clot retracts, the edges of the broken blood vessel are pulled together, thus contributing still further to hemostasis.

Positive Feedback of Clot Formation

Once a blood clot has started to develop, it normally extends within minutes into the surrounding blood. That is, the clot itself initiates a positive feedback to promote more clotting. One of the most important causes of this is the fact that the proteolytic action of thrombin allows it to act on many of the other blood-clotting factors in addition to fibrinogen. For instance, thrombin has a direct proteolytic effect on prothrombin itself, tending to convert this into still more thrombin, and it acts on some of the blood-clotting factors responsible for formation of prothrombin activator. (These effects, discussed in subsequent paragraphs, include acceleration of the actions of Factors VIII, IX, X, XI, and XII and aggregation of platelets.) Once a critical amount of thrombin is formed, a positive feedback develops that causes still more blood clotting and more and more thrombin to be formed; thus, the blood clot continues to grow until blood leakage ceases.

Initiation of Coagulation: Formation of Prothrombin Activator

Now that we have discussed the clotting process, we turn to the more complex mechanisms that initiate clotting in the first place. These mechanisms are set into play by (1) trauma to the vascular wall and adjacent tissues, (2) trauma to the blood, or (3) contact of the blood with damaged endothelial cells or with collagen and other tissue elements outside the blood vessel. In each instance, this leads to the formation of *prothrombin activator*, which then causes prothrombin conversion to thrombin and all the subsequent clotting steps.

Prothrombin activator is generally considered to be formed in two ways, although, in reality, the two ways interact constantly with each other: (1) by the *extrinsic pathway* that begins with trauma to the vascular wall and surrounding tissues and (2) by the *intrinsic pathway* that begins in the blood itself.

In both the extrinsic and the intrinsic pathways, a series of different plasma proteins called *blood-clotting factors* plays a major role. Most of these proteins are *inactive* forms of proteolytic enzymes. When converted to the active forms, their enzymatic actions cause the successive, cascading reactions of the clotting process.

Most of the clotting factors, which are listed in Table 36-1, are designated by Roman numerals. To indicate the activated form of the factor, a small letter "a" is added after the Roman numeral, such as Factor VIIIa to indicate the activated state of Factor VIII.

Extrinsic Pathway for Initiating Clotting

The extrinsic pathway for initiating the formation of prothrombin activator begins with a traumatized vascular wall or traumatized extravascular tissues that come in contact with the blood. This leads to the following steps, as shown in Figure 36-3:

1. *Release of tissue factor.* Traumatized tissue releases a complex of several factors called *tissue factor* or *tissue thromboplastin.* This factor is composed especially of *phospholipids* from the membranes of the tissue plus a *lipoprotein complex* that functions mainly as a *proteolytic enzyme.*

2. *Activation of Factor X—role of Factor VII and tissue factor.* The lipoprotein complex of tissue factor further complexes with blood coagulation Factor VII and, in the presence of calcium ions, acts enzymatically on Factor X to form *activated Factor X* (Xa).

3. *Effect of Xa to form prothrombin activator—role of Factor V.* The activated Factor X combines immediately with tissue phospholipids that are part of tissue factors or with additional phospholipids released from platelets, as well as with Factor V to form the complex called *prothrombin activator.* Within a few seconds, in the presence of calcium ions (Ca^{++}), this splits

prothrombin to form thrombin, and the clotting process proceeds as already explained. At first, the Factor V in the prothrombin activator complex is inactive, but once clotting begins and thrombin begins to form, the proteolytic action of thrombin activates Factor V. This then becomes an additional strong accelerator of prothrombin activation. Thus, in the final prothrombin activator complex, activated Factor X is the actual protease that causes splitting of prothrombin to form thrombin; activated Factor V greatly accelerates this protease activity, and platelet phospholipids act as a vehicle that further accelerates the process. Note especially the *positive feedback* effect of thrombin, acting through Factor V, to accelerate the entire process once it begins.

Intrinsic Pathway for Initiating Clotting

The second mechanism for initiating formation of prothrombin activator, and therefore for initiating clotting, *begins with trauma to the blood or exposure of the blood to collagen* from a traumatized blood vessel wall. Then the process continues through the series of cascading reactions shown in Figure 36-4.

1. *Blood trauma causes (1) activation of Factor XII and (2) release of platelet phospholipids.* Trauma to the blood or exposure of the blood to vascular wall collagen alters two important clotting factors in the blood: Factor XII and the platelets. When Factor XII is disturbed, such as by coming into contact with collagen or with a wettable surface such as glass, it takes on a new molecular configuration that converts it into a proteolytic enzyme called "activated Factor XII." Simultaneously, the blood trauma also damages the platelets because of adherence to either collagen or a wettable surface (or by damage in other ways), and this releases platelet phospholipids that contain the lipoprotein called *platelet factor 3,* which also plays a role in subsequent clotting reactions.

2. *Activation of Factor XI.* The activated Factor XII acts enzymatically on Factor XI to activate this factor as well, which is the second step in the intrinsic pathway. This reaction also requires *HMW (high-molecular-weight) kininogen* and is accelerated by prekallikrein.

3. *Activation of Factor IX by activated Factor XI.* The activated Factor XI then acts enzymatically on Factor IX to activate this factor as well.

4. *Activation of Factor X—role of Factor VIII.* The activated Factor IX, acting in concert with activated Factor VIII and with the platelet phospholipids and factor 3 from the traumatized platelets, activates Factor X. It is clear that when either Factor VIII or platelets are in short supply, this step is deficient. Factor VIII is the factor that is missing in a person who has classic *hemophilia,* for which reason it is called *antihemophilic factor.* Platelets are the clotting factor that is lacking in the bleeding disease called *thrombocytopenia.*

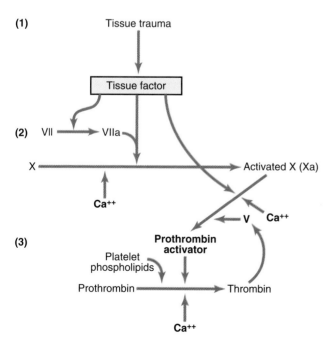

Figure 36-3 Extrinsic pathway for initiating blood clotting.

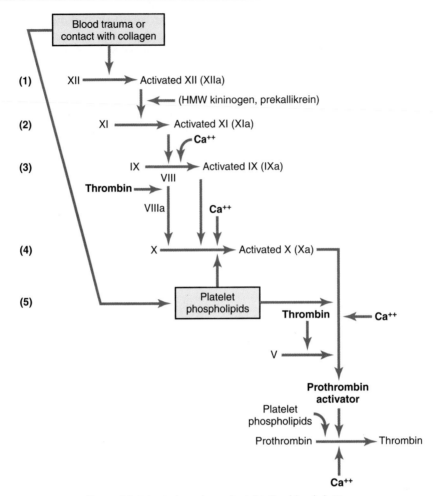

Figure 36-4 Intrinsic pathway for initiating blood clotting.

5. *Action of activated Factor X to form prothrombin activator—role of Factor V.* This step in the intrinsic pathway is the same as the last step in the extrinsic pathway. That is, activated Factor X combines with Factor V and platelet or tissue phospholipids to form the complex called *prothrombin activator.* The prothrombin activator in turn initiates within seconds the cleavage of prothrombin to form thrombin, thereby setting into motion the final clotting process, as described earlier.

Role of Calcium Ions in the Intrinsic and Extrinsic Pathways

Except for the first two steps in the intrinsic pathway, calcium ions are required for promotion or acceleration of all the blood-clotting reactions. Therefore, in the absence of calcium ions, blood clotting by either pathway does not occur.

In the living body, the calcium ion concentration seldom falls low enough to significantly affect the kinetics of blood clotting. But, when blood is removed from a person, it can be prevented from clotting by reducing the calcium ion concentration below the threshold level for clotting, either by deionizing the calcium by causing it to react with substances such as *citrate ion* or by precipitating the calcium with substances such as *oxalate ion.*

Interaction Between the Extrinsic and Intrinsic Pathways—Summary of Blood-Clotting Initiation

It is clear from the schemas of the intrinsic and extrinsic systems that after blood vessels rupture, clotting occurs by both pathways simultaneously. Tissue factor initiates the extrinsic pathway, whereas contact of Factor XII and platelets with collagen in the vascular wall initiates the intrinsic pathway.

An especially important difference between the extrinsic and intrinsic pathways is that *the extrinsic pathway* can be explosive; once initiated, its speed of completion to the final clot is limited only by the amount of tissue factor released from the traumatized tissues and by the quantities of Factors X, VII, and V in the blood. With severe tissue trauma, clotting can occur in as little as 15 seconds. The intrinsic pathway is much slower to proceed, usually requiring 1 to 6 minutes to cause clotting.

Prevention of Blood Clotting in the Normal Vascular System—Intravascular Anticoagulants

Endothelial Surface Factors. Probably the most important factors for preventing clotting in the normal vascular system are (1) the *smoothness* of the endothelial cell surface, which prevents contact activation of the intrinsic clotting system; (2) a layer of *glycocalyx* on the endothelium (glycocalyx is a mucopolysaccharide adsorbed to the surfaces of the endothelial cells), which repels clotting factors and platelets, thereby preventing activation of clotting; and (3) a protein bound with the endothelial membrane, *thrombomodulin,* which binds thrombin. Not only does the binding of thrombin with thrombomodulin slow the clotting process by removing thrombin, but the thrombomodulin-thrombin complex also activates a plasma protein, *protein C,* that acts as an anticoagulant by *inactivating* activated Factors V and VIII.

When the endothelial wall is damaged, its smoothness and its glycocalyx-thrombomodulin layer are lost, which activates both Factor XII and the platelets, thus setting off the intrinsic pathway of clotting. If Factor XII and platelets come in contact with the subendothelial collagen, the activation is even more powerful.

Antithrombin Action of Fibrin and Antithrombin III.

Among the most important *anticoagulants* in the blood are those that remove thrombin from the blood. The most powerful of these are (1) the *fibrin fibers* that are formed during the process of clotting and (2) an alpha-globulin called *antithrombin III* or *antithrombin-heparin cofactor.*

While a clot is forming, about 85 to 90 percent of the thrombin formed from the prothrombin becomes adsorbed to the fibrin fibers as they develop. This helps prevent the spread of thrombin into the remaining blood and, therefore, prevents excessive spread of the clot.

The thrombin that does not adsorb to the fibrin fibers soon combines with antithrombin III, which further blocks the effect of the thrombin on the fibrinogen and then also inactivates the thrombin itself during the next 12 to 20 minutes.

Heparin.

Heparin is another powerful anticoagulant, but its concentration in the blood is normally low, so only under special physiologic conditions does it have significant anticoagulant effects. However, heparin is used widely as a pharmacological agent in medical practice in much higher concentrations to prevent intravascular clotting.

The heparin molecule is a highly negatively charged conjugated polysaccharide. By itself, it has little or no anticoagulant properties, but when it combines with antithrombin III, the effectiveness of antithrombin III for removing thrombin increases by a hundredfold to a thousandfold, and thus it acts as an anticoagulant. Therefore, in the presence of excess heparin, removal of free thrombin from the circulating blood by antithrombin III is almost instantaneous.

The complex of heparin and antithrombin III removes several other activated coagulation factors in addition to thrombin, further enhancing the effectiveness of anticoagulation. The others include activated Factors XII, XI, X, and IX.

Heparin is produced by many different cells of the body, but especially large quantities are formed by the basophilic *mast cells* located in the pericapillary connective tissue throughout the body. These cells continually secrete small quantities of heparin that diffuse into the circulatory system. The *basophil cells* of the blood, which are functionally almost identical to the mast cells, release small quantities of heparin into the plasma.

Mast cells are abundant in tissue surrounding the capillaries of the lungs and, to a lesser extent, capillaries of the liver. It is easy to understand why large quantities of heparin might be needed in these areas because the capillaries of the lungs and liver receive many embolic clots formed in slowly flowing venous blood; sufficient formation of heparin prevents further growth of the clots.

Lysis of Blood Clots—Plasmin

The plasma proteins contain a euglobulin called *plasminogen* (or *profibrinolysin*) that, when activated, becomes a substance called *plasmin* (or *fibrinolysin*). Plasmin is a proteolytic enzyme that resembles trypsin, the most important proteolytic digestive enzyme of pancreatic secretion. Plasmin digests fibrin fibers and some other protein coagulants such as fibrinogen, Factor V, Factor VIII, prothrombin, and Factor XII. Therefore, whenever plasmin is formed, it can cause lysis of a clot by destroying many of the clotting factors, thereby sometimes even causing hypocoagulability of the blood.

Activation of Plasminogen to Form Plasmin, Then Lysis of Clots.

When a clot is formed, a large amount of plasminogen is trapped in the clot along with other plasma proteins. This will not become plasmin or cause lysis of the clot until it is activated. The injured tissues and vascular endothelium very slowly release a powerful activator called *tissue plasminogen activator* (t-PA) that a few days later, after the clot has stopped the bleeding, eventually converts plasminogen to plasmin, which in turn removes the remaining unnecessary blood clot. In fact, many small blood vessels in which blood flow has been blocked by clots are reopened by this mechanism. Thus, an especially important function of the plasmin system is to remove minute clots from millions of tiny peripheral vessels that eventually would become occluded were there no way to clear them.

Conditions That Cause Excessive Bleeding in Humans

Excessive bleeding can result from deficiency of any one of the many blood-clotting factors. Three particular types of bleeding tendencies that have been studied to the greatest extent are discussed here: bleeding caused by (1) vitamin K deficiency, (2) hemophilia, and (3) thrombocytopenia (platelet deficiency).

Decreased Prothrombin, Factor VII, Factor IX, and Factor X Caused by Vitamin K Deficiency

With few exceptions, almost all the blood-clotting factors are formed by the liver. Therefore, diseases of the liver such as *hepatitis, cirrhosis,* and *acute yellow atrophy* can sometimes depress the clotting system so greatly that the patient develops a severe tendency to bleed.

Another cause of depressed formation of clotting factors by the liver is vitamin K deficiency. Vitamin K is an essential factor to a liver carboxylase that adds a carboxyl group to glutamic acid residues on five of the important clotting factors: *prothrombin, Factor VII, Factor IX, Factor X*, and *protein C*. In adding the carboxyl group to glutamic acid residues on the immature clotting factors, vitamin K is oxidized and becomes inactive. Another enzyme, *vitamin K epoxide reductase complex 1 (VKOR c1)*, reduces vitamin K back to its active form.

In the absence of active vitamin K, subsequent insufficiency of these coagulation factors in the blood can lead to serious bleeding tendencies.

Vitamin K is continually synthesized in the intestinal tract by bacteria, so vitamin K deficiency seldom occurs in the normal person as a result of vitamin K absence from the diet (except in neonates before they establish their intestinal bacterial flora). However, in gastrointestinal disease, vitamin K deficiency often occurs as a result of poor absorption of fats from the gastrointestinal tract. The reason is that vitamin K is fat soluble and ordinarily absorbed into the blood along with the fats.

One of the most prevalent causes of vitamin K deficiency is failure of the liver to secrete bile into the gastrointestinal tract (which occurs either as a result of obstruction of the bile ducts or as a result of liver disease). Lack of bile prevents adequate fat digestion and absorption and, therefore, depresses vitamin K absorption as well. Thus, liver disease often causes decreased production of prothrombin and some other clotting factors both because of poor vitamin K absorption and because of the diseased liver cells. Because of this, vitamin K is injected into surgical patients with liver disease or with obstructed bile ducts before performing the surgical procedure. Ordinarily, if vitamin K is given to a deficient patient 4 to 8 hours before the operation and the liver parenchymal cells are at least one-half normal in function, sufficient clotting factors will be produced to prevent excessive bleeding during the operation.

Hemophilia

Hemophilia is a bleeding disease that occurs almost exclusively in males. In 85 percent of cases, it is caused by an *abnormality or deficiency of Factor VIII*; this type of hemophilia is called *hemophilia A* or *classic hemophilia*. About 1 of every 10,000 males in the United States has classic hemophilia. In the other 15 percent of hemophilia patients, the bleeding tendency is caused by deficiency of Factor IX. Both of these factors are transmitted genetically by way of the female chromosome. Therefore, almost never will a woman have hemophilia because at least one of her two X chromosomes will have the appropriate genes. If one of her X chromosomes is deficient, she will be a *hemophilia carrier*, transmitting the disease to half of her male offspring and transmitting the carrier state to half of her female offspring.

The bleeding trait in hemophilia can have various degrees of severity, depending on the character of the genetic deficiency. Bleeding usually does not occur except after trauma, but in some patients, the degree of trauma required to cause severe and prolonged bleeding may be so mild that it is hardly noticeable. For instance, bleeding can often last for days after extraction of a tooth.

Factor VIII has two active components, a large component with a molecular weight in the millions and a smaller component with a molecular weight of about 230,000. The smaller component is most important in the intrinsic pathway for clotting, and it is deficiency of this part of Factor VIII that causes classic hemophilia. Another bleeding disease with somewhat different characteristics, called *von Willebrand's disease*, results from loss of the large component.

When a person with classic hemophilia experiences severe prolonged bleeding, almost the only therapy that is truly effective is injection of purified Factor VIII. The cost of Factor VIII is high, because it is gathered from human blood and only in extremely small quantities. However, increasing production and use of recombinant Factor VIII will make this treatment available to more patients with classic hemophilia.

Thrombocytopenia

Thrombocytopenia means the presence of very low numbers of platelets in the circulating blood. People with thrombocytopenia have a tendency to bleed, as do hemophiliacs, except that the bleeding is usually from many small venules or capillaries, rather than from larger vessels, as in hemophilia. As a result, small punctate hemorrhages occur throughout all the body tissues. The skin of such a person displays many small, purplish blotches, giving the disease the name *thrombocytopenic purpura*. As stated earlier, platelets are especially important for repair of minute breaks in capillaries and other small vessels.

Ordinarily, bleeding will not occur until the number of platelets in the blood falls below 50,000/μl, rather than the normal 150,000 to 300,000. Levels as low as 10,000/μl are frequently lethal.

Even without making specific platelet counts in the blood, sometimes one can suspect the existence of thrombocytopenia if the person's blood fails to retract, because, as pointed out earlier, clot retraction is normally dependent on release of multiple coagulation factors from the large numbers of platelets entrapped in the fibrin mesh of the clot.

Most people with thrombocytopenia have the disease known as *idiopathic thrombocytopenia*, which means thrombocytopenia of unknown cause. In most of these people, it has been discovered that, for unknown reasons, specific antibodies have formed and react against the platelets themselves to destroy them. Relief from bleeding for 1 to 4 days can often be effected in a patient with thrombocytopenia by giving *fresh whole blood transfusions* that contain large numbers of platelets. Also, *splenectomy* is often helpful, sometimes effecting almost complete cure because the spleen normally removes large numbers of platelets from the blood.

Thromboembolic Conditions in the Human Being

Thrombi and Emboli. An abnormal clot that develops in a blood vessel is called a *thrombus.* Once a clot has developed, continued flow of blood past the clot is likely to break it away from its attachment and cause the clot to flow with the blood; such freely flowing clots are known as *emboli.* Also, emboli that originate in large arteries or in the left side of the heart can flow peripherally and plug arteries or arterioles in the brain, kidneys, or elsewhere. Emboli that originate in the venous system or in the right side of the heart generally flow into the lungs to cause pulmonary arterial embolism.

Cause of Thromboembolic Conditions. The causes of thromboembolic conditions in the human being are usually twofold: (1) Any *roughened endothelial surface of a vessel*—as may be caused by arteriosclerosis, infection, or trauma—is likely to initiate the clotting process. (2) Blood often clots *when it flows very slowly* through blood vessels, where small quantities of thrombin and other procoagulants are always being formed.

Use of t-PA in Treating Intravascular Clots. Genetically engineered t-PA (tissue plasminogen activator) is available. When delivered directly to a thrombosed area through a catheter, it is effective in activating plasminogen to plasmin, which in turn can dissolve some intravascular clots. For instance, if used within the first hour or so after thrombotic occlusion of a coronary artery, the heart is often spared serious damage.

Femoral Venous Thrombosis and Massive Pulmonary Embolism

Because clotting almost always occurs when blood flow is blocked for many hours in any vessel of the body, the immobility of patients confined to bed plus the practice of propping the knees with pillows often causes intravascular clotting because of blood stasis in one or more of the leg veins for hours at a time. Then the clot grows, mainly in the direction of the slowly moving venous blood, sometimes growing the entire length of the leg veins and occasionally even up into the common iliac vein and inferior vena cava. Then, about 1 time out of every 10, a large part of the clot disengages from its attachments to the vessel wall and flows freely with the venous blood through the right side of the heart and into the pulmonary arteries to cause massive blockage of the pulmonary arteries, called *massive pulmonary embolism.* If the clot is large enough to occlude both of the pulmonary arteries at the same time, immediate death ensues. If only one pulmonary artery is blocked, death may not occur, or the embolism may lead to death a few hours to several days later because of further growth of the clot within the pulmonary vessels. But, again, t-PA therapy can be a lifesaver.

Disseminated Intravascular Coagulation

Occasionally the clotting mechanism becomes activated in widespread areas of the circulation, giving rise to the condition called *disseminated intravascular coagulation.* This often results from the presence of large amounts of traumatized or dying tissue in the body that releases great quantities of tissue factor into the blood. Frequently, the clots are small but numerous, and they plug a large share of the small peripheral blood vessels. This occurs especially in patients with widespread septicemia, in which either circulating bacteria or bacterial toxins—especially *endotoxins*—activate the clotting mechanisms. Plugging of small peripheral vessels greatly diminishes delivery of oxygen and other nutrients to the tissues—a situation that leads to or exacerbates circulatory shock. It is partly for this reason that *septicemic shock* is lethal in 85 percent or more of patients.

A peculiar effect of disseminated intravascular coagulation is that the patient on occasion begins to bleed. The reason for this is that so many of the clotting factors are removed by the widespread clotting that too few procoagulants remain to allow normal hemostasis of the remaining blood.

Anticoagulants for Clinical Use

In some thromboembolic conditions, it is desirable to delay the coagulation process. Various anticoagulants have been developed for this purpose. The ones most useful clinically are *heparin* and the *coumarins.*

Heparin as an Intravenous Anticoagulant

Commercial heparin is extracted from several different animal tissues and prepared in almost pure form. Injection of relatively small quantities, about 0.5 to 1 mg/kg of body weight, causes the blood-clotting time to increase from a normal of about 6 minutes to 30 or more minutes. Furthermore, this change in clotting time occurs instantaneously, thereby immediately preventing or slowing further development of a thromboembolic condition.

The action of heparin lasts about 1.5 to 4 hours. The injected heparin is destroyed by an enzyme in the blood known as *heparinase.*

Coumarins as Anticoagulants

When a coumarin, such as *warfarin,* is given to a patient, the amounts of active prothrombin and Factors VII, IX, and X, all formed by the liver, begin to fall. Warfarin causes this effect by inhibiting the enzyme, *vitamin K epoxide reductase complex 1 (VKOR c1).* As discussed previously, this enzyme converts the inactive, oxidized form of vitamin K to its active, reduced form. By inhibiting VKOR c1, warfarin decreases the available active form of vitamin K in the tissues. When this occurs, the coagulation factors are no longer carboxylated and are biologically inactive. Over several days the body stores of the active coagulation factors degrade and are replaced by inactive factors. Although the coagulation factors continue to be produced, they have greatly decreased coagulant activity.

After administration of an effective dose of warfarin, the coagulant activity of the blood decreases to about 50 percent of normal by the end of 12 hours and to about 20 percent of normal by the end of 24 hours. In other words, the coagulation process is not blocked immediately but must await the degradation of the active prothrombin and the other affected coagulation factors already present in the plasma. Normal coagulation usually returns 1 to 3 days after discontinuing coumarin therapy.

Prevention of Blood Coagulation Outside the Body

Although blood removed from the body and held in a glass test tube normally clots in about 6 minutes, blood collected in *siliconized containers* often does not clot for 1 hour or more. The reason for this delay is that preparing the surfaces of the containers with silicone prevents contact activation of platelets and Factor XII, the two principal factors that initiate the intrinsic clotting mechanism. Conversely, untreated glass containers allow contact activation of the platelets and Factor XII, with rapid development of clots.

Heparin can be used for preventing coagulation of blood outside the body, as well as in the body. Heparin is especially used in surgical procedures in which the blood must be passed through a heart-lung machine or artificial kidney machine and then back into the person.

Various substances that *decrease the concentration of calcium ions* in the blood can also be used for preventing blood coagulation *outside* the body. For instance, a soluble *oxalate* compound mixed in a very small quantity with a sample of blood causes precipitation of calcium oxalate from the plasma and thereby decreases the ionic calcium level so much that blood coagulation is blocked.

Any substance that deionizes the blood calcium will prevent coagulation. The negatively charged *citrate ion* is especially valuable for this purpose, mixed with blood usually in the form of *sodium, ammonium,* or *potassium citrate.* The citrate ion combines with calcium in the blood to cause an un-ionized calcium compound, and the lack of *ionic* calcium prevents coagulation. Citrate anticoagulants have an important advantage over the oxalate anticoagulants because oxalate is toxic to the body, whereas moderate quantities of citrate can be injected intravenously. After injection, the citrate ion is removed from the blood within a few minutes by the liver and is polymerized into glucose or metabolized directly for energy. Consequently, 500 milliliters of blood that has been rendered incoagulable by citrate can ordinarily be transfused into a recipient within a few minutes without dire consequences. But if the liver is damaged or if large quantities of citrated blood or plasma are given too rapidly (within fractions of a minute), the citrate ion may not be removed quickly enough, and the citrate can, under these conditions, greatly depress the level of calcium ion in the blood, which can result in tetany and convulsive death.

Blood Coagulation Tests

Bleeding Time

When a sharp-pointed knife is used to pierce the tip of the finger or lobe of the ear, bleeding ordinarily lasts for 1 to 6 minutes. The time depends largely on the depth of the wound and the degree of hyperemia in the finger or ear lobe at the time of the test. Lack of any one of several of the clotting factors can prolong the bleeding time, but it is especially prolonged by lack of platelets.

Clotting Time

Many methods have been devised for determining blood clotting times. The one most widely used is to collect blood in a chemically clean glass test tube and then to tip the tube back and forth about every 30 seconds until the blood has clotted. By this method, the normal clotting time is 6 to 10 minutes. Procedures using multiple test tubes have also been devised for determining clotting time more accurately.

Unfortunately, the clotting time varies widely, depending on the method used for measuring it, so it is no longer used in many clinics. Instead, measurements of the clotting factors themselves are made, using sophisticated chemical procedures.

Prothrombin Time and International Normalized Ratio

Prothrombin time gives an indication of the concentration of prothrombin in the blood. Figure 36-5 shows the relation of prothrombin concentration to prothrombin

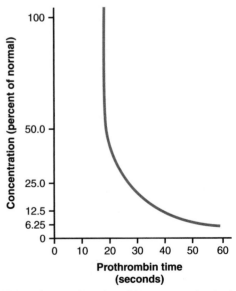

Figure 36-5 Relation of prothrombin concentration in the blood to "prothrombin time."

time. The method for determining prothrombin time is the following.

Blood removed from the patient is immediately oxalated so that none of the prothrombin can change into thrombin. Then, a large excess of calcium ion and tissue factor is quickly mixed with the oxalated blood. The excess calcium nullifies the effect of the oxalate, and the tissue factor activates the prothrombin-to-thrombin reaction by means of the extrinsic clotting pathway. The time required for coagulation to take place is known as the *prothrombin time.* The *shortness of the time* is determined mainly by prothrombin concentration. The normal prothrombin time is about 12 seconds. In each laboratory, a curve relating prothrombin concentration to prothrombin time, such as that shown in Figure 36-5, is drawn for the method used so that the prothrombin in the blood can be quantified.

The results obtained for prothrombin time may vary considerably even in the same individual if there are differences in activity of the tissue factor and the analytical system used to perform the test. Tissue factor is isolated from human tissues, such as placental tissue, and different batches may have different activity. The *international normalized ratio (INR)* was devised as a way to standardize measurements of prothrombin time. For each batch of tissue factor, the manufacturer assigns an international sensitivity index (ISI), which indicates the activity of the tissue factor with a standardized sample. The ISI usually varies between 1.0 and 2.0. The INR is the ratio of the person's prothrombin time to a normal control sample raised to the power of the ISI:

$$INR = \left(\frac{PT_{test}}{PT_{normal}}\right)^{ISI}$$

The normal range for INR in a healthy person is 0.9 to 1.3. A high INR level (e.g., 4 or 5) indicates a high risk of bleeding, whereas a low INR (e.g., 0.5) suggests that there is a chance of having a clot. Patients on warfarin therapy usually have an INR of 2.0 to 3.0.

Tests similar to that for prothrombin time and INR have been devised to determine the quantities of other blood clotting factors. In each of these tests, excesses of calcium ions and all the other factors *besides the one being tested* are added to oxalated blood all at once. Then the time required for coagulation is determined in the same manner as for prothrombin time. If the factor being tested is deficient, the coagulation time is prolonged. The time itself can then be used to quantitate the concentration of the factor.

Bibliography

Andrews RK, Berndt MC: Platelet adhesion: a game of catch and release, *J Clin Invest* 118:3009, 2008.

Brass LF, Zhu L, Stalker TJ: Minding the gaps to promote thrombus growth and stability, *J Clin Invest* 115:3385, 2005.

Crawley JT, Lane DA: The haemostatic role of tissue factor pathway inhibitor, *Arterioscler Thromb Vasc Biol* 28:233, 2008.

Furie B, Furie BC: Mechanisms of thrombus formation, *N Engl J Med* 359:938, 2008.

Gailani D, Renné T: Intrinsic pathway of coagulation and arterial thrombosis, *Arterioscler Thromb Vasc Biol* 27:2507, 2007.

Jennings LK: Role of platelets in atherothrombosis, *Am J Cardiol* 103(3 Suppl):4A, 2009.

Koreth R, Weinert C, Weisdorf DJ, et al: Measurement of bleeding severity: a critical review, *Transfusion* 44:605, 2004.

Nachman RL, Rafii S: Platelets, petechiae, and preservation of the vascular wall, *N Engl J Med* 359:1261, 2008.

Pabinger I, Ay C: Biomarkers and venous thromboembolism, *Arterioscler Thromb Vasc Biol* 29:332, 2009.

Rijken DC, Lijnen HR: New insights into the molecular mechanisms of the fibrinolytic system, *J Thromb Haemost* 7:4, 2009.

Schmaier AH: The elusive physiologic role of Factor XII, *J Clin Invest* 118:3006, 2008.

Smyth SS, Woulfe DS, Weitz JI, et al: 2008 Platelet Colloquium Participants. G-protein-coupled receptors as signaling targets for antiplatelet therapy, *Arterioscler Thromb Vasc Biol.* 29:449, 2009.

Tapson VF: Acute pulmonary embolism, *N Engl J Med* 358:1037, 2008.

Toh CH, Dennis M: Disseminated intravascular coagulation: old disease, new hope, *BMJ* 327:974, 2003.

Tsai HM: Advances in the pathogenesis, diagnosis, and treatment of thrombotic thrombocytopenic purpura, *J Am Soc Nephrol* 14:1072, 2003.

Tsai HM: Platelet activation and the formation of the platelet plug: deficiency of ADAMTS13 causes thrombotic thrombocytopenic purpura, *Arterioscler Thromb Vasc Biol* 23:388, 2003.

VandenDriessche T, Collen D, Chuah MK: Gene therapy for the hemophilias, *J Thromb Haemost* 1:1550, 2003.

UNIT VII

Respiration

37. Pulmonary Ventilation

38. Pulmonary Circulation, Pulmonary Edema, Pleural Fluid

39. Physical Principles of Gas Exchange; Diffusion of Oxygen and Carbon Dioxide Through the Respiratory Membrane

40. Transport of Oxygen and Carbon Dioxide in Blood and Tissue Fluids

41. Regulation of Respiration

42. Respiratory Insufficiency— Pathophysiology, Diagnosis, Oxygen Therapy

CHAPTER 37

Pulmonary Ventilation

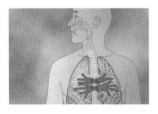

Respiration provides oxygen to the tissues and removes carbon dioxide. The four major functions of respiration are (1) *pulmonary ventilation*, which means the inflow and outflow of air between the atmosphere and the lung alveoli; (2) *diffusion of oxygen and carbon dioxide between the alveoli and the blood*; (3) *transport of oxygen and carbon dioxide in the blood and body fluids* to and from the body's tissue cells; and (4) *regulation of ventilation* and other facets of respiration. This chapter is a discussion of pulmonary ventilation, and the subsequent five chapters cover other respiratory functions plus the physiology of special respiratory abnormalities.

Mechanics of Pulmonary Ventilation

Muscles That Cause Lung Expansion and Contraction

The lungs can be expanded and contracted in two ways: (1) by downward and upward movement of the diaphragm to lengthen or shorten the chest cavity, and (2) by elevation and depression of the ribs to increase and decrease the anteroposterior diameter of the chest cavity. Figure 37-1 shows these two methods.

Normal quiet breathing is accomplished almost entirely by the first method, that is, by movement of the diaphragm. During inspiration, contraction of the diaphragm pulls the lower surfaces of the lungs downward. Then, during expiration, the diaphragm simply relaxes, and the *elastic recoil* of the lungs, chest wall, and abdominal structures compresses the lungs and expels the air. During heavy breathing, however, the elastic forces are not powerful enough to cause the necessary rapid expiration, so extra force is achieved mainly by contraction of the *abdominal muscles*, which pushes the abdominal contents upward against the bottom of the diaphragm, thereby compressing the lungs.

The second method for expanding the lungs is to raise the rib cage. This expands the lungs because, in the natural resting position, the ribs slant downward, as shown on the left side of Figure 37-1, thus allowing the sternum to fall backward toward the vertebral column. When the rib cage is elevated, however, the ribs project almost directly forward, so the sternum also moves forward, away from the spine, making the anteroposterior thickness of the chest about 20 percent greater during maximum inspiration than during expiration. Therefore, all the muscles that elevate the chest cage are classified as muscles of inspiration, and those muscles that depress the chest cage are classified as muscles of expiration. The most important muscles that raise the rib cage are the *external intercostals*, but others that help are the (1) *sternocleidomastoid* muscles, which lift upward on the sternum; (2) *anterior serrati*, which lift many of the ribs; and (3) *scaleni*, which lift the first two ribs.

The muscles that pull the rib cage downward during expiration are mainly the (1) *abdominal recti*, which have the powerful effect of pulling downward on the lower ribs at the same time that they and other abdominal muscles also compress the abdominal contents upward against the diaphragm, and (2) *internal intercostals*.

Figure 37-1 also shows the mechanism by which the external and internal intercostals act to cause inspiration and expiration. To the left, the ribs during expiration are angled downward, and the external intercostals are elongated forward and downward. As they contract, they pull the upper ribs forward in relation to the lower ribs, and this causes leverage on the ribs to raise them upward, thereby causing inspiration. The internal intercostals function exactly in the opposite manner, functioning as expiratory muscles because they angle between the ribs in the opposite direction and cause opposite leverage.

Pressures That Cause the Movement of Air In and Out of the Lungs

The lung is an elastic structure that collapses like a balloon and expels all its air through the trachea whenever there is no force to keep it inflated. Also, there are no attachments between the lung and the walls of the chest cage, except where it is suspended at its hilum from the *mediastinum*, the middle section of the chest cavity. Instead, the lung "floats" in the thoracic cavity, surrounded by a thin layer of *pleural fluid* that lubricates movement of the lungs

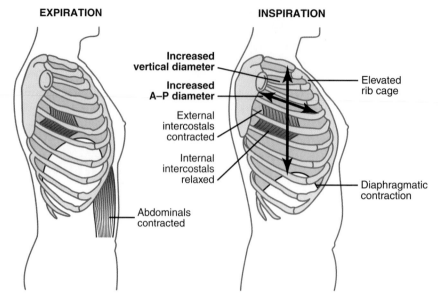

EXPIRATION   **INSPIRATION**

Increased
vertical diameter

Increased
A–P diameter

External
intercostals
contracted

Internal
intercostals
relaxed

Abdominals
contracted

Elevated
rib cage

Diaphragmatic
contraction

Figure 37-1 Contraction and expansion of the thoracic cage during expiration and inspiration, demonstrating diaphragmatic contraction, function of the intercostal muscles, and elevation and depression of the rib cage.

within the cavity. Further, continual suction of excess fluid into lymphatic channels maintains a slight suction between the visceral surface of the lung pleura and the parietal pleural surface of the thoracic cavity. Therefore, the lungs are held to the thoracic wall as if glued there, except that they are well lubricated and can slide freely as the chest expands and contracts.

Pleural Pressure and Its Changes During Respiration

Pleural pressure is the pressure of the fluid in the thin space between the lung pleura and the chest wall pleura. As noted earlier, this is normally a slight suction, which means a slightly *negative* pressure. The normal pleural pressure at the beginning of inspiration is about −5 centimeters of water, which is the amount of suction required to hold the lungs open to their resting level. Then, during normal inspiration, expansion of the chest cage pulls outward on the lungs with greater force and creates more negative pressure, to an average of about −7.5 centimeters of water.

These relationships between pleural pressure and changing lung volume are demonstrated in Figure 37-2, showing in the lower panel the increasing negativity of the pleural pressure from −5 to −7.5 during inspiration and in the upper panel an increase in lung volume of 0.5 liter. Then, during expiration, the events are essentially reversed.

Alveolar Pressure

Alveolar pressure is the pressure of the air inside the lung alveoli. When the glottis is open and no air is flowing into or out of the lungs, the pressures in all parts of the respiratory tree, all the way to the alveoli, are equal to atmospheric pressure, which is considered to be zero reference pressure in the airways—that is, 0 cm water pressure. To cause inward flow of air into the alveoli

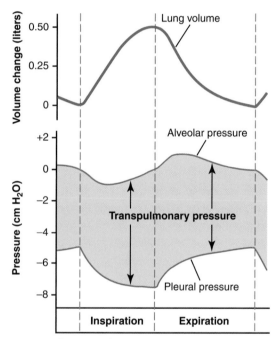

Figure 37-2 Changes in lung volume, alveolar pressure, pleural pressure, and transpulmonary pressure during normal breathing.

during inspiration, the pressure in the alveoli must fall to a value slightly below atmospheric pressure (below 0). The second curve (labeled "alveolar pressure") of Figure 37-2 demonstrates that during normal inspiration, alveolar pressure decreases to about −1 centimeters of water. This slight negative pressure is enough to pull 0.5 liter of air into the lungs in the 2 seconds required for normal quiet inspiration.

During expiration, opposite pressures occur: The alveolar pressure rises to about +1 centimeter of water, and this forces the 0.5 liter of inspired air out of the lungs during the 2 to 3 seconds of expiration.

Transpulmonary Pressure. Finally, note in Figure 37-2 the difference between the alveolar pressure and the pleural pressure. This is called the *transpulmonary pressure*. It is the pressure difference between that in the alveoli and that on the outer surfaces of the lungs, and it is a measure of the elastic forces in the lungs that tend to collapse the lungs at each instant of respiration, called the *recoil pressure*.

Compliance of the Lungs

The extent to which the lungs will expand for each unit increase in transpulmonary pressure (if enough time is allowed to reach equilibrium) is called the *lung compliance*. The total compliance of both lungs together in the normal adult human being averages about 200 milliliters of air per centimeter of water transpulmonary pressure. That is, every time the transpulmonary pressure increases 1 centimeter of water, the lung volume, after 10 to 20 seconds, will expand 200 milliliters.

Compliance Diagram of the Lungs. Figure 37-3 is a diagram relating lung volume changes to changes in transpulmonary pressure. Note that the relation is different for inspiration and expiration. Each curve is recorded by changing the transpulmonary pressure in small steps and allowing the lung volume to come to a steady level between successive steps. The two curves are called, respectively, the *inspiratory compliance curve* and the *expiratory compliance curve*, and the entire diagram is called the *compliance diagram of the lungs*.

The characteristics of the compliance diagram are determined by the elastic forces of the lungs. These can be divided into two parts: (1) *elastic forces of the lung tissue* and (2) *elastic forces caused by surface tension of the fluid that lines the inside walls of the alveoli* and other lung air spaces.

The elastic forces of the lung tissue are determined mainly by *elastin* and *collagen* fibers interwoven among the lung parenchyma. In deflated lungs, these fibers are in an elastically contracted and kinked state; then, when the

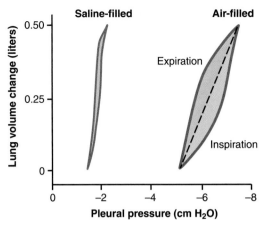

Figure 37-4 Comparison of the compliance diagrams of saline-filled and air-filled lungs when the alveolar pressure is maintained at atmospheric pressure (0 cm H_2O) and pleural pressure is changed.

lungs expand, the fibers become stretched and unkinked, thereby elongating and exerting even more elastic force.

The elastic forces caused by surface tension are much more complex. The significance of surface tension is shown in Figure 37-4, which compares the compliance diagram of the lungs when filled with saline solution and when filled with air. When the lungs are filled with air, there is an interface between the alveolar fluid and the air in the alveoli. In the case of the saline solution–filled lungs, there is no air-fluid interface; therefore, the surface tension effect is not present—only tissue elastic forces are operative in the saline solution–filled lung.

Note that transpleural pressures required to expand air-filled lungs are about three times as great as those required to expand saline solution–filled lungs. Thus, one can conclude that *the tissue elastic forces tending to cause collapse of the air-filled lung represent only about one third of the total lung elasticity, whereas the fluid-air surface tension forces in the alveoli represent about two thirds.*

The fluid-air surface tension elastic forces of the lungs also increase tremendously when the substance called *surfactant* is *not* present in the alveolar fluid. Let us now discuss surfactant and its relation to the surface tension forces.

Surfactant, Surface Tension, and Collapse of the Alveoli

Principle of Surface Tension. When water forms a surface with air, the water molecules on the surface of the water have an especially strong attraction for one another. As a result, the water surface is always attempting to contract. This is what holds raindrops together—a tight contractile membrane of water molecules around the entire surface of the raindrop. Now let us reverse these principles and see what happens on the inner surfaces of the alveoli. Here, the water surface is also attempting to contract. This results in an attempt to force the air out of the alveoli through the bronchi and, in doing so, causes the alveoli to try to collapse. The net effect is to cause an

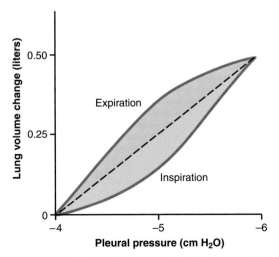

Figure 37-3 Compliance diagram in a healthy person. This diagram shows compliance of the lungs alone.

elastic contractile force of the entire lungs, which is called the *surface tension elastic force.*

Surfactant and Its Effect on Surface Tension. Surfactant is a *surface active agent in water*, which means that it greatly reduces the surface tension of water. It is secreted by special surfactant-secreting epithelial cells called *type II alveolar epithelial cells*, which constitute about 10 percent of the surface area of the alveoli. These cells are granular, containing lipid inclusions that are secreted in the surfactant into the alveoli.

Surfactant is a complex mixture of several phospholipids, proteins, and ions. The most important components are the phospholipid *dipalmitoylphosphatidylcholine,* *surfactant apoproteins*, and *calcium ions*. The dipalmitoylphosphatidylcholine and several less important phospholipids are responsible for reducing the surface tension. They do this by not dissolving uniformly in the fluid lining the alveolar surface. Instead, part of the molecule dissolves while the remainder spreads over the surface of the water in the alveoli. This surface has from one-twelfth to one-half the surface tension of a pure water surface.

In quantitative terms, the surface tension of different water fluids is approximately the following: pure water, 72 dynes/cm; normal fluids lining the alveoli but without surfactant, 50 dynes/cm; normal fluids lining the alveoli and *with* normal amounts of surfactant included, between 5 and 30 dynes/cm.

Pressure in Occluded Alveoli Caused by Surface Tension. If the air passages leading from the alveoli of the lungs are blocked, the surface tension in the alveoli tends to collapse the alveoli. This creates positive pressure in the alveoli, attempting to push the air out. The amount of pressure generated in this way in an alveolus can be calculated from the following formula:

$$\text{Pressure} = \frac{2 \times \text{Surface tension}}{\text{Radius of alveolus}}$$

For the average-sized alveolus with a radius of about 100 micrometers and lined with *normal surfactant*, this calculates to be about 4 centimeters of water pressure (3 mm Hg). If the alveoli were lined with pure water without any surfactant, the pressure would calculate to be about 18 centimeters of water pressure, 4.5 times as great. Thus, one sees how important surfactant is in reducing alveolar surface tension and therefore also reducing the effort required by the respiratory muscles to expand the lungs.

Effect of Alveolar Radius on the Pressure Caused by Surface Tension. Note from the preceding formula that the pressure generated as a result of surface tension in the alveoli is *inversely* affected by the radius of the alveolus, which means that the smaller the alveolus, the greater the alveolar pressure caused by the surface tension. Thus, when the alveoli have half the normal radius (50 instead of 100 micrometers), the pressures noted earlier are doubled. This is especially significant in small premature babies, many of whom have alveoli with radii less than one quarter that of an adult person. Further, surfactant does not normally begin to be secreted into the alveoli until between the sixth and seventh months of gestation, and in some cases, even later than that. Therefore, many premature babies have little or

---

no surfactant in the alveoli when they are born, and their lungs have an extreme tendency to collapse, sometimes as great as six to eight times that in a normal adult person. This causes the condition called *respiratory distress syndrome of the newborn*. It is fatal if not treated with strong measures, especially properly applied continuous positive pressure breathing.

Effect of the Thoracic Cage on Lung Expansibility

Thus far, we have discussed the expansibility of the lungs alone, without considering the thoracic cage. The thoracic cage has its own elastic and viscous characteristics, similar to those of the lungs; even if the lungs were not present in the thorax, muscular effort would still be required to expand the thoracic cage.

Compliance of the Thorax and the Lungs Together

The compliance of the entire pulmonary system (the lungs and thoracic cage together) is measured while expanding the lungs of a totally relaxed or paralyzed person. To do this, air is forced into the lungs a little at a time while recording lung pressures and volumes. To inflate this total pulmonary system, almost twice as much pressure as to inflate the same lungs after removal from the chest cage is necessary. Therefore, the compliance of the combined lung-thorax system is almost exactly one half that of the lungs alone— 110 milliliters of volume per centimeter of water pressure for the combined system, compared with 200 ml/cm for the lungs alone. Furthermore, when the lungs are expanded to high volumes or compressed to low volumes, the limitations of the chest become extreme; when near these limits, the compliance of the combined lung-thorax system can be less than one fifth that of the lungs alone.

"Work" of Breathing
We have already pointed out that during normal quiet breathing, all respiratory muscle contraction occurs during inspiration; expiration is almost entirely a passive process caused by elastic recoil of the lungs and chest cage. Thus, under resting conditions, the respiratory muscles normally perform "work" to cause inspiration but not to cause expiration.

The work of inspiration can be divided into three fractions: (1) that required to expand the lungs against the lung and chest elastic forces, called *compliance work* or *elastic work*; (2) that required to overcome the viscosity of the lung and chest wall structures, called *tissue resistance work*; and (3) that required to overcome airway resistance to movement of air into the lungs, called *airway resistance work*.

Energy Required for Respiration. During normal quiet respiration, only 3 to 5 percent of the total energy expended by the body is required for pulmonary ventilation. But during heavy exercise, the amount of energy required can increase as much as 50-fold, especially if the person has any degree of increased airway resistance or decreased pulmonary compliance. Therefore, one of the major limitations on the intensity of exercise that can be performed is the person's ability to provide enough muscle energy for the respiratory process alone.

Pulmonary Volumes and Capacities

Recording Changes in Pulmonary Volume—Spirometry

Pulmonary ventilation can be studied by recording the volume movement of air into and out of the lungs, a method called *spirometry*. A typical basic spirometer is shown in Figure 37-5. It consists of a drum inverted over a chamber of water, with the drum counterbalanced by a weight. In the drum is a breathing gas, usually air or oxygen; a tube connects the mouth with the gas chamber. When one breathes into and out of the chamber, the drum rises and falls, and an appropriate recording is made on a moving sheet of paper.

Figure 37-6 shows a spirogram indicating changes in lung volume under different conditions of breathing. For ease in describing the events of pulmonary ventilation, the air in the lungs has been subdivided in this diagram into four *volumes* and four *capacities*, which are the average for a *young adult man*.

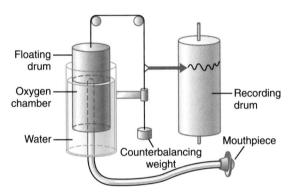

Figure 37-5 Spirometer.

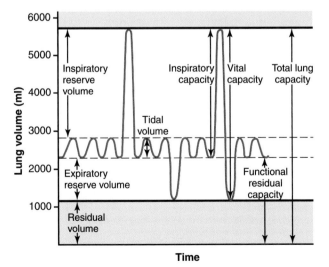

Figure 37-6 Diagram showing respiratory excursions during normal breathing and during maximal inspiration and maximal expiration.

Pulmonary Volumes

To the left in Figure 37-6 are listed four pulmonary lung volumes that, when added together, equal the maximum volume to which the lungs can be expanded. The significance of each of these volumes is the following:

1. The *tidal volume* is the volume of air inspired or expired with each normal breath; it amounts to about 500 milliliters in the adult male.

2. The *inspiratory reserve volume* is the extra volume of air that can be inspired over and above the normal tidal volume when the person inspires with full force; it is usually equal to about 3000 milliliters.

3. The *expiratory reserve volume* is the maximum extra volume of air that can be expired by forceful expiration after the end of a normal tidal expiration; this normally amounts to about 1100 milliliters.

4. The *residual volume* is the volume of air remaining in the lungs after the most forceful expiration; this volume averages about 1200 milliliters.

Pulmonary Capacities

In describing events in the pulmonary cycle, it is sometimes desirable to consider two or more of the volumes together. Such combinations are called *pulmonary capacities*. To the right in Figure 37-6 are listed the important pulmonary capacities, which can be described as follows:

1. The *inspiratory capacity* equals the *tidal volume* plus the *inspiratory reserve volume*. This is the amount of air (about 3500 milliliters) a person can breathe in, beginning at the normal expiratory level and distending the lungs to the maximum amount.

2. The *functional residual capacity* equals the *expiratory reserve volume* plus the *residual volume*. This is the amount of air that remains in the lungs at the end of normal expiration (about 2300 milliliters).

3. The *vital capacity* equals the *inspiratory reserve volume* plus the *tidal volume* plus the *expiratory reserve volume*. This is the maximum amount of air a person can expel from the lungs after first filling the lungs to their maximum extent and then expiring to the maximum extent (about 4600 milliliters).

4. The *total lung capacity* is the maximum volume to which the lungs can be expanded with the greatest possible effort (about 5800 milliliters); it is equal to the *vital capacity* plus the *residual volume*.

All pulmonary volumes and capacities are about 20 to 25 percent less in women than in men, and they are greater in large and athletic people than in small and asthenic people.

Abbreviations and Symbols Used in Pulmonary Function Studies

Spirometry is only one of many measurement procedures that the pulmonary physician uses daily. Many of these measurement procedures depend heavily on mathematical computations. To simplify these calculations, as well as the presentation of pulmonary function data, several abbreviations and symbols have become standardized. The more important of these are given in Table 37-1. Using these symbols, we present here a few simple algebraic exercises showing some of the interrelations among the pulmonary volumes and capacities; the student should think through and verify these interrelations.

$$VC = IRV + V_T + ERV$$

$$VC = IC + ERV$$

$$TLC = VC + RV$$

$$TLC = IC + FRC$$

$$FRC = ERV + RV$$

Determination of Functional Residual Capacity, Residual Volume, and Total Lung Capacity— Helium Dilution Method

The functional residual capacity (FRC), which is the volume of air that remains in the lungs at the end of each normal expiration, is important to lung function. Because its value changes markedly in some types of pulmonary disease, it is often desirable to measure this capacity. The spirometer cannot be used in a direct way to measure the functional residual capacity because the air in the residual volume of the lungs cannot be expired into the spirometer, and this volume constitutes about one half of the functional residual capacity. To measure functional residual capacity, the spirometer must be used in an indirect manner, usually by means of a helium dilution method, as follows.

A spirometer of known volume is filled with air mixed with helium at a known concentration. Before breathing from the spirometer, the person expires normally. At the end of this expiration, the remaining volume in the lungs is equal to the functional residual capacity. At this point, the subject immediately begins to breathe from the spirometer, and the gases of the spirometer mix with the gases of the lungs. As a result, the helium becomes diluted by the functional residual capacity gases, and the volume of the functional residual capacity can be calculated from the degree of dilution of the helium, using the following formula:

$$FRC = \left(\frac{Ci_{He}}{Cf_{He}} - 1\right)Vi_{Spir}$$

where FRC is functional residual capacity, Ci_{He} is initial concentration of helium in the spirometer, Cf_{He} is final concentration of helium in the spirometer, and Vi_{Spir} is initial volume of the spirometer.

Table 37-1 Abbreviations and Symbols for Pulmonary Function

V_T	tidal volume		P_B	atmospheric pressure
FRC	functional residual capacity		Palv	alveolar pressure
ERV	expiratory reserve volume		Ppl	pleural pressure
RV	residual volume		Po_2	partial pressure of oxygen
IC	inspiratory capacity		Pco_2	partial pressure of carbon dioxide
IRV	inspiratory reserve volume		PN_2	partial pressure of nitrogen
TLC	total lung capacity		Pao_2	partial pressure of oxygen in arterial blood
VC	vital capacity		$Paco_2$	partial pressure of carbon dioxide in arterial blood
Raw	resistance of the airways to flow of air into the lung		PAo_2	partial pressure of oxygen in alveolar gas
C	compliance		$PAco_2$	partial pressure of carbon dioxide in alveolar gas
V_D	volume of dead space gas		PAH_2O	partial pressure of water in alveolar gas
V_A	volume of alveolar gas		R	respiratory exchange ratio
$\dot{V}_I$	inspired volume of ventilation per minute		$\dot{Q}$	cardiac output
$\dot{V}_E$	expired volume of ventilation per minute			
$\dot{V}_s$	shunt flow			
$\dot{V}_A$	alveolar ventilation per minute		Cao_2	concentration of oxygen in arterial blood
$\dot{V}O_2$	rate of oxygen uptake per minute		$C\bar{v}o_2$	concentration of oxygen in mixed venous blood
$\dot{V}CO_2$	amount of carbon dioxide eliminated per minute		So_2	percentage saturation of hemoglobin with oxygen
$\dot{V}CO$	rate of carbon monoxide uptake per minute		Sao_2	percentage saturation of hemoglobin with oxygen in arterial blood
DLO_2	diffusing capacity of the lungs for oxygen			
DL_{CO}	diffusing capacity of the lungs for carbon monoxide			

Once the FRC has been determined, the residual volume (RV) can be determined by subtracting expiratory reserve volume (ERV), as measured by normal spirometry, from the FRC. Also, the total lung capacity (TLC) can be determined by adding the inspiratory capacity (IC) to the FRC. That is,

$$RV = FRC - ERV$$

and

$$TLC = FRC + IC$$

Minute Respiratory Volume Equals Respiratory Rate Times Tidal Volume

The *minute respiratory volume* is the total amount of new air moved into the respiratory passages each minute; this is equal to the *tidal volume* times the *respiratory rate per minute*. The normal tidal volume is about 500 milliliters, and the normal respiratory rate is about 12 breaths per minute. Therefore, the *minute respiratory volume averages about 6 L/min*. A person can live for a short period with a minute respiratory volume as low as 1.5 L/min and a respiratory rate of only 2 to 4 breaths per minute.

The respiratory rate occasionally rises to 40 to 50 per minute, and the tidal volume can become as great as the vital capacity, about 4600 milliliters in a young adult man. This can give a minute respiratory volume greater than 200 L/min, or more than 30 times normal. Most people cannot sustain more than one half to two thirds of these values for longer than 1 minute.

Alveolar Ventilation

The ultimate importance of pulmonary ventilation is to continually renew the air in the gas exchange areas of the lungs, where air is in proximity to the pulmonary blood. These areas include the alveoli, alveolar sacs, alveolar ducts, and respiratory bronchioles. The rate at which new air reaches these areas is called *alveolar ventilation*.

"Dead Space" and Its Effect on Alveolar Ventilation

Some of the air a person breathes never reaches the gas exchange areas but simply fills respiratory passages where gas exchange does not occur, such as the nose, pharynx, and trachea. This air is called *dead space air* because it is not useful for gas exchange.

On expiration, the air in the dead space is expired first, before any of the air from the alveoli reaches the atmosphere. Therefore, the dead space is very disadvantageous for removing the expiratory gases from the lungs.

Measurement of the Dead Space Volume. A simple method for measuring dead space volume is demonstrated by the graph in Figure 37-7. In making this measurement, the subject suddenly takes a deep breath of oxygen. This fills the entire dead space with pure oxygen. Some oxygen also mixes

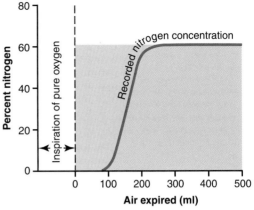

Figure 37-7 Record of the changes in nitrogen concentration in the expired air after a single previous inspiration of pure oxygen. This record can be used to calculate dead space, as discussed in the text.

with the alveolar air but does not completely replace this air. Then the person expires through a rapidly recording nitrogen meter, which makes the record shown in the figure. The first portion of the expired air comes from the dead space regions of the respiratory passageways, where the air has been completely replaced by oxygen. Therefore, in the early part of the record, only oxygen appears, and the nitrogen concentration is zero. Then, when alveolar air begins to reach the nitrogen meter, the nitrogen concentration rises rapidly, because alveolar air containing large amounts of nitrogen begins to mix with the dead space air. After still more air has been expired, all the dead space air has been washed from the passages and only alveolar air remains. Therefore, the recorded nitrogen concentration reaches a plateau level equal to its concentration in the alveoli, as shown to the right in the figure. With a little thought, the student can see that the gray area represents the air that has no nitrogen in it; this area is a measure of the volume of dead space air. For exact quantification, the following equation is used:

$$V_D = \frac{\text{Gray area} \times V_E}{\text{Pink area} + \text{Gray area}}$$

where V_D is dead space air and V_E is the total volume of expired air.

Let us assume, for instance, that the gray area on the graph is 30 square centimeters, the pink area is 70 square centimeters, and the total volume expired is 500 milliliters. The dead space would be

$$\frac{30}{30 + 70} \times 500 = 150 \, \text{ml}$$

Normal Dead Space Volume. The normal dead space air in a young adult man is about 150 milliliters. This increases slightly with age.

Anatomic Versus Physiologic Dead Space. The method just described for measuring the dead space measures the volume of all the space of the respiratory system other than the alveoli and their other closely related gas exchange areas; this space is called the *anatomic dead space*. On occasion, some of the alveoli themselves are nonfunctional or only partially functional because of absent or poor blood flow through the adjacent pulmonary capillaries. Therefore, from a functional point of view, these alveoli must also be considered dead space. When the alveolar dead space is included in the total measurement of dead space, this is called the *physiologic dead space*, in contradistinction to the anatomic dead space. In a normal person, the anatomic and physiologic dead spaces are nearly equal because all alveoli are functional in the normal lung, but in a person with partially functional or nonfunctional alveoli in some parts of the lungs, the physiologic dead space may be as much as 10 times the volume of the anatomic dead space, or 1 to 2 liters. These problems are discussed further in Chapter 39 in relation to pulmonary gaseous exchange and in Chapter 42 in relation to certain pulmonary diseases.

Rate of Alveolar Ventilation

Alveolar ventilation per minute is the total volume of new air entering the alveoli and adjacent gas exchange areas each minute. It is equal to the respiratory rate times the amount of new air that enters these areas with each breath.

$$\dot{V}_A = \text{Freq} \times (V_T - V_D)$$

where $\dot{V}_A$ is the volume of alveolar ventilation per minute, Freq is the frequency of respiration per minute, V_T is the tidal volume, and V_D is the physiologic dead space volume.

Thus, with a normal tidal volume of 500 milliliters, a normal dead space of 150 milliliters, and a respiratory rate of 12 breaths per minute, alveolar ventilation equals $12 \times (500 - 150)$, or 4200 ml/min.

Alveolar ventilation is one of the major factors determining the concentrations of oxygen and carbon dioxide in the alveoli. Therefore, almost all discussions of gaseous exchange in the following chapters on the respiratory system emphasize alveolar ventilation.

Functions of the Respiratory Passageways

Trachea, Bronchi, and Bronchioles

Figure 37-8 shows the respiratory system, demonstrating especially the respiratory passageways. The air is distributed to the lungs by way of the trachea, bronchi, and bronchioles.

One of the most important challenges in the respiratory passageways is to keep them open and allow easy passage of air to and from the alveoli. To keep the trachea from collapsing, multiple cartilage rings extend about five sixths of the way around the trachea. In the walls of the bronchi, less extensive curved cartilage plates also maintain a reasonable amount of rigidity yet allow sufficient motion for the lungs to expand and contract. These plates become progressively less extensive in the later generations of bronchi and are gone in the bronchioles, which usually have diameters less than 1.5 millimeters. The bronchioles are not prevented from collapsing by the rigidity of their walls. Instead, they are kept expanded mainly by the same transpulmonary pressures that expand the alveoli. That is, as the alveoli enlarge, the bronchioles also enlarge, but not as much.

Muscular Wall of the Bronchi and Bronchioles and Its Control. In all areas of the *trachea* and *bronchi* not occupied by cartilage plates, the walls are composed mainly of smooth muscle. Also, the walls of the *bronchioles* are almost entirely smooth muscle, with the exception of the most terminal bronchiole, called the *respiratory bronchiole*, which is mainly pulmonary epithelium and underlying fibrous tissue plus a few smooth muscle fibers. Many obstructive diseases of the lung result from narrowing of the smaller bronchi and

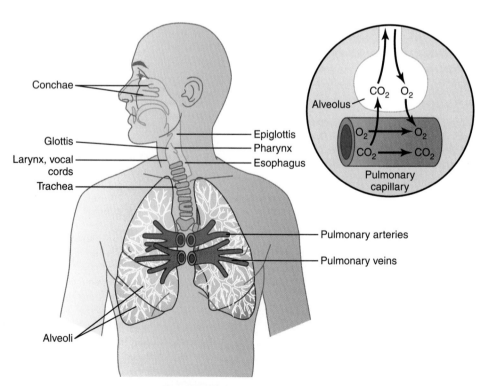

Figure 37-8 Respiratory passages.

larger bronchioles, often because of excessive contraction of the smooth muscle itself.

Resistance to Airflow in the Bronchial Tree. Under *normal respiratory conditions*, air flows through the respiratory passageways so easily that less than 1 centimeter of water pressure gradient from the alveoli to the atmosphere is sufficient to cause enough airflow for quiet breathing. The greatest amount of resistance to airflow occurs not in the minute air passages of the terminal bronchioles but in some of the larger bronchioles and bronchi near the trachea. The reason for this high resistance is that there are relatively few of these larger bronchi in comparison with the approximately 65,000 parallel terminal bronchioles, through each of which only a minute amount of air must pass.

Yet in disease conditions, the smaller bronchioles often play a far greater role in determining airflow resistance because of their small size and because they are easily occluded by (1) muscle contraction in their walls, (2) edema occurring in the walls, or (3) mucus collecting in the lumens of the bronchioles.

Nervous and Local Control of the Bronchiolar Musculature— "Sympathetic" Dilation of the Bronchioles. Direct control of the bronchioles by sympathetic nerve fibers is relatively weak because few of these fibers penetrate to the central portions of the lung. However, the bronchial tree is very much exposed to *norepinephrine* and *epinephrine* released into the blood by sympathetic stimulation of the adrenal gland medullae. Both these hormones, especially epinephrine because of its greater stimulation of *beta-adrenergic receptors*, cause dilation of the bronchial tree.

Parasympathetic Constriction of the Bronchioles. A few parasympathetic nerve fibers derived from the vagus nerves penetrate the lung parenchyma. These nerves secrete *acetylcholine* and, when activated, cause mild to moderate constriction of the bronchioles. When a disease process such as asthma has already caused some bronchiolar constriction, superimposed parasympathetic nervous stimulation often worsens the condition. When this occurs, administration of drugs that block the effects of acetylcholine, such as *atropine*, can sometimes relax the respiratory passages enough to relieve the obstruction.

Sometimes the parasympathetic nerves are also activated by reflexes that originate in the lungs. Most of these begin with irritation of the epithelial membrane of the respiratory passageways themselves, initiated by noxious gases, dust, cigarette smoke, or bronchial infection. Also, a bronchiolar constrictor reflex often occurs when microemboli occlude small pulmonary arteries.

Local Secretory Factors Often Cause Bronchiolar Constriction. Several substances formed in the lungs are often quite active in causing bronchiolar constriction. Two of the most important of these are *histamine* and *slow reactive substance of anaphylaxis*. Both of these are released in the lung tissues by *mast cells* during allergic reactions, especially those caused by pollen in the air. Therefore, they play key roles in causing the airway obstruction that occurs in allergic asthma; this is especially true of the slow reactive substance of anaphylaxis.

The same irritants that cause parasympathetic constrictor reflexes of the airways—smoke, dust, sulfur dioxide, and some of the acidic elements in smog—often act directly on the lung tissues to initiate local, non-nervous reactions that cause obstructive constriction of the airways.

Mucus Lining the Respiratory Passageways, and Action of Cilia to Clear the Passageways

All the respiratory passages, from the nose to the terminal bronchioles, are kept moist by a layer of mucus that coats the entire surface. The mucus is secreted partly by individual mucous goblet cells in the epithelial lining of the passages and partly by small submucosal glands. In addition to keeping the surfaces moist, the mucus traps small particles out of the inspired air and keeps most of these from ever reaching the alveoli. The mucus itself is removed from the passages in the following manner.

The entire surface of the respiratory passages, both in the nose and in the lower passages down as far as the terminal bronchioles, is lined with ciliated epithelium, with about 200 cilia on each epithelial cell. These cilia beat continually at a rate of 10 to 20 times per second by the mechanism explained in Chapter 2, and the direction of their "power stroke" is always toward the pharynx. That is, the cilia in the lungs beat upward, whereas those in the nose beat downward. This continual beating causes the coat of mucus to flow slowly, at a velocity of a few millimeters per minute, toward the pharynx. Then the mucus and its entrapped particles are either swallowed or coughed to the exterior.

Cough Reflex

The bronchi and trachea are so sensitive to light touch that slight amounts of foreign matter or other causes of irritation initiate the cough reflex. The larynx and carina (the point where the trachea divides into the bronchi) are especially sensitive, and the terminal bronchioles and even the alveoli are sensitive to corrosive chemical stimuli such as sulfur dioxide gas or chlorine gas. Afferent nerve impulses pass from the respiratory passages mainly through the vagus nerves to the medulla of the brain. There, an automatic sequence of events is triggered by the neuronal circuits of the medulla, causing the following effect.

First, up to 2.5 liters of air are rapidly inspired. Second, the epiglottis closes, and the vocal cords shut tightly to entrap the air within the lungs. Third, the abdominal muscles contract forcefully, pushing against the diaphragm while other expiratory muscles, such as the internal intercostals, also contract forcefully. Consequently, the pressure in the lungs rises rapidly to as much as 100 mm Hg or more. Fourth, the vocal cords and the epiglottis suddenly open widely, so that air under this high pressure in the lungs *explodes* outward. Indeed, sometimes this air is expelled at velocities ranging from 75 to 100 miles per hour. Importantly, the strong compression of the lungs collapses the bronchi and trachea by causing their noncartilaginous parts to invaginate inward, so the exploding air actually passes through *bronchial* and *tracheal slits*. The rapidly moving air usually carries with it any foreign matter that is present in the bronchi or trachea.

Sneeze Reflex

The sneeze reflex is very much like the cough reflex, except that it applies to the nasal passageways instead of the lower respiratory passages. The initiating stimulus of the sneeze reflex is irritation in the nasal passageways; the afferent impulses pass in the fifth cranial nerve to the medulla, where the reflex is triggered. A series of reactions similar to those for the cough reflex takes place; however, the uvula is depressed, so large amounts of air pass rapidly through the nose, thus helping to clear the nasal passages of foreign matter.

Normal Respiratory Functions of the Nose

As air passes through the nose, three distinct normal respiratory functions are performed by the nasal cavities: (1) the air is *warmed* by the extensive surfaces of the conchae and septum, a total area of about 160 square centimeters (see Figure 37-8); (2) the air is *almost completely humidified* even before it passes beyond the nose; and (3) the air is *partially filtered*. These functions together are called the *air conditioning function* of the upper respiratory passageways. Ordinarily, the temperature of the inspired air rises to within 1°F of body temperature and to within 2 to 3 percent of full saturation with water vapor before it reaches the trachea. When a person breathes air through a tube directly into the trachea (as through a tracheostomy), the cooling and especially the drying effect in the lower lung can lead to serious lung crusting and infection.

Filtration Function of the Nose. The hairs at the entrance to the nostrils are important for filtering out large particles. Much more important, though, is the removal of particles by *turbulent precipitation*. That is, the air passing through the nasal passageways hits many obstructing vanes: the *conchae* (also called *turbinates*, because they cause turbulence of the air); the septum; and the pharyngeal wall. Each time air hits one of these obstructions, it must change its direction of movement. The particles suspended in the air, having far more mass and momentum than air, cannot change their direction of travel as rapidly as the air can. Therefore, they continue forward, striking the surfaces of the obstructions, and are entrapped in the mucous coating and transported by the cilia to the pharynx to be swallowed.

Size of Particles Entrapped in the Respiratory Passages. The nasal turbulence mechanism for removing particles from air is so effective that almost no particles larger than 6 micrometers in diameter enter the lungs through the nose. This size is smaller than the size of red blood cells.

Of the remaining particles, many that are between 1 and 5 micrometers *settle* in the smaller bronchioles as a result of *gravitational precipitation*. For instance, terminal bronchiolar disease is common in coal miners because of settled dust particles. Some of the still smaller particles (smaller than 1 micrometer in diameter) *diffuse* against the walls of the alveoli and adhere to the alveolar fluid. But many particles smaller than 0.5 micrometer in diameter remain suspended in the alveolar air and are expelled by expiration. For instance, the particles of cigarette smoke are about 0.3 micrometer. Almost none of these particles are precipitated

in the respiratory passageways before they reach the alveoli. Unfortunately, up to one third of them do precipitate in the alveoli by the diffusion process, with the balance remaining suspended and expelled in the expired air.

Many of the particles that become entrapped in the alveoli are removed by *alveolar macrophages*, as explained in Chapter 33, and others are carried away by the lung lymphatics. An excess of particles can cause growth of fibrous tissue in the alveolar septa, leading to permanent debility.

Vocalization

Speech involves not only the respiratory system but also (1) specific speech nervous control centers in the cerebral cortex, which are discussed in Chapter 57; (2) respiratory control centers of the brain; and (3) the articulation and resonance structures of the mouth and nasal cavities. Speech is composed of two mechanical functions: (1) *phonation*, which is achieved by the larynx, and (2) *articulation*, which is achieved by the structures of the mouth.

Phonation. The larynx, shown in Figure 37-9A, is especially adapted to act as a vibrator. The vibrating element is the *vocal folds*, commonly called the *vocal cords*. The vocal cords protrude from the lateral walls of the larynx toward the center of the glottis; they are stretched and positioned by several specific muscles of the larynx itself.

Figure 37-9B shows the vocal cords as they are seen when looking into the glottis with a laryngoscope. During normal breathing, the cords are wide open to allow easy passage of air. During phonation, the cords move together so that passage of air between them will cause vibration. The pitch of the vibration is determined mainly by the degree of stretch of the cords, but also by how tightly the cords are approximated to one another and by the mass of their edges.

Figure 37-9A shows a dissected view of the vocal folds after removal of the mucous epithelial lining. Immediately inside each cord is a strong elastic ligament called the *vocal ligament*. This is attached anteriorly to the large *thyroid cartilage*, which is the cartilage that projects forward from the anterior surface of the neck and is called the "Adam's apple." Posteriorly, the vocal ligament is attached to the *vocal processes* of two *arytenoid cartilages*. The thyroid cartilage and the arytenoid cartilages articulate from below with another cartilage not shown in Figure 37-9, the *cricoid cartilage*.

The vocal cords can be stretched by either forward rotation of the thyroid cartilage or posterior rotation of the arytenoid cartilages, activated by muscles stretching from

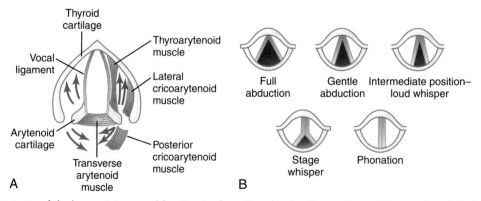

Figure 37-9 *A,* Anatomy of the larynx. *B,* Laryngeal function in phonation, showing the positions of the vocal cords during different types of phonation. (Modified from Greene MC: The Voice and Its Disorders, 4th ed. Philadelphia: JB Lippincott, 1980.)

the thyroid cartilage and arytenoid cartilages to the cricoid cartilage. Muscles located within the vocal cords lateral to the vocal ligaments, the thyroarytenoid muscles, can pull the arytenoid cartilages toward the thyroid cartilage and, therefore, loosen the vocal cords. Also, slips of these muscles *within* the vocal cords can change the *shapes and masses of the vocal cord edges*, sharpening them to emit high-pitched sounds and blunting them for the more bass sounds.

Several other sets of small laryngeal muscles lie between the arytenoid cartilages and the cricoid cartilage and can rotate these cartilages inward or outward or pull their bases together or apart to give the various configurations of the vocal cords shown in Figure 37-9*B*.

Articulation and Resonance. The three major organs of articulation are the *lips, tongue,* and *soft palate*. They need not be discussed in detail because we are all familiar with their movements during speech and other vocalizations.

The resonators include the *mouth*, the *nose* and *associated nasal sinuses*, the *pharynx*, and even the *chest cavity*. Again, we are all familiar with the resonating qualities of these structures. For instance, the function of the nasal resonators is demonstrated by the change in voice quality when a person has a severe cold that blocks the air passages to these resonators.

Bibliography

Anthony M: The obesity hypoventilation syndrome, *Respir Care* 53:1723, 2008.

Daniels CB, Orgeig S: Pulmonary surfactant: the key to the evolution of air breathing, *News Physiol Sci* 18:151, 2003.

Hilaire G, Duron B: Maturation of the mammalian respiratory system, *Physiol Rev* 79:325, 1999.

Lai-Fook SJ: Pleural mechanics and fluid exchange, *Physiol Rev* 84:385, 2004.

Mason RJ, Greene K, Voelker DR: Surfactant protein A and surfactant protein D in health and disease, *Am J Physiol Lung Cell Mol Physiol* 275:L1, 1998.

McConnell AK, Romer LM: Dyspnoea in health and obstructive pulmonary disease: the role of respiratory muscle function and training, *Sports Med* 34:117, 2004.

Paton JF, Dutschmann M: Central control of upper airway resistance regulating respiratory airflow in mammals, *J Anat* 201:319, 2002.

Pavord ID, Chung KF: Management of chronic cough, *Lancet* 371:1375, 2008.

Powell FL, Hopkins SR: Comparative physiology of lung complexity: implications for gas exchange, *News Physiol Sci* 19:55, 2004.

Sant'Ambrogio G, Widdicombe J: Reflexes from airway rapidly adapting receptors, *Respir Physiol* 125:33, 2001.

Uhlig S, Taylor AE: *Methods in Pulmonary Research*, Basel, 1998, Birkhauser Verlag.

Voynow JA, Rubin BK: Mucins, mucus, and sputum, *Chest* 135:505, 2009.

West JB: *Respiratory Physiology*, New York, 1996, Oxford University Press.

West JB: Why doesn't the elephant have a pleural space? *News Physiol Sci* 17:47, 2002.

Widdicombe J: Reflexes from the lungs and airways: historical perspective, *J Appl Physiol* 101:628, 2006.

Widdicombe J: Neuroregulation of cough: implications for drug therapy, *Curr Opin Pharmacol* 2:256, 2002.

Wright JR: Pulmonary surfactant: a front line of lung host defense, *J Clin Invest* 111:1453, 2003.

Zeitels SM, Healy GB: Laryngology and phonosurgery. *N Engl J Med* 349:882, 2003.

Pulmonary Circulation, Pulmonary Edema, Pleural Fluid

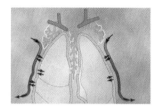 The lung has two circulations: (1) *A high-pressure, low-flow circulation* supplies systemic arterial blood to the trachea, the bronchial tree including the terminal bronchioles, the supporting tissues of the lung, and the outer coats (adventia) of the pulmonary arteries and veins. The *bronchial arteries*, which are branches of the thoracic aorta, supply most of this systemic arterial blood at a pressure that is only slightly lower than the aortic pressure. (2) *A low-pressure, high-flow circulation* that supplies venous blood from all parts of the body to the alveolar capillaries where oxygen is added and carbon dioxide is removed. The *pulmonary artery*, which receives blood from the right ventricle, and its arterial branches carry blood to the alveolar capillaries for gas exchange and the pulmonary veins then return the blood to the left atrium to be pumped by the left ventricle though the systemic circulation.

In this chapter we discuss the special aspects of blood flow distribution and other hemodynamics of the pulmonary circulation that are especially important for gas exchange in the lungs.

Physiologic Anatomy of the Pulmonary Circulatory System

Pulmonary Vessels. The pulmonary artery extends only 5 centimeters beyond the apex of the right ventricle and then divides into right and left main branches that supply blood to the two respective lungs.

The pulmonary artery is thin, with a wall thickness one third that of the aorta. The pulmonary arterial branches are very short, and all the pulmonary arteries, even the smaller arteries and arterioles, have larger diameters than their counterpart systemic arteries. This, combined with the fact that the vessels are thin and distensible, gives the pulmonary arterial tree a *large compliance*, averaging almost 7 ml/mm Hg, which is similar to that of the entire systemic arterial tree. This large compliance allows the pulmonary arteries to accommodate the stroke volume output of the right ventricle.

The pulmonary veins, like the pulmonary arteries, are also short. They immediately empty their effluent blood into the left atrium.

Bronchial Vessels. Blood also flows to the lungs through small bronchial arteries that originate from the systemic circulation, amounting to about 1 to 2 percent of the total cardiac output. This bronchial arterial blood is *oxygenated* blood, in contrast to the partially deoxygenated blood in the pulmonary arteries. It supplies the supporting tissues of the lungs, including the connective tissue, septa, and large and small bronchi. After this bronchial and arterial blood has passed through the supporting tissues, it empties into the pulmonary veins and *enters the left atrium*, rather than passing back to the right atrium. Therefore, the flow into the left atrium and the left ventricular output are about 1 to 2 percent greater than that of the right ventricular output.

Lymphatics. Lymph vessels are present in all the supportive tissues of the lung, beginning in the connective tissue spaces that surround the terminal bronchioles, coursing to the hilum of the lung, and then mainly into the *right thoracic lymph duct*. Particulate matter entering the alveoli is partly removed by way of these channels, and plasma protein leaking from the lung capillaries is also removed from the lung tissues, thereby helping to prevent pulmonary edema.

Pressures in the Pulmonary System

Pressure Pulse Curve in the Right Ventricle. The pressure pulse curves of the right ventricle and pulmonary artery are shown in the lower portion of Figure 38-1. These curves are contrasted with the much higher aortic pressure curve shown in the upper portion of the figure. The systolic pressure in the right ventricle of the normal human being averages about 25 mm Hg, and the diastolic pressure averages about 0 to 1 mm Hg, values that are only one-fifth those for the left ventricle.

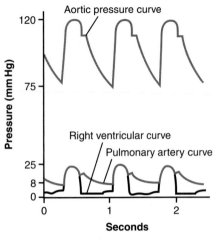

Figure 38-1 Pressure pulse contours in the right ventricle, pulmonary artery, and aorta.

Pressures in the Pulmonary Artery. During *systole*, the pressure in the pulmonary artery is essentially equal to the pressure in the right ventricle, as also shown in Figure 38-1. However, after the pulmonary valve closes at the end of systole, the ventricular pressure falls precipitously, whereas the pulmonary arterial pressure falls more slowly as blood flows through the capillaries of the lungs.

As shown in Figure 38-2, the *systolic pulmonary arterial pressure* averages about 25 mm Hg in the normal human being, the *diastolic pulmonary arterial pressure* is about 8 mm Hg, and the *mean pulmonary arterial pressure* is 15 mm Hg.

Pulmonary Capillary Pressure. The mean pulmonary capillary pressure, as diagrammed in Figure 38-2, is about 7 mm Hg. The importance of this low capillary pressure is discussed in detail later in the chapter in relation to fluid exchange functions of the pulmonary capillaries.

Left Atrial and Pulmonary Venous Pressures. The mean pressure in the left atrium and the major pulmonary veins averages about 2 mm Hg in the recumbent

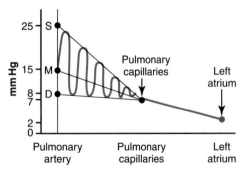

Figure 38-2 Pressures in the different vessels of the lungs. D, diastolic; M, mean; S, systolic; red curve, arterial pulsations.

human being, varying from as low as 1 mm Hg to as high as 5 mm Hg. It usually is not feasible to measure a human being's left atrial pressure using a direct measuring device because it is difficult to pass a catheter through the heart chambers into the left atrium. However, the left atrial pressure can often be estimated with moderate accuracy by measuring the so-called *pulmonary wedge pressure*. This is achieved by inserting a catheter first through a peripheral vein to the right atrium, then through the right side of the heart and through the pulmonary artery into one of the small branches of the pulmonary artery, finally pushing the catheter until it *wedges tightly in the small branch*.

The pressure measured through the catheter, called the "wedge pressure," is about 5 mm Hg. Because all blood flow has been stopped in the small wedged artery, and because the blood vessels extending beyond this artery make a direct connection with the pulmonary capillaries, this wedge pressure is usually only 2 to 3 mm Hg greater than the left atrial pressure. When the left atrial pressure rises to high values, the pulmonary wedge pressure also rises. Therefore, wedge pressure measurements can be used to clinically study changes in pulmonary capillary pressure and left atrial pressure in patients with congestive heart failure.

Blood Volume of the Lungs

The blood volume of the lungs is about 450 milliliters, about 9 percent of the total blood volume of the entire circulatory system. Approximately 70 milliliters of this pulmonary blood volume is in the pulmonary capillaries, and the remainder is divided about equally between the pulmonary arteries and the veins.

The Lungs Serve as a Blood Reservoir. Under various physiological and pathological conditions, the quantity of blood in the lungs can vary from as little as one-half normal up to twice normal. For instance, when a person blows out air so hard that high pressure is built up in the lungs—such as when blowing a trumpet—as much as 250 milliliters of blood can be expelled from the pulmonary circulatory system into the systemic circulation. Also, loss of blood from the systemic circulation by hemorrhage can be partly compensated for by the automatic shift of blood from the lungs into the systemic vessels.

Cardiac Pathology May Shift Blood from the Systemic Circulation to the Pulmonary Circulation. Failure of the left side of the heart or increased resistance to blood flow through the mitral valve as a result of mitral stenosis or mitral regurgitation causes blood to dam up in the pulmonary circulation, sometimes increasing the pulmonary blood volume as much as 100 percent and causing large increases in the pulmonary vascular pressures. Because the volume of the systemic circulation is about nine times that of the pulmonary system, a shift of blood from one system to the other affects the pulmonary system greatly but usually has only mild systemic circulatory effects.

Blood Flow Through the Lungs and Its Distribution

The blood flow through the lungs is essentially equal to the cardiac output. Therefore, the factors that control cardiac output—mainly peripheral factors, as discussed in Chapter 20—also control pulmonary blood flow. Under most conditions, the pulmonary vessels act as passive, distensible tubes that enlarge with increasing pressure and narrow with decreasing pressure. For adequate aeration of the blood to occur, it is important for the blood to be distributed to those segments of the lungs where the alveoli are best oxygenated. This is achieved by the following mechanism.

Decreased Alveolar Oxygen Reduces Local Alveolar Blood Flow and Regulates Pulmonary Blood Flow Distribution. When the concentration of oxygen in the air of the alveoli decreases below normal, especially when it falls below 70 percent of normal (below 73 mm Hg Po_2), the adjacent blood vessels constrict, with the vascular resistance increasing more than fivefold at extremely low oxygen levels. This is *opposite to the effect observed in systemic vessels*, which dilate rather than constrict in response to low oxygen. It is believed that the low oxygen concentration causes some yet undiscovered vasoconstrictor substance to be released from the lung tissue; this substance promotes constriction of the small arteries and arterioles. It has been suggested that this vasoconstrictor might be secreted by the alveolar epithelial cells when they become hypoxic.

This effect of low oxygen on pulmonary vascular resistance has an important function: to distribute blood flow where it is most effective. That is, if some alveoli are poorly ventilated so that their oxygen concentration becomes low, the local vessels constrict. This causes the blood to flow through other areas of the lungs that are better aerated, thus providing an automatic control system for distributing blood flow to the pulmonary areas in proportion to their alveolar oxygen pressures.

Effect of Hydrostatic Pressure Gradients in the Lungs on Regional Pulmonary Blood Flow

In Chapter 15, it was pointed out that the blood pressure in the foot of a standing person can be as much as 90 mm Hg greater than the pressure at the level of the heart. This is caused by *hydrostatic pressure*—that is, by the weight of the blood itself in the blood vessels. The same effect, but to a lesser degree, occurs in the lungs. In the normal, upright adult, the lowest point in the lungs is about 30 cm below the highest point. This represents a 23 mm Hg pressure difference, about 15 mm Hg of which is above the heart and 8 below. That is, the pulmonary arterial pressure in the uppermost portion of the lung of a standing person is about 15 mm Hg less than the pulmonary arterial pressure at the level of the heart, and the pressure in the lowest portion of the lungs is about 8 mm Hg greater. Such pressure differences have profound effects on blood flow through the different areas of the lungs. This is demonstrated by the lower curve in Figure 38-3, which depicts blood flow per unit of lung tissue at different levels of the lung in the upright person. Note that in the standing position at rest, there is little flow in the top of the lung but about five times as much flow in the bottom. To help explain these differences, one often describes the lung as being divided into three zones, as shown in Figure 38-4. In each zone, the patterns of blood flow are quite different.

Zones 1, 2, and 3 of Pulmonary Blood Flow

The capillaries in the alveolar walls are distended by the blood pressure inside them, but simultaneously they are compressed by the alveolar air pressure on their outsides. Therefore, any time the lung alveolar air pressure becomes greater than the capillary blood pressure, the capillaries close and there is no blood flow. Under different normal and pathological lung conditions, one may find any one of three possible zones (patterns) of pulmonary blood flow, as follows:

Zone 1: No blood flow during all portions of the cardiac cycle because the local alveolar capillary pressure in that area of the lung never rises higher than the alveolar air pressure during any part of the cardiac cycle

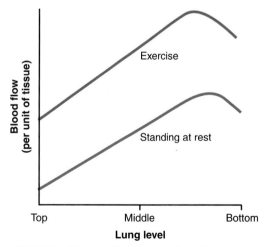

Figure 38-3 Blood flow at different levels in the lung of an upright person *at rest* and *during exercise*. Note that when the person is at rest, the blood flow is very low at the top of the lungs; most of the flow is through the bottom of the lung.

479

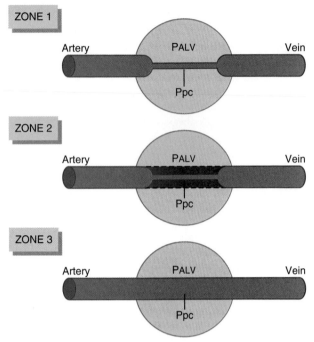

ZONE 1

Artery   PALV   Vein

Ppc

ZONE 2

Artery   PALV   Vein

Ppc

ZONE 3

Artery   PALV   Vein

Ppc

Figure 38-4 Mechanics of blood flow in the three blood flow zones of the lung: *zone 1, no flow*—alveolar air pressure (PALV) is greater than arterial pressure; *zone 2, intermittent flow*—systolic arterial pressure rises higher than alveolar air pressure, but diastolic arterial pressure falls below alveolar air pressure; and *zone 3, continuous flow*—arterial pressure and pulmonary capillary pressure (Ppc) remain greater than alveolar air pressure at all times.

Zone 2: Intermittent blood flow only during the peaks of pulmonary arterial pressure because the systolic pressure is then greater than the alveolar air pressure, but the diastolic pressure is less than the alveolar air pressure

Zone 3: Continuous blood flow because the alveolar capillary pressure remains greater than alveolar air pressure during the entire cardiac cycle

Normally, the lungs have only zones 2 and 3 blood flow—zone 2 (intermittent flow) in the apices and zone 3 (continuous flow) in all the lower areas. For example, when a person is in the upright position, the pulmonary arterial pressure at the lung apex is about 15 mm Hg less than the pressure at the level of the heart. Therefore, the apical systolic pressure is only 10 mm Hg (25 mm Hg at heart level minus 15 mm Hg hydrostatic pressure difference). This 10 mm Hg apical blood pressure is greater than the zero alveolar air pressure, so blood flows through the pulmonary apical capillaries during cardiac systole. Conversely, during diastole, the 8 mm Hg diastolic pressure at the level of the heart is not sufficient to push the blood up the 15 mm Hg hydrostatic pressure gradient required to cause diastolic capillary flow. Therefore, blood flow through the apical part of the lung is intermittent, with flow during systole but cessation of flow during diastole; this is called *zone 2 blood flow*. Zone 2 blood flow begins in the normal lungs about 10 cm above the midlevel of the heart and extends from there to the top of the lungs.

In the lower regions of the lungs, from about 10 cm above the level of the heart all the way to the bottom of the lungs, the pulmonary arterial pressure during both systole and diastole remains greater than the zero alveolar air pressure. Therefore, there is continuous flow through the alveolar capillaries, or zone 3 blood flow. Also, when a person is lying down, no part of the lung is more than a few centimeters above the level of the heart. In this case, blood flow in a normal person is entirely zone 3 blood flow, including the lung apices.

Zone 1 Blood Flow Occurs Only Under Abnormal Conditions. Zone 1 blood flow, which means no blood flow at any time during the cardiac cycle, occurs when either the pulmonary systolic arterial pressure is too low or the alveolar pressure is too high to allow flow. For instance, if an upright person is breathing against a positive air pressure so that the intra-alveolar air pressure is at least 10 mm Hg greater than normal but the pulmonary systolic blood pressure is normal, one would expect zone 1 blood flow— no blood flow—in the lung apices. Another instance in which zone 1 blood flow occurs is in an upright person whose pulmonary systolic arterial pressure is exceedingly low, as might occur after severe blood loss.

Effect of Exercise on Blood Flow Through the Different Parts of the Lungs. Referring again to Figure 38-3, one sees that the blood flow in all parts of the lung increases during exercise. The increase in flow in the top of the lung may be 700 to 800 percent, whereas the increase in the lower part of the lung may be no more than 200 to 300 percent. The reason for these differences is that the pulmonary vascular pressures rise enough during exercise to convert the lung apices from a zone 2 pattern into a zone 3 pattern of flow.

Increased Cardiac Output During Heavy Exercise Is Normally Accommodated by the Pulmonary Circulation Without Large Increases in Pulmonary Artery Pressure

During heavy exercise, blood flow through the lungs increases fourfold to sevenfold. This extra flow is accommodated in the lungs in three ways: (1) by increasing the number of open capillaries, sometimes as much as threefold; (2) by distending all the capillaries and increasing the rate of flow through each capillary more than twofold; and (3) by increasing the pulmonary arterial pressure. In the normal person, the first two changes decrease pulmonary vascular resistance so much that the pulmonary arterial pressure rises very little, even during maximum exercise; this effect is shown in Figure 38-5.

The ability of the lungs to accommodate greatly increased blood flow during exercise without increasing the pulmonary arterial pressure conserves the energy of the right side of the heart. This ability also prevents a significant rise in pulmonary capillary pressure, thus also preventing the development of pulmonary edema.

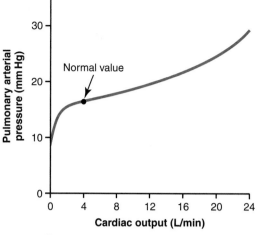

Figure 38-5 Effect on mean pulmonary arterial pressure caused by increasing the cardiac output during exercise.

Function of the Pulmonary Circulation When the Left Atrial Pressure Rises as a Result of Left-Sided Heart Failure

The left atrial pressure in a healthy person almost never rises above +6 mm Hg, even during the most strenuous exercise. These small changes in left atrial pressure have virtually no effect on pulmonary circulatory function because this merely expands the pulmonary venules and opens up more capillaries so that blood continues to flow with almost equal ease from the pulmonary arteries.

When the left side of the heart fails, however, blood begins to dam up in the left atrium. As a result, the left atrial pressure can rise on occasion from its normal value of 1 to 5 mm Hg all the way up to 40 to 50 mm Hg. The initial rise in atrial pressure, up to about 7 mm Hg, has very little effect on pulmonary circulatory function. But when the left atrial pressure rises to greater than 7 or 8 mm Hg, further increases in left atrial pressure above these levels cause almost equally great increases in pulmonary arterial pressure, thus causing a concomitant increased load on the right heart. Any increase in left atrial pressure above 7 or 8 mm Hg increases the capillary pressure almost equally as much. When the left atrial pressure has risen above 30 mm Hg, causing similar increases in capillary pressure, pulmonary edema is likely to develop, as we discuss later in the chapter.

Pulmonary Capillary Dynamics

Exchange of gases between the alveolar air and the pulmonary capillary blood is discussed in the next chapter. However, it is important for us to note here that the alveolar walls are lined with so many capillaries that, in most places, the capillaries almost touch one another side by side. Therefore, it is often said that the capillary blood flows in the alveolar walls as a "sheet of flow," rather than in individual capillaries.

Pulmonary Capillary Pressure. No direct measurements of pulmonary capillary pressure have ever been made. However, "isogravimetric" measurement of pulmonary capillary pressure, using a technique described in Chapter 16, has given a value of 7 mm Hg. This is probably nearly correct because the mean left atrial pressure is about 2 mm Hg and the mean pulmonary arterial pressure is only 15 mm Hg, so the mean pulmonary capillary pressure must lie somewhere between these two values.

Length of Time Blood Stays in the Pulmonary Capillaries. From histological study of the total cross-sectional area of all the pulmonary capillaries, it can be calculated that when the cardiac output is normal, blood passes through the pulmonary capillaries in about 0.8 second. When the cardiac output increases, this can shorten to as little as 0.3 second. The shortening would be much greater were it not for the fact that additional capillaries, which normally are collapsed, open up to accommodate the increased blood flow. Thus, in only a fraction of a second, blood passing through the alveolar capillaries becomes oxygenated and loses its excess carbon dioxide.

Capillary Exchange of Fluid in the Lungs and Pulmonary Interstitial Fluid Dynamics

The dynamics of fluid exchange across the lung capillary membranes are *qualitatively* the same as for peripheral tissues. However, *quantitatively*, there are important differences, as follows:

1. The pulmonary capillary pressure is low, about 7 mm Hg, in comparison with a considerably higher functional capillary pressure in the peripheral tissues of about 17 mm Hg.

2. The interstitial fluid pressure in the lung is slightly more negative than that in the peripheral subcutaneous tissue. (This has been measured in two ways: by a micropipette inserted into the pulmonary interstitium, giving a value of about −5 mm Hg, and by measuring the absorption pressure of fluid from the alveoli, giving a value of about −8 mm Hg.)

3. The pulmonary capillaries are relatively leaky to protein molecules, so the colloid osmotic pressure of the pulmonary interstitial fluid is about 14 mm Hg, in comparison with less than half this value in the peripheral tissues.

4. The alveolar walls are extremely thin, and the alveolar epithelium covering the alveolar surfaces is so weak that it can be ruptured by any positive pressure in the interstitial spaces greater than alveolar air pressure (>0 mm Hg), which allows dumping of fluid from the interstitial spaces into the alveoli.

Now let us see how these quantitative differences affect pulmonary fluid dynamics.

Interrelations Between Interstitial Fluid Pressure and Other Pressures in the Lung. Figure 38-6 shows a pulmonary capillary, a pulmonary alveolus, and a lymphatic capillary draining the interstitial space between the blood capillary and the alveolus. Note the balance of forces at the blood capillary membrane, as follows:

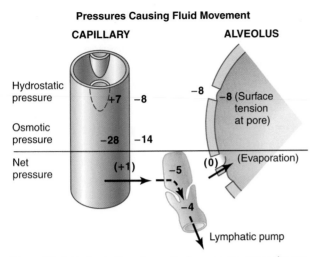

Pressures Causing Fluid Movement

Figure 38-6 Hydrostatic and osmotic forces in mm Hg at the capillary (*left*) and alveolar membrane (*right*) of the lungs. Also shown is the tip end of a lymphatic vessel (*center*) that pumps fluid from the pulmonary interstitial spaces. (Modified from Guyton AC, Taylor AE, Granger HJ: Circulatory Physiology II: Dynamics and Control of the Body Fluids. Philadelphia: WB Saunders, 1975.)

	mm Hg
Forces tending to cause movement of fluid outward from the capillaries and into the pulmonary interstitium:	
Capillary pressure	7
Interstitial fluid colloid osmotic pressure	14
Negative interstitial fluid pressure	8
TOTAL OUTWARD FORCE	29
Forces tending to cause absorption of fluid into the capillaries:	
Plasma colloid osmotic pressure	28
TOTAL INWARD FORCE	28

Thus, the normal outward forces are slightly greater than the inward forces, providing a *mean filtration pressure* at the pulmonary capillary membrane; this can be calculated as follows:

	mm Hg
Total outward force	+29
Total inward force	−28
MEAN FILTRATION PRESSURE	+1

This filtration pressure causes a slight continual flow of fluid from the pulmonary capillaries into the interstitial spaces, and except for a small amount that evaporates in the alveoli, this fluid is pumped back to the circulation through the pulmonary lymphatic system.

Negative Pulmonary Interstitial Pressure and the Mechanism for Keeping the Alveoli "Dry."

What keeps the alveoli from filling with fluid under normal conditions? One's first inclination is to think that the alveolar epithelium is strong enough and continuous enough to keep fluid from leaking out of the interstitial spaces into the alveoli. This is not true because experiments have shown that there are always openings between the alveolar epithelial cells through which even large protein molecules, as well as water and electrolytes, can pass.

However, if one remembers that the pulmonary capillaries and the pulmonary lymphatic system normally maintain a slight *negative pressure* in the interstitial spaces, it is clear that whenever extra fluid appears in the alveoli, it will simply be sucked mechanically into the lung interstitium through the small openings between the alveolar epithelial cells. Then the excess fluid is either carried away through the pulmonary lymphatics or absorbed into the pulmonary capillaries. Thus, under normal conditions, the alveoli are kept "dry," except for a small amount of fluid that seeps from the epithelium onto the lining surfaces of the alveoli to keep them moist.

Pulmonary Edema

Pulmonary edema occurs in the same way that edema occurs elsewhere in the body. Any factor that increases fluid filtration out of the pulmonary capillaries or that impedes pulmonary lymphatic function and causes the pulmonary interstitial fluid pressure to rise from the negative range into the positive range will cause rapid filling of the pulmonary interstitial spaces and alveoli with large amounts of free fluid.

The most common causes of pulmonary edema are as follows:

1. Left-sided heart failure or mitral valve disease, with consequent great increases in pulmonary venous pressure and pulmonary capillary pressure and flooding of the interstitial spaces and alveoli.
2. Damage to the pulmonary blood capillary membranes caused by infections such as pneumonia or by breathing noxious substances such as chlorine gas or sulfur dioxide gas. Each of these causes rapid leakage of both plasma proteins and fluid out of the capillaries and into both the lung interstitial spaces and the alveoli.

"Pulmonary Edema Safety Factor." Experiments in animals have shown that the pulmonary capillary pressure normally must rise to a value at least equal to the colloid osmotic pressure of the plasma inside the capillaries before significant pulmonary edema will occur. To give an example, Figure 38-7 shows how different levels of left atrial

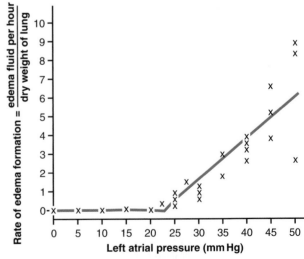

Figure 38-7 Rate of fluid loss into the lung tissues when the left atrial pressure (and pulmonary capillary pressure) is increased. (From Guyton AC, Lindsey AW: Effect of elevated left atrial pressure and decreased plasma protein concentration on the development of pulmonary edema. Circ Res 7:649, 1959.)

pressure increase the rate of pulmonary edema formation in dogs. Remember that every time the left atrial pressure rises to high values, the pulmonary capillary pressure rises to a level 1 to 2 mm Hg greater than the left atrial pressure. In these experiments, as soon as the left atrial pressure rose above 23 mm Hg (causing the pulmonary capillary pressure to rise above 25 mm Hg), fluid began to accumulate in the lungs. This fluid accumulation increased even more rapidly with further increases in capillary pressure. The plasma colloid osmotic pressure during these experiments was equal to this 25 mm Hg critical pressure level. Therefore, in the human being, whose normal plasma colloid osmotic pressure is 28 mm Hg, one can predict that the pulmonary capillary pressure must rise from the normal level of 7 mm Hg to more than 28 mm Hg to cause pulmonary edema, giving an *acute safety factor against pulmonary edema* of 21 mm Hg.

Safety Factor in Chronic Conditions. When the pulmonary capillary pressure remains elevated chronically (for at least 2 weeks), the lungs become even more resistant to pulmonary edema because the lymph vessels expand greatly, increasing their capability of carrying fluid away from the interstitial spaces perhaps as much as 10-fold. Therefore, in patients with chronic mitral stenosis, pulmonary capillary pressures of 40 to 45 mm Hg have been measured without the development of lethal pulmonary edema.

Rapidity of Death in Acute Pulmonary Edema. When the pulmonary capillary pressure rises even slightly above the safety factor level, lethal pulmonary edema can occur within hours, or even within 20 to 30 minutes if the capillary pressure rises 25 to 30 mm Hg above the safety factor level. Thus, in acute left-sided heart failure, in which the pulmonary capillary pressure occasionally does rise to 50 mm Hg, death frequently ensues in less than 30 minutes from acute pulmonary edema.

Fluid in the Pleural Cavity

When the lungs expand and contract during normal breathing, they slide back and forth within the pleural cavity. To facilitate this, a thin layer of mucoid fluid lies between the parietal and visceral pleurae.

Figure 38-8 shows the dynamics of fluid exchange in the pleural space. The pleural membrane is a porous, mesenchymal, serous membrane through which small amounts of interstitial fluid transude continually into the pleural space. These fluids carry with them tissue proteins, giving the pleural fluid a mucoid characteristic, which is what allows extremely easy slippage of the moving lungs.

The total amount of fluid in each pleural cavity is normally slight, only a few milliliters. Whenever the quantity becomes more than barely enough to begin flowing in the pleural cavity, the excess fluid is pumped away by lymphatic vessels opening directly from the pleural cavity into (1) the mediastinum, (2) the superior surface of the diaphragm, and (3) the lateral surfaces of the parietal pleura. Therefore, the *pleural space*—the space between the parietal and visceral pleurae—is called a *potential space* because it normally is so narrow that it is not obviously a physical space.

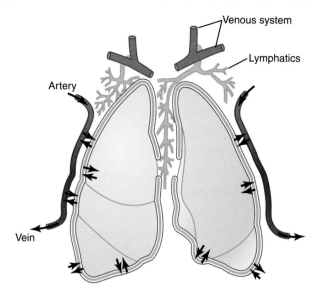

Figure 38-8 Dynamics of fluid exchange in the intrapleural space.

"Negative Pressure" in Pleural Fluid. A negative force is always required on the outside of the lungs to keep the lungs expanded. This is provided by negative pressure in the normal pleural space. The basic cause of this negative pressure is pumping of fluid from the space by the lymphatics (which is also the basis of the negative pressure found in most tissue spaces of the body). Because the normal collapse tendency of the lungs is about −4 mm Hg, the pleural fluid pressure must always be at least as negative as −4 mm Hg to keep the lungs expanded. Actual measurements have shown that the pressure is usually about −7 mm Hg, which is a few millimeters of mercury more negative than the collapse pressure of the lungs. Thus, the negativity of the pleural fluid keeps the normal lungs pulled against the parietal pleura of the chest cavity, except for an extremely thin layer of mucoid fluid that acts as a lubricant.

Pleural Effusion—Collection of Large Amounts of Free Fluid in the Pleural Space. Pleural effusion is analogous to edema fluid in the tissues and can be called "edema of the pleural cavity." The causes of the effusion are the same as the causes of edema in other tissues (discussed in Chapter 25), including (1) blockage of lymphatic drainage from the pleural cavity; (2) cardiac failure, which causes excessively high peripheral and pulmonary capillary pressures, leading to excessive transudation of fluid into the pleural cavity; (3) greatly reduced plasma colloid osmotic pressure, thus allowing excessive transudation of fluid; and (4) infection or any other cause of inflammation of the surfaces of the pleural cavity, which breaks down the capillary membranes and allows rapid dumping of both plasma proteins and fluid into the cavity.

Bibliography

Bogaard HJ, Abe K, Vonk Noordegraaf A, et al: The right ventricle under pressure: cellular and molecular mechanisms of right-heart failure in pulmonary hypertension, *Chest* 135:794, 2009.

Effros RM, Parker JC: Pulmonary vascular heterogeneity and the Starling hypothesis, *Microvasc Res* 78:71, 2009.

Effros RM, Pornsuriyasak P, Porszasz J, et al: Indicator dilution measurements of extravascular lung water: basic assumptions and observations, *Am J Physiol Lung Cell Mol Physiol* 294:L1023, 2008.

Guyton AC, Lindsey AW: Effect of elevated left atrial pressure and decreased plasma protein concentration on the development of pulmonary edema, *Circ Res* 7:649, 1959.

Guyton AC, Taylor AE, Granger HJ: *Circulatory Physiology. II. Dynamics and Control of the Body Fluids*, Philadelphia, 1975, WB Saunders.

Hoschele S, Mairbaurl H: Alveolar flooding at high altitude: failure of reabsorption? *News Physiol Sci* 18:55, 2003.

Hughes M, West JB: Gravity is the major factor determining the distribution of blood flow in the human lung, *J Appl Physiol* 104:1531, 2008.

Lai-Fook SJ: Pleural mechanics and fluid exchange, *Physiol Rev* 84:385, 2004.

Michelakis ED, Wilkins MR, Rabinovitch M: Emerging concepts and translational priorities in pulmonary arterial hypertension, *Circulation* 118:1486, 2008.

Miserocchi G, Negrini D, Passi A, et al: Development of lung edema: interstitial fluid dynamics and molecular structure, *News Physiol Sci* 16:66, 2001.

Parker JC: Hydraulic conductance of lung endothelial phenotypes and Starling safety factors against edema, *Am J Physiol Lung Cell Mol Physiol* 292:L378, 2007.

Parker JC, Townsley MI: Physiological determinants of the pulmonary filtration coefficient, *Am J Physiol Lung Cell Mol Physiol* 295:L235, 2008.

Peinado VI, Pizarro S, Barberà JA: Pulmonary vascular involvement in COPD, *Chest* 134:808, 2008.

Robertson HT, Hlastala MP: Microsphere maps of regional blood flow and regional ventilation, *J Appl Physiol* 102:1265, 2007.

West JB: *Respiratory Physiology—The Essentials*, ed 8, Baltimore, Lippincott, Williams & Wilkins, 2008.

Physical Principles of Gas Exchange; Diffusion of Oxygen and Carbon Dioxide Through the Respiratory Membrane

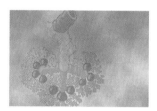

After the alveoli are ventilated with fresh air, the next step in the respiratory process is *diffusion* of oxygen from the alveoli into the pulmonary blood and diffusion of carbon dioxide in the opposite direction, out of the blood. The process of diffusion is simply the random motion of molecules in all directions through the respiratory membrane and adjacent fluids. However, in respiratory physiology, one is concerned not only with the basic mechanism by which diffusion occurs but also with the *rate* at which it occurs; this is a much more complex problem, requiring a deeper understanding of the physics of diffusion and gas exchange.

Physics of Gas Diffusion and Gas Partial Pressures

Molecular Basis of Gas Diffusion

All the gases of concern in respiratory physiology are simple molecules that are free to move among one another, a process called "diffusion." This is also true of gases dissolved in the fluids and tissues of the body.

For diffusion to occur there must be a source of energy. This is provided by the kinetic motion of the molecules themselves. Except at absolute zero temperature, all molecules of all matter are continually undergoing motion. For free molecules that are not physically attached to others, this means linear movement at high velocity until they strike other molecules. Then they bounce away in new directions and continue until striking other molecules again. In this way, the molecules move rapidly and randomly among one another.

Net Diffusion of a Gas in One Direction—Effect of a Concentration Gradient. If a gas chamber or a solution has a high concentration of a particular gas at one end of the chamber and a low concentration at the other end, as shown in Figure 39-1, net diffusion of the gas will occur from the high-concentration area toward the low-concentration area. The reason is obvious: There are far more molecules at end A of the chamber to diffuse toward end B than there are molecules to diffuse in the opposite direction. Therefore, the rates of diffusion in each of the two directions are proportionately different, as demonstrated by the lengths of the arrows in the figure.

Gas Pressures in a Mixture of Gases—"Partial Pressures" of Individual Gases

Pressure is caused by multiple impacts of moving molecules against a surface. Therefore, the pressure of a gas acting on the surfaces of the respiratory passages and alveoli is proportional to the summated force of impact of all the molecules of that gas striking the surface at any given instant. This means that *the pressure is directly proportional to the concentration of the gas molecules.*

In respiratory physiology, one deals with mixtures of gases, mainly of *oxygen, nitrogen,* and *carbon dioxide.* The rate of diffusion of each of these gases is directly proportional to the pressure caused by that gas alone, which is called the *partial pressure* of that gas. The concept of partial pressure can be explained as follows.

Consider air, which has an approximate composition of 79 percent nitrogen and 21 percent oxygen. The total pressure of this mixture at sea level averages 760 mm Hg. It is clear from the preceding description of the molecular basis of pressure that each gas contributes to the total pressure in direct proportion to its concentration. Therefore, 79 percent of the 760 mm Hg is caused by nitrogen (600 mm Hg) and 21 percent by oxygen (160 mm Hg). Thus, the "partial pressure" of nitrogen in the mixture is 600 mm Hg, and the "partial pressure" of oxygen is 160 mm Hg; the total pressure is 760 mm Hg, the sum of the individual partial pressures. The partial pressures of individual gases in a mixture are designated by the symbols P_{O_2}, P_{CO_2}, P_{N_2}, P_{He}, and so forth.

Pressures of Gases Dissolved in Water and Tissues

Gases dissolved in water or in body tissues also exert pressure because the dissolved gas molecules are moving randomly and have kinetic energy. Further, when the gas dissolved in fluid encounters a surface, such as the membrane of a cell, it exerts its own partial pressure in the same way that a gas in the gas phase does. The partial pressures of the separate dissolved gases are designated the same as the partial pressures in the gas state, that is, P_{O_2}, P_{CO_2}, P_{N_2}, P_{He}, and so forth.

Factors That Determine the Partial Pressure of a Gas Dissolved in a Fluid. The partial pressure of a gas in a solution is determined not only by its concentration but also by the *solubility coefficient* of the gas. That is, some types of molecules, especially carbon dioxide, are physically or chemically attracted to water molecules, whereas others are repelled. When molecules are attracted, far more of them can be dissolved without building up excess partial pressure

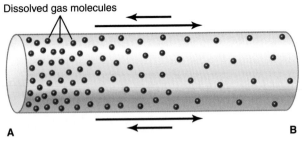

Dissolved gas molecules

A   **B**

Figure 39-1 Diffusion of oxygen from one end of a chamber (*A*) to the other (*B*). The difference between the lengths of the arrows represents *net diffusion*.

within the solution. Conversely, in the case of those that are repelled, high partial pressure will develop with fewer dissolved molecules. These relations are expressed by the following formula, which is *Henry's law:*

$$\text{Partial pressure} = \frac{\text{Concentration of dissolved gas}}{\text{Solubility coefficient}}$$

When partial pressure is expressed in atmospheres (1 atmosphere pressure equals 760 mm Hg) and concentration is expressed in volume of gas dissolved in each volume of water, the solubility coefficients for important respiratory gases at body temperature are the following:

Oxygen	0.024
Carbon dioxide	0.57
Carbon monoxide	0.018
Nitrogen	0.012
Helium	0.008

From this table, one can see that carbon dioxide is more than 20 times as soluble as oxygen. Therefore, the partial pressure of carbon dioxide (for a given concentration) is less than one-twentieth that exerted by oxygen.

Diffusion of Gases Between the Gas Phase in the Alveoli and the Dissolved Phase in the Pulmonary Blood. The partial pressure of each gas in the alveolar respiratory gas mixture tends to force molecules of that gas into solution in the blood of the alveolar capillaries. Conversely, the molecules of the same gas that are already dissolved in the blood are bouncing randomly in the fluid of the blood, and some of these bouncing molecules escape back into the alveoli. The rate at which they escape is directly proportional to their partial pressure in the blood.

But in which direction will *net diffusion* of the gas occur? The answer is that net diffusion is determined by the difference between the two partial pressures. If the partial pressure is greater in the gas phase in the alveoli, as is normally true for oxygen, then more molecules will diffuse into the blood than in the other direction. Alternatively, if the partial pressure of the gas is greater in the dissolved state in the blood, which is normally true for carbon dioxide, then net diffusion will occur toward the gas phase in the alveoli.

Vapor Pressure of Water

When nonhumidified air is breathed into the respiratory passageways, water immediately evaporates from the surfaces of these passages and humidifies the air. This results from the fact that water molecules, like the different dissolved gas molecules, are continually escaping from the water surface into the gas phase. The partial pressure that the water molecules exert to escape through the surface is called the *vapor pressure* of the water. At normal body temperature, 37°C, this vapor pressure is 47 mm Hg. Therefore, once the gas mixture has become fully humidified—that is, once it is in "equilibrium" with the water—the partial pressure of the water vapor in the gas mixture is 47 mm Hg. This partial pressure, like the other partial pressures, is designated P_{H_2O}.

The vapor pressure of water depends entirely on the temperature of the water. The greater the temperature, the greater the kinetic activity of the molecules and, therefore, the greater the likelihood that the water molecules will escape from the surface of the water into the gas phase. For instance, the water vapor pressure at 0°C is 5 mm Hg, and at 100°C it is 760 mm Hg. But the most important value to remember is the *vapor pressure at body temperature, 47 mm Hg*; this value appears in many of our subsequent discussions.

Diffusion of Gases Through Fluids—Pressure Difference Causes Net Diffusion

From the preceding discussion, it is clear that when the partial pressure of a gas is greater in one area than in another area, there will be net diffusion from the high-pressure area toward the low-pressure area. For instance, returning to Figure 39-1, one can readily see that the molecules in the area of high pressure, because of their greater number, have a greater chance of moving randomly into the area of low pressure than do molecules attempting to go in the other direction. However, some molecules do bounce randomly from the area of low pressure toward the area of high pressure. Therefore, the *net diffusion* of gas from the area of high pressure to the area of low pressure is equal to the number of molecules bouncing in this forward direction *minus* the number bouncing in the opposite direction; this is proportional to the gas partial pressure difference between the two areas, called simply the *pressure difference for causing diffusion.*

Quantifying the Net Rate of Diffusion in Fluids. In addition to the pressure difference, several other factors affect the rate of gas diffusion in a fluid. They are (1) the solubility of the gas in the fluid, (2) the cross-sectional area of the fluid, (3) the distance through which the gas must diffuse, (4) the molecular weight of the gas, and (5) the temperature of the fluid. In the body, the last of these factors, the temperature, remains reasonably constant and usually need not be considered.

The greater the solubility of the gas, the greater the number of molecules available to diffuse for any given partial pressure difference. The greater the cross-sectional area of the diffusion pathway, the greater the total number of molecules that diffuse. Conversely, the greater the distance the molecules must diffuse, the longer it will take the molecules to diffuse the entire distance. Finally, the greater the velocity of kinetic movement of the molecules, which is inversely proportional to the square root of the molecular weight, the greater the rate of diffusion of the gas. All these factors can be expressed in a single formula, as follows:

$$D \propto \frac{\Delta P \times A \times S}{d \times \sqrt{MW}},$$

in which D is the diffusion rate, ΔP is the partial pressure difference between the two ends of the diffusion pathway, A is the cross-sectional area of the pathway, S is the solubility of the gas, d is the distance of diffusion, and MW is the molecular weight of the gas.

It is obvious from this formula that the characteristics of the gas itself determine two factors of the formula: solubility and molecular weight. Together, these two factors determine the *diffusion coefficient of the gas*, which is proportional to $S/\sqrt{MW}$ that is, the relative rates at which different gases at the same partial pressure levels will diffuse are proportional to their diffusion coefficients. Assuming that the diffusion coefficient for oxygen is 1, the *relative* diffusion coefficients for different gases of respiratory importance in the body fluids are as follows:

Oxygen	1.0
Carbon dioxide	20.3
Carbon monoxide	0.81
Nitrogen	0.53
Helium	0.95

Diffusion of Gases Through Tissues

The gases that are of respiratory importance are all highly soluble in lipids and, consequently, are highly soluble in cell membranes. Because of this, the major limitation to the movement of gases in tissues is the rate at which the gases can diffuse through the tissue water instead of through the cell membranes. Therefore, diffusion of gases through the tissues, including through the respiratory membrane, is almost equal to the diffusion of gases in water, as given in the preceding list.

Compositions of Alveolar Air and Atmospheric Air Are Different

Alveolar air does not have the same concentrations of gases as atmospheric air by any means, which can readily be seen by comparing the alveolar air composition in Table 39-1 with that of atmospheric air. There are several reasons for the differences. First, the alveolar air is only partially replaced by atmospheric air with each breath. Second, oxygen is constantly being absorbed into the pulmonary blood from the alveolar air. Third, carbon dioxide is constantly diffusing from the pulmonary

blood into the alveoli. And fourth, dry atmospheric air that enters the respiratory passages is humidified even before it reaches the alveoli.

Humidification of the Air in the Respiratory Passages. Table 39-1 shows that atmospheric air is composed almost entirely of nitrogen and oxygen; it normally contains almost no carbon dioxide and little water vapor. However, as soon as the atmospheric air enters the respiratory passages, it is exposed to the fluids that cover the respiratory surfaces. Even before the air enters the alveoli, it becomes (for all practical purposes) totally humidified.

The partial pressure of water vapor at a normal body temperature of 37°C is 47 mm Hg, which is therefore the partial pressure of water vapor in the alveolar air. Because the total pressure in the alveoli cannot rise to more than the atmospheric pressure (760 mm Hg at sea level), this water vapor simply *dilutes* all the other gases in the inspired air. Table 39-1 also shows that humidification of the air dilutes the oxygen partial pressure at sea level from an average of 159 mm Hg in atmospheric air to 149 mm Hg in the humidified air, and it dilutes the nitrogen partial pressure from 597 to 563 mm Hg.

Rate at Which Alveolar Air Is Renewed by Atmospheric Air

In Chapter 37, it was pointed out that the average male *functional residual capacity* of the lungs (the volume of air remaining in the lungs at the end of normal expiration) measures about 2300 milliliters. Yet only 350 milliliters of new air is brought into the alveoli with each normal inspiration, and this same amount of old alveolar air is expired. Therefore, the volume of alveolar air replaced by new atmospheric air with each breath is only one seventh of the total, so multiple breaths are required to exchange most of the alveolar air. Figure 39-2 shows this slow rate of renewal of the alveolar air. In the first alveolus of the figure, excess gas is present in the alveoli, but note that even at the end of 16 breaths, the excess gas still has not been completely removed from the alveoli.

Figure 39-3 demonstrates graphically the rate at which excess gas in the alveoli is normally removed, showing that with normal alveolar ventilation, about one-half the gas is

Table 39-1 Partial Pressures of Respiratory Gases as They Enter and Leave the Lungs (at Sea Level)

	Atmospheric Air* (mm Hg)		Humidified Air (mm Hg)		Alveolar Air (mm Hg)		Expired Air (mm Hg)	
N_2	597.0	(78.62%)	563.4	(74.09%)	569.0	(74.9%)	566.0	(74.5%)
O_2	159.0	(20.84%)	149.3	(19.67%)	104.0	(13.6%)	120.0	(15.7%)
CO_2	0.3	(0.04%)	0.3	(0.04%)	40.0	(5.3%)	27.0	(3.6%)
H_2O	3.7	(0.50%)	47.0	(6.20%)	47.0	(6.2%)	47.0	(6.2%)
TOTAL	760.0	(100.0%)	760.0	(100.0%)	760.0	(100.0%)	760.0	(100.0%)

*On an average cool, clear day.

487

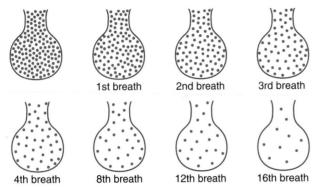

Figure 39-2 Expiration of a gas from an alveolus with successive breaths.

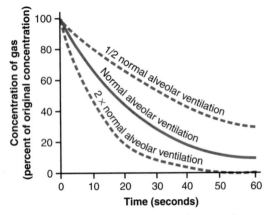

Figure 39-3 Rate of removal of excess gas from alveoli.

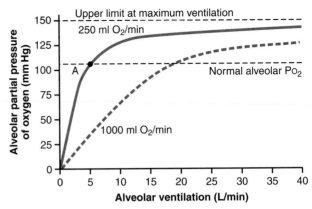

Figure 39-4 Effect of alveolar ventilation on the alveolar P_{O_2} at two rates of oxygen absorption from the alveoli—250 ml/min and 1000 ml/min. *Point A* is the normal operating point.

removed in 17 seconds. When a person's rate of alveolar ventilation is only one-half normal, one-half the gas is removed in 34 seconds, and when the rate of ventilation is twice normal, one half is removed in about 8 seconds.

Importance of the Slow Replacement of Alveolar Air.

The slow replacement of alveolar air is of particular importance in preventing sudden changes in gas concentrations in the blood. This makes the respiratory control mechanism much more stable than it would be otherwise, and it helps prevent excessive increases and decreases in tissue oxygenation, tissue carbon dioxide concentration, and tissue pH when respiration is temporarily interrupted.

Oxygen Concentration and Partial Pressure in the Alveoli

Oxygen is continually being absorbed from the alveoli into the blood of the lungs, and new oxygen is continually being breathed into the alveoli from the atmosphere. The more rapidly oxygen is absorbed, the lower its concentration in the alveoli becomes; conversely, the more rapidly new oxygen is breathed into the alveoli from the atmosphere, the higher its concentration becomes. Therefore, oxygen concentration in the alveoli, as well as its partial pressure, is controlled by (1) the rate of absorption of oxygen into the blood and (2) the rate of entry of new oxygen into the lungs by the ventilatory process.

Figure 39-4 shows the effect of both alveolar ventilation and rate of oxygen absorption into the blood on the alveolar partial pressure of oxygen (P_{O_2}). One curve represents oxygen absorption at a rate of 250 ml/min, and the other curve represents a rate of 1000 ml/min. At a normal ventilatory rate of 4.2 L/min and an oxygen consumption of 250 ml/min, the normal operating point in Figure 39-4 is point A. The figure also shows that when 1000 milliliters of oxygen is being absorbed each minute, as occurs during moderate exercise, the rate of alveolar ventilation must increase fourfold to maintain the alveolar P_{O_2} at the normal value of 104 mm Hg.

Another effect shown in Figure 39-4 is that an extremely marked increase in alveolar ventilation can never increase the alveolar P_{O_2} above 149 mm Hg as long as the person is breathing normal atmospheric air at sea level pressure, because this is the maximum P_{O_2} in humidified air at this pressure. If the person breathes gases that contain partial pressures of oxygen higher than 149 mm Hg, the alveolar P_{O_2} can approach these higher pressures at high rates of ventilation.

CO_2 Concentration and Partial Pressure in the Alveoli

Carbon dioxide is continually being formed in the body and then carried in the blood to the alveoli; it is continually being removed from the alveoli by ventilation. Figure 39-5 shows the effects on the alveolar partial pressure of carbon dioxide (P_{CO_2}) of both alveolar ventilation and two rates of carbon dioxide excretion, 200 and 800 ml/min. One curve represents a normal rate of carbon dioxide excretion of 200 ml/min. At the normal rate of alveolar ventilation of 4.2 L/min, the operating point for alveolar P_{CO_2} is at point A in Figure 39-5 (i.e., 40 mm Hg).

Two other facts are also evident from Figure 39-5: First, *the alveolar P_{CO_2} increases directly in proportion to the rate of carbon dioxide excretion*, as represented by the fourfold elevation of the curve (when 800 milliliters of CO_2 are excreted per minute). Second, *the alveolar P_{CO_2} decreases in inverse proportion to alveolar ventilation.*

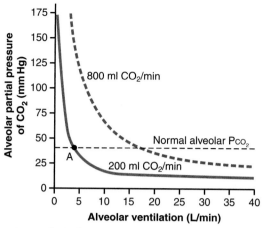

Figure 39-5 Effect of alveolar ventilation on the alveolar P_{CO_2} at two rates of carbon dioxide excretion from the blood—800 ml/min and 200 ml/min. *Point A* is the normal operating point.

Therefore, the concentrations and partial pressures of both oxygen and carbon dioxide in the alveoli are determined by the rates of absorption or excretion of the two gases and by the amount of alveolar ventilation.

Expired Air Is a Combination of Dead Space Air and Alveolar Air

The overall composition of expired air is determined by (1) the amount of the expired air that is dead space air and (2) the amount that is alveolar air. Figure 39-6 shows the progressive changes in oxygen and carbon dioxide partial pressures in the expired air during the course of expiration. The first portion of this air, the dead space air from the respiratory passageways, is typical humidified air, as shown in Table 39-1. Then, progressively more and more alveolar air becomes mixed with the dead space air until all the dead space air has finally been washed out and nothing but alveolar air is expired at the end of expiration. Therefore, the method of collecting alveolar air for study is simply to collect a sample of the last portion of the expired air after forceful expiration has removed all the dead space air.

Normal expired air, containing both dead space air and alveolar air, has gas concentrations and partial pressures

approximately as shown in Table 39-1 (i.e., concentrations between those of alveolar air and humidified atmospheric air).

Diffusion of Gases Through the Respiratory Membrane

Respiratory Unit. Figure 39-7 shows the *respiratory unit* (also called "respiratory lobule"), which is composed of a *respiratory bronchiole, alveolar ducts, atria,* and *alveoli.* There are about 300 million alveoli in the two lungs, and each alveolus has an average diameter of about 0.2 millimeter. The alveolar walls are extremely thin, and between the alveoli is an almost solid network of interconnecting capillaries, shown in Figure 39-8. Indeed, because of the extensiveness of the capillary plexus, the flow of blood in the alveolar wall has been described as a "sheet" of flowing blood. Thus, it is obvious that the alveolar gases are in very close proximity to the blood of the pulmonary capillaries. Further, gas exchange between the alveolar air and the pulmonary blood occurs through the membranes of all the terminal portions of the lungs, not merely in the alveoli themselves. All these membranes are collectively known as the *respiratory membrane,* also called the *pulmonary membrane.*

Respiratory Membrane. Figure 39-9 shows the ultrastructure of the respiratory membrane drawn in cross section on the left and a red blood cell on the right. It also shows the diffusion of oxygen from the alveolus into the red blood cell and diffusion of carbon dioxide in

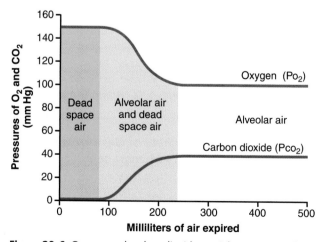

Figure 39-6 Oxygen and carbon dioxide partial pressures in the various portions of normal expired air.

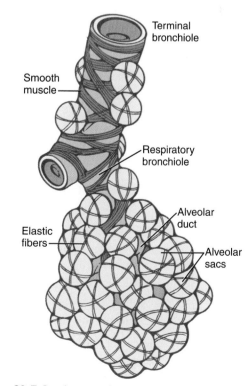

Figure 39-7 Respiratory unit.

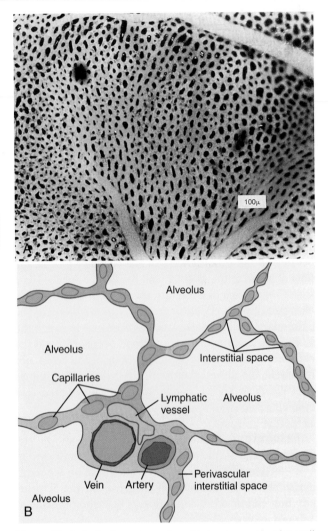

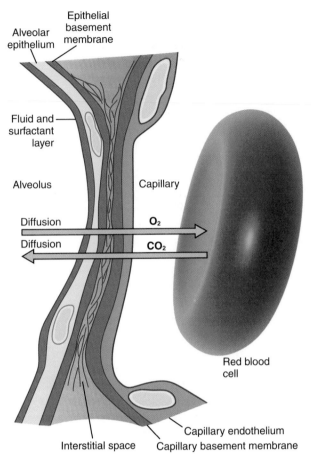

Figure 39-9 Ultrastructure of the alveolar respiratory membrane, shown in cross section.

Figure 39-8 *A,* Surface view of capillaries in an alveolar wall. *B,* Cross-sectional view of alveolar walls and their vascular supply. (*A,* From Maloney JE, Castle BL: Pressure-diameter relations of capillaries and small blood vessels in frog lung. Respir Physiol 7:150, 1969. Reproduced by permission of ASP Biological and Medical Press, North-Holland Division.)

the opposite direction. Note the following different layers of the respiratory membrane:

1. A layer of fluid lining the alveolus and containing surfactant that reduces the surface tension of the alveolar fluid

2. The alveolar epithelium composed of thin epithelial cells

3. An epithelial basement membrane

4. A thin interstitial space between the alveolar epithelium and the capillary membrane

5. A capillary basement membrane that in many places fuses with the alveolar epithelial basement membrane

6. The capillary endothelial membrane

Despite the large number of layers, the overall thickness of the respiratory membrane in some areas is as little as 0.2 micrometer, and it averages about 0.6 micrometer, except where there are cell nuclei. From histological

studies, it has been estimated that the total surface area of the respiratory membrane is about 70 square meters in the normal adult human male. This is equivalent to the floor area of a 25-by-30-foot room. The total quantity of blood in the capillaries of the lungs at any given instant is 60 to 140 milliliters. Now imagine this small amount of blood spread over the entire surface of a 25-by-30-foot floor, and it is easy to understand the rapidity of the respiratory exchange of oxygen and carbon dioxide.

The average diameter of the pulmonary capillaries is only about 5 micrometers, which means that red blood cells must squeeze through them. The red blood cell membrane usually touches the capillary wall, so oxygen and carbon dioxide need not pass through significant amounts of plasma as they diffuse between the alveolus and the red cell. This, too, increases the rapidity of diffusion.

Factors That Affect the Rate of Gas Diffusion Through the Respiratory Membrane

Referring to the earlier discussion of diffusion of gases in water, one can apply the same principles and mathematical formulas to diffusion of gases through the respiratory membrane. Thus, the factors that determine how rapidly a gas will pass through the membrane are (1) the *thickness of the membrane,* (2) the *surface area of the membrane,*

(3) the *diffusion coefficient* of the gas in the substance of the membrane, and (4) the *partial pressure difference* of the gas between the two sides of the membrane.

The *thickness of the respiratory membrane* occasionally increases—for instance, as a result of edema fluid in the interstitial space of the membrane and in the alveoli—so the respiratory gases must then diffuse not only through the membrane but also through this fluid. Also, some pulmonary diseases cause fibrosis of the lungs, which can increase the thickness of some portions of the respiratory membrane. Because the rate of diffusion through the membrane is inversely proportional to the thickness of the membrane, any factor that increases the thickness to more than two to three times normal can interfere significantly with normal respiratory exchange of gases.

The *surface area of the respiratory membrane* can be greatly decreased by many conditions. For instance, removal of an entire lung decreases the total surface area to one half normal. Also, in *emphysema*, many of the alveoli coalesce, with dissolution of many alveolar walls. Therefore, the new alveolar chambers are much larger than the original alveoli, but the total surface area of the respiratory membrane is often decreased as much as fivefold because of loss of the alveolar walls. When the total surface area is decreased to about one-third to one-fourth normal, exchange of gases through the membrane is impeded to a significant degree, *even under resting conditions*, and during competitive sports and other strenuous exercise even the slightest decrease in surface area of the lungs can be a serious detriment to respiratory exchange of gases.

The *diffusion coefficient* for transfer of each gas through the respiratory membrane depends on the gas's *solubility* in the membrane and, inversely, on the *square root* of the gas's *molecular weight*. The rate of diffusion in the respiratory membrane is almost exactly the same as that in water, for reasons explained earlier. Therefore, for a given pressure difference, carbon dioxide diffuses about 20 times as rapidly as oxygen. Oxygen diffuses about twice as rapidly as nitrogen.

The *pressure difference* across the respiratory membrane is the difference between the partial pressure of the gas in the alveoli and the partial pressure of the gas in the pulmonary capillary blood. The partial pressure represents a measure of the total number of molecules of a particular gas striking a unit area of the alveolar surface of the membrane in unit time, and the pressure of the gas in the blood represents the number of molecules that attempt to escape from the blood in the opposite direction. Therefore, the difference between these two pressures is a measure of the *net tendency* for the gas molecules to move through the membrane.

When the partial pressure of a gas in the alveoli is greater than the pressure of the gas in the blood, as is true for oxygen, net diffusion from the alveoli into the blood occurs; when the pressure of the gas in the blood is greater than the partial pressure in the alveoli, as is true for carbon dioxide, net diffusion from the blood into the alveoli occurs.

Diffusing Capacity of the Respiratory Membrane

The ability of the respiratory membrane to exchange a gas between the alveoli and the pulmonary blood is expressed in quantitative terms by the *respiratory membrane's diffusing capacity*, which is defined as the *volume of a gas that will diffuse through the membrane each minute for a partial pressure difference of 1 mm Hg*. All the factors discussed earlier that affect diffusion through the respiratory membrane can affect this diffusing capacity.

Diffusing Capacity for Oxygen. In the average young man, the *diffusing capacity for oxygen* under resting conditions averages *21 ml/min/mm Hg*. In functional terms, what does this mean? The mean oxygen pressure difference across the respiratory membrane during normal, quiet breathing is about 11 mm Hg. Multiplication of this pressure by the diffusing capacity (11 × 21) gives a total of about 230 milliliters of oxygen diffusing through the respiratory membrane each minute; this is equal to the rate at which the resting body uses oxygen.

Increased Oxygen Diffusing Capacity During Exercise. During strenuous exercise or other conditions that greatly increase pulmonary blood flow and alveolar ventilation, the diffusing capacity for oxygen increases in young men to a maximum of about 65 ml/min/mm Hg, which is three times the diffusing capacity under resting conditions. This increase is caused by several factors, among which are (1) opening up of many previously dormant pulmonary capillaries or extra dilation of already open capillaries, thereby increasing the surface area of the blood into which the oxygen can diffuse; and (2) a better match between the ventilation of the alveoli and the perfusion of the alveolar capillaries with blood, called the *ventilation-perfusion ratio*, which is explained in detail later in this chapter. Therefore, during exercise, oxygenation of the blood is increased not only by increased alveolar ventilation but also by greater diffusing capacity of the respiratory membrane for transporting oxygen into the blood.

Diffusing Capacity for Carbon Dioxide. The diffusing capacity for carbon dioxide has never been measured because of the following technical difficulty: Carbon dioxide diffuses through the respiratory membrane so rapidly that the average P_{CO_2} in the pulmonary blood is not far different from the P_{CO_2} in the alveoli—the average difference is less than 1 mm Hg—and with the available techniques, this difference is too small to be measured.

Nevertheless, measurements of diffusion of other gases have shown that the diffusing capacity varies directly with the diffusion coefficient of the particular gas. Because the diffusion coefficient of carbon dioxide is slightly more than 20 times that of oxygen, one would expect a diffusing capacity for carbon dioxide under resting conditions of about 400 to 450 ml/min/mm Hg and during exercise of about 1200 to 1300 ml/min/mm Hg. Figure 39-10

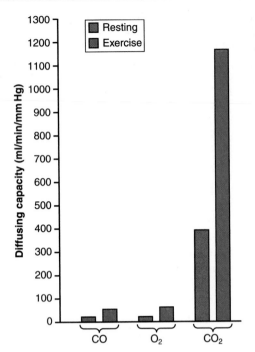

Figure 39-10 *Diffusing capacities* for carbon monoxide, oxygen, and carbon dioxide in the normal lungs under resting conditions and during exercise.

compares the measured or calculated diffusing capacities of carbon monoxide, oxygen, and carbon dioxide at rest and during exercise, showing the extreme diffusing capacity of carbon dioxide and the effect of exercise on the diffusing capacity of each of these gases.

Measurement of Diffusing Capacity—the Carbon Monoxide Method. The oxygen diffusing capacity can be calculated from measurements of (1) alveolar P_{O_2}, (2) P_{O_2} in the pulmonary capillary blood, and (3) the rate of oxygen uptake by the blood. However, measuring the P_{O_2} in the pulmonary capillary blood is so difficult and so imprecise that it is not practical to measure oxygen diffusing capacity by such a direct procedure, except on an experimental basis.

To obviate the difficulties encountered in measuring oxygen diffusing capacity directly, physiologists usually measure carbon monoxide diffusing capacity instead and then calculate the oxygen diffusing capacity from this. The principle of the carbon monoxide method is the following: A small amount of carbon monoxide is breathed into the alveoli, and the partial pressure of the carbon monoxide in the alveoli is measured from appropriate alveolar air samples. The carbon monoxide pressure in the blood is essentially zero because hemoglobin combines with this gas so rapidly that its pressure never has time to build up. Therefore, the pressure difference of carbon monoxide across the respiratory membrane is equal to its partial pressure in the alveolar air sample. Then, by measuring the volume of carbon monoxide absorbed in a short period and dividing this by the alveolar carbon monoxide partial pressure, one can determine accurately the carbon monoxide diffusing capacity.

To convert carbon monoxide diffusing capacity to oxygen diffusing capacity, the value is multiplied by a factor of 1.23 because the diffusion coefficient for oxygen is 1.23 times that for carbon monoxide. Thus, the average diffusing capacity for carbon monoxide in young men at rest is 17 ml/min/mm Hg, and the diffusing capacity for oxygen is 1.23 times this, or 21 ml/min/mm Hg.

Effect of the Ventilation-Perfusion Ratio on Alveolar Gas Concentration

In the early part of this chapter, we learned that two factors determine the P_{O_2} and the P_{CO_2} in the alveoli: (1) the rate of alveolar ventilation and (2) the rate of transfer of oxygen and carbon dioxide through the respiratory membrane. These earlier discussions made the assumption that all the alveoli are ventilated equally and that blood flow through the alveolar capillaries is the same for each alveolus. However, even normally to some extent, and especially in many lung diseases, some areas of the lungs are well ventilated but have almost no blood flow, whereas other areas may have excellent blood flow but little or no ventilation. In either of these conditions, gas exchange through the respiratory membrane is seriously impaired, and the person may suffer severe respiratory distress despite both normal *total* ventilation and normal *total* pulmonary blood flow, but with the ventilation and blood flow going to different parts of the lungs. Therefore, a highly quantitative concept has been developed to help us understand respiratory exchange when there is imbalance between alveolar ventilation and alveolar blood flow. This concept is called the *ventilation-perfusion ratio*.

In quantitative terms, the ventilation-perfusion ratio is expressed as $\dot{V}_A/\dot{Q}$. When $\dot{V}_A$ (alveolar ventilation) is normal for a given alveolus and $\dot{Q}$ (blood flow) is also normal for the same alveolus, the ventilation-perfusion ratio ($\dot{V}_A/\dot{Q}$) is also said to be normal. When the ventilation ($\dot{V}_A$) is zero, yet there is still perfusion ($\dot{Q}$) of the alveolus, the $\dot{V}_A/\dot{Q}$ is zero. Or, at the other extreme, when there is adequate ventilation ($\dot{V}_A$) but zero perfusion ($\dot{Q}$), the ratio $\dot{V}_A/\dot{Q}$ is infinity. At a ratio of either zero or infinity, there is no exchange of gases through the respiratory membrane of the affected alveoli, which explains the importance of this concept. Therefore, let us explain the respiratory consequences of these two extremes.

Alveolar Oxygen and Carbon Dioxide Partial Pressures When $\dot{V}_A/\dot{Q}$ Equals Zero. When $\dot{V}_A/\dot{Q}$ is equal to zero—that is, without any alveolar ventilation—the air in the alveolus comes to equilibrium with the blood oxygen and carbon dioxide because these gases diffuse between the blood and the alveolar air. Because the blood that perfuses the capillaries is venous blood returning to the lungs from the systemic circulation, it is the gases in this blood with which the alveolar gases equilibrate. In Chapter 40, we describe how the normal venous blood ($\bar{v}$) has a P_{O_2} of 40 mm Hg and a P_{CO_2} of 45 mm Hg. Therefore, these are also the normal partial pressures of these two gases in alveoli that have blood flow but no ventilation.

Alveolar Oxygen and Carbon Dioxide Partial Pressures When $\dot{V}_A/\dot{Q}$ Equals Infinity. The effect on the alveolar gas partial pressures when $\dot{V}_A/\dot{Q}$ equals infinity is entirely different from the effect when $\dot{V}_A/\dot{Q}$ equals zero because now there is no capillary blood flow to carry oxygen away or to bring carbon dioxide to the alveoli. Therefore, instead of the alveolar gases coming to equilibrium with the venous blood, the alveolar air becomes equal to the humidified inspired air.

That is, the air that is inspired loses no oxygen to the blood and gains no carbon dioxide from the blood. And because normal inspired and humidified air has a P_{O_2} of 149 mm Hg and a P_{CO_2} of 0 mm Hg, these will be the partial pressures of these two gases in the alveoli.

Gas Exchange and Alveolar Partial Pressures When $\dot{V}_A/\dot{Q}$ Is Normal. When there is both normal alveolar ventilation and normal alveolar capillary blood flow (normal alveolar perfusion), exchange of oxygen and carbon dioxide through the respiratory membrane is nearly optimal, and alveolar P_{O_2} is normally at a level of 104 mm Hg, which lies between that of the inspired air (149 mm Hg) and that of venous blood (40 mm Hg). Likewise, alveolar P_{CO_2} lies between two extremes; it is normally 40 mm Hg, in contrast to 45 mm Hg in venous blood and 0 mm Hg in inspired air. Thus, under normal conditions, the alveolar air P_{O_2} averages 104 mm Hg and the P_{CO_2} averages 40 mm Hg.

P_{O_2}-P_{CO_2}, $\dot{V}_A/\dot{Q}$ Diagram

The concepts presented in the preceding sections can be shown in graphical form, as demonstrated in Figure 39-11, called the P_{O_2}-P_{CO_2}, $\dot{V}_A/\dot{Q}$ diagram. The curve in the diagram represents all possible P_{O_2} and P_{CO_2} combinations between the limits of $\dot{V}_A/\dot{Q}$ equals zero and $\dot{V}_A/\dot{Q}$ equals infinity when the gas pressures in the venous blood are normal and the person is breathing air at sea-level pressure. Thus, point $\bar{v}$ is the plot of P_{O_2} and P_{CO_2} when $\dot{V}_A/\dot{Q}$ equals zero. At this point, the P_{O_2} is 40 mm Hg and the P_{CO_2} is 45 mm Hg, which are the values in normal venous blood.

At the other end of the curve, when $\dot{V}_A/\dot{Q}$ equals infinity, point I represents inspired air, showing P_{O_2} to be 149 mm Hg while P_{CO_2} is zero. Also plotted on the curve is the point that represents normal alveolar air when $\dot{V}_A/\dot{Q}$ is normal. At this point, P_{O_2} is 104 mm Hg and P_{CO_2} is 40 mm Hg.

Concept of "Physiologic Shunt" (When $\dot{V}_A/\dot{Q}$ Is Below Normal)

Whenever $\dot{V}_A/\dot{Q}$ is below normal, there is inadequate ventilation to provide the oxygen needed to fully oxygenate the blood flowing through the alveolar capillaries. Therefore, a certain fraction of the venous blood passing through the pulmonary capillaries does not become oxygenated. This fraction is called *shunted blood*. Also, some additional blood flows through bronchial vessels rather than through alveolar

capillaries, normally about 2 percent of the cardiac output; this, too, is unoxygenated, shunted blood.

The total quantitative amount of shunted blood per minute is called the *physiologic shunt*. This physiologic shunt is measured in clinical pulmonary function laboratories by analyzing the concentration of oxygen in both mixed venous blood and arterial blood, along with simultaneous measurement of cardiac output. From these values, the physiologic shunt can be calculated by the following equation:

$$\frac{\dot{Q}_{PS}}{\dot{Q}_T} = \frac{Ci_{O_2} - Ca_{O_2}}{Ci_{O_2} - C\bar{v}_{O_2}}.$$

in which $\dot{Q}_{PS}$ is the physiologic shunt blood flow per minute, $\dot{Q}_T$ is cardiac output per minute, Ci_{O_2} is the concentration of oxygen in the arterial blood if there is an "ideal" ventilation-perfusion ratio, Ca_{O_2} is the measured concentration of oxygen in the arterial blood, and $C\bar{v}_{O_2}$ is the measured concentration of oxygen in the mixed venous blood.

The greater the physiologic shunt, the greater the *amount of blood that fails to be oxygenated* as it passes through the lungs.

Concept of the "Physiologic Dead Space" (When $\dot{V}_A/\dot{Q}$ Is Greater Than Normal)

When ventilation of some of the alveoli is great but alveolar blood flow is low, there is far more available oxygen in the alveoli than can be transported away from the alveoli by the flowing blood. Thus, the ventilation of these alveoli is said to be *wasted*. The ventilation of the anatomical dead space areas of the respiratory passageways is also wasted. The sum of these two types of wasted ventilation is called the *physiologic dead space*. This is measured in the clinical pulmonary function laboratory by making appropriate blood and expiratory gas measurements and using the following equation, called the Bohr equation:

$$\frac{\dot{V}_{D_{phys}}}{\dot{V}_T} = \frac{Pa_{CO_2} - P\bar{e}_{CO_2}}{Pa_{CO_2}},$$

in which $\dot{V}_{D_{phys}}$ is the physiologic dead space, $\dot{V}_T$ is the tidal volume, Pa_{CO_2} is the partial pressure of carbon dioxide in the arterial blood, and $P\bar{e}_{CO_2}$ is the average partial pressure of carbon dioxide in the entire expired air.

When the physiologic dead space is great, much of the *work of ventilation* is wasted effort because so much of the ventilating air never reaches the blood.

Abnormalities of Ventilation-Perfusion Ratio

Abnormal $\dot{V}_A/\dot{Q}$ in the Upper and Lower Normal Lung. In a normal person in the upright position, both pulmonary capillary blood flow and alveolar ventilation are considerably less in the upper part of the lung than in the lower part; however, blood flow is decreased considerably more than ventilation is. Therefore, at the top of the lung, $\dot{V}_A/\dot{Q}$ is as much as 2.5 times as great as the ideal value, which causes a moderate degree of *physiologic dead space* in this area of the lung.

At the other extreme, in the bottom of the lung, there is slightly too little ventilation in relation to blood flow, with $\dot{V}_A/\dot{Q}$ as low as 0.6 times the ideal value. In this area, a small fraction of the blood fails to become normally oxygenated, and this represents a *physiologic shunt*.

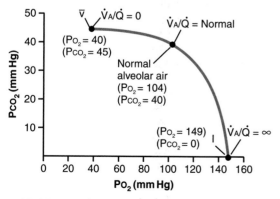

Figure 39-11 Normal P_{O_2}-P_{CO_2}, $\dot{V}_A/\dot{Q}$ diagram.

In both extremes, inequalities of ventilation and perfusion decrease slightly the lung's effectiveness for exchanging oxygen and carbon dioxide. However, during exercise, blood flow to the upper part of the lung increases markedly, so far less physiologic dead space occurs, and the effectiveness of gas exchange now approaches optimum.

Abnormal $\dot{V}_A/\dot{Q}$ in Chronic Obstructive Lung Disease. Most people who smoke for many years develop various degrees of bronchial obstruction; in a large share of these persons, this condition eventually becomes so severe that they develop serious alveolar air trapping and resultant *emphysema*. The emphysema in turn causes many of the alveolar walls to be destroyed. Thus, two abnormalities occur in smokers to cause abnormal $\dot{V}_A/\dot{Q}$. First, because many of the small bronchioles are obstructed, the alveoli beyond the obstructions are unventilated, causing a $\dot{V}_A/\dot{Q}$ that approaches zero. Second, in those areas of the lung where the alveolar walls have been mainly destroyed but there is still alveolar ventilation, most of the ventilation is wasted because of inadequate blood flow to transport the blood gases.

Thus, in chronic obstructive lung disease, some areas of the lung exhibit *serious physiologic shunt*, and other areas exhibit *serious physiologic dead space*. Both conditions tremendously decrease the effectiveness of the lungs as gas exchange organs, sometimes reducing their effectiveness to as little as one-tenth normal. In fact, this is the most prevalent cause of pulmonary disability today.

Bibliography

Albert R, Spiro S, Jett J: *Comprehensive Respiratory Medicine*, Philadelphia, 2002, Mosby.

Guazzi M: Alveolar-capillary membrane dysfunction in heart failure: evidence of a pathophysiologic role, *Chest* 124:1090, 2003.

Hughes JM: Assessing gas exchange, *Chron Respir Dis* 4:205, 2007.

Hopkins SR, Levin DL, Emami K, et al: Advances in magnetic resonance imaging of lung physiology, *J Appl Physiol* 102:1244, 2007.

MacIntyre NR: Mechanisms of functional loss in patients with chronic lung disease, *Respir Care* 53:1177, 2008.

Moon RE, Cherry AD, Stolp BW, et al: Pulmonary gas exchange in diving, *J Appl Physiol* 106:668, 2009.

Otis AB: Quantitative relationships in steady-state gas exchange. In Fenn WQ, Rahn H, eds. *Handbook of Physiology*, Sec 3, vol 1, Baltimore, 1964, Williams & Wilkins, pp 681.

Powell FL, Hopkins SR: Comparative physiology of lung complexity: implications for gas exchange, *News Physiol Sci* 19:55, 2004.

Rahn H, Farhi EE: Ventilation, perfusion, and gas exchange-the Va/Q concept. In Fenn WO, Rahn H, eds. *Handbook of Physiology*, Sec 3, vol 1, Baltimore, 1964, Williams & Wilkins, pp 125.

Robertson HT, Hlastala MP: Microsphere maps of regional blood flow and regional ventilation, *J Appl Physiol* 102:1265, 2007.

Wagner PD: Assessment of gas exchange in lung disease: balancing accuracy against feasibility, *Crit Care* 11:182, 2007.

Wagner PD: The multiple inert gas elimination technique (MIGET), *Intensive Care Med* 34:994, 2008.

West JB: *Pulmonary Physiology-The Essentials*, Baltimore, 2003, Lippincott Williams & Wilkins.

Transport of Oxygen and Carbon Dioxide in Blood and Tissue Fluids

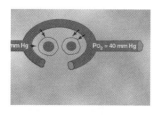

Once *oxygen* has diffused from the alveoli into the pulmonary blood, it is transported to the peripheral tissue capillaries almost entirely in combination with hemoglobin. The presence of hemoglobin in the red blood cells allows the blood to transport 30 to 100 times as much oxygen as could be transported in the form of dissolved oxygen in the water of the blood.

In the body's tissue cells, oxygen reacts with various foodstuffs to form large quantities of *carbon dioxide*. This carbon dioxide enters the tissue capillaries and is transported back to the lungs. Carbon dioxide, like oxygen, also combines with chemical substances in the blood that increase carbon dioxide transport 15- to 20-fold.

The purpose of this chapter is to present both qualitatively and quantitatively the physical and chemical principles of oxygen and carbon dioxide transport in the blood and tissue fluids.

Transport of Oxygen from the Lungs to the Body Tissues

In Chapter 39, we pointed out that gases can move from one point to another by diffusion and that the cause of this movement is always a partial pressure difference from the first point to the next. Thus, oxygen diffuses from the alveoli into the pulmonary capillary blood because the oxygen partial pressure (P_{O_2}) in the alveoli is greater than the P_{O_2} in the pulmonary capillary blood. In the other tissues of the body, a higher P_{O_2} in the capillary blood than in the tissues causes oxygen to diffuse into the surrounding cells.

Conversely, when oxygen is metabolized in the cells to form carbon dioxide, the intracellular carbon dioxide pressure (P_{CO_2}) rises to a high value, which causes carbon dioxide to diffuse into the tissue capillaries. After blood flows to the lungs, the carbon dioxide diffuses out of the blood into the alveoli, because the P_{CO_2} in the pulmonary capillary blood is greater than that in the alveoli.

Thus, the transport of oxygen and carbon dioxide by the blood depends on both diffusion and the flow of blood. We now consider quantitatively the factors responsible for these effects.

Diffusion of Oxygen from the Alveoli to the Pulmonary Capillary Blood

The top part of Figure 40-1 shows a pulmonary alveolus adjacent to a pulmonary capillary, demonstrating diffusion of oxygen molecules between the alveolar air and the pulmonary blood. The P_{O_2} of the gaseous oxygen in the alveolus averages 104 mm Hg, whereas the P_{O_2} of the venous blood entering the pulmonary capillary at its arterial end averages only 40 mm Hg because a large amount of oxygen was removed from this blood as it passed through the peripheral tissues. Therefore, the *initial* pressure difference that causes oxygen to diffuse into the pulmonary capillary is 104 − 40, or 64 mm Hg. In the graph at the bottom of the figure, the curve shows the rapid rise in blood P_{O_2} as the blood passes through the capillary; the blood P_{O_2} rises almost to that of the alveolar air by the time the blood has moved a third of the distance through the capillary, becoming almost 104 mm Hg.

Uptake of Oxygen by the Pulmonary Blood During Exercise. During strenuous exercise, a person's body may require as much as 20 times the normal amount of oxygen. Also, because of increased cardiac output during exercise, the time that the blood remains in the pulmonary capillary may be reduced to less than one-half normal. Yet because of the great *safety factor* for diffusion of oxygen through the pulmonary membrane, the blood still becomes *almost saturated* with oxygen by the time it leaves the pulmonary capillaries. This can be explained as follows.

First, it was pointed out in Chapter 39 that the diffusing capacity for oxygen increases almost threefold during exercise; this results mainly from increased surface area of capillaries participating in the diffusion and also from a more nearly ideal ventilation-perfusion ratio in the upper part of the lungs.

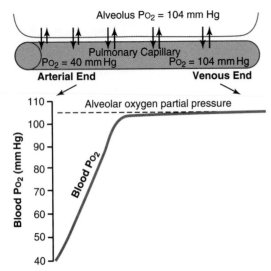

Figure 40-1 Uptake of oxygen by the pulmonary capillary blood. (The curve in this figure was constructed from data in Milhorn HT Jr, Pulley PE Jr: A theoretical study of pulmonary capillary gas exchange and venous admixture. Biophys J 8:337, 1968.)

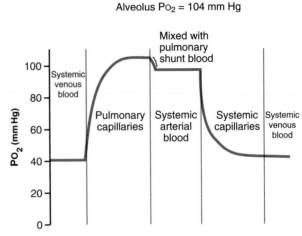

Figure 40-2 Changes in P_{O_2} in the pulmonary capillary blood, systemic arterial blood, and systemic capillary blood, demonstrating the effect of "venous admixture."

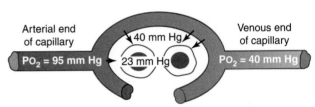

Figure 40-3 Diffusion of oxygen from a peripheral tissue capillary to the cells. (P_{O_2} in interstitial fluid = 40 mm Hg, and in tissue cells = 23 mm Hg.)

Second, note in the curve of Figure 40-1 that under nonexercising conditions, the blood becomes almost saturated with oxygen by the time it has passed through one third of the pulmonary capillary, and little additional oxygen normally enters the blood during the latter two thirds of its transit. That is, the blood normally stays in the lung capillaries about three times as long as needed to cause full oxygenation. Therefore, during exercise, even with a shortened time of exposure in the capillaries, the blood can still become fully oxygenated, or nearly so.

Transport of Oxygen in the Arterial Blood

About 98 percent of the blood that enters the left atrium from the lungs has just passed through the alveolar capillaries and has become oxygenated up to a P_{O_2} of about 104 mm Hg. Another 2 percent of the blood has passed from the aorta through the bronchial circulation, which supplies mainly the deep tissues of the lungs and is not exposed to lung air. This blood flow is called "shunt flow," meaning that blood is shunted past the gas exchange areas. On leaving the lungs, the P_{O_2} of the shunt blood is about that of normal systemic venous blood, about 40 mm Hg. When this blood combines in the pulmonary veins with the oxygenated blood from the alveolar capillaries, this so-called *venous admixture of blood* causes the P_{O_2} of the blood entering the left heart and pumped into the aorta to fall to about 95 mm Hg. These changes in blood P_{O_2} at different points in the circulatory system are shown in Figure 40-2.

Diffusion of Oxygen from the Peripheral Capillaries into the Tissue Fluid

When the arterial blood reaches the peripheral tissues, its P_{O_2} in the capillaries is still 95 mm Hg. Yet, as shown in Figure 40-3, the P_{O_2} in the *interstitial fluid* that surrounds the tissue cells averages only 40 mm Hg. Thus, there is a tremendous initial pressure difference that causes oxygen to diffuse rapidly from the capillary blood into the tissues—so rapidly that the capillary P_{O_2} falls almost to equal the 40 mm Hg pressure in the interstitium. Therefore, the P_{O_2} of the blood leaving the tissue capillaries and entering the systemic veins is also about 40 mm Hg.

Effect of Rate of Blood Flow on Interstitial Fluid P_{O_2}. If the blood flow through a particular tissue is increased, greater quantities of oxygen are transported into the tissue and the tissue P_{O_2} becomes correspondingly higher. This is shown in Figure 40-4. Note that an increase in flow to 400 percent of normal increases the P_{O_2} from 40 mm Hg (at point A in the figure) to 66 mm Hg (at point B). However, the upper limit

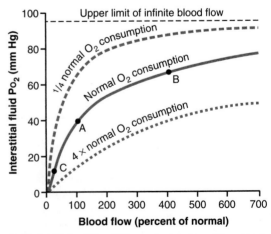

Figure 40-4 Effect of blood flow and rate of oxygen consumption on tissue P_{O_2}.

to which the Po_2 can rise, even with maximal blood flow, is 95 mm Hg because this is the oxygen pressure in the arterial blood. Conversely, if blood flow through the tissue decreases, the tissue Po_2 also decreases, as shown at point C.

Effect of Rate of Tissue Metabolism on Interstitial Fluid Po_2. If the cells use more oxygen for metabolism than normally, this reduces the interstitial fluid Po_2. Figure 40-4 also demonstrates this effect, showing reduced interstitial fluid Po_2 when the cellular oxygen consumption is increased and increased Po_2 when consumption is decreased.

In summary, tissue Po_2 is determined by a balance between (1) the rate of oxygen transport to the tissues in the blood and (2) the rate at which the oxygen is used by the tissues.

Diffusion of Oxygen from the Peripheral Capillaries to the Tissue Cells

Oxygen is always being used by the cells. Therefore, the intracellular Po_2 in the peripheral tissue cells remains lower than the Po_2 in the peripheral capillaries. Also, in many instances, there is considerable physical distance between the capillaries and the cells. Therefore, the normal intracellular Po_2 ranges from as low as 5 mm Hg to as high as 40 mm Hg, averaging (by direct measurement in lower animals) 23 mm Hg. Because only 1 to 3 mm Hg of oxygen pressure is normally required for full support of the chemical processes that use oxygen in the cell, one can see that even this low intracellular Po_2 of 23 mm Hg is more than adequate and provides a large safety factor.

Diffusion of Carbon Dioxide from the Peripheral Tissue Cells into the Capillaries and from the Pulmonary Capillaries into the Alveoli

When oxygen is used by the cells, virtually all of it becomes carbon dioxide, and this increases the intracellular Pco_2; because of this high tissue cell Pco_2, carbon dioxide diffuses from the cells into the tissue capillaries and is then carried by the blood to the lungs. In the lungs, it diffuses from the pulmonary capillaries into the alveoli and is expired.

Thus, at each point in the gas transport chain, carbon dioxide diffuses in the direction exactly opposite to the diffusion of oxygen. Yet there is one major difference between diffusion of carbon dioxide and of oxygen: *carbon dioxide can diffuse about 20 times as rapidly as oxygen.* Therefore, the pressure differences required to cause carbon dioxide diffusion are, in each instance, far less than the pressure differences required to cause oxygen diffusion. The CO_2 pressures are approximately the following:

1. Intracellular Pco_2, 46 mm Hg; interstitial Pco_2, 45 mm Hg. Thus, there is only a 1 mm Hg pressure differential, as shown in Figure 40-5.

2. Pco_2 of the arterial blood entering the tissues, 40 mm Hg; Pco_2 of the venous blood leaving the tissues, 45 mm Hg. Thus, as shown in Figure 40-5, the tissue capillary blood comes almost exactly to equilibrium with the interstitial Pco_2 of 45 mm Hg.

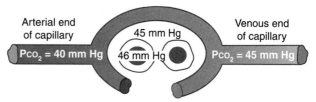

Figure 40-5 Uptake of carbon dioxide by the blood in the tissue capillaries. (Pco_2 in tissue cells = 46 mm Hg, and in interstitial fluid = 45 mm Hg.)

3. Pco_2 of the blood entering the pulmonary capillaries at the arterial end, 45 mm Hg; Pco_2 of the alveolar air, 40 mm Hg. Thus, only a 5 mm Hg pressure difference causes all the required carbon dioxide diffusion out of the pulmonary capillaries into the alveoli. Furthermore, as shown in Figure 40-6, the Pco_2 of the pulmonary capillary blood falls to almost exactly equal the alveolar Pco_2 of 40 mm Hg before it has passed more than about one third the distance through the capillaries. This is the same effect that was observed earlier for oxygen diffusion, except that it is in the opposite direction.

Effect of Rate of Tissue Metabolism and Tissue Blood Flow on Interstitial Pco_2. Tissue capillary blood flow and tissue metabolism affect the Pco_2 in ways exactly opposite to their effect on tissue Po_2. Figure 40-7 shows these effects, as follows:

1. A decrease in blood flow from normal (point A) to one quarter-normal (point B) increases peripheral tissue Pco_2 from the normal value of 45 mm Hg to an elevated level of 60 mm Hg. Conversely, increasing the blood flow to six times normal (point C) decreases the interstitial Pco_2 from the normal value of 45 mm Hg to 41 mm Hg, down to a level almost equal to the Pco_2 in the arterial blood (40 mm Hg) entering the tissue capillaries.

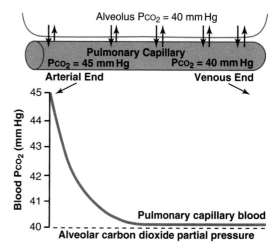

Figure 40-6 Diffusion of carbon dioxide from the pulmonary blood into the alveolus. (This curve was constructed from data in Milhorn HT Jr, Pulley PE Jr: A theoretical study of pulmonary capillary gas exchange and venous admixture. Biophys J 8:337, 1968.)

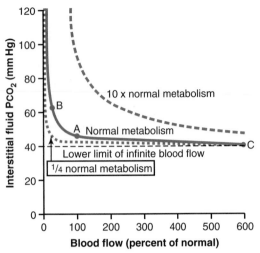

Figure 40-7 Effect of blood flow and metabolic rate on peripheral tissue P_{CO_2}.

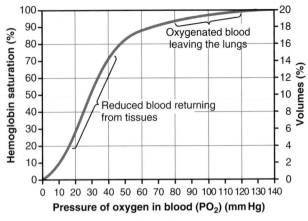

Figure 40-8 Oxygen-hemoglobin dissociation curve.

2. Note also that a 10-fold increase in tissue metabolic rate greatly elevates the interstitial fluid P_{CO_2} at all rates of blood flow, whereas decreasing the metabolism to one-quarter normal causes the interstitial fluid P_{CO_2} to fall to about 41 mm Hg, closely approaching that of the arterial blood, 40 mm Hg.

Role of Hemoglobin in Oxygen Transport

Normally, about 97 percent of the oxygen transported from the lungs to the tissues is carried in chemical combination with hemoglobin in the red blood cells. The remaining 3 percent is transported in the dissolved state in the water of the plasma and blood cells. Thus, *under normal conditions*, oxygen is carried to the tissues almost entirely by hemoglobin.

Reversible Combination of Oxygen with Hemoglobin

The chemistry of hemoglobin is presented in Chapter 32, where it was pointed out that the oxygen molecule combines loosely and reversibly with the heme portion of hemoglobin. When P_{O_2} is high, as in the pulmonary capillaries, oxygen binds with the hemoglobin, but when P_{O_2} is low, as in the tissue capillaries, oxygen is released from the hemoglobin. This is the basis for almost all oxygen transport from the lungs to the tissues.

Oxygen-Hemoglobin Dissociation Curve. Figure 40-8 shows the oxygen-hemoglobin dissociation curve, which demonstrates a progressive increase in the percentage of hemoglobin bound with oxygen as blood P_{O_2} increases, which is called the *percent saturation of hemoglobin*. Because the blood leaving the lungs and entering the systemic arteries usually has a P_{O_2} of about 95 mm Hg, one can see from the dissociation curve that the *usual oxygen saturation of systemic arterial blood averages 97 percent*. Conversely, in normal venous blood returning from the peripheral tissues, the P_{O_2} is about 40 mm Hg, and *the saturation of hemoglobin averages 75 percent*.

Maximum Amount of Oxygen That Can Combine with the Hemoglobin of the Blood. The blood of a normal person contains about 15 grams of hemoglobin in each 100 milliliters of blood, and each gram of hemoglobin can bind with a maximum of 1.34 milliliters of oxygen (1.39 milliliters when the hemoglobin is chemically pure, but impurities such as methemoglobin reduce this). Therefore, 15 times 1.34 equals 20.1, which means that, on average, the 15 grams of hemoglobin in 100 milliliter of blood can combine with a total of about 20 milliliters of oxygen if the hemoglobin is 100 percent saturated. This is usually expressed as *20 volumes percent*. The oxygen-hemoglobin dissociation curve for the normal person can also be expressed in terms of volume percent of oxygen, as shown by the far right scale in Figure 40-8, instead of percent saturation of hemoglobin.

Amount of Oxygen Released from the Hemoglobin When Systemic Arterial Blood Flows Through the Tissues. The total quantity of oxygen *bound with hemoglobin* in normal systemic arterial blood, which is 97 percent saturated, is about 19.4 milliliters per 100 milliliters of blood. This is shown in Figure 40-9. On passing through the tissue capillaries, this amount is reduced, on average, to 14.4 milliliters (P_{O_2} of 40 mm Hg, 75 percent saturated hemoglobin). Thus, *under normal conditions, about 5 milliliters of oxygen are transported from the lungs to the tissues by each 100 milliliters of blood flow*.

Transport of Oxygen During Strenuous Exercise. During heavy exercise, the muscle cells use oxygen at a rapid rate, which, in extreme cases, can cause the muscle interstitial fluid P_{O_2} to fall from the normal 40 mm Hg to as low as 15 mm Hg. At this low pressure, only 4.4 milliliters of oxygen remain bound with hemoglobin in each 100 milliliters of blood, as shown in Figure 40-9. Thus, 19.4 − 4.4, or 15 milliliters, is the quantity of oxygen actually delivered to the tissues by each 100 milliliters of blood flow. Thus, three times as much oxygen as normal is delivered in each volume of blood that passes through the tissues. And keep in mind that the cardiac output can increase to six to seven times normal

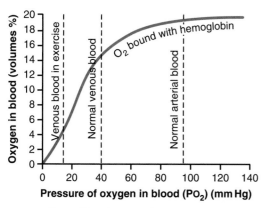

Figure 40-9 Effect of blood PO_2 on the quantity of oxygen bound with hemoglobin in each 100 milliliters of blood.

in well-trained marathon runners. Thus, multiplying the increase in cardiac output (6- to 7-fold) by the increase in oxygen transport in each volume of blood (3-fold) gives a 20-fold increase in oxygen transport to the tissues. We see later in the chapter that several other factors facilitate delivery of oxygen into muscles during exercise, so muscle tissue PO_2 often falls on slightly below normal even during very strenuous exercise.

Utilization Coefficient. The percentage of the blood that gives up its oxygen as it passes through the tissue capillaries is called the *utilization coefficient*. The normal value for this is about 25 percent, as is evident from the preceding discussion—that is, 25 percent of the oxygenated hemoglobin gives its oxygen to the tissues. During strenuous exercise, the utilization coefficient in the entire body can increase to 75 to 85 percent. And in local tissue areas where blood flow is extremely slow or the metabolic rate is very high, utilization coefficients approaching 100 percent have been recorded—that is, essentially all the oxygen is given to the tissues.

Effect of Hemoglobin to "Buffer" the Tissue PO_2

Although hemoglobin is necessary for the transport of oxygen to the tissues, it performs another function essential to life. This is its function as a "tissue oxygen buffer" system. That is, the hemoglobin in the blood is mainly responsible for stabilizing the oxygen pressure in the tissues. This can be explained as follows.

Role of Hemoglobin in Maintaining Nearly Constant PO_2 in the Tissues. Under basal conditions, the tissues require about 5 milliliters of oxygen from each 100 milliliters of blood passing through the tissue capillaries. Referring to the oxygen-hemoglobin dissociation curve in Figure 40-9, one can see that for the normal 5 milliliters of oxygen to be released per 100 milliliters of blood flow, the PO_2 must fall to about 40 mm Hg. Therefore, the tissue PO_2 normally cannot rise above this 40 mm Hg level because, if it did, the amount of oxygen needed by the tissues would not be released from the hemoglobin. In this

way, the hemoglobin normally sets an upper limit on the oxygen pressure in the tissues at about 40 mm Hg.

Conversely, during heavy exercise, extra amounts of oxygen (as much as 20 times normal) must be delivered from the hemoglobin to the tissues. But this can be achieved with little further decrease in tissue PO_2 because of (1) the steep slope of the dissociation curve and (2) the increase in tissue blood flow caused by the decreased PO_2; that is, a very small fall in PO_2 causes large amounts of extra oxygen to be released from the hemoglobin. It can be seen, then, that the hemoglobin in the blood automatically delivers oxygen to the tissues at a pressure that is held rather tightly between about 15 and 40 mm Hg.

When Atmospheric Oxygen Concentration Changes Markedly, the Buffer Effect of Hemoglobin Still Maintains Almost Constant Tissue PO_2. The normal PO_2 in the alveoli is about 104 mm Hg, but as one ascends a mountain or ascends in an airplane, the PO_2 can easily fall to less than half this amount. Alternatively, when one enters areas of compressed air, such as deep in the sea or in pressurized chambers, the PO_2 may rise to 10 times this level. Even so, the tissue PO_2 changes little.

It can be seen from the oxygen-hemoglobin dissociation curve in Figure 40-8 that when the alveolar PO_2 is decreased to as low as 60 mm Hg, the arterial hemoglobin is still 89 percent saturated with oxygen—only 8 percent below the normal saturation of 97 percent. Further, the tissues still remove about 5 milliliters of oxygen from each 100 milliliter of blood passing through the tissues; to remove this oxygen, the PO_2 of the venous blood falls to 35 mm Hg—only 5 mm Hg below the normal value of 40 mm Hg. Thus, the tissue PO_2 hardly changes, despite the marked fall in alveolar PO_2 from 104 to 60 mm Hg.

Conversely, when the alveolar PO_2 rises as high as 500 mm Hg, the maximum oxygen saturation of hemoglobin can never rise above 100 percent, which is only 3 percent above the normal level of 97 percent. Only a small amount of additional oxygen dissolves in the fluid of the blood, as will be discussed subsequently. Then, when the blood passes through the tissue capillaries and loses several milliliters of oxygen to the tissues, this reduces the PO_2 of the capillary blood to a value only a few milliliters greater than the normal 40 mm Hg. Consequently, the level of alveolar oxygen may vary greatly—from 60 to more than 500 mm Hg PO_2—and still the PO_2 in the peripheral tissues does not vary more than a few milliliters from normal, *demonstrating beautifully the tissue "oxygen buffer" function of the blood hemoglobin system.*

Factors That Shift the Oxygen-Hemoglobin Dissociation Curve—Their Importance for Oxygen Transport

The oxygen-hemoglobin dissociation curves of Figures 40-8 and 40-9 are for normal, average blood. However, a number of factors can displace the dissociation curve in

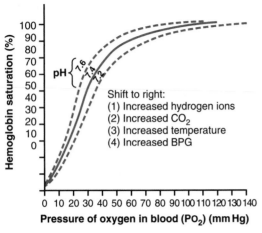

Figure 40-10 Shift of the oxygen-hemoglobin dissociation curve to the right caused by an increase in hydrogen ion concentration (decrease in pH). BPG, 2,3-biphosphoglycerate.

one direction or the other in the manner shown in Figure 40-10. This figure shows that when the blood becomes slightly acidic, with the pH decreasing from the normal value of 7.4 to 7.2, the oxygen-hemoglobin dissociation curve shifts, on average, about 15 percent to the right. Conversely, an increase in pH from the normal 7.4 to 7.6 shifts the curve a similar amount to the left.

In addition to pH changes, several other factors are known to shift the curve. Three of these, all of which shift the curve to the *right*, are (1) increased carbon dioxide concentration, (2) increased blood temperature, and (3) increased 2,3-biphosphoglycerate (BPG), a metabolically important phosphate compound present in the blood in different concentrations under different metabolic conditions.

Increased Delivery of Oxygen to the Tissues When Carbon Dioxide and Hydrogen Ions Shift the Oxygen-Hemoglobin Dissociation Curve—The Bohr Effect.

A shift of the oxygen-hemoglobin dissociation curve to the right in response to increases in blood carbon dioxide and hydrogen ions has a significant effect by enhancing the release of oxygen from the blood in the tissues and enhancing oxygenation of the blood in the lungs. This is called the *Bohr effect,* which can be explained as follows: As the blood passes through the tissues, carbon dioxide diffuses from the tissue cells into the blood. This increases the blood P_{CO_2}, which in turn raises the blood H_2CO_3 (carbonic acid) and the hydrogen ion concentration. These effects shift the oxygen-hemoglobin dissociation curve to the right and downward, as shown in Figure 40-10, forcing oxygen away from the hemoglobin and therefore delivering increased amounts of oxygen to the tissues.

Exactly the opposite effects occur in the lungs, where carbon dioxide diffuses from the blood into the alveoli. This reduces the blood P_{CO_2} and decreases the hydrogen ion concentration, shifting the oxygen-hemoglobin dissociation curve to the left and upward. Therefore, the quantity of oxygen that binds with the hemoglobin at any given alveolar P_{O_2} becomes considerably increased, thus allowing greater oxygen transport to the tissues.

Effect of BPG to Cause Rightward Shift of the Oxygen-Hemoglobin Dissociation Curve.

The normal BPG in the blood keeps the oxygen-hemoglobin dissociation curve shifted slightly to the right all the time. In hypoxic conditions that last longer than a few hours, the quantity of BPG in the blood increases considerably, thus shifting the oxygen-hemoglobin dissociation curve even farther to the right. This causes oxygen to be released to the tissues at as much as 10 mm Hg higher tissue oxygen pressure than would be the case without this increased BPG. Therefore, under some conditions, the BPG mechanism can be important for adaptation to hypoxia, especially to hypoxia caused by poor tissue blood flow.

Rightward Shift of the Oxygen-Hemoglobin Dissociation Curve During Exercise.

During exercise, several factors shift the dissociation curve considerably to the right, thus delivering extra amounts of oxygen to the active, exercising muscle fibers. The exercising muscles, in turn, release large quantities of carbon dioxide; this and several other acids released by the muscles increase the hydrogen ion concentration in the muscle capillary blood. In addition, the temperature of the muscle often rises 2° to 3°C, which can increase oxygen delivery to the muscle fibers even more. All these factors act together to shift the oxygen-hemoglobin dissociation curve *of the muscle capillary blood* considerably to the right. This rightward shift of the curve forces oxygen to be released from the blood hemoglobin to the muscle at P_{O_2} levels as great as 40 mm Hg, even when 70 percent of the oxygen has already been removed from the hemoglobin. Then, in the lungs, the shift occurs in the opposite direction, allowing the pickup of extra amounts of oxygen from the alveoli.

Metabolic Use of Oxygen by the Cells

Effect of Intracellular P_{O_2} on Rate of Oxygen Usage.

Only a minute level of oxygen pressure is required in the cells for normal intracellular chemical reactions to take place. The reason for this is that the respiratory enzyme systems of the cell, which are discussed in Chapter 67, are geared so that when the cellular P_{O_2} is more than 1 mm Hg, oxygen availability is no longer a limiting factor in the rates of the chemical reactions. Instead, the main limiting factor is the *concentration of adenosine diphosphate* (ADP) in the cells. This effect is demonstrated in Figure 40-11, which shows the relation between intracellular P_{O_2} and the rate of oxygen usage at different concentrations of ADP. Note that whenever the intracellular P_{O_2} is above 1 mm Hg, the rate of oxygen usage becomes constant for any given concentration of ADP in the cell. Conversely, when the ADP concentration is altered, the rate of oxygen usage changes in proportion to the change in ADP concentration.

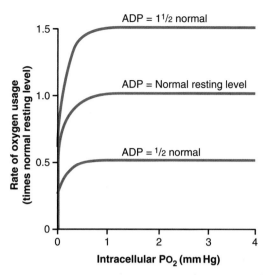

Figure 40-11 Effect of intracellular adenosine diphosphate (ADP) and Po$_2$ on rate of oxygen usage by the cells. Note that as long as the intracellular Po$_2$ remains above 1 mm Hg, the controlling factor for the rate of oxygen usage is the intracellular concentration of ADP.

As explained in Chapter 3, when adenosine triphosphate (ATP) is used in the cells to provide energy, it is converted into ADP. The increasing concentration of ADP increases the metabolic usage of oxygen as it combines with the various cell nutrients, releasing energy that reconverts the ADP back to ATP. *Under normal operating conditions, the rate of oxygen usage by the cells is controlled ultimately by the rate of energy expenditure within the cells—that is, by the rate at which ADP is formed from ATP.*

Effect of Diffusion Distance from the Capillary to the Cell on Oxygen Usage. Tissue cells are seldom more than 50 micrometers away from a capillary, and oxygen normally can diffuse readily enough from the capillary to the cell to supply all the required amounts of oxygen for metabolism. However, occasionally, cells are located farther from the capillaries, and the rate of oxygen diffusion to these cells can become so low that intracellular Po$_2$ falls below the critical level required to maintain maximal intracellular metabolism. Thus, under these conditions, oxygen usage by the cells is said to be *diffusion limited* and is no longer determined by the amount of ADP formed in the cells. But this almost never occurs, except in pathological states.

Effect of Blood Flow on Metabolic Use of Oxygen. The total amount of oxygen available each minute for use in any given tissue is determined by (1) the quantity of oxygen that can be transported to the tissue in each 100 ml of blood and (2) the rate of blood flow. If the rate of blood flow falls to zero, the amount of available oxygen also falls to zero. Thus, there are times when the rate of blood flow through a tissue can be so low that tissue Po$_2$ falls below the critical 1 mm Hg required for intracellular metabolism. Under these conditions, the rate of tissue usage of oxygen

is *blood flow limited.* Neither diffusion-limited nor blood flow–limited oxygen states can continue for long, because the cells receive less oxygen than is required to continue the life of the cells.

Transport of Oxygen in the Dissolved State

At the normal arterial Po$_2$ of 95 mm Hg, about 0.29 milliliter of oxygen is dissolved in every 100 milliliters of water in the blood, and when the Po$_2$ of the blood falls to the normal 40 mm Hg in the tissue capillaries, only 0.12 milliliters of oxygen remains dissolved. In other words, 0.17 milliliters of oxygen is normally transported in the dissolved state to the tissues by each 100 milliliters of arterial blood flow. This compares with almost 5 milliliters of oxygen transported by the red cell hemoglobin. Therefore, the amount of oxygen transported to the tissues in the dissolved state is normally slight, only about 3 percent of the total, as compared with 97 percent transported by the hemoglobin.

During strenuous exercise, when hemoglobin release of oxygen to the tissues increases another threefold, the relative quantity of oxygen transported in the dissolved state falls to as little as 1.5 percent. But if a person breathes oxygen at very high alveolar Po$_2$ levels, the amount transported in the dissolved state can become much greater, sometimes so much so that a serious excess of oxygen occurs in the tissues, and "oxygen poisoning" ensues. This often leads to brain convulsions and even death, as discussed in detail in Chapter 44 in relation to the high-pressure breathing of oxygen among deep-sea divers.

Combination of Hemoglobin with Carbon Monoxide—Displacement of Oxygen

Carbon monoxide combines with hemoglobin at the same point on the hemoglobin molecule as does oxygen; it can therefore displace oxygen from the hemoglobin, thereby decreasing the oxygen-carrying capacity of blood. Further, it binds with about 250 times as much tenacity as oxygen, which is demonstrated by the carbon monoxide–hemoglobin dissociation curve in Figure 40-12. This curve is almost identical to the oxygen-hemoglobin dissociation curve, except that the carbon monoxide partial pressures, shown on the abscissa, are at a level $\frac{1}{250}$ of those for the oxygen-hemoglobin dissociation curve of Figure 40-8. Therefore,

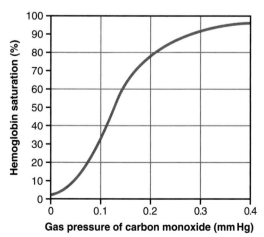

Figure 40-12 Carbon monoxide–hemoglobin dissociation curve. Note the extremely low carbon monoxide pressures at which carbon monoxide combines with hemoglobin.

a carbon monoxide partial pressure of only 0.4 mm Hg in the alveoli, ½₂₅₀ that of normal alveolar oxygen (100 mm Hg Po_2), allows the carbon monoxide to compete equally with the oxygen for combination with the hemoglobin and causes half the hemoglobin in the blood to become bound with carbon monoxide instead of with oxygen. Therefore, a carbon monoxide pressure of only 0.6 mm Hg (a volume concentration of less than one part per thousand in air) can be lethal.

Even though the oxygen content of blood is greatly reduced in carbon monoxide poisoning, the Po_2 of the blood may be normal. This makes exposure to carbon monoxide especially dangerous because the blood is bright red and there are no obvious signs of hypoxemia, such as a bluish color of the fingertips or lips (cyanosis). Also, Po_2 is not reduced, and the feedback mechanism that usually stimulates increased respiration rate in response to lack of oxygen (usually reflected by a low Po_2) is absent. Because the brain is one of the first organs affected by lack of oxygen, the person may become disoriented and unconscious before becoming aware of the danger.

A patient severely poisoned with carbon monoxide can be treated by administering pure oxygen because oxygen at high alveolar pressure can displace carbon monoxide rapidly from its combination with hemoglobin. The patient can also benefit from simultaneous administration of 5 percent carbon dioxide because this strongly stimulates the respiratory center, which increases alveolar ventilation and reduces the alveolar carbon monoxide. With intensive oxygen and carbon dioxide therapy, carbon monoxide can be removed from the blood as much as 10 times as rapidly as without therapy.

Transport of Carbon Dioxide in the Blood

Transport of carbon dioxide by the blood is not nearly as problematical as transport of oxygen is because even in the most abnormal conditions, carbon dioxide can usually be transported in far greater quantities than oxygen can be. However, the amount of carbon dioxide in the blood has a lot to do with the acid-base balance of the body fluids, which is discussed in Chapter 30. Under normal resting conditions, *an average of 4 milliliters of carbon dioxide is transported from the tissues to the lungs in each 100 milliliters of blood.*

Chemical Forms in Which Carbon Dioxide Is Transported

To begin the process of carbon dioxide transport, carbon dioxide diffuses out of the tissue cells in the dissolved molecular carbon dioxide form. On entering the tissue capillaries, the carbon dioxide initiates a host of almost instantaneous physical and chemical reactions, shown in Figure 40-13, which are essential for carbon dioxide transport.

Transport of Carbon Dioxide in the Dissolved State. A small portion of the carbon dioxide is transported in the dissolved state to the lungs. Recall that the

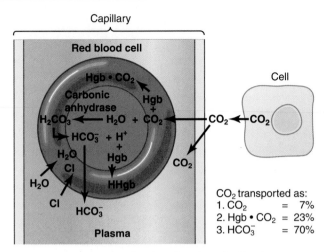

Figure 40-13 Transport of carbon dioxide in the blood.

Pco_2 of venous blood is 45 mm Hg and that of arterial blood is 40 mm Hg. The amount of carbon dioxide dissolved in the fluid of the blood at 45 mm Hg is about 2.7 ml/dl (2.7 volumes percent). The amount dissolved at 40 mm Hg is about 2.4 milliliters, or a difference of 0.3 milliliter. Therefore, only about 0.3 milliliter of carbon dioxide is transported in the dissolved form by each 100 milliliters of blood flow. This is about 7 percent of all the carbon dioxide normally transported.

Transport of Carbon Dioxide in the Form of Bicarbonate Ion

Reaction of Carbon Dioxide with Water in the Red Blood Cells—Effect of Carbonic Anhydrase. The dissolved carbon dioxide in the blood reacts with water to form *carbonic acid*. This reaction would occur much too slowly to be of importance were it not for the fact that inside the red blood cells is a protein enzyme called *carbonic anhydrase*, which catalyzes the reaction between carbon dioxide and water and accelerates its reaction rate about 5000-fold. Therefore, instead of requiring many seconds or minutes to occur, as is true in the plasma, the reaction occurs so rapidly in the red blood cells that it reaches almost complete equilibrium within a very small fraction of a second. This allows tremendous amounts of carbon dioxide to react with the red blood cell water even before the blood leaves the tissue capillaries.

Dissociation of Carbonic Acid into Bicarbonate and Hydrogen Ions. In another fraction of a second, the carbonic acid formed in the red cells (H_2CO_3) dissociates into *hydrogen* and *bicarbonate ions* (H^+ and HCO_3^-). Most of the H^+ ions then combine with the hemoglobin in the red blood cells because the hemoglobin protein is a powerful acid-base buffer. In turn, many of the HCO_3^- ions diffuse from the red cells into the plasma, while chloride ions diffuse into the red cells to take their place. This is made possible by the presence of a special *bicarbonate-chloride carrier protein* in the red cell membrane that shuttles these two ions in opposite directions at rapid velocities. Thus, the chloride content of venous red blood cells is greater than that of arterial red cells, a phenomenon called the *chloride shift.*

The reversible combination of carbon dioxide with water in the red blood cells under the influence of carbonic anhydrase accounts for about 70 percent of the carbon dioxide transported from the tissues to the lungs. Thus, this means of transporting carbon dioxide is by far the most important. Indeed, when a carbonic anhydrase inhibitor (acetazolamide) is administered to an animal to block the action of carbonic anhydrase in the red blood cells, carbon dioxide transport from the tissues becomes so poor that the tissue P_{CO_2} can be made to rise to 80 mm Hg instead of the normal 45 mm Hg.

Transport of Carbon Dioxide in Combination with Hemoglobin and Plasma Proteins—Carbaminohemoglobin. In addition to reacting with water, carbon dioxide reacts directly with amine radicals of the hemoglobin molecule to form the compound *carbaminohemoglobin* (CO_2Hgb). This combination of carbon dioxide and hemoglobin is a reversible reaction that occurs with a loose bond, so the carbon dioxide is easily released into the alveoli, where the P_{CO_2} is lower than in the pulmonary capillaries.

A small amount of carbon dioxide also reacts in the same way with the plasma proteins in the tissue capillaries. This is much less significant for the transport of carbon dioxide because the quantity of these proteins in the blood is only one fourth as great as the quantity of hemoglobin.

The quantity of carbon dioxide that can be carried from the peripheral tissues to the lungs by carbamino combination with hemoglobin and plasma proteins is about 30 percent of the total quantity transported— that is, normally about 1.5 milliliters of carbon dioxide in each 100 milliliters of blood. However, because this reaction is much slower than the reaction of carbon dioxide with water inside the red blood cells, it is doubtful that under normal conditions this carbamino mechanism transports more than 20 percent of the total carbon dioxide.

Carbon Dioxide Dissociation Curve

The curve shown in Figure 40-14—called the *carbon dioxide dissociation curve*—depicts the dependence of total blood carbon dioxide in all its forms on P_{CO_2}. Note that the normal blood P_{CO_2} ranges between the limits of 40 mm Hg in arterial blood and 45 mm Hg in venous blood, which is a very narrow range. Note also that the normal concentration of carbon dioxide in the blood in all its different forms is about 50 volumes percent, but only 4 volumes percent of this is exchanged during normal transport of carbon dioxide from the tissues to the lungs. That is, the concentration rises to about 52 volumes percent as the blood passes through the tissues and falls to about 48 volumes percent as it passes through the lungs.

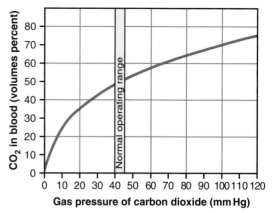

Figure 40-14 Carbon dioxide dissociation curve.

When Oxygen Binds with Hemoglobin, Carbon Dioxide Is Released (the Haldane Effect) to Increase CO₂ Transport

Earlier in the chapter, it was pointed out that an increase in carbon dioxide in the blood causes oxygen to be displaced from the hemoglobin (the Bohr effect), which is an important factor in increasing oxygen transport. The reverse is also true: binding of oxygen with hemoglobin tends to displace carbon dioxide from the blood. Indeed, this effect, called the *Haldane effect*, is quantitatively far more important in promoting carbon dioxide transport than is the Bohr effect in promoting oxygen transport.

The Haldane effect results from the simple fact that the combination of oxygen with hemoglobin in the lungs causes the hemoglobin to become a stronger acid. This displaces carbon dioxide from the blood and into the alveoli in two ways: (1) The more highly acidic hemoglobin has less tendency to combine with carbon dioxide to form carbaminohemoglobin, thus displacing much of the carbon dioxide that is present in the carbamino form from the blood. (2) The increased acidity of the hemoglobin also causes it to release an excess of hydrogen ions, and these bind with bicarbonate ions to form carbonic acid; this then dissociates into water and carbon dioxide, and the carbon dioxide is released from the blood into the alveoli and, finally, into the air.

Figure 40-15 demonstrates quantitatively the significance of the Haldane effect on the transport of carbon dioxide from the tissues to the lungs. This figure shows small portions of two carbon dioxide dissociation curves: (1) when the P_{O_2} is 100 mm Hg, which is the case in the blood capillaries of the lungs, and (2) when the P_{O_2} is 40 mm Hg, which is the case in the tissue capillaries. Point A shows that the normal P_{CO_2} of 45 mm Hg in the tissues causes 52 volumes percent of carbon dioxide to combine with the blood. On entering the lungs, the P_{CO_2} falls to 40 mm Hg and the P_{O_2} rises to 100 mm Hg. If the carbon dioxide dissociation curve did not shift because of the Haldane effect, the carbon dioxide content of the blood would fall only to 50 volumes percent, which would be a loss of only 2 volumes percent of carbon dioxide. However,

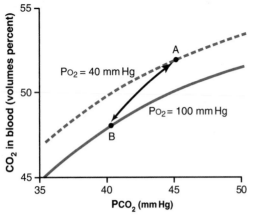

Figure 40-15 Portions of the carbon dioxide dissociation curve when the Po_2 is 100 mm Hg or 40 mm Hg. The arrow represents the Haldane effect on the transport of carbon dioxide, as discussed in the text.

the increase in Po_2 in the lungs lowers the carbon dioxide dissociation curve from the top curve to the lower curve of the figure, so the carbon dioxide content falls to 48 volumes percent (point B). This represents an additional two volumes percent loss of carbon dioxide. Thus, the Haldane effect approximately doubles the amount of carbon dioxide released from the blood in the lungs and approximately doubles the pickup of carbon dioxide in the tissues.

Change in Blood Acidity During Carbon Dioxide Transport

The carbonic acid formed when carbon dioxide enters the blood in the peripheral tissues decreases the blood pH. However, reaction of this acid with the acid-base buffers of the blood prevents the H^+ concentration from rising greatly (and the pH from falling greatly). Ordinarily, arterial blood has a pH of about 7.41, and as the blood acquires carbon dioxide in the tissue capillaries, the pH falls to a venous value of about 7.37. In other words, a pH change of 0.04 unit takes place. The reverse occurs when carbon dioxide is released from the blood in the lungs, with the pH rising to the arterial value of 7.41 once again. In heavy exercise or other conditions of high metabolic activity, or when blood flow through the tissues is sluggish, the decrease in pH in the tissue blood (and in the tissues themselves) can be as much as 0.50, about 12 times normal, thus causing significant tissue acidosis.

Respiratory Exchange Ratio

The discerning student will have noted that normal transport of oxygen from the lungs to the tissues by each 100 milliliters of blood is about 5 milliliters, whereas normal transport of carbon dioxide from the tissues to the lungs

is about 4 milliliters. Thus, under normal resting conditions, only about 82 percent as much carbon dioxide is expired from the lungs as oxygen is taken up by the lungs. The ratio of carbon dioxide output to oxygen uptake is called the *respiratory exchange ratio* (R). That is,

$$R = \frac{\text{Rate of carbon dioxide output}}{\text{Rate of oxygen uptake}}$$

The value for R changes under different metabolic conditions. When a person is using exclusively carbohydrates for body metabolism, R rises to 1.00. Conversely, when a person is using exclusively fats for metabolic energy, the R level falls to as low as 0.7. The reason for this difference is that when oxygen is metabolized with carbohydrates, one molecule of carbon dioxide is formed for each molecule of oxygen consumed; when oxygen reacts with fats, a large share of the oxygen combines with hydrogen atoms from the fats to form water instead of carbon dioxide. In other words, when fats are metabolized, the *respiratory quotient of the chemical reactions* in the tissues is about 0.70 instead of 1.00. (The tissue respiratory quotient is discussed in Chapter 71.) For a person on a normal diet consuming average amounts of carbohydrates, fats, and proteins, the average value for R is considered to be 0.825.

Bibliography

Albert R, Spiro S, Jett J: *Comprehensive Respiratory Medicine*, Philadelphia, 2002, Mosby.

Amann M, Calbet JA: Convective oxygen transport and fatigue, *J Appl Physiol* 104:861, 2008.

Geers C, Gros G: Carbon dioxide transport and carbonic anhydrase in blood and muscle, *Physiol Rev* 80:681, 2000.

Hopkins SR, Levin DL, Emami K, et al: Advances in magnetic resonance imaging of lung physiology, *J Appl Physiol* 102:1244, 2007.

Hughes JM: Assessing gas exchange, *Chron Respir Dis* 4:205, 2007.

Jensen FB: Red blood cell pH, the Bohr effect, and other oxygenation-linked phenomena in blood O_2 and CO_2 transport, *Acta Physiol Scand* 182:215, 2004.

Maina JN, West JB: Thin and strong! The bioengineering dilemma in the structural and functional design of the blood-gas barrier, *Physiol Rev* 85:811, 2005.

Piiper J: Perfusion, diffusion and their heterogeneities limiting blood-tissue O_2 transfer in muscle, *Acta Physiol Scand* 168:603, 2000.

Richardson RS: Oxygen transport and utilization: an integration of the muscle systems, *Adv Physiol Educ* 27:183, 2003.

Sonveaux P, Lobysheva II, Feron O, et al: Transport and peripheral bioactivities of nitrogen oxides carried by red blood cell hemoglobin: role in oxygen delivery, *Physiology (Bethesda)* 22:97, 2007.

Tsai AG, Johnson PC, Intaglietta M: Oxygen gradients in the microcirculation, *Physiol Rev* 83:933, 2003.

West JB: *Respiratory Physiology-The Essentials*, ed 8, Baltimore, 2008, Lippincott, Williams & Wilkins.

Regulation of Respiration

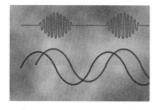

The nervous system normally adjusts the rate of alveolar ventilation almost exactly to the demands of the body so that the oxygen pressure (P_{O_2}) and carbon dioxide pressure (P_{CO_2}) in the arterial blood are hardly altered, even during heavy exercise and most other types of respiratory stress. This chapter describes the function of this neurogenic system for regulation of respiration.

Respiratory Center

The *respiratory center* is composed of several groups of neurons located *bilaterally* in the *medulla oblongata* and pons of the brain stem, as shown in Figure 41-1. It is divided into three major collections of neurons: (1) a *dorsal respiratory group*, located in the dorsal portion of the medulla, which mainly causes inspiration; (2) a *ventral respiratory group*, located in the ventrolateral part of the medulla, which mainly causes expiration; and (3) the *pneumotaxic center*, located dorsally in the superior portion of the pons, which mainly controls rate and depth of breathing.

Dorsal Respiratory Group of Neurons—Its Control of Inspiration and of Respiratory Rhythm

The dorsal respiratory group of neurons plays the most fundamental role in the control of respiration and extends most of the length of the medulla. Most of its neurons are located within the *nucleus of the tractus solitarius (NTS)*, although additional neurons in the adjacent reticular substance of the medulla also play important roles in respiratory control. The NTS is the sensory termination of both the vagal and the glossopharyngeal nerves, which transmit sensory signals into the respiratory center from (1) peripheral chemoreceptors, (2) baroreceptors, and (3) several types of receptors in the lungs.

Rhythmical Inspiratory Discharges from the Dorsal Respiratory Group. The basic rhythm of respiration is generated mainly in the dorsal respiratory group of neurons. Even when all the peripheral nerves entering the medulla have been sectioned and the brain stem transected both above and below the medulla, this group of neurons still emits repetitive bursts of *inspiratory neuronal action potentials*. The basic cause of these repetitive discharges is unknown. In primitive animals, neural networks have been found in which activity of one set of neurons excites a second set, which in turn inhibits the first. Then, after a period of time, the mechanism repeats itself, continuing throughout the life of the animal. Therefore, most respiratory physiologists believe that some similar network of neurons is present in the human being, located entirely within the medulla; it probably involves not only the dorsal respiratory group but adjacent areas of the medulla as well, and it is responsible for the basic rhythm of respiration.

Inspiratory "Ramp" Signal. The nervous signal that is transmitted to the inspiratory muscles, mainly the diaphragm, is not an instantaneous burst of action potentials. Instead, it begins weakly and increases steadily in a ramp manner for about 2 seconds in normal respiration. Then it ceases abruptly for approximately the next 3 seconds, which turns off the excitation of the diaphragm and allows elastic recoil of the lungs and the chest wall to cause expiration. Next, the inspiratory signal begins again for another cycle; this cycle repeats again and again, with expiration occurring in between. Thus, the inspiratory signal is a *ramp signal*. The obvious advantage of the ramp is that it causes a steady increase in the volume of the lungs during inspiration, rather than inspiratory gasps.

There are two qualities of the inspiratory ramp that are controlled, as follows:

1. Control of the *rate of increase of the ramp signal* so that during heavy respiration, the ramp increases rapidly and therefore fills the lungs rapidly.

2. Control of the *limiting point at which the ramp suddenly ceases*. This is the usual method for controlling the rate of respiration; that is, the earlier the ramp ceases, the

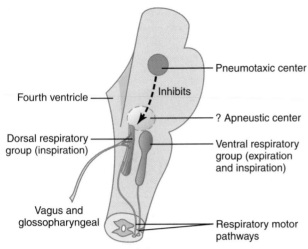

Figure 41-1 Organization of the respiratory center.

shorter the duration of inspiration. This also shortens the duration of expiration. Thus, the frequency of respiration is increased.

A Pneumotaxic Center Limits the Duration of Inspiration and Increases the Respiratory Rate

A *pneumotaxic center*, located dorsally in the *nucleus parabrachialis* of the upper pons, transmits signals to the inspiratory area. The primary effect of this center is to control the "switch-off" point of the inspiratory ramp, thus controlling the duration of the filling phase of the lung cycle. When the pneumotaxic signal is strong, inspiration might last for as little as 0.5 second, thus filling the lungs only slightly; when the pneumotaxic signal is weak, inspiration might continue for 5 or more seconds, thus filling the lungs with a great excess of air.

The function of the pneumotaxic center is primarily to limit inspiration. This has a secondary effect of increasing the rate of breathing because limitation of inspiration also shortens expiration and the entire period of each respiration. A strong pneumotaxic signal can increase the rate of breathing to 30 to 40 breaths per minute, whereas a weak pneumotaxic signal may reduce the rate to only 3 to 5 breaths per minute.

Ventral Respiratory Group of Neurons—Functions in Both Inspiration and Expiration

Located in each side of the medulla, about 5 millimeters anterior and lateral to the dorsal respiratory group of neurons, is the *ventral respiratory group of neurons*, found in the *nucleus ambiguus* rostrally and the *nucleus retroambiguus* caudally. The function of this neuronal group differs from that of the dorsal respiratory group in several important ways:

1. The neurons of the ventral respiratory group remain almost totally *inactive* during normal quiet respiration. Therefore, normal quiet breathing is caused only by repetitive inspiratory signals from the dorsal respiratory group transmitted mainly to the diaphragm, and expiration results from elastic recoil of the lungs and thoracic cage.

2. The ventral respiratory neurons do not appear to participate in the basic rhythmical oscillation that controls respiration.

3. When the respiratory drive for increased pulmonary ventilation becomes greater than normal, respiratory signals spill over into the ventral respiratory neurons from the basic oscillating mechanism of the dorsal respiratory area. As a consequence, the ventral respiratory area contributes extra respiratory drive as well.

4. Electrical stimulation of a few of the neurons in the ventral group causes inspiration, whereas stimulation of others causes expiration. Therefore, these neurons contribute to both inspiration and expiration. They are especially important in providing the powerful expiratory signals to the abdominal muscles during very heavy expiration. Thus, this area operates more or less as an overdrive mechanism when high levels of pulmonary ventilation are required, especially during heavy exercise.

Lung Inflation Signals Limit Inspiration—The Hering-Breuer Inflation Reflex

In addition to the central nervous system respiratory control mechanisms operating entirely within the brain stem, sensory nerve signals from the lungs also help control respiration. Most important, located in the muscular portions of the walls of the bronchi and bronchioles throughout the lungs are *stretch receptors* that transmit signals through the *vagi* into the dorsal respiratory group of neurons when the lungs become overstretched. These signals affect inspiration in much the same way as signals from the pneumotaxic center; that is, when the lungs become overly inflated, the stretch receptors activate an appropriate feedback response that "switches off" the inspiratory ramp and thus stops further inspiration. This is called the *Hering-Breuer inflation reflex*. This reflex also increases the rate of respiration, as is true for signals from the pneumotaxic center.

In humans, the Hering-Breuer reflex probably is not activated until the tidal volume increases to more than three times normal ($>\approx$ 1.5 liters per breath). Therefore, this reflex appears to be mainly a protective mechanism for preventing excess lung inflation rather than an important ingredient in normal control of ventilation.

Control of Overall Respiratory Center Activity

Up to this point, we have discussed the basic mechanisms for causing inspiration and expiration, but it is also important to know how the intensity of the respiratory control signals is increased or decreased to match the ventilatory needs of the body. For example, during heavy exercise, the rates of oxygen usage and carbon dioxide formation are often increased to as much as 20 times normal, requiring commensurate increases in pulmonary ventilation. The major purpose of the remainder of this chapter is to discuss this control of ventilation in accord with the respiratory needs of the body.

Chemical Control of Respiration

The ultimate goal of respiration is to maintain proper concentrations of oxygen, carbon dioxide, and hydrogen ions in the tissues. It is fortunate, therefore, that respiratory activity is highly responsive to changes in each of these.

Excess carbon dioxide or excess hydrogen ions in the blood mainly act directly on the respiratory center itself, causing greatly increased strength of both the inspiratory and the expiratory motor signals to the respiratory muscles.

Oxygen, in contrast, does not have a significant *direct* effect on the respiratory center of the brain in controlling respiration. Instead, it acts almost entirely on peripheral *chemoreceptors* located in the *carotid* and *aortic bodies*, and these in turn transmit appropriate nervous signals to the respiratory center for control of respiration.

Direct Chemical Control of Respiratory Center Activity by Carbon Dioxide and Hydrogen Ions

Chemosensitive Area of the Respiratory Center. We have discussed mainly three areas of the respiratory center: the dorsal respiratory group of neurons, the ventral respiratory group, and the pneumotaxic center. It is believed that none of these is affected directly by changes in blood carbon dioxide concentration or hydrogen ion concentration. Instead, an additional neuronal area, a *chemosensitive area*, shown in Figure 41-2, is located bilaterally, lying only 0.2 millimeter beneath the ventral surface of the medulla. This area is highly sensitive to changes in either

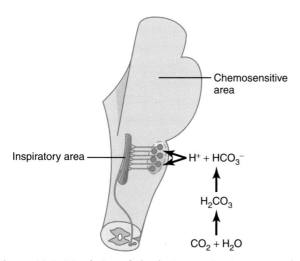

Figure 41-2 Stimulation of the *brain stem inspiratory* area by signals from the *chemosensitive area* located bilaterally in the medulla, lying only a fraction of a millimeter beneath the ventral medullary surface. Note also that hydrogen ions stimulate the chemosensitive area, but carbon dioxide in the fluid gives rise to most of the hydrogen ions.

blood P_{CO_2} or hydrogen ion concentration, and it in turn excites the other portions of the respiratory center.

Excitation of the Chemosensitive Neurons by Hydrogen Ions Is Likely the Primary Stimulus

The sensor neurons in the chemosensitive area are especially excited by hydrogen ions; in fact, it is believed that hydrogen ions may be the only important direct stimulus for these neurons. However, hydrogen ions do not easily cross the blood-brain barrier. For this reason, changes in hydrogen ion concentration in the blood have considerably less effect in stimulating the chemosensitive neurons than do changes in blood carbon dioxide, even though carbon dioxide is believed to stimulate these neurons secondarily by changing the hydrogen ion concentration, as explained in the following section.

Carbon Dioxide Stimulates the Chemosensitive Area

Although carbon dioxide has little direct effect in stimulating the neurons in the chemosensitive area, it does have a potent indirect effect. It does this by reacting with the water of the tissues to form carbonic acid, which dissociates into hydrogen and bicarbonate ions; the hydrogen ions then have a potent direct stimulatory effect on respiration. These reactions are shown in Figure 41-2.

Why does blood carbon dioxide have a more potent effect in stimulating the chemosensitive neurons than do blood hydrogen ions? The answer is that the blood-brain barrier is not very permeable to hydrogen ions, but carbon dioxide passes through this barrier almost as if the barrier did not exist. Consequently, whenever the blood P_{CO_2} increases, so does the P_{CO_2} of both the interstitial fluid of the medulla and the cerebrospinal fluid. In both these fluids, the carbon dioxide immediately reacts with the water to form new hydrogen ions. Thus, paradoxically, more hydrogen ions are released into the respiratory chemosensitive sensory area of the medulla when the blood carbon dioxide concentration increases than when the blood hydrogen ion concentration increases. For this reason, respiratory center activity is increased very strongly by changes in blood carbon dioxide, a fact that we subsequently discuss quantitatively.

Decreased Stimulatory Effect of Carbon Dioxide After the First 1 to 2 Days. Excitation of the respiratory center by carbon dioxide is great the first few hours after the blood carbon dioxide first increases, but then it gradually declines over the next 1 to 2 days, decreasing to about one-fifth the initial effect. Part of this decline results from renal readjustment of the hydrogen ion concentration in the circulating blood back toward normal after the carbon dioxide first increases the hydrogen concentration. The kidneys achieve this by increasing the blood bicarbonate, which binds with the hydrogen ions in the blood and cerebrospinal fluid to reduce their concentrations. But even more important, over a period of hours, the bicarbonate ions also slowly diffuse through the blood-brain and blood-cerebrospinal fluid barriers and combine directly with the hydrogen ions adjacent to the respiratory neurons as well, thus reducing the hydrogen ions back to near normal. A change in blood carbon dioxide concentration therefore has a potent *acute* effect on controlling respiratory drive but only a weak *chronic* effect after a few days' adaptation.

Quantitative Effects of Blood PCO₂ and Hydrogen Ion Concentration on Alveolar Ventilation

Figure 41-3 shows quantitatively the approximate effects of blood P_{CO_2} and blood pH (which is an inverse logarithmic measure of hydrogen ion concentration) on alveolar ventilation. Note especially the very marked increase in ventilation caused by an increase in P_{CO_2} *in the normal range* between 35 and 75 mm Hg. This demonstrates the tremendous effect that carbon dioxide changes have in controlling respiration. By contrast, the change in respiration in the normal blood pH range between 7.3 and 7.5 is less than one-tenth as great.

Changes in Oxygen Have Little Direct Effect on Control of the Respiratory Center

Changes in oxygen concentration have virtually no *direct* effect on the respiratory center itself to alter respiratory drive (although oxygen changes do have an indirect effect, acting through the peripheral chemoreceptors, as explained in the next section).

We learned in Chapter 40 that the hemoglobin-oxygen buffer system delivers almost exactly normal amounts of oxygen to the tissues even when the pulmonary P_{O_2} changes

from a value as low as 60 mm Hg up to a value as high as 1000 mm Hg. Therefore, except under special conditions, adequate delivery of oxygen can occur despite changes in lung ventilation ranging from slightly below one-half normal to as high as 20 or more times normal. This is not true for carbon dioxide because both the blood and tissue P_{CO_2} change inversely with the rate of pulmonary ventilation; thus, the processes of animal evolution have made carbon dioxide the major controller of respiration, not oxygen.

Yet for those special conditions in which the tissues get into trouble for lack of oxygen, the body has a special mechanism for respiratory control located in the peripheral chemoreceptors, outside the brain respiratory center; this mechanism responds when the blood oxygen falls too low, mainly below a P_{O_2} of 70 mm Hg, as explained in the next section.

Peripheral Chemoreceptor System for Control of Respiratory Activity—Role of Oxygen in Respiratory Control

In addition to control of respiratory activity by the respiratory center itself, still another mechanism is available for controlling respiration. This is the *peripheral chemoreceptor system*, shown in Figure 41-4. Special nervous chemical receptors, called *chemoreceptors*, are located in several areas outside the brain. They are especially important for detecting changes in oxygen in the blood, although they also respond to a lesser extent to changes in carbon dioxide and hydrogen ion concentrations. The chemoreceptors transmit nervous signals to the respiratory center in the brain to help regulate respiratory activity.

Most of the chemoreceptors are in the *carotid bodies*. However, a few are also in the *aortic bodies*, shown in the lower part of Figure 41-4, and a very few are located elsewhere in association with other arteries of the thoracic and abdominal regions.

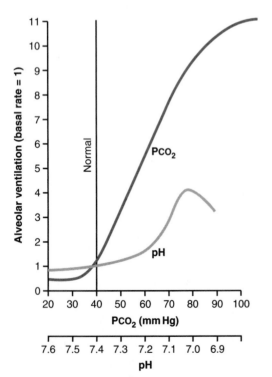

Figure 41-3 Effects of increased arterial blood P_{CO_2} and decreased arterial pH (increased hydrogen ion concentration) on the rate of alveolar ventilation.

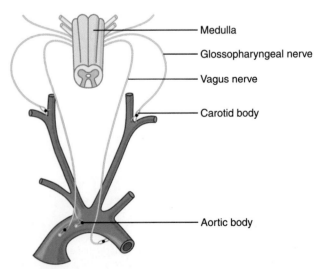

Figure 41-4 Respiratory control by peripheral chemoreceptors in the carotid and aortic bodies.

The *carotid bodies* are located bilaterally in the bifurcations of the common carotid arteries. Their afferent nerve fibers pass through Hering's nerves to the *glossopharyngeal nerves* and then to the dorsal respiratory area of the medulla. The *aortic bodies* are located along the arch of the aorta; their afferent nerve fibers pass through the *vagi*, also to the dorsal medullary respiratory area.

Each of the chemoreceptor bodies receives its own special blood supply through a minute artery directly from the adjacent arterial trunk. Further, blood flow through these bodies is extreme, 20 times the weight of the bodies themselves each minute. Therefore, the percentage of oxygen removed from the flowing blood is virtually zero. This means that *the chemoreceptors are exposed at all times to arterial blood*, not venous blood, and their Po_2s are arterial Po_2s.

Decreased Arterial Oxygen Stimulates the Chemoreceptors. When the oxygen concentration in the arterial blood falls below normal, the chemoreceptors become strongly stimulated. This is demonstrated in Figure 41-5, which shows the effect of different levels of *arterial* Po_2 on the rate of nerve impulse transmission from a carotid body. Note that the impulse rate is particularly sensitive to changes in arterial Po_2 in the range of 60 down to 30 mm Hg, a range in which hemoglobin saturation with oxygen decreases rapidly.

Increased Carbon Dioxide and Hydrogen Ion Concentration Stimulates the Chemoreceptors. An increase in either carbon dioxide concentration or hydrogen ion concentration also excites the chemoreceptors and, in this way, indirectly increases respiratory activity. However, the direct effects of both these factors in the respiratory center itself are much more powerful than their effects mediated through the chemoreceptors (about seven times as powerful). Yet there is one difference between the peripheral and central effects of carbon dioxide: The stimulation by way of the peripheral chemoreceptors occurs as much as five times as rapidly as central stimulation, so the peripheral chemoreceptors might be especially important in increasing the rapidity of response to carbon dioxide at the onset of exercise.

Basic Mechanism of Stimulation of the Chemoreceptors by Oxygen Deficiency. The exact means by which low Po_2 excites the nerve endings in the carotid and aortic bodies are still unknown. However, these bodies have multiple highly characteristic glandular-like cells, called *glomus cells*, which synapse directly or indirectly with the nerve endings. Some investigators have suggested that these glomus cells might function as the chemoreceptors and then stimulate the nerve endings. But other studies suggest that the nerve endings themselves are directly sensitive to the low Po_2.

Effect of Low Arterial Po_2 to Stimulate Alveolar Ventilation When Arterial Carbon Dioxide and Hydrogen Ion Concentrations Remain Normal

Figure 41-6 shows the effect of low arterial Po_2 on alveolar ventilation when the Pco_2 and the hydrogen ion concentration are kept constant at their normal levels. In other words, in this figure, only the ventilatory drive, due to the effect of low oxygen on the chemoreceptors, is active. The figure shows almost no effect on ventilation as long as the arterial Po_2 remains greater than 100 mm Hg. But at pressures lower than 100 mm Hg, ventilation approximately doubles when the arterial Po_2 falls to 60 mm Hg and can increase as much as five-fold at very low Po_2s. Under these conditions, low arterial Po_2 obviously drives the ventilatory process quite strongly.

Because the effect of hypoxia on ventilation is modest for Po_2s greater than 60 to 80 mm Hg, the Pco_2 and the hydrogen ion response are mainly responsible for regulating ventilation in healthy humans at sea level.

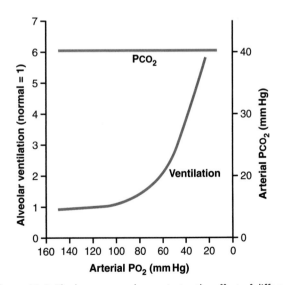

Figure 41-6 The lower curve demonstrates the effect of different levels of arterial Po_2 on alveolar ventilation, showing a sixfold increase in ventilation as the Po_2 decreases from the normal level of 100 mm Hg to 20 mm Hg. The upper line shows that the arterial Pco_2 was kept at a constant level during the measurements of this study; pH also was kept constant.

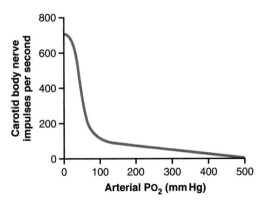

Figure 41-5 Effect of arterial Po_2 on impulse rate from the carotid body.

Chronic Breathing of Low Oxygen Stimulates Respiration Even More—The Phenomenon of "Acclimatization"

Mountain climbers have found that when they ascend a mountain slowly, over a period of days rather than a period of hours, they breathe much more deeply and therefore can withstand far lower atmospheric oxygen concentrations than when they ascend rapidly. This is called *acclimatization.*

The reason for acclimatization is that, within 2 to 3 days, the respiratory center in the brain stem loses about four fifths of its sensitivity to changes in Pco_2 and hydrogen ions. Therefore, the excess ventilatory blow-off of carbon dioxide that normally would inhibit an increase in respiration fails to occur, and low oxygen can drive the respiratory system to a much higher level of alveolar ventilation than under acute conditions. Instead of the 70 percent increase in ventilation that might occur after acute exposure to low oxygen, the alveolar ventilation often increases 400 to 500 percent after 2 to 3 days of low oxygen; this helps immensely in supplying additional oxygen to the mountain climber.

Composite Effects of Pco_2, pH, and Po_2 on Alveolar Ventilation

Figure 41-7 gives a quick overview of the manner in which the chemical factors Po_2, Pco_2, and pH together affect alveolar ventilation. To understand this diagram, first observe the four red curves. These curves were recorded at different levels of arterial Po_2—40 mm Hg, 50 mm Hg, 60 mm Hg, and 100 mm Hg. For each of these curves, the Pco_2 was changed from lower to higher levels. Thus, this "family" of red curves represents the combined effects of alveolar Pco_2 and Po_2 on ventilation.

Now observe the green curves. The red curves were measured at a blood pH of 7.4; the green curves were measured at a pH of 7.3. We now have two families of curves repre-

senting the combined effects of Pco_2 and Po_2 on ventilation at two different pH values. Still other families of curves would be displaced to the right at higher pHs and displaced to the left at lower pHs. Thus, using this diagram, one can predict the level of alveolar ventilation for most combinations of alveolar Pco_2, alveolar Po_2, and arterial pH.

Regulation of Respiration During Exercise

In strenuous exercise, oxygen consumption and carbon dioxide formation can increase as much as 20-fold. Yet, as illustrated in Figure 41-8, in the healthy athlete, alveolar ventilation ordinarily increases almost exactly in step with the increased level of oxygen metabolism. The arterial Po_2, Pco_2, and pH remain *almost exactly normal.*

In trying to analyze what causes the increased ventilation during exercise, one is tempted to ascribe this to increases in blood carbon dioxide and hydrogen ions, plus a decrease in blood oxygen. However, this is questionable because measurements of arterial Pco_2, pH, and Po_2 show that none of these values changes significantly during exercise, so none of them becomes abnormal enough to stimulate respiration so vigorously as observed during strenuous exercise. Therefore, the question must be asked: What causes intense ventilation during exercise? At least one effect seems to be predominant. The brain, on transmitting motor impulses to the exercising muscles, is believed to transmit at the same time collateral impulses into the brain stem to excite the respiratory center. This is analogous to the stimulation of the vasomotor center of the brain stem during exercise that causes a simultaneous increase in arterial pressure.

Actually, when a person begins to exercise, a large share of the total increase in ventilation begins immediately on initiation of the exercise, before any blood chemicals have had time to change. It is likely that most of the increase in respiration results from neurogenic signals transmitted directly into the brain stem respiratory center at the same time that signals go to the body muscles to cause muscle contraction.

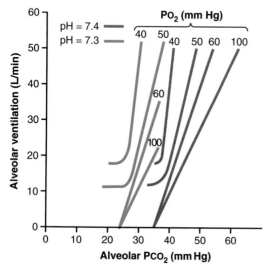

Figure 41-7   Composite diagram showing the interrelated effects of Pco_2, Po_2, and pH on alveolar ventilation. (Drawn from data in Cunningham DJC, Lloyd BB: The Regulation of Human Respiration. Oxford: Blackwell Scientific Publications, 1963.)

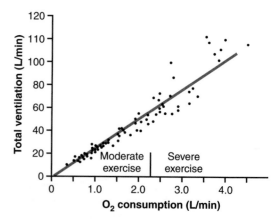

Figure 41-8   Effect of exercise on oxygen consumption and ventilatory rate. (From Gray JS: Pulmonary Ventilation and Its Physiological Regulation. Springfield, Ill: Charles C Thomas, 1950.)

Interrelation Between Chemical Factors and Nervous Factors in the Control of Respiration During Exercise.

When a person exercises, direct nervous signals presumably stimulate the respiratory center *almost* the proper amount to supply the extra oxygen required for exercise and to blow off extra carbon dioxide. Occasionally, however, the nervous respiratory control signals are either too strong or too weak. Then chemical factors play a significant role in bringing about the final adjustment of respiration required to keep the oxygen, carbon dioxide, and hydrogen ion concentrations of the body fluids as nearly normal as possible.

This is demonstrated in Figure 41-9, which shows in the lower curve changes in alveolar ventilation during a 1-minute period of exercise and in the upper curve changes in arterial P_{CO_2}. Note that at the onset of exercise, the alveolar ventilation increases almost instantaneously, without an initial increase in arterial P_{CO_2}. In fact, this increase in ventilation is usually great enough so that at first it actually *decreases* arterial P_{CO_2} below normal, as shown in the figure. The presumed reason that the ventilation forges ahead of the buildup of blood carbon dioxide is that the brain provides an "anticipatory" stimulation of respiration at the onset of exercise, causing extra alveolar ventilation even before it is necessary. However, after about 30 to 40 seconds, the amount of carbon dioxide released into the blood from the active muscles approximately matches the increased rate of ventilation, and the arterial P_{CO_2} returns essentially to normal even as the exercise continues, as shown toward the end of the 1-minute period of exercise in the figure.

Figure 41-10 summarizes the control of respiration during exercise in still another way, this time more quantitatively. The lower curve of this figure shows the

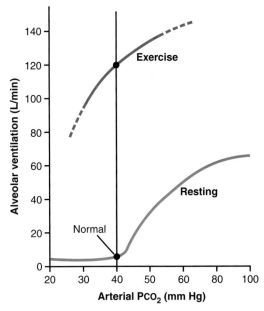

Figure 41-10 Approximate effect of maximum exercise in an athlete to shift the alveolar P_{CO_2}-ventilation response curve to a level much higher than normal. The shift, believed to be caused by neurogenic factors, is almost exactly the right amount to maintain arterial P_{CO_2} at the normal level of 40 mm Hg both in the resting state and during heavy exercise.

effect of different levels of arterial P_{CO_2} on alveolar ventilation when the body is at rest—that is, not exercising. The upper curve shows the approximate shift of this ventilatory curve caused by neurogenic drive from the respiratory center that occurs during heavy exercise. The points indicated on the two curves show the arterial P_{CO_2} first in the resting state and then in the exercising state. Note in both instances that the P_{CO_2} is at the normal level of 40 mm Hg. In other words, the neurogenic factor shifts the curve about 20-fold in the upward direction, so ventilation almost matches the rate of carbon dioxide release, thus keeping arterial P_{CO_2} near its normal value. The upper curve of Figure 41-10 also shows that if, during exercise, the arterial P_{CO_2} does change from its normal value of 40 mm Hg, it has an extra stimulatory effect on ventilation at a P_{CO_2} greater than 40 mm Hg and a depressant effect at a P_{CO_2} less than 40 mm Hg.

Neurogenic Control of Ventilation During Exercise May Be Partly a Learned Response.

Many experiments suggest that the brain's ability to shift the ventilatory response curve during exercise, as shown in Figure 41-10, is at least partly a *learned* response. That is, with repeated periods of exercise, the brain becomes progressively more able to provide the proper signals required to keep the blood P_{CO_2} at its normal level. Also, there is reason to believe that even the cerebral cortex is involved in this learning because experiments that block only the cortex also block the learned response.

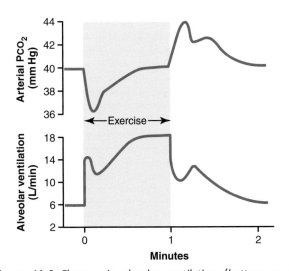

Figure 41-9 Changes in alveolar ventilation (*bottom curve*) and arterial PCO_2 (*top curve*) during a 1-minute period of exercise and also after termination of exercise. (Extrapolated to the human from data in dogs in Bainton CR: Effect of speed vs grade and shivering on ventilation in dogs during active exercise. J Appl Physiol 33:778, 1972.)

Other Factors That Affect Respiration

Voluntary Control of Respiration. Thus far, we have discussed the involuntary system for the control of respiration. However, we all know that for short periods of time, respiration can be controlled voluntarily and that one can hyperventilate or hypoventilate to such an extent that serious derangements in Pco_2, pH, and Po_2 can occur in the blood.

Effect of Irritant Receptors in the Airways. The epithelium of the trachea, bronchi, and bronchioles is supplied with sensory nerve endings called *pulmonary irritant receptors* that are stimulated by many incidents. These cause coughing and sneezing, as discussed in Chapter 39. They may also cause bronchial constriction in such diseases as asthma and emphysema.

Function of Lung "J Receptors". A few sensory nerve endings have been described in the alveolar walls in *juxtaposition* to the pulmonary capillaries—hence the name "J receptors." They are stimulated especially when the pulmonary capillaries become engorged with blood or when pulmonary edema occurs in such conditions as congestive heart failure. Although the functional role of the J receptors is not clear, their excitation may give the person a feeling of dyspnea.

Brain Edema Depresses the Respiratory Center. The activity of the respiratory center may be depressed or even inactivated by acute brain edema resulting from brain concussion. For instance, the head might be struck against some solid object, after which the damaged brain tissues swell, compressing the cerebral arteries against the cranial vault and thus partially blocking cerebral blood supply.

Occasionally, respiratory depression resulting from brain edema can be relieved temporarily by intravenous injection of hypertonic solutions such as highly concentrated mannitol solution. These solutions osmotically remove some of the fluids of the brain, thus relieving intracranial pressure and sometimes re-establishing respiration within a few minutes.

Anesthesia. Perhaps the most prevalent cause of respiratory depression and respiratory arrest is overdosage with anesthetics or narcotics. For instance, sodium pentobarbital depresses the respiratory center considerably more than many other anesthetics, such as halothane. At one time, morphine was used as an anesthetic, but this drug is now used only as an adjunct to anesthetics because it greatly depresses the respiratory center while having less ability to anesthetize the cerebral cortex.

Periodic Breathing. An abnormality of respiration called *periodic breathing* occurs in a number of disease conditions. The person breathes deeply for a short interval and then breathes slightly or not at all for an additional interval, with the cycle repeating itself over and over. One type of periodic breathing, *Cheyne-Stokes breathing*, is characterized by slowly waxing and waning respiration occurring about every 40 to 60 seconds, as illustrated in Figure 41-11.

Basic Mechanism of Cheyne-Stokes Breathing. The basic cause of Cheyne-Stokes breathing is the following: When a person overbreathes, thus blowing off too much carbon dioxide from the pulmonary blood while at the same time increasing blood oxygen, it takes several seconds before the changed pulmonary blood can be transported to the brain and inhibit the excess ventilation. By this time, the person has already overventilated for an extra few seconds.

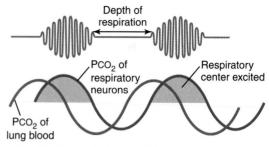

Figure 41-11 Cheyne-Stokes breathing, showing changing Pco_2 in the pulmonary blood (*red line*) and delayed changes in the Pco_2 of the fluids of the respiratory center (*blue line*).

Therefore, when the overventilated blood finally reaches the brain respiratory center, the center becomes depressed to an excessive amount. Then the opposite cycle begins. That is, carbon dioxide increases and oxygen decreases in the alveoli. Again, it takes a few seconds before the brain can respond to these new changes. When the brain does respond, the person breathes hard once again and the cycle repeats.

The basic cause of Cheyne-Stokes breathing occurs in everyone. However, under normal conditions, this mechanism is highly "damped." That is, the fluids of the blood and the respiratory center control areas have large amounts of dissolved and chemically bound carbon dioxide and oxygen. Therefore, normally, the lungs cannot build up enough extra carbon dioxide or depress the oxygen sufficiently in a few seconds to cause the next cycle of the periodic breathing. But under two separate conditions, the damping factors can be overridden and Cheyne-Stokes breathing does occur:

1. When a *long delay occurs for transport of blood from the lungs to the brain,* changes in carbon dioxide and oxygen in the alveoli can continue for many more seconds than usual. Under these conditions, the storage capacities of the alveoli and pulmonary blood for these gases are exceeded; then, after a few more seconds, the periodic respiratory drive becomes extreme and Cheyne-Stokes breathing begins. This type of Cheyne-Stokes breathing often occurs in patients with *severe cardiac failure* because blood flow is slow, thus delaying the transport of blood gases from the lungs to the brain. In fact, in patients with chronic heart failure, Cheyne-Stokes breathing can sometimes occur on and off for months.

2. A second cause of Cheyne-Stokes breathing is *increased negative feedback gain* in the respiratory control areas. This means that a change in blood carbon dioxide or oxygen causes a far greater change in ventilation than normally. For instance, instead of the normal 2- to 3-fold increase in ventilation that occurs when the Pco_2 rises 3 mm Hg, the same 3 mm Hg rise might increase ventilation 10- to 20-fold. The brain feedback tendency for periodic breathing is now strong enough to cause Cheyne-Stokes breathing without extra blood flow delay between the lungs and brain. This type of Cheyne-Stokes breathing occurs mainly in patients with *brain damage.* The brain damage often turns off the respiratory drive entirely for a few seconds; then an extra intense increase in blood carbon dioxide turns it back on with great force. Cheyne-Stokes breathing of this type is frequently a prelude to death from brain malfunction.

Typical records of changes in pulmonary and respiratory center P_{CO_2} during Cheyne-Stokes breathing are shown in Figure 41-11. Note that the P_{CO_2} of the pulmonary blood changes *in advance* of the P_{CO_2} of the respiratory neurons. But the depth of respiration corresponds with the P_{CO_2} in the brain, not with the P_{CO_2} in the pulmonary blood where the ventilation is occurring.

Sleep Apnea

The term *apnea* means absence of spontaneous breathing. Occasional apneas occur during normal sleep, but in persons with *sleep apnea*, the frequency and duration are greatly increased, with episodes of apnea lasting for 10 seconds or longer and occurring 300 to 500 times each night. Sleep apneas can be caused by obstruction of the upper airways, especially the pharynx, or by impaired central nervous system respiratory drive.

Obstructive Sleep Apnea Is Caused by Blockage of the Upper Airway. The muscles of the pharynx normally keep this passage open to allow air to flow into the lungs during inspiration. During sleep, these muscles usually relax, but the airway passage remains open enough to permit adequate airflow. Some individuals have an especially narrow passage, and relaxation of these muscles during sleep causes the pharynx to completely close so that air cannot flow into the lungs.

In persons with sleep apnea, loud *snoring* and *labored breathing* occur soon after falling asleep. The snoring proceeds, often becoming louder, and is then interrupted by a long silent period during which no breathing (apnea) occurs. These periods of apnea result in significant decreases in P_{O_2} and increases in P_{CO_2}, which greatly stimulate respiration. This, in turn, causes sudden attempts to breathe, which result in loud snorts and gasps followed by snoring and repeated episodes of apnea. The periods of apnea and labored breathing are repeated several hundred times during the night, resulting in fragmented, restless sleep. Therefore, patients with sleep apnea usually have excessive daytime *drowsiness*, as well as other disorders, including increased sympathetic activity, high heart rates, pulmonary and systemic hypertension, and a greatly elevated risk for cardiovascular disease.

Obstructive sleep apnea most commonly occurs in older, obese persons in whom there is increased fat deposition in the soft tissues of the pharynx or compression of the pharynx due to excessive fat masses in the neck. In a few individuals, sleep apnea may be associated with nasal obstruction, a very large tongue, enlarged tonsils, or certain shapes of the palate that greatly increase resistance to the flow of air to the lungs during inspiration. The most common treatments of obstructive sleep apnea include (1) surgery to remove excess fat tissue at the back of the throat (a procedure called *uvulopalatopharyngoplasty*), to remove enlarged tonsils or adenoids, or to create an opening in the trachea (tracheostomy) to bypass the obstructed airway during sleep, and (2) nasal ventilation with *continuous positive airway pressure* (CPAP).

"Central" Sleep Apnea Occurs When the Neural Drive to Respiratory Muscles Is Transiently Abolished. In a few persons with sleep apnea, the central nervous system drive to the ventilatory muscles transiently ceases. Disorders that can cause cessation of the ventilatory drive during sleep include *damage to the central respiratory centers or abnormalities of the respiratory neuromuscular apparatus*. Patients affected by central sleep apnea may have decreased ventilation when they are awake, although they are fully capable of normal voluntary breathing. During sleep, their breathing disorders usually worsen, resulting in more frequent episodes of apnea that decrease P_{O_2} and increase P_{CO_2} until a critical level is reached that eventually stimulates respiration. These transient instabilities of respiration cause restless sleep and clinical features similar to those observed in obstructive sleep apnea.

In most patients the cause of central sleep apnea is unknown, although instability of the respiratory drive can result from strokes or other disorders that make the respiratory centers of the brain less responsive to the stimulatory effects of carbon dioxide and hydrogen ions. Patients with this disease are extremely sensitive to even small doses of sedatives or narcotics, which further reduce the responsiveness of the respiratory centers to the stimulatory effects of carbon dioxide. Medications that stimulate the respiratory centers can sometimes be helpful, but ventilation with CPAP at night is usually necessary.

Bibliography

Albert R, Spiro S, Jett J: *Comprehensive Respiratory Medicine*, Philadelphia, 2002, Mosby.

Bradley TD, Floras JS: Obstructive sleep apnoea and its cardiovascular consequences, *Lancet* 373:82, 2009.

Datta A, Tipton M: Respiratory responses to cold water immersion: neural pathways, interactions, and clinical consequences awake and asleep, *J Appl Physiol* 100:2057, 2006.

Dean JB, Ballantyne D, Cardone DL, et al: Role of gap junctions in CO_2 chemoreception and respiratory control, *Am J Physiol Lung Cell Mol Physiol* 283:L665, 2002.

Dempsey JA, McKenzie DC, Haverkamp HC, et al: Update in the understanding of respiratory limitations to exercise performance in fit, active adults, *Chest* 134:613, 2008.

Eckert DJ, Jordan AS, Merchia P, et al: Central sleep apnea: Pathophysiology and treatment, *Chest* 131:595, 2007.

Forster HV: Plasticity in the control of breathing following sensory denervation, *J Appl Physiol* 94:784, 2003.

Gaultier C, Gallego J: Neural control of breathing: insights from genetic mouse models, *J Appl Physiol* 104:1522, 2008.

Gray PA: Transcription factors and the genetic organization of brain stem respiratory neurons, *J Appl Physiol* 104:1513, 2008.

Guyenet PG: The 2008 Carl Ludwig Lecture: retrotrapezoid nucleus, CO2 homeostasis, and breathing automaticity, *J Appl Physiol* 105:404, 2008.

Hilaire G, Pasaro R: Genesis and control of the respiratory rhythm in adult mammals, *News Physiol Sci* 18:23, 2003.

Horner RL, Bradley TD: Update in sleep and control of ventilation 2008, *Am J Respir Crit Care Med* 179:528, 2009.

Morris KF, Baekey DM, Nuding SC, et al: Neural network plasticity in respiratory control, *J Appl Physiol* 94:1242, 2003.

Somers VK, White DP, Amin R, et al: *J Am Coll Cardiol* 52:686, 2008.

Sharp FR, Bernaudin M: HIF1 and oxygen sensing in the brain, *Nat Rev Neurosci* 5:437, 2004.

Thach BT: Some aspects of clinical relevance in the maturation of respiratory control in infants, *J Appl Physiol* 104:1828, 2008.

West JB: *Pulmonary Physiology-The Essentials*, Baltimore, 2003, Lippincott Williams & Wilkins.

Younes M: Role of respiratory control mechanisms in the pathogenesis of obstructive sleep disorders, *J Appl Physiol* 105:1389, 2008.

Young T, Skatrud J, Peppard PE: Risk factors for obstructive sleep apnea in adults, *JAMA* 291:2013, 2004.

CHAPTER 42

Respiratory Insufficiency—Pathophysiology, Diagnosis, Oxygen Therapy

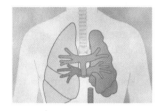

Diagnosis and treatment of most respiratory disorders depend heavily on understanding the basic physiologic principles of respiration and gas exchange. Some respiratory diseases result from inadequate ventilation. Others result from abnormalities of diffusion through the pulmonary membrane or abnormal blood transport of gases between the lungs and tissues. Therapy is often entirely different for these diseases, so it is no longer satisfactory simply to make a diagnosis of "respiratory insufficiency."

Useful Methods for Studying Respiratory Abnormalities

In the previous few chapters, we have discussed several methods for studying respiratory abnormalities, including measuring vital capacity, tidal air, functional residual capacity, dead space, physiologic shunt, and physiologic dead space. This array of measurements is only part of the armamentarium of the clinical pulmonary physiologist. Some other tools are described here.

Study of Blood Gases and Blood pH

Among the most fundamental of all tests of pulmonary performance are determinations of the blood P_{O_2}, CO_2, and pH. It is often important to make these measurements rapidly as an aid in determining appropriate therapy for acute respiratory distress or acute abnormalities of acid-base balance. Several simple and rapid methods have been developed to make these measurements within minutes, using no more than a few drops of blood. They are the following.

Determination of Blood pH. Blood pH is measured using a glass pH electrode of the type used in all chemical laboratories. However, the electrodes used for this purpose are miniaturized. The voltage generated by the glass electrode is a direct measure of pH, and this is generally read directly from a voltmeter scale, or it is recorded on a chart.

Determination of Blood CO_2. A glass electrode pH meter can also be used to determine blood CO_2 in the following way: When a weak solution of sodium bicarbonate is exposed to carbon dioxide gas, the carbon dioxide dissolves in the solution until an equilibrium state is established. In this equilibrium state, the pH of the solution is a function of the carbon dioxide and bicarbonate ion concentrations in accordance with the Henderson-Hasselbalch equation that is explained in Chapter 30; that is,

$$pH = 6.1 + \log \frac{HCO_3^-}{CO_2}$$

When the glass electrode is used to measure CO_2 in blood, a miniature glass electrode is surrounded by a thin plastic membrane. In the space between the electrode and plastic membrane is a solution of sodium bicarbonate of known concentration. Blood is then superfused onto the outer surface of the plastic membrane, allowing carbon dioxide to diffuse from the blood into the bicarbonate solution. Only a drop or so of blood is required. Next, the pH is measured by the glass electrode, and the CO_2 is calculated by use of the previously given formula.

Determination of Blood P_{O_2}. The concentration of oxygen in a fluid can be measured by a technique called *polarography*. Electric current is made to flow between a small negative electrode and the solution. If the voltage of the electrode is more than −0.6 volt different from the voltage of the solution, oxygen will deposit on the electrode. Furthermore, the rate of current flow through the electrode will be directly proportional to the concentration of oxygen (and therefore to P_{O_2} as well). In practice, a negative platinum electrode with a surface area of about 1 square millimeter is used, and this is separated from the blood by a thin plastic membrane that allows diffusion of oxygen but not diffusion of proteins or other substances that will "poison" the electrode.

Often all three of the measuring devices for pH, CO_2, and P_{O_2} are built into the same apparatus, and all these

515

measurements can be made within a minute or so using a single, droplet-size sample of blood. Thus, changes in the blood gases and pH can be followed almost moment by moment at the bedside.

Measurement of Maximum Expiratory Flow

In many respiratory diseases, particularly in asthma, the resistance to airflow becomes especially great during expiration, sometimes causing tremendous difficulty in breathing. This has led to the concept called *maximum expiratory flow*, which can be defined as follows: When a person expires with great force, the expiratory airflow reaches a maximum flow beyond which the flow cannot be increased any more, even with greatly increased additional force. This is the maximum expiratory flow. The maximum expiratory flow is much greater when the lungs are filled with a large volume of air than when they are almost empty. These principles can be understood by referring to Figure 42-1.

Figure 42-1*A* shows the effect of increased pressure applied to the outsides of the alveoli and air passageways caused by compressing the chest cage. The arrows indicate that the same pressure compresses the outsides of both the alveoli and the bronchioles. Therefore, not only does this pressure force air from the alveoli toward the bronchioles, but it also tends to collapse the bronchioles at the same time, which will oppose movement of air to the exterior. Once the bronchioles have almost completely collapsed, further expiratory force can still greatly increase the alveolar pressure, but it also increases the degree of bronchiolar collapse and airway resistance by an equal amount, thus preventing further increase in flow.

Therefore, beyond a critical degree of expiratory force, a maximum expiratory flow has been reached.

Figure 42-1*B* shows the effect of different degrees of lung collapse (and therefore of bronchiolar collapse as well) on the maximum expiratory flow. The curve recorded in this section shows the maximum expiratory flow at all levels of lung volume after a healthy person first inhales as much air as possible and then expires with maximum expiratory effort until he or she can expire at no greater rate. Note that the person quickly reaches a *maximum expiratory airflow* of more than 400 L/min. But regardless of how much additional expiratory effort the person exerts, this is still the maximum flow rate that he or she can achieve.

Note also that as the lung volume becomes smaller, the maximum expiratory flow rate also becomes less. The main reason for this is that in the enlarged lung the bronchi and bronchioles are held open partially by way of elastic pull on their outsides by lung structural elements; however, as the lung becomes smaller, these structures are relaxed so that the bronchi and bronchioles are collapsed more easily by external chest pressure, thus progressively reducing the maximum expiratory flow rate as well.

Abnormalities of the Maximum Expiratory Flow-Volume Curve. Figure 42-2 shows the normal maximum expiratory flow-volume curve, along with two additional flow-volume curves recorded in two types of lung diseases: constricted lungs and partial airway obstruction. Note that the *constricted lungs* have both reduced total lung capacity (TLC) and reduced residual volume (RV). Furthermore, because the lung cannot expand to a normal maximum volume, even with the greatest possible expiratory effort, the maximal expiratory flow cannot rise to equal that of the normal curve. Constricted lung diseases include fibrotic diseases of the lung itself, such as *tuberculosis* and *silicosis*, and diseases that constrict the chest cage, such as *kyphosis*, *scoliosis*, and *fibrotic pleurisy*.

In diseases with *airway obstruction*, it is usually much more difficult to expire than to inspire because the closing tendency of the airways is greatly increased by the extra

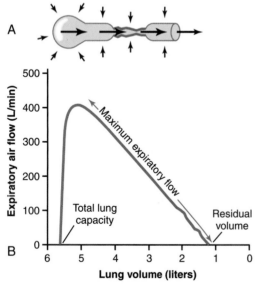

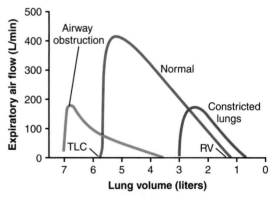

Figure 42-1 *A*, Collapse of the respiratory passageway during maximum expiratory effort, an effect that limits expiratory flow rate. *B*, Effect of lung volume on the maximum expiratory air flow, showing decreasing maximum expiratory air flow as the lung volume becomes smaller.

Figure 42-2 Effect of two respiratory abnormalities—constricted lungs and airway obstruction—on the maximum expiratory flow-volume curve. TLC, total lung capacity; RV, residual volume.

positive pressure required in the chest to cause expiration. By contrast, the extra negative pleural pressure that occurs during inspiration actually "pulls" the airways open at the same time that it expands the alveoli. Therefore, air tends to enter the lung easily but then becomes trapped in the lungs. Over a period of months or years, this effect increases both the TLC and the RV, as shown by the green curve in Figure 42-2. Also, because of the obstruction of the airways and because they collapse more easily than normal airways, the maximum expiratory flow rate is greatly reduced.

The classic disease that causes severe airway obstruction is *asthma*. Serious airway obstruction also occurs in some stages of *emphysema*.

Forced Expiratory Vital Capacity and Forced Expiratory Volume

Another exceedingly useful clinical pulmonary test, and one that is also simple, is to record on a spirometer the *forced expiratory vital capacity* (FVC). Such a recording is shown in Figure 42-3A for a person with normal lungs and in Figure 42-3B for a person with partial airway obstruction. In performing the FVC maneuver, the person first inspires maximally to the total lung capacity and then exhales into the spirometer with maximum expiratory effort as rapidly and as completely as possible. The total distance of the downslope of the lung volume record represents the FVC, as shown in the figure.

Now, study the difference between the two records (1) for normal lungs and (2) for *partial* airway obstruction. The total volume changes of the FVCs are not greatly different, indicating only a moderate difference in basic lung volumes in the two persons. There is, however, a *major difference in the amounts of air that these persons can expire each second*, especially during the first second. Therefore, it is customary to compare the recorded forced expiratory volume during the first second (FEV$_1$) with the normal. In the normal person (see Figure 42-3A), the percentage of the FVC that is expired in the first second divided by the total FVC (FEV$_1$/FVC%) is 80 percent. However, note in Figure 42-3B that, with airway obstruction, this value decreased to only 47 percent. In serious airway obstruction, as often occurs in acute asthma, this can decrease to less than 20 percent.

Pathophysiology of Specific Pulmonary Abnormalities

Chronic Pulmonary Emphysema

The term *pulmonary emphysema* literally means excess air in the lungs. However, this term is usually used to describe complex obstructive and destructive process of the lungs caused by many years of smoking. It results from the following major pathophysiologic changes in the lungs:

1. *Chronic infection*, caused by inhaling smoke or other substances that irritate the bronchi and bronchioles. The chronic infection seriously deranges the normal protective mechanisms of the airways, including partial paralysis of the cilia of the respiratory epithelium, an effect caused by nicotine. As a result, mucus cannot be moved easily out of the passageways. Also, stimulation of excess mucus secretion occurs, which further exacerbates the condition. Inhibition of the alveolar macrophages also occurs, so they become less effective in combating infection.

2. The infection, excess mucus, and inflammatory edema of the bronchiolar epithelium together cause *chronic obstruction* of many of the smaller airways.

3. The obstruction of the airways makes it especially difficult to expire, thus causing *entrapment of air in the alveoli* and overstretching them. This, combined with the lung infection, causes *marked destruction of as much as 50 to 80 percent of the alveolar walls*. Therefore, the final picture of the emphysematous lung is that shown in Figures 42-4 *(top)* and 42-5.

The physiologic effects of chronic emphysema are variable, depending on the severity of the disease and the relative degrees of bronchiolar obstruction versus lung parenchymal destruction. Among the different abnormalities are the following:

1. The bronchiolar obstruction *increases airway resistance* and results in greatly increased work of breathing. It is especially difficult for the person to move air through the bronchioles during expiration because the compressive force on the outside of the lung not only compresses the alveoli but also compresses the bronchioles, which further increases their resistance during expiration.

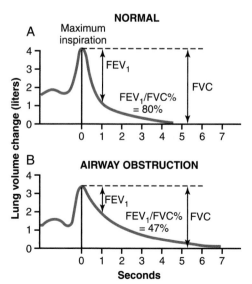

Figure 42-3 Recordings during the forced vital capacity maneuver: *A*, in a healthy person and *B*, in a person with partial airway obstruction. (The "zero" on the volume scale is residual volume.)

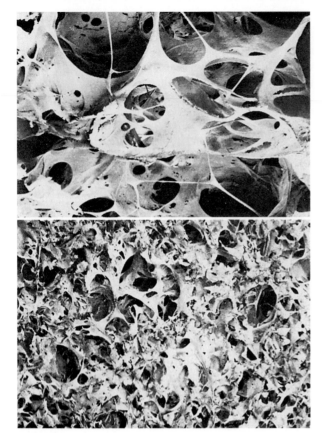

Figure 42-4 Contrast of the emphysematous lung (*top figure*) with the normal lung (*bottom figure*), showing extensive alveolar destruction in emphysema. (Reproduced with permission of Patricia Delaney and the Department of Anatomy, The Medical College of Wisconsin.)

2. The marked loss of alveolar walls greatly *decreases the diffusing capacity* of the lung, which reduces the ability of the lungs to oxygenate the blood and remove carbon dioxide from the blood.

3. The obstructive process is frequently much worse in some parts of the lungs than in other parts, so some portions of the lungs are well ventilated, whereas other portions are poorly ventilated. This often causes *extremely abnormal ventilation-perfusion ratios*, with a very low $\dot{V}a/\dot{Q}$ in some parts *(physiologic shunt)*, result-ing in poor aeration of the blood, and very high $\dot{V}a/\dot{Q}$ in other parts *(physiologic dead space)*, resulting in wasted ventilation, both effects occurring in the same lungs.

4. Loss of large portions of the alveolar walls also decreases the number of pulmonary capillaries through which blood can pass. As a result, the pulmonary vascular resistance often increases markedly, causing *pulmonary hypertension*. This in turn overloads the right side of the heart and frequently causes right-sided heart failure.

Chronic emphysema usually progresses slowly over many years. The person develops both hypoxia and hypercapnia because of hypoventilation of many alveoli plus loss of alveolar walls. The net result of all these effects is severe, prolonged, devastating *air hunger* that can last for years until the hypoxia and hypercapnia cause death—a high penalty to pay for smoking.

Pneumonia

The term *pneumonia* includes any inflammatory condition of the lung in which some or all of the alveoli are filled with fluid and blood cells, as shown in Figure 42-5. A common type of pneumonia is *bacterial pneumonia*, caused most frequently by *pneumococci*. This disease begins with infection in the alveoli; the pulmonary membrane becomes inflamed and highly porous so that fluid and even red and white blood cells leak out of the blood into the alveoli. Thus, the infected alveoli become progressively filled with fluid and cells, and the infection spreads by extension of bacteria or virus from alveolus to alveolus. Eventually, large areas of the lungs, sometimes whole lobes or even a whole lung, become "consolidated," which means that they are filled with fluid and cellular debris.

In pneumonia, the gas exchange functions of the lungs decline in different stages of the disease. In early stages, the pneumonia process might well be localized to only one lung, with alveolar ventilation reduced while blood flow through the lung continues normally. This causes two major pulmonary abnormalities: (1) reduction in the total available surface area of the respiratory membrane

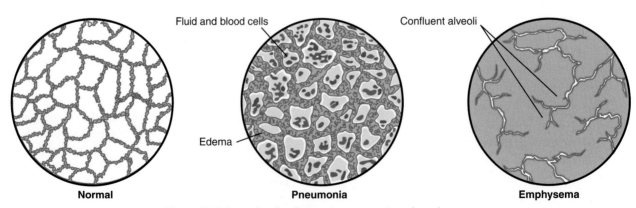

Figure 42-5 Lung alveolar changes in pneumonia and emphysema.

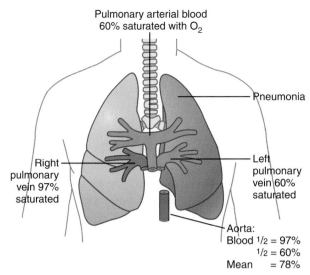

Figure 42-6 Effect of pneumonia on percentage saturation of oxygen in the pulmonary artery, the right and left pulmonary veins, and the aorta.

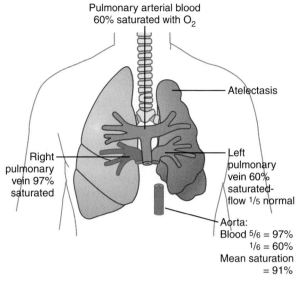

Figure 42-7 Effect of atelectasis on aortic blood oxygen saturation.

and (2) decreased ventilation-perfusion ratio. Both these effects cause *hypoxemia* (low blood oxygen) and *hypercapnia* (high blood carbon dioxide).

Figure 42-6 shows the effect of the decreased ventilation-perfusion ratio in pneumonia, showing that the blood passing through the aerated lung becomes 97 percent saturated with oxygen, whereas that passing through the unaerated lung is about 60 percent saturated. Therefore, the average saturation of the blood pumped by the left heart into the aorta is only about 78 percent, which is far below normal.

Atelectasis

Atelectasis means collapse of the alveoli. It can occur in localized areas of a lung or in an entire lung. Common causes of atelectasis are (1) total obstruction of the airway or (2) lack of surfactant in the fluids lining the alveoli.

Airway Obstruction Causes Lung Collapse. The airway obstruction type of atelectasis usually results from (1) blockage of many small bronchi with mucus or (2) obstruction of a major bronchus by either a large mucus plug or some solid object such as a tumor. The air entrapped beyond the block is absorbed within minutes to hours by the blood flowing in the pulmonary capillaries. If the lung tissue is pliable enough, this will lead simply to collapse of the alveoli. However, if the lung is rigid because of fibrotic tissue and cannot collapse, absorption of air from the alveoli creates very negative pressures within the alveoli, which pull fluid out of the pulmonary capillaries into the alveoli, thus causing the alveoli to fill completely with edema fluid. This almost always is the effect that occurs when an entire lung becomes atelectatic, a condition called *massive collapse* of the lung.

The effects on overall pulmonary function caused by *massive collapse* (atelectasis) of an entire lung are

shown in Figure 42-7. Collapse of the lung tissue not only occludes the alveoli but also almost always increases the *resistance to blood flow* through the pulmonary vessels of the collapsed lung. This resistance increase occurs partially because of the lung collapse itself, which compresses and folds the vessels as the volume of the lung decreases. In addition, hypoxia in the collapsed alveoli causes additional vasoconstriction, as explained in Chapter 38.

Because of the vascular constriction, blood flow through the atelectatic lung is greatly reduced. Fortunately, most of the blood is routed through the ventilated lung and therefore becomes well aerated. In the situation shown in Figure 42-7, five sixths of the blood passes through the aerated lung and only one sixth through the unaerated lung. As a result, the overall ventilation-perfusion ratio is only moderately compromised, so the aortic blood has only mild oxygen desaturation despite total loss of ventilation in an entire lung.

Lack of "Surfactant" as a Cause of Lung Collapse. The secretion and function of *surfactant* in the alveoli were discussed in Chapter 37. It was pointed out that the surfactant is secreted by special alveolar epithelial cells into the fluids that coat the inside surface of the alveoli. The surfactant in turn decreases the surface tension in the alveoli 2- to 10-fold, which normally plays a major role in preventing alveolar collapse. However, in a number of conditions, such as in *hyaline membrane disease* (also called *respiratory distress syndrome*), which often occurs in newborn premature babies, the quantity of surfactant secreted by the alveoli is so greatly depressed that the surface tension of the alveolar fluid becomes several times normal. This causes a serious tendency for the lungs of these babies to collapse or to become filled with fluid. As explained in Chapter 37, many of these infants die of suffocation when large portions of the lungs become atelectatic.

Asthma—Spasmodic Contraction of Smooth Muscles in Bronchioles

Asthma is characterized by spastic contraction of the smooth muscle in the bronchioles, which partially obstructs the bronchioles and causes extremely difficult breathing. It occurs in 3 to 5 percent of all people at some time in life.

The usual cause of asthma is contractile hypersensitivity of the bronchioles in response to foreign substances in the air. In about 70 percent of patients younger than age 30 years, the asthma is caused by allergic hypersensitivity, especially sensitivity to plant pollens. In older people, the cause is almost always hypersensitivity to nonallergenic types of irritants in the air, such as irritants in smog.

The allergic reaction that occurs in the allergic type of asthma is believed to occur in the following way: The typical allergic person tends to form abnormally large amounts of IgE antibodies, and these antibodies cause allergic reactions when they react with the specific antigens that have caused them to develop in the first place, as explained in Chapter 34. In asthma, these *antibodies are mainly attached to mast cells* that are present in the lung interstitium in close association with the bronchioles and small bronchi. When the asthmatic person breathes in pollen to which he or she is sensitive (i.e., to which the person has developed IgE antibodies), the pollen reacts with the mast cell–attached antibodies and causes the mast cells to release several different substances. Among them are (a) *histamine*, (b) *slow-reacting substance of anaphylaxis* (which is a mixture of leukotrienes), (c) *eosinophilic chemotactic factor*, and (d) *bradykinin*. The combined effects of all these factors, especially the slow-reacting substance of anaphylaxis, are to produce (1) localized edema in the walls of the small bronchioles, as well as secretion of thick mucus into the bronchiolar lumens, and (2) spasm of the bronchiolar smooth muscle. Therefore, the airway resistance increases greatly.

As discussed earlier in this chapter, the bronchiolar diameter becomes more reduced during expiration than during inspiration in asthma, caused by bronchiolar collapse during expiratory effort that compresses the outsides of the bronchioles. Because the bronchioles of the asthmatic lungs are already partially occluded, further occlusion resulting from the external pressure creates especially severe obstruction during expiration. That is, the asthmatic person often can inspire quite adequately but has great difficulty expiring. Clinical measurements show (1) greatly reduced maximum expiratory rate and (2) reduced timed expiratory volume. Also, all of this together results in dyspnea, or "air hunger," which is discussed later in this chapter.

The *functional residual capacity* and *residual volume* of the lung become especially increased during the acute asthmatic attack because of the difficulty in expiring air from the lungs. Also, over a period of years, the chest cage becomes permanently enlarged, causing a "barrel chest," and both the functional residual capacity and lung residual volume become permanently increased.

Tuberculosis

In tuberculosis, the tubercle bacilli cause a peculiar tissue reaction in the lungs, including (1) invasion of the infected tissue by macrophages and (2) "walling off" of the lesion by fibrous tissue to form the so-called *tubercle*. This walling-off process helps to limit further transmission of the tubercle bacilli in the lungs and therefore is part of the protective process against extension of the infection. However, in about 3 percent of all people who develop tuberculosis, if untreated, the walling-off process fails and tubercle bacilli spread throughout the lungs, often causing extreme destruction of lung tissue with formation of large abscess cavities.

Thus, tuberculosis in its late stages is characterized by many areas of fibrosis throughout the lungs, as well as reduced total amount of functional lung tissue. These effects cause (1) *increased "work"* on the part of the respiratory muscles to cause pulmonary ventilation and *reduced vital capacity and breathing capacity*; (2) *reduced total respiratory membrane surface area* and *increased thickness of the respiratory membrane*, causing progressively *diminished pulmonary diffusing capacity*; and (3) *abnormal ventilation-perfusion ratio* in the lungs, further reducing overall pulmonary diffusion of oxygen and carbon dioxide.

Hypoxia and Oxygen Therapy

Almost any of the conditions discussed in the past few sections of this chapter can cause serious degrees of cellular hypoxia throughout the body. Sometimes, oxygen therapy is of great value; other times, it is of moderate value; and, at still other times, it is of almost no value. Therefore, it is important to understand the different types of hypoxia; then we can discuss the physiologic principles of oxygen therapy. The following is a descriptive classification of the causes of hypoxia:

1. Inadequate oxygenation of the blood in the lungs because of extrinsic reasons
   a. Deficiency of oxygen in the atmosphere
   b. Hypoventilation (neuromuscular disorders)
2. Pulmonary disease
   a. Hypoventilation caused by increased airway resistance or decreased pulmonary compliance
   b. Abnormal alveolar ventilation-perfusion ratio (including either increased physiologic dead space or increased physiologic shunt)
   c. Diminished respiratory membrane diffusion
3. Venous-to-arterial shunts ("right-to-left" cardiac shunts)
4. Inadequate oxygen transport to the tissues by the blood
   a. Anemia or abnormal hemoglobin
   b. General circulatory deficiency

c. Localized circulatory deficiency (peripheral, cerebral, coronary vessels)

d. Tissue edema

5. Inadequate tissue capability of using oxygen

a. Poisoning of cellular oxidation enzymes

b. Diminished cellular metabolic capacity for using oxygen, because of toxicity, vitamin deficiency, or other factors

This classification of the types of hypoxia is mainly self-evident from the discussions earlier in the chapter. Only one type of hypoxia in the classification needs further elaboration: the hypoxia caused by inadequate capability of the body's tissue cells to use oxygen.

Inadequate Tissue Capability to Use Oxygen. The classic cause of inability of the tissues to use oxygen is *cyanide poisoning*, in which the action of the enzyme *cytochrome oxidase* is completely blocked by the cyanide—to such an extent that the tissues simply cannot use oxygen even when plenty is available. Also, deficiencies of some of the *tissue cellular oxidative enzymes* or of other elements in the tissue oxidative system can lead to this type of hypoxia. A special example occurs in the disease *beriberi*, in which several important steps in tissue utilization of oxygen and formation of carbon dioxide are compromised because of *vitamin B deficiency*.

Effects of Hypoxia on the Body. Hypoxia, if severe enough, can cause death of cells throughout the body, but in less severe degrees it causes principally (1) depressed mental activity, sometimes culminating in coma, and (2) reduced work capacity of the muscles. These effects are specifically discussed in Chapter 43 in relation to high-altitude physiology.

Oxygen Therapy in Different Types of Hypoxia

Oxygen can be administered by (1) placing the patient's head in a "tent" that contains air fortified with oxygen, (2) allowing the patient to breathe either pure oxygen or high concentrations of oxygen from a mask, or (3) administering oxygen through an intranasal tube.

Recalling the basic physiologic principles of the different types of hypoxia, one can readily decide when oxygen therapy will be of value and, if so, how valuable.

In *atmospheric hypoxia*, oxygen therapy can completely correct the depressed oxygen level in the inspired gases and, therefore, provide 100 percent effective therapy.

In *hypoventilation hypoxia*, a person breathing 100 percent oxygen can move five times as much oxygen into the alveoli with each breath as when breathing normal air. Therefore, here again oxygen therapy can be extremely beneficial. (However, this provides no benefit for the excess blood carbon dioxide also caused by the hypoventilation.)

In *hypoxia caused by impaired alveolar membrane diffusion*, essentially the same result occurs as in hypoventilation hypoxia because oxygen therapy can increase the

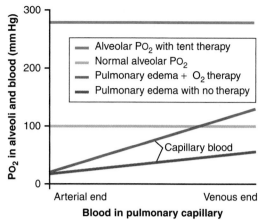

Figure 42-8 Absorption of oxygen into the pulmonary capillary blood in pulmonary edema with and without oxygen tent therapy.

P_{O_2} in the lung alveoli from the normal value of about 100 mm Hg to as high as 600 mm Hg. This raises the oxygen pressure gradient for diffusion of oxygen from the alveoli to the blood from the normal value of 60 mm Hg to as high as 560 mm Hg, an increase of more than 800 percent. This highly beneficial effect of oxygen therapy in diffusion hypoxia is demonstrated in Figure 42-8, which shows that the pulmonary blood in this patient with pulmonary edema picks up oxygen three to four times as rapidly as would occur with no therapy.

In *hypoxia caused by anemia, abnormal hemoglobin transport of oxygen, circulatory deficiency, or physiologic shunt*, oxygen therapy is of much less value because normal oxygen is already available in the alveoli. The problem instead is that one or more of the mechanisms for transporting oxygen from the lungs to the tissues are deficient. Even so, a small amount of extra oxygen, between 7 and 30 percent, can be *transported in the dissolved state* in the blood when alveolar oxygen is increased to maximum even though the amount transported by the hemoglobin is hardly altered. This small amount of extra oxygen may be the difference between life and death.

In the different types of *hypoxia caused by inadequate tissue use of oxygen*, there is abnormality neither of oxygen pickup by the lungs nor of transport to the tissues. Instead, the tissue metabolic enzyme system is simply incapable of using the oxygen that is delivered. Therefore, oxygen therapy provides no measurable benefit.

Cyanosis

The term *cyanosis* means blueness of the skin, and its cause is excessive amounts of deoxygenated hemoglobin in the skin blood vessels, especially in the capillaries. This deoxygenated hemoglobin has an intense dark blue–purple color that is transmitted through the skin.

In general, definite cyanosis appears whenever the *arterial blood* contains more than 5 grams of deoxygenated hemoglobin in each 100 milliliters of blood. A person with *anemia* almost never becomes cyanotic because there is not enough hemoglobin for 5 grams to be deoxygenated in 100 milliliters of arterial blood. Conversely, in a person with excess red blood cells, as occurs in *polycythemia vera*, the great excess of available hemoglobin that can become deoxygenated leads frequently to cyanosis, even under otherwise normal conditions.

Hypercapnia—Excess Carbon Dioxide in the Body Fluids

One might suspect, on first thought, that any respiratory condition that causes hypoxia would also cause hypercapnia. However, hypercapnia usually occurs in association with hypoxia only when the hypoxia is caused by *hypoventilation* or *circulatory deficiency*. The reasons for this are the following.

Hypoxia caused by *too little oxygen in the air, too little hemoglobin*, or *poisoning of the oxidative enzymes* has to do only with the availability of oxygen or use of oxygen by the tissues. Therefore, it is readily understandable that hypercapnia is *not* a concomitant of these types of hypoxia.

In hypoxia resulting from poor diffusion through the pulmonary membrane or through the tissues, serious hypercapnia usually does not occur at the same time because carbon dioxide diffuses 20 times as rapidly as oxygen. If hypercapnia does begin to occur, this immediately stimulates pulmonary ventilation, which corrects the hypercapnia but not necessarily the hypoxia.

Conversely, in hypoxia caused by hypoventilation, carbon dioxide transfer between the alveoli and the atmosphere is affected as much as is oxygen transfer. Hypercapnia then occurs along with the hypoxia. And in circulatory deficiency, diminished flow of blood decreases carbon dioxide removal from the tissues, resulting in tissue hypercapnia in addition to tissue hypoxia. However, the transport capacity of the blood for carbon dioxide is more than three times that for oxygen, so that the resulting tissue hypercapnia is much less than the tissue hypoxia.

When the alveolar P_{CO_2} rises above about 60 to 75 mm Hg, an otherwise normal person by then is breathing about as rapidly and deeply as he or she can, and "air hunger," also called *dyspnea*, becomes severe.

If the P_{CO_2} rises to 80 to 100 mm Hg, the person becomes lethargic and sometimes even semicomatose. Anesthesia and death can result when the P_{CO_2} rises to 120 to 150 mm Hg. At these higher levels of P_{CO_2}, the excess carbon dioxide now begins to depress respiration rather than stimulate it, thus causing a vicious circle: (1) more carbon dioxide, (2) further decrease in respiration, (3) then more carbon dioxide, and so forth—culminating rapidly in a respiratory death.

Dyspnea

Dyspnea means mental anguish associated with inability to ventilate enough to satisfy the demand for air. A common synonym is *air hunger*.

At least three factors often enter into the development of the sensation of dyspnea. They are (1) abnormality of respiratory gases in the body fluids, especially hypercapnia and, to a much less extent, hypoxia; (2) the amount of work that must be performed by the respiratory muscles to provide adequate ventilation; and (3) state of mind.

A person becomes very dyspneic, especially from excess buildup of carbon dioxide in the body fluids. At times, however, the levels of both carbon dioxide and oxygen in the body fluids are normal, but to attain this normality of the respiratory gases, the person has to breathe forcefully. In these instances, the forceful activity of the respiratory muscles frequently gives the person a sensation of dyspnea.

Finally, the person's respiratory functions may be normal and still dyspnea may be experienced because of an abnormal state of mind. This is called *neurogenic dyspnea* or *emotional dyspnea*. For instance, almost anyone momentarily thinking about the act of breathing may suddenly start taking breaths a little more deeply than ordinarily because of a feeling of mild dyspnea. This feeling is greatly enhanced in people who have a psychological fear of not being able to receive a sufficient quantity of air, such as on entering small or crowded rooms.

Artificial Respiration

Resuscitator. Many types of respiratory resuscitators are available, and each has its own characteristic principles of operation. The resuscitator shown in Figure 42-9A consists of a tank supply of oxygen or air; a mechanism for applying intermittent positive pressure and, with some

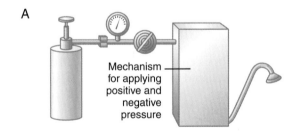

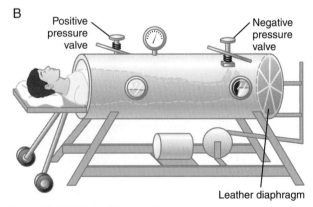

Figure 42-9 *A*, Resuscitator. *B*, Tank respirator.

machines, negative pressure as well; and a mask that fits over the face of the patient or a connector for joining the equipment to an endotracheal tube. This apparatus forces air through the mask or endotracheal tube into the lungs of the patient during the positive-pressure cycle of the resuscitator and then usually allows the air to flow passively out of the lungs during the remainder of the cycle.

Earlier resuscitators often caused damage to the lungs because of excessive positive pressure. Their usage was at one time greatly decried. However, resuscitators now have adjustable positive-pressure limits that are commonly set at 12 to 15 cm H_2O pressure for normal lungs (but sometimes much higher for noncompliant lungs).

Tank Respirator (the "Iron-Lung"). Figure 42-9*B* shows the tank respirator with a patient's body inside the tank and the head protruding through a flexible but airtight collar. At the end of the tank opposite the patient's head, a motor-driven leather diaphragm moves back and forth with sufficient excursion to raise and lower the pressure inside the tank. As the leather diaphragm moves inward, positive pressure develops around the body and causes expiration; as the diaphragm moves outward, negative pressure causes inspiration. Check valves on the respirator control the positive and negative pressures. Ordinarily these pressures are adjusted so that the negative pressure that causes inspiration falls to −10 to −20 cm H_2O and the positive pressure rises to 0 to +5 cm H_2O.

Effect of the Resuscitator and the Tank Respirator on Venous Return. When air is forced into the lungs under positive pressure by a resuscitator, or when the pressure around the patient's body is *reduced* by the tank respirator, the pressure inside the lungs becomes greater than pressure everywhere else in the body. Flow of blood into the chest and heart from the peripheral veins becomes impeded. As a result, use of excessive pressures with either the resuscitator or the tank respirator can reduce the cardiac output—sometimes to lethal levels.

For instance, continuous exposure for more than a few minutes to greater than 30 mm Hg positive pressure in the lungs can cause death because of inadequate venous return to the heart.

Bibliography

Albert R, Spiro S, Jett J: *Comprehensive Respiratory Medicine*, Philadelphia, 2002, Mosby.

Barnes PJ: The cytokine network in asthma and chronic obstructive pulmonary disease, *J Clin Invest* 118:3546, 2008.

Cardoso WV: Molecular regulation of lung development, *Annu Rev Physiol* 63:471, 2001.

Casey KR, Cantillo KO, Brown LK: Sleep-related hypoventilation/hypoxemic syndromes, *Chest* 131:1936, 2007.

Eder W, Ege MJ, von Mutius E: The asthma epidemic, *N Engl J Med* 355:2226, 2006.

Herzog EL, Brody AR, Colby TV, et al: Knowns and unknowns of the alveolus, *Proc Am Thorac Soc* 5:778, 2008.

Knight DA, Holgate ST: The airway epithelium: structural and functional properties in health and disease, *Respirology* 8:432, 2003.

McConnell AK, Romer LM: Dyspnoea in health and obstructive pulmonary disease: the role of respiratory muscle function and training, *Sports Med* 34:117, 2004.

Mühlfeld C, Rothen-Rutishauser B, Blank F, et al: Interactions of nanoparticles with pulmonary structures and cellular responses, *Am J Physiol Lung Cell Mol Physiol* 294:L817, 2008.

Naureckas ET, Solway J: Clinical practice. Mild asthma, *N Engl J Med* 345:1257, 2001.

Ramanathan R: Optimal ventilatory strategies and surfactant to protect the preterm lungs, *Neonatology* 93:302, 2008.

Sharafkhaneh A, Hanania NA, Kim V: Pathogenesis of emphysema: from the bench to the bedside, *Proc Am Thorac Soc* 5:475, 2008.

Sin DD, McAlister FA, Man SF, et al: Contemporary management of chronic obstructive pulmonary disease: scientific review, *JAMA* 290:2301, 2003.

Soni N, Williams P: Positive pressure ventilation: what is the real cost? *Br J Anaesth* 101:446, 2008.

Taraseviciene-Stewart L, Voelkel NF: Molecular pathogenesis of emphysema, *J Clin Invest* 118:394, 2008.

Whitsett JA, Weaver TE: Hydrophobic surfactant proteins in lung function and disease, *N Engl J Med* 347:2141, 2002.

Wills-Karp M, Ewart SL: Time to draw breath: asthma-susceptibility genes are identified, *Nat Rev Genet* 5:376, 2004.

Wright JL, Cosio M, Churg A: Animal models of chronic obstructive pulmonary disease, *Am J Physiol Lung Cell Mol Physiol* 295:L1, 2008.

VIII

Aviation, Space, and Deep-Sea Diving Physiology

43. Aviation, High Altitude, and Space Physiology

44. Physiology of Deep-Sea Diving and Other Hyperbaric Conditions

Aviation, High Altitude, and Space Physiology

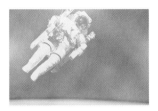

As humans have ascended to higher and higher altitudes in aviation, mountain climbing, and space vehicles, it has become progressively more important to understand the effects of altitude and low gas pressures on the human body. This chapter deals with these problems, as well as acceleratory forces, weightlessness, and other challenges to body homeostasis that occur at high altitude and in space flight.

Effects of Low Oxygen Pressure on the Body

Barometric Pressures at Different Altitudes. Table 43-1 gives the approximate *barometric* and *oxygen pressures* at different altitudes, showing that at sea level, the barometric pressure is 760 mm Hg; at 10,000 feet, only 523 mm Hg; and at 50,000 feet, 87 mm Hg. This decrease in barometric pressure is the basic cause of all the hypoxia problems in high-altitude physiology because, as the barometric pressure decreases, the atmospheric oxygen partial pressure (Po_2) decreases proportionately, remaining at all times slightly less than 21 percent of the total barometric pressure; at sea level Po_2 is about 159 mm Hg, but at 50,000 feet Po_2 is only 18 mm Hg.

Alveolar Po_2 at Different Elevations

Carbon Dioxide and Water Vapor Decrease the Alveolar Oxygen. Even at high altitudes, carbon dioxide is continually excreted from the pulmonary blood into the alveoli. Also, water vaporizes into the inspired air from the respiratory surfaces. These two gases dilute the oxygen in the alveoli, thus reducing the oxygen concentration. Water vapor pressure in the alveoli remains at 47 mm Hg as long as the body temperature is normal, regardless of altitude.

In the case of carbon dioxide, during exposure to very high altitudes, the alveolar Pco_2 falls from the sea-level value of 40 mm Hg to lower values. In the *acclimatized* person, who increases his or her ventilation about fivefold, the Pco_2 falls to about 7 mm Hg because of increased respiration.

Now let us see how the pressures of these two gases affect the alveolar oxygen. For instance, assume that the barometric pressure falls from the normal sea-level value of 760 mm Hg to 253 mm Hg, which is the usual measured value at the top of 29,028-foot Mount Everest. Forty-seven mm Hg of this must be water vapor, leaving only 206 mm Hg for all the other gases. In the *acclimatized* person, 7 mm of the 206 mm Hg must be carbon dioxide, leaving only 199 mm Hg. If there were no use of oxygen by the body, one fifth of this 199 mm Hg would be oxygen and four fifths would be nitrogen; that is, the Po_2 in the alveoli would be 40 mm Hg. However, some of this remaining alveolar oxygen is continually being absorbed into the blood, leaving about 35 mm Hg oxygen pressure in the alveoli. At the summit of Mount Everest, only the best of acclimatized people can barely survive when breathing air. But the effect is very different when the person is breathing pure oxygen, as we see in the following discussions.

Alveolar Po_2 at Different Altitudes. The fifth column of Table 43-1 shows the approximate Po_2s in the alveoli at different altitudes when one is breathing air for both the *unacclimatized* and the *acclimatized* person. At sea level, the alveolar Po_2 is 104 mm Hg; at 20,000 feet altitude, it falls to about 40 mm Hg in the unacclimatized person but only to 53 mm Hg in the acclimatized person. The difference between these two is that alveolar ventilation increases much more in the acclimatized person than in the unacclimatized person, as we discuss later.

Saturation of Hemoglobin with Oxygen at Different Altitudes. Figure 43-1 shows arterial blood oxygen saturation at different altitudes while a person is breathing air and while breathing oxygen. Up to an altitude of about 10,000 feet, even when air is breathed, the arterial oxygen saturation remains at least as high as 90 percent. Above 10,000 feet, the arterial oxygen saturation falls rapidly, as shown by the blue curve of the figure, until it is slightly less than 70 percent at 20,000 feet and much less at still higher altitudes.

Table 43-1 Effects of Acute Exposure to Low Atmospheric Pressures on Alveolar Gas Concentrations and Arterial Oxygen Saturation*

Altitude (ft/meters)	Barometric Pressure (mm Hg)	Po₂ in Air (mm Hg)	Breathing Air			Breathing Pure Oxygen		
			Pco₂ in Alveoli (mm Hg)	Po₂ in Alveoli (mm Hg)	Arterial Oxygen Saturation (%)	Pco₂ in Alveoli (mm Hg)	Po₂ in Alveoli (mm Hg)	Arterial Oxygen Saturation (%)
0	760	159	40 (40)	104 (104)	97 (97)	40	673	100
10,000/3048	523	110	36 (23)	67 (77)	90 (92)	40	436	100
20,000/6096	349	73	24 (10)	40 (53)	73 (85)	40	262	100
30,000/9144	226	47	24 (7)	18 (30)	24 (38)	40	139	99
40,000/12,192	141	29				36	58	84
50,000/15,240	87	18				24	16	15

*Numbers in parentheses are acclimatized values.

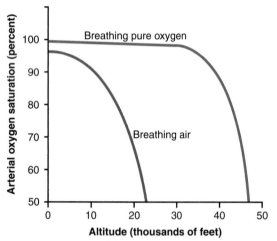

Figure 43-1 Effect of high altitude on arterial oxygen saturation when breathing air and when breathing pure oxygen.

Effect of Breathing Pure Oxygen on Alveolar Po₂ at Different Altitudes

When a person breathes pure oxygen instead of air, most of the space in the alveoli formerly occupied by nitrogen becomes occupied by oxygen. At 30,000 feet, an aviator could have an alveolar Po₂ as high as 139 mm Hg instead of the 18 mm Hg when breathing air (see Table 43-1).

The red curve of Figure 43-1 shows arterial blood hemoglobin oxygen saturation at different altitudes when one is breathing pure oxygen. Note that the saturation remains above 90 percent until the aviator ascends to about 39,000 feet; then it falls rapidly to about 50 percent at about 47,000 feet.

The "Ceiling" When Breathing Air and When Breathing Oxygen in an Unpressurized Airplane

Comparing the two arterial blood oxygen saturation curves in Figure 43-1, one notes that an aviator breathing pure oxygen in an unpressurized airplane can ascend to far higher altitudes than one breathing air. For instance,

the arterial saturation at 47,000 feet when one is breathing oxygen is about 50 percent and is equivalent to the arterial oxygen saturation at 23,000 feet when one is breathing air. In addition, because an unacclimatized person usually can remain conscious until the arterial oxygen saturation falls to 50 percent, for short exposure times the ceiling for an aviator in an unpressurized airplane when breathing air is about 23,000 feet and when breathing pure oxygen is about 47,000 feet, provided the oxygen-supplying equipment operates perfectly.

Acute Effects of Hypoxia

Some of the important acute effects of hypoxia in the unacclimatized person breathing air, beginning at an altitude of about 12,000 feet, are drowsiness, lassitude, mental and muscle fatigue, sometimes headache, occasionally nausea, and sometimes euphoria. These effects progress to a stage of twitchings or seizures above 18,000 feet and end, above 23,000 feet in the unacclimatized person, in coma, followed shortly thereafter by death.

One of the most important effects of hypoxia is decreased mental proficiency, which decreases judgment, memory, and performance of discrete motor movements. For instance, if an unacclimatized aviator stays at 15,000 feet for 1 hour, mental proficiency ordinarily falls to about 50 percent of normal, and after 18 hours at this level it falls to about 20 percent of normal.

Acclimatization to Low Po₂

A person remaining at high altitudes for days, weeks, or years becomes more and more *acclimatized* to the low Po₂, so it causes fewer deleterious effects on the body. And it becomes possible for the person to work harder without hypoxic effects or to ascend to still higher altitudes.

The principal means by which acclimatization comes about are (1) a great increase in pulmonary ventilation, (2) increased numbers of red blood cells, (3) increased diffusing capacity of the lungs, (4) increased vascularity of the peripheral tissues, and (5) increased ability of the tissue cells to use oxygen despite low P_{O_2}.

Increased Pulmonary Ventilation—Role of Arterial Chemoreceptors.

Immediate exposure to low P_{O_2} stimulates the arterial chemoreceptors, and this increases alveolar ventilation to a maximum of about 1.65 times normal. Therefore, compensation occurs within seconds for the high altitude, and it alone allows the person to rise several thousand feet higher than would be possible without the increased ventilation. Then, if the person remains at very high altitude for several days, the chemoreceptors increase ventilation still more, up to about five times normal.

The immediate increase in pulmonary ventilation on rising to a high altitude blows off large quantities of carbon dioxide, reducing the P_{CO_2} and increasing the pH of the body fluids. These changes *inhibit* the brain stem respiratory center and thereby *oppose the effect of low P_{O_2} to stimulate respiration by way of the peripheral arterial chemoreceptors in the carotid and aortic bodies.* But during the ensuing 2 to 5 days, this inhibition fades away, allowing the respiratory center to respond with full force to the peripheral chemoreceptor stimulus from hypoxia, and ventilation increases to about five times normal.

The cause of this fading inhibition is believed to be mainly a reduction of bicarbonate ion concentration in the cerebrospinal fluid, as well as in the brain tissues. This in turn decreases the pH in the fluids surrounding the chemosensitive neurons of the respiratory center, thus increasing the respiratory stimulatory activity of the center.

An important mechanism for the gradual decrease in bicarbonate concentration is compensation by the kidneys for the respiratory alkalosis, as discussed in Chapter 30. The kidneys respond to decreased P_{CO_2} by reducing hydrogen ion secretion and increasing bicarbonate excretion. This metabolic compensation for the respiratory alkalosis gradually reduces plasma and cerebrospinal fluid bicarbonate concentration and pH toward normal and removes part of the inhibitory effect on respiration of low hydrogen ion concentration. Thus, the respiratory centers are much more responsive to the peripheral chemoreceptor stimulus caused by the hypoxia after the kidneys compensate for the alkalosis.

Increase in Red Blood Cells and Hemoglobin Concentration During Acclimatization.

As discussed in Chapter 32, hypoxia is the principal stimulus for causing an increase in red blood cell production. Ordinarily, when a person remains exposed to low oxygen for weeks at a time, the hematocrit rises slowly from a normal value of 40 to 45 to an average of about 60, with an average increase in whole blood hemoglobin concentration from normal of 15 g/dl to about 20 g/dl.

In addition, the blood volume also increases, often by 20 to 30 percent, and this increase times the increased blood hemoglobin concentration gives an increase in total body hemoglobin of 50 or more percent.

Increased Diffusing Capacity After Acclimatization.

The normal diffusing capacity for oxygen through the pulmonary membrane is about 21 ml/mm Hg/min, and this diffusing capacity can increase as much as threefold during exercise. A similar increase in diffusing capacity occurs at high altitude.

Part of the increase results from increased pulmonary capillary blood volume, which expands the capillaries and increases the surface area through which oxygen can diffuse into the blood. Another part results from an increase in lung air volume, which expands the surface area of the alveolar-capillary interface still more. A final part results from an increase in pulmonary arterial blood pressure; this forces blood into greater numbers of alveolar capillaries than normally—especially in the upper parts of the lungs, which are poorly perfused under usual conditions.

Peripheral Circulatory System Changes During Acclimatization—Increased Tissue Capillarity.

The cardiac output often increases as much as 30 percent immediately after a person ascends to high altitude but then decreases back toward normal *over a period of weeks as the blood hematocrit increases,* so the amount of oxygen transported to the peripheral body tissues remains about normal.

Another circulatory adaptation is *growth of increased numbers of systemic circulatory capillaries* in the nonpulmonary tissues, which is called *increased tissue capillarity* (or *angiogenesis*). This occurs especially in animals born and bred at high altitudes but less so in animals that later in life become exposed to high altitude.

In active tissues exposed to chronic hypoxia, the increase in capillarity is especially marked. For instance, capillary density in right ventricular muscle increases markedly because of the combined effects of hypoxia and excess workload on the right ventricle caused by pulmonary hypertension at high altitude.

Cellular Acclimatization.

In animals native to altitudes of 13,000 to 17,000 feet, cell mitochondria and cellular oxidative enzyme systems are slightly more plentiful than in sea-level inhabitants. Therefore, it is presumed that the tissue cells of high altitude–acclimatized human beings also can use oxygen more effectively than can their sea-level counterparts.

Natural Acclimatization of Native Human Beings Living at High Altitudes

Many native human beings in the Andes and in the Himalayas live at altitudes above 13,000 feet—one group in the Peruvian Andes lives at an altitude of 17,500 feet and works a mine at an altitude of 19,000 feet. Many of these natives are born at these altitudes and live there all their lives. In all aspects of acclimatization, the natives are superior to even the best-acclimatized lowlanders, even though the lowlanders might also have lived at high altitudes for 10 or more years. Acclimatization of the natives

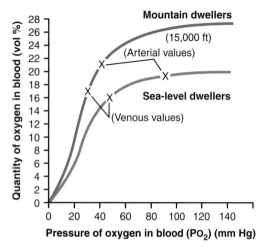

Figure 43-2 Oxygen-hemoglobin dissociation curves for blood of high-altitude residents (*red curve*) and sea-level residents (*blue curve*), showing the respective arterial and venous P_{O_2} levels and oxygen contents as recorded in their native surroundings. (Data from Oxygen-dissociation curves for bloods of high-altitude and sea-level residents. PAHO Scientific Publication No. 140, Life at High Altitudes, 1966.)

begins in infancy. The chest size, especially, is greatly increased, whereas the body size is somewhat decreased, giving a high ratio of ventilatory capacity to body mass. In addition, their hearts, which from birth onward pump extra amounts of cardiac output, are considerably larger than the hearts of lowlanders.

Delivery of oxygen by the blood to the tissues is also highly facilitated in these natives. For instance, Figure 43-2 shows oxygen-hemoglobin dissociation curves for natives who live at sea level and for their counterparts who live at 15,000 feet. Note that the arterial oxygen P_{O_2} in the natives at high altitude is only 40 mm Hg, but because of the greater quantity of hemoglobin, the quantity of oxygen in their arterial blood is greater than that in the blood of the natives at the lower altitude. Note also that the venous P_{O_2} in the high-altitude natives is only 15 mm Hg less than the venous P_{O_2} for the lowlanders, despite the very low arterial P_{O_2}, indicating that oxygen transport to the tissues is exceedingly effective in the naturally acclimatized high-altitude natives.

Reduced Work Capacity at High Altitudes and Positive Effect of Acclimatization

In addition to the mental depression caused by hypoxia, as discussed earlier, the work capacity of all muscles is greatly decreased in hypoxia. This includes not only skeletal muscles but also cardiac muscles.

In general, work capacity is reduced in direct proportion to the decrease in maximum rate of oxygen uptake that the body can achieve.

To give an idea of the importance of acclimatization in increasing work capacity, consider the large differences in work capacities as percent of normal for unacclimatized and acclimatized people at an altitude of 17,000 feet:

	Work capacity (percent of normal)
Unacclimatized	50
Acclimatized for 2 months	68
Native living at 13,200 feet but working at 17,000 feet	87

Thus, naturally acclimatized native persons can achieve a daily work output even at high altitude almost equal to that of a lowlander at sea level, but even well-acclimatized lowlanders can almost never achieve this result.

Acute Mountain Sickness and High-Altitude Pulmonary Edema

A small percentage of people who ascend rapidly to high altitudes become acutely sick and can die if not given oxygen or removed to a low altitude. The sickness begins from a few hours up to about 2 days after ascent. Two events frequently occur:

1. *Acute cerebral edema.* This is believed to result from local vasodilation of the cerebral blood vessels, caused by the hypoxia. Dilation of the arterioles increases blood flow into the capillaries, thus increasing capillary pressure, which in turn causes fluid to leak into the cerebral tissues. The cerebral edema can then lead to severe disorientation and other effects related to cerebral dysfunction.

2. *Acute pulmonary edema.* The cause of this is still unknown, but one explanation is the following: The severe hypoxia causes the pulmonary arterioles to constrict potently, but the constriction is much greater in some parts of the lungs than in other parts, so more and more of the pulmonary blood flow is forced through fewer and fewer still unconstricted pulmonary vessels. The postulated result is that the capillary pressure in these areas of the lungs becomes especially high and local edema occurs. Extension of the process to progressively more areas of the lungs leads to spreading pulmonary edema and severe pulmonary dysfunction that can be lethal. Allowing the person to breathe oxygen usually reverses the process within hours.

Chronic Mountain Sickness

Occasionally, a person who remains at high altitude too long develops *chronic mountain sickness*, in which the following effects occur: (1) The red cell mass and hematocrit become exceptionally high, (2) the pulmonary arterial pressure becomes elevated even more than the normal elevation that occurs during acclimatization, (3) the right side of the heart becomes greatly enlarged, (4) the peripheral arterial pressure begins to fall, (5) congestive heart failure ensues, and (6) death often follows unless the person is removed to a lower altitude.

The causes of this sequence of events are probably threefold: First, the red cell mass becomes so great that the blood viscosity increases severalfold; this increased viscosity tends to *decrease* tissue blood flow so that oxygen delivery also begins to decrease. Second, the pulmonary arterioles become vasoconstricted because of the lung hypoxia. This results from the hypoxic vascular constrictor effect that normally operates to divert blood flow from low-oxygen to high-oxygen alveoli, as explained in Chapter 38. But because *all* the alveoli are now in the low-oxygen state, all the arterioles become constricted, the pulmonary arterial pressure rises excessively, and the right side of the heart fails. Third, the alveolar arteriolar spasm diverts much of the blood flow through nonalveolar pulmonary vessels, thus causing an excess of pulmonary shunt blood flow where the blood is poorly oxygenated; this further compounds the problem. Most of these people recover within days or weeks when they are moved to a lower altitude.

Effects of Acceleratory Forces on the Body in Aviation and Space Physiology

Because of rapid changes in velocity and direction of motion in airplanes or spacecraft, several types of acceleratory forces affect the body during flight. At the beginning of flight, simple linear acceleration occurs; at the end of flight, deceleration; and every time the vehicle turns, centrifugal acceleration.

Centrifugal Acceleratory Forces

When an airplane makes a turn, the force of centrifugal acceleration is determined by the following relation:

$$f = \frac{mv^2}{r}$$

in which f is centrifugal acceleratory force, m is the mass of the object, v is velocity of travel, and r is radius of curvature of the turn. From this formula, it is obvious that as the velocity increases, the *force of centrifugal acceleration increases in proportion to the square of the velocity.* It is also obvious that the force of acceleration is *directly proportional to the sharpness of the turn (the less the radius).*

Measurement of Acceleratory Force—"G." When an aviator is simply sitting in his seat, the force with which he is pressing against the seat results from the pull of gravity and is equal to his weight. The intensity of this force is said to be +1G because it is equal to the pull of gravity. If the force with which he presses against the seat becomes five times his normal weight during pull-out from a dive, the force acting on the seat is +5 G.

If the airplane goes through an outside loop so that the person is held down by his seat belt, *negative G* is applied to his body; if the force with which he is held down by his belt is equal to the weight of his body, the negative force is −1G.

Effects of Centrifugal Acceleratory Force on the Body—(Positive G)

Effects on the Circulatory System. The most important effect of centrifugal acceleration is on the circulatory system, because blood is mobile and can be translocated by centrifugal forces.

When an aviator is subjected to *positive G*, blood is centrifuged toward the lowermost part of the body. Thus, if the centrifugal acceleratory force is +5 G and the person is in an immobilized standing position, the pressure in the veins of the feet becomes greatly increased (to about 450 mm Hg). In the sitting position, the pressure becomes nearly 300 mm Hg. And, as pressure in the vessels of the lower body increases, these vessels passively dilate so that a major portion of the blood from the upper body is translocated into the lower vessels. Because the heart cannot pump unless blood returns to it, the greater the quantity of blood "pooled" in this way in the lower body, the less that is available for the cardiac output.

Figure 43-3 shows the changes in systolic and diastolic arterial pressures (top and bottom curves, respectively) in the upper body when a centrifugal acceleratory force of +3.3 G is suddenly applied to a sitting person. Note that both these pressures fall below 22 mm Hg for the first few seconds after the acceleration begins but then return to a systolic pressure of about 55 mm Hg and a diastolic pressure of 20 mm Hg within another 10 to 15 seconds. This secondary recovery is caused mainly by activation of the baroreceptor reflexes.

Acceleration greater than 4 to 6 G causes "blackout" of vision within a few seconds and unconsciousness shortly thereafter. If this great degree of acceleration is continued, the person will die.

Effects on the Vertebrae. Extremely high acceleratory forces for even a fraction of a second can fracture the vertebrae. The degree of positive acceleration that the average person can withstand in the sitting position before vertebral fracture occurs is about 20 G.

Negative G. The effects of negative G on the body are less dramatic acutely but possibly more damaging permanently than the effects of positive G. An aviator can

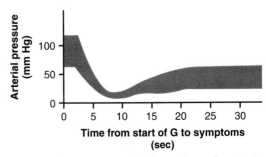

Figure 43-3 Changes in systolic (*top of curve*) and diastolic (*bottom of curve*) arterial pressures after abrupt and continuing exposure of a sitting person to an acceleratory force from top to bottom of 3.3 G. (Data from Martin EE, Henry JP: Effects of time and temperature upon tolerance to positive acceleration. J Aviation Med 22:382, 1951.)

usually go through outside loops up to negative acceleratory forces of −4 to −5 G without causing permanent harm, although causing intense momentary hyperemia of the head. Occasionally, psychotic disturbances lasting for 15 to 20 minutes occur as a result of brain edema.

Occasionally, negative G forces can be so great (−20 G, for instance) and centrifugation of the blood into the head is so great that the cerebral blood pressure reaches 300 to 400 mm Hg, sometimes causing small vessels on the surface of the head and in the brain to rupture. However, the vessels inside the cranium show less tendency for rupture than would be expected for the following reason: The cerebrospinal fluid is centrifuged toward the head at the same time that blood is centrifuged toward the cranial vessels, and the greatly increased pressure of the cerebrospinal fluid acts as a cushioning buffer on the outside of the brain to prevent intracerebral vascular rupture.

Because the eyes are not protected by the cranium, intense hyperemia occurs in them during strong negative G. As a result, the eyes often become temporarily blinded with "red-out."

Protection of the Body Against Centrifugal Acceleratory Forces. Specific procedures and apparatus have been developed to protect aviators against the circulatory collapse that might occur during positive G. First, if the aviator tightens his or her abdominal muscles to an extreme degree and leans forward to compress the abdomen, some of the pooling of blood in the large vessels of the abdomen can be prevented, delaying the onset of blackout. Also, special "anti-G" suits have been devised to prevent pooling of blood in the lower abdomen and legs. The simplest of these applies positive pressure to the legs and abdomen by inflating compression bags as the G increases. Theoretically, a pilot submerged in a tank or suit of water might experience little effect of G forces on the circulation because the pressures developed in the water pressing on the outside of the body during centrifugal acceleration would almost exactly balance the forces acting in the body. However, the presence of air in the lungs still allows displacement of the heart, lung tissues, and diaphragm into seriously abnormal positions despite submersion in water. Therefore, even if this procedure were used, the limit of safety almost certainly would still be less than 10 G.

Effects of Linear Acceleratory Forces on the Body

Acceleratory Forces in Space Travel. Unlike an airplane, a spacecraft cannot make rapid turns; therefore, centrifugal acceleration is of little importance except when the spacecraft goes into abnormal gyrations. However, blast-off acceleration and landing deceleration can be tremendous; both of these are types of *linear acceleration,* one positive and the other negative.

Figure 43-4 shows an approximate profile of acceleration during blast-off in a three-stage spacecraft, demonstrating that the first-stage booster causes acceleration as high as 9 G, and the second-stage booster as high as 8 G. In the standing position, the human body could not

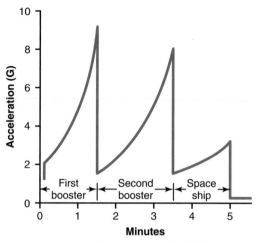

Figure 43-4 Acceleratory forces during takeoff of a spacecraft.

withstand this much acceleration, but in a semireclining position *transverse to the axis of acceleration,* this amount of acceleration can be withstood with ease despite the fact that the acceleratory forces continue for as long as several minutes at a time. Therefore, we see the reason for the reclining seats used by astronauts.

Problems also occur during deceleration when the spacecraft re-enters the atmosphere. A person traveling at Mach 1 (the speed of sound and of fast airplanes) can be safely decelerated in a distance of about 0.12 mile, whereas a person traveling at a speed of Mach 100 (a speed possible in interplanetary space travel) would require a distance of about 10,000 miles for safe deceleration. The principal reason for this difference is that the total amount of energy that must be dispelled during deceleration is proportional to the *square* of the velocity, which alone increases the required distance for decelerations between Mach 1 versus Mach 100 about 10,000-fold. Therefore, deceleration must be accomplished much more slowly from high velocities than is necessary at lower velocities.

Deceleratory Forces Associated with Parachute Jumps. When the parachuting aviator leaves the airplane, his velocity of fall is at first exactly 0 feet per second. However, because of the acceleratory force of gravity, within 1 second his velocity of fall is 32 feet per second (if there is no air resistance); in 2 seconds it is 64 feet per second; and so on. As the velocity of fall increases, the air resistance tending to slow the fall also increases. Finally, the deceleratory force of the air resistance exactly balances the acceleratory force of gravity, so after falling for about 12 seconds, the person will be falling at a "terminal velocity" of 109 to 119 miles per hour (175 feet per second). If the parachutist has already reached terminal velocity before opening his parachute, an "opening shock load" of up to 1200 pounds can occur on the parachute shrouds.

The usual-sized parachute slows the fall of the parachutist to about one-ninth the terminal velocity. In other words, the speed of landing is about 20 feet per second, and the force of impact against the earth is 1/81 the impact force without a parachute. Even so, the force of impact is still great enough to cause considerable damage to the body unless the parachutist is properly trained in landing. Actually, the force of impact with the earth is about the same as that which would be experienced by jumping without a parachute from a height of about 6 feet. Unless forewarned, the parachutist will be tricked by his senses into striking the earth with extended legs, and this will result in tremendous deceleratory forces along the skeletal axis of the body, resulting in fracture of his pelvis, vertebrae, or leg. Consequently, the trained parachutist strikes the earth with knees bent but muscles taut to cushion the shock of landing.

"Artificial Climate" in the Sealed Spacecraft

Because there is no atmosphere in outer space, an artificial atmosphere and climate must be produced in a spacecraft. Most important, the oxygen concentration must remain high enough and the carbon dioxide concentration low enough to prevent suffocation. In some earlier space missions, a capsule atmosphere containing pure oxygen at about 260 mm Hg pressure was used, but in the modern space shuttle, gases about equal to those in normal air are used, with four times as much nitrogen as oxygen and a total pressure of 760 mm Hg. The presence of nitrogen in the mixture greatly diminishes the likelihood of fire and explosion. It also protects against development of local patches of lung atelectasis that often occur when breathing pure oxygen because oxygen is absorbed rapidly when small bronchi are temporarily blocked by mucous plugs.

For space travel lasting more than several months, it is impractical to carry along an adequate oxygen supply. For this reason, recycling techniques have been proposed for use of the same oxygen over and over again. Some recycling processes depend on purely physical procedures, such as electrolysis of water to release oxygen. Others depend on biological methods, such as use of algae with their large store of chlorophyll to release oxygen from carbon dioxide by the process of photosynthesis. A completely satisfactory system for recycling has yet to be achieved.

Weightlessness in Space

A person in an orbiting satellite or a nonpropelled spacecraft experiences *weightlessness*, or a state of near-zero G force, which is sometimes called *microgravity*. That is, the person is not drawn toward the bottom, sides, or top of the spacecraft but simply floats inside its chambers. The cause of this is not failure of gravity to pull on the body because gravity from any nearby heavenly body is still active. However, the gravity acts on both the spacecraft and the person at the same time so that both are pulled with exactly the same acceleratory forces and in the same direction. For this reason, the person simply is not attracted toward any specific wall of the spacecraft.

Physiologic Problems of Weightlessness (Microgravity). The physiologic problems of weightlessness have not proved to be of much significance, as long as the period of weightlessness is not too long. Most of the problems that do occur are related to three effects of the weightlessness: (1) motion sickness during the first few days of travel, (2) translocation of fluids within the body because of failure of gravity to cause normal hydrostatic pressures, and (3) diminished physical activity because no strength of muscle contraction is required to oppose the force of gravity.

Almost 50 percent of astronauts experience motion sickness, with nausea and sometimes vomiting, during the first 2 to 5 days of space travel. This probably results from an unfamiliar pattern of motion signals arriving in the equilibrium centers of the brain, and at the same time lack of gravitational signals.

The observed effects of prolonged stay in space are the following: (1) decrease in blood volume, (2) decrease in red blood cell mass, (3) decrease in muscle strength and work capacity, (4) decrease in maximum cardiac output, and (5) loss of calcium and phosphate from the bones, as well as loss of bone mass. Most of these same effects also occur in people who lie in bed for an extended period of time. For this reason, exercise programs are carried out by astronauts during prolonged space missions.

In previous space laboratory expeditions in which the exercise program had been less vigorous, the astronauts had severely decreased work capacities for the first few days after returning to earth. They also tended to faint (and still do, to some extent) when they stood up during the first day or so after return to gravity because of diminished blood volume and diminished responses of the arterial pressure control mechanisms.

Cardiovascular, Muscle, and Bone "Deconditioning" During Prolonged Exposure to Weightlessness. During very long space flights and prolonged exposure to microgravity, gradual "deconditioning" effects occur on the cardiovascular system, skeletal muscles, and bone despite rigorous exercise during the flight. Studies of astronauts on space flights lasting several months have shown that they may lose as much 1.0 percent of their bone mass each month even though they continue to exercise. Substantial atrophy of cardiac and skeletal muscles also occurs during prolonged exposure to a microgravity environment.

One of the most serious effects is cardiovascular "deconditioning," which includes decreased work capacity, reduced blood volume, impaired baroreceptor reflexes, and reduced orthostatic tolerance. These changes greatly limit the astronauts' ability to stand upright or perform normal daily activities after returning to the full gravity of Earth.

Astronauts returning from space flights lasting 4 to 6 months are also susceptible to bone fractures and may require several weeks before they return to preflight cardiovascular, bone, and muscle fitness. As space flights become longer in preparation for possible human exploration of other planets, such as Mars, the effects of prolonged microgravity could pose a very serious threat to astronauts after they land, especially in the event of an emergency landing. Therefore, considerable research effort has been directed toward developing countermeasures, in addition to exercise, that can prevent or more effectively attenuate these changes. One such countermeasure that is being tested is the application of intermittent "artificial gravity" caused by short periods (e.g., 1 hour each day) of centrifugal acceleration of the astronauts while they sit in specially designed short-arm centrifuges that create forces of up to 2 to 3 G.

Bibliography

Adams GR, Caiozzo VJ, Baldwin KM: Skeletal muscle unweighting: space-flight and ground-based models, *J Appl Physiol* 95:2185, 2003.

Bärtsch P, Mairbäurl H, Maggiorini M, et al: Physiological aspects of high-altitude pulmonary edema, *J Appl Physiol* 98:1101, 2005.

Basnyat B, Murdoch DR: High-altitude illness, *Lancet* 361:1967, 2003.

Convertino VA: Mechanisms of microgravity induced orthostatic intolerance: implications for effective countermeasures, *J Gravit Physiol* 9:1, 2002.

Diedrich A, Paranjape SY, Robertson D: Plasma and blood volume in space, *Am J Med Sci* 334:80, 2007.

Di Rienzo M, Castiglioni P, Iellamo F, et al: Dynamic adaptation of cardiac baroreflex sensitivity to prolonged exposure to microgravity: data from a 16-day spaceflight, *J Appl Physiol* 105:1569, 2008.

Hackett PH, Roach RC: High-altitude illness, *N Engl J Med* 345:107, 2001.

Hainsworth R, Drinkhill MJ: Cardiovascular adjustments for life at high altitude, *Respir Physiol Neurobiol* 158:204, 2007.

Hoschele S, Mairbaurl H: Alveolar flooding at high altitude: failure of reabsorption? *News Physiol Sci* 18:55, 2003.

LeBlanc AD, Spector ER, Evans HJ, et al: Skeletal responses to space flight and the bed rest analog: a review, *J Musculoskelet Neuronal Interact* 7:33, 2007.

Penaloza D, Arias-Stella J: The heart and pulmonary circulation at high altitudes: healthy highlanders and chronic mountain sickness, *Circulation* 115:1132, 2007.

Smith SM, Heer M: Calcium and bone metabolism during space flight, *Nutrition* 18:849, 2002.

West JB: Man in space, *News Physiol Sci* 1:198, 1986.

West JB: George I. Finch and his pioneering use of oxygen for climbing at extreme altitudes, *J Appl Physiol* 94:1702, 2003.

CHAPTER 44

Physiology of Deep-Sea Diving and Other Hyperbaric Conditions

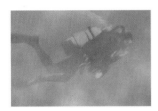

When human beings descend beneath the sea, the pressure around them increases tremendously. To keep the lungs from collapsing, air must be supplied at very high pressure to keep them inflated. This exposes the blood in the lungs to extremely high alveolar gas pressure, a condition called *hyperbarism*. Beyond certain limits, these high pressures cause tremendous alterations in body physiology and can be lethal.

Relationship of Pressure to Sea Depth. A column of seawater 33 feet (10.1 meters) deep exerts the same pressure at its bottom as the pressure of the atmosphere above the sea. Therefore, a person 33 feet beneath the ocean surface is exposed to 2 atmospheres pressure, 1 atmosphere of pressure caused by the weight of the air above the water and the second atmosphere by the weight of the water itself. At 66 feet the pressure is 3 atmospheres, and so forth, in accord with the table in Figure 44-1.

Effect of Sea Depth on the Volume of Gases— Boyle's Law. Another important effect of depth is compression of gases to smaller and smaller volumes. The lower part of Figure 44-1 shows a bell jar at sea level containing 1 liter of air. At 33 feet beneath the sea, where the pressure is 2 atmospheres, the volume has been compressed to only one-half liter, and at 8 atmospheres (233 feet) to one-eighth liter. Thus, the volume to which a given quantity of gas is compressed is inversely proportional to the pressure. This is a principle of physics called *Boyle's law*, which is extremely important in diving physiology because increased pressure can collapse the air chambers of the diver's body, especially the lungs, and often causes serious damage.

Many times in this chapter it is necessary to refer to *actual volume* versus *sea-level volume*. For instance, we might speak of an actual volume of 1 liter at a depth of 300 feet; this is the same *quantity* of air as a sea-level volume of 10 liters.

Effect of High Partial Pressures of Individual Gases on the Body

The individual gases to which a diver is exposed when breathing air are *nitrogen*, *oxygen*, and *carbon dioxide*; each of these at times can cause significant physiologic effects at high pressures.

Nitrogen Narcosis at High Nitrogen Pressures

About four fifths of the air is nitrogen. At sea-level pressure, the nitrogen has no significant effect on bodily function, but at high pressures it can cause varying degrees of narcosis. When the diver remains beneath the sea for an hour or more and is breathing compressed air, the depth at which the first symptoms of mild narcosis appear is about 120 feet. At this level the diver begins to exhibit joviality and to lose many of his or her cares. At 150 to 200 feet, the diver becomes drowsy. At 200 to 250 feet, his or her strength wanes considerably, and the diver often becomes too clumsy to perform the work required. Beyond 250 feet (8.5 atmospheres pressure), the diver usually becomes almost useless as a result of nitrogen narcosis if he or she remains at these depths too long.

Nitrogen narcosis has characteristics similar to those of alcohol intoxication, and for this reason it has frequently been called "raptures of the depths." The mechanism of the narcotic effect is believed to be the same as that of most other gas anesthetics. That is, it dissolves in the fatty substances in neuronal membranes and, because of its *physical* effect on altering ionic conductance through the membranes, reduces neuronal excitability.

Oxygen Toxicity at High Pressures

Effect of Very High P_{O_2} on Blood Oxygen Transport. When the P_{O_2} in the blood rises above 100 mm Hg, the amount of oxygen dissolved in the water of the blood increases markedly. This is shown in Figure 44-2, which depicts the same oxygen-hemoglobin dissociation curve as that shown in Chapter 40 but with the alveolar P_{O_2} extended to more than 3000 mm Hg. Also depicted by the lowest curve in the figure is the *volume of oxygen dissolved in the fluid of the blood* at each P_{O_2} level. Note that

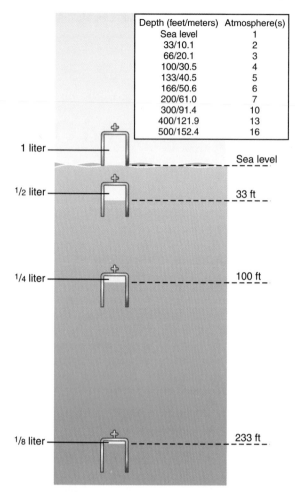

Depth (feet/meters)	Atmosphere(s)
Sea level	1
33/10.1	2
66/20.1	3
100/30.5	4
133/40.5	5
166/50.6	6
200/61.0	7
300/91.4	10
400/121.9	13
500/152.4	16

Figure 44-1 Effect of sea depth on pressure (*top table*) and on gas volume (*bottom*).

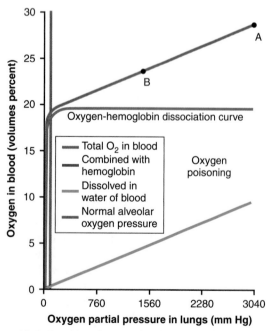

Figure 44-2 Quantity of oxygen dissolved in the fluid of the blood and in combination with hemoglobin at very high P_{O_2}s.

in the normal range of alveolar P_{O_2} (below 120 mm Hg), almost none of the total oxygen in the blood is accounted for by dissolved oxygen, but as the oxygen pressure rises into the thousands of millimeters of mercury, a large portion of the total oxygen is then dissolved in the water of the blood, in addition to that bound with hemoglobin.

Effect of High Alveolar P_{O_2} on Tissue P_{O_2}. Let us assume that the P_{O_2} in the lungs is about 3000 mm Hg (4 atmospheres pressure). Referring to Figure 44-2, one finds that this represents a total oxygen content in each 100 milliliters of blood of about 29 volumes percent, as demonstrated by point A in the figure—this means 20 volumes percent bound with hemoglobin and 9 volumes percent dissolved in the blood water. As this blood passes through the tissue capillaries and the tissues use their normal amount of oxygen, about 5 milliliters from each 100 milliliters of blood, the oxygen content on leaving the tissue capillaries is still 24 volumes percent (point B in the figure). At this point, the P_{O_2} is approximately 1200 mm Hg, which means that oxygen is delivered to the tissues at this extremely high pressure instead of at the normal value of 40 mm Hg. Thus, once the alveolar P_{O_2} rises above a critical level, the hemoglobin-oxygen buffer mechanism (discussed in Chapter 40) is no longer capable of keeping the tissue P_{O_2} in the normal, safe range between 20 and 60 mm Hg.

Acute Oxygen Poisoning. The extremely high tissue P_{O_2} that occurs when oxygen is breathed at very high alveolar oxygen pressure can be detrimental to many of the body's tissues. For instance, breathing oxygen at 4 atmospheres pressure of oxygen (P_{O_2} = 3040 mm Hg) will cause brain *seizures followed by coma* in most people within 30 to 60 minutes. The seizures often occur without warning and, for obvious reasons, are likely to be lethal to divers submerged beneath the sea.

Other symptoms encountered in acute oxygen poisoning include nausea, muscle twitchings, dizziness, disturbances of vision, irritability, and disorientation. Exercise greatly increases the diver's susceptibility to oxygen toxicity, causing symptoms to appear much earlier and with far greater severity than in the resting person.

Excessive Intracellular Oxidation as a Cause of Nervous System Oxygen Toxicity—"Oxidizing Free Radicals." Molecular oxygen (O_2) has little capability of oxidizing other chemical compounds. Instead, it must first be converted into an "active" form of oxygen. There are several forms of active oxygen called *oxygen free radicals*. One of the most important of these is the *superoxide free radical* O_2^-, and another is the *peroxide radical* in the form of *hydrogen peroxide*. Even when the tissue P_{O_2} is normal at the level of 40 mm Hg, small amounts of free radicals are continually being formed from the dissolved molecular oxygen. Fortunately, the tissues also contain multiple enzymes that rapidly remove these free radicals, including *peroxidases, catalases,* and *superoxide* *dismutases*. Therefore, so long as the hemoglobin-oxygen buffering mechanism maintains a normal tissue P_{O_2}, the oxidizing free radicals are removed rapidly enough that they have little or no effect in the tissues.

Above a critical alveolar P_{O_2} (above about 2 atmospheres P_{O_2}), the hemoglobin-oxygen buffering mechanism fails, and the tissue P_{O_2} can then rise to hundreds or thousands of millimeters of mercury. At these high levels, the amounts of oxidizing free radicals literally swamp the enzyme systems designed to remove them, and now they can have serious destructive and even lethal effects on the cells. One of the principal effects is to oxidize the polyunsaturated fatty acids that are essential components of many of the cell membranes. Another effect is to oxidize some of the cellular enzymes, thus damaging severely the cellular metabolic systems. The nervous tissues are especially susceptible because of their high lipid content. Therefore, most of the acute lethal effects of acute oxygen toxicity are caused by brain dysfunction.

Chronic Oxygen Poisoning Causes Pulmonary Disability. A person can be exposed to only 1 atmosphere pressure of oxygen almost indefinitely without developing the *acute* oxygen toxicity of the nervous system just described. However, after only about 12 hours of 1 atmosphere oxygen exposure, *lung passageway congestion, pulmonary edema*, and *atelectasis* caused by damage to the linings of the bronchi and alveoli begin to develop. The reason for this effect in the lungs but not in other tissues is that the air spaces of the lungs are directly exposed to the high oxygen pressure, but oxygen is delivered to the other body tissues at almost normal P_{O_2} because of the hemoglobin-oxygen buffer system.

Carbon Dioxide Toxicity at Great Depths in the Sea

If the diving gear is properly designed and functions properly, the diver has no problem due to carbon dioxide toxicity because depth alone does not increase the carbon dioxide partial pressure in the alveoli. This is true because depth does not increase the rate of carbon dioxide production in the body, and as long as the diver continues to breathe a normal tidal volume and expires the carbon dioxide as it is formed, alveolar carbon dioxide pressure will be maintained at a normal value.

In certain types of diving gear, however, such as the diving helmet and some types of rebreathing apparatuses, carbon dioxide can build up in the dead space air of the apparatus and be rebreathed by the diver. Up to an alveolar carbon dioxide pressure (P_{CO_2}) of about 80 mm Hg, twice that in normal alveoli, the diver usually tolerates this buildup by increasing the minute respiratory volume a maximum of 8- to 11-fold to compensate for the increased carbon dioxide. Beyond 80 mm Hg alveolar P_{CO_2}, the situation becomes intolerable, and eventually the respiratory center begins to be depressed, rather than excited, because of the negative tissue metabolic effects of high P_{CO_2}. The diver's respiration then begins to fail rather than to compensate. In addition, the diver develops severe respiratory acidosis and varying degrees of lethargy, narcosis, and finally even anesthesia, as discussed in Chapter 42.

Decompression of the Diver After Excess Exposure to High Pressure

When a person breathes air under high pressure for a long time, the amount of nitrogen dissolved in the body fluids increases. The reason for this is the following: Blood flowing through the pulmonary capillaries becomes saturated with nitrogen to the same high pressure as that in the alveolar breathing mixture. And over several more hours, enough nitrogen is carried to all the tissues of the body to raise their tissue P_{N_2} also to equal the P_{N_2} in the breathing air.

Because nitrogen is not metabolized by the body, it remains dissolved in all the body tissues until the nitrogen pressure in the lungs is decreased back to some lower level, at which time the nitrogen can be removed by the reverse respiratory process; however, this removal often takes hours to occur and is the source of multiple problems collectively called *decompression sickness*.

Volume of Nitrogen Dissolved in the Body Fluids at Different Depths. At sea level, almost exactly 1 liter of nitrogen is dissolved in the entire body. Slightly less than one half of this is dissolved in the water of the body and a little more than one half in the fat of the body. This is true because nitrogen is five times as soluble in fat as in water.

After the diver has become saturated with nitrogen, the *sea-level volume of nitrogen* dissolved in the body at different depths is as follows:

Feet	Liters
0	1
33	2
100	4
200	7
300	10

Several hours are required for the gas pressures of nitrogen in all the body tissues to come nearly to equilibrium with the gas pressure of nitrogen in the alveoli. The reason for this is that the blood does not flow rapidly enough and the nitrogen does not diffuse rapidly enough to cause instantaneous equilibrium. The nitrogen dissolved in the water of the body comes to almost complete equilibrium in less than 1 hour, but the fat tissue, requiring five times as much transport of nitrogen and having a relatively poor blood supply, reaches equilibrium only after several hours. For this reason, if a person remains at deep levels for only a few minutes, not much nitrogen dissolves in the body fluids and tissues, whereas if the person remains at a deep level for several hours, both the body water and body fat become saturated with nitrogen.

Decompression Sickness (Synonyms: Bends, Compressed Air Sickness, Caisson Disease, Diver's Paralysis, Dysbarism). If a diver has been beneath the sea long enough that large amounts of nitrogen have dissolved in his or her body and the diver then suddenly comes back to the surface of the sea, significant quantities of nitrogen bubbles can develop in the body fluids either intracellularly or extracellularly and can cause minor or serious damage in almost any area of the body, depending on the number and sizes of bubbles formed; this is called *decompression sickness.*

The principles underlying bubble formation are shown in Figure 44-3. In Figure 44-3*A*, the diver's tissues have become equilibrated to a high *dissolved nitrogen pressure* (Pn_2 = 3918 mm Hg), about 6.5 times the normal amount of nitrogen in the tissues. As long as the diver remains deep beneath the sea, the pressure against the outside of his or her body (5000 mm Hg) compresses all the body tissues sufficiently to keep the excess nitrogen gas dissolved. But when the diver suddenly rises to sea level (Figure 44-3*B*), the pressure on the outside of the body becomes only 1 atmosphere (760 mm Hg), while the gas pressure inside the body fluids is the sum of the pressures of water vapor, carbon dioxide, oxygen, and nitrogen, or a total of 4065 mm Hg, 97 percent of which is caused by the nitrogen. Obviously, this total value of 4065 mm Hg is far greater than the 760 mm Hg pressure on the outside of the body. Therefore, the gases can escape from the dissolved state and form actual bubbles, composed almost entirely of nitrogen, both in the tissues and in the blood where they plug many small blood vessels. The bubbles may not appear for many minutes to hours because sometimes the gases can remain dissolved in the "supersaturated" state for hours before bubbling.

Symptoms of Decompression Sickness ("Bends").

The symptoms of decompression sickness are caused by gas bubbles blocking many blood vessels in different tissues. At first, only the smallest vessels are blocked by minute bubbles, but as the bubbles coalesce, progressively larger vessels are affected. Tissue ischemia and sometimes tissue death result.

In most people with decompression sickness, the symptoms are pain in the joints and muscles of the legs and arms, affecting 85 to 90 percent of those persons who develop decompression sickness. The joint pain accounts for the term "bends" that is often applied to this condition.

In 5 to 10 percent of people with decompression sickness, nervous system symptoms occur, ranging from dizziness in about 5 percent to paralysis or collapse and unconsciousness in as many as 3 percent. The paralysis may be temporary, but in some instances, damage is permanent.

Finally, about 2 percent of people with decompression sickness develop "the chokes," caused by massive numbers of microbubbles plugging the capillaries of the lungs; this is characterized by serious shortness of breath, often followed by severe pulmonary edema and, occasionally, death.

Nitrogen Elimination from the Body; Decompression Tables.

If a diver is brought to the surface slowly, enough of the dissolved nitrogen can usually be eliminated by expiration through the lungs to prevent decompression sickness. About two thirds of the total nitrogen is liberated in 1 hour and about 90 percent in 6 hours.

Decompression tables that detail procedures for safe decompression have been prepared by the U.S. Navy. To give the student an idea of the decompression process, a diver who has been breathing air and has been on the sea bottom for 60 minutes at a depth of 190 feet is decompressed according to the following schedule:

10 minutes at 50 feet depth

17 minutes at 40 feet depth

19 minutes at 30 feet depth

50 minutes at 20 feet depth

84 minutes at 10 feet depth

Thus, for a work period on the bottom of only 1 hour, the total time for decompression is about 3 hours.

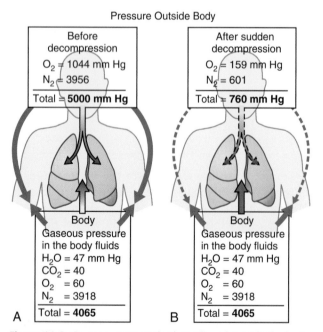

Figure 44-3 Gaseous pressures both inside and outside the body, showing (*A*) saturation of the body to high gas pressures when breathing air at a total pressure of 5000 mm Hg, and (*B*) the great excesses of intrabody pressures that are responsible for bubble formation in the tissues when the lung intra-alveolar pressure body is suddenly returned from 5000 mm Hg to normal pressure of 760 mm Hg.

Tank Decompression and Treatment of Decompression Sickness.

Another procedure widely used for decompression of professional divers is to put the diver into a pressurized tank and then to lower the pressure gradually back to normal atmospheric pressure, using essentially the same time schedule as noted earlier.

Tank decompression is even more important for treating people in whom symptoms of decompression sickness develop minutes or even hours after they have returned to the surface. In this case, the diver is recompressed immediately to a deep level. Then decompression is carried out over a period several times as long as the usual decompression period.

"Saturation Diving" and Use of Helium-Oxygen Mixtures in Deep Dives. When divers must work at very deep levels—between 250 feet and nearly 1000 feet—they frequently live in a large compression tank for days or weeks at a time, remaining compressed at a pressure level near that at which they will be working. This keeps the tissues and fluids of the body saturated with the gases to which they will be exposed while diving. Then, when they return to the same tank after working, there are no significant changes in pressure, so decompression bubbles do not occur.

In very deep dives, especially during saturation diving, helium is usually used in the gas mixture instead of nitrogen for three reasons: (1) it has only about one-fifth the narcotic effect of nitrogen; (2) only about one half as much volume of helium dissolves in the body tissues as nitrogen, and the volume that does dissolve diffuses out of the tissues during decompression several times as rapidly as does nitrogen, thus reducing the problem of decompression sickness; and (3) the low density of helium (one seventh the density of nitrogen) keeps the airway resistance for breathing at a minimum, which is very important because highly compressed nitrogen is so dense that airway resistance can become extreme, sometimes making the work of breathing beyond endurance.

Finally, in very deep dives it is important to reduce the oxygen concentration in the gaseous mixture because otherwise oxygen toxicity would result. For instance, at a depth of 700 feet (22 atmospheres of pressure), a 1 percent oxygen mixture will provide all the oxygen required by the diver, whereas a 21 percent mixture of oxygen (the percentage in air) delivers a P_{O_2} to the lungs of more than 4 atmospheres, a level very likely to cause seizures in as little as 30 minutes.

Scuba (Self-Contained Underwater Breathing Apparatus) Diving

Before the 1940s, almost all diving was done using a diving helmet connected to a hose through which air was pumped to the diver from the surface. Then, in 1943, French explorer Jacques Cousteau popularized a *self-contained underwater breathing apparatus*, known as the SCUBA apparatus. The type of SCUBA apparatus used in more than 99 percent of all sports and commercial diving is the *open-circuit demand system* shown in Figure 44-4. This system consists of the following components: (1) one or more tanks of compressed air or

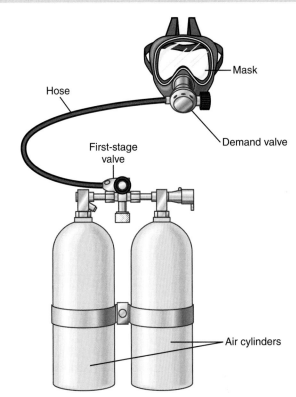

Figure 44-4 Open-circuit demand type of SCUBA apparatus.

some other breathing mixture, (2) a first-stage "reducing" valve for reducing the very high pressure from the tanks to a low pressure level, (3) a combination inhalation "demand" valve and exhalation valve that allows air to be pulled into the lungs with slight negative pressure of breathing and then to be exhaled into the sea at a pressure level slightly positive to the surrounding water pressure, and (4) a mask and tube system with small "dead space."

The demand system operates as follows: The first-stage reducing valve reduces the pressure from the tanks so that the air delivered to the mask has a pressure only a few mm Hg greater than the surrounding water pressure. The breathing mixture does not flow continually into the mask. Instead, with each inspiration, slight extra negative pressure in the demand valve of the mask pulls the diaphragm of the valve open, and this automatically releases air from the tank into the mask and lungs. In this way, only the amount of air needed for inhalation enters the mask. Then, on expiration, the air cannot go back into the tank but instead is expired into the sea.

The most important problem in use of the self-contained underwater breathing apparatus is the limited amount of time one can remain beneath the sea surface; for instance, only a few minutes are possible at a 200-foot depth. The reason for this is that tremendous airflow from the tanks is required to wash carbon dioxide out of the lungs—the greater the depth, the greater the airflow in terms of *quantity* of air per minute that is required, because the *volumes* have been compressed to small sizes.

Special Physiologic Problems in Submarines

Escape from Submarines. Essentially the same problems encountered in deep-sea diving are often met in relation to submarines, especially when it is necessary to escape from a submerged submarine. Escape is possible from as deep as 300 feet without using any apparatus. However, proper use of rebreathing devices, especially when using helium, theoretically can allow escape from as deep as 600 feet or perhaps more.

One of the major problems of escape is prevention of air embolism. As the person ascends, the gases in the lungs expand and sometimes rupture a pulmonary blood vessel, forcing the gases to enter the vessel and cause air embolism of the circulation. Therefore, as the person ascends, he or she must make a special effort to exhale continually.

Health Problems in the Submarine Internal Environment. Except for escape, submarine medicine generally centers on several engineering problems to keep hazards out of the internal environment. First, in atomic submarines, there exists the problem of radiation hazards, but with appropriate shielding, the amount of radiation received by the crew submerged beneath the sea has been less than normal radiation received above the surface of the sea from cosmic rays.

Second, poisonous gases on occasion escape into the atmosphere of the submarine and must be controlled rapidly. For instance, during several weeks' submergence, cigarette smoking by the crew can liberate enough carbon monoxide, if not removed rapidly, to cause carbon monoxide poisoning. And, on occasion, even Freon gas has been found to diffuse out of refrigeration systems in sufficient quantity to cause toxicity.

Hyperbaric Oxygen Therapy

The intense oxidizing properties of high-pressure oxygen (*hyperbaric oxygen*) can have valuable therapeutic effects in several important clinical conditions. Therefore, large pressure tanks are now available in many medical centers into which patients can be placed and treated with hyperbaric oxygen. The oxygen is usually administered at Po_2s of 2 to 3 atmospheres of pressure through a mask or intratracheal tube, whereas the gas around the body is normal air compressed to the same high-pressure level.

It is believed that the same oxidizing free radicals responsible for oxygen toxicity are also responsible for at least some of the therapeutic benefits. Some of the conditions in which hyperbaric oxygen therapy has been especially beneficial follow.

Probably the most successful use of hyperbaric oxygen has been for treatment of *gas gangrene*. The bacteria that cause this condition, *clostridial organisms*, grow best under anaerobic conditions and stop growing at oxygen pressures greater than about 70 mm Hg. Therefore, hyperbaric oxygenation of the tissues can frequently stop the infectious process entirely and thus convert a condition that formerly was almost 100 percent fatal into one that is cured in most instances by early treatment with hyperbaric therapy.

Other conditions in which hyperbaric oxygen therapy has been either valuable or possibly valuable include decompression sickness, arterial gas embolism, carbon monoxide poisoning, osteomyelitis, and myocardial infarction.

Bibliography

Butler PJ: Diving beyond the limits, *News Physiol Sci* 16:222, 2001.

Leach RM, Rees PJ, Wilmshurst P: Hyperbaric oxygen therapy, *BMJ* 317:1140, 1998.

Lindholm P, Lundgren CE: The physiology and pathophysiology of human breath-hold diving, *J Appl Physiol* 106:284, 2009.

Moon RE, Cherry AD, Stolp BW, et al: Pulmonary Gas Exchange in Diving, *J Appl Physiol* 2008 [Epub ahead of print].

Neuman TS: Arterial gas embolism and decompression sickness, *News Physiol Sci* 17:77, 2002.

Pendergast DR, Lundgren CEG: The physiology and pathophysiology of the hyperbaric and diving environments, *J Appl Physiol* 106:274, 2009.

Thom SR: Oxidative stress is fundamental to hyperbaric oxygen therapy, *J Appl Physiol* 2008 doi:10.1152/japplphysiol.91004.

IX

The Nervous System: A. General Principles and Sensory Physiology

45. Organization of the Nervous System, Basic Functions of Synapses, and Neurotransmitters

46. Sensory Receptors, Neuronal Circuits for Processing Information

47. Somatic Sensations: I. General Organization, the Tactile and Position Senses

48. Somatic Sensations: II. Pain, Headache, and Thermal Sensations

Organization of the Nervous System, Basic Functions of Synapses, and Neurotransmitters

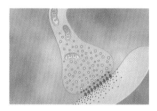

The nervous system is unique in the vast complexity of thought processes and control actions it can perform. It receives each minute literally millions of bits of information from the different sensory nerves and sensory organs and then integrates all these to determine responses to be made by the body.

Before beginning this discussion of the nervous system, the reader should review Chapters 5 and 7, which present the principles of membrane potentials and transmission of signals in nerves and through neuromuscular junctions.

General Design of the Nervous System

Central Nervous System Neuron: The Basic Functional Unit

The central nervous system contains more than 100 billion neurons. Figure 45-1 shows a typical neuron of a type found in the brain motor cortex. Incoming signals enter this neuron through synapses located mostly on the neuronal dendrites, but also on the cell body. For different types of neurons, there may be only a few hundred or as many as 200,000 such synaptic connections from input fibers. Conversely, the output signal travels by way of a single axon leaving the neuron. Then, this axon has many separate branches to other parts of the nervous system or peripheral body.

A special feature of most synapses is that the signal normally passes only in the forward direction, from the axon of a preceding neuron to dendrites on cell membranes of subsequent neurons. This forces the signal to travel in required directions for performing specific nervous functions.

Sensory Part of the Nervous System—Sensory Receptors

Most activities of the nervous system are initiated by sensory experiences that excite *sensory receptors*, whether visual receptors in the eyes, auditory receptors in the

ears, tactile receptors on the surface of the body, or other kinds of receptors. These sensory experiences can either cause immediate reactions from the brain, or memories of the experiences can be stored in the brain for minutes, weeks, or years and determine bodily reactions at some future date.

Figure 45-2 shows the *somatic* portion of the sensory system, which transmits sensory information from the receptors of the entire body surface and from some deep structures. This information enters the central nervous system through peripheral nerves and is conducted immediately to multiple sensory areas in (1) the spinal cord at all levels; (2) the reticular substance of the medulla, pons, and mesencephalon of the brain; (3) the cerebellum; (4) the thalamus; and (5) areas of the cerebral cortex.

Motor Part of the Nervous System—Effectors

The most important eventual role of the nervous system is to control the various bodily activities. This is achieved by controlling (1) contraction of appropriate skeletal muscles throughout the body, (2) contraction of smooth muscle in the internal organs, and (3) secretion of active chemical substances by both exocrine and endocrine glands in many parts of the body. These activities are collectively called *motor functions* of the nervous system, and the muscles and glands are called *effectors* because they are the actual anatomical structures that perform the functions dictated by the nerve signals.

Figure 45-3 shows the *"skeletal" motor nerve axis* of the nervous system for controlling skeletal muscle contraction. Operating parallel to this axis is another system, called the *autonomic nervous system,* for controlling smooth muscles, glands, and other internal bodily systems; this is discussed in Chapter 60.

Note in Figure 45-3 that the skeletal muscles can be controlled from many levels of the central nervous system, including (1) the spinal cord; (2) the reticular substance of the medulla, pons, and mesencephalon; (3) the basal ganglia; (4) the cerebellum; and (5) the motor cortex. Each of these areas plays its own specific role, the lower regions concerned primarily with automatic, instantaneous muscle responses to sensory stimuli, and the higher regions

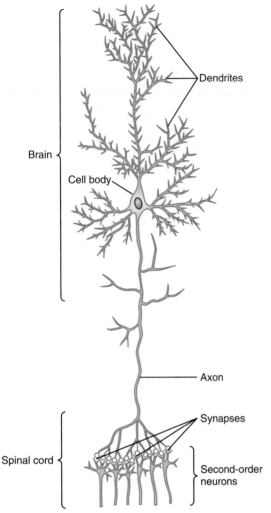

Figure 45-1 Structure of a large neuron in the brain, showing its important functional parts. (Redrawn from Guyton AC: Basic Neuroscience: Anatomy and Physiology. Philadelphia: WB Saunders, 1987.)

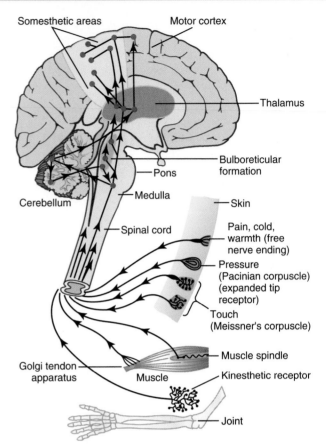

Figure 45-2 Somatosensory axis of the nervous system.

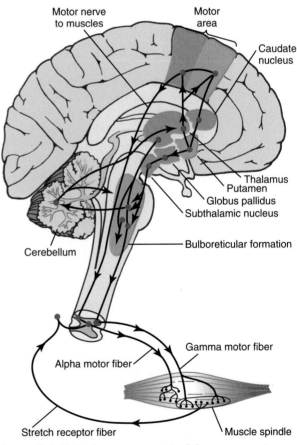

Figure 45-3 Skeletal motor nerve axis of the nervous system.

with deliberate complex muscle movements controlled by the thought processes of the brain.

Processing of Information—"Integrative" Function of the Nervous System

One of the most important functions of the nervous system is to process incoming information in such a way that *appropriate* mental and motor responses will occur. More than 99 percent of all sensory information is discarded by the brain as irrelevant and unimportant. For instance, one is ordinarily unaware of the parts of the body that are in contact with clothing, as well as of the seat pressure when sitting. Likewise, attention is drawn only to an occasional object in one's field of vision, and even the perpetual noise of our surroundings is usually relegated to the subconscious.

But, when important sensory information excites the mind, it is immediately channeled into proper integrative and motor regions of the brain to cause desired responses. This channeling and processing of information is called the *integrative function* of the nervous system. Thus, if a person places a hand on a hot stove, the desired instantaneous response is to lift the hand. And other associated responses follow, such as moving the entire body away from the stove and perhaps even shouting with pain.

Role of Synapses in Processing Information. The synapse is the junction point from one neuron to the next. Later in this chapter, we discuss the details of synaptic function. However, it is important to point out here that synapses determine the directions that the nervous signals will spread through the nervous system. Some synapses transmit signals from one neuron to the next with ease, whereas others transmit signals only with difficulty. Also, *facilitatory* and *inhibitory* signals from other areas in the nervous system can control synaptic transmission, sometimes opening the synapses for transmission and at other times closing them. In addition, some postsynaptic neurons respond with large numbers of output impulses, and others respond with only a few. Thus, the synapses perform a selective action, often blocking weak signals while allowing strong signals to pass, but at other times selecting and amplifying certain weak signals, and often channeling these signals in many directions rather than in only one direction.

Storage of Information—Memory

Only a small fraction of even the most important sensory information usually causes immediate motor response. But much of the information is stored for future control of motor activities and for use in the thinking processes. Most storage occurs in the *cerebral cortex,* but even the basal regions of the brain and the spinal cord can store small amounts of information.

The storage of information is the process we call *memory,* and this, too, is a function of the synapses. Each time certain types of sensory signals pass through sequences of synapses, these synapses become more capable of transmitting the same type of signal the next time, a process called *facilitation.* After the sensory signals have passed through the synapses a large number of times, the synapses become so facilitated that signals generated within the brain itself can also cause transmission of impulses through the same sequences of synapses, even when the sensory input is not excited. This gives the person a perception of experiencing the original sensations, although the perceptions are only memories of the sensations.

The precise mechanisms by which long-term facilitation of synapses occurs in the memory process are still uncertain, but what is known about this and other details of the sensory memory process is discussed in Chapter 57.

Once memories have been stored in the nervous system, they become part of the brain processing mechanism for future "thinking." That is, the thinking processes of the brain compare new sensory experiences with stored memories; the memories then help to select the important new sensory information and to channel this into appropriate memory storage areas for future use or into motor areas to cause immediate bodily responses.

Major Levels of Central Nervous System Function

The human nervous system has inherited special functional capabilities from each stage of human evolutionary development. From this heritage, three major levels of the central nervous system have specific functional characteristics: (1) the *spinal cord level,* (2) the *lower brain* or *subcortical level,* and (3) the *higher brain* or *cortical level.*

Spinal Cord Level

We often think of the spinal cord as being only a conduit for signals from the periphery of the body to the brain, or in the opposite direction from the brain back to the body. This is far from the truth. Even after the spinal cord has been cut in the high neck region, many highly organized spinal cord functions still occur. For instance, neuronal circuits in the cord can cause (1) walking movements, (2) reflexes that withdraw portions of the body from painful objects, (3) reflexes that stiffen the legs to support the body against gravity, and (4) reflexes that control local blood vessels, gastrointestinal movements, or urinary excretion. In fact, the upper levels of the nervous system often operate not by sending signals directly to the periphery of the body but by sending signals to the control centers of the cord, simply "commanding" the cord centers to perform their functions.

Lower Brain or Subcortical Level

Many, if not most, of what we call subconscious activities of the body are controlled in the lower areas of the brain—in the medulla, pons, mesencephalon, hypothalamus, thalamus, cerebellum, and basal ganglia. For instance, subconscious control of arterial pressure and respiration is achieved mainly in the medulla and pons. Control of equilibrium is a combined function of the older portions of the cerebellum and the reticular substance of the medulla, pons, and mesencephalon. Feeding reflexes, such as salivation and licking of the lips in response to the taste of food, are controlled by areas in the medulla, pons, mesencephalon, amygdala, and hypothalamus. And many emotional patterns, such as anger, excitement, sexual response, reaction to pain, and reaction to pleasure, can still occur after destruction of much of the cerebral cortex.

Higher Brain or Cortical Level

After the preceding account of the many nervous system functions that occur at the cord and lower brain levels, one may ask, what is left for the cerebral cortex to do? The answer to this is complex, but it begins with the fact that the cerebral cortex is an extremely large memory storehouse. The cortex never functions alone but always in association with lower centers of the nervous system.

Without the cerebral cortex, the functions of the lower brain centers are often imprecise. The vast storehouse of cortical information usually converts these functions to determinative and precise operations.

Finally, the cerebral cortex is essential for most of our thought processes, but it cannot function by itself. In fact, it is the lower brain centers, not the cortex, that initiate *wakefulness* in the cerebral cortex, thus opening its bank of memories to the thinking machinery of the brain. Thus, each portion of the nervous system performs specific functions. But it is the cortex that opens a world of stored information for use by the mind.

Comparison of the Nervous System with a Computer

When computers were first developed, it soon became apparent that these machines have many features in common with the nervous system. First, all computers have input circuits that are comparable to the sensory portion of the nervous system, as well as output circuits that are comparable to the motor portion of the nervous system.

In simple computers, the output signals are controlled directly by the input signals, operating in a manner similar to that of simple reflexes of the spinal cord. In more complex computers, the output is determined both by input signals and by information that has already been stored in memory in the computer, which is analogous to the more complex reflex and processing mechanisms of our higher nervous system. Furthermore, as computers become even more complex, it is necessary to add still another unit, called the *central processing unit,* which determines the sequence of all operations. This unit is analogous to the control mechanisms in our brain that direct our attention first to one thought or sensation or motor activity, then to another, and so forth, until complex sequences of thought or action take place.

Figure 45-4 is a simple block diagram of a computer. Even a rapid study of this diagram demonstrates its similarity to the nervous system. The fact that the basic components of the general-purpose computer are analogous to those of the human nervous system demonstrates that the brain is basically a computer that continuously collects

sensory information and uses this along with stored information to compute the daily course of bodily activity.

Central Nervous System Synapses

Information is transmitted in the central nervous system mainly in the form of nerve action potentials, called simply "nerve impulses," through a succession of neurons, one after another. However, in addition, each impulse (1) may be blocked in its transmission from one neuron to the next, (2) may be changed from a single impulse into repetitive impulses, or (3) may be integrated with impulses from other neurons to cause highly intricate patterns of impulses in successive neurons. All these functions can be classified as *synaptic functions of neurons.*

Types of Synapses—Chemical and Electrical

There are two major types of synapses: (1) the *chemical synapse* and (2) the *electrical synapse.*

Almost all the synapses used for signal transmission in the central nervous system of the human being are *chemical synapses.* In these, the first neuron secretes at its nerve ending synapse a chemical substance called a *neurotransmitter* (or often called simply *transmitter substance*), and this transmitter in turn acts on receptor proteins in the membrane of the next neuron to excite the neuron, inhibit it, or modify its sensitivity in some other way. More than 40 important transmitter substances have been discovered thus far. Some of the best known are acetylcholine, norepinephrine, epinephrine, histamine, gamma-aminobutyric acid (GABA), glycine, serotonin, and glutamate.

Electrical synapses, in contrast, are characterized by direct open fluid channels that conduct electricity from one cell to the next. Most of these consist of small protein tubular structures called *gap junctions* that allow free movement of ions from the interior of one cell to the interior of the next. Such junctions were discussed in Chapter 4. Only a few examples of gap junctions have been found in the central nervous system. However, it is by way of gap junctions and other similar junctions that action potentials are transmitted from one smooth muscle fiber to the next in visceral smooth muscle (Chapter 8) and from one cardiac muscle cell to the next in cardiac muscle (Chapter 10).

"One-Way" Conduction at Chemical Synapses. Chemical synapses have one exceedingly important characteristic that makes them highly desirable for transmitting most nervous system signals. They always transmit the signals in one direction: that is, from the neuron that secretes the transmitter substance, called the *presynaptic neuron,* to the neuron on which the transmitter acts, called the *postsynaptic neuron.* This is the *principle of one-way conduction* at chemical synapses, and it is quite different from conduction through electrical synapses, which often transmit signals in either direction.

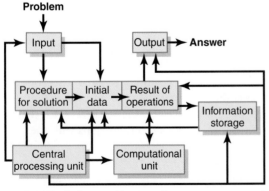

Figure 45-4 Block diagram of a general-purpose computer, showing the basic components and their interrelations.

Think for a moment about the extreme importance of the one-way conduction mechanism. It allows signals to be directed toward specific goals. Indeed, it is this specific transmission of signals to discrete and highly focused areas both within the nervous system and at the terminals of the peripheral nerves that allows the nervous system to perform its myriad functions of sensation, motor control, memory, and many others.

Physiologic Anatomy of the Synapse

Figure 45-5 shows a typical *anterior motor neuron* in the anterior horn of the spinal cord. It is composed of three major parts: the *soma,* which is the main body of the neuron; a single *axon,* which extends from the soma into a peripheral nerve that leaves the spinal cord; and the *dendrites,* which are great numbers of branching projections of the soma that extend as much as 1 millimeter into the surrounding areas of the cord.

As many as 10,000 to 200,000 minute synaptic knobs called *presynaptic terminals* lie on the surfaces of the dendrites and soma of the motor neuron, about 80 to 95 percent of them on the dendrites and only 5 to 20 percent on the soma. These presynaptic terminals are the ends of nerve fibrils that originate from many other neurons. Many of these presynaptic terminals are *excitatory*—that is, they secrete a transmitter substance that excites the postsynaptic neuron. But other presynaptic terminals are *inhibitory*—they secrete a transmitter substance that inhibits the postsynaptic neuron.

Neurons in other parts of the cord and brain differ from the anterior motor neuron in (1) the size of the cell body; (2) the length, size, and number of dendrites, ranging in length from almost zero to many centimeters; (3) the length and size of the axon; and (4) the number of presynaptic terminals, which may range from only a few to as many as 200,000. These differences make neurons in different parts of the nervous system react differently to incoming synaptic signals and, therefore, perform many different functions.

Presynaptic Terminals. Electron microscopic studies of the presynaptic terminals show that they have varied anatomical forms, but most resemble small round or oval knobs and, therefore, are sometimes called *terminal knobs, boutons, end-feet,* or *synaptic knobs.*

Figure 45-6 illustrates the basic structure of a synapse, showing a single presynaptic terminal on the membrane surface of a postsynaptic neuron. The presynaptic terminal is separated from the postsynaptic neuronal soma by a *synaptic cleft* having a width usually of 200 to 300 angstroms. The terminal has two internal structures important to the excitatory or inhibitory function of the synapse: the *transmitter vesicles* and the *mitochondria.* The transmitter vesicles contain the *transmitter substance* that, when released into the synaptic cleft, either *excites* or *inhibits* the postsynaptic neuron—excites if the neuronal membrane contains *excitatory receptors,* inhibits if the membrane contains *inhibitory receptors.* The mitochondria provide adenosine triphosphate (ATP), which in turn supplies the energy for synthesizing new transmitter substance.

When an action potential spreads over a presynaptic terminal, depolarization of its membrane causes a small number of vesicles to empty into the cleft. The released

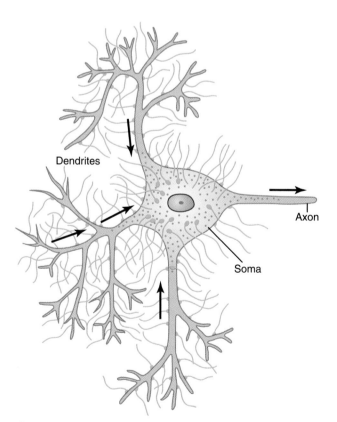

Dendrites

Axon

Soma

Figure 45-5 Typical anterior motor neuron, showing presynaptic terminals on the neuronal soma and dendrites. Note also the single axon.

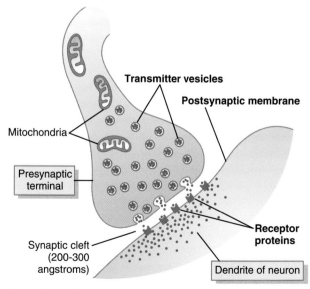

Transmitter vesicles

Postsynaptic membrane

Mitochondria

Presynaptic terminal

Synaptic cleft (200-300 angstroms)

Receptor proteins

Dendrite of neuron

Figure 45-6 Physiologic anatomy of the synapse.

transmitter in turn causes an immediate change in permeability characteristics of the postsynaptic neuronal membrane, and this leads to excitation or inhibition of the postsynaptic neuron, depending on the neuronal receptor characteristics.

Mechanism by Which an Action Potential Causes Transmitter Release from the Presynaptic Terminals—Role of Calcium Ions

The membrane of the presynaptic terminal is called the *presynaptic membrane.* It contains large numbers of *voltage-gated calcium channels.* When an action potential depolarizes the presynaptic membrane, these calcium channels open and allow large numbers of calcium ions to flow into the terminal. The quantity of transmitter substance that is then released from the terminal into the synaptic cleft is directly related to the number of calcium ions that enter. The precise mechanism by which the calcium ions cause this release is not known, but it is believed to be the following.

When the calcium ions enter the presynaptic terminal, it is believed that they bind with special protein molecules on the inside surface of the presynaptic membrane, called *release sites.* This binding in turn causes the release sites to open through the membrane, allowing a few transmitter vesicles to release their transmitter into the cleft after each single action potential. For those vesicles that store the neurotransmitter acetylcholine, between 2000 and 10,000 molecules of acetylcholine are present in each vesicle, and there are enough vesicles in the presynaptic terminal to transmit from a few hundred to more than 10,000 action potentials.

Action of the Transmitter Substance on the Postsynaptic Neuron—Function of "Receptor Proteins"

The membrane of the postsynaptic neuron contains large numbers of *receptor proteins,* also shown in Figure 45-6. The molecules of these receptors have two important components: (1) a *binding component* that protrudes outward from the membrane into the synaptic cleft—here it binds the neurotransmitter coming from the presynaptic terminal—and (2) an *ionophore component* that passes all the way through the postsynaptic membrane to the interior of the postsynaptic neuron. The ionophore in turn is one of two types: (1) an *ion channel* that allows passage of specified types of ions through the membrane or (2) a *"second messenger" activator* that is not an ion channel but instead is a molecule that protrudes into the cell cytoplasm and activates one or more substances inside the postsynaptic neuron. These substances in turn serve as "second messengers" to increase or decrease specific cellular functions.

Ion Channels. The ion channels in the postsynaptic neuronal membrane are usually of two types: (1) *cation channels* that most often allow sodium ions to pass when opened, but sometimes allow potassium and/or calcium

ions as well, and (2) *anion channels* that allow mainly chloride ions to pass but also minute quantities of other anions.

The *cation channels* that conduct sodium ions are lined with negative charges. These charges attract the positively charged sodium ions into the channel when the channel diameter increases to a size larger than that of the hydrated sodium ion. But those same negative charges *repel chloride ions and other anions* and prevent their passage.

For the *anion channels,* when the channel diameters become large enough, chloride ions pass into the channels and on through to the opposite side, whereas sodium, potassium, and calcium cations are blocked, mainly because their hydrated ions are too large to pass.

We will learn later that when cation channels open and allow positively charged sodium ions to enter, the positive electrical charges of the sodium ions will in turn excite this neuron. Therefore, a transmitter substance that opens cation channels is called an *excitatory transmitter.* Conversely, opening anion channels allows negative electrical charges to enter, which inhibits the neuron. Therefore, transmitter substances that open these channels are called *inhibitory transmitters.*

When a transmitter substance activates an ion channel, the channel usually opens within a fraction of a millisecond; when the transmitter substance is no longer present, the channel closes equally rapidly. The opening and closing of ion channels provide a means for very rapid control of postsynaptic neurons.

"Second Messenger" System in the Postsynaptic Neuron. Many functions of the nervous system—for instance, the process of memory—require prolonged changes in neurons for seconds to months after the initial transmitter substance is gone. The ion channels are not suitable for causing prolonged postsynaptic neuronal changes because these channels close within milliseconds after the transmitter substance is no longer present. However, in many instances, prolonged postsynaptic neuronal excitation or inhibition is achieved by activating a "second messenger" chemical system inside the postsynaptic neuronal cell itself, and then it is the second messenger that causes the prolonged effect.

There are several types of second messenger systems. One of the most common types uses a group of proteins called *G-proteins.* Figure 45-7 shows in the upper left corner a membrane receptor protein. A G-protein is attached to the portion of the receptor that protrudes into the interior of the cell. The G-protein in turn consists of three components: an alpha (α) component that is the *activator* portion of the G-protein and beta (β) and gamma (γ) components that are attached to the alpha component and also to the inside of the cell membrane adjacent to the receptor protein. On activation by a nerve impulse, the alpha portion of the G-protein separates from the beta and gamma portions and then is free to move within the cytoplasm of the cell.

Inside the cytoplasm, the separated alpha component performs one or more of multiple functions, depending on

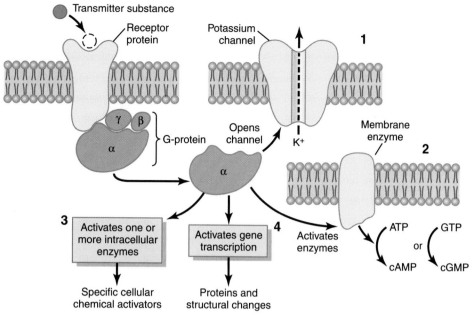

Figure 45-7 "Second messenger" system by which a transmitter substance from an initial neuron can activate a second neuron by first releasing a "G-protein" into the second neuron's cytoplasm. Four subsequent possible effects of the G-protein are shown, including *1*, opening an ion channel in the membrane of the second neuron; *2*, activating an enzyme system in the neuron's membrane; *3*, activating an intracellular enzyme system; and/or *4*, causing gene transcription in the second neuron.

the specific characteristic of each type of neuron. Shown in Figure 45-7 are four changes that can occur. They are as follows:

1. *Opening specific ion channels through the postsynaptic cell membrane.* Shown in the upper right of the figure is a potassium channel that is opened in response to the G-protein; this channel often stays open for a prolonged time, in contrast to rapid closure of directly activated ion channels that do not use the second messenger system.

2. *Activation of cyclic adenosine monophosphate (cAMP) or cyclic guanosine monophosphate (cGMP) in the neuronal cell.* Recall that either cyclic AMP or cyclic GMP can activate highly specific metabolic machinery in the neuron and, therefore, can initiate any one of many chemical results, including long-term changes in cell structure itself, which in turn alters long-term excitability of the neuron.

3. *Activation of one or more intracellular enzymes.* The G-protein can directly activate one or more intracellular enzymes. In turn the enzymes can cause any one of many specific chemical functions in the cell.

4. *Activation of gene transcription.* This is one of the most important effects of activation of the second messenger systems because gene transcription can cause formation of new proteins within the neuron, thereby changing its metabolic machinery or its structure. Indeed, it is well known that structural changes of appropriately activated neurons do occur, especially in long-term memory processes.

It is clear that activation of second messenger systems within the neuron, whether they be of the G-protein type

or of other types, is extremely important for changing the long-term response characteristics of different neuronal pathways. We will return to this subject in more detail in Chapter 57 when we discuss memory functions of the nervous system.

Excitatory or Inhibitory Receptors in the Postsynaptic Membrane

Some postsynaptic receptors, when activated, cause excitation of the postsynaptic neuron, and others cause inhibition. The importance of having inhibitory, as well as excitatory, types of receptors is that this gives an additional dimension to nervous function, allowing restraint of nervous action and excitation.

The different molecular and membrane mechanisms used by the different receptors to cause excitation or inhibition include the following.

Excitation

1. Opening of sodium channels to allow large numbers of positive electrical charges to flow to the interior of the postsynaptic cell. This raises the intracellular membrane potential in the positive direction up toward the threshold level for excitation. It is by far the most widely used means for causing excitation.

2. Depressed conduction through chloride or potassium channels, or both. This decreases the diffusion of negatively charged chloride ions to the inside of the postsynaptic neuron or decreases the diffusion of positively charged potassium ions to the outside. In either instance, the effect is to make the internal membrane potential more positive than normal, which is excitatory.

3. Various changes in the internal metabolism of the postsynaptic neuron to excite cell activity or, in some instances, to increase the number of excitatory membrane receptors or decrease the number of inhibitory membrane receptors.

Inhibition

1. *Opening of chloride ion channels through the postsynaptic neuronal membrane.* This allows rapid diffusion of negatively charged chloride ions from outside the postsynaptic neuron to the inside, thereby carrying negative charges inward and increasing the negativity inside, which is inhibitory.

2. *Increase in conductance of potassium ions out of the neuron.* This allows positive ions to diffuse to the exterior, which causes increased negativity inside the neuron; this is inhibitory.

3. *Activation of receptor enzymes* that inhibit cellular metabolic functions that increase the number of inhibitory synaptic receptors or decrease the number of excitatory receptors.

Chemical Substances That Function as Synaptic Transmitters

More than 50 chemical substances have been proved or postulated to function as synaptic transmitters. Many of them are listed in Tables 45-1 and 45-2, which give two groups of synaptic transmitters. One group comprises *small-molecule, rapidly acting transmitters*. The other is made up of a large number of *neuropeptides* of much larger molecular size that are usually much more slowly acting.

Table 45-1 Small-Molecule, Rapidly Acting Transmitters

Class I
Acetylcholine
Class II: The Amines
Norepinephrine
Epinephrine
Dopamine
Serotonin
Histamine
Class III: Amino Acids
Gamma-aminobutyric acid (GABA)
Glycine
Glutamate
Aspartate
Class IV
Nitric oxide (NO)

Table 45-2 Neuropeptide, Slowly Acting Transmitters or Growth Factors

Hypothalamic-releasing hormones
Thyrotropin-releasing hormone
Luteinizing hormone–releasing hormone
Somatostatin (growth hormone inhibitory factor)
Pituitary peptides
Adrenocorticotropic hormone (ACTH)
β-Endorphin
α-Melanocyte-stimulating hormone
Prolactin
Luteinizing hormone
Thyrotropin
Growth hormone
Vasopressin
Oxytocin
Peptides that act on gut and brain
Leucine enkephalin
Methionine enkephalin
Substance P
Gastrin
Cholecystokinin
Vasoactive intestinal polypeptide (VIP)
Nerve growth factor
Brain-derived neurotropic factor
Neurotensin
Insulin
Glucagon
From other tissues
Angiotensin II
Bradykinin
Carnosine
Sleep peptides
Calcitonin

The small-molecule, rapidly acting transmitters are the ones that cause most acute responses of the nervous system, such as transmission of sensory signals to the brain and of motor signals back to the muscles. The neuropeptides, in contrast, usually cause more prolonged actions, such as long-term changes in numbers of neuronal receptors, long-term opening or closure of certain ion channels, and possibly even long-term changes in numbers of synapses or sizes of synapses.

Small-Molecule, Rapidly Acting Transmitters

In most cases, the small-molecule types of transmitters are synthesized in the cytosol of the presynaptic terminal and are absorbed by means of active transport into the many transmitter vesicles in the terminal. Then, each time an action potential reaches the presynaptic terminal, a few vesicles at a time release their transmitter into the synaptic cleft. This usually occurs within a millisecond or less by the mechanism described earlier. The subsequent action of the small-molecule type of transmitter on the membrane receptors of the postsynaptic neuron usually also occurs within another millisecond or less. Most often the effect is to increase or decrease conductance through ion channels; an example is to increase sodium conductance, which causes excitation, or to increase potassium or chloride conductance, which causes inhibition.

Recycling of the Small-Molecule Types of Vesicles. Vesicles that store and release small-molecule transmitters are continually recycled and used over and over again. After they fuse with the synaptic membrane and open to release their transmitter substance, the vesicle membrane at first simply becomes part of the synaptic membrane. However, within seconds to minutes, the vesicle portion of the membrane invaginates back to the inside of the presynaptic terminal and pinches off to form a new vesicle. And the new vesicular membrane still contains appropriate enzyme proteins or transport proteins required for synthesizing and/or concentrating new transmitter substance inside the vesicle.

Acetylcholine is a typical small-molecule transmitter that obeys the principles of synthesis and release stated earlier. This transmitter substance is synthesized in the presynaptic terminal from acetyl coenzyme A and choline in the presence of the enzyme *choline acetyltransferase.* Then it is transported into its specific vesicles. When the vesicles later release the acetylcholine into the synaptic cleft during synaptic neuronal signal transmission, the acetylcholine is rapidly split again to acetate and choline by the enzyme *cholinesterase,* which is present in the proteoglycan reticulum that fills the space of the synaptic cleft. And then again, inside the presynaptic terminal, the vesicles are recycled; choline is actively transported back into the terminal to be used again for synthesis of new acetylcholine.

Characteristics of Some of the More Important Small-Molecule Transmitters. The most important of the small-molecule transmitters are the following.

Acetylcholine is secreted by neurons in many areas of the nervous system but specifically by (1) the terminals of the large pyramidal cells from the motor cortex, (2) several different types of neurons in the basal ganglia, (3) the motor neurons that innervate the skeletal muscles, (4) the preganglionic neurons of the autonomic nervous system, (5) the postganglionic neurons of the parasympathetic nervous system, and (6) some of the postganglionic neurons of the sympathetic nervous system. In most instances, acetylcholine has an excitatory effect; however, it is known to have inhibitory effects at some peripheral parasympathetic nerve endings, such as inhibition of the heart by the vagus nerves.

Norepinephrine is secreted by the terminals of many neurons whose cell bodies are located in the brain stem and hypothalamus. Specifically, norepinephrine-secreting neurons located in the *locus ceruleus* in the pons send nerve fibers to widespread areas of the brain to help control overall activity and mood of the mind, such as increasing the level of wakefulness. In most of these areas, norepinephrine probably activates excitatory receptors, but in a few areas, it activates inhibitory receptors instead. Norepinephrine is also secreted by most postganglionic neurons of the sympathetic nervous system, where it excites some organs but inhibits others.

Dopamine is secreted by neurons that originate in the substantia nigra. The termination of these neurons is mainly in the striatal region of the basal ganglia. The effect of dopamine is usually inhibition.

Glycine is secreted mainly at synapses in the spinal cord. It is believed to always act as an inhibitory transmitter.

GABA (gamma-aminobutyric acid) is secreted by nerve terminals in the spinal cord, cerebellum, basal ganglia, and many areas of the cortex. It is believed always to cause inhibition.

Glutamate is secreted by the presynaptic terminals in many of the sensory pathways entering the central nervous system, as well as in many areas of the cerebral cortex. It probably always causes excitation.

Serotonin is secreted by nuclei that originate in the median raphe of the brain stem and project to many brain and spinal cord areas, especially to the dorsal horns of the spinal cord and to the hypothalamus. Serotonin acts as an inhibitor of pain pathways in the cord, and an inhibitor action in the higher regions of the nervous system is believed to help control the mood of the person, perhaps even to cause sleep.

Nitric oxide is especially secreted by nerve terminals in areas of the brain responsible for long-term behavior and for memory. Therefore, this transmitter system might in the future explain some behavior and memory functions that thus far have defied understanding. Nitric oxide is different from other small-molecule transmitters in its mechanism of formation in the presynaptic terminal and in its actions on the postsynaptic neuron. It is not preformed and stored in vesicles in the presynaptic terminal as are other transmitters. Instead, it is synthesized almost instantly as needed, and it then diffuses out of the presynaptic terminals over a period of seconds rather than being released in vesicular packets. Next, it diffuses into postsynaptic neurons nearby. In the postsynaptic neuron, it usually does not greatly alter the membrane potential but instead changes intracellular metabolic functions that modify neuronal excitability for seconds, minutes, or perhaps even longer.

Neuropeptides

Neuropeptides are synthesized differently and have actions that are usually slow and in other ways quite different from those of the small-molecule transmitters. The neuropeptides are not synthesized in the cytosol of the presynaptic terminals. Instead, they are synthesized as integral parts of large-protein molecules by ribosomes in the neuronal cell body.

The protein molecules then enter the spaces inside the endoplasmic reticulum of the cell body and subsequently inside the Golgi apparatus, where two changes occur: First, the neuropeptide-forming protein is enzymatically split into smaller fragments, some of which are either the neuropeptide itself or a precursor of it. Second, the Golgi apparatus packages the neuropeptide into minute transmitter vesicles that are released into the cytoplasm. Then the transmitter vesicles are transported all the way to the tips of the nerve fibers by *axonal streaming* of the axon cytoplasm, traveling at the slow rate of only a few centimeters per day. Finally, these vesicles release their transmitter at the neuronal terminals in response to action potentials in the same manner as for small-molecule transmitters. However, the vesicle is autolyzed and is not reused.

Because of this laborious method of forming the neuropeptides, much smaller quantities of them are usually released than of the small-molecule transmitters. This is partly compensated for by the fact that the neuropeptides are generally a thousand or more times as potent as the small-molecule transmitters. Another important characteristic of the neuropeptides is that they often cause much more prolonged actions. Some of these actions include prolonged closure of calcium channels, prolonged changes in the metabolic machinery of cells, prolonged changes in activation or deactivation of specific genes in the cell nucleus, and/or prolonged alterations in numbers of excitatory or inhibitory receptors. Some of these effects last for days, but others perhaps for months or years. Our knowledge of the functions of the neuropeptides is only beginning to develop.

Electrical Events During Neuronal Excitation

The electrical events in neuronal excitation have been studied especially in the large motor neurons of the anterior horns of the spinal cord. Therefore, the events described in the next few sections pertain essentially to these neurons. Except for quantitative differences, they apply to most other neurons of the nervous system as well.

Resting Membrane Potential of the Neuronal Soma.

Figure 45-8 shows the soma of a spinal motor neuron, indicating a *resting membrane potential* of about −65 millivolts. This is somewhat less negative than the −90 millivolts found in large peripheral nerve fibers and in skeletal muscle fibers; the lower voltage is important because it allows both positive and negative control of the degree of excitability of the neuron. That is, decreasing the voltage to a less negative value makes the membrane of the neuron more excitable, whereas increasing this voltage to a more negative value makes the neuron less excitable. This is the basis for the two modes of function of the neuron—either excitation or inhibition—as explained in detail in the next sections.

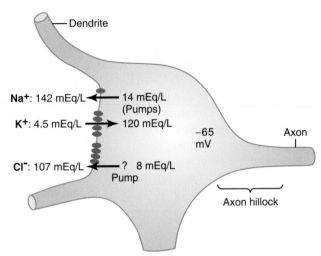

Figure 45-8 Distribution of sodium, potassium, and chloride ions across the neuronal somal membrane; origin of the intrasomal membrane potential.

Concentration Differences of Ions Across the Neuronal Somal Membrane. Figure 45-8 also shows the concentration differences across the neuronal somal membrane of the three ions that are most important for neuronal function: sodium ions, potassium ions, and chloride ions. At the top, the *sodium ion concentration* is shown to be *high in the extracellular fluid* (142 mEq/L) but *low inside the neuron* (14 mEq/L). This sodium concentration gradient is caused by a strong somal membrane sodium pump that continually pumps sodium out of the neuron.

The figure also shows that *potassium ion concentration is high inside the neuronal soma* (120 mEq/L) but *low in the extracellular fluid* (4.5 mEq/L). It shows that there is a potassium pump (the other half of the Na⁺ – K⁺ pump) that pumps potassium to the interior.

Figure 45-8 shows the *chloride ion* to be of *high concentration in the extracellular fluid* but *low concentration inside the neuron.* The membrane may be somewhat permeable to chloride ions and there may be a weak chloride pump. Yet most of the reason for the low concentration of chloride ions inside the neuron is the −65 millivolts in the neuron. That is, this negative voltage repels the negatively charged chloride ions, forcing them outward through the pores until the concentration is much less inside the membrane than outside.

Let us recall from Chapters 4 and 5 that an electrical potential across the cell membrane can oppose movement of ions through a membrane if the potential is of proper polarity and magnitude. A potential that *exactly* opposes movement of an ion is called the *Nernst potential* for that ion; the equation for this is the following:

$$\text{EMF (mV)} = \pm 61 \times \log\left(\frac{\text{Concentration inside}}{\text{Concentration outside}}\right)$$

where EMF is the Nernst potential in millivolts on the *inside of the membrane.* The potential will be negative (−) for positive ions and positive (+) for negative ions.

Now, let us calculate the Nernst potential that will exactly oppose the movement of each of the three separate ions: sodium, potassium, and chloride.

For the sodium concentration difference shown in Figure 45-8, 142 mEq/L on the exterior and 14 mEq/L on the interior, the membrane potential that will exactly oppose sodium ion movement through the sodium channels calculates to be +61 millivolts. However, the actual membrane potential is –65 millivolts, not +61 millivolts. Therefore, those sodium ions that leak to the interior are immediately pumped back to the exterior by the sodium pump, thus maintaining the –65 millivolt negative potential inside the neuron.

For potassium ions, the concentration gradient is 120 mEq/L inside the neuron and 4.5 mEq/L outside. This calculates to be a Nernst potential of –86 millivolts inside the neuron, which is more negative than the –65 that actually exists. Therefore, because of the high intracellular potassium ion concentration, there is a net tendency for potassium ions to diffuse to the outside of the neuron, but this is opposed by continual pumping of these potassium ions back to the interior.

Finally, the chloride ion gradient, 107 mEq/L outside and 8 mEq/L inside, yields a Nernst potential of –70 millivolts inside the neuron, which is only *slightly* more negative than the actual measured value of –65 millivolts. Therefore, chloride ions tend to leak very slightly to the interior of the neuron, but those few that do leak are moved back to the exterior, perhaps by an active chloride pump.

Keep these three Nernst potentials in mind and remember the direction in which the different ions tend to diffuse because this information is important in understanding both excitation and inhibition of the neuron by synapse activation or inactivation of ion channels.

Uniform Distribution of Electrical Potential Inside the Soma. The interior of the neuronal soma contains a highly conductive electrolytic solution, the *intracellular fluid* of the neuron. Furthermore, the diameter of the neuronal soma is large (from 10 to 80 micrometers), causing almost no resistance to conduction of electric current from one part of the somal interior to another part. Therefore, any change in potential in any part of the intrasomal fluid causes an almost exactly equal change in potential at all other points inside the soma (i.e., as long as the neuron is not transmitting an action potential). This is an important principle because it plays a major role in "summation" of signals entering the neuron from multiple sources, as we shall see in subsequent sections of this chapter.

Effect of Synaptic Excitation on the Postsynaptic Membrane—Excitatory Postsynaptic Potential. Figure 45-9A shows the resting neuron with an unexcited presynaptic terminal resting on its surface. The resting membrane potential everywhere in the soma is –65 millivolts.

Figure 45-9B shows a presynaptic terminal that has secreted an excitatory transmitter into the cleft between the terminal and the neuronal somal membrane. This

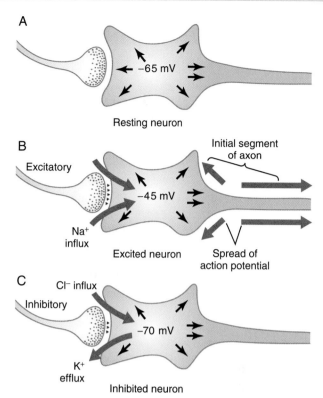

Figure 45-9 Three states of a neuron. *A, Resting neuron*, with a normal intraneuronal potential of –65 millivolts. *B*, Neuron in an *excited state*, with a less negative intraneuronal potential (–45 millivolts) caused by sodium influx. *C*, Neuron in an *inhibited state*, with a more negative intraneuronal membrane potential (–70 millivolts) caused by potassium ion efflux, chloride ion influx, or both.

transmitter acts on the membrane excitatory receptor *to increase the membrane's permeability to Na^+*. Because of the large sodium concentration gradient and large electrical negativity inside the neuron, sodium ions diffuse rapidly to the inside of the membrane.

The rapid influx of positively charged sodium ions to the interior neutralizes part of the negativity of the resting membrane potential. Thus, in Figure 45-9B, the resting membrane potential has increased in the positive direction from –65 to –45 millivolts. This positive increase in voltage above the normal resting neuronal potential— that is, to a less negative value—is called the *excitatory postsynaptic potential* (or EPSP) because if this potential rises high enough in the positive direction, it will elicit an action potential in the postsynaptic neuron, thus exciting it. (In this case, the EPSP is +20 millivolts—i.e., 20 millivolts more positive than the resting value.)

However, we must issue a word of warning. Discharge of a single presynaptic terminal can never increase the neuronal potential from –65 millivolts all the way up to –45 millivolts. An increase of this magnitude requires simultaneous discharge of many terminals—about 40 to 80 for the usual anterior motor neuron—at the same time or in rapid succession. This occurs by a process called *summation*, which is discussed in detail in the next sections.

Generation of Action Potentials in the Initial Segment of the Axon Leaving the Neuron—Threshold for Excitation. When the EPSP rises high enough in the positive direction, there comes a point at which this initiates an action potential in the neuron. However, the action potential does not begin adjacent to the excitatory synapses. Instead, *it begins in the initial segment of the axon* where the axon leaves the neuronal soma. The main reason for this point of origin of the action potential is that the soma has relatively few voltage-gated sodium channels in its membrane, which makes it difficult for the EPSP to open the required number of sodium channels to elicit an action potential. Conversely, *the membrane of the initial segment* has seven times as great a concentration of voltage-gated sodium channels as does the soma and, therefore, can generate an action potential with much greater ease than can the soma. The EPSP that will elicit an action potential in the axon initial segment is between +10 and +20 millivolts. This is in contrast to the +30 or +40 millivolts or more required on the soma.

Once the action potential begins, it travels peripherally along the axon and usually also backward over the soma. In some instances it travels backward into the dendrites but not into all of them because they, like the neuronal soma, have very few voltage-gated sodium channels and therefore frequently cannot generate action potentials at all. Thus, in Figure 45-9B, the *threshold* for excitation of the neuron is shown to be about −45 millivolts, which represents an EPSP of +20 millivolts—that is, 20 millivolts more positive than the normal resting neuronal potential of −65 millivolts.

Electrical Events During Neuronal Inhibition

Effect of Inhibitory Synapses on the Postsynaptic Membrane—Inhibitory Postsynaptic Potential. The inhibitory synapses *open mainly chloride channels*, allowing easy passage of chloride ions. Now, to understand how the inhibitory synapses inhibit the postsynaptic neuron, we must recall what we learned about the Nernst potential for chloride ions. We calculated the Nernst potential for chloride ions to be about −70 millivolts. This potential is more negative than the −65 millivolts normally present inside the resting neuronal membrane. Therefore, opening the chloride channels will allow negatively charged chloride ions to move from the extracellular fluid to the interior, which will make the interior membrane potential more negative than normal, approaching the −70 millivolt level.

Opening potassium channels will allow positively charged potassium ions to move to the exterior, and this will also make the interior membrane potential more negative than usual. Thus, both chloride influx and potassium efflux increase the degree of intracellular negativity, which is called *hyperpolarization*. This inhibits the neuron because the membrane potential is even more negative than the normal intracellular potential. Therefore, an increase in negativity beyond the normal resting membrane potential level is called an *inhibitory postsynaptic potential* (IPSP).

Figure 45-9C shows the effect on the membrane potential caused by activation of inhibitory synapses, allowing chloride influx into the cell and/or potassium efflux out of the cell, with the membrane potential decreasing from its normal value of −65 millivolts to the more negative value of −70 millivolts. This membrane potential is 5 millivolts more negative than normal and is therefore an IPSP of −5 millivolts, which inhibits transmission of the nerve signal through the synapse.

Presynaptic Inhibition

In addition to inhibition caused by inhibitory synapses operating at the neuronal membrane, which is called *postsynaptic inhibition*, another type of inhibition often occurs at the presynaptic terminals before the signal ever reaches the synapse. This type of inhibition, called *presynaptic inhibition*, occurs in the following way.

Presynaptic inhibition is caused by release of an inhibitory substance onto the outsides of the presynaptic nerve fibrils before their own endings terminate on the postsynaptic neuron. *In most instances, the inhibitory transmitter substance is GABA (gamma-aminobutyric acid).* This has a specific effect of opening anion channels, allowing large numbers of chloride ions to diffuse into the terminal fibril. The negative charges of these ions inhibit synaptic transmission because they cancel much of the excitatory effect of the positively charged sodium ions that also enter the terminal fibrils when an action potential arrives.

Presynaptic inhibition occurs in many of the sensory pathways in the nervous system. In fact, adjacent sensory nerve fibers often mutually inhibit one another, which minimizes sideways spread and mixing of signals in sensory tracts. We discuss the importance of this phenomenon more fully in subsequent chapters.

Time Course of Postsynaptic Potentials

When an excitatory synapse excites the anterior motor neuron, the neuronal membrane becomes highly permeable to sodium ions for 1 to 2 milliseconds. During this very short time, enough sodium ions diffuse rapidly to the interior of the postsynaptic motor neuron to increase its intraneuronal potential by a few millivolts, thus creating the excitatory postsynaptic potential (EPSP) shown by the blue and green curves of Figure 45-10. This potential then slowly declines over the next 15 milliseconds because this is the time required for the excess positive charges to leak out of the excited neuron and to re-establish the normal resting membrane potential.

Precisely the opposite effect occurs for an IPSP; that is, the inhibitory synapse increases the permeability of the membrane to potassium or chloride ions, or both, for 1 to 2 milliseconds, and this decreases the intraneuronal potential to a more negative value than normal, thereby creating the IPSP. This potential also dies away in about 15 milliseconds.

Other types of transmitter substances can excite or inhibit the postsynaptic neuron for much longer

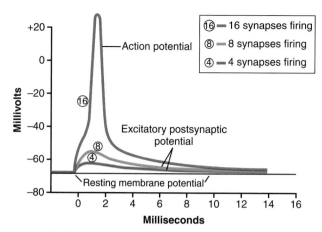

Figure 45-10 Excitatory postsynaptic potentials, showing that simultaneous firing of only a few synapses will not cause sufficient summated potential to elicit an action potential, but that simultaneous firing of many synapses will raise the summated potential to threshold for excitation and cause a superimposed action potential.

periods—for hundreds of milliseconds or even for seconds, minutes, or hours. This is especially true for some of the neuropeptide transmitters.

"Spatial Summation" in Neurons—Threshold for Firing

Excitation of a single presynaptic terminal on the surface of a neuron almost never excites the neuron. The reason for this is that the amount of transmitter substance released by a single terminal to cause an EPSP is usually no greater than 0.5 to 1 millivolt, instead of the 10 to 20 millivolts normally required to reach threshold for excitation.

However, many presynaptic terminals are usually stimulated at the same time. Even though these terminals are spread over wide areas of the neuron, their effects can still *summate;* that is, they can add to one another until neuronal excitation does occur. The reason for this is the following: It was pointed out earlier that a change in potential at any single point within the soma will cause the potential to change everywhere inside the soma almost equally. This is true because of the very high electrical conductivity inside the large neuronal cell body. Therefore, for each excitatory synapse that discharges simultaneously, the total intrasomal potential becomes more positive by 0.5 to 1.0 millivolt. When the EPSP becomes great enough, the *threshold for firing* will be reached and an action potential will develop spontaneously in the initial segment of the axon. This is demonstrated in Figure 45-10. The bottom postsynaptic potential in the figure was caused by simultaneous stimulation of 4 synapses; the next higher potential was caused by stimulation of 8 synapses; finally, a still higher EPSP was caused by stimulation of 16 synapses. In this last instance, the firing threshold had been reached, and an action potential was generated in the axon.

This effect of summing simultaneous postsynaptic potentials by activating multiple terminals on widely spaced areas of the neuronal membrane is called *spatial summation.*

"Temporal Summation" Caused by Successive Discharges of a Presynaptic Terminal

Each time a presynaptic terminal fires, the released transmitter substance opens the membrane channels for at most a millisecond or so. But the changed postsynaptic potential lasts up to 15 milliseconds after the synaptic membrane channels have already closed. Therefore, a second opening of the same channels can increase the postsynaptic potential to a still greater level, and the more rapid the rate of stimulation, the greater the postsynaptic potential becomes. Thus, successive discharges from a single presynaptic terminal, if they occur rapidly enough, can add to one another; that is, they can "summate." This type of summation is called *temporal summation.*

Simultaneous Summation of Inhibitory and Excitatory Postsynaptic Potentials. If an IPSP is tending to *decrease* the membrane potential to a more negative value while an EPSP is tending to *increase* the potential at the same time, these two effects can either completely or partially nullify each other. Thus, if a neuron is being excited by an EPSP, an inhibitory signal from another source can often reduce the postsynaptic potential to less than threshold value for excitation, thus turning off the activity of the neuron.

"Facilitation" of Neurons

Often the summated postsynaptic potential is excitatory but has not risen high enough to reach the threshold for firing by the postsynaptic neuron. When this happens, the neuron is said to be *facilitated.* That is, its membrane potential is nearer the threshold for firing than normal, but not yet at the firing level. Consequently, another excitatory signal entering the neuron from some other source can then excite the neuron very easily. Diffuse signals in the nervous system often do facilitate large groups of neurons so that they can respond quickly and easily to signals arriving from other sources.

Special Functions of Dendrites for Exciting Neurons

Large Spatial Field of Excitation of the Dendrites. The dendrites of the anterior motor neurons often extend 500 to 1000 micrometers in all directions from the neuronal soma. And these dendrites can receive signals from a large spatial area around the motor neuron. This provides a vast opportunity for summation of signals from many separate presynaptic nerve fibers.

It is also important that between 80 and 95 percent of all the presynaptic terminals of the anterior motor neuron terminate on dendrites, in contrast to only 5 to 20 percent terminating on the neuronal soma. Therefore, a large share of the excitation is provided by signals transmitted by way of the dendrites.

Most Dendrites Cannot Transmit Action Potentials, but They Can Transmit Signals Within the Same Neuron by Electrotonic Conduction. Most dendrites fail to transmit action potentials because their membranes have relatively few voltage-gated sodium channels, and their thresholds for excitation are too high for action potentials to occur. Yet they do transmit *electrotonic current* down the dendrites to the soma. Transmission of electrotonic current means direct spread of electrical current by ion conduction in the fluids of the dendrites but without generation of action potentials. Stimulation (or inhibition) of the neuron by this current has special characteristics, as follows.

Decrement of Electrotonic Conduction in the Dendrites—Greater Excitatory (or Inhibitory) Effect by Synapses Located Near the Soma. In Figure 45-11, multiple excitatory and inhibitory synapses are shown stimulating the dendrites of a neuron. On the two dendrites to the left, there are excitatory effects near the tip ends; note the high levels of excitatory postsynaptic potentials at these ends—that is, note the *less negative* membrane potentials at these points. However, a large share of the excitatory postsynaptic potential is lost before it reaches the soma. The reason is that the dendrites are long, and their membranes are thin and at least partially permeable to potassium and chloride ions, making them "leaky" to electric current. Therefore, before the excitatory potentials can reach the soma, a large share of the potential is lost by leakage through the membrane. This decrease in membrane potential as it spreads electrotonically along dendrites toward the soma is called *decremental conduction.*

The farther the excitatory synapse is from the soma of the neuron, the greater will be the decrement and the lesser will be excitatory signal reaching the soma. Therefore, those synapses that lie near the soma have far more effect in causing neuron excitation or inhibition than those that lie far away from the soma.

Summation of Excitation and Inhibition in Dendrites. The uppermost dendrite of Figure 45-11 is shown to be stimulated by both excitatory and inhibitory synapses. At the tip of the dendrite is a strong excitatory postsynaptic potential, but nearer the soma are two inhibitory synapses acting on the same dendrite. These inhibitory synapses provide a hyperpolarizing voltage that completely nullifies the excitatory effect and indeed transmits a small amount of inhibition by electrotonic conduction toward the soma. Thus, dendrites can summate excitatory and inhibitory postsynaptic potentials in the same way that the soma can. Also shown in the figure are several inhibitory synapses located directly on the axon hillock and initial axon segment. This location provides especially powerful inhibition because it has the direct effect of increasing the threshold for excitation at the very point where the action potential is normally generated.

Relation of State of Excitation of the Neuron to Rate of Firing

"Excitatory State." The "excitatory state" of a neuron is defined as the summated degree of excitatory drive to the neuron. If there is a higher degree of excitation than inhibition of the neuron at any given instant, then it is said that there is an *excitatory state.* Conversely, if there is more inhibition than excitation, then it is said that there is an *inhibitory state.*

When the excitatory state of a neuron rises above the threshold for excitation, the neuron will fire repetitively as long as the excitatory state remains at that level. Figure 45-12 shows responses of three types of neurons

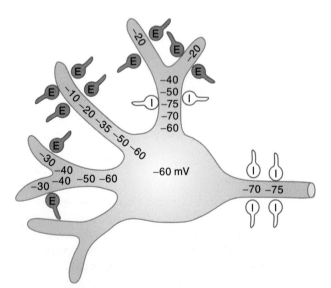

Figure 45-11 Stimulation of a neuron by presynaptic terminals located on dendrites, showing, especially, decremental conduction of excitatory (*E*) electrotonic potentials in the two dendrites to the left and inhibition (*I*) of dendritic excitation in the dendrite that is uppermost. A powerful effect of inhibitory synapses at the initial segment of the axon is also shown.

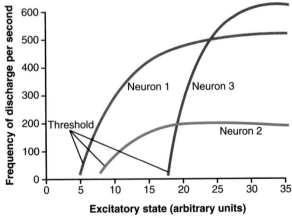

Figure 45-12 Response characteristics of different types of neurons to different levels of excitatory state.

to varying levels of excitatory state. Note that neuron 1 has a low threshold for excitation, whereas neuron 3 has a high threshold. But note also that neuron 2 has the lowest maximum frequency of discharge, whereas neuron 3 has the highest maximum frequency.

Some neurons in the central nervous system fire continuously because even the normal excitatory state is above the threshold level. Their frequency of firing can usually be increased still more by further increasing their excitatory state. The frequency can be decreased, or firing can even be stopped, by superimposing an inhibitory state on the neuron. Thus, different neurons respond differently, have different thresholds for excitation, and have widely differing maximum frequencies of discharge. With a little imagination, one can readily understand the importance of having different neurons with these many types of response characteristics to perform the widely varying functions of the nervous system.

Some Special Characteristics of Synaptic Transmission

Fatigue of Synaptic Transmission. When excitatory synapses are repetitively stimulated at a rapid rate, the number of discharges by the postsynaptic neuron is at first very great, but the firing rate becomes progressively less in succeeding milliseconds or seconds. This is called *fatigue* of synaptic transmission.

Fatigue is an exceedingly important characteristic of synaptic function because when areas of the nervous system become overexcited, fatigue causes them to lose this excess excitability after a while. For example, fatigue is probably the most important means by which the excess excitability of the brain during an epileptic seizure is finally subdued so that the seizure ceases. Thus, the development of fatigue is a protective mechanism against excess neuronal activity. This is discussed further in the description of reverberating neuronal circuits in Chapter 46.

The mechanism of fatigue is mainly exhaustion or partial exhaustion of the stores of transmitter substance in the presynaptic terminals. The excitatory terminals on many neurons can store enough excitatory transmitter to cause only about 10,000 action potentials, and the transmitter can be exhausted in only a few seconds to a few minutes of rapid stimulation. Part of the fatigue process probably results from two other factors as well: (1) progressive inactivation of many of the postsynaptic membrane receptors and (2) slow development of abnormal concentrations of ions inside the *postsynaptic* neuronal cell.

Effect of Acidosis or Alkalosis on Synaptic Transmission. Most neurons are highly responsive to changes in pH of the surrounding interstitial fluids. *Normally, alkalosis greatly increases neuronal excitability.* For instance, a rise in arterial blood pH from the 7.4 norm to 7.8 to 8.0 often causes cerebral epileptic seizures because of increased excitability of some or all of the cerebral neurons. This can be demonstrated especially well by asking a person who is predisposed to epileptic seizures to overbreathe. The overbreathing blows off carbon dioxide and therefore elevates the pH of the blood momentarily, but even this short time can often precipitate an epileptic attack.

Conversely, *acidosis greatly depresses neuronal activity;* a fall in pH from 7.4 to below 7.0 usually causes a comatose state. For instance, in very severe diabetic or uremic acidosis, coma virtually always develops.

Effect of Hypoxia on Synaptic Transmission. Neuronal excitability is also highly dependent on an adequate supply of oxygen. Cessation of oxygen for only a few seconds can cause complete inexcitability of some neurons. This is observed when the brain's blood flow is temporarily interrupted because within 3 to 7 seconds, the person becomes unconscious.

Effect of Drugs on Synaptic Transmission. Many drugs are known to increase the excitability of neurons, and others are known to decrease excitability. For instance, *caffeine, theophylline,* and *theobromine,* which are found in coffee, tea, and cocoa, respectively, all *increase* neuronal excitability, presumably by reducing the threshold for excitation of neurons.

Strychnine is one of the best known of all agents that increase excitability of neurons. However, it does not do this by reducing the threshold for excitation of the neurons; instead, it *inhibits the action of some normally inhibitory transmitter substances,* especially the inhibitory effect of glycine in the spinal cord. Therefore, the effects of the excitatory transmitters become overwhelming, and the neurons become so excited that they go into rapidly repetitive discharge, resulting in severe tonic muscle spasms.

Most anesthetics increase the neuronal membrane threshold for excitation and thereby decrease synaptic transmission at many points in the nervous system. Because many of the anesthetics are especially lipid soluble, it has been reasoned that some of them might change the physical characteristics of the neuronal membranes, making them less responsive to excitatory agents.

Synaptic Delay. During transmission of a neuronal signal from a presynaptic neuron to a postsynaptic neuron, a certain amount of time is consumed in the process of (1) discharge of the transmitter substance by the presynaptic terminal, (2) diffusion of the transmitter to the postsynaptic neuronal membrane, (3) action of the transmitter on the membrane receptor, (4) action of the receptor to increase the membrane permeability, and (5) inward diffusion of sodium to raise the excitatory postsynaptic potential to a high enough level to elicit an action potential. The *minimal* period of time required for all these events to take place, even when large numbers of excitatory synapses are stimulated simultaneously, is about 0.5 millisecond. This is called the *synaptic delay.* Neurophysiologists can measure the *minimal* delay time between an input volley of impulses into a pool of neurons and the consequent output volley. From the measure of delay time, one can then estimate the number of series neurons in the circuit.

Bibliography

Alberini CM: Transcription factors in long-term memory and synaptic plasticity, *Physiol Rev* 89:121, 2009.

Bloodgood BL, Sabatini BL: Regulation of synaptic signalling by postsynaptic, non-glutamate receptor ion channels, *J Physiol* 586:1475, 2008.

Ben-Ari Y, Gaiarsa JL, Tyzio R, et al: GABA: a pioneer transmitter that excites immature neurons and generates primitive oscillations, *Physiol Rev* 87:1215, 2007.

Boehning D, Snyder SH: Novel neural modulators, *Annu Rev Neurosci* 26:105, 2003.

Brasnjo G, Otis TS: Glycine transporters not only take out the garbage, they recycle, *Neuron* 40:667, 2003.

Conde C, Cáceres A: Microtubule assembly, organization and dynamics in axons and dendrites, *Nat Rev Neurosci* 10:319, 2009.

Dalva MB, McClelland AC, Kayser MS: Cell adhesion molecules: signalling functions at the synapse, *Nat Rev Neurosci* 8:206, 2007.

Deeg KE: Synapse-specific homeostatic mechanisms in the hippocampus, *J Neurophysiol* 101:503, 2009.

Engelman HS, MacDermott AB: Presynaptic inotropic receptors and control of transmitter release, *Nat Rev Neurosci* 5:135, 2004.

Haines DE, Lancon JA: *Review of Neuroscience*, New York, 2003, Churchill Livingstone.

Jacob TC, Moss SJ, Jurd R: GABA(A) receptor trafficking and its role in the dynamic modulation of neuronal inhibition, *Nat Rev Neurosci* 9(5):331–343, 2008 May.

Kandel ER: The molecular biology of memory storage: a dialogue between genes and synapses, *Science* 294:1030, 2001.

Kandel ER, Schwartz JH, Jessell TM: *Principles of Neural Science*, ed 4, New York, 2000, McGraw-Hill.

Kerchner GA, Nicoll RA: Silent synapses and the emergence of a postsynaptic mechanism for LTP, *Nat Rev Neurosci* 9:813, 2008.

Klein R: Bidirectional modulation of synaptic functions by Eph/ephrin signaling, *Nat Neurosci* 12:15, 2009.

Lisman JE, Raghavachari S, Tsien RW: The sequence of events that underlie quantal transmission at central glutamatergic synapses, *Nat Rev Neurosci* 8:597, 2007.

Magee JC: Dendritic integration of excitatory synaptic input, *Nat Rev Neurosci* 1:181, 2000.

Migliore M, Shepherd GM: Emerging rules for the distributions of active dendritic conductances, *Nat Rev Neurosci* 3:362, 2002.

Muller D, Nikonenko I: Dynamic presynaptic varicosities: a role in activity-dependent synaptogenesis, *Trends Neurosci* 26:573, 2003.

Prast H, Philippu A: Nitric oxide as modulator of neuronal function, *Prog Neurobiol* 64:51, 2001.

Reid CA, Bekkers JM, Clements JD: Presynaptic Ca^{2+} channels: a functional patchwork, *Trends Neurosci* 26:683, 2003.

Robinson RB, Siegelbaum SA: Hyperpolarization-activated cation currents: from molecules to physiological function, *Annu Rev Physiol* 65:453, 2003.

Ruff RL: Neurophysiology of the neuromuscular junction: overview, *Ann N Y Acad Sci* 998:1, 2003.

Schmolesky MT, Weber JT, De Zeeuw CI, et al: The making of a complex spike: ionic composition and plasticity, *Ann N Y Acad Sci* 978:359, 2002.

Semyanov A, Walker MC, Kullmann DM, et al: Tonically active GABA A receptors: modulating gain and maintaining the tone, *Trends Neurosci* 27:262, 2004.

Sjöström PJ, Rancz EA, Roth A, et al: Dendritic excitability and synaptic plasticity, *Physiol Rev* 88:769, 2008.

Spruston N: Pyramidal neurons: dendritic structure and synaptic integration, *Nat Rev Neurosci* 9:206, 2008.

Williams SR, Wozny C, Mitchell SJ: The back and forth of dendritic plasticity, *Neuron* 56:947, 2007.

Zucker RS, Regehr WG: Short-term synaptic plasticity, *Annu Rev Physiol* 64:355, 2002.

Sensory Receptors, Neuronal Circuits for Processing Information

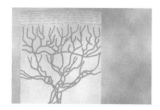

Input to the nervous system is provided by sensory receptors that detect such sensory stimuli as touch, sound, light, pain, cold, and warmth. The purpose of this chapter is to discuss the basic mechanisms by which these receptors change sensory stimuli into nerve signals that are then conveyed to and processed in the central nervous system.

Types of Sensory Receptors and the Stimuli They Detect

Table 46-1 lists and classifies five basic types of sensory receptors: (1) *mechanoreceptors,* which detect mechanical compression or stretching of the receptor or of tissues adjacent to the receptor; (2) *thermoreceptors,* which detect changes in temperature, with some receptors detecting cold and others warmth; (3) *nociceptors* (pain receptors), which detect damage occurring in the tissues, whether physical damage or chemical damage; (4) *electromagnetic receptors,* which detect light on the retina of the eye; and (5) *chemoreceptors,* which detect taste in the mouth, smell in the nose, oxygen level in the arterial blood, osmolality of the body fluids, carbon dioxide concentration, and other factors that make up the chemistry of the body.

In this chapter, we discuss the function of a few specific types of receptors, primarily peripheral mechanoreceptors, to illustrate some of the principles by which receptors operate. Other receptors are discussed in other chapters in relation to the sensory systems that they subserve. Figure 46-1 shows some of the types of mechanoreceptors found in the skin or in deep tissues of the body.

Differential Sensitivity of Receptors

How do two types of sensory receptors detect different types of sensory stimuli? The answer is, by *"differential sensitivities."* That is, each type of receptor is highly sensitive to one type of stimulus for which it is designed and yet is almost nonresponsive to other types of sensory stimuli. Thus, the rods and cones of the eyes are highly responsive to light but are almost completely nonresponsive to normal ranges of heat, cold, pressure on the eyeballs, or chemical changes in the blood. The osmoreceptors of the supraoptic nuclei in the hypothalamus detect minute changes in the osmolality of the body fluids but have never been known to respond to sound. Finally, pain receptors in the skin are almost never stimulated by usual touch or pressure stimuli but do become highly active the moment tactile stimuli become severe enough to damage the tissues.

Modality of Sensation—The "Labeled Line" Principle

Each of the principal types of sensation that we can experience—pain, touch, sight, sound, and so forth—is called a *modality* of sensation. Yet despite the fact that we experience these different modalities of sensation, nerve fibers transmit only impulses. Therefore, how do different nerve fibers transmit different modalities of sensation?

The answer is that each nerve tract terminates at a specific point in the central nervous system, and the type of sensation felt when a nerve fiber is stimulated is determined by the point in the nervous system to which the fiber leads. For instance, if a pain fiber is stimulated, the person perceives pain regardless of what type of stimulus excites the fiber. The stimulus can be electricity, overheating of the fiber, crushing of the fiber, or stimulation of the pain nerve ending by damage to the tissue cells. In all these instances, the person perceives pain. Likewise, if a touch fiber is stimulated by electrical excitation of a touch receptor or in any other way, the person perceives touch because touch fibers lead to specific touch areas in the brain. Similarly, fibers from the retina of the eye terminate in the vision areas of the brain, fibers from the ear terminate in the auditory areas of the brain, and temperature fibers terminate in the temperature areas.

This specificity of nerve fibers for transmitting only one modality of sensation is called the *labeled line principle.*

Table 46-1 Classification of Sensory Receptors

I. Mechanoreceptors
  Skin tactile sensibilities (epidermis and dermis)
    Free nerve endings
    Expanded tip endings
      Merkel's discs
      Plus several other variants
    Spray endings
      Ruffini's endings
    Encapsulated endings
      Meissner's corpuscles
      Krause's corpuscles
    Hair end-organs
  Deep tissue sensibilities
    Free nerve endings
    Expanded tip endings
    Spray endings
      Ruffini's endings
    Encapsulated endings
      Pacinian corpuscles
      Plus a few other variants
    Muscle endings
      Muscle spindles
      Golgi tendon receptors
  Hearing
    Sound receptors of cochlea
  Equilibrium
    Vestibular receptors
  Arterial pressure
    Baroreceptors of carotid sinuses and aorta
II. Thermoreceptors
  Cold
    Cold receptors
  Warmth
    Warm receptors
III. Nociceptors
  Pain
    Free nerve endings
IV. Electromagnetic receptors
  Vision
    Rods
    Cones
V. Chemoreceptors
  Taste
    Receptors of taste buds
  Smell
    Receptors of olfactory epithelium
  Arterial oxygen
    Receptors of aortic and carotid bodies
  Osmolality
    Neurons in or near supraoptic nuclei
  Blood CO_2
    Receptors in or on surface of medulla and in
    aortic and carotid bodies
  Blood glucose, amino acids, fatty acids
    Receptors in hypothalamus

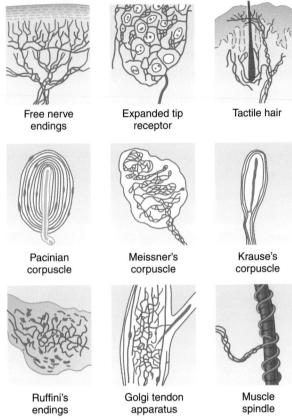

Free nerve endings   Expanded tip receptor   Tactile hair

Pacinian corpuscle   Meissner's corpuscle   Krause's corpuscle

Ruffini's endings   Golgi tendon apparatus   Muscle spindle

Figure 46-1 Several types of somatic sensory nerve endings.

Transduction of Sensory Stimuli into Nerve Impulses

Local Electrical Currents at Nerve Endings—Receptor Potentials

All sensory receptors have one feature in common. Whatever the type of stimulus that excites the receptor, its immediate effect is to change the membrane electrical potential of the receptor. This change in potential is called a *receptor potential.*

Mechanisms of Receptor Potentials. Different receptors can be excited in one of several ways to cause receptor potentials: (1) by mechanical deformation of the receptor, which stretches the receptor membrane and opens ion channels; (2) by application of a chemical to the membrane, which also opens ion channels; (3) by change of the temperature of the membrane, which alters the permeability of the membrane; or (4) by the effects of electromagnetic radiation, such as light on a retinal visual receptor, which either directly or indirectly changes the receptor membrane characteristics and allows ions to flow through membrane channels.

These four means of exciting receptors correspond in general with the different types of known sensory receptors. In all instances, the basic cause of the change in membrane potential is a change in membrane permeability of the receptor, which allows ions to diffuse more or less readily through the membrane and thereby to change the *transmembrane potential.*

Maximum Receptor Potential Amplitude. The maximum amplitude of most sensory receptor potentials is about 100 millivolts, but this level occurs only at an extremely high intensity of sensory stimulus. This is about the same maximum voltage recorded in action potentials and is also the change in voltage when the membrane becomes maximally permeable to sodium ions.

Relation of the Receptor Potential to Action Potentials. When the receptor potential rises above the *threshold* for eliciting action potentials in the nerve fiber attached to the receptor, then action potentials occur, as illustrated in Figure 46-2. Note also that the more the receptor potential rises above the threshold level, the greater becomes the *action potential frequency.*

Receptor Potential of the Pacinian Corpuscle—An Example of Receptor Function

The student should at this point restudy the anatomical structure of the pacinian corpuscle shown in Figure 46-1. Note that the corpuscle has a central nerve fiber extending through its core. Surrounding this are multiple concentric capsule layers, so compression anywhere on the outside of the corpuscle will elongate, indent, or otherwise deform the central fiber.

Now study Figure 46-3, which shows only the central fiber of the pacinian corpuscle after all capsule layers but one have been removed. The tip of the central fiber inside the capsule is unmyelinated, but the fiber does become myelinated (the blue sheath shown in the figure) shortly before leaving the corpuscle to enter a peripheral sensory nerve.

The figure also shows the mechanism by which a receptor potential is produced in the pacinian corpuscle. Observe the small area of the terminal fiber that has been deformed by compression of the corpuscle, and note that ion channels have opened in the membrane, allowing

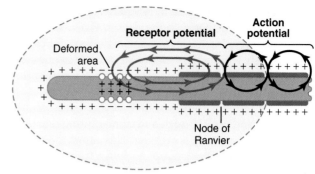

Figure 46-3 Excitation of a sensory nerve fiber by a receptor potential produced in a pacinian corpuscle. (Modified from Loëwenstein WR: Excitation and inactivation in a receptor membrane. Ann N Y Acad Sci 94:510, 1961.)

positively charged sodium ions to diffuse to the interior of the fiber. This creates increased positivity inside the fiber, which is the "receptor potential." The receptor potential in turn induces a *local circuit* of current flow, shown by the arrows, that spreads along the nerve fiber. At the first node of Ranvier, which itself lies inside the capsule of the pacinian corpuscle, the local current flow depolarizes the fiber membrane at this node, which then sets off typical action potentials that are transmitted along the nerve fiber toward the central nervous system.

Relation Between Stimulus Intensity and the Receptor Potential. Figure 46-4 shows the changing amplitude of the receptor potential caused by progressively stronger mechanical compression (increasing "stimulus strength") applied experimentally to the central core of a pacinian corpuscle. Note that the amplitude increases rapidly at first but then progressively less rapidly at high stimulus strength.

In turn, the *frequency of repetitive action potentials* transmitted from sensory receptors increases approximately in

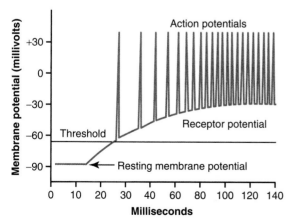

Figure 46-2 Typical relation between receptor potential and action potentials when the receptor potential rises above threshold level.

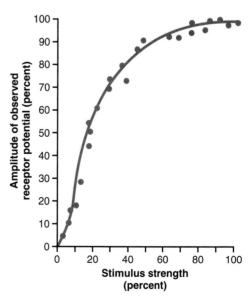

Figure 46-4 Relation of amplitude of receptor potential to strength of a mechanical stimulus applied to a pacinian corpuscle. (Data from Loëwenstein WR: Excitation and inactivation in a receptor membrane. Ann N Y Acad Sci 94:510, 1961.)

proportion to the increase in receptor potential. Putting this principle together with the data in Figure 46-4, one can see that very intense stimulation of the receptor causes progressively less and less additional increase in numbers of action potentials. This is an exceedingly important principle that is applicable to almost all sensory receptors. It allows the receptor to be sensitive to very weak sensory experience and yet not reach a maximum firing rate until the sensory experience is extreme. This allows the receptor to have an extreme range of response, from very weak to very intense.

Adaptation of Receptors

Another characteristic of all sensory receptors is that they *adapt* either partially or completely to any constant stimulus after a period of time. That is, when a continuous sensory stimulus is applied, the receptor responds at a high impulse rate at first and then at a progressively slower rate until finally the rate of action potentials decreases to very few or often to none at all.

Figure 46-5 shows typical adaptation of certain types of receptors. Note that the pacinian corpuscle adapts very rapidly, hair receptors adapt within a second or so, and some joint capsule and muscle spindle receptors adapt slowly.

Furthermore, some sensory receptors adapt to a far greater extent than others. For example, the pacinian corpuscles adapt to "extinction" within a few hundredths of a second, and the receptors at the bases of the hairs adapt to extinction within a second or more. It is probable that all other *mechanoreceptors* eventually adapt almost completely, but some require hours or days to do so, for which reason they are called "nonadapting" receptors. The longest measured time for almost complete adaptation of a mechanoreceptor is about 2 days, which is the adaptation time for many carotid and aortic baroreceptors. Conversely, some of the nonmechanoreceptors—the chemoreceptors and pain receptors, for instance—probably never adapt completely.

Mechanisms by Which Receptors Adapt. The mechanism of receptor adaptation is different for each type of receptor, in much the same way that development of a receptor potential is an individual property. For instance, in the eye, the rods and cones adapt by changing the concentrations of their light-sensitive chemicals (which is discussed in Chapter 50).

In the case of the mechanoreceptors, the receptor that has been studied in greatest detail is the pacinian corpuscle. Adaptation occurs in this receptor in two ways. First, the pacinian corpuscle is a viscoelastic structure, so that when a distorting force is suddenly applied to one side of the corpuscle, this force is instantly transmitted by the viscous component of the corpuscle directly to the same side of the central nerve fiber, thus eliciting a receptor potential. However, within a few hundredths of a second, the fluid within the corpuscle redistributes and the receptor potential is no longer elicited. Thus, the receptor potential appears at the onset of compression but disappears within a small fraction of a second even though the compression continues.

The second mechanism of adaptation of the pacinian corpuscle, but a much slower one, results from a process called *accommodation,* which occurs in the nerve fiber itself. That is, even if by chance the central core fiber should continue to be distorted, the tip of the nerve fiber itself gradually becomes "accommodated" to the stimulus. This probably results from progressive "inactivation" of the sodium channels in the nerve fiber membrane, which means that sodium current flow through the channels causes them gradually to close, an effect that seems to occur for all or most cell membrane sodium channels, as was explained in Chapter 5.

Presumably, these same two general mechanisms of adaptation apply also to the other types of mechanoreceptors. That is, part of the adaptation results from readjustments in the structure of the receptor itself, and part from an electrical type of accommodation in the terminal nerve fibril.

Slowly Adapting Receptors Detect Continuous Stimulus Strength—The "Tonic" Receptors. Slowly adapting receptors continue to transmit impulses to the brain as long as the stimulus is present (or at least for many minutes or hours). Therefore, they keep the brain constantly apprised of the status of the body and its relation to its surroundings. For instance, impulses from the muscle spindles and Golgi tendon apparatuses allow the nervous system to know the status of muscle contraction and load on the muscle tendon at each instant.

Other slowly adapting receptors include (1) receptors of the macula in the vestibular apparatus, (2) pain receptors, (3) baroreceptors of the arterial tree, and (4) chemoreceptors of the carotid and aortic bodies.

Because the slowly adapting receptors can continue to transmit information for many hours, they are called *tonic* receptors.

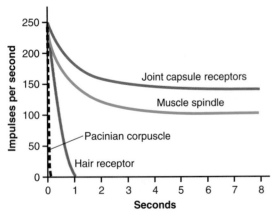

Figure 46-5 Adaptation of different types of receptors, showing rapid adaptation of some receptors and slow adaptation of others.

Rapidly Adapting Receptors Detect Change in Stimulus Strength—The "Rate Receptors," "Movement Receptors," or "Phasic Receptors." Receptors that adapt rapidly cannot be used to transmit a continuous signal because these receptors are stimulated only when the stimulus strength changes. Yet they react strongly *while a change is actually taking place*. Therefore, these receptors are called *rate* receptors, *movement* receptors, or *phasic* receptors. Thus, in the case of the pacinian corpuscle, sudden pressure applied to the tissue excites this receptor for a few milliseconds, and then its excitation is over even though the pressure continues. But later, it transmits a signal again when the pressure is released. In other words, the pacinian corpuscle is exceedingly important in apprising the nervous system of rapid tissue deformations, but it is useless for transmitting information about constant conditions in the body.

Importance of the Rate Receptors—Their Predictive Function. If one knows the rate at which some change in bodily status is taking place, one can predict in one's mind the state of the body a few seconds or even a few minutes later. For instance, the receptors of the semicircular canals in the vestibular apparatus of the ear detect the rate at which the head begins to turn when one runs around a curve. Using this information, a person can predict how much he or she will turn within the next 2 seconds and can adjust the motion of the legs *ahead of time* to keep from losing balance. Likewise, receptors located in or near the joints help detect the rates of movement of the different parts of the body. For instance, when one is running, information from the joint rate receptors allows the nervous system to predict where the feet will be during any precise fraction of the next second. Therefore, appropriate motor signals can be transmitted to the muscles of the legs to make any necessary anticipatory corrections in position so that the person will not fall. Loss of this predictive function makes it impossible for the person to run.

Nerve Fibers That Transmit Different Types of Signals and Their Physiologic Classification

Some signals need to be transmitted to or from the central nervous system extremely rapidly; otherwise, the information would be useless. An example of this is the sensory signals that apprise the brain of the momentary positions of the legs at each fraction of a second during running. At the other extreme, some types of sensory information, such as that depicting prolonged, aching pain, do not need to be transmitted rapidly, so slowly conducting fibers will suffice. As shown in Figure 46-6, nerve fibers come in all sizes between 0.5 and 20 micrometers in diameter—the larger the diameter, the greater the conducting velocity. The range of conducting velocities is between 0.5 and 120 m/sec.

General Classification of Nerve Fibers. Shown in Figure 46-6 is a "general classification" and a "sensory nerve classification" of the different types of nerve fibers. In the

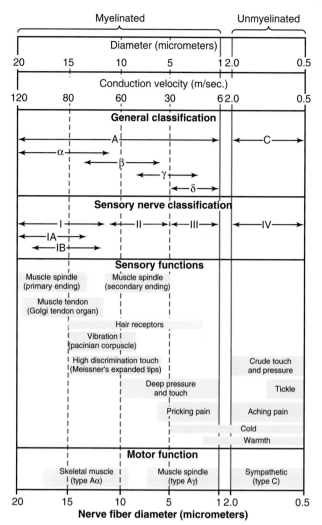

Figure 46-6 Physiologic classifications and functions of nerve fibers.

general classification, the fibers are divided into types A and C, and the type A fibers are further subdivided into α, β, γ, and δ fibers.

Type A fibers are the typical large and medium-sized *myelinated* fibers of spinal nerves. Type C fibers are the small *unmyelinated* nerve fibers that conduct impulses at low velocities. The C fibers constitute more than one half of the sensory fibers in most peripheral nerves, as well as all the postganglionic autonomic fibers.

The sizes, velocities of conduction, and functions of the different nerve fiber types are also given in Figure 46-6. Note that a few large myelinated fibers can transmit impulses at velocities as great as 120 m/sec, a distance in 1 second that is longer than a football field. Conversely, the smallest fibers transmit impulses as slowly as 0.5 m/sec, requiring about 2 seconds to go from the big toe to the spinal cord.

Alternative Classification Used by Sensory Physiologists. Certain recording techniques have made it possible to separate the type Aα fibers into two subgroups; yet these same recording techniques cannot distinguish easily between Aβ and Aγ fibers. Therefore, the following classification is frequently used by sensory physiologists:

Group Ia

Fibers from the annulospiral endings of muscle spindles (average about 17 microns in diameter; these are α-type A fibers in the general classification).

Group Ib

Fibers from the Golgi tendon organs (average about 16 micrometers in diameter; these also are α-type A fibers).

Group II

Fibers from most discrete cutaneous tactile receptors and from the flower-spray endings of the muscle spindles (average about 8 micrometers in diameter; these are β- and γ-type A fibers in the general classification).

Group III

Fibers carrying temperature, crude touch, and pricking pain sensations (average about 3 micrometers in diameter; they are δ-type A fibers in the general classification).

Group IV

Unmyelinated fibers carrying pain, itch, temperature, and crude touch sensations (0.5 to 2 micrometers in diameter; they are type C fibers in the general classification).

Transmission of Signals of Different Intensity in Nerve Tracts—Spatial and Temporal Summation

One of the characteristics of each signal that always must be conveyed is signal intensity—for instance, the intensity of pain. The different gradations of intensity can be transmitted either by using increasing numbers of parallel fibers or by sending more action potentials along a single fiber. These two mechanisms are called, respectively, *spatial summation* and *temporal summation*.

Spatial Summation. Figure 46-7 shows the phenomenon of *spatial summation,* whereby increasing signal strength is transmitted by using progressively greater numbers of fibers. This figure shows a section of skin innervated by a large number of parallel pain fibers. Each of these arborizes into hundreds of minute *free nerve endings* that serve as pain receptors. The entire cluster of fibers from one pain fiber frequently covers an area of skin as large as 5 centimeters in diameter. This area is called the *receptor field* of that fiber. The number of endings is large in the center of the field but diminishes toward the periphery. One can also see from the figure that the arborizing fibrils overlap those from other pain fibers. Therefore, a pinprick of the skin usually stimulates endings from many different pain fibers simultaneously. When the pinprick is in the center of the receptive field of a particular pain fiber, the degree of stimulation of that fiber is far greater than when it is in the periphery of the field because the number of free nerve endings in the middle of the field is much greater than at the periphery.

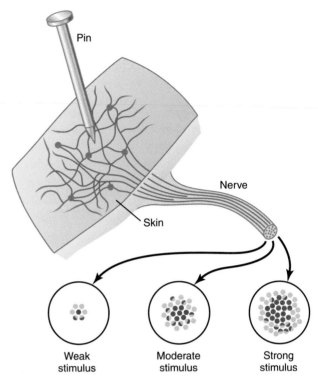

Figure 46-7 Pattern of stimulation of pain fibers in a nerve leading from an area of skin pricked by a pin. This is an example of *spatial summation.*

Thus, the lower part of Figure 46-7 shows three views of the cross section of the nerve bundle leading from the skin area. To the left is the effect of a weak stimulus, with only a single nerve fiber in the middle of the bundle stimulated strongly (represented by the red-colored fiber), whereas several adjacent fibers are stimulated weakly (half-red fibers). The other two views of the nerve cross section show the effect of a moderate stimulus and a strong stimulus, with progressively more fibers being stimulated. Thus, the stronger signals spread to more and more fibers. This is the phenomenon of *spatial summation.*

Temporal Summation. A second means for transmitting signals of increasing strength is by increasing the *frequency* of nerve impulses in each fiber, which is called *temporal summation.* Figure 46-8 demonstrates this, showing in the upper part a changing strength of signal and in the lower part the actual impulses transmitted by the nerve fiber.

Transmission and Processing of Signals in Neuronal Pools

The central nervous system is composed of thousands to millions of neuronal pools; some of these contain few neurons, whereas others have vast numbers. For instance, the entire cerebral cortex could be considered to be a single large neuronal pool. Other neuronal pools include the different basal ganglia and the specific nuclei in the thalamus,

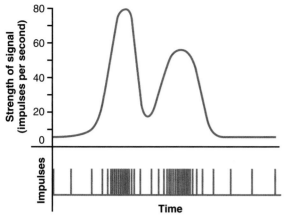

Figure 46-8 Translation of signal strength into a frequency-modulated series of nerve impulses, showing the strength of signal (*above*) and the separate nerve impulses (*below*). This is an example of *temporal summation*.

cerebellum, mesencephalon, pons, and medulla. Also, the entire dorsal gray matter of the spinal cord could be considered one long pool of neurons.

Each neuronal pool has its own special organization that causes it to process signals in its own unique way, thus allowing the total consortium of pools to achieve the multitude of functions of the nervous system. Yet despite their differences in function, the pools also have many similar principles of function, described in the following pages.

Relaying of Signals Through Neuronal Pools

Organization of Neurons for Relaying Signals. Figure 46-9 is a schematic diagram of several neurons in a neuronal pool, showing "input" fibers to the left and

"output" fibers to the right. Each input fiber divides hundreds to thousands of times, providing a thousand or more terminal fibrils that spread into a large area in the pool to synapse with dendrites or cell bodies of the neurons in the pool. The dendrites usually also arborize and spread hundreds to thousands of micrometers in the pool.

The neuronal area stimulated by each incoming nerve fiber is called its *stimulatory field.* Note in Figure 46-9 that large numbers of the terminals from each input fiber lie on the nearest neuron in its "field," but progressively fewer terminals lie on the neurons farther away.

Threshold and Subthreshold Stimuli—Excitation or Facilitation. From the discussion of synaptic function in Chapter 45, it will be recalled that discharge of a single excitatory presynaptic terminal almost never causes an action potential in a postsynaptic neuron. Instead, large numbers of input terminals must discharge on the same neuron either simultaneously or in rapid succession to cause excitation. For instance, in Figure 46-9, let us assume that six terminals must discharge almost simultaneously to excite any one of the neurons. If the student counts the number of terminals on each one of the neurons from each input fiber, he or she will see that *input fiber 1* has more than enough terminals to cause *neuron a* to discharge. The stimulus from input fiber 1 to this neuron is said to be an *excitatory stimulus*; it is also called a *suprathreshold stimulus* because it is above the threshold required for excitation.

Input fiber 1 also contributes terminals to neurons b and c, but not enough to cause excitation. Nevertheless, discharge of these terminals makes both these neurons more likely to be excited by signals arriving through other incoming nerve fibers. Therefore, the stimuli to these neurons are said to be *subthreshold*, and the neurons are said to be *facilitated.*

Similarly, for *input fiber 2*, the stimulus to *neuron d* is a suprathreshold stimulus, and the stimuli to *neurons b* and c are subthreshold, but facilitating, stimuli.

Figure 46-9 represents a highly condensed version of a neuronal pool because each input nerve fiber usually provides massive numbers of branching terminals to hundreds or thousands of neurons in its distribution "field," as shown in Figure 46-10. In the central portion of the field in this figure, designated by the circled area, all the neurons are stimulated by the incoming fiber. Therefore, this is said to be the *discharge zone* of the incoming fiber, also called the *excited zone* or *liminal zone.* To each side,

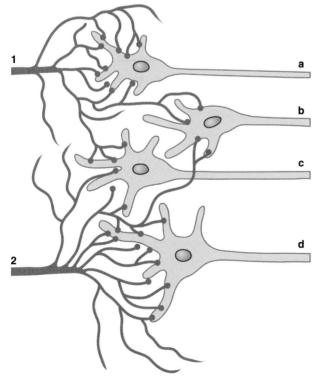

Figure 46-9 Basic organization of a neuronal pool.

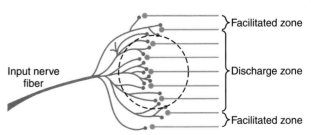

Figure 46-10 "Discharge" and "facilitated" zones of a neuronal pool.

the neurons are facilitated but not excited, and these areas are called the *facilitated zone,* also called the *subthreshold zone* or *subliminal zone.*

Inhibition of a Neuronal Pool. We must also remember that some incoming fibers inhibit neurons, rather than exciting them. This is the opposite of facilitation, and the entire field of the inhibitory branches is called the *inhibitory zone.* The degree of inhibition in the center of this zone is great because of large numbers of endings in the center; it becomes progressively less toward its edges.

Divergence of Signals Passing Through Neuronal Pools

Often it is important for weak signals entering a neuronal pool to excite far greater numbers of nerve fibers leaving the pool. This phenomenon is called *divergence.* Two major types of divergence occur and have entirely different purposes.

An *amplifying* type of divergence is shown in Figure 46-11A. This means simply that an input signal spreads to an increasing number of neurons as it passes through successive orders of neurons in its path. This type of divergence is characteristic of the corticospinal pathway in its control of skeletal muscles, with a single large pyramidal cell in the motor cortex capable, under highly facilitated conditions, of exciting as many as 10,000 muscle fibers.

The second type of divergence, shown in Figure 46-11B, is *divergence into multiple tracts.* In this case, the signal is transmitted in two directions from the pool. For instance, information transmitted up the dorsal columns of the spinal cord takes two courses in the lower part of the brain: (1) into the cerebellum and (2) on through the lower regions of the brain to the thalamus and cerebral cortex. Likewise, in the thalamus, almost all sensory information is relayed both into still deeper structures of the thalamus and at the same time to discrete regions of the cerebral cortex.

Convergence of Signals

Convergence means signals from multiple inputs uniting to excite a single neuron. Figure 46-12A shows *convergence from a single source.* That is, multiple terminals from a single incoming fiber tract terminate on the same neuron. The importance of this is that neurons are almost never excited by an action potential from a single input terminal. But action potentials converging on the neuron from multiple terminals provide enough spatial summation to bring the neuron to the threshold required for discharge.

Convergence can also result from input signals (excitatory or inhibitory) *from multiple sources,* as shown in Figure 46-12B. For instance, the interneurons of the spinal cord receive converging signals from (1) peripheral nerve fibers entering the cord, (2) propriospinal fibers passing from one segment of the cord to another, (3) corticospinal fibers from the cerebral cortex, and (4) several other long pathways descending from the brain into the spinal cord. Then the signals from the interneurons converge on the anterior motor neurons to control muscle function.

Such convergence allows *summation* of information from different sources, and the resulting response is a summated effect of all the different types of information. Convergence is one of the important means by which the central nervous system correlates, summates, and sorts different types of information.

Neuronal Circuit with both Excitatory and Inhibitory Output Signals

Sometimes an incoming signal to a neuronal pool causes an output excitatory signal going in one direction and at the same time an inhibitory signal going elsewhere. For instance, at the same time that an excitatory signal is transmitted by one set of neurons in the spinal cord to cause forward movement of a leg, an inhibitory signal is transmitted through a separate set of neurons to inhibit the muscles on the back of the leg so that they will not oppose the forward movement. This type of circuit is characteristic for controlling all antagonistic pairs of muscles, and it is called the *reciprocal inhibition circuit.*

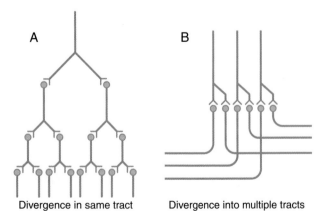

Divergence in same tract   Divergence into multiple tracts

Figure 46-11 "Divergence" in neuronal pathways. *A,* Divergence within a pathway to cause "amplification" of the signal. *B,* Divergence into multiple tracts to transmit the signal to separate areas.

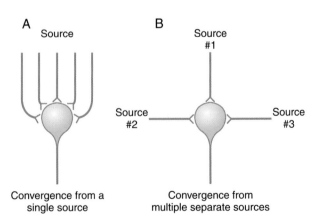

Convergence from a single source   Convergence from multiple separate sources

Figure 46-12 "Convergence" of multiple input fibers onto a single neuron. *A,* Multiple input fibers from a single source. *B,* Input fibers from multiple separate sources.

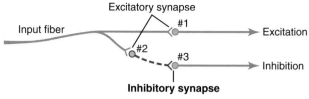

Figure 46-13 Inhibitory circuit. Neuron 2 is an inhibitory neuron.

Figure 46-13 shows the means by which the inhibition is achieved. The input fiber directly excites the excitatory output pathway, but it stimulates an intermediate *inhibitory neuron* (neuron 2), which secretes a different type of transmitter substance to inhibit the second output pathway from the pool. This type of circuit is also important in preventing overactivity in many parts of the brain.

Prolongation of a Signal by a Neuronal Pool—"Afterdischarge"

Thus far, we have considered signals that are merely relayed through neuronal pools. However, in many instances, a signal entering a pool causes a prolonged output discharge, called *afterdischarge*, lasting a few milliseconds to as long as many minutes after the incoming signal is over. The most important mechanisms by which afterdischarge occurs are the following.

Synaptic Afterdischarge. When excitatory synapses discharge on the surfaces of dendrites or soma of a neuron, a postsynaptic electrical potential develops in the neuron and lasts for many milliseconds, especially when some of the long-acting synaptic transmitter substances are involved. As long as this potential lasts, it can continue to excite the neuron, causing it to transmit a continuous train of output impulses, as was explained in Chapter 45. Thus, as a result of this synaptic "afterdischarge" mechanism alone, it is possible for a single instantaneous input signal to cause a sustained signal output (a series of repetitive discharges) lasting for many milliseconds.

Reverberatory (Oscillatory) Circuit as a Cause of Signal Prolongation. One of the most important of all circuits in the entire nervous system is the *reverberatory,* or *oscillatory, circuit.* Such circuits are caused by positive feedback within the neuronal circuit that feeds back to re-excite the input of the same circuit. Consequently, once stimulated, the circuit may discharge repetitively for a long time.

Several possible varieties of reverberatory circuits are shown in Figure 46-14. The simplest, shown in Figure 46-14*A*, involves only a single neuron. In this case, the output neuron simply sends a collateral nerve fiber back to its own dendrites or soma to restimulate itself. Although this type of circuit probably is not an important one, theoretically, once the neuron discharges, the feedback stimuli could keep the neuron discharging for a protracted time thereafter.

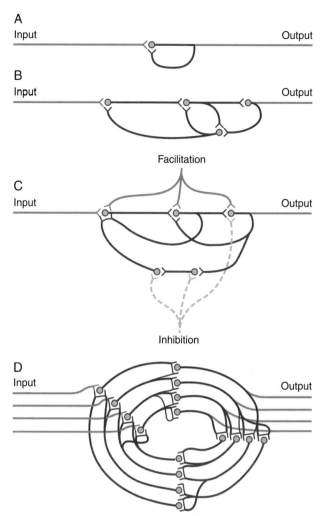

Figure 46-14 Reverberatory circuits of increasing complexity.

Figure 46-14*B* shows a few additional neurons in the feedback circuit, which causes a longer delay between initial discharge and the feedback signal. Figure 46-14*C* shows a still more complex system in which both facilitatory and inhibitory fibers impinge on the reverberating circuit. A facilitatory signal enhances the intensity and frequency of reverberation, whereas an inhibitory signal depresses or stops the reverberation.

Figure 46-14*D* shows that most reverberating pathways are constituted of many parallel fibers. At each cell station, the terminal fibrils spread widely. In such a system, the total reverberating signal can be either weak or strong, depending on how many parallel nerve fibers are momentarily involved in the reverberation.

Characteristics of Signal Prolongation from a Reverberatory Circuit. Figure 46-15 shows output signals from a typical reverberatory circuit. The input stimulus may last only 1 millisecond or so, and yet the output can last for many milliseconds or even minutes. The figure demonstrates that the intensity of the output signal usually increases to a high value early in reverberation and then decreases to a critical point, at which it suddenly ceases entirely. The cause of this sudden cessation of

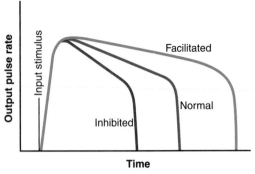

Figure 46-15 Typical pattern of the output signal from a reverberatory circuit after a single input stimulus, showing the effects of facilitation and inhibition.

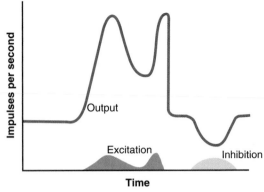

Figure 46-16 Continuous output from either a reverberating circuit or a pool of intrinsically discharging neurons. This figure also shows the effect of excitatory or inhibitory input signals.

reverberation is fatigue of synaptic junctions in the circuit. Fatigue beyond a certain critical level lowers the stimulation of the next neuron in the circuit below threshold level so that the circuit feedback is suddenly broken.

The duration of the total signal before cessation can also be controlled by signals from other parts of the brain that inhibit or facilitate the circuit. Almost these exact patterns of output signals are recorded from the motor nerves exciting a muscle involved in a flexor reflex after pain stimulation of the foot (as shown later in Figure 46-18).

Continuous Signal Output from Some Neuronal Circuits

Some neuronal circuits emit output signals continuously, even without excitatory input signals. At least two mechanisms can cause this effect: (1) continuous intrinsic neuronal discharge and (2) continuous reverberatory signals.

Continuous Discharge Caused by Intrinsic Neuronal Excitability. Neurons, like other excitable tissues, discharge repetitively if their level of excitatory membrane potential rises above a certain threshold level. The membrane potentials of many neurons even normally are high enough to cause them to emit impulses continually. This occurs especially in many of the neurons of the cerebellum, as well as in most of the interneurons of the spinal cord. The rates at which these cells emit impulses can be increased by excitatory signals or decreased by inhibitory signals; inhibitory signals often can decrease the rate of firing to zero.

Continuous Signals Emitted from Reverberating Circuits as a Means for Transmitting Information. A reverberating circuit that does not fatigue enough to stop reverberation is a source of continuous impulses. And excitatory impulses entering the reverberating pool can increase the output signal, whereas inhibition can decrease or even extinguish the signal.

Figure 46-16 shows a continuous output signal from a pool of neurons. The pool may be emitting impulses because of intrinsic neuronal excitability or as a result of reverberation. Note that an excitatory input signal greatly increases the output signal, whereas an inhibitory input signal greatly decreases the output. Those students

who are familiar with radio transmitters will recognize this to be a *carrier wave* type of information transmission. That is, the excitatory and inhibitory control signals are not the *cause* of the output signal, but they do *control* its changing level of intensity. Note that this carrier wave system allows a *decrease* in signal intensity, as well as an increase, whereas up to this point, the types of information transmission we have discussed have been mainly positive information rather than negative information. This type of information transmission is used by the autonomic nervous system to control such functions as vascular tone, gut tone, degree of constriction of the iris in the eye, and heart rate. That is, the nerve excitatory signal to each of these can be either increased or decreased by accessory input signals into the reverberating neuronal pathway.

Rhythmical Signal Output

Many neuronal circuits emit rhythmical output signals—for instance, a rhythmical respiratory signal originates in the respiratory centers of the medulla and pons. This respiratory rhythmical signal continues throughout life. Other rhythmical signals, such as those that cause scratching movements by the hind leg of a dog or the walking movements of any animal, require input stimuli into the respective circuits to initiate the rhythmical signals.

All or almost all rhythmical signals that have been studied experimentally have been found to result from reverberating circuits or a succession of sequential reverberating circuits that feed excitatory or inhibitory signals in a circular pathway from one neuronal pool to the next.

Excitatory or inhibitory signals can also increase or decrease the amplitude of the rhythmical signal output. Figure 46-17, for instance, shows changes in the respiratory signal output in the phrenic nerve. When the carotid body is stimulated by arterial oxygen deficiency, both the frequency and the amplitude of the respiratory rhythmical output signal increase progressively.

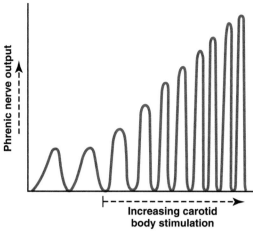

Figure 46-17 The rhythmical output of summated nerve impulses from the respiratory center, showing that progressively increasing stimulation of the carotid body increases both the intensity and the frequency of the phrenic nerve signal to the diaphragm to increase respiration.

Instability and Stability of Neuronal Circuits

Almost every part of the brain connects either directly or indirectly with every other part, and this creates a serious problem. If the first part excites the second, the second the third, the third the fourth, and so on until finally the signal re-excites the first part, it is clear that an excitatory signal entering any part of the brain would set off a continuous cycle of re-excitation of all parts. If this should occur, the brain would be inundated by a mass of uncontrolled reverberating signals—signals that would be transmitting no information but, nevertheless, would be consuming the circuits of the brain so that none of the informational signals could be transmitted. Such an effect occurs in widespread areas of the brain during *epileptic seizures.* How does the central nervous system prevent this from happening all the time? The answer lies mainly in two basic mechanisms that function throughout the central nervous system: (1) inhibitory circuits and (2) fatigue of synapses.

Inhibitory Circuits as a Mechanism for Stabilizing Nervous System Function

Two types of inhibitory circuits in widespread areas of the brain help prevent excessive spread of signals: (1) inhibitory feedback circuits that return from the termini of pathways back to the initial excitatory neurons of the same pathways—these circuits occur in virtually all sensory nervous pathways and inhibit either the input neurons or the intermediate neurons in the sensory pathway when the termini become overly excited; and (2) some neuronal pools that exert gross inhibitory control over widespread areas of the brain—for instance, many of the basal ganglia exert inhibitory influences throughout the muscle control system.

Synaptic Fatigue as a Means of Stabilizing the Nervous System

Synaptic fatigue means simply that synaptic transmission becomes progressively weaker the more prolonged and more intense the period of excitation. Figure 46-18 shows three successive records of a flexor reflex elicited in an animal caused by inflicting pain in the footpad of the paw. Note in each record that the strength of contraction progressively "decrements"—that is, its strength diminishes; much of this effect is caused by *fatigue* of synapses in the flexor reflex circuit. Furthermore, the shorter the interval between successive flexor reflexes, the less the intensity of the subsequent reflex response.

Automatic Short-Term Adjustment of Pathway Sensitivity by the Fatigue Mechanism. Now let us apply this phenomenon of fatigue to other pathways in the brain. Those that are overused usually become fatigued, so their sensitivities decrease. Conversely, those that are underused become rested and their sensitivities increase. Thus, fatigue and recovery from fatigue constitute an important short-term means of moderating the sensitivities of the different nervous system circuits. These help to keep the circuits operating in a range of sensitivity that allows effective function.

Long-Term Changes in Synaptic Sensitivity Caused by Automatic Down-regulation or Up-regulation of Synaptic Receptors. The long-term sensitivities of synapses can be changed tremendously by up-regulating the number of receptor proteins at the synaptic sites when there is underactivity and down-regulating the receptors when there is overactivity. The mechanism for this is the following: Receptor proteins are being formed constantly by the endoplasmic reticular–Golgi apparatus system and are constantly being inserted into the receptor neuron synaptic membrane. However, when the synapses are overused so that excesses of transmitter substance combine with the receptor proteins, many of these receptors are inactivated and removed from the synaptic membrane.

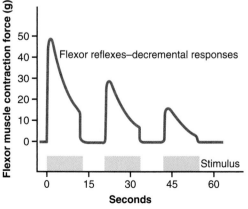

Figure 46-18 Successive flexor reflexes showing fatigue of conduction through the reflex pathway.

It is indeed fortunate that up-regulation and down-regulation of receptors, as well as other control mechanisms for adjusting synaptic sensitivity, continually adjust the sensitivity in each circuit to almost the exact level required for proper function. Think for a moment how serious it would be if the sensitivities of only a few of these circuits were abnormally high; one might then expect almost continual muscle cramps, seizures, psychotic disturbances, hallucinations, mental tension, or other nervous disorders. But fortunately, the automatic controls normally readjust the sensitivities of the circuits back to controllable ranges of reactivity any time the circuits begin to be too active or too depressed.

Bibliography

Bensmaia SJ: Tactile intensity and population codes, *Behav Brain Res* 190:165, 2008.

Buzsaki G: Large-scale recording of neuronal ensembles, *Nat Neurosci* 7:446, 2004.

Faisal AA, Selen LP, Wolpert DM: Noise in the nervous system, *Nat Rev Neurosci* 9:292, 2008.

Fontanini A, Katz DB: Behavioral states, network states, and sensory response variability, *J Neurophysiol* 100:1160, 2008.

Gandevia SC: Spinal and supraspinal factors in human muscle fatigue, *Physiol Rev* 81:1725, 2001.

Gebhart GF: Descending modulation of pain, *Neurosci Biobehav Rev* 27:729, 2004.

Hamill OP, Martinac B: Molecular basis of mechanotransduction in living cells, *Physiol Rev* 81:685, 2001.

Housley GD, Bringmann A: Reichenbach A Purinergic signaling in special senses, *Trends Neurosci* 32:128, 2009.

Kandel ER, Schwartz JH, Jessell TM: *Principles of Neural Science*, ed 4, New York, 2000, McGraw-Hill.

Katz DB, Matsunami H, Rinberg D, et al: Receptors, circuits, and behaviors: new directions in chemical senses, *J Neurosci* 28:11802, 2008.

Lumpkin EA, Caterina MJ: Mechanisms of sensory transduction in the skin, *Nature* 445:858, 2007.

Pearson KG: Neural adaptation in the generation of rhythmic behavior, *Annu Rev Physiol* 62:723, 2000.

Pugh JR, Raman IM: Nothing can be coincidence: synaptic inhibition and plasticity in the cerebellar nuclei, *Trends Neurosci* 32:170, 2009.

Ramocki MB, Zoghbi HY: Failure of neuronal homeostasis results in common neuropsychiatric phenotypes, *Nature* 455:912, 2008.

Richerson GB, Wu Y: Dynamic equilibrium of neurotransmitter transporters: not just for reuptake anymore, *J Neurophysiol* 90:1363, 2003.

Schepers RJ, Ringkamp M: Thermoreceptors and thermosensitive afferents, *Neurosci Biobehav Rev* 33:205, 2009.

Schoppa NE: Making scents out of how olfactory neurons are ordered in space, *Nat Neurosci* 12:103, 2009.

Sjöström PJ, Rancz EA, Roth A, et al: Dendritic excitability and synaptic plasticity, *Physiol Rev* 88:769, 2008.

Stein BE, Stanford TR: Multisensory integration: current issues from the perspective of the single neuron, *Nat Rev Neurosci* 9:255, 2008.

Somatic Sensations: I. General Organization, the Tactile and Position Senses

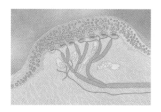

The *somatic senses* are the nervous mechanisms that collect sensory information from all over the body. These senses are in contradistinction to the *special senses*, which mean specifically vision, hearing, smell, taste, and equilibrium.

Classification of Somatic Senses

The somatic senses can be classified into three physiologic types: (1) the *mechanoreceptive somatic senses*, which include both *tactile* and *position* sensations that are stimulated by mechanical displacement of some tissue of the body; (2) the *thermoreceptive senses*, which detect heat and cold; and (3) the *pain sense*, which is activated by factors that damage the tissues.

This chapter deals with the mechanoreceptive tactile and position senses. Chapter 48 discusses the thermoreceptive and pain senses. The tactile senses include *touch, pressure, vibration,* and *tickle* senses, and the position senses include *static position* and *rate of movement* senses.

Other Classifications of Somatic Sensations.
Somatic sensations are also often grouped together in other classes, as follows.

Exteroreceptive sensations are those from the surface of the body. *Proprioceptive sensations* are those relating to the physical state of the body, including position sensations, tendon and muscle sensations, pressure sensations from the bottom of the feet, and even the sensation of equilibrium (which is often considered a "special" sensation rather than a somatic sensation).

Visceral sensations are those from the viscera of the body; in using this term, one usually refers specifically to sensations from the internal organs.

Deep sensations are those that come from deep tissues, such as from fasciae, muscles, and bone. These include mainly "deep" pressure, pain, and vibration.

Detection and Transmission of Tactile Sensations

Interrelations Among the Tactile Sensations of Touch, Pressure, and Vibration. Although touch, pressure, and vibration are frequently classified as separate sensations, they are all detected by the same types of receptors. There are three principal differences among them: (1) touch sensation generally results from stimulation of tactile receptors in the skin or in tissues immediately beneath the skin; (2) pressure sensation generally results from deformation of deeper tissues; and (3) vibration sensation results from rapidly repetitive sensory signals, but some of the same types of receptors as those for touch and pressure are used.

Tactile Receptors. There are at least six entirely different types of tactile receptors, but many more similar to these also exist. Some were shown in Figure 46-1 of the previous chapter; their special characteristics are the following.

First, some *free nerve endings*, which are found everywhere in the skin and in many other tissues, can detect touch and pressure. For instance, even light contact with the cornea of the eye, which contains no other type of nerve ending besides free nerve endings, can nevertheless elicit touch and pressure sensations.

Second, a touch receptor with great sensitivity is the *Meissner's corpuscle* (illustrated in Figure 46-1), an elongated encapsulated nerve ending of a large (type Aβ) myelinated sensory nerve fiber. Inside the capsulation are many branching terminal nerve filaments. These corpuscles are present in the nonhairy parts of the skin and are particularly abundant in the fingertips, lips, and other areas of the skin where one's ability to discern spatial locations of touch sensations is highly developed. Meissner's corpuscles adapt in a fraction of a second after they are stimulated, which means that they are particularly sensitive to movement of objects over the surface of the skin, as well as to low-frequency vibration.

Third, the fingertips and other areas that contain large numbers of Meissner's corpuscles usually also contain large numbers of *expanded tip tactile receptors,* one type of which is *Merkel's discs,* shown in Figure 47-1. The hairy parts of the skin also contain moderate numbers of expanded tip receptors, even though they have almost no Meissner's corpuscles. These receptors differ from Meissner's corpuscles in that they transmit an initially strong but partially adapting signal and then a continuing weaker signal that adapts only slowly. Therefore, they are responsible for giving steady-state signals that allow one to determine continuous touch of objects against the skin.

Merkel's discs are often grouped together in a receptor organ called the *Iggo dome receptor,* which projects upward against the underside of the epithelium of the skin, as also shown in Figure 47-1. This causes the epithelium at this point to protrude outward, thus creating a dome and constituting an extremely sensitive receptor. Also note that the entire group of Merkel's discs is innervated by a single large myelinated nerve fiber (type Aβ). These receptors, along with the Meissner's corpuscles discussed earlier, play extremely important roles in localizing touch sensations to specific surface areas of the body and in determining the texture of what is felt.

Fourth, slight movement of any hair on the body stimulates a nerve fiber entwining its base. Thus, each hair and its basal nerve fiber, called the *hair end-organ,* are also touch receptors. A receptor adapts readily and, like Meissner's corpuscles, detects mainly (a) movement of objects on the surface of the body or (b) initial contact with the body.

Fifth, located in the deeper layers of the skin and also in still deeper internal tissues are many *Ruffini's endings,* which are multibranched, encapsulated endings, as shown in Figure 46-1. These endings adapt very slowly and, therefore, are important for signaling continuous states of deformation of the tissues, such as heavy prolonged touch and pressure signals. They are also found in joint capsules and help to signal the degree of joint rotation.

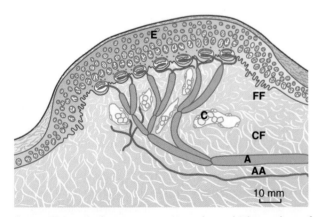

Figure 47-1 Iggo dome receptor. Note the multiple numbers of Merkel's discs connecting to a single large myelinated fiber and abutting tightly the undersurface of the epithelium. (From Iggo A, Muir AR: The structure and function of a slowly adapting touch corpuscle in hairy skin. J Physiol 200:763, 1969.)

Sixth, pacinian corpuscles, which were discussed in detail in Chapter 46, lie both immediately beneath the skin and deep in the fascial tissues of the body. They are stimulated only by rapid local compression of the tissues because they adapt in a few hundredths of a second. Therefore, they are particularly important for detecting tissue vibration or other rapid changes in the mechanical state of the tissues.

Transmission of Tactile Signals in Peripheral Nerve Fibers. Almost all specialized sensory receptors, such as Meissner's corpuscles, Iggo dome receptors, hair receptors, pacinian corpuscles, and Ruffini's endings, transmit their signals in type Aβ nerve fibers that have transmission velocities ranging from 30 to 70 m/sec. Conversely, free nerve ending tactile receptors transmit signals mainly by way of the small type Aδ myelinated fibers that conduct at velocities of only 5 to 30 m/sec.

Some tactile free nerve endings transmit by way of type C unmyelinated fibers at velocities from a fraction of a meter up to 2 m/sec; these send signals into the spinal cord and lower brain stem, probably subserving mainly the sensation of tickle.

Thus, the more critical types of sensory signals—those that help to determine precise localization on the skin, minute gradations of intensity, or rapid changes in sensory signal intensity—are all transmitted in more rapidly conducting types of sensory nerve fibers. Conversely, the cruder types of signals, such as pressure, poorly localized touch, and especially tickle, are transmitted by way of much slower, very small nerve fibers that require much less space in the nerve bundle than the fast fibers.

Detection of Vibration

All tactile receptors are involved in detection of vibration, although different receptors detect different frequencies of vibration. Pacinian corpuscles can detect signal vibrations from 30 to 800 cycles per second because they respond extremely rapidly to minute and rapid deformations of the tissues, and they also transmit their signals over type Aβ nerve fibers, which can transmit as many as 1000 impulses per second. Low-frequency vibrations from 2 up to 80 cycles per second, in contrast, stimulate other tactile receptors, especially Meissner's corpuscles, which are less rapidly adapting than pacinian corpuscles.

Detection of Tickle and Itch by Mechanoreceptive Free Nerve Endings

Neurophysiologic studies have demonstrated the existence of very sensitive, rapidly adapting mechanoreceptive free nerve endings that elicit only the tickle and itch sensations. Furthermore, these endings are found almost exclusively in superficial layers of the skin, which is also the only tissue from which the tickle and itch sensations usually can be elicited. These sensations are transmitted by very small type C, unmyelinated fibers similar to those that transmit the aching, slow type of pain.

The purpose of the itch sensation is presumably to call attention to mild surface stimuli such as a flea crawling on the skin or a fly about to bite, and the elicited signals then activate the scratch reflex or other maneuvers that rid the host of the irritant. Itch can be relieved by scratching if this removes the irritant or if the scratch is strong enough to elicit pain. The pain signals are believed to suppress the itch signals in the cord by lateral inhibition, as described in Chapter 48.

Sensory Pathways for Transmitting Somatic Signals into the Central Nervous System

Almost all sensory information from the somatic segments of the body enters the spinal cord through the dorsal roots of the spinal nerves. However, from the entry point into the cord and then to the brain, the sensory signals are carried through one of two alternative sensory pathways: (1) the *dorsal column*–medial lemniscal system or (2) the *anterolateral system*. These two systems come back together partially at the level of the thalamus.

The dorsal column–medial lemniscal system, as its name implies, carries signals upward to the medulla of the brain mainly in the *dorsal columns* of the cord. Then, after the signals synapse and cross to the opposite side in the medulla, they continue upward through the brain stem to the thalamus by way of the *medial lemniscus.*

Conversely, signals in the anterolateral system, immediately after entering the spinal cord from the dorsal spinal nerve roots, synapse in the dorsal horns of the spinal gray matter, then cross to the opposite side of the cord and ascend through the anterior and lateral white columns of the cord. They terminate at all levels of the lower brain stem and in the thalamus.

The dorsal column–medial lemniscal system is composed of large, myelinated nerve fibers that transmit signals to the brain at velocities of 30 to 110 m/sec, whereas the anterolateral system is composed of smaller myelinated fibers that transmit signals at velocities ranging from a few meters per second up to 40 m/sec.

Another difference between the two systems is that the dorsal column–medial lemniscal system has a high degree of spatial orientation of the nerve fibers with respect to their origin, while the anterolateral system has much less spatial orientation. These differences immediately characterize the types of sensory information that can be transmitted by the two systems. That is, sensory information that must be transmitted rapidly and with temporal and spatial fidelity is transmitted mainly in the dorsal column–medial lemniscal system; that which does not need to be transmitted rapidly or with great spatial fidelity is transmitted mainly in the anterolateral system.

The anterolateral system has a special capability that the dorsal system does not have: the ability to transmit a broad spectrum of sensory modalities—pain, warmth, cold, and crude tactile sensations; most of these are discussed in detail in Chapter 48. The dorsal system is limited to discrete types of mechanoreceptive sensations.

With this differentiation in mind, we can now list the types of sensations transmitted in the two systems.

Dorsal Column—Medial Lemniscal System
1. Touch sensations requiring a high degree of localization of the stimulus
2. Touch sensations requiring transmission of fine gradations of intensity
3. Phasic sensations, such as vibratory sensations
4. Sensations that signal movement against the skin
5. Position sensations from the joints
6. Pressure sensations related to fine degrees of judgment of pressure intensity

Anterolateral System
1. Pain
2. Thermal sensations, including both warmth and cold sensations
3. Crude touch and pressure sensations capable only of crude localizing ability on the surface of the body
4. Tickle and itch sensations
5. Sexual sensations

Transmission in the Dorsal Column–Medial Lemniscal System

Anatomy of the Dorsal Column–Medial Lemniscal System

On entering the spinal cord through the spinal nerve dorsal roots, the large myelinated fibers from the specialized mechanoreceptors divide almost immediately to form a *medial branch* and a *lateral branch*, shown by the right-hand fiber entering through the spinal root in Figure 47-2.

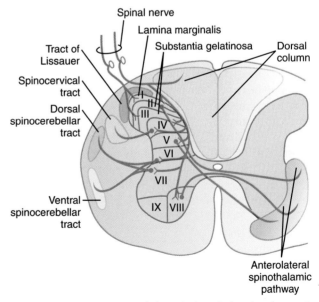

Figure 47-2 Cross section of the spinal cord, showing the anatomy of the cord gray matter and of ascending sensory tracts in the white columns of the spinal cord.

The medial branch turns medially first and then upward in the dorsal column, proceeding by way of the dorsal column pathway all the way to the brain.

The lateral branch enters the dorsal horn of the cord gray matter, then divides many times to provide terminals that synapse with local neurons in the intermediate and anterior portions of the cord gray matter. These local neurons in turn serve three functions: (1) A major share of them give off fibers that enter the dorsal columns of the cord and then travel upward to the brain. (2) Many of the fibers are very short and terminate locally in the spinal cord gray matter to elicit local spinal cord reflexes, which are discussed in Chapter 54. (3) Others give rise to the spinocerebellar tracts, which we discuss in Chapter 56 in relation to the function of the cerebellum.

Dorsal Column—Medial Lemniscal Pathway. Note in Figure 47-3 that nerve fibers entering the dorsal columns pass uninterrupted up to the dorsal medulla, where they synapse in the *dorsal column nuclei* (the *cuneate* and *gracile nuclei*). From there, *second-order neurons* decussate immediately to the opposite side of the brain stem and continue upward through the *medial lemnisci* to the thalamus. In this pathway through the brain stem, each medial lemniscus is joined by additional fibers from the *sensory nuclei of the trigeminal nerve;* these fibers subserve the same sensory functions for the head that the dorsal column fibers subserve for the body.

In the thalamus, the medial lemniscal fibers terminate in the thalamic sensory relay area, called the *ventrobasal complex.* From the ventrobasal complex, *third-order nerve fibers* project, as shown in Figure 47-4, mainly to the *postcentral gyrus* of the *cerebral cortex,* which is called *somatic sensory area I* (as shown in Figure 47-6, these fibers also project to a smaller area in the lateral parietal cortex called *somatic sensory area II*).

Spatial Orientation of the Nerve Fibers in the Dorsal Column–Medial Lemniscal System

One of the distinguishing features of the dorsal column–medial lemniscal system is a distinct spatial orientation of nerve fibers from the individual parts of the body that is maintained throughout. For instance, in the dorsal columns of the spinal cord, the fibers from the lower parts of the body lie toward the center of the cord, whereas those that enter the cord at progressively higher segmental levels form successive layers laterally.

In the thalamus, distinct spatial orientation is still maintained, with the tail end of the body represented by the most lateral portions of the ventrobasal complex and the head and face represented by the medial areas of the complex. Because of the crossing of the medial lemnisci in the medulla, the left side of the body is represented in the right side of the thalamus, and the right side of the body in the left side of the thalamus.

Somatosensory Cortex

Before discussing the role of the cerebral cortex in somatic sensation, we need to give an orientation to the various areas of the cortex. Figure 47-5 is a map of the human

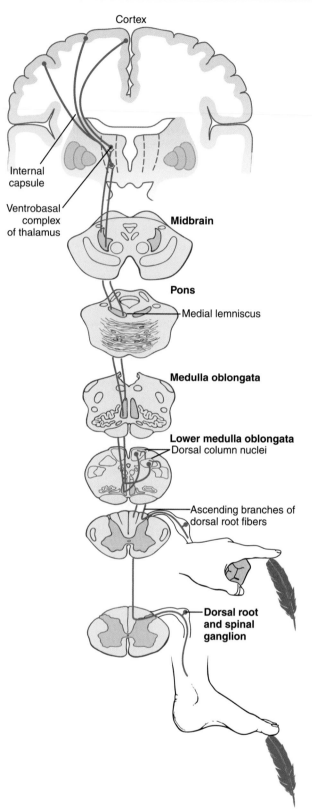

Figure 47-3 The dorsal column–medial lemniscal pathway for transmitting critical types of tactile signals.

cerebral cortex, showing that it is divided into about 50 distinct areas called *Brodmann's areas* based on histological structural differences. This map is important because virtually all neurophysiologists and neurologists use it to

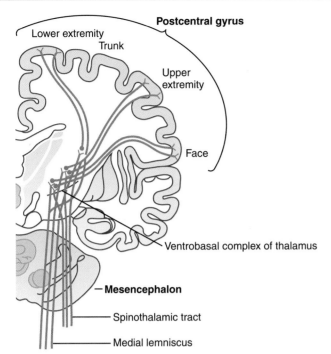

Figure 47-4 Projection of the dorsal column–medial lemniscal system through the thalamus to the somatosensory cortex. (Modified from Brodal A: Neurological Anatomy in Relation to Clinical Medicine. New York: Oxford University Press, 1969, by permission of Oxford University Press.)

refer by number to many of the different functional areas of the human cortex.

Note in the figure the large *central fissure* (also called *central sulcus*) that extends horizontally across the brain. In general, sensory signals from all modalities of sensation terminate in the cerebral cortex immediately posterior to the central fissure. And, generally, the anterior half of the *parietal lobe* is concerned almost entirely with reception and interpretation of *somatosensory signals*. But the posterior half of the parietal lobe provides still higher levels of interpretation.

Visual signals terminate in the *occipital lobe*, and *auditory signals* terminate in the *temporal lobe*.

Conversely, that portion of the cerebral cortex anterior to the central fissure and constituting the posterior half of the frontal lobe is called the *motor cortex* and is devoted almost entirely to control of muscle contractions and body movements. A major share of this motor control is in response to somatosensory signals received from the sensory portions of the cortex, which keep the motor cortex informed at each instant about the positions and motions of the different body parts.

Somatosensory Areas I and II. Figure 47-6 shows two separate sensory areas in the anterior parietal lobe called *somatosensory area I* and *somatosensory area II*. The reason for this division into two areas is that a distinct and separate spatial orientation of the different parts of the body is found in each of these two areas. However, somatosensory area I is so much more extensive and so much more important than somatosensory area II that in popular usage, the term "somatosensory cortex" almost always means area I.

Somatosensory area I has a high degree of localization of the different parts of the body, as shown by the names of virtually all parts of the body in Figure 47-6. By contrast, localization is poor in somatosensory area II, although roughly, the face is represented anteriorly, the arms centrally, and the legs posteriorly.

Little is known about the function of somatosensory area II. It is known that signals enter this area from the brain stem, transmitted upward from both sides of the body. In addition, many signals come secondarily from somatosensory area I, as well as from other sensory areas of the brain, even from the visual and auditory areas. Projections from somatosensory area I are required for function of somatosensory area II. However, removal of parts of somatosensory area II has no apparent effect on the response of neurons in somatosensory area I. Thus, much of what we know about somatic sensation appears to be explained by the functions of somatosensory area I.

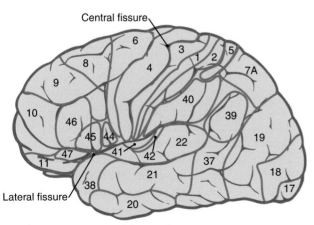

Figure 47-5 Structurally distinct areas, called *Brodmann's areas*, of the human cerebral cortex. Note specifically areas *1, 2,* and *3,* which constitute *primary somatosensory area I*, and areas 5 and 7, which constitute the *somatosensory association area.*

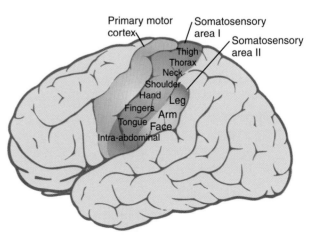

Figure 47-6 Two somatosensory cortical areas, somatosensory areas I and II.

Spatial Orientation of Signals from Different Parts of the Body in Somatosensory Area I. Somatosensory area I lies immediately behind the central fissure, located in the postcentral gyrus of the human cerebral cortex (in Brodmann's areas 3, 1, and 2).

Figure 47-7 shows a cross section through the brain at the level of the *postcentral gyrus*, demonstrating representations of the different parts of the body in separate regions of somatosensory area I. Note, however, that each lateral side of the cortex receives sensory information almost exclusively from the opposite side of the body.

Some areas of the body are represented by large areas in the somatic cortex—the lips the greatest of all, followed by the face and thumb—whereas the trunk and lower part of the body are represented by relatively small areas. The sizes of these areas are directly proportional to the number of specialized sensory receptors in each respective peripheral area of the body. For instance, a great number of specialized nerve endings are found in the lips and thumb, whereas only a few are present in the skin of the body trunk.

Note also that the head is represented in the most lateral portion of somatosensory area I, and the lower part of the body is represented medially.

Layers of the Somatosensory Cortex and Their Function

The cerebral cortex contains *six* layers of neurons, beginning with layer I next to the brain surface and extending progressively deeper to layer VI, shown in Figure 47-8.

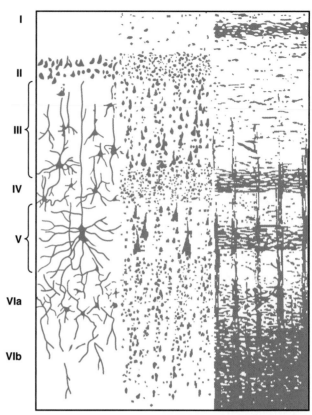

Figure 47-8 Structure of the cerebral cortex, showing I, molecular layer; II, external granular layer; III, layer of small pyramidal cells; IV, internal granular layer; V, large pyramidal cell layer; and VI, layer of fusiform or polymorphic cells. (From Ranson SW, Clark SL [after Brodmann]: Anatomy of the Nervous System. Philadelphia: WB Saunders, 1959.)

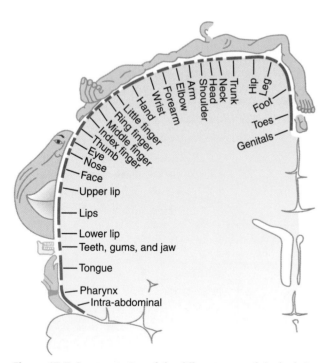

Figure 47-7 Representation of the different areas of the body in somatosensory area I of the cortex. (From Penfield W, Rasmussen T: Cerebral Cortex of Man: A Clinical Study of Localization of Function. New York: Hafner, 1968.)

As would be expected, the neurons in each layer perform functions different from those in other layers. Some of these functions are:

1. The incoming sensory signal excites neuronal layer IV first; then the signal spreads toward the surface of the cortex and also toward deeper layers.

2. Layers I and II receive diffuse, nonspecific input signals from lower brain centers that facilitate specific regions of the cortex; this system is described in Chapter 57. This input mainly controls the overall level of excitability of the respective regions stimulated.

3. The neurons in layers II and III send axons to related portions of the cerebral cortex on the opposite side of the brain through the *corpus callosum.*

4. The neurons in layers V and VI send axons to the deeper parts of the nervous system. Those in layer V are generally larger and project to more distant areas, such as to the basal ganglia, brain stem, and spinal cord, where they control signal transmission. From layer VI, especially large numbers of axons extend to the thalamus, providing signals from the cerebral cortex that interact with and help to control the excitatory levels of incoming sensory signals entering the thalamus.

The Sensory Cortex Is Organized in Vertical Columns of Neurons; Each Column Detects a Different Sensory Spot on the Body with a Specific Sensory Modality

Functionally, the neurons of the somatosensory cortex are arranged in vertical columns extending all the way through the six layers of the cortex, each column having a diameter of 0.3 to 0.5 millimeter and containing perhaps 10,000 neuronal cell bodies. Each of these columns serves a single specific sensory modality, some columns responding to stretch receptors around joints, some to stimulation of tactile hairs, others to discrete localized pressure points on the skin, and so forth. At layer IV, where the input sensory signals first enter the cortex, the columns of neurons function almost entirely separately from one another. At other levels of the columns, interactions occur that initiate analysis of the meanings of the sensory signals.

In the most anterior 5 to 10 millimeters of the postcentral gyrus, located deep in the central fissure in Brodmann's area 3a, an especially large share of the vertical columns respond to muscle, tendon, and joint stretch receptors. Many of the signals from these sensory columns then spread anteriorly, directly to the motor cortex located immediately forward of the central fissure. These signals play a major role in controlling the effluent motor signals that activate sequences of muscle contraction.

As one moves posteriorly in somatosensory area I, more and more of the vertical columns respond to slowly adapting cutaneous receptors, and then still farther posteriorly, greater numbers of the columns are sensitive to deep pressure.

In the most posterior portion of somatosensory area I, about 6 percent of the vertical columns respond only when a stimulus moves across the skin in a particular direction. Thus, this is a still higher order of interpretation of sensory signals; the process becomes even more complex as the signals spread farther backward from somatosensory area I into the parietal cortex, an area called the *somatosensory association area*, as we discuss subsequently.

Functions of Somatosensory Area I

Widespread bilateral excision of somatosensory area I causes loss of the following types of sensory judgment:

1. The person is unable to localize discretely the different sensations in the different parts of the body. However, he or she can localize these sensations crudely, such as to a particular hand, to a major level of the body trunk, or to one of the legs. Thus, it is clear that the brain stem, thalamus, or parts of the cerebral cortex not normally considered to be concerned with somatic sensations can perform some degree of localization.

2. The person is unable to judge critical degrees of pressure against the body.

3. The person is unable to judge the weights of objects.

4. The person is unable to judge shapes or forms of objects. This is called *astereognosis.*

5. The person is unable to judge texture of materials because this type of judgment depends on highly critical sensations caused by movement of the fingers over the surface to be judged.

Note that in the list nothing has been said about loss of pain and temperature sense. In specific absence of only somatosensory area I, appreciation of these sensory modalities is still preserved both in quality and intensity. But the sensations are poorly localized, indicating that pain and temperature *localization* depend greatly on the topographical map of the body in somatosensory area I to localize the source.

Somatosensory Association Areas

Brodmann's areas 5 and 7 of the cerebral cortex, located in the parietal cortex behind somatosensory area I (see Figure 47-5), play important roles in deciphering deeper meanings of the sensory information in the somatosensory areas. Therefore, these areas are called *somatosensory association areas.*

Electrical stimulation in a somatosensory association area can occasionally cause an awake person to experience a complex body sensation, sometimes even the "feeling" of an object such as a knife or a ball. Therefore, it seems clear that the somatosensory association area combines information arriving from multiple points in the primary somatosensory area to decipher its meaning. This also fits with the anatomical arrangement of the neuronal tracts that enter the somatosensory association area because it receives signals from (1) somatosensory area I, (2) the ventrobasal nuclei of the thalamus, (3) other areas of the thalamus, (4) the visual cortex, and (5) the auditory cortex.

Effect of Removing the Somatosensory Association Area—Amorphosynthesis. When the somatosensory association area is removed on one side of the brain, the person loses ability to recognize complex objects and complex forms felt on the opposite side of the body. In addition, he or she loses most of the sense of form of his or her own body or body parts on the opposite side. In fact, the person is mainly oblivious to the opposite side of the body—that is, forgets that it is there. Therefore, he or she also often forgets to use the other side for motor functions as well. Likewise, when feeling objects, the person tends to recognize only one side of the object and forgets that the other side even exists. This complex sensory deficit is called *amorphosynthesis.*

Overall Characteristics of Signal Transmission and Analysis in the Dorsal Column–Medial Lemniscal System

Basic Neuronal Circuit in the Dorsal Column–Medial Lemniscal System. The lower part of Figure 47-9 shows the basic organization of the neuronal circuit of the spinal cord dorsal column pathway, demonstrating that at each synaptic stage, divergence occurs. The upper

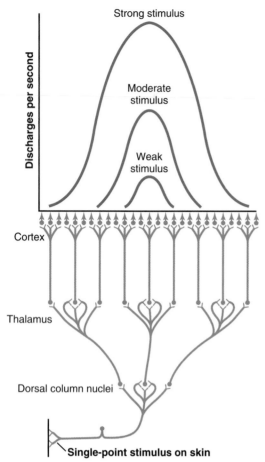

Figure 47-9 Transmission of a pinpoint stimulus signal to the cerebral cortex.

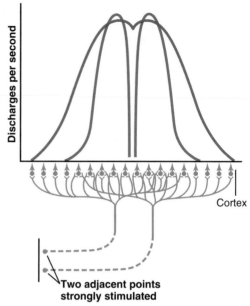

Figure 47-10 Transmission of signals to the cortex from two adjacent pinpoint stimuli. The blue curve represents the pattern of cortical stimulation without "surround" inhibition, and the two red curves represent the pattern when "surround" inhibition does occur.

curves of the figure show that the cortical neurons that discharge to the greatest extent are those in a central part of the cortical "field" for each respective receptor. Thus, a weak stimulus causes only the centralmost neurons to fire. A stronger stimulus causes still more neurons to fire, but those in the center discharge at a considerably more rapid rate than do those farther away from the center.

Two-Point Discrimination. A method frequently used to test tactile discrimination is to determine a person's so-called "two-point" discriminatory ability. In this test, two needles are pressed lightly against the skin at the same time, and the person determines whether two points of stimulus are felt or one point. On the tips of the fingers, a person can normally distinguish two separate points even when the needles are as close together as 1 to 2 millimeters. However, on the person's back, the needles must usually be as far apart as 30 to 70 millimeters before two separate points can be detected. The reason for this difference is the different numbers of specialized tactile receptors in the two areas.

Figure 47-10 shows the mechanism by which the dorsal column pathway (as well as all other sensory pathways) transmits two-point discriminatory information. This figure shows two adjacent points on the skin that are strongly stimulated, as well as the areas of the somatosensory

cortex (greatly enlarged) that are excited by signals from the two stimulated points. The blue curve shows the spatial pattern of cortical excitation when both skin points are stimulated simultaneously. Note that the resultant zone of excitation has two separate peaks. These two peaks, separated by a valley, allow the sensory cortex to detect the presence of two stimulatory points, rather than a single point. The capability of the sensorium to distinguish this presence of two points of stimulation is strongly influenced by another mechanism, *lateral inhibition,* as explained in the next section.

Effect of Lateral Inhibition (Also Called *Surround Inhibition*) to Increase the Degree of Contrast in the Perceived Spatial Pattern. As pointed out in Chapter 46, virtually every sensory pathway, when excited, gives rise simultaneously to lateral *inhibitory* signals; these spread to the sides of the excitatory signal and inhibit adjacent neurons. For instance, consider an excited neuron in a dorsal column nucleus. Aside from the central excitatory signal, short lateral pathways transmit inhibitory signals to the surrounding neurons. That is, these signals pass through additional interneurons that secrete an inhibitory transmitter.

The importance of *lateral inhibition* is that it blocks lateral spread of the excitatory signals and, therefore, increases the degree of contrast in the sensory pattern perceived in the cerebral cortex.

In the case of the dorsal column system, lateral inhibitory signals occur at each synaptic level—for instance, in (1) the dorsal column nuclei of the medulla, (2) the ventrobasal nuclei of the thalamus, and (3) the cortex itself. At each of these levels, the lateral inhibition helps to block lateral spread of the excitatory signal. As a result, the peaks of excitation stand out, and much of the surrounding diffuse stimulation is blocked. This effect is demonstrated by the two red curves in Figure 47-10, showing complete separation of the peaks when the intensity of lateral inhibition is great.

Transmission of Rapidly Changing and Repetitive Sensations. The dorsal column system is also of particular importance in apprising the sensorium of rapidly changing peripheral conditions. Based on recorded action potentials, this system can recognize changing stimuli that occur in as little as 1/400 of a second.

Vibratory Sensation. Vibratory signals are rapidly repetitive and can be detected as vibration up to 700 cycles per second. The higher-frequency vibratory signals originate from the pacinian corpuscles in the skin and deeper tissues, but lower-frequency signals (below about 200 per second) can originate from Meissner's corpuscles as well. These signals are transmitted only in the dorsal column pathway. For this reason, application of vibration (e.g., from a "tuning fork") to different peripheral parts of the body is an important tool used by neurologists for testing functional integrity of the dorsal columns.

Interpretation of Sensory Stimulus Intensity

The ultimate goal of most sensory stimulation is to apprise the psyche of the state of the body and its surroundings. Therefore, it is important that we discuss briefly some of the principles related to transmission of sensory *stimulus intensity* to the higher levels of the nervous system.

One question that comes to mind is, how is it possible for the sensory system to transmit sensory experiences of tremendously varying intensities? For instance, the auditory system can detect the weakest possible whisper but can also discern the meanings of an explosive sound, even though the sound intensities of these two experiences can vary more than 10 billion times; the eyes can see visual images with light intensities that vary as much as a half million times; and the skin can detect pressure differences of 10,000 to 100,000 times.

As a partial explanation of these effects, Figure 46-4 in the previous chapter shows the relation of the receptor potential produced by the pacinian corpuscle to the intensity of the sensory stimulus. At low stimulus intensity, slight changes in intensity increase the potential markedly, whereas at high levels of stimulus intensity, further increases in receptor potential are slight. Thus, the pacinian corpuscle is capable of accurately measuring extremely minute *changes* in stimulus at low-intensity levels, but at high-intensity levels, the change in stimulus must be much greater to cause the same amount of *change* in receptor potential.

The transduction mechanism for detecting sound by the cochlea of the ear demonstrates still another method for separating gradations of stimulus intensity. When sound stimulates a specific point on the basilar membrane, weak sound stimulates only those hair cells at the point of maximum sound vibration. But as the sound intensity increases, many more hair cells in each direction farther away from the maximum vibratory point also become stimulated. Thus, signals are transmitted over progressively increasing numbers of nerve fibers, which is another mechanism by which stimulus intensity is transmitted to the central nervous system. This mechanism, plus the direct effect of stimulus intensity on impulse rate in each nerve fiber, as well as several other mechanisms, makes it possible for some sensory systems to operate reasonably faithfully at stimulus intensity levels changing as much as millions of times.

Importance of the Tremendous Intensity Range of Sensory Reception. Were it not for the tremendous intensity range of sensory reception that we can experience, the various sensory systems would more often than not be operating in the wrong range. This is demonstrated by the attempts of most people, when taking photographs with a camera, to adjust the light exposure without using a light meter. Left to intuitive judgment of light intensity, a person almost always overexposes the film on bright days and greatly underexposes the film at twilight. Yet that person's own eyes are capable of discriminating with great detail visual objects in bright sunlight or at twilight; the camera cannot do this without very special manipulation because of the narrow critical range of light intensity required for proper exposure of film.

Judgment of Stimulus Intensity

Weber-Fechner Principle—Detection of "Ratio" of Stimulus Strength. In the mid-1800s, Weber first and Fechner later proposed the principle that *gradations of stimulus strength are discriminated approximately in proportion to the logarithm of stimulus strength.* That is, a person already holding 30 grams weight in his or her hand can barely detect an additional 1-gram increase in weight. And, when already holding 300 grams, he or she can barely detect a 10-gram increase in weight. Thus, in this instance, the *ratio* of the change in stimulus strength required for detection remains essentially constant, about 1 to 30, which is what the logarithmic principle means. To express this mathematically.

$$\text{Interpreted signal strength} = \text{Log (Stimulus)} + \text{Constant}$$

More recently, it has become evident that the Weber-Fechner principle is quantitatively accurate only for higher intensities of visual, auditory, and cutaneous sensory experience and applies only poorly to most other types of sensory experience. Yet the Weber-Fechner principle is still a good one to remember because it emphasizes that the greater the background sensory intensity, the greater an additional change must be for the psyche to detect the change.

Power Law. Another attempt by physiopsychologists to find a good mathematical relation is the following formula, known as the power law.

$$\text{Interpreted signal strength} = \text{K} \times (\text{Stimulus} - \text{k})^y$$

In this formula, the exponent y and the constants K and k are different for each type of sensation.

When this power law relation is plotted on a graph using double logarithmic coordinates, as shown in Figure 47-11, and when appropriate quantitative values for the constants y, K, and k are found, a linear relation can be attained between interpreted stimulus strength and actual stimulus strength over a large range for almost any type of sensory perception.

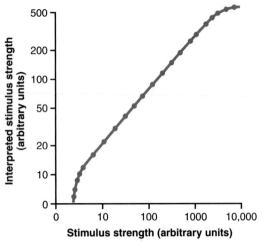

Figure 47-11 Graphical demonstration of the "power law" relation between actual stimulus strength and strength that the psyche interprets it to be. Note that the power law does not hold at either very weak or very strong stimulus strengths.

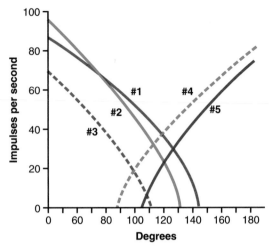

Figure 47-12 Typical responses of five different thalamic neurons in the thalamic ventrobasal complex when the knee joint is moved through its range of motion. (Data from Mountcastle VB, Poggie GF, Werner G: The relation of thalamic cell response to peripheral stimuli varied over an intensive continuum. J Neurophysiol 26:807, 1963.)

Position Senses

The *position senses* are frequently also called *proprioceptive senses*. They can be divided into two subtypes: (1) *static position sense*, which means conscious perception of the orientation of the different parts of the body with respect to one another, and (2) *rate of movement sense*, also called *kinesthesia* or *dynamic proprioception*.

Position Sensory Receptors. Knowledge of position, both static and dynamic, depends on knowing the degrees of angulation of all joints in all planes and their rates of change. Therefore, multiple different types of receptors help to determine joint angulation and are used together for position sense. Both skin tactile receptors and deep receptors near the joints are used. In the case of the fingers, where skin receptors are in great abundance, as much as half of position recognition is believed to be detected through the skin receptors. Conversely, for most of the larger joints of the body, deep receptors are more important.

For determining joint angulation in midranges of motion, among the most important receptors are the *muscle spindles*. They are also exceedingly important in helping to control muscle movement, as we shall see in Chapter 54. When the angle of a joint is changing, some muscles are being stretched while others are loosened, and the net stretch information from the spindles is transmitted into the computational system of the spinal cord and higher regions of the dorsal column system for deciphering joint angulations.

At the extremes of joint angulation, stretch of the ligaments and deep tissues around the joints is an additional important factor in determining position. Types of sensory endings used for this are the pacinian corpuscles, Ruffini's endings, and receptors similar to the Golgi tendon receptors found in muscle tendons.

The pacinian corpuscles and muscle spindles are especially adapted for detecting rapid rates of change. It is likely that these are the receptors most responsible for detecting rate of movement.

Processing of Position Sense Information in the Dorsal Column–Medial Lemniscal Pathway. Referring to Figure 47-12, one sees that *thalamic neurons* responding to joint rotation are of two categories: (1) those maximally stimulated when the joint is at full rotation and (2) those maximally stimulated when the joint is at minimal rotation. Thus, the signals from the individual joint receptors are used to tell the psyche how much each joint is rotated.

Transmission of Less Critical Sensory Signals in the Anterolateral Pathway

The anterolateral pathway for transmitting sensory signals up the spinal cord and into the brain, in contrast to the dorsal column pathway, transmits sensory signals that do not require highly discrete localization of the signal source and do not require discrimination of fine gradations of intensity. These types of signals include pain, heat, cold, crude tactile, tickle, itch, and sexual sensations. In Chapter 48, pain and temperature sensations are discussed specifically.

Anatomy of the Anterolateral Pathway

The *spinal cord anterolateral fibers* originate mainly in dorsal horn laminae I, IV, V, and VI (see Figure 47-2). These laminae are where many of the dorsal root sensory nerve fibers terminate after entering the cord.

As shown in Figure 47-13, the anterolateral fibers cross immediately in the *anterior commissure* of the cord to the opposite *anterior* and *lateral white columns*, where they turn upward toward the brain by way of the *anterior spinothalamic* and *lateral spinothalamic tracts*.

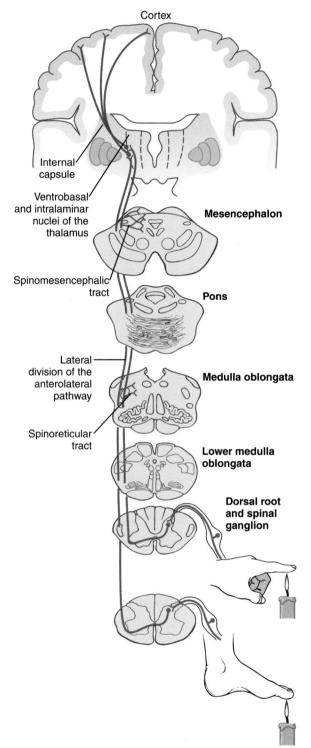

Cortex

Internal capsule

Ventrobasal and intralaminar nuclei of the thalamus

Mesencephalon

Spinomesencephalic tract

Pons

Lateral division of the anterolateral pathway

Medulla oblongata

Spinoreticular tract

Lower medulla oblongata

Dorsal root and spinal ganglion

Figure 47-13 Anterior and lateral divisions of the anterolateral sensory pathway.

The upper terminus of the two spinothalamic tracts is mainly twofold: (1) throughout the *reticular nuclei of the brain stem* and (2) in two different nuclear complexes of the thalamus, the *ventrobasal complex* and the *intralaminar nuclei*. In general, the tactile signals are transmitted mainly into the ventrobasal complex, terminating in some of the same thalamic nuclei where the dorsal column tactile signals terminate. From here, the signals are transmitted to the somatosensory cortex along with the signals from the dorsal columns.

Conversely, only a small fraction of the pain signals project directly to the ventrobasal complex of the thalamus. Instead, most pain signals terminate in the reticular nuclei of the brain stem and from there are relayed to the intralaminar nuclei of the thalamus where the pain signals are further processed, as discussed in greater detail in Chapter 48.

Characteristics of Transmission in the Anterolateral Pathway. In general, the same principles apply to transmission in the anterolateral pathway as in the dorsal column–medial lemniscal system, except for the following differences: (1) the velocities of transmission are only one-third to one-half those in the dorsal column–medial lemniscal system, ranging between 8 and 40 m/sec; (2) the degree of spatial localization of signals is poor; (3) the gradations of intensities are also far less accurate, most of the sensations being recognized in 10 to 20 gradations of strength, rather than as many as 100 gradations for the dorsal column system; and (4) the ability to transmit rapidly changing or rapidly repetitive signals is poor.

Thus, it is evident that the anterolateral system is a cruder type of transmission system than the dorsal column–medial lemniscal system. Even so, certain modalities of sensation are transmitted only in this system and not at all in the dorsal column–medial lemniscal system. They are pain, temperature, tickle, itch, and sexual sensations, in addition to crude touch and pressure.

Some Special Aspects of Somatosensory Function

Function of the Thalamus in Somatic Sensation

When the somatosensory cortex of a human being is destroyed, that person loses most critical tactile sensibilities, but a slight degree of crude tactile sensibility does return. Therefore, it must be assumed that the thalamus (as well as other lower centers) has a slight ability to discriminate tactile sensation, even though the thalamus normally functions mainly to relay this type of information to the cortex.

Conversely, loss of the somatosensory cortex has little effect on one's perception of pain sensation and only a moderate effect on the perception of temperature. Therefore, there is much reason to believe that the lower brain stem, the thalamus, and other associated basal regions of the brain play dominant roles in discrimination of these sensibilities. It is interesting that these sensibilities appeared very early in the phylogenetic development of animals, whereas the critical tactile sensibilities and the somatosensory cortex were late developments.

Cortical Control of Sensory Sensitivity—"Corticofugal" Signals

In addition to somatosensory signals transmitted from the periphery to the brain, *corticofugal* signals are transmitted in the backward direction from the cerebral cortex to the lower sensory relay stations of the thalamus, medulla, and spinal cord; they control the intensity of sensitivity of the sensory input.

Corticofugal signals are almost entirely inhibitory, so when sensory input intensity becomes too great, the corticofugal signals automatically decrease transmission in

UNIT IX

the relay nuclei. This does two things: First, it decreases lateral spread of the sensory signals into adjacent neurons and, therefore, increases the degree of sharpness in the signal pattern. Second, it keeps the sensory system operating in a range of sensitivity that is not so low that the signals are ineffectual nor so high that the system is swamped beyond its capacity to differentiate sensory patterns. This principle of corticofugal sensory control is used by all sensory systems, not only the somatic system, as explained in subsequent chapters.

Segmental Fields of Sensation—Dermatomes

Each spinal nerve innervates a "segmental field" of the skin called a *dermatome*. The different dermatomes are shown in Figure 47-14. They are shown in the figure as if there were distinct borders between the adjacent dermatomes, which is far from true because much overlap exists from segment to segment.

The figure shows that the anal region of the body lies in the dermatome of the most distal cord segment, dermatome S5. In the embryo, this is the tail region and the most distal portion of the body. The legs originate embryologically from the lumbar and upper sacral segments (L2 to S3), rather than from the distal sacral segments, which is evident from the dermatomal map. One can use a dermatomal map as shown in Figure 47-14 to determine the level in the spinal cord at which a cord injury has occurred when the peripheral sensations are disturbed by the injury.

Bibliography

Alonso JM, Swadlow HA: Thalamocortical specificity and the synthesis of sensory cortical receptive fields, *J Neurophysiol* 94:26, 2005.

Baker SN: Oscillatory interactions between sensorimotor cortex and the periphery, *Curr Opin Neurobiol* 17:649, 2007.

Bosco G, Poppele RE: Proprioception from a spinocerebellar perspective, *Physiol Rev* 81:539, 2001.

Chalfie M: Neurosensory mechanotransduction, *Nat Rev Mol Cell Biol* 10:44, 2009.

Cohen YE, Andersen RA: A common reference frame for movement plans in the posterior parietal cortex, *Nat Rev Neurosci* 3:553, 2002.

Craig AD: Pain mechanisms: labeled lines versus convergence in central processing, *Annu Rev Neurosci* 26:1, 2003.

Fontanini A, Katz DB: Behavioral states, network states, and sensory response variability, *J Neurophysiol* 100:1160, 2008.

Fox K: Experience-dependent plasticity mechanisms for neural rehabilitation in somatosensory cortex, *Philos Trans R Soc Lond B Biol Sci* 364:369, 2009.

Haines DE: *Fundamental Neuroscience for Basic and Clinical Applications*, ed 3, Philadelphia, 2006, Churchill Livingstone, Elsevier.

Hsiao S: Central mechanisms of tactile shape perception, *Curr Opin Neurobiol* 18:418, 2008.

Johansson RS, Flanagan JR: Coding and use of tactile signals from the fingertips in object manipulation tasks, *Nat Rev Neurosci* 10:345, 2009.

Kaas JH: The evolution of the complex sensory and motor systems of the human brain, *Brain Res Bull* 75:384, 2008.

Kaas JH, Qi HX, Burish MJ, et al: Cortical and subcortical plasticity in the brains of humans, primates, and rats after damage to sensory afferents in the dorsal columns of the spinal cord, *Exp Neurol* 209:407, 2008.

Kandel ER, Schwartz JH, Jessell TM: *Principles of Neural Science*, ed 4, New York, 2000, McGraw-Hill.

Knutsen PM, Ahissar E: Orthogonal coding of object location, *Trends Neurosci* 32:101, 2009.

Pelli DG, Tillman KA: The uncrowded window of object recognition, *Nat Neurosci* 11:1129, 2008.

Suga N, Ma X: Multiparametric corticofugal modulation and plasticity in the auditory system, *Nat Rev Neurosci* 4:783, 2003.

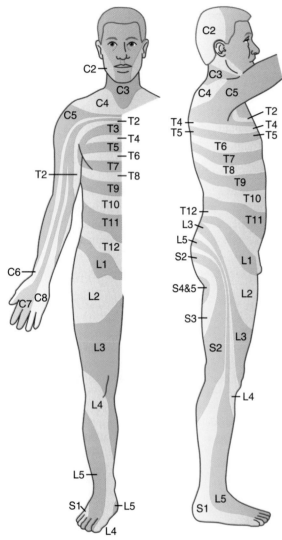

Figure 47-14 Dermatomes. (Modified from Grinker RR, Sahs AL: Neurology, 6th ed. Springfield, Ill: Charles C Thomas, 1966. Courtesy Charles C Thomas, Publisher, Ltd., Springfield, Ill.)

CHAPTER 48

Somatic Sensations: II. Pain, Headache, and Thermal Sensations

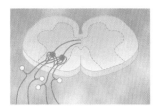 Many, if not most, ailments of the body cause pain. Furthermore, the ability to diagnose different diseases depends to a great extent on a physician's knowledge of the different qualities of pain. For these reasons, the first part of this chapter is devoted mainly to pain and to the physiologic bases of some associated clinical phenomena.

Pain Is a Protective Mechanism. Pain occurs whenever tissues are being damaged, and it causes the individual to react to remove the pain stimulus. Even such simple activities as sitting for a long time on the ischia can cause tissue destruction because of lack of blood flow to the skin where it is compressed by the weight of the body. When the skin becomes painful as a result of the ischemia, the person normally shifts weight subconsciously. But a person who has lost the pain sense, as after spinal cord injury, fails to feel the pain and, therefore, fails to shift. This soon results in total breakdown and desquamation of the skin at the areas of pressure.

Types of Pain and Their Qualities—Fast Pain and Slow Pain

Pain has been classified into two major types: *fast pain* and *slow pain.* Fast pain is felt within about 0.1 second after a pain stimulus is applied, whereas slow pain begins only after 1 second or more and then increases slowly over many seconds and sometimes even minutes. During the course of this chapter, we shall see that the conduction pathways for these two types of pain are different and that each of them has specific qualities.

Fast pain is also described by many alternative names, such as *sharp pain, pricking pain, acute pain,* and *electric pain.* This type of pain is felt when a needle is stuck into the skin, when the skin is cut with a knife, or when the skin is acutely burned. It is also felt when the skin is subjected to electric shock. Fast-sharp pain is not felt in most deeper tissues of the body.

Slow pain also goes by many names, such as *slow burning pain, aching pain, throbbing pain, nauseous pain,* and *chronic pain.* This type of pain is usually associated with *tissue destruction.* It can lead to prolonged, almost unbearable suffering. It can occur both in the skin and in almost any deep tissue or organ.

Pain Receptors and Their Stimulation

Pain Receptors Are Free Nerve Endings. The pain receptors in the skin and other tissues are all free nerve endings. They are widespread in the superficial layers of the *skin,* as well as in certain internal tissues, such as the *periosteum,* the *arterial walls,* the *joint surfaces,* and the *falx* and *tentorium* in the cranial vault. Most other deep tissues are only sparsely supplied with pain endings; nevertheless, any widespread tissue damage can summate to cause the slow-chronic-aching type of pain in most of these areas.

Three Types of Stimuli Excite Pain Receptors— Mechanical, Thermal, and Chemical. Pain can be elicited by multiple types of stimuli. They are classified as *mechanical, thermal,* and *chemical pain stimuli.* In general, fast pain is elicited by the mechanical and thermal types of stimuli, whereas slow pain can be elicited by all three types.

Some of the chemicals that excite the chemical type of pain are *bradykinin, serotonin, histamine, potassium ions, acids, acetylcholine,* and *proteolytic enzymes.* In addition, *prostaglandins* and *substance P* enhance the sensitivity of pain endings but do not directly excite them. The chemical substances are especially important in stimulating the slow, suffering type of pain that occurs after tissue injury.

Nonadapting Nature of Pain Receptors. In contrast to most other sensory receptors of the body, pain receptors adapt very little and sometimes not at all. In fact, under some conditions, excitation of pain fibers becomes progressively greater, especially so for slow-aching-nauseous pain, as the pain stimulus continues. This increase in sensitivity of the pain receptors is called *hyperalgesia.*

One can readily understand the importance of this failure of pain receptors to adapt because it allows the pain to keep the person apprised of a tissue-damaging stimulus as long as it persists.

Rate of Tissue Damage as a Stimulus for Pain

The average person begins to perceive pain when the skin is heated above 45 °C, as shown in Figure 48-1. This is also the temperature at which the tissues begin to be damaged by heat; indeed, the tissues are eventually destroyed if the temperature remains above this level indefinitely. Therefore, it is immediately apparent that pain resulting from heat is closely correlated with the *rate at which damage to the tissues is occurring* and not with the total damage that has already occurred.

The intensity of pain is also closely correlated with the *rate of tissue damage* from causes other than heat, such as bacterial infection, tissue ischemia, tissue contusion, and so forth.

Special Importance of Chemical Pain Stimuli During Tissue Damage. Extracts from damaged tissue cause intense pain when injected beneath the normal skin. Most of the chemicals listed earlier that excite the chemical pain receptors can be found in these extracts. One chemical that seems to be more painful than others is *bradykinin.* Many researchers have suggested that bradykinin might be the agent most responsible for causing pain following tissue damage. Also, the intensity of the pain felt correlates with the local increase in potassium ion concentration or the increase in proteolytic enzymes that directly attack the nerve endings and excite pain by making the nerve membranes more permeable to ions.

Tissue Ischemia as a Cause of Pain.   When blood flow to a tissue is blocked, the tissue often becomes very painful within a few minutes. The greater the rate of metabolism of the tissue, the more rapidly the pain appears. For instance, if a blood pressure cuff is placed around the upper arm and inflated until the arterial blood flow ceases, exercise of the forearm muscles sometimes can cause muscle pain within 15 to 20 seconds. In the absence of muscle exercise, the pain may not appear for 3 to 4 minutes even though the muscle blood flow remains zero.

One of the suggested causes of pain during ischemia is accumulation of large amounts of lactic acid in the tissues, formed as a consequence of anaerobic metabolism (metabolism without oxygen). It is also probable that other chemical agents, such as bradykinin and proteolytic enzymes, are formed in the tissues because of cell damage and that these, in addition to lactic acid, stimulate the pain nerve endings.

Muscle Spasm as a Cause of Pain.   Muscle spasm is also a common cause of pain, and it is the basis of many clinical pain syndromes. This pain probably results partially from the direct effect of muscle spasm in stimulating mechanosensitive pain receptors, but it might also result from the indirect effect of muscle spasm to compress the blood vessels and cause ischemia. Also, the spasm increases the rate of metabolism in the muscle tissue, thus making the relative ischemia even greater, creating ideal conditions for the release of chemical pain-inducing substances.

Dual Pathways for Transmission of Pain Signals into the Central Nervous System

Even though all pain receptors are free nerve endings, these endings use two separate pathways for transmitting pain signals into the central nervous system. The two pathways mainly correspond to the two types of pain—a *fast-sharp pain pathway* and a *slow-chronic pain pathway.*

Peripheral Pain Fibers—"Fast" and "Slow" Fibers. The fast-sharp pain signals are elicited by either mechanical or thermal pain stimuli; they are transmitted in the peripheral nerves to the spinal cord by small type Aδ fibers at velocities between 6 and 30 m/sec. Conversely, the slow-chronic type of pain is elicited mostly by chemical types of pain stimuli but sometimes by persisting mechanical or thermal stimuli. This slow-chronic pain is transmitted to the spinal cord by type C fibers at velocities between 0.5 and 2 m/sec.

Because of this double system of pain innervation, a sudden painful stimulus often gives a "double" pain sensation: a fast-sharp pain that is transmitted to the brain by the Aδ fiber pathway, followed a second or so later by a slow pain that is transmitted by the C fiber pathway. The sharp pain apprises the person rapidly of a damaging influence and, therefore, plays an important role in making the person react immediately to remove himself or herself from the stimulus. The slow pain tends to become greater over time. This sensation eventually produces intolerable

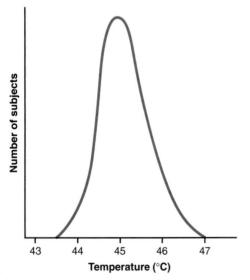

Figure 48-1 Distribution curve obtained from a large number of persons showing the minimal skin temperature that will cause pain. (Modified from Hardy DJ: Nature of pain. J Clin Epidemiol 4:22, 1956.)

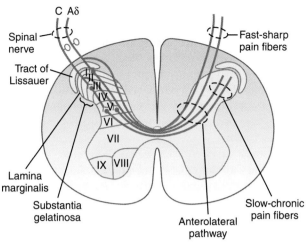

Figure 48-2 Transmission of both "fast-sharp" and "slow-chronic" pain signals into and through the spinal cord on their way to the brain.

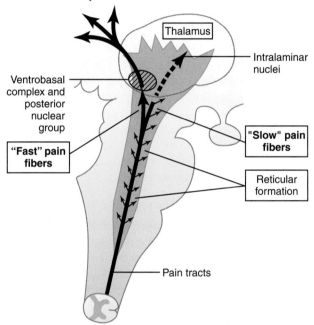

Figure 48-3 Transmission of pain signals into the brain stem, thalamus, and cerebral cortex by way of the *fast pricking pain pathway* and the *slow burning pain pathway*.

pain and makes the person keep trying to relieve the cause of the pain.

On entering the spinal cord from the dorsal spinal roots, the pain fibers terminate on relay neurons in the dorsal horns. Here again, there are two systems for processing the pain signals on their way to the brain, as shown in Figures 48-2 and 48-3.

Dual Pain Pathways in the Cord and Brain Stem—The Neospinothalamic Tract and the Paleospinothalamic Tract

On entering the spinal cord, the pain signals take two pathways to the brain, through (1) the *neospinothalamic tract* and (2) the *paleospinothalamic tract.*

Neospinothalamic Tract for Fast Pain. The fast type Aδ pain fibers transmit mainly mechanical and acute thermal pain. They terminate mainly in lamina I (lamina marginalis) of the dorsal horns, as shown in Figure 48-2, and there excite second-order neurons of the neospinothalamic tract. These give rise to long fibers that cross immediately to the opposite side of the cord through the anterior commissure and then turn upward, passing to the brain in the anterolateral columns.

Termination of the Neospinothalamic Tract in the Brain Stem and Thalamus. A few fibers of the neospinothalamic tract terminate in the reticular areas of the brain stem, but most pass all the way to the thalamus without interruption, terminating in the *ventrobasal complex* along with the dorsal column–medial lemniscal tract for tactile sensations, as was discussed in Chapter 47. A few fibers also terminate in the posterior nuclear group of the thalamus. From these thalamic areas, the signals are transmitted to other basal areas of the brain, as well as to the somatosensory cortex.

Capability of the Nervous System to Localize Fast Pain in the Body. The fast-sharp type of pain can be localized much more exactly in the different parts of the body than can slow-chronic pain. However, when only pain receptors are stimulated, without the simultaneous stimulation of tactile receptors, even fast pain may be poorly localized, often only within 10 centimeters or so of the stimulated area. Yet when tactile receptors that excite the dorsal column–medial lemniscal system are simultaneously stimulated, the localization can be nearly exact.

Glutamate, the Probable Neurotransmitter of the Type Aδ Fast Pain Fibers. It is believed that *glutamate* is the neurotransmitter substance secreted in the spinal cord at the type Aδ pain nerve fiber endings. This is one of the most widely used excitatory transmitters in the central nervous system, usually having a duration of action lasting for only a few milliseconds.

Paleospinothalamic Pathway for Transmitting Slow-Chronic Pain. The paleospinothalamic pathway is a much older system and transmits pain mainly from the peripheral slow-chronic type C pain fibers, although it does transmit some signals from type Aδ fibers as well. In this pathway, the peripheral fibers terminate in the spinal cord almost entirely in laminae II and III of the dorsal horns, which together are called the *substantia gelatinosa,* as shown by the lateral most dorsal root type C fiber in Figure 48-2. Most of the signals then pass through one or more additional short fiber neurons within the dorsal horns themselves before entering mainly lamina V, also in the dorsal horn. Here the last neurons in the series give rise to long axons that mostly join the fibers from the fast pain pathway, passing first through the anterior commissure to the opposite side of the cord, then upward to the brain in the anterolateral pathway.

Substance P, the Probable Slow-Chronic Neuro-transmitter of Type C Nerve Endings. Research suggests that type C pain fiber terminals entering the spinal cord release both glutamate transmitter and substance P transmitter. The glutamate transmitter acts instantaneously and lasts for only a few milliseconds. Substance P is released much more slowly, building up in concentration over a period of seconds or even minutes. In fact, it has been suggested that the "double" pain sensation one feels after a pinprick might result partly from the fact that the glutamate transmitter gives a faster pain sensation, whereas the substance P transmitter gives a more lagging sensation. Regardless of the yet unknown details, it seems clear that glutamate is the neurotransmitter most involved in transmitting fast pain into the central nervous system, and substance P is concerned with slow-chronic pain.

Projection of the Paleospinothalamic Pathway (Slow-Chronic Pain Signals) into the Brain Stem and Thalamus. The slow-chronic paleospinothalamic pathway terminates widely in the brain stem, in the large shaded area shown in Figure 48-3. Only one tenth to one fourth of the fibers pass all the way to the thalamus. Instead, most terminate in one of three areas: (1) the *reticular nuclei* of the medulla, pons, and mesencephalon; (2) the *tectal area* of the mesencephalon deep to the superior and inferior colliculi; or (3) the *periaqueductal gray region* surrounding the aqueduct of Sylvius. These lower regions of the brain appear to be important for feeling the suffering types of pain, because animals whose brains have been sectioned above the mesencephalon to block pain signals from reaching the cerebrum still evince undeniable evidence of suffering when any part of the body is traumatized. From the brain stem pain areas, multiple short-fiber neurons relay the pain signals upward into the intralaminar and ventrolateral nuclei of the thalamus and into certain portions of the hypothalamus and other basal regions of the brain.

Very Poor Capability of the Nervous System to Localize Precisely the Source of Pain Transmitted in the Slow-Chronic Pathway. Localization of pain transmitted by way of the paleospinothalamic pathway is imprecise. For instance, slow-chronic pain can usually be localized only to a major part of the body, such as to one arm or leg but not to a specific point on the arm or leg. This is in keeping with the multisynaptic, diffuse connectivity of this pathway. It explains why patients often have serious difficulty in localizing the source of some chronic types of pain.

Function of the Reticular Formation, Thalamus, and Cerebral Cortex in the Appreciation of Pain. Complete removal of the somatic sensory areas of the cerebral cortex does not destroy an animal's ability to perceive pain. Therefore, it is likely that pain impulses entering the brain stem reticular formation, the thalamus, and other lower brain centers cause conscious perception of pain. This does not mean that the cerebral cortex has nothing to do with normal pain appreciation; electrical stimulation of cortical somatosensory areas does cause a human being to perceive mild pain from about 3 percent of the points stimulated. However, it is believed that the cortex plays an especially important role in interpreting pain quality, even though pain perception might be principally the function of lower centers.

Special Capability of Pain Signals to Arouse Overall Brain Excitability. Electrical stimulation in the *reticular areas of the brain stem* and in the *intralaminar nuclei of the thalamus,* the areas where the slow-suffering type of pain terminates, has a strong arousal effect on nervous activity throughout the entire brain. In fact, these two areas constitute part of the brain's principal "arousal system," which is discussed in Chapter 59. This explains why it is almost impossible for a person to sleep when he or she is in severe pain.

Surgical Interruption of Pain Pathways. When a person has severe and intractable pain (sometimes resulting from rapidly spreading cancer), it is necessary to relieve the pain. To do this, the pain nervous pathways can be cut at any one of several points. If the pain is in the lower part of the body, a *cordotomy* in the thoracic region of the spinal cord often relieves the pain for a few weeks to a few months. To do this, the spinal cord on the side opposite to the pain is partially cut in its *anterolateral quadrant* to interrupt the anterolateral sensory pathway.

A cordotomy, however, is not always successful in relieving pain, for two reasons. First, many pain fibers from the upper part of the body do not cross to the opposite side of the spinal cord until they have reached the brain, so the cordotomy does not transect these fibers. Second, pain frequently returns several months later, partly as a result of sensitization of other pathways that normally are too weak to be effectual (e.g., sparse pathways in the dorsolateral cord). Another experimental operative procedure to relieve pain has been to cauterize specific pain areas in the intralaminar nuclei in the thalamus, which often relieves suffering types of pain while leaving intact one's appreciation of "acute" pain, an important protective mechanism.

Pain Suppression ("Analgesia") System in the Brain and Spinal Cord

The degree to which a person reacts to pain varies tremendously. This results partly from a capability of the brain itself to suppress input of pain signals to the nervous system by activating a pain control system, called an *analgesia system.*

The analgesia system is shown in Figure 48-4. It consists of three major components: (1) The *periaqueductal gray* and *periventricular areas* of the mesencephalon and upper pons surround the aqueduct of Sylvius and

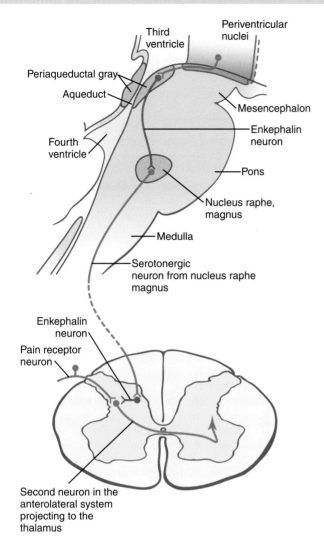

Figure 48-4 Analgesia system of the brain and spinal cord, showing (1) inhibition of incoming pain signals at the cord level and (2) presence of *enkephalin-secreting neurons* that suppress pain signals in both the cord and the brain stem.

Labels in figure:
- Third ventricle
- Periventricular nuclei
- Periaqueductal gray
- Aqueduct
- Mesencephalon
- Enkephalin neuron
- Fourth ventricle
- Pons
- Nucleus raphe, magnus
- Medulla
- Serotonergic neuron from nucleus raphe magnus
- Enkephalin neuron
- Pain receptor neuron
- Second neuron in the anterolateral system projecting to the thalamus

portions of the third and fourth ventricles. Neurons from these areas send signals to (2) the *raphe magnus nucleus,* a thin midline nucleus located in the lower pons and upper medulla, and the *nucleus reticularis paragigantocellularis,* located laterally in the medulla. From these nuclei, second-order signals are transmitted down the dorsolateral columns in the spinal cord to (3) a *pain inhibitory complex located in the dorsal horns of the spinal cord.* At this point, the analgesia signals can block the pain before it is relayed to the brain.

Electrical stimulation either in the periaqueductal gray area or in the raphe magnus nucleus can suppress many strong pain signals entering by way of the dorsal spinal roots. Also, stimulation of areas at still higher levels of the brain that excite the periaqueductal gray area can also suppress pain. Some of these areas are (1) the *periventricular nuclei in the hypothalamus,* lying adjacent to the third ventricle, and (2) to a lesser extent, the *medial forebrain bundle,* also in the hypothalamus.

Several transmitter substances are involved in the analgesia system; especially involved are *enkephalin* and

serotonin. Many nerve fibers derived from the periventricular nuclei and from the periaqueductal gray area secrete enkephalin at their endings. Thus, as shown in Figure 48-4, the endings of many fibers in the raphe magnus nucleus release enkephalin when stimulated.

Fibers originating in this area send signals to the dorsal horns of the spinal cord to secrete serotonin at their endings. The serotonin causes local cord neurons to secrete enkephalin as well. The enkephalin is believed to cause both *presynaptic* and *postsynaptic inhibition* of incoming type C and type Aδ pain fibers where they synapse in the dorsal horns.

Thus, the analgesia system can block pain signals at the initial entry point to the spinal cord. In fact, it can also block many local cord reflexes that result from pain signals, especially withdrawal reflexes described in Chapter 54.

Brain's Opiate System—Endorphins and Enkephalins

More than 40 years ago it was discovered that injection of minute quantities of morphine either into the periventricular nucleus around the third ventricle or into the periaqueductal gray area of the brain stem causes an extreme degree of analgesia. In subsequent studies, it has been found that morphine-like agents, mainly the opiates, also act at many other points in the analgesia system, including the dorsal horns of the spinal cord. Because most drugs that alter excitability of neurons do so by acting on synaptic receptors, it was assumed that the "morphine receptors" of the analgesia system must be receptors for some morphine-like neurotransmitter that is naturally secreted in the brain. Therefore, an extensive search was undertaken for the natural opiate of the brain. About a dozen such opiate-like substances have now been found at different points of the nervous system; all are breakdown products of three large protein molecules: *pro-opiomelanocortin, proenkephalin,* and *prodynorphin.* Among the more important of these opiate-like substances are β-endorphin, met-enkephalin, *leu-enkephalin,* and *dynorphin.*

The two enkephalins are found in the brain stem and spinal cord, in the portions of the analgesia system described earlier, and β-endorphin is present in both the hypothalamus and the pituitary gland. Dynorphin is found mainly in the same areas as the enkephalins, but in much lower quantities.

Thus, although the fine details of the brain's opiate system are not understood, *activation of the analgesia system* by nervous signals entering the periaqueductal gray and periventricular areas, or *inactivation of pain pathways* by morphine-like drugs, can almost totally suppress many pain signals entering through the peripheral nerves.

Inhibition of Pain Transmission by Simultaneous Tactile Sensory Signals

Another important event in the saga of pain control was the discovery that stimulation of large-type Aβ sensory fibers from peripheral tactile receptors can depress transmission of pain signals from the same body area. This presumably results from local lateral inhibition in the spinal cord. It explains why such simple maneuvers as rubbing the skin near painful areas is often effective in relieving pain. And it probably also explains why liniments are often useful for pain relief.

This mechanism and the simultaneous psychogenic excitation of the central analgesia system are probably also the basis of pain relief by *acupuncture.*

Treatment of Pain by Electrical Stimulation

Several clinical procedures have been developed for suppressing pain by electrical stimulation. Stimulating electrodes are placed on selected areas of the skin or, on occasion, implanted over the spinal cord, supposedly to stimulate the dorsal sensory columns.

In some patients, electrodes have been placed stereotaxically in appropriate intralaminar nuclei of the thalamus or in the periventricular or periaqueductal area of the diencephalon. The patient can then personally control the degree of stimulation. Dramatic relief has been reported in some instances. Also, pain relief has been reported to last for as long as 24 hours after only a few minutes of stimulation.

Referred Pain

Often a person feels pain in a part of the body that is fairly remote from the tissue causing the pain. This is called *referred pain.* For instance, pain in one of the visceral organs often is referred to an area on the body surface. Knowledge of the different types of referred pain is important in clinical diagnosis because in many visceral ailments the only clinical sign is referred pain.

Mechanism of Referred Pain. Figure 48-5 shows the probable mechanism by which most pain is referred. In the figure, branches of visceral pain fibers are shown to synapse in the spinal cord on the same second-order neurons (1 and 2) that receive pain signals from the skin. When the visceral pain fibers are stimulated, pain signals from the viscera are conducted through at least some of the same neurons that conduct pain signals from the

skin, and the person has the feeling that the sensations originate in the skin itself.

Visceral Pain

Pain from the different viscera of the abdomen and chest is one of the few criteria that can be used for diagnosing visceral inflammation, visceral infectious disease, and other visceral ailments. Often, the viscera have sensory receptors for no other modalities of sensation besides pain. Also, visceral pain differs from surface pain in several important aspects.

One of the most important differences between surface pain and visceral pain is that highly localized types of damage to the viscera seldom cause severe pain. For instance, a surgeon can cut the gut entirely in two in a patient who is awake without causing significant pain. Conversely, any stimulus that causes *diffuse stimulation of pain nerve endings* throughout a viscus causes pain that can be severe. For instance, ischemia caused by occluding the blood supply to a large area of gut stimulates many diffuse pain fibers at the same time and can result in extreme pain.

Causes of True Visceral Pain

Any stimulus that excites pain nerve endings in diffuse areas of the viscera can cause visceral pain. Such stimuli include ischemia of visceral tissue, chemical damage to the surfaces of the viscera, spasm of the smooth muscle of a hollow viscus, excess distention of a hollow viscus, and stretching of the connective tissue surrounding or within the viscus. Essentially all visceral pain that originates in the thoracic and abdominal cavities is transmitted through small type C pain fibers and, therefore, can transmit only the chronic-aching-suffering type of pain.

Ischemia. Ischemia causes visceral pain in the same way that it does in other tissues, presumably because of the formation of acidic metabolic end products or tissue-degenerative products such as bradykinin, proteolytic enzymes, or others that stimulate pain nerve endings.

Chemical Stimuli. On occasion, damaging substances leak from the gastrointestinal tract into the peritoneal cavity. For instance, proteolytic acidic gastric juice may leak through a ruptured gastric or duodenal ulcer. This juice causes widespread digestion of the visceral peritoneum, thus stimulating broad areas of pain fibers. The pain is usually excruciatingly severe.

Spasm of a Hollow Viscus. Spasm of a portion of the gut, the gallbladder, a bile duct, a ureter, or any other hollow viscus can cause pain, possibly by mechanical stimulation of the pain nerve endings. Or the spasm might cause diminished blood flow to the muscle, combined with the muscle's increased metabolic need for nutrients, thus causing severe pain.

Often pain from a spastic viscus occurs in the form of *cramps,* with the pain increasing to a high degree of severity and then subsiding. This process continues intermittently, once every few minutes. The intermittent cycles result from periods of contraction of smooth muscle. For instance, each time a peristaltic wave travels along an overly excitable spastic gut, a cramp occurs. The cramping type of pain frequently occurs in appendicitis, gastroenteritis, constipation,

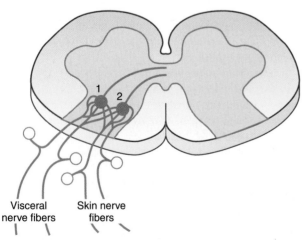

Figure 48-5 Mechanism of referred pain and referred hyperalgesia.

menstruation, parturition, gallbladder disease, or ureteral obstruction.

Overdistention of a Hollow Viscus. Extreme overfilling of a hollow viscus also can result in pain, presumably because of overstretch of the tissues themselves. Overdistention can also collapse the blood vessels that encircle the viscus or that pass into its wall, thus perhaps promoting ischemic pain.

Insensitive Viscera. A few visceral areas are almost completely insensitive to pain of any type. These include the parenchyma of the liver and the alveoli of the lungs. Yet the liver *capsule* is extremely sensitive to both direct trauma and stretch, and the *bile ducts* are also sensitive to pain. In the lungs, even though the alveoli are insensitive, both the *bronchi* and the *parietal pleura* are very sensitive to pain.

"Parietal Pain" Caused by Visceral Disease

When a disease affects a viscus, the disease process often spreads to the parietal peritoneum, pleura, or pericardium. These parietal surfaces, like the skin, are supplied with extensive pain innervation from the peripheral spinal nerves. Therefore, pain from the parietal wall overlying a viscus is frequently sharp. An example can emphasize the difference between this pain and true visceral pain: a knife incision through the *parietal* peritoneum is very painful, whereas a similar cut through the visceral peritoneum or through a gut wall is not very painful, if painful at all.

Localization of Visceral Pain—"Visceral" and the "Parietal" Pain Transmission Pathways

Pain from the different viscera is frequently difficult to localize, for a number of reasons. First, the patient's brain does not know from firsthand experience that the different internal organs exist; therefore, any pain that originates internally can be localized only generally. Second, sensations from the abdomen and thorax are transmitted through two pathways to the central nervous system—the *true visceral pathway* and the *parietal pathway*. True visceral pain is transmitted via pain sensory fibers within the autonomic nerve bundles, and the sensations are *referred* to surface areas of the body often far from the painful organ. Conversely, parietal sensations are conducted *directly* into local spinal nerves from the parietal peritoneum, pleura, or pericardium, and these sensations are usually *localized directly over the painful area*.

Localization of Referred Pain Transmitted via Visceral Pathways. When visceral pain is referred to the surface of the body, the person generally localizes it in the dermatomal segment from which the visceral organ originated in the embryo, not necessarily where the visceral organ now lies. For instance, the heart originated in the neck and upper thorax, so the heart's visceral pain fibers pass upward along the sympathetic sensory nerves and enter the spinal cord between segments C-3 and T-5. Therefore, as shown in Figure 48-6, pain from the heart is referred to the side of the neck, over the shoulder, over the pectoral muscles, down the arm, and into the substernal area of the upper chest. These are the areas of the body surface that send their own somatosensory nerve fibers into the C-3 to T-5 cord segments. Most frequently, the pain is on the left side rather than on the right because the left side of the heart is much more frequently involved in coronary disease than the right.

The stomach originated approximately from the seventh to ninth thoracic segments of the embryo. Therefore, stomach

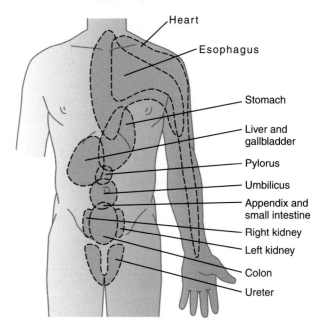

Figure 48-6 Surface areas of referred pain from different visceral organs.

pain is referred to the anterior epigastrium above the umbilicus, which is the surface area of the body subserved by the seventh through ninth thoracic segments. Figure 48-6 shows several other surface areas to which visceral pain is referred from other organs, representing in general the areas in the embryo from which the respective organs originated.

Parietal Pathway for Transmission of Abdominal and Thoracic Pain. Pain from the viscera is frequently localized to two surface areas of the body at the same time because of the dual transmission of pain through the referred visceral pathway and the direct parietal pathway. Thus, Figure 48-7 shows dual transmission from an inflamed appendix. Pain impulses pass first from the appendix through visceral

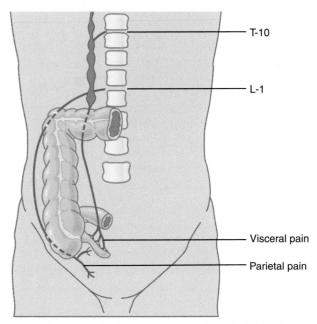

Figure 48-7 Visceral and parietal transmission of pain signals from the appendix.

pain fibers located within sympathetic nerve bundles, and then into the spinal cord at about T-10 or T-11; this pain is referred to an area around the umbilicus and is of the aching, cramping type. Pain impulses also often originate in the parietal peritoneum where the inflamed appendix touches or is adherent to the abdominal wall. These cause pain of the sharp type directly over the irritated peritoneum in the right lower quadrant of the abdomen.

Some Clinical Abnormalities of Pain and Other Somatic Sensations

Hyperalgesia

A pain nervous pathway sometimes becomes excessively excitable; this gives rise to *hyperalgesia*, which means hypersensitivity to pain. Possible causes of hyperalgesia are (1) excessive sensitivity of the pain receptors themselves, which is called *primary hyperalgesia*, and (2) facilitation of sensory transmission, which is called *secondary hyperalgesia*.

An example of primary hyperalgesia is the extreme sensitivity of sunburned skin, which results from sensitization of the skin pain endings by local tissue products from the burn—perhaps histamine, and prostaglandins, and others. Secondary hyperalgesia frequently results from lesions in the spinal cord or the thalamus. Several of these lesions are discussed in subsequent sections.

Herpes Zoster (Shingles)

Occasionally *herpesvirus* infects a dorsal root ganglion. This causes severe pain in the dermatomal segment subserved by the ganglion, thus eliciting a segmental type of pain that circles halfway around the body. The disease is called *herpes zoster,* or "shingles," because of a skin eruption that often ensues.

The cause of the pain is presumably infection of the pain neuronal cells in the dorsal root ganglion by the virus. In addition to causing pain, the virus is carried by neuronal cytoplasmic flow outward through the neuronal peripheral axons to their cutaneous origins. Here the virus causes a rash that vesiculates within a few days and then crusts over within another few days, all of this occurring within the dermatomal area served by the infected dorsal root.

Tic Douloureux

Lancinating pain occasionally occurs in some people over one side of the face in the sensory distribution area (or part of the area) of the fifth or ninth nerves; this phenomenon is called *tic douloureux* (or *trigeminal neuralgia* or *glossopharyngeal neuralgia*). The pain feels like sudden electrical shocks, and it may appear for only a few seconds at a time or may be almost continuous. Often it is set off by exceedingly sensitive trigger areas on the surface of the face, in the mouth, or inside the throat—almost always by a mechanoreceptive stimulus rather than a pain stimulus. For instance, when the patient swallows a bolus of food, as the food touches a tonsil, it might set off a severe lancinating pain in the mandibular portion of the fifth nerve.

The pain of tic douloureux can usually be blocked by surgically cutting the peripheral nerve from the hypersensitive area. The sensory portion of the fifth nerve is often sectioned immediately inside the cranium, where the motor and sensory roots of the fifth nerve separate from each other, so that the motor portions, which are necessary for many jaw movements, can be spared while the sensory elements are destroyed. This operation leaves the side of the face anesthetic, which in itself may be annoying. Furthermore, sometimes the operation is unsuccessful, indicating that the lesion that causes the pain might be in the sensory nucleus in the brain stem and not in the peripheral nerves.

Brown-Séquard Syndrome

If the spinal cord is transected entirely, all sensations and motor functions distal to the segment of transection are blocked, but if the spinal cord is transected on only one side, the *Brown-Séquard syndrome* occurs. The effects of such transection can be predicted from knowledge of the cord fiber tracts shown in Figure 48-8. All motor functions are blocked on the side of the transection in all segments below the level of the transection. Yet only some of the modalities of sensation are lost on the transected side, and others are lost on the opposite side. The sensations of pain, heat, and cold—sensations served by the spinothalamic pathway—are lost *on the opposite side of the body* in all dermatomes two to six segments below the level of the transection. By contrast, the sensations that are transmitted only in the dorsal and dorsolateral columns—kinesthetic and position sensations, vibration sensation, discrete localization, and two-point discrimination—are lost *on the side of the transection* in all dermatomes below the level of the transection. Discrete "light touch" is impaired on the side of the transection because the principal pathway for the transmission of light touch, the dorsal column, is transected. That is, the fibers in this column do not cross to the opposite side until they reach the medulla of the brain. "Crude touch," which is poorly localized, still persists because of partial transmission in the opposite spinothalamic tract.

Headache

Headaches are a type of pain referred to the surface of the head from deep head structures. Some headaches result from pain stimuli arising inside the cranium, but others result from pain arising outside the cranium, such as from the nasal sinuses.

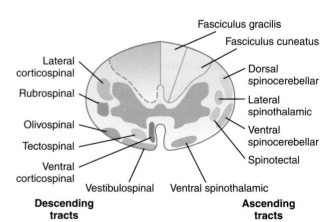

Figure 48-8 Cross section of the spinal cord, showing principal ascending tracts on the right and principal descending tracts on the left.

Headache of Intracranial Origin

Pain-Sensitive Areas in the Cranial Vault. The brain tissues themselves are almost totally insensitive to pain. Even cutting or electrically stimulating the sensory areas of the cerebral cortex only occasionally causes pain; instead, it causes prickly types of paresthesias on the area of the body represented by the portion of the sensory cortex stimulated. Therefore, it is likely that much or most of the pain of headache is not caused by damage within the brain itself.

Conversely, *tugging on the venous sinuses around the brain, damaging the tentorium,* or *stretching the dura at the base of the brain* can cause intense pain that is recognized as headache. Also, almost any type of traumatizing, crushing, or stretching stimulus to the *blood vessels of the meninges* can cause headache. An especially sensitive structure is the middle meningeal artery, and neurosurgeons are careful to anesthetize this artery specifically when performing brain operations under local anesthesia.

Areas of the Head to Which Intracranial Headache Is Referred. Stimulation of pain receptors in the cerebral vault above the tentorium, including the upper surface of the tentorium itself, initiates pain impulses in the cerebral portion of the fifth nerve and, therefore, causes referred headache to the front half of the head in the surface areas supplied by this somatosensory portion of the fifth cranial nerve, as shown in Figure 48-9.

Conversely, pain impulses from beneath the tentorium enter the central nervous system mainly through the glossopharyngeal, vagal, and second cervical nerves, which also supply the scalp above, behind, and slightly below the ear. Subtentorial pain stimuli cause "occipital headache" referred to the posterior part of the head.

Types of Intracranial Headache

Headache of Meningitis. One of the most severe headaches of all is that resulting from meningitis, which causes inflammation of all the meninges, including the sensitive areas of the dura and the sensitive areas around the venous sinuses. Such intense damage can cause extreme headache pain referred over the entire head.

Headache Caused by Low Cerebrospinal Fluid Pressure. Removing as little as 20 milliliters of fluid from the spinal canal, particularly if the person remains in an upright position, often causes intense intracranial headache. Removing this quantity of fluid removes part of the flotation for the brain that is normally provided by the cerebrospinal fluid. The weight of the brain stretches and otherwise distorts the various dural surfaces and thereby elicits the pain that causes the headache.

Migraine Headache. Migraine headache is a special type of headache that may result from abnormal vascular phenomena, although the exact mechanism is unknown. Migraine headaches often begin with various prodromal sensations, such as nausea, loss of vision in part of the field of vision, visual aura, and other types of sensory hallucinations. Ordinarily, the prodromal symptoms begin 30 minutes to 1 hour before the beginning of the headache. Any theory that explains migraine headache must also explain the prodromal symptoms.

One theory of migraine headaches is that prolonged emotion or tension causes reflex vasospasm of some of the arteries of the head, including arteries that supply the brain. The vasospasm theoretically produces ischemia of portions of the brain, and this is responsible for the prodromal symptoms. Then, as a result of the intense ischemia, something happens to the vascular walls, perhaps exhaustion of smooth muscle contraction, to allow the blood vessels to become flaccid and incapable of maintaining normal vascular tone for 24 to 48 hours. The blood pressure in the vessels causes them to dilate and pulsate intensely, and it is postulated that the excessive stretching of the walls of the arteries—including some extracranial arteries, such as the temporal artery—causes the actual pain of migraine headaches. Other theories of the cause of migraine headaches include spreading cortical depression, psychological abnormalities, and vasospasm caused by excess local potassium in the cerebral extracellular fluid.

There may be a genetic predisposition to migraine headaches because a positive family history for migraine has been reported in 65 to 90 percent of cases. Migraine headaches also occur about twice as frequently in women as in men.

Alcoholic Headache.. As many people have experienced, a headache often follows excessive alcohol consumption. It is likely that alcohol, because it is toxic to tissues, directly irritates the meninges and causes the intracranial pain. Dehydration may also play a role in the "hangover" that follows an alcoholic binge; hydration usually attenuates but does not abolish headache and other symptoms of hangover.

Extracranial Types of Headache

Headache Resulting from Muscle Spasm. Emotional tension often causes many of the muscles of the head, especially those muscles attached to the scalp and the neck muscles attached to the occiput, to become spastic, and it is postulated that this is one of the common causes of headache. The pain of the spastic head muscles supposedly is referred to the overlying areas of the head and gives one the same type of headache as intracranial lesions do.

Headache Caused by Irritation of Nasal and Accessory Nasal Structures. The mucous membranes of the nose and nasal sinuses are sensitive to pain, but not intensely so. Nevertheless, infection or other irritative processes in widespread areas of the nasal structures often summate and cause headache that is referred behind the eyes or, in the case of

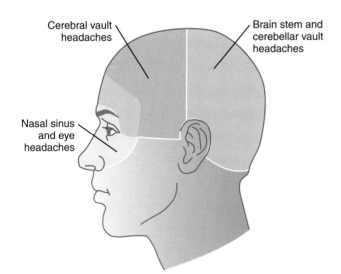

Figure 48-9 Areas of headache resulting from different causes.

Cerebral vault headaches

Brain stem and cerebellar vault headaches

Nasal sinus and eye headaches

frontal sinus infection, to the frontal surfaces of the forehead and scalp, as shown in Figure 48-9. Also, pain from the lower sinuses, such as from the maxillary sinuses, can be felt in the face.

Headache Caused by Eye Disorders. Difficulty in focusing one's eyes clearly may cause excessive contraction of the eye ciliary muscles in an attempt to gain clear vision. Even though these muscles are extremely small, it is believed that tonic contraction of them can cause retro-orbital headache. Also, excessive attempts to focus the eyes can result in reflex spasm in various facial and extraocular muscles, which is a possible cause of headache.

A second type of headache that originates in the eyes occurs when the eyes are exposed to excessive irradiation by light rays, especially ultraviolet light. Looking at the sun or the arc of an arc-welder for even a few seconds may result in headache that lasts from 24 to 48 hours. The headache sometimes results from "actinic" irritation of the conjunctivae, and the pain is referred to the surface of the head or retro-orbitally. However, focusing intense light from an arc or the sun on the retina can also burn the retina, and this could be the cause of the headache.

Thermal Sensations

Thermal Receptors and Their Excitation

The human being can perceive different gradations of cold and heat, from *freezing cold* to *cold* to *cool* to *indifferent* to *warm* to *hot* to *burning hot.*

Thermal gradations are discriminated by at least three types of sensory receptors: cold receptors, warmth receptors, and pain receptors. The pain receptors are stimulated only by extreme degrees of heat or cold and, therefore, are responsible, along with the cold and warmth receptors, for "freezing cold" and "burning hot" sensations.

The cold and warmth receptors are located immediately under the skin at discrete separated *spots*. In most areas of the body, there are 3 to 10 times as many cold spots as warmth spots, and the number in different areas of the body varies from 15 to 25 cold spots per square centimeter in the lips to 3 to 5 cold spots per square centimeter in the finger to less than 1 cold spot per square centimeter in some broad surface areas of the trunk.

Although the existence of distinctive warmth nerve endings is quite certain, on the basis of psychological tests, they have not been identified histologically. They are presumed to be free nerve endings because warmth signals are transmitted mainly over type C nerve fibers at transmission velocities of only 0.4 to 2 m/sec.

A definitive cold receptor, however, has been identified. It is a special, small type Aδ myelinated nerve ending that branches several times, the tips of which protrude into the bottom surfaces of basal epidermal cells. Signals are transmitted from these receptors via type Aδ nerve fibers at velocities of about 20 m/sec. Some cold sensations are believed to be transmitted in type C nerve fibers as well, which suggests that some free nerve endings also might function as cold receptors.

Stimulation of Thermal Receptors—Sensations of Cold, Cool, Indifferent, Warm, and Hot. Figure 48-10 shows the effects of different temperatures on the responses of four types of nerve fibers: (1) a pain fiber stimulated by cold, (2) a cold fiber, (3) a warmth fiber, and (4) a pain fiber stimulated by heat. Note especially that these fibers respond differently at different levels of temperature. For instance, in the *very* cold region, only the cold-pain fibers are stimulated (if the skin becomes even colder so that it nearly freezes or actually does freeze, these fibers cannot be stimulated). As the temperature rises to +10° to 15°C, the cold-pain impulses cease, but the cold receptors begin to be stimulated, reaching peak stimulation at about 24°C and fading out slightly above 40°C. Above about 30°C, the warmth receptors begin to be stimulated, but these also fade out at about 49°C. Finally, at around 45°C, the heat-pain fibers begin to be stimulated by heat and, paradoxically, some of the cold fibers begin to be stimulated again, possibly because of damage to the cold endings caused by the excessive heat.

One can understand from Figure 48-10 that a person determines the different gradations of thermal sensations by the relative degrees of stimulation of the different types of endings. One can also understand why extreme degrees of both cold and heat can be painful and why both these sensations, when intense enough, may give almost the same quality of sensation—that is, freezing cold and burning hot sensations feel almost alike.

Stimulatory Effects of Rising and Falling Temperature—Adaptation of Thermal Receptors. When a cold receptor is suddenly subjected to an abrupt fall in temperature, it becomes strongly stimulated at first, but this stimulation fades rapidly during the first few seconds and progressively more slowly during the next 30 minutes or more. In other words, the receptor "adapts" to a great extent, but never 100 percent.

Thus, it is evident that the thermal senses respond markedly to *changes in temperature*, in addition to being able to respond to steady states of temperature. This means that when the temperature of the skin is actively

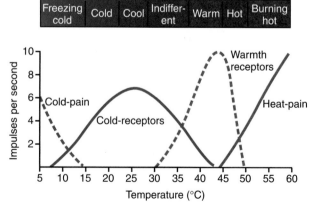

Figure 48-10 Discharge frequencies at different skin temperatures of a *cold-pain fiber*, a *cold fiber*, a *warmth fiber*, and a *heat-pain fiber.*

falling, a person feels much colder than when the temperature remains cold at the same level. Conversely, if the temperature is actively rising, the person feels much warmer than he or she would at the same temperature if it were constant. The response to changes in temperature explains the extreme degree of heat one feels on first entering a tub of hot water and the extreme degree of cold felt on going from a heated room to the out-of-doors on a cold day.

Mechanism of Stimulation of Thermal Receptors

It is believed that the cold and warmth receptors are stimulated by changes in their metabolic rates, and that these changes result from the fact that temperature alters the rate of intracellular chemical reactions more than twofold for each 10°C change. In other words, thermal detection probably results not from direct physical effects of heat or cold on the nerve endings but from chemical stimulation of the endings as modified by temperature.

Spatial Summation of Thermal Sensations. Because the number of cold or warm endings in any one surface area of the body is slight, it is difficult to judge gradations of temperature when small skin areas are stimulated. However, when a large skin area is stimulated all at once, the thermal signals from the entire area summate. For instance, rapid changes in temperature as little as 0.01°C can be detected if this change affects the entire surface of the body simultaneously. Conversely, temperature changes 100 times as great often will not be detected when the affected skin area is only 1 square centimeter in size.

Transmission of Thermal Signals in the Nervous System

In general, thermal signals are transmitted in pathways parallel to those for pain signals. On entering the spinal cord, the signals travel for a few segments upward or downward in the *tract of Lissauer* and then terminate mainly in laminae I, II, and III of the dorsal horns—the same as for pain. After a small amount of processing by one or more cord neurons, the signals enter long, ascending thermal fibers that cross to the opposite anterolateral sensory tract and terminate in both (1) the reticular areas of the brain stem and (2) the ventrobasal complex of the thalamus.

A few thermal signals are also relayed to the cerebral somatic sensory cortex from the ventrobasal complex. Occasionally a neuron in cortical somatic sensory area I

has been found by microelectrode studies to be directly responsive to either cold or warm stimuli on a specific area of the skin. However, removal of the entire cortical postcentral gyrus in the human being reduces but does not abolish the ability to distinguish gradations of temperature.

Bibliography

Almeida TF, Roizenblatt S, Tufik S: Afferent pain pathways: a neuroanatomical review, *Brain Res* 1000:40, 2004.

Ballantyne JC, Mao J: Opioid therapy for chronic pain, *N Engl J Med* 349:1943, 2003.

Bandell M, Macpherson LJ, Patapoutian A: From chills to chilis: mechanisms for thermosensation and chemesthesis via thermoTRPs, *Curr Opin Neurobiol* 17:490, 2007.

Benarroch EE: Descending monoaminergic pain modulation: bidirectional control and clinical relevance, *Neurology* 71:217, 2008.

Bingel U, Tracey I: Imaging CNS modulation of pain in humans, *Physiology (Bethesda)* 23:371, 2008.

Borsook D, Becerra L: Pain imaging: future applications to integrative clinical and basic neurobiology, *Adv Drug Deliv Rev* 55:967, 2003.

Bromm B: Brain images of pain, *News Physiol Sci* 16:244, 2001.

Franks NP: General anaesthesia: from molecular targets to neuronal pathways of sleep and arousal, *Nat Rev Neurosci* 9:370, 2008.

Gebhart GF: Descending modulation of pain, *Neurosci Biobehav Rev* 27:729, 2004.

Kandel ER, Schwartz JH, Jessell TM: *Principles of Neural Science*, ed 4, New York, 2000, McGraw-Hill.

Lumpkin EA, Caterina MJ: Mechanisms of sensory transduction in the skin, *Nature* 445:858, 2007.

McKemy DD: Temperature sensing across species, *Pflugers Arch* 454:777, 2007.

Mendell JR, Sahenk Z: Clinical practice: painful sensory neuropathy, *N Engl J Med* 348:1243, 2003.

Milligan ED, Watkins LR: Pathological and protective roles of glia in chronic pain, *Nat Rev Neurosci* 10:23, 2009.

Montell C: Thermosensation: hot findings make TRPNs very cool, *Curr Biol* 13:R476, 2003.

Sanchez-del-Rio M, Reuter U: Migraine aura: new information on underlying mechanisms, *Curr Opin Neurol* 17:289, 2004.

Sandkühler J: Models and mechanisms of hyperalgesia and allodynia, *Physiol Rev* 89:707, 2009.

Schaible HG, Ebersberger A, Von Banchet GS: Mechanisms of pain in arthritis, *Ann N Y Acad Sci* 966:343, 2002.

Schepers RJ, Ringkamp M: Thermoreceptors and thermosensitive afferents, *Neurosci Biobehav Rev* 33:205, 2009.

Silberstein SD: Recent developments in migraine, *Lancet* 372:1369, 2008.

Stein BE, Stanford TR: Multisensory integration: current issues from the perspective of the single neuron, *Nat Rev Neurosci* 9:255, 2008.

Watkins LR, Maier SF: Beyond neurons: evidence that immune and glial cells contribute to pathological pain states, *Physiol Rev* 82:981, 2002.

White FA, Jung H, Miller RJ: Chemokines and the pathophysiology of neuropathic pain, *Proc Natl Acad Sci U S A* 104:20151, 2007.

Zubrzycka M, Janecka A: Substance P: transmitter of nociception (minireview), *Endocr Regul* 34:195, 2000.

The Nervous System: B. The Special Senses

49. The Eye: I. Optics of Vision

50. The Eye: II. Receptor and Neural Function of the Retina

51. The Eye: III. Central Neurophysiology of Vision

52. The Sense of Hearing

53. The Chemical Senses—Taste and Smell

The Eye: I. Optics of Vision

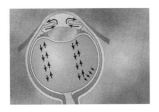

Physical Principles of Optics

Before it is possible to understand the optical system of the eye, the student must first be thoroughly familiar with the basic principles of optics, including the physics of light refraction, focusing, depth of focus, and so forth. A brief review of these physical principles is presented; then the optics of the eye is discussed.

Refraction of Light

Refractive Index of a Transparent Substance. Light rays travel through air at a velocity of about 300,000 km/sec, but they travel much slower through transparent solids and liquids. The refractive index of a transparent substance is the *ratio* of the velocity of light in air to the velocity in the substance. The refractive index of air itself is 1.00. Thus, if light travels through a particular type of glass at a velocity of 200,000 km/sec, the refractive index of this glass is 300,000 divided by 200,000, or 1.50.

Refraction of Light Rays at an Interface Between Two Media with Different Refractive Indices. When light rays traveling forward in a beam (as shown in Figure 49-1A) strike an interface that is *perpendicular* to the beam, the rays enter the second medium without deviating from their course. The only effect that occurs is decreased velocity of transmission and shorter wavelength, as shown in the figure by the shorter distances between wave fronts.

If the light rays pass through an angulated interface as shown in Figure 49-1B, the rays bend if the refractive indices of the two media are different from each other. In this particular figure, the light rays are leaving air, which has a refractive index of 1.00, and are entering a block of glass having a refractive index of 1.50. When the beam first strikes the angulated interface, the lower edge of the beam enters the glass ahead of the upper edge. The wave front in the upper portion of the beam continues to travel at a velocity of 300,000 km/sec, while that which entered the glass travels at a velocity of 200,000 km/sec. This causes the upper portion of the wave front to move ahead of the lower portion so that the wave front is no longer vertical but angulated to the right. Because *the direction in which light travels is always perpendicular to the plane of the wave front,* the direction of travel of the light beam bends downward.

This bending of light rays at an angulated interface is known as *refraction.* Note particularly that the degree of refraction increases as a function of (1) the ratio of the two refractive indices of the two transparent media and (2) the degree of angulation between the interface and the entering wave front.

Application of Refractive Principles to Lenses

Convex Lens Focuses Light Rays. Figure 49-2 shows parallel light rays entering a convex lens. The light rays passing through the center of the lens strike the lens exactly perpendicular to the lens surface and, therefore, pass through the lens without being refracted. Toward either edge of the lens,

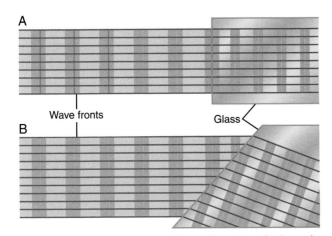

Figure 49-1 Light rays entering a glass surface perpendicular to the light rays (*A*) and a glass surface angulated to the light rays (*B*). This figure demonstrates that the distance between waves after they enter the glass is shortened to about two-thirds that in air. It also shows that light rays striking an angulated glass surface are bent.

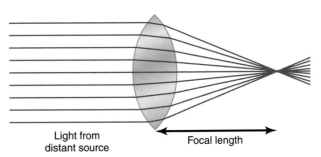

Figure 49-2 Bending of light rays at each surface of a convex spherical lens, showing that parallel light rays are focused to a *focal point.*

however, the light rays strike a progressively more angulated interface. The outer rays bend more and more toward the center, which is called *convergence* of the rays. Half the bending occurs when the rays enter the lens, and half as they exit from the opposite side. If the lens has exactly the proper curvature, parallel light rays passing through each part of the lens will be bent exactly enough so that all the rays will pass through a single point, which is called the *focal point*.

Concave Lens Diverges Light Rays. Figure 49-3 shows the effect of a concave lens on parallel light rays. The rays that enter the center of the lens strike an interface that is perpendicular to the beam and, therefore, do not refract. The rays at the edge of the lens enter the lens ahead of the rays in the center. This is opposite to the effect in the convex lens, and it causes the peripheral light rays to *diverge* from the light rays that pass through the center of the lens. Thus, the concave lens *diverges* light rays, but the convex lens *converges* light rays.

Cylindrical Lens Bends Light Rays in Only One Plane—Comparison with Spherical Lenses. Figure 49-4 shows both a convex *spherical* lens and a convex *cylindrical* lens. Note that the cylindrical lens bends light rays from the two sides of the lens but not from the top or the bottom. That is, bending occurs in one plane but not the other. Thus, parallel light rays are bent to a *focal line*. Conversely, light rays that pass through the spherical lens are refracted at all edges of the lens (in both planes) toward the central ray, and all the rays come to a *focal point*.

The cylindrical lens is well demonstrated by a test tube full of water. If the test tube is placed in a beam of sunlight and a piece of paper is brought progressively closer to the opposite side of the tube, a certain distance will be found at which the light rays come to a *focal line*. The spherical lens is demonstrated by an ordinary magnifying glass. If such a lens is placed in a beam of sunlight and a piece of paper is brought progressively closer to the lens, the light rays will impinge on a common focal point at an appropriate distance.

Concave cylindrical lenses *diverge* light rays in only one plane in the same manner that *convex* cylindrical lenses *converge* light rays in one plane.

Combination of Two Cylindrical Lenses at Right Angles Equals a Spherical Lens. Figure 49-5B shows two convex cylindrical lenses at right angles to each other. The vertical cylindrical lens converges the light rays that pass through the

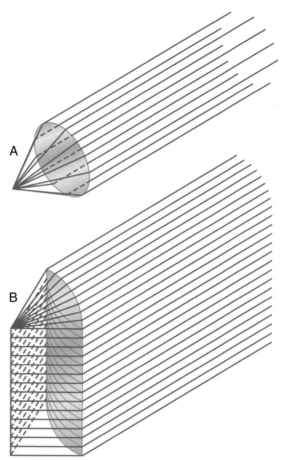

Figure 49-4 *A, Point focus* of parallel light rays by a spherical convex lens. *B, Line focus* of parallel light rays by a cylindrical convex lens.

two sides of the lens, and the horizontal lens converges the top and bottom rays. Thus, all the light rays come to a single-point focus. In other words, *two cylindrical lenses crossed at right angles to each other perform the same function as one spherical lens of the same refractive power.*

Focal Length of a Lens

The distance beyond a convex lens at which *parallel* rays converge to a common focal point is called the *focal length* of the lens. The diagram at the top of Figure 49-6 demonstrates this focusing of parallel light rays.

In the middle diagram, the light rays that enter the convex lens are not parallel but are *diverging* because the origin of the light is a point source not far away from the lens itself. Because these rays are diverging outward from the point source, it can be seen from the diagram that they do not focus at the same distance away from the lens as do parallel rays. In other words, when rays of light that are already diverging enter a convex lens, the distance of focus on the other side of the lens is farther from the lens than is the focal length of the lens for parallel rays.

The bottom diagram of Figure 49-6 shows light rays that are diverging toward a convex lens that has far greater curvature than that of the other two lenses in the figure. In this diagram, the distance from the lens at which the light rays come to focus is exactly the same as that from the lens in the first diagram, in which the lens is less convex but the rays entering it are parallel. This demonstrates that both parallel rays and

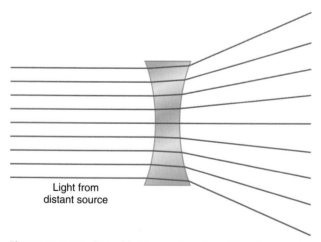

Light from
distant source

Figure 49-3 Bending of light rays at each surface of a concave spherical lens, showing that parallel light rays are *diverged*.

A

Line focus

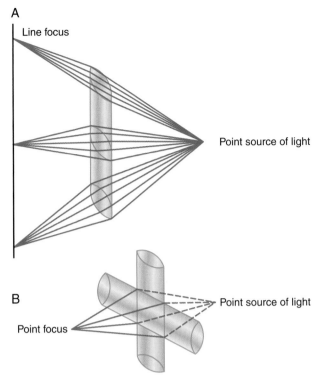

Point source of light

B

Point focus

Point source of light

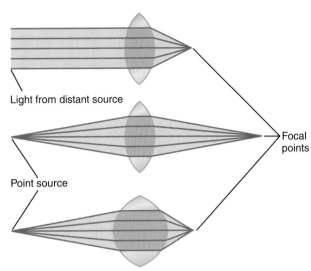

Light from distant source

Point source

Focal points

Figure 49-6 The two upper lenses of this figure have the same focal length, but the light rays entering the top lens are parallel, whereas those entering the middle lens are diverging; the effect of parallel versus diverging rays on the focal distance is shown. The bottom lens has far more refractive power than either of the other two lenses (i.e., has a much shorter focal length), demonstrating that the stronger the lens is, the nearer to the lens the point focus is.

Figure 49-5 *A,* Focusing of light from a point source to a line focus by a cylindrical lens. *B,* Two cylindrical convex lenses at right angles to each other, demonstrating that one lens converges light rays in one plane and the other lens converges light rays in the plane at a right angle. The two lenses combined give the same point focus as that obtained with a single spherical convex lens.

in which *f* is the focal length of the lens for parallel rays, *a* is the distance of the point source of light from the lens, and *b* is the distance of focus on the other side of the lens.

Formation of an Image by a Convex Lens

Figure 49-7*A* shows a convex lens with two point sources of light to the left. Because light rays pass through the center of a convex lens without being refracted in either direction, the light rays from each point source of light are shown to come to a point focus on the opposite side of the lens *directly in line with the point source and the center of the lens.*

Any object in front of the lens is, in reality, a mosaic of point sources of light. Some of these points are very bright,

diverging rays can be focused at the same distance beyond a lens, provided the lens changes its convexity.

The relation of focal length of the lens, distance of the point source of light, and distance of focus is expressed by the following formula:

$$\frac{1}{f} = \frac{1}{a} + \frac{1}{b}$$

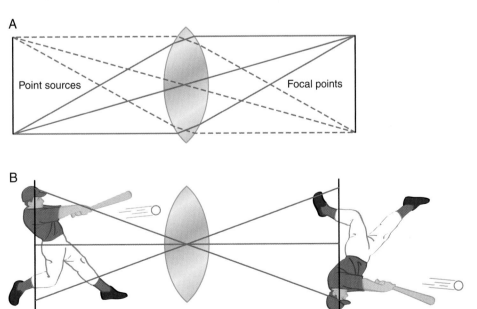

A

Point sources

Focal points

B

Figure 49-7 *A,* Two point sources of light focused at two separate points on opposite sides of the lens. *B,* Formation of an image by a convex spherical lens.

some are very weak, and they vary in color. Each point source of light on the object comes to a separate point focus on the opposite side of the lens in line with the lens center. If a white sheet of paper is placed at the focus distance from the lens, one can see an image of the object, as demonstrated in Figure 49-7B. However, this image is upside down with respect to the original object, and the two lateral sides of the image are reversed. This is the method by which the lens of a camera focuses images on film.

Measurement of the Refractive Power of a Lens—"Diopter"

The more a lens bends light rays, the greater is its "refractive power." This refractive power is measured in terms of *diopters*. The refractive power in diopters of a convex lens is equal to 1 meter divided by its focal length. Thus, a spherical lens that converges parallel light rays to a focal point 1 meter beyond the lens has a refractive power of +1 diopter, as shown in Figure 49-8. If the lens is capable of bending parallel light rays twice as much as a lens with a power of +1 diopter, it is said to have a strength of +2 diopters, and the light rays come to a focal point 0.5 meter beyond the lens. A lens capable of converging parallel light rays to a focal point only 10 centimeters (0.10 meter) beyond the lens has a refractive power of +10 diopters.

The refractive power of concave lenses cannot be stated in terms of the focal distance beyond the lens because the light rays diverge, rather than focus to a point. However, if a concave lens diverges light rays at the same rate that a 1-diopter convex lens converges them, the concave lens is said to have a dioptric strength of –1. Likewise, if the concave lens diverges light rays as much as a +10-diopter lens converges them, this lens is said to have a strength of –10 diopters.

Concave lenses "neutralize" the refractive power of convex lenses. Thus, placing a 1-diopter concave lens immediately in front of a 1-diopter convex lens results in a lens system with zero refractive power.

The strengths of cylindrical lenses are computed in the same manner as the strengths of spherical lenses, except that the *axis* of the cylindrical lens must be stated in addition to its strength. If a cylindrical lens focuses parallel light rays to a line focus 1 meter beyond the lens, it has a strength of +1 diopter. Conversely, if a cylindrical lens of a concave type *diverges* light rays as much as a +1-diopter cylindrical lens *converges* them, it has a strength of –1 diopter. If the focused line is horizontal, its axis is said to be 0 degrees. If it is vertical, its axis is 90 degrees.

Optics of the Eye

The Eye as a Camera

The eye, shown in Figure 49-9, is optically equivalent to the usual photographic camera. It has a lens system, a variable aperture system (the pupil), and a retina that corresponds to the film. The lens system of the eye is composed of four refractive interfaces: (1) the interface between air and the anterior surface of the cornea, (2) the interface between the posterior surface of the cornea and the aqueous humor, (3) the interface between the aqueous humor and the anterior surface of the lens of the eye, and (4) the interface between the posterior surface of the lens and the vitreous humor. The internal index of air is 1; the cornea, 1.38; the aqueous humor, 1.33; the crystalline lens (on average), 1.40; and the vitreous humor, 1.34.

Consideration of All Refractive Surfaces of the Eye as a Single Lens—The "Reduced" Eye. If all the refractive surfaces of the eye are algebraically added together and then considered to be one single lens, the optics of the normal eye may be simplified and represented schematically as a "reduced eye." This is useful in simple calculations. In the reduced eye, a single refractive surface is considered to exist, with its central point 17 millimeters in front of the retina and a total refractive power of 59 diopters when the lens is accommodated for distant vision.

About two thirds of the 59 diopters of refractive power of the eye is provided by the anterior surface of the cornea (*not* by the eye lens). The principal reason for this is that the refractive index of the cornea is markedly different from that of air, whereas the refractive index of the eye lens is not greatly different from the indices of the aqueous humor and vitreous humor.

The total refractive power of the internal lens of the eye, as it normally lies in the eye surrounded by fluid on each side, is only 20 diopters, about one-third the total refractive power of the eye. But the importance of the internal lens is that, in response to nervous signals from the brain, *its curvature can be increased* markedly to provide "accommodation," which is discussed later in the chapter.

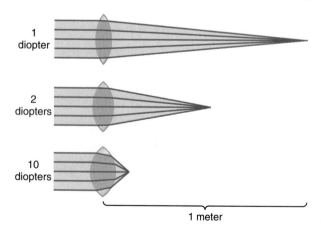

1 diopter

2 diopters

10 diopters

1 meter

Figure 49-8 Effect of lens strength on the focal distance.

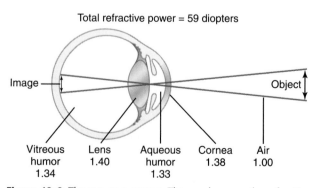

Total refractive power = 59 diopters

Image

Object

Vitreous humor 1.34

Lens 1.40

Aqueous humor 1.33

Cornea 1.38

Air 1.00

Figure 49-9 The eye as a camera. The numbers are the refractive indices.

Formation of an Image on the Retina. In the same manner that a glass lens can focus an image on a sheet of paper, the lens system of the eye can focus an image on the retina. The image is inverted and reversed with respect to the object. However, the mind perceives objects in the upright position despite the upside-down orientation on the retina because the brain is trained to consider an inverted image as normal.

Mechanism of "Accommodation"

In children, the refractive power of the lens of the eye can be increased voluntarily from 20 diopters to about 34 diopters; this in an "accommodation" of 14 diopters. To do this, the shape of the lens is changed from that of a moderately convex lens to that of a very convex lens. The mechanism is as follows.

In a young person, the lens is composed of a strong elastic capsule filled with viscous, proteinaceous, but transparent fluid. When the lens is in a relaxed state with no tension on its capsule, it assumes an almost spherical shape, owing mainly to the elastic retraction of the lens capsule. However, as shown in Figure 49-10, about 70 *suspensory ligaments* attach radially around the lens, pulling the lens edges toward the outer circle of the eyeball. These ligaments are constantly tensed by their attachments at the anterior border of the choroid and retina. The tension on the ligaments causes the lens to remain relatively flat under normal conditions of the eye.

However, also located at the lateral attachments of the lens ligaments to the eyeball is the *ciliary muscle,* which itself has two separate sets of smooth muscle fibers—*meridional fibers* and *circular fibers.* The meridional fibers extend from the peripheral ends of the suspensory ligaments to the corneoscleral junction. When these muscle fibers contract, the *peripheral insertions* of the lens ligaments are pulled medially toward the edges of the cornea,

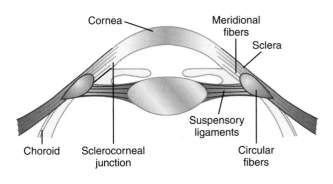

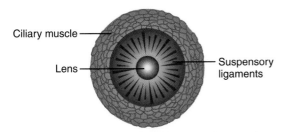

Figure 49-10 Mechanism of accommodation (focusing).

Labels: Cornea; Meridional fibers; Sclera; Suspensory ligaments; Choroid; Sclerocorneal junction; Circular fibers; Ciliary muscle; Lens; Suspensory ligaments

thereby releasing the ligaments' tension on the lens. The circular fibers are arranged circularly all the way around the ligament attachments so that when they contract, a sphincter-like action occurs, decreasing the diameter of the circle of ligament attachments; this also allows the ligaments to pull less on the lens capsule.

Thus, contraction of either set of smooth muscle fibers in the ciliary muscle relaxes the ligaments to the lens capsule, and the lens assumes a more spherical shape, like that of a balloon, because of the natural elasticity of the lens capsule.

Accommodation Is Controlled by Parasympathetic Nerves. The ciliary muscle is controlled almost entirely by parasympathetic nerve signals transmitted to the eye through the third cranial nerve from the third nerve nucleus in the brain stem, as explained in Chapter 51. Stimulation of the parasympathetic nerves contracts both sets of ciliary muscle fibers, which relaxes the lens ligaments, thus allowing the lens to become thicker and increase its refractive power. With this increased refractive power, the eye focuses on objects nearer than when the eye has less refractive power. Consequently, as a distant object moves toward the eye, the number of parasympathetic impulses impinging on the ciliary muscle must be progressively increased for the eye to keep the object constantly in focus. (Sympathetic stimulation has an additional effect in relaxing the ciliary muscle, but this effect is so weak that it plays almost no role in the normal accommodation mechanism; the neurology of this is discussed in Chapter 51.)

Presbyopia—Loss of Accommodation by the Lens. As a person grows older, the lens grows larger and thicker and becomes far less elastic, partly because of progressive denaturation of the lens proteins. The ability of the lens to change shape decreases with age. The power of accommodation decreases from about 14 diopters in a child to less than 2 diopters by the time a person reaches 45 to 50 years; it then decreases to essentially 0 diopters at age 70 years. Thereafter, the lens remains almost totally nonaccommodating, a condition known as "presbyopia."

Once a person has reached the state of presbyopia, each eye remains focused permanently at an almost constant distance; this distance depends on the physical characteristics of each person's eyes. The eyes can no longer accommodate for both near and far vision. To see clearly both in the distance and nearby, an older person must wear bifocal glasses with the upper segment focused for far-seeing and the lower segment focused for near-seeing (e.g., for reading).

Pupillary Diameter

The major function of the iris is to increase the amount of light that enters the eye during darkness and to decrease the amount of light that enters the eye in daylight. The reflexes for controlling this mechanism are considered in the discussion of the neurology of the eye in Chapter 51.

The amount of light that enters the eye through the pupil is proportional to the *area* of the pupil or to the *square of the diameter* of the pupil. The pupil of the human eye can become as small as about 1.5 millimeters and as large as 8 millimeters in diameter. The quantity of light entering the eye can change about 30-fold as a result of changes in pupillary aperture.

"Depth of Focus" of the Lens System Increases with Decreasing Pupillary Diameter. Figure 49-11 shows two eyes that are exactly alike except for the diameters of the pupillary apertures. In the upper eye, the pupillary aperture is small, and in the lower eye, the aperture is large. In front of each of these two eyes are two small point sources of light; light from each passes through the pupillary aperture and focuses on the retina. Consequently, in both eyes, the retina sees two spots of light in perfect focus. It is evident from the diagrams, however, that if the retina is moved forward or backward to an out-of-focus position, the size of each spot will not change much in the upper eye, but in the lower eye the size of each spot will increase greatly, becoming a "blur circle." In other words, the upper lens system has far greater *depth of focus* than the bottom lens system. When a lens system has great depth of focus, the retina can be displaced considerably from the focal plane or the lens strength can change considerably from normal and the image will still remain nearly in sharp focus, whereas when a lens system has a "shallow" depth of focus, moving the retina only slightly away from the focal plane causes extreme blurring.

The greatest possible depth of focus occurs when the pupil is extremely small. The reason for this is that, with a very small aperture, almost all the rays pass through the center of the lens, and the central-most rays are always in focus, as explained earlier.

Errors of Refraction

Emmetropia (Normal Vision). As shown in Figure 49-12, the eye is considered to be normal, or "emmetropic," if parallel light rays *from distant objects* are in sharp focus on the retina

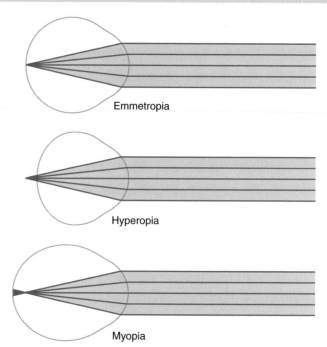

Figure 49-12 Parallel light rays focus on the retina in emmetropia, behind the retina in hyperopia, and in front of the retina in myopia.

when the ciliary muscle is completely relaxed. This means that the emmetropic eye can see all distant objects clearly with its ciliary muscle relaxed. However, to focus objects at close range, the eye must contract its ciliary muscle and thereby provide appropriate degrees of accommodation.

Hyperopia (Farsightedness). Hyperopia, which is also known as "farsightedness," is usually due to either an eyeball that is too short or, occasionally, a lens system that is too weak. In this condition, as seen in the middle panel of Figure 49-12, parallel light rays are not bent sufficiently by the relaxed lens system to come to focus by the time they reach the retina. To overcome this abnormality, the ciliary muscle must contract to increase the strength of the lens. By using the mechanism of accommodation, a farsighted person is capable of focusing distant objects on the retina. If the person has used only a small amount of strength in the ciliary muscle to accommodate for the distant objects, he or she still has much accommodative power left, and objects closer and closer to the eye can also be focused sharply until the ciliary muscle has contracted to its limit. In old age, when the lens becomes "presbyopic," a farsighted person is often unable to accommodate the lens sufficiently to focus even distant objects, much less near objects.

Myopia (Nearsightedness). In myopia, or "nearsightedness," when the ciliary muscle is completely relaxed, the light rays coming from distant objects are focused in front of the retina, as shown in the bottom panel of Figure 49-12. This is usually due to too long an eyeball, but it can result from too much refractive power in the lens system of the eye.

No mechanism exists by which the eye can decrease the strength of its lens to less than that which exists when the ciliary muscle is completely relaxed. A myopic person has no mechanism by which to focus distant objects sharply on the retina. However, as an object moves nearer to the person's eye, it finally gets close enough that its image can be focused. Then, when the object comes still closer to the eye,

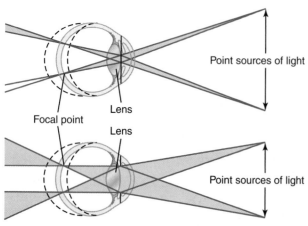

Point sources of light

Lens

Focal point

Lens

Point sources of light

Figure 49-11 Effect of small (*top*) and large (*bottom*) pupillary apertures on "depth of focus."

the person can use the mechanism of accommodation to keep the image focused clearly. A myopic person has a definite limiting "far point" for clear vision.

Correction of Myopia and Hyperopia by Use of Lenses. It will be recalled that light rays passing through a concave lens diverge. If the refractive surfaces of the eye have too much refractive power, as in *myopia,* this excessive refractive power can be neutralized by placing in front of the eye a concave spherical lens, which will diverge rays. Such correction is demonstrated in the upper diagram of Figure 49-13.

Conversely, in a person who has *hyperopia*—that is, someone who has too weak a lens system—the abnormal vision can be corrected by adding refractive power using a convex lens in front of the eye. This correction is demonstrated in the lower diagram of Figure 49-13.

One usually determines the strength of the concave or convex lens needed for clear vision by "trial and error"—that is, by trying first a strong lens and then a stronger or weaker lens until the one that gives the best visual acuity is found.

Astigmatism. Astigmatism is a refractive error of the eye that causes the visual image in one plane to focus at a different distance from that of the plane at right angles. This most often results from too great a curvature of the cornea in one plane of the eye. An example of an astigmatic lens would be a lens surface like that of an egg lying sidewise to the incoming light. The degree of curvature in the plane through the long axis of the egg is not nearly as great as the degree of curvature in the plane through the short axis.

Because the curvature of the astigmatic lens along one plane is less than the curvature along the other plane, light rays striking the peripheral portions of the lens in one plane are not bent nearly as much as the rays striking the peripheral portions of the other plane. This is demonstrated in Figure 49-14, which shows rays of light originating from a point source and passing through an oblong, astigmatic lens. The light rays in the vertical plane, indicated by plane BD, are refracted greatly by the astigmatic lens because of the greater curvature in the vertical direction than in the horizontal direction. By contrast, the light rays in the horizontal plane, indicated by plane AC,

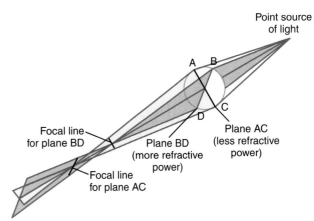

Figure 49-14 Astigmatism, demonstrating that light rays focus at one focal distance in one focal plane (*plane AC*) and at another focal distance in the plane at a right angle (*plane BD*).

are not bent nearly as much as the light rays in vertical plane BD. It is obvious that light rays passing through an astigmatic lens do not all come to a common focal point because the light rays passing through one plane focus far in front of those passing through the other plane.

The accommodative power of the eye can never compensate for astigmatism because, during accommodation, the curvature of the eye lens changes approximately equally in both planes; therefore, in astigmatism, each of the two planes requires a different degree of accommodation. Thus, without the aid of glasses, a person with astigmatism never sees in sharp focus.

Correction of Astigmatism with a Cylindrical Lens. One may consider an astigmatic eye as having a lens system made up of two cylindrical lenses of different strengths and placed at right angles to each other. To correct for astigmatism, the usual procedure is to find a spherical lens by trial and error that corrects the focus in one of the two planes of the astigmatic lens. Then an additional cylindrical lens is used to correct the remaining error in the remaining plane. To do this, both the *axis* and the *strength* of the required cylindrical lens must be determined.

Several methods exist for determining the axis of the abnormal cylindrical component of the lens system of an eye. One of these methods is based on the use of parallel black bars of the type shown in Figure 49-15. Some of these parallel bars are vertical, some horizontal, and some at various angles to the vertical and horizontal axes. After placing various spherical lenses in front of the astigmatic eye, a strength of lens that causes sharp focus of one set of parallel bars but does not correct the fuzziness of the set of bars at right angles to the sharp bars is usually found. It can be shown from the physical principles of optics discussed earlier in this chapter that the *axis* of the *out-of-focus* cylindrical component of the optical system is parallel to the bars that are fuzzy. Once this axis is found, the examiner tries progressively stronger and weaker positive or negative *cylindrical* lenses, the axes of which are placed in line with the out-of-focus bars, until the patient sees all the crossed bars with equal clarity. When this has been accomplished, the examiner directs the optician to grind a special lens combining both the spherical correction and the cylindrical correction at the appropriate axis.

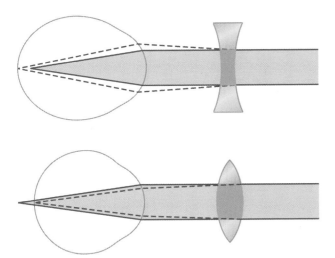

Figure 49-13 Correction of myopia with a concave lens, and correction of hyperopia with a convex lens.

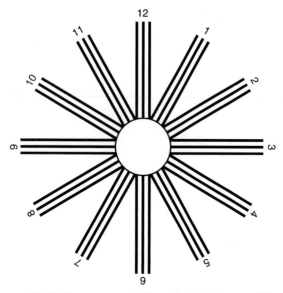

Figure 49-15 Chart composed of parallel black bars at different angular orientations for determining the axis of astigmatism.

Correction of Optical Abnormalities by Use of Contact Lenses

Glass or plastic contact lenses that fit snugly against the anterior surface of the cornea can be inserted. These lenses are held in place by a thin layer of tear fluid that fills the space between the contact lens and the anterior eye surface.

A special feature of the contact lens is that it nullifies almost entirely the refraction that normally occurs at the anterior surface of the cornea. The reason for this is that the tears between the contact lens and the cornea have a refractive index almost equal to that of the cornea, so the anterior surface of the cornea no longer plays a significant role in the eye's optical system. Instead, the outer surface of the contact lens plays the major role. Thus, the refraction of this surface of the contact lens substitutes for the cornea's usual refraction. This is especially important in people whose eye refractive errors are caused by an abnormally shaped cornea, such as those who have an odd-shaped, bulging cornea—a condition called *keratoconus.* Without the contact lens, the bulging cornea causes such severe abnormality of vision that almost no glasses can correct the vision satisfactorily; when a contact lens is used, however, the corneal refraction is neutralized and normal refraction by the outer surface of the contact lens is substituted.

The contact lens has several other advantages as well, including (1) the lens turns with the eye and gives a broader field of clear vision than glasses do, and (2) the contact lens has little effect on the size of the object the person sees through the lens, whereas lenses placed 1 centimeter or so in front of the eye do affect the size of the image, in addition to correcting the focus.

Cataracts—Opaque Areas in the Lens

"Cataracts" are an especially common eye abnormality that occurs mainly in older people. A cataract is a cloudy or opaque area or areas in the lens. In the early stage of cataract formation, the proteins in some of the lens fibers become denatured. Later, these same proteins coagulate to form opaque areas in place of the normal transparent protein fibers.

When a cataract has obscured light transmission so greatly that it seriously impairs vision, the condition can be corrected by surgical removal of the lens. When this is done, the eye loses a large portion of its refractive power, which must be replaced by a powerful convex lens in front of the eye; usually, however, an artificial plastic lens is implanted in the eye in place of the removed lens.

Visual Acuity

Theoretically, light from a distant point source, when focused on the retina, should be infinitely small. However, because the lens system of the eye is never perfect, such a retinal spot ordinarily has a total diameter of about 11 micrometers, even with maximal resolution of the normal eye optical system. The spot is brightest in its center and shades off gradually toward the edges, as shown by the two-point images in Figure 49-16.

The average diameter of the cones in the *fovea* of the retina—the central part of the retina, where vision is most highly developed—is about 1.5 micrometers, which is one-seventh the diameter of the spot of light. Nevertheless, because the spot of light has a bright center point and shaded edges, a person can normally distinguish two separate points if their centers lie up to 2 micrometers apart on the retina, which is slightly greater than the width of a foveal cone. This discrimination between points is also shown in Figure 49-16.

The normal visual acuity of the human eye for discriminating between point sources of light is about 25 seconds of arc. That is, when light rays from two separate points strike the eye with an angle of at least 25 seconds between them, they can usually be recognized as two points instead of one. This means that a person with normal visual acuity looking at two bright pinpoint spots of light 10 meters away can barely distinguish the spots as separate entities when they are 1.5 to 2 millimeters apart.

The fovea is less than 0.5 millimeter (<500 micrometers) in diameter, which means that maximum visual acuity occurs in less than 2 degrees of the visual field. Outside this foveal area, the visual acuity becomes progressively poorer, decreasing more than 10-fold as the periphery is approached. This is caused by the connection of more and more rods and cones to each optic nerve fiber in the

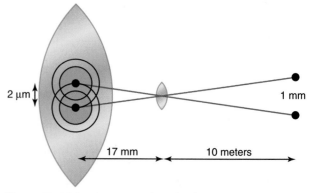

Figure 49-16 Maximum visual acuity for two-point sources of light.

nonfoveal, more peripheral parts of the retina, as discussed in Chapter 51.

Clinical Method for Stating Visual Acuity. The chart for testing eyes usually consists of letters of different sizes placed 20 feet away from the person being tested. If the person can see well the letters of a size that he or she should be able to see at 20 feet, the person is said to have 20/20 vision—that is, normal vision. If the person can see only letters that he or she should be able to see at 200 feet, the person is said to have 20/200 vision. In other words, the clinical method for expressing visual acuity is to use a mathematical fraction that expresses the ratio of two distances, which is also the ratio of one's visual acuity to that of a person with normal visual acuity.

Determination of Distance of an Object from the Eye—"Depth Perception"

A person normally perceives distance by three major means: (1) the sizes of the images of known objects on the retina, (2) the phenomenon of moving parallax, and (3) the phenomenon of stereopsis. This ability to determine distance is called *depth perception.*

Determination of Distance by Sizes of Retinal Images of Known Objects. If one knows that a person being viewed is 6 feet tall, one can determine how far away the person is simply by the size of the person's image on the retina. One does not consciously think about the size, but the brain has learned to calculate automatically from image sizes the distances of objects when the dimensions are known.

Determination of Distance by Moving Parallax. Another important means by which the eyes determine distance is that of moving parallax. If an individual looks off into the distance with the eyes completely still, he or she perceives no moving parallax, but when the person moves his or her head to one side or the other, the images of close-by objects move rapidly across the retinas, while the images of distant objects remain almost completely stationary. For instance, by moving the head 1 inch to the side when the object is only 1 inch in front of the eye, the image moves almost all the way across the retinas, whereas the image of an object 200 feet away from the eyes does not move perceptibly. Thus, by using this mechanism of moving parallax, one can tell the *relative distances* of different objects even though only one eye is used.

Determination of Distance by Stereopsis—Binocular Vision. Another method by which one perceives parallax is that of "binocular vision." Because one eye is a little more than 2 inches to one side of the other eye, the images on the two retinas are different from each other. For instance, an object 1 inch in front of the nose forms an image on the left side of the retina of the left eye but on the right side of the retina of the right eye, whereas

a small object 20 feet in front of the nose has its image at closely corresponding points in the centers of the two retinas. This type of parallax is demonstrated in Figure 49-17, which shows the images of a red spot and a yellow square actually reversed on the two retinas because they are at different distances in front of the eyes. This gives a type of parallax that is present all the time when both eyes are being used. It is almost entirely this binocular parallax (or *stereopsis*) that gives a person with two eyes far greater ability to judge relative distances *when objects are nearby* than a person who has only one eye. However, stereopsis is virtually useless for depth perception at distances beyond 50 to 200 feet.

Ophthalmoscope

The ophthalmoscope is an instrument through which an observer can look into another person's eye and see the retina with clarity. Although the ophthalmoscope appears to be a relatively complicated instrument, its principles are simple. The basic components are shown in Figure 49-18 and can be explained as follows.

If a bright spot of light is on the retina of an *emmetropic eye,* light rays from this spot diverge toward the lens system of the eye. After passing through the lens system, they are parallel with one another because the retina is located one focal length distance behind the lens system. Then, when

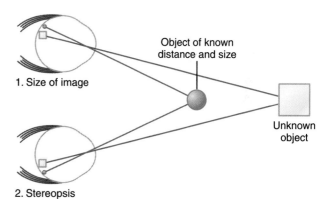

Figure 49-17 Perception of distance (*1*) by the size of the image on the retina and (*2*) as a result of stereopsis.

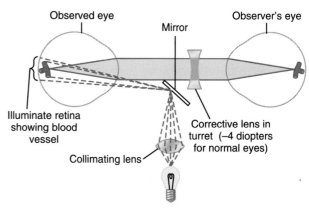

Figure 49-18 Optical system of the ophthalmoscope.

these parallel rays pass into an emmetropic eye of another person, they focus again to a point focus on the retina of the second person, because his or her retina is also one focal length distance behind the lens. Any spot of light on the retina of the observed eye projects to a focal spot on the retina of the observing eye. Thus, if the retina of one person is made to emit light, the image of his or her retina will be focused on the retina of the observer, provided the two eyes are emmetropic and are simply looking into each other.

To make an ophthalmoscope, one need only devise a means for illuminating the retina to be examined. Then, the reflected light from that retina can be seen by the observer simply by putting the two eyes close to each other. To illuminate the retina of the observed eye, an angulated mirror or a segment of a prism is placed in front of the observed eye in such a manner, as shown in Figure 49-18, that light from a bulb is reflected into the observed eye. Thus, the retina is illuminated through the pupil, and the observer sees into the subject's pupil by looking over the edge of the mirror or prism or *through* an appropriately designed prism.

It is clear that these principles apply only to people with completely emmetropic eyes. If the refractive power of either the observed eye or the observer's eye is abnormal, it is necessary to correct the refractive power for the observer to see a sharp image of the observed retina. The usual ophthalmoscope has a series of very small lenses mounted on a turret so that the turret can be rotated from one lens to another until the correction for abnormal refraction is made by selecting a lens of appropriate strength. In normal young adults, natural accommodative reflexes occur, causing an approximate +2-diopter increase in strength of the lens of each eye. To correct for this, it is necessary that the lens turret be rotated to approximately –4-diopter correction.

Fluid System of the Eye—Intraocular Fluid

The eye is filled with *intraocular fluid,* which maintains sufficient pressure in the eyeball to keep it distended. Figure 49-19 demonstrates that this fluid can be divided into two portions—*aqueous humor,* which lies in front of the lens, and *vitreous humor,* which is between the posterior surface of the lens and the retina. The aqueous humor is a freely flowing fluid, whereas the vitreous humor, sometimes called the *vitreous body,* is a gelatinous mass held together by a fine fibrillar network composed primarily of greatly elongated proteoglycan molecules. Both water and dissolved substances can *diffuse* slowly in the vitreous humor, but there is little *flow* of fluid.

Aqueous humor is continually being formed and reabsorbed. The balance between formation and reabsorption of aqueous humor regulates the total volume and pressure of the intraocular fluid.

Formation of Aqueous Humor by the Ciliary Body

Aqueous humor is formed in the eye *at an average rate of 2 to 3 microliters each minute.* Essentially all of it is secreted by the *ciliary processes,* which are linear folds projecting from the *ciliary body* into the space behind the iris where the lens ligaments and ciliary muscle attach to the eyeball. A cross section of these ciliary processes is shown in Figure 49-20, and their relation to the fluid chambers of the eye can be seen in Figure 49-19. Because of their folded architecture, the total surface area of the ciliary processes is about 6 square centimeters in each eye—a large area, considering the small size of the ciliary body. The surfaces of these processes are covered by highly secretory epithelial cells, and immediately beneath them is a highly vascular area.

Aqueous humor is formed almost entirely as an active secretion by the epithelium of the ciliary processes. Secretion begins with active transport of sodium ions into the spaces between the epithelial cells. The sodium ions pull chloride and bicarbonate ions along with them to maintain electrical neutrality. Then all these ions together cause osmosis of water from the blood capillaries lying below into the same epithelial intercellular spaces, and the resulting solution washes from the spaces of the ciliary processes into the anterior chamber of the eye. In addition, several nutrients are transported across the epithelium by active transport or facilitated diffusion; they include amino acids, ascorbic acid, and glucose.

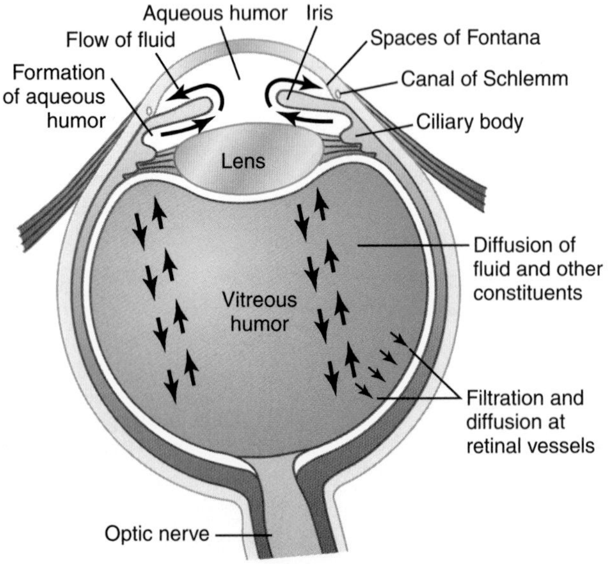

Figure 49-19 Formation and flow of fluid in the eye.

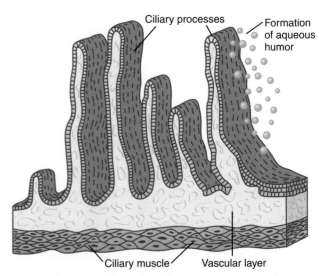

Figure 49-20 Anatomy of the ciliary processes. Aqueous humor is formed on surfaces.

Outflow of Aqueous Humor from the Eye

After aqueous humor is formed by the ciliary processes, it first flows, as shown in Figure 49-19, *through the pupil into the anterior chamber of the eye.* From here, the fluid flows *anterior to the lens and* into the *angle between the cornea and the iris,* then through a meshwork of *trabeculae,* finally entering the *canal of Schlemm,* which empties into extraocular veins. Figure 49-21 demonstrates the anatomical structures at this iridocorneal angle, showing that the spaces between the trabeculae extend all the way from the anterior chamber to the canal of Schlemm. The canal of Schlemm is a thin-walled vein that extends circumferentially all the way around the eye. Its endothelial membrane is so porous that even large protein molecules, as well as small particulate matter up to the size of red blood cells, can pass from the anterior chamber into the canal of Schlemm. Even though the canal of Schlemm is actually a venous blood vessel, so much aqueous humor normally flows into it that it is filled only with aqueous humor rather than with blood. The small veins that lead from the canal of Schlemm to the larger veins of the eye usually contain only aqueous humor, and they are called *aqueous veins.*

Intraocular Pressure

The average normal intraocular pressure is about 15 mm Hg, with a range from 12 to 20 mm Hg.

Tonometry. Because it is impractical to pass a needle into a patient's eye to measure intraocular pressure, this pressure is measured clinically by using a "tonometer," the principle of which is shown in Figure 49-22. The cornea of the eye is anesthetized with a local anesthetic, and the footplate of the tonometer is placed on the cornea. A small force is then applied to a central plunger, causing the part of the cornea beneath the plunger to be displaced inward. The amount of displacement is recorded on the scale of the tonometer, and this is calibrated in terms of intraocular pressure.

Regulation of Intraocular Pressure. Intraocular pressure remains constant in the normal eye, usually within ±2 mm Hg of its normal level, which averages about 15 mm Hg. The level of this pressure is determined mainly by the resistance to

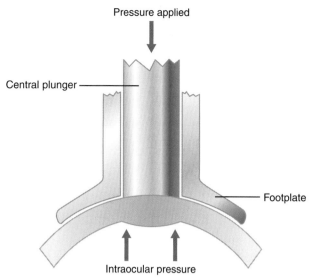

Figure 49-22   Principles of the tonometer.

outflow of aqueous humor from the anterior chamber into the canal of Schlemm. This outflow resistance results from the meshwork of trabeculae through which the fluid must percolate on its way from the lateral angles of the anterior chamber to the wall of the canal of Schlemm. These trabeculae have minute openings of only 2 to 3 micrometers. The rate of fluid flow into the canal increases markedly as the pressure rises. At about 15 mm Hg in the normal eye, the amount of fluid leaving the eye by way of the canal of Schlemm usually averages 2.5 μl/min and equals the inflow of fluid from the ciliary body. The pressure normally remains at about this level of 15 mm Hg.

Mechanism for Cleansing the Trabecular Spaces and Intraocular Fluid. When large amounts of debris are present in the aqueous humor, as occurs after hemorrhage into the eye or during intraocular infection, the debris is likely to accumulate in the trabecular spaces leading from the anterior chamber to the canal of Schlemm; this debris can prevent adequate reabsorption of fluid from the anterior chamber, sometimes causing "glaucoma," as explained subsequently. However, on the surfaces of the trabecular plates are large numbers of phagocytic cells. Immediately outside the canal of Schlemm is a layer of interstitial gel that contains large numbers of reticuloendothelial cells that have an extremely high capacity for engulfing debris and digesting it into small molecular substances that can then be absorbed. Thus, this phagocytic system keeps the trabecular spaces cleaned. The surface of the iris and other surfaces of the eye behind the iris are covered with an epithelium that is capable of phagocytizing proteins and small particles from the aqueous humor, thereby helping to maintain a clear fluid.

"Glaucoma"—a Principal Cause of Blindness. Glaucoma is one of the most common causes of blindness. It is a disease of the eye in which the intraocular pressure becomes pathologically high, sometimes rising acutely to 60 to 70 mm Hg. Pressures above 25 to 30 mm Hg can cause loss of vision when maintained for long periods. Extremely high pressures can cause blindness within days or even hours. As the pressure rises, the axons of the optic nerve are compressed where they leave the eyeball at the optic disc. This compression is believed to block axonal flow of cytoplasm from the retinal neuronal cell bodies into the optic nerve fibers leading to the brain. The result is lack of appropriate nutrition of the fibers,

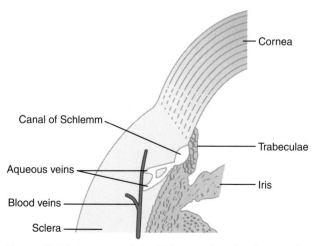

Figure 49-21 Anatomy of the iridocorneal angle, showing the system for outflow of aqueous humor from the eyeball into the conjunctival veins.

which eventually causes death of the involved fibers. It is possible that compression of the retinal artery, which enters the eyeball at the optic disc, also adds to the neuronal damage by reducing nutrition to the retina.

In most cases of glaucoma, the abnormally high pressure results from increased resistance to fluid outflow through the trabecular spaces into the canal of Schlemm at the iridocorneal junction. For instance, in acute eye inflammation, white blood cells and tissue debris can block these trabecular spaces and cause an acute increase in intraocular pressure. In chronic conditions, especially in older individuals, fibrous occlusion of the trabecular spaces appears to be the likely culprit.

Glaucoma can sometimes be treated by placing drops in the eye that contain a drug that diffuses into the eyeball and reduces the secretion or increases the absorption of aqueous humor. When drug therapy fails, operative techniques to open the spaces of the trabeculae or to make channels to allow fluid to flow directly from the fluid space of the eyeball into the subconjunctival space outside the eyeball can often effectively reduce the pressure.

Bibliography

Buisseret P: Influence of extraocular muscle proprioception on vision, *Physiol Rev* 75:323, 1995.

Buznego C, Trattler WB: Presbyopia-correcting intraocular lenses, *Curr Opin Ophthalmol* 20:13, 2009.

Candia OA, Alvarez LJ: Fluid transport phenomena in ocular epithelia, *Prog Retin Eye Res* 27:197, 2008.

Congdon NG, Friedman DS, Lietman T: Important causes of visual impairment in the world today, *JAMA* 290:2057, 2003.

Doane JF: Accommodating intraocular lenses, *Curr Opin Ophthalmol* 15:16, 2004.

Khaw PT, Shah P, Elkington AR: Glaucoma-1: diagnosis, *BMJ* 328:97, 2004.

Krag S, Andreassen TT: Mechanical properties of the human lens capsule, *Prog Retin Eye Res* 22:749, 2003.

Kwon YH, Fingert JH, Kuehn MH, et al: Primary open-angle glaucoma, *N Engl J Med* 360:1113, 2009.

Mathias RT, Rae JL, Baldo GJ: Physiological properties of the normal lens, *Physiol Rev* 77:21, 1997.

Sakimoto T, Rosenblatt MI, Azar DT: Laser eye surgery for refractive errors, *Lancet* 367:1432, 2006.

Schaeffel F, Simon P, Feldkaemper M, et al: Molecular biology of myopia, *Clin Exp Optom* 86:295, 2003.

Schwartz K, Budenz D: Current management of glaucoma, *Curr Opin Ophthalmol* 15:119, 2004.

Smith G: The optical properties of the crystalline lens and their significance, *Clin Exp Optom* 86:3, 2003.

Tan JC, Peters DM, Kaufman PL: Recent developments in understanding the pathophysiology of elevated intraocular pressure, *Curr Opin Ophthalmol* 17:168, 2006.

Weber AJ, Harman CD, Viswanathan S: Effects of optic nerve injury, glaucoma, and neuroprotection on the survival, structure, and function of ganglion cells in the mammalian retina, *J Physiol* 586:4393, 2008.

Weinreb RN, Khaw PT: Primary open-angle glaucoma, *Lancet* 363:1711, 2004.

The Eye: II. Receptor and Neural Function of the Retina

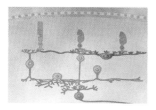

The retina is the light-sensitive portion of the eye that contains (1) the *cones,* which are responsible for color vision, and (2) the *rods,* which can detect dim light and are mainly responsible for black and white vision and vision in the dark. When either rods or cones are excited, signals are transmitted first through successive layers of neurons in the retina and, finally, into optic nerve fibers and the cerebral cortex. The purpose of this chapter is to explain the mechanisms by which the rods and cones detect light and color and convert the visual image into optic nerve signals.

Anatomy and Function of the Structural Elements of the Retina

Layers of the Retina. Figure 50-1 shows the functional components of the retina, which are arranged in layers from the outside to the inside as follows: (1) pigmented layer, (2) layer of rods and cones projecting to the pigment, (3) outer nuclear layer containing the cell bodies of the rods and cones, (4) outer plexiform layer, (5) inner nuclear layer, (6) inner plexiform layer, (7) ganglionic layer, (8) layer of optic nerve fibers, and (9) inner limiting membrane.

After light passes through the lens system of the eye and then through the vitreous humor, it *enters the retina from the inside of the eye* (see Figure 50-1); that is, it passes first through the ganglion cells and then through the plexiform and nuclear layers before it finally reaches the layer of rods and cones located all the way on the outer edge of the retina. This distance is a thickness of several hundred micrometers; visual acuity is decreased by this passage through such non-homogeneous tissue. However, in the *central foveal region of the retina,* as discussed subsequently, the inside layers are pulled aside to decrease this loss of acuity.

Foveal Region of the Retina and Its Importance in Acute Vision. The *fovea* is a minute area in the center of the retina, shown in Figure 50-2, occupying a total area a little more than 1 square millimeter; it is especially capable of acute and detailed vision. The *central fovea,* only 0.3 millimeter in diameter, is composed almost entirely of cones; these cones have a special structure that aids their detection of detail in

the visual image. That is, the foveal cones have especially long and slender bodies, in contradistinction to the much fatter cones located more peripherally in the retina. Also, in the foveal region, the blood vessels, ganglion cells, inner nuclear layer of cells, and plexiform layers are all displaced to one side rather than resting directly on top of the cones. This allows light to pass unimpeded to the cones.

Rods and Cones. Figure 50-3 is a diagrammatic representation of the essential components of a photoreceptor (either a rod or a cone). As shown in Figure 50-4, the outer segment of the cone is conical in shape. In general, the rods are narrower and longer than the cones, but this is not always the case. In the peripheral portions of the retina, the rods are 2 to 5 micrometers in diameter, whereas the cones are 5 to 8 micrometers in diameter; in the central part of the retina, in the fovea, there are rods, and the cones are slender and have a diameter of only 1.5 micrometers.

The major functional segments of either a rod or cone are shown in Figure 50-3: (1) the *outer segment,* (2) the *inner segment,* (3) the *nucleus,* and (4) the *synaptic body.* The light-sensitive photochemical is found in the outer segment. In the case of the rods, this is *rhodopsin;* in the cones, it is one of three "color" photochemicals, usually called simply *color pigments,* that function almost exactly the same as rhodopsin except for differences in spectral sensitivity.

Note in the *outer segments* of the rods and cones in Figures 50-3 and 50-4 the large numbers of *discs.* Each disc is actually an infolded shelf of cell membrane. There are as many as 1000 discs in each rod or cone.

Both rhodopsin and the color pigments are conjugated proteins. They are incorporated into the membranes of the discs in the form of transmembrane proteins. The concentrations of these photosensitive pigments in the discs are so great that the pigments themselves constitute about 40 percent of the entire mass of the outer segment.

The *inner segment* of the rod or cone contains the usual cytoplasm with cytoplasmic organelles. Especially important are the mitochondria, which, as explained later, play the important role of providing energy for function of the photoreceptors.

The *synaptic body* is the portion of the rod or cone that connects with subsequent neuronal cells, the *horizontal* and *bipolar cells,* which represent the next stages in the vision chain.

Pigment Layer of the Retina. The black pigment *melanin* in the pigment layer prevents light reflection throughout the globe of the eyeball; this is extremely important for clear

Figure 50-1 Layers of retina.

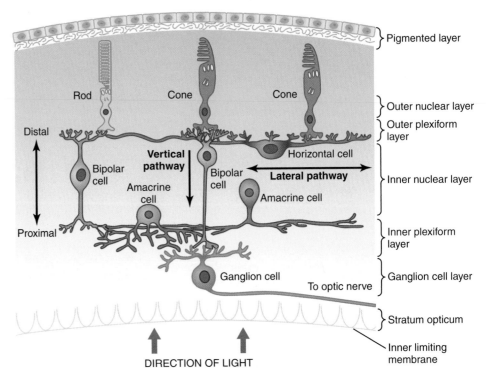

Pigmented layer

Outer nuclear layer

Outer plexiform layer

Inner nuclear layer

Inner plexiform layer

Ganglion cell layer

Stratum opticum

Inner limiting membrane

Rod

Cone

Cone

Distal

Bipolar cell

Amacrine cell

Vertical pathway

Bipolar cell

Horizontal cell

Lateral pathway

Amacrine cell

Proximal

Ganglion cell

To optic nerve

DIRECTION OF LIGHT

Figure 50-2 Photomicrograph of the macula and of the fovea in its center. Note that the inner layers of the retina are pulled to the side to decrease interference with light transmission. (From Fawcett DW: Bloom and Fawcett: A Textbook of Histology, 11th ed. Philadelphia: WB Saunders, 1986; courtesy H. Mizoguchi.)

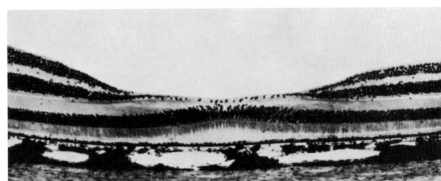

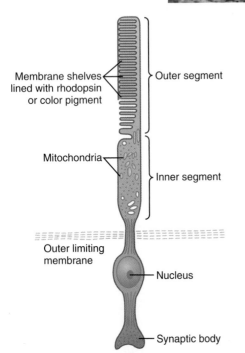

Membrane shelves lined with rhodopsin or color pigment

Outer segment

Mitochondria

Inner segment

Outer limiting membrane

Nucleus

Synaptic body

Figure 50-3 Schematic drawing of the functional parts of the rods and cones.

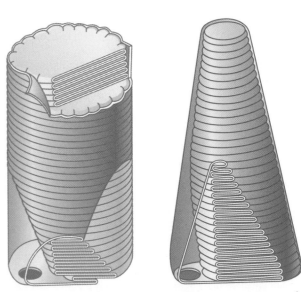

Figure 50-4 Membranous structures of the outer segments of a rod (*left*) and a cone (*right*). (Courtesy Dr. Richard Young.)

vision. This pigment performs the same function in the eye as the black coloring inside the bellows of a camera. Without it, light rays would be reflected in all directions within the eyeball and would cause diffuse lighting of the retina rather than the normal contrast between dark and light spots required for formation of precise images.

The importance of melanin in the pigment layer is well illustrated by its absence in *albinos,* people who are hereditarily lacking in melanin pigment in all parts of their bodies. When an albino enters a bright room, light that impinges on the retina is reflected in all directions inside the eyeball by the unpigmented surfaces of the retina and by the underlying sclera, so a single discrete spot of light that would normally excite only a few rods or cones is reflected everywhere and excites many receptors. Therefore, the visual acuity of albinos, even with the best optical correction, is seldom better than 20/100 to 20/200 rather than the normal 20/20 values.

The pigment layer also stores large quantities of *vitamin A.* This vitamin A is exchanged back and forth through the cell membranes of the outer segments of the rods and cones, which themselves are embedded in the pigment. We show later that vitamin A is an important precursor of the photosensitive chemicals of the rods and cones.

Blood Supply of the Retina—The Central Retinal Artery and the Choroid. The nutrient blood supply for the internal layers of the retina is derived from the central retinal artery, which enters the eyeball through the center of the optic nerve and then divides *to supply the entire inside retinal surface.* Thus, the inner layers of the retina have their own blood supply independent of the other structures of the eye.

However, the outermost layer of the retina is adherent to the *choroid,* which is also a highly vascular tissue lying between the retina and the sclera. The outer layers of the retina, especially the outer segments of the rods and cones, depend mainly on diffusion from the choroid blood vessels for their nutrition, especially for their oxygen.

Retinal Detachment. The neural retina occasionally *detaches from the pigment epithelium.* In some instances, the cause of such detachment is injury to the eyeball that allows fluid or blood to collect between the neural retina and the pigment epithelium. Detachment is occasionally caused by contracture of fine collagenous fibrils in the vitreous humor, which pull areas of the retina toward the interior of the globe.

Partly because of diffusion across the detachment gap and partly because of the independent blood supply to the neural retina through the retinal artery, the detached retina can resist degeneration for days and can become functional again if it is surgically replaced in its normal relation with the pigment epithelium. If it is not replaced soon, however, the retina will be destroyed and will be unable to function even after surgical repair.

Photochemistry of Vision

Both rods and cones contain chemicals that decompose on exposure to light and, in the process, excite the nerve fibers leading from the eye. The light-sensitive chemical in the *rods* is called *rhodopsin;* the light-sensitive chemicals in the *cones,* called *cone pigments* or *color pigments,* have compositions only slightly different from that of rhodopsin.

In this section, we discuss principally the photochemistry of rhodopsin, but the same principles can be applied to the cone pigments.

Rhodopsin-Retinal Visual Cycle, and Excitation of the Rods

Rhodopsin and Its Decomposition by Light Energy. The outer segment of the rod that projects into the pigment layer of the retina has a concentration of about 40 percent of the light-sensitive pigment called *rhodopsin,* or *visual purple.* This substance is a combination of the protein *scotopsin* and the carotenoid pigment *retinal* (also called "retinene"). Furthermore, the retinal is a particular type called 11-*cis* retinal. This *cis* form of retinal is important because only this form can bind with scotopsin to synthesize rhodopsin.

When light energy is absorbed by rhodopsin, the rhodopsin begins to decompose within a very small fraction of a second, as shown at the top of Figure 50-5. The cause of this is photoactivation of electrons in the retinal portion of the rhodopsin, which leads to instantaneous change of the *cis* form of retinal into an all-*trans* form that still has the same chemical structure as the *cis* form but has a different physical structure—a straight molecule rather than an angulated molecule. Because the three-dimensional orientation of the reactive sites of the all-*trans* retinal no longer fits with the orientation of the reactive sites on the protein *scotopsin,* the all-*trans* retinal begins to pull away from the scotopsin. The immediate product is *bathorhodopsin,* which is a partially split combination of the all-*trans* retinal and scotopsin. Bathorhodopsin is extremely unstable and decays in nanoseconds to *lumirhodopsin.* This then decays in microseconds to *metarhodopsin I,* then in about a millisecond to *metarhodopsin II,* and finally, much more slowly

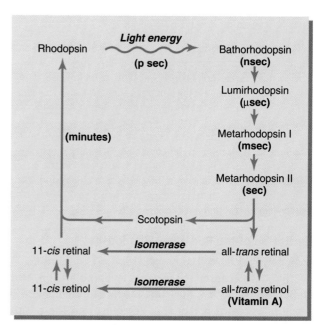

Figure 50-5 Rhodopsin-retinal visual cycle in the rod, showing decomposition of rhodopsin during exposure to light and subsequent slow re-formation of rhodopsin by the chemical processes.

(in seconds), into the completely split products *scotopsin* and all-*trans* retinal.

It is the metarhodopsin II, also called *activated rhodopsin*, that excites electrical changes in the rods, and the rods then transmit the visual image into the central nervous system in the form of optic nerve action potential, as we discuss later.

Re-formation of Rhodopsin. The first stage in re-formation of rhodopsin, as shown in Figure 50-5, is to reconvert the all-*trans* retinal into 11-*cis* retinal. This process requires metabolic energy and is catalyzed by the enzyme *retinal isomerase*. Once the 11-*cis* retinal is formed, it automatically recombines with the scotopsin to re-form rhodopsin, which then remains stable until its decomposition is again triggered by absorption of light energy.

Role of Vitamin A for Formation of Rhodopsin. Note in Figure 50-5 that there is a second chemical route by which all-*trans* retinal can be converted into 11-*cis* retinal. This is by conversion of the all-*trans* retinal first into all-*trans* retinol, which is one form of vitamin A. Then the all-*trans* retinol is converted into 11-*cis* retinol under the influence of the enzyme isomerase. Finally, the 11-*cis* retinol is converted into 11-*cis* retinal, which combines with scotopsin to form new rhodopsin.

Vitamin A is present both in the cytoplasm of the rods and in the pigment layer of the retina. Therefore, vitamin A is normally always available to form new retinal when needed. Conversely, when there is excess retinal in the retina, it is converted back into vitamin A, thus reducing the amount of light-sensitive pigment in the retina. We shall see later that this interconversion between retinal and vitamin A is especially important in long-term adaptation of the retina to different light intensities.

Night Blindness. Night blindness occurs in any person with severe vitamin A deficiency. The reason for this is that without vitamin A, the amounts of retinal and rhodopsin that can be formed are severely depressed. This condition is called *night blindness* because the amount of light available at night is too little to permit adequate vision in vitamin A–deficient persons.

For night blindness to occur, a person usually must remain on a vitamin A–deficient diet for months because large quantities of vitamin A are normally stored in the liver and can be made available to the eyes. Once night blindness develops, it can sometimes be reversed in less than 1 hour by intravenous injection of vitamin A.

Excitation of the Rod When Rhodopsin Is Activated by Light

The Rod Receptor Potential Is Hyperpolarizing, Not Depolarizing. When the rod is exposed to light, the resulting receptor potential is different from the receptor potentials in almost all other sensory receptors. That is, excitation of the rod causes *increased negativity* of the intrarod membrane potential, which is a state of *hyperpolarization*, meaning that there is more negativity than normal *inside* the rod membrane. This is exactly opposite to the decreased negativity (the process of "depolarization") that occurs in almost all other sensory receptors.

How does activation of rhodopsin cause hyperpolarization? The answer is that *when rhodopsin decomposes, it decreases the rod membrane conductance for sodium ions in the outer segment of the rod.* This causes hyperpolarization of the entire rod membrane in the following way.

Figure 50-6 shows movement of sodium and potassium ions in a complete electrical circuit through the inner and outer segments of the rod. The inner segment continually pumps sodium from inside the rod to the outside and potassium ions are pumped to the inside of the

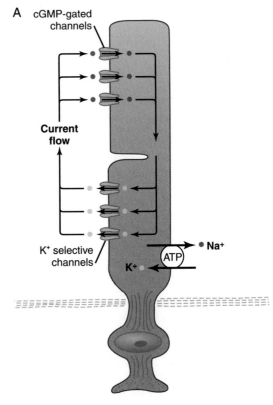

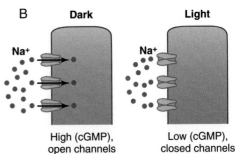

Figure 50-6 Sodium flows into a photoreceptor (e.g., rod) through cGMP-gated channels. Potassium flows out of the cell through nongated potassium channels. A sodium-potassium pump maintains steady levels of sodium and potassium inside the cell. In the dark, cGMP levels are high and the sodium channels are open. In the light, cGMP levels are reduced and the sodium channels close, causing the cell to hyperpolarize.

cell. Potassium ions leak out of the cell through non-gated potassium channels that are confined to the inner segment of the rod. As in other cells, this sodium-potassium pump creates a negative potential on the inside of the entire cell. However, the outer segment of the rod, where the photoreceptor discs are located, is entirely different; here, the rod membrane, in the *dark* state, is leaky to sodium ions that flow through cGMP-gated channels. In the dark state, cGMP levels are high, permitting positively charged sodium ions to continually leak back to the inside of the rod and thereby neutralize much of the negativity on the inside of the entire cell. Thus, *under normal dark conditions, when the rod is not excited, there is reduced electronegativity* inside the membrane of the rod, measuring about –40 millivolts rather than the usual –70 to –80 millivolts found in most sensory receptors.

Then, when the rhodopsin in the outer segment of the rod is exposed to light, it is activated and begins to decompose, the cGMP gated sodium channels are closed, and the outer segment membrane conductance of sodium to the interior of the rod is reduced by a three-step process (Figure 50-7): (1) Light is absorbed by the rhodopsin, causing photoactivation of the electrons in the retinal portion, as previously described; (2) the activated rhodopsin stimulates a G-protein called *transducin,* which then activates cGMP phosphodiesterase; this enzyme catalyzes the breakdown of cGMP to 5′-cGMP; and (3) the reduction in cGMP closes the cGMP-gated sodium channels and reduces the inward sodium current. Sodium ions continue to be pumped outward through the membrane of the inner segment. Thus, more sodium ions now leave the rod than leak back in. Because they are positive ions, their loss from inside the rod creates increased negativity

inside the membrane, and the greater the amount of light energy striking the rod, the greater the electronegativity becomes—that is, the greater is the degree of *hyperpolarization.* At maximum light intensity, the membrane potential approaches –70 to –80 millivolts, which is near the equilibrium potential for potassium ions across the membrane.

Duration of the Receptor Potential, and Logarithmic Relation of the Receptor Potential to Light Intensity. When a sudden pulse of light strikes the retina, the transient hyperpolarization that occurs in the rods—that is, the *receptor potential* that occurs—reaches a peak in about 0.3 second and lasts for more than a second. In cones, the change occurs four times as fast as in the rods. A visual image impinged on the rods of the retina for only one millionth of a second can sometimes cause the sensation of seeing the image for longer than a second.

Another characteristic of the receptor potential is that it is approximately proportional to the logarithm of the light intensity. This is exceedingly important because it allows the eye to discriminate light intensities through a range many thousand times as great as would be possible otherwise.

Mechanism by Which Rhodopsin Decomposition *Decreases* **Membrane Sodium Conductance—The Excitation "Cascade."** Under optimal conditions, a single photon of light, the smallest possible quantal unit of light energy, can cause a measurable receptor potential in a rod of about 1 millivolt. Only 30 photons of light will cause half saturation of the rod. How can such a small amount of light cause such great excitation? The answer is that the photoreceptors have an extremely sensitive chemical cascade that amplifies the stimulatory effects about a millionfold, as follows:

1. The *photon activates an electron* in the 11-*cis* retinal portion of the rhodopsin; this leads to the formation of *metarhodopsin II,* which is the active form of rhodopsin, as already discussed and shown in Figure 50-5.

2. The *activated rhodopsin* functions as an enzyme to activate many molecules of *transducin,* a protein present in an inactive form in the membranes of the discs and cell membrane of the rod.

3. The *activated transducin* activates many more molecules of *phosphodiesterase.*

4. *Activated phosphodiesterase* is another enzyme; it immediately hydrolyzes many molecules of *cyclic guanosine monophosphate* (cGMP), thus destroying it. Before being destroyed, the cGMP had been bound with the sodium channel protein of the rod's outer membrane in a way that "splints" it in the open state. But in light, when phosphodiesterase hydrolyzes the cGMP, this removes the splinting and allows the sodium channels to close. Several hundred channels close for each originally activated molecule of rhodopsin. Because the sodium flux through each of these channels has been extremely rapid, flow of more than a million sodium

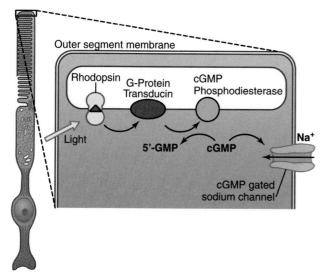

Figure 50-7 Phototransduction in the outer segment of the photoreceptor (rod or cone) membrane. When light hits the photoreceptor (e.g., rod cell), the light-absorbing retinal portion of rhodopsin is activated. This stimulates transducin, a G-protein, which then activates cGMP phosphodiesterase. This enzyme catalyzes the degradation of cGMP into 5′-GMP. The reduction in cGMP then causes closure of the sodium channels, which, in turn, causes hyperpolarization of the photoreceptor.

ions is blocked by the channel closure before the channel opens again. This diminution of sodium ion flow is what excites the rod, as already discussed.

5. Within about a second, another enzyme, *rhodopsin kinase,* which is always present in the rod, inactivates the activated rhodopsin (the metarhodopsin II), and the entire cascade reverses back to the normal state with open sodium channels.

Thus, the rods have developed an important chemical cascade that amplifies the effect of a single photon of light to cause movement of millions of sodium ions. This explains the extreme sensitivity of the rods under dark conditions.

The cones are about 30 to 300 times less sensitive than the rods, but even this allows color vision at any intensity of light greater than extremely dim twilight.

Photochemistry of Color Vision by the Cones

It was pointed out at the outset of this discussion that the photochemicals in the cones have almost exactly the same chemical composition as that of rhodopsin in the rods. The only difference is that the protein portions, or the opsins—called *photopsins* in the cones—are slightly different from the scotopsin of the rods. The *retinal* portion of all the visual pigments is exactly the same in the cones as in the rods. The color-sensitive pigments of the cones, therefore, are combinations of retinal and photopsins.

In the discussion of color vision later in the chapter, it will become evident that only one of three types of color pigments is present in each of the different cones, thus making the cones selectively sensitive to different colors: blue, green, or red. These color pigments are called, respectively, *blue-sensitive pigment, green-sensitive pigment,* and *red-sensitive pigment.* The absorption characteristics of the pigments in the three types of cones show peak absorbencies at light wavelengths of 445, 535, and 570 nanometers, respectively. These are also the wavelengths for peak light sensitivity for each type of cone, which begins to explain how the retina differentiates the colors. The approximate absorption curves for these three pigments are shown in Figure 50-8. Also shown is the absorption curve for the rhodopsin of the rods, with a peak at 505 nanometers.

Automatic Regulation of Retinal Sensitivity— Light and Dark Adaptation

Light and Dark Adaptation. If a person has been in bright light for hours, large portions of the photochemicals in both the rods and the cones will have been reduced to retinal and opsins. Furthermore, much of the retinal of both the rods and the cones will have been converted into vitamin A. Because of these two effects, the concentrations of the photosensitive chemicals remaining in the rods and cones are considerably reduced, and the sensitivity of the eye to light is correspondingly reduced. This is called *light adaptation.*

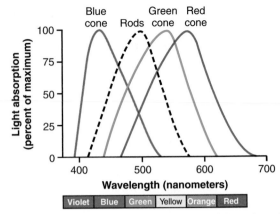

Figure 50-8 Light absorption by the pigment of the rods and by the pigments of the three color-receptive cones of the human retina. (Drawn from curves recorded by Marks WB, Dobelle WH, MacNichol EF Jr: Visual pigments of single primate cones. Science 143:1181, 1964, and by Brown PK, Wald G: Visual pigments in single rods and cones of the human retina: direct measurements reveal mechanisms of human night and color vision. Science 144:45, 1964. ©1964 by the American Association for the Advancement of Science.)

Conversely, if a person remains in darkness for a long time, the retinal and opsins in the rods and cones are converted back into the light-sensitive pigments. Furthermore, vitamin A is converted back into retinal to increase light-sensitive pigments, the final limit being determined by the amount of opsins in the rods and cones to combine with the retinal. This is called *dark adaptation.*

Figure 50-9 shows the course of dark adaptation when a person is exposed to total darkness after having been exposed to bright light for several hours. Note that the sensitivity of the retina is very low on first entering the darkness, but within 1 minute, the sensitivity has already increased 10-fold—that is, the retina can respond to light of one tenth the previously required intensity. At the end of 20 minutes, the sensitivity has increased about 6000-fold, and at the end of 40 minutes, about 25,000-fold.

The resulting curve of Figure 50-9 is called the *dark adaptation curve.* Note, however, the inflection in the

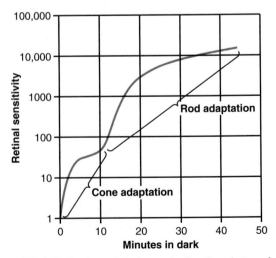

Figure 50-9 Dark adaptation, demonstrating the relation of cone adaptation to rod adaptation.

curve. The early portion of the curve is caused by adaptation of the cones because all the chemical events of vision, including adaptation, occur about four times as rapidly in cones as in rods. However, the cones do not achieve anywhere near the same degree of sensitivity change in darkness as the rods do. Therefore, despite rapid adaptation, the cones cease adapting after only a few minutes, while the slowly adapting rods continue to adapt for many minutes and even hours, their sensitivity increasing tremendously. In addition, still more sensitivity of the rods is caused by neuronal signal convergence of 100 or more rods onto a single ganglion cell in the retina; these rods summate to increase their sensitivity, as discussed later in the chapter.

> **Other Mechanisms of Light and Dark Adaptation.** In addition to adaptation caused by changes in concentrations of rhodopsin or color photochemicals, the eye has two other mechanisms for light and dark adaptation. The first of these is a *change in pupillary size,* as discussed in Chapter 49. This can cause adaptation of approximately 30-fold within a fraction of a second because of changes in the amount of light allowed through the pupillary opening.
>
> The other mechanism is *neural adaptation,* involving the neurons in the successive stages of the visual chain in the retina itself and in the brain. That is, when light intensity first increases, the signals transmitted by the bipolar cells, horizontal cells, amacrine cells, and ganglion cells are all intense. However, most of these signals decrease rapidly at different stages of transmission in the neural circuit. Although the degree of adaptation is only a fewfold rather than the many thousandfold that occurs during adaptation of the photochemical system, neural adaptation occurs in a fraction of a second, in contrast to the many minutes to hours required for full adaptation by the photochemicals.

Value of Light and Dark Adaptation in Vision. Between the limits of maximal dark adaptation and maximal light adaptation, the eye can change its sensitivity to light as much as 500,000 to 1 million times, the sensitivity automatically adjusting to changes in illumination.

Because registration of images by the retina requires detection of both dark and light spots in the image, it is essential that the sensitivity of the retina always be adjusted so that the receptors respond to the lighter areas but not to the darker areas. An example of maladjustment of retinal adaptation occurs when a person leaves a movie theater and enters the bright sunlight. Then, even the dark spots in the images seem exceedingly bright, and as a consequence, the entire visual image is bleached, having little contrast among its different parts. This is poor vision, and it remains poor until the retina has adapted sufficiently so that the darker areas of the image no longer stimulate the receptors excessively.

Conversely, when a person first enters darkness, the sensitivity of the retina is usually so slight that even the light spots in the image cannot excite the retina. After dark adaptation, the light spots begin to register. As an example of the extremes of light and dark adaptation, the intensity of sunlight is about 10 billion times that of starlight,

yet the eye can function both in bright sunlight after light adaptation and in starlight after dark adaptation.

Color Vision

From the preceding sections, we have learned that different cones are sensitive to different colors of light. This section is a discussion of the mechanisms by which the retina detects the different gradations of color in the visual spectrum.

Tricolor Mechanism of Color Detection

All theories of color vision are based on the well-known observation that the human eye can detect almost all gradations of colors when only red, green, and blue monochromatic lights are appropriately mixed in different combinations.

Spectral Sensitivities of the Three Types of Cones. On the basis of color vision tests, the spectral sensitivities of the three types of cones in humans have proved to be essentially the same as the light absorption curves for the three types of pigment found in the cones. These curves are shown in Figure 50-8 and slightly differently in Figure 50-10. They can explain most of the phenomena of color vision.

Interpretation of Color in the Nervous System. Referring to Figure 50-10, one can see that an orange monochromatic light with a wavelength of 580 nanometers stimulates the red cones to a value of about 99 (99 percent of the peak stimulation at optimum wavelength); it stimulates the green cones to a value of about 42, but the blue cones not at all. Thus, the ratios of stimulation of the three types of cones in this instance are 99:42:0. The nervous system interprets this set of ratios as the sensation of orange. Conversely, a monochromatic blue light with a wavelength of 450 nanometers stimulates the red cones to a stimulus value of 0, the green cones to

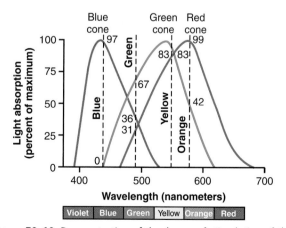

Figure 50-10 Demonstration of the degree of stimulation of the different color-sensitive cones by monochromatic lights of four colors: blue, green, yellow, and orange.

a value of 0, and the blue cones to a value of 97. This set of ratios—0:0:97—is interpreted by the nervous system as blue. Likewise, ratios of 83:83:0 are interpreted as yellow, and 31:67:36 as green.

Perception of White Light. About equal stimulation of all the red, green, and blue cones gives one the sensation of seeing white. Yet there is no single wavelength of light corresponding to white; instead, white is a combination of all the wavelengths of the spectrum. Furthermore, the perception of white can be achieved by stimulating the retina with a proper combination of only three chosen colors that stimulate the respective types of cones about equally.

Color Blindness

Red-Green Color Blindness. When a single group of color-receptive cones is missing from the eye, the person is unable to distinguish some colors from others. For instance, one can see in Figure 50-10 that green, yellow, orange, and red colors, which are the colors between the wavelengths of 525 and 675 nanometers, are normally distinguished from one another by the red and green cones. If either of these two cones is missing, the person cannot use this mechanism for distinguishing these four colors; the person is especially unable to distinguish red from green and is therefore said to have *red-green color blindness.*

A person with loss of red cones is called a *protanope;* the overall visual spectrum is noticeably shortened at the long wavelength end because of a lack of the red cones. A color-blind person who lacks green cones is called a *deuteranope;* this person has a perfectly normal visual spectral width because red cones are available to detect the long wavelength red color.

Red-green color blindness is a genetic disorder that occurs almost exclusively in males. That is, genes in the female X chromosome code for the respective cones. Yet color blindness almost never occurs in females because at least one of the two X chromosomes almost always has a normal gene for each type of cone. Because the male has only one X chromosome, a missing gene can lead to color blindness.

Because the X chromosome in the male is always inherited from the mother, never from the father, color blindness is passed from mother to son, and the mother is said to be a *color blindness carrier;* this is true in about 8 percent of all women.

Blue Weakness. Only rarely are blue cones missing, although sometimes they are underrepresented, which is a genetically inherited state giving rise to the phenomenon called *blue weakness.*

Color Test Charts. A rapid method for determining color blindness is based on the use of spot charts such as those shown in Figure 50-11. These charts are arranged with a confusion of spots of several different colors. In the top chart, the person with normal color vision reads "74," whereas the red-green color-blind person reads "21." In the bottom chart, the person with normal color vision reads "42," whereas the red-blind person reads "2," and the green-blind person reads "4."

If one studies these charts while at the same time observing the spectral sensitivity curves of the different cones depicted in Figure 50-10, it can be readily understood how excessive emphasis can be placed on spots of certain colors by color-blind people.

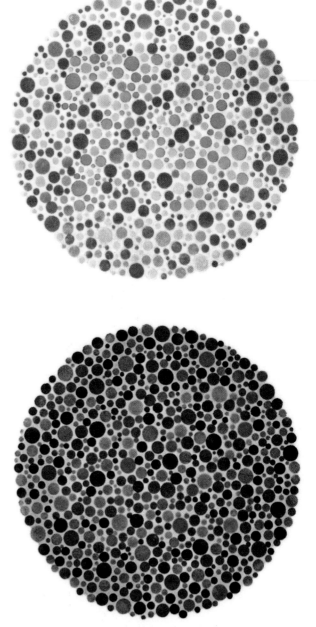

Figure 50-11 Two Ishihara charts. *Upper:* In this chart, the normal person reads "74," but the red-green color-blind person reads "21." *Lower:* In this chart, the red-blind person (protanope) reads "2," but the green-blind person (deuteranope) reads "4." The normal person reads "42." (Reproduced from Ishihara's Tests for Colour Blindness. Tokyo: Kanehara & Co., but tests for color blindness cannot be conducted with this material. For accurate testing, the original plates should be used.)

Neural Function of the Retina

Neural Circuitry of the Retina

Figure 50-12 presents the essentials of the retina's neural connections, showing at the left the circuit in the peripheral retina and at the right the circuit in the foveal retina. The different neuronal cell types are as follows:

1. The photoreceptors themselves—the *rods* and *cones*—which transmit signals to the outer plexiform

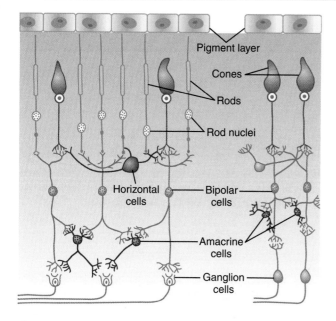

Figure 50-12 Neural organization of the retina: peripheral area to the left, foveal area to the right.

layer, where they synapse with bipolar cells and horizontal cells

2. The *horizontal cells*, which transmit signals horizontally in the outer plexiform layer from the rods and cones to bipolar cells

3. The *bipolar cells*, which transmit signals vertically from the rods, cones, and horizontal cells to the inner plexiform layer, where they synapse with ganglion cells and amacrine cells

4. The *amacrine cells*, which transmit signals in two directions, either directly from bipolar cells to ganglion cells or horizontally within the inner plexiform layer from axons of the bipolar cells to dendrites of the ganglion cells or to other amacrine cells

5. The *ganglion cells*, which transmit output signals from the retina through the optic nerve into the brain

A sixth type of neuronal cell in the retina, not very prominent and not shown in the figure, is the *interplexiform* cell. This cell transmits signals in the retrograde direction from the inner plexiform layer to the outer plexiform layer. These signals are inhibitory and are believed to control lateral spread of visual signals by the horizontal cells in the outer plexiform layer. Their role may be to help control the degree of contrast in the visual image.

The Visual Pathway from the Cones to the Ganglion Cells Functions Differently from the Rod Pathway. As is true for many of our other sensory systems, the retina has both an old type of vision based on rod vision and a new type of vision based on cone vision. The neurons and nerve fibers that conduct the visual signals for cone vision are considerably larger than those that conduct the visual signals for rod vision, and the signals are conducted to the brain two to five times as

rapidly. Also, the circuitry for the two systems is slightly different, as follows.

To the right in Figure 50-12 is the visual pathway from the *foveal portion of the retina*, representing the new, fast cone system. This shows three neurons in the direct pathway: (1) cones, (2) bipolar cells, and (3) ganglion cells. In addition, horizontal cells transmit inhibitory signals laterally in the outer plexiform layer, and amacrine cells transmit signals laterally in the inner plexiform layer.

To the left in Figure 50-12 are the neural connections for the peripheral retina, where both rods and cones are present. Three bipolar cells are shown; the middle of these connects only to rods, representing the type of visual system present in many lower animals. The output from the bipolar cell passes only to amacrine cells, which relay the signals to the ganglion cells. Thus, for pure rod vision, there are four neurons in the direct visual pathway: (1) rods, (2) bipolar cells, (3) amacrine cells, and (4) ganglion cells. Also, horizontal and amacrine cells provide lateral connectivity.

The other two bipolar cells shown in the peripheral retinal circuitry of Figure 50-12 connect with both rods and cones; the outputs of these bipolar cells pass both directly to ganglion cells and by way of amacrine cells.

Neurotransmitters Released by Retinal Neurons. Not all the neurotransmitter chemical substances used for synaptic transmission in the retina have been entirely delineated. However, both the rods and the cones release *glutamate* at their synapses with the bipolar cells.

Histological and pharmacological studies have proven there are many types of amacrine cells secreting at least eight types of transmitter substances, including *gamma-aminobutyric acid, glycine, dopamine, acetylcholine,* and *indolamine,* all of which normally function as inhibitory transmitters. The transmitters of the bipolar, horizontal, and interplexiform cells are unclear, but at least some of the horizontal cells release inhibitory transmitters.

Transmission of Most Signals Occurs in the Retinal Neurons by Electrotonic Conduction, Not by Action Potentials. The only retinal neurons that always transmit visual signals by means of action potentials are the ganglion cells, and they send their signals all the way to the brain through the optic nerve. Occasionally, action potentials have also been recorded in amacrine cells, although the importance of these action potentials is questionable. Otherwise, all the retinal neurons conduct their visual signals by *electrotonic conduction*, which can be explained as follows.

Electrotonic conduction means direct flow of electric current, not action potentials, in the neuronal cytoplasm and nerve axons from the point of excitation all the way to the output synapses. Even in the rods and cones, conduction from their outer segments, where the visual signals are generated, to the synaptic bodies is by electrotonic conduction. That is, when hyperpolarization occurs in response to light in the outer segment of a rod or a cone, almost the same degree of hyperpolarization is conducted by direct electric current flow in the cytoplasm all the way to the synaptic body, and no action potential is required. Then, when the transmitter from a rod or cone stimulates a bipolar cell or horizontal cell, once again the signal is transmitted from the input to the output by direct electric current flow, not by action potentials.

The importance of electrotonic conduction is that it allows *graded conduction* of signal strength. Thus, for the rods and cones, the strength of the hyperpolarizing output signal is directly related to the intensity of illumination; the signal is not all or none, as would be the case for each action potential.

Lateral Inhibition to Enhance Visual Contrast—Function of the Horizontal Cells

The horizontal cells, shown in Figure 50-12, connect laterally between the synaptic bodies of the rods and cones, as well as connecting with the dendrites of the bipolar cells. The outputs of the horizontal cells *are always inhibitory.* Therefore, this lateral connection provides the same phenomenon of lateral inhibition that is important in all other sensory systems—that is, helping to ensure transmission of visual patterns with proper visual contrast. This phenomenon is demonstrated in Figure 50-13, which shows a minute spot of light focused on the retina. The visual pathway from the central most area where the light strikes is excited, whereas an area to the side is inhibited. In other words, instead of the excitatory signal spreading widely in the retina because of spreading dendritic and axonal trees in the plexiform layers, transmission through the horizontal cells puts a stop to this by providing lateral inhibition in the surrounding areas. This is essential to allow high visual accuracy in transmitting contrast borders in the visual image.

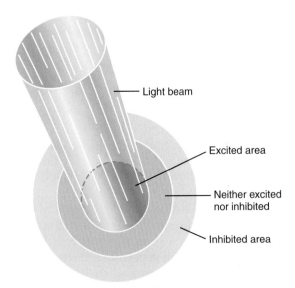

Figure 50-13 Excitation and inhibition of a retinal area caused by a small beam of light, demonstrating the principle of lateral inhibition.

Light beam

Excited area

Neither excited nor inhibited

Inhibited area

Some of the amacrine cells probably provide additional lateral inhibition and further enhancement of visual contrast in the inner plexiform layer of the retina as well.

Excitation of Some Bipolar Cells and Inhibition of Others—The Depolarizing and Hyperpolarizing Bipolar Cells

Two types of bipolar cells provide opposing excitatory and inhibitory signals in the visual pathway: (1) the *depolarizing bipolar cell* and (2) the *hyperpolarizing bipolar cell.* That is, some bipolar cells depolarize when the rods and cones are excited, and others hyperpolarize.

There are two possible explanations for this difference. One explanation is that the two bipolar cells are of entirely different types—one responding by depolarizing in response to the glutamate neurotransmitter released by the rods and cones, and the other responding by hyperpolarizing. The other possibility is that one of the bipolar cells receives direct excitation from the rods and cones, whereas the other receives its signal indirectly through a horizontal cell. Because the horizontal cell is an inhibitory cell, this would reverse the polarity of the electrical response.

Regardless of the mechanism for the two types of bipolar responses, the importance of this phenomenon is that it allows half the bipolar cells to transmit positive signals and the other half to transmit negative signals. We shall see later that both positive and negative signals are used in transmitting visual information to the brain.

Another important aspect of this reciprocal relation between depolarizing and hyperpolarizing bipolar cells is that it provides a second mechanism for lateral inhibition, in addition to the horizontal cell mechanism. Because depolarizing and hyperpolarizing bipolar cells lie immediately against each other, this provides a mechanism for separating contrast borders in the visual image, even when the border lies exactly between two adjacent photoreceptors. In contrast, the horizontal cell mechanism for lateral inhibition operates over a much greater distance.

Amacrine Cells and Their Functions

About 30 types of amacrine cells have been identified by morphological or histochemical means. The functions of about half a dozen types of amacrine cells have been characterized, and all of them are different. One type of amacrine cell is part of the direct pathway for rod vision—that is, from rod to bipolar cells to amacrine cells to ganglion cells.

Another type of amacrine cell responds strongly at the onset of a continuing visual signal, but the response dies rapidly.

Other amacrine cells respond strongly at the offset of visual signals, but again, the response fades quickly.

Still other amacrine cells respond when a light is turned either on or off, signaling simply a change in illumination, irrespective of direction.

Still another type of amacrine cell responds to movement of a spot across the retina in a specific direction;

therefore, these amacrine cells are said to be *directional sensitive.*

In a sense, then, many or most amacrine cells are interneurons that help analyze visual signals before they ever leave the retina.

Ganglion Cells and Optic Nerve Fibers

Each retina contains about 100 million rods and 3 million cones; yet the number of ganglion cells is only about 1.6 million. Thus, an average of 60 rods and 2 cones converge on each ganglion cell and the optic nerve fiber leading from the ganglion cell to the brain.

However, major differences exist between the peripheral retina and the central retina. As one approaches the fovea, fewer rods and cones converge on each optic fiber, and the rods and cones also become more slender. These effects progressively increase the acuity of vision in the central retina. In the center, in the *central fovea,* there are only slender cones—about 35,000 of them—and no rods. Also, the number of optic nerve fibers leading from this part of the retina is almost exactly equal to the number of cones, as shown to the right in Figure 50-12. This explains the high degree of visual acuity in the central retina in comparison with the much poorer acuity peripherally.

Another difference between the peripheral and central portions of the retina is the much greater sensitivity of the peripheral retina to weak light. This results partly from the fact that rods are 30 to 300 times more sensitive to light than cones are, but it is further magnified by the fact that as many as 200 rods converge on a single optic nerve fiber in the more peripheral portions of the retina, so signals from the rods summate to give even more intense stimulation of the peripheral ganglion cells and their optic nerve fibers.

Three Types of Retinal Ganglion Cells and Their Respective Fields

There are three distinct types of ganglion cells, designated W, X, and Y cells. Each of these serves a different function.

Transmission of Rod Vision by the W Cells. The W cells, constituting about 40 percent of all the ganglion cells, are small, having a diameter less than 10 micrometers, and they transmit signals in their optic nerve fibers at the slow velocity of only 8 m/sec. These ganglion cells receive most of their excitation from rods, transmitted by way of small bipolar cells and amacrine cells. They have broad fields in the peripheral retina because the dendrites of the ganglion cells spread widely in the inner plexiform layer, receiving signals from broad areas.

On the basis of histology, as well as physiological experiments, the W cells seem to be especially sensitive for detecting directional movement in the field of vision, and they are probably important for much of our crude rod vision under dark conditions.

Transmission of the Visual Image and Color by the X Cells. The most numerous of the ganglion cells are the X cells, representing 55 percent of the total. They are of medium diameter, between 10 and 15 micrometers, and transmit signals in their optic nerve fibers at about 14 m/sec.

The X cells have small fields because their dendrites do not spread widely in the retina. Because of this, their signals represent discrete retinal locations. Therefore, it is mainly through the X cells that the fine details of the visual image are transmitted. Also, because every X cell receives input from at least one cone, X cell transmission is probably responsible for all color vision.

Function of the Y Cells to Transmit Instantaneous Changes in the Visual Image. The Y cells are the largest of all, up to 35 micrometers in diameter, and they transmit their signals to the brain at 50 m/sec or faster. They are the least numerous of all the ganglion cells, representing only 5 percent of the total. Also, they have broad dendritic fields, so signals are picked up by these cells from widespread retinal areas.

The Y ganglion cells respond, like many of the amacrine cells, to rapid changes in the visual image—either rapid movement or rapid change in light intensity—sending bursts of signals for only small fractions of a second. These ganglion cells presumably apprise the central nervous system almost instantaneously when a new visual event occurs anywhere in the visual field, but without specifying with great accuracy the location of the event, other than to give appropriate clues that make the eyes move toward the exciting vision.

Excitation of the Ganglion Cells

Spontaneous, Continuous Action Potentials in the Ganglion Cells. It is from the ganglion cells that the long fibers of the optic nerve lead into the brain. Because of the distance involved, the electrotonic method of conduction employed in the rods, cones, and bipolar cells within the retina is no longer appropriate; therefore, ganglion cells transmit their signals by means of repetitive action potentials instead. Furthermore, even when unstimulated, they still transmit continuous impulses at rates varying between 5 and 40 per second. The visual signals, in turn, are superimposed onto this background ganglion cell firing.

Transmission of Changes in Light Intensity—The On-Off Response. As noted previously, many ganglion cells are specifically excited by *changes* in light intensity. This is demonstrated by the records of nerve impulses in Figure 50-14. The upper panel shows rapid impulses for a fraction of a second when a light is first turned on, but decreasing rapidly in the next fraction of a second. The lower tracing is from a ganglion cell located lateral to the spot of light; this cell is markedly inhibited when the light is turned on because of lateral inhibition. Then, when the light is turned off, opposite effects occur. Thus, these records are called "on-off" and "off-on" responses. The opposite directions of these responses to light are caused, respectively, by the depolarizing and hyperpolarizing bipolar cells, and

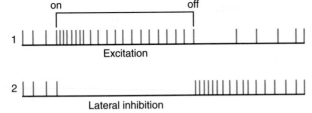

Figure 50-14 Responses of a ganglion cell to light in (*1*) an area excited by a spot of light and (*2*) an area adjacent to the excited spot; the ganglion cell in this area is inhibited by the mechanism of *lateral inhibition*. (Modified from Granit R: Receptors and Sensory Perception: A Discussion of Aims, Means, and Results of Electrophysiological Research into the Process of Reception. New Haven, Conn: Yale University Press, 1955.)

the transient nature of the responses is probably at least partly generated by the amacrine cells, many of which have similar transient responses themselves.

This capability of the eyes to detect *change* in light intensity is strongly developed in both the peripheral retina and the central retina. For instance, a minute gnat flying across the field of vision is instantaneously detected. Conversely, the same gnat sitting quietly remains below the threshold of visual detection.

Transmission of Signals Depicting Contrasts in the Visual Scene—The Role of Lateral Inhibition

Many ganglion cells respond mainly to contrast borders in the scene. Because this seems to be the major means by which the pattern of a scene is transmitted to the brain, let us explain how this process occurs.

When flat light is applied to the entire retina—that is, when all the photoreceptors are stimulated equally by the incident light—the contrast type of ganglion cell is neither stimulated nor inhibited. The reason for this is that signals transmitted *directly* from the photoreceptors through depolarizing bipolar cells are excitatory, whereas the signals transmitted *laterally* through hyperpolarizing bipolar cells, as well as through horizontal cells, are mainly inhibitory. Thus, the direct excitatory signal through one pathway is likely to be neutralized by inhibitory signals through lateral pathways. One circuit for this is demonstrated in Figure 50-15, which shows at the top three photoreceptors. The central receptor excites a depolarizing bipolar cell. The two receptors on each side are connected to the same bipolar cell through inhibitory horizontal cells that neutralize the direct excitatory signal if all three receptors are stimulated simultaneously by light.

Now, let us examine what happens when a contrast border occurs in the visual scene. Referring again to Figure 50-15, assume that the central photoreceptor is stimulated by a bright spot of light while one of the two lateral receptors is in the dark. The bright spot of light excites the direct pathway through the bipolar cell. The fact that one of the lateral photoreceptors is in the dark causes one of the horizontal cells to remain unstimulated. Therefore, this cell does not inhibit the bipolar cell, and this allows extra excitation of the bipolar cell. Thus, where

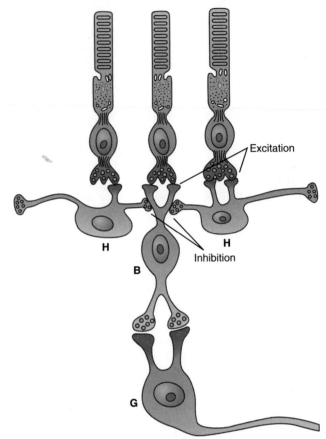

Figure 50-15 Typical arrangement of rods, horizontal cells (H), a bipolar cell (B), and a ganglion cell (G) in the retina, showing excitation at the synapses between the rods and the bipolar cell and horizontal cells, but inhibition from the horizontal cells to the bipolar cell.

visual contrasts occur, the signals through the direct and lateral pathways accentuate one another.

In summary, the mechanism of lateral inhibition functions in the eye in the same way that it functions in most other sensory systems—to provide contrast detection and enhancement.

Transmission of Color Signals by the Ganglion Cells

A single ganglion cell may be stimulated by several cones or by only a few. When all three types of cones—the red, blue, and green types—stimulate the same ganglion cell, the signal transmitted through the ganglion cell is the same for any color of the spectrum. Therefore, the signal from the ganglion cell plays no role in the detection of different colors. Instead, it is a "white" signal.

Conversely, some of the ganglion cells are excited by only one color type of cone but inhibited by a second type. For instance, this frequently occurs for the red and green cones, with red causing excitation and green causing inhibition, or vice versa.

The same type of reciprocal effect occurs between blue cones on the one hand and a combination of red and green cones (both of which are excited by yellow) on the other hand, giving a reciprocal excitation-inhibition relation between the blue and yellow colors.

The mechanism of this opposing effect of colors is the following: One color type of cone excites the ganglion cell by the direct excitatory route through a depolarizing bipolar cell, whereas the other color type inhibits the ganglion cell by the indirect inhibitory route through a hyperpolarizing bipolar cell.

The importance of these color-contrast mechanisms is that they represent a means by which the retina itself begins to differentiate colors. Thus, each color-contrast type of ganglion cell is excited by one color but inhibited by the "opponent" color. Therefore, color analysis begins in the retina and is not entirely a function of the brain.

Bibliography

Artemyev NO: Light-dependent compartmentalization of transducin in rod photoreceptors, *Mol Neurobiol* 37:44, 2008.

Bloomfield SA, Völgyi B: The diverse functional roles and regulation of neuronal gap junctions in the retina, *Nat Rev Neurosci* 10:495, 2009.

Bowmaker JK: Evolution of vertebrate visual pigments, *Vision Res* 48:2022, 2008.

Carroll J: Focus on molecules: the cone opsins, *Exp Eye Res* 86:865, 2008.

D'Amico DJ: Clinical practice. Primary retinal detachment, *N Engl J Med* 359:2346, 2008.

Fain GL, Matthews HR, Cornwall MC, Koutalos Y: Adaptation in vertebrate photoreceptors, *Physiol Rev* 81:117, 2001.

Garriga P, Manyosa J: The eye photoreceptor protein rhodopsin: structural implications for retinal disease, *FEBS Lett* 528:17, 2002.

Gegenfurtner KR: Cortical mechanisms of colour vision, *Nat Rev Neurosci* 4:563, 2003.

Gegenfurtner KR, Kiper DC: Color vision, *Annu Rev Neurosci* 26:181, 2003.

Hankins MW, Peirson SN, Foster RG: Melanopsin: an exciting photopigment, *Trends Neurosci* 31:27, 2008.

Hardie RC: Phototransduction: shedding light on translocation, *Curr Biol* 13:R775, 2003.

Hartzell HC, Qu Z, Yu K, et al: Molecular physiology of bestrophins: multifunctional membrane proteins linked to Best disease and other retinopathies, *Physiol Rev* 88:639, 2008.

Kandel ER, Schwartz JH, Jessell TM: *Principles of Neural Science*, 4th ed, New York, 2000, McGraw-Hill.

Kolb H, Nelson R, Ahnelt P, Cuenca N: Cellular organization of the vertebrate retina, *Prog Brain Res* 131:3, 2001.

Luo DG, Xue T, Yau KW: How vision begins: an odyssey, *Proc Natl Acad Sci U S A* 105:9855, 2008.

Masland RH: The fundamental plan of the retina, *Nat Neurosci* 4:877, 2001.

Okawa H, Sampath AP: Optimization of single-photon response transmission at the rod-to-rod bipolar synapse, *Physiology (Bethesda)* 22:279, 2007.

Schwartz EA: Transport-mediated synapses in the retina, *Physiol Rev* 82:875, 2002.

Solomon SG, Lennie P: The machinery of colour vision, *Nat Rev Neurosci* 8:276, 2007.

Taylor WR, Vaney DI: New directions in retinal research, *Trends Neurosci* 26:379, 2003.

Wensel TG: Signal transducing membrane complexes of photoreceptor outer segments, *Vision Res* 48:2052, 2008.

Westheimer G: The ON-OFF dichotomy in visual processing: from receptors to perception, *Prog Retin Eye Res* 26:636, 2007.

CHAPTER 51

The Eye: III. Central Neurophysiology of Vision

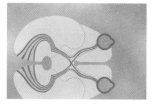

Visual Pathways

Figure 51-1 shows the principal visual pathways from the two retinas to the *visual cortex*. The visual nerve signals leave the retinas through the *optic nerves*. At the *optic chiasm*, the optic nerve fibers from the nasal halves of the retinas cross to the opposite sides, where they join the fibers from the opposite temporal retinas to form the *optic tracts*. The fibers of each optic tract then synapse in the *dorsal lateral geniculate nucleus* of the thalamus, and from there, *geniculocalcarine fibers* pass by way of the *optic radiation* (also called the *geniculocalcarine tract*) to the *primary visual cortex* in the *calcarine fissure* area of the medial occipital lobe.

Visual fibers also pass to several older areas of the brain: (1) from the optic tracts to the *suprachiasmatic nucleus of the hypothalamus*, presumably to control circadian rhythms that synchronize various physiologic changes of the body with night and day; (2) into the *pretectal nuclei* in the midbrain, to elicit reflex movements of the eyes to focus on objects of importance and to activate the pupillary light reflex; (3) into the *superior colliculus*, to control rapid directional movements of the two eyes; and (4) into the *ventral lateral geniculate nucleus* of the thalamus and surrounding basal regions of the brain, presumably to help control some of the body's behavioral functions.

Thus, the visual pathways can be divided roughly into an *old system* to the midbrain and base of the forebrain and a *new system* for direct transmission of visual signals into the visual cortex located in the occipital lobes. In humans, the new system is responsible for perception of virtually all aspects of visual form, colors, and other conscious vision. Conversely, in many primitive animals, even visual form is detected by the older system, using the superior colliculus in the same manner that the visual cortex is used in mammals.

Function of the Dorsal Lateral Geniculate Nucleus of the Thalamus

The optic nerve fibers of the new visual system terminate in the *dorsal lateral geniculate nucleus*, located at the dorsal end of the thalamus and also called the *lateral geniculate body*, as shown in Figure 51-1. The dorsal lateral geniculate nucleus serves two principal functions: First, it relays visual information from the optic tract to the *visual cortex* by way of the *optic radiation* (also called the *geniculocalcarine tract*). This relay function is so accurate that there is exact point-to-point transmission with a high degree of spatial fidelity all the way from the retina to the visual cortex.

Half the fibers in each optic tract after passing the optic chiasm are derived from one eye and half from the other eye, representing corresponding points on the two retinas. However, the signals from the two eyes are kept apart in the dorsal lateral geniculate nucleus. This nucleus is composed of six nuclear layers. Layers II, III, and V (from ventral to dorsal) receive signals from the lateral half of the ipsilateral retina, whereas layers I, IV, and VI receive signals from the medial half of the retina of the opposite eye. The respective retinal areas of the two eyes connect with neurons that are superimposed over one another in

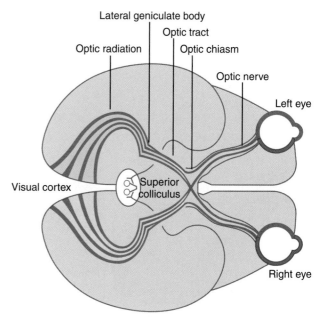

Figure 51-1 Principal visual pathways from the eyes to the visual cortex. (Modified from Polyak SL: The Retina. Chicago: University of Chicago, 1941.)

the paired layers, and similar parallel transmission is preserved all the way to the visual cortex.

The second major function of the dorsal lateral geniculate nucleus is to "gate" the transmission of signals to the visual cortex—that is, to control how much of the signal is allowed to pass to the cortex. The nucleus receives gating control signals from two major sources: (1) *corticofugal fibers* returning in a backward direction from the primary visual cortex to the lateral geniculate nucleus, and (2) *reticular areas of the mesencephalon*. Both of these are inhibitory and, when stimulated, can turn off transmission through selected portions of the dorsal lateral geniculate nucleus. Both of these gating circuits help highlight the visual information that is allowed to pass.

Finally, the dorsal lateral geniculate nucleus is divided in another way: (1) Layers I and II are called *magnocellular layers* because they contain large neurons. These receive their input almost entirely from the large *type Y retinal ganglion cells*. This magnocellular system provides a *rapidly conducting* pathway to the visual cortex. However, this system is color blind, transmitting only black-and-white information. Also, its point-to-point transmission is poor because there are not many Y ganglion cells, and their dendrites spread widely in the retina. (2) Layers III through VI are called *parvocellular layers* because they contain large numbers of small to medium-sized neurons. These neurons receive their input almost entirely from the *type X retinal ganglion cells* that transmit color and convey accurate point-to-point spatial information, but at only a moderate velocity of conduction rather than at high velocity.

Organization and Function of the Visual Cortex

Figures 51-2 and 51-3 show the *visual cortex* located primarily on the medial aspect of the occipital lobes. Like the cortical representations of the other sensory systems, the

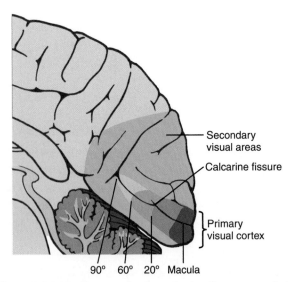

Figure 51-2 Visual cortex in the *calcarine fissure area* of the *medial* occipital cortex.

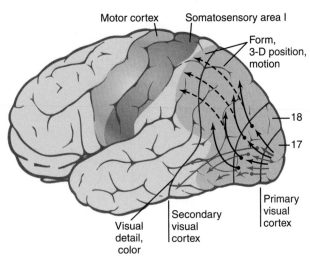

Figure 51-3 Transmission of visual signals from the primary visual cortex into secondary visual areas on the lateral surfaces of the occipital and parietal cortices. Note that the signals representing form, third-dimensional position, and motion are transmitted mainly into the superior portions of the occipital lobe and posterior portions of the parietal lobe. By contrast, the signals for visual detail and color are transmitted mainly into the anteroventral portion of the occipital lobe and the ventral portion of the posterior temporal lobe.

visual cortex is divided into a *primary visual cortex* and *secondary visual areas.*

Primary Visual Cortex. The primary visual cortex (see Figure 51-2) lies in the *calcarine fissure area*, extending forward from the *occipital pole* on the *medial* aspect of each occipital cortex. This area is the terminus of direct visual signals from the eyes. Signals from the macular area of the retina terminate near the occipital pole, as shown in Figure 51-2, whereas signals from the more peripheral retina terminate at or in concentric half circles anterior to the pole but still along the calcarine fissure on the medial occipital lobe. The upper portion of the retina is represented superiorly and the lower portion inferiorly.

Note in the figure the large area that represents the macula. It is to this region that the retinal fovea transmits its signals. The fovea is responsible for the highest degree of visual acuity. Based on retinal area, the fovea has several hundred times as much representation in the primary visual cortex as do the most peripheral portions of the retina.

The primary visual cortex is also called *visual area I.* Still another name is the *striate cortex* because this area has a grossly striated appearance.

Secondary Visual Areas of the Cortex. The secondary visual areas, also called *visual association areas*, lie lateral, anterior, superior, and inferior to the primary visual cortex. Most of these areas also fold outward over the lateral surfaces of the occipital and parietal cortex, as shown in Figure 51-3. Secondary signals are transmitted to these areas for analysis of visual meanings. For instance, on all sides of the primary visual cortex is *Brodmann's area 18* (see Figure 51-3), which is where virtually all signals from the primary visual cortex pass next. Therefore, Brodmann's area 18 is called *visual area II*, or simply V-2. The other, more distant secondary visual areas have specific designations—V-3, V-4, and so forth—up to more than a dozen areas. The importance of all these areas is that various aspects of the visual image are progressively dissected and analyzed.

The Primary Visual Cortex Has Six Major Layers

Like almost all other portions of the cerebral cortex, the primary visual cortex has six distinct layers, as shown in Figure 51-4. Also, as is true for the other sensory systems, the geniculocalcarine fibers terminate mainly in layer IV. But this layer, too, is organized into subdivisions. The rapidly conducted signals from the Y retinal ganglion cells terminate in layer IVcα, and from there they are relayed vertically both outward toward the cortical surface and inward toward deeper levels.

The visual signals from the medium-sized optic nerve fibers, derived from the X ganglion cells in the retina, also terminate in layer IV, but at points different from

the Y signals. They terminate in layers IVa and IVcβ, the shallowest and deepest portions of layer IV, shown to the right in Figure 51-4. From there, these signals are transmitted vertically both toward the surface of the cortex and to deeper layers. It is these X ganglion pathways that transmit the accurate point-to-point type of vision, as well as color vision.

Vertical Neuronal Columns in the Visual Cortex. The visual cortex is organized structurally into several million vertical columns of neuronal cells, each column having a diameter of 30 to 50 micrometers. The same vertical columnar organization is found throughout the cerebral cortex for the other senses as well (and also in the motor and analytical cortical regions). Each column represents a functional unit. One can roughly calculate that each of the visual vertical columns has perhaps 1000 or more neurons.

After the optic signals terminate in layer IV, they are further processed as they spread both outward and inward along each vertical column unit. This processing is believed to decipher separate bits of visual information at successive stations along the pathway. The signals that pass outward to layers I, II, and III eventually transmit signals for short distances laterally in the cortex. Conversely, the signals that pass inward to layers V and VI excite neurons that transmit signals much greater distances.

"Color Blobs" in the Visual Cortex. Interspersed among the primary visual columns, as well as among the columns of some of the secondary visual areas, are special column-like areas called *color blobs*. They receive lateral signals from adjacent visual columns and are activated specifically by color signals. Therefore, these blobs are presumably the primary areas for deciphering color.

Interaction of Visual Signals from the Two Separate Eyes. Recall that visual signals from the two separate eyes are relayed through separate neuronal layers in the lateral geniculate nucleus. These signals still remain separated from each other when they arrive in layer IV of the primary visual cortex. In fact, layer IV is interlaced with stripes of neuronal columns, each stripe about 0.5 millimeter wide; the signals from one eye enter the columns of every other stripe, alternating with signals from the second eye. This cortical area deciphers whether the respective areas of the two visual images from the two separate eyes are "in register" with each other—that is, whether corresponding points from the two retinas fit with each other. In turn, the deciphered information is used to adjust the directional gaze of the separate eyes so that they will fuse with each other (be brought into "register"). The information observed about degree of register of images from the two eyes also allows a person to distinguish the distance of objects by the mechanism of *stereopsis*.

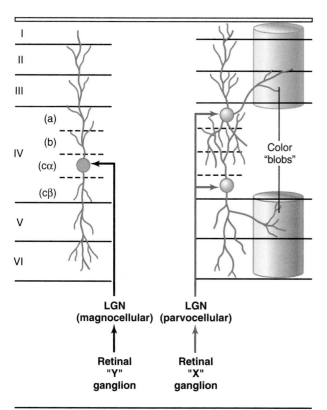

Fast, Black and White   Very Accurate, Color

Figure 51-4 Six layers of the primary visual cortex. The connections shown on the left side of the figure originate in the magnocellular layers of the lateral geniculate nucleus (LGN) and transmit rapidly changing black-and-white visual signals. The pathways to the right originate in the parvocellular layers (layers III through VI) of the LGN; they transmit signals that depict accurate spatial detail, as well as color. Note especially the areas of the visual cortex called "color blobs," which are necessary for detection of color.

Two Major Pathways for Analysis of Visual Information—(1) The Fast "Position" and "Motion" Pathway; (2) The Accurate Color Pathway

Figure 51-3 shows that after leaving the primary visual cortex, the visual information is analyzed in two major pathways in the secondary visual areas.

1. **Analysis of Third-Dimensional Position, Gross Form, and Motion of Objects.** One of the analytical pathways, demonstrated in Figure 51-3 by the black arrows, analyzes the third-dimensional positions of visual objects in the space around the body. This pathway also analyzes the gross physical form of the visual scene, as well as motion in the scene. In other words, this pathway tells where every object is during each instant and whether it is moving. After leaving the primary visual cortex, the signals flow generally into the *posterior midtemporal area* and upward into the broad *occipitoparietal cortex*. At the anterior border of the parietal cortex, the signals overlap with signals from the posterior somatic association areas that analyze three-dimensional aspects of somatosensory signals. The signals transmitted in this *position-form-motion* pathway are mainly from the large Y optic nerve fibers of the retinal Y ganglion cells, transmitting rapid signals but depicting only black and white with no color.

2. **Analysis of Visual Detail and Color.** The red arrows in Figure 51-3, passing from the primary visual cortex into secondary visual areas of the *inferior, ventral,* and *medial regions* of the *occipital* and *temporal cortex,* show the principal pathway for analysis of visual detail. Separate portions of this pathway specifically dissect out color as well. Therefore, this pathway is concerned with such visual feats as recognizing letters, reading, determining the texture of surfaces, determining detailed colors of objects, and deciphering from all this information what the object is and what it means.

Neuronal Patterns of Stimulation During Analysis of the Visual Image

Analysis of Contrasts in the Visual Image. If a person looks at a blank wall, only a few neurons in the primary visual cortex will be stimulated, regardless of whether the illumination of the wall is bright or weak. Therefore, what does the primary visual cortex detect? To answer this, let us now place on the wall a large solid cross, as shown to the left in Figure 51-5. To the right is shown the spatial pattern of the most excited neurons in the visual cortex. *Note that the areas of maximum excitation occur along the sharp borders of the visual pattern.* Thus, the visual signal in the primary visual cortex is concerned mainly with *contrasts* in the visual scene, rather than with noncontrasting areas. We noted in Chapter 50 that this is also true of most of the retinal ganglion because equally

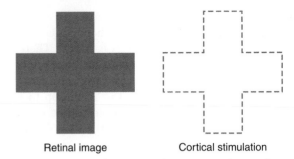

Retinal image   Cortical stimulation

Figure 51-5 Pattern of excitation that occurs in the visual cortex in response to a retinal image of a dark cross.

stimulated adjacent retinal receptors mutually inhibit one another. But at any border in the visual scene where there is a change from dark to light or light to dark, mutual inhibition does not occur, and the intensity of stimulation of most neurons is proportional to the *gradient of contrast*—that is, the greater the sharpness of contrast and the greater the intensity difference between light and dark areas, the greater the degree of stimulation.

Visual Cortex Also Detects Orientation of Lines and Borders—"Simple" Cells. The visual cortex detects not only the existence of lines and borders in the different areas of the retinal image but also the direction of orientation of each line or border—that is, whether it is vertical or horizontal or lies at some degree of inclination. This is believed to result from linear organizations of mutually inhibiting cells that excite second-order neurons when inhibition occurs all along a line of cells where there is a contrast edge. Thus, for each such orientation of a line, specific neuronal cells are stimulated. A line oriented in a different direction excites a different set of cells. These neuronal cells are called *simple cells*. They are found mainly in layer IV of the primary visual cortex.

Detection of Line Orientation When a Line Is Displaced Laterally or Vertically in the Visual Field—"Complex" Cells. As the visual signal progresses farther away from layer IV, some neurons respond to lines that are oriented in the same direction but are not position specific. That is, even if a line is displaced moderate distances laterally or vertically in the field, the same few neurons will still be stimulated if the line has the same direction. These cells are called *complex cells*.

Detection of Lines of Specific Lengths, Angles, or Other Shapes. Some neurons in the outer layers of the primary visual columns, as well as neurons in some secondary visual areas, are stimulated only by lines or borders of specific lengths, by specific angulated shapes, or by images that have other characteristics. That is, these neurons detect still higher orders of information from the visual scene. Thus, as one goes farther into the analytical pathway of the visual cortex, progressively more characteristics of each visual scene are deciphered.

Detection of Color

Color is detected in much the same way that lines are detected: by means of color contrast. For instance, a red area is often contrasted against a green area, a blue area against a red area, or a green area against a yellow area. All these colors can also be contrasted against a white area within the visual scene. In fact, this contrasting against white is believed to be mainly responsible for the phenomenon called "color constancy"; that is, when the color of an illuminating light changes, the color of the "white" changes with the light, and appropriate computation in the brain allows red to be interpreted as red even though the illuminating light has changed the color entering the eyes.

The mechanism of color contrast analysis depends on the fact that contrasting colors, called "opponent colors," excite specific neuronal cells. It is presumed that the initial details of color contrast are detected by simple cells, whereas more complex contrasts are detected by complex and hypercomplex cells.

Effect of Removing the Primary Visual Cortex

Removal of the primary visual cortex in the human being causes loss of conscious vision, that is, blindness. However, psychological studies demonstrate that such "blind" people can still, at times, react subconsciously to changes in light intensity, to movement in the visual scene, or, rarely, even to some gross patterns of vision. These reactions include turning the eyes, turning the head, and avoidance. This vision is believed to be subserved by neuronal pathways that pass from the optic tracts mainly into the superior colliculi and other portions of the older visual system.

Fields of Vision; Perimetry

The *field of vision* is the visual area seen by an eye at a given instant. The area seen to the nasal side is called the *nasal field of vision*, and the area seen to the lateral side is called the *temporal field of vision*.

To diagnose blindness in specific portions of the retina, one charts the field of vision for each eye by a process called *perimetry*. This is done by having the subject look with one eye closed and the other eye looking toward a central spot directly in front of the eye. Then a small dot of light or a small object is moved back and forth in all areas of the field of vision, and the subject indicates when the spot of light or object can be seen and when it cannot. Thus, the field of vision for the left eye is plotted as shown in Figure 51-6. In all perimetry charts, a *blind spot* caused by lack of rods and cones in the retina over the *optic disc* is found about 15 degrees lateral to the central point of vision, as shown in the figure.

Abnormalities in the Fields of Vision. Occasionally, blind spots are found in portions of the field of vision other than the optic disc area. Such blind spots are called *scotomata*; they frequently are caused by damage to the optic nerve resulting from glaucoma (too much fluid pressure in the eyeball), from allergic reactions in the retina, or from toxic conditions such as lead poisoning or excessive use of tobacco.

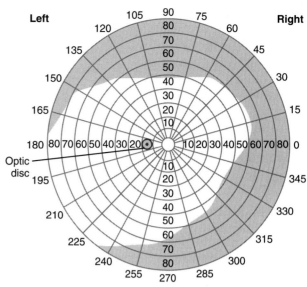

Figure 51-6 Perimetry chart, showing the field of vision for the left eye.

Another condition that can be diagnosed by perimetry is *retinitis pigmentosa*. In this disease, portions of the retina degenerate, and excessive melanin pigment deposits in the degenerated areas. Retinitis pigmentosa usually causes blindness in the peripheral field of vision first and then gradually encroaches on the central areas.

Effect of Lesions in the Optic Pathway on the Fields of Vision. Destruction of an entire *optic nerve* causes blindness of the affected eye.

Destruction of the *optic chiasm* prevents the crossing of impulses from the nasal half of each retina to the opposite optic tract. Therefore, the nasal half of each retina is blinded, which means that the person is blind in the temporal field of vision for each eye *because the image of the field of vision is inverted on the retina* by the optical system of the eye; this condition is called *bitemporal hemianopsia*. Such lesions frequently result from tumors of the pituitary gland pressing upward from the sella turcica on the bottom of the optic chiasm.

Interruption of an *optic tract* denervates the corresponding half of each retina on the same side as the lesion; as a result, neither eye can see objects to the opposite side of the head. This condition is known as *homonymous hemianopsia*.

Eye Movements and Their Control

To make full use of the visual abilities of the eyes, almost equally as important as interpretation of the visual signals from the eyes is the cerebral control system for directing the eyes toward the object to be viewed.

Muscular Control of Eye Movements. The eye movements are controlled by three pairs of muscles, shown in Figure 51-7: (1) the *medial* and *lateral recti*, (2) the *superior* and *inferior recti*, and (3) the *superior* and

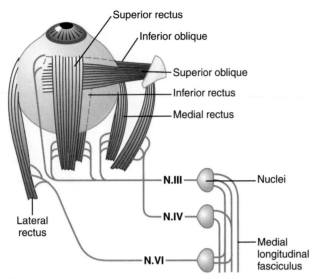

Figure 51-7 Extraocular muscles of the eye and their innervation.

inferior obliques. The medial and lateral recti contract to move the eyes from side to side. The superior and inferior recti contract to move the eyes upward or downward. The oblique muscles function mainly to rotate the eyeballs to keep the visual fields in the upright position.

Neural Pathways for Control of Eye Movements.

Figure 51-7 also shows brain stem nuclei for the third, fourth, and sixth cranial nerves and their connections with the peripheral nerves to the ocular muscles. Shown,

too, are interconnections among the brain stem nuclei by way of the nerve tract called the *medial longitudinal fasciculus.* Each of the three sets of muscles to each eye is *reciprocally* innervated so that one muscle of the pair relaxes while the other contracts.

Figure 51-8 demonstrates cortical control of the oculomotor apparatus, showing spread of signals from visual areas in the occipital cortex through occipitotectal and occipitocollicular tracts to the pretectal and superior colliculus areas of the brain stem. From both the pretectal and the superior colliculus areas, the oculomotor control signals pass to the brain stem nuclei of the oculomotor nerves. Strong signals are also transmitted from the body's equilibrium control centers in the brain stem into the oculomotor system (from the vestibular nuclei by way of the medial longitudinal fasciculus).

Fixation Movements of the Eyes

Perhaps the most important movements of the eyes are those that cause the eyes to "fix" on a discrete portion of the field of vision. Fixation movements are controlled by two neuronal mechanisms. The first of these allows a person to move the eyes voluntarily to find the object on which he or she wants to fix the vision; this is called the *voluntary fixation mechanism.* The second is an involuntary mechanism that holds the eyes firmly on the object once it has been found; this is called the *involuntary fixation mechanism.*

The voluntary fixation movements are controlled by a cortical field located bilaterally in the premotor

Figure 51-8 Neural pathways for control of conjugate movement of the eyes.

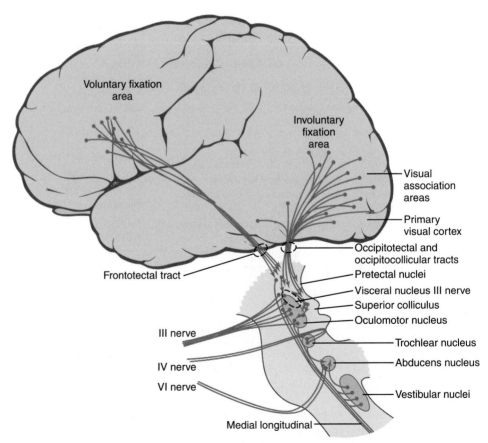

cortical regions of the frontal lobes, as shown in Figure 51-8. Bilateral dysfunction or destruction of these areas makes it difficult for a person to "unlock" the eyes from one point of fixation and move them to another point. It is usually necessary to blink the eyes or put a hand over the eyes for a short time, which then allows the eyes to be moved.

Conversely, the fixation mechanism that causes the eyes to "lock" on the object of attention once it is found is controlled by *secondary visual areas in the occipital cortex*, located mainly anterior to the primary visual cortex. When this fixation area is destroyed bilaterally in an animal, the animal has difficulty keeping its eyes directed toward a given fixation point or may become totally unable to do so.

To summarize, posterior "involuntary" occipital cortical eye fields automatically "lock" the eyes on a given spot of the visual field and thereby prevent movement of the image across the retinas. To unlock this visual fixation, voluntary signals must be transmitted from cortical "voluntary" eye fields located in the frontal cortices.

Mechanism of Involuntary Locking Fixation—Role of the Superior Colliculi.

The involuntary locking type of fixation discussed in the previous section results from a negative feedback mechanism that prevents the object of attention from leaving the foveal portion of the retina. The eyes normally have three types of continuous but almost imperceptible movements: (1) a *continuous tremor* at a rate of 30 to 80 cycles per second caused by successive contractions of the motor units in the ocular muscles, (2) a *slow drift* of the eyeballs in one direction or another, and (3) sudden *flicking movements* that are controlled by the involuntary fixation mechanism.

When a spot of light has become fixed on the foveal region of the retina, the tremulous movements cause the spot to move back and forth at a rapid rate across the cones, and the drifting movements cause the spot to drift slowly across the cones. Each time the spot drifts as far as the edge of the fovea, a sudden reflex reaction occurs, producing a flicking movement that moves the spot away from this edge back toward the center of the fovea. Thus, an automatic response moves the image back toward the central point of vision.

These drifting and flicking motions are demonstrated in Figure 51-9, which shows by the dashed lines the slow drifting across the fovea and by the solid lines the flicks that keep the image from leaving the foveal region. This involuntary fixation capability is mostly lost when the superior colliculi are destroyed.

Saccadic Movement of the Eyes—A Mechanism of Successive Fixation Points.

When a visual scene is moving continually before the eyes, such as when a person is riding in a car, the eyes fix on one highlight after another in the visual field, jumping from one to the next at a rate of two to three jumps per second. The jumps are called *saccades*, and the movements are called *opticokinetic*

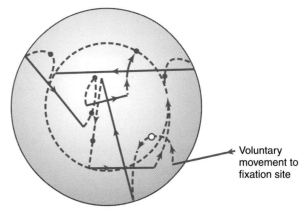

Figure 51-9 Movements of a spot of light on the fovea, showing sudden "flicking" eye movements that move the spot back toward the center of the fovea whenever it drifts to the foveal edge. (The *dashed lines* represent slow drifting movements, and the *solid lines* represent sudden flicking movements.) (Modified from Whitteridge D: Central control of the eye movements. In Field J, Magoun HW, Hall VE (eds): Handbook of Physiology. vol. 2, sec. 1. Washington, DC: American Physiological Society, 1960.)

Voluntary movement to fixation site

movements. The saccades occur so rapidly that no more than 10 percent of the total time is spent in moving the eyes, with 90 percent of the time being allocated to the fixation sites. Also, the brain suppresses the visual image during saccades, so the person is not conscious of the movements from point to point.

Saccadic Movements During Reading.

During the process of reading, a person usually makes several saccadic movements of the eyes for each line. In this case, the visual scene is not moving past the eyes, but the eyes are trained to move by means of several successive saccades across the visual scene to extract the important information. Similar saccades occur when a person observes a painting, except that the saccades occur in upward, sideways, downward, and angulated directions one after another from one highlight of the painting to another, and so forth.

Fixation on Moving Objects—"Pursuit Movement."

The eyes can also remain fixed on a moving object, which is called *pursuit movement*. A highly developed cortical mechanism automatically detects the course of movement of an object and then rapidly develops a similar course of movement for the eyes. For instance, if an object is moving up and down in a wavelike form at a rate of several times per second, the eyes at first may be unable to fixate on it. However, after a second or so, the eyes begin to jump by means of saccades in approximately the same wavelike pattern of movement as that of the object. Then, after another few seconds, the eyes develop progressively smoother movements and finally follow the wave movement almost exactly. This represents a high degree of automatic subconscious computational ability by the pursuit system for controlling eye movements.

Superior Colliculi Are Mainly Responsible for Turning the Eyes and Head Toward a Visual Disturbance

Even after the visual cortex has been destroyed, a sudden visual disturbance in a lateral area of the visual field often causes immediate turning of the eyes in that direction. This does not occur if the superior colliculi have also been destroyed. To support this function, the various points of the retina are represented topographically in the superior colliculi in the same way as in the primary visual cortex, although with less accuracy. Even so, the principal direction of a flash of light in a peripheral retinal field is mapped by the colliculi, and secondary signals are transmitted to the oculomotor nuclei to turn the eyes. To help in this directional movement of the eyes, the superior colliculi also have topological maps of somatic sensations from the body and acoustic signals from the ears.

The optic nerve fibers from the eyes to the colliculi, which are responsible for these rapid turning movements, are branches from the rapidly conducting Y fibers, with one branch going to the visual cortex and the other going to the superior colliculi. (The superior colliculi and other regions of the brain stem are also strongly supplied with visual signals transmitted in type W optic nerve fibers. These represent the oldest visual pathway, but their function is unclear.)

In addition to causing the eyes to turn toward a visual disturbance, signals are relayed from the superior colliculi through the *medial longitudinal fasciculus* to other levels of the brain stem to cause turning of the whole head and even of the whole body toward the direction of the disturbance. Other types of nonvisual disturbances, such as strong sounds or even stroking of the side of the body, cause similar turning of the eyes, head, and body, but only if the superior colliculi are intact. Therefore, the superior colliculi play a global role in orienting the eyes, head, and body with respect to external disturbances, whether they are visual, auditory, or somatic.

"Fusion" of the Visual Images from the Two Eyes

To make the visual perceptions more meaningful, the visual images in the two eyes normally *fuse* with each other on "corresponding points" of the two retinas. The visual cortex plays an important role in fusion. It was pointed out earlier in the chapter that corresponding points of the two retinas transmit visual signals to different neuronal layers of the lateral geniculate body, and these signals in turn are relayed to parallel neurons in the visual cortex. Interactions occur between these cortical neurons to cause *interference excitation* in specific neurons when the two visual images are not "in register"—that is, are not precisely "fused." This excitation presumably provides the signal that is transmitted to the oculomotor apparatus to cause convergence or divergence or rotation of the eyes so that fusion can be re-established. Once the corresponding points of the two retinas are in register, excitation of the specific "interference" neurons in the visual cortex disappears.

Neural Mechanism of Stereopsis for Judging Distances of Visual Objects

In Chapter 49, it is pointed out that because the two eyes are more than 2 inches apart, the images on the two retinas are not exactly the same. That is, the right eye sees a little more of the right-hand side of the object, and the left eye a little more of the left-hand side, and the closer the object, the greater the disparity. Therefore, even when the two eyes are fused with each other, it is still impossible for all corresponding points in the two visual images to be exactly in register at the same time. Furthermore, the nearer the object is to the eyes, the less the degree of register. This degree of nonregister provides the neural mechanism for *stereopsis*, an important mechanism for judging the distances of visual objects up to about 200 feet (60 meters).

The neuronal cellular mechanism for stereopsis is based on the fact that some of the fiber pathways from the retinas to the visual cortex stray 1 to 2 degrees on each side of the central pathway. Therefore, some optic pathways from the two eyes are exactly in register for objects 2 meters away; still another set of pathways is in register for objects 25 meters away. Thus, the distance is determined by which set or sets of pathways are excited by nonregister or register. This phenomenon is called *depth perception*, which is another name for stereopsis.

Strabismus—Lack of Fusion of the Eyes

Strabismus, also called *squint* or *cross-eye*, means lack of fusion of the eyes in one or more of the visual coordinates: horizontal, vertical, or rotational. The basic types of strabismus are shown in Figure 51-10: (1) *horizontal strabismus*, (2) *torsional strabismus*, and (3) *vertical strabismus*. Combinations of two or even all three of the different types of strabismus often occur.

Strabismus is often caused by abnormal "set" of the fusion mechanism of the visual system. That is, in a young child's early efforts to fixate the two eyes on the same object, one of the eyes fixates satisfactorily while the other fails do so, or they both fixate satisfactorily but never simultaneously. Soon the patterns of conjugate movements of the eyes become abnormally "set" in the neuronal control pathways themselves, so the eyes never fuse.

Suppression of the Visual Image from a Repressed Eye. In a few patients with strabismus, the eyes alternate in fixing on the object of attention. In other patients, one eye alone is used all the time, and the other eye becomes repressed and is never used for precise vision. The visual acuity of the repressed eye develops only slightly, sometimes remaining 20/400 or less. If the dominant eye then becomes blinded,

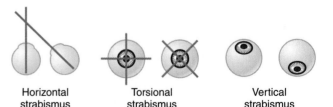

Horizontal strabismus   Torsional strabismus   Vertical strabismus

Figure 51-10 Basic types of strabismus.

vision in the repressed eye can develop only to a slight extent in adults but far more in young children. This demonstrates that visual acuity is highly dependent on proper development of central nervous system synaptic connections from the eyes. In fact, even anatomically, the numbers of neuronal connections diminish in the visual cortex areas that would normally receive signals from the repressed eye.

Autonomic Control of Accommodation and Pupillary Aperture

Autonomic Nerves to the Eyes. The eye is innervated by both parasympathetic and sympathetic nerve fibers, as shown in Figure 51-11. The parasympathetic preganglionic fibers arise in the *Edinger-Westphal nucleus* (the visceral nucleus portion of the third cranial nerve) and then pass in the *third nerve* to the *ciliary ganglion*, which lies immediately behind the eye. There, the preganglionic fibers synapse with postganglionic parasympathetic neurons, which in turn send fibers through *ciliary nerves* into the eyeball. These nerves excite (1) the ciliary muscle that controls focusing of the eye lens and (2) the sphincter of the iris that constricts the pupil.

The sympathetic innervation of the eye originates in the *intermediolateral horn cells* of the first thoracic segment of the spinal cord. From there, sympathetic fibers enter the sympathetic chain and pass upward to the *superior cervical ganglion*, where they synapse with postganglionic

neurons. Postganglionic sympathetic fibers from these then spread along the surfaces of the carotid artery and successively smaller arteries until they reach the eye. There, the sympathetic fibers innervate the radial fibers of the iris (which open the pupil), as well as several extraocular muscles of the eye, which are discussed subsequently in relation to Horner's syndrome.

Control of Accommodation (Focusing the Eyes)

The accommodation mechanism—that is, the mechanism that focuses the lens system of the eye—is essential for a high degree of visual acuity. Accommodation results from contraction or relaxation of the eye ciliary muscle. Contraction causes increased refractive power of the lens, as explained in Chapter 49, and relaxation causes decreased power. How does a person adjust accommodation to keep the eyes in focus all the time?

Accommodation of the lens is regulated by a negative feedback mechanism that automatically adjusts the refractive power of the lens to achieve the highest degree of visual acuity. When the eyes have been focused on some far object and must then suddenly focus on a near object, the lens usually accommodates for best acuity of vision within less than 1 second. Although the precise control mechanism that causes this rapid and accurate focusing of the eye is unclear, some of the known features are the following.

First, when the eyes suddenly change distance of the fixation point, the lens changes its strength in the proper direction to achieve a new state of focus within a fraction of a second. Second, different types of clues help to change the lens strength in the proper direction:

1. *Chromatic aberration* appears to be important. That is, red light rays focus slightly posteriorly to blue light rays because the lens bends blue rays more than red rays. The eyes appear to be able to detect which of these two types of rays is in better focus, and this clue relays information to the accommodation mechanism whether to make the lens stronger or weaker.

2. When the eyes fixate on a near object, the eyes must converge. The neural mechanisms for *convergence cause a simultaneous signal to strengthen the lens of the eye.*

3. *Because the fovea lies in a hollowed-out depression that is slightly deeper than the remainder of the retina, the clarity of focus in the depth of the fovea is different from the clarity of focus on the edges.* This may also give clues about which way the strength of the lens needs to be changed.

4. *The degree of accommodation of the lens oscillates slightly* all the time at a frequency up to twice per second. The visual image becomes clearer when the oscillation of the lens strength is changing in the appropriate direction and becomes poorer when the lens strength is changing in the wrong direction. This could give a rapid clue as to which way the strength of the lens needs to change to provide appropriate focus.

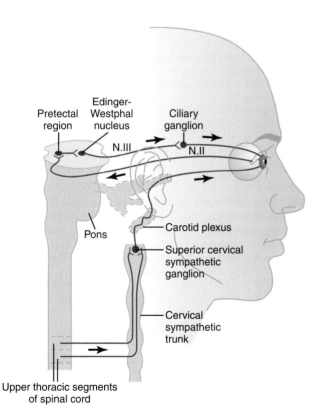

Figure 51-11 Autonomic innervation of the eye, showing also the reflex arc of the light reflex. (Modified from Ranson SW, Clark SL: Anatomy of the Nervous System: Its Development and Function, 10th ed. Philadelphia: WB Saunders, 1959.)

The brain cortical areas that control accommodation closely parallel those that control fixation movements of the eyes, with analysis of the visual signals in Brodmann's cortical areas 18 and 19 and transmission of motor signals to the ciliary muscle through the pretectal area in the brain stem, then through the *Edinger-Westphal nucleus*, and finally by way of parasympathetic nerve fibers to the eyes.

Control of Pupillary Diameter

Stimulation of the parasympathetic nerves also excites the pupillary sphincter muscle, thereby decreasing the pupillary aperture; this is called *miosis*. Conversely, stimulation of the sympathetic nerves excites the radial fibers of the iris and causes pupillary dilation, called *mydriasis*.

Pupillary Light Reflex. When light is shone into the eyes, the pupils constrict, a reaction called the *pupillary light reflex*. The neuronal pathway for this reflex is demonstrated by the upper two black arrows in Figure 51-11. When light impinges on the retina, a few of the resulting impulses pass from the optic nerves to the pretectal nuclei. From here, secondary impulses pass to the *Edinger-Westphal nucleus* and, finally, back through *parasympathetic nerves* to constrict the sphincter of the iris. Conversely, in darkness, the reflex becomes inhibited, which results in dilation of the pupil.

The function of the light reflex is to help the eye adapt extremely rapidly to changing light conditions, as explained in Chapter 50. The limits of pupillary diameter are about 1.5 millimeters on the small side and 8 millimeters on the large side. Therefore, because light brightness on the retina increases with the square of pupillary diameter, the range of light and dark adaptation that can be brought about by the pupillary reflex is about 30 to 1—that is, up to as much as 30 times change in the amount of light entering the eye.

Pupillary Reflexes or Reactions in Central Nervous System Disease. A few central nervous system diseases damage nerve transmission of visual signals from the retinas to the Edinger-Westphal nucleus, thus sometimes blocking the pupillary reflexes. Such blocks may occur as a result of *central nervous system syphilis, alcoholism, encephalitis,* and so forth. The block usually occurs in the pretectal region of the brain stem, although it can result from destruction of some small fibers in the optic nerves.

The final nerve fibers in the pathway through the pretectal area to the Edinger-Westphal nucleus are mostly of the inhibitory type. When their inhibitory effect is lost, the nucleus becomes chronically active, causing the pupils to remain mostly constricted, in addition to their failure to respond to light.

Yet the pupils can constrict a little more if the Edinger-Westphal nucleus is stimulated through some other pathway. For instance, when the eyes fixate on a near object, the signals that cause accommodation of the lens and those that cause convergence of the two eyes cause a mild degree of pupillary constriction at the same time. This is called the *pupillary reaction to accommodation*. A pupil that fails to respond to light but does respond to accommodation and is also very small (an *Argyll Robertson pupil*) is an important diagnostic sign of central nervous system disease such as syphilis.

Horner's Syndrome. The sympathetic nerves to the eye are occasionally interrupted. Interruption frequently occurs in the cervical sympathetic chain. This causes the clinical condition called *Horner's syndrome*, which consists of the following effects: First, because of interruption of sympathetic nerve fibers to the pupillary dilator muscle, the pupil remains persistently constricted to a smaller diameter than the pupil of the opposite eye. Second, the superior eyelid droops because it is normally maintained in an open position during waking hours partly by contraction of smooth muscle fibers embedded in the superior eyelid and innervated by the sympathetics. Therefore, destruction of the sympathetic nerves makes it impossible to open the superior eyelid as widely as normally. Third, the blood vessels on the corresponding side of the face and head become persistently dilated. Fourth, sweating (which requires sympathetic nerve signals) cannot occur on the side of the face and head affected by Horner's syndrome.

Bibliography

Bridge H, Cumming BG: Representation of binocular surfaces by cortical neurons, *Curr Opin Neurobiol* 18:425, 2008.

Buttner-Ennever JA, Eberhorn A, Horn AK: Motor and sensory innervation of extraocular eye muscles, *Ann N Y Acad Sci* 1004:40, 2003.

Collewijn H, Kowler E: The significance of microsaccades for vision and oculomotor control, *J Vis* 8:20, 1–21, 2008.

Crawford JD, Martinez-Trujillo JC, Klier EM: Neural control of three-dimensional eye and head movements, *Curr Opin Neurobiol* 13:655, 2003.

Derrington AM, Webb BS: Visual system: how is the retina wired up to the cortex? *Curr Biol* 14:R14, 2004.

Guyton DL: Ocular torsion reveals the mechanisms of cyclovertical strabismus: the Weisenfeld lecture, *Invest Ophthalmol Vis Sci* 49:847, 2008.

Hikosaka O, Takikawa Y, Kawagoe R: Role of the basal ganglia in the control of purposive saccadic eye movements, *Physiol Rev* 80:953, 2000.

Kandel ER, Schwartz JH, Jessell TM: *Principles of Neural Science*, ed 4, New York, 2000, McGraw-Hill.

Kingdom FA: Perceiving light versus material, *Vision Res* 48:2090, 2008.

Klier EM, Angelaki DE: Spatial updating and the maintenance of visual constancy, *Neuroscience* 156:801, 2008.

Krauzlis RJ: Recasting the smooth pursuit eye movement system, *J Neurophysiol* 91:591, 2004.

Luna B, Velanova K, Geier CF: Development of eye-movement control, *Brain Cogn* 68:293, 2008.

Martinez-Conde S, Macknik SL, Hubel DH: The role of fixational eye movements in visual perception, *Nat Rev Neurosci* 5:229, 2004.

Munoz DP, Everling S: Look away: the anti-saccade task and the voluntary control of eye movement, *Nat Rev Neurosci* 5:218, 2004.

Nassi JJ, Callaway EM: Parallel processing strategies of the primate visual system, *Nat Rev Neurosci* 10:360, 2009.

Parker AJ: Binocular depth perception and the cerebral cortex, *Nat Rev Neurosci* 8:379, 2007.

Peelen MV, Downing PE: The neural basis of visual body perception, *Nat Rev Neurosci* 8:636, 2007.

Pelli DG: Crowding: a cortical constraint on object recognition, *Curr Opin Neurobiol* 18:445, 2008.

Pierrot-Deseilligny C, Milea D, Muri RM: Eye movement control by the cerebral cortex, *Curr Opin Neurol* 17:17, 2004.

Roe AW, Parker AJ, Born RT, et al: Disparity channels in early vision, *J Neurosci* 27:11820, 2007.

Sharpe JA: Neurophysiology and neuroanatomy of smooth pursuit: lesion studies, *Brain Cogn* 68:241, 2008.

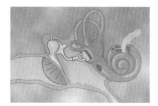

CHAPTER 52

The Sense of Hearing

This chapter describes the mechanisms by which the ear receives sound waves, discriminates their frequencies, and transmits auditory information into the central nervous system, where its meaning is deciphered.

Tympanic Membrane and the Ossicular System

Conduction of Sound from the Tympanic Membrane to the Cochlea

Figure 52-1 shows the *tympanic membrane* (commonly called the *eardrum*) and the *ossicles*, which conduct sound from the tympanic membrane through the middle ear to the *cochlea* (the inner ear). Attached to the tympanic membrane is the *handle* of the *malleus*. The malleus is bound to the *incus* by minute ligaments, so whenever the malleus moves, the incus moves with it. The opposite end of the incus articulates with the stem of the *stapes*, and the *faceplate* of the stapes lies against the *membranous labyrinth* of the cochlea in the opening of the *oval window*.

The tip end of the handle of the malleus is attached to the center of the tympanic membrane, and this point of attachment is constantly pulled by the *tensor tympani muscle*, which keeps the tympanic membrane tensed. This allows sound vibrations on *any* portion of the tympanic membrane to be transmitted to the ossicles, which would not be true if the membrane were lax.

The ossicles of the middle ear are suspended by ligaments in such a way that the combined malleus and incus act as a single lever, having its fulcrum approximately at the border of the tympanic membrane.

The articulation of the incus with the stapes causes the stapes to push forward on the oval window and on the cochlear fluid on the other side of window every time the tympanic membrane moves inward, and to pull backward on the fluid every time the malleus moves outward.

"Impedance Matching" by the Ossicular System. The amplitude of movement of the stapes faceplate with each sound vibration is only three fourths as much as the amplitude of the handle of the malleus. Therefore, the ossicular lever system does not increase the movement distance of the stapes, as is commonly believed. Instead, the system actually reduces the distance but increases the *force* of movement about 1.3 times. In addition, the surface area of the tympanic membrane is about 55 square millimeters, whereas the surface area of the stapes averages 3.2 square millimeters. This 17-fold difference times the 1.3-fold ratio of the lever system causes about 22 times as much *total force* to be exerted on the fluid of the cochlea as is exerted by the sound waves against the tympanic membrane. Because fluid has far greater inertia than air does, increased amounts of force are necessary to cause vibration in the fluid. Therefore, the tympanic membrane and ossicular system provide *impedance matching* between the sound waves in air and the sound vibrations in the fluid of the cochlea. Indeed, the impedance matching is about 50 to 75 percent of perfect for sound frequencies between 300 and 3000 cycles per second, which allows utilization of most of the energy in the incoming sound waves.

In the absence of the ossicular system and tympanic membrane, sound waves can still travel directly through the air of the middle ear and enter the cochlea at the oval window. However, the sensitivity for hearing is then

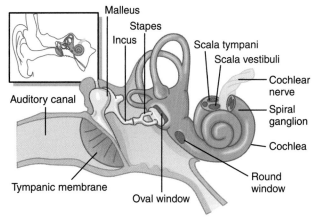

Figure 52-1 Tympanic membrane, ossicular system of the middle ear, and inner ear.

15 to 20 decibels less than for ossicular transmission— equivalent to a decrease from a medium to a barely perceptible voice level.

Attenuation of Sound by Contraction of the Tensor Tympani and Stapedius Muscles. When loud sounds are transmitted through the ossicular system and from there into the central nervous system, a reflex occurs after a latent period of only 40 to 80 milliseconds to cause contraction of the *stapedius muscle* and, to a lesser extent, the *tensor tympani muscle.* The tensor tympani muscle pulls the handle of the malleus inward while the stapedius muscle pulls the stapes outward. These two forces oppose each other and thereby cause the entire ossicular system to develop increased rigidity, thus greatly reducing the ossicular conduction of low-frequency sound, mainly frequencies below 1000 cycles per second.

This *attenuation reflex* can reduce the intensity of lower-frequency sound transmission by 30 to 40 decibels, which is about the same difference as that between a loud voice and a whisper. The function of this mechanism is believed to be twofold:

1. To *protect* the cochlea from damaging vibrations caused by excessively loud sound.
2. To *mask* low-frequency sounds in loud environments. This usually removes a major share of the background noise and allows a person to concentrate on sounds above 1000 cycles per second, where most of the pertinent information in voice communication is transmitted.

Another function of the tensor tympani and stapedius muscles is to decrease a person's hearing sensitivity to his or her own speech. This effect is activated by collateral nerve signals transmitted to these muscles at the same time that the brain activates the voice mechanism.

Transmission of Sound Through Bone

Because the inner ear, the *cochlea*, is embedded in a bony cavity in the temporal bone, called the *bony labyrinth,*

vibrations of the entire skull can cause fluid vibrations in the cochlea itself. Therefore, under appropriate conditions, a tuning fork or an electronic vibrator placed on any bony protuberance of the skull, but especially on the mastoid process near the ear, causes the person to hear the sound. However, the energy available even in loud sound in the air is not sufficient to cause hearing via bone conduction unless a special electromechanical sound-amplifying device is applied to the bone.

Cochlea

Functional Anatomy of the Cochlea

The cochlea is a system of coiled tubes, shown in Figure 52-1 and in cross section in Figures 52-2 and 52-3. It consists of three tubes coiled side by side: (1) the *scala vestibuli*, (2) the *scala media*, and (3) the *scala tympani.* The scala vestibuli and scala media are separated from each

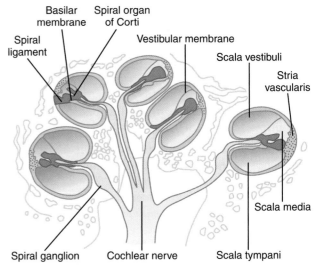

Figure 52-2 Cochlea. (Redrawn from Gray H, Goss CM [eds]: Gray's Anatomy of the Human Body. Philadelphia: Lea & Febiger, 1948.)

Figure 52-3 Section through one of the turns of the cochlea.

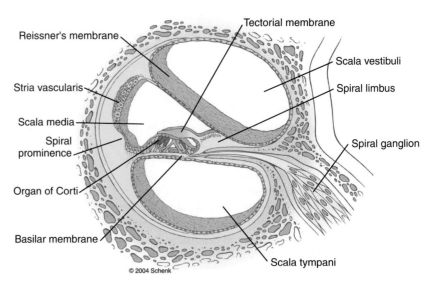

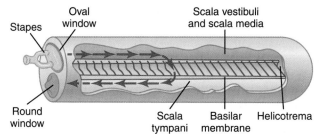

Figure 52-4 Movement of fluid in the cochlea after forward thrust of the stapes.

other by *Reissner's membrane* (also called the *vestibular membrane*), shown in Figure 52-3; the scala tympani and scala media are separated from each other by the *basilar membrane*. On the surface of the basilar membrane lies the *organ of Corti*, which contains a series of electromechanically sensitive cells, the *hair cells*. They are the receptive end organs that generate nerve impulses in response to sound vibrations.

Figure 52-4 diagrams the functional parts of the uncoiled cochlea for conduction of sound vibrations. First, note that Reissner's membrane is missing from this figure. This membrane is so thin and so easily moved that it does not obstruct the passage of sound vibrations from the scala vestibuli into the scala media. Therefore, as far as fluid conduction of sound is concerned, the scala vestibuli and scala media are considered to be a single chamber. (The importance of Reissner's membrane is to maintain a special kind of fluid in the scala media that is required for normal function of the sound-receptive hair cells, as discussed later in the chapter.)

Sound vibrations enter the scala vestibuli from the faceplate of the stapes at the oval window. The faceplate covers this window and is connected with the window's edges by a loose annular ligament so that it can move inward and outward with the sound vibrations. Inward movement causes the fluid to move forward in the scala vestibuli and scala media, and outward movement causes the fluid to move backward.

Basilar Membrane and Resonance in the Cochlea. The basilar membrane is a fibrous membrane that separates the scala media from the scala tympani. It contains 20,000 to 30,000 *basilar fibers* that project from the bony center of the cochlea, the *modiolus*, toward the outer wall. These fibers are stiff, elastic, reedlike structures that are fixed at their basal ends in the central bony structure of the cochlea (the modiolus) but are not fixed at their distal ends, except that the distal ends are embedded in the loose basilar membrane. Because the fibers are stiff and free at one end, they can vibrate like the reeds of a harmonica.

The *lengths* of the basilar fibers *increase* progressively beginning at the oval window and going from the base of the cochlea to the apex, increasing from a length of about 0.04 millimeter near the oval and round windows to 0.5 millimeter at the tip of the cochlea (the "helicotrema"), a 12-fold increase in length.

The *diameters* of the fibers, however, *decrease* from the oval window to the helicotrema, so their overall stiffness decreases more than 100-fold. As a result, the stiff, short fibers near the oval window of the cochlea vibrate best at a very high frequency, whereas the long, limber fibers near the tip of the cochlea vibrate best at a low frequency.

Thus, *high-frequency resonance* of the basilar membrane occurs near the base, where the sound waves enter the cochlea through the oval window. But *low-frequency resonance* occurs near the helicotrema, mainly because of the less stiff fibers but also because of increased "loading" with extra masses of fluid that must vibrate along the cochlear tubules.

Transmission of Sound Waves in the Cochlea—"Traveling Wave"

When the foot of the stapes moves inward against the *oval* window, the *round* window must bulge outward because the cochlea is bounded on all sides by bony walls. The initial effect of a sound wave entering at the oval window is to cause the basilar membrane at the base of the cochlea to bend in the direction of the round window. However, the elastic tension that is built up in the basilar fibers as they bend toward the round window initiates a fluid wave that "travels" along the basilar membrane toward the helicotrema, as shown in Figure 52-5. Figure 52-5*A* shows movement of a high-frequency wave down the basilar membrane; Figure 52-5*B*, a medium-frequency wave; and Figure 52-5*C*, a very low frequency wave. Movement of the wave along the basilar membrane is comparable to the movement of a pressure wave along the arterial walls, which is discussed in Chapter 15; it is also comparable to a wave that travels along the surface of a pond.

Pattern of Vibration of the Basilar Membrane for Different Sound Frequencies. Note in Figure 52-5 the different patterns of transmission for sound waves of different frequencies. Each wave is relatively weak at the

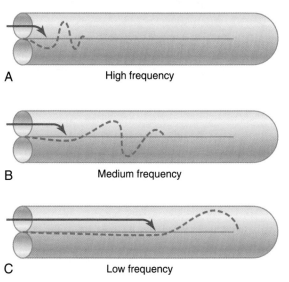

A   High frequency

B   Medium frequency

C   Low frequency

Figure 52-5 "Traveling waves" along the basilar membrane for high-, medium-, and low-frequency sounds.

outset but becomes strong when it reaches that portion of the basilar membrane that has a natural resonant frequency equal to the respective sound frequency. At this point, the basilar membrane can vibrate back and forth with such ease that the energy in the wave is dissipated. Consequently, the wave dies at this point and fails to travel the remaining distance along the basilar membrane. Thus, a high-frequency sound wave travels only a short distance along the basilar membrane before it reaches its resonant point and dies, a medium-frequency sound wave travels about halfway and then dies, and a very low frequency sound wave travels the entire distance along the membrane.

Another feature of the traveling wave is that it travels fast along the initial portion of the basilar membrane but becomes progressively slower as it goes farther into the cochlea. The cause of this is the high coefficient of elasticity of the basilar fibers near the oval window and a progressively decreasing coefficient farther along the membrane. This rapid initial transmission of the wave allows the high-frequency sounds to travel far enough into the cochlea to spread out and separate from one another on the basilar membrane. Without this, all the high-frequency waves would be bunched together within the first millimeter or so of the basilar membrane, and their frequencies could not be discriminated from one another.

Amplitude Pattern of Vibration of the Basilar Membrane. The dashed curves of Figure 52-6*A* show the position of a sound wave on the basilar membrane when the stapes (a) is all the way inward, (b) has moved back to the neutral point, (c) is all the way outward, and (d) has moved back again to the neutral point but

is moving inward. The shaded area around these different waves shows the extent of vibration of the basilar membrane during a complete vibratory cycle. This is the *amplitude pattern of vibration* of the basilar membrane for this particular sound frequency.

Figure 52-6*B* shows the amplitude patterns of vibration for different frequencies, demonstrating that the maximum amplitude for sound at 8000 cycles per second occurs near the base of the cochlea, whereas that for frequencies less than 200 cycles per second is all the way at the tip of the basilar membrane near the helicotrema, where the scala vestibuli opens into the scala tympani.

The principal method by which sound frequencies are discriminated from one another is based on the "place" of maximum stimulation of the nerve fibers from the organ of Corti lying on the basilar membrane, as explained in the next section.

Function of the Organ of Corti

The organ of Corti, shown in Figures 52-3, and 52-7, is the receptor organ that generates nerve impulses in response to vibration of the basilar membrane. Note that the organ of Corti lies on the surface of the basilar fibers and basilar membrane. The actual sensory receptors in the organ of Corti are two specialized types of nerve cells called *hair cells*—a single row of *internal* (or "inner") *hair cells*, numbering about 3500 and measuring about 12 micrometers in diameter, and three or four rows of *external* (or "outer") *hair cells*, numbering about 12,000 and having diameters of only about 8 micrometers. The bases and sides of the hair cells synapse with a network of cochlea nerve endings. Between 90 and 95 percent of these endings terminate on the inner hair cells, which emphasizes their special importance for the detection of sound.

The nerve fibers stimulated by the hair cells lead to the *spiral ganglion of Corti*, which lies in the modiolus (center) of the cochlea. The spiral ganglion neuronal cells send axons—a total of about 30,000—into the *cochlear nerve* and then into the central nervous system at the level of

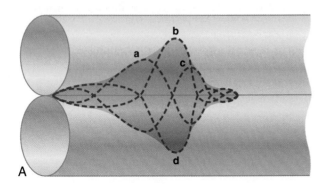

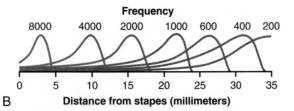

Figure 52-6 *A,* Amplitude pattern of vibration of the basilar membrane for a medium-frequency sound. *B,* Amplitude patterns for sounds of frequencies between 200 and 8000 cycles per second, showing the points of maximum amplitude on the basilar membrane for the different frequencies.

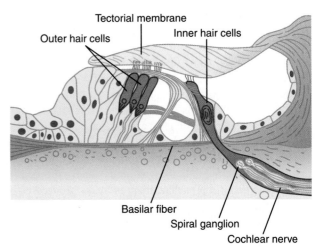

Figure 52-7 Organ of Corti, showing especially the hair cells and the tectorial membrane pressing against the projecting hairs.

the upper medulla. The relation of the organ of Corti to the spiral ganglion and to the cochlear nerve is shown in Figure 52-2.

Excitation of the Hair Cells. Note in Figure 52-7 that minute hairs, or *stereocilia*, project upward from the hair cells and either touch or are embedded in the surface gel coating of the *tectorial membrane*, which lies above the stereocilia in the scala media. These hair cells are similar to the hair cells found in the macula and cristae ampullaris of the vestibular apparatus, which are discussed in Chapter 55. Bending of the hairs in one direction depolarizes the hair cells, and bending in the opposite direction hyperpolarizes them. This in turn excites the auditory nerve fibers synapsing with their bases.

Figure 52-8 shows the mechanism by which vibration of the basilar membrane excites the hair endings. The outer ends of the hair cells are fixed tightly in a rigid structure composed of a flat plate, called the *reticular lamina*, supported by triangular *rods of Corti*, which are attached tightly to the basilar fibers. The basilar fibers, the rods of Corti, and the reticular lamina move as a rigid unit.

Upward movement of the basilar fiber rocks the reticular lamina upward and *inward* toward the modiolus. Then, when the basilar membrane moves downward, the reticular lamina rocks downward and *outward*. The inward and outward motion causes the hairs on the hair cells to shear back and forth against the tectorial membrane. Thus, the hair cells are excited whenever the basilar membrane vibrates.

Auditory Signals Are Transmitted Mainly by the Inner Hair Cells. Even though there are three to four times as many outer hair cells as inner hair cells, about 90 percent of the auditory nerve fibers are stimulated by the inner cells rather than by the outer cells. Yet, despite this, if the outer cells are damaged while the inner cells remain fully functional, a large amount of hearing loss occurs. Therefore, it has been proposed that the outer hair cells in some way control the sensitivity of the inner hair cells at different sound pitches, a phenomenon called "tuning" of the receptor system. In support of this concept, a large number of retrograde nerve fibers pass from the brain stem to the vicinity of the outer hair cells. Stimulating these nerve fibers can actually cause shortening of the outer hair cells and possibly also change their degree of stiffness. These effects suggest a retrograde nervous mechanism for control of the ear's sensitivity to different sound pitches, activated through the outer hair cells.

Hair Cell Receptor Potentials and Excitation of Auditory Nerve Fibers. The stereocilia (the "hairs" protruding from the ends of the hair cells) are stiff structures because each has a rigid protein framework. Each hair cell has about 100 stereocilia on its apical border. These become progressively longer on the side of the hair cell away from the modiolus, and the tops of the shorter stereocilia are attached by thin filaments to the back sides of their adjacent longer stereocilia. Therefore, whenever the cilia are bent in the direction of the longer ones, the tips of the smaller stereocilia are tugged outward from the surface of the hair cell. This causes a mechanical transduction that opens 200 to 300 cation-conducting channels, allowing rapid movement of positively charged potassium ions from the surrounding scala media fluid into the stereocilia, which causes depolarization of the hair cell membrane.

Thus, when the basilar fibers bend toward the scala vestibuli, the hair cells depolarize, and in the opposite direction they hyperpolarize, thereby generating an alternating hair cell receptor potential. This, in turn, stimulates the cochlear nerve endings that synapse with the bases of the hair cells. It is believed that a rapidly acting neurotransmitter is released by the hair cells at these synapses during depolarization. It is possible that the transmitter substance is glutamate, but this is not certain.

Endocochlear Potential. To explain even more fully the electrical potentials generated by the hair cells, we need to explain another electrical phenomenon called the *endocochlear potential*: The scala media is filled with a fluid called *endolymph*, in contradistinction to the *perilymph* present in the scala vestibuli and scala tympani. The scala vestibuli and scala tympani communicate directly with the subarachnoid space around the brain, so the perilymph is almost identical to cerebrospinal fluid. Conversely, the endolymph that fills the scala media is an entirely different fluid secreted by the *stria vascularis*, a highly vascular area on the outer wall of the scala media. Endolymph contains a high concentration of potassium and a low concentration of sodium, which is exactly opposite to the contents of perilymph.

An electrical potential of about +80 millivolts exists all the time between endolymph and perilymph, with positivity inside the scala media and negativity outside. This is called the *endocochlear potential*, and it is generated by continual secretion of positive potassium ions into the scala media by the stria vascularis.

The importance of the endocochlear potential is that the tops of the hair cells project through the reticular lamina and are bathed by the endolymph of the scala media, whereas perilymph bathes the lower bodies of the hair cells. Furthermore, the hair cells have a negative intracellular potential of –70 millivolts with respect to the perilymph but –150 millivolts with respect to the endolymph at their upper

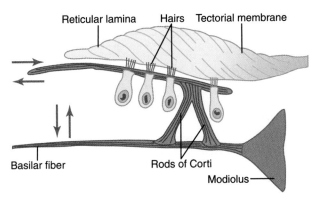

Figure 52-8 Stimulation of the hair cells by to-and-fro movement of the hairs projecting into the gel coating of the tectorial membrane.

surfaces where the hairs project through the reticular lamina and into the endolymph. It is believed that this high electrical potential at the tips of the stereocilia sensitizes the cell an extra amount, thereby increasing its ability to respond to the slightest sound.

Determination of Sound Frequency—The "Place" Principle

From earlier discussions in this chapter, it is apparent that low-frequency sounds cause maximal activation of the basilar membrane near the apex of the cochlea, and high-frequency sounds activate the basilar membrane near the base of the cochlea. Intermediate-frequency sounds activate the membrane at intermediate distances between the two extremes. Furthermore, there is spatial organization of the nerve fibers in the cochlear pathway, all the way from the cochlea to the cerebral cortex. Recording of signals in the auditory tracts of the brain stem and in the auditory receptive fields of the cerebral cortex shows that specific brain neurons are activated by specific sound frequencies. Therefore, the *major* method used by the nervous system to detect different sound frequencies is to determine the positions along the basilar membrane that are most stimulated. This is called the *place principle* for the determination of sound frequency.

Yet, referring again to Figure 52-6, one can see that the distal end of the basilar membrane at the helicotrema is stimulated by all sound frequencies below 200 cycles per second. Therefore, it has been difficult to understand from the place principle how one can differentiate between low sound frequencies in the range of 200 down to 20. These low frequencies have been postulated to be discriminated mainly by the so-called *volley* or *frequency principle*. That is, low-frequency sounds, from 20 to 1500 to 2000 cycles per second, can cause volleys of nerve impulses synchronized at the same frequencies, and these volleys are transmitted by the cochlear nerve into the cochlear nuclei of the brain. It is further suggested that the cochlear nuclei can distinguish the different frequencies of the volleys. In fact, destruction of the entire apical half of the cochlea, which destroys the basilar membrane where all lower-frequency sounds are normally detected, does not totally eliminate discrimination of the lower-frequency sounds.

Determination of Loudness

Loudness is determined by the auditory system in at least three ways.

First, as the sound becomes louder, the amplitude of vibration of the basilar membrane and hair cells also increases so that the hair cells excite the nerve endings at more rapid rates.

Second, as the amplitude of vibration increases, it causes more and more of the hair cells on the fringes of the resonating portion of the basilar membrane to become stimulated, thus causing *spatial summation* of impulses— that is, transmission through many nerve fibers rather than through only a few.

Third, the outer hair cells do not become stimulated significantly until vibration of the basilar membrane reaches high intensity, and stimulation of these cells presumably apprises the nervous system that the sound is loud.

Detection of Changes in Loudness—The Power Law. As pointed out in Chapter 46, a person interprets changes in intensity of sensory stimuli approximately in proportion to an inverse power function of the actual intensity. In the case of sound, the interpreted sensation changes approximately in proportion to the cube root of the actual sound intensity. To express this in another way, the ear can discriminate differences in sound intensity from the softest whisper to the loudest possible noise, representing an *approximately 1 trillion times* increase in sound energy or 1 million times increase in amplitude of movement of the basilar membrane. Yet the ear interprets this much difference in sound level as approximately a 10,000-fold change. Thus, the scale of intensity is greatly "compressed" by the sound perception mechanisms of the auditory system. This allows a person to interpret differences in sound intensities over a far wider range than would be possible were it not for compression of the intensity scale.

Decibel Unit. Because of the extreme changes in sound intensities that the ear can detect and discriminate, sound intensities are usually expressed in terms of the logarithm of their actual intensities. A 10-fold increase in sound energy is called 1 *bel*, and 0.1 bel is called 1 *decibel*. One decibel represents an actual increase in sound energy of 1.26 times.

Another reason for using the decibel system to express changes in loudness is that, in the usual sound intensity range for communication, the ears can barely distinguish an approximately 1-decibel *change* in sound intensity.

Threshold for Hearing Sound at Different Frequencies. Figure 52-9 shows the pressure thresholds at which sounds of different frequencies can barely be heard by the ear. This figure demonstrates that a 3000-cycle-per-second sound can be heard even when its intensity is as low as 70 decibels below

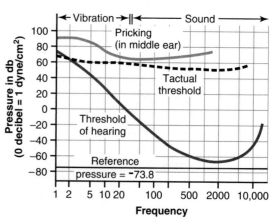

Figure 52-9 Relation of the threshold of hearing and of somesthetic perception (pricking and tactual threshold) to the sound energy level at each sound frequency.

1 dyne/cm² sound pressure level, which is one ten-millionth microwatt per square centimeter. Conversely, a 100-cycle-per-second sound can be detected only if its intensity is 10,000 times as great as this.

Frequency Range of Hearing. The frequencies of sound that a young person can hear are between 20 and 20,000 cycles per second. However, referring again to Figure 52-9, we see that the sound range depends to a great extent on loudness. If the loudness is 60 decibels below 1 dyne/cm² sound pressure level, the sound range is 500 to 5000 cycles per second; only with intense sounds can the complete range of 20 to 20,000 cycles be achieved. In old age, this frequency range is usually shortened to 50 to 8000 cycles per second or less, as discussed later in the chapter.

Central Auditory Mechanisms

Auditory Nervous Pathways

Figure 52-10 shows the major auditory pathways. It shows that nerve fibers from the *spiral ganglion of Corti* enter the *dorsal* and *ventral cochlear nuclei* located in the upper part of the medulla. At this point, all the fibers synapse, and second-order neurons pass mainly to the opposite side of the brain stem to terminate in the *superior olivary nucleus*. A few second-order fibers also pass to the superior olivary nucleus on the same side.

From the superior olivary nucleus, the auditory pathway passes upward through the *lateral lemniscus*. Some of the fibers terminate in the *nucleus of the lateral lemniscus*, but many bypass this nucleus and travel on to the inferior colliculus, where all or almost all the auditory fibers synapse. From there, the pathway passes to the *medial geniculate nucleus*, where all the fibers do synapse. Finally, the pathway proceeds by way of the *auditory radiation* to the *auditory cortex*, located mainly in the superior gyrus of the temporal lobe.

Several important points should be noted. First, signals from both ears are transmitted through the pathways of both sides of the brain, with a preponderance of transmission in the contralateral pathway. In at least three places in the brain stem, crossing over occurs between the two pathways: (1) in the trapezoid body, (2) in the commissure between the two nuclei of the lateral lemnisci, and (3) in the commissure connecting the two inferior colliculi.

Second, many collateral fibers from the auditory tracts pass directly into the *reticular activating system of the brain stem*. This system projects diffusely upward in the brain stem and downward into the spinal cord and activates the entire nervous system in response to loud sounds. Other collaterals go to the *vermis of the cerebellum*, which is also activated instantaneously in the event of a sudden noise.

Third, a high degree of spatial orientation is maintained in the fiber tracts from the cochlea all the way to the cortex. In fact, there are *three spatial patterns* for termination of the different sound frequencies in the cochlear nuclei, *two patterns* in the inferior colliculi, *one precise pattern*

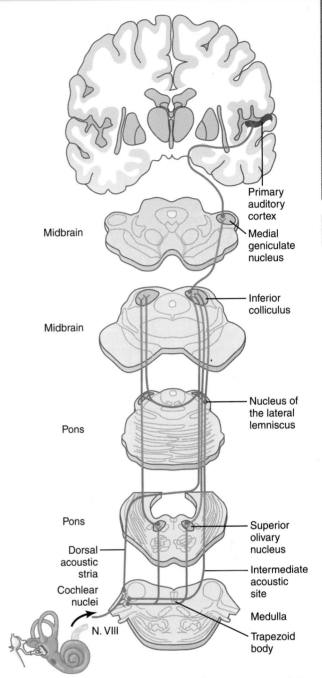

Figure 52-10 Auditory nervous pathways. (Modified from Brodal A: The auditory system. In Neurological Anatomy in Relation to Clinical Medicine, 3rd ed. New York: Oxford University Press, 1981.)

for discrete sound frequencies in the auditory cortex, and *at least five other less precise patterns* in the auditory cortex and auditory association areas.

Firing Rates at Different Levels of the Auditory Pathways. Single nerve fibers entering the cochlear nuclei from the auditory nerve can fire at rates up to at least 1000 per second, the rate being determined mainly by the loudness of the sound. At sound frequencies up to 2000 to 4000 cycles per second, the auditory nerve impulses are often synchronized with the sound waves, but they do not necessarily occur with every wave.

In the auditory tracts of the brain stem, the firing is usually no longer synchronized with the sound frequency, except at sound frequencies below 200 cycles per second. Above the level of the inferior colliculi, even this synchronization is mainly lost. These findings demonstrate that the sound signals are not transmitted unchanged directly from the ear to the higher levels of the brain; instead, information from the sound signals begins to be dissected from the impulse traffic at levels as low as the cochlear nuclei. We will have more to say about this later, especially in relation to perception of direction from which sound comes.

Function of the Cerebral Cortex in Hearing

The projection area of auditory signals to the cerebral cortex is shown in Figure 52-11, which demonstrates that the auditory cortex lies principally on the *supratemporal plane of the superior temporal gyrus* but also extends onto the *lateral side of the temporal lobe*, over much of the *insular cortex*, and even onto the lateral portion of the *parietal operculum*.

Two separate subdivisions are shown in Figure 52-11: the *primary auditory cortex* and the *auditory association cortex* (also called the *secondary auditory cortex*). The primary auditory cortex is directly excited by projections from the medial geniculate body, whereas the auditory association areas are excited secondarily by impulses from the primary auditory cortex, as well as by some projections from thalamic association areas adjacent to the medial geniculate body.

Sound Frequency Perception in the Primary Auditory Cortex. At least six *tonotopic maps* have been found in the primary auditory cortex and auditory association areas. In each of these maps, high-frequency sounds

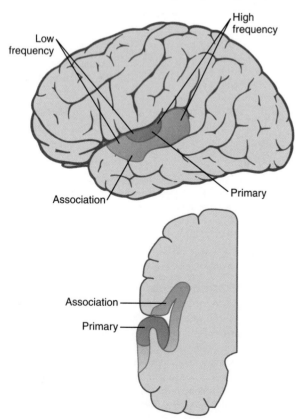

Figure 52-11 Auditory cortex.

excite neurons at one end of the map, whereas low-frequency sounds excite neurons at the opposite end. In most, the low-frequency sounds are located anteriorly, as shown in Figure 52-11, and the high-frequency sounds are located posteriorly. This is not true for all the maps.

Why does the auditory cortex have so many different tonotopic maps? The answer, presumably, is that each of the separate areas dissects out some specific feature of the sounds. For instance, one of the large maps in the primary auditory cortex almost certainly discriminates the sound frequencies themselves and gives the person the psychic sensation of sound pitches. Another map is probably used to detect the direction from which the sound comes. Other auditory cortex areas detect special qualities, such as the sudden onset of sounds, or perhaps special modulations, such as noise versus pure frequency sounds.

The frequency range to which each individual neuron in the auditory cortex responds is much narrower than that in the cochlear and brain stem relay nuclei. Referring to Figure 52-6B, note that the basilar membrane near the base of the cochlea is stimulated by sounds of all frequencies, and in the cochlear nuclei, this same breadth of sound representation is found. Yet, by the time the excitation has reached the cerebral cortex, most sound-responsive neurons respond to only a narrow range of frequencies rather than to a broad range. Therefore, somewhere along the pathway, processing mechanisms "sharpen" the frequency response. It is believed that this sharpening effect is caused mainly by the phenomenon of lateral inhibition, which is discussed in Chapter 46 in relation to mechanisms for transmitting information in nerves. That is, stimulation of the cochlea at one frequency inhibits sound frequencies on both sides of this primary frequency; this is caused by collateral fibers angling off the primary signal pathway and exerting inhibitory influences on adjacent pathways. The same effect has been demonstrated to be important in sharpening patterns of somesthetic images, visual images, and other types of sensations.

Many of the neurons in the auditory cortex, *especially in the auditory association cortex,* do not respond only to specific sound frequencies in the ear. It is believed that these neurons "associate" different sound frequencies with one another or associate sound information with information from other sensory areas of the cortex. Indeed, the parietal portion of the auditory association cortex partly overlaps somatosensory area II, which could provide an easy opportunity for the association of auditory information with somatosensory information.

Discrimination of Sound "Patterns" by the Auditory Cortex. Complete bilateral removal of the auditory cortex does not prevent a cat or monkey from detecting sounds or reacting in a crude manner to sounds. However, it does greatly reduce or sometimes even abolish the animal's ability to discriminate different sound pitches and especially *patterns of sound*. For instance, an animal that has been trained to recognize a combination or sequence of tones, one following the other in a particular pattern, loses this ability when the auditory cortex is destroyed; furthermore, the animal cannot relearn this type of response. Therefore, the auditory cortex is especially important in the discrimination of *tonal* and *sequential sound patterns*.

Destruction of both primary auditory cortices in the human being greatly reduces one's sensitivity for hearing. Destruction of one side only slightly reduces hearing in the opposite ear; it does not cause deafness in the ear because of many crossover connections from side to side in the auditory neural pathway. However, it does affect one's ability to localize the source of a sound, because comparative signals in both cortices are required for the localization function.

Lesions that affect the auditory association areas but not the primary auditory cortex do not decrease a person's ability to hear and differentiate sound tones, or even to interpret at least simple patterns of sound. However, the person is often unable to interpret the *meaning* of the sound heard. For instance, lesions in the posterior portion of the superior temporal gyrus, which is called Wernicke's area and is part of the auditory association cortex, often make it impossible for a person to interpret the meanings of words even though he or she hears them perfectly well and can even repeat them. These functions of the auditory association areas and their relation to the overall intellectual functions of the brain are discussed in more detail in Chapter 57.

Determination of the Direction from Which Sound Comes

A person determines the horizontal direction from which sound comes by two principal means: (1) the time lag between the entry of sound into one ear and its entry into the opposite ear, and (2) the difference between the intensities of the sounds in the two ears.

The first mechanism functions best at frequencies below 3000 cycles per second, and the second mechanism operates best at higher frequencies because the head is a greater sound barrier at these frequencies. The time lag mechanism discriminates direction much more exactly than the intensity mechanism because it does not depend on extraneous factors but only on the exact interval of time between two acoustical signals. If a person is looking straight toward the source of the sound, the sound reaches both ears at exactly the same instant, whereas if the right ear is closer to the sound than the left ear is, the sound signals from the right ear enter the brain ahead of those from the left ear.

The two aforementioned mechanisms cannot tell whether the sound is emanating from in front of or behind the person or from above or below. This discrimination is achieved mainly by the *pinnae* of the two ears. The shape of the pinna changes the *quality* of the sound entering the ear, depending on the direction from which the sound comes. It does this by emphasizing specific sound frequencies from the different directions.

Neural Mechanisms for Detecting Sound Direction. Destruction of the auditory cortex on both sides of the brain, whether in human beings or in lower mammals, causes loss of almost all ability to detect the direction from which sound comes. Yet, the neural analyses for this detection process begin in the *superior olivary nuclei* in the brain stem, even though the neural pathways all the way from these nuclei to the cortex are required for interpretation of the signals. The mechanism is believed to be the following.

The superior olivary nucleus is divided into two sections: (1) the *medial superior olivary nucleus* and (2) the *lateral superior olivary nucleus*. The lateral nucleus is concerned with detecting the direction from which the sound is coming, presumably by simply comparing the *difference in intensities of the sound* reaching the two ears and sending an appropriate signal to the auditory cortex to estimate the direction.

The *medial superior olivary nucleus*, however, has a specific mechanism for *detecting the time lag between acoustical signals entering the two ears*. This nucleus contains large numbers of neurons that have two major dendrites, one projecting to the right and the other to the left. The acoustical signal from the right ear impinges on the right dendrite, and the signal from the left ear impinges on the left dendrite. The intensity of excitation of each neuron is highly sensitive to a specific time lag between the two acoustical signals from the two ears. The neurons near one border of the nucleus respond maximally to a short time lag, whereas those near the opposite border respond to a long time lag; those in between respond to intermediate time lags. Thus, a spatial pattern of neuronal stimulation develops in the medial superior olivary nucleus, with sound from directly in front of the head stimulating one set of olivary neurons maximally and sounds from different side angles stimulating other sets of neurons on opposite sides. This spatial orientation of signals is then transmitted to the auditory cortex, where sound direction is determined by the locus of the maximally stimulated neurons. It is believed that all these signals for determining sound direction are transmitted through a different pathway and excite a different locus in the cerebral cortex from the transmission pathway and termination locus for tonal patterns of sound.

This mechanism for detection of sound direction indicates again how specific information in sensory signals is dissected out as the signals pass through different levels of neuronal activity. In this case, the "quality" of sound direction is separated from the "quality" of sound tones at the level of the superior olivary nuclei.

Centrifugal Signals from the Central Nervous System to Lower Auditory Centers

Retrograde pathways have been demonstrated at each level of the auditory nervous system from the cortex to the cochlea in the ear itself. The final pathway is mainly from the superior olivary nucleus to the sound-receptor hair cells in the organ of Corti.

These retrograde fibers are inhibitory. Indeed, direct stimulation of discrete points in the olivary nucleus has been shown to inhibit specific areas of the organ of Corti, reducing their sound sensitivities 15 to 20 decibels. One can readily understand how this could allow a person to direct his or her attention to sounds of particular qualities while rejecting sounds of other qualities. This is readily demonstrated when one listens to a single instrument in a symphony orchestra.

Hearing Abnormalities

Types of Deafness

Deafness is usually divided into two types: (1) that caused by impairment of the cochlea, the auditory nerve, or the central nervous system circuits from the ear, which is usually classified as "nerve deafness," and (2) that caused by impairment of the physical structures of the ear that conduct sound itself to the cochlea, which is usually called "conduction deafness."

If either the cochlea or the auditory nerve is destroyed, the person becomes permanently deaf. However, if the cochlea and nerve are still intact but the tympanum-ossicular system has been destroyed or ankylosed ("frozen" in place by fibrosis or calcification), sound waves can still be conducted into the cochlea by means of bone conduction from a sound generator applied to the skull over the ear.

Audiometer. To determine the nature of hearing disabilities, the "audiometer" is used. Simply an earphone connected to an electronic oscillator capable of emitting pure tones ranging from low frequencies to high frequencies, the instrument is calibrated so that zero-intensity-level sound at each frequency is the loudness that can barely be heard by the normal ear. A calibrated volume control can increase the loudness above the zero level. If the loudness must be increased to 30 decibels above normal before it can be heard, the person is said to have a *hearing loss* of 30 decibels at that particular frequency.

In performing a hearing test using an audiometer, one tests about 8 to 10 frequencies covering the auditory spectrum, and the hearing loss is determined for each of these frequencies. Then the so-called *audiogram* is plotted, as shown in Figures 52-12 and 52-13, depicting hearing loss at each of the frequencies in the auditory spectrum. The audiometer, in addition to being equipped with an earphone for testing air conduction by the ear, is equipped with a mechanical vibrator for testing bone conduction from the mastoid process of the skull into the cochlea.

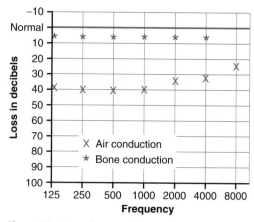

Figure 52-13 Audiogram of air conduction deafness resulting from middle ear sclerosis.

Audiogram in Nerve Deafness. In nerve deafness, which includes damage to the cochlea, the auditory nerve, or the central nervous system circuits from the ear, the person has decreased or total loss of ability to hear sound as tested by both air conduction and bone conduction. An audiogram depicting partial nerve deafness is shown in Figure 52-12. In this figure, the deafness is mainly for high-frequency sound. Such deafness could be caused by damage to the base of the cochlea. This type of deafness occurs to some extent in almost all older people.

Other patterns of nerve deafness frequently occur as follows: (1) deafness for low-frequency sounds caused by excessive and prolonged exposure to very loud sounds (a rock band or a jet airplane engine), because low-frequency sounds are usually louder and more damaging to the organ of Corti, and (2) deafness for all frequencies caused by drug sensitivity of the organ of Corti—in particular, sensitivity to some antibiotics such as streptomycin, kanamycin, and chloramphenicol.

Audiogram for Middle Ear Conduction Deafness. A common type of deafness is caused by fibrosis in the middle ear following repeated infection or by fibrosis that occurs in the hereditary disease called *otosclerosis*. In either case, the sound waves cannot be transmitted easily through the ossicles from the tympanic membrane to the oval window. Figure 52-13 shows an audiogram from a person with "middle ear air conduction deafness." In this case, bone conduction is essentially normal, but conduction through the ossicular system is greatly depressed at all frequencies, but more so at low frequencies. In some instances of conduction deafness, the faceplate of the stapes becomes "ankylosed" by bone overgrowth to the edges of the oval window. In this case, the person becomes totally deaf for ossicular conduction but can regain almost normal hearing by the surgical removal of the stapes and its replacement with a minute Teflon or metal prosthesis that transmits the sound from the incus to the oval window.

Bibliography

Dahmen JC, King AJ: Learning to hear: plasticity of auditory cortical processing, *Curr Opin Neurobiol* 17:456, 2007.

Dallos P: Cochlear amplification, outer hair cells and prestin, *Curr Opin Neurobiol* 18:370, 2008.

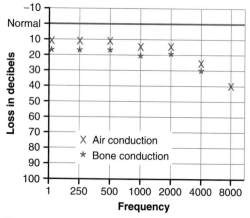

Figure 52-12 Audiogram of the old-age type of nerve deafness.

Frolenkov GI, Belyantseva IA, Friedman TB, et al: Genetic insights into the morphogenesis of inner ear hair cells, *Nat Rev Genet* 5:489, 2004.

Glowatzki E, Grant L, Fuchs P: Hair cell afferent synapses, *Curr Opin Neurobiol* 18:389, 2008.

Griffiths TD, Warren JD, Scott SK, et al: Cortical processing of complex sound: a way forward? *Trends Neurosci* 27:181, 2004.

Grothe B: New roles for synaptic inhibition in sound localization, *Nat Rev Neurosci* 4:540, 2003.

Hudspeth AJ: Making an effort to listen: mechanical amplification in the ear, *Neuron* 59:530, 2008.

Joris PX, Schreiner CE, Rees A: Neural processing of amplitude-modulated sounds, *Physiol Rev* 84:541, 2004.

Kandler K, Clause A, Noh J: Tonotopic reorganization of developing auditory brainstem circuits, *Nat Neurosci* 12:711, 2009.

Kandler K, Gillespie DC: Developmental refinement of inhibitory sound-localization circuits, *Trends Neurosci* 28:290, 2005.

King AJ, Nelken I: Unraveling the principles of auditory cortical processing: can we learn from the visual system? *Nat Neurosci* 12:698, 2009.

Nelken I: Processing of complex sounds in the auditory system, *Curr Opin Neurobiol* 18:413, 2008.

Papsin BC, Gordon KA: Cochlear implants for children with severe-to-profound hearing loss, *N Engl J Med* 357:2380, 2007.

Rauch SD: Clinical practice. Idiopathic sudden sensorineural hearing loss, *N Engl J Med* 359:833, 2008.

Rauschecker JP, Shannon RV: Sending sound to the brain, *Science* 295:1025, 2002.

Read HL, Winer JA, Schreiner CE: Functional architecture of auditory cortex, *Curr Opin Neurobiol* 12:433, 2002.

Robles L, Ruggero MA: Mechanics of the mammalian cochlea, *Physiol Rev* 81:1305, 2001.

Sajjadi H, Paparella MM: Meniere's disease, *Lancet* 372:406, 2008.

Smith RJ, Bale JF Jr, White KR: Sensorineural hearing loss in children, *Lancet* 365:879, 2005.

Syka J: Plastic changes in the central auditory system after hearing loss, restoration of function, and during learning, *Physiol Rev* 82:601, 2002.

Weinberger NM: Specific long-term memory traces in primary auditory cortex, *Nat Rev Neurosci* 5:279, 2004.

UNIT X

The Chemical Senses—Taste and Smell

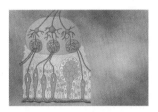 The senses of taste and smell allow us to separate undesirable or even lethal foods from those that are pleasant to eat and nutritious. They also elicit physiological responses that are involved in digestion and utilization of foods. The sense of smell also allows animals to recognize the proximity of other animals or even individuals among animals. Finally, both senses are strongly tied to primitive emotional and behavioral functions of our nervous systems. In this chapter, we discuss how taste and smell stimuli are detected and how they are encoded in neural signals transmitted to the brain.

Sense of Taste

Taste is mainly a function of the *taste buds* in the mouth, but it is common experience that one's sense of smell also contributes strongly to taste perception. In addition, the texture of food, as detected by tactual senses of the mouth, and the presence of substances in the food that stimulate pain endings, such as pepper, greatly alter the taste experience. The importance of taste lies in the fact that it allows a person to select food in accord with desires and often in accord with the body tissues' metabolic need for specific substances.

Primary Sensations of Taste

The identities of the specific chemicals that excite different taste receptors are not all known. Even so, psychophysiologic and neurophysiologic studies have identified at least 13 possible or probable chemical receptors in the taste cells, as follows: 2 sodium receptors, 2 potassium receptors, 1 chloride receptor, 1 adenosine receptor, 1 inosine receptor, 2 sweet receptors, 2 bitter receptors, 1 glutamate receptor, and 1 hydrogen ion receptor.

For practical analysis of taste, the aforementioned receptor capabilities have also been grouped into five general categories called the *primary sensations of taste*. They are *sour, salty, sweet, bitter*, and "*umami.*"

A person can perceive hundreds of different tastes. They are all supposed to be combinations of the elementary taste sensations, just as all the colors we can see are combinations of the three primary colors, as described in Chapter 50.

Sour Taste. The sour taste is caused by acids, that is, by the hydrogen ion concentration, and the intensity of this taste sensation is approximately proportional to the *logarithm of the hydrogen ion concentration*. That is, the more acidic the food, the stronger the sour sensation becomes.

Salty Taste. The salty taste is elicited by ionized salts, mainly by the sodium ion concentration. The quality of the taste varies somewhat from one salt to another because some salts elicit other taste sensations in addition to saltiness. The cations of the salts, especially sodium cations, are mainly responsible for the salty taste, but the anions also contribute to a lesser extent.

Sweet Taste. The sweet taste is not caused by any single class of chemicals. Some of the types of chemicals that cause this taste include sugars, glycols, alcohols, aldehydes, ketones, amides, esters, some amino acids, some small proteins, sulfonic acids, halogenated acids, and inorganic salts of lead and beryllium. Note specifically that most of the substances that cause a sweet taste are organic chemicals. It is especially interesting that slight changes in the chemical structure, such as addition of a simple radical, can often change the substance from sweet to bitter.

Bitter Taste. The bitter taste, like the sweet taste, is not caused by any single type of chemical agent. Here again, the substances that give the bitter taste are almost entirely organic substances. Two particular classes of substances are especially likely to cause bitter taste sensations: (1) long-chain organic substances that contain nitrogen and (2) alkaloids. The alkaloids include many of the drugs used in medicines, such as quinine, caffeine, strychnine, and nicotine.

Some substances that at first taste sweet have a bitter aftertaste. This is true of saccharin, which makes this substance objectionable to some people.

The bitter taste, when it occurs in high intensity, usually causes the person or animal to reject the food. This is undoubtedly an important function of the bitter taste sensation because many deadly toxins found in poisonous plants are alkaloids, and virtually all of these cause intensely bitter taste, usually followed by rejection of the food.

Umami Taste. *Umami* is a Japanese word (meaning "delicious") designating a pleasant taste sensation that is qualitatively different from sour, salty, sweet, or bitter. Umami is the dominant taste of food containing L-*glutamate,* such as meat extracts and aging cheese, and some physiologists consider it to be a separate, fifth category of primary taste stimuli.

A taste receptor for L-glutamate may be related to one of the glutamate receptors that are also expressed in neuronal synapses of the brain. However, the precise molecular mechanisms responsible for umami taste are still unclear.

Threshold for Taste

The threshold for stimulation of the sour taste by hydrochloric acid averages 0.0009 N; for stimulation of the salty taste by sodium chloride, 0.01 M; for the sweet taste by sucrose, 0.01 M; and for the bitter taste by quinine, 0.000008 M. Note especially how much more sensitive is the bitter taste sense than all the others, which would be expected, because this sensation provides an important protective function against many dangerous toxins in food.

Table 53-1 gives the relative taste indices (the reciprocals of the taste thresholds) of different substances. In this table, the intensities of four of the primary sensations of taste are referred, respectively, to the intensities of the taste of hydrochloric acid, quinine, sucrose, and sodium chloride, each of which is arbitrarily chosen to have a taste index of 1.

Taste Blindness. Some people are taste blind for certain substances, especially for different types of thiourea compounds. A substance used frequently by psychologists for demonstrating taste blindness is *phenylthiocarbamide,* for which about 15 to 30 percent of all people exhibit taste blindness; the exact percentage depends on the method of testing and the concentration of the substance.

Taste Bud and Its Function

Figure 53-1 shows a taste bud, which has a diameter of about $1/30$ millimeter and a length of about $1/16$ millimeter. The taste bud is composed of about 50 modified epithelial cells, some of which are supporting cells called *sustentacular cells* and others of which are *taste cells.* The taste cells are continually being replaced by mitotic division of surrounding epithelial cells, so some taste cells are young cells. Others are mature cells that lie toward the center of the bud; these soon break up and dissolve. The life span of each taste cell is about 10 days in lower mammals but is unknown for humans.

The outer tips of the taste cells are arranged around a minute *taste pore,* shown in Figure 53-1. From the tip of each taste cell, several *microvilli,* or *taste hairs,* protrude outward into the taste pore to approach the cavity of the mouth. These microvilli provide the receptor surface for taste.

Table 53-1 Relative Taste Indices of Different Substances

Sour Substances	Index	Bitter Substances	Index	Sweet Substances	Index	Salty Substances	Index
Hydrochloric acid	1	Quinine	1	Sucrose	1	NaCl	1
Formic acid	1.1	Brucine	11	1-Propoxy-2-amino-4-nitrobenzene	5000	NaF	2
Chloracetic acid	0.9	Strychnine	3.1	Saccharin	675	$CaCl_2$	1
Acetylacetic acid	0.85	Nicotine	1.3	Chloroform	40	NaBr	0.4
Lactic acid	0.85	Phenylthiourea	0.9	Fructose	1.7	NaI	0.35
Tartaric acid	0.7	Caffeine	0.4	Alanine	1.3	LiCl	0.4
Malic acid	0.6	Veratrine	0.2	Glucose	0.8	NH_4Cl	2.5
Potassium H tartrate	0.58	Pilocarpine	0.16	Maltose	0.45	KCl	0.6
Acetic acid	0.55	Atropine	0.13	Galactose	0.32		
Citric acid	0.46	Cocaine	0.02	Lactose	0.3		
Carbonic acid	0.06	Morphine	0.02				

Data from Pfaffman C: Handbook of Physiology, vol 1. Baltimore: Williams & Wilkins, 1959, p 507.

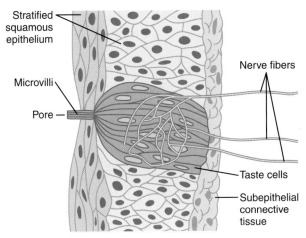

Stratified squamous epithelium

Nerve fibers

Microvilli

Pore

Taste cells

Subepithelial connective tissue

Figure 53-1 Taste bud.

Interwoven around the bodies of the taste cells is a branching terminal network of *taste nerve fibers* that are stimulated by the taste receptor cells. Some of these fibers invaginate into folds of the taste cell membranes. Many vesicles form beneath the cell membrane near the fibers. It is believed that these vesicles contain a neurotransmitter substance that is released through the cell membrane to excite the nerve fiber endings in response to taste stimulation.

Location of the Taste Buds. The taste buds are found on three types of papillae of the tongue, as follows: (1) A large number of taste buds are on the walls of the troughs that surround the circumvallate papillae, which form a V line on the surface of the posterior tongue. (2) Moderate numbers of taste buds are on the fungiform papillae over the flat anterior surface of the tongue. (3) Moderate numbers are on the foliate papillae located in the folds along the lateral surfaces of the tongue. Additional taste buds are located on the palate, and a few are found on the tonsillar pillars, on the epiglottis, and even in the proximal esophagus. Adults have 3000 to 10,000 taste buds, and children have a few more. Beyond the age of 45 years, many taste buds degenerate, causing taste sensitivity to decrease in old age.

Specificity of Taste Buds for a Primary Taste Stimulus. Microelectrode studies from single taste buds show that each taste bud usually *responds mostly to one of the five primary taste stimuli when the taste substance is in low concentration.* But at high concentration, most buds can be excited by two or more of the primary taste stimuli, as well as by a few other taste stimuli that do not fit into the "primary" categories.

Mechanism of Stimulation of Taste Buds

Receptor Potential. The membrane of the taste cell, like that of most other sensory receptor cells, is negatively charged on the inside with respect to the outside. Application of a taste substance to the taste hairs causes partial loss of this negative potential—that is, the taste cell

becomes *depolarized.* In most instances, the decrease in potential, within a wide range, is approximately proportional to the logarithm of concentration of the stimulating substance. This *change in electrical potential* in the taste cell is called the *receptor potential* for taste.

The mechanism by which most stimulating substances react with the taste villi to initiate the receptor potential is by binding of the taste chemical to a protein receptor molecule that lies on the outer surface of the taste receptor cell near to or protruding through a villus membrane. This, in turn, opens ion channels, which allows positively charged sodium ions or hydrogen ions to enter and depolarize the normal negativity of the cell. Then the taste chemical itself is gradually washed away from the taste villus by the saliva, which removes the stimulus.

The type of receptor protein in each taste villus determines the type of taste that will be perceived. For sodium ions and hydrogen ions, which elicit salty and sour taste sensations, respectively, the receptor proteins open specific ion channels in the apical membranes of the taste cells, thereby activating the receptors. However, for the sweet and bitter taste sensations, the portions of the receptor protein molecules that protrude through the apical membranes activate *second-messenger transmitter substances* inside the taste cells, and these second messengers cause intracellular chemical changes that elicit the taste signals.

Generation of Nerve Impulses by the Taste Bud. On first application of the taste stimulus, the rate of discharge of the nerve fibers from taste buds rises to a peak in a small fraction of a second but then adapts within the next few seconds back to a lower, steady level as long as the taste stimulus remains. Thus, a strong immediate signal is transmitted by the taste nerve, and a weaker continuous signal is transmitted as long as the taste bud is exposed to the taste stimulus.

Transmission of Taste Signals into the Central Nervous System

Figure 53-2 shows the neuronal pathways for transmission of taste signals from the tongue and pharyngeal region into the central nervous system. Taste impulses from the anterior two thirds of the tongue pass first into the *lingual nerve,* then through the *chorda tympani* into the *facial nerve,* and finally into the *tractus solitarius* in the brain stem. Taste sensations from the circumvallate papillae on the back of the tongue and from other posterior regions of the mouth and throat are transmitted through the *glossopharyngeal nerve* also into the *tractus solitarius,* but at a slightly more posterior level. Finally, a few taste signals are transmitted into the *tractus solitarius* from the base of the tongue and other parts of the pharyngeal region by way of the *vagus nerve.*

All taste fibers synapse in the posterior brain stem in the *nuclei of the tractus solitarius.* These nuclei send second-order neurons to a small area of the *ventral posterior medial nucleus of the thalamus,* located slightly medial

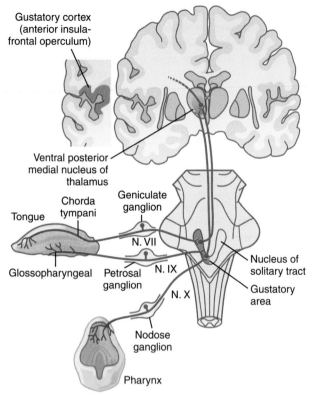

Figure 53-2 Transmission of taste signals into the central nervous system.

to the thalamic terminations of the facial regions of the dorsal column-medial lemniscal system. From the thalamus, third-order neurons are transmitted to the *lower tip of the postcentral gyrus in the parietal cerebral cortex*, where it curls *deep into the sylvian fissure*, and into the adjacent *opercular insular area*. This lies slightly lateral, ventral, and rostral to the area for tongue tactile signals in cerebral somatic area I. From this description of the taste pathways, it is evident that they closely parallel the somatosensory pathways from the tongue.

Taste Reflexes Are Integrated in the Brain Stem. From the tractus solitarius, many taste signals are transmitted within the brain stem itself directly into the *superior* and *inferior salivatory nuclei*, and these areas transmit signals to the submandibular, sublingual, and parotid glands to help control the secretion of saliva during the ingestion and digestion of food.

Rapid Adaptation of Taste. Everyone is familiar with the fact that taste sensations adapt rapidly, often almost completely within a minute or so of continuous stimulation. Yet from electrophysiologic studies of taste nerve fibers, it is clear that adaptation of the taste buds themselves usually accounts for no more than about half of this. Therefore, the final extreme degree of adaptation that occurs in the sensation of taste almost certainly occurs in the central nervous system itself, although the mechanism and site of this are not known. At any rate, it is a mechanism different from that of most other sensory systems, which adapt almost entirely at the receptors.

Taste Preference and Control of the Diet

Taste preference simply means that an animal will choose certain types of food in preference to others, and the animal automatically uses this to help control the diet it eats. Furthermore, its taste preferences often change in accord with the body's need for certain specific substances.

The following experiments demonstrate this ability of animals to choose food in accord with the needs of their bodies. First, adrenalectomized, *salt-depleted* animals automatically select drinking water with a high concentration of sodium chloride in preference to pure water, and this is often sufficient to supply the needs of the body and prevent salt-depletion death. Second, an animal given injections of excessive amounts of insulin develops a depleted blood sugar, and the animal automatically chooses the sweetest food from among many samples. Third, calcium-depleted parathyroidectomized animals automatically choose drinking water with a high concentration of calcium chloride.

The same phenomena are also observed in everyday life. For instance, the "salt licks" of desert regions are known to attract animals from far and wide. Also, human beings reject any food that has an unpleasant affective sensation, which in many instances protects our bodies from undesirable substances.

The phenomenon of taste preference almost certainly results from some mechanism located in the central nervous system and not from a mechanism in the taste receptors themselves, although the receptors often become sensitized in favor of a needed nutrient. An important reason for believing that taste preference is mainly a central nervous system phenomenon is that previous experience with unpleasant or pleasant tastes plays a major role in determining one's taste preferences. For instance, if a person becomes sick soon after eating a particular type of food, the person generally develops a negative taste preference, or *taste aversion*, for that particular food thereafter; the same effect can be demonstrated in lower animals.

Sense of Smell

Smell is the least understood of our senses. This results partly from the fact that the sense of smell is a subjective phenomenon that cannot be studied with ease in lower animals. Another complicating problem is that the sense of smell is poorly developed in human beings in comparison with the sense of smell in many lower animals.

Olfactory Membrane

The olfactory membrane, the histology of which is shown in Figure 53-3, lies in the superior part of each nostril. Medially, the olfactory membrane folds downward along the surface of the superior septum; laterally, it folds over the superior turbinate and even over a small portion of the upper surface of the middle turbinate. In each nostril, the olfactory membrane has a surface area of about 2.4 square centimeters.

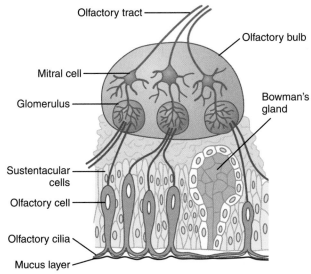

Figure 53-3 Organization of the olfactory membrane and olfactory bulb, and connections to the olfactory tract.

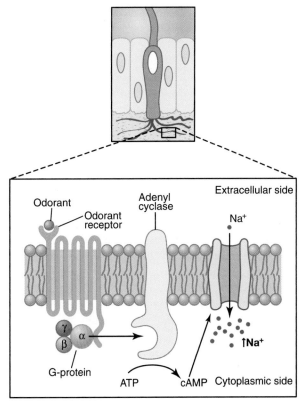

Figure 53-4 Summary of olfactory signal transduction. Binding of the odorant to a G-coupled protein receptor causes activation of adenylate cyclase, which converts adenosine triphosphate (ATP) to cyclic adenosine monophosphate (cAMP). The cAMP activates a gated sodium channel that increases sodium influx and depolarizes the cell, exciting the olfactory neuron and transmitting action potentials to the central nervous system.

Olfactory Cells. The receptor cells for the smell sensation are the *olfactory cells* (see Figure 53-3), which are actually bipolar nerve cells derived originally from the central nervous system itself. There are about 100 million of these cells in the olfactory epithelium interspersed among *sustentacular cells*, as shown in Figure 53-3. The mucosal end of the olfactory cell forms a knob from which 4 to 25 *olfactory hairs* (also called *olfactory cilia*), measuring 0.3 micrometer in diameter and up to 200 micrometers in length, project into the mucus that coats the inner surface of the nasal cavity. These projecting olfactory cilia form a dense mat in the mucus, and it is these cilia that react to odors in the air and stimulate the olfactory cells, as discussed later. Spaced among the olfactory cells in the olfactory membrane are many small *Bowman's glands* that secrete mucus onto the surface of the olfactory membrane.

Stimulation of the Olfactory Cells

Mechanism of Excitation of the Olfactory Cells. The portion of each olfactory cell that responds to the olfactory chemical stimuli is the *olfactory cilia*. The odorant substance, on coming in contact with the olfactory membrane surface, first diffuses into the mucus that covers the cilia. Then it binds with *receptor proteins* in the membrane of each cilium (Figure 53-4). Each receptor protein is actually a long molecule that threads its way through the membrane about seven times, folding inward and outward. The odorant binds with the portion of the receptor protein that folds to the outside. The inside of the folding protein, however, is coupled to a *G-protein*, itself a combination of three subunits. On excitation of the receptor protein, an *alpha* subunit breaks away from the G-protein and immediately activates *adenylyl cyclase*, which is attached to the inside of the ciliary membrane near the receptor cell body. The activated cyclase, in turn, converts many molecules of intracellular *adenosine triphosphate*

into *cyclic adenosine monophosphate* (cAMP). Finally, this cAMP activates another nearby membrane protein, a *gated sodium ion channel*, that opens its "gate" and allows large numbers of sodium ions to pour through the membrane into the receptor cell cytoplasm. The sodium ions increase the electrical potential in the positive direction inside the cell membrane, thus exciting the olfactory neuron and transmitting action potentials into the central nervous system by way of the *olfactory nerve*.

The importance of this mechanism for activating olfactory nerves is that it greatly multiplies the excitatory effect of even the weakest odorant. To summarize: (1) Activation of the receptor protein by the odorant substance activates the G-protein complex. (2) This, in turn, activates multiple molecules of adenylyl cyclase inside the olfactory cell membrane. (3) This causes the formation of many times more molecules of cAMP. (4) Finally, the cAMP opens still many times more sodium ion channels. Therefore, even the most minute concentration of a specific odorant initiates a cascading effect that opens extremely large numbers of sodium channels. This accounts for the exquisite sensitivity of the olfactory neurons to even the slightest amount of odorant.

In addition to the basic chemical mechanism by which the olfactory cells are stimulated, several physical factors affect the degree of stimulation. First, only volatile substances that can be sniffed into the nostrils can be smelled. Second, the stimulating substance must be at least slightly water soluble so that it can pass through the mucus to reach the olfactory cilia. Third, it is helpful for the substance to be at least slightly lipid soluble, presumably because lipid constituents of the cilium itself are a weak barrier to non-lipid-soluble odorants.

Membrane Potentials and Action Potentials in Olfactory Cells. The membrane potential inside unstimulated olfactory cells, as measured by microelectrodes, averages about –55 millivolts. At this potential, most of the cells generate continuous action potentials at a very slow rate, varying from once every 20 seconds up to two or three per second.

Most odorants cause *depolarization* of the olfactory cell membrane, decreasing the negative potential in the cell from the normal level of –55 millivolts to –30 millivolts or less—that is, changing the voltage in the positive direction. Along with this, the number of action potentials increases to 20 to 30 per second, which is a high rate for the minute olfactory nerve fibers.

Over a wide range, the rate of olfactory nerve impulses changes approximately in proportion to the logarithm of the stimulus strength, which demonstrates that the olfactory receptors obey principles of transduction similar to those of other sensory receptors.

Rapid Adaptation of Olfactory Sensations. The olfactory receptors adapt about 50 percent in the first second or so after stimulation. Thereafter, they adapt very little and very slowly. Yet we all know from our own experience that smell sensations adapt almost to extinction within a minute or so after entering a strongly odorous atmosphere. Because this psychological adaptation is far greater than the degree of adaptation of the receptors themselves, it is almost certain that most of the additional adaptation occurs within the central nervous system. This seems to be true for the adaptation of taste sensations as well.

A postulated neuronal mechanism for the adaptation is the following: Large numbers of centrifugal nerve fibers pass from the olfactory regions of the brain backward along the olfactory tract and terminate on special inhibitory cells in the olfactory bulb, the *granule cells*. It has been postulated that after the onset of an olfactory stimulus, the central nervous system quickly develops strong feedback inhibition to suppress relay of the smell signals through the olfactory bulb.

Search for the Primary Sensations of Smell

In the past, most physiologists were convinced that the many smell sensations are subserved by a few rather discrete primary sensations, in the same way that vision and taste are subserved by a few select primary sensations.

On the basis of psychological studies, one attempt to classify these sensations is the following:

1. Camphoraceous
2. Musky
3. Floral
4. Pepperminty
5. Ethereal
6. Pungent
7. Putrid

It is certain that this list does not represent the true primary sensations of smell. In recent years, multiple clues, including specific studies of the genes that encode for the receptor proteins, suggest the existence of at least 100 primary sensations of smell—a marked contrast to only three primary sensations of color detected by the eyes and only four or five primary sensations of taste detected by the tongue. Some studies suggest that there may be as many as 1000 different types of odorant receptors. Further support for the many primary sensations of smell is that people have been found who have *odor blindness* for single substances; such discrete odor blindness has been identified for more than 50 different substances. It is presumed that odor blindness for each substance represents lack of the appropriate receptor protein in olfactory cells for that particular substance.

"Affective Nature of Smell." Smell, even more so than taste, has the affective quality of either *pleasantness* or *unpleasantness*. Because of this, smell is probably even more important than taste for the selection of food. Indeed, a person who has previously eaten food that disagreed with him or her is often nauseated by the smell of that same food on a second occasion. Conversely, perfume of the right quality can be a powerful stimulant of human emotions. In addition, in some lower animals, odors are the primary excitant of sexual drive.

Threshold for Smell. One of the principal characteristics of smell is the minute quantity of stimulating agent in the air that can elicit a smell sensation. For instance, the substance *methylmercaptan* can be smelled when only one 25 trillionth of a gram is present in each milliliter of air. Because of this very low threshold, this substance is mixed with natural gas to give the gas an odor that can be detected when even small amounts of gas leak from a pipeline.

Gradations of Smell Intensities. Although the threshold concentrations of substances that evoke smell are extremely slight, for many (if not most) odorants, concentrations only 10 to 50 times above the threshold evoke maximum intensity of smell. This is in contrast to most other sensory systems of the body, in which the ranges of intensity discrimination are tremendous—for example, 500,000 to 1 in the case of the eyes and 1 trillion to 1 in the case of the ears. This difference might be explained by the fact that smell is concerned more with detecting the presence or absence of odors rather than with quantitative detection of their intensities.

Transmission of Smell Signals into the Central Nervous System

The olfactory portions of the brain were among the first brain structures developed in primitive animals, and much of the remainder of the brain developed around these olfactory beginnings. In fact, part of the brain that originally subserved olfaction later evolved into the basal brain structures that control emotions and other aspects of human behavior; this is the system we call the *limbic system*, discussed in Chapter 58.

Transmission of Olfactory Signals into the Olfactory Bulb. The *olfactory bulb* is shown in Figure 53-5. The olfactory nerve fibers leading backward from the bulb are called *cranial nerve I*, or the *olfactory tract*. However, in reality, both the tract and the bulb are an anterior outgrowth of brain tissue from the base of the brain; the bulbous enlargement at its end, the *olfactory bulb*, lies over the *cribriform plate*, separating the brain cavity from the upper reaches of the nasal cavity. The cribriform plate has multiple small perforations through which an equal number of small nerves pass upward from the olfactory membrane in the nasal cavity to enter the olfactory bulb in the cranial cavity. Figure 53-3 demonstrates the close relation between the *olfactory cells* in the olfactory membrane and the olfactory bulb, showing short axons from the olfactory cells terminating in multiple globular structures within the olfactory bulb called *glomeruli*. Each bulb has several thousand such glomeruli, each of which is the terminus for about 25,000 axons from olfactory cells. Each glomerulus also is the terminus for dendrites from about 25 large *mitral cells* and about 60 smaller *tufted cells*, the cell bodies of which lie in the olfactory bulb superior to the glomeruli. These dendrites receive synapses from the olfactory cell neurons, and the mitral and tufted cells send axons through the olfactory tract to transmit olfactory signals to higher levels in the central nervous system.

Some research has suggested that different glomeruli respond to different odors. It is possible that specific

glomeruli are the real clue to the analysis of different odor signals transmitted into the central nervous system.

The Very Old, the Less Old, and the Newer Olfactory Pathways into the Central Nervous System

The olfactory tract enters the brain at the anterior junction between the mesencephalon and cerebrum; there, the tract divides into two pathways, as shown in Figure 53-5, one passing medially into the *medial olfactory area* of the brain stem, and the other passing laterally into the *lateral olfactory area*. The medial olfactory area represents a very old olfactory system, whereas the lateral olfactory area is the input to (1) a less old olfactory system and (2) a newer system.

The Very Old Olfactory System—The Medial Olfactory Area. The medial olfactory area consists of a group of nuclei located in the midbasal portions of the brain immediately anterior to the hypothalamus. Most conspicuous are the *septal nuclei*, which are midline nuclei that feed into the hypothalamus and other primitive portions of the brain's limbic system. This is the brain area most concerned with basic behavior (described in Chapter 58).

The importance of this medial olfactory area is best understood by considering what happens in animals when the lateral olfactory areas on both sides of the brain are removed and only the medial system remains. The answer is that this hardly affects the more primitive responses to olfaction, such as licking the lips, salivation, and other feeding responses caused by the smell of food or by primitive emotional drives associated with smell. Conversely, removal of the lateral areas abolishes the more complicated olfactory conditioned reflexes.

The Less Old Olfactory System—The Lateral Olfactory Area. The lateral olfactory area is composed mainly of the *prepyriform* and *pyriform cortex* plus the *cortical portion of the amygdaloid nuclei*. From these areas, signal pathways pass into almost all portions of the limbic system, especially into less primitive portions such as the hippocampus, which seem to be most important for learning to like or dislike certain foods depending on one's experiences with them. For instance, it is believed that this lateral olfactory area and its many connections with the limbic behavioral system cause a person to develop an absolute aversion to foods that have caused nausea and vomiting.

An important feature of the lateral olfactory area is that many signal pathways from this area also feed directly into an *older part of the cerebral cortex* called the *paleocortex* in the *anteromedial portion of the temporal lobe*. This is the only area of the entire cerebral cortex where sensory signals pass directly to the cortex without passing first through the thalamus.

The Newer Pathway. A newer olfactory pathway that passes through the thalamus, passing to the dorsomedial thalamic nucleus and then to the lateroposterior quadrant of the orbitofrontale cortex, has been found. On the basis of studies in monkeys, this newer system probably helps in the conscious analysis of odor.

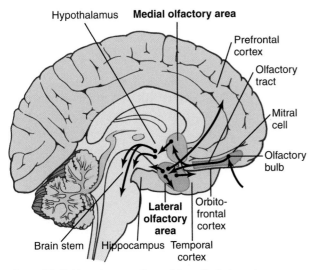

Figure 53-5 Neural connections of the olfactory system.

Summary. Thus, there appear to be a *very old* olfactory system that subserves the basic olfactory reflexes, a *less old* system that provides automatic but partially learned control of food intake and aversion to toxic and unhealthy foods, and a *newer* system that is comparable to most of the other cortical sensory systems and is used for conscious perception and analysis of olfaction.

Centrifugal Control of Activity in the Olfactory Bulb by the Central Nervous System. Many nerve fibers that originate in the olfactory portions of the brain pass from the brain in the outward direction into the olfactory tract to the olfactory bulb (i.e., "centrifugally" from the brain to the periphery). These terminate on a large number of small *granule cells* located among the mitral and tufted cells in the olfactory bulb. The granule cells send inhibitory signals to the mitral and tufted cells. It is believed that this inhibitory feedback might be a means for sharpening one's specific ability to distinguish one odor from another.

Bibliography

Bermudez-Rattoni F: Molecular mechanisms of taste-recognition memory, *Nat Rev Neurosci* 5:209, 2004.

Chandrashekar J, Hoon MA, Ryba NJ, et al: The receptors and cells for mammalian taste, *Nature* 444:288, 2006.

Frank ME, Lundy RF Jr, Contreras RJ: Cracking taste codes by tapping into sensory neuron impulse traffic, *Prog Neurobiol* 86:245, 2008.

Gaillard D, Passilly-Degrace P, Besnard P: Molecular mechanisms of fat preference and overeating, *Ann N Y Acad Sci* 1141:163, 2008.

Housley GD, Bringmann A, Reichenbach A: Purinergic signaling in special senses, *Trends Neurosci* 32:128, 2009.

Keller A, Vosshall LB: Better smelling through genetics: mammalian odor perception, *Curr Opin Neurobiol* 18:364, 2008.

Lowe G: Electrical signaling in the olfactory bulb, *Curr Opin Neurobiol* 13:476, 2003.

Mandairon N, Linster C: Odor perception and olfactory bulb plasticity in adult mammals, *J Neurophysiol* 101:2204, 2009.

Margolskee RF: Molecular mechanisms of bitter and sweet taste transduction, *J Biol Chem* 277:1, 2002.

Matthews HR, Reisert J: Calcium, the two-faced messenger of olfactory transduction and adaptation, *Curr Opin Neurobiol* 13:469, 2003.

Menini A, Lagostena L, Boccaccio A: Olfaction: from odorant molecules to the olfactory cortex, *News Physiol Sci* 19:101, 2004.

Mombaerts P: Genes and ligands for odorant, vomeronasal and taste receptors, *Nat Rev Neurosci* 5:263, 2004.

Montmayeur JP, Matsunami H: Receptors for bitter and sweet taste, *Curr Opin Neurobiol* 12:366, 2002.

Mori K, Takahashi YK, Igarashi KM, et al: Maps of odorant molecular features in the mammalian olfactory bulb, *Physiol Rev* 86:409, 2006.

Nei M, Niimura Y, Nozawa M: The evolution of animal chemosensory receptor gene repertoires: roles of chance and necessity, *Nat Rev Genet* 9:951, 2008.

Roper SD: Signal transduction and information processing in mammalian taste buds, *Pflugers Arch* 454:759, 2007.

Simon SA, de Araujo IE, Gutierrez R, et al: The neural mechanisms of gustation: a distributed processing code, *Nat Rev Neurosci* 7:890, 2006.

Smith DV, Margolskee RF: Making sense of taste, *Sci Am* 284:32, 2001.

The Nervous System: C. Motor and Integrative Neurophysiology

54. Motor Functions of the Spinal Cord; the Cord Reflexes

55. Cortical and Brain Stem Control of Motor Function

56. Contributions of the Cerebellum and Basal Ganglia to Overall Motor Control

57. Cerebral Cortex, Intellectual Functions of the Brain, Learning, and Memory

58. Behavioral and Motivational Mechanisms of the Brain—The Limbic System and the Hypothalamus

59. States of Brain Activity—Sleep, Brain Waves, Epilepsy, Psychoses

60. The Autonomic Nervous System and the Adrenal Medulla

61. Cerebral Blood Flow, Cerebrospinal Fluid, and Brain Metabolism

Motor Functions of the Spinal Cord; the Cord Reflexes

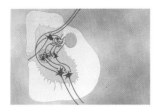

Sensory information is integrated at all levels of the nervous system and causes appropriate motor responses that begin in the spinal cord with relatively simple muscle reflexes, extend into the brain stem with more complicated responses, and finally extend to the cerebrum, where the most complicated muscle skills are controlled.

In this chapter, we discuss the control of muscle function by the spinal cord. Without the special neuronal circuits of the cord, even the most complex motor control systems in the brain could not cause any purposeful muscle movement. For example, there is no neuronal circuit anywhere in the brain that causes the specific to-and-fro movements of the legs that are required in walking. Instead, the circuits for these movements are in the cord and the brain simply sends *command* signals to the spinal cord to set into motion the walking process.

Let us not belittle the role of the brain, however, because the brain gives directions that control the sequential cord activities—to promote turning movements when they are required, to lean the body forward during acceleration, to change the movements from walking to jumping as needed, and to monitor continuously and control equilibrium. All this is done through "analytical" and "command" signals generated in the brain. But it also requires the many neuronal circuits of the spinal cord that are the objects of the commands. These circuits provide all but a small fraction of the direct control of the muscles.

Organization of the Spinal Cord for Motor Functions

The cord gray matter is the integrative area for the cord reflexes. Figure 54-1 shows the typical organization of the cord gray matter in a single cord segment. Sensory signals enter the cord almost entirely through the sensory (posterior) roots. After entering the cord, every sensory signal travels to two separate destinations: (1) One branch of the sensory nerve terminates almost immediately in the gray matter of the cord and elicits local segmental cord reflexes and other local effects. (2) Another branch transmits signals to higher levels of the nervous system—to higher levels in the cord itself, to the brain stem, or even to the cerebral cortex, as described in earlier chapters.

Each segment of the spinal cord (at the level of each spinal nerve) has several million neurons in its gray matter. Aside from the sensory relay neurons discussed in Chapters 47 and 48, the other neurons are of two types: (1) *anterior motor neurons* and (2) *interneurons.*

Anterior Motor Neurons. Located in each segment of the anterior horns of the cord gray matter are several thousand neurons that are 50 to 100 percent larger than most of the others and are called *anterior motor neurons* (Figure 54-2). They give rise to the nerve fibers that leave the cord by way of the anterior roots and directly innervate the skeletal muscle fibers. The neurons are of two types, *alpha motor neurons* and *gamma motor neurons.*

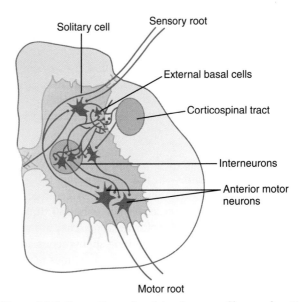

Figure 54-1 Connections of peripheral sensory fibers and corticospinal fibers with the interneurons and anterior motor neurons of the spinal cord.

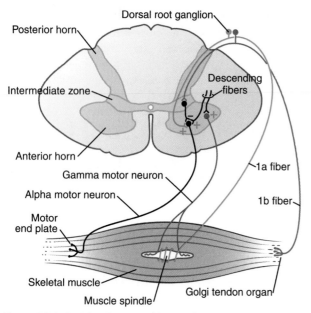

Figure 54-2 Peripheral sensory fibers and anterior motor neurons innervating skeletal muscle.

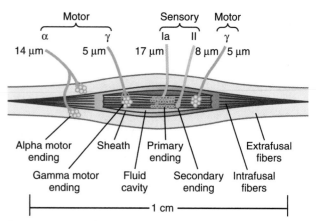

Figure 54-3 Muscle spindle, showing its relation to the large extrafusal skeletal muscle fibers. Note also both motor and sensory innervation of the muscle spindle.

Alpha Motor Neurons. The alpha motor neurons give rise to large type A alpha (Aα) motor nerve fibers, averaging 14 micrometers in diameter; these fibers branch many times after they enter the muscle and innervate the large skeletal muscle fibers. Stimulation of a single alpha nerve fiber excites anywhere from three to several hundred skeletal muscle fibers, which are collectively called the *motor unit.* Transmission of nerve impulses into skeletal muscles and their stimulation of the muscle motor units are discussed in Chapters 6 and 7.

Gamma Motor Neurons. Along with the alpha motor neurons, which excite contraction of the skeletal muscle fibers, about one half as many much smaller *gamma motor neurons* are located in the spinal cord anterior horns. These gamma motor neurons transmit impulses through much smaller type A gamma (Aγ) motor nerve fibers, averaging 5 micrometers in diameter, which go to small, special skeletal muscle fibers called *intrafusal fibers,* shown in Figures 54-2 and 54-3. These fibers constitute the middle of the *muscle spindle,* which helps control basic muscle "tone," as discussed later in this chapter.

Interneurons. Interneurons are present in all areas of the cord gray matter—in the dorsal horns, the anterior horns, and the intermediate areas between them, as shown in Figure 54-1. These cells are about 30 times as numerous as the anterior motor neurons. They are small and highly excitable, often exhibiting spontaneous activity and capable of firing as rapidly as 1500 times per second. They have many interconnections with one another, and many of them also synapse directly with the anterior motor neurons, as shown in Figure 54-1. The interconnections among the interneurons and anterior motor neurons are responsible for most of the integrative func-

tions of the spinal cord that are discussed in the remainder of this chapter.

Essentially all the different types of neuronal circuits described in Chapter 46 are found in the interneuron pool of cells of the spinal cord, including *diverging, converging, repetitive-discharge,* and other types of circuits. In this chapter, we examine many applications of these different circuits in the performance of specific reflex acts by the spinal cord.

Only a few incoming sensory signals from the spinal nerves or signals from the brain terminate directly on the anterior motor neurons. Instead, almost all these signals are transmitted first through interneurons, where they are appropriately processed. Thus, in Figure 54-1, the corticospinal tract from the brain is shown to terminate almost entirely on spinal interneurons, where the signals from this tract are combined with signals from other spinal tracts or spinal nerves before finally converging on the anterior motor neurons to control muscle function.

Renshaw Cells Transmit Inhibitory Signals to Surrounding Motor Neurons. Also located in the anterior horns of the spinal cord, in close association with the motor neurons, are a large number of small neurons called *Renshaw cells.* Almost immediately after the anterior motor neuron axon leaves the body of the neuron, collateral branches from the axon pass to adjacent Renshaw cells. These are *inhibitory cells* that transmit inhibitory signals to the surrounding motor neurons. Thus, stimulation of each motor neuron tends to inhibit adjacent motor neurons, an effect called *lateral inhibition.* This effect is important for the following major reason: The motor system uses this lateral inhibition to focus, or sharpen, its signals in the same way that the sensory system uses the same principle to allow unabated transmission of the primary signal in the desired direction while suppressing the tendency for signals to spread laterally.

Multisegmental Connections from One Spinal Cord Level to Other Levels—Propriospinal Fibers

More than half of all the nerve fibers that ascend and descend in the spinal cord are *propriospinal fibers.* These fibers run from one segment of the cord to another. In addition, as the sensory fibers enter the cord from the posterior cord roots, they bifurcate and branch both up and down the spinal cord; some of the branches transmit signals to only a segment or two, while others transmit signals to many segments. These ascending and descending propriospinal fibers of the cord provide pathways for the multisegmental reflexes described later in this chapter, including reflexes that coordinate simultaneous movements in the forelimbs and hindlimbs.

Muscle Sensory Receptors—Muscle Spindles and Golgi Tendon Organs—and Their Roles in Muscle Control

Proper control of muscle function requires not only excitation of the muscle by spinal cord anterior motor neurons but also continuous feedback of sensory information from each muscle to the spinal cord, indicating the functional status of each muscle at each instant. That is, what is the length of the muscle, what is its instantaneous tension, and how rapidly is its length or tension changing? To provide this information, the muscles and their tendons are supplied abundantly with two special types of sensory receptors: (1) *muscle spindles* (see Figure 54-2), which are distributed throughout the belly of the muscle and send information to the nervous system about muscle length or rate of change of length, and (2) *Golgi tendon organs* (see Figures 54-2 and 54-8), which are located in the muscle tendons and transmit information about tendon tension or rate of change of tension.

The signals from these two receptors are either entirely or almost entirely for the purpose of intrinsic muscle control. They operate almost completely at a subconscious level. Even so, they transmit tremendous amounts of information not only to the spinal cord but also to the cerebellum and even to the cerebral cortex, helping each of these portions of the nervous system function to control muscle contraction.

Receptor Function of the Muscle Spindle

Structure and Motor Innervation of the Muscle Spindle. The organization of the muscle spindle is shown in Figure 54-3. Each spindle is 3 to 10 millimeters long. It is built around 3 to 12 tiny *intrafusal muscle fibers* that are pointed at their ends and attached to the glycocalyx of the surrounding large *extrafusal* skeletal muscle fibers.

Each intrafusal muscle fiber is a tiny skeletal muscle fiber. However, the central region of each of these fibers—that is, the area midway between its two ends—has few or no actin and myosin filaments. Therefore, this central portion does not contract when the ends do. Instead, it functions as a sensory receptor, as described later. The end portions that do contract are excited by small *gamma motor nerve fibers* that originate from small type A gamma motor neurons in the anterior horns of the spinal cord, as described earlier. These gamma motor nerve fibers are also called *gamma efferent fibers,* in contradistinction to the large *alpha efferent fibers* (type A alpha nerve fibers) that innervate the extrafusal skeletal muscle.

Sensory Innervation of the Muscle Spindle. The receptor portion of the muscle spindle is its central portion. In this area, the intrafusal muscle fibers do not have myosin and actin contractile elements. As shown in Figure 54-3 and in more detail in Figure 54-4, sensory fibers originate in this area. They are stimulated by stretching of this midportion of the spindle. One can readily see that the muscle spindle receptor can be excited in two ways:

1. Lengthening the whole muscle stretches the midportion of the spindle and, therefore, excites the receptor.
2. Even if the length of the entire muscle does not change, contraction of the end portions of the spindle's intrafusal fibers stretches the midportion of the spindle and therefore excites the receptor.

Two types of sensory endings are found in this central receptor area of the muscle spindle. They are the *primary ending* and the *secondary ending.*

Primary Ending. In the center of the receptor area, a large sensory nerve fiber encircles the central portion of each intrafusal fiber, forming the so-called *primary ending* or *annulospiral ending.* This nerve fiber is a type Ia fiber averaging 17 micrometers in diameter, and it transmits sensory signals to the spinal cord at a velocity of 70 to 120 m/sec, as rapidly as any type of nerve fiber in the entire body.

Secondary Ending. Usually one but sometimes two smaller sensory nerve fibers—type II fibers with an average diameter of 8 micrometers—innervate the receptor region on one or both sides of the primary ending, as shown in Figures 54-3 and 54-4. This sensory ending is called the *secondary ending;* sometimes it encircles the intrafusal fibers in the same way that the type Ia fiber does, but often it spreads like branches on a bush.

Division of the Intrafusal Fibers into Nuclear Bag and Nuclear Chain Fibers—Dynamic and Static Responses of the Muscle Spindle. There are also two types of muscle spindle intrafusal fibers: (1) *nuclear bag muscle fibers* (one to three in each spindle), in which several

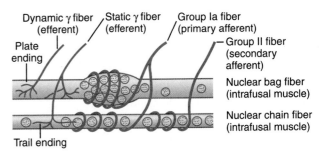

Figure 54-4 Details of nerve connections from the nuclear bag and nuclear chain muscle spindle fibers. (Modified from Stein RB: Peripheral control of movement. Physiol Rev 54:225, 1974.)

muscle fiber nuclei are congregated in expanded "bags" in the central portion of the receptor area, as shown by the top fiber in Figure 54-4, and (2) *nuclear chain fibers* (three to nine), which are about half as large in diameter and half as long as the nuclear bag fibers and have nuclei aligned in a chain throughout the receptor area, as shown by the bottom fiber in the figure. The primary sensory nerve ending (the 17-micrometer sensory fiber) is excited by both the nuclear bag intrafusal fibers *and* the nuclear chain fibers. Conversely, the secondary ending (the 8-micrometer sensory fiber) is usually excited only by nuclear chain fibers. These relations are shown in Figure 54-4.

Response of Both the Primary and the Secondary Endings to the Length of the Receptor—"Static" Response.

When the receptor portion of the muscle spindle is stretched *slowly*, the number of impulses transmitted from both the primary and the secondary endings increases almost directly in proportion to the degree of stretching and the endings continue to transmit these impulses for several minutes. This effect is called the *static response* of the spindle receptor, meaning simply that both the primary and secondary endings continue to transmit their signals for at least several minutes if the muscle spindle itself remains stretched.

Response of the Primary Ending (but Not the Secondary Ending) to Rate of Change of Receptor Length—"Dynamic" Response.

When the length of the spindle receptor increases suddenly, the primary ending (but not the secondary ending) is stimulated powerfully. This excess stimulus of the primary ending is called the *dynamic response*, which means that the primary ending responds extremely actively to a rapid *rate of change* in spindle length. Even when the length of a spindle receptor increases only a fraction of a micrometer for only a fraction of a second, the primary receptor transmits tremendous numbers of excess impulses to the large 17-micrometer sensory nerve fiber, *but only while the length is actually increasing*. As soon as the length stops increasing, this extra rate of impulse discharge returns to the level of the much smaller static response that is still present in the signal.

Conversely, when the spindle receptor shortens, exactly opposite sensory signals occur. Thus, the primary ending sends extremely strong, either positive or negative, signals to the spinal cord to apprise it of any change in length of the spindle receptor.

Control of Intensity of the Static and Dynamic Responses by the Gamma Motor Nerves.

The gamma motor nerves to the muscle spindle can be divided into two types: *gamma-dynamic (gamma-d)* and *gamma-static (gamma-s)*. The first of these excites mainly the nuclear bag intrafusal fibers, and the second excites mainly the nuclear chain intrafusal fibers. When the gamma-d fibers excite the nuclear bag fibers, the dynamic response of the muscle spindle becomes tremendously enhanced, whereas the static response is hardly affected. Conversely, stimulation of the gamma-s fibers, which excite the nuclear chain fibers, enhances the static response while having little influence on the dynamic response. Subsequent paragraphs illustrate that these two types of muscle spindle responses are important in different types of muscle control.

Continuous Discharge of the Muscle Spindles Under Normal Conditions.

Normally, particularly when there is some degree of gamma nerve excitation, the muscle spindles emit sensory nerve impulses continuously. Stretching the muscle spindles increases the rate of firing, whereas shortening the spindle decreases the rate of firing. Thus, the spindles can send to the spinal cord either *positive signals*—that is, increased numbers of impulses to indicate stretch of a muscle—or *negative signals*—below-normal numbers of impulses to indicate that the muscle is unstretched.

Muscle Stretch Reflex

The simplest manifestation of muscle spindle function is the *muscle stretch reflex.* Whenever a muscle is stretched suddenly, excitation of the spindles causes reflex contraction of the large skeletal muscle fibers of the stretched muscle and also of closely allied synergistic muscles.

Neuronal Circuitry of the Stretch Reflex.

Figure 54-5 demonstrates the basic circuit of the muscle spindle stretch reflex, showing a type Ia proprioceptor nerve fiber originating in a muscle spindle and entering a dorsal root of the spinal cord. A branch of this fiber then goes directly to the anterior horn of the cord gray matter and synapses with anterior motor neurons that send motor nerve fibers back to the same muscle from which the muscle spindle fiber originated. Thus, this is a *monosynaptic pathway* that allows a reflex signal to return with the shortest possible time delay back to the muscle after excitation of

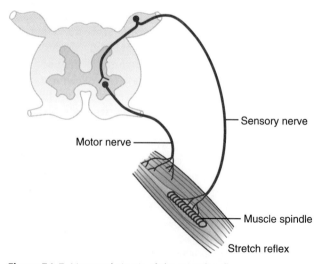

Sensory nerve

Motor nerve

Muscle spindle

Stretch reflex

Figure 54-5 Neuronal circuit of the stretch reflex.

the spindle. Most type II fibers from the muscle spindle terminate on multiple interneurons in the cord gray matter, and these transmit delayed signals to the anterior motor neurons or serve other functions.

Dynamic Stretch Reflex and Static Stretch Reflexes. The stretch reflex can be divided into two components: the dynamic stretch reflex and the static stretch reflex. The *dynamic stretch reflex* is elicited by the potent dynamic signal transmitted from the primary sensory endings of the muscle spindles, caused by rapid stretch or unstretch. That is, when a muscle is suddenly stretched or unstretched, a strong signal is transmitted to the spinal cord; this causes an instantaneous strong reflex contraction (or decrease in contraction) of the same muscle from which the signal originated. Thus, *the reflex functions to oppose sudden changes in muscle length.*

The dynamic stretch reflex is over within a fraction of a second after the muscle has been stretched (or unstretched) to its new length, but then a weaker *static stretch reflex* continues for a prolonged period thereafter. This reflex is elicited by the continuous static receptor signals transmitted by both primary and secondary endings. The importance of the static stretch reflex is that it causes the degree of muscle contraction to remain reasonably constant, except when the person's nervous system specifically wills otherwise.

"Damping" Function of the Dynamic and Static Stretch Reflexes

An especially important function of the stretch reflex is its ability to prevent oscillation or jerkiness of body movements. This is a *damping*, or smoothing, function, as explained in the following paragraph.

Damping Mechanism in Smoothing Muscle Contraction. Signals from the spinal cord are often transmitted to a muscle in an unsmooth form, increasing in intensity for a few milliseconds, then decreasing in intensity, then changing to another intensity level, and so forth. When the muscle spindle apparatus is not functioning satisfactorily, the muscle contraction is jerky during the course of such a signal. This effect is demonstrated in Figure 54-6. In curve A, the muscle spindle reflex of the excited muscle is intact. Note that the contraction is relatively smooth, even though the motor nerve to the muscle is excited at a slow frequency of only eight signals per second. Curve B illustrates the same experiment in an animal whose muscle spindle sensory nerves had been sectioned 3 months earlier. Note the unsmooth muscle contraction. Thus, curve A graphically demonstrates the damping mechanism's ability to smooth muscle contractions, even though the primary input signals to the muscle motor system may themselves be jerky. This effect can also be called a *signal averaging* function of the muscle spindle reflex.

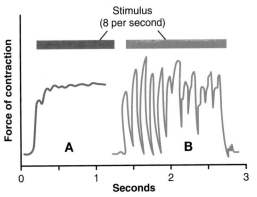

Figure 54-6 Muscle contraction caused by a spinal cord signal under two conditions: *curve A*, in a normal muscle, and *curve B*, in a muscle whose muscle spindles were denervated by section of the posterior roots of the cord 82 days previously. Note the smoothing effect of the muscle spindle reflex in *curve A*. (Modified from Creed RS et al: Reflex Activity of the Spinal Cord. New York: Oxford University Press, 1932.)

Role of the Muscle Spindle in Voluntary Motor Activity

To understand the importance of the gamma efferent system, one should recognize that 31 percent of all the motor nerve fibers to the muscle are the small type A gamma efferent fibers rather than large type A alpha motor fibers. Whenever signals are transmitted from the motor cortex or from any other area of the brain to the alpha motor neurons, in most instances the gamma motor neurons are stimulated simultaneously, an effect called *coactivation* of the alpha and gamma motor neurons. This causes both the extrafusal skeletal muscle fibers and the muscle spindle intrafusal muscle fibers to contract at the same time.

The purpose of contracting the muscle spindle intrafusal fibers at the same time that the large skeletal muscle fibers contract is twofold: First, it keeps the length of the receptor portion of the muscle spindle from changing during the course of the whole muscle contraction. Therefore, coactivation keeps the muscle spindle reflex from opposing the muscle contraction. Second, it maintains the proper damping function of the muscle spindle, regardless of any change in muscle length. For instance, if the muscle spindle did not contract and relax along with the large muscle fibers, the receptor portion of the spindle would sometimes be flail and sometimes be overstretched, in neither instance operating under optimal conditions for spindle function.

Brain Areas for Control of the Gamma Motor System

The gamma efferent system is excited specifically by signals from the *bulboreticular facilitatory* region of the brain stem and, secondarily, by impulses transmitted into the bulboreticular area from (1) the *cerebellum*, (2) the *basal ganglia*, and (3) the *cerebral cortex*.

Little is known about the precise mechanisms of control of the gamma efferent system. However, because the bulboreticular facilitatory area is particularly concerned with antigravity contractions, and because the antigravity muscles have an especially high density of muscle spindles, emphasis is given to the importance of the gamma efferent mechanism for damping the movements of the different body parts during walking and running.

Muscle Spindle System Stabilizes Body Position During Tense Action

One of the most important functions of the muscle spindle system is to stabilize body position during tense motor action. To do this, the bulboreticular facilitatory region and its allied areas of the brain stem transmit excitatory signals through the gamma nerve fibers to the intrafusal muscle fibers of the muscle spindles. This shortens the ends of the spindles and stretches the central receptor regions, thus increasing their signal output. However, if the spindles on both sides of each joint are activated at the same time, reflex excitation of the skeletal muscles on both sides of the joint also increases, producing tight, tense muscles opposing each other at the joint. The net effect is that the position of the joint becomes strongly stabilized, and any force that tends to move the joint from its current position is opposed by highly sensitized stretch reflexes operating on both sides of the joint.

Any time a person must perform a muscle function that requires a high degree of delicate and exact positioning, excitation of the appropriate muscle spindles by signals from the bulboreticular facilitatory region of the brain stem stabilizes the positions of the major joints. This aids tremendously in performing the additional detailed voluntary movements (of fingers or other body parts) required for intricate motor procedures.

Clinical Applications of the Stretch Reflex
Almost every time a clinician performs a physical examination on a patient, he or she elicits multiple stretch reflexes. The purpose is to determine how much background excitation, or "tone," the brain is sending to the spinal cord. This reflex is elicited as follows.

Knee Jerk and Other Muscle Jerks Can Be Used to Assess Sensitivity of Stretch Reflexes. Clinically, a method used to determine the sensitivity of the stretch reflexes is to elicit the knee jerk and other muscle jerks. The knee jerk can be elicited by simply striking the patellar tendon with a reflex hammer; this instantaneously stretches the quadriceps muscle and excites a *dynamic stretch reflex* that causes the lower leg to "jerk" forward. The upper part of Figure 54-7 shows a myogram from the quadriceps muscle recorded during a knee jerk.

Similar reflexes can be obtained from almost any muscle of the body either by striking the tendon of the muscle or by striking the belly of the muscle itself. In other words, sudden stretch of muscle spindles is all that is required to elicit a dynamic stretch reflex.

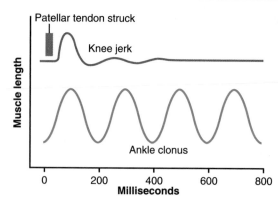

Figure 54-7 Myograms recorded from the quadriceps muscle during elicitation of the knee jerk (*above*) and from the gastrocnemius muscle during ankle clonus (*below*).

The muscle jerks are used by neurologists to assess the degree of facilitation of spinal cord centers. When large numbers of facilitatory impulses are being transmitted from the upper regions of the central nervous system into the cord, the muscle jerks are greatly exaggerated. Conversely, if the facilitatory impulses are depressed or abrogated, the muscle jerks are considerably weakened or absent. These reflexes are used most frequently in determining the presence or absence of muscle spasticity caused by lesions in the motor areas of the brain or diseases that excite the bulboreticular facilitatory area of the brain stem. Ordinarily, large *lesions in the motor areas of the cerebral cortex* but not in the lower motor control areas (especially lesions caused by strokes or brain tumors) cause greatly exaggerated muscle jerks in the muscles on the opposite side of the body.

Clonus—Oscillation of Muscle Jerks. Under some conditions, the muscle jerks can oscillate, a phenomenon called *clonus* (see lower myogram, Figure 54-7). Oscillation can be explained particularly well in relation to ankle clonus, as follows.

If a person standing on the tip ends of the feet suddenly drops his or her body downward and stretches the gastrocnemius muscles, stretch reflex impulses are transmitted from the muscle spindles into the spinal cord. These impulses reflexively excite the stretched muscle, which lifts the body up again. After a fraction of a second, the reflex contraction of the muscle dies out and the body falls again, thus stretching the spindles a second time. Again, a dynamic stretch reflex lifts the body, but this too dies out after a fraction of a second, and the body falls once more to begin a new cycle. In this way, the stretch reflex of the gastrocnemius muscle continues to oscillate, often for long periods; this is clonus.

Clonus ordinarily occurs only when the stretch reflex is highly sensitized by facilitatory impulses from the brain. For instance, in a decerebrate animal, in which the stretch reflexes are highly facilitated, clonus develops readily. To determine the degree of facilitation of the spinal cord, neurologists test patients for clonus by suddenly stretching a muscle and applying a steady stretching force to it. If clonus occurs, the degree of facilitation is certain to be high.

Golgi Tendon Reflex

Golgi Tendon Organ Helps Control Muscle Tension. The Golgi tendon organ, shown in Figure 54-8, is an encapsulated sensory receptor through which muscle tendon fibers pass. About 10 to 15 muscle fibers are usually connected to each Golgi tendon organ, and the organ is stimulated when this small bundle of muscle fibers is "tensed" by contracting or stretching the muscle. Thus, the major difference in excitation of the Golgi tendon organ versus the muscle spindle is that *the spindle detects muscle length and changes in muscle length,* whereas *the tendon organ detects muscle tension* as reflected by the tension in itself.

The tendon organ, like the primary receptor of the muscle spindle, has both a *dynamic response* and a *static response,* reacting intensely when the muscle tension suddenly increases (the dynamic response) but settling down within a fraction of a second to a lower level of steady-state firing that is almost directly proportional to the muscle tension (the static response). Thus, Golgi tendon organs provide the nervous system with instantaneous information on the degree of tension in each small segment of each muscle.

Transmission of Impulses from the Tendon Organ into the Central Nervous System. Signals from the tendon organ are transmitted through large, rapidly conducting type Ib nerve fibers that average 16 micrometers in diameter, only slightly smaller than those from the primary endings of the muscle spindle. These fibers, like those from the primary spindle endings, transmit signals both into local areas of the cord and, after synapsing in a dorsal horn of the cord, through long fiber pathways such as the spinocerebellar tracts into the cerebellum and through still other tracts to the cerebral cortex. The local cord signal excites a single *inhibitory* interneuron that inhibits the anterior motor neuron. This local circuit directly inhibits the individual muscle without affecting adjacent muscles. The relation between signals to the brain and function of the cerebellum and other parts of the brain for muscle control is discussed in Chapter 56.

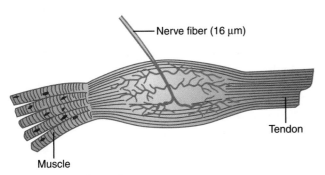

Figure 54-8 Golgi tendon organ.

Inhibitory Nature of the Tendon Reflex and Its Importance

When the Golgi tendon organs of a muscle tendon are stimulated by increased tension in the connecting muscle, signals are transmitted to the spinal cord to cause reflex effects in the respective muscle. This reflex is entirely *inhibitory.* Thus, this reflex provides a *negative feedback* mechanism that prevents the development of too much tension on the muscle.

When tension on the muscle and, therefore, on the tendon becomes extreme, the inhibitory effect from the tendon organ can be so great that it leads to a sudden reaction in the spinal cord that causes instantaneous relaxation of the entire muscle. This effect is called the *lengthening reaction;* it is probably a protective mechanism to prevent tearing of the muscle or avulsion of the tendon from its attachments to the bone. We know, for instance, that direct electrical stimulation of muscles in the laboratory, which cannot be opposed by this negative reflex, can occasionally cause such destructive effects.

Possible Role of the Tendon Reflex to Equalize Contractile Force Among the Muscle Fibers. Another likely function of the Golgi tendon reflex is to equalize contractile forces of the separate muscle fibers. That is, those fibers that exert excess tension become inhibited by the reflex, whereas those that exert too little tension become more excited because of absence of reflex inhibition. This spreads the muscle load over all the fibers and prevents damage in isolated areas of a muscle where small numbers of fibers might be overloaded.

Function of the Muscle Spindles and Golgi Tendon Organs in Conjunction with Motor Control from Higher Levels of the Brain

Although we have emphasized the function of the muscle spindles and Golgi tendon organs in spinal cord control of motor function, these two sensory organs also apprise the higher motor control centers of instantaneous changes taking place in the muscles. For instance, the dorsal spinocerebellar tracts carry instantaneous information from both the muscle spindles and the Golgi tendon organs directly to the cerebellum at conduction velocities approaching 120 m/sec, the most rapid conduction anywhere in the brain or spinal cord. Additional pathways transmit similar information into the reticular regions of the brain stem and, to a lesser extent, all the way to the motor areas of the cerebral cortex. As discussed in Chapters 55 and 56, the information from these receptors is crucial for feedback control of motor signals that originate in all these areas.

Flexor Reflex and the Withdrawal Reflexes

In the spinal or decerebrate animal, almost any type of cutaneous sensory stimulus from a limb is likely to cause the flexor muscles of the limb to contract, thereby withdrawing the limb from the stimulating object. This is called the *flexor reflex.*

In the figure: Nerve fiber (16 μm), Tendon, Muscle

In its classic form, the flexor reflex is elicited most powerfully by stimulation of pain endings, such as by a pinprick, heat, or a wound, for which reason it is also called a *nociceptive reflex*, or simply a *pain reflex*. Stimulation of touch receptors can also elicit a weaker and less prolonged flexor reflex.

If some part of the body other than one of the limbs is painfully stimulated, that part will similarly be *withdrawn from the stimulus*, but the reflex may not be confined to flexor muscles, even though it is basically the same type of reflex. Therefore, the many patterns of these reflexes in the different areas of the body are called *withdrawal reflexes*.

Neuronal Mechanism of the Flexor Reflex.

The left-hand portion of Figure 54-9 shows the neuronal pathways for the flexor reflex. In this instance, a painful stimulus is applied to the hand; as a result, the flexor muscles of the upper arm become excited, thus withdrawing the hand from the painful stimulus.

The pathways for eliciting the flexor reflex do not pass directly to the anterior motor neurons but instead pass first into the spinal cord interneuron pool of neurons and only secondarily to the motor neurons. The shortest possible circuit is a three- or four-neuron pathway; however, most of the signals of the reflex traverse many more neurons and involve the following basic types of circuits: (1) diverging circuits to spread the reflex to the necessary muscles for withdrawal; (2) circuits to inhibit the antagonist muscles, called *reciprocal inhibition circuits;* and (3) circuits to cause *afterdischarge* lasting many fractions of a second after the stimulus is over.

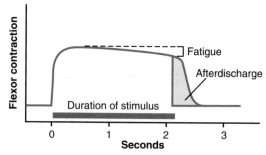

Figure 54-10 Myogram of the flexor reflex showing rapid onset of the reflex, an interval of fatigue, and, finally, afterdischarge after the input stimulus is over.

Figure 54-10 shows a typical myogram from a flexor muscle during a flexor reflex. Within a few milliseconds after a pain nerve begins to be stimulated, the flexor response appears. Then, in the next few seconds, the reflex begins to *fatigue*, which is characteristic of essentially all complex integrative reflexes of the spinal cord. Finally, after the stimulus is over, the contraction of the muscle returns toward the baseline, but because of afterdischarge, it takes many milliseconds for this to occur. The duration of afterdischarge depends on the intensity of the sensory stimulus that elicited the reflex; a weak tactile stimulus causes almost no afterdischarge, but after a strong pain stimulus, the afterdischarge may last for a second or more.

The afterdischarge that occurs in the flexor reflex almost certainly results from both types of repetitive discharge circuits discussed in Chapter 46. Electrophysiologic studies indicate that immediate afterdischarge, lasting for about 6 to 8 milliseconds, results from repetitive firing of the excited interneurons themselves. Also, prolonged afterdischarge occurs after strong pain stimuli, almost certainly resulting from recurrent pathways that initiate oscillation in reverberating interneuron circuits. These, in turn, transmit impulses to the anterior motor neurons, sometimes for several seconds after the incoming sensory signal is over.

Thus, the flexor reflex is appropriately organized to withdraw a pained or otherwise irritated part of the body from a stimulus. Further, because of afterdischarge, the reflex can hold the irritated part away from the stimulus for 0.1 to 3 seconds after the irritation is over. During this time, other reflexes and actions of the central nervous system can move the entire body away from the painful stimulus.

Pattern of Withdrawal.

The pattern of withdrawal that results when the flexor reflex is elicited depends on which sensory nerve is stimulated. Thus, a pain stimulus on the inward side of the arm elicits not only contraction of the flexor muscles of the arm but also contraction of abductor muscles to pull the arm

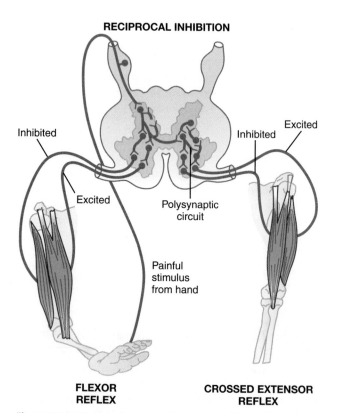

Figure 54-9 Flexor reflex, crossed extensor reflex, and reciprocal inhibition.

outward. In other words, the integrative centers of the cord cause those muscles to contract that can most effectively remove the pained part of the body away from the object causing the pain. Although this principle, called the principle of "local sign," applies to any part of the body, it is especially applicable to the limbs because of their highly developed flexor reflexes.

Crossed Extensor Reflex

About 0.2 to 0.5 second after a stimulus elicits a flexor reflex in one limb, the opposite limb begins to extend. This is called the *crossed extensor reflex.* Extension of the opposite limb can push the entire body away from the object causing the painful stimulus in the withdrawn limb.

Neuronal Mechanism of the Crossed Extensor Reflex. The right-hand portion of Figure 54-9 shows the neuronal circuit responsible for the crossed extensor reflex, demonstrating that signals from sensory nerves cross to the opposite side of the cord to excite extensor muscles. Because the crossed extensor reflex usually does not begin until 200 to 500 milliseconds after onset of the initial pain stimulus, it is certain that many interneurons are involved in the circuit between the incoming sensory neuron and the motor neurons of the opposite side of the cord responsible for the crossed extension. After the painful stimulus is removed, the crossed extensor reflex has an even longer period of afterdischarge than does the flexor reflex. Again, it is presumed that this prolonged afterdischarge results from reverberating circuits among the interneuronal cells.

Figure 54-11 shows a typical myogram recorded from a muscle involved in a crossed extensor reflex. This demonstrates the relatively long latency before the reflex begins and the long afterdischarge at the end of the stimulus. The prolonged afterdischarge is of benefit in holding the pained area of the body away from the painful object until other nervous reactions cause the entire body to move away.

Reciprocal Inhibition and Reciprocal Innervation

We previously pointed out several times that excitation of one group of muscles is often associated with inhibition of another group. For instance, when a stretch reflex excites one muscle, it often simultaneously inhibits the antagonist muscles. This is the phenomenon of *reciprocal inhibition,* and the neuronal circuit that causes this reciprocal relation is called *reciprocal innervation.* Likewise, reciprocal relations often exist between the muscles on the two sides of the body, as exemplified by the flexor and extensor muscle reflexes described earlier.

Figure 54-12 shows a typical example of reciprocal inhibition. In this instance, a moderate but prolonged flexor reflex is elicited from one limb of the body; while this reflex is still being elicited, a stronger flexor reflex is elicited in the limb on the opposite side of the body. This stronger reflex sends reciprocal inhibitory signals to the first limb and depresses its degree of flexion. Finally, removal of the stronger reflex allows the original reflex to reassume its previous intensity.

Reflexes of Posture and Locomotion

Postural and Locomotive Reflexes of the Cord

Positive Supportive Reaction. Pressure on the footpad of a decerebrate animal causes the limb to extend against the pressure applied to the foot. Indeed, this reflex is so strong that if an animal whose spinal cord has been transected for several months—that is, after the reflexes have become exaggerated—is placed on its feet, the reflex often stiffens the limbs sufficiently to support the weight of the body. This reflex is called the *positive supportive reaction.*

The positive supportive reaction involves a complex circuit in the interneurons similar to the circuits responsible for the flexor and cross extensor reflexes. The locus of the pressure on the pad of the foot determines the direction in which the limb will extend; pressure on one side causes extension in that direction, an effect called the *magnet reaction.* This helps keep an animal from falling to that side.

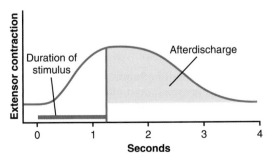

Figure 54-11 Myogram of a crossed extensor reflex showing slow onset but prolonged afterdischarge.

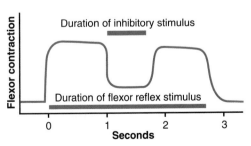

Figure 54-12 Myogram of a flexor reflex showing reciprocal inhibition caused by an inhibitory stimulus from a stronger flexor reflex on the opposite side of the body.

Cord "Righting" Reflexes. When a spinal animal is laid on its side, it will make uncoordinated movements trying to raise itself to the standing position. This is called the *cord righting reflex.* Such a reflex demonstrates that some relatively complex reflexes associated with posture are integrated in the spinal cord. Indeed, an animal with a well-healed transected thoracic cord between the levels for forelimb and hindlimb innervation can right itself from the lying position and even walk using its hindlimbs in addition to its forelimbs. In the case of an opossum with a similar transection of the thoracic cord, the walking movements of the hindlimbs are hardly different from those in a normal opossum—except that the hindlimb walking movements are not synchronized with those of the forelimbs.

Stepping and Walking Movements

Rhythmical Stepping Movements of a Single Limb. Rhythmical stepping movements are frequently observed in the limbs of spinal animals. Indeed, even when the lumbar portion of the spinal cord is separated from the remainder of the cord and a longitudinal section is made down the center of the cord to block neuronal connections between the two sides of the cord and between the two limbs, each hindlimb can still perform individual stepping functions. Forward flexion of the limb is followed a second or so later by backward extension. Then flexion occurs again, and the cycle is repeated over and over.

This oscillation back and forth between flexor and extensor muscles can occur even after the sensory nerves have been cut, and it seems to result mainly from mutually reciprocal inhibition circuits within the matrix of the cord itself, oscillating between the neurons controlling agonist and antagonist muscles.

The sensory signals from the footpads and from the position sensors around the joints play a strong role in controlling foot pressure and frequency of stepping when the foot is allowed to walk along a surface. In fact, the cord mechanism for control of stepping can be even more complex. For instance, if the top of the foot encounters an obstruction during forward thrust, the forward thrust will stop temporarily; then, in rapid sequence, the foot will be lifted higher and proceed forward to be placed over the obstruction. This is the *stumble reflex.* Thus, the cord is an intelligent walking controller.

Reciprocal Stepping of Opposite Limbs. If the lumbar spinal cord is not split down its center, every time stepping occurs in the forward direction in one limb, the opposite limb ordinarily moves backward. This effect results from reciprocal innervation between the two limbs.

Diagonal Stepping of All Four Limbs—"Mark Time" Reflex. If a well-healed spinal animal (with spinal transection in the neck above the forelimb area of the cord) is held up from the floor and its legs are allowed to dangle, the stretch on the limbs occasionally elicits stepping reflexes that involve all four limbs. In general, stepping occurs diagonally between the forelimbs and hindlimbs. This diagonal response is another manifestation of reciprocal innervation, this time occurring the entire distance up and down the cord between the forelimbs and hindlimbs. Such a walking pattern is called a *mark time reflex.*

Galloping Reflex. Another type of reflex that occasionally develops in a spinal animal is the galloping reflex, in which both forelimbs move backward in unison while both hindlimbs move forward. This often occurs when almost equal stretch or pressure stimuli are applied to the limbs on both sides of the body at the same time; unequal stimulation elicits the diagonal walking reflex. This is in keeping with the normal patterns of walking and galloping because in walking, only one forelimb and one hindlimb at a time are stimulated, which would predispose the animal to continue walking. Conversely, when the animal strikes the ground during galloping, both forelimbs and both hindlimbs are stimulated about equally; this predisposes the animal to keep galloping and, therefore, continues this pattern of motion.

Scratch Reflex

An especially important cord reflex in some animals is the scratch reflex, which is initiated by *itch* or *tickle sensation.* It involves two functions: (1) a *position sense* that allows the paw to find the exact point of irritation on the surface of the body and (2) a *to-and-fro scratching movement.*

The *position sense* of the scratch reflex is a highly developed function. If a flea is crawling as far forward as the shoulder of a spinal animal, the hind paw can still find its position, even though 19 muscles in the limb must be contracted simultaneously in a precise pattern to bring the paw to the position of the crawling flea. To make the reflex even more complicated, when the flea crosses the midline, the first paw stops scratching and the opposite paw begins the to-and-fro motion and eventually finds the flea.

The *to-and-fro movement*, like the stepping movements of locomotion, involves reciprocal innervation circuits that cause oscillation.

Spinal Cord Reflexes That Cause Muscle Spasm

In human beings, local muscle spasm is often observed. In many, if not most, instances, localized pain is the cause of the local spasm.

Muscle Spasm Resulting from a Broken Bone. One type of clinically important spasm occurs in muscles that surround a broken bone. The spasm results from pain impulses initiated from the broken edges of the bone, which cause the muscles that surround the area to contract tonically. Pain relief obtained by injecting a local anesthetic at the broken edges of the bone relieves the spasm; a deep general anesthetic of the entire body, such as ether anesthesia, also relieves the spasm. One of these two anesthetic procedures is often necessary before the spasm can be overcome sufficiently for the two ends of the bone to be set back into their appropriate positions.

Abdominal Muscle Spasm in Peritonitis. Another type of local spasm caused by cord reflexes is abdominal spasm resulting from irritation of the parietal peritoneum by peritonitis. Here again, relief of the pain caused by the peritonitis allows the spastic muscle to relax. The same type of spasm often occurs during surgical operations; for instance, during abdominal operations, pain impulses from the parietal peritoneum often cause the abdominal muscles to contract extensively, sometimes extruding the intestines through the surgical wound. For this reason, deep anesthesia is usually required for intra-abdominal operations.

Muscle Cramps. Still another type of local spasm is the typical muscle cramp. Electromyographic studies indicate that the cause of at least some muscle cramps is as follows: Any local irritating factor or metabolic abnormality of a muscle, such as severe cold, lack of blood flow, or overexercise, can elicit pain or other sensory signals transmitted from the muscle to the spinal cord, which in turn cause reflex feedback muscle contraction. The contraction is believed to stimulate the same sensory receptors even more, which causes the spinal cord to increase the intensity of contraction. Thus, positive feedback develops, so a small amount of initial irritation causes more and more contraction until a full-blown muscle cramp ensues.

Autonomic Reflexes in the Spinal Cord

Many types of segmental autonomic reflexes are integrated in the spinal cord, most of which are discussed in other chapters. Briefly, these include (1) changes in vascular tone resulting from changes in local skin heat (see Chapter 73); (2) sweating, which results from localized heat on the surface of the body (see Chapter 73); (3) intestinointestinal reflexes that control some motor functions of the gut (see Chapter 62); (4) peritoneointestinal reflexes that inhibit gastrointestinal motility in response to peritoneal irritation (see Chapter 66); and (5) evacuation reflexes for emptying the full bladder (see Chapter 31) or the colon (see Chapter 63). In addition, all the segmental reflexes can at times be elicited simultaneously in the form of the so-called *mass reflex*, described next.

Mass Reflex. In a spinal animal or human being, sometimes the spinal cord suddenly becomes excessively active, causing massive discharge in large portions of the cord. The usual stimulus that causes this is a strong pain stimulus to the skin or excessive filling of a viscus, such as overdistention of the bladder or the gut. Regardless of the type of stimulus, the resulting reflex, called the *mass reflex*, involves large portions or even all of the cord. The effects are (1) a major portion of the body's skeletal muscles goes into strong flexor spasm; (2) the colon and bladder are likely to evacuate; (3) the arterial pressure often rises to maximal values, sometimes to a systolic

pressure well over 200 mm Hg; and (4) large areas of the body break out into profuse sweating.

Because the mass reflex can last for minutes, it presumably results from activation of great numbers of reverberating circuits that excite large areas of the cord at once. This is similar to the mechanism of epileptic seizures, which involve reverberating circuits that occur in the brain instead of in the cord.

Spinal Cord Transection and Spinal Shock

When the spinal cord is suddenly transected in the upper neck, at first, essentially all cord functions, including the cord reflexes, immediately become depressed to the point of total silence, a reaction called *spinal shock*. The reason for this is that normal activity of the cord neurons depends to a great extent on continual tonic excitation by the discharge of nerve fibers entering the cord from higher centers, particularly discharge transmitted through the reticulospinal tracts, vestibulospinal tracts, and corticospinal tracts.

After a few hours to a few weeks, the spinal neurons gradually regain their excitability. This seems to be a natural characteristic of neurons everywhere in the nervous system—that is, after they lose their source of facilitatory impulses, they increase their own natural degree of excitability to make up at least partially for the loss. In most nonprimates, excitability of the cord centers returns essentially to normal within a few hours to a day or so, but in human beings, the return is often delayed for several weeks and occasionally is never complete; conversely, sometimes recovery is excessive, with resultant hyperexcitability of some or all cord functions.

Some of the spinal functions specifically affected during or after spinal shock are the following:

1. At onset of spinal shock, the arterial blood pressure falls instantly and drastically—sometimes to as low as 40 mm Hg—thus demonstrating that sympathetic nervous system activity becomes blocked almost to extinction. The pressure ordinarily returns to normal within a few days, even in human beings.

2. All skeletal muscle reflexes integrated in the spinal cord are blocked during the initial stages of shock. In lower animals, a few hours to a few days are required for these reflexes to return to normal; in human beings, 2 weeks to several months are sometimes required. In both animals and humans, some reflexes may eventually become hyperexcitable, particularly if a few facilitatory pathways remain intact between the brain and the cord while the remainder of the spinal cord is transected. The first reflexes to return are the stretch reflexes, followed in order by the progressively more complex reflexes: flexor reflexes, postural antigravity reflexes, and remnants of stepping reflexes.

3. The sacral reflexes for control of bladder and colon evacuation are suppressed in human beings for the first few weeks after cord transection, but in most cases they eventually return. These effects are discussed in Chapters 31 and 66.

Bibliography

Alvarez FJ, Fyffe RE: The continuing case for the Renshaw cell, *J Physiol* 584:31, 2007.

Buffelli M, Busetto G, Bidoia C, et al: Activity-dependent synaptic competition at mammalian neuromuscular junctions, *News Physiol Sci* 19:85, 2004.

Dietz V, Sinkjaer T: Spastic movement disorder: impaired reflex function and altered muscle mechanics, *Lancet Neurol* 6:725, 2007.

Dietz V: Proprioception and locomotor disorders, *Nat Rev Neurosci* 3:781, 2002.

Duysens J, Clarac F, Cruse H: Load-regulating mechanisms in gait and posture: comparative aspects, *Physiol Rev* 80:83, 2000.

Frigon A: Reconfiguration of the spinal interneuronal network during locomotion in vertebrates, *J Neurophysiol* 101:2201, 2009.

Glover JC: Development of specific connectivity between premotor neurons and motoneurons in the brain stem and spinal cord, *Physiol Rev* 80:615, 2000.

Goulding M: Circuits controlling vertebrate locomotion: moving in a new direction, *Nat Rev Neurosci* 10:507, 2009.

Grillner S: The motor infrastructure: from ion channels to neuronal networks, *Nat Rev Neurosci* 4:573, 2003.

Grillner S: Muscle twitches during sleep shape the precise muscles of the withdrawal reflex, *Trends Neurosci* 27:169, 2004.

Heckman CJ, Hyngstrom AS, Johnson MD: Active properties of motoneurone dendrites: diffuse descending neuromodulation, focused local inhibition, *J Physiol* 586:1225, 2008.

Ivanenko YP, Poppele RE, Lacquaniti F: Distributed neural networks for controlling human locomotion: lessons from normal and SCI subjects, *Brain Res Bull* 78:13, 2009.

Kandel ER, Schwartz JH, Jessell TM: *Principles of Neural Science*, ed 4, New York, 2000, McGraw-Hill.

Kiehn O: Locomotor circuits in the mammalian spinal cord, *Annu Rev Neurosci* 29:279, 2006.

Marchand-Pauvert V, Iglesias C: Properties of human spinal interneurones: normal and dystonic control, *J Physiol* 586:1247, 2008.

Marder E, Goaillard JM: Variability, compensation and homeostasis in neuron and network function, *Nat Rev Neurosci* 7:563, 2006.

Pearson KG: Generating the walking gait: role of sensory feedback, *Prog Brain Res* 143:123, 2004.

Rekling JC, Funk GD, Bayliss DA, et al: Synaptic control of motoneuronal excitability, *Physiol Rev* 80:767, 2000.

Rossignol S, Barrière G, Alluin O, et al: Re-expression of locomotor function after partial spinal cord injury, *Physiology (Bethesda)* 24:127, 2009.

Rossignol S, Barrière G, Frigon A, et al: Plasticity of locomotor sensorimotor interactions after peripheral and/or spinal lesions, *Brain Res Rev* 57:228, 2008.

Cortical and Brain Stem Control of Motor Function

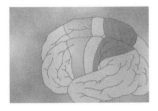

Most "voluntary" movements initiated by the cerebral cortex are achieved when the cortex activates "patterns" of function stored in lower brain areas—the cord, brain stem, basal ganglia, and cerebellum. These lower centers, in turn, send specific control signals to the muscles.

For a few types of movements, however, the cortex has almost a direct pathway to the anterior motor neurons of the cord, bypassing some motor centers on the way. This is especially true for control of the fine dexterous movements of the fingers and hands. This chapter and Chapter 56 explain the interplay among the different motor areas of the brain and spinal cord to provide overall synthesis of voluntary motor function.

Motor Cortex and Corticospinal Tract

Figure 55-1 shows the functional areas of the cerebral cortex. Anterior to the central cortical sulcus, occupying approximately the posterior one third of the frontal lobes, is the *motor cortex*. Posterior to the central sulcus is the *somatosensory cortex* (an area discussed in detail in earlier chapters), which feeds the motor cortex many of the signals that initiate motor activities.

The motor cortex itself is divided into three subareas, each of which has its own topographical representation of muscle groups and specific motor functions: (1) the *primary motor cortex*, (2) the *premotor area*, and (3) the *supplementary motor area.*

Primary Motor Cortex

The primary motor cortex, shown in Figure 55-1, lies in the first convolution of the frontal lobes anterior to the central sulcus. It begins laterally in the sylvian fissure, spreads superiorly to the uppermost portion of the brain, and then dips deep into the longitudinal fissure. (This area is the same as area 4 in Brodmann's classification of the brain cortical areas, shown in Figure 47-5.)

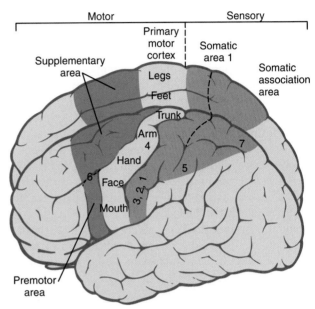

Figure 55-1 Motor and somatosensory functional areas of the cerebral cortex. The numbers *4, 5, 6,* and *7* are Brodmann's cortical areas, as explained in Chapter 47.

Figure 55-1 lists the approximate topographical representations of the different muscle areas of the body in the primary motor cortex, beginning with the face and mouth region near the sylvian fissure; the arm and hand area, in the midportion of the primary motor cortex; the trunk, near the apex of the brain; and the leg and foot areas, in the part of the primary motor cortex that dips into the longitudinal fissure. This topographical organization is demonstrated even more graphically in Figure 55-2, which shows the degrees of representation of the different muscle areas as mapped by Penfield and Rasmussen. This mapping was done by electrically stimulating the different areas of the motor cortex in human beings who were undergoing neurosurgical operations. Note that more than one half of the entire primary motor cortex is concerned with controlling the muscles of the hands and the muscles of speech. Point stimulation in these hand and speech motor areas on rare occasion causes contraction of a single muscle; most often, stimulation contracts a group of muscles instead. To express this in another way, excitation of a single motor cortex neuron usually excites a specific movement rather than one specific muscle. To do this, it excites a "pattern" of separate muscles, each of which contributes its own direction and strength of muscle movement.

Premotor Area

The premotor area, also shown in Figure 55-1, lies 1 to 3 centimeters anterior to the primary motor cortex, extending inferiorly into the sylvian fissure and superiorly into the longitudinal fissure, where it abuts the supplementary motor area, which has functions similar to those of the premotor area. The topographical organization of the premotor cortex is roughly the same as that of the primary motor cortex, with the mouth and face areas located most laterally; as one moves upward, the hand, arm, trunk, and leg areas are encountered.

Nerve signals generated in the premotor area cause much more complex "patterns" of movement than the discrete patterns generated in the primary motor cortex. For instance, the pattern may be to position the shoulders and arms so that the hands are properly oriented to perform specific tasks. To achieve these results, the most anterior part of the premotor area first develops a "motor image" of the total muscle movement that is to be performed. Then, in the posterior premotor cortex, this image excites each successive pattern of muscle activity required to achieve the image. This posterior part of the premotor cortex sends its signals either directly to the primary motor cortex to excite specific muscles or, often, by way of the basal ganglia and thalamus back to the primary motor cortex.

A special class of neurons called *mirror neurons* becomes active when a person performs a specific motor task or when he or she observes the same task performed by others. Thus, the activity of these neurons "mirrors" the behavior of another person as though the observer was performing the specific motor task. Mirror neurons are located in the premotor cortex and the inferior parietal cortex (and perhaps in other regions of the brain) and were first discovered in monkeys. However, brain imaging studies indicate that these neurons are also present in humans and may serve the same functions as observed in monkeys—to transform sensory representations of acts that are heard or seen into motor representations of these acts. Many neurophysiologists believe that these mirror neurons may be important for understanding the actions of other people and for learning new skills by imitation. Thus, the premotor cortex, basal ganglia, thalamus, and primary motor cortex constitute a complex overall system for the control of complex patterns of coordinated muscle activity.

Supplementary Motor Area

The supplementary motor area has yet another topographical organization for the control of motor function. It lies mainly in the longitudinal fissure but extends a few centimeters onto the superior frontal cortex. Contractions elicited by stimulating this area are often bilateral rather than unilateral. For instance, stimulation frequently leads to bilateral grasping movements of both hands simultaneously; these movements are perhaps rudiments of the hand functions required for climbing. In general, this area functions in concert with the premotor area to provide body-wide attitudinal movements, fixation movements of the different segments of the body, positional movements of the head and eyes, and so forth, as background for the finer motor control of the arms and hands by the premotor area and primary motor cortex.

Some Specialized Areas of Motor Control Found in the Human Motor Cortex

A few highly specialized motor regions of the human cerebral cortex (shown in Figure 55-3) control specific motor functions. These regions have been localized either by electrical stimulation or by noting the loss of motor function when destructive lesions occur in specific cortical areas. Some of the more important regions are the following.

Broca's Area and Speech. Figure 55-3 shows a premotor area labeled "word formation" lying immediately anterior to the primary motor cortex and immediately above the sylvian fissure. This region is called *Broca's area.* Damage to it does not prevent a person from vocalizing but makes it impossible for the person to speak whole words rather than uncoordinated utterances or an occasional simple word such as "no" or "yes." A closely associated cortical area also causes appropriate respiratory function, so respiratory activation of the vocal cords can occur simultaneously with the movements of the mouth

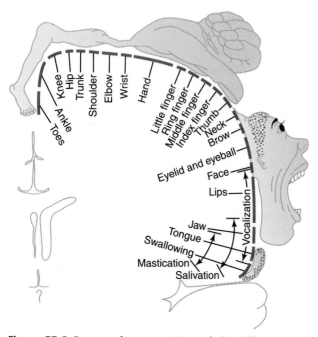

Figure 55-2 Degree of representation of the different muscles of the body in the motor cortex. (Redrawn from Penfield W, Rasmussen T: The Cerebral Cortex of Man: A Clinical Study of Localization of Function. New York: Hafner, 1968.)

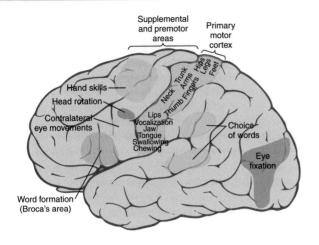

Figure 55-3 Representation of the different muscles of the body in the motor cortex and location of other cortical areas responsible for specific types of motor movements.

and tongue during speech. Thus, the premotor neuronal activities related to speech are highly complex.

"Voluntary" Eye Movement Field. In the premotor area immediately above Broca's area is a locus for controlling voluntary eye movements. Damage to this area prevents a person from *voluntarily* moving the eyes toward different objects. Instead, the eyes tend to lock involuntarily onto specific objects, an effect controlled by signals from the occipital visual cortex, as explained in Chapter 51. This frontal area also controls eyelid movements such as blinking.

Head Rotation Area. Slightly higher in the motor association area, electrical stimulation elicits head rotation. This area is closely associated with the eye movement field; it directs the head toward different objects.

Area for Hand Skills. In the premotor area immediately anterior to the primary motor cortex for the hands and fingers is a region that is important for "hand skills." That is, when tumors or other lesions cause destruction in this area, hand movements become uncoordinated and nonpurposeful, a condition called *motor apraxia.*

Transmission of Signals from the Motor Cortex to the Muscles

Motor signals are transmitted directly from the cortex to the spinal cord through the *corticospinal tract* and indirectly through multiple accessory pathways that involve the *basal ganglia, cerebellum,* and various *nuclei of the brain stem.* In general, the direct pathways are concerned more with discrete and detailed movements, especially of the distal segments of the limbs, particularly the hands and fingers.

Corticospinal (Pyramidal) Tract

The most important output pathway from the motor cortex is the *corticospinal tract,* also called the *pyramidal tract,* shown in Figure 55-4. The corticospinal tract originates about 30 percent from the primary motor cortex, 30 percent from the premotor and supplementary motor areas, and 40 percent from the somatosensory areas posterior to the central sulcus.

After leaving the cortex, it passes through the posterior limb of the internal capsule (between the caudate nucleus and the putamen of the basal ganglia) and then downward through the brain stem, forming the *pyramids of the medulla.* The majority of the pyramidal fibers then cross in the lower medulla to the opposite side and descend into the *lateral corticospinal tracts* of the cord, finally terminating principally on the interneurons in the intermediate regions of the cord gray matter; a few terminate on sensory relay neurons in the dorsal horn, and a very few terminate directly on the anterior motor neurons that cause muscle contraction.

A few of the fibers do not cross to the opposite side in the medulla but pass ipsilaterally down the cord in the *ventral corticospinal tracts.* Many, if not most, of these fibers eventually cross to the opposite side of the cord either in the neck or in the upper thoracic region. These fibers may be concerned with control of bilateral postural movements by the supplementary motor cortex.

The most impressive fibers in the pyramidal tract are a population of large myelinated fibers with a mean diameter of 16 micrometers. These fibers originate from *giant pyramidal cells,* called *Betz cells,* that are found only in the primary motor cortex. The Betz cells are about 60 micrometers in diameter, and their fibers transmit nerve impulses to the spinal cord at a velocity of about 70 m/sec, the most rapid rate of transmission of any signals from the brain to the cord. There are about 34,000 of these large Betz cell fibers in each corticospinal tract. The total number of fibers in each corticospinal tract is more than 1 million, so these large fibers represent only 3 percent of the total. The other 97 percent are mainly fibers smaller than 4 micrometers in diameter that conduct background tonic signals to the motor areas of the cord.

Other Fiber Pathways from the Motor Cortex. The motor cortex gives rise to large numbers of additional, mainly small, fibers that go to deep regions in the cerebrum and brain stem, including the following:

1. The axons from the giant Betz cells send short collaterals back to the cortex itself. These collaterals are believed to inhibit adjacent regions of the cortex when the Betz cells discharge, thereby "sharpening" the boundaries of the excitatory signal.

2. A large number of fibers pass from the motor cortex into the *caudate nucleus* and *putamen.* From there, additional pathways extend into the brain stem and spinal cord, as discussed in the next chapter, mainly to control body postural muscle contractions.

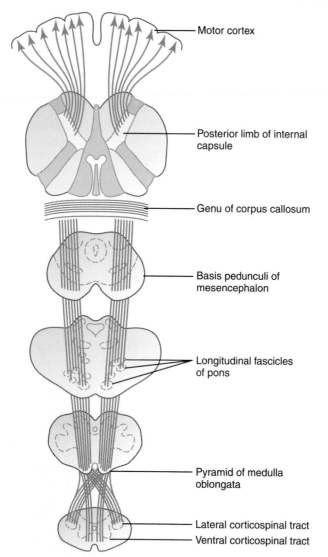

Figure 55-4 Corticospinal (pyramidal) tract. (Modified from Ranson SW, Clark SL: Anatomy of the Nervous System. Philadelphia: WB Saunders, 1959.)

Labels in figure:
- Motor cortex
- Posterior limb of internal capsule
- Genu of corpus callosum
- Basis pedunculi of mesencephalon
- Longitudinal fascicles of pons
- Pyramid of medulla oblongata
- Lateral corticospinal tract
- Ventral corticospinal tract

3. A moderate number of motor fibers pass to *red nuclei* of the midbrain. From these, additional fibers pass down the cord through the *rubrospinal tract.*

4. A moderate number of motor fibers deviate into the *reticular substance* and *vestibular nuclei* of the brain stem; from there, signals go to the cord by way of *reticulospinal* and *vestibulospinal tracts,* and others go to the cerebellum by way of *reticulocerebellar* and *vestibulocerebellar tracts.*

5. A tremendous number of motor fibers synapse in the pontile nuclei, which give rise to the *pontocerebellar fibers,* carrying signals into the cerebellar hemispheres.

6. Collaterals also terminate in the *inferior olivary nuclei,* and from there, secondary *olivocerebellar fibers* transmit signals to multiple areas of the cerebellum.

Thus, the basal ganglia, brain stem, and cerebellum all receive strong motor signals from the corticospinal system every time a signal is transmitted down the spinal cord to cause a motor activity.

Incoming Sensory Fiber Pathways to the Motor Cortex

The functions of the motor cortex are controlled mainly by nerve signals from the somatosensory system but also, to some degree, from other sensory systems such as hearing and vision. Once the sensory information is received, the motor cortex operates in association with the basal ganglia and cerebellum to excite an appropriate course of motor action. The more important incoming fiber pathways to the motor cortex are the following:

1. Subcortical fibers from adjacent regions of the cerebral cortex, especially from (a) the somatosensory areas of the parietal cortex, (b) the adjacent areas of the frontal cortex anterior to the motor cortex, and (c) the visual and auditory cortices.

2. Subcortical fibers that arrive through the corpus callosum from the opposite cerebral hemisphere. These fibers connect corresponding areas of the cortices in the two sides of the brain.

3. Somatosensory fibers that arrive directly from the ventrobasal complex of the thalamus. These relay mainly cutaneous tactile signals and joint and muscle signals from the peripheral body.

4. Tracts from the ventrolateral and ventroanterior nuclei of the thalamus, which in turn receive signals from the cerebellum and basal ganglia. These tracts provide signals that are necessary for coordination among the motor control functions of the motor cortex, basal ganglia, and cerebellum.

5. Fibers from the intralaminar nuclei of the thalamus. These fibers control the general level of excitability of the motor cortex in the same way they control the general level of excitability of most other regions of the cerebral cortex.

Red Nucleus Serves as an Alternative Pathway for Transmitting Cortical Signals to the Spinal Cord

The *red nucleus,* located in the mesencephalon, functions in close association with the corticospinal tract. As shown in Figure 55-5, it receives a large number of direct fibers from the primary motor cortex through the *corticorubral tract,* as well as branching fibers from the corticospinal tract as it passes through the mesencephalon. These fibers synapse in the lower portion of the red nucleus, the *magnocellular portion,* which contains large neurons similar in size to the Betz cells in the motor cortex. These large neurons then give rise to the *rubrospinal tract,* which crosses to the opposite side in the lower brain stem and follows a course immediately adjacent and anterior to the corticospinal tract into the lateral columns of the spinal cord.

The rubrospinal fibers terminate mostly on the interneurons of the intermediate areas of the cord gray matter, along with the corticospinal fibers, but some of the rubrospinal fibers terminate directly on anterior motor neurons, along with some corticospinal fibers. The red nucleus also has close connections with the cerebellum, similar to the connections between the motor cortex and the cerebellum.

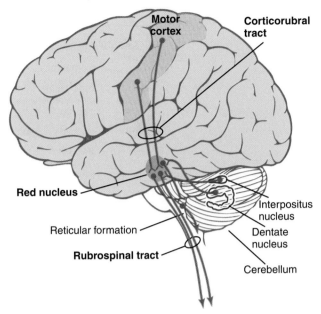

Figure 55-5 Corticorubrospinal pathway for motor control, showing also the relation of this pathway to the cerebellum.

Function of the Corticorubrospinal System. The magnocellular portion of the red nucleus has a somatographic representation of all the muscles of the body, as is true of the motor cortex. Therefore, stimulation of a single point in this portion of the red nucleus causes contraction of either a single muscle or a small group of muscles. However, the fineness of representation of the different muscles is far less developed than in the motor cortex. This is especially true in human beings, who have relatively small red nuclei.

The corticorubrospinal pathway serves as an accessory route for transmission of relatively discrete signals from the motor cortex to the spinal cord. When the corticospinal fibers are destroyed but the corticorubrospinal pathway is intact, discrete movements can still occur, except that the movements for fine control of the fingers and hands are considerably impaired. Wrist movements are still functional, which is not the case when the corticorubrospinal pathway is also blocked.

Therefore, the pathway through the red nucleus to the spinal cord is associated with the corticospinal system. Further, the rubrospinal tract lies in the lateral columns of the spinal cord, along with the corticospinal tract, and terminates on the interneurons and motor neurons that control the more distal muscles of the limbs. Therefore, the corticospinal and rubrospinal tracts together are called the *lateral motor system of the cord,* in contradistinction to a vestibuloreticulospinal system, which lies mainly medially in the cord and is called the *medial motor system of the cord,* as discussed later in this chapter.

"Extrapyramidal" System

The term *extrapyramidal motor system* is widely used in clinical circles to denote all those portions of the brain and brain stem that contribute to motor control but are not part of the direct corticospinal-pyramidal system. These include pathways through the basal ganglia, the reticular formation of the brain stem, the vestibular nuclei, and often the red nuclei. This is such an all-inclusive and diverse group of motor control areas that it is difficult to ascribe specific neurophysiologic functions to the so-called extrapyramidal system as a whole. In fact, the pyramidal and extrapyramidal systems are extensively interconnected and interact to control movement. For these reasons, the term "extrapyramidal" is being used less often both clinically and physiologically.

Excitation of the Spinal Cord Motor Control Areas by the Primary Motor Cortex and Red Nucleus

Vertical Columnar Arrangement of the Neurons in the Motor Cortex. In Chapters 47 and 51, we pointed out that the cells in the somatosensory cortex and visual cortex are organized in *vertical columns of cells.* In like manner, the cells of the motor cortex are organized in vertical columns a fraction of a millimeter in diameter, with thousands of neurons in each column.

Each column of cells functions as a unit, usually stimulating a group of synergistic muscles, but sometimes stimulating just a single muscle. Also, each column has six distinct layers of cells, as is true throughout nearly all the cerebral cortex. The pyramidal cells that give rise to the corticospinal fibers all lie in the fifth layer of cells from the cortical surface. Conversely, the input signals all enter by way of layers 2 through 4. And the sixth layer gives rise mainly to fibers that communicate with other regions of the cerebral cortex itself.

Function of Each Column of Neurons. The neurons of each column operate as an integrative processing system, using information from multiple input sources to determine the output response from the column. In addition, each column can function as an amplifying system to stimulate large numbers of pyramidal fibers to the same muscle or to synergistic muscles simultaneously. This is important because stimulation of a single pyramidal cell can seldom excite a muscle. Usually, 50 to 100 pyramidal cells need to be excited simultaneously or in rapid succession to achieve definitive muscle contraction.

Dynamic and Static Signals Are Transmitted by the Pyramidal Neurons. If a strong signal is sent to a muscle to cause initial rapid contraction, then a much weaker continuing signal can maintain the contraction for long periods thereafter. This is the usual manner in which excitation is provided to cause muscle contractions. To do this, each column of cells excites two populations of pyramidal cell neurons, one called *dynamic neurons* and the other *static neurons.* The dynamic neurons are excited at a high rate for a short period at the beginning of a contraction, causing the initial rapid *development of force.* Then the static neurons fire at a much slower rate, but they continue firing at this slow rate to *maintain the force* of contraction as long as the contraction is required.

The neurons of the red nucleus have similar dynamic and static characteristics, except that a greater percentage of dynamic neurons is in the red nucleus and a greater percentage of static neurons is in the primary motor cortex. This may be related to the fact that the red nucleus is closely allied with the cerebellum, and the cerebellum plays an important role in rapid initiation of muscle contraction, as explained in the next chapter.

Somatosensory Feedback to the Motor Cortex Helps Control the Precision of Muscle Contraction

When nerve signals from the motor cortex cause a muscle to contract, somatosensory signals return all the way from the activated region of the body to the neurons in the motor cortex that are initiating the action. Most of these somatosensory signals arise in (1) the muscle spindles, (2) the tendon organs of the muscle tendons, or (3) the tactile receptors of the skin overlying the muscles. These somatic signals often cause positive feedback enhancement of the muscle contraction in the following ways: In the case of the muscle spindles, if the fusimotor muscle fibers in the spindles contract more than the large skeletal muscle fibers contract, the central portions of the spindles become stretched and, therefore, excited. Signals from these spindles then return rapidly to the pyramidal cells in the motor cortex to signal them that the large muscle fibers have not contracted enough. The pyramidal cells further excite the muscle, helping its contraction to catch up with the contraction of the muscle spindles. In the case of the tactile receptors, if the muscle contraction causes compression of the skin against an object, such as compression of the fingers around an object being grasped, the signals from the skin receptors can, if necessary, cause further excitation of the muscles and, therefore, increase the tightness of the hand grasp.

Stimulation of the Spinal Motor Neurons

Figure 55-6 shows a cross section of a spinal cord segment demonstrating (1) multiple motor and sensorimotor control tracts entering the cord segment and (2) a representative anterior motor neuron in the middle of the anterior horn gray matter. The corticospinal tract and the rubrospinal tract lie in the dorsal portions of the lateral white columns. Their fibers terminate mainly on interneurons in the intermediate area of the cord gray matter.

In the cervical enlargement of the cord where the hands and fingers are represented, large numbers of both corticospinal and rubrospinal fibers also terminate directly on the anterior motor neurons, thus allowing a direct route from the brain to activate muscle contraction. This is in keeping with the fact that the primary motor cortex has an extremely high degree of representation for fine control of hand, finger, and thumb actions.

Patterns of Movement Elicited by Spinal Cord Centers. From Chapter 54, recall that the spinal cord can

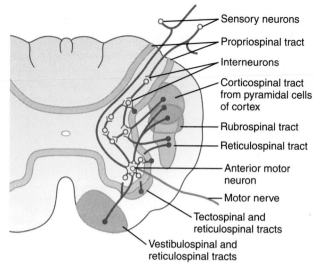

Figure 55-6 Convergence of different motor control pathways on the anterior motor neurons.

provide certain specific reflex patterns of movement in response to sensory nerve stimulation. Many of these same patterns are also important when the cord's anterior motor neurons are excited by signals from the brain. For example, the stretch reflex is functional at all times, helping to damp any oscillations of the motor movements initiated from the brain, and probably also providing at least part of the motive power required to cause muscle contractions when the intrafusal fibers of the muscle spindles contract more than the large skeletal muscle fibers do, thus eliciting reflex "servo-assist" stimulation of the muscle, in addition to the direct stimulation by the corticospinal fibers.

Also, when a brain signal excites a muscle, it is usually unnecessary to transmit an inverse signal to relax the antagonist muscle at the same time; this is achieved by the *reciprocal innervation* circuit that is always present in the cord for coordinating the function of antagonistic pairs of muscles.

Finally, other cord reflex mechanisms, such as withdrawal, stepping and walking, scratching, and postural mechanisms, can each be activated by "command" signals from the brain. Thus, simple command signals from the brain can initiate many normal motor activities, particularly for such functions as walking and attaining different postural attitudes of the body.

Effect of Lesions in the Motor Cortex or in the Corticospinal Pathway—The "Stroke"

The motor control system can be damaged by the common abnormality called a "stroke." This is caused by either a ruptured blood vessel that hemorrhages into the brain or by thrombosis of one of the major arteries supplying the brain. In either case, the result is loss of blood supply to the cortex or to the corticospinal tract where it passes through the internal capsule between the caudate nucleus and the putamen. Also, experiments have been performed in animals to selectively remove different parts of the motor cortex.

Removal of the Primary Motor Cortex (Area Pyramidalis). Removal of a portion of the primary motor cortex—the area that contains the giant Betz pyramidal cells—causes varying degrees of paralysis of the represented muscles. If the sublying caudate nucleus and adjacent premotor and supplementary motor areas are not damaged, gross postural and limb "fixation" movements can still occur, but there is *loss of voluntary control of discrete movements of the distal segments of the limbs, especially of the hands and fingers.* This does not mean that the hand and finger muscles themselves cannot contract; rather, the *ability to control the fine movements is gone.* From these observations, one can conclude that the area pyramidalis is essential for voluntary initiation of finely controlled movements, especially of the hands and fingers.

Muscle Spasticity Caused by Lesions That Damage Large Areas Adjacent to the Motor Cortex. The primary motor cortex normally exerts a continual tonic stimulatory effect on the motor neurons of the spinal cord; when this stimulatory effect is removed, *hypotonia* results. Most lesions of the motor cortex, especially those caused by a *stroke,* involve not only the primary motor cortex but also adjacent parts of the brain such as the basal ganglia. In these instances, *muscle spasm* almost invariably occurs in the afflicted muscle areas on the *opposite side* of the body (because the motor pathways cross to the opposite side). This spasm results mainly from damage to accessory pathways from the nonpyramidal portions of the motor cortex. These pathways normally inhibit the vestibular and reticular brain stem motor nuclei. When these nuclei cease their state of inhibition (i.e., are "disinhibited"), they become spontaneously active and cause excessive spastic tone in the involved muscles, as we discuss more fully later in the chapter. This is the spasticity that normally accompanies a "stroke" in a human being.

Role of the Brain Stem in Controlling Motor Function

The brain stem consists of the *medulla, pons,* and *mesencephalon.* In one sense, it is an extension of the spinal cord upward into the cranial cavity because it contains motor and sensory nuclei that perform motor and sensory functions for the face and head regions in the same way that the spinal cord performs these functions from the neck down. But in another sense, the brain stem is its own master because it provides many special control functions, such as the following:

1. Control of respiration
2. Control of the cardiovascular system
3. Partial control of gastrointestinal function
4. Control of many stereotyped movements of the body
5. Control of equilibrium
6. Control of eye movements

Finally, the brain stem serves as a way station for "command signals" from higher neural centers. In the following sections, we discuss the role of the brain stem in controlling whole-body movement and equilibrium. Especially important for these purposes are the brain stem's *reticular nuclei* and *vestibular nuclei.*

Support of the Body Against Gravity—Roles of the Reticular and Vestibular Nuclei

Figure 55-7 shows the locations of the reticular and vestibular nuclei in the brain stem.

Excitatory-Inhibitory Antagonism Between Pontine and Medullary Reticular Nuclei

The reticular nuclei are divided into two major groups: (1) *pontine reticular nuclei,* located slightly posteriorly and laterally in the pons and extending into the mesencephalon, and (2) *medullary reticular nuclei,* which extend through the entire medulla, lying ventrally and medially near the midline. These two sets of nuclei function mainly antagonistically to each other, with the pontine exciting the antigravity muscles and the medullary relaxing these same muscles.

Pontine Reticular System. The pontine reticular nuclei transmit excitatory signals downward into the cord through the *pontine reticulospinal tract* in the anterior column of the cord, as shown in Figure 55-8. The fibers of this pathway terminate on the medial anterior motor neurons that excite the axial muscles of the body, which support the body against gravity—that is, the muscles of the vertebral column and the extensor muscles of the limbs.

The pontine reticular nuclei have a high degree of natural excitability. In addition, they receive strong excitatory signals from the vestibular nuclei, as well as from deep nuclei of the cerebellum. Therefore, when the pontine reticular excitatory system is unopposed by the medullary reticular system, it causes powerful excitation of antigravity muscles throughout the body, so much so that

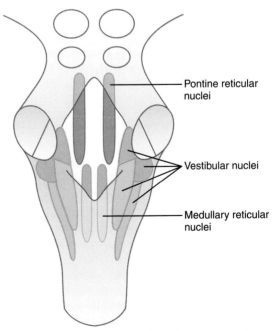

Figure 55-7 Locations of the reticular and vestibular nuclei in the brain stem.

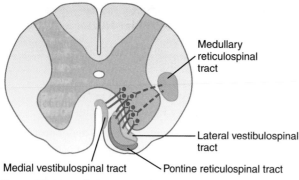

Figure 55-8 Vestibulospinal and reticulospinal tracts descending in the spinal cord to excite (*solid lines*) or inhibit (*dashed lines*) the anterior motor neurons that control the body's axial musculature.

four-legged animals can be placed in a standing position, supporting the body against gravity without any signals from higher levels of the brain.

Medullary Reticular System. The medullary reticular nuclei transmit *inhibitory* signals to the same antigravity anterior motor neurons by way of a different tract, the *medullary reticulospinal tract*, located in the lateral column of the cord, as also shown in Figure 55-8. The medullary reticular nuclei receive strong input collaterals from (1) the corticospinal tract, (2) the rubrospinal tract, and (3) other motor pathways. These normally activate the medullary reticular inhibitory system to counterbalance the excitatory signals from the pontine reticular system, so under normal conditions the body muscles are not abnormally tense.

Yet some signals from higher areas of the brain can "disinhibit" the medullary system when the brain wishes to excite the pontine system to cause standing. At other times, excitation of the medullary reticular system can inhibit antigravity muscles in certain portions of the body to allow those portions to perform special motor activities. The excitatory and inhibitory reticular nuclei constitute a controllable system that is manipulated by motor signals from the cerebral cortex and elsewhere to provide necessary background muscle contractions for standing against gravity and to inhibit appropriate groups of muscles as needed so that other functions can be performed.

Role of the Vestibular Nuclei to Excite the Antigravity Muscles

All the *vestibular nuclei*, shown in Figure 55-7, function in association with the pontine reticular nuclei to control the antigravity muscles. The vestibular nuclei transmit strong excitatory signals to the antigravity muscles by way of the *lateral* and *medial vestibulospinal tracts* in the anterior columns of the spinal cord, as shown in Figure 55-8. Without this support of the vestibular nuclei, the pontine reticular system would lose much of its excitation of the axial antigravity muscles.

The specific role of the vestibular nuclei, however, is to *selectively* control the excitatory signals to the different antigravity muscles to maintain equilibrium *in response*

to signals from the vestibular apparatus. We discuss this more fully later in the chapter.

The Decerebrate Animal Develops Spastic Rigidity

When the brain stem of an animal is sectioned below the midlevel of the mesencephalon, but the pontine and medullary reticular systems, as well as the vestibular system, are left intact, the animal develops a condition called *decerebrate rigidity.* This rigidity does not occur in all muscles of the body but does occur in the antigravity muscles—the muscles of the neck and trunk and the extensors of the legs.

The cause of decerebrate rigidity is blockage of normally strong input to the medullary reticular nuclei from the cerebral cortex, the red nuclei, and the basal ganglia. Lacking this input, the medullary reticular inhibitor system becomes nonfunctional; full overactivity of the pontine excitatory system occurs, and rigidity develops. We shall see later that other causes of rigidity occur in other neuromotor diseases, especially lesions of the basal ganglia.

Vestibular Sensations and Maintenance of Equilibrium

Vestibular Apparatus

The vestibular apparatus, shown in Figure 55-9, is the sensory organ for detecting sensations of equilibrium. It is encased in a system of bony tubes and chambers located in the petrous portion of the temporal bone, called the *bony labyrinth*. Within this system are membranous tubes and chambers called the *membranous labyrinth*. The membranous labyrinth is the functional part of the vestibular apparatus.

The top of Figure 55-9 shows the membranous labyrinth. It is composed mainly of the *cochlea* (ductus cochlearis); three *semicircular canals;* and two large chambers, the *utricle* and *saccule*. The cochlea is the major sensory organ for hearing (see Chapter 52) and has little to do with equilibrium. However, the *semicircular canals*, the *utricle*, and the *saccule* are all integral parts of the equilibrium mechanism.

"Maculae"—Sensory Organs of the Utricle and Saccule for Detecting Orientation of the Head with Respect to Gravity. Located on the inside surface of each utricle and saccule, shown in the top diagram of Figure 55-9, is a small sensory area slightly over 2 millimeters in diameter called a *macula*. The *macula of the utricle* lies mainly in the *horizontal plane* on the inferior surface of the utricle and plays an important role in determining orientation of the head when the head is upright. Conversely, the *macula of the saccule* is located mainly in a *vertical plane* and signals head orientation when the person is lying down.

Each macula is covered by a gelatinous layer in which many small calcium carbonate crystals called *statoconia* are embedded. Also in the macula are thousands of *hair cells*, one of which is shown in Figure 55-10; these project *cilia* up into the gelatinous layer. The bases and sides of

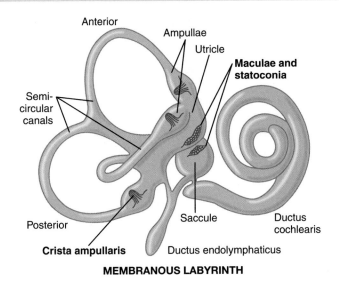

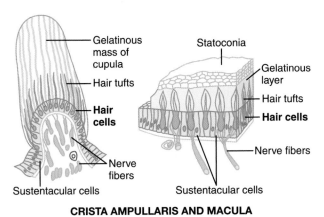

CRISTA AMPULLARIS AND MACULA

Figure 55-9 Membranous labyrinth and organization of the crista ampullaris and the macula.

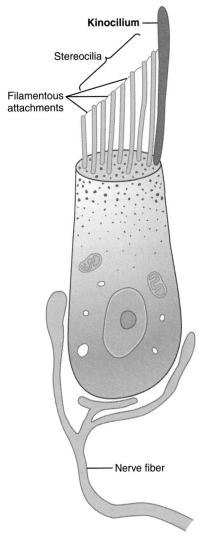

Figure 55-10 Hair cell of the equilibrium apparatus and its synapses with the vestibular nerve.

the hair cells synapse with sensory endings of the *vestibular nerve.*

The calcified statoconia have a *specific gravity* two to three times the specific gravity of the surrounding fluid and tissues. The weight of the statoconia bends the cilia in the direction of gravitational pull.

Directional Sensitivity of the Hair Cells— Kinocilium. Each hair cell has 50 to 70 small cilia called *stereocilia,* plus one large cilium, the *kinocilium,* as shown in Figure 55-10. The kinocilium is always located to one side, and the stereocilia become progressively shorter toward the other side of the cell. Minute filamentous attachments, almost invisible even to the electron microscope, connect the tip of each stereocilium to the next longer stereocilium and, finally, to the kinocilium.

Because of these attachments, when the stereocilia and kinocilium bend in the direction of the kinocilium, the filamentous attachments tug in sequence on the stereocilia, pulling them outward from the cell body. This opens several hundred fluid channels in the neuronal cell membrane around the bases of the stereocilia, and these channels are capable of conducting large numbers

of positive ions. Therefore, positive ions pour into the cell from the surrounding endolymphatic fluid, causing *receptor membrane depolarization.* Conversely, bending the pile of stereocilia in the opposite direction (backward to the kinocilium) reduces the tension on the attachments; this closes the ion channels, thus causing *receptor hyperpolarization.*

Under normal resting conditions, the nerve fibers leading from the hair cells transmit continuous nerve impulses at a rate of about 100 per second. When the stereocilia are bent toward the kinocilium, the impulse traffic increases, often to several hundred per second; conversely, bending the cilia away from the kinocilium decreases the impulse traffic, often turning it off completely. Therefore, as the orientation of the head in space changes and the weight of the statoconia bends the cilia, appropriate signals are transmitted to the brain to control equilibrium.

In each macula, each of the hair cells is oriented in a different direction so that some of the hair cells are stimulated when the head bends forward, some are stimulated when it bends backward, others are stimulated when it bends to one side, and so forth. Therefore, a different pattern of excitation occurs in the macular nerve fibers for each orientation of the head in the gravitational field. It is this "pattern" that apprises the brain of the head's orientation in space.

Semicircular Ducts. The three semicircular ducts in each vestibular apparatus, known as the *anterior, posterior,* and *lateral (horizontal) semicircular ducts,* are arranged at right angles to one another so that they represent all three planes in space. When the head is bent forward about 30 degrees, the lateral semicircular ducts are approximately horizontal with respect to the surface of the earth; the anterior ducts are in vertical planes that project *forward and 45 degrees outward,* whereas the posterior ducts are in vertical planes that project *backward and 45 degrees outward.*

Each semicircular duct has an enlargement at one of its ends called the *ampulla,* and the ducts and ampulla are filled with a fluid called *endolymph.* Flow of this fluid through one of the ducts and through its ampulla excites the sensory organ of the ampulla in the following manner: Figure 55-11 shows in each ampulla a small crest called a *crista ampullaris.* On top of this crista is a loose gelatinous tissue mass, the *cupula.* When a person's head begins to rotate in any direction, the inertia of the fluid in one or more of the semicircular ducts causes the fluid to remain stationary while the semicircular duct rotates with the head. This causes fluid to flow from the duct and through the ampulla, bending the cupula to one side, as demonstrated by the position of the colored cupula in Figure 55-11. Rotation of the head in the opposite direction causes the cupula to bend to the opposite side.

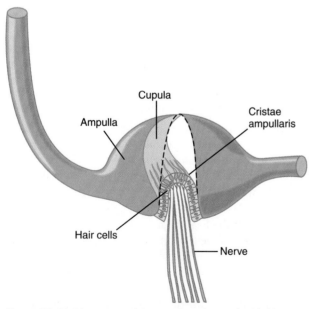

Figure 55-11 Movement of the cupula and its embedded hairs at the onset of rotation.

Ampulla
Cupula
Cristae ampullaris
Hair cells
Nerve

Into the cupula are projected hundreds of cilia from hair cells located on the ampullary crest. The kinocilia of these hair cells are all oriented in the same direction in the cupula, and bending the cupula in that direction causes depolarization of the hair cells, whereas bending it in the opposite direction hyperpolarizes the cells. Then, from the hair cells, appropriate signals are sent by way of the *vestibular nerve* to apprise the central nervous system of a *change in rotation* of the head and the *rate of change* in each of the three planes of space.

Function of the Utricle and Saccule in the Maintenance of Static Equilibrium

It is especially important that the hair cells are all oriented in different directions in the maculae of the utricles and saccules so that with different positions of the head, different hair cells become stimulated. The "patterns" of stimulation of the different hair cells apprise the brain of the position of the head with respect to the pull of gravity. In turn, the vestibular, cerebellar, and reticular motor nerve systems of the brain excite appropriate postural muscles to maintain proper equilibrium.

This utricle and saccule system functions extremely effectively for maintaining equilibrium when the head is in the near-vertical position. Indeed, a person can determine as little as half a degree of dysequilibrium when the body leans from the precise upright position.

Detection of Linear Acceleration by the Utricle and Saccule Maculae. When the body is suddenly thrust forward—that is, when the body accelerates—the statoconia, which have greater mass inertia than the surrounding fluid, fall backward on the hair cell cilia, and information of dysequilibrium is sent into the nervous centers, causing the person to feel as though he or she were falling backward. This automatically causes the person to lean forward until the resulting anterior shift of the statoconia exactly equals the tendency for the statoconia to fall backward because of the acceleration. At this point, the nervous system senses a state of proper equilibrium and leans the body forward no farther. Thus, the maculae operate to maintain equilibrium during linear acceleration in exactly the same manner as they operate during static equilibrium.

The maculae *do not* operate for the detection of linear *velocity.* When runners first begin to run, they must lean far forward to keep from falling backward because of initial *acceleration,* but once they have achieved running speed, if they were running in a vacuum, they would not have to lean forward. When running in air, they lean forward to maintain equilibrium only because of air resistance against their bodies; in this instance, it is not the maculae that make them lean but air pressure acting on pressure end-organs in the skin, which initiate appropriate equilibrium adjustments to prevent falling.

Detection of Head Rotation by the Semicircular Ducts

When the head suddenly begins to rotate in any direction (called *angular acceleration*), the endolymph in the semicircular ducts, because of its inertia, tends to remain stationary while the semicircular ducts turn. This causes relative fluid flow in the ducts in the direction opposite to head rotation.

Figure 55-12 shows a typical discharge signal from a single hair cell in the crista ampullaris when an animal is rotated for 40 seconds, demonstrating that (1) even when the cupula is in its resting position, the hair cell emits a tonic discharge of about 100 impulses per second; (2) when the animal begins to rotate, the hairs bend to one side and the rate of discharge increases greatly; and (3) with continued rotation, the excess discharge of the hair cell gradually subsides back to the resting level during the next few seconds.

The reason for this adaptation of the receptor is that within the first few seconds of rotation, back resistance to the flow of fluid in the semicircular duct and past the bent cupula causes the endolymph to begin rotating as rapidly as the semicircular canal itself; then, in another 5 to 20 seconds, the cupula slowly returns to its resting position in the middle of the ampulla because of its own elastic recoil.

When the rotation suddenly stops, exactly opposite effects take place: The endolymph continues to rotate while the semicircular duct stops. This time, the cupula bends in the opposite direction, causing the hair cell to stop discharging entirely. After another few seconds, the endolymph stops moving and the cupula gradually returns to its resting position, thus allowing hair cell discharge to return to its normal tonic level, as shown to the right in Figure 55-12. Thus, the semicircular duct transmits a signal of one polarity when the head *begins* to rotate and of opposite polarity when it *stops* rotating.

"Predictive" Function of the Semicircular Duct System in the Maintenance of Equilibrium. Because the semicircular ducts do not detect that the body is off balance in the forward direction, in the side direction, or in the backward direction, one might ask: What is the semicircular ducts' function in the maintenance of equilibrium? All they detect is that the person's head is *beginning* or *stopping* to rotate in one direction or another. Therefore, the function of the semicircular ducts is not to maintain static equilibrium or to maintain equilibrium during steady directional or rotational movements. Yet loss of function of the semicircular ducts does cause a person to have poor equilibrium when attempting to perform *rapid, intricate changing* body movements.

The function of the semicircular ducts can be explained by the following illustration: If a person is running forward rapidly and then suddenly begins to turn to one side, *he or she will fall off balance a fraction of a second later* unless appropriate corrections are made *ahead of time.* But the maculae of the utricle and saccule cannot detect that he or she is off balance until *after* this has occurred. The semicircular ducts, however, will have already detected that the person is turning, and this information can easily apprise the central nervous system of the fact that the person *will* fall off balance within the next fraction of a second or so unless some *anticipatory correction* is made.

In other words, the semicircular duct mechanism *predicts* that dysequilibrium is going to occur and thereby causes the equilibrium centers to make appropriate anticipatory preventive adjustments. This helps the person maintain balance before the situation can be corrected.

Removal of the flocculonodular lobes of the cerebellum prevents normal detection of semicircular duct signals but has less effect on detecting macular signals. It is especially interesting that the cerebellum serves as a "predictive" organ for most rapid movements of the body, as well as for those having to do with equilibrium. These other functions of the cerebellum are discussed in the following chapter.

Vestibular Mechanisms for Stabilizing the Eyes

When a person changes his or her direction of movement rapidly or even leans the head sideways, forward, or backward, it would be impossible to maintain a stable image on the retinas unless the person had some automatic control mechanism to stabilize the direction of the eyes' gaze. In addition, the eyes would be of little use in detecting an image unless they remained "fixed" on each object long enough to gain a clear image. Fortunately, each time the head is suddenly rotated, signals from the semicircular ducts cause the eyes to rotate in a direction equal and opposite to the rotation of the head. This results from reflexes transmitted through the *vestibular nuclei* and the *medial longitudinal fasciculus* to the *oculomotor nuclei*. These reflexes are described in Chapter 51.

Other Factors Concerned with Equilibrium

Neck Proprioceptors. The vestibular apparatus detects the orientation and movement *only of the head.* Therefore, it is essential that the nervous centers also receive appropriate information about the orientation of the head with respect to the body. This information is transmitted from the proprioceptors of the neck and body directly to the vestibular

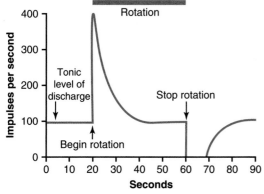

Figure 55-12 Response of a hair cell when a semicircular canal is stimulated first by the onset of head rotation and then by stopping rotation.

and reticular nuclei in the brain stem and indirectly by way of the cerebellum.

Among the most important proprioceptive information needed for the maintenance of equilibrium is that transmitted by *joint receptors of the neck.* When the head is leaned in one direction by bending the neck, impulses from the neck proprioceptors keep the signals originating in the vestibular apparatus from giving the person a sense of dysequilibrium. They do this by transmitting signals that exactly oppose the signals transmitted from the vestibular apparatus. However, *when the entire body* leans in one direction, the impulses from the vestibular apparatus *are not opposed* by signals from the neck proprioceptors; therefore, in this case, the person does perceive a change in equilibrium status of the entire body.

Proprioceptive and Exteroceptive Information from Other Parts of the Body. Proprioceptive information from parts of the body other than the neck is also important in the maintenance of equilibrium. For instance, pressure sensations from the footpads tell one (1) whether weight is distributed equally between the two feet and (2) whether weight on the feet is more forward or backward.

Exteroceptive information is especially necessary for the maintenance of equilibrium when a person is running. The air pressure against the front of the body signals that a force is opposing the body in a direction different from that caused by gravitational pull; as a result, the person leans forward to oppose this.

Importance of Visual Information in the Maintenance of Equilibrium. After destruction of the vestibular apparatus, and even after loss of most proprioceptive information from the body, a person can still use the visual mechanisms reasonably effectively for maintaining equilibrium. Even a slight linear or rotational movement of the body instantaneously shifts the visual images on the retina, and this information is relayed to the equilibrium centers. Some people with bilateral destruction of the vestibular apparatus have almost normal equilibrium as long as their eyes are open and all motions are performed slowly. But when moving rapidly or when the eyes are closed, equilibrium is immediately lost.

Neuronal Connections of the Vestibular Apparatus with the Central Nervous System

Figure 55-13 shows the connections in the hindbrain of the vestibular nerve. Most of the vestibular nerve fibers terminate in the brain stem in the *vestibular nuclei,* which are located approximately at the junction of the medulla and the pons. Some fibers pass directly to the brain stem reticular nuclei without synapsing and also to the cerebellar fastigial, uvular, and flocculonodular lobe nuclei. The fibers that end in the brain stem vestibular nuclei synapse with second-order neurons that also send fibers into the cerebellum, the vestibulospinal tracts, the medial longitudinal fasciculus, and other areas of the brain stem, particularly the reticular nuclei.

The primary pathway for the equilibrium reflexes begins in the vestibular nerves, where the nerves are excited by the vestibular apparatus. The pathway then passes to the vestibular nuclei and cerebellum. Next, signals are sent into the reticular nuclei of the brain stem, as well as down the spinal cord by way of the vestibulospinal and reticulospinal tracts. The signals to the cord control the interplay between facili-

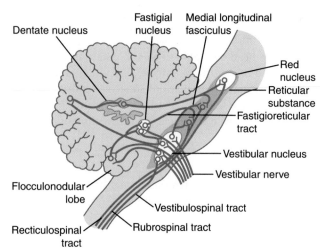

Figure 55-13 Connections of vestibular nerves through the vestibular nuclei (*large oval white area*) with other areas of the central nervous system.

tation and inhibition of the many antigravity muscles, thus automatically controlling equilibrium.

The *flocculonodular* lobes of the cerebellum are especially concerned with dynamic equilibrium signals from the semicircular ducts. In fact, destruction of these lobes results in almost exactly the same clinical symptoms as destruction of the semicircular ducts themselves. That is, severe injury to either the lobes or the ducts causes loss of dynamic equilibrium during *rapid changes in direction of motion* but does not seriously disturb equilibrium under static conditions. It is believed that the *uvula* of the cerebellum plays a similar important role in static equilibrium.

Signals transmitted upward in the brain stem from both the vestibular nuclei and the cerebellum by way of the *medial longitudinal fasciculus* cause corrective movements of the eyes every time the head rotates, so the eyes remain fixed on a specific visual object. Signals also pass upward (either through this same tract or through reticular tracts) to the cerebral cortex, terminating in a primary cortical center for equilibrium located in the parietal lobe deep in the sylvian fissure on the opposite side of the fissure from the auditory area of the superior temporal gyrus. These signals apprise the psyche of the equilibrium status of the body.

Functions of Brain Stem Nuclei in Controlling Subconscious, Stereotyped Movements

Rarely, a baby is born without brain structures above the mesencephalic region, a condition called *anencephaly.* Some of these babies have been kept alive for many months. They are able to perform some stereotyped movements for feeding, such as suckling, extrusion of unpleasant food from the mouth, and moving the hands to the mouth to suck the fingers. In addition, they can yawn and stretch. They can cry and can follow objects with movements of the eyes and head. Also, placing pressure on the upper anterior parts of their legs causes them to pull to the sitting position. It is clear that many of the stereotyped motor functions of the human being are integrated in the brain stem.

Bibliography

Angelaki DE, Cullen KE: Vestibular system: the many facets of a multimodal sense, *Annu Rev Neurosci* 31:125, 2008.

Baker SN: Oscillatory interactions between sensorimotor cortex and the periphery, *Curr Opin Neurobiol* 17:649, 2007.

Briggs F, Usrey WM: Emerging views of corticothalamic function, *Curr Opin Neurobiol* 18:403, 2008.

Cullen KE, Roy JE: Signal processing in the vestibular system during active versus passive head movements, *J Neurophysiol* 91:1919, 2004.

Fabbri-Destro M, Rizzolatti G: Mirror neurons and mirror systems in monkeys and humans, *Physiology (Bethesda)* 23:171, 2008.

Holtmaat A, Svoboda K: Experience-dependent structural synaptic plasticity in the mammalian brain, *Nat Rev Neurosci* 10:647, 2009.

Horak FB: Postural compensation for vestibular loss, *Ann N Y Acad Sci* 1164:76, 2009.

Klier EM, Angelaki DE: Spatial updating and the maintenance of visual constancy, *Neuroscience* 156:801, 2008.

Lemon RN: Descending pathways in motor control, *Annu Rev Neurosci* 31:195, 2008.

Müller U: Cadherins and mechanotransduction by hair cells, *Curr Opin Cell Biol* 5:557, 2008.

Nachev P, Kennard C, Husain M: Functional role of the supplementary and pre-supplementary motor areas, *Nat Rev Neurosci* 9:856, 2008.

Nishitani N, Schürmann M, Amunts K, et al: Broca's region: from action to language, *Physiology (Bethesda)* 20:60, 2005.

Nielsen JB, Cohen LG: The Olympic brain. Does corticospinal plasticity play a role in acquisition of skills required for high-performance sports? *J Physiol* 586:65, 2008.

Pierrot-Deseilligny C: Effect of gravity on vertical eye position, *Ann N Y Acad Sci* 1164:155, 2009.

Raineteau O: Plastic responses to spinal cord injury, *Behav Brain Res* 192:114, 2008.

Robles L, Ruggero MA: Mechanics of the mammalian cochlea, *Physiol Rev* 81:1305, 2001.

Schieber MH: Motor control: basic units of cortical output? *Curr Biol* 14:R353, 2004.

Scott SH: Inconvenient truths about neural processing in primary motor cortex, *J Physiol* 586:1217, 2008.

Scott SK, McGettigan C, Eisner F: A little more conversation, a little less action—candidate roles for the motor cortex in speech perception, *Nat Rev Neurosci* 10:295, 2009.

Stepien AE, Arber S: Probing the locomotor conundrum: descending the 'V' interneuron ladder, *Neuron* 60:1, 2008.

Umilta MA: Frontal cortex: goal-relatedness and the cortical motor system, *Curr Biol* 14:R204, 2004.

Contributions of the Cerebellum and Basal Ganglia to Overall Motor Control

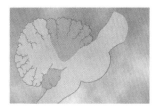

Aside from the areas in the cerebral cortex that stimulate muscle contraction, two other brain structures are also essential for normal motor function. They are the *cerebellum* and the *basal ganglia*. Yet neither of these two can control muscle function by themselves. Instead, *they always function in association with other systems of motor control.*

The cerebellum plays major roles in the timing of motor activities and in rapid, smooth progression from one muscle movement to the next. It also helps to control the intensity of muscle contraction when the muscle load changes and controls the necessary instantaneous interplay between agonist and antagonist muscle groups.

The basal ganglia help to plan and control complex patterns of muscle movement, controlling relative intensities of the separate movements, directions of movements, and sequencing of multiple successive and parallel movements for achieving specific complicated motor goals. This chapter explains the basic functions of the cerebellum and basal ganglia and discusses the overall brain mechanisms for achieving intricate coordination of total motor activity.

Cerebellum and Its Motor Functions

The cerebellum, illustrated in Figures 56-1 and 56-2, has long been called a *silent area* of the brain, principally because electrical excitation of the cerebellum does not cause any conscious sensation and rarely causes any motor movement. Removal of the cerebellum, however, causes body movements to become highly abnormal. The cerebellum is especially vital during rapid muscular activities such as running, typing, playing the piano, and even talking. Loss of this area of the brain can cause almost total incoordination of these activities even though its loss causes paralysis of no muscles.

But how is it that the cerebellum can be so important when it has no direct ability to cause muscle contrac-

tion? The answer is that it helps to *sequence the motor activities* and also *monitors and makes corrective adjustments in the body's motor activities while they are being executed so that they will conform to the motor signals directed by the cerebral motor cortex and other parts of the brain.*

The cerebellum receives continuously updated information about the desired sequence of muscle contractions from the brain motor control areas; it also receives continuous sensory information from the peripheral parts of the body, giving sequential changes in the status of each part of the body—its position, rate of movement, forces acting on it, and so forth. The cerebellum then *compares* the actual movements as depicted by the peripheral sensory feedback information with the movements intended by the motor system. If the two do not compare favorably, then instantaneous subconscious corrective signals are transmitted back into the motor system to increase or decrease the levels of activation of specific muscles.

The cerebellum also aids the cerebral cortex in planning the next sequential movement a fraction of a second in advance while the current movement is still being executed, thus helping the person to progress smoothly from one movement to the next. Also, it learns by its mistakes—that is, if a movement does not occur exactly as intended, the cerebellar circuit learns to make a stronger or weaker movement the next time. To do this, *changes occur in the excitability of appropriate cerebellar neurons, thus bringing subsequent muscle contractions into better correspondence with the intended movements.*

Anatomical Functional Areas of the Cerebellum
Anatomically, the cerebellum is divided into three lobes by two deep fissures, as shown in Figures 56-1 and 56-2: (1) the *anterior lobe,* (2) the *posterior lobe,* and (3) the *flocculonodular lobe.* The flocculonodular lobe is the oldest of all portions of the cerebellum; it developed along with (and functions with) the vestibular system in controlling body equilibrium, as discussed in Chapter 55.

Longitudinal Functional Divisions of the Anterior and Posterior Lobes. From a functional point of view, the anterior and posterior lobes are organized not by lobes but along

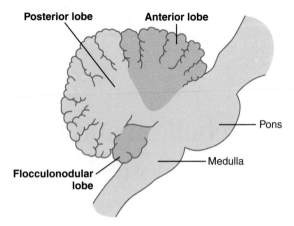

Figure 56-1 Anatomical lobes of the cerebellum as seen from the lateral side.

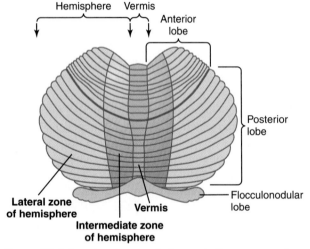

Figure 56-2 Functional parts of the cerebellum as seen from the posteroinferior view, with the inferiormost portion of the cerebellum rolled outward to flatten the surface.

the longitudinal axis, as demonstrated in Figure 56-2, which shows a posterior view of the human cerebellum after the lower end of the posterior cerebellum has been rolled downward from its normally hidden position. Note down the center of the cerebellum a narrow band called the *vermis*, separated from the remainder of the cerebellum by shallow grooves. In this area, most cerebellar control functions for muscle movements of the *axial body, neck, shoulders, and hips* are located.

To each side of the vermis is a large, laterally protruding *cerebellar hemisphere*, and each of these hemispheres is divided into an *intermediate zone* and a *lateral zone.*

The intermediate zone of the hemisphere is concerned with controlling muscle contractions in the distal portions of the upper and lower limbs, especially the hands and fingers and feet and toes.

The lateral zone of the hemisphere operates at a much more remote level because this area joins with the cerebral cortex in the overall planning of sequential motor movements. Without this lateral zone, most discrete motor activities of the body lose their appropriate timing and sequencing and therefore become incoordinate, as we discuss more fully later.

Topographical Representation of the Body in the Vermis and Intermediate Zones. In the same manner that the cerebral sensory cortex, motor cortex, basal ganglia, red nuclei, and reticular formation all have topographical representations of the different parts of the body, so also is this true for the vermis and intermediate zones of the cerebellum. Figure 56-3 shows two such representations. Note that the axial portions of the body lie in the vermis part of the cerebellum, whereas the limbs and facial regions lie in the intermediate zones. These topographical representations receive afferent nerve signals from all the respective parts of the body, as well as from corresponding topographical motor areas in the cerebral cortex and brain stem. In turn, they send motor signals back to the same respective topographical areas of the cerebral motor cortex, as well as to topographical areas of the red nucleus and reticular formation in the brain stem.

Note that the large lateral portions of the cerebellar hemispheres *do not* have topographical representations of the body. These areas of the cerebellum receive their input signals almost exclusively from the cerebral cortex, especially from the premotor areas of the frontal cortex and from the somatosensory and other sensory association areas of the parietal cortex. It is believed that this connectivity with the cerebral cortex allows the lateral portions of the cerebellar hemispheres to play important roles in planning and coordinating the body's *rapid* sequential muscular activities that occur one after another within fractions of a second.

Neuronal Circuit of the Cerebellum

The human cerebellar cortex is actually a large folded sheet, about 17 centimeters wide by 120 centimeters long, with the folds lying crosswise, as shown in Figures 56-2 and 56-3. Each fold is called a *folium.* Lying deep beneath the folded mass of cerebellar cortex are *deep cerebellar nuclei.*

Input Pathways to the Cerebellum

Afferent Pathways from Other Parts of the Brain. The basic input pathways to the cerebellum are shown in Figure 56-4. An extensive and important afferent pathway is the *corticopontocerebellar pathway,* which originates in the *cerebral motor* and *premotor cortices* and also in the *cerebral somatosensory cortex.* It passes by way of the *pontile nuclei* and *pontocerebellar tracts* mainly to the lateral divisions of the cerebellar hemispheres on the opposite side of the brain from the cerebral areas.

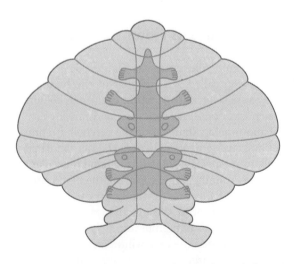

Figure 56-3 Somatosensory projection areas in the cerebellar cortex.

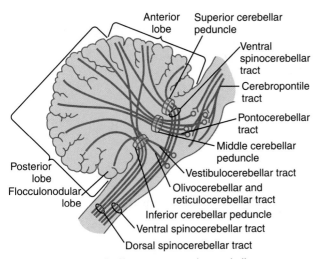

Figure 56-4 Principal *afferent* tracts to the cerebellum.

In addition, important afferent tracts originate in each side of the brain stem; they include (1) an extensive *olivocerebellar tract,* which passes from the *inferior olive* to all parts of the cerebellum and is excited in the olive by fibers from the *cerebral motor cortex, basal ganglia,* widespread areas of the *reticular formation,* and *spinal cord;* (2) *vestibulocerebellar fibers,* some of which originate in the vestibular apparatus itself and others from the brain stem vestibular nuclei—almost all of these terminate in the *flocculonodular lobe* and *fastigial nucleus* of the cerebellum; and (3) *reticulocerebellar fibers,* which originate in different portions of the brain stem reticular formation and terminate in the midline cerebellar areas (mainly in the vermis).

Afferent Pathways from the Periphery. The cerebellum also receives important sensory signals directly from the peripheral parts of the body mainly through four tracts on each side, two of which are located dorsally in the cord and two ventrally. The two most important of these tracts are shown in Figure 56-5: the *dorsal spinocerebellar tract* and

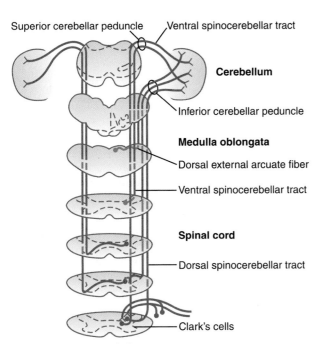

Figure 56-5 Spinocerebellar tracts.

the *ventral spinocerebellar tract.* The dorsal tract enters the cerebellum through the inferior cerebellar peduncle and terminates in the vermis and intermediate zones of the cerebellum on the same side as its origin. The ventral tract enters the cerebellum through the superior cerebellar peduncle, but it terminates in both sides of the cerebellum.

The signals transmitted in the dorsal spinocerebellar tracts come mainly from the muscle spindles and to a lesser extent from other somatic receptors throughout the body, such as Golgi tendon organs, large tactile receptors of the skin, and joint receptors. All these signals apprise the cerebellum of the momentary status of (1) muscle contraction, (2) degree of tension on the muscle tendons, (3) positions and rates of movement of the parts of the body, and (4) forces acting on the surfaces of the body.

The ventral spinocerebellar tracts receive much less information from the peripheral receptors. Instead, they are excited mainly by motor signals arriving in the anterior horns of the spinal cord from (1) the brain through the corticospinal and rubrospinal tracts and (2) the internal motor pattern generators in the cord itself. Thus, this ventral fiber pathway tells the cerebellum which motor signals have arrived at the anterior horns; this feedback is called the *efference copy* of the anterior horn motor drive.

The spinocerebellar pathways can transmit impulses at velocities up to 120 m/sec, which is the most rapid conduction in any pathway in the central nervous system. This extremely rapid conduction is important for instantaneous apprisal of the cerebellum of changes in peripheral muscle actions.

In addition to signals from the spinocerebellar tracts, signals are transmitted into the cerebellum from the body periphery through the spinal dorsal columns to the dorsal column nuclei of the medulla and then relayed to the cerebellum. Likewise, signals are transmitted up the spinal cord through the *spinoreticular pathway* to the reticular formation of the brain stem and also through the *spino-olivary pathway* to the inferior olivary nucleus. Then signals are relayed from both of these areas to the cerebellum. Thus, the cerebellum continually collects information about the movements and positions of all parts of the body even though it is operating at a subconscious level.

Output Signals from the Cerebellum

Deep Cerebellar Nuclei and the Efferent Pathways. Located deep in the cerebellar mass on each side are three *deep cerebellar nuclei*—the *dentate, interposed,* and *fastigial.* (The *vestibular nuclei* in the medulla also function in some respects as if they were deep cerebellar nuclei because of their direct connections with the cortex of the flocculonodular lobe.) All the deep cerebellar nuclei receive signals from two sources: (1) the cerebellar cortex and (2) the deep sensory afferent tracts to the cerebellum.

Each time an input signal arrives in the cerebellum, it divides and goes in two directions: (1) directly to one of the cerebellar deep nuclei and (2) to a corresponding area of the cerebellar cortex overlying the deep nucleus. Then, a fraction of a second later, the cerebellar cortex relays an *inhibitory* output signal to the deep nucleus. Thus, all input signals that enter the cerebellum eventually end in the deep nuclei in the form of initial excitatory signals followed a fraction of a second later by inhibitory signals. From the deep nuclei, output signals leave the cerebellum and are distributed to other parts of the brain.

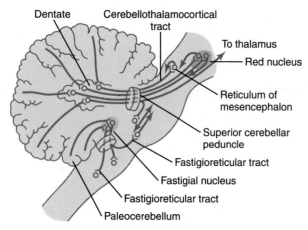

Figure 56-6 Principal *efferent* tracts from the cerebellum.

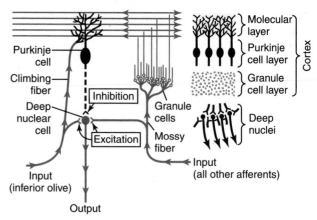

Figure 56-7 The left side of this figure shows the basic neuronal circuit of the cerebellum, with excitatory neurons shown in *red* and the Purkinje cell (an inhibitory neuron) shown in *black*. To the right is shown the physical relationship of the deep cerebellar nuclei to the cerebellar cortex with its three layers.

The general plan of the major efferent pathways leading out of the cerebellum is shown in Figure 56-6 and consists of the following:

1. A pathway that originates in the *midline structures of the cerebellum* (the *vermis*) and then passes through the *fastigial nuclei* into the *medullary* and *pontile regions of the brain stem.* This circuit functions in close association with the equilibrium apparatus and brain stem vestibular nuclei to control equilibrium, as well as in association with the reticular formation of the brain stem to control the postural attitudes of the body. It was discussed in detail in Chapter 55 in relation to equilibrium.

2. A pathway that originates in (1) the intermediate zone of the cerebellar hemisphere and then passes through (2) the interposed nucleus to (3) the ventrolateral and ventroanterior nuclei of the thalamus and then to (4) the cerebral cortex, to (5) several midline structures of the thalamus and then to (6) the basal ganglia and (7) the red nucleus and reticular formation of the upper portion of the brain stem. This complex circuit helps to coordinate mainly the reciprocal contractions of agonist and antagonist muscles in the peripheral portions of the limbs, especially in the hands, fingers, and thumbs.

3. A pathway that begins in the cerebellar cortex of the lateral zone of the cerebellar hemisphere and then passes to the dentate nucleus, next to the ventrolateral and ventroanterior nuclei of the thalamus, and, finally, to the cerebral cortex. This pathway plays an important role in helping coordinate sequential motor activities initiated by the cerebral cortex.

Functional Unit of the Cerebellar Cortex— the Purkinje Cell and the Deep Nuclear Cell

The cerebellum has about 30 million nearly identical functional units, one of which is shown to the left in Figure 56-7. This functional unit centers on a single, very large *Purkinje cell* and on a corresponding *deep nuclear cell.*

To the top and right in Figure 56-7, the three major layers of the cerebellar cortex are shown: the *molecular layer, Purkinje cell layer,* and *granule cell layer.* Beneath these cortical layers, in the center of the cerebellar mass, are the deep cerebellar nuclei that send output signals to other parts of the nervous system.

Neuronal Circuit of the Functional Unit. Also shown in the left half of Figure 56-7 is the neuronal circuit of the functional unit, which is repeated with little variation 30 million times in the cerebellum. The output from the functional unit is from a *deep nuclear cell.* This cell is continually under both excitatory and inhibitory influences. The excitatory influences arise from direct connections with afferent fibers that enter the cerebellum from the brain or the periphery. The inhibitory influence arises entirely from the Purkinje cell in the cortex of the cerebellum.

The afferent inputs to the cerebellum are mainly of two types, one called the *climbing fiber type* and the other called the *mossy fiber type.*

The climbing fibers *all originate from the inferior olives of the medulla.* There is one climbing fiber for about 5 to 10 Purkinje cells. After sending branches to several deep nuclear cells, the climbing fiber continues all the way to the outer layers of the cerebellar cortex, where it makes about 300 synapses with the soma and dendrites of each Purkinje cell. This climbing fiber is distinguished by the fact that a single impulse in it will always cause a single, prolonged (up to 1 second), peculiar type of action potential in each Purkinje cell with which it connects, beginning with a strong spike and followed by a trail of weakening secondary spikes. This action potential is called the *complex spike.*

The mossy fibers are all the other fibers that enter the cerebellum from multiple sources: from the higher brain, brain stem, and spinal cord. These fibers also send collaterals to excite the deep nuclear cells. Then they proceed to the granule cell layer of the cortex, where they, too, synapse with hundreds to thousands of *granule cells.* In turn, the granule cells send extremely small axons, less than 1 micrometer in diameter, up to the molecular layer on the outer surface of the cerebellar cortex. Here the axons divide into two branches that extend 1 to 2 millimeters in each direction parallel to the folia. There are many millions of these *parallel nerve fibers* because there are some 500 to 1000 granule cells for every 1 Purkinje cell. It is into this molecular layer that the dendrites of the Purkinje cells project and 80,000 to 200,000 of the parallel fibers synapse with each Purkinje cell.

The mossy fiber input to the Purkinje cell is quite different from the climbing fiber input because the synaptic connections are weak, so large numbers of mossy fibers must be stimulated simultaneously to excite the Purkinje cell. Furthermore, activation usually takes the form of a much weaker short-duration Purkinje cell action potential called a *simple spike*, rather than the prolonged complex action potential caused by climbing fiber input.

Purkinje Cells and Deep Nuclear Cells Fire Continuously Under Normal Resting Conditions. One characteristic of both Purkinje cells and deep nuclear cells is that normally both of them fire continuously; the Purkinje cell fires at about 50 to 100 action potentials per second, and the deep nuclear cells at much higher rates. Furthermore, the output activity of both these cells can be modulated upward or downward.

Balance Between Excitation and Inhibition at the Deep Cerebellar Nuclei. Referring again to the circuit of Figure 56-7, note that direct stimulation of the deep nuclear cells by both the climbing and the mossy fibers excites them. By contrast, signals arriving from the Purkinje cells inhibit them. Normally, the balance between these two effects is slightly in favor of excitation so that under quiet conditions, output from the deep nuclear cell remains relatively constant at a moderate level of continuous stimulation.

In execution of a rapid motor movement, the initiating signal from the cerebral motor cortex or brain stem at first greatly increases deep nuclear cell excitation. Then, another few milliseconds later, feedback inhibitory signals from the Purkinje cell circuit arrive. In this way, there is first a rapid excitatory signal sent by the deep nuclear cells into the motor output pathway to enhance the motor movement, but this is followed within another small fraction of a second by an inhibitory signal. This inhibitory signal resembles a "delay-line" negative feedback signal of the type that is effective in providing *damping*. That is, when the motor system is excited, a negative feedback signal occurs after a short delay to stop the muscle movement from overshooting its mark. Otherwise, oscillation of the movement would occur.

Other Inhibitory Cells in the Cerebellum. In addition to the deep nuclear cells, granule cells, and Purkinje cells, two other types of neurons are located in the cerebellum: *basket cells* and *stellate cells*. These are inhibitory cells with short axons. Both the basket cells and the stellate cells are located in the molecular layer of the cerebellar cortex, lying among and stimulated by the small parallel fibers. These cells in turn send their axons at right angles across the parallel fibers and cause *lateral inhibition* of adjacent Purkinje cells, thus sharpening the signal in the same manner that lateral inhibition sharpens contrast of signals in many other neuronal circuits of the nervous system.

Turn-On/Turn-Off and Turn-Off/Turn-On Output Signals from the Cerebellum

The typical function of the cerebellum is to help provide rapid turn-on signals for the agonist muscles and simultaneous reciprocal turn-off signals for the antagonist muscles at the onset of a movement. Then on approaching termination of the movement, the cerebellum is mainly responsible for timing and executing the turn-off signals to the agonists and turn-on signals to the antagonists. Although the exact details are not fully known, one can speculate from the basic cerebellar circuit of Figure 56-7 how this might work, as follows.

Let us suppose that the turn-on/turn-off pattern of agonist/antagonist contraction at the onset of movement begins with signals from the cerebral cortex. These signals pass through noncerebellar brain stem and cord pathways directly to the agonist muscle to begin the initial contraction.

At the same time, parallel signals are sent by way of the pontile mossy fibers into the cerebellum. One branch of each mossy fiber goes directly to deep nuclear cells in the dentate or other deep cerebellar nuclei; this instantly sends an excitatory signal back into the cerebral corticospinal motor system, either by way of return signals through the thalamus to the cerebral cortex or by way of neuronal circuitry in the brain stem, to support the muscle contraction signal that had already been begun by the cerebral cortex. As a consequence, the turn-on signal, after a few milliseconds, becomes even more powerful than it was at the start because it becomes the sum of both the cortical and the cerebellar signals. This is the normal effect when the cerebellum is intact, but in the absence of the cerebellum, the secondary extra supportive signal is missing. This cerebellar support makes the turn-on muscle contraction much stronger than it would be if the cerebellum did not exist.

Now, what causes the turn-off signal for the agonist muscles at the termination of the movement? Remember that all mossy fibers have a second branch that transmits signals by way of the granule cells to the cerebellar cortex and eventually, by way of "parallel" fibers, to the Purkinje cells. The Purkinje cells in turn *inhibit* the deep nuclear cells. This pathway passes through some of the smallest, slowest-conducting nerve fibers in the nervous system: that is, the parallel fibers of the cerebellar cortical molecular layer, which have diameters of only a fraction of a millimeter. Also, the signals from these fibers are weak, so they require a finite period of time to build up enough excitation in the dendrites of the Purkinje cell to excite it. But once the Purkinje cell is excited, it in turn sends a strong *inhibitory signal* to the same deep nuclear cell that had originally turned on the movement. Therefore, this helps *to turn off* the movement after a short time.

Thus, one can see how the complete cerebellar circuit could cause a rapid turn-on agonist muscle contraction at the beginning of a movement and yet cause also a *precisely timed* turn-off of the same agonist contraction after a given time period.

Now let us speculate on the circuit for the antagonist muscles. Most important, remember that throughout the spinal cord there are reciprocal agonist/antagonist circuits for virtually every movement that the cord can initiate. Therefore, these circuits are part of the basis for antagonist turn-off at the onset of movement and then turn-on at termination of movement, mirroring whatever occurs in the agonist muscles. But we must remember, too, that the cerebellum contains several other types of inhibitory cells besides Purkinje cells. The functions of some of these are still to be determined; they, too, could play roles in the initial inhibition of the antagonist muscles at onset of a movement and subsequent excitation at the end of a movement.

All these mechanisms are still partly speculation. They are presented here especially to illustrate ways by which the cerebellum could cause exaggerated turn-on and turn-off signals, controlling the agonist and antagonist muscles, as well as the timing.

The Purkinje Cells "Learn" to Correct Motor Errors— Role of the Climbing Fibers

The degree to which the cerebellum supports onset and offset of muscle contractions, as well as timing of contractions, must be learned by the cerebellum. Typically, when a person first performs a new motor act, the degree of motor enhancement by the cerebellum at the onset of contraction, the degree or inhibition at the end of contraction, and the timing of these are almost always incorrect for precise performance of the movement. But after the act has been performed many times, the individual events become progressively more precise, sometimes requiring only a few movements before the desired result is achieved, but at other times requiring hundreds of movements.

How do these adjustments come about? The exact answer is not known, although it is known that sensitivity levels of cerebellar circuits themselves progressively adapt during the training process, especially the sensitivity of the Purkinje cells to respond to the granule cell excitation. Furthermore, this sensitivity change is brought about by signals from the climbing fibers entering the cerebellum from the inferior olivary complex.

Under resting conditions, the climbing fibers fire about once per second. But they cause extreme depolarization of the entire dendritic tree of the Purkinje cell, lasting for up to a second, each time they fire. During this time, the Purkinje cell fires with one initial strong output spike followed by a series of diminishing spikes. When a person performs a new movement for the first time, feedback signals from the muscle and joint proprioceptors will usually denote to the cerebellum how much the actual movement fails to match the intended movement. And the climbing fiber signals in some way alter long-term sensitivity of the Purkinje cells. Over a period of time, this change in sensitivity, along with other possible "learning" functions of the cerebellum, is believed to make the timing and other aspects of cerebellar control of movements

approach perfection. When this has been achieved, the climbing fibers no longer need to send "error" signals to the cerebellum to cause further change.

Function of the Cerebellum in Overall Motor Control

The nervous system uses the cerebellum to coordinate motor control functions at three levels, as follows:

1. The *vestibulocerebellum.* This consists principally of the small flocculonodular cerebellar lobes that lie under the posterior cerebellum and adjacent portions of the vermis. It provides neural circuits for most of the body's equilibrium movements.

2. The *spinocerebellum.* This consists of most of the vermis of the posterior and anterior cerebellum plus the adjacent intermediate zones on both sides of the vermis. It provides the circuitry for coordinating mainly movements of the distal portions of the limbs, especially the hands and fingers.

3. The *cerebrocerebellum.* This consists of the large lateral zones of the cerebellar hemispheres, lateral to the intermediate zones. It receives virtually all its input from the cerebral motor cortex and adjacent premotor and somatosensory cortices of the cerebrum. It transmits its output information in the upward direction back to the brain, functioning in a feedback manner with the cerebral cortical sensorimotor system to plan sequential voluntary body and limb movements, planning these as much as tenths of a second in advance of the actual movements. This is called development of "motor imagery" of movements to be performed.

Vestibulocerebellum Functions in Association with the Brain Stem and Spinal Cord to Control Equilibrium and Postural Movements

The vestibulocerebellum originated phylogenetically at about the same time that the vestibular apparatus in the inner ear developed. Furthermore, as discussed in Chapter 55, loss of the flocculonodular lobes and adjacent portions of the vermis of the cerebellum, which constitute the vestibulocerebellum, causes extreme disturbance of equilibrium and postural movements.

We still must ask the question, what role does the vestibulocerebellum play in equilibrium that cannot be provided by other neuronal machinery of the brain stem? A clue is the fact that in people with vestibulocerebellar dysfunction, equilibrium is far more disturbed *during performance of rapid motions* than during stasis, especially when these movements involve *changes in direction* of movement and stimulate the semicircular ducts. This suggests that the vestibulocerebellum is important in controlling balance between agonist and antagonist muscle contractions of the spine, hips, and shoulders during *rapid changes* in body positions as required by the vestibular apparatus.

One of the major problems in controlling balance is the amount of time required to transmit position signals and velocity of movement signals from the different parts of the body to the brain. Even when the most rapidly conducting sensory pathways are used, up to 120 m/sec in the spinocerebellar afferent tracts, the delay for transmission from the feet to the brain is still 15 to 20 milliseconds. The feet of a person running rapidly can move as much as 10 inches during that time. Therefore, it is never possible for return signals from the peripheral parts of the body to reach the brain at the same time that the movements actually occur. How, then, is it possible for the brain to know when to stop a movement and to perform the next sequential act when the movements are performed rapidly? The answer is that the signals from the periphery tell the brain how rapidly and in which directions the body parts are moving. It is then the function of the vestibulocerebellum to *calculate in advance* from these rates and directions where the different parts will be during the next few milliseconds. The results of these calculations are the key to the brain's progression to the next sequential movement.

Thus, during control of equilibrium, it is presumed that information from both the body periphery and the vestibular apparatus is used in a typical feedback control circuit to provide *anticipatory correction* of postural motor signals necessary for maintaining equilibrium even during extremely rapid motion, including rapidly changing directions of motion.

Spinocerebellum—Feedback Control of Distal Limb Movements by Way of the Intermediate Cerebellar Cortex and the Interposed Nucleus

As shown in Figure 56-8, the intermediate zone of each cerebellar hemisphere receives two types of information when a movement is performed: (1) information from the cerebral motor cortex and from the midbrain red nucleus, telling the cerebellum the *intended sequential plan of movement* for the next few fractions of a second, and (2) feedback information from the peripheral parts of the body, especially from the distal proprioceptors of the limbs, telling the cerebellum what *actual movements* result.

After the intermediate zone of the cerebellum has compared the intended movements with the actual movements, the deep nuclear cells of the interposed nucleus send *corrective* output signals (1) back to the *cerebral motor cortex* through relay nuclei in the *thalamus* and (2) to the *magnocellular portion* (the lower portion) *of the red nucleus* that gives rise to the *rubrospinal tract.* The rubrospinal tract in turn joins the corticospinal tract in innervating the lateral most motor neurons in the anterior horns of the spinal cord gray matter, the neurons that control the distal parts of the limbs, particularly the hands and fingers.

This part of the cerebellar motor control system provides smooth, coordinate movements of the agonist and antagonist muscles of the distal limbs for performing

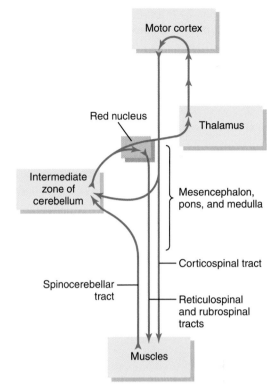

Figure 56-8 Cerebral and cerebellar control of voluntary movements, involving especially the intermediate zone of the cerebellum.

acute purposeful patterned movements. The cerebellum seems to compare the "intentions" of the higher levels of the motor control system, as transmitted to the intermediate cerebellar zone through the corticopontocerebellar tract, with the "performance" by the respective parts of the body, as transmitted back to the cerebellum from the periphery. In fact, the ventral spinocerebellar tract even transmits back to the cerebellum an "efference" copy of the actual motor control signals that reach the anterior motor neurons, and this is also integrated with the signals arriving from the muscle spindles and other proprioceptor sensory organs, transmitted principally in the dorsal spinocerebellar tract. Similar comparator signals also go to the inferior olivary complex; if the signals do not compare favorably, the olivary-Purkinje cell system along with possibly other cerebellar learning mechanisms eventually corrects the motions until they perform the desired function.

Function of the Cerebellum to Prevent Overshoot of Movements and to "Damp" Movements. Almost all movements of the body are "pendular." For instance, when an arm is moved, momentum develops, and the momentum must be overcome before the movement can be stopped. Because of momentum, all pendular movements have a tendency to *overshoot.* If overshooting does occur in a person whose cerebellum has been destroyed, the conscious centers of the cerebrum eventually recognize this and initiate a movement in the reverse direction attempting to bring the arm to its intended position. But the arm, by virtue of its momentum, overshoots once more in the opposite direction, and appropriate corrective signals must again be instituted. Thus, the arm oscillates back and forth past its intended point for several cycles before it finally fixes on its mark. This effect is called an *action tremor,* or *intention tremor.*

But, if the cerebellum is intact, appropriate learned, subconscious signals stop the movement precisely at the intended point, thereby preventing the overshoot and the tremor. *This is the basic characteristic of a damping system.* All control systems regulating pendular elements that have inertia must have damping circuits built into the mechanisms. For motor control by the nervous system, the cerebellum provides most of this damping function.

Cerebellar Control of Ballistic Movements. Most rapid movements of the body, such as the movements of the fingers in typing, occur so rapidly that it is not possible to receive feedback information either from the periphery to the cerebellum or from the cerebellum back to the motor cortex before the movements are over. These movements are called *ballistic movements,* meaning that the entire movement is preplanned and set into motion to go a specific distance and then to stop. Another important example is the saccadic movements of the eyes, in which the eyes jump from one position to the next when reading or when looking at successive points along a road as a person is moving in a car.

Much can be understood about the function of the cerebellum by studying the changes that occur in these ballistic movements when the cerebellum is removed. Three major changes occur: (1) The movements are slow to develop and do not have the extra onset surge that the cerebellum usually provides, (2) the force developed is weak, and (3) the movements are slow to turn off, usually allowing the movement to go well beyond the intended mark. Therefore, in the absence of the cerebellar circuit, the motor cortex has to think extra hard to turn ballistic movements on and again has to think hard and take extra time to turn the movement off. Thus, the automatism of ballistic movements is lost.

Considering once again the circuitry of the cerebellum, one sees that it is beautifully organized to perform this biphasic, first excitatory and then delayed inhibitory function that is required for preplanned rapid ballistic movements. One also sees that the built-in timing circuits of the cerebellar cortex are fundamental to this particular ability of the cerebellum.

Cerebrocerebellum—Function of the Large Lateral Zone of the Cerebellar Hemisphere to Plan, Sequence, and Time Complex Movements

In human beings, the lateral zones of the two cerebellar hemispheres are highly developed and greatly enlarged. This goes along with human abilities to plan and perform intricate sequential patterns of movement, especially with the hands and fingers, and to speak. Yet the large lateral zones of the cerebellar hemispheres have no direct input of information from the peripheral parts of the body. Also, almost all communication between these lateral cerebellar areas and the cerebral cortex is not with the primary cerebral motor cortex itself but instead with the *premotor area* and *primary* and *association somatosensory areas.*

Even so, destruction of the lateral zones of the cerebellar hemispheres along with their deep nuclei, the dentate nuclei, can lead to extreme incoordination of complex purposeful movements of the hands, fingers, and feet and of the speech apparatus. This has been difficult to understand because of lack of direct communication between this part of the cerebellum and the primary motor cortex. However, experimental studies suggest that these portions of the cerebellum are concerned with two other important but indirect aspects of motor control: (1) the planning of sequential movements and (2) the "timing" of the sequential movements.

Planning of Sequential Movements. The planning of sequential movements requires that the lateral zones of the hemispheres communicate with both the premotor and the sensory portions of the cerebral cortex, and it requires two-way communication between these cerebral cortex areas with corresponding areas of the basal ganglia. It seems that the "plan" of sequential movements actually begins in the sensory and premotor areas of the cerebral cortex, and from there the plan is transmitted to the lateral zones of the cerebellar hemispheres. Then, amid much two-way traffic between cerebellum and cerebral cortex, appropriate motor signals provide transition from one sequence of movements to the next.

An interesting observation that supports this view is that many neurons in the cerebellar dentate nuclei display the activity pattern for the sequential movement that is yet to come while the present movement is still occurring. Thus, the lateral cerebellar zones appear to be involved not with what movement is happening at a given moment but with *what will be happening during the next sequential movement* a fraction of a second or perhaps even seconds later.

To summarize, one of the most important features of normal motor function is one's ability to progress smoothly from one movement to the next in orderly succession. In the absence of the large lateral zones of the cerebellar hemispheres, this capability is seriously disturbed for rapid movements.

Timing Function. Another important function of the lateral zones of the cerebellar hemispheres is to provide appropriate timing for each succeeding movement. In the absence of these cerebellar zones, one loses the subconscious ability to predict how far the different parts of the body will move in a given time. Without this timing capability, the person becomes unable to determine when the next sequential movement needs to begin. As a result, the succeeding movement may begin too early or, more likely, too late. Therefore, lesions in the lateral zones of the cerebellum cause complex movements (such as those required for writing, running, or even talking) to become incoordinate and lacking ability to progress in orderly sequence from one movement to the next. Such cerebellar lesions are said to cause *failure of smooth progression of movements.*

Extramotor Predictive Functions of the Cerebrocerebellum. The cerebrocerebellum (the large lateral lobes) also helps to "time" events other than movements of the body. For instance, the rates of progression of both auditory and visual phenomena can be predicted by the brain, but both of these require cerebellar participation. As an example, a person can predict from the changing visual scene how rapidly he or she is approaching an object. A striking experiment that demonstrates the importance of the cerebellum in this ability is the effects of removing the large lateral portions of the cerebellum in monkeys. Such a monkey occasionally charges the wall of a corridor and literally bashes its brains because it is unable to predict when it will reach the wall.

We are only now beginning to learn about these extramotor predictive functions of the cerebellum. It is quite possible that the cerebellum provides a "time-base," perhaps using time-delay circuits, against which signals from other parts of the central nervous system can be compared; it is often stated that the cerebellum is particularly helpful in interpreting *rapidly changing spatiotemporal relations* in sensory information.

Clinical Abnormalities of the Cerebellum

Destruction of small portions of the lateral cerebellar *cortex* seldom causes detectable abnormalities in motor function. In fact, several months after as much as one half of the lateral cerebellar cortex on one side of the brain has been removed, if the deep cerebellar nuclei are not removed along with the cortex, the motor functions of the animal appear to be almost normal *as long as the animal performs all movements slowly.* Thus, the remaining portions of the motor control system are capable of compensating tremendously for loss of parts of the cerebellum.

To cause serious and continuing dysfunction of the cerebellum, the cerebellar lesion usually must involve one or more of the deep cerebellar nuclei—the *dentate, interposed,* or *fastigial nuclei.*

Dysmetria and Ataxia. Two of the most important symptoms of cerebellar disease are *dysmetria* and *ataxia.* In the absence of the cerebellum, the subconscious motor control system cannot predict how far movements will go. Therefore, the movements ordinarily overshoot their intended mark; then the conscious portion of the brain overcompensates in the opposite direction for the succeeding compensatory movement. This effect is called *dysmetria,* and it results in uncoordinated movements that are called *ataxia.* Dysmetria and ataxia can also result from *lesions in the spinocerebellar tracts* because feedback information from the moving parts of the body to the cerebellum is essential for cerebellar timing of movement termination.

Past Pointing. *Past pointing* means that in the absence of the cerebellum, a person ordinarily moves the hand or some other moving part of the body considerably beyond the point of intention. This results from the fact that normally the cerebellum initiates most of the motor signal that turns off a movement after it is begun; if the cerebellum is not available to do this, the movement ordinarily goes beyond the intended mark. Therefore, past pointing is actually a manifestation of dysmetria.

Failure of Progression

Dysdiadochokinesia—Inability to Perform Rapid Alternating Movements. When the motor control system fails to predict where the different parts of the body will be at a given time, it "loses" perception of the parts during rapid motor movements. As a result, the succeeding movement may begin much too early or much too late, so no orderly "progression of movement" can occur. One can demonstrate this readily by having a patient with cerebellar damage turn one hand upward and downward at a rapid rate. The patient rapidly "loses" all perception of the instantaneous position of the hand during any portion of the movement. As a result, a series of stalled attempted but jumbled movements occurs instead of the normal coordinate upward and downward motions. This is called *dysdiadochokinesia.*

Dysarthria—Failure of Progression in Talking. Another example in which failure of progression occurs is in talking because the formation of words depends on rapid and orderly succession of individual muscle movements in the larynx, mouth, and respiratory system. Lack of coordination among these and inability to adjust in advance either the intensity of sound or duration of each successive sound causes jumbled vocalization, with some syllables loud, some weak, some held for long intervals, some held for short intervals, and resultant speech that is often unintelligible. This is called *dysarthria.*

Intention Tremor. When a person who has lost the cerebellum performs a voluntary act, the movements tend to oscillate, especially when they approach the intended mark, first overshooting the mark and then vibrating back and forth several times before settling on the mark. This reaction is called an *intention tremor* or an *action tremor,* and it results from cerebellar overshooting and failure of the cerebellar system to "damp" the motor movements.

Cerebellar Nystagmus—Tremor of the Eyeballs. *Cerebellar nystagmus* is tremor of the eyeballs that occurs usually when one attempts to fixate the eyes on a scene to one side of the head. This off-center type of fixation results in rapid, tremulous movements of the eyes rather than steady fixation, and it is another manifestation of failure of damping by the cerebellum. It occurs especially when the flocculonodular lobes of the cerebellum are damaged; in this instance it is also associated with loss of equilibrium because of dysfunction of the pathways through the flocculonodular cerebellum from the semicircular ducts.

Hypotonia—Decreased Tone of the Musculature. Loss of the deep cerebellar nuclei, particularly of the dentate and interposed nuclei, causes decreased tone of the peripheral body musculature on the side of the cerebellar lesion. The hypotonia results from loss of cerebellar facilitation of the motor cortex and brain stem motor nuclei by tonic signals from the deep cerebellar nuclei.

Basal Ganglia—Their Motor Functions

The basal ganglia, like the cerebellum, constitute another *accessory motor system* that functions usually not by itself but in close association with the cerebral cortex and corticospinal motor control system. In fact, the basal ganglia receive most of their input signals from the cerebral cortex itself and also return almost all their output signals back to the cortex.

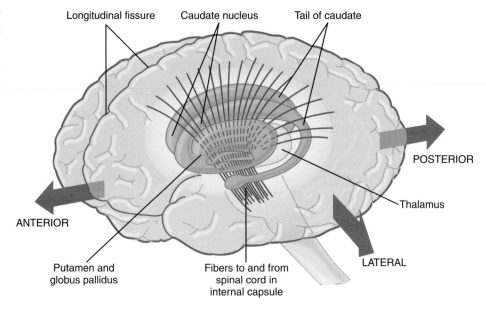

Figure 56-9 Anatomical relations of the basal ganglia to the cerebral cortex and thalamus, shown in three-dimensional view. (Redrawn from Guyton AC: Basic Neuroscience: Anatomy and Physiology. Philadelphia: WB Saunders, 1992.)

Longitudinal fissure   Caudate nucleus   Tail of caudate

POSTERIOR

Thalamus

ANTERIOR

Putamen and globus pallidus

Fibers to and from spinal cord in internal capsule

LATERAL

Figure 56-9 shows the anatomical relations of the basal ganglia to other structures of the brain. On each side of the brain, these ganglia consist of the *caudate nucleus, putamen, globus pallidus, substantia nigra,* and *subthalamic nucleus.* They are located mainly lateral to and surrounding the thalamus, occupying a large portion of the interior regions of both cerebral hemispheres. Note also that almost all motor and sensory nerve fibers connecting the cerebral cortex and spinal cord pass through the space that lies between the major masses of the basal ganglia, the *caudate nucleus* and the *putamen.* This space is called the *internal capsule* of the brain. It is important for our current discussion because of the intimate association between the basal ganglia and the corticospinal system for motor control.

Neuronal Circuitry of the Basal Ganglia. The anatomical connections between the basal ganglia and the other brain elements that provide motor control are complex, as shown in Figure 56-10. To the left is shown the motor cortex, thalamus, and associated brain stem and cerebellar circuitry. To the right is the major circuitry of the basal ganglia system, showing the tremendous interconnections among the basal ganglia themselves plus extensive input and output pathways between the other motor regions of the brain and the basal ganglia.

In the next few sections we concentrate especially on two major circuits, the *putamen circuit* and the *caudate circuit.*

Function of the Basal Ganglia in Executing Patterns of Motor Activity—the Putamen Circuit

One of the principal roles of the basal ganglia in motor control is to function in association with the corticospinal system to control *complex patterns of motor activity.* An example is the writing of letters of the alphabet. When there is serious damage to the basal ganglia, the cortical system of motor control can no longer provide these patterns. Instead, one's writing becomes crude, as if one were learning for the first time how to write.

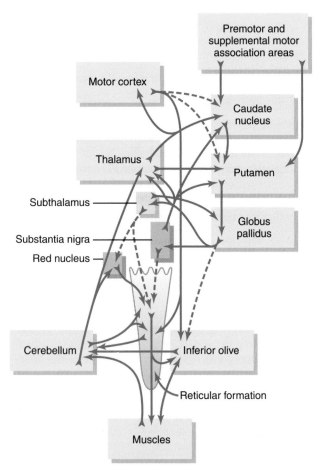

Figure 56-10 Relation of the basal ganglial circuitry to the corticospinal-cerebellar system for movement control.

Other patterns that require the basal ganglia are cutting paper with scissors, hammering nails, shooting a basketball through a hoop, passing a football, throwing a baseball, the movements of shoveling dirt, most aspects of vocalization, controlled movements of the eyes, and virtually any other of our skilled movements, most of them performed subconsciously.

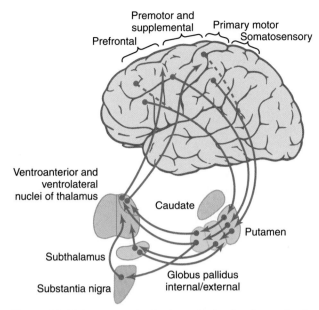

Figure 56-11 Putamen circuit through the basal ganglia for subconscious execution of learned patterns of movement.

Neural Pathways of the Putamen Circuit.

Figure 56-11 shows the principal pathways through the basal ganglia for executing learned patterns of movement. They begin mainly in the premotor and supplementary areas of the motor cortex and in the somatosensory areas of the sensory cortex. Next they pass to the putamen (mainly bypassing the caudate nucleus), then to the internal portion of the globus pallidus, next to the ventroanterior and ventrolateral relay nuclei of the thalamus, and finally return to the cerebral primary motor cortex and to portions of the premotor and supplementary cerebral areas closely associated with the primary motor cortex. Thus, the putamen circuit has its inputs mainly from those parts of the brain adjacent to the primary motor cortex but not much from the primary motor cortex itself. Then its outputs do go mainly back to the primary motor cortex or closely associated premotor and supplementary cortex. Functioning in close association with this primary putamen circuit are ancillary circuits that pass from the putamen through the external globus pallidus, the subthalamus, and the substantia nigra—finally returning to the motor cortex by way of the thalamus.

Abnormal Function in the Putamen Circuit: Athetosis, Hemiballismus, and Chorea.

How does the putamen circuit function to help execute patterns of movement? The answer is poorly known. However, when a portion of the circuit is damaged or blocked, certain patterns of movement become severely abnormal. For instance, lesions in the *globus pallidus* frequently lead to spontaneous and often continuous *writhing movements* of a hand, an arm, the neck, or the face—movements called *athetosis*.

A lesion in the *subthalamus* often leads to sudden *flailing movements* of an entire limb, a condition called *hemiballismus*.

Multiple small lesions in the *putamen* lead to *flicking movements* in the hands, face, and other parts of the body, called *chorea*.

Lesions of the *substantia nigra* lead to the common and extremely severe disease of *rigidity, akinesia,* and *tremors* known as *Parkinson's disease,* which we discuss in more detail later.

Role of the Basal Ganglia for Cognitive Control of Sequences of Motor Patterns—the Caudate Circuit

The term *cognition* means the thinking processes of the brain, using both sensory input to the brain plus information already stored in memory. Most of our motor actions occur as a consequence of thoughts generated in the mind, a process called *cognitive control of motor activity.* The caudate nucleus plays a major role in this cognitive control of motor activity.

The neural connections between the caudate nucleus and the corticospinal motor control system, shown in Figure 56-12, are somewhat different from those of the putamen circuit. Part of the reason for this is that the caudate nucleus, as shown in Figure 56-9, extends into all lobes of the cerebrum, beginning anteriorly in the frontal lobes, then passing posteriorly through the parietal and occipital lobes, and finally curving forward again like the letter "C" into the temporal lobes. Furthermore, the caudate nucleus receives large amounts of its input from the *association areas* of the cerebral cortex overlying the caudate nucleus, mainly areas that also integrate the different types of sensory and motor information into usable thought patterns.

After the signals pass from the cerebral cortex to the caudate nucleus, they are next transmitted to the internal globus pallidus, then to the relay nuclei of the

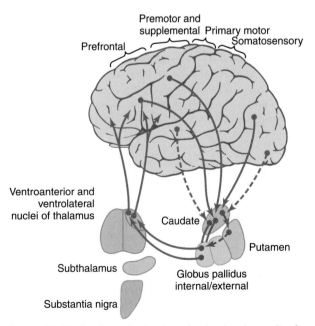

Figure 56-12 Caudate circuit through the basal ganglia for cognitive planning of sequential and parallel motor patterns to achieve specific conscious goals.

ventroanterior and ventrolateral thalamus, and finally back to the prefrontal, premotor, and supplementary motor areas of the cerebral cortex, but with almost none of the returning signals passing directly to the primary motor cortex. Instead, the returning signals go to those accessory motor regions in the premotor and supplementary motor areas that are concerned with putting together sequential patterns of movement lasting 5 or more seconds instead of exciting individual muscle movements.

A good example of this would be a person seeing a lion approach and then responding instantaneously and automatically by (1) turning away from the lion, (2) beginning to run, and (3) even attempting to climb a tree. Without the cognitive functions, the person might not have the instinctive knowledge, without thinking for too long a time, to respond quickly and appropriately. Thus, cognitive control of motor activity determines subconsciously, and within seconds, which patterns of movement will be used together to achieve a complex goal that might itself last for many seconds.

Function of the Basal Ganglia to Change the Timing and to Scale the Intensity of Movements

Two important capabilities of the brain in controlling movement are (1) to determine how rapidly the movement is to be performed and (2) to control how large the movement will be. For instance, a person may write the letter "a" slowly or rapidly. Also, he or she may write a small "a" on a piece of paper or a large "a" on a chalkboard. Regardless of the choice, the proportional characteristics of the letter remain nearly the same.

In patients with severe lesions of the basal ganglia, these timing and scaling functions are poor; in fact, sometimes they are nonexistent. Here again, the basal ganglia do not function alone; they function in close association with the cerebral cortex. One especially important cortical area is the posterior parietal cortex, which is the locus of the spatial coordinates for motor control of all parts of the body, as well as for the relation of the body and its parts to all its surroundings. Damage to this area does not produce simple deficits of sensory perception, such as loss of tactile sensation, blindness, or deafness. Instead, lesions of the posterior parietal cortex produce an inability to accurately perceive objects through normally functioning sensory mechanisms, a condition called *agnosia*. Figure 56-13 shows the way in which a person with a lesion in the right posterior parietal cortex might try to copy drawings. In these cases, the patient's ability to copy the left side of the drawings is severely impaired. Also, such a person will always try to avoid using his or her left arm, left hand, or other portions of his or her left body for the performance of tasks, or even wash this side of the body *(personal neglect syndrome)*, almost not knowing that these parts of his or her body exist.

Because the caudate circuit of the basal ganglial system functions mainly with association areas of the cerebral cortex such as the posterior parietal cortex, presumably

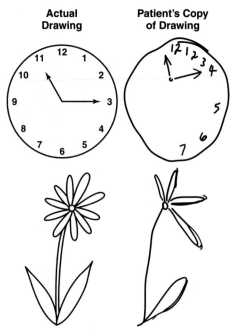

Actual Drawing   **Patient's Copy of Drawing**

Figure 56-13 Illustration of drawings that might be made by a person who has *neglect syndrome* caused by severe damage in his or her right posterior parietal cortex compared with the actual drawing the patient was requested to copy. Note that the person's ability to copy the left side of the drawings is severely impaired.

the timing and scaling of movements are functions of this caudate cognitive motor control circuit. However, our understanding of function in the basal ganglia is still so imprecise that much of what is conjectured in the last few sections is analytical deduction rather than proven fact.

Functions of Specific Neurotransmitter Substances in the Basal Ganglial System

Figure 56-14 demonstrates the interplay of several specific neurotransmitters that are known to function within the

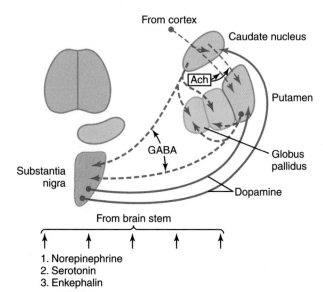

From cortex
Caudate nucleus
Ach
Putamen
GABA
Substantia nigra
Globus pallidus
Dopamine
From brain stem

1. Norepinephrine
2. Serotonin
3. Enkephalin

Figure 56-14 Neuronal pathways that secrete different types of neurotransmitter substances in the basal ganglia. Ach, acetylcholine; GABA, gamma-aminobutyric acid.

basal ganglia, showing (1) *dopamine* pathways from the substantia nigra to the caudate nucleus and putamen, (2) *gamma-aminobutyric acid (GABA)* pathways from the caudate nucleus and putamen to the globus pallidus and substantia nigra, (3) *acetylcholine* pathways from the cortex to the caudate nucleus and putamen, and (4) multiple general pathways from the brain stem that secrete *norepinephrine, serotonin, enkephalin,* and several other neurotransmitters in the basal ganglia, as well as in other parts of the cerebrum. In addition to all these are *multiple glutamate pathways* that provide most of the excitatory signals (not shown in the figure) that balance out the large numbers of inhibitory signals transmitted especially by the dopamine, GABA, and serotonin inhibitory transmitters. We have more to say about some of these neurotransmitter and hormonal systems in subsequent sections when we discuss diseases of the basal ganglia, as well as in subsequent chapters when we discuss behavior, sleep, wakefulness, and functions of the autonomic nervous system.

For the present, it should be remembered that the neurotransmitter GABA always functions as an inhibitory agent. Therefore, GABA neurons in the feedback loops from the cortex through the basal ganglia and then back to the cortex make virtually all these loops *negative feedback loops,* rather than positive feedback loops, thus lending stability to the motor control systems. Dopamine also functions as an inhibitory neurotransmitter in most parts of the brain, so it also functions as a stabilizer under some conditions.

Clinical Syndromes Resulting from Damage to the Basal Ganglia

Aside from *athetosis* and *hemiballismus,* which have already been mentioned in relation to lesions in the globus pallidus and subthalamus, two other major diseases result from damage in the basal ganglia. These are Parkinson's disease and Huntington's disease.

Parkinson's Disease

Parkinson's disease, known also as *paralysis agitans,* results from widespread destruction of that portion of the substantia nigra (the pars compacta) that sends dopamine-secreting nerve fibers to the caudate nucleus and putamen. The disease is characterized by (1) rigidity of much of the musculature of the body; (2) involuntary tremor of the involved areas even when the person is resting at a fixed rate of three to six cycles per second; and (3) serious difficulty in initiating movement, called *akinesia;* (4) postural instability caused by impaired postural reflexes, leading to poor balance and falls; and (5) other motor symptoms including dysphagia (impaired ability to swallow), speech disorders, gait disturbances, and fatigue.

The causes of these abnormal motor effects are unknown. However, the dopamine secreted in the caudate nucleus and putamen is an inhibitory transmitter; therefore, destruction of the dopaminergic neurons in the substantia nigra of the parkinsonian patient theoretically would allow the caudate nucleus and putamen to become overly active and possibly cause continuous output of excitatory signals to the corticospinal motor control system. These signals could overly excite many or all of the muscles of the body, thus leading to *rigidity.*

Some of the feedback circuits might easily *oscillate* because of high feedback gains after loss of their inhibition, leading to the *tremor* of Parkinson's disease. This tremor is quite different from that of cerebellar disease because it occurs during all waking hours and therefore is an *involuntary tremor,* in contradistinction to cerebellar tremor, which occurs only when the person performs intentionally initiated movements and therefore is called *intention tremor.*

The *akinesia* that occurs in Parkinson's disease is often much more distressing to the patient than are the symptoms of muscle rigidity and tremor, because to perform even the simplest movement in severe parkinsonism, the person must exert the highest degree of concentration. The mental effort, even mental anguish, that is necessary to make the desired movements is often at the limit of the patient's willpower. Then, when the movements do occur, they are usually stiff and staccato in character instead of smooth. The cause of this akinesia is still speculative. However, dopamine secretion in the limbic system, especially in the *nucleus accumbens,* is often decreased along with its decrease in the basal ganglia. It has been suggested that this might reduce the psychic drive for motor activity so greatly that akinesia results.

Treatment with L-Dopa. Administration of the drug *L-dopa* to patients with Parkinson's disease usually ameliorates many of the symptoms, especially the rigidity and akinesia. The reason for this is believed to be that L-dopa is converted in the brain into dopamine, and the dopamine then restores the normal balance between inhibition and excitation in the caudate nucleus and putamen. Administration of dopamine itself does not have the same effect because dopamine has a chemical structure that will not allow it to pass through the blood-brain barrier, even though the slightly different structure of L-dopa does allow it to pass.

Treatment with L-Deprenyl. Another treatment for Parkinson's disease is the drug L-deprenyl. This drug inhibits monoamine oxidase, which is responsible for destruction of most of the dopamine after it has been secreted. Therefore, any dopamine that is released remains in the basal ganglial tissues for a longer time. In addition, for reasons not understood, this treatment helps to slow destruction of the dopamine-secreting neurons in the substantia nigra. Therefore, appropriate combinations of L-dopa therapy along with L-deprenyl therapy usually provide much better treatment than use of one of these drugs alone.

Treatment with Transplanted Fetal Dopamine Cells. Transplantation of dopamine-secreting cells (cells obtained from the brains of aborted fetuses) into the caudate nuclei and putamen has been used with some short-term success to treat Parkinson's disease. However, the cells do not live for more than a few months. If persistence could be achieved, perhaps this would become the treatment of the future.

Treatment by Destroying Part of the Feedback Circuitry in the Basal Ganglia. Because abnormal signals from the basal ganglia to the motor cortex cause most of the abnormalities in Parkinson's disease, multiple attempts have been made to treat these patients by blocking these signals surgically. For a number of years, surgical lesions were made in the ventrolateral and ventroanterior nuclei of the thalamus, which blocked part of the feedback circuit from the basal ganglia to the cortex; variable degrees of success were achieved, as well as sometimes serious neurological damage. In monkeys with Parkinson's disease, lesions placed in the subthalamus have been used, sometimes with surprisingly good results.

Huntington's Disease (Huntington's Chorea)

Huntington's disease is a hereditary disorder that usually begins causing symptoms at age 30 to 40 years. It is characterized at first by flicking movements in individual muscles and then progressive severe distortional movements of the entire body. In addition, severe dementia develops along with the motor dysfunctions.

The abnormal movements of Huntington's disease are believed to be caused by loss of most of the cell bodies of the GABA-secreting neurons in the caudate nucleus and putamen and of acetylcholine-secreting neurons in many parts of the brain. The axon terminals of the GABA neurons normally inhibit portions of the globus pallidus and substantia nigra. This loss of inhibition is believed to allow spontaneous outbursts of globus pallidus and substantia nigra activity that cause the distortional movements.

The dementia in Huntington's disease probably does not result from the loss of GABA neurons but from the loss of acetylcholine-secreting neurons, perhaps especially in the thinking areas of the cerebral cortex.

The abnormal gene that causes Huntington's disease has been found; it has a many-times-repeating codon, CAG, that codes for multiple extra *glutamine* amino acids in the molecular structure of an abnormal neuronal cell protein called *huntington* that causes the symptoms. How this protein causes the disease effects is now the question for major research effort.

Integration of the Many Parts of the Total Motor Control System

Finally, we need to summarize as best we can what is known about overall control of movement. To do this, let us first give a synopsis of the different levels of control.

Spinal Level

Programmed in the spinal cord are local patterns of movement for all muscle areas of the body—for instance, programmed withdrawal reflexes that pull any part of the body away from a source of pain. The cord is the locus also of complex patterns of rhythmical motions such as to-and-fro movement of the limbs for walking, plus reciprocal motions on opposite sides of the body or of the hindlimbs versus the forelimbs in four-legged animals.

All these programs of the cord can be commanded into action by higher levels of motor control, or they can be inhibited while the higher levels take over control.

Hindbrain Level

The hindbrain provides two major functions for general motor control of the body: (1) maintenance of axial tone of the body for the purpose of standing and (2) continuous modification of the degrees of tone in the different muscles in response to information from the vestibular apparatuses for the purpose of maintaining body equilibrium.

Motor Cortex Level

The motor cortex system provides most of the activating motor signals to the spinal cord. It functions partly by issuing sequential and parallel commands that set into motion various cord patterns of motor action. It can also change the intensities of the different patterns or modify their timing or other characteristics. When needed, the corticospinal system can bypass the cord patterns, replacing them with higher-level patterns from the brain stem or cerebral cortex. The cortical patterns are usually complex; also, they can be "learned," whereas cord patterns are mainly determined by heredity and are said to be "hard wired."

Associated Functions of the Cerebellum. The cerebellum functions with all levels of muscle control. It functions with the spinal cord especially to enhance the stretch reflex, so when a contracting muscle encounters an unexpectedly heavy load, a long stretch reflex signal transmitted all the way through the cerebellum and back again to the cord strongly enhances the load-resisting effect of the basic stretch reflex.

At the brain stem level, the cerebellum functions to make the postural movements of the body, especially the rapid movements required by the equilibrium system, smooth and continuous and without abnormal oscillations.

At the cerebral cortex level, the cerebellum operates in association with the cortex to provide many accessory motor functions, especially to provide extra motor force for turning on muscle contraction rapidly at the start of a movement. Near the end of each movement, the *cerebellum* turns on antagonist muscles at exactly the right time and with proper force to stop the movement at the intended point. Furthermore, there is good physiologic evidence that all aspects of this turn-on/turn-off patterning by the cerebellum can be learned with experience.

The cerebellum functions with the cerebral cortex at still another level of motor control: it helps to program in advance muscle contractions that are required for smooth progression from a present rapid movement in one direction to the next rapid movement in another direction, all this occurring in a fraction of a second. The neural circuit for this passes from the cerebral cortex to the large lateral zones of the cerebellar hemispheres and then back to the cerebral cortex.

The cerebellum functions mainly when muscle movements have to be rapid. Without the cerebellum, slow and calculated movements can still occur, but it is difficult for the corticospinal system to achieve rapid and changing intended movements to execute a particular goal or especially to progress smoothly from one rapid movement to the next.

Associated Functions of the Basal Ganglia. The basal ganglia are essential to motor control in ways entirely different from those of the cerebellum. Their most important functions are (1) to help the cortex execute subconscious but *learned patterns of movement* and (2) to help plan multiple parallel and sequential patterns of movement that the mind must put together to accomplish a purposeful task.

The types of motor patterns that require the basal ganglia include those for writing all the different letters of the alphabet, for throwing a ball, and for typing. Also, the basal ganglia are required to modify these patterns for writing small or writing very large, thus controlling dimensions of the patterns.

At a still higher level of control is another combined cerebral and basal ganglia circuit, beginning in the thinking processes of the cerebrum to provide overall sequential steps of action for responding to each new situation, such as planning one's immediate motor response to an assailant who hits the person in the face or one's sequential response to an unexpectedly fond embrace.

What Drives Us to Action?

What is it that arouses us from inactivity and sets into play our trains of movement? We are beginning to learn about the motivational systems of the brain. Basically, the brain has an older core located beneath, anterior, and lateral to the thalamus—including the hypothalamus, amygdala, hippocampus, septal region anterior to the hypothalamus and thalamus, and even old regions of the thalamus and cerebral cortex themselves—all of which function together to initiate most motor and other functional activities of the brain. These areas are collectively called the *limbic system* of the brain. We discuss this system in detail in Chapter 58.

Bibliography

Bastian AJ: Learning to predict the future: the cerebellum adapts feedforward movement control, *Curr Opin Neurobiol* 16:645, 2006.

Bloom F, Lazerson A: *Brain, Mind and Behavior*, ed 2, New York, 1988, W.H. Freeman, p 300.

Breakefield XO, Blood AJ, Li Y, et al: The pathophysiological basis of dystonias, *Nat Rev Neurosci* 9:222, 2008.

Cheron G, Servais L, Dan B: Cerebellar network plasticity: from genes to fast oscillation, *Neuroscience* 153:1, 2008.

DeKosky ST, Marek K: Looking backward to move forward: early detection of neurodegenerative disorders, *Science* 302:830, 2003.

Fuentes CT, Bastian AJ: 'Motor cognition'—what is it and is the cerebellum involved? *Cerebellum* 6:232, 2007.

Gibson AR, Horn KM, Pong M: Inhibitory control of olivary discharge, *Ann N Y Acad Sci* 978:219, 2002.

Hasnain M, Vieweg WV, Baron MS, et al: Pharmacological management of psychosis in elderly patients with parkinsonism, *Am J Med* 122:614, 2009.

Ito M: Cerebellar long-term depression: characterization, signal transduction, and functional roles, *Physiol Rev* 81:1143, 2001.

Kandel ER, Schwartz JH, Jessell TM: *Principles of Neural Science*, ed 4, New York, 2000, McGraw-Hill.

Kreitzer AC, Malenka RC: Striatal plasticity and basal ganglia circuit function, *Neuron* 60:543, 2008.

Lees AJ, Hardy J, Revesz T: Parkinson's disease, *Lancet* 373:2055, 2009.

Li JY, Plomann M, Brundin P: Huntington's disease: a synaptopathy? *Trends Mol Med* 9:414, 2003.

Mustari MJ, Ono S, Das VE: Signal processing and distribution in cortical-brainstem pathways for smooth pursuit eye movements, *Ann N Y Acad Sci* 1164:147, 2009.

Nambu A: Seven problems on the basal ganglia, *Curr Opin Neurobiol* 18:595, 2008.

Pugh JR, Raman IM: Nothing can be coincidence: synaptic inhibition and plasticity in the cerebellar nuclei, *Trends Neurosci* 32:170, 2009.

Ramnani N: The primate cortico-cerebellar system: anatomy and function, *Nat Rev Neurosci* 7:511, 2006.

Rosas HD, Salat DH, Lee SY, et al: Complexity and heterogeneity: what drives the ever-changing brain in Huntington's disease? *Ann N Y Acad Sci* 1147:196, 2008.

Spruston N: Pyramidal neurons: dendritic structure and synaptic integration, *Nat Rev Neurosci* 9:206, 2008.

Sethi KD: Tremor, *Curr Opin Neurol* 16:481, 2003.

Cerebral Cortex, Intellectual Functions of the Brain, Learning, and Memory

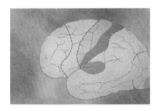

It is ironic that of all the parts of the brain, we know the least about the functions of the cerebral cortex, even though it is by far the largest portion of the nervous system. But we do know the effects of damage or specific stimulation in various portions of the cortex. In the first part of this chapter, the known cortical functions are discussed; then basic theories of neuronal mechanisms involved in thought processes, memory, analysis of sensory information, and so forth are presented briefly.

Physiologic Anatomy of the Cerebral Cortex

The functional part of the cerebral cortex is a thin layer of neurons covering the surface of all the convolutions of the cerebrum. This layer is only 2 to 5 millimeters thick, with a total area of about one quarter of a square meter. The total cerebral cortex contains about 100 *billion* neurons.

Figure 57-1 shows the typical histological structure of the neuronal surface of the cerebral cortex, with its successive layers of different types of neurons. Most of the neurons are of three types: (1) *granular* (also called *stellate*), (2) *fusiform,* and (3) *pyramidal,* the last named for their characteristic pyramidal shape.

The *granular* neurons generally have short axons and, therefore, function mainly as interneurons that transmit neural signals only short distances within the cortex itself. Some are excitatory, releasing mainly the excitatory neurotransmitter *glutamate;* others are inhibitory and release mainly the inhibitory neurotransmitter *gamma-aminobutyric acid* (GABA). The sensory areas of the cortex, as well as the association areas between sensory and motor areas, have large concentrations of these granule cells, suggesting a high degree of intracortical processing of incoming sensory signals within the sensory areas and association areas.

The *pyramidal* and *fusiform cells* give rise to almost all the output fibers from the cortex. The pyramidal cells are larger and more numerous than the fusiform cells. They are the source of the long, large nerve fibers that go all the way to the spinal cord. They also give rise to most of the large subcortical association fiber bundles that pass from one major part of the brain to another.

To the right in Figure 57-1 is shown the typical organization of nerve fibers within the different layers of the cerebral cortex. Note particularly the large number of

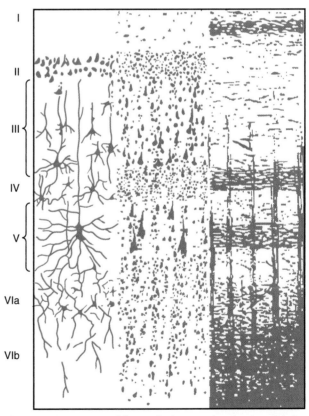

Figure 57-1 Structure of the cerebral cortex, showing: *I*, molecular layer; *II*, external granular layer; *III*, layer of pyramidal cells; *IV*, internal granular layer; *V*, large pyramidal cell layer; and *VI*, layer of fusiform or polymorphic cells. (Redrawn from Ranson SW, Clark SL [after Brodmann]: Anatomy of the Nervous System. Philadelphia: WB Saunders, 1959.)

horizontal fibers that extend between adjacent areas of the cortex, but note also the *vertical fibers* that extend to and from the cortex to lower areas of the brain and some all the way to the spinal cord or to distant regions of the cerebral cortex through long association bundles.

The functions of the specific layers of the cerebral cortex are discussed in Chapters 47 and 51. By way of review, let us recall that most incoming specific sensory signals from the body terminate in cortical layer IV. Most of the output signals leave the cortex through neurons located in layers V and VI; the very large fibers to the brain stem and cord arise generally in layer V; and the tremendous numbers of fibers to the thalamus arise in layer VI. Layers I, II, and III perform most of the intracortical association functions, with especially large numbers of neurons in layers II and III making short horizontal connections with adjacent cortical areas.

Anatomical and Functional Relations of the Cerebral Cortex to the Thalamus and Other Lower Centers. All areas of the cerebral cortex have extensive to-and-fro efferent and afferent connections with deeper structures of the brain. It is important to emphasize the relation between the cerebral cortex and the thalamus. When the thalamus is damaged along with the cortex, the loss of cerebral function is far greater than when the cortex alone is damaged because thalamic excitation of the cortex is necessary for almost all cortical activity.

Figure 57-2 shows the areas of the cerebral cortex that connect with specific parts of the thalamus. These connections act in *two* directions, both from the thalamus to the cortex and then from the cortex back to essentially the same area of the thalamus. Furthermore, when the thalamic connections are cut, the functions of the corresponding cortical area become almost entirely lost. Therefore, the cortex operates in close association with the thalamus and can almost be considered both anatomically and functionally a unit with the thalamus: for this reason, the thalamus and the cortex together are sometimes called the *thalamocortical system*. Almost all pathways from the sensory receptors and sensory organs to the cortex pass through the thalamus, with the principal exception of some sensory pathways of olfaction.

Functions of Specific Cortical Areas

Studies in human beings have shown that different cerebral cortical areas have separate functions. Figure 57-3 is a map of some of these functions as determined from electrical stimulation of the cortex in awake patients or during neurological examination of patients after portions of the cortex had been removed. The electrically stimulated patients told their thoughts evoked by the stimulation, and sometimes they experienced movements. Occasionally they spontaneously emitted a sound or even a word or gave some other evidence of the stimulation.

Putting large amounts of information together from many different sources gives a more general map, as shown in Figure 57-4. This figure shows the major primary and secondary premotor and supplementary motor areas of the cortex, as well as the major primary and secondary sensory areas for somatic sensation, vision, and hearing, all of which are discussed in earlier chapters. The primary motor areas have direct connections with specific muscles for causing discrete muscle movements. The primary sensory areas detect specific sensations—visual, auditory, or somatic—transmitted directly to the brain from peripheral sensory organs.

The secondary areas make sense out of the signals in the primary areas. For instance, the supplementary and premotor areas function along with the primary motor cortex and basal ganglia to provide "patterns" of motor activity. On the sensory side, the secondary sensory areas, located within a few centimeters of the primary areas, begin to analyze the meanings of the specific sensory signals, such as (1) interpretation of the shape or texture of an object in one's hand; (2) interpretation of color, light intensity, directions of lines and angles, and other aspects of vision; and (3) interpretations of the meanings of sound tones and sequence of tones in the auditory signals.

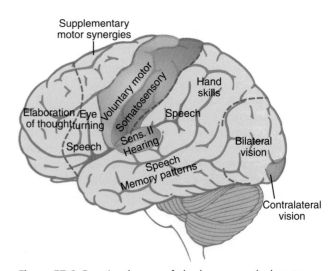

Figure 57-3 Functional areas of the human cerebral cortex as determined by electrical stimulation of the cortex during neurosurgical operations and by neurological examinations of patients with destroyed cortical regions. (Redrawn from Penfield W, Rasmussen T: The Cerebral Cortex of Man: A Clinical Study of Localization of Function. New York: Hafner, 1968.)

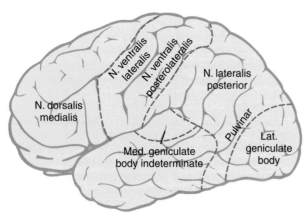

Figure 57-2 Areas of the cerebral cortex that connect with specific portions of the thalamus.

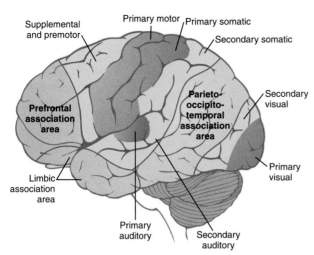

Figure 57-4 Locations of major association areas of the cerebral cortex, as well as primary and secondary motor and sensory areas.

Association Areas

Figure 57-4 also shows several large areas of the cerebral cortex that do not fit into the rigid categories of primary and secondary motor and sensory areas. These areas are called *association areas* because they receive and analyze signals simultaneously from multiple regions of both the motor and sensory cortices, as well as from subcortical structures. Yet even the association areas have their specializations. Important association areas include (1) the *parieto-occipitotemporal association area*, (2) the *prefrontal association area*, and (3) the *limbic association area*. Following are explanations of the functions of these areas.

Parieto-occipitotemporal Association Area. This association area lies in the large parietal and occipital cortical space bounded by the somatosensory cortex anteriorly, the visual cortex posteriorly, and the auditory cortex laterally. As would be expected, it provides a high level of interpretative meaning for signals from all the surrounding sensory areas. However, even the parieto-occipitotemporal association area has its own functional subareas, which are shown in Figure 57-5.

1. Analysis of the Spatial Coordinates of the Body. An area beginning in the posterior parietal cortex and extending into the superior occipital cortex provides continuous analysis of the spatial coordinates of all parts of the body, as well as of the surroundings of the body. This area receives visual sensory information from the posterior occipital cortex and simultaneous somatosensory information from the anterior parietal cortex. From all this information, it computes the coordinates of the visual, auditory, and body surroundings.

2. Wernicke's Area Is Important for Language Comprehension. The major area for language comprehension, called *Wernicke's area,* lies behind *the primary auditory cortex in the posterior part of the superior gyrus of the temporal lobe.* We discuss this area much more fully later; it is the most important region of the entire brain for higher intellectual function because almost all such intellectual functions are language based.

3. Angular Gyrus Area Is Needed for Initial Processing of Visual Language (Reading). Posterior to the language comprehension area, lying mainly in the anterolateral region of the occipital lobe, is a visual association area that feeds visual information conveyed by words read from a book into Wernicke's area, the language comprehension area. This so-called *angular gyrus area* is needed to make meaning out of the visually perceived words. In its absence, a person can still have excellent language comprehension through hearing but not through reading.

4. Area for Naming Objects. *In the most lateral portions of the anterior occipital lobe and posterior temporal lobe is an area for naming objects.* The names are learned mainly through auditory input, whereas the physical

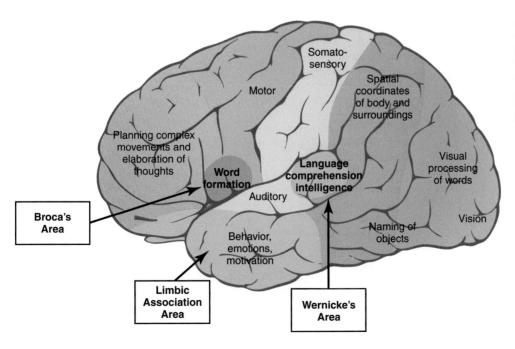

Figure 57-5 Map of specific functional areas in the cerebral cortex, showing especially Wernicke's and Broca's areas for language comprehension and speech production, which in 95 percent of all people are located in the left hemisphere.

natures of the objects are learned mainly through visual input. In turn, the names are essential for both auditory and visual language comprehension (*functions performed in Wernicke's area* located immediately superior to the auditory "names" region and anterior to the visual word processing area).

Prefrontal Association Area. As discussed in Chapter 56, the prefrontal association area functions in close association with the motor cortex to plan complex patterns and sequences of motor movements. To aid in this function, it receives strong input through a massive subcortical bundle of nerve fibers connecting the parieto-occipitotemporal association area with the prefrontal association area. Through this bundle, the prefrontal cortex receives much preanalyzed sensory information, especially information on the spatial coordinates of the body that is necessary for planning effective movements. Much of the output from the prefrontal area into the motor control system passes through the caudate portion of the basal ganglia–thalamic feedback circuit for motor planning, which provides many of the sequential and parallel components of movement stimulation.

The *prefrontal association area* is also *essential to carrying out "thought" processes in the mind.* This presumably results from some of the same capabilities of the prefrontal cortex that allow it to plan motor activities. It seems to be capable of processing nonmotor and motor information from widespread areas of the brain and therefore to achieve nonmotor types of thinking, as well as motor types. In fact, the prefrontal association area is frequently described simply as important for *elaboration of thoughts,* and it is said to store on a short-term basis "working memories" that are used to combine new thoughts while they are entering the brain.

Broca's Area Provides the Neural Circuitry for Word Formation. *Broca's area,* shown in Figure 57-5, is located partly in the posterior lateral prefrontal cortex and partly in the premotor area. It is here that plans and motor patterns for expressing individual words or even short phrases are initiated and executed. This area also works in close association with the Wernicke's language comprehension center in the temporal association cortex, as we discuss more fully later in the chapter.

An especially interesting discovery is the following: When a person has already learned one language and then learns a new language, the area in the brain where the new language is stored is slightly removed from the storage area for the first language. If both languages are learned simultaneously, they are stored together in the same area of the brain.

Limbic Association Area. Figures 57-4 and 57-5 show still another association area called the *limbic association area.* This area is found in the anterior pole of the temporal lobe, in the ventral portion of the frontal lobe, and in the cingulate gyrus lying deep in the longitudinal fissure on the midsurface of each cerebral hemisphere. It

is concerned primarily with *behavior, emotions,* and *motivation.* We discuss in Chapter 58 that the limbic cortex is part of a much more extensive system, the *limbic system,* that includes a complex set of neuronal structures in the midbasal regions of the brain. This limbic system provides most of the emotional drives for activating other areas of the brain and even provides motivational drive for the process of learning itself.

Area for Recognition of Faces

An interesting type of brain abnormality called *prosopagnosia* is inability to recognize faces. This occurs in people who have extensive damage on the medial undersides of both occipital lobes and along the medioventral surfaces of the temporal lobes, as shown in Figure 57-6. Loss of these face recognition areas, strangely enough, results in little other abnormality of brain function.

One wonders why so much of the cerebral cortex should be reserved for the simple task of face recognition. Most of our daily tasks involve associations with other people, and one can see the importance of this intellectual function.

The occipital portion of this facial recognition area is contiguous with the visual cortex, and the temporal portion is closely associated with the limbic system that has to do with emotions, brain activation, and control of one's behavioral response to the environment, as we see in Chapter 58.

Comprehensive Interpretative Function of the Posterior Superior Temporal Lobe—"Wernicke's Area" (a General Interpretative Area)

The somatic, visual, and auditory association areas all meet one another in the posterior part of the superior temporal lobe, shown in Figure 57-7, where the temporal, parietal, and occipital lobes all come together. This area of confluence of the different sensory interpretative areas

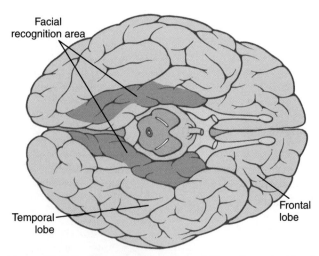

Figure 57-6 Facial recognition areas located on the underside of the brain in the medial occipital and temporal lobes. (Redrawn from Geschwind N: Specializations of the human brain. Sci Am 241:180, 1979. ® 1979 by Scientific American, Inc. All rights reserved.)

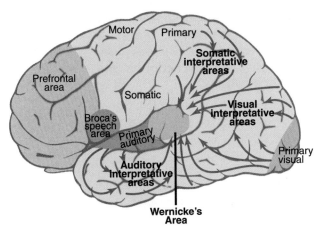

Figure 57-7 Organization of the somatic auditory and visual association areas into a general mechanism for interpretation of sensory experience. All of these feed also into *Wernicke's area,* located in the posterosuperior portion of the temporal lobe. Note also the prefrontal area and *Broca's speech area* in the frontal lobe.

is especially highly developed in the *dominant* side of the brain—the *left side* in almost all right-handed people—and it plays the greatest single role of any part of the cerebral cortex for the higher comprehension levels of brain function that we call *intelligence.* Therefore, this region has been called by different names suggestive of an area that has almost global importance: the *general interpretative area,* the *gnostic area,* the *knowing* area, the *tertiary association area,* and so forth. It is best known as *Wernicke's area* in honor of the neurologist who first described its special significance in intellectual processes.

After severe damage in Wernicke's area, a person might hear perfectly well and even recognize different words but still be unable to arrange these words into a coherent thought. Likewise, the person may be able to read words from the printed page but be unable to recognize the thought that is conveyed.

Electrical stimulation in Wernicke's area of a conscious person occasionally causes a highly complex thought. This is particularly true when the stimulation electrode is passed deep enough into the brain to approach the corresponding connecting areas of the thalamus. The types of thoughts that might be experienced include complicated visual scenes that one might remember from childhood, auditory hallucinations such as a specific musical piece, or even a statement made by a specific person. For this reason, it is believed that activation of Wernicke's area can call forth complicated memory patterns that involve more than one sensory modality even though most of the individual memories may be stored elsewhere. This belief is in accord with the importance of Wernicke's area in interpreting the complicated meanings of different patterns of sensory experiences.

Angular Gyrus—Interpretation of Visual Information. The *angular gyrus* is the most inferior portion of the posterior parietal lobe, lying immediately behind Wernicke's area and fusing posteriorly into the visual areas

of the occipital lobe as well. If this region is destroyed while Wernicke's area in the temporal lobe is still intact, the person can still interpret auditory experiences as usual, but the stream of visual experiences passing into Wernicke's area from the visual cortex is mainly blocked. Therefore, the person may be able to see words and even know that they are words but not be able to interpret their meanings. This is the condition called *dyslexia,* or *word blindness.*

Let us again emphasize the global importance of Wernicke's area for processing most intellectual functions of the brain. Loss of this area in an adult usually leads thereafter to a lifetime of almost demented existence.

Concept of the Dominant Hemisphere

The general interpretative functions of Wernicke's area and the angular gyrus, as well as the functions of the speech and motor control areas, are usually much more highly developed in one cerebral hemisphere than in the other. Therefore, this hemisphere is called the *dominant hemisphere.* In about 95 percent of all people, the left hemisphere is the dominant one.

Even at birth, the area of the cortex that will eventually become Wernicke's area is as much as 50 percent larger in the left hemisphere than in the right in more than one half of neonates. Therefore, it is easy to understand why the left side of the brain might become dominant over the right side. However, if for some reason this left side area is damaged or removed in very early childhood, the opposite side of the brain will usually develop dominant characteristics.

A theory that can explain the capability of one hemisphere to dominate the other hemisphere is the following. The attention of the "mind" seems to be directed to one principal thought at a time. Presumably, because the left posterior temporal lobe at birth is usually slightly larger than the right, the left side normally begins to be used to a greater extent than the right. Thereafter, because of the tendency to direct one's attention to the better developed region, the rate of learning in the cerebral hemisphere that gains the first start increases rapidly, whereas in the opposite, less-used side, learning remains slight. Therefore, the left side normally becomes dominant over the right.

In about 95 percent of all people, the left temporal lobe and angular gyrus become dominant, and in the remaining 5 percent, either both sides develop simultaneously to have dual function or, more rarely, the right side alone becomes highly developed, with full dominance.

As discussed later in the chapter, the premotor speech area (Broca's area), located far laterally in the intermediate frontal lobe, is also almost always dominant on the left side of the brain. This speech area is responsible for formation of words by exciting simultaneously the laryngeal muscles, respiratory muscles, and muscles of the mouth.

The motor areas for controlling hands are also dominant in the left side of the brain in about 9 of 10 persons, thus causing right-handedness in most people.

Although the interpretative areas of the temporal lobe and angular gyrus, as well as many of the motor areas, are usually highly developed in only the left hemisphere, these areas receive sensory information from both hemispheres and are capable also of controlling motor activities in both hemispheres. For this purpose, they use mainly fiber pathways in the *corpus callosum* for communication between the two hemispheres. This unitary, cross-feeding organization prevents interference between the two sides of the brain; such interference could create havoc with both mental thoughts and motor responses.

Role of Language in the Function of Wernicke's Area and in Intellectual Functions

A major share of our sensory experience is converted into its language equivalent before being stored in the memory areas of the brain and before being processed for other intellectual purposes. For instance, when we read a book, we do not store the visual images of the printed words but instead store the words themselves or their conveyed thoughts often in language form.

The sensory area of the dominant hemisphere for interpretation of language is Wernicke's area, and this is closely associated with both the primary and secondary hearing areas of the temporal lobe. This close relation probably results from the fact that the first introduction to language is by way of hearing. Later in life, when visual perception of language through the medium of reading develops, the visual information conveyed by written words is then presumably channeled through the angular gyrus, a visual association area, into the already developed Wernicke's language interpretative area of the dominant temporal lobe.

Functions of the Parieto-occipitotemporal Cortex in the Nondominant Hemisphere

When Wernicke's area in the dominant hemisphere of an adult person is destroyed, the person normally loses almost all intellectual functions associated with language or verbal symbolism, such as the ability to read, the ability to perform mathematical operations, and even the ability to think through logical problems. Many other types of interpretative capabilities, some of which use the temporal lobe and angular gyrus regions of the opposite hemisphere, are retained.

Psychological studies in patients with damage to the nondominant hemisphere have suggested that this hemisphere may be especially important for understanding and interpreting music, nonverbal visual experiences (especially visual patterns), spatial relations between the person and their surroundings, the significance of "body language" and intonations of people's voices, and probably many somatic experiences related to use of the limbs and hands. Thus, even though we speak of the "dominant" hemisphere, this is primarily for language-based intellectual functions; the so-called nondominant hemisphere might actually be dominant for some other types of intelligence.

Higher Intellectual Functions of the Prefrontal Association Areas

For years, it has been taught that the prefrontal cortex is the locus of "higher intellect" in the human being, principally because the main difference between the brains of monkeys and of human beings is the great prominence of the human prefrontal areas. Yet efforts to show that the prefrontal cortex is more important in higher intellectual functions than other portions of the brain have not been successful. Indeed, destruction of the language comprehension area in the posterior superior temporal lobe (Wernicke's area) and the adjacent angular gyrus region in the dominant hemisphere causes much more harm to the intellect than does destruction of the prefrontal areas. The prefrontal areas do, however, have less definable but nevertheless important intellectual functions of their own. These functions can best be explained by describing what happens to patients in whom the prefrontal areas have become damaged, as follows.

Several decades ago, before the advent of modern drugs for treating psychiatric conditions, it was found that some patients could receive significant relief from severe psychotic depression by severing the neuronal connections between the prefrontal areas of the brain and the remainder of the brain, that is, by a procedure called *prefrontal lobotomy*. This was done by inserting a blunt, thin-bladed knife through a small opening in the lateral frontal skull on each side of the head and slicing the brain at the back edge of the prefrontal lobes from top to bottom. Subsequent studies in these patients showed the following mental changes:

1. The patients lost their ability to solve complex problems.
2. They became unable to string together sequential tasks to reach complex goals.
3. They became unable to learn to do several parallel tasks at the same time.
4. Their level of aggressiveness was decreased, sometimes markedly, and, in general, they lost ambition.
5. Their social responses were often inappropriate for the occasion, often including loss of morals and little reticence in relation to sexual activity and excretion.
6. The patients could still talk and comprehend language, but they were unable to carry through any long trains of thought, and their moods changed rapidly from sweetness to rage to exhilaration to madness.
7. The patients could also still perform most of the usual patterns of motor function that they had performed throughout life, but often without purpose.

From this information, let us try to piece together a coherent understanding of the function of the prefrontal association areas.

Decreased Aggressiveness and Inappropriate Social Responses. These two characteristics probably result from loss of the ventral parts of the frontal lobes on the underside of the brain. As explained earlier and shown in Figures 57-4 and 57-5, this area is part of the limbic association cortex, rather than of the prefrontal association cortex. This limbic area helps to control behavior, which is discussed in detail in Chapter 58.

Inability to Progress Toward Goals or to Carry Through Sequential Thoughts. We learned earlier in this chapter that the prefrontal association areas have the capability of calling forth information from widespread areas of the brain and using this information to achieve deeper thought patterns for attaining goals.

Although people without prefrontal cortices can still think, they show little concerted thinking in logical sequence for longer than a few seconds or a minute or so at most. One of the results is that people without prefrontal cortices are *easily distracted from their central theme of thought,* whereas people with functioning prefrontal cortices can drive themselves to completion of their thought goals irrespective of distractions.

Elaboration of Thought, Prognostication, and Performance of Higher Intellectual Functions by the Prefrontal Areas—Concept of a "Working Memory." Another function that has been ascribed to the prefrontal areas is *elaboration of thought.* This means simply an increase in depth and abstractness of the different thoughts put together from multiple sources of information. Psychological tests have shown that prefrontal lobectomized lower animals presented with successive bits of sensory information fail to keep track of these bits even in temporary memory, probably because they are distracted so easily that they cannot hold thoughts long enough for memory storage to take place.

This ability of the prefrontal areas to keep track of many bits of information simultaneously and to cause recall of this information instantaneously as it is needed for subsequent thoughts is called the brain's "working memory." This may explain the many functions of the brain that we associate with higher intelligence. In fact, studies have shown that the prefrontal areas are divided into separate segments for storing different types of temporary memory, such as one area for storing shape and form of an object or a part of the body and another for storing movement.

By combining all these temporary bits of working memory, we have the abilities to (1) prognosticate; (2) plan for the future; (3) delay action in response to incoming sensory signals so that the sensory information can be weighed until the best course of response is decided; (4) consider the consequences of motor actions before they are performed; (5) solve complicated mathematical, legal, or philosophical problems; (6) correlate all avenues of information in diagnosing rare diseases; and (7) control our activities in accord with moral laws.

Function of the Brain in Communication—Language Input and Language Output

One of the most important differences between human beings and lower animals is the facility with which human beings can communicate with one another. Furthermore, because neurological tests can easily assess the ability of a person to communicate with others, we know more about the sensory and motor systems related to communication than about any other segment of brain cortex function. Therefore, we will review, with the help of anatomical maps of neural pathways in Figure 57-8, function of the cortex in communication. From this, one will see immediately how the principles of sensory analysis and motor control apply to this art.

There are two aspects to communication: first, the *sensory aspect* (language input), involving the ears and eyes, and, second, the *motor aspect* (language output), involving vocalization and its control.

Sensory Aspects of Communication. We noted earlier in the chapter that destruction of portions of the *auditory* or *visual association areas* of the cortex can result in inability to understand the spoken word or the written word. These effects are called, respectively, *auditory receptive aphasia* and *visual receptive aphasia* or, more commonly, *word deafness* and *word blindness* (also called *dyslexia*).

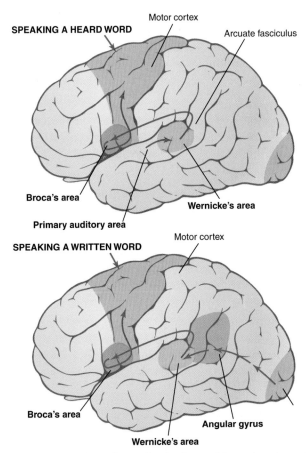

Figure 57-8 Brain pathways for (*top*) perceiving a heard word and then speaking the same word and (*bottom*) perceiving a written word and then speaking the same word. (Redrawn from Geschwind N: Specializations of the human brain. Sci Am 241:180, 1979. ® 1979 by Scientific American, Inc. All rights reserved.)

Wernicke's Aphasia and Global Aphasia. Some people are capable of understanding either the spoken word or the written word but are *unable to interpret the thought* that is expressed. This results most frequently when *Wernicke's area* in the *posterior superior temporal gyrus in the dominant hemisphere* is damaged or destroyed. Therefore, this type of aphasia is called *Wernicke's aphasia.*

When the lesion in Wernicke's area is widespread and extends (1) backward into the angular gyrus region, (2) inferiorly into the lower areas of the temporal lobe, and (3) superiorly into the superior border of the sylvian fissure, the person is likely to be almost totally demented for language understanding or communication and therefore is said to have *global aphasia.*

Motor Aspects of Communication. The process of speech involves two principal stages of mentation: (1) formation in the mind of thoughts to be expressed, as well as choice of words to be used, and then (2) motor control of vocalization and the actual act of vocalization itself.

The formation of thoughts and even most choices of words are the function of sensory association areas of the brain. Again, it is Wernicke's area in the posterior part of the superior temporal gyrus that is most important for this ability. Therefore, a person with either Wernicke's aphasia or global aphasia is unable to formulate the thoughts that are to be communicated. Or, if the lesion is less severe, the person may be able to formulate the thoughts but unable to put together appropriate sequences of words to express the thought. The person sometimes is even fluent with words but the words are jumbled.

Loss of Broca's Area Causes Motor Aphasia. Sometimes a person is capable of deciding what he or she wants to say but cannot make the vocal system emit words instead of noises. This effect, called *motor aphasia,* results from damage to *Broca's speech area,* which lies in the *prefrontal* and *premotor* facial region of the cerebral cortex—about 95 percent of the time in the left hemisphere, as shown in Figures 57-5 and 57-8. Therefore, the *skilled motor patterns* for control of the larynx, lips, mouth, respiratory system, and other accessory muscles of speech are all initiated from this area.

Articulation. Finally, we have the act of articulation, which means the muscular movements of the mouth, tongue, larynx, vocal cords, and so forth that are responsible for the intonations, timing, and rapid changes in intensities of the sequential sounds. The *facial and laryngeal regions of the motor cortex* activate these muscles, and the *cerebellum, basal ganglia,* and *sensory cortex* all help to control the sequences and intensities of muscle contractions, making liberal use of basal ganglial and cerebellar feedback mechanisms described in Chapters 55 and 56. Destruction of any of these regions can cause either total or partial inability to speak distinctly.

Summary. Figure 57-8 shows two principal pathways for communication. The upper half of the figure shows the pathway involved in hearing and speaking. This sequence is the following: (1) reception in the primary auditory area of the sound signals that encode the words; (2) interpretation of the words in Wernicke's area; (3) determination, also in Wernicke's area, of the thoughts and the words to be spoken; (4) transmission of signals from Wernicke's area to Broca's area by way of the *arcuate fasciculus;* (5) activation of the skilled motor programs in Broca's area for control of word formation; and (6) transmission of appropriate signals into the motor cortex to control the speech muscles.

The lower figure illustrates the comparable steps in reading and then speaking in response. The initial receptive area for the words is in the primary visual area rather than in the primary auditory area. Then the information passes through early stages of interpretation in the *angular gyrus region* and finally reaches its full level of recognition in Wernicke's area. From here, the sequence is the same as for speaking in response to the spoken word.

Function of the Corpus Callosum and Anterior Commissure to Transfer Thoughts, Memories, Training, and Other Information Between the Two Cerebral Hemispheres

Fibers in the *corpus callosum* provide abundant bidirectional neural connections between most of the respective cortical areas of the two cerebral hemispheres except for the anterior portions of the temporal lobes; these temporal areas, including especially the *amygdala,* are interconnected by fibers that pass through the *anterior commissure.*

Because of the tremendous number of fibers in the corpus callosum, it was assumed from the beginning that this massive structure must have some important function to correlate activities of the two cerebral hemispheres. However, when the corpus callosum was destroyed in laboratory animals, it was at first difficult to discern deficits in brain function. Therefore, for a long time, the function of the corpus callosum was a mystery.

Properly designed experiments have now demonstrated extremely important functions for the corpus callosum and anterior commissure. These functions can best be explained by describing one of the experiments: A monkey is first prepared by cutting the corpus callosum and splitting the optic chiasm longitudinally so that signals from each eye can go only to the cerebral hemisphere on the side of the eye. Then the monkey is taught to recognize different objects with its right eye while its left eye is covered. Next, the right eye is covered and the monkey is tested to determine whether its left eye can recognize the same objects. The answer to this is that the left eye *cannot* recognize the objects. However, on repeating the same experiment in another monkey with the optic chiasm split but the corpus callosum intact, it is found invariably that recognition in one hemisphere of the brain creates recognition in the opposite hemisphere.

Thus, one of the functions of the corpus callosum and the anterior commissure is to make information stored in the cortex of one hemisphere available to corresponding cortical areas of the opposite hemisphere. Important examples of such cooperation between the two hemispheres are the following.

1. Cutting the corpus callosum blocks transfer of information from Wernicke's area of the dominant hemisphere to the motor cortex on the opposite side of the brain. Therefore, the intellectual functions of Wernicke's area, located in the left hemisphere, lose control over the right

motor cortex that initiates voluntary motor functions of the left hand and arm, even though the usual subconscious movements of the left hand and arm are normal.

2. Cutting the corpus callosum prevents transfer of somatic and visual information from the right hemisphere into Wernicke's area in the left dominant hemisphere. Therefore, somatic and visual information from the left side of the body frequently fails to reach this general interpretative area of the brain and therefore cannot be used for decision making.

3. Finally, people whose corpus callosum is completely sectioned have two entirely separate conscious portions of the brain. For example, in a teenage boy with a sectioned corpus callosum, only the left half of his brain could understand both the written word and the spoken word because the left side was the dominant hemisphere. Conversely, the right side of the brain could understand the written word but not the spoken word. Furthermore, the right cortex could elicit a motor action response to the written word without the left cortex ever knowing why the response was performed.

The effect was quite different when an emotional response was evoked in the right side of the brain: In this case, a subconscious emotional response occurred in the left side of the brain as well. This undoubtedly occurred because the areas of the two sides of the brain for emotions, the anterior temporal cortices and adjacent areas, were still communicating with each other through the anterior commissure that was not sectioned. For instance, when the command "kiss" was written for the right half of his brain to see, the boy immediately and with full emotion said, "No way!" This response required function of Wernicke's area and the motor areas for speech in the left hemisphere because these left-side areas were necessary to speak the words "No way!" But when questioned why he said this, the boy could not explain. Thus, the two halves of the brain have independent capabilities for consciousness, memory storage, communication, and control of motor activities. The corpus callosum is required for the two sides to operate cooperatively at the superficial subconscious level, and the anterior commissure plays an important additional role in unifying the emotional responses of the two sides of the brain.

Thoughts, Consciousness, and Memory

Our most difficult problem in discussing consciousness, thoughts, memory, and learning is that we do not know the neural mechanisms of a thought and we know little about the mechanisms of memory. We know that destruction of large portions of the cerebral cortex does not prevent a person from having thoughts, but it does reduce the *depth* of the thoughts and also the *degree* of awareness of the surroundings.

Each thought certainly involves simultaneous signals in many portions of the cerebral cortex, thalamus, limbic system, and reticular formation of the brain stem. Some basic thoughts probably depend almost entirely on lower centers; the thought of pain is probably a good example because electrical stimulation of the human cortex seldom elicits anything more than mild pain, whereas stimulation of certain areas of the hypothalamus, amygdala, and mesencephalon can cause excruciating pain. Conversely, a type of thought pattern that does require large involvement of the cerebral cortex is that of vision because loss of the visual cortex causes complete inability to perceive visual form or color.

We might formulate a provisional definition of a thought in terms of neural activity as follows: A thought results from a "pattern" of stimulation of many parts of the nervous system at the same time, probably involving most importantly the cerebral cortex, thalamus, limbic system, and upper reticular formation of the brain stem. This is called the *holistic theory* of thoughts. The stimulated areas of the limbic system, thalamus, and reticular formation are believed to determine the general nature of the thought, giving it such qualities as pleasure, displeasure, pain, comfort, crude modalities of sensation, localization to gross areas of the body, and other general characteristics. However, specific stimulated areas of the cerebral cortex determine discrete characteristics of the thought, such as (1) specific localization of sensations on the surface of the body and of objects in the fields of vision, (2) the feeling of the texture of silk, (3) visual recognition of the rectangular pattern of a concrete block wall, and (4) other individual characteristics that enter into one's overall awareness of a particular instant. *Consciousness* can perhaps be described as our continuing stream of awareness of either our surroundings or our sequential thoughts.

Memory—Roles of Synaptic Facilitation and Synaptic Inhibition

Memories are stored in the brain by changing the basic sensitivity of synaptic transmission between neurons as a result of previous neural activity. The new or facilitated pathways are called *memory traces*. They are important because once the traces are established, they can be selectively activated by the thinking mind to reproduce the memories.

Experiments in lower animals have demonstrated that memory traces can occur at all levels of the nervous system. Even spinal cord reflexes can change at least slightly in response to repetitive cord activation, and these reflex changes are part of the memory process. Also, long-term memories result from changed synaptic conduction in lower brain centers. However, most memory that we associate with intellectual processes is based on memory traces in the cerebral cortex.

Positive and Negative Memory—"Sensitization" or "Habituation" of Synaptic Transmission. Although we often think of memories as being *positive* recollections of previous thoughts or experiences, probably the greater share of our memories is *negative,* not positive. That is, our brain is inundated with sensory information from all our senses. If our minds attempted to remember all this information, the memory capacity of the brain would be rapidly exceeded. Fortunately, the brain has the capability to learn to ignore information that is of no consequence. This results from *inhibition* of the synaptic pathways for this type of information; the resulting effect is called *habituation.* This is a type of *negative* memory.

Conversely, for incoming information that causes important consequences such as pain or pleasure, the brain has a different automatic capability of enhancing and storing the memory traces. This is *positive* memory. It results from *facilitation* of the synaptic pathways, and the process is called *memory sensitization.* We discuss later that special areas in the basal limbic regions of the brain determine whether information is important or unimportant and make the subconscious decision whether to store the thought as a *sensitized* memory trace or to suppress it.

Classification of Memories. We know that some memories last for only a few seconds, whereas others last for hours, days, months, or years. For the purpose of discussing these, let us use a common classification of memories that divides memories into (1) *short-term memory,* which includes memories that last for seconds or at most minutes unless they are converted into longer-term memories; (2) *intermediate long-term memories,* which last for days to weeks but then fade away; and (3) *long-term memory,* which, once stored, can be recalled up to years or even a lifetime later.

In addition to this general classification of memories, we also discussed earlier (in connection with the prefrontal lobes) another type of memory, called "working memory," which includes mainly short-term memory that is used during the course of intellectual reasoning but is terminated as each stage of the problem is resolved.

Memories are frequently classified according to the type of information that is stored. One of these classifications divides memory into *declarative memory* and *skill memory,* as follows:

1. *Declarative memory* basically means memory of the various details of an integrated thought, such as memory of an important experience that includes (1) memory of the surroundings, (2) memory of time relationships, (3) memory of causes of the experience, (4) memory of the meaning of the experience, and (5) memory of one's deductions that were left in the person's mind.

2. *Skill memory* is frequently associated with motor activities of the person's body, such as all the skills developed for hitting a tennis ball, including automatic memories to (1) sight the ball, (2) calculate the relationship and speed of the ball to the racquet, and (3) deduce rapidly the motions of the body, the arms, and the racquet required to hit the ball as desired—all of these activated instantly based on previous learning of the game of tennis—then moving on to the next stroke of the game while forgetting the details of the previous stroke.

Short-Term Memory

Short-term memory is typified by one's memory of 7 to 10 numerals in a telephone number (or 7 to 10 other discrete facts) for a few seconds to a few minutes at a time but lasting only as long as the person continues to think about the numbers or facts.

Many physiologists have suggested that this short-term memory is caused by continual neural activity resulting from nerve signals that travel around and around a temporary memory trace in a *circuit of reverberating neurons.* It has not yet been possible to prove this theory. Another possible explanation of short-term memory is *presynaptic facilitation or inhibition.* This occurs at synapses that lie on terminal nerve fibrils immediately before these fibrils synapse with a subsequent neuron. The neurotransmitter chemicals secreted at such terminals frequently cause facilitation or inhibition lasting for seconds up to several minutes. Circuits of this type could lead to short-term memory.

Intermediate Long-Term Memory

Intermediate long-term memories may last for many minutes or even weeks. They will eventually be lost unless the memory traces are activated enough to become more permanent; then they are classified as long-term memories. Experiments in primitive animals have demonstrated that memories of the intermediate long-term type can result from temporary chemical or physical changes, or both, in either the synapse presynaptic terminals or the synapse postsynaptic membrane, changes that can persist for a few minutes up to several weeks. These mechanisms are so important that they deserve special description.

Memory Based on Chemical Changes in the Presynaptic Terminal or Postsynaptic Neuronal Membrane

Figure 57-9 shows a mechanism of memory studied especially by Kandel and his colleagues that can cause memories lasting from a few minutes up to 3 weeks in the large snail *Aplysia.* In this figure, there are two synaptic terminals. One terminal is from a sensory input neuron and terminates directly on the surface of the neuron that is to be stimulated; this is called the *sensory terminal.* The other terminal is a *presynaptic ending* that lies on the surface of the sensory terminal, and it is called the *facilitator terminal.* When the sensory terminal is stimulated repeatedly but without stimulation of the facilitator terminal, signal transmission at first is great, but it becomes less and less intense with repeated stimulation until transmission almost ceases. This phenomenon is *habituation,* as was explained previously. It is a type of *negative* memory that causes the neuronal circuit to lose its response to repeated events that are insignificant.

Conversely, if a noxious stimulus excites the facilitator terminal at the same time that the sensory terminal is stimulated, then instead of the transmitted signal into

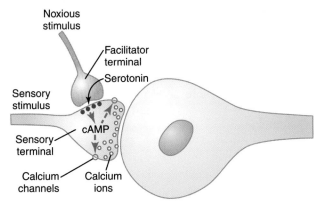

Figure 57-9 Memory system that has been discovered in the snail *Aplysia*.

the postsynaptic neuron becoming progressively weaker, the ease of transmission becomes stronger and stronger; and it will remain strong for minutes, hours, days, or, with more intense training, up to about 3 weeks even without further stimulation of the facilitator terminal. Thus, the noxious stimulus causes the memory pathway through the sensory terminal to become *facilitated* for days or weeks thereafter. It is especially interesting that even after habituation has occurred, this pathway can be converted back to a facilitated pathway with only a few noxious stimuli.

Molecular Mechanism of Intermediate Memory

Mechanism for Habituation. At the molecular level, the habituation effect in the sensory terminal results from progressive closure of calcium channels through the terminal membrane, though the cause of this calcium channel closure is not fully known. Nevertheless, much smaller than normal amounts of calcium ions can diffuse into the habituated terminal, and much less sensory terminal transmitter is therefore released because calcium entry is the principal stimulus for transmitter release (as was discussed in Chapter 45).

Mechanism for Facilitation. In the case of facilitation, at least part of the molecular mechanism is believed to be the following:

1. Stimulation of the facilitator presynaptic terminal at the same time that the sensory terminal is stimulated causes *serotonin* release at the facilitator synapse on the surface of the sensory terminal.

2. The serotonin acts on *serotonin receptors* in the sensory terminal membrane, and these receptors activate the enzyme *adenyl cyclase* inside the membrane. The adenyl cyclase then causes formation of *cyclic adenosine monophosphate (cAMP)* also inside the sensory presynaptic terminal.

3. The cyclic AMP activates a *protein kinase* that causes phosphorylation of a protein that itself is part of the potassium channels in the sensory synaptic terminal membrane; this in turn blocks the channels for potassium

conductance. The blockage can last for minutes up to several weeks.

4. Lack of potassium conductance causes a greatly prolonged action potential in the synaptic terminal because flow of potassium ions out of the terminal is necessary for rapid recovery from the action potential.

5. The prolonged action potential causes prolonged activation of the calcium channels, allowing tremendous quantities of calcium ions to enter the sensory synaptic terminal. These calcium ions cause greatly increased transmitter release by the synapse, thereby markedly facilitating synaptic transmission to the subsequent neuron.

Thus, in a very indirect way, the associative effect of stimulating the facilitator terminal at the same time that the sensory terminal is stimulated causes prolonged increase in excitatory sensitivity of the sensory terminal, and this establishes the memory trace. Studies by Byrne and colleagues, also in the snail *Aplysia*, have suggested still another mechanism of synaptic memory. Their studies have shown that stimuli from separate sources acting on a single neuron, under appropriate conditions, can cause long-term changes in *membrane properties of the postsynaptic neuron* instead of in the presynaptic neuronal membrane, but leading to essentially the same memory effects.

Long-Term Memory

There is no obvious demarcation between the more prolonged types of intermediate long-term memory and true long-term memory. The distinction is one of degree. However, long-term memory is generally believed to result from actual *structural changes*, instead of only chemical changes, at the synapses, and these enhance or suppress signal conduction. Again, let us recall experiments in primitive animals (where the nervous systems are much easier to study) that have aided immensely in understanding possible mechanisms of long-term memory.

Structural Changes Occur in Synapses During the Development of Long-Term Memory

Electron microscopic pictures taken from invertebrate animals have demonstrated multiple physical structural changes in many synapses during development of long-term memory traces. The structural changes will not occur if a drug is given that blocks DNA stimulation of protein replication in the presynaptic neuron; nor will the permanent memory trace develop. Therefore, it appears that development of true long-term memory depends on physically restructuring the synapses themselves in a way that changes their sensitivity for transmitting nervous signals.

The most important of the physical structural changes that occur are the following:

1. Increase in vesicle release sites for secretion of transmitter substance

2. Increase in number of transmitter vesicles released

3. Increase in number of presynaptic terminals

4. Changes in structures of the dendritic spines that permit transmission of stronger signals

Thus, in several different ways, the structural capability of synapses to transmit signals appears to increase during establishment of true long-term memory traces.

Number of Neurons and Their Connectivities Often Change Significantly During Learning

During the first few weeks, months, and perhaps even year or so of life, many parts of the brain produce a great excess of neurons and the neurons send out numerous axon branches to make connections with other neurons. If the new axons fail to connect with appropriate neurons, muscle cells, or gland cells, the new axons themselves will dissolute within a few weeks. Thus, the number of neuronal connections is determined by specific *nerve growth factors* released retrogradely from the stimulated cells. Furthermore, when insufficient connectivity occurs, the entire neuron that is sending out the axon branches might eventually disappear.

Therefore, soon after birth, there is a principle of "use it or lose it" that governs the final number of neurons and their connectivities in respective parts of the human nervous system. This is a type of learning. For example, if one eye of a newborn animal is covered for many weeks after birth, neurons in alternate stripes of the cerebral visual cortex—neurons normally connected to the covered eye—will degenerate, and the covered eye will remain either partially or totally blind for the remainder of life. Until recently, it was believed that very little "learning" is achieved in adult human beings and animals by modification of numbers of neurons in the memory circuits; however, recent research suggests that even adults use this mechanism to at least some extent.

Consolidation of Memory

For short-term memory to be converted into long-term memory that can be recalled weeks or years later, it must become "consolidated." That is, the short-term memory if activated repeatedly will initiate chemical, physical, and anatomical changes in the synapses that are responsible for the long-term type of memory. This process requires 5 to 10 minutes for minimal consolidation and 1 hour or more for strong consolidation. For instance, if a strong sensory impression is made on the brain but is then followed within a minute or so by an electrically induced brain convulsion, the sensory experience will not be remembered. Likewise, brain concussion, sudden application of deep general anesthesia, or any other effect that temporarily blocks the dynamic function of the brain can prevent consolidation.

Consolidation and the time required for it to occur can probably be explained by the phenomenon of rehearsal of the short-term memory as follows.

Rehearsal Enhances the Transference of Short-Term Memory into Long-Term Memory. Studies have shown that rehearsal of the same information again and again in the mind accelerates and potentiates the degree of transfer of short-term memory into long-term memory and therefore accelerates and enhances consolidation. The brain has a natural tendency to rehearse newfound information, especially newfound information that catches the mind's attention. Therefore, over a period of time, the important features of sensory experiences become progressively more and more fixed in the memory stores. This explains why a person can remember small amounts of information studied in depth far better than large amounts of information studied only superficially. It also explains why a person who is wide awake can consolidate memories far better than a person who is in a state of mental fatigue.

New Memories Are Codified During Consolidation. One of the most important features of consolidation is that new memories are *codified* into different classes of information. During this process, similar types of information are pulled from the memory storage bins and used to help process the new information. The new and old are compared for similarities and differences, and part of the storage process is to store the information about these similarities and differences, rather than to store the new information unprocessed. Thus, during consolidation, the new memories are not stored randomly in the brain but are stored in direct association with other memories of the same type. This is necessary if one is to be able to "search" the memory store at a later date to find the required information.

Role of Specific Parts of the Brain in the Memory Process

Hippocampus Promotes Storage of Memories—Anterograde Amnesia After Hippocampal Lesions. The hippocampus is the most medial portion of the temporal lobe cortex, where it folds first medially underneath the brain and then upward into the lower, inside surface of the lateral ventricle. The two hippocampi have been removed for the treatment of epilepsy in a few patients. This procedure does not seriously affect the person's memory for information stored in the brain before removal of the hippocampi. However, after removal, these people have virtually no capability thereafter for storing *verbal and symbolic types* of memories (declarative types of memory) in long-term memory, or even in intermediate memory lasting longer than a few minutes. Therefore, these people are unable to establish new long-term memories of those types of information that are the basis of intelligence. This is called *anterograde amnesia*.

But why are the hippocampi so important in helping the brain to store new memories? The probable answer is that the hippocampi are among the most important output pathways from the "reward" and "punishment" areas of the limbic system, as explained in Chapter 58. Sensory stimuli or thoughts that cause pain or aversion excite the limbic *punishment centers,* and stimuli that cause pleasure, happiness, or sense of reward excite the limbic *reward centers.* All these together provide the background mood and motivations of the person. Among these motivations is the drive in the brain to remember those experiences and thoughts that are either pleasant or unpleasant. The hippocampi especially and to a lesser degree the dorsal medial nuclei of the thalamus, another limbic structure, have proved especially important in making the decision about which of our thoughts are important enough on a basis of reward or punishment to be worthy of memory.

Retrograde Amnesia—Inability to Recall Memories from the Past. When retrograde amnesia occurs, the degree of amnesia for recent events is likely to be much greater than for events of the distant past. The reason for this difference is probably that the distant memories have been rehearsed so many times that the memory traces are deeply ingrained, and elements of these memories are stored in widespread areas of the brain.

In some people who have hippocampal lesions, some degree of retrograde amnesia occurs along with anterograde amnesia, which suggests that these two types of amnesia are at least partially related and that hippocampal lesions can cause both. However, damage in some thalamic areas may lead specifically to retrograde amnesia without causing significant anterograde amnesia. A possible explanation of this is that the thalamus may play a role in helping the person "search" the memory storehouses and thus "read out" the memories. That is, the memory process not only requires the storing of memories but also an ability to search and find the memory at a later date. The possible function of the thalamus in this process is discussed further in Chapter 58.

Hippocampi Are Not Important in Reflexive Learning. People with hippocampal lesions usually do not have difficulty in learning physical skills that do not involve verbalization or symbolic types of intelligence. For instance, these people can still learn the rapid hand and physical skills required in many types of sports. This type of learning is called *skill learning* or *reflexive learning;* it depends on physically repeating the required tasks over and over again, rather than on symbolical rehearsing in the mind.

Bibliography

Bailey CH, Kandel ER: Synaptic remodeling, synaptic growth and the storage of long-term memory in Aplysia, *Prog Brain Res* 169:179, 2008.

Glickstein M: Paradoxical inter-hemispheric transfer after section of the cerebral commissures, *Exp Brain Res* 192:425, 2009.

Haggard P: Human volition: towards a neuroscience of will, *Nat Rev Neurosci* 9:934, 2008.

Hickok G, Poeppel D: The cortical organization of speech processing, *Nat Rev Neurosci* 8:393, 2007.

Kandel ER: The molecular biology of memory storage: a dialogue between genes and synapses, *Science* 294:1030, 2001.

Kandel ER, Schwartz JH, Jessell TM: *Principles of Neural Science*, ed 4, New York, 2000, McGraw-Hill.

LaBar KS, Cabeza R: Cognitive neuroscience of emotional memory, *Nat Rev Neurosci* 7:54, 2006.

Lee YS, Silva AJ: The molecular and cellular biology of enhanced cognition, *Nat Rev Neurosci* 10:126, 2009.

Lynch MA: Long-term potentiation and memory, *Physiol Rev* 84:87, 2004.

Mansouri FA, Tanaka K, Buckley MJ: Conflict-induced behavioural adjustment: a clue to the executive functions of the prefrontal cortex, *Nat Rev Neurosci* 10:141, 2009.

Nader K, Hardt O: A single standard for memory: the case for reconsolidation, *Nat Rev Neurosci* 10:224, 2009.

Osada T, Adachi Y, Kimura HM, et al: Towards understanding of the cortical network underlying associative memory, *Philos Trans R Soc Lond B Biol Sci* 363:2187, 2008.

Roth TL, Sweatt JD: Rhythms of memory, *Nat Neurosci* 11:993, 2008.

Shirvalkar PR: Hippocampal neural assemblies and conscious remembering, *J Neurophysiol* 101:2197, 2009.

Tanji J, Hoshi E: Role of the lateral prefrontal cortex in executive behavioral control, *Physiol Rev* 88:37, 2008.

Tronson NC, Taylor JR: Molecular mechanisms of memory reconsolidation, *Nat Rev Neurosci* 8:262, 2007.

van Strien NM, Cappaert NL, Witter MP: The anatomy of memory: an interactive overview of the parahippocampal-hippocampal network, *Nat Rev Neurosci* 10:272, 2009.

Wilson DA, Linster C: Neurobiology of a simple memory, *J Neurophysiol* 100:2, 2008.

Zamarian L, Ischebeck A, Delazer M: Neuroscience of learning arithmetic—evidence from brain imaging studies, *Neurosci Biobehav Rev* 33:909, 2009.

Behavioral and Motivational Mechanisms of the Brain—The Limbic System and the Hypothalamus

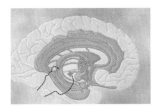

Control of behavior is a function of the entire nervous system. Even the wakefulness and sleep cycle discussed in Chapter 59 is one of our most important behavioral patterns.

In this chapter, we deal first with those mechanisms that control levels of activity in the different parts of the brain. Then we discuss the causes of motivational drives, especially motivational control of the learning process and feelings of pleasure and punishment. These functions of the nervous system are performed mainly by the basal regions of the brain, which together are loosely called the *limbic system*, meaning the "border" system.

Activating—Driving Systems of the Brain

Without continuous transmission of nerve signals from the lower brain into the cerebrum, the cerebrum becomes useless. In fact, severe compression of the brain stem at the juncture between the mesencephalon and cerebrum, as sometimes results from a pineal tumor, often causes the person to go into unremitting coma lasting for the remainder of his or her life.

Nerve signals in the brain stem activate the cerebral part of the brain in two ways: (1) by directly stimulating a background level of neuronal activity in wide areas of the brain and (2) by activating neurohormonal systems that release specific facilitory or inhibitory hormone-like neurotransmitter substances into selected areas of the brain.

Control of Cerebral Activity by Continuous Excitatory Signals from the Brain Stem
Reticular Excitatory Area of the Brain Stem

Figure 58-1 shows a general system for controlling the level of activity of the brain. The central driving component of this system is an excitatory area located in the *reticular substance of the pons and mesencephalon*. This area is also known by the name *bulboreticular facilitory area*. We also discuss this area in Chapter 55 because it is the same brain stem reticular area that transmits facilitory signals *downward to the spinal cord* to maintain tone in the antigravity muscles and to control levels of activity of the spinal cord reflexes. In addition to these downward signals, this area also sends a profusion of signals in the upward direction. Most of these go first to the thalamus, where they excite a different set of neurons that transmit nerve signals to all regions of the cerebral cortex, as well as to multiple subcortical areas.

The signals passing through the thalamus are of two types. One type is rapidly transmitted action potentials that excite the cerebrum for only a few milliseconds. These originate from large neuronal cell bodies that lie throughout the brain stem reticular area. Their nerve endings release the neurotransmitter substance *acetylcholine*, which serves as an excitatory agent, lasting for only a few milliseconds before it is destroyed.

The second type of excitatory signal originates from large numbers of small neurons spread throughout the brain stem reticular excitatory area. Again, most of these pass to the thalamus, but this time through small, slowly conducting fibers that synapse mainly in the intralaminar nuclei of the thalamus and in the reticular nuclei over the surface of the thalamus. From here, additional small fibers are distributed everywhere in the cerebral cortex. The excitatory effect caused by this system of fibers can build up progressively for many seconds to a minute or more, which suggests that its signals are especially important for controlling longer-term background excitability level of the brain.

Excitation of the Excitatory Area by Peripheral Sensory Signals. The level of activity of the excitatory area in the brain stem, and therefore the level of activity of the entire brain, is determined to a great extent by the number and type of sensory signals that enter the brain from the periphery. Pain signals in particular increase activity in this excitatory area and therefore strongly excite the brain to attention.

The importance of sensory signals in activating the excitatory area is demonstrated by the effect of cutting the brain stem above the point where the fifth cerebral nerves enter the pons. These nerves are the highest nerves entering the brain that transmit significant numbers of somatosensory signals into the brain. When all these

711

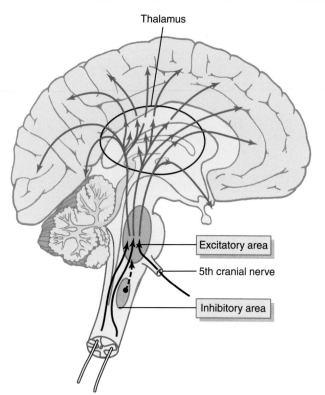

Thalamus

Excitatory area

5th cranial nerve

Inhibitory area

Figure 58-1 *Excitatory-activating system* of the brain. Also shown is an *inhibitory area* in the medulla that can inhibit or depress the activating system.

input sensory signals are gone, the level of activity in the brain excitatory area diminishes abruptly, and the brain proceeds instantly to a state of greatly reduced activity, approaching a permanent state of coma. But when the brain stem is transected *below* the fifth nerves, which leaves much input of sensory signals from the facial and oral regions, the coma is averted.

Increased Activity of the Excitatory Area Caused by Feedback Signals Returning from the Cerebral Cortex. Not only do excitatory signals pass to the cerebral cortex from the bulboreticular excitatory area of the brain stem, but feedback signals also return from the cerebral cortex back to this same area. Therefore, any time the cerebral cortex becomes activated by either brain thought processes or motor processes, signals are sent from the cortex to the brain stem excitatory area, which in turn sends still more excitatory signals to the cortex. This helps to maintain the level of excitation of the cerebral cortex or even to enhance it. This is a general mechanism of *positive feedback* that allows any beginning activity in the cerebral cortex to support still more activity, thus leading to an "awake" mind.

Thalamus Is a Distribution Center That Controls Activity in Specific Regions of the Cortex. As pointed out in Chapter 57 and shown in Figure 57-2, almost every area of the cerebral cortex connects with its own highly specific area in the thalamus. Therefore, electrical stimulation of a specific point in the thalamus generally activates its own specific small region of the cortex. Furthermore, signals regularly reverberate back and forth between the thalamus and the cerebral cortex, the thalamus exciting the cortex and the cortex then re-exciting the thalamus by

way of return fibers. It has been suggested that the thinking process establishes long-term memories by activating such back-and-forth reverberation of signals.

Can the thalamus also function to call forth specific memories from the cortex or to activate specific thought processes? Proof of this is still lacking, but the thalamus does have appropriate neuronal circuitry for these purposes.

A Reticular Inhibitory Area Is Located in the Lower Brain Stem

Figure 58-1 shows still another area that is important in controlling brain activity. This is the reticular *inhibitory area*, located medially and ventrally in the medulla. In Chapter 55, we learned that this area can inhibit the reticular facilitory area of the upper brain stem and thereby decrease activity in the superior portions of the brain as well. One of the mechanisms for this is to excite *serotonergic neurons*; these in turn secrete the inhibitory neurohormone *serotonin* at crucial points in the brain; we discuss this in more detail later.

Neurohormonal Control of Brain Activity

Aside from direct control of brain activity by specific transmission of nerve signals from the lower brain areas to the cortical regions of the brain, still another physiologic mechanism is very often used to control brain activity. This is to secrete *excitatory* or *inhibitory neurotransmitter hormonal agents* into the substance of the brain. These neurohormones often persist for minutes or hours and thereby provide long periods of control, rather than just instantaneous activation or inhibition.

Figure 58-2 shows three neurohormonal systems that have been studied in detail in the rat brain: (1) a *norepinephrine system*, (2) a *dopamine system*, and (3) a *serotonin system*. Norepinephrine usually functions as an excitatory hormone, whereas serotonin is usually inhibitory and dopamine is excitatory in some areas but inhibitory in others. As would be expected, these three systems have different effects on levels of excitability in different parts of the brain. The norepinephrine system spreads to virtually every area of the brain, whereas the serotonin and dopamine systems are directed much more to specific brain regions—the dopamine system mainly into the basal ganglial regions and the serotonin system more into the midline structures.

Neurohormonal Systems in the Human Brain. Figure 58-3 shows the brain stem areas in the human brain for activating four neurohormonal systems, the same three discussed for the rat and one other, the *acetylcholine system*. Some of the specific functions of these are as follows:

1. *The locus ceruleus and the norepinephrine system.* The locus ceruleus is a small area located bilaterally and posteriorly at the juncture between the pons and mesencephalon. Nerve fibers from this area spread throughout the brain, the same as shown for the rat in the top frame of Figure 58-2, and they secrete

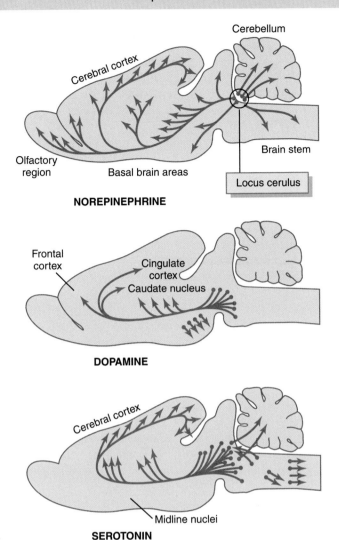

Figure 58-2 Three neurohormonal systems that have been mapped in the rat brain: a *norepinephrine system,* a *dopamine system,* and a *serotonin system.* (Adapted from Kelly, after Cooper, Bloom, and Roth: In: Kandel ER, Schwartz JH (eds): Principles of Neural Science, 2nd ed. New York: Elsevier, 1985.)

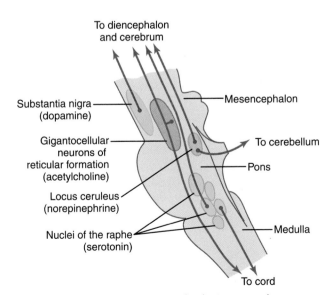

Figure 58-3 Multiple centers in the brain stem, the neurons of which secrete different transmitter substances (specified in parentheses). These neurons send control signals upward into the diencephalon and cerebrum and downward into the spinal cord.

norepinephrine. The norepinephrine generally excites the brain to increased activity. However, it has inhibitory effects in a few brain areas because of inhibitory receptors at certain neuronal synapses. Chapter 59 covers how this system probably plays an important role in causing dreaming, thus leading to a type of sleep called rapid eye movement sleep *(REM sleep).*

2. *The substantia nigra and the dopamine system.* The substantia nigra is discussed in Chapter 56 in relation to the basal ganglia. It lies anteriorly in the superior mesencephalon, and its neurons send nerve endings mainly to the caudate nucleus and putamen of the cerebrum, where they secrete *dopamine.* Other neurons located in adjacent regions also secrete dopamine, but they send their endings into more ventral areas of the brain, especially to the hypothalamus and the limbic system. The dopamine is believed to act as an inhibitory transmitter in the basal ganglia, but in some other areas of the brain it is possibly excitatory. Also, remember from Chapter 56 that destruction of the dopaminergic neurons in the substantia nigra is the basic cause of Parkinson's disease.

3. *The raphe nuclei and the serotonin system.* In the midline of the pons and medulla are several thin nuclei called the raphe nuclei. Many of the neurons in these nuclei secrete *serotonin.* They send fibers into the diencephalon and a few fibers to the cerebral cortex; still other fibers descend to the spinal cord. The serotonin secreted at the cord fiber endings has the ability to suppress pain, which was discussed in Chapter 48. The serotonin released in the diencephalon and cerebrum almost certainly plays an essential inhibitory role to help cause normal sleep, as we discuss in Chapter 59.

4. *The gigantocellular neurons of the reticular excitatory area and the acetylcholine system.* Earlier we discussed the gigantocellular neurons *(giant cells)* in the reticular excitatory area of the pons and mesencephalon. The fibers from these large cells divide immediately into two branches, one passing upward to the higher levels of the brain and the other passing downward through the reticulospinal tracts into the spinal cord. The neurohormone secreted at their terminals is *acetylcholine.* In most places, the acetylcholine functions as an excitatory neurotransmitter. Activation of these acetylcholine neurons leads to an acutely awake and excited nervous system.

Other Neurotransmitters and Neurohormonal Substances Secreted in the Brain. Without describing their function, the following is a partial list of still other neurohormonal substances that function either at specific synapses or by release into the fluids of the brain: enkephalins, gamma-aminobutyric acid, glutamate, vasopressin, adrenocorticotropic hormone, α-melanocyte stimulating hormone (α-MSH), neuropeptide-Y (NPY), epinephrine, histamine, endorphins, angiotensin II, and neurotensin. Thus, there are multiple neurohormonal systems in the brain, the activation of each of which plays its own role in controlling a different quality of brain function.

Limbic System

The word "limbic" means "border." Originally, the term "limbic" was used to describe the border structures around the basal regions of the cerebrum, but as we have learned more about the functions of the limbic system, the term *limbic system* has been expanded to mean the entire neuronal circuitry that controls emotional behavior and motivational drives.

A major part of the limbic system is the *hypothalamus,* with its related structures. In addition to their roles in behavioral control, these areas control many internal conditions of the body, such as body temperature, osmolality of the body fluids, and the drives to eat and drink and to control body weight. These internal functions are collectively called *vegetative functions* of the brain, and their control is closely related to behavior.

Functional Anatomy of the Limbic System; Key Position of the Hypothalamus

Figure 58-4 shows the anatomical structures of the limbic system, demonstrating that they are an interconnected complex of basal brain elements. Located in the middle of all these is the extremely small *hypothalamus,* which from a physiologic point of view is one of the central elements of the limbic system. Figure 58-5 illustrates schematically

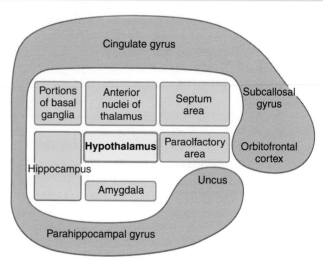

Figure 58-5 Limbic system, showing the key position of the hypothalamus.

this key position of the hypothalamus in the limbic system and shows surrounding it other subcortical structures of the limbic system, including the *septum, paraolfactory area, anterior nucleus of the thalamus, portions of the basal ganglia, hippocampus,* and *amygdala.*

And surrounding the subcortical limbic areas is the *limbic cortex,* composed of a ring of cerebral cortex in each side of the brain (1) beginning in the *orbitofrontal area* on the ventral surface of the frontal lobes, (2) extending upward into the *subcallosal gyrus,* (3) then over the

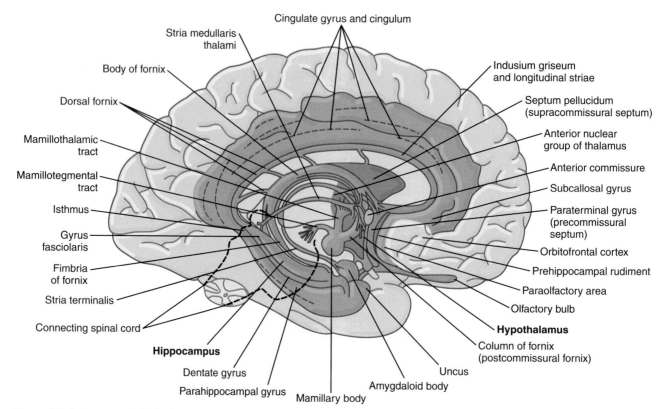

Figure 58-4 Anatomy of the limbic system, shown in the dark pink area. (Redrawn from Warwick R, Williams PL: Gray's Anatomy, 35th Br. ed. London: Longman Group Ltd, 1973.)

top of the corpus callosum onto the medial aspect of the cerebral hemisphere in the *cingulate gyrus,* and finally (4) passing behind the corpus callosum and downward onto the ventromedial surface of the temporal lobe to the *parahippocampal gyrus* and *uncus.*

Thus, on the medial and ventral surfaces of each cerebral hemisphere is a ring of mostly *paleocortex* that surrounds a group of deep structures intimately associated with overall behavior and emotions. In turn, this ring of limbic cortex functions as a two-way communication and association linkage between the *neocortex* and the lower limbic structures.

Many of the behavioral functions elicited from the hypothalamus and other limbic structures are also mediated through the reticular nuclei in the brain stem and their associated nuclei. It was pointed out in Chapter 55, as well as earlier in this chapter, that stimulation of the excitatory portion of this reticular formation can cause high degrees of cerebral excitability while also increasing the excitability of much of the spinal cord synapses. In Chapter 60, we see that most of the hypothalamic signals for controlling the autonomic nervous system are also transmitted through synaptic nuclei located in the brain stem.

An important route of communication between the limbic system and the brain stem is the *medial forebrain bundle,* which extends from the septal and orbitofrontal regions of the cerebral cortex downward through the middle of the hypothalamus to the brain stem reticular formation. This bundle carries fibers in both directions, forming a trunk line communication system. A second route of communication is through short pathways among the reticular formation of the brain stem, thalamus, hypothalamus, and most other contiguous areas of the basal brain.

Hypothalamus, a Major Control Headquarters for the Limbic System

The hypothalamus, despite its small size of only a few cubic centimeters, has two-way communicating pathways with all levels of the limbic system. In turn, the hypothalamus and its closely allied structures send output signals in three directions: (1) backward and downward to the brain stem, mainly into the reticular areas of the mesencephalon, pons, and medulla and from these areas into the peripheral nerves of the autonomic nervous system; (2) upward toward many higher areas of the diencephalon and cerebrum, especially to the anterior thalamus and limbic portions of the cerebral cortex; and (3) into the hypothalamic infundibulum to control or partially control most of the secretory functions of both the posterior and the anterior pituitary glands.

Thus, the hypothalamus, which represents less than 1 percent of the brain mass, is one of the most important of the control pathways of the limbic system. It controls most of the vegetative and endocrine functions of the body and

many aspects of emotional behavior. Let us discuss first the vegetative and endocrine control functions and then return to the behavioral functions of the hypothalamus to see how these operate together.

Vegetative and Endocrine Control Functions of the Hypothalamus

The different hypothalamic mechanisms for controlling multiple functions of the body are so important that they are discussed in multiple chapters throughout this text. For instance, the role of the hypothalamus to help regulate arterial pressure is discussed in Chapter 18, thirst and water conservation in Chapter 29, appetite and energy expenditure in Chapter 71, temperature regulation in Chapter 73, and endocrine control in Chapter 75. To illustrate the organization of the hypothalamus as a functional unit, let us summarize the more important of its vegetative and endocrine functions here as well.

Figures 58-6 and 58-7 show enlarged sagittal and coronal views of the hypothalamus, which represents only a small area in Figure 58-4. Take a few minutes to study these diagrams, especially to see in Figure 58-6 the multiple activities that are excited or inhibited when respective hypothalamic nuclei are stimulated. In addition to the centers shown in Figure 58-6, a large *lateral hypothalamic* area (shown in Figure 58-7) is present on each side of the hypothalamus. The lateral areas are especially important in controlling thirst, hunger, and many of the emotional drives.

A word of caution must be issued for studying these diagrams because the areas that cause specific activities are not nearly as accurately localized as suggested in the figures. Also, it is not known whether the effects noted in the figures result from stimulation of specific control nuclei or whether they result merely from activation of fiber tracts leading from or to control nuclei located elsewhere. With this caution in mind, we can give the following general description of the vegetative and control functions of the hypothalamus.

Cardiovascular Regulation. Stimulation of different areas throughout the hypothalamus can cause many neurogenic effects on the cardiovascular system, including increased arterial pressure, decreased arterial pressure, increased heart rate, and decreased heart rate. In general, stimulation in the *posterior* and *lateral hypothalamus* increases the arterial pressure and heart rate, whereas stimulation in the *preoptic area* often has opposite effects, causing a decrease in both heart rate and arterial pressure. These effects are transmitted mainly through specific cardiovascular control centers in the reticular regions of the pons and medulla.

Regulation of Body Temperature. The anterior portion of the hypothalamus, especially the *preoptic area,* is concerned with regulation of body temperature. An increase in the temperature of the blood flowing through this area increases the activity of temperature-sensitive neurons, whereas a decrease in temperature decreases their activity. In turn, these neurons control mechanisms for increasing or decreasing body temperature, as discussed in Chapter 73.

Figure 58-6 Control centers of the hypothalamus (sagittal view).

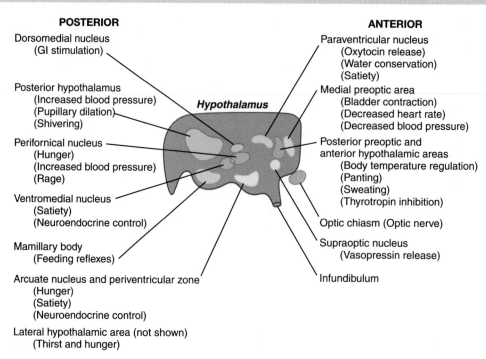

POSTERIOR

Dorsomedial nucleus
(GI stimulation)

Posterior hypothalamus
(Increased blood pressure)
(Pupillary dilation)
(Shivering)

Periformical nucleus
(Hunger)
(Increased blood pressure)
(Rage)

Ventromedial nucleus
(Satiety)
(Neuroendocrine control)

Mamillary body
(Feeding reflexes)

Arcuate nucleus and periventricular zone
(Hunger)
(Satiety)
(Neuroendocrine control)

Lateral hypothalamic area (not shown)
(Thirst and hunger)

Hypothalamus

ANTERIOR

Paraventricular nucleus
(Oxytocin release)
(Water conservation)
(Satiety)

Medial preoptic area
(Bladder contraction)
(Decreased heart rate)
(Decreased blood pressure)

Posterior preoptic and
anterior hypothalamic areas
(Body temperature regulation)
(Panting)
(Sweating)
(Thyrotropin inhibition)

Optic chiasm (Optic nerve)

Supraoptic nucleus
(Vasopressin release)

Infundibulum

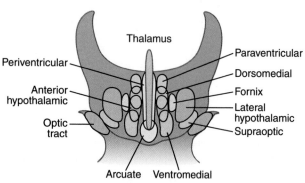

Thalamus

Periventricular

Anterior
hypothalamic

Optic
tract

Paraventricular

Dorsomedial

Fornix

Lateral
hypothalamic

Supraoptic

Arcuate   Ventromedial

Figure 58-7 Coronal view of the hypothalamus, showing the mediolateral positions of the respective hypothalamic nuclei.

Regulation of Body Water. The hypothalamus regulates body water in two ways: (1) by creating the sensation of thirst, which drives the animal or person to drink water, and (2) by controlling the excretion of water into the urine. An area called the *thirst center* is located in the lateral hypothalamus. When the fluid electrolytes in either this center or closely allied areas become too concentrated, the animal develops an intense desire to drink water; it will search out the nearest source of water and drink enough to return the electrolyte concentration of the thirst center to normal.

Control of renal excretion of water is vested mainly in the *supraoptic* nuclei. When the body fluids become too concentrated, the neurons of these areas become stimulated. Nerve fibers from these neurons project downward through the infundibulum of the hypothalamus into the posterior pituitary gland, where the nerve endings secrete the hormone *antidiuretic hormone* (also called *vasopressin*). This hormone is then absorbed into the blood and transported to the kidneys, where it acts on the collecting ducts of the kidneys to cause increased reabsorption of water. This decreases loss of water into the urine but allows continuing excretion of electrolytes, thus decreasing the concentration of the body fluids back toward normal. These functions are presented in Chapter 28.

Regulation of Uterine Contractility and of Milk Ejection from the Breasts. Stimulation of the *paraventricular nuclei* causes their neuronal cells to secrete the hormone *oxytocin*. This in turn causes increased contractility of the uterus, as well as contraction of the myoepithelial cells surrounding the alveoli of the breasts, which then causes the alveoli to empty their milk through the nipples.

At the end of pregnancy, especially large quantities of oxytocin are secreted and this secretion helps to promote labor contractions that expel the baby. Then, whenever the baby suckles the mother's breast, a reflex signal from the nipple to the posterior hypothalamus also causes oxytocin release and the oxytocin now performs the necessary function of contracting the ductules of the breast, thereby expelling milk through the nipples so that the baby can nourish itself. These functions are discussed in Chapter 82.

Gastrointestinal and Feeding Regulation. Stimulation of several areas of the hypothalamus causes an animal to experience extreme hunger, a voracious appetite, and an intense desire to search for food. One area associated with hunger is the *lateral hypothalamic area*. Conversely, damage to this area on both sides of the hypothalamus causes the animal to lose desire for food, sometimes causing lethal starvation as discussed in Chapter 71.

A center that opposes the desire for food, called the *satiety center*, is located in the *ventromedial nuclei*. When this center is stimulated electrically, an animal that is eating food suddenly stops eating and shows complete indifference to food. However, if this area is destroyed bilaterally, the animal cannot be satiated; instead, its hypothalamic hunger centers become overactive, so it has a voracious appetite, resulting eventually in tremendous obesity. Another area of the hypothalamus that enters into overall control of gastrointestinal activity is the *mamillary bodies;* these control at least partially the patterns of many feeding reflexes, such as licking the lips and swallowing.

Hypothalamic Control of Endocrine Hormone Secretion by the Anterior Pituitary Gland. Stimulation of certain areas of the hypothalamus also causes the *anterior* pituitary gland to secrete its endocrine hormones. This subject is discussed in detail in Chapter 74 in relation to neural control of the endocrine glands. Briefly, the basic mechanisms are the following.

The anterior pituitary gland receives its blood supply mainly from blood that flows first through the lower part of the hypothalamus and then through the anterior pituitary vascular sinuses. As the blood courses through the hypothalamus before reaching the anterior pituitary, specific *releasing* and *inhibitory hormones* are secreted into the blood by various hypothalamic nuclei. These hormones are then transported via the blood to the anterior pituitary gland, where they act on the glandular cells to control release of specific anterior pituitary hormones.

Summary. Several areas of the hypothalamus control specific vegetative and endocrine functions. These areas are still poorly delimited, so the specification given earlier of different areas for different hypothalamic functions is still partially tentative.

Behavioral Functions of the Hypothalamus and Associated Limbic Structures

Effects Caused by Stimulation of the Hypothalamus.
In addition to the vegetative and endocrine functions of the hypothalamus, stimulation of or lesions in the hypothalamus often have profound effects on emotional behavior of animals and human beings.

Some of the behavioral effects of stimulation are the following:

1. Stimulation in the *lateral hypothalamus* not only causes thirst and eating, as discussed earlier, but also increases the general level of activity of the animal, sometimes leading to overt rage and fighting, as discussed subsequently.

2. Stimulation in the *ventromedial nucleus* and surrounding areas mainly causes effects opposite to those caused by lateral hypothalamic stimulation—that is, a sense of *satiety, decreased eating,* and *tranquility.*

3. Stimulation of a *thin zone of periventricular nuclei,* located immediately adjacent to the third ventricle (or also stimulation of the central gray area of the mesencephalon that is continuous with this portion of the hypothalamus), usually leads to *fear* and *punishment reactions.*

4. *Sexual drive* can be stimulated from several areas of the hypothalamus, especially the most anterior and most posterior portions of the hypothalamus.

Effects Caused by Hypothalamic Lesions.
Lesions in the hypothalamus, in general, cause effects opposite to those caused by stimulation. For instance:

1. Bilateral lesions in the lateral hypothalamus will decrease drinking and eating almost to zero, often leading to lethal starvation. These lesions cause extreme *passivity* of the animal as well, with loss of most of its overt drives.

2. Bilateral lesions of the ventromedial areas of the hypothalamus cause effects that are mainly opposite to those caused by lesions of the lateral hypothalamus:

excessive drinking and eating, as well as hyperactivity and often continuous savagery along with frequent bouts of extreme rage on the slightest provocation.

Stimulation or lesions in other regions of the limbic system, especially in the amygdala, the septal area, and areas in the mesencephalon, often cause effects similar to those elicited from the hypothalamus. We discuss some of these in more detail later.

"Reward" and "Punishment" Function of the Limbic System

From the discussion thus far, it is already clear that several limbic structures are particularly concerned with the *affective* nature of sensory sensations—that is, whether the sensations are *pleasant* or *unpleasant.* These affective qualities are also called *reward* or *punishment,* or *satisfaction* or *aversion.* Electrical stimulation of certain limbic areas pleases or satisfies the animal, whereas electrical stimulation of other regions causes terror, pain, fear, defense, escape reactions, and all the other elements of punishment. The degrees of stimulation of these two oppositely responding systems greatly affect the behavior of the animal.

Reward Centers

Experimental studies in monkeys have used electrical stimulators to map out the reward and punishment centers of the brain. The technique that has been used is to implant electrodes in different areas of the brain so that the animal can stimulate the area by pressing a lever that makes electrical contact with a stimulator. If stimulating the particular area gives the animal a sense of reward, then it will press the lever again and again, sometimes as much as hundreds or even thousands of times per hour. Furthermore, when offered the choice of eating some delectable food as opposed to the opportunity to stimulate the reward center, the animal often chooses the electrical stimulation.

By using this procedure, the major reward centers have been found to be located *along the course of the medial forebrain bundle,* especially in the *lateral* and *ventromedial nuclei of the hypothalamus.* It is strange that the lateral nucleus should be included among the reward areas—indeed, it is one of the most potent of all—because even stronger stimuli in this area can cause rage. But this is true in many areas, with weaker stimuli giving a sense of reward and stronger ones a sense of punishment. Less potent reward centers, which are perhaps secondary to the major ones in the hypothalamus, are found in the septum, the amygdala, certain areas of the thalamus and basal ganglia, and extending downward into the basal tegmentum of the mesencephalon.

Punishment Centers

The stimulator apparatus discussed earlier can also be connected so that the stimulus to the brain continues all the time *except* when the lever is pressed. In this case, the animal will not press the lever to turn the stimulus off when the electrode is in one of the reward areas; but when it is in certain other areas, the animal immediately learns to turn it off. Stimulation in these areas causes the animal to show all the signs of displeasure, fear, terror, pain, punishment, and even sickness.

By means of this technique, the most potent areas for punishment and escape tendencies have been found in the central gray area surrounding the aqueduct of Sylvius in the mesencephalon and extending upward into the periventricular zones of the hypothalamus and thalamus. Less potent punishment areas are found in some locations in the amygdala and hippocampus. It is particularly interesting that stimulation in the punishment centers can frequently inhibit the reward and pleasure centers completely, demonstrating that *punishment and fear can take precedence over pleasure and reward.*

Rage—Its Association with Punishment Centers

An emotional pattern that involves the punishment centers of the hypothalamus and other limbic structures, and has also been well characterized, is the *rage pattern,* described as follows.

Strong stimulation of the punishment centers of the brain, especially in the *periventricular zone of the hypothalamus* and in the *lateral hypothalamus,* causes the animal to (1) develop a defense posture, (2) extend its claws, (3) lift its tail, (4) hiss, (5) spit, (6) growl, and (7) develop piloerection, wide-open eyes, and dilated pupils. Furthermore, even the slightest provocation causes an immediate savage attack. This is approximately the behavior that one would expect from an animal being severely punished, and it is a pattern of behavior that is called *rage.*

Fortunately, in the normal animal, the rage phenomenon is held in check mainly by inhibitory signals from the ventromedial nuclei of the hypothalamus. In addition, portions of the hippocampi and anterior limbic cortex, especially in the anterior cingulate gyri and subcallosal gyri, help suppress the rage phenomenon.

Placidity and Tameness. Exactly the opposite emotional behavior patterns occur when the reward centers are stimulated: placidity and tameness.

Importance of Reward or Punishment on Behavior

Almost everything that we do is related in some way to reward and punishment. If we are doing something that is rewarding, we continue to do it; if it is punishing, we cease to do it. Therefore, the reward and punishment centers undoubtedly constitute one of the most important of all the controllers of our bodily activities, our drives, our aversions, our motivations.

Effect of Tranquilizers on the Reward or Punishment Centers. Administration of a tranquilizer, such as chlorpromazine, usually inhibits both the reward and the punishment centers, thereby decreasing the affective reactivity of the animal. Therefore, it is presumed that tranquilizers function in psychotic states by suppressing many of the important behavioral areas of the hypothalamus and its associated regions of the limbic brain.

Importance of Reward or Punishment in Learning and Memory—Habituation Versus Reinforcement

Animal experiments have shown that a sensory experience that causes neither reward nor punishment is hardly remembered at all. Electrical recordings from the brain show that a newly experienced sensory stimulus almost always excites multiple areas in the cerebral cortex. But if the sensory experience does not elicit a sense of either reward or punishment, repetition of the stimulus over and over leads to almost complete extinction of the cerebral cortical response. That is, the animal becomes *habituated* to that specific sensory stimulus and thereafter ignores it.

If the stimulus *does* cause either reward or punishment rather than indifference, the cerebral cortical response becomes progressively more and more intense during repeated stimulation instead of fading away, and the response is said to be *reinforced.* An animal builds up strong memory traces for sensations that are either rewarding or punishing but, conversely, develops complete habituation to indifferent sensory stimuli.

It is evident that the reward and punishment centers of the limbic system have much to do with selecting the information that we learn, usually throwing away more than 99 percent of it and selecting less than 1 percent for retention.

Specific Functions of Other Parts of the Limbic System

Functions of the Hippocampus

The hippocampus is the elongated portion of the cerebral cortex that folds inward to form the ventral surface of much of the inside of the lateral ventricle. One end of the hippocampus abuts the amygdaloid nuclei, and along its lateral border it fuses with the parahippocampal gyrus, which is the cerebral cortex on the ventromedial outside surface of the temporal lobe.

The hippocampus (and its adjacent temporal and parietal lobe structures, all together called the *hippocampal formation*) has numerous but mainly indirect connections with many portions of the cerebral cortex, as well as with the basal structures of the limbic system—the amygdala, hypothalamus, septum, and mamillary bodies. Almost any type of sensory experience causes activation of at least some part of the hippocampus, and the hippocampus in turn distributes many outgoing signals to the anterior thalamus, hypothalamus, and other parts of the limbic system, especially through the *fornix,* a major communicating pathway. Thus, the hippocampus is an additional channel through which incoming sensory signals can initiate behavioral reactions for different purposes. As in other limbic structures, stimulation of different areas in the hippocampus can cause almost any of the different behavioral patterns such as pleasure, rage, passivity, or excess sex drive.

Another feature of the hippocampus is that it can become hyperexcitable. For instance, weak electrical stimuli can cause focal epileptic seizures in small areas of the hippocampi. These often persist for many seconds after the stimulation is over, suggesting that the hippocampi can perhaps give off prolonged output signals even under normal functioning conditions. During hippocampal seizures, the person experiences various psychomotor effects, including olfactory, visual, auditory, tactile, and other types of hallucinations that cannot be suppressed as long as the seizure persists even though the person has not lost consciousness and knows these hallucinations to be unreal. Probably one of the reasons for this hyperexcitability of the hippocampi is that they have a different type of cortex from that elsewhere in the cerebrum, with only three nerve cell layers in some of its areas instead of the six layers found elsewhere.

Role of the Hippocampus in Learning

Effect of Bilateral Removal of the Hippocampi— Inability to Learn. Portions of the hippocampi have been surgically removed bilaterally in a few human beings for treatment of epilepsy. These people can recall most previously learned memories satisfactorily. However, they often can learn essentially no new information that is based on verbal symbolism. In fact, they often cannot even learn the names of people with whom they come in contact every day. Yet they can remember for a moment or so what transpires during the course of their activities. Thus, they are capable of short-term memory for seconds up to a minute or two, although their ability to establish memories lasting longer than a few minutes is either completely or almost completely abolished. This is the phenomenon called *anterograde amnesia* that was discussed in Chapter 57.

Theoretical Function of the Hippocampus in Learning. The hippocampus originated as part of the olfactory cortex. In many lower animals, this cortex plays essential roles in determining whether the animal will eat a particular food, whether the smell of a particular object suggests danger, or whether the odor is sexually inviting, thus making decisions that are of life-or-death importance. Very early in evolutionary development of the brain, the hippocampus presumably became a critical decision-making neuronal mechanism, determining the importance of the incoming sensory signals. Once this critical decision-making capability had been established, presumably the remainder of the brain also began to call on the hippocampus for decision making. Therefore, if the hippocampus signals that a neuronal input is important, the information is likely to be committed to memory.

Thus, a person rapidly becomes habituated to indifferent stimuli but learns assiduously any sensory experience that causes either pleasure or pain. But what is the mechanism by which this occurs? It has been suggested that the hippocampus provides the drive that causes translation of short-term memory into long-term memory—that is, the hippocampus transmits some signal or signals that seem to make the mind *rehearse over and over* the new information until permanent storage takes place. Whatever the mechanism, without the hippocampi, *consolidation* of long-term memories of the verbal or symbolic thinking type is poor or does not take place.

Functions of the Amygdala

The amygdala is a complex of multiple small nuclei located immediately beneath the cerebral cortex of the medial anterior pole of each temporal lobe. It has abundant bidirectional connections with the hypothalamus, as well as with other areas of the limbic system.

In lower animals, the amygdala is concerned to a great extent with olfactory stimuli and their interrelations with the limbic brain. Indeed, it is pointed out in Chapter 53 that one of the major divisions of the olfactory tract terminates in a portion of the amygdala called the *corticomedial nuclei*, which lies immediately beneath the cerebral cortex in the olfactory pyriform area of the temporal lobe. In the human being, another portion of the amygdala, the *basolateral nuclei*, has become much more highly developed than the olfactory portion and plays important roles in many behavioral activities not generally associated with olfactory stimuli.

The amygdala receives neuronal signals from all portions of the limbic cortex, as well as from the neocortex of the temporal, parietal, and occipital lobes—especially from the auditory and visual association areas. Because of these multiple connections, the amygdala has been called the "window" through which the limbic system sees the place of the person in the world. In turn, the amygdala transmits signals (1) back into these same cortical areas, (2) into the hippocampus, (3) into the septum, (4) into the thalamus, and (5) especially into the hypothalamus.

Effects of Stimulating the Amygdala. In general, stimulation in the amygdala can cause almost all the same effects as those elicited by direct stimulation of the hypothalamus, plus other effects. Effects initiated from the amygdala and then sent through the hypothalamus include (1) increases or decreases in arterial pressure; (2) increases or decreases in heart rate; (3) increases or decreases in gastrointestinal motility and secretion; (4) defecation or micturition; (5) pupillary dilation or, rarely, constriction; (6) piloerection; and (7) secretion of various anterior pituitary hormones, especially the gonadotropins and adrenocorticotropic hormone.

Aside from these effects mediated through the hypothalamus, amygdala stimulation can also cause several types of involuntary movement. These include (1) tonic movements, such as raising the head or bending the body; (2) circling movements; (3) occasionally clonic, rhythmical movements; and (4) different types of movements associated with olfaction and eating, such as licking, chewing, and swallowing.

In addition, stimulation of certain amygdaloid nuclei can cause a pattern of rage, escape, punishment, severe pain, and fear similar to the rage pattern elicited from the hypothalamus, as described earlier. Stimulation of other amygdaloid nuclei can give reactions of reward and pleasure.

Finally, excitation of still other portions of the amygdala can cause sexual activities that include erection, copulatory movements, ejaculation, ovulation, uterine activity, and premature labor.

Effects of Bilateral Ablation of the Amygdala—the Klüver-Bucy Syndrome. When the anterior parts of both temporal lobes are destroyed in a monkey, this removes not only portions of temporal cortex but also of the amygdalas that lie inside these parts of the temporal lobes. This causes changes in behavior called the *Klüver-Bucy syndrome,* which is demonstrated by an animal that (1) is not afraid of anything, (2) has extreme curiosity about everything, (3) forgets rapidly, (4) has a tendency to place everything in its mouth and sometimes even tries to eat solid objects, and (5) often has a sex drive so strong that it attempts to copulate with immature animals, animals of the wrong sex, or even animals of a different species. Although similar lesions in human beings are rare, afflicted people respond in a manner not too different from that of the monkey.

Overall Function of the Amygdalas. The amygdalas seem to be behavioral awareness areas that operate at a semiconscious level. They also seem to project into the limbic system one's current status in relation to both surroundings and thoughts. On the basis of this information, the amygdala is believed to make the person's behavioral response appropriate for each occasion.

Function of the Limbic Cortex

The most poorly understood portion of the limbic system is the ring of cerebral cortex called the *limbic cortex* that surrounds the subcortical limbic structures. This cortex functions as a transitional zone through which signals are transmitted from the remainder of the brain cortex into the limbic system and also in the opposite direction. Therefore, the limbic cortex in effect functions as a cerebral *association area for control of behavior.*

Stimulation of the different regions of the limbic cortex has failed to give any real idea of their functions. However, as is true of so many other portions of the limbic system, essentially all behavioral patterns can be elicited by stimulation of specific portions of the limbic cortex. Likewise, ablation of some limbic cortical areas can cause persistent changes in an animal's behavior, as follows.

Ablation of the Anterior Temporal Cortex. When the anterior temporal cortex is ablated bilaterally, the amygdalas are almost invariably damaged as well. This was discussed earlier in this chapter; it was pointed out that the Klüver-Bucy syndrome occurs. The animal especially develops consummatory behavior: it investigates any and all objects, has intense sex drives toward inappropriate animals or even inanimate objects, and loses all fear—and thus develops tameness as well.

Ablation of the Posterior Orbital Frontal Cortex. Bilateral removal of the posterior portion of the orbital frontal cortex often causes an animal to develop insomnia associated with intense motor restlessness, becoming unable to sit still and moving about continuously.

Ablation of the Anterior Cingulate Gyri and Subcallosal Gyri. The anterior cingulate gyri and the subcallosal gyri are the portions of the limbic cortex that communicate between the prefrontal cerebral cortex and the subcortical limbic structures. Destruction of these gyri bilaterally releases the rage centers of the septum and hypothalamus from prefrontal inhibitory influence. Therefore, the animal can become vicious and much more subject to fits of rage than normally.

Summary. Until further information is available, it is perhaps best to state that the cortical regions of the limbic system occupy intermediate associative positions between the functions of the specific areas of the cerebral cortex and functions of the subcortical limbic structures for control of behavioral patterns. Thus, in the anterior temporal cortex, one especially finds gustatory and olfactory behavioral associations. In the parahippocampal gyri, there is a tendency for complex auditory associations and complex thought associations derived from Wernicke area of the posterior temporal lobe. In the middle and posterior cingulate cortex, there is reason to believe that sensorimotor behavioral associations occur.

Bibliography

Adell A, Celada P, Abellan MT, et al: Origin and functional role of the extracellular serotonin in the midbrain raphe nuclei, *Brain Res Brain Res Rev* 39:154, 2002.

Bechara A, Damasio H, Damasio AR: Role of the amygdala in decision-making, *Ann N Y Acad Sci* 985:356, 2003.

Bird CM, Burgess N: The hippocampus and memory: insights from spatial processing, *Nat Rev Neurosci* 9:182, 2008.

Ehrlich I, Humeau Y, Grenier F, et al: Amygdala inhibitory circuits and the control of fear memory, *Neuron* 62:757, 2009.

Guillery RW: Branching thalamic afferents link action and perception, *J Neurophysiol* 90:539, 2003.

Heinricher MM, Tavares I, Leith JL, et al: Descending control of nociception: Specificity, recruitment and plasticity, *Brain Res Rev* 60:214, 2009.

Holland PC, Gallagher M: Amygdala—frontal interactions and reward expectancy, *Curr Opin Neurobiol* 14:148, 2004.

Joels M, Verkuyl JM, Van Riel E: Hippocampal and hypothalamic function after chronic stress, *Ann N Y Acad Sci* 1007:367, 2003.

Jones EG: Synchrony in the interconnected circuitry of the thalamus and cerebral cortex, *Ann N Y Acad Sci* 1157:10, 2009.

Kandel ER, Schwartz JH, Jessell TM: *Principles of Neural Science*, ed 4, New York, 2000, McGraw-Hill.

LeDoux JE: Emotion circuits in the brain, *Annu Rev Neurosci* 23:155, 2000.

Lumb BM: Hypothalamic and midbrain circuitry that distinguishes between escapable and inescapable pain, *News Physiol Sci* 19:22, 2004.

Neves G, Cooke SF, Bliss TV: Synaptic plasticity, memory and the hippocampus: a neural network approach to causality, *Nat Rev Neurosci* 9:65, 2008.

Pessoa L: On the relationship between emotion and cognition, *Nat Rev Neurosci* 9:148, 2008.

Phelps EA, LeDoux JE: Contributions of the amygdala to emotion processing: from animal models to human behavior, *Neuron* 48:175, 2005.

Roozendaal B, McEwen BS, Chattarji S: Stress, memory and the amygdala, *Nat Rev Neurosci* 10:423, 2009.

Sah P, Faber ES, Lopez De Armentia M, et al: The amygdaloid complex: anatomy and physiology, *Physiol Rev* 83:803, 2003.

Sara SJ: The locus coeruleus and noradrenergic modulation of cognition, *Nat Rev Neurosci* 10:211, 2009.

Ulrich-Lai YM, Herman JP: Neural regulation of endocrine and autonomic stress responses, *Nat Rev Neurosci* 10:397, 2009.

Vann SD, Aggleton JP: The mammillary bodies: two memory systems in one? *Nat Rev Neurosci* 5:35, 2004.

Woods SC, D'Alessio DA: Central control of body weight and appetite, *J Clin Endocrinol Metab* 93(11 Suppl 1):S37, 2008.

States of Brain Activity—Sleep, Brain Waves, Epilepsy, Psychoses

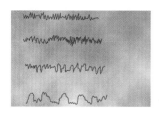

All of us are aware of the many different states of brain activity, including sleep, wakefulness, extreme excitement, and even different levels of mood such as exhilaration, depression, and fear. All these states result from different activating or inhibiting forces generated usually within the brain itself. In Chapter 58, we began a partial discussion of this subject when we described different systems that are capable of activating large portions of the brain. In this chapter, we present brief surveys of specific states of brain activity, beginning with sleep.

Sleep

Sleep is defined as unconsciousness from which the person can be aroused by sensory or other stimuli. It is to be distinguished from *coma,* which is unconsciousness from which the person cannot be aroused. There are multiple stages of sleep, from very light sleep to very deep sleep; sleep researchers also divide sleep into two entirely different types of sleep that have different qualities, as follows.

Two Types of Sleep—Slow-Wave Sleep and Rapid Eye Movement (REM) Sleep. During each night, a person goes through stages of two types of sleep that alternate with each other. They are called (1) *slow-wave sleep,* in which the brain waves are strong and of low frequency, as we discuss later, and (2) *rapid eye movement sleep* (REM sleep), in which the eyes undergo rapid movements despite the fact that the person is still asleep.

Most sleep during each night is of the slow-wave variety; this is the deep, restful sleep that the person experiences during the first hour of sleep after having been awake for many hours. REM sleep, on the other hand, occurs in episodes that occupy about 25 percent of the sleep time in young adults; each episode normally recurs about every 90 minutes. This type of sleep is not so restful, and it is usually associated with vivid dreaming.

Slow-Wave Sleep

Most of us can understand the characteristics of deep slow-wave sleep by remembering the last time we were kept awake for more than 24 hours and then the deep sleep that occurred during the first hour after going to sleep. This sleep is exceedingly restful and is associated with decreases in both peripheral vascular tone and many other vegetative functions of the body. For instance, there are 10 to 30 percent decreases in blood pressure, respiratory rate, and basal metabolic rate.

Although slow-wave sleep is frequently called "dreamless sleep," dreams and sometimes even nightmares do occur during slow-wave sleep. The difference between the dreams that occur in slow-wave sleep and those that occur in REM sleep is that those of REM sleep are associated with more bodily muscle activity. Also, the dreams of slow-wave sleep are usually not remembered because consolidation of the dreams in memory does not occur.

REM Sleep (Paradoxical Sleep, Desynchronized Sleep)

In a normal night of sleep, bouts of REM sleep lasting 5 to 30 minutes usually appear on the average every 90 minutes. When the person is extremely sleepy, each bout of REM sleep is short and may even be absent. Conversely, as the person becomes more rested through the night, the durations of the REM bouts increase.

REM sleep has several important characteristics:

1. It is an active form of sleep usually associated with dreaming and active bodily muscle movements.

2. The person is even more difficult to arouse by sensory stimuli than during deep slow-wave sleep, and yet people usually awaken spontaneously in the morning during an episode of REM sleep.

3. Muscle tone throughout the body is exceedingly depressed, indicating strong inhibition of the spinal muscle control areas.

4. Heart rate and respiratory rate usually become irregular, which is characteristic of the dream state.

5. Despite the extreme inhibition of the peripheral muscles, irregular muscle movements do occur. These are in addition to the rapid movements of the eyes.

6. The brain is highly active in REM sleep, and overall brain metabolism may be increased as much as 20 percent. The electroencephalogram (EEG) shows a pattern of brain waves similar to those that occur during wakefulness. This type of sleep is also called *paradoxical sleep* because it is a paradox that a person can still be asleep despite marked activity in the brain.

In summary, REM sleep is a type of sleep in which the brain is quite active. However, the brain activity is not channeled in the proper direction for the person to be fully aware of his or her surroundings, and therefore the person is truly asleep.

Basic Theories of Sleep

Sleep Is Believed to Be Caused by an Active Inhibitory Process. An earlier theory of sleep was that the excitatory areas of the upper brain stem, the *reticular activating system*, simply fatigued during the waking day and became inactive as a result. This was called the *passive theory of sleep*. An important experiment changed this view to the current belief that *sleep is caused by an active inhibitory process:* it was discovered that transecting the brain stem at the level of the midpons creates a brain whose cortex never goes to sleep. In other words, a center located below the midpontile level of the brain stem appears to be required to cause sleep by inhibiting other parts of the brain.

Neuronal Centers, Neurohumoral Substances, and Mechanisms That Can Cause Sleep—A Possible Specific Role for Serotonin

Stimulation of several specific areas of the brain can produce sleep with characteristics near those of natural sleep. Some of these areas are the following:

1. The most conspicuous stimulation area for causing almost natural sleep is the *raphe nuclei in the lower half of the pons and in the medulla*. These nuclei comprise a thin sheet of special neurons located in the midline. Nerve fibers from these nuclei spread locally in the brain stem reticular formation and also upward into the thalamus, hypothalamus, most areas of the limbic system, and even the neocortex of the cerebrum. In addition, fibers extend downward into the spinal cord, terminating in the posterior horns, where they can inhibit incoming sensory signals, including pain, as discussed in Chapter 48. Many nerve endings of fibers from these raphe neurons secrete *serotonin.* When a drug that blocks the formation of serotonin is administered to an animal, the animal often cannot sleep for the next several days. Therefore, it has been assumed that serotonin is a transmitter substance associated with production of sleep.

2. Stimulation of some areas in the *nucleus of the tractus solitarius* can also cause sleep. This nucleus is the termination in the medulla and pons for visceral sensory signals entering by way of the vagus and glossopharyngeal nerves.

3. Sleep can be promoted by stimulation of several regions in the diencephalon, including (1) the rostral part of the hypothalamus, mainly in the suprachiasmal area, and (2) an occasional area in the diffuse nuclei of the thalamus.

Lesions in Sleep-Promoting Centers Can Cause Intense Wakefulness. Discrete lesions in the *raphe nuclei* lead to a high state of wakefulness. This is also true of bilateral lesions in the *medial rostral suprachiasmal area in the anterior hypothalamus.* In both instances, the excitatory reticular nuclei of the mesencephalon and upper pons seem to become released from inhibition, thus causing the intense wakefulness. Indeed, sometimes lesions of the anterior hypothalamus can cause such intense wakefulness that the animal actually dies of exhaustion.

Other Possible Transmitter Substances Related to Sleep. Experiments have shown that the cerebrospinal fluid and the blood or urine of animals that have been kept awake for several days contain a substance or substances that will cause sleep when injected into the brain ventricular system of another animal. One likely substance has been identified as *muramyl peptide,* a low-molecular-weight substance that accumulates in the cerebrospinal fluid and urine in animals kept awake for several days. When only micrograms of this sleep-producing substance are injected into the third ventricle, almost natural sleep occurs within a few minutes and the animal may stay asleep for several hours. Another substance that has similar effects in causing sleep is a nonapeptide isolated from the blood of sleeping animals. And still a third sleep factor, not yet identified molecularly, has been isolated from the neuronal tissues of the brain stem of animals kept awake for days. It is possible that prolonged wakefulness causes progressive accumulation of a sleep factor or factors in the brain stem or cerebrospinal fluid that lead to sleep.

Possible Cause of REM Sleep. Why slow-wave sleep is broken periodically by REM sleep is not understood. However, drugs that mimic the action of acetylcholine increase the occurrence of REM sleep. Therefore, it has been postulated that the large acetylcholine-secreting neurons in the upper brain stem reticular formation might, through their extensive efferent fibers, activate many portions of the brain. This theoretically could cause the excess activity that occurs in certain brain regions in REM sleep, even though the signals are not channeled appropriately in the brain to cause normal conscious awareness that is characteristic of wakefulness.

Cycle Between Sleep and Wakefulness

The preceding discussions have merely identified neuronal areas, transmitters, and mechanisms that are related to sleep. They have not explained the cyclical, reciprocal operation of the sleep-wakefulness cycle. There is as yet no definitive explanation. Therefore, we might suggest the following possible mechanism for causing the sleep-wakefulness cycle.

When the sleep centers are *not* activated, the mesencephalic and upper pontile reticular activating nuclei are released from inhibition, which allows the reticular activating nuclei to become spontaneously active. This in turn excites both the cerebral cortex and the peripheral nervous system, both of which send numerous *positive feedback* signals back to the same reticular activating nuclei to activate them still further. Therefore, once wakefulness begins, it has a natural tendency to sustain itself because of all this positive feedback activity.

Then, after the brain remains activated for many hours, even the neurons themselves in the activating system presumably become fatigued. Consequently, the positive feedback cycle between the mesencephalic reticular nuclei and the cerebral cortex fades and the sleep-promoting effects of the sleep centers take over, leading to rapid transition from wakefulness back to sleep.

This overall theory could explain the rapid transitions from sleep to wakefulness and from wakefulness to sleep. It could also explain arousal, the insomnia that occurs when a person's mind becomes preoccupied with a thought, and the wakefulness that is produced by bodily physical activity.

Physiologic Functions of Sleep Are Not Yet Known

There is little doubt that sleep has important functions. It exists in all mammals and after total deprivation there is usually a period of "catch-up" or "rebound" sleep; after selective deprivation of REM or slow-wave sleep, there is also a selective rebound of these specific stages of sleep. Even mild sleep restriction over a few days may degrade cognitive and physical performance, overall productivity, and health of a person. The essential role of sleep in homeostasis is perhaps most vividly demonstrated by the fact that rats deprived of sleep for 2 to 3 weeks may actually die. Despite the obvious importance of sleep, our understanding of why sleep is an essential part of life is still limited.

Sleep causes two major types of physiologic effects: first, effects on the nervous system itself, and second, effects on other functional systems of the body. The nervous system effects seem to be by far the more important because any person who has a transected spinal cord in the neck (and therefore has no sleep-wakefulness cycle below the transection) shows no harmful effects in the body beneath the level of transection that can be attributed directly to a sleep-wakefulness cycle.

Lack of sleep certainly does, however, affect the functions of the central nervous system. Prolonged wakefulness is often associated with progressive malfunction of the thought processes and sometimes even causes abnormal behavioral activities. We are all familiar with the increased sluggishness of thought that occurs toward the end of a prolonged wakeful period, but in addition, a person can become irritable or even psychotic after forced wakefulness. Therefore, we can assume that sleep in multiple ways restores both normal levels of brain activity and normal "balance" among the different functions of the central nervous system. This might be likened to the "rezeroing" of electronic analog computers after prolonged use because computers of this type gradually lose their "baseline" of operation; it is reasonable to assume that the same effect occurs in the central nervous system because overuse of some brain areas during wakefulness could easily throw these areas out of balance with the remainder of the nervous system.

Sleep has been postulated to serve many functions including (1) neural maturation, (2) facilitation of learning or memory, (3) cognition, and (4) conservation of metabolic energy. There is some evidence for each of these functions, as well as physiologic purposes of sleep, but evidence supporting each of these ideas has been challenged. We might postulate that *the principal value of sleep is to restore natural balances among the neuronal centers.* The specific physiologic functions of sleep, however, remain a mystery, and they are the subject of much research.

Brain Waves

Electrical recordings from the surface of the brain or even from the outer surface of the head demonstrate that there is continuous electrical activity in the brain. Both the intensity and the patterns of this electrical activity are determined by the level of excitation of different parts of the brain resulting from *sleep, wakefulness,* or brain diseases such as *epilepsy* or even *psychoses.* The undulations in the recorded electrical potentials, shown in Figure 59-1, are called *brain waves,* and the entire record is called an EEG (electroencephalogram).

The intensities of brain waves recorded from the surface of the scalp range from 0 to 200 microvolts, and their frequencies range from once every few seconds to 50 or more per second. The character of the waves is dependent on the degree of activity in respective parts of the cerebral cortex, and the waves change markedly between the states of wakefulness and sleep and coma.

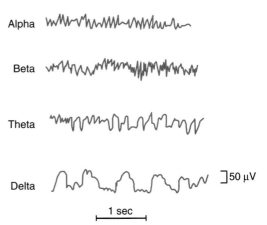

Figure 59-1 Different types of *brain waves* in the normal electroencephalogram.

Much of the time, the brain waves are irregular and no specific pattern can be discerned in the EEG. At other times, distinct patterns do appear, some of which are characteristic of specific abnormalities of the brain such as epilepsy, which is discussed later.

In healthy people, most waves in the EEG can be classified as *alpha, beta, theta,* and *delta waves,* which are shown in Figure 59-1.

Alpha waves are rhythmical waves that occur at frequencies between 8 and 13 cycles per second and are found in the EEGs of almost all normal adults when they are awake and in a quiet, resting state of cerebration. These waves occur most intensely in the occipital region but can also be recorded from the parietal and frontal regions of the scalp. Their voltage is usually about 50 microvolts. During deep sleep, the alpha waves disappear.

When the awake person's attention is directed to some specific type of mental activity, the alpha waves are replaced by asynchronous, higher-frequency but lower-voltage *beta waves.* Figure 59-2 shows the effect on the alpha waves of simply opening the eyes in bright light and then closing the eyes. Note that the visual sensations cause immediate cessation of the alpha waves and that these are replaced by low-voltage, asynchronous beta waves.

Beta waves occur at frequencies greater than 14 cycles per second and as high as 80 cycles per second. They are recorded mainly from the parietal and frontal regions during specific activation of these parts of the brain.

Theta waves have frequencies between four and seven cycles per second. They occur normally in the parietal and temporal regions in children, but they also occur during emotional stress in some adults, particularly during disappointment and frustration. Theta waves also occur in many brain disorders, often in degenerative brain states.

Delta waves include all the waves of the EEG with frequencies less than 3.5 cycles per second, and they often have voltages two to four times greater than most other types of brain waves. They occur in very deep sleep, in infancy, and in serious organic brain disease. They also occur in the cortex of animals that have had subcortical transections separating the cerebral cortex from the thalamus. Therefore, delta waves can occur strictly in the cortex independent of activities in lower regions of the brain.

Origin of Brain Waves

The discharge of a single neuron or single nerve fiber in the brain can never be recorded from the surface of the head. Instead, many thousands or even millions of neurons or fibers *must fire synchronously;* only then will the potentials from the individual neurons or fibers summate enough to be recorded all the way through the skull. Thus, the intensity of the brain waves from the scalp is determined mainly by the numbers of neurons and fibers that

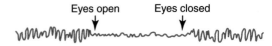

Figure 59-2 Replacement of the *alpha* rhythm by an asynchronous, low-voltage *beta* rhythm when the eyes are opened.

fire *in synchrony* with one another, not by the total level of electrical activity in the brain. In fact, strong *nonsynchronous* nerve signals often nullify one another in the recorded brain waves because of opposing polarities. This is demonstrated in Figure 59-2, which shows, when the eyes were closed, synchronous discharge of many neurons in the cerebral cortex at a frequency of about 12 per second, thus causing *alpha waves.* Then, when the eyes were opened, the activity of the brain increased greatly, but synchronization of the signals became so little that the brain waves mainly nullified one another. The resultant effect was low voltage waves of generally high but irregular frequency, the *beta waves.*

Origin of Alpha Waves. Alpha waves will *not* occur in the cerebral cortex without cortical connections with the thalamus. Conversely, stimulation in the nonspecific layer of *reticular nuclei* that surround the thalamus or in "diffuse" nuclei deep inside the thalamus often sets up electrical waves in the thalamocortical system at a frequency between 8 and 13 per second, which is the natural frequency of the alpha waves. Therefore, it is believed that the alpha waves result from spontaneous feedback oscillation in this diffuse thalamocortical system, possibly including the reticular activating system in the brain stem as well. This oscillation presumably causes both the periodicity of the alpha waves and the synchronous activation of literally millions of cortical neurons during each wave.

Origin of Delta Waves. Transection of the fiber tracts from the thalamus to the cerebral cortex, which blocks thalamic activation of the cortex and thereby eliminates the alpha waves, nevertheless does not block delta waves in the cortex. This indicates that some synchronizing mechanism can occur in the cortical neuronal system by itself—mainly independent of lower structures in the brain—to cause the delta waves.

Delta waves also occur during deep slow-wave sleep; this suggests that the cortex then is mainly released from the activating influences of the thalamus and other lower centers.

Effect of Varying Levels of Cerebral Activity on the Frequency of the EEG

There is a general correlation between level of cerebral activity and average frequency of the EEG rhythm, the average frequency increasing progressively with higher degrees of activity. This is demonstrated in Figure 59-3, which shows

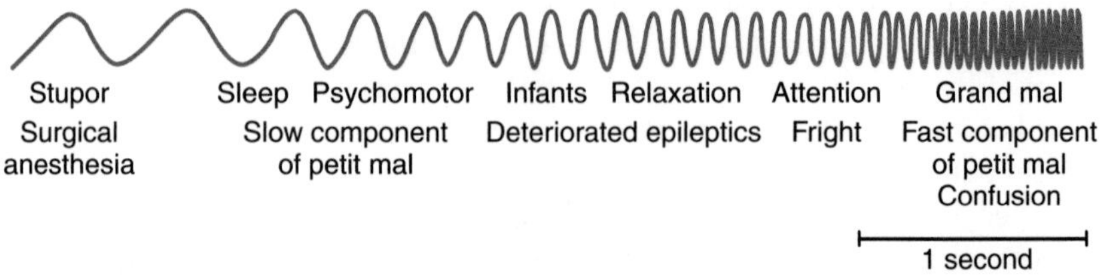

Figure 59-3 Effect of varying degrees of cerebral activity on the basic rhythm of the electroencephalogram. (Redrawn from Gibbs FA, Gibbs EL: Atlas of Electroencephalography, 2nd ed, vol I: Methodology and Controls.® 1974. Reprinted by permission of Prentice-Hall, Inc., Upper Saddle River, NJ.)

| Stupor | Sleep | Psychomotor | Infants | Relaxation | Attention | Grand mal |
| Surgical anesthesia | Slow component of petit mal | Deteriorated epileptics | | Fright | Fast component of petit mal Confusion |

1 second

the existence of delta waves in stupor, surgical anesthesia, and deep sleep; theta waves in psychomotor states and in infants; alpha waves during relaxed states; and beta waves during periods of intense mental activity. *During periods of mental activity, the waves usually become asynchronous rather than synchronous, so the voltage falls considerably despite markedly increased cortical activity,* as shown in Figure 59-2.

Changes in the EEG at Different Stages of Wakefulness and Sleep

Figure 59-4 shows EEG patterns from a typical person in different stages of wakefulness and sleep. Alert wakefulness is characterized by high-frequency *beta waves,* whereas quiet wakefulness is usually associated with *alpha waves,* as demonstrated by the first two EEGs of the figure.

Slow-wave sleep is divided into four stages. In the first stage, a stage of light sleep, the voltage of the EEG waves becomes low. This is broken by *"sleep spindles"* (i.e,, short spindle-shaped bursts of alpha waves that occur periodically). In stages 2, 3, and 4 of slow-wave sleep, the frequency of the EEG becomes progressively slower until it reaches a frequency of only one to three waves per second in stage 4; these are *delta waves.*

Finally, the bottom record in Figure 59-4 shows the EEG during REM sleep. It is often difficult to tell the difference between this brain wave pattern and that of an awake, active person. The waves are irregular and of high frequency, which are normally suggestive of desynchronized nervous activity as found in the awake state. Therefore, REM sleep is frequently called *desynchronized sleep* because there is lack of synchrony in the firing of the neurons despite significant brain activity.

Epilepsy

Epilepsy (also called "seizures") is characterized by *uncontrolled* excessive activity of either part or all of the central nervous system. A person who is predisposed to epilepsy has attacks when the basal level of excitability of the nervous system (or of the part that is susceptible to the epileptic state) rises above a certain critical threshold. As long as the degree of excitability is held below this threshold, no attack occurs.

Epilepsy can be classified into three major types: *grand mal epilepsy, petit mal epilepsy,* and *focal epilepsy.*

Grand Mal Epilepsy

Grand mal epilepsy is characterized by extreme neuronal discharges in all areas of the brain—in the cerebral cortex, in the deeper parts of the cerebrum, and even in the brain stem. Also, discharges transmitted all the way into the spinal cord sometimes cause generalized *tonic seizures* of the entire body, followed toward the end of the attack by alternating tonic and spasmodic muscle contractions called *tonic-clonic seizures.* Often the person bites or "swallows" his or her tongue and may have difficulty breathing, sometimes to the extent that cyanosis occurs. Also, signals transmitted from the brain to the viscera frequently cause urination and defecation.

The usual grand mal seizure lasts from a few seconds to 3 to 4 minutes. It is also characterized by *postseizure depression* of the entire nervous system; the person remains in stupor for 1 to many minutes after the seizure attack is over and then often remains severely fatigued and asleep for hours thereafter.

The top recording of Figure 59-5 shows a typical EEG from almost any region of the cortex during the tonic phase of a grand mal attack. This demonstrates that high-voltage, high-frequency discharges occur over the entire cortex. Furthermore, the same type of discharge occurs on both sides of the brain at the same time, demonstrating that the abnormal neuronal circuitry responsible for the attack strongly involves the basal regions of the brain that drive the two halves of the cerebrum simultaneously.

In laboratory animals and even in human beings, grand mal attacks can be initiated by administering a neuronal stimulant such as the drug pentylenetetrazol. They can also be caused by insulin hypoglycemia or passage of alternating electrical current directly through the brain. Electrical recordings from the thalamus, as well as from the reticular formation of the brain stem during the grand mal attack, show typical high-voltage activity in both of these areas similar to that recorded from the cerebral cortex. Therefore, a grand mal attack presumably involves not only abnormal activation of the thalamus and cerebral cortex but also abnormal activation in the subthalamic brain stem portions of the brain-activating system itself.

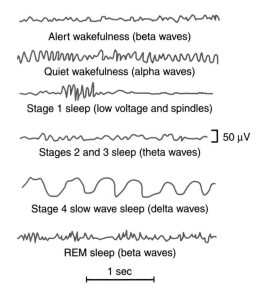

Alert wakefulness (beta waves)

Quiet wakefulness (alpha waves)

Stage 1 sleep (low voltage and spindles)

Stages 2 and 3 sleep (theta waves) ⟩ 50 μV

Stage 4 slow wave sleep (delta waves)

REM sleep (beta waves)

1 sec

Figure 59-4 Progressive change in the characteristics of the brain waves during different stages of wakefulness and sleep.

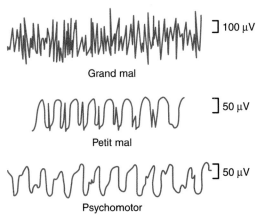

Grand mal ⟩ 100 μV

Petit mal ⟩ 50 μV

Psychomotor ⟩ 50 μV

Figure 59-5 Electroencephalograms in different types of epilepsy.

What Initiates a Grand Mal Attack? Most people who have grand mal attacks have a hereditary predisposition to epilepsy, a predisposition that occurs in about 1 of every 50 to 100 persons. In such people, factors that can increase the excitability of the abnormal "epileptogenic" circuitry enough to precipitate attacks include (1) strong emotional stimuli, (2) alkalosis caused by overbreathing, (3) drugs, (4) fever, and (5) loud noises or flashing lights.

Even in people who are not genetically predisposed, certain types of traumatic lesions in almost any part of the brain can cause excess excitability of local brain areas, as we discuss shortly; these, too, sometimes transmit signals into the activating systems of the brain to elicit grand mal seizures.

What Stops the Grand Mal Attack? The cause of the extreme neuronal overactivity during a grand mal attack is presumed to be massive simultaneous activation of many reverberating neuronal pathways throughout the brain. Presumably, the major factor that stops the attack after a few minutes is *neuronal fatigue.* A second factor is probably *active inhibition* by inhibitory neurons that have been activated by the attack.

Petit Mal Epilepsy

Petit mal epilepsy almost certainly involves the thalamo-cortical brain activating system. It is usually characterized by 3 to 30 seconds of unconsciousness (or diminished consciousness) during which time the person has twitchlike contractions of muscles usually in the head region, especially blinking of the eyes; this is followed by return of consciousness and resumption of previous activities. This total sequence is called the *absence syndrome* or absence epilepsy. The patient may have one such attack in many months or, in rare instances, may have a rapid series of attacks, one after the other. The usual course is for the petit mal attacks to appear first during late childhood and then to disappear by the age of 30. On occasion, a petit mal epileptic attack will initiate a grand mal attack.

The brain wave pattern in petit mal epilepsy is demonstrated by the middle recording of Figure 59-5, which is typified by a *spike and dome pattern.* The spike and dome can be recorded over most or all of the cerebral cortex, showing that the seizure involves much or most of the thalamocortical activating system of the brain. In fact, animal studies suggest that it results from oscillation of (1) inhibitory thalamic reticular neurons (which are *inhibitory* gamma-aminobutyric acid [GABA]-producing neurons) and (2) *excitatory* thalamocortical and cortico-thalamic neurons.

Focal Epilepsy

Focal epilepsy can involve almost any local part of the brain, either localized regions of the cerebral cortex or deeper structures of both the cerebrum and brain stem. Most often, focal epilepsy results from some localized organic lesion or functional abnormality, such as (1) scar tissue in the brain that pulls on the adjacent neuronal tissue, (2) a tumor that compresses an area of the brain, (3) a destroyed area of brain tissue, or (4) congenitally deranged local circuitry.

Lesions such as these can promote extremely rapid discharges in the local neurons; when the discharge rate rises above several hundred per second, synchronous waves begin to spread over adjacent cortical regions. These waves

presumably result from *localized reverberating circuits* that gradually recruit adjacent areas of the cortex into the epileptic discharge zone. The process spreads to adjacent areas at a rate as slow as a few millimeters a minute to as fast as several centimeters per second. When such a wave of excitation spreads over the motor cortex, it causes progressive "march" of muscle contractions throughout the opposite side of the body, beginning most characteristically in the mouth region and marching progressively downward to the legs but at other times marching in the opposite direction. This is called *jacksonian epilepsy.*

A focal epileptic attack may remain confined to a single area of the brain, but in many instances, the strong signals from the convulsing cortex excite the mesencephalic portion of the brain-activating system so greatly that a grand mal epileptic attack ensues as well.

Another type of focal epilepsy is the so-called *psychomotor seizure,* which may cause (1) a short period of amnesia; (2) an attack of abnormal rage; (3) sudden anxiety, discomfort, or fear; and/or (4) a moment of incoherent speech or mumbling of some trite phrase. Sometimes the person cannot remember his or her activities during the attack, but at other times he or she is conscious of everything that he or she is doing but unable to control it. Attacks of this type frequently involve part of the limbic portion of the brain, such as the hippocampus, the amygdala, the septum, and/or portions of the temporal cortex.

The lowest tracing of Figure 59-5 demonstrates a typical EEG during a psychomotor seizure, showing a low-frequency rectangular wave with a frequency between 2 and 4 per second and with occasional superimposed 14-per-second waves.

Surgical Excision of Epileptic Foci Can Often Prevent Seizures. The EEG can be used to localize abnormal spiking waves originating in areas of organic brain disease that predispose to focal epileptic attacks. Once such a focal point is found, surgical excision of the focus frequently prevents future attacks.

Psychotic Behavior and Dementia—Roles of Specific Neurotransmitter Systems

Clinical studies of patients with different psychoses or different types of dementia have suggested that many of these conditions result from diminished function of neurons that secrete a specific neurotransmitter. Use of appropriate drugs to counteract loss of the respective neurotransmitter has been successful in treating some patients.

In Chapter 56, we discussed the cause of Parkinson's disease. This disease results from loss of neurons in the substantia nigra whose nerve endings secrete *dopamine* in the caudate nucleus and putamen. Also in Chapter 56, we pointed out that in Huntington's disease, loss of GABA-secreting neurons and acetylcholine-secreting neurons is associated with *specific abnormal motor patterns* plus *dementia* occurring in the same patient.

Depression and Manic-Depressive Psychoses—Decreased Activity of the Norepinephrine and Serotonin Neurotransmitter Systems

Much evidence has accumulated suggesting that *mental depression psychosis,* which occurs in about 8 million people in the United States, might be caused by *diminished formation in the brain of norepinephrine or serotonin, or both.* (New evidence has implicated still other neurotransmitters.) Depressed patients experience symptoms of grief, unhappiness, despair, and misery. In addition, they often lose their appetite and sex drive and have severe insomnia. Often associated with these is a state of psychomotor agitation despite the depression.

Moderate numbers of *norepinephrine-secreting neurons* are located in the brain stem, especially in the *locus ceruleus.* These neurons send fibers upward to most parts of the brain limbic system, thalamus, and cerebral cortex. Also, many *serotonin-producing neurons* located in the *midline raphe nuclei* of the lower pons and medulla send fibers to many areas of the limbic system and to some other areas of the brain.

A principal reason for believing that depression might be caused by diminished activity of norepinephrine- and serotonin-secreting neurons is that drugs that block secretion of norepinephrine and serotonin, such as reserpine, frequently cause depression. Conversely, about 70 percent of depressive patients can be treated effectively with drugs that increase the excitatory effects of norepinephrine and serotonin at the nerve endings—for instance, (1) *monoamine oxidase inhibitors,* which block destruction of norepinephrine and serotonin once they are formed, and (2) *tricyclic antidepressants,* such as *imipramine* and *amitriptyline,* which block reuptake of norepinephrine and serotonin by nerve endings so that these transmitters remain active for longer periods after secretion.

Mental depression can be treated by electroconvulsive therapy—commonly called "shock therapy." In this therapy, electrical current is passed through the brain to cause a generalized seizure similar to that of an epileptic attack. This has been shown to enhance norepinephrine activity.

Some patients with mental depression alternate between depression and mania, which is called either *bipolar disorder* or *manic-depressive psychosis,* and fewer patients exhibit only mania without the depressive episodes. Drugs that diminish the formation or action of norepinephrine and serotonin, such as lithium compounds, can be effective in treating the manic phase of the condition.

It is presumed that the norepinephrine and serotonin systems normally provide drive to the limbic areas of the brain to increase a person's sense of well-being, to create happiness, contentment, good appetite, appropriate sex drive, and psychomotor balance—although too much of a good thing can cause mania. In support of this concept is the fact that pleasure and reward centers of the hypothalamus and surrounding areas receive large numbers of nerve endings from the norepinephrine and serotonin systems.

Schizophrenia—Possible Exaggerated Function of Part of the Dopamine System

Schizophrenia comes in many varieties. One of the most common types is seen in the person who hears voices and has delusions of grandeur, intense fear, or other types of feelings that are unreal. Many schizophrenics are highly paranoid, with a sense of persecution from outside sources. They may develop incoherent speech, dissociation of ideas, and abnormal sequences of thought, and they are often withdrawn, sometimes with abnormal posture and even rigidity.

There are reasons to believe that schizophrenia results from one or more of three possibilities: (1) multiple areas in the cerebral cortex *prefrontal lobes* in which neural signals have become blocked or where processing of the signals becomes dysfunctional because many synapses normally excited by the neurotransmitter *glutamate* lose their responsiveness to this transmitter; (2) excessive excitement of a group of neurons that secrete *dopamine* in the behavioral centers of the brain, including in the frontal lobes; and/or (3) abnormal function of a crucial part of the brain's *limbic behavioral control system centered around the hippocampus.*

The reason for believing that the prefrontal lobes are involved in schizophrenia is that a schizophrenic-like pattern of mental activity can be induced in monkeys by making multiple minute lesions in widespread areas of the prefrontal lobes.

Dopamine has been implicated as a possible cause of schizophrenia because many patients with Parkinson's disease develop schizophrenic-like symptoms when they are treated with the drug called L-dopa. This drug releases dopamine in the brain, which is advantageous for treating Parkinson's disease, but at the same time it depresses various portions of the prefrontal lobes and other related areas.

It has been suggested that in schizophrenia excess dopamine is secreted by a group of dopamine-secreting neurons whose cell bodies lie in the ventral tegmentum of the mesencephalon, medial and superior to the substantia nigra. These neurons give rise to the so-called *mesolimbic dopaminergic system* that projects nerve fibers and dopamine secretion into the medial and anterior portions of the limbic system, especially into the hippocampus, amygdala, anterior caudate nucleus, and portions of the prefrontal lobes. All of these are powerful behavioral control centers.

An even more compelling reason for believing that schizophrenia might be caused by excess production of dopamine is that many drugs that are effective in treating schizophrenia—such as chlorpromazine, haloperidol, and thiothixene—all either decrease secretion of dopamine at dopaminergic nerve endings or decrease the effect of dopamine on subsequent neurons.

Finally, possible involvement of the hippocampus in schizophrenia was discovered recently when it was learned that *in schizophrenia, the hippocampus is often reduced in size,* especially in the dominant hemisphere.

Alzheimer's Disease—Amyloid Plaques and Depressed Memory

Alzheimer's disease is defined as premature aging of the brain, usually beginning in midadult life and progressing rapidly to extreme loss of mental powers—similar to that seen in very, very old age. The clinical features of Alzheimer's disease include (1) an amnesic type of memory impairment, (2) deterioration of language, and (3) visuospatial deficits. Motor and sensory abnormalities, gait disturbances, and seizures are uncommon until the late phases of the disease. One consistent finding in Alzheimer's disease is loss of neurons in that part of the limbic pathway that drives the memory process. Loss of this memory function is devastating.

Alzheimer's disease is a progressive and fatal neurodegenerative disorder that results in impairment of the person's ability to perform activities of daily living, as well as a variety of neuropsychiatric symptoms and behavioral disturbances in the later stages of the disease. Patients with Alzheimer's disease usually require continuous care within a few years after the disease begins.

Alzheimer's disease is the most common form of dementia in the elderly, and more than 5 million people in the United States are estimated to be afflicted by this disorder. The percentage of persons with Alzheimer's disease approximately doubles with every 5 years of age, with about 1 percent of 60-year-olds and about 30 percent of 85-year-olds having the disease.

Alzheimer's Disease Is Associated with Accumulation of Brain Beta-Amyloid Peptide. Pathologically, one finds increased amounts of beta-amyloid peptide in the brains of patients with Alzheimer's disease. The peptide accumulates in amyloid plaques, which range in diameter from 10 micrometers to several hundred micrometers and are found in widespread areas of the brain, including in the cerebral cortex, hippocampus, basal ganglia, thalamus, and even the cerebellum. Thus, Alzheimer's disease appears to be a metabolic degenerative disease.

A key role for excess accumulation of beta-amyloid peptide in the pathogenesis of Alzheimer's disease is suggested by the following observations: (1) all currently known mutations associated with Alzheimer's disease increase the production of beta-amyloid peptide; (2) patients with trisomy 21 (Down syndrome) have three copies of the gene for amyloid precursor protein and develop neurological characteristics of Alzheimer's disease by midlife; (3) patients who have abnormality of a gene that controls apolipoprotein E, a blood protein that transports cholesterol to the tissues, have accelerated deposition of amyloid and greatly increased risk for Alzheimer's disease; (4) transgenic mice that overproduce the human amyloid precursor protein have learning and memory deficits in association with the accumulation of amyloid plaques; and (5) generation of anti-amyloid antibodies in humans with Alzheimer's disease appears to attenuate the disease process.

Vascular Disorders May Contribute to Progression of Alzheimer's Disease. There is also accumulating evidence that cerebrovascular disease caused by *hypertension* and *atherosclerosis* may play a role in Alzheimer's disease. Cerebrovascular disease is the second most common cause of acquired cognitive impairment and dementia and likely contributes to cognitive decline in Alzheimer's disease. In fact, many of the common risk factors for cerebrovascular disease, such as hypertension, diabetes, and hyperlipidemia, are also recognized to greatly increase the risk for developing Alzheimer's disease.

Bibliography

Beenhakker MP, Huguenard JR: Neurons that fire together also conspire together: is normal sleep circuitry hijacked to generate epilepsy? *Neuron* 62:612, 2009.

Brayne C: The elephant in the room—healthy brains in later life, epidemiology and public health, *Nat Rev Neurosci* 8:233, 2007.

Canli T, Lesch KP: Long story short: the serotonin transporter in emotion regulation and social cognition, *Nat Neurosci* 10:1103, 2007.

Casserly I, Topol E: Convergence of atherosclerosis and Alzheimer's disease: inflammation, cholesterol, and misfolded proteins, *Lancet* 363:1139, 2004.

Cirelli C: The genetic and molecular regulation of sleep: from fruit flies to humans, *Nat Rev Neurosci* 10:549, 2009.

Cummings JL: Alzheimer's disease, *N Engl J Med* 351:56, 2004.

de la Torre JC: Is Alzheimer's disease a neurodegenerative or a vascular disorder? Data, dogma, and dialectics, *Lancet Neurol* 3:184, 2004.

Golde TE: Alzheimer disease therapy: can the amyloid cascade be halted?, *J Clin Invest* 111:11, 2003.

Iadecola C, Park L, Capone C: Threats to the mind: aging, amyloid, and hypertension, *Stroke* 40(3 Suppl):S40, 2009.

Iadecola C: Neurovascular regulation in the normal brain and in Alzheimer's disease, *Nat Rev Neurosci* 5:347–360, 2004.

Jacob TC, Moss SJ, Jurd R: GABA(A) receptor trafficking and its role in the dynamic modulation of neuronal inhibition, *Nat Rev Neurosci* 9:331, 2008.

Kilduff TS, Lein ES, de la Iglesia H, et al: New developments in sleep research: molecular genetics, gene expression, and systems neurobiology, *J Neurosci* 28:11814, 2008.

Krueger JM, Rector DM, Roy S, et al: Sleep as a fundamental property of neuronal assemblies, *Nat Rev Neurosci* 9:910, 2008.

McCormick DA, Contreras D: On the cellular and network bases of epileptic seizures, *Annu Rev Physiol* 63:815, 2001.

Ressler KJ, Mayberg HS: Targeting abnormal neural circuits in mood and anxiety disorders: from the laboratory to the clinic, *Nat Neurosci* 10:1116, 2007.

Seeman P: Glutamate and dopamine components in schizophrenia, *J Psychiatry Neurosci* 34:143, 2009.

Selkoe DJ: Alzheimer disease: mechanistic understanding predicts novel therapies, *Ann Intern Med* 140:627, 2004.

Smith EE, Greenberg SM: *Beta-amyloid, blood vessels, and brain function* 40:2601, 2009.

Steinlein OK: Genetic mechanisms that underlie epilepsy, *Nat Rev Neurosci* 5:400–408, 2004.

Tononi G, Cirelli C: Staying awake puts pressure on brain arousal systems, *J Clin Invest* 117:3648, 2007.

Viswanathan A, Rocca WA, Tzourio C: Vascular risk factors and dementia: how to move forward? *Neurology* 72:368, 2009.

Zacchigna S, Lambrechts D, Carmeliet P: Neurovascular signalling defects in neurodegeneration, *Nat Rev Neurosci* 9:169, 2008.

The Autonomic Nervous System and the Adrenal Medulla

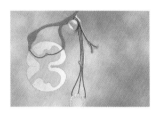

The *autonomic nervous system* is the portion of the nervous system that controls most visceral functions of the body. This system helps to control arterial pressure, gastrointestinal motility, gastrointestinal secretion, urinary bladder emptying, sweating, body temperature, and many other activities, some of which are controlled almost entirely and some only partially by the autonomic nervous system.

One of the most striking characteristics of the autonomic nervous system is the rapidity and intensity with which it can change visceral functions. For instance, within 3 to 5 seconds it can increase the heart rate to twice normal, and within 10 to 15 seconds the arterial pressure can be doubled; or, at the other extreme, the arterial pressure can be decreased low enough within 10 to 15 seconds to cause fainting. Sweating can begin within seconds, and the urinary bladder may empty involuntarily, also within seconds.

General Organization of the Autonomic Nervous System

The autonomic nervous system is activated mainly by centers located in the *spinal cord, brain stem,* and *hypothalamus.* Also, portions of the cerebral cortex, especially of the limbic cortex, can transmit signals to the lower centers and in this way influence autonomic control.

The autonomic nervous system also often operates through *visceral reflexes.* That is, subconscious sensory signals from a visceral organ can enter the autonomic ganglia, the brain stem, or the hypothalamus and then return *subconscious reflex responses* directly back to the visceral organ to control its activities.

The efferent autonomic signals are transmitted to the various organs of the body through two major subdivisions called the *sympathetic nervous system* and the *parasympathetic nervous system,* the characteristics and functions of which follow.

Physiologic Anatomy of the Sympathetic Nervous System

Figure 60-1 shows the general organization of the peripheral portions of the sympathetic nervous system. Shown specifically in the figure are (1) one of the two *paravertebral sympathetic chains of ganglia* that are interconnected with the spinal nerves on the side of the vertebral column, (2) two *prevertebral ganglia* (the *celiac* and *hypogastric*), and (3) nerves extending from the ganglia to the different internal organs.

The sympathetic nerve fibers originate in the spinal cord along with spinal nerves between cord segments T-1 and L-2 and pass first into the *sympathetic chain* and then to the tissues and organs that are stimulated by the sympathetic nerves.

Preganglionic and Postganglionic Sympathetic Neurons

The sympathetic nerves are different from skeletal motor nerves in the following way: Each sympathetic pathway from the cord to the stimulated tissue is composed of two neurons, a *preganglionic neuron* and a *postganglionic neuron,* in contrast to only a single neuron in the skeletal motor pathway. The cell body of each preganglionic neuron lies in the *intermediolateral horn* of the spinal cord; its fiber passes, as shown in Figure 60-2, through an *anterior root* of the cord into the corresponding *spinal nerve.*

Immediately after the spinal nerve leaves the spinal canal, the preganglionic sympathetic fibers leave the spinal nerve and pass through a *white ramus* into one of the *ganglia* of the *sympathetic chain.* Then the course of the fibers can be one of the following three: (1) It can synapse with postganglionic sympathetic neurons in the ganglion that it enters; (2) it can pass upward or downward in the chain and synapse in one of the other ganglia of the chain; or (3) it can pass for variable distances through the chain and then through one of the *sympathetic nerves* radiating outward from the chain, finally synapsing in a *peripheral sympathetic ganglion.*

The postganglionic sympathetic neuron thus originates either in one of the sympathetic chain ganglia or in one of the peripheral sympathetic ganglia. From either of these two sources, the postganglionic fibers then travel to their destinations in the various organs.

Sympathetic Nerve Fibers in the Skeletal Nerves. Some of the postganglionic fibers pass back from the sympathetic chain into the spinal nerves through *gray rami* at all levels of the cord, as shown in Figure 60-2. These sympathetic fibers are all very small type C fibers, and they extend to all parts

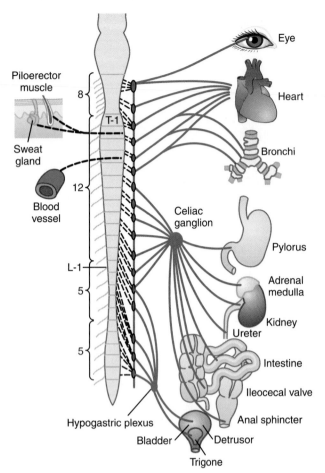

Figure 60-1 Sympathetic nervous system. The *black dashed lines* represent postganglionic fibers in the gray rami leading from the sympathetic chains into spinal nerves for distribution to blood vessels, sweat glands, and piloerector muscles.

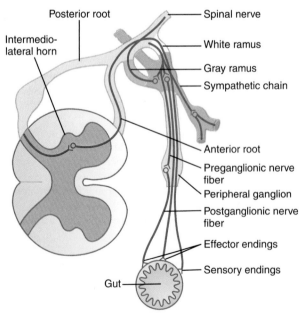

Figure 60-2 Nerve connections among the spinal cord, spinal nerves, sympathetic chain, and peripheral sympathetic nerves.

of the body by way of the skeletal nerves. They control the blood vessels, sweat glands, and piloerector muscles of the hairs. About 8 percent of the fibers in the average skeletal nerve are sympathetic fibers, a fact that indicates their great importance.

Segmental Distribution of the Sympathetic Nerve Fibers. The sympathetic pathways that originate in the different segments of the spinal cord are not necessarily distributed to the same part of the body as the somatic spinal nerve fibers from the same segments. Instead, the *sympathetic fibers from cord segment T-1 generally pass up the sympathetic chain to terminate in the head; from T-2 to terminate in the neck; from T-3, T-4, T-5, and T-6 into the thorax; from T-7, T-8, T-9, T-10, and T-11 into the abdomen; and from T-12, L-1, and L-2 into the legs.* This distribution is only approximate and overlaps greatly.

The distribution of sympathetic nerves to each organ is determined partly by the locus in the embryo from which the organ originated. For instance, the heart receives many sympathetic nerve fibers from the neck portion of the sympathetic chain because the heart originated in the neck of the embryo before translocating into the thorax. Likewise, the abdominal organs receive most of their sympathetic innervation from the lower thoracic spinal cord segments because most of the primitive gut originated in this area.

Special Nature of the Sympathetic Nerve Endings in the Adrenal Medullae. Preganglionic sympathetic nerve fibers pass, *without synapsing,* all the way from the intermediolateral horn cells of the spinal cord, through the sympathetic chains, then through the splanchnic nerves, and finally into the two adrenal medullae. There they end directly on modified neuronal cells that secrete *epinephrine* and *norepinephrine* into the blood stream. These secretory cells embryologically are derived from nervous tissue and are actually themselves postganglionic neurons; indeed, they even have rudimentary nerve fibers, and it is the endings of these fibers that secrete the adrenal hormones *epinephrine* and *norepinephrine.*

Physiologic Anatomy of the Parasympathetic Nervous System

The *parasympathetic nervous system* is shown in Figure 60-3, demonstrating that parasympathetic fibers leave the central nervous system through cranial nerves III, VII, IX, and X; additional parasympathetic fibers leave the lowermost part of the spinal cord through the second and third sacral spinal nerves and occasionally the first and fourth sacral nerves. About 75 percent of all parasympathetic nerve fibers are in the *vagus nerves* (cranial nerve X), passing to the entire thoracic and abdominal regions of the body. Therefore, a physiologist speaking of the parasympathetic nervous system often thinks mainly of the two vagus nerves. The vagus nerves supply parasympathetic nerves to the heart, lungs, esophagus, stomach, entire small intestine, proximal half of the colon, liver, gallbladder, pancreas, kidneys, and upper portions of the ureters.

Parasympathetic fibers in the *third cranial nerve* go to the pupillary sphincter and ciliary muscle of the eye. Fibers from the *seventh cranial nerve* pass to the lacrimal, nasal, and

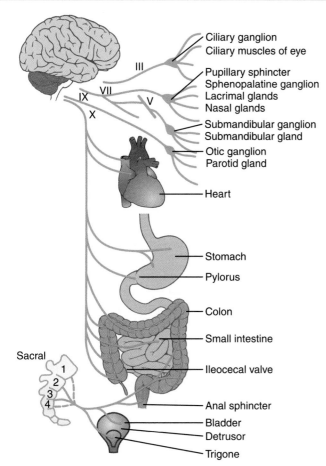

Figure 60-3 Parasympathetic nervous system.

submandibular glands. And fibers from the *ninth cranial nerve* go to the parotid gland.

The sacral parasympathetic fibers are in the *pelvic nerves,* which pass through the spinal nerve sacral plexus on each side of the cord at the S-2 and S-3 levels. These fibers then distribute to the descending colon, rectum, urinary bladder, and lower portions of the ureters. Also, this sacral group of parasympathetics supplies nerve signals to the external genitalia to cause erection.

Preganglionic and Postganglionic Parasympathetic Neurons. The parasympathetic system, like the sympathetic, has both preganglionic and postganglionic neurons. However, except in the case of a few cranial parasympathetic nerves, the *preganglionic fibers* pass uninterrupted all the way to the organ that is to be controlled. In the wall of the organ are located the *postganglionic neurons.* The preganglionic fibers synapse with these, and extremely short postganglionic fibers, a fraction of a millimeter to several centimeters in length, leave the neurons to innervate the tissues of the organ. This location of the parasympathetic postganglionic neurons in the visceral organ itself is quite different from the arrangement of the sympathetic ganglia because the cell bodies of the sympathetic postganglionic neurons are almost

always located in the ganglia of the sympathetic chain or in various other discrete ganglia in the abdomen, rather than in the excited organ itself.

Basic Characteristics of Sympathetic and Parasympathetic Function

Cholinergic and Adrenergic Fibers—Secretion of Acetylcholine or Norepinephrine

The sympathetic and parasympathetic nerve fibers secrete mainly one or the other of two synaptic transmitter substances, *acetylcholine* or *norepinephrine.* Those fibers that secrete acetylcholine are said to be *cholinergic.* Those that secrete norepinephrine are said to be *adrenergic,* a term derived from *adrenalin,* which is an alternate name for epinephrine.

All *preganglionic neurons* are *cholinergic* in both the sympathetic and the parasympathetic nervous systems. Acetylcholine or acetylcholine-like substances, when applied to the ganglia, will excite both sympathetic and parasympathetic postganglionic neurons. Either *all or almost all of the postganglionic neurons of the parasympathetic system are also cholinergic.* Conversely, *most of the postganglionic sympathetic neurons are adrenergic.* However, the postganglionic sympathetic nerve fibers to the sweat glands, to the piloerector muscles of the hairs, and to a very few blood vessels are cholinergic.

Thus, the terminal nerve endings of the parasympathetic system *all or virtually all* secrete *acetylcholine.* Almost all of the sympathetic nerve endings secrete *norepinephrine,* but a few secrete acetylcholine. These neurotransmitters in turn act on the different organs to cause respective parasympathetic or sympathetic effects. Therefore, acetylcholine is called a *parasympathetic transmitter* and norepinephrine is called a *sympathetic transmitter.*

The molecular structures of acetylcholine and norepinephrine are the following:

Acetylcholine

Norepinephrine

Mechanisms of Transmitter Secretion and Subsequent Removal of the Transmitter at the Postganglionic Endings

Secretion of Acetylcholine and Norepinephrine by Postganglionic Nerve Endings. A few of the postganglionic autonomic nerve endings, especially those of the parasympathetic nerves, are similar to but much smaller than those of the skeletal neuromuscular junction. However, many of the parasympathetic nerve fibers and almost all the sympathetic fibers merely touch the effector cells of the organs that they innervate as they pass by; or in some instances, they terminate in connective tissue located adjacent to the cells that are to be stimulated. Where these filaments touch or pass over or near the cells to be stimulated, they usually have bulbous enlargements called *varicosities;* it is in these varicosities that the transmitter vesicles of acetylcholine or norepinephrine are synthesized and stored. Also in the varicosities are large numbers of mitochondria that supply adenosine triphosphate, which is required to energize acetylcholine or norepinephrine synthesis.

When an action potential spreads over the terminal fibers, the depolarization process increases the permeability of the fiber membrane to calcium ions, allowing these ions to diffuse into the nerve terminals or nerve varicosities. The calcium ions in turn cause the terminals or varicosities to empty their contents to the exterior. Thus, the transmitter substance is secreted.

Synthesis of Acetylcholine, Its Destruction After Secretion, and Its Duration of Action. Acetylcholine is synthesized in the terminal endings and varicosities of the cholinergic nerve fibers where it is stored in vesicles in highly concentrated form until it is released. The basic chemical reaction of this synthesis is the following:

$$\text{Acetyl-CoA + Choline} \xrightarrow{\text{Choline acetyl-transferase}} \text{Acetylcholine}$$

Once acetylcholine is secreted into a tissue by a cholinergic nerve ending, it persists in the tissue for a few seconds while it performs its nerve signal transmitter function. Then it is split into an *acetate ion* and *choline*, catalyzed by the enzyme *acetylcholinesterase* that is bound with collagen and glycosaminoglycans in the local connective tissue. This is the same mechanism for acetylcholine signal transmission and subsequent acetylcholine destruction that occurs at the neuromuscular junctions of skeletal nerve fibers. The choline that is formed is then transported back into the terminal nerve ending, where it is used again and again for synthesis of new acetylcholine.

Synthesis of Norepinephrine, Its Removal, and Its Duration of Action. Synthesis of norepinephrine begins in the axoplasm of the terminal nerve endings of adrenergic nerve fibers but is completed inside the secretory vesicles. The basic steps are the following:

1. $\text{Tyrosine} \xrightarrow{\text{Hydroxylation}} \text{Dopa}$

2. $\text{Dopa} \xrightarrow{\text{Decarboxylation}} \text{Dopamine}$

3. Transport of dopamine into the vesicles

4. $\text{Dopamine} \xrightarrow{\text{Hydroxylation}} \text{Norepinephrine}$

In the adrenal medulla, this reaction goes still one step further to transform about 80 per cent of the norepinephrine into epinephrine, as follows:

5. $\text{Norepinephrine} \xrightarrow{\text{Methylation}} \text{Epinephrine}$

After secretion of norepinephrine by the terminal nerve endings, it is removed from the secretory site in three ways: (1) reuptake into the adrenergic nerve endings by an active transport process—accounting for removal of 50 to 80 percent of the secreted norepinephrine; (2) diffusion away from the nerve endings into the surrounding body fluids and then into the blood—accounting for removal of most of the remaining norepinephrine; and (3) destruction of small amounts by tissue enzymes (one of these enzymes is *monoamine oxidase*, which is found in the nerve endings, and another is *catechol-O-methyl transferase*, which is present diffusely in all tissues).

Ordinarily, the norepinephrine secreted directly into a tissue remains active for only a few seconds, demonstrating that its reuptake and diffusion away from the tissue are rapid. However, the norepinephrine and epinephrine secreted into the blood by the adrenal medullae remain active until they diffuse into some tissue, where they can be destroyed by catechol-O-methyl transferase; this occurs mainly in the liver. Therefore, when secreted into the blood, both norepinephrine and epinephrine remain active for 10 to 30 seconds; but their activity declines to extinction over 1 to several minutes.

Receptors on the Effector Organs

Before acetylcholine, norepinephrine, or epinephrine secreted at an autonomic nerve ending can stimulate an effector organ, it must first bind with specific *receptors* on the effector cells. The receptor is on the outside of the cell membrane, bound as a prosthetic group to a protein molecule that penetrates all the way through the cell membrane. When the transmitter substance binds with the receptor, this causes a conformational change in the structure of the protein molecule. In turn, the altered protein molecule excites or inhibits the cell, most often by (1) causing a change in cell membrane permeability to one or more ions or (2) activating or inactivating an enzyme attached to the other end of the receptor protein, where it protrudes into the interior of the cell.

Excitation or Inhibition of the Effector Cell by Changing Its Membrane Permeability. Because the receptor protein is an integral part of the cell membrane, a conformational change in structure of the receptor protein often *opens or closes an ion channel* through the interstices of the protein molecule, thus altering the permeability of the cell membrane to various ions. For instance, sodium and/or calcium ion channels frequently become opened and allow rapid influx of the respective ions into the cell, usually depolarizing the cell membrane and *exciting* the cell. At other times, potassium channels are opened, allowing potassium ions to diffuse out of the cell, and this usually *inhibits* the cell because loss of electropositive potassium ions creates hypernegativity inside the cell. In some cells, the changed intracellular ion environment will cause an internal cell action, such as a direct effect of calcium ions to promote smooth muscle contraction.

Receptor Action by Altering Intracellular "Second Messenger" Enzymes. Another way a receptor often functions is to activate or inactivate an enzyme (or other intracellular chemical) inside the cell. The enzyme often is attached to the receptor protein where the receptor protrudes into the interior of the cell. For instance, binding of norepinephrine with its receptor on the outside of many cells increases the activity of the enzyme *adenylyl cyclase* on the inside of the cell, and this causes formation of *cyclic adenosine monophosphate* (cAMP). The cAMP in turn can initiate any one of many different intracellular actions, the exact effect depending on the chemical machinery of the effector cell.

It is easy to understand how an autonomic transmitter substance can cause inhibition in some organs or excitation in others. This is usually determined by the nature of the receptor protein in the cell membrane and the effect of receptor binding on its conformational state. In each organ, the resulting effects are likely to be different from those in other organs.

Two Principal Types of Acetylcholine Receptors— Muscarinic and Nicotinic Receptors

Acetylcholine activates mainly two types of *receptors*. They are called *muscarinic* and *nicotinic* receptors. The reason for these names is that muscarine, a poison from toadstools, activates only muscarinic receptors and will not activate nicotinic receptors, whereas nicotine activates only nicotinic receptors; acetylcholine activates both of them.

Muscarinic receptors are found on all effector cells that are stimulated by the postganglionic cholinergic neurons of either the parasympathetic nervous system or the sympathetic system.

Nicotinic receptors are found in the autonomic ganglia at the synapses between the preganglionic and postganglionic neurons of both the sympathetic and parasympathetic systems. (Nicotinic receptors are also present at many nonautonomic nerve endings—for instance, at the neuromuscular junctions in skeletal muscle [discussed in Chapter 7].)

An understanding of the two types of receptors is especially important because specific drugs are frequently used as medicine to stimulate or block one or the other of the two types of receptors.

Adrenergic Receptors—Alpha and Beta Receptors

There are also two major types of adrenergic receptors, *alpha receptors* and *beta receptors*. The beta receptors in turn are divided into *beta$_1$*, *beta$_2$* and *beta$_3$* receptors because certain chemicals affect only certain beta receptors. Also, there is a division of alpha receptors into alpha$_1$ and alpha$_2$ receptors.

Norepinephrine and epinephrine, both of which are secreted into the blood by the adrenal medulla, have slightly different effects in exciting the alpha and beta receptors. Norepinephrine excites mainly alpha receptors but excites the beta receptors to a lesser extent as well. Conversely, epinephrine excites both types of receptors approximately equally. Therefore, the relative effects of norepinephrine and epinephrine on different effector organs are determined by the types of receptors in the organs. If they are all beta receptors, epinephrine will be the more effective excitant.

Table 60-1 gives the distribution of alpha and beta receptors in some of the organs and systems controlled by the sympathetics. Note that certain alpha functions are excitatory, whereas others are inhibitory. Likewise, certain beta functions are excitatory and others are inhibitory. Therefore, alpha and beta receptors are not necessarily associated with excitation or inhibition but simply with the affinity of the hormone for the receptors in the given effector organ.

A synthetic hormone chemically similar to epinephrine and norepinephrine, *isopropyl norepinephrine*, has an extremely strong action on beta receptors but essentially no action on alpha receptors.

Excitatory and Inhibitory Actions of Sympathetic and Parasympathetic Stimulation

Table 60-2 lists the effects on different visceral functions of the body caused by stimulating either the parasympathetic nerves or the sympathetic nerves. From this table, it can be seen again that *sympathetic stimulation causes excitatory effects in some organs but inhibitory effects in others. Likewise, parasympathetic stimulation causes excitation in some but inhibition in others.* Also, when sympathetic stimulation excites a particular organ, parasympathetic stimulation sometimes inhibits it, demonstrating that the

Table 60-1 Adrenergic Receptors and Function

Alpha Receptor	Beta Receptor
Vasoconstriction	Vasodilation (β_2)
Iris dilation	Cardioacceleration (β_1)
Intestinal relaxation	Increased myocardial strength (β_1)
Intestinal sphincter contraction	Intestinal relaxation (β_2) Uterus relaxation (β_2)
Pilomotor contraction	Bronchodilation (β_2)
Bladder sphincter contraction	Calorigenesis (β_2)
Inhibits neurotransmitter release (α_2)	Glycogenolysis (β_2) Lipolysis (β_1) Bladder wall relaxation (β_2) Thermogenesis (β_3)

Table 60-2 Autonomic Effects on Various Organs of the Body

Organ	Effect of Sympathetic Stimulation	Effect of Parasympathetic Stimulation
Eye		
Pupil	Dilated	Constricted
Ciliary muscle	Slight relaxation (far vision)	Constricted (near vision)
Glands	Vasoconstriction and slight secretion	Stimulation of copious secretion (containing many enzymes for enzyme-secreting glands)
Nasal		
Lacrimal		
Parotid		
Submandibular		
Gastric		
Pancreatic		
Sweat glands	Copious sweating (cholinergic)	Sweating on palms of hands
Apocrine glands	Thick, odoriferous secretion	None
Blood vessels	Most often constricted	Most often little or no effect
Heart		
Muscle	Increased rate	Slowed rate
	Increased force of contraction	Decreased force of contraction (especially of atria)
Coronaries	Dilated (β_2); constricted (α)	Dilated
Lungs		
Bronchi	Dilated	Constricted
Blood vessels	Mildly constricted	? Dilated
Gut		
Lumen	Decreased peristalsis and tone	Increased peristalsis and tone
Sphincter	Increased tone (most times)	Relaxed (most times)
Liver	Glucose released	Slight glycogen synthesis
Gallbladder and bile ducts	Relaxed	Contracted
Kidney	Decreased urine output and increased renin secretion	None
Bladder		
Detrusor	Relaxed (slight)	Contracted
Trigone	Contracted	Relaxed
Penis	Ejaculation	Erection
Systemic arterioles		
Abdominal viscera	Constricted	None
Muscle	Constricted (adrenergic α)	None
	Dilated (adrenergic β_2)	
	Dilated (cholinergic)	
Skin	Constricted	None
Blood		
Coagulation	Increased	None
Glucose	Increased	None
Lipids	Increased	None
Basal metabolism	Increased up to 100%	None
Adrenal medullary secretion	Increased	None
Mental activity	Increased	None
Piloerector muscles	Contracted	None
Skeletal muscle	Increased glycogenolysis	None
	Increased strength	
Fat cells	Lipolysis	None

two systems occasionally act reciprocally to each other. But most organs are dominantly controlled by one or the other of the two systems.

There is no generalization one can use to explain whether sympathetic or parasympathetic stimulation will cause excitation or inhibition of a particular organ. Therefore, to understand sympathetic and parasympathetic function, one must learn all the separate functions of these two nervous systems on each organ, as listed in Table 60-2. Some of these functions need to be clarified in still greater detail, as follows.

Effects of Sympathetic and Parasympathetic Stimulation on Specific Organs

Eyes. Two functions of the eyes are controlled by the autonomic nervous system. They are (1) the pupillary opening and (2) the focus of the lens.

Sympathetic stimulation *contracts the meridional fibers of the iris that dilate* the pupil, whereas parasympathetic stimulation contracts the *circular muscle of the iris to constrict* the pupil.

The parasympathetics that control the pupil are reflexly stimulated when excess light enters the eyes, which is explained in Chapter 51; this reflex reduces the pupillary opening and decreases the amount of light that strikes the retina. Conversely, the sympathetics become stimulated during periods of excitement and increase pupillary opening at these times.

Focusing of the lens is controlled almost entirely by the parasympathetic nervous system. The lens is normally held in a flattened state by intrinsic elastic tension of its radial ligaments. Parasympathetic excitation contracts the *ciliary muscle*, which is a ringlike body of smooth muscle fibers that encircles the outside ends of the lens radial ligaments. This contraction releases the tension on the ligaments and allows the lens to become more convex, causing the eye to focus on objects near at hand. The detailed focusing mechanism is discussed in Chapters 49 and 51 in relation to function of the eyes.

Glands of the Body. The *nasal, lacrimal, salivary,* and many *gastrointestinal glands* are strongly stimulated by the parasympathetic nervous system, usually resulting in copious quantities of watery secretion. The glands of the alimentary tract most strongly stimulated by the parasympathetics are those of the upper tract, especially those of the mouth and stomach. On the other hand, the glands of the small and large intestines are controlled principally by local factors in the intestinal tract itself and by the *intestinal enteric nervous system* and much less by the autonomic nerves.

Sympathetic stimulation has a direct effect on most alimentary gland cells to cause formation of a concentrated secretion that contains high percentages of enzymes and mucus. But it also causes vasoconstriction of the blood vessels that supply the glands and in this way sometimes reduces their rates of secretion.

The *sweat glands* secrete large quantities of sweat when the sympathetic nerves are stimulated, but no effect is caused by stimulating the parasympathetic nerves. However, the sympathetic fibers to most sweat glands are *cholinergic* (except for a few adrenergic fibers to the palms and soles), in contrast to almost all other sympathetic fibers, which are adrenergic. Furthermore, the sweat glands are stimulated primarily by centers in the hypothalamus that are usually considered to be parasympathetic centers. Therefore, sweating could be called a parasympathetic function, even though it is controlled by nerve fibers that anatomically are distributed through the sympathetic nervous system.

The *apocrine glands* in the axillae secrete a thick, odoriferous secretion as a result of sympathetic stimulation, but they do not respond to parasympathetic stimulation. This secretion actually functions as a lubricant to allow easy sliding motion of the inside surfaces under the shoulder joint. The apocrine glands, despite their close embryological relation to sweat glands, are activated by adrenergic fibers rather than by cholinergic fibers and are also controlled by the sympathetic centers of the central nervous system rather than by the parasympathetic centers.

Intramural Nerve Plexus of the Gastrointestinal System. The gastrointestinal system has its own intrinsic set of nerves known as the *intramural plexus* or the *intestinal enteric nervous system,* located in the walls of the gut. Also, both parasympathetic and sympathetic stimulation originating in the brain can affect gastrointestinal activity mainly by increasing or decreasing specific actions in the gastrointestinal intramural plexus. Parasympathetic stimulation, in general, increases overall degree of activity of the gastrointestinal tract by promoting peristalsis and relaxing the sphincters, thus allowing rapid propulsion of contents along the tract. This propulsive effect is associated with simultaneous increases in rates of secretion by many of the gastrointestinal glands, described earlier.

Normal function of the gastrointestinal tract is not very dependent on sympathetic stimulation. However, strong sympathetic stimulation inhibits peristalsis and increases the tone of the sphincters. The net result is greatly slowed propulsion of food through the tract and sometimes decreased secretion as well—even to the extent of sometimes causing constipation.

Heart. In general, sympathetic stimulation increases the overall activity of the heart. This is accomplished by increasing both the rate and force of heart contraction.

Parasympathetic stimulation causes mainly opposite effects—decreased heart rate and strength of contraction. To express these effects in another way, sympathetic stimulation increases the effectiveness of the heart as a pump, as required during heavy exercise, whereas parasympathetic stimulation decreases heart pumping, allowing the heart to rest between bouts of strenuous activity.

Systemic Blood Vessels. Most systemic blood vessels, especially those of the abdominal viscera and skin of the limbs, are constricted by sympathetic stimulation. Parasympathetic stimulation has almost no effects on most blood vessels except to dilate vessels in certain restricted areas, such as in the blush area of the face. Under some conditions, the beta function of the sympathetics causes vascular dilation instead of the usual sympathetic vascular constriction, but this occurs rarely except after drugs have paralyzed the sympathetic alpha vasoconstrictor effects, which, in most blood vessels, are usually far dominant over the beta effects.

Effect of Sympathetic and Parasympathetic Stimulation on Arterial Pressure. The arterial pressure is determined by two factors: propulsion of blood by the heart and resistance to flow of blood through the peripheral blood vessels. Sympathetic stimulation increases both propulsion by the heart and resistance to flow, which usually causes a marked *acute* increase in arterial pressure but often very little change in long-term pressure unless the sympathetics stimulate the kidneys to retain salt and water at the same time.

Conversely, moderate parasympathetic stimulation via the vagal nerves decreases pumping by the heart but has virtually no effect on vascular peripheral resistance. Therefore, the usual effect is a slight decrease in arterial pressure. But *very strong vagal parasympathetic* stimulation can almost stop or occasionally actually stop the heart entirely for a few seconds and cause temporary loss of all or most arterial pressure.

Effects of Sympathetic and Parasympathetic Stimulation on Other Functions of the Body. Because of the great importance of the sympathetic and parasympathetic control systems, they are discussed many times in this text in relation to multiple body functions. In general, most of the entodermal structures, such as the ducts of the liver, gallbladder, ureter, urinary bladder, and bronchi, are inhibited by sympathetic stimulation but excited by parasympathetic stimulation. Sympathetic stimulation also has multiple metabolic effects such as release of glucose from the liver, increase in blood glucose concentration, increase in glycogenolysis in both liver and muscle, increase in skeletal muscle strength, increase in basal metabolic rate, and increase in mental activity. Finally, the sympathetics and parasympathetics are involved in execution of the male and female sexual acts, as explained in Chapters 80 and 81.

Function of the Adrenal Medullae

Stimulation of the sympathetic nerves to the adrenal medullae causes large quantities of epinephrine and norepinephrine to be released into the circulating blood, and these two hormones in turn are carried in the blood to all tissues of the body. On average, about 80 percent of the secretion is epinephrine and 20 percent is norepinephrine, although the relative proportions can change considerably under different physiologic conditions.

The circulating epinephrine and norepinephrine have almost the same effects on the different organs as the effects caused by direct sympathetic stimulation, except that *the effects last 5 to 10 times as long* because both of these hormones are removed from the blood slowly over a period of 2 to 4 minutes.

The circulating norepinephrine causes constriction of most of the blood vessels of the body; it also causes increased activity of the heart, inhibition of the gastrointestinal tract, dilation of the pupils of the eyes, and so forth.

Epinephrine causes almost the same effects as those caused by norepinephrine, but the effects differ in the following respects: First, epinephrine, because of its greater effect in stimulating the beta receptors, has a greater effect on cardiac stimulation than does norepinephrine. Second, epinephrine causes only weak constriction of the blood vessels in the muscles, in comparison with much stronger constriction caused by norepinephrine. Because the muscle vessels represent a major segment of the vessels of the body, this difference is of special importance because norepinephrine greatly increases the total peripheral resistance and elevates arterial pressure, whereas epinephrine raises the arterial pressure to a lesser extent but increases the cardiac output more.

A third difference between the actions of epinephrine and norepinephrine relates to their effects on tissue metabolism. Epinephrine has 5 to 10 times as great a metabolic effect as norepinephrine. Indeed, the epinephrine secreted by the adrenal medullae can increase the metabolic rate of the whole body often to as much as 100 percent above normal, in this way increasing the activity and excitability of the body. It also increases the rates of other metabolic activities, such as glycogenolysis in the liver and muscle, and glucose release into the blood.

In summary, stimulation of the adrenal medullae causes release of the hormones epinephrine and norepinephrine, which together have almost the same effects throughout the body as direct sympathetic stimulation, except that the effects are greatly prolonged, lasting 2 to 4 minutes after the stimulation is over.

Value of the Adrenal Medullae to the Function of the Sympathetic Nervous System. Epinephrine and norepinephrine are almost always released by the adrenal medullae at the same time that the different organs are stimulated directly by generalized sympathetic activation. Therefore, the organs are actually stimulated in two ways: directly by the sympathetic nerves and indirectly by the adrenal medullary hormones. The two means of stimulation support each other, and either can, in most instances, substitute for the other. For instance, destruction of the direct sympathetic pathways to the different body organs does not abrogate sympathetic excitation of the organs because norepinephrine and epinephrine are still released into the circulating blood and indirectly cause stimulation. Likewise, loss of the two adrenal medullae usually has little effect on the operation of the sympathetic nervous system because the direct pathways can still perform almost all the necessary duties. Thus, the dual mechanism of sympathetic stimulation provides a safety factor, one mechanism substituting for the other if it is missing.

Another important value of the adrenal medullae is the capability of epinephrine and norepinephrine to stimulate structures of the body that are not innervated by direct sympathetic fibers. For instance, the metabolic rate of every cell of the body is increased by these hormones, especially by epinephrine, even though only a small proportion of all the cells in the body are innervated directly by sympathetic fibers.

Relation of Stimulus Rate to Degree of Sympathetic and Parasympathetic Effect

A special difference between the autonomic nervous system and the skeletal nervous system is that only a low frequency of stimulation is required for full activation of autonomic effectors. In general, only one nerve impulse every few seconds suffices to maintain normal sympathetic or parasympathetic effect, and full activation occurs when the nerve fibers discharge 10 to 20 times per second. This compares with full activation in the skeletal nervous system at 50 to 500 or more impulses per second.

Sympathetic and Parasympathetic "Tone"

Normally, the sympathetic and parasympathetic systems are continually active, and the basal rates of activity are known, respectively, as *sympathetic tone* and *parasympathetic tone.*

The value of tone is that *it allows a single nervous system both to increase and decrease the activity of a stimulated organ.* For instance, sympathetic tone normally keeps almost all the systemic arterioles constricted to about one-half their maximum diameter. By increasing the degree of sympathetic stimulation above normal, these vessels can be constricted even more; conversely, by decreasing the stimulation below normal, the arterioles can be dilated. If it were not for the continual background sympathetic tone, the sympathetic system could cause only vasoconstriction, never vasodilation.

Another interesting example of tone is the background "tone" of the parasympathetics in the gastrointestinal tract. Surgical removal of the parasympathetic supply to most of the gut by cutting the vagus nerves can cause serious and prolonged gastric and intestinal "atony" with resulting blockage of much of the normal gastrointestinal propulsion and consequent serious constipation, thus demonstrating that parasympathetic tone to the gut is normally very much required. This tone can be decreased by the brain, thereby inhibiting gastrointestinal motility, or it can be increased, thereby promoting increased gastrointestinal activity.

Tone Caused by Basal Secretion of Epinephrine and Norepinephrine by the Adrenal Medullae. The normal resting rate of secretion by the adrenal medullae is about 0.2 μg/kg/min of epinephrine and about 0.05 μg/kg/min of norepinephrine. These quantities are considerable—indeed, enough to maintain the blood pressure almost up to normal even if all direct sympathetic pathways to the cardiovascular system are removed. Therefore, it is obvious that much of the overall tone of the sympathetic nervous system results from basal secretion of epinephrine and norepinephrine in addition to the tone resulting from direct sympathetic stimulation.

Effect of Loss of Sympathetic or Parasympathetic Tone After Denervation. Immediately after a sympathetic or parasympathetic nerve is cut, the innervated organ loses its sympathetic or parasympathetic tone. In the case of the blood vessels, for instance, cutting the sympathetic nerves results within 5 to 30 seconds in almost maximal vasodilation. However, over minutes, hours, days, or weeks, *intrinsic tone* in the smooth muscle of the vessels increases—that is, increased tone caused by increased smooth muscle contractile force that is *not* the result of sympathetic stimulation but of chemical adaptations in the smooth muscle fibers themselves. This intrinsic tone eventually restores almost normal vasoconstriction.

Essentially the same effects occur in most other effector organs whenever sympathetic or parasympathetic tone is lost. That is, intrinsic compensation soon develops to return the function of the organ almost to its normal basal level. However, in the parasympathetic system, the compensation sometimes requires many months. For instance, loss of parasympathetic tone to the heart after cardiac vagotomy increases the heart rate to 160 beats per minute in a dog, and this will still be partially elevated 6 months later.

Denervation Supersensitivity of Sympathetic and Parasympathetic Organs After Denervation

During the first week or so after a sympathetic or parasympathetic nerve is destroyed, the innervated organ becomes more sensitive to injected norepinephrine or acetylcholine, respectively. This effect is demonstrated in Figure 60-4, showing blood flow in the forearm before removal of the sympathetics to be about 200 ml/min; a test dose of norepinephrine causes only a slight depression in flow lasting a minute or so. Then the stellate ganglion is removed, and normal sympathetic tone is lost. At first, the blood flow rises markedly because of the lost vascular tone, but over a period of days to weeks the blood flow returns much of the way back toward normal because of progressive increase in intrinsic tone of the vascular musculature itself, thus partially compensating for the loss of sympathetic tone. Then another test dose of norepinephrine is administered, and the blood flow decreases much more than before, demonstrating that the blood vessels have become about two to four times as responsive to norepinephrine as previously. This phenomenon is called *denervation supersensitivity*. It occurs in both sympathetic and parasympathetic organs but to far greater extent in some organs than in others, occasionally increasing the response more than 10-fold.

Mechanism of Denervation Supersensitivity. The cause of denervation supersensitivity is only partially known. Part of the answer is that the number of receptors in the postsynaptic membranes of the effector cells increases—sometimes manyfold—when norepinephrine or acetylcholine is no longer released at the synapses, a process called "up-regulation" of the receptors. Therefore, when a dose of the hormone is now injected into the circulating blood, the effector reaction is vastly enhanced.

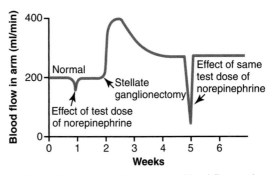

Figure 60-4 Effect of sympathectomy on blood flow in the arm, and effect of a test dose of norepinephrine before and after sympathectomy, showing *supersensitization* of the vasculature to norepinephrine.

Autonomic Reflexes

Many visceral functions of the body are regulated by *autonomic reflexes.* Throughout this text, the functions of these reflexes are discussed in relation to individual organ systems; to illustrate their importance, a few are presented here briefly.

Cardiovascular Autonomic Reflexes. Several reflexes in the cardiovascular system help to control the arterial blood pressure and the heart rate. One of these is the *baroreceptor reflex,* which is described in Chapter 18 along with other cardiovascular reflexes. Briefly, stretch receptors called *baroreceptors* are located in the walls of several major arteries, including especially the internal carotid arteries and the arch of the aorta. When these become stretched by high pressure, signals are transmitted to the brain stem, where they inhibit the sympathetic impulses to the heart and blood vessels and excite the parasympathetics; this allows the arterial pressure to fall back toward normal.

Gastrointestinal Autonomic Reflexes. The uppermost part of the gastrointestinal tract and the rectum are controlled principally by autonomic reflexes. For instance, the smell of appetizing food or the presence of food in the mouth initiates signals from the nose and mouth to the vagal, glossopharyngeal, and salivatory nuclei of the brain stem. These in turn transmit signals through the parasympathetic nerves to the secretory glands of the mouth and stomach, causing secretion of digestive juices sometimes even before food enters the mouth.

When fecal matter fills the rectum at the other end of the alimentary canal, sensory impulses initiated by stretching the rectum are sent to the sacral portion of the spinal cord, and a reflex signal is transmitted back through the sacral parasympathetics to the distal parts of the colon; these result in strong peristaltic contractions that cause defecation.

Other Autonomic Reflexes. Emptying of the urinary bladder is controlled in the same way as emptying the rectum; stretching of the bladder sends impulses to the sacral cord, and this in turn causes reflex contraction of the bladder and relaxation of the urinary sphincters, thereby promoting micturition.

Also important are the sexual reflexes, which are initiated both by psychic stimuli from the brain and by stimuli from the sexual organs. Impulses from these sources converge on the sacral cord and, in the male, result first in *erection, mainly a parasympathetic function,* and then *ejaculation, partially a sympathetic function.*

Other autonomic control functions include reflex contributions to the regulation of pancreatic secretion, gallbladder emptying, kidney excretion of urine, sweating, blood glucose concentration, and many other visceral functions, all of which are discussed in detail at other points in this text.

Stimulation of Discrete Organs in Some Instances and Mass Stimulation in Other Instances by the Sympathetic and Parasympathetic Systems

Sympathetic System Sometimes Responds by Mass Discharge. In some instances, almost all portions of the sympathetic nervous system discharge simultaneously as a complete unit, a phenomenon called *mass discharge.* This frequently occurs when the hypothalamus is activated by fright or fear or severe pain. The result is a widespread reaction throughout the body called the *alarm* or *stress response,* which is discussed shortly.

At other times, activation occurs in isolated portions of the sympathetic nervous system. Important examples are the following: (1) During the process of heat regulation, the sympathetics control sweating and blood flow in the skin without affecting other organs innervated by the sympathetics. (2) Many "local reflexes" involving sensory afferent fibers travel centrally in the peripheral nerves to the sympathetic ganglia and spinal cord and cause highly localized reflex responses. For instance, heating a skin area causes local vasodilation and enhanced local sweating, whereas cooling causes opposite effects. (3) Many of the sympathetic reflexes that control gastrointestinal functions operate by way of nerve pathways that do not even enter the spinal cord, merely passing from the gut mainly to the paravertebral ganglia, and then back to the gut through sympathetic nerves to control motor or secretory activity.

Parasympathetic System Usually Causes Specific Localized Responses. Control functions by the parasympathetic system are often highly specific. For instance, parasympathetic cardiovascular reflexes usually act only on the heart to increase or decrease its rate of beating. Likewise, other parasympathetic reflexes cause secretion mainly by the mouth glands and in other instances secretion is mainly by the stomach glands. Finally, the rectal emptying reflex does not affect other parts of the bowel to a major extent.

Yet there is often association between closely allied parasympathetic functions. For instance, although salivary secretion can occur independently of gastric secretion, these two also often occur together, and pancreatic secretion frequently occurs at the same time. Also, the rectal emptying reflex often initiates a urinary bladder emptying reflex, resulting in simultaneous emptying of both the bladder and the rectum. Conversely, the bladder emptying reflex can help initiate rectal emptying.

"Alarm" or "Stress" Response of the Sympathetic Nervous System

When large portions of the sympathetic nervous system discharge at the same time—that is, a *mass discharge*—this increases in many ways the ability of the body to perform vigorous muscle activity. Let us summarize these ways:

1. Increased arterial pressure

2. Increased blood flow to active muscles concurrent with decreased blood flow to organs such as the gastrointestinal tract and the kidneys that are not needed for rapid motor activity

3. Increased rates of cellular metabolism throughout the body

4. Increased blood glucose concentration

5. Increased glycolysis in the liver and in muscle

6. Increased muscle strength

7. Increased mental activity

8. Increased rate of blood coagulation

The sum of these effects permits a person to perform far more strenuous physical activity than would otherwise be possible. Because either *mental* or *physical stress* can excite the sympathetic system, it is frequently said that the purpose of the sympathetic system is to provide extra activation of the body in states of stress: this is called the sympathetic *stress response.*

The sympathetic system is especially strongly activated in many emotional states. For instance, in the state of *rage,* which is elicited to a great extent by stimulating the hypothalamus, signals are transmitted downward through the reticular formation of the brain stem and into the spinal cord to cause massive sympathetic discharge; most aforementioned sympathetic events ensue immediately. This is called the sympathetic *alarm reaction.* It is also called the *fight or flight reaction* because an animal in this state decides almost instantly whether to stand and fight or to run. In either event, the sympathetic alarm reaction makes the animal's subsequent activities vigorous.

Medullary, Pontine, and Mesencephalic Control of the Autonomic Nervous System

Many neuronal areas in the brain stem reticular substance and along the course of the tractus solitarius of the medulla, pons, and mesencephalon, as well as in many special nuclei (Figure 60-5), control different autonomic functions such as arterial pressure, heart rate, glandular secretion in the gastrointestinal tract, gastrointestinal peristalsis, and degree of contraction of the urinary bladder. Control of each of these is discussed at appropriate points in this text. Some of the *most important factors controlled in the brain stem are arterial pressure, heart rate, and respiratory rate.* Indeed, transection of the brain stem above the midpontine

level allows basal control of arterial pressure to continue as before but prevents its modulation by higher nervous centers such as the hypothalamus. Conversely, transection immediately below the medulla causes the arterial pressure to fall to less than one-half normal.

Closely associated with the cardiovascular regulatory centers in the brain stem are the medullary and pontine centers for regulation of respiration, which are discussed in Chapter 41. Although this is not considered to be an autonomic function, it is one of the *involuntary* functions of the body.

Control of Brain Stem Autonomic Centers by Higher Areas. Signals from the hypothalamus and even from the cerebrum can affect the activities of almost all the brain stem autonomic control centers. For instance, stimulation in appropriate areas mainly of the posterior hypothalamus can activate the medullary cardiovascular control centers strongly enough to increase arterial pressure to more than twice normal. Likewise, other hypothalamic centers control body temperature, increase or decrease salivation and gastrointestinal activity, and cause bladder emptying. To some extent, therefore, the autonomic centers in the brain stem act as relay stations for control activities initiated at higher levels of the brain, especially in the hypothalamus.

In Chapters 58 and 59, it is pointed out also that many of our behavioral responses are mediated through (1) the hypothalamus, (2) the reticular areas of the brain stem, and (3) the autonomic nervous system. Indeed, some higher areas of the brain can alter function of the whole autonomic nervous system or of portions of it strongly enough to cause severe autonomic-induced disease such as peptic ulcer of the stomach or duodenum, constipation, heart palpitation, or even heart attack.

Pharmacology of the Autonomic Nervous System

Drugs That Act on Adrenergic Effector Organs— Sympathomimetic Drugs

From the foregoing discussion, it is obvious that intravenous injection of norepinephrine causes essentially the same effects throughout the body as sympathetic stimulation. Therefore, norepinephrine is called a *sympathomimetic* or *adrenergic drug. Epinephrine* and *methoxamine* are also sympathomimetic drugs, and there are many others. They differ from one another in the degree to which they stimulate different sympathetic effector organs and in their duration of action. Norepinephrine and epinephrine have actions as short as 1 to 2 minutes, whereas the actions of some other commonly used sympathomimetic drugs last for 30 minutes to 2 hours.

Important drugs that stimulate specific adrenergic receptors are *phenylephrine* (alpha receptors), *isoproterenol* (beta receptors), and *albuterol* (only beta$_2$ receptors).

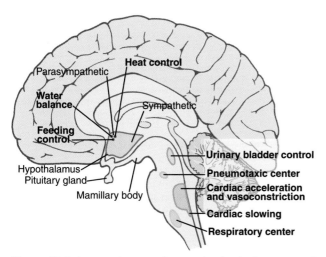

Figure 60-5 Autonomic control areas in the brain stem and hypothalamus.

Drugs That Cause Release of Norepinephrine from Nerve Endings. Certain drugs have an indirect sympathomimetic action instead of directly exciting adrenergic effector organs. These drugs include *ephedrine, tyramine,* and *amphetamine.* Their effect is to cause release of norepinephrine from its storage vesicles in the sympathetic nerve endings. The released norepinephrine in turn causes the sympathetic effects.

Drugs That Block Adrenergic Activity. Adrenergic activity can be blocked at several points in the stimulatory process, as follows:

1. The synthesis and storage of norepinephrine in the sympathetic nerve endings can be prevented. The best known drug that causes this effect is *reserpine.*

2. Release of norepinephrine from the sympathetic endings can be blocked. This can be caused by *guanethidine.*

3. The sympathetic *alpha* receptors can be blocked. Two drugs that cause this effect are *phenoxybenzamine* and *phentolamine.*

4. The sympathetic *beta* receptors can be blocked. A drug that blocks beta$_1$ and beta$_2$ receptors is *propranolol.* One that blocks mainly beta$_1$ receptors is *metoprolol.*

5. Sympathetic activity can be blocked by drugs that block transmission of nerve impulses through the autonomic ganglia. They are discussed in a later section, but an important drug for blockade of both sympathetic and parasympathetic transmission through the ganglia is *hexamethonium.*

Drugs That Act on Cholinergic Effector Organs

Parasympathomimetic Drugs (Cholinergic Drugs). Acetylcholine injected intravenously usually does not cause exactly the same effects throughout the body as parasympathetic stimulation because most of the acetylcholine is destroyed by cholinesterase in the blood and body fluids before it can reach all the effector organs. Yet a number of other drugs that are not so rapidly destroyed can produce typical widespread parasympathetic effects, and they are called *parasympathomimetic drugs.*

Two commonly used parasympathomimetic drugs are *pilocarpine* and *methacholine.* They act directly on the muscarinic type of cholinergic receptors.

Drugs That Have a Parasympathetic Potentiating Effect—Anticholinesterase Drugs. Some drugs do not have a direct effect on parasympathetic effector organs but do potentiate the effects of the naturally secreted acetylcholine at the parasympathetic endings. They are the same drugs as those discussed in Chapter 7 that potentiate the effect of acetylcholine at the neuromuscular junction. They include *neostigmine, pyridostigmine,* and *ambenonium.* These drugs inhibit acetylcholinesterase, thus *preventing rapid destruction of the acetylcholine* liberated at parasympathetic nerve endings. As a consequence, the quantity of acetylcholine increases with successive stimuli and the degree of action also increases.

Drugs That Block Cholinergic Activity at Effector Organs—Antimuscarinic Drugs. *Atropine* and similar drugs, such as *homatropine* and *scopolamine, block the action of acetylcholine on the muscarinic type of cholinergic effector organs.*

These drugs *do not* affect the nicotinic action of acetylcholine on the postganglionic neurons or on skeletal muscle.

Drugs That Stimulate or Block Sympathetic and Parasympathetic Postganglionic Neurons

Drugs That Stimulate Autonomic Postganglionic Neurons. The preganglionic neurons of both the parasympathetic and the sympathetic nervous systems secrete acetylcholine at their endings, and this acetylcholine in turn stimulates the postganglionic neurons. Furthermore, injected acetylcholine can also stimulate the postganglionic neurons of both systems, thereby causing at the same time both sympathetic and parasympathetic effects throughout the body.

Nicotine is another drug that can stimulate postganglionic neurons in the same manner as acetylcholine because the membranes of these neurons all contain the *nicotinic type of acetylcholine receptor.* Therefore, drugs that cause autonomic effects by stimulating postganglionic neurons are called *nicotinic drugs.* Some other drugs, such as *methacholine,* have both nicotinic and muscarinic actions, whereas *pilocarpine* has only muscarinic actions.

Nicotine excites both the sympathetic and parasympathetic postganglionic neurons at the same time, resulting in strong sympathetic vasoconstriction in the abdominal organs and limbs but at the same time resulting in parasympathetic effects such as increased gastrointestinal activity and, sometimes, slowing of the heart.

Ganglionic Blocking Drugs. Many important drugs block impulse transmission from the autonomic preganglionic neurons to the postganglionic neurons, including *tetraethyl ammonium ion, hexamethonium ion,* and *pentolinium.* These drugs block acetylcholine stimulation of the postganglionic neurons in both the sympathetic and the parasympathetic systems simultaneously. They are often used for blocking sympathetic activity but seldom for blocking parasympathetic activity because their effects of sympathetic blockade usually far overshadow the effects of parasympathetic blockade. The ganglionic blocking drugs especially can reduce the arterial pressure in many patients with hypertension, but these drugs are not useful clinically because their effects are difficult to control.

Bibliography

Cannon WB: Organization for physiological homeostasis, *Physiol Rev* 9:399, 1929.

Dajas-Bailador F, Wonnacott S: Nicotinic acetylcholine receptors and the regulation of neuronal signalling, *Trends Pharmacol Sci* 25:317, 2004.

Dampney RA, Horiuchi J, McDowall LM: Hypothalamic mechanisms coordinating cardiorespiratory function during exercise and defensive behaviour, *Auton Neurosci* 142:3, 2008.

DiBona GF: Physiology in perspective: The Wisdom of the Body. Neural control of the kidney, *Am J Physiol Regul Integr Comp Physiol* 2005.

Eisenhofer G, Kopin IJ, Goldstein DS: Catecholamine metabolism: a contemporary view with implications for physiology and medicine, *Pharmacol Rev* 56:331, 2004.

Goldstein DS, Sharabi Y: Neurogenic orthostatic hypotension: a pathophysiological approach, *Circulation* 119:139, 2009.

Goldstein DS, Robertson D, Esler M, et al: Dysautonomias: clinical disorders of the autonomic nervous system, *Ann Intern Med* 137:753, 2002.

Guyenet PG: The 2008 Carl Ludwig Lecture: retrotrapezoid nucleus, CO2 homeostasis, and breathing automaticity, *J Appl Physiol* 105:404, 2008.

Guyenet PG: The sympathetic control of blood pressure, *Nat Rev Neurosci* 7:335, 2006.

Hall JE, Hildebrandt DA, Kuo J: Obesity hypertension: role of leptin and sympathetic nervous system, *Am J Hypertens* 14:103S, 2001.

Kvetnansky R, Sabban EL, Palkovits M: Catecholaminergic systems in stress: structural and molecular genetic approaches, *Physiol Rev* 89:535, 2009.

Lohmeier TE: The sympathetic nervous system and long-term blood pressure regulation, *Am J Hypertens* 14:147S, 2001.

Lohmeier TE, Hildebrandt DA, Warren S, et al: Recent insights into the interactions between the baroreflex and the kidneys in hypertension, *Am J Physiol Regul Integr Comp Physiol* 288:R828, 2005.

Olshansky B, Sabbah HN, Hauptman PJ, et al: Parasympathetic nervous system and heart failure: pathophysiology and potential implications for therapy, *Circulation* 118:863, 2008.

Saper CB: The central autonomic nervous system: conscious visceral perception and autonomic pattern generation, *Annu Rev Neurosci* 25:433, 2002.

Taylor EW, Jordan D, Coote JH: Central control of the cardiovascular and respiratory systems and their interactions in vertebrates, *Physiol Rev* 79:855, 1999.

Ulrich-Lai YM, Herman JP: Neural regulation of endocrine and autonomic stress responses, *Nat Rev Neurosci* 10:397, 2009.

Wess J: Novel insights into muscarinic acetylcholine receptor function using gene targeting technology, *Trends Pharmacol Sci* 24:414, 2003.

UNIT XI

CHAPTER 61

Cerebral Blood Flow, Cerebrospinal Fluid, and Brain Metabolism

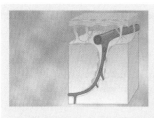

Thus far, we have discussed the function of the brain as if it were independent of its blood flow, its metabolism, and its fluids. However, this is far from true because abnormalities of any of these can profoundly affect brain function. For instance, total cessation of blood flow to the brain causes unconsciousness within 5 to 10 seconds. This occurs because lack of oxygen delivery to the brain cells nearly shuts down metabolism in these cells. Also, on a longer time scale, abnormalities of the cerebrospinal fluid, either its composition or its fluid pressure, can have equally severe effects on brain function.

Cerebral Blood Flow

Blood flow of the brain is supplied by four large arteries—two carotid and two vertebral arteries—which merge to form the *circle of Willis* at the base of the brain. The arteries arising from the circle of Willis travel along the brain surface and give rise to *pial* arteries, which branch out into smaller vessels called *penetrating arteries and arterioles* (Figure 61-1). The penetrating vessels are separated slightly from the brain tissue by an extension of the subarachnoid space called the *Virchow-Robin space.* The penetrating vessels dive down into the brain tissue, giving rise to intracerebral arterioles, which eventually branch into capillaries where exchange among the blood and the tissues of oxygen, nutrients, carbon dioxide, and metabolites occurs.

Normal Rate of Cerebral Blood Flow
Normal blood flow through the brain of the adult person averages 50 to 65 milliliters per 100 grams of brain tissue per minute. For the entire brain, this amounts to 750 to 900 ml/min. Thus, the brain comprises only about 2 percent of the body weight but receives 15 percent of the resting cardiac output.

Regulation of Cerebral Blood Flow
As in most other vascular areas of the body, cerebral blood flow is highly related to metabolism of the tissue. Several metabolic factors are believed to contribute to cerebral blood flow regulation: (1) carbon dioxide concentration,

(2) hydrogen ion concentration, (3) oxygen concentration, and (4) substances released from *astrocytes*, which are specialized, non-neuronal cells that appear to couple neuronal activity with local blood flow regulation.

Increase of Cerebral Blood Flow in Response to Excess Carbon Dioxide or Excess Hydrogen Ion Concentration. An increase in carbon dioxide concentration in the arterial blood perfusing the brain greatly increases cerebral blood flow. This is demonstrated in Figure 61-2, which shows that a 70 percent increase in arterial P_{CO_2} approximately doubles cerebral blood flow.

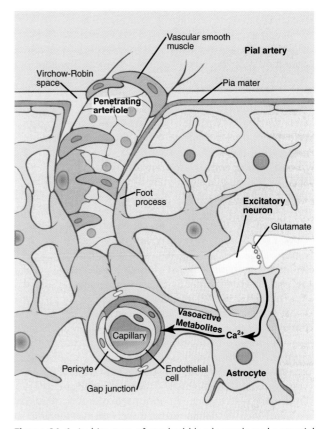

Figure 61-1 Architecture of cerebral blood vessels and potential mechanism for blood flow regulation by astrocytes. The pial arteries lie on the glia limitans and the penetrating arteries are surrounded by astrocyte foot processes. Note that the astrocytes also have fine processes that are closely associated with synapses.

743

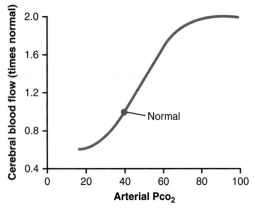

Figure 61-2 Relationship between arterial P_{CO_2} and cerebral blood flow.

Carbon dioxide is believed to increase cerebral blood flow by combining first with water in the body fluids to form carbonic acid, with subsequent dissociation of this acid to form hydrogen ions. The hydrogen ions then cause vasodilation of the cerebral vessels—the dilation being almost directly proportional to the increase in hydrogen ion concentration up to a blood flow limit of about twice normal.

Other substances that increase the acidity of the brain tissue and therefore increase hydrogen ion concentration will likewise increase cerebral blood flow. Such substances include lactic acid, pyruvic acid, and any other acidic material formed during the course of tissue metabolism.

Importance of Cerebral Blood Flow Control by Carbon Dioxide and Hydrogen Ions. Increased hydrogen ion concentration greatly depresses neuronal activity. Therefore, it is fortunate that increased hydrogen ion concentration also causes increased blood flow, which in turn carries hydrogen ions, carbon dioxide, and other acid-forming substances away from the brain tissues. Loss of carbon dioxide removes carbonic acid from the tissues; this, along with removal of other acids, reduces the hydrogen ion concentration back toward normal. Thus, this mechanism helps maintain a constant hydrogen ion concentration in the cerebral fluids and thereby helps to maintain a normal, constant level of neuronal activity.

Oxygen Deficiency as a Regulator of Cerebral Blood Flow. Except during periods of intense brain activity, the rate of utilization of oxygen by the brain tissue remains within narrow limits—almost exactly 3.5 ($\pm$0.2) milliliters of oxygen per 100 grams of brain tissue per minute. If blood flow to the brain ever becomes insufficient to supply this needed amount of oxygen, the oxygen deficiency almost immediately causes vasodilation, returning the brain blood flow and transport of oxygen to the cerebral tissues to near normal. Thus, this local blood flow regulatory mechanism is almost exactly the same in the brain as in coronary blood vessels, in skeletal muscle, and in most other circulatory areas of the body.

Experiments have shown that a decrease in cerebral *tissue* P_{O_2} below about 30 mm Hg (normal value is 35 to 40 mm Hg) immediately begins to increase cerebral blood flow. This is fortuitous because brain function becomes deranged at lower values of P_{O_2}, especially so at P_{O_2} levels below 20 mm Hg. Even coma can result at these low levels. Thus, the oxygen mechanism for local regulation of cerebral blood flow is an important protective response against diminished cerebral neuronal activity and, therefore, against derangement of mental capability.

Substances Released from *Astrocytes* as Regulators of Cerebral Blood Flow. Increasing evidence suggests that the close coupling between neuronal activity and cerebral blood flow is due, in part, to substances released from *astrocytes* (also called *astroglial cells*) that surround blood vessels of the central nervous system. Astrocytes are star-shaped *non-neuronal cells* that support and protect neurons, as well as provide nutrition. They have numerous projections that make contact with neurons and the surrounding blood vessels, providing a potential mechanism for neurovascular communication. Gray matter astrocytes (*protoplasmic astrocytes*) extend fine processes that cover most synapses and large *foot processes* that are closely apposed to the vascular wall (see Figure 61-1).

Experimental studies have shown that electrical stimulation of excitatory glutaminergic neurons leads to increases in intracellular calcium ion concentration in astrocyte foot processes and vasodilation of nearby arterioles. Additional studies have suggested that the vasodilation is mediated by several vasoactive metabolites released from astrocytes. Although the precise mediators are still unclear, nitric oxide, metabolites of arachidonic acid, potassium ions, adenosine, and other substances generated by astrocytes in response to stimulation of adjacent excitatory neurons have all been suggested to be important in mediating local vasodilation.

Measurement of Cerebral Blood Flow, and Effect of Brain Activity on the Flow. A method has been developed to record blood flow in as many as 256 isolated segments of the human cerebral cortex simultaneously. To do this, *a radioactive substance, such as radioactive xenon, is injected into the carotid artery; then the radioactivity of each segment of the cortex is recorded as the radioactive substance passes through the brain tissue. For this purpose, 256 small radioactive scintillation detectors are pressed against the surface of the cortex.* The rapidity of rise and decay of radioactivity in each tissue segment is a direct measure of the rate of blood flow through that segment.

Using this technique, it has become clear that blood flow in each individual segment of the brain changes as much as 100 to 150 percent within seconds in response to changes in local neuronal activity. For instance, simply making a fist of the hand causes an immediate increase in blood flow in the motor cortex of the opposite side of the brain. Reading a book increases the blood flow, especially in the visual areas of the occipital cortex and in the language perception areas of the temporal cortex. This measuring procedure can also be used for localizing the origin of epileptic attacks because local brain blood flow increases acutely and markedly at the focal point of each attack.

Demonstrating the effect of local neuronal activity on cerebral blood flow, Figure 61-3 shows a typical increase in occipital blood flow recorded in a cat's brain when intense light is shined into its eyes for one-half minute.

Cerebral Blood Flow Autoregulation Protects the Brain From Fluctuations in Arterial Pressure Changes. During normal daily activities, arterial pressure can fluctuate widely, rising to high levels during states of excitement or

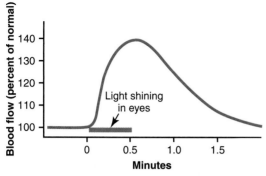

Figure 61-3 Increase in blood flow to the occipital regions of a cat's brain when light is shined into its eyes.

strenuous activity and falling to low levels during sleep. However, cerebral blood flow is "autoregulated" extremely well between arterial pressure limits of 60 and 140 mm Hg. That is, mean arterial pressure can be decreased acutely to as low as 60 mm Hg or increased to as high as 140 mm Hg without significant change in cerebral blood flow. And, in people who have hypertension, autoregulation of cerebral blood flow occurs even when the mean arterial pressure rises to as high as 160 to 180 mm Hg. This is demonstrated in Figure 61-4, which shows cerebral blood flow measured in both persons with normal blood pressure and hypertensive and hypotensive patients. Note the extreme constancy of cerebral blood flow between the limits of 60 and 180 mm Hg mean arterial pressure. But, if the arterial pressure falls below 60 mm Hg, cerebral blood flow becomes severely decreased.

Role of the Sympathetic Nervous System in Controlling Cerebral Blood Flow. The cerebral circulatory system has strong sympathetic innervation that passes upward from the superior cervical sympathetic ganglia in the neck and then into the brain along with the cerebral arteries. This innervation supplies both the large brain arteries and the arteries that penetrate into the substance of the brain. However, transection of the sympathetic nerves or mild to moderate stimulation of them usually causes little change in cerebral blood flow because the blood flow autoregulation mechanism can override the nervous effects.

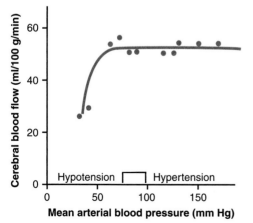

Figure 61-4 Effect of differences in mean arterial pressure, from hypotensive to hypertensive level, on cerebral blood flow in different human beings. (Modified from Lassen NA: Cerebral blood flow and oxygen consumption in man. Physiol Rev 39:183, 1959.)

When mean arterial pressure rises acutely to an exceptionally high level, such as during strenuous exercise or during other states of excessive circulatory activity, the sympathetic nervous system normally constricts the large- and intermediate-sized brain arteries enough to prevent the high pressure from reaching the smaller brain blood vessels. This is important in preventing vascular hemorrhages into the brain—that is, for preventing the occurrence of "cerebral stroke."

Cerebral Microcirculation

As is true for almost all other tissues of the body, the number of blood capillaries in the brain is greatest where the metabolic needs are greatest. The overall metabolic rate of the brain gray matter where the neuronal cell bodies lie is about four times as great as that of white matter; correspondingly, the number of capillaries and rate of blood flow are also about four times as great in the gray matter.

An important structural characteristic of the brain capillaries is that most of them are much less "leaky" than the blood capillaries in almost any other tissue of the body. One reason for this is that the capillaries are supported on all sides by "glial feet," which are small projections from the surrounding glial cells (e.g. astroglial cells) that abut against all surfaces of the capillaries and provide physical support to prevent overstretching of the capillaries in case of high capillary blood pressure.

The walls of the small arterioles leading to the brain capillaries become greatly thickened in people who develop high blood pressure, and these arterioles remain significantly constricted all the time to prevent transmission of the high pressure to the capillaries. We shall see later in the chapter that whenever these systems for protecting against transudation of fluid into the brain break down, serious brain edema ensues, which can lead rapidly to coma and death.

Cerebral "Stroke" Occurs When Cerebral Blood Vessels Are Blocked

Almost all elderly people have blockage of some small arteries in the brain, and up to 10 percent eventually have enough blockage to cause serious disturbance of brain function, a condition called a "stroke."

Most strokes are caused by arteriosclerotic plaques that occur in one or more of the feeder arteries to the brain. The plaques can activate the clotting mechanism of the blood, causing a blood clot to occur and block blood flow in the artery, thereby leading to acute loss of brain function in a localized area.

In about one quarter of people who develop strokes, high blood pressure makes one of the blood vessels burst; hemorrhage then occurs, compressing the local brain tissue and further compromising its functions. The neurological effects of a stroke are determined by the brain area affected. One of the most common types of stroke is blockage of the *middle cerebral artery* that supplies the midportion of one brain hemisphere. For instance, if the middle cerebral artery is blocked on the left side of the brain, the person is likely to become almost totally demented because of lost function in Wernicke's speech comprehension area in the left cerebral hemisphere, and he or she also becomes unable to speak words because of loss of Broca's motor area for word formation. In addition, loss of function of neural motor control areas of the left hemisphere can create spastic paralysis of most muscles on the opposite side of the body.

In a similar manner, blockage of a *posterior cerebral artery* will cause infarction of the occipital pole of the hemisphere on the same side as the blockage, which causes loss of vision in both eyes in the half of the retina on the same side as the stroke lesion. Especially devastating are strokes that involve the blood supply to the midbrain because this can block nerve conduction in major pathways between the brain and spinal cord, causing *both sensory and motor abnormalities.*

Cerebrospinal Fluid System

The entire cerebral cavity enclosing the brain and spinal cord has a capacity of about 1600 to 1700 milliliters; about 150 milliliters of this capacity is occupied by *cerebrospinal fluid* and the remainder by the brain and cord. This fluid, as shown in Figure 61-5, is present in the *ventricles of the brain,* in the *cisterns around the outside of the brain,* and in the *subarachnoid space around both the brain and the spinal cord.* All these chambers are connected with one another, and the pressure of the fluid is maintained at a surprisingly constant level.

Cushioning Function of the Cerebrospinal Fluid

A major function of the cerebrospinal fluid is to cushion the brain within its solid vault. The brain and the cerebrospinal fluid have about the same specific gravity (only about 4 percent different), so the brain simply floats in the fluid. Therefore, a blow to the head, if it is not too intense, moves the entire brain simultaneously with the skull, causing no one portion of the brain to be momentarily contorted by the blow.

Contrecoup.   When a blow to the head is extremely severe, it may not damage the brain on the side of the head where the blow is struck but on the opposite side. This phenomenon is known as "contrecoup," and the reason for this effect is the following: When the blow is struck, the fluid on the struck side is so incompressible that as the skull moves, the fluid pushes the brain at the same time in unison with the skull. On the side opposite to the area that is struck, the sudden movement of the whole skull causes the skull to pull away from the brain momentarily because of the brain's inertia,

creating for a split second a vacuum space in the cranial vault in the area opposite to the blow. Then, when the skull is no longer being accelerated by the blow, the vacuum suddenly collapses and the brain strikes the inner surface of the skull.

The poles and the inferior surfaces of the frontal and temporal lobes, where the brain comes into contact with bony protuberances in the base of the skull, are often the sites of injury and *contusions* (bruises) after a severe blow to the head, such as that experienced by a boxer. If the contusion occurs on the same side as the impact injury, it is a *coup injury;* if it occurs on the opposite side, the contusion is a *contrecoup injury.*

Coup and contrecoup injuries can also be caused by rapid acceleration or deceleration alone in the absence of physical impact due to a blow to the head. In these instances the brain may bounce off the wall of the skull causing a coup injury and then also bounce off the opposite side causing a contrecoup contusion. Such injuries are thought to occur, for example, in "shaken baby syndrome" or sometimes in vehicular accidents.

Formation, Flow, and Absorption of Cerebrospinal Fluid

Cerebrospinal fluid is formed at a rate of about 500 milliliters each day, which is three to four times as much as the total volume of fluid in the entire cerebrospinal fluid system. About two thirds or more of this fluid originates as *secretion from the choroid plexuses* in the four ventricles, *mainly in the two lateral ventricles.* Additional small amounts of fluid are secreted by the ependymal surfaces of all the ventricles and by the arachnoidal membranes. A small amount comes from the brain itself through the perivascular spaces that surround the blood vessels passing through the brain.

The arrows in Figure 61-5 show that the main channels of fluid flow from the *choroid plexuses* and then through the cerebrospinal fluid system. The fluid secreted in the *lateral ventricles* passes first into the *third ventricle;* then, after addition of minute amounts of fluid from the third ventricle, it flows downward along the *aqueduct of Sylvius* into the *fourth ventricle,* where still another minute amount of fluid is added. Finally, the fluid passes out of the fourth ventricle through three small openings, *two lateral foramina of Luschka* and a *midline foramen of Magendie,* entering the *cisterna magna,* a fluid space that lies behind the medulla and beneath the cerebellum.

Figure 61-5 The arrows show the pathway of cerebrospinal fluid flow from the choroid plexuses in the lateral ventricles to the arachnoidal villi protruding into the dural sinuses.

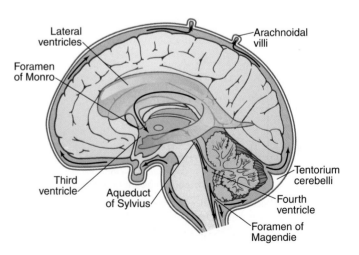

The cisterna magna is continuous with the *subarachnoid space* that surrounds the entire brain and spinal cord. Almost all the cerebrospinal fluid then flows upward from the cisterna magna through the subarachnoid spaces surrounding the cerebrum. From here, the fluid flows into and through multiple *arachnoidal villi* that project into the large sagittal venous sinus and other venous sinuses of the cerebrum. Thus, any extra fluid empties into the venous blood through pores of these villi.

Secretion by the Choroid Plexus. The *choroid plexus,* a section of which is shown in Figure 61-6, is a cauliflower-like growth of blood vessels covered by a thin layer of epithelial cells. This plexus projects into the temporal horn of each lateral ventricle, the posterior portion of the third ventricle, and the roof of the fourth ventricle.

Secretion of fluid into the ventricles by the choroid plexus depends mainly on active transport of sodium ions through the epithelial cells lining the outside of the plexus. The sodium ions in turn pull along large amounts of chloride ions as well because the positive charge of the sodium ion attracts the chloride ion's negative charge. The two ions combined increase the quantity of osmotically active sodium chloride in the cerebrospinal fluid, which then causes almost immediate osmosis of water through the membrane, thus providing the fluid of the secretion.

Less important transport processes move small amounts of glucose into the cerebrospinal fluid and both potassium and bicarbonate ions out of the cerebrospinal fluid into the capillaries. Therefore, the resulting characteristics of the cerebrospinal fluid become the following: osmotic pressure, approximately equal to that of plasma; sodium ion concentration, also approximately equal to that of plasma; chloride ion, about 15 percent greater than in plasma; potassium ion, approximately 40 percent less; and glucose, about 30 percent less.

Absorption of Cerebrospinal Fluid Through the Arachnoidal Villi. The *arachnoidal villi* are microscopic fingerlike inward projections of the arachnoidal membrane through the walls and into the venous sinuses. Conglomerates of these villi form macroscopic structures called *arachnoidal granulations* that can be seen protruding into the sinuses. The endothelial cells covering the villi have been shown by electron microscopy to have vesicular passages directly through the bodies of the cells large enough to allow relatively free flow of (1) cerebrospinal fluid, (2) dissolved protein molecules, and (3) even particles as large as red and white blood cells into the venous blood.

Perivascular Spaces and Cerebrospinal Fluid. The large arteries and veins of the brain lie on the surface of the brain but their ends penetrate inward, carrying with them a layer of *pia mater,* the membrane that covers the brain, as shown in Figure 61-7. The pia is only loosely adherent to the vessels, so a space, the *perivascular space,* exists between it and each vessel. Therefore, perivascular spaces follow both the arteries and the veins into the brain as far as the arterioles and venules go.

Lymphatic Function of the Perivascular Spaces. As is true elsewhere in the body, a small amount of protein leaks out of the brain capillaries into the interstitial spaces of the brain. Because no true lymphatics are present in brain tissue, excess protein in the brain tissue leaves the tissue flowing with fluid through the perivascular spaces into the subarachnoid spaces. On reaching the subarachnoid spaces, the protein then flows with the cerebrospinal fluid, to be absorbed through the *arachnoidal villi* into the large cerebral veins. Therefore, perivascular spaces, in effect, are a specialized lymphatic system for the brain.

In addition to transporting fluid and proteins, the perivascular spaces transport extraneous particulate matter out of the brain. For instance, whenever infection occurs in the brain, dead white blood cells and other infectious debris are carried away through the perivascular spaces.

Cerebrospinal Fluid Pressure

The normal pressure in the cerebrospinal fluid system *when one is lying in a horizontal position* averages 130 mm of water (10 mm Hg), although this may be as low as 65 mm of water or as high as 195 mm of water even in the normal healthy person.

Regulation of Cerebrospinal Fluid Pressure by the Arachnoidal Villi. The normal rate of cerebrospinal fluid formation remains nearly constant, so changes in fluid

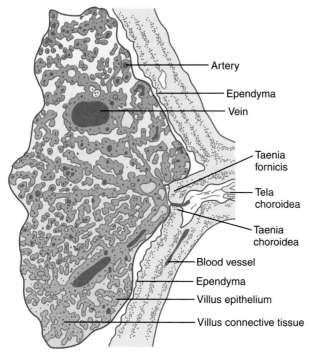

Artery
Ependyma
Vein
Taenia fornicis
Tela choroidea
Taenia choroidea
Blood vessel
Ependyma
Villus epithelium
Villus connective tissue

Figure 61-6 Choroid plexus in a lateral ventricle.

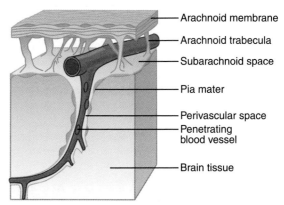

Arachnoid membrane
Arachnoid trabecula
Subarachnoid space
Pia mater
Perivascular space
Penetrating blood vessel
Brain tissue

Figure 61-7 Drainage of a perivascular space into the subarachnoid space. (Redrawn from Ranson SW, Clark SL: Anatomy of the Nervous System. Philadelphia: WB Saunders, 1959.)

formation are seldom a factor in pressure control. Conversely, the arachnoidal villi function like "valves" that allow cerebrospinal fluid and its contents to flow readily into the blood of the venous sinuses while not allowing blood to flow backward in the opposite direction. Normally, this valve action of the villi allows cerebrospinal fluid to begin to flow into the blood when cerebrospinal fluid pressure is about 1.5 mm Hg greater than the pressure of the blood in the venous sinuses. Then, if the cerebrospinal fluid pressure rises still higher, the valves open more widely. Under normal conditions, the cerebrospinal fluid pressure almost never rises more than a few millimeters of mercury higher than the pressure in the cerebral venous sinuses.

Conversely, in disease states, the villi sometimes become blocked by large particulate matter, by fibrosis, or by excesses of blood cells that have leaked into the cerebrospinal fluid in brain diseases. Such blockage can cause high cerebrospinal fluid pressure, as follows.

High Cerebrospinal Fluid Pressure in Pathological Conditions of the Brain. Often a large *brain tumor* elevates the cerebrospinal fluid pressure by decreasing reabsorption of the cerebrospinal fluid back into the blood. As a result, the cerebrospinal fluid pressure can rise to as much as 500 mm of water (37 mm Hg) or about four times normal.

The cerebrospinal fluid pressure also rises considerably when *hemorrhage* or *infection* occurs in the cranial vault. In both these conditions, large numbers of red and/or white blood cells suddenly appear in the cerebrospinal fluid and can cause serious blockage of the small absorption channels through the arachnoidal villi. This also sometimes elevates the cerebrospinal fluid pressure to 400 to 600 mm of water (about four times normal).

Some babies are born with high cerebrospinal fluid pressure. This is often caused by abnormally high resistance to fluid reabsorption through the arachnoidal villi, resulting either from too few arachnoidal villi or from villi with abnormal absorptive properties. This is discussed later in connection with *hydrocephalus.*

Measurement of Cerebrospinal Fluid Pressure. The usual procedure for measuring cerebrospinal fluid pressure is simple: First, the person lies exactly horizontally on his or her side so that the fluid pressure in the spinal canal is equal to the pressure in the cranial vault. A spinal needle is then inserted into the lumbar spinal canal below the lower end of the cord, and the needle is connected to a vertical glass tube that is open to the air at its top. The spinal fluid is allowed to rise in the tube as high as it will. If it rises to a level 136 mm above the level of the needle, the pressure is said to be 136 mm of water pressure or, dividing this by 13.6, which is the specific gravity of mercury, about 10 mm Hg pressure.

High Cerebrospinal Fluid Pressure Causes Edema of the Optic Disc—Papilledema. Anatomically, the dura of the brain extends as a sheath around the optic nerve and then connects with the sclera of the eye. When the pressure rises in the cerebrospinal fluid system, it also rises inside the optic nerve sheath. The retinal artery and vein pierce this sheath a few millimeters behind the eye and then pass along with the optic nerve fibers into the eye itself. Therefore, (1) high cerebrospinal fluid pressure pushes fluid first into the optic nerve sheath and then along the spaces between the optic nerve fibers to the interior of the eyeball; (2) the high pressure decreases outward fluid flow in the optic nerves, causing accumulation of excess fluid in the optic disc at the center of the retina; and (3) the pressure in the sheath also impedes flow of blood in the retinal vein, thereby increasing the retinal capillary pressure throughout the eye, which results in still more retinal edema.

The tissues of the optic disc are much more distensible than those of the remainder of the retina, so the disc becomes far more edematous than the remainder of the retina and swells into the cavity of the eye. The swelling of the disc can be observed with an ophthalmoscope and is called *papilledema.* Neurologists can estimate the cerebrospinal fluid pressure by assessing the extent to which the edematous optic disc protrudes into the eyeball.

Obstruction to Flow of Cerebrospinal Fluid Can Cause Hydrocephalus

"Hydrocephalus" means excess water in the cranial vault. This condition is frequently divided into *communicating hydrocephalus* and *noncommunicating hydrocephalus.* In communicating hydrocephalus fluid flows readily from the ventricular system into the subarachnoid space, whereas in noncommunicating hydrocephalus fluid flow out of one or more of the ventricles is blocked.

Usually the *noncommunicating* type of hydrocephalus is caused by a *block in the aqueduct of Sylvius,* resulting from *atresia* (closure) before birth in many babies or from blockage by a brain tumor at any age. As fluid is formed by the choroid plexuses in the two lateral and the third ventricles, the volumes of these three ventricles increase greatly. This flattens the brain into a thin shell against the skull. In neonates, the increased pressure also causes the whole head to swell because the skull bones have not yet fused.

The *communicating* type of hydrocephalus is usually caused by blockage of fluid flow in the subarachnoid spaces around the basal regions of the brain or by blockage of the arachnoidal villi where the fluid is normally absorbed into the venous sinuses. Fluid therefore collects both on the outside of the brain and to a lesser extent inside the ventricles. This will also cause the head to swell tremendously if it occurs in infancy when the skull is still pliable and can be stretched, and it can damage the brain at any age. A therapy for many types of hydrocephalus is surgical placement of a silicone tube shunt all the way from one of the brain ventricles to the peritoneal cavity where the excess fluid can be absorbed into the blood.

Blood-Cerebrospinal Fluid and Blood-Brain Barriers

It has already been pointed out that the concentrations of several important constituents of cerebrospinal fluid are not the same as in extracellular fluid elsewhere in the body. Furthermore, many large molecular substances hardly pass at all from the blood into the cerebrospinal fluid or into the interstitial fluids of the brain, even though these same substances pass readily into the usual interstitial fluids of the body. Therefore, it is said that barriers, called the *blood-cerebrospinal fluid barrier* and the *blood-brain barrier,* exist between the blood and the cerebrospinal fluid and brain fluid, respectively.

Barriers exist both at the choroid plexus and at the tissue capillary membranes in essentially all areas of the brain parenchyma *except in some areas of the hypothalamus, pineal gland,* and *area postrema,* where substances diffuse with greater ease into the tissue spaces. The ease of diffusion in these areas is important because they have sensory receptors that respond to specific changes in the body fluids, such as changes in osmolality and in glucose concentration, as well as receptors for peptide hormones that regulate thirst, such as angiotensin II. The blood-brain barrier also has specific carrier molecules that facilitate transport of hormones, such as leptin, from the blood into the hypothalamus where they bind to specific receptors that control other functions such as appetite and sympathetic nervous system activity.

In general, the blood-cerebrospinal fluid and blood-brain barriers are highly permeable to water, carbon dioxide, oxygen, and most lipid-soluble substances such as alcohol and anesthetics; slightly permeable to electrolytes such as sodium, chloride, and potassium; and almost totally impermeable to plasma proteins and most non-lipid-soluble large organic molecules. Therefore, the blood-cerebrospinal fluid and blood-brain barriers often make it impossible to achieve effective concentrations of therapeutic drugs, such as protein antibodies and non-lipid-soluble drugs, in the cerebrospinal fluid or parenchyma of the brain.

The cause of the low permeability of the blood-cerebrospinal fluid and blood-brain barriers is the manner in which the endothelial cells of the brain tissue capillaries are joined to one another. They are joined by so-called *tight junctions.* That is, the membranes of the adjacent endothelial cells are tightly fused rather than having large slit-pores between them, as is the case for most other capillaries of the body.

Brain Edema

One of the most serious complications of abnormal cerebral fluid dynamics is the development of *brain edema.* Because the brain is encased in a solid cranial vault, accumulation of extra edema fluid compresses the blood vessels, often causing seriously decreased blood flow and destruction of brain tissue.

The usual cause of brain edema is either greatly increased capillary pressure or damage to the capillary wall that makes the wall leaky to fluid. A common cause is a serious blow to the head, leading to *brain concussion,* in which the brain tissues and capillaries are traumatized and capillary fluid leaks into the traumatized tissues.

Once brain edema begins, it often initiates two vicious circles because of the following positive feedbacks: (1) Edema compresses the vasculature. This in turn decreases blood flow and causes brain ischemia. The ischemia in turn causes arteriolar dilation with still further increase in capillary pressure. The increased capillary pressure then causes more edema fluid, so the edema becomes progressively worse. (2) The decreased cerebral blood flow also decreases oxygen delivery. This increases the permeability of the capillaries, allowing still more fluid leakage. It also turns off the sodium pumps of the neuronal tissue cells, thus allowing these cells to swell in addition.

Once these two vicious circles have begun, heroic measures must be used to prevent total destruction of the brain. One such measure is to infuse intravenously a concentrated osmotic substance, such as a concentrated mannitol solution. This pulls fluid by osmosis from the brain tissue and breaks up the vicious circles. Another procedure is to remove fluid quickly from the lateral ventricles of the brain by means of ventricular needle puncture, thereby relieving the intracerebral pressure.

Brain Metabolism

Like other tissues, the brain requires oxygen and food nutrients to supply its metabolic needs. However, there are special peculiarities of brain metabolism that require mention.

Total Brain Metabolic Rate and Metabolic Rate of Neurons. Under resting but awake conditions, the metabolism of the brain accounts for about 15 percent of the total metabolism in the body, even though the mass of the brain is only 2 percent of the total body mass. Therefore, under resting conditions, brain metabolism per unit mass of tissue is about 7.5 times the average metabolism in non-nervous system tissues.

Most of this excess metabolism of the brain occurs in the neurons, not in the glial supportive tissues. The major need for metabolism in the neurons is to pump ions through their membranes, mainly to transport sodium and calcium ions to the outside of the neuronal membrane and potassium ions to the interior. Each time a neuron conducts an action potential, these ions move through the membranes, increasing the need for additional membrane transport to restore proper ionic concentration differences across the neuron membranes. Therefore, during high levels of brain activity, neuronal metabolism can increase as much as 100 to 150 percent.

Special Requirement of the Brain for Oxygen—Lack of Significant Anaerobic Metabolism. Most tissues of the body can live without oxygen for several minutes and some for as long as 30 minutes. During this time, the tissue cells obtain their energy through processes of anaerobic metabolism, which means release of energy by partially breaking down glucose and glycogen but without combining these with oxygen. This delivers energy only at the expense of consuming tremendous amounts of glucose and glycogen. However, it does keep the tissues alive.

The brain is not capable of much anaerobic metabolism. One of the reasons for this is the high metabolic rate of the neurons, so most neuronal activity depends on second-by-second delivery of oxygen from the blood. Putting these factors together, one can understand why sudden cessation of blood flow to the brain or sudden total lack of oxygen in the blood can cause unconsciousness within 5 to 10 seconds.

Under Normal Conditions Most Brain Energy Is Supplied by Glucose. Under normal conditions, almost all the energy used by the brain cells is supplied by glucose derived from the blood. As is true for oxygen, most of this is derived minute by minute and second by second from the capillary blood, with a total of only about a 2-minute supply of glucose normally stored as glycogen in the neurons at any given time.

A special feature of glucose delivery to the neurons is that its transport into the neurons through the cell membrane is not dependent on insulin, even though insulin is required for glucose transport into most other body cells. Therefore, in patients who have serious diabetes with essentially zero secretion of insulin, glucose still diffuses readily into the neurons, which is most fortunate in preventing loss of mental function in diabetic patients. Yet when a diabetic patient is overtreated with insulin, the blood glucose concentration can fall extremely low because the excess insulin causes almost all the glucose in the blood to be transported rapidly into the vast numbers of insulin-sensitive non-neural cells throughout the body, especially into muscle and liver cells. When this happens, not enough glucose is left in the blood to supply the neurons properly and mental function becomes seriously deranged, leading sometimes to coma and even more often to mental imbalances and psychotic disturbances—all caused by overtreatment with insulin.

Bibliography

Ainslie PN, Duffin J: Integration of cerebrovascular CO_2 reactivity and chemoreflex control of breathing: mechanisms of regulation, measurement, and interpretation, *Am J Physiol Regul Integr Comp Physiol* 296:R1473, 2009.

Alawneh JA, Moustafa RR, Baron JC: Hemodynamic factors and perfusion abnormalities in early neurological deterioration, *Stroke* 40:e443–e450, 2009.

Barres BA: The mystery and magic of glia: a perspective on their roles in health and disease, *Neuron* 60:430, 2008.

Chesler M: Regulation and modulation of pH in the brain, *Physiol Rev* 83:1183, 2003.

Duelli R, Kuschinsky W: Brain glucose transporters: relationship to local energy demand, *News Physiol Sci* 16:71, 2001.

Faraci FM: Reactive oxygen species: influence on cerebral vascular tone, *J Appl Physiol* 100:739, 2006.

Gore JC: Principles and practice of functional MRI of the human brain, *J Clin Invest* 112:4, 2003.

Haydon PG, Carmignoto G: Astrocyte control of synaptic transmission and neurovascular coupling, *Physiol Rev* 86:1009, 2006.

Iadecola C, Davisson RL: Hypertension and cerebrovascular dysfunction, *Cell Metab* 7:476, 2008.

Iadecola C, Nedergaard M: Glial regulation of the cerebral microvasculature, *Nat Neurosci* 10:1369, 2007.

Iadecola C, Park L, Capone C: Threats to the mind: aging, amyloid, and hypertension, *Stroke* 40(Suppl 3):S40, 2009.

Johnston M, Papaiconomou C: Cerebrospinal fluid transport: a lymphatic perspective, *News Physiol Sci* 17:227, 2002.

Koehler RC, Roman RJ, Harder DR: Astrocytes and the regulation of cerebral blood flow, *Trends Neurosci* 32:160, 2009.

Moore CI, Cao R: The hemo-neural hypothesis: on the role of blood flow in information processing, *J Neurophysiol* 99:2035, 2008.

Murkin JM: Cerebral autoregulation: the role of CO_2 in metabolic homeostasis, *Semin Cardiothorac Vasc Anesth* 11:269, 2007.

Paulson OB: Blood-brain barrier, brain metabolism and cerebral blood flow, *Eur Neuropsychopharmacol* 12:495, 2002.

Syková E, Nicholson C: Diffusion in brain extracellular space, *Physiol Rev* 88:1277, 2008.

Toda N, Ayajiki K, Okamura T: Cerebral blood flow regulation by nitric oxide: recent advances, *Pharmacol Rev* 61:62, 2009.

Yenari M, Kitagawa K, Lyden P, Perez-Pinzon M: Metabolic downregulation: a key to successful neuroprotection?, *Stroke* 39:2910, 2008.

XII

UNIT

Gastrointestinal Physiology

62. General Principles of Gastrointestinal Function—Motility, Nervous Control, and Blood Circulation

63. Propulsion and Mixing of Food in the Alimentary Tract

64. Secretory Functions of the Alimentary Tract

65. Digestion and Absorption in the Gastrointestinal Tract

66. Physiology of Gastrointestinal Disorders

General Principles of Gastrointestinal Function— Motility, Nervous Control, and Blood Circulation

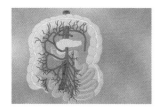

The alimentary tract provides the body with a continual supply of water, electrolytes, vitamins, and nutrients. To achieve this requires (1) movement of food through the alimentary tract; (2) secretion of digestive juices and digestion of the food; (3) absorption of water, various electrolytes, vitamins, and digestive products; (4) circulation of blood through the gastrointestinal organs to carry away the absorbed substances; and (5) control of all these functions by local, nervous, and hormonal systems.

Figure 62-1 shows the entire alimentary tract. Each part is adapted to its specific functions: some to simple passage of food, such as the esophagus; others to temporary storage of food, such as the stomach; and others to digestion and absorption, such as the small intestine. In this chapter, we discuss the basic principles of function in the entire alimentary tract; in the following chapters, we discuss the specific functions of different segments of the tract.

General Principles of Gastrointestinal Motility

Physiologic Anatomy of the Gastrointestinal Wall

Figure 62-2 shows a typical cross section of the intestinal wall, including the following layers from outer surface inward: (1) the *serosa*, (2) a *longitudinal smooth muscle layer*, (3) a *circular smooth muscle layer*, (4) the *submucosa*, and (5) the *mucosa*. In addition, sparse bundles of smooth muscle fibers, the *mucosal muscle*, lie in the deeper layers of the mucosa. The motor functions of the gut are performed by the different layers of smooth muscle.

The general characteristics of smooth muscle and its function are discussed in Chapter 8, which should be reviewed as a background for the following sections of this chapter. The specific characteristics of smooth muscle in the gut are the following.

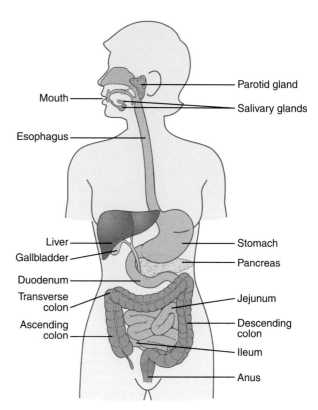

Figure 62-1 Alimentary tract.

Gastrointestinal Smooth Muscle Functions as a Syncytium. The individual smooth muscle fibers in the gastrointestinal tract are 200 to 500 micrometers in length and 2 to 10 micrometers in diameter, and they are arranged in bundles of as many as 1000 parallel fibers. In the *longitudinal muscle layer*, the bundles extend longitudinally down the intestinal tract; in the *circular muscle layer*, they extend around the gut.

Within each bundle, the muscle fibers are electrically connected with one another through large numbers of *gap junctions* that allow low-resistance movement of ions from one muscle cell to the next. Therefore, electrical signals that initiate muscle contractions can travel readily from one fiber to the next within each bundle but more rapidly along the length of the bundle than sideways.

753

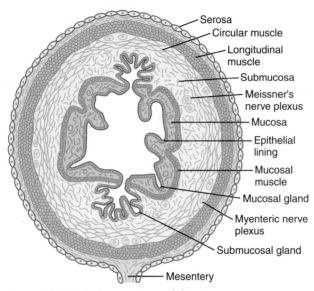

Figure 62-2 Typical cross section of the gut.

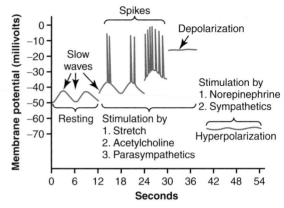

Figure 62-3 Membrane potentials in intestinal smooth muscle. Note the slow waves, the spike potentials, total depolarization, and hyperpolarization, all of which occur under different physiologic conditions of the intestine.

Each bundle of smooth muscle fibers is partly separated from the next by loose connective tissue, but the muscle bundles fuse with one another at many points, so in reality each muscle layer represents a branching latticework of smooth muscle bundles. Therefore, each muscle layer functions as a *syncytium*; that is, when an action potential is elicited anywhere within the muscle mass, it generally travels in all directions in the muscle. The distance that it travels depends on the excitability of the muscle; sometimes it stops after only a few millimeters and at other times it travels many centimeters or even the entire length and breadth of the intestinal tract.

Also, a few connections exist between the longitudinal and circular muscle layers, so excitation of one of these layers often excites the other as well.

Electrical Activity of Gastrointestinal Smooth Muscle

The smooth muscle of the gastrointestinal tract is excited by almost continual slow, intrinsic electrical activity along the membranes of the muscle fibers. This activity has two basic types of electrical waves: (1) *slow waves* and (2) *spikes*, both of which are shown in Figure 62-3. In addition, the voltage of the resting membrane potential of the gastrointestinal smooth muscle can be made to change to different levels, and this, too, can have important effects in controlling motor activity of the gastrointestinal tract.

Slow Waves. Most gastrointestinal contractions occur rhythmically, and this rhythm is determined mainly by the frequency of so-called "slow waves" of smooth muscle membrane potential. These waves, shown in Figure 62-3, are not action potentials. Instead, they are slow, undulating changes in the resting membrane potential. Their intensity usually varies between 5 and 15 millivolts, and their frequency ranges in different parts of the human gastrointestinal tract from 3 to 12 per minute: about 3

in the body of the stomach, as much as 12 in the duodenum, and about 8 or 9 in the terminal ileum. Therefore, the rhythm of contraction of the body of the stomach is usually about 3 per minute, of the duodenum about 12 per minute, and of the ileum 8 to 9 per minute.

The precise cause of the slow waves is not completely understood, although they appear to be caused by complex interactions among the smooth muscle cells and specialized cells, called the *interstitial cells of Cajal,* that are believed to act as *electrical pacemakers* for smooth muscle cells. These interstitial cells form a network with each other and are interposed between the smooth muscle layers, with synaptic-like contacts to smooth muscle cells. The interstitial cells of Cajal undergo cyclic changes in membrane potential due to unique ion channels that periodically open and produce inward (pacemaker) currents that may generate slow wave activity.

The slow waves usually do not by themselves cause muscle contraction in most parts of the gastrointestinal tract, *except perhaps in the stomach.* Instead, they mainly excite the appearance of intermittent spike potentials, and the spike potentials in turn actually excite the muscle contraction.

Spike Potentials. The spike potentials are true action potentials. They occur automatically when the resting membrane potential of the gastrointestinal smooth muscle becomes more positive than about −40 millivolts (the normal resting membrane potential in the smooth muscle fibers of the gut is between −50 and −60 millivolts). Note in Figure 62-3 that each time the peaks of the slow waves temporarily become more positive than −40 millivolts, spike potentials appear on these peaks. The higher the slow wave potential rises, the greater the frequency of the spike potentials, usually ranging between 1 and 10 spikes per second. The spike potentials last 10 to 40 times as long in gastrointestinal muscle as the action potentials in large nerve fibers, each gastrointestinal spike lasting as long as 10 to 20 milliseconds.

Another important difference between the action potentials of the gastrointestinal smooth muscle and those of nerve fibers is the manner in which they are generated. In nerve fibers, the action potentials are caused almost entirely by rapid entry of sodium ions through sodium channels to the interior of the fibers. In gastrointestinal smooth muscle fibers, the channels responsible for the action potentials are somewhat different; they allow especially large numbers of calcium ions to enter along with smaller numbers of sodium ions and therefore are called *calcium-sodium channels.* These channels are much slower to open and close than are the rapid sodium channels of large nerve fibers. The slowness of opening and closing of the calcium-sodium channels accounts for the long duration of the action potentials. Also, the movement of large amounts of calcium ions to the interior of the muscle fiber during the action potential plays a special role in causing the intestinal muscle fibers to contract, as we discuss shortly.

Changes in Voltage of the Resting Membrane Potential. In addition to the slow waves and spike potentials, the baseline voltage level of the smooth muscle resting membrane potential can also change. Under normal conditions, the resting membrane potential averages about –56 millivolts, but multiple factors can change this level. When the potential becomes less negative, which is called *depolarization* of the membrane, the muscle fibers become more excitable. When the potential becomes more negative, which is called *hyperpolarization,* the fibers become less excitable.

Factors that depolarize the membrane—that is, make it more excitable—are (1) *stretching* of the muscle, (2) stimulation by *acetylcholine* released from the endings of *parasympathetic nerves,* and (3) stimulation by several *specific gastrointestinal hormones.*

Important factors that make the membrane potential more negative—that is, hyperpolarize the membrane and make the muscle fibers less excitable—are (1) the effect of *norepinephrine* or *epinephrine* on the fiber membrane and (2) stimulation of the sympathetic nerves that secrete mainly norepinephrine at their endings.

Calcium Ions and Muscle Contraction. Smooth muscle contraction occurs in response to entry of calcium ions into the muscle fiber. As explained in Chapter 8, calcium ions, acting through a calmodulin control mechanism, activate the myosin filaments in the fiber, causing attractive forces to develop between the myosin filaments and the actin filaments, thereby causing the muscle to contract.

The slow waves do not cause calcium ions to enter the smooth muscle fiber (only sodium ions). Therefore, the slow waves by themselves usually cause no muscle contraction. Instead, it is during the spike potentials, generated at the peaks of the slow waves, that significant quantities of calcium ions do enter the fibers and cause most of the contraction.

Tonic Contraction of Some Gastrointestinal Smooth Muscle. Some smooth muscle of the gastrointestinal tract exhibits *tonic contraction,* as well as, or instead of, rhythmical contractions. Tonic contraction is continu-ous, not associated with the basic electrical rhythm of the slow waves but often lasting several minutes or even hours. The tonic contraction often increases or decreases in intensity but continues.

Tonic contraction is sometimes caused by continuous repetitive spike potentials—the greater the frequency, the greater the degree of contraction. At other times, tonic contraction is caused by hormones or other factors that bring about continuous partial depolarization of the smooth muscle membrane without causing action potentials. A third cause of tonic contraction is continuous entry of calcium ions into the interior of the cell brought about in ways not associated with changes in membrane potential. The details of these mechanisms are still unclear.

Neural Control of Gastrointestinal Function—Enteric Nervous System

The gastrointestinal tract has a nervous system all its own called the *enteric nervous system.* It lies entirely in the wall of the gut, beginning in the esophagus and extending all the way to the anus. The number of neurons in this enteric system is about 100 million, almost exactly equal to the number in the entire spinal cord. This highly developed enteric nervous system is especially important in controlling gastrointestinal movements and secretion.

The enteric nervous system is composed mainly of two plexuses, shown in Figure 62-4: (1) an outer plexus lying between the longitudinal and circular muscle layers, called the *myenteric plexus* or *Auerbach's plexus,* and (2) an inner plexus, called the *submucosal plexus* or *Meissner's plexus,* that lies in the submucosa. The nervous connections within and between these two plexuses are also shown in Figure 62-4.

The myenteric plexus controls mainly the gastrointestinal movements, and the submucosal plexus controls mainly gastrointestinal secretion and local blood flow.

Note especially in Figure 62-4 the extrinsic sympathetic and parasympathetic fibers that connect to both the myenteric and submucosal plexuses. Although the enteric nervous system can function independently of these extrinsic nerves, stimulation by the parasympathetic and sympathetic systems can greatly enhance or inhibit gastrointestinal functions, as we discuss later.

Also shown in Figure 62-4 are sensory nerve endings that originate in the gastrointestinal epithelium or gut wall and send afferent fibers to both plexuses of the enteric system, as well as (1) to the prevertebral ganglia of the sympathetic nervous system, (2) to the spinal cord, and (3) in the vagus nerves all the way to the brain stem. These sensory nerves can elicit local reflexes within the gut wall itself and still other reflexes that are relayed to the gut from either the prevertebral ganglia or the basal regions of the brain.

Figure 62-4 Neural control of the gut wall, showing (1) the myenteric and submucosal plexuses (*black fibers*); (2) extrinsic control of these plexuses by the sympathetic and parasympathetic nervous systems (*red fibers*); and (3) sensory fibers passing from the luminal epithelium and gut wall to the enteric plexuses, then to the prevertebral ganglia of the spinal cord and directly to the spinal cord and brain stem (*dashed fibers*).

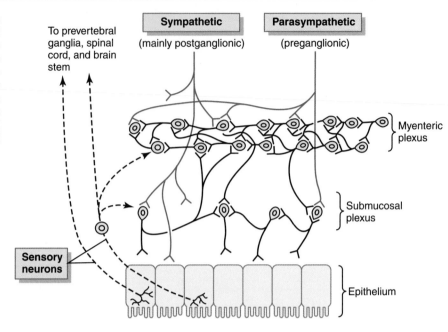

Differences Between the Myenteric and Submucosal Plexuses

The *myenteric plexus* consists mostly of a linear chain of many interconnecting neurons that extends the entire length of the gastrointestinal tract. A section of this chain is shown in Figure 62-4.

Because the myenteric plexus extends all the way along the intestinal wall and because it lies between the longitudinal and circular layers of intestinal smooth muscle, it is concerned mainly with controlling muscle activity along the length of the gut. When this plexus is stimulated, its principal effects are (1) increased tonic contraction, or "tone," of the gut wall; (2) increased intensity of the rhythmical contractions; (3) slightly increased rate of the rhythm of contraction; and (4) increased velocity of conduction of excitatory waves along the gut wall, causing more rapid movement of the gut peristaltic waves.

The *myenteric plexus* should not be considered entirely excitatory because some of its neurons are *inhibitory*; their fiber endings secrete an inhibitory transmitter, possibly *vasoactive intestinal polypeptide* or some other inhibitory peptide. The resulting inhibitory signals are especially useful for inhibiting some of the intestinal sphincter muscles that impede movement of food along successive segments of the gastrointestinal tract, such as the *pyloric sphincter,* which controls emptying of the stomach into the duodenum, and the *sphincter of the ileocecal valve,* which controls emptying from the small intestine into the cecum.

The *submucosal plexus,* in contrast to the myenteric plexus, is mainly concerned with controlling function within the inner wall of each minute segment of the intestine. For instance, many sensory signals originate from the gastrointestinal epithelium and are then integrated in the submucosal plexus to help control local *intestinal secretion,* local *absorption,* and local *contraction of the submucosal muscle* that causes various degrees of infolding of the gastrointestinal mucosa.

Types of Neurotransmitters Secreted by Enteric Neurons

In an attempt to understand better the multiple functions of the gastrointestinal enteric nervous system, research workers the world over have identified a dozen or more different neurotransmitter substances that are released by the nerve endings of different types of enteric neurons. Two of them with which we are already familiar are (1) *acetylcholine* and (2) *norepinephrine.* Others are (3) *adenosine triphosphate,* (4) *serotonin,* (5) *dopamine,* (6) *cholecystokinin,* (7) *substance P,* (8) *vasoactive intestinal polypeptide,* (9) *somatostatin,* (10) *leu-enkephalin,* (11) *met-enkephalin,* and (12) *bombesin.* The specific functions of many of these are not known well enough to justify discussion here, other than to point out the following.

Acetylcholine most often excites gastrointestinal activity. *Norepinephrine* almost always inhibits gastrointestinal activity. This is also true of *epinephrine,* which reaches the gastrointestinal tract mainly by way of the blood after it is secreted by the adrenal medullae into the circulation. The other aforementioned transmitter substances are a mixture of excitatory and inhibitory agents, some of which we discuss in the following chapter.

Autonomic Control of the Gastrointestinal Tract

Parasympathetic Stimulation Increases Activity of the Enteric Nervous System. The parasympathetic supply to the gut is divided into *cranial* and *sacral divisions,* which were discussed in Chapter 60.

Except for a few parasympathetic fibers to the mouth and pharyngeal regions of the alimentary tract, the *cranial parasympathetic* nerve fibers are almost entirely in the *vagus nerves.* These fibers provide extensive innervation to the esophagus, stomach, and pancreas and somewhat less to the intestines down through the first half of the large intestine.

The *sacral parasympathetics* originate in the second, third, and fourth sacral segments of the spinal cord and pass through the *pelvic nerves* to the distal half of the large intestine and all the way to the anus. The sigmoidal, rectal, and anal regions are considerably better supplied with parasympathetic fibers than are the other intestinal areas. These fibers function especially to execute the defecation reflexes, discussed in Chapter 63.

The *postganglionic neurons* of the gastrointestinal parasympathetic system are located mainly in the myenteric and submucosal plexuses. Stimulation of these parasympathetic nerves causes general increase in activity of the entire enteric nervous system. This in turn enhances activity of most gastrointestinal functions.

Sympathetic Stimulation Usually Inhibits Gastrointestinal Tract Activity. The sympathetic fibers to the gastrointestinal tract originate in the spinal cord between segments T5 and L2. Most of the preganglionic fibers that innervate the gut, after leaving the cord, enter the *sympathetic chains* that lie lateral to the spinal column, and many of these fibers then pass on through the chains to outlying ganglia such as to the *celiac ganglion* and various *mesenteric ganglia.* Most of the *postganglionic sympathetic neuron bodies* are in these ganglia, and postganglionic fibers then spread through postganglionic sympathetic nerves to all parts of the gut. The sympathetics innervate essentially all of the gastrointestinal tract, rather than being more extensive nearest the oral cavity and anus, as is true of the parasympathetics. The sympathetic nerve endings secrete mainly *norepinephrine* but also small amounts of *epinephrine.*

In general, stimulation of the sympathetic nervous system *inhibits* activity of the gastrointestinal tract, causing many effects opposite to those of the parasympathetic system. It exerts its effects in two ways: (1) to a slight extent by direct effect of secreted norepinephrine to inhibit intestinal tract smooth muscle (except the mucosal muscle, which it excites) and (2) to a major extent by an inhibitory effect of norepinephrine on the neurons of the entire enteric nervous system.

Strong stimulation of the sympathetic system can inhibit motor movements of the gut so greatly that this can literally block movement of food through the gastrointestinal tract.

Afferent *Sensory* Nerve Fibers from the Gut

Many afferent sensory nerve fibers innervate the gut. Some of them have their cell bodies in the enteric nervous system itself and some in the dorsal root ganglia of the spinal cord. These sensory nerves can be stimulated by (1) irritation of the gut mucosa, (2) excessive distention of the gut, or (3) presence of specific chemical substances in the gut. Signals transmitted through the fibers can then cause *excitation* or, under other conditions, *inhibition* of intestinal movements or intestinal secretion.

In addition, other sensory signals from the gut go all the way to multiple areas of the spinal cord and even the brain stem. For example, 80 percent of the nerve fibers in the vagus nerves are afferent rather than efferent. These afferent fibers transmit sensory signals from the gastrointestinal tract into the brain medulla, which in turn initiates vagal reflex signals that return to the gastrointestinal tract to control many of its functions.

Gastrointestinal Reflexes

The anatomical arrangement of the enteric nervous system and its connections with the sympathetic and parasympathetic systems support three types of gastrointestinal reflexes that are essential to gastrointestinal control. They are the following:

1. *Reflexes that are integrated entirely within the gut wall enteric nervous system.* These include reflexes that control much gastrointestinal secretion, peristalsis, mixing contractions, local inhibitory effects, and so forth.

2. *Reflexes from the gut to the prevertebral sympathetic ganglia and then back to the gastrointestinal tract.* These reflexes transmit signals long distances to other areas of the gastrointestinal tract, such as signals from the stomach to cause evacuation of the colon (the *gastrocolic reflex*), signals from the colon and small intestine to inhibit stomach motility and stomach secretion (the *enterogastric reflexes*), and reflexes from the colon to inhibit emptying of ileal contents into the colon (the *colonoileal reflex*).

3. *Reflexes from the gut to the spinal cord or brain stem and then back to the gastrointestinal tract.* These include especially (1) reflexes from the stomach and duodenum to the brain stem and back to the stomach—by way of the vagus nerves—to control gastric motor and secretory activity; (2) pain reflexes that cause general inhibition of the entire gastrointestinal tract; and (3) defecation reflexes that travel from the colon and rectum to the spinal cord and back again to produce the powerful colonic, rectal, and abdominal contractions required for defecation (the defecation reflexes).

Hormonal Control of Gastrointestinal Motility

The gastrointestinal hormones are released into the portal circulation and exert physiological actions on target cells with specific receptors for the hormone. The effects of the hormones persist even after all nervous connections between the site of release and the site of action have been severed. Table 62-1 outlines the actions of each gastrointestinal hormone, as well as the stimuli for secretion and sites at which secretion takes place.

In Chapter 64, we discuss the extreme importance of several hormones for controlling gastrointestinal secretion. Most of these same hormones also affect motility in some parts of the gastrointestinal tract. Although the

Table 62-1 Gastrointestinal Hormone Actions, Stimuli for Secretion, and Site of Secretion

Hormone	Stimuli for Secretion	Site of Secretion	Actions

Gastrin	Protein
	Distention
	Nerve
	(Acid inhibits release)
		G cells of the antrum, duodenum, and jejunum	Stimulates
			  Gastric acid secretion
			  Mucosal growth

Cholecystokinin	Protein
	Fat
	Acid
		I cells of the duodenum, jejunum, and ileum	Stimulates
			  Pancreatic enzyme secretion
			  Pancreatic bicarbonate secretion
			  Gallbladder contraction
			  Growth of exocrine pancreas
			Inhibits
			  Gastric emptying

Secretin	Acid
	Fat
		S cells of the duodenum, jejunum, and ileum	Stimulates
			  Pepsin secretion
			  Pancreatic bicarbonate secretion
			  Biliary bicarbonate secretion
			  Growth of exocrine pancreas
			Inhibits
			  Gastric acid secretion

Gastric inhibitory peptide	Protein
	Fat
	Carbohydrate
		K cells of the duodenum and jejunum	Stimulates
			  Insulin release
			Inhibits
			  Gastric acid secretion

Motilin	Fat
	Acid
	Nerve
		M cells of the duodenum and jejunum	Stimulates
			  Gastric motility
			  Intestinal motility

motility effects are usually less important than the secretory effects of the hormones, some of the more important of them are the following.

Gastrin is secreted by the "G" cells of the *antrum of the stomach* in response to stimuli associated with ingestion of a meal, such as distention of the stomach, the products of proteins, and *gastrin releasing peptide*, which is released by the nerves of the gastric mucosa during vagal stimulation. The primary actions of gastrin are (1) *stimulation of gastric acid secretion* and (2) *stimulation of growth of the gastric mucosa.*

Cholecystokinin (CCK) is secreted by "I" cells in the *mucosa of the duodenum and jejunum* mainly in response to digestive products of fat, fatty acids, and monoglycerides in the intestinal contents. This hormone strongly contracts the gallbladder, expelling bile into the small intestine, where the bile in turn plays important roles in emulsifying fatty substances, and allowing them to be digested and absorbed. CCK also inhibits stomach contraction moderately. Therefore, at the same time that this hormone causes emptying of the gallbladder, it also slows the emptying of food from the stomach to give adequate time for digestion of the fats in the upper intestinal tract. CCK also inhibits appetite to prevent overeating during meals by stimulating sensory afferent nerve fibers in the duodenum; these fibers, in turn, send signals by way of the vagus nerve to inhibit feeding centers in the brain as discussed in Chapter 71.

Secretin was the first gastrointestinal hormone discovered and is secreted by the "S" cells in the *mucosa of the duodenum* in response to acidic gastric juice emptying into the duodenum from the pylorus of the stomach. Secretin has a mild effect on motility of the gastrointestinal tract and acts to promote pancreatic secretion of bicarbonate, which in turn helps to neutralize the acid in the small intestine.

Gastric inhibitory peptide (GIP) is secreted by the *mucosa of the upper small intestine,* mainly in response to fatty acids and amino acids but to a lesser extent in response to carbohydrate. It has a mild effect in decreasing motor activity of the stomach and therefore slows emptying of gastric contents into the duodenum when the upper small intestine is already overloaded with food products. GIP, at blood levels even lower than those needed to inhibit gastric motility, also stimulates insulin secretion and for this reason is also known as *glucose-dependent insulinotropic peptide.*

Motilin is secreted by the stomach and *upper duodenum* during fasting, and the only known function of this hormone is to *increase gastrointestinal motility.* Motilin is released cyclically and stimulates waves of gastrointestinal motility called *interdigestive myoelectric complexes* that move through the stomach and small intestine every

90 minutes in a fasted person. Motilin secretion is inhibited after ingestion by mechanisms that are not fully understood.

Functional Types of Movements in the Gastrointestinal Tract

Two types of movements occur in the gastrointestinal tract: (1) *propulsive movements,* which cause food to move forward along the tract at an appropriate rate to accommodate digestion and absorption, and (2) *mixing movements,* which keep the intestinal contents thoroughly mixed at all times.

Propulsive Movements—Peristalsis

The basic propulsive movement of the gastrointestinal tract is *peristalsis,* which is illustrated in Figure 62-5. A contractile ring appears around the gut and then moves forward; this is analogous to putting one's fingers around a thin distended tube, then constricting the fingers and sliding them forward along the tube. Any material in front of the contractile ring is moved forward.

Peristalsis is an inherent property of many syncytial smooth muscle tubes; stimulation at any point in the gut can cause a contractile ring to appear in the circular muscle, and this ring then spreads along the gut tube. (Peristalsis also occurs in the bile ducts, glandular ducts, ureters, and many other smooth muscle tubes of the body.)

The usual stimulus for intestinal peristalsis is *distention of the gut.* That is, if a large amount of food collects at any point in the gut, the stretching of the gut wall stimulates the enteric nervous system to contract the gut wall 2 to 3 centimeters behind this point, and a contractile ring appears that initiates a peristaltic movement. Other stimuli that can initiate peristalsis include chemical or physical irritation of the epithelial lining in the gut. Also, strong parasympathetic nervous signals to the gut will elicit strong peristalsis.

Function of the Myenteric Plexus in Peristalsis. Peristalsis occurs only weakly or not at all in any portion of the gastrointestinal tract that has congenital absence of the myenteric plexus. Also, it is greatly depressed or completely blocked in the entire gut when a person is treated with atropine to paralyze the cholinergic nerve endings of the myenteric plexus. Therefore, *effectual* peristalsis requires an active myenteric plexus.

Directional Movement of Peristaltic Waves Toward the Anus. Peristalsis, theoretically, can occur in either direction from a stimulated point, but it normally dies out rapidly in the orad (toward the mouth) direction while continuing for a considerable distance toward the anus. The exact cause of this directional transmission of peristalsis has never been ascertained, although it probably results mainly from the fact that the myenteric plexus itself is "polarized" in the anal direction, which can be explained as follows.

Peristaltic Reflex and the "Law of the Gut". When a segment of the intestinal tract is excited by distention and thereby initiates peristalsis, the contractile ring causing the peristalsis normally begins on the orad side of the distended segment and moves toward the distended segment, pushing the intestinal contents in the anal direction for 5 to 10 centimeters before dying out. At the same time, the gut sometimes relaxes several centimeters downstream toward the anus, which is called "receptive relaxation," thus allowing the food to be propelled more easily toward the anus than toward the mouth.

This complex pattern does not occur in the absence of the myenteric plexus. Therefore, the complex is called the *myenteric reflex* or the *peristaltic reflex.* The peristaltic reflex plus the anal direction of movement of the peristalsis is called the "law of the gut."

Mixing Movements

Mixing movements differ in different parts of the alimentary tract. In some areas, the peristaltic contractions themselves cause most of the mixing. This is especially true when forward progression of the intestinal contents is blocked by a sphincter so that a peristaltic wave can then only churn the intestinal contents, rather than propelling them forward. At other times, *local intermittent constrictive contractions* occur every few centimeters in the gut wall. These constrictions usually last only 5 to 30 seconds; then new constrictions occur at other points in the gut, thus "chopping" and "shearing" the contents first here and then there. These peristaltic and constrictive movements are modified in different parts of the gastrointestinal tract for proper propulsion and mixing, as discussed for each portion of the tract in Chapter 63.

Gastrointestinal Blood Flow—"Splanchnic Circulation"

The blood vessels of the gastrointestinal system are part of a more extensive system called the *splanchnic circulation,* shown in Figure 62-6. It includes the blood flow

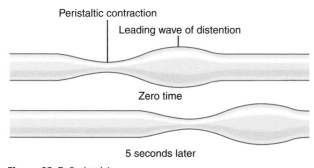

Peristaltic contraction

Leading wave of distention

Zero time

5 seconds later

Figure 62-5 Peristalsis.

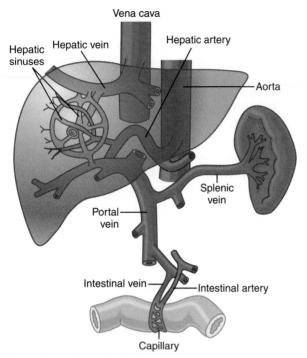

Figure 62-6 Splanchnic circulation.

millions of minute *liver sinusoids* and finally leaves the liver by way of *hepatic veins* that empty into the vena cava of the general circulation. This flow of blood through the liver, before it empties into the vena cava, allows the *reticuloendothelial cells* that line the liver sinusoids to remove bacteria and other particulate matter that might enter the blood from the gastrointestinal tract, thus preventing direct transport of potentially harmful agents into the remainder of the body.

The *nonfat, water-soluble nutrients* absorbed from the gut (such as carbohydrates and proteins) are transported in the portal venous blood to the same liver sinusoids. Here, both the reticuloendothelial cells and the principal parenchymal cells of the liver, the *hepatic cells,* absorb and store temporarily from one half to three quarters of the nutrients. Also, much chemical intermediary processing of these nutrients occurs in the liver cells. We discuss these nutritional functions of the liver in Chapters 67 through 71. Almost all of the *fats* absorbed from the intestinal tract *are not carried in the portal blood* but instead are absorbed into the intestinal lymphatics and then conducted to the systemic circulating blood by way of the *thoracic duct,* bypassing the liver.

through the gut itself plus blood flows through the spleen, pancreas, and liver. The design of this system is such that all the blood that courses through the gut, spleen, and pancreas then flows immediately into the liver by way of the *portal vein.* In the liver, the blood passes through

Anatomy of the Gastrointestinal Blood Supply

Figure 62-7 shows the general plan of the arterial blood supply to the gut, including the superior mesenteric and inferior mesenteric arteries supplying the walls of the

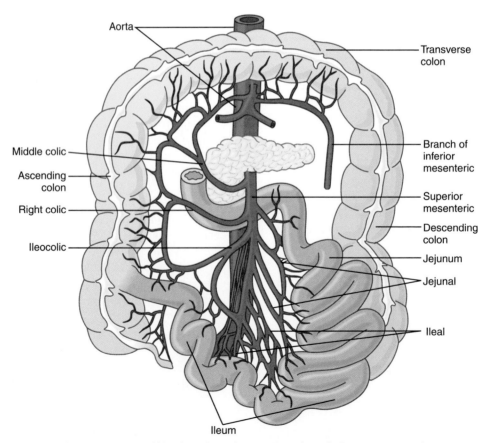

Figure 62-7 Arterial blood supply to the intestines through the mesenteric web.

small and large intestines by way of an arching arterial system. Not shown in the figure is the celiac artery, which provides a similar blood supply to the stomach.

On entering the wall of the gut, the arteries branch and send smaller arteries circling in both directions around the gut, with the tips of these arteries meeting on the side of the gut wall opposite the mesenteric attachment. From the circling arteries, still much smaller arteries penetrate into the intestinal wall and spread (1) along the muscle bundles, (2) into the intestinal villi, and (3) into submucosal vessels beneath the epithelium to serve the secretory and absorptive functions of the gut.

Figure 62-8 shows the special organization of the blood flow through an intestinal villus, including a small arteriole and venule that interconnect with a system of multiple looping capillaries. The walls of the arterioles are highly muscular and are highly active in controlling villus blood flow.

Effect of Gut Activity and Metabolic Factors on Gastrointestinal Blood Flow

Under normal conditions, the blood flow in each area of the gastrointestinal tract, as well as in each layer of the gut wall, is directly related to the level of local activity. For instance, during active absorption of nutrients, blood

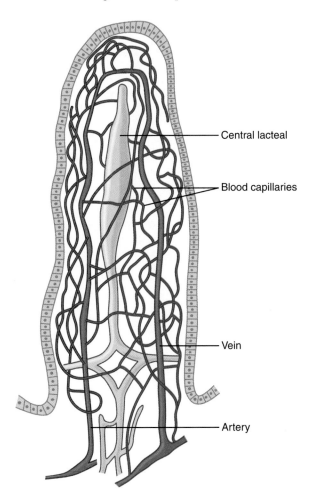

Figure 62-8 Microvasculature of the villus, showing a countercurrent arrangement of blood flow in the arterioles and venules.

Central lacteal

Blood capillaries

Vein

Artery

flow in the villi and adjacent regions of the submucosa is increased as much as eightfold. Likewise, blood flow in the muscle layers of the intestinal wall increases with increased motor activity in the gut. For instance, after a meal, the motor activity, secretory activity, and absorptive activity all increase; likewise, the blood flow increases greatly but then decreases back to the resting level over another 2 to 4 hours.

Possible Causes of the Increased Blood Flow During Gastrointestinal Activity. Although the precise causes of the increased blood flow during increased gastrointestinal activity are still unclear, some facts are known.

First, several vasodilator substances are released from the mucosa of the intestinal tract during the digestive process. Most of these are peptide hormones, including *cholecystokinin, vasoactive intestinal peptide, gastrin,* and *secretin.* These same hormones control specific motor and secretory activities of the gut, as discussed in Chapters 63 and 64.

Second, some of the gastrointestinal glands also release into the gut wall two kinins, *kallidin* and *bradykinin,* at the same time that they secrete other substances into the lumen. These kinins are powerful vasodilators that are believed to cause much of the increased mucosal vasodilation that occurs along with secretion.

Third, *decreased oxygen concentration* in the gut wall can increase intestinal blood flow at least 50 to 100 percent; therefore, the increased mucosal and gut wall metabolic rate during gut activity probably lowers the oxygen concentration enough to cause much of the vasodilation. The decrease in oxygen can also lead to as much as a fourfold increase of *adenosine,* a well-known vasodilator that could be responsible for much of the increased flow.

Thus, the increased blood flow during increased gastrointestinal activity is probably a combination of many of the aforementioned factors plus still others yet undiscovered.

"Countercurrent" Blood Flow in the Villi. Note in Figure 62-8 that the arterial flow into the villus and the venous flow out of the villus are in directions opposite to each other, and that the vessels lie in close apposition to each other. Because of this vascular arrangement, much of the blood oxygen diffuses out of the arterioles directly into the adjacent venules without ever being carried in the blood to the tips of the villi. As much as 80 percent of the oxygen may take this short-circuit route and therefore not be available for local metabolic functions of the villi. The reader will recognize that this type of countercurrent mechanism in the villi is analogous to the countercurrent mechanism in the vasa recta of the kidney medulla, discussed in detail in Chapter 28.

Under normal conditions, this shunting of oxygen from the arterioles to the venules is not harmful to the villi, but in disease conditions in which blood flow to the gut becomes greatly curtailed, such as in circulatory shock, the oxygen deficit in the tips of the villi can become so great that the villus tip or even the whole villus suffers ischemic death and can disintegrate. Therefore, for this reason and others, in many gastrointestinal diseases the villi become seriously blunted, leading to greatly diminished intestinal absorptive capacity.

Nervous Control of Gastrointestinal Blood Flow

Stimulation of the parasympathetic nerves going to the *stomach* and *lower colon* increases local blood flow at the same time that it increases glandular secretion. This increased flow probably results secondarily from the increased glandular activity and not as a direct effect of the nervous stimulation.

Sympathetic stimulation, by contrast, has a direct effect on essentially all the gastrointestinal tract to cause intense vasoconstriction of the arterioles with greatly decreased blood flow. After a few minutes of this vasoconstriction, the flow often returns to near normal by means of a mechanism called "autoregulatory escape." That is, the local metabolic vasodilator mechanisms that are elicited by ischemia override the sympathetic vasoconstriction, returning toward normal the necessary nutrient blood flow to the gastrointestinal glands and muscle.

Importance of Nervous Depression of Gastrointestinal Blood Flow When Other Parts of the Body Need Extra Blood Flow. A major value of sympathetic vasoconstriction in the gut is that it allows shutoff of gastrointestinal and other splanchnic blood flow for short periods of time during heavy exercise, when the skeletal muscle and heart need increased flow. Also, in circulatory shock, when all the body's vital tissues are in danger of cellular death for lack of blood flow—especially the brain and the heart—sympathetic stimulation can decrease splanchnic blood flow to very little for many hours.

Sympathetic stimulation also causes strong vasoconstriction of the large-volume *intestinal* and *mesenteric veins.* This decreases the volume of these veins, thereby displacing large amounts of blood into other parts of the circulation. In hemorrhagic shock or other states of low blood volume, this mechanism can provide as much as 200 to 400 milliliters of extra blood to sustain the general circulation.

Bibliography

Adelson DW, Million M: Tracking the moveable feast: sonomicrometry and gastrointestinal motility, *News Physiol Sci* 19:27, 2004.

Daniel EE: Physiology and pathophysiology of the interstitial cell of Cajal: from bench to bedside. III. Interaction of interstitial cells of Cajal with neuromediators: an interim assessment, *Am J Physiol Gastrointest Liver Physiol* 281:G1329, 2001.

Grundy D, Al-Chaer ED, Aziz Q, et al: Fundamentals of neurogastroenterology: basic science, *Gastroenterology* 130:1391, 2006.

Hobson AR, Aziz Q: Central nervous system processing of human visceral pain in health and disease, *News Physiol Sci* 18:109, 2003.

Holst JJ: The physiology of glucagon-like peptide 1, *Physiol Rev* 87:1409, 2009.

Huizinga JD: Physiology and pathophysiology of the interstitial cell of Cajal: from bench to bedside. II. Gastric motility: lessons from mutant mice on slow waves and innervation, *Am J Physiol Gastrointest Liver Physiol* 281:G1129, 2001.

Huizinga JD, Lammers WJ: Gut peristalsis is governed by a multitude of cooperating mechanisms, *Am J Physiol Gastrointest Liver Physiol* 296:G1, 2009.

Jeays AD, Lawford PV, Gillott R, et al: A framework for the modeling of gut blood flow regulation and postprandial hyperaemia, *World J Gastroenterol* 13:1393, 2007.

Johnson LR: *Gastrointestinal Physiology*, ed 3, St. Louis, 2001, Mosby.

Kim W, Egan JM: The role of incretins in glucose homeostasis and diabetes treatment, *Pharmacol Rev* 60:470, 2009.

Kolkman JJ, Bargeman M, Huisman AB, Geelkerken RH: Diagnosis and management of splanchnic ischemia, *World J Gastroenterol* 14:7309, 2008.

Lammers WJ, Slack JR: Of slow waves and spike patches, *News Physiol Sci* 16:138, 2001.

Moran TH, Dailey MJ: Minireview: Gut peptides: targets for antiobesity drug development? *Endocrinology* 150:2526, 2009.

Nauck MA: Unraveling the science of incretin biology, *Am J Med* 122(Suppl 6):S3, 2009.

Powley TL, Phillips RJ: Musings on the wanderer: what's new in our understanding of vago-vagal reflexes? I. Morphology and topography of vagal afferents innervating the GI tract, *Am J Physiol Gastrointest Liver Physiol* 283:G1217, 2002.

Phillips RJ, Powley TL: Innervation of the gastrointestinal tract: patterns of aging, *Auton Neurosci* 136:1, 2007.

Sanders KM, Ordog T, Ward SM: Physiology and pathophysiology of the interstitial cells of Cajal: from bench to bedside. IV. Genetic and animal models of GI motility disorders caused by loss of interstitial cells of Cajal, *Am J Physiol Gastrointest Liver Physiol* 282:G747, 2002.

Schubert ML, Peura DA: Control of gastric acid secretion in health and disease, *Gastroenterology* 134:1842, 2008.

Vanden Berghe P, Tack J, Boesmans W: Highlighting synaptic communication in the enteric nervous system, *Gastroenterology* 135:20, 2008.

Propulsion and Mixing of Food in the Alimentary Tract

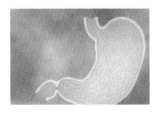

The time that food remains in each part of the alimentary tract is critical for optimal processing and absorption of nutrients. Also, appropriate mixing must be provided. Because the requirements for mixing and propulsion are quite different at each stage of processing, multiple automatic nervous and hormonal mechanisms control the timing of each of these so that they will occur optimally, not too rapidly, not too slowly.

The purpose of this chapter is to discuss these movements, especially the automatic mechanisms of this control.

Ingestion of Food

The amount of food that a person ingests is determined principally by intrinsic desire for food called *hunger*. The type of food that a person preferentially seeks is determined by *appetite*. These mechanisms are extremely important for maintaining an adequate nutritional supply for the body and are discussed in Chapter 71 in relation to nutrition of the body. The current discussion of food ingestion is confined to the mechanics of ingestion, especially *mastication* and *swallowing*.

Mastication (Chewing)

The teeth are admirably designed for chewing. The anterior teeth (incisors) provide a strong cutting action and the posterior teeth (molars) a grinding action. All the jaw muscles working together can close the teeth with a force as great as 55 pounds on the incisors and 200 pounds on the molars.

Most of the muscles of chewing are innervated by the motor branch of the fifth cranial nerve, and the chewing process is controlled by nuclei in the brain stem. Stimulation of specific reticular areas in the brain stem taste centers will cause rhythmical chewing movements. Also, stimulation of areas in the hypothalamus, amygdala, and even the cerebral cortex near the sensory areas for taste and smell can often cause chewing.

Much of the chewing process is caused by a *chewing reflex*. The presence of a bolus of food in the mouth at first initiates reflex inhibition of the muscles of mastication, which allows the lower jaw to drop. The drop in turn initiates a stretch reflex of the jaw muscles that leads to *rebound* contraction. This automatically raises the jaw to cause closure of the teeth, but it also compresses the bolus again against the linings of the mouth, which inhibits the jaw muscles once again, allowing the jaw to drop and rebound another time; this is repeated again and again.

Chewing is important for digestion of all foods, but especially important for most fruits and raw vegetables because these have indigestible cellulose membranes around their nutrient portions that must be broken before the food can be digested. Also, chewing aids the digestion of food for still another simple reason: *Digestive enzymes act only on the surfaces of food particles*; therefore, the rate of digestion is absolutely dependent on the total surface area exposed to the digestive secretions. In addition, grinding the food to a very fine particulate consistency prevents excoriation of the gastrointestinal tract and increases the ease with which food is emptied from the stomach into the small intestine, then into all succeeding segments of the gut.

Swallowing (Deglutition)

Swallowing is a complicated mechanism, principally because the pharynx subserves respiration and swallowing. The pharynx is converted for only a few seconds at a time into a tract for propulsion of food. It is especially important that respiration not be compromised because of swallowing.

In general, swallowing can be divided into (1) a *voluntary stage*, which initiates the swallowing process; (2) a *pharyngeal stage*, which is involuntary and constitutes passage of food through the pharynx into the esophagus; and (3) an *esophageal stage*, another involuntary phase that transports food from the pharynx to the stomach.

Voluntary Stage of Swallowing. When the food is ready for swallowing, it is "voluntarily" squeezed or rolled posteriorly into the pharynx by pressure of the tongue upward and backward against the palate, as shown in

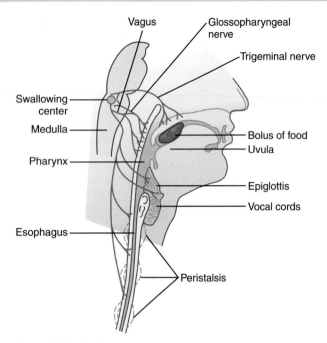

Figure 63-1 Swallowing mechanism.

Figure 63-1. From here on, swallowing becomes entirely—or almost entirely—automatic and ordinarily cannot be stopped.

Pharyngeal Stage of Swallowing. As the bolus of food enters the posterior mouth and pharynx, it stimulates *epithelial swallowing receptor areas* all around the opening of the pharynx, especially on the tonsillar pillars, and impulses from these pass to the brain stem to initiate a series of automatic pharyngeal muscle contractions as follows:

1. The soft palate is pulled upward to close the posterior nares, to prevent reflux of food into the nasal cavities.

2. The palatopharyngeal folds on each side of the pharynx are pulled medially to approximate each other. In this way, these folds form a sagittal slit through which the food must pass into the posterior pharynx. This slit performs a selective action, allowing food that has been masticated sufficiently to pass with ease. Because this stage of swallowing lasts less than 1 second, any large object is usually impeded too much to pass into the esophagus.

3. The vocal cords of the larynx are strongly approximated, and the larynx is pulled upward and anteriorly by the neck muscles. These actions, combined with the presence of ligaments that prevent upward movement of the epiglottis, cause the epiglottis to swing backward over the opening of the larynx. All these effects acting together prevent passage of food into the nose and trachea. Most essential is the tight approximation of the vocal cords, but the epiglottis helps to prevent food from ever getting as far as the vocal cords. Destruction of the vocal cords or of the muscles that approximate them can cause strangulation.

4. The upward movement of the larynx also pulls up and enlarges the opening to the esophagus. At the same time, the upper 3 to 4 centimeters of the esophageal muscular wall, called the *upper esophageal sphincter* (also called the *pharyngoesophageal sphincter*), relaxes. Thus, food moves easily and freely from the posterior pharynx into the upper esophagus. Between swallows, this sphincter remains strongly contracted, thereby preventing air from going into the esophagus during respiration. The upward movement of the larynx also lifts the glottis out of the main stream of food flow, so the food mainly passes on each side of the epiglottis rather than over its surface; this adds still another protection against entry of food into the trachea.

5. Once the larynx is raised and the pharyngoesophageal sphincter becomes relaxed, the entire muscular wall of the pharynx contracts, beginning in the superior part of the pharynx, then spreading downward over the middle and inferior pharyngeal areas, which propels the food by peristalsis into the esophagus.

To summarize the mechanics of the pharyngeal stage of swallowing: The trachea is closed, the esophagus is opened, and a fast peristaltic wave initiated by the nervous system of the pharynx forces the bolus of food into the upper esophagus, the entire process occurring in less than 2 seconds.

Nervous Initiation of the Pharyngeal Stage of Swallowing. The most sensitive tactile areas of the posterior mouth and pharynx for initiating the pharyngeal stage of swallowing lie in a ring around the pharyngeal opening, with greatest sensitivity on the tonsillar pillars. Impulses are transmitted from these areas through the sensory portions of the trigeminal and glossopharyngeal nerves into the medulla oblongata, either into or closely associated with the *tractus solitarius*, which receives essentially all sensory impulses from the mouth.

The successive stages of the swallowing process are then automatically initiated in orderly sequence by neuronal areas of the reticular substance of the medulla and lower portion of the pons. The sequence of the swallowing reflex is the same from one swallow to the next, and the timing of the entire cycle also remains constant from one swallow to the next. The areas in the medulla and lower pons that control swallowing are collectively called the *deglutition* or *swallowing center.*

The motor impulses from the swallowing center to the pharynx and upper esophagus that cause swallowing are transmitted successively by the fifth, ninth, tenth, and twelfth cranial nerves and even a few of the superior cervical nerves.

In summary, the pharyngeal stage of swallowing is principally a reflex act. It is almost always initiated by voluntary movement of food into the back of the mouth, which in turn excites involuntary pharyngeal sensory receptors to elicit the swallowing reflex.

Effect of the Pharyngeal Stage of Swallowing on Respiration.

The entire pharyngeal stage of swallowing usually occurs in less than 6 seconds, thereby interrupting respiration for only a fraction of a usual respiratory cycle. The swallowing center specifically inhibits the respiratory center of the medulla during this time, halting respiration at any point in its cycle to allow swallowing to proceed. Yet even while a person is talking, swallowing interrupts respiration for such a short time that it is hardly noticeable.

Esophageal Stage of Swallowing.

The esophagus functions primarily to conduct food rapidly from the pharynx to the stomach, and its movements are organized specifically for this function.

The esophagus normally exhibits two types of peristaltic movements: *primary peristalsis* and *secondary peristalsis.* Primary peristalsis is simply continuation of the peristaltic wave that begins in the pharynx and spreads into the esophagus during the pharyngeal stage of swallowing. This wave passes all the way from the pharynx to the stomach in about 8 to 10 seconds. Food swallowed by a person who is in the upright position is usually transmitted to the lower end of the esophagus even more rapidly than the peristaltic wave itself, in about 5 to 8 seconds, because of the additional effect of gravity pulling the food downward.

If the primary peristaltic wave fails to move into the stomach all the food that has entered the esophagus, *secondary peristaltic waves* result from distention of the esophagus itself by the retained food; these waves continue until all the food has emptied into the stomach. The secondary peristaltic waves are initiated partly by intrinsic neural circuits in the myenteric nervous system and partly by reflexes that begin in the pharynx and are then transmitted upward through *vagal afferent fibers* to the medulla and back again to the esophagus through *glossopharyngeal* and *vagal efferent nerve fibers.*

The musculature of the pharyngeal wall and upper third of the esophagus is *striated muscle.* Therefore, the peristaltic waves in these regions are controlled by skeletal nerve impulses from the glossopharyngeal and vagus nerves. In the lower two thirds of the esophagus, the musculature is *smooth muscle,* but this portion of the esophagus is also strongly controlled by the vagus nerves acting through connections with the esophageal myenteric nervous system. When the vagus nerves to the esophagus are cut, the myenteric nerve plexus of the esophagus becomes excitable enough after several days to cause strong secondary peristaltic waves even without support from the vagal reflexes. Therefore, even after paralysis of the brain stem swallowing reflex, food fed by tube or in some other way into the esophagus still passes readily into the stomach.

Receptive Relaxation of the Stomach.

When the esophageal peristaltic wave approaches toward the stomach, a wave of relaxation, transmitted through myenteric inhibitory neurons, precedes the peristalsis. Furthermore, the entire stomach and, to a lesser extent, even the duodenum become relaxed as this wave reaches the lower end of the esophagus and thus are prepared ahead of time to receive the food propelled into the esophagus during the swallowing act.

Function of the Lower Esophageal Sphincter (Gastroesophageal Sphincter).

At the lower end of the esophagus, extending upward about 3 centimeters above its juncture with the stomach, the esophageal circular muscle functions as a broad *lower esophageal sphincter,* also called the *gastroesophageal sphincter.* This sphincter normally remains tonically constricted with an intraluminal pressure at this point in the esophagus of about 30 mm Hg, in contrast to the midportion of the esophagus, which normally remains relaxed. When a peristaltic swallowing wave passes down the esophagus, there is "receptive relaxation" of the lower esophageal sphincter ahead of the peristaltic wave, which allows easy propulsion of the swallowed food into the stomach. Rarely, the sphincter does not relax satisfactorily, resulting in a condition called *achalasia.* This is discussed in Chapter 66.

The stomach secretions are highly acidic and contain many proteolytic enzymes. The esophageal mucosa, except in the lower one eighth of the esophagus, is not capable of resisting for long the digestive action of gastric secretions. Fortunately, the tonic constriction of the lower esophageal sphincter helps to prevent significant reflux of stomach contents into the esophagus except under abnormal conditions.

Additional Prevention of Esophageal Reflux by Valvelike Closure of the Distal End of the Esophagus.

Another factor that helps to prevent reflux is a valvelike mechanism of a short portion of the esophagus that extends slightly into the stomach. Increased intra-abdominal pressure caves the esophagus inward at this point. Thus, this valvelike closure of the lower esophagus helps to prevent high intra-abdominal pressure from forcing stomach contents backward into the esophagus. Otherwise, every time we walked, coughed, or breathed hard, we might expel stomach acid into the esophagus.

Motor Functions of the Stomach

The motor functions of the stomach are threefold: (1) storage of large quantities of food until the food can be processed in the stomach, duodenum, and lower intestinal tract; (2) mixing of this food with gastric secretions until it forms a semifluid mixture called *chyme;* and (3) slow emptying of the chyme from the stomach into the small intestine at a rate suitable for proper digestion and absorption by the small intestine.

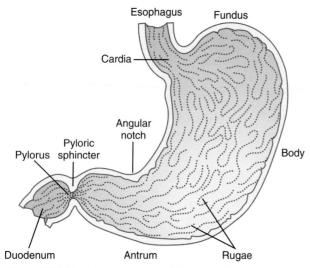

Esophagus   Fundus

Cardia

Angular
notch

Pyloric
Pylorus sphincter

Body

Duodenum   Antrum   Rugae

Figure 63-2 Physiologic anatomy of the stomach.

Figure 63-2 shows the basic anatomy of the stomach. Anatomically, the stomach is usually divided into two major parts: (1) the *body* and (2) the *antrum*. Physiologically, it is more appropriately divided into (1) the *"orad"* portion, comprising about the first two thirds of the body, and (2) the *"caudad"* portion, comprising the remainder of the body plus the antrum.

Storage Function of the Stomach

As food enters the stomach, it forms concentric circles of the food in the orad portion of the stomach, the newest food lying closest to the esophageal opening and the oldest food lying nearest the outer wall of the stomach. Normally, when food stretches the stomach, a "vagovagal reflex" from the stomach to the brain stem and then back to the stomach reduces the tone in the muscular wall of the body of the stomach so that the wall bulges progressively outward, accommodating greater and greater quantities of food up to a limit in the completely relaxed stomach of 0.8 to 1.5 liters. The pressure in the stomach remains low until this limit is approached.

Mixing and Propulsion of Food in the Stomach— Basic Electrical Rhythm of the Stomach Wall

The digestive juices of the stomach are secreted by *gastric glands,* which are present in almost the entire wall of the body of the stomach except along a narrow strip on the lesser curvature of the stomach. These secretions come immediately into contact with that portion of the stored food lying against the mucosal surface of the stomach. As long as food is in the stomach, weak peristaltic *constrictor waves,* called *mixing waves,* begin in the mid to upper portions of the stomach wall and move toward the antrum about once every 15 to 20 seconds. These waves are initiated by the gut wall *basic electrical rhythm,* which was discussed in Chapter 62, consisting of electrical "slow waves" that occur spontaneously in the stomach

wall. As the constrictor waves progress from the body of the stomach into the antrum, they become more intense, some becoming extremely intense and providing powerful *peristaltic action potential*–driven constrictor rings that force the antral contents under higher and higher pressure toward the pylorus.

These constrictor rings also play an important role in mixing the stomach contents in the following way: Each time a peristaltic wave passes down the antral wall toward the pylorus, it digs deeply into the food contents in the antrum. Yet the opening of the pylorus is still small enough that only a few milliliters or less of antral contents are expelled into the duodenum with each peristaltic wave. Also, as each peristaltic wave approaches the pylorus, the pyloric muscle itself often contracts, which further impedes emptying through the pylorus. Therefore, most of the antral contents are squeezed upstream through the peristaltic ring toward the body of the stomach, not through the pylorus. Thus, the moving peristaltic constrictive ring, combined with this upstream squeezing action, called "retropulsion," is an exceedingly important mixing mechanism in the stomach.

Chyme. After food in the stomach has become thoroughly mixed with the stomach secretions, the resulting mixture that passes down the gut is called *chyme.* The degree of fluidity of the chyme leaving the stomach depends on the relative amounts of food, water, and stomach secretions and on the degree of digestion that has occurred. The appearance of chyme is that of a murky semifluid or paste.

Hunger Contractions. Besides the peristaltic contractions that occur when food is present in the stomach, another type of intense contractions, called *hunger contractions,* often occurs *when the stomach has been empty* for several hours or more. They are rhythmical peristaltic contractions in the *body* of the stomach. When the successive contractions become extremely strong, they often fuse to cause a continuing tetanic contraction that sometimes lasts for 2 to 3 minutes.

Hunger contractions are most intense in young, healthy people who have high degrees of gastrointestinal tonus; they are also greatly increased by the person's having lower than normal levels of blood sugar. When hunger contractions occur in the stomach, the person sometimes experiences mild pain in the pit of the stomach, called *hunger pangs.* Hunger pangs usually do not begin until 12 to 24 hours after the last ingestion of food; in starvation, they reach their greatest intensity in 3 to 4 days and gradually weaken in succeeding days.

Stomach Emptying

Stomach emptying is promoted by intense peristaltic contractions in the stomach antrum. At the same time, emptying is opposed by varying degrees of resistance to passage of chyme at the pylorus.

Intense Antral Peristaltic Contractions During Stomach Emptying—"Pyloric Pump."

Most of the time, the rhythmical stomach contractions are weak and function mainly to cause mixing of food and gastric secretions. However, for about 20 percent of the time while food is in the stomach, the contractions become intense, beginning in midstomach and spreading through the caudad stomach; these contractions are strong peristaltic, very tight ringlike constrictions that can cause stomach emptying. As the stomach becomes progressively more and more empty, these constrictions begin farther and farther up the body of the stomach, gradually pinching off the food in the body of the stomach and adding this food to the chyme in the antrum. These intense peristaltic contractions often create 50 to 70 centimeters of water pressure, which is about six times as powerful as the usual mixing type of peristaltic waves.

When pyloric tone is normal, each strong peristaltic wave forces up to several milliliters of chyme into the duodenum. Thus, the peristaltic waves, in addition to causing mixing in the stomach, also provide a pumping action called the "pyloric pump."

Role of the Pylorus in Controlling Stomach Emptying.

The distal opening of the stomach is the *pylorus*. Here the thickness of the circular wall muscle becomes 50 to 100 percent greater than in the earlier portions of the stomach antrum, and it remains slightly tonically contracted almost all the time. Therefore, the pyloric circular muscle is called the *pyloric sphincter*.

Despite normal tonic contraction of the pyloric sphincter, the pylorus usually is open enough for water and other fluids to empty from the stomach into the duodenum with ease. Conversely, the constriction usually prevents passage of food particles until they have become mixed in the chyme to almost fluid consistency. The degree of constriction of the pylorus is increased or decreased under the influence of nervous and humoral reflex signals from both the stomach and the duodenum, as discussed shortly.

Regulation of Stomach Emptying

The rate at which the stomach empties is regulated by signals from both the stomach and the duodenum. However, the duodenum provides by far the more potent of the signals, controlling the emptying of chyme into the duodenum at a rate no greater than the rate at which the chyme can be digested and absorbed in the small intestine.

Gastric Factors That Promote Emptying

Effect of Gastric Food Volume on Rate of Emptying.

Increased food volume in the stomach promotes increased emptying from the stomach. But this increased emptying does not occur for the reasons that one would expect. It is not increased storage pressure of the food in the stomach that causes the increased emptying because, in the usual normal range of volume, the increase in volume does not increase the pressure much. However, stretching of the stomach wall does elicit local myenteric reflexes in the wall that greatly accentuate activity of the pyloric pump and at the same time inhibit the pylorus.

Effect of the Hormone *Gastrin* on Stomach Emptying.

In Chapter 64, we discuss how stomach wall stretch and the presence of certain types of foods in the stomach—particularly digestive products of meat—elicit release of the hormone *gastrin* from the antral mucosa. This has potent effects to cause secretion of highly acidic gastric juice by the stomach glands. Gastrin also has mild to moderate stimulatory effects on motor functions in the body of the stomach. Most important, it seems to enhance the activity of the pyloric pump. Thus, gastrin likely promotes stomach emptying.

Powerful Duodenal Factors That Inhibit Stomach Emptying

Inhibitory Effect of Enterogastric Nervous Reflexes from the Duodenum.

When food enters the duodenum, multiple nervous reflexes are initiated from the duodenal wall. They pass back to the stomach to slow or even stop stomach emptying if the volume of chyme in the duodenum becomes too much. These reflexes are mediated by three routes: (1) directly from the duodenum to the stomach through the enteric nervous system in the gut wall, (2) through extrinsic nerves that go to the prevertebral sympathetic ganglia and then back through inhibitory sympathetic nerve fibers to the stomach, and (3) probably to a slight extent through the vagus nerves all the way to the brain stem, where they inhibit the normal excitatory signals transmitted to the stomach through the vagi. All these parallel reflexes have two effects on stomach emptying: First, they strongly inhibit the "pyloric pump" propulsive contractions, and second, they increase the tone of the pyloric sphincter.

The types of factors that are continually monitored in the duodenum and that can initiate enterogastric inhibitory reflexes include the following:

1. The degree of distention of the duodenum
2. The presence of any degree of irritation of the duodenal mucosa
3. The degree of acidity of the duodenal chyme
4. The degree of osmolality of the chyme
5. The presence of certain breakdown products in the chyme, especially breakdown products of proteins and, perhaps to a lesser extent, of fats

The enterogastric inhibitory reflexes are especially sensitive to the presence of irritants and acids in the duodenal chyme, and they often become strongly activated within as little as 30 seconds. For instance, whenever the pH of the chyme in the duodenum falls below about 3.5 to 4, the reflexes frequently block further release of acidic stomach contents into the duodenum until the duodenal chyme can be neutralized by pancreatic and other secretions.

Breakdown products of protein digestion also elicit inhibitory enterogastric reflexes; by slowing the rate of stomach emptying, sufficient time is ensured for adequate protein digestion in the duodenum and small intestine.

Finally, either hypotonic or hypertonic fluids (especially hypertonic) elicit the inhibitory reflexes. Thus, too rapid flow of nonisotonic fluids into the small intestine is prevented, thereby also preventing rapid changes in electrolyte concentrations in the whole-body extracellular fluid during absorption of the intestinal contents.

Hormonal Feedback from the Duodenum Inhibits Gastric Emptying—Role of Fats and the Hormone Cholecystokinin. Not only do nervous reflexes from the duodenum to the stomach inhibit stomach emptying, but hormones released from the upper intestine do so as well. The stimulus for releasing these inhibitory hormones is mainly fats entering the duodenum, although other types of foods can increase the hormones to a lesser degree.

On entering the duodenum, the fats extract several different hormones from the duodenal and jejunal epithelium, either by binding with "receptors" on the epithelial cells or in some other way. In turn, the hormones are carried by way of the blood to the stomach, where they inhibit the pyloric pump and at the same time increase the strength of contraction of the pyloric sphincter. These effects are important because fats are much slower to be digested than most other foods.

Precisely which hormones cause the hormonal feedback inhibition of the stomach is not fully clear. The most potent appears to be *cholecystokinin* (CCK), which is released from the mucosa of the jejunum in response to fatty substances in the chyme. This hormone acts as an inhibitor to block increased stomach motility caused by gastrin.

Other possible inhibitors of stomach emptying are the hormones *secretin* and *gastric inhibitory peptide* (GIP), also called *glucose-dependent insulinotropic peptide.* Secretin is released mainly from the duodenal mucosa in response to gastric acid passed from the stomach through the pylorus. GIP has a general but weak effect of decreasing gastrointestinal motility.

GIP is released from the upper small intestine in response mainly to fat in the chyme, but to a lesser extent to carbohydrates as well. Although GIP inhibits gastric motility under some conditions, its main effect at physiologic concentrations is probably mainly to stimulate secretion of insulin by the pancreas.

These hormones are discussed at greater length elsewhere in this text, especially in Chapter 64 in relation to control of gallbladder emptying and control of rate of pancreatic secretion.

In summary, hormones, especially CCK, can inhibit gastric emptying when excess quantities of chyme, especially acidic or fatty chyme, enter the duodenum from the stomach.

Summary of the Control of Stomach Emptying

Emptying of the stomach is controlled only to a moderate degree by stomach factors such as the degree of filling in the stomach and the excitatory effect of gastrin on stomach peristalsis. Probably the more important control of stomach emptying resides in inhibitory feedback signals from the duodenum, including both enterogastric inhibitory nervous feedback reflexes and hormonal feedback by CCK. These feedback inhibitory mechanisms work together to slow the rate of emptying when (1) too much chyme is already in the small intestine or (2) the chyme is excessively acidic, contains too much unprocessed protein or fat, is hypotonic or hypertonic, or is irritating. In this way, the rate of stomach emptying is limited to that amount of chyme that the small intestine can process.

Movements of the Small Intestine

The movements of the small intestine, like those elsewhere in the gastrointestinal tract, can be divided into *mixing contractions* and *propulsive contractions.* To a great extent, this separation is artificial because essentially all movements of the small intestine cause at least some degree of both mixing and propulsion. The usual classification of these processes is the following.

Mixing Contractions (Segmentation Contractions)

When a portion of the small intestine becomes distended with chyme, stretching of the intestinal wall elicits localized concentric contractions spaced at intervals along the intestine and lasting a fraction of a minute. The contractions cause "segmentation" of the small intestine, as shown in Figure 63-3. That is, they divide the intestine into spaced segments that have the appearance of a chain of sausages. As one set of segmentation contractions relaxes, a new set often begins, but the contractions this time occur mainly at new points between the previous contractions. Therefore, the segmentation contractions "chop" the chyme two to three times per minute, in this way promoting progressive mixing of the food with secretions of the small intestine.

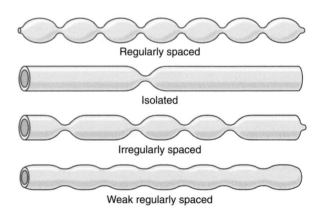

Figure 63-3 Segmentation movements of the small intestine.

The maximum frequency of the segmentation contractions in the small intestine is determined by the frequency of *electrical slow waves* in the intestinal wall, which is the basic electrical rhythm described in Chapter 62. Because this frequency normally is not over 12 per minute in the duodenum and proximal jejunum, the *maximum* frequency of the segmentation contractions in these areas is also about 12 per minute, but this occurs only under extreme conditions of stimulation. In the terminal ileum, the maximum frequency is usually eight to nine contractions per minute.

The segmentation contractions become exceedingly weak when the excitatory activity of the enteric nervous system is blocked by the drug atropine. Therefore, even though it is the slow waves in the smooth muscle itself that cause the segmentation contractions, these contractions are not effective without background excitation mainly from the myenteric nerve plexus.

Propulsive Movements

Peristalsis in the Small Intestine. Chyme is propelled through the small intestine by *peristaltic waves.* These can occur in any part of the small intestine, and they move toward the anus at a velocity of 0.5 to 2.0 cm/sec, faster in the proximal intestine and slower in the terminal intestine. They are normally weak and usually die out after traveling only 3 to 5 centimeters, rarely farther than 10 centimeters, so forward movement of the chyme is very slow, so slow that *net* movement along the small intestine normally averages only 1 cm/min. This means that 3 to 5 hours are required for passage of chyme from the pylorus to the ileocecal valve.

Control of Peristalsis by Nervous and Hormonal Signals. Peristaltic activity of the small intestine is greatly increased after a meal. This is caused partly by the beginning entry of chyme into the duodenum causing stretch of the duodenal wall. Also, peristaltic activity is increased by the so-called *gastroenteric reflex* that is initiated by distention of the stomach and conducted principally through the myenteric plexus from the stomach down along the wall of the small intestine.

In addition to the nervous signals that may affect small intestinal peristalsis, several hormonal factors also affect peristalsis. They include *gastrin, CCK, insulin, motilin,* and *serotonin,* all of which enhance intestinal motility and are secreted during various phases of food processing. Conversely, *secretin* and *glucagon* inhibit small intestinal motility. The physiologic importance of each of these hormonal factors for controlling motility is still questionable.

The function of the peristaltic waves in the small intestine is not only to cause progression of chyme toward the ileocecal valve but also to spread out the chyme along the intestinal mucosa. As the chyme enters the intestines from the stomach and elicits peristalsis, this immediately spreads the chyme along the intestine; and this process intensifies as additional chyme enters the duodenum. On reaching the ileocecal valve, the chyme is sometimes blocked for several hours until the person eats another meal; at that time, a *gastroileal* reflex intensifies peristalsis in the ileum and forces the remaining chyme through the ileocecal valve into the cecum of the large intestine.

Propulsive Effect of the Segmentation Movements. The segmentation movements, although lasting for only a few seconds at a time, often also travel 1 centimeter or so in the anal direction and during that time help propel the food down the intestine. The difference between the segmentation and the peristaltic movements is not as great as might be implied by their separation into these two classifications.

Peristaltic Rush. Although peristalsis in the small intestine is normally weak, intense irritation of the intestinal mucosa, as occurs in some severe cases of infectious diarrhea, can cause both powerful and rapid peristalsis, called the *peristaltic rush.* This is initiated partly by nervous reflexes that involve the autonomic nervous system and brain stem and partly by intrinsic enhancement of the myenteric plexus reflexes within the gut wall itself. The powerful peristaltic contractions travel long distances in the small intestine within minutes, sweeping the contents of the intestine into the colon and thereby relieving the small intestine of irritative chyme and excessive distention.

> **Movements Caused by the Muscularis Mucosae and Muscle Fibers of the Villi** The *muscularis mucosae* can cause short folds to appear in the intestinal mucosa. In addition, individual fibers from this muscle extend into the intestinal villi and cause them to contract intermittently. The mucosal folds increase the surface area exposed to the chyme, thereby increasing absorption. Also, contractions of the villi—shortening, elongating, and shortening again—"milk" the villi so that lymph flows freely from the central lacteals of the villi into the lymphatic system. These mucosal and villous contractions are initiated mainly by local nervous reflexes in the submucosal nerve plexus that occur in response to chyme in the small intestine.

Function of the Ileocecal Valve

A principal function of the ileocecal valve is to prevent backflow of fecal contents from the colon into the small intestine. As shown in Figure 63-4, the ileocecal valve itself protrudes into the lumen of the cecum and therefore is forcefully closed when excess pressure builds up in the cecum and tries to push cecal contents backward against the valve lips. The valve usually can resist reverse pressure of at least 50 to 60 centimeters of water.

In addition, the wall of the ileum for several centimeters immediately upstream from the ileocecal valve has a thickened circular muscle called the *ileocecal sphincter.* This sphincter normally remains mildly constricted and slows emptying of ileal contents into the cecum. However, immediately after a meal, a gastroileal reflex (described

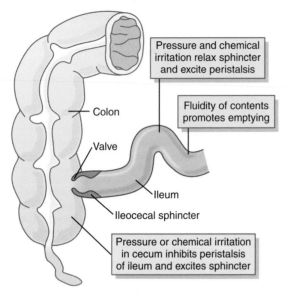

Figure 63-4 Emptying at the ileocecal valve.

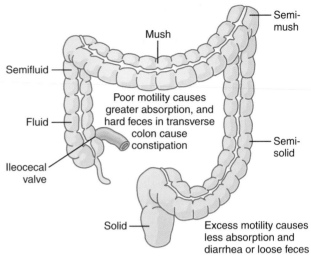

Figure 63-5 Absorptive and storage functions of the large intestine.

earlier) intensifies peristalsis in the ileum, and emptying of ileal contents into the cecum proceeds.

Resistance to emptying at the ileocecal valve prolongs the stay of chyme in the ileum and thereby facilitates absorption. Normally, only 1500 to 2000 milliliters of chyme empty into the cecum each day.

Feedback Control of the Ileocecal Sphincter. The degree of contraction of the ileocecal sphincter and the intensity of peristalsis in the terminal ileum are controlled significantly by reflexes from the cecum. When the cecum is distended, contraction of the ileocecal sphincter becomes intensified and ileal peristalsis is inhibited, both of which greatly delay emptying of additional chyme into the cecum from the ileum. Also, any irritant in the cecum delays emptying. For instance, when a person has an inflamed appendix, the irritation of this vestigial remnant of the cecum can cause such intense spasm of the ileocecal sphincter and partial paralysis of the ileum that these effects together block emptying of the ileum into the cecum. The reflexes from the cecum to the ileocecal sphincter and ileum are mediated both by way of the myenteric plexus in the gut wall itself and of the extrinsic autonomic nerves, especially by way of the prevertebral sympathetic ganglia.

Movements of the Colon

The principal functions of the colon are (1) absorption of water and electrolytes from the chyme to form solid feces and (2) storage of fecal matter until it can be expelled. The proximal half of the colon, shown in Figure 63-5, is concerned principally with absorption, and the distal half with storage. Because intense colon wall movements are not required for these functions, the movements of the colon are normally sluggish. Yet in a sluggish manner, the movements still have characteristics similar to those of the small intestine and can be divided once again into mixing movements and propulsive movements.

Mixing Movements—"Haustrations." In the same manner that segmentation movements occur in the small intestine, large circular constrictions occur in the large intestine. At each of these constrictions, about 2.5 centimeters of the circular muscle contract, sometimes constricting the lumen of the colon almost to occlusion. At the same time, the longitudinal muscle of the colon, which is aggregated into three longitudinal strips called the *teniae coli*, contracts. These combined contractions of the circular and longitudinal strips of muscle cause the unstimulated portion of the large intestine to bulge outward into baglike sacs called *haustrations*.

Each haustration usually reaches peak intensity in about 30 seconds and then disappears during the next 60 seconds. They also at times move slowly toward the anus during contraction, especially in the cecum and ascending colon, and thereby provide a minor amount of forward propulsion of the colonic contents. After another few minutes, new haustral contractions occur in other areas nearby. Therefore, the fecal material in the large intestine is slowly *dug into and rolled over* in much the same manner that one spades the earth. In this way, all the fecal material is gradually exposed to the mucosal surface of the large intestine, and fluid and dissolved substances are progressively absorbed until only 80 to 200 milliliters of feces are expelled each day.

Propulsive Movements—"Mass Movements." Much of the propulsion in the cecum and ascending colon results from the slow but persistent haustral contractions, requiring as many as 8 to 15 hours to move the chyme from the ileocecal valve through the colon, while the chyme itself becomes fecal in quality, a semisolid slush instead of semifluid.

From the cecum to the sigmoid, *mass movements* can, for many minutes at a time, take over the propulsive role. These movements usually occur only one to three times each day, in many people especially for about 15 minutes during the first hour after eating breakfast.

A mass movement is a modified type of peristalsis characterized by the following sequence of events: First, a *constrictive ring* occurs in response to a distended or irritated point in the colon, usually in the transverse colon. Then, rapidly, the 20 or more centimeters of colon *distal to the constrictive ring* lose their haustrations and instead contract as a unit, propelling the fecal material in this segment *en masse* further down the colon. The contraction develops progressively more force for about 30 seconds, and relaxation occurs during the next 2 to 3 minutes. Then, another mass movement occurs, this time perhaps farther along the colon.

A series of mass movements usually persists for 10 to 30 minutes. Then they cease but return perhaps a half day later. When they have forced a mass of feces into the rectum, the desire for defecation is felt.

Initiation of Mass Movements by Gastrocolic and Duodenocolic Reflexes.
Appearance of mass movements after meals is facilitated by *gastrocolic* and *duodenocolic reflexes.* These reflexes result from distention of the stomach and duodenum. They occur either not at all or hardly at all when the extrinsic autonomic nerves to the colon have been removed; therefore, the reflexes almost certainly are transmitted by way of the autonomic nervous system.

Irritation in the colon can also initiate intense mass movements. For instance, a person who has an ulcerated condition of the colon mucosa *(ulcerative colitis)* frequently has mass movements that persist almost all the time.

Defecation

Most of the time, the rectum is empty of feces. This results partly from the fact that a weak functional sphincter exists about 20 centimeters from the anus at the juncture between the sigmoid colon and the rectum. There is also a sharp angulation here that contributes additional resistance to filling of the rectum.

When a mass movement forces feces into the rectum, the desire for defecation occurs immediately, including reflex contraction of the rectum and relaxation of the anal sphincters.

Continual dribble of fecal matter through the anus is prevented by tonic constriction of (1) an *internal anal sphincter,* a several-centimeters-long thickening of the circular smooth muscle that lies immediately inside the anus, and (2) an *external anal sphincter,* composed of striated voluntary muscle that both surrounds the internal sphincter and extends distal to it. The external sphincter is controlled by nerve fibers in the *pudendal nerve,* which is part of the somatic nervous system and therefore is under *voluntary, conscious,* or at least *subconscious con-* trol; subconsciously, the external sphincter is usually kept continuously constricted unless conscious signals inhibit the constriction.

Defecation Reflexes.
Ordinarily, defecation is initiated by *defecation reflexes.* One of these reflexes is an *intrinsic reflex* mediated by the local enteric nervous system in the rectal wall. This can be described as follows: When feces enter the rectum, distention of the rectal wall initiates afferent signals that spread through the *myenteric plexus* to initiate peristaltic waves in the descending colon, sigmoid, and rectum, forcing feces toward the anus. As the peristaltic wave approaches the anus, the *internal* anal sphincter is relaxed by inhibitory signals from the myenteric plexus; if the *external* anal sphincter is also consciously, voluntarily relaxed at the same time, defecation occurs.

The intrinsic myenteric defecation reflex functioning by itself normally is relatively weak. To be effective in causing defecation, it usually must be fortified by another type of defecation reflex, a *parasympathetic defecation reflex* that involves the sacral segments of the spinal cord, shown in Figure 63-6. When the nerve endings in the rectum are stimulated, signals are transmitted first into the spinal cord and then reflexly back to the descending colon, sigmoid, rectum, and anus by way of parasympathetic nerve fibers in the *pelvic nerves.* These parasympathetic signals greatly intensify the peristaltic waves and relax the internal anal sphincter, thus converting the intrinsic myenteric defecation reflex from a weak effort into a powerful process of defecation that is sometimes effective in emptying the large bowel all the way from the splenic flexure of the colon to the anus.

Defecation signals entering the spinal cord initiate other effects, such as taking a deep breath, closure of the glottis, and contraction of the abdominal wall muscles to force the fecal contents of the colon downward and at the same time cause the pelvic floor to relax downward and pull outward on the anal ring to evaginate the feces.

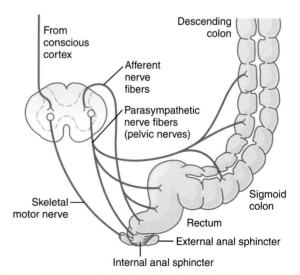

Figure 63-6 Afferent and efferent pathways of the parasympathetic mechanism for enhancing the defecation reflex.

When it becomes convenient for the person to defecate, the defecation reflexes can purposely be activated by taking a deep breath to move the diaphragm downward and then contracting the abdominal muscles to increase the pressure in the abdomen, thus forcing fecal contents into the rectum to cause new reflexes. Reflexes initiated in this way are almost never as effective as those that arise naturally, for which reason people who too often inhibit their natural reflexes are likely to become severely constipated.

In newborn babies and in some people with transected spinal cords, the defecation reflexes cause automatic emptying of the lower bowel at inconvenient times during the day because of lack of conscious control exercised through voluntary contraction or relaxation of the external anal sphincter.

Other Autonomic Reflexes That Affect Bowel Activity

Aside from the duodenocolic, gastrocolic, gastroileal, enterogastric, and defecation reflexes that have been discussed in this chapter, several other important nervous reflexes also can affect the overall degree of bowel activity. They are the peritoneointestinal reflex, renointestinal reflex, and vesicointestinal reflex.

The *peritoneointestinal reflex* results from irritation of the peritoneum; it strongly inhibits the excitatory enteric nerves and thereby can cause intestinal paralysis, especially in patients with peritonitis. The *renointestinal* and *vesicointestinal reflexes* inhibit intestinal activity as a result of kidney or bladder irritation, respectively.

Bibliography

Adelson DW, Million M: Tracking the moveable feast: sonomicrometry and gastrointestinal motility, *News Physiol Sci* 19:27, 2004.

Cooke HJ, Wunderlich J, Christofi FL: "The force be with you": ATP in gut mechanosensory transduction, *News Physiol Sci* 18:43, 2003.

Gonella J, Bouvier M, Blanquet F: Extrinsic nervous control of motility of small and large intestines and related sphincters, *Physiol Rev* 67:902, 1987.

Grundy D, Al-Chaer ED, Aziz Q, et al: Fundamentals of neurogastroenterology: basic science, *Gastroenterology* 130:1391, 2006.

Hall KE: Aging and neural control of the GI tract. II. Neural control of the aging gut: can an old dog learn new tricks? *Am J Physiol Gastrointest Liver Physiol* 283:G827, 2002.

Hatoum OA, Miura H, Binion DG: The vascular contribution in the pathogenesis of inflammatory bowel disease, *Am J Physiol Heart Circ Physiol* 285:H1791, 2003.

Huizinga JD, Lammers WJ: Gut peristalsis is governed by a multitude of cooperating mechanisms, *Am J Physiol Gastrointest Liver Physiol* 296:G1, 2009.

Laroux FS, Pavlick KP, Wolf RE, Grisham MB: Dysregulation of intestinal mucosal immunity: implications in inflammatory bowel disease, *News Physiol Sci* 16:272, 2001.

Orr WC, Chen CL: Aging and neural control of the GI tract: IV. Clinical and physiological aspects of gastrointestinal motility and aging, *Am J Physiol Gastrointest Liver Physiol* 283:G1226, 2002.

Parkman HP, Jones MP: Tests of gastric neuromuscular function, *Gastroenterology* 136:1526, 2009.

Sanders KM, Ordog T, Koh SD, Ward SM: A novel pacemaker mechanism drives gastrointestinal rhythmicity, *News Physiol Sci* 15:291, 2000.

Sarna SK: Molecular, functional, and pharmacological targets for the development of gut promotility drugs, *Am J Physiol Gastrointest Liver Physiol* 291:G545, 2006.

Sarna SK: Are interstitial cells of Cajal plurifunction cells in the gut? *Am J Physiol Gastrointest Liver Physiol* 294:G372, 2008.

Sharma A, Lelic D, Brock C, Paine P, Aziz Q: New technologies to investigate the brain-gut axis, *World J Gastroenterol* 15:182, 2009.

Szarka LA, Camilleri M: Methods for measurement of gastric motility, *Am J Physiol Gastrointest Liver Physiol* 296:G461, 2009.

Timmons S, Liston R, Moriarty KJ: Functional dyspepsia: motor abnormalities, sensory dysfunction, and therapeutic options, *Am J Gastroenterol* 99:739, 2004.

Wood JD: Neuropathophysiology of functional gastrointestinal disorders, *World J Gastroenterol* 13:1313, 2007.

Xue J, Askwith C, Javed NH, Cooke HJ: Autonomic nervous system and secretion across the intestinal mucosal surface, *Auton Neurosci* 133:55, 2007.

CHAPTER 64

Secretory Functions of the Alimentary Tract

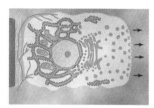

Throughout the gastrointestinal tract, secretory glands subserve two primary functions: First, *digestive enzymes* are secreted in most areas of the alimentary tract, from the mouth to the distal end of the ileum. Second, mucous glands, from the mouth to the anus, provide *mucus* for lubrication and protection of all parts of the alimentary tract.

Most digestive secretions are formed only in response to the presence of food in the alimentary tract, and the quantity secreted in each segment of the tract is usually the precise amount needed for proper digestion. Furthermore, in some portions of the gastrointestinal tract, even the *types of enzymes* and other constituents of the secretions are varied in accordance with the types of food present. The purpose of this chapter is to describe the different alimentary secretions, their functions, and regulation of their production.

General Principles of Alimentary Tract Secretion

Anatomical Types of Glands

Several types of glands provide the different types of alimentary tract secretions. First, on the surface of the epithelium in most parts of the gastrointestinal tract are billions of *single-cell mucous glands* called simply *mucous cells* or sometimes *goblet cells* because they look like goblets. They function mainly in response to local irritation of the epithelium: They extrude *mucus* directly onto the epithelial surface to act as a lubricant that also protects the surfaces from excoriation and digestion.

Second, many surface areas of the gastrointestinal tract are lined by *pits* that represent invaginations of the epithelium into the submucosa. In the small intestine, these pits, called *crypts of Lieberkühn*, are deep and contain specialized secretory cells. One of these cells is shown in Figure 64-1.

Third, in the stomach and upper duodenum are large numbers of deep *tubular glands*. A typical tubular gland can be seen in Figure 64-4, which shows an acid- and pepsinogen-secreting gland of the stomach (oxyntic gland).

Fourth, also associated with the alimentary tract are several complex glands—the *salivary glands, pancreas,* and

liver—that provide secretions for digestion or emulsification of food. The liver has a highly specialized structure that is discussed in Chapter 70. The salivary glands and the pancreas are compound acinous glands of the type shown in Figure 64-2. These glands lie outside the walls of the alimentary tract and, in this, differ from all other alimentary glands. They contain millions of *acini* lined with secreting glandular cells; these acini feed into a system of ducts that finally empty into the alimentary tract itself.

Basic Mechanisms of Stimulation of the Alimentary Tract Glands

Contact of Food with the Epithelium Stimulates Secretion—Function of Enteric Nervous Stimuli. The mechanical presence of food in a particular segment of the gastrointestinal tract usually causes the glands of that region and adjacent regions to secrete moderate to large quantities of juices. Part of this local effect, especially the secretion of mucus by mucous cells, results from direct contact stimulation of the surface glandular cells by the food.

In addition, local epithelial stimulation also activates the *enteric nervous system* of the gut wall. The types of stimuli that do this are (1) tactile stimulation, (2) chemical irritation, and (3) distention of the gut wall. The resulting nervous reflexes stimulate both the mucous cells on the gut epithelial surface and the deep glands in the gut wall to increase their secretion.

Autonomic Stimulation of Secretion

Parasympathetic Stimulation Increases Alimentary Tract Glandular Secretion Rate. Stimulation of the parasympathetic nerves to the alimentary tract almost invariably increases the rates of alimentary glandular secretion. This is especially true of the glands in the upper portion of the tract (innervated by the glossopharyngeal and vagus parasympathetic nerves) such as the salivary glands, esophageal glands, gastric glands, pancreas, and Brunner's glands in the duodenum. It is also true of some glands in the distal portion of the large intestine, innervated by pelvic parasympathetic nerves. Secretion in the remainder of the small intestine and in the first two thirds of the large intestine occurs mainly

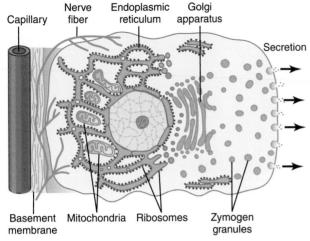

Figure 64-1 Typical function of a glandular cell for formation and secretion of enzymes and other secretory substances.

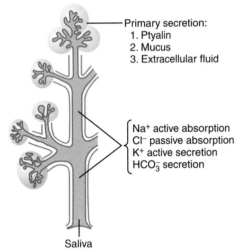

Primary secretion:
1. Ptyalin
2. Mucus
3. Extracellular fluid

Na^+ active absorption
Cl^- passive absorption
K^+ active secretion
HCO_3^- secretion

Saliva

Figure 64-2 Formation and secretion of saliva by a submandibular salivary gland.

in response to local neural and hormonal stimuli in each segment of the gut.

Sympathetic Stimulation Has a Dual Effect on Alimentary Tract Glandular Secretion Rate. Stimulation of the sympathetic nerves going to the gastrointestinal tract causes a slight to moderate increase in secretion by some of the local glands. But sympathetic stimulation also results in constriction of the blood vessels that supply the glands. Therefore, sympathetic stimulation can have a dual effect: (1) sympathetic stimulation alone usually slightly increases secretion and (2) if parasympathetic or hormonal stimulation is already causing copious secretion by the glands, superimposed sympathetic stimulation usually reduces the secretion, sometimes significantly so, mainly because of vasoconstrictive reduction of the blood supply.

Regulation of Glandular Secretion by Hormones. In the stomach and intestine, several different *gastrointestinal hormones* help regulate the volume and character of the secretions. These hormones are liberated from the gastrointestinal mucosa in response to the presence of food in the lumen of the gut. The hormones are then absorbed into the blood and carried to the glands, where they stimulate secretion. This type of stimulation is particularly valuable to increase the output of gastric juice and pancreatic juice when food enters the stomach or duodenum.

Chemically, the gastrointestinal hormones are polypeptides or polypeptide derivatives.

Basic Mechanism of Secretion by Glandular Cells

Secretion of Organic Substances. Although all the basic mechanisms by which glandular cells function are not known, experimental evidence points to the following principles of secretion, as shown in Figure 64-1.

1. The nutrient material needed for formation of the secretion must first diffuse or be actively transported by the blood in the capillaries into the base of the glandular cell.

2. Many *mitochondria* located inside the glandular cell near its base use oxidative energy to form adenosine triphosphate (ATP).

3. Energy from the ATP, along with appropriate substrates provided by the nutrients, is then used to synthesize the organic secretory substances; this synthesis occurs almost entirely in the *endoplasmic reticulum* and *Golgi complex* of the glandular cell. *Ribosomes* adherent to the reticulum are specifically responsible for formation of the proteins that are secreted.

4. The secretory materials are transported through the tubules of the endoplasmic reticulum, passing in about 20 minutes all the way to the vesicles of the Golgi complex.

5. In the Golgi complex, the materials are modified, added to, concentrated, and discharged into the cytoplasm in the form of *secretory vesicles,* which are stored in the apical ends of the secretory cells.

6. These vesicles remain stored until nervous or hormonal control signals cause the cells to extrude the vesicular contents through the cells' surface. This probably occurs in the following way: The control signal first *increases the cell membrane permeability to calcium ions,* and calcium enters the cell. The *calcium* in turn causes many of the vesicles to fuse with the apical cell membrane. Then the apical cell membrane breaks open, thus emptying the vesicles to the exterior; this process is called *exocytosis.*

Water and Electrolyte Secretion. A second necessity for glandular secretion is secretion of sufficient water and electrolytes to go along with the organic substances. Secretion by the salivary glands, discussed in more detail later, provides an example of how nervous stimulation causes water and salts to pass through the glandular cells in great profusion, washing the organic substances through the secretory border of the cells at the same time. Hormones acting on the cell membrane of some glandular cells are believed also to cause secretory effects similar to those caused by nervous stimulation.

Lubricating and Protective Properties of Mucus, and Importance of Mucus in the Gastrointestinal Tract

Mucus is a thick secretion composed mainly of water, electrolytes, and a mixture of several glycoproteins, which themselves are composed of large polysaccharides bound with much smaller quantities of protein. Mucus is slightly different in different parts of the gastrointestinal tract, but everywhere it has several important characteristics that make it both an excellent lubricant and a protectant for the wall of the gut. *First,* mucus has adherent qualities that make it adhere tightly to the food or other particles and to spread as a thin film over the surfaces. *Second,* it has sufficient *body* that it coats the wall of the gut and prevents actual contact of most food particles with the mucosa. *Third,* mucus has a low resistance for slippage, so the particles can slide along the epithelium with great ease. *Fourth,* mucus causes fecal particles to adhere to one another to form the feces that are expelled during a bowel movement. *Fifth,* mucus is strongly resistant to digestion by the gastrointestinal enzymes. And *sixth,* the glycoproteins of mucus have amphoteric properties, which means that they are capable of buffering small amounts of either acids or alkalies; also, mucus often contains moderate quantities of bicarbonate ions, which specifically neutralize acids.

In summary, mucus has the ability to allow easy slippage of food along the gastrointestinal tract and to prevent excoriative or chemical damage to the epithelium. A person becomes acutely aware of the lubricating qualities of mucus when the salivary glands fail to secrete saliva, because then it is difficult to swallow solid food even when it is eaten along with large amounts of water.

Secretion of Saliva

Saliva Contains a Serous Secretion and a Mucus Secretion.

The principal glands of salivation are the *parotid, submandibular,* and *sublingual glands;* in addition, there are many tiny *buccal* glands. Daily secretion of saliva normally ranges between 800 and 1500 milliliters, as shown by the average value of 1000 milliliters in Table 64-1.

Saliva contains two major types of protein secretion: (1) a *serous secretion* that contains *ptyalin* (an α-amylase), which is an enzyme for digesting starches, and (2) *mucus secretion* that contains *mucin* for lubricating and for surface protective purposes.

The parotid glands secrete almost entirely the serous type of secretion, whereas the submandibular and sublingual glands secrete both serous secretion and mucus. The buccal glands secrete only mucus. Saliva has a pH between 6.0 and 7.0, a favorable range for the digestive action of ptyalin.

Table 64-1 Daily Secretion of Intestinal Juices

	Daily Volume (ml)	pH
Saliva	1000	6.0–7.0
Gastric secretion	1500	1.0–3.5
Pancreatic secretion	1000	8.0–8.3
Bile	1000	7.8
Small intestine secretion	1800	7.5–8.0
Brunner's gland secretion	200	8.0–8.9
Large intestinal secretion	200	7.5–8.0
Total	6700	

Secretion of Ions in Saliva. Saliva contains especially large quantities of potassium and bicarbonate ions. Conversely, the concentrations of both sodium and chloride ions are several times less in saliva than in plasma. One can understand these special concentrations of ions in the saliva from the following description of the mechanism for secretion of saliva.

Figure 64-2 shows secretion by the submandibular gland, a typical compound gland that contains *acini* and *salivary ducts.* Salivary secretion is a two-stage operation: The first stage involves the acini, and the second, the salivary ducts. The acini secrete a *primary secretion* that contains ptyalin and/or mucin in a solution of ions in concentrations not greatly different from those of typical extracellular fluid. As the primary secretion flows through the ducts, two major active transport processes take place that markedly modify the ionic composition of the fluid in the saliva.

First, *sodium ions* are actively reabsorbed from all the salivary ducts and *potassium ions* are actively secreted in exchange for the sodium. Therefore, the sodium ion concentration of the saliva becomes greatly reduced, whereas the potassium ion concentration becomes increased. However, there is excess sodium reabsorption over potassium secretion, and this creates electrical negativity of about −70 millivolts in the salivary ducts; this in turn causes chloride ions to be reabsorbed passively. Therefore, the chloride ion concentration in the salivary fluid falls to a very low level, matching the ductal decrease in sodium ion concentration.

Second, *bicarbonate ions* are secreted by the ductal epithelium into the lumen of the duct. This is at least partly caused by passive exchange of bicarbonate for chloride ions, but it may also result partly from an active secretory process.

The net result of these transport processes is that *under resting conditions,* the concentrations of sodium and chloride ions in the saliva are only about 15 mEq/L each, about one-seventh to one-tenth their concentrations in plasma. Conversely, the concentration of potassium ions is about 30 mEq/L, seven times as great as in plasma, and the concentration of bicarbonate ions is 50 to 70 mEq/L, about two to three times that of plasma.

During maximal salivation, the salivary ionic concentrations change considerably because the rate of formation of primary secretion by the acini can increase as much as 20-fold. This acinar secretion then flows through the ducts so rapidly that the ductal reconditioning of the secretion is considerably reduced. Therefore, when copious quantities of saliva are being secreted, the sodium chloride concentration is about one-half or two-thirds that of plasma, and the potassium concentration rises to only four times that of plasma.

Function of Saliva for Oral Hygiene. Under basal awake conditions, about 0.5 milliliter of saliva, almost entirely of the mucous type, is secreted each minute; but during sleep, little secretion occurs. This secretion plays an exceedingly important role for maintaining healthy oral tissues. The mouth is loaded with pathogenic bacteria that can easily destroy tissues and cause dental caries. Saliva helps prevent the deteriorative processes in several ways.

First, the flow of saliva itself helps wash away pathogenic bacteria, as well as food particles that provide their metabolic support.

Second, saliva contains several factors that destroy bacteria. One of these is *thiocyanate ions* and another is several *proteolytic enzymes*—most important, *lysozyme*—that (a) attack the bacteria, (b) aid the thiocyanate ions in entering the bacteria where these ions in turn become bactericidal, and (c) digest food particles, thus helping further to remove the bacterial metabolic support.

Third, saliva often contains significant amounts of protein antibodies that can destroy oral bacteria, including some that cause dental caries. In the absence of salivation, oral tissues often become ulcerated and otherwise infected, and caries of the teeth can become rampant.

Nervous Regulation of Salivary Secretion

Figure 64-3 shows the parasympathetic nervous pathways for regulating salivation, demonstrating that the salivary glands are controlled mainly by *parasympathetic nervous signals* all the way from the *superior* and *inferior salivatory nuclei* in the brain stem.

The salivatory nuclei are located approximately at the juncture of the medulla and pons and are excited by both taste and tactile stimuli from the tongue and other areas of the mouth and pharynx. Many taste stimuli, especially the sour taste (caused by acids), elicit copious secretion of saliva—often 8 to 20 times the basal rate of secretion. Also, certain tactile stimuli, such as the presence of smooth objects in the mouth (e.g., a pebble), cause marked salivation, whereas rough objects cause less salivation and occasionally even inhibit salivation.

Salivation can also be stimulated or inhibited by nervous signals arriving in the salivatory nuclei from higher centers of the central nervous system. For instance, when a person smells or eats favorite foods, salivation is greater than when disliked food is smelled or eaten. The *appetite area* of the brain, which partially regulates these effects, is located in proximity to the parasympathetic centers of the anterior hypothalamus, and it functions to a great extent in response to signals from the taste and smell areas of the cerebral cortex or amygdala.

Salivation also occurs in response to reflexes originating in the stomach and upper small intestines—particularly when irritating foods are swallowed or when a person is nauseated because of some gastrointestinal abnormality. The saliva, when swallowed, helps to remove the irritating factor in the gastrointestinal tract by diluting or neutralizing the irritant substances.

Sympathetic stimulation can also increase salivation a slight amount, much less so than does parasympathetic stimulation. The sympathetic nerves originate from the superior cervical ganglia and travel along the surfaces of the blood vessel walls to the salivary glands.

A secondary factor that also affects salivary secretion is the *blood supply to the glands* because secretion always requires adequate nutrients from the blood. The parasympathetic nerve signals that induce copious salivation also moderately dilate the blood vessels. In addition, salivation itself directly dilates the blood vessels, thus providing increased salivary gland nutrition as needed by the secreting cells. Part of this additional vasodilator effect is caused by *kallikrein* secreted by the activated salivary cells, which in turn acts as an enzyme to split one of the blood proteins, an alpha2-globulin, to form *bradykinin,* a strong vasodilator.

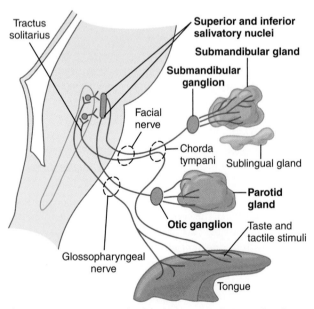

Figure 64-3 Parasympathetic nervous regulation of salivary secretion.

Tractus solitarius

Superior and inferior salivatory nuclei

Submandibular gland

Submandibular ganglion

Facial nerve

Chorda tympani   Sublingual gland

Parotid gland

Otic ganglion   Taste and tactile stimuli

Glossopharyngeal nerve

Tongue

Esophageal Secretion

The esophageal secretions are entirely mucous and mainly provide lubrication for swallowing. The main body of the esophagus is lined with many *simple mucous glands.* At the gastric end and to a lesser extent in the initial portion of the esophagus, there are also many *compound mucous glands.* The mucus secreted by the compound glands in the upper esophagus prevents mucosal excoriation by newly entering food, whereas the compound glands located near the esophagogastric junction protect the esophageal wall from digestion by acidic gastric juices that often reflux from the stomach back into the lower esophagus. Despite this protection, a peptic ulcer at times can still occur at the gastric end of the esophagus.

Gastric Secretion

Characteristics of the Gastric Secretions

In addition to mucus-secreting cells that line the entire surface of the stomach, the stomach mucosa has two important types of tubular glands: *oxyntic glands* (also called *gastric* glands) and *pyloric glands.* The oxyntic (acid-forming) glands secrete *hydrochloric acid, pepsinogen, intrinsic factor,* and *mucus.* The pyloric glands secrete mainly *mucus* for protection of the pyloric mucosa from the stomach acid. They also secrete the hormone *gastrin.*

The oxyntic glands are located on the inside surfaces of the body and fundus of the stomach, constituting the proximal 80 percent of the stomach. The pyloric glands are located in the antral portion of the stomach, the distal 20 percent of the stomach.

Secretions from the Oxyntic (Gastric) Glands

A typical stomach oxyntic gland is shown in Figure 64-4. It is composed of three types of cells: (1) *mucous neck cells,* which secrete mainly *mucus;* (2) *peptic* (or *chief*) *cells,* which secrete large quantities of *pepsinogen;* and (3) *parietal* (or *oxyntic*) *cells,* which secrete *hydrochloric acid* and *intrinsic factor.* Secretion of hydrochloric acid by the parietal cells involves special mechanisms, as follows.

Basic Mechanism of Hydrochloric Acid Secretion. When stimulated, the parietal cells secrete an acid solution that contains about 160 mmol/L of hydrochloric acid, which is nearly isotonic with the body fluids. The pH of this acid is about 0.8, demonstrating its extreme acidity. At this pH, the hydrogen ion concentration is about

3 million times that of the arterial blood. To concentrate the hydrogen ions this tremendous amount requires more than 1500 calories of energy per liter of gastric juice. At the same time that hydrogen ions are secreted, bicarbonate ions diffuse into the blood so that gastric venous blood has a higher pH than arterial blood when the stomach is secreting acid.

Figure 64-5 shows schematically the functional structure of a parietal cell (also called *oxyntic cell*), demonstrating that it contains large branching intracellular *canaliculi.* The hydrochloric acid is formed at the villus-like projections inside these canaliculi and is then conducted through the canaliculi to the secretory end of the cell.

The main driving force for hydrochloric acid secretion by the parietal cells is a *hydrogen-potassium pump (H^+-K^+ ATPase).* The chemical mechanism of hydrochloric acid formation is shown in Figure 64-6 and consists of the following steps:

1. Water inside the parietal cell becomes dissociated into H^+ and OH^- in the cell cytoplasm. The H^+ is then actively secreted into the canaliculus in exchange for K^+, an active exchange process that is catalyzed by H^+-K^+ ATPase. Potassium ions transported into the cell by the Na^+-K^+ ATPase pump on the basolateral (extracellular) side of the membrane tend to leak into the lumen but are recycled back into the cell by the H^+-K^+ ATPase. The basolateral Na^+-K^+ ATPase creates low intracellular Na^+, which contributes to Na^+ reabsorption from the lumen of the canaliculus. Thus, most of the K^+ and Na^+ in the canaliculus is reabsorbed into the cell cytoplasm, and hydrogen ions take their place in the canaliculus.

2. The pumping of H^+ out of the cell by the H^+-K^+ ATPase permits OH^- to accumulate and form HCO_3^- from CO_2, either formed during metabolism in the cell or entering

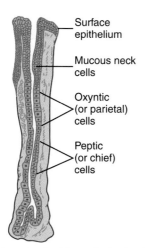

Figure 64-4 Oxyntic gland from the body of the stomach.

Surface epithelium

Mucous neck cells

Oxyntic (or parietal) cells

Peptic (or chief) cells

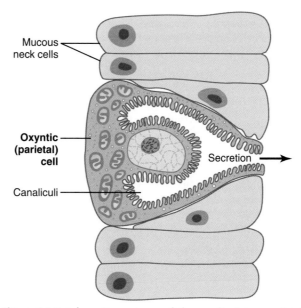

Figure 64-5 Schematic anatomy of the canaliculi in a parietal (oxyntic) cell.

Mucous neck cells

Oxyntic (parietal) cell

Canaliculi

Secretion

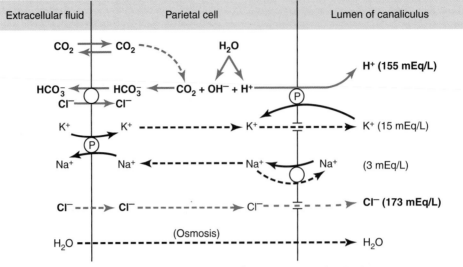

Figure 64-6 Postulated mechanism for secretion of hydrochloric acid. (The points labeled *"P"* indicate active pumps, and the *dashed lines* represent free diffusion and osmosis.)

the cell from the blood. This reaction is catalyzed by *carbonic anhydrase*. The HCO_3^- is then transported across the basolateral membrane into the extracellular fluid in exchange for chloride ions, which enter the cell and are secreted through chloride channels into the canaliculus, giving a strong solution of hydrochloric acid in the canaliculus. The hydrochloric acid is then secreted outward through the open end of the canaliculus into the lumen of the gland.

3. Water passes into the canaliculus by osmosis because of extra ions secreted into the canaliculus. Thus, the final secretion from the canaliculus contains water, hydrochloric acid at a concentration of about 150 to 160 mEq/L, potassium chloride at a concentration of 15 mEq/L, and a small amount of sodium chloride.

To produce a concentration of hydrogen ions as great as that found in gastric juice requires minimal back leak into the mucosa of the secreted acid. A major part of the stomach's ability to prevent back leak of acid can be attributed to the *gastric barrier* due to the formation of alkaline mucus and to tight junctions between epithelia cells as described later. If this barrier is damaged by toxic substances, such as occurs with excessive use of aspirin or alcohol, the secreted acid does leak down an electrochemical gradient into the mucosa, causing stomach mucosal damage.

Basic Factors That Stimulate Gastric Secretion Are Acetylcholine, Gastrin, and Histamine. Acetylcholine released by parasympathetic stimulation excites secretion of pepsinogen by peptic cells, hydrochloric acid by parietal cells, and mucus by mucous cells. In comparison, both gastrin and histamine strongly stimulate secretion of acid by parietal cells but have little effect on the other cells.

Secretion and Activation of Pepsinogen. Several slightly different types of pepsinogen are secreted by the

peptic and mucous cells of the gastric glands. Even so, all the pepsinogens perform the same functions.

When pepsinogen is first secreted, it has no digestive activity. However, as soon as it comes in contact with hydrochloric acid, it is activated to form active *pepsin*. In this process, the pepsinogen molecule, having a molecular weight of about 42,500, is split to form a pepsin molecule, having a molecular weight of about 35,000.

Pepsin functions as an active proteolytic enzyme in a highly acid medium (optimum pH 1.8 to 3.5), but above a pH of about 5 it has almost no proteolytic activity and becomes completely inactivated in a short time. Hydrochloric acid is as necessary as pepsin for protein digestion in the stomach, as discussed in Chapter 65.

Secretion of Intrinsic Factor by Parietal Cells. The substance *intrinsic factor*, essential for absorption of vitamin B_{12} in the ileum, is secreted by the *parietal cells* along with the secretion of hydrochloric acid. When the acid-producing parietal cells of the stomach are destroyed, which frequently occurs in chronic gastritis, the person develops not only *achlorhydria* (lack of stomach acid secretion) but often also *pernicious anemia* because of failure of maturation of the red blood cells in the absence of vitamin B_{12} stimulation of the bone marrow. This is discussed in detail in Chapter 32.

Pyloric Glands—Secretion of Mucus and Gastrin

The pyloric glands are structurally similar to the oxyntic glands but contain few peptic cells and almost no parietal cells. Instead, they contain mostly mucous cells that are identical with the mucous neck cells of the oxyntic glands. These cells secrete a small amount of pepsinogen, as discussed earlier, and an especially large amount of thin mucus that helps to lubricate food movement, as well as to protect the stomach wall from digestion by the gastric enzymes. The pyloric glands also secrete the hormone *gastrin*, which plays a key role in controlling gastric secretion, as we discuss shortly.

Surface Mucous Cells

The entire surface of the stomach mucosa between glands has a continuous layer of a special type of mucous cells called simply "surface mucous cells." They secrete large quantities of *viscid mucus* that coats the stomach mucosa with a gel layer of mucus often more than 1 millimeter thick, thus providing a major shell of protection for the stomach wall, as well as contributing to lubrication of food transport.

Another characteristic of this mucus is that *it is alkaline.* Therefore, the *normal* underlying stomach wall is not directly exposed to the highly acidic, proteolytic stomach secretion. Even the slightest contact with food or any irritation of the mucosa directly stimulates the surface mucous cells to secrete additional quantities of this thick, alkaline, viscid mucus.

Stimulation of Gastric Acid Secretion

Parietal Cells of the Oxyntic Glands Are the Only Cells That Secrete Hydrochloric Acid.

The *parietal cells,* located deep in the oxyntic glands of the main body of the stomach, are the only cells that secrete hydrochloric acid. As noted earlier in the chapter, the acidity of the fluid secreted by these cells can be great, with pH as low as 0.8. However, secretion of this acid is under continuous control by both endocrine and nervous signals. Furthermore, the parietal cells operate in close association with another type of cell called *enterochromaffin-like cells* (ECL cells), the primary function of which is to secrete *histamine.*

The ECL cells lie in the deep recesses of the oxyntic glands and therefore release histamine in direct contact with the parietal cells of the glands. The rate of formation and secretion of hydrochloric acid by the parietal cells is directly related to the amount of histamine secreted by the ECL cells. In turn, the ECL cells are stimulated to secrete histamine by the hormonal substance *gastrin,* which is formed almost entirely in the antral portion of the stomach mucosa in response to proteins in the foods being digested. The ECL cells may also be stimulated by hormonal substances secreted by the enteric nervous system of the stomach wall. Let us discuss first the gastrin mechanism for control of the ECL cells and their subsequent control of parietal cell secretion of hydrochloric acid.

Stimulation of Acid Secretion by Gastrin.

Gastrin is itself a hormone secreted by *gastrin cells,* also called *G cells.* These cells are located in the *pyloric glands* in the distal end of the stomach. Gastrin is a large polypeptide secreted in two forms: a large form called G-34, which contains 34 amino acids, and a smaller form, G-17, which contains 17 amino acids. Although both of these are important, the smaller is more abundant.

When meats or other protein-containing foods reach the antral end of the stomach, some of the proteins from these foods have a special stimulatory effect on the *gastrin cells in the pyloric glands* to cause release of *gastrin* into the blood to be transported to the ECL cells of the stomach. The vigorous mixing of the gastric juices transports the gastrin rapidly to the ECL cells in the body of the stomach, causing release of *histamine directly into the deep oxyntic glands.* The histamine then acts quickly to stimulate gastric hydrochloric acid secretion.

Regulation of Pepsinogen Secretion

Regulation of *pepsinogen* secretion by the peptic cells in the oxyntic glands occurs in response to two main types of signals: (1) stimulation of the *peptic cells* by *acetylcholine* released from the *vagus nerves* or from the *gastric enteric nervous plexus,* and (2) stimulation of peptic cell secretion in response to acid in the stomach. The acid probably does not stimulate the peptic cells directly but instead elicits additional enteric nervous reflexes that support the original nervous signals to the peptic cells. Therefore, the rate of secretion of *pepsinogen,* the precursor of the enzyme *pepsin* that causes protein digestion, is strongly influenced by the amount of acid in the stomach. In people who have lost the ability to secrete normal amounts of acid, secretion of pepsinogen is also decreased, even though the peptic cells may otherwise appear to be normal.

Phases of Gastric Secretion

Gastric secretion is said to occur in three "phases" (as shown in Figure 64-7): a *cephalic phase,* a *gastric phase,* and an *intestinal phase.*

Cephalic Phase. The cephalic phase of gastric secretion occurs even before food enters the stomach, especially while it is being eaten. It results from the sight, smell, thought, or taste of food, and the greater the appetite, the more intense is the stimulation. Neurogenic signals that cause the cephalic phase of gastric secretion originate in the cerebral cortex and in the appetite centers of the amygdala and hypothalamus. They are transmitted through the dorsal motor nuclei of the vagi and thence through the vagus nerves to the stomach. This phase of secretion normally accounts for about 30 percent of the gastric secretion associated with eating a meal.

Gastric Phase. Once food enters the stomach, it excites (1) long vagovagal reflexes from the stomach to the brain and back to the stomach, (2) local enteric reflexes, and (3) the gastrin mechanism, all of which in turn cause secretion of gastric juice during several hours while food remains in the stomach. The gastric phase of secretion accounts for about 60 percent of the total gastric secretion associated with eating a meal and therefore accounts for most of the total daily gastric secretion of about 1500 milliliters.

Intestinal Phase. The presence of food in the upper portion of the small intestine, particularly in the duodenum, will continue to cause stomach secretion of small amounts of gastric juice, probably partly because of small amounts of gastrin released by the duodenal mucosa. This accounts for about 10 percent of the acid response to a meal.

Figure 64-7 Phases of gastric secretion and their regulation.

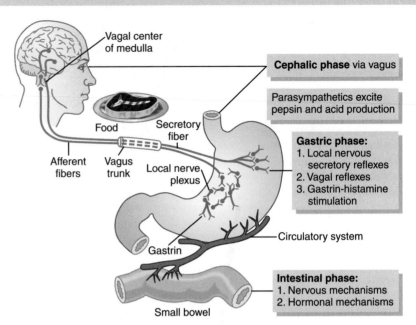

Vagal center of medulla

Cephalic phase via vagus

Parasympathetics excite pepsin and acid production

Food   Secretory fiber

Gastric phase:
1. Local nervous secretory reflexes
2. Vagal reflexes
3. Gastrin-histamine stimulation

Afferent fibers   Vagus trunk   Local nerve plexus

Circulatory system

Gastrin

Intestinal phase:
1. Nervous mechanisms
2. Hormonal mechanisms

Small bowel

Inhibition of Gastric Secretion by Other Post-Stomach Intestinal Factors

Although intestinal chyme slightly stimulates gastric secretion during the early intestinal phase of stomach secretion, it paradoxically inhibits gastric secretion at other times. This inhibition results from at least two influences.

1. The presence of food in the small intestine initiates a *reverse enterogastric reflex,* transmitted through the myenteric nervous system and extrinsic sympathetic and vagus nerves, that inhibits stomach secretion. This reflex can be initiated by distending the small bowel, by the presence of acid in the upper intestine, by the presence of protein breakdown products, or by irritation of the mucosa. This is part of the complex mechanism discussed in Chapter 63 for slowing stomach emptying when the intestines are already filled.

2. The presence of acid, fat, protein breakdown products, hyperosmotic or hypo-osmotic fluids, or any irritating factor in the upper small intestine causes release of several intestinal hormones. One of these is *secretin,* which is especially important for control of pancreatic secretion. However, secretin opposes stomach secretion. Three other hormones—*gastric inhibitory peptide (glucose-dependent insulinotropic peptide), vasoactive intestinal polypeptide,* and *somatostatin*—also have slight to moderate effects in inhibiting gastric secretion.

The functional purpose of intestinal factors that inhibit gastric secretion is presumably to slow passage of chyme from the stomach when the small intestine is already filled or already overactive. In fact, the enterogastric inhibitory reflexes plus inhibitory hormones usually also reduce stomach motility at the same time that they reduce gastric secretion, as was discussed in Chapter 63.

Gastric Secretion During the Interdigestive Period. The stomach secretes a few milliliters of gastric juice each hour during the "interdigestive period," when little or no digestion is occurring anywhere in the gut. The secretion that does occur is usually almost entirely of the nonoxyntic type, composed mainly of *mucus* but little pepsin and almost no acid.

Unfortunately, emotional stimuli frequently increase interdigestive gastric secretion (highly peptic and acidic) to 50 milliliters or more per hour, in much the same way that the cephalic phase of gastric secretion excites secretion at the onset of a meal. This increase of secretion in response to emotional stimuli is believed to be one of the causative factors in development of peptic ulcers, as discussed in Chapter 66.

Chemical Composition of Gastrin and Other Gastrointestinal Hormones

Gastrin, cholecystokinin (CCK), and *secretin* are all large polypeptides with approximate molecular weights, respectively, of 2000, 4200, and 3400. The terminal five amino acids in the gastrin and CCK molecular chains are the same. The functional activity of gastrin resides in the terminal four amino acids, and the activity for CCK resides in the terminal eight amino acids. All the amino acids in the secretin molecule are essential.

A synthetic gastrin, composed of the terminal four amino acids of natural gastrin plus the amino acid alanine, has all the same physiologic properties as the natural gastrin. This synthetic product is called *pentagastrin.*

Pancreatic Secretion

The pancreas, which lies parallel to and beneath the stomach (illustrated in Figure 64-10), is a large compound gland with most of its internal structure similar to that of the salivary glands shown in Figure 64-2. The pancreatic digestive enzymes are secreted by *pancreatic acini,* and large volumes of sodium bicarbonate solution are secreted by the small ductules and larger ducts leading from the acini. The combined product of enzymes and sodium bicarbonate then flows through a long *pancreatic duct* that normally joins the hepatic duct immediately before it empties into the duodenum through the *papilla of Vater,* surrounded by the *sphincter of Oddi.*

Pancreatic juice is secreted most abundantly in response to the presence of chyme in the upper portions of the small intestine, and the characteristics of the pancreatic juice are determined to some extent by the types of food in the chyme. (The pancreas also secretes *insulin,* but this is not secreted by the same pancreatic tissue that secretes intestinal pancreatic juice. Instead, insulin is secreted directly into the *blood*—not into the intestine—by the *islets of Langerhans* that occur in islet patches throughout the pancreas. These are discussed in detail in Chapter 78.)

Pancreatic Digestive Enzymes

Pancreatic secretion contains multiple enzymes for digesting all of the three major types of food: proteins, carbohydrates, and fats. It also contains large quantities of bicarbonate ions, which play an important role in neutralizing the acidity of the chyme emptied from the stomach into the duodenum.

The most important of the pancreatic enzymes for digesting proteins are *trypsin, chymotrypsin,* and *carboxypolypeptidase.* By far the most abundant of these is trypsin.

Trypsin and chymotrypsin split whole and partially digested proteins into peptides of various sizes but do not cause release of individual amino acids. However, carboxypolypeptidase splits some peptides into individual amino acids, thus completing digestion of some proteins all the way to the amino acid state.

The pancreatic enzyme for digesting carbohydrates is *pancreatic amylase,* which hydrolyzes starches, glycogen, and most other carbohydrates (except cellulose) to form mostly disaccharides and a few trisaccharides.

The main enzymes for fat digestion are (1) *pancreatic lipase,* which is capable of hydrolyzing neutral fat into fatty acids and monoglycerides; (2) *cholesterol esterase,* which causes hydrolysis of cholesterol esters; and (3) *phospholipase,* which splits fatty acids from phospholipids.

When first synthesized in the pancreatic cells, the proteolytic digestive enzymes are in the inactive forms *trypsinogen, chymotrypsinogen,* and *procarboxypolypeptidase,* which are all inactive enzymatically. They become activated only after they are secreted into the intestinal tract. Trypsinogen is activated by an enzyme called *enterokinase,* which is secreted by the intestinal mucosa when chyme comes in contact with the mucosa. Also, trypsinogen can be autocatalytically activated by trypsin that has already been formed from previously secreted trypsinogen. Chymotrypsinogen is activated by trypsin to form chymotrypsin, and procarboxypolypeptidase is activated in a similar manner.

Secretion of Trypsin Inhibitor Prevents Digestion of the Pancreas Itself. It is important that the proteolytic enzymes of the pancreatic juice not become activated until after they have been secreted into the intestine because the trypsin and the other enzymes would digest the pancreas itself. Fortunately, the same cells that secrete proteolytic enzymes into the acini of the pancreas secrete simultaneously another substance called *trypsin inhibitor.* This substance is formed in the cytoplasm of the glandular cells, and it prevents activation of trypsin both inside the secretory cells and in the acini and ducts of the pancreas. And, because it is trypsin that activates the other pancreatic proteolytic enzymes, trypsin inhibitor prevents activation of the others as well.

When the pancreas becomes severely damaged or when a duct becomes blocked, large quantities of pancreatic secretion sometimes become pooled in the damaged areas of the pancreas. Under these conditions, the effect of trypsin inhibitor is often overwhelmed, in which case the pancreatic secretions rapidly become activated and can literally digest the entire pancreas within a few hours, giving rise to the condition called *acute pancreatitis.* This is sometimes lethal because of accompanying circulatory shock; even if not lethal, it usually leads to a subsequent lifetime of pancreatic insufficiency.

Secretion of Bicarbonate Ions

Although the enzymes of the pancreatic juice are secreted entirely by the acini of the pancreatic glands, the other two important components of pancreatic juice, bicarbonate ions and water, are secreted mainly by the epithelial cells of the ductules and ducts that lead from the acini. When the pancreas is stimulated to secrete copious quantities of pancreatic juice, the bicarbonate ion concentration can rise to as high as 145 mEq/L, a value about five times that of bicarbonate ions in the plasma. This provides a large quantity of alkali in the pancreatic juice that serves to neutralize the hydrochloric acid emptied into the duodenum from the stomach.

The basic steps in the cellular mechanism for secreting sodium bicarbonate solution into the pancreatic ductules and ducts are shown in Figure 64-8. They are the following:

1. Carbon dioxide diffuses to the interior of the cell from the blood and, under the influence of carbonic anhydrase, combines with water to form carbonic acid (H_2CO_3). The carbonic acid in turn dissociates into bicarbonate ions and hydrogen ions (HCO_3^- and H^+). Then the bicarbonate ions are actively transported in association with sodium ions (Na^+) through the *luminal border* of the cell into the lumen of the duct.

2. The hydrogen ions formed by dissociation of carbonic acid inside the cell are *exchanged for sodium ions through the blood border* of the cell by a secondary active transport process. This supplies the sodium ions (Na^+) that are transported through the *luminal border* into the pancreatic duct lumen to provide electrical neutrality for the secreted bicarbonate ions.

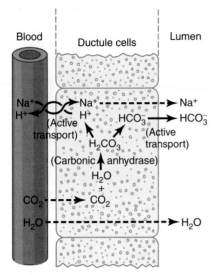

Figure 64-8 Secretion of isosmotic sodium bicarbonate solution by the pancreatic ductules and ducts.

3. The overall movement of sodium and bicarbonate ions from the blood into the duct lumen creates an osmotic pressure gradient that causes osmosis of water also into the pancreatic duct, thus forming an almost completely isosmotic bicarbonate solution.

Regulation of Pancreatic Secretion

Basic Stimuli That Cause Pancreatic Secretion

Three basic stimuli are important in causing pancreatic secretion:

1. *Acetylcholine,* which is released from the parasympathetic vagus nerve endings and from other cholinergic nerves in the enteric nervous system

2. *Cholecystokinin,* which is secreted by the duodenal and upper jejunal mucosa when food enters the small intestine

3. *Secretin,* which is also secreted by the duodenal and jejunal mucosa when highly acidic food enters the small intestine

The first two of these stimuli, acetylcholine and cholecystokinin, stimulate the acinar cells of the pancreas, causing production of large quantities of pancreatic digestive enzymes but relatively small quantities of water and electrolytes to go with the enzymes. Without the water, most of the enzymes remain temporarily stored in the acini and ducts until more fluid secretion comes along to wash them into the duodenum. Secretin, in contrast to the first two basic stimuli, stimulates secretion of large quantities of water solution of sodium bicarbonate by the pancreatic ductal epithelium.

Multiplicative Effects of Different Stimuli. When all the different stimuli of pancreatic secretion occur at once, the total secretion is far greater than the sum of the secretions caused by each one separately. Therefore, the various stimuli are said to "multiply," or "potentiate," one

another. Thus, pancreatic secretion normally results from the combined effects of the multiple basic stimuli, not from one alone.

Phases of Pancreatic Secretion

Pancreatic secretion occurs in three phases, the same as for gastric secretion: the *cephalic phase,* the *gastric phase,* and the *intestinal phase.* Their characteristics are as follows.

Cephalic and Gastric Phases. During the cephalic phase of pancreatic secretion, the same nervous signals from the brain that cause secretion in the stomach also cause acetylcholine release by the vagal nerve endings in the pancreas. This causes moderate amounts of enzymes to be secreted into the pancreatic acini, accounting for about 20 percent of the total secretion of pancreatic enzymes after a meal. But little of the secretion flows immediately through the pancreatic ducts into the intestine because only small amounts of water and electrolytes are secreted along with the enzymes.

During the gastric phase, the nervous stimulation of enzyme secretion continues, accounting for another 5 to 10 percent of pancreatic enzymes secreted after a meal. But, again, only small amounts reach the duodenum because of continued lack of significant fluid secretion.

Intestinal Phase. After chyme leaves the stomach and enters the small intestine, pancreatic secretion becomes copious, mainly in response to the hormone *secretin.*

Secretin Stimulates Copious Secretion of Bicarbonate Ions, Which Neutralizes Acidic Stomach Chyme. Secretin is a polypeptide, containing 27 amino acids (molecular weight about 3400), present in an inactive form, prosecretin, in so-called S cells in the mucosa of the duodenum and jejunum. When acid chyme with pH less than 4.5 to 5.0 enters the duodenum from the stomach, it causes duodenal mucosal release and activation of secretin, which is then absorbed into the blood. The one truly potent constituent of chyme that causes this secretin release is the hydrochloric acid from the stomach.

Secretin in turn causes the pancreas to secrete large quantities of fluid containing a high concentration of bicarbonate ion (up to 145 mEq/L) but a low concentration of chloride ion. The secretin mechanism is especially important for two reasons: First, secretin begins to be released from the mucosa of the small intestine when the pH of the duodenal contents falls below 4.5 to 5.0, and its release increases greatly as the pH falls to 3.0. This immediately causes copious secretion of pancreatic juice containing abundant amounts of sodium bicarbonate. The net result is then the following reaction in the duodenum:

$$HCl + NaHCO_3 \rightarrow NaCl + H_2CO_3$$

Then the carbonic acid immediately dissociates into carbon dioxide and water. The carbon dioxide is absorbed into the blood and expired through the lungs, thus leaving a neutral solution of sodium chloride in the duodenum.

In this way, the acid contents emptied into the duodenum from the stomach become neutralized, so further peptic digestive activity by the gastric juices in the duodenum is immediately blocked. Because the mucosa of the small intestine cannot withstand the digestive action of acid gastric juice, this is an essential protective mechanism to prevent development of duodenal ulcers, as is discussed in further detail in Chapter 66.

Bicarbonate ion secretion by the pancreas provides an appropriate pH for action of the pancreatic digestive enzymes, which function optimally in a slightly alkaline or neutral medium, at a pH of 7.0 to 8.0. Fortunately, the pH of the sodium bicarbonate secretion averages 8.0.

Cholecystokinin—Its Contribution to Control of Digestive Enzyme Secretion by the Pancreas. The presence of food in the upper small intestine also causes a second hormone, *CCK,* a polypeptide containing 33 amino acids, to be released from yet another group of cells, the *I cells,* in the mucosa of the duodenum and upper jejunum. This release of CCK results especially from the presence of *proteoses* and *peptones* (products of partial protein digestion) and *long-chain fatty acids* in the chyme coming from the stomach.

CCK, like secretin, passes by way of the blood to the pancreas but instead of causing sodium bicarbonate secretion causes mainly secretion of still much more pancreatic digestive enzymes by the acinar cells. This effect is similar to that caused by vagal stimulation but even more pronounced, accounting for 70 to 80 percent of the total secretion of the pancreatic digestive enzymes after a meal.

The differences between the pancreatic stimulatory effects of secretin and CCK are shown in Figure 64-9, which demonstrates (1) intense sodium bicarbonate secretion in response to acid in the duodenum, stimulated by secretin; (2) a dual effect in response to soap (a fat); and (3) intense digestive enzyme secretion (when peptones enter the duodenum) stimulated by CCK.

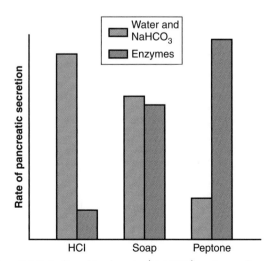

Figure 64-9 Sodium bicarbonate (NaHCO₃), water, and enzyme secretion by the pancreas, caused by the presence of acid (HCl), fat (soap), or peptone solutions in the duodenum.

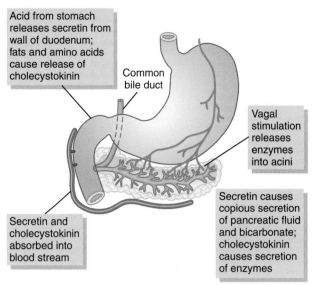

Figure 64-10 Regulation of pancreatic secretion.

Figure 64-10 summarizes the more important factors in the regulation of pancreatic secretion. The total amount secreted each day is about 1 liter.

Secretion of Bile by the Liver; Functions of the Biliary Tree

One of the many functions of the liver is to secrete *bile,* normally between 600 and 1000 ml/day. Bile serves two important functions.

First, bile plays an important role in fat digestion and absorption, not because of any enzymes in the bile that cause fat digestion, but because *bile acids* in the bile do two things: (1) They help to emulsify the large fat particles of the food into many minute particles, the surface of which can then be attacked by lipase enzymes secreted in pancreatic juice, and (2) they aid in absorption of the digested fat end products through the intestinal mucosal membrane.

Second, bile serves as a means for excretion of several important waste products from the blood. These include especially *bilirubin,* an end product of hemoglobin destruction, and excesses of *cholesterol.*

Physiologic Anatomy of Biliary Secretion

Bile is secreted in two stages by the liver: (1) The initial portion is secreted by the principal functional cells of the liver, the *hepatocytes;* this initial secretion contains large amounts of bile acids, cholesterol, and other organic constituents. It is secreted into minute *bile canaliculi* that originate between the hepatic cells.

(2) Next, the bile flows in the canaliculi toward the interlobular septa, where the canaliculi empty into *terminal bile ducts* and then into progressively larger ducts, finally reaching the *hepatic duct* and *common bile duct.*

Figure 64-11 Liver secretion and gallbladder emptying.

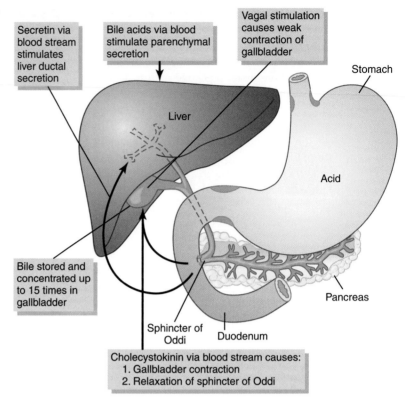

From these the bile either empties directly into the duodenum or is diverted for minutes up to several hours through the *cystic duct* into the *gallbladder*, shown in Figure 64-11.

In its course through the bile ducts, a second portion of liver secretion is added to the initial bile. This additional secretion is a watery solution of sodium and bicarbonate ions secreted by secretory epithelial cells that line the ductules and ducts. This second secretion sometimes increases the total quantity of bile by as much as an additional 100 percent. The second secretion is stimulated especially by *secretin*, which causes release of additional quantities of bicarbonate ions to supplement the bicarbonate ions in pancreatic secretion (for neutralizing acid that empties into the duodenum from the stomach).

Storing and Concentrating Bile in the Gallbladder.
Bile is secreted continually by the liver cells, but most of it is normally stored in the gallbladder until needed in the duodenum. The maximum volume that the gallbladder can hold is only 30 to 60 milliliters. Nevertheless, as much as 12 hours of bile secretion (usually about 450 milliliters) can be stored in the gallbladder because water, sodium, chloride, and most other small electrolytes are continually absorbed through the gallbladder mucosa, concentrating the remaining bile constituents that contain the bile salts, cholesterol, lecithin, and bilirubin.

Most of this gallbladder absorption is caused by active transport of sodium through the gallbladder epithelium, and this is followed by secondary absorption of chloride ions, water, and most other diffusible constituents. Bile is normally concentrated in this way about 5-fold, but it can be concentrated up to a maximum of 20-fold.

Composition of Bile. Table 64-2 gives the composition of bile when it is first secreted by the liver and then after it has been concentrated in the gallbladder. This table shows that by far the most abundant substances secreted in the bile are *bile salts*, which account for about one half of the total solutes also in the bile. Also secreted or excreted in large concentrations are *bilirubin, cholesterol, lecithin,* and the usual *electrolytes* of plasma.

Table 64-2 Composition of Bile

	Liver Bile	Gallbladder Bile
Water	97.5 g/dl	92 g/dl
Bile salts	1.1 g/dl	6 g/dl
Bilirubin	0.04 g/dl	0.3 g/dl
Cholesterol	0.1 g/dl	0.3 to 0.9 g/dl
Fatty acids	0.12 g/dl	0.3 to 1.2 g/dl
Lecithin	0.04 g/dl	0.3 g/dl
Na^+	145 mEq/L	130 mEq/L
K^+	5 mEq/L	12 mEq/L
Ca^{++}	5 mEq/L	23 mEq/L
Cl^-	100 mEq/L	25 mEq/L
HCO_3^-	28 mEq/L	10 mEq/L

In the concentrating process in the gallbladder, water and large portions of the electrolytes (except calcium ions) are reabsorbed by the gallbladder mucosa; essentially all other constituents, especially the bile salts and the lipid substances cholesterol and lecithin, are not reabsorbed and, therefore, become highly concentrated in the gallbladder bile.

Emptying of the Gallbladder—Stimulatory Role of Cholecystokinin.

When food begins to be digested in the upper gastrointestinal tract, the gallbladder begins to empty, especially when fatty foods reach the duodenum about 30 minutes after a meal. The mechanism of gallbladder emptying is rhythmical contractions of the wall of the gallbladder, but effective emptying also requires simultaneous relaxation of the *sphincter of Oddi,* which guards the exit of the common bile duct into the duodenum.

By far the most potent stimulus for causing the gallbladder contractions is the hormone *CCK.* This is the same CCK discussed earlier that causes increased secretion of digestive enzymes by the acinar cells of the pancreas. The stimulus for CCK entry into the blood from the duodenal mucosa is mainly the presence of fatty foods in the duodenum.

The gallbladder is also stimulated less strongly by acetylcholine-secreting nerve fibers from both the vagi and the intestinal enteric nervous system. They are the same nerves that promote motility and secretion in other parts of the upper gastrointestinal tract.

In summary, the gallbladder empties its store of concentrated bile into the duodenum mainly in response to the CCK stimulus that itself is initiated mainly by fatty foods. When fat is not in the food, the gallbladder empties poorly, but when significant quantities of fat are present, the gallbladder normally empties completely in about 1 hour. Figure 64-11 summarizes the secretion of bile, its storage in the gallbladder, and its ultimate release from the bladder to the duodenum.

Function of Bile Salts in Fat Digestion and Absorption

The liver cells synthesize about 6 grams of *bile salts* daily. The precursor of the bile salts is *cholesterol,* which is either present in the diet or synthesized in the liver cells during the course of fat metabolism. The cholesterol is first converted to *cholic acid* or *chenodeoxycholic acid* in about equal quantities. These acids in turn combine principally with glycine and to a lesser extent with taurine to form *glyco-* and *tauro-conjugated bile acids.* The salts of these acids, mainly sodium salts, are then secreted in the bile.

The bile salts have two important actions in the intestinal tract:

First, they have a detergent action on the fat particles in the food. This decreases the surface tension of the particles and allows agitation in the intestinal tract to break the fat globules into minute sizes. This is called the *emulsifying* or *detergent function* of bile salts.

Second, and even more important than the emulsifying function, bile salts help in the absorption of (1) fatty acids, (2) monoglycerides, (3) cholesterol, and (4) other lipids from the intestinal tract. They do this by forming small physical complexes with these lipids; the complexes are called *micelles,* and they are semisoluble in the chyme because of the electrical charges of the bile salts. The intestinal lipids are "ferried" in this form to the intestinal mucosa, where they are then absorbed into the blood, as will be described in detail in Chapter 65. Without the presence of bile salts in the intestinal tract, up to 40 percent of the ingested fats are lost into the feces and the person often develops a metabolic deficit because of this nutrient loss.

Enterohepatic Circulation of Bile Salts.

About 94 percent of the bile salts are reabsorbed into the blood from the small intestine, about one half of this by *diffusion* through the mucosa in the early portions of the small intestine and the remainder by an *active transport* process through the intestinal mucosa in the distal ileum. They then enter the portal blood and pass back to the liver. On reaching the liver, on first passage through the venous sinusoids these salts are absorbed almost entirely back into the hepatic cells and then resecreted into the bile.

In this way, about 94 percent of all the bile salts are recirculated into the bile, so on the average these salts make the entire circuit some 17 times before being carried out in the feces. The small quantities of bile salts lost into the feces are replaced by new amounts formed continually by the liver cells. This recirculation of the bile salts is called the *enterohepatic circulation of bile salts.*

The quantity of bile secreted by the liver each day is highly dependent on the availability of bile salts—the greater the quantity of bile salts in the enterohepatic circulation (usually a total of only about 2.5 grams), the greater the rate of bile secretion. Indeed, ingestion of supplemental bile salts can increase bile secretion by several hundred milliliters per day.

If a bile fistula empties the bile salts to the exterior for several days to several weeks so that they cannot be reabsorbed from the ileum, the liver increases its production of bile salts 6- to 10-fold, which increases the rate of bile secretion most of the way back to normal. This demonstrates that the daily rate of liver bile salt secretion is actively controlled by the availability (or lack of availability) of bile salts in the enterohepatic circulation.

Role of Secretin in Controlling Bile Secretion.

In addition to the strong stimulating effect of bile acids to cause bile secretion, the hormone *secretin* that also stimulates pancreatic secretion increases bile secretion, sometimes more than doubling its secretion for several hours after a meal. This increase in secretion is almost entirely secretion of a sodium bicarbonate–rich watery solution by the epithelial cells of the bile ductules and ducts, and not increased secretion by the liver parenchymal cells themselves. The bicarbonate in turn passes into the small intestine and joins the bicarbonate from the pancreas in neutralizing the hydrochloric acid from the stomach. Thus, the secretin feedback mechanism for neutralizing duodenal acid operates not only through its effects on pancreatic secretion but also to a lesser extent through its effect on secretion by the liver ductules and ducts.

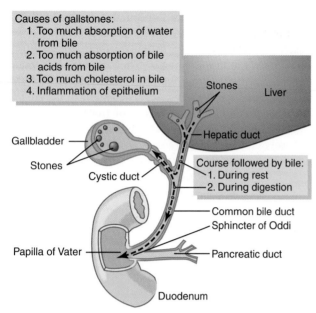

Causes of gallstones:
1. Too much absorption of water from bile
2. Too much absorption of bile acids from bile
3. Too much cholesterol in bile
4. Inflammation of epithelium

Stones

Liver

Hepatic duct

Gallbladder

Stones

Cystic duct

Course followed by bile:
1. During rest
2. During digestion

Common bile duct

Sphincter of Oddi

Papilla of Vater

Pancreatic duct

Duodenum

Figure 64-12 Formation of gallstones.

Liver Secretion of Cholesterol and Gallstone Formation

Bile salts are formed in the hepatic cells from cholesterol in the blood plasma. In the process of secreting the bile salts, about 1 to 2 grams of cholesterol are removed from the blood plasma and secreted into the bile each day.

Cholesterol is almost completely insoluble in pure water, but the bile salts and lecithin in bile combine physically with the cholesterol to form ultramicroscopic *micelles* in the form of a colloidal solution, as explained in more detail in Chapter 65. When the bile becomes concentrated in the gallbladder, the bile salts and lecithin become concentrated along with the cholesterol, which keeps the cholesterol in solution.

Under abnormal conditions, the cholesterol may precipitate in the gallbladder, resulting in the formation of *cholesterol gallstones*, as shown in Figure 64-12. The amount of cholesterol in the bile is determined partly by the quantity of fat that the person eats, because liver cells synthesize cholesterol as one of the products of fat metabolism in the body. For this reason, people on a high-fat diet over a period of years are prone to the development of gallstones.

Inflammation of the gallbladder epithelium, often resulting from low-grade chronic infection, may also change the absorptive characteristics of the gallbladder mucosa, sometimes allowing excessive absorption of water and bile salts but leaving behind the cholesterol in the gallbladder in progressively greater concentrations. Then the cholesterol begins to precipitate, first forming many small crystals of cholesterol on the surface of the inflamed mucosa, but then progressing to large gallstones.

Secretions of the Small Intestine

Secretion of Mucus by Brunner's Glands in the Duodenum

An extensive array of compound mucous glands, called *Brunner's glands*, is located in the wall of the first few centimeters of the duodenum, mainly between the pylorus

of the stomach and the papilla of Vater, where pancreatic secretion and bile empty into the duodenum. These glands secrete large amounts of alkaline mucus in response to (1) tactile or irritating stimuli on the duodenal mucosa; (2) vagal stimulation, which causes increased Brunner's glands secretion concurrently with increase in stomach secretion; and (3) gastrointestinal hormones, especially *secretin*.

The function of the mucus secreted by Brunner's glands is to protect the duodenal wall from digestion by the highly acidic gastric juice emptying from the stomach. In addition, the mucus contains a large excess of bicarbonate ions, which add to the bicarbonate ions from pancreatic secretion and liver bile in neutralizing the hydrochloric acid entering the duodenum from the stomach.

Brunner's glands are inhibited by sympathetic stimulation; therefore, such stimulation in very excitable persons is likely to leave the duodenal bulb unprotected and is perhaps one of the factors that cause this area of the gastrointestinal tract to be the site of peptic ulcers in about 50 percent of ulcer patients.

Secretion of Intestinal Digestive Juices by the Crypts of Lieberkühn

Located over the entire surface of the small intestine are small pits called *crypts of Lieberkühn*, one of which is illustrated in Figure 64-13. These crypts lie between the intestinal villi. The surfaces of both the crypts and the villi are covered by an epithelium composed of two types of cells: (1) a moderate number of *goblet cells*, which secrete *mucus* that lubricates and protects the intestinal surfaces, and (2) a large number of *enterocytes*, which, in the crypts, secrete large quantities of water and electrolytes and, over the surfaces of adjacent villi, reabsorb the water and electrolytes along with end products of digestion.

The intestinal secretions are formed by the enterocytes of the crypts at a rate of about 1800 ml/day. These secretions are almost pure extracellular fluid and have a slightly alkaline pH in the range of 7.5 to 8.0. The secretions are

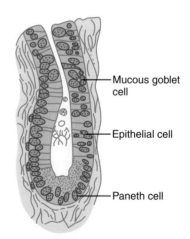

Mucous goblet cell

Epithelial cell

Paneth cell

Figure 64-13 A *crypt of Lieberkühn*, found in all parts of the small intestine between the villi, which secretes almost pure extracellular fluid.

also rapidly reabsorbed by the villi. This flow of fluid from the crypts into the villi supplies a watery vehicle for absorption of substances from chyme when it comes in contact with the villi. Thus, the primary function of the small intestine is to absorb nutrients and their digestive products into the blood.

Mechanism of Secretion of the Watery Fluid. The exact mechanism that controls the marked secretion of watery fluid by the crypts of Lieberkühn is still unclear, but it is believed to involve at least two active secretory processes: (1) active secretion of chloride ions into the crypts and (2) active secretion of bicarbonate ions. The secretion of both ions causes electrical drag of positively charged sodium ions through the membrane and into the secreted fluid as well. Finally, all these ions together cause osmotic movement of water.

Digestive Enzymes in the Small Intestinal Secretion. When secretions of the small intestine are collected without cellular debris, they have almost no enzymes. The enterocytes of the mucosa, especially those that cover the villi, contain digestive enzymes that digest specific food substances *while they are being absorbed* through the epithelium. These enzymes are the following: (1) several *peptidases* for splitting small peptides into amino acids; (2) four enzymes—*sucrase, maltase, isomaltase,* and *lactase*—for splitting disaccharides into monosaccharides; and (3) small amounts of *intestinal lipase* for splitting neutral fats into glycerol and fatty acids.

The epithelial cells deep in the crypts of Lieberkühn continually undergo mitosis, and new cells migrate along the basement membrane upward out of the crypts toward the tips of the villi, thus continually replacing the villus epithelium and also forming new digestive enzymes. As the villus cells age, they are finally shed into the intestinal secretions. The life cycle of an intestinal epithelial cell is about 5 days. This rapid growth of new cells also allows rapid repair of excoriations that occur in the mucosa.

Regulation of Small Intestine Secretion—Local Stimuli

By far the most important means for regulating small intestine secretion are local enteric nervous reflexes, especially reflexes initiated by tactile or irritative stimuli from the chyme in the intestines.

Secretion of Mucus by the Large Intestine

Mucus Secretion. The mucosa of the large intestine, like that of the small intestine, has many crypts of Lieberkühn; however, unlike the small intestine, there are no villi. The epithelial cells secrete almost no digestive enzymes. Instead, they contain mucous cells that secrete only *mucus.* This mucus contains moderate amounts of bicarbonate ions secreted by a few non-mucus-secreting epithelial cells. The rate of secretion of mucus is regulated principally by direct, tactile stimulation of the epithelial cells lining the large intestine and by local nervous reflexes to the mucous cells in the crypts of Lieberkühn.

Stimulation of the *pelvic nerves* from the spinal cord, which carry *parasympathetic innervation* to the distal one half to two thirds of the large intestine, also can cause marked increase in mucus secretion. This occurs along with increase in peristaltic motility of the colon, which was discussed in Chapter 63.

During extreme parasympathetic stimulation, often caused by emotional disturbances, so much mucus can occasionally be secreted into the large intestine that the person has a bowel movement of ropy mucus as often as every 30 minutes; this mucus often contains little or no fecal material.

Mucus in the large intestine protects the intestinal wall against excoriation, but in addition, it provides an adherent medium for holding fecal matter together. Furthermore, it protects the intestinal wall from the great amount of bacterial activity that takes place inside the feces, and, finally, the mucus plus the alkalinity of the secretion (pH of 8.0 caused by large amounts of sodium bicarbonate) provides a barrier to keep acids formed in the feces from attacking the intestinal wall.

Diarrhea Caused by Excess Secretion of Water and Electrolytes in Response to Irritation.

Whenever a segment of the large intestine becomes intensely irritated, as occurs when bacterial infection becomes rampant during *enteritis,* the mucosa secretes extra large quantities of water and electrolytes in addition to the normal viscid alkaline mucus. This acts to dilute the irritating factors and to cause rapid movement of the feces toward the anus. The result is *diarrhea,* with loss of large quantities of water and electrolytes. But the diarrhea also washes away irritant factors, which promotes earlier recovery from the disease than might otherwise occur.

Bibliography

Allen A, Flemström G: Gastroduodenal mucus bicarbonate barrier: protection against acid and pepsin, *Am J Physiol Cell Physiol* 288:C1, 2005.

Barrett KE: New ways of thinking about (and teaching about) intestinal epithelial function, *Adv Physiol Educ* 32:25, 2008.

Barrett KE, Keely SJ: Chloride secretion by the intestinal epithelium: molecular basis and regulatory aspects, *Annu Rev Physiol* 62:535, 2000.

Chen D, Aihara T, Zhao CM, Håkanson R, Okabe S: Differentiation of the gastric mucosa. I. Role of histamine in control of function and integrity of oxyntic mucosa: understanding gastric physiology through disruption of targeted genes, *Am J Physiol Gastrointest Liver Physiol* 291:G539, 2006.

Dockray GJ: Cholecystokinin and gut-brain signalling, *Regul Pept* 155:6, 2009.

Dockray GJ, Varro A, Dimaline R, Wang T: The gastrins: their production and biological activities, *Annu Rev Physiol* 63:119, 2001.

Flemstrom G, Isenberg JI: Gastroduodenal mucosal alkaline secretion and mucosal protection, *News Physiol Sci* 16:23, 2001.

Flemstrom G, Sjöblom M: Epithelial cells and their neighbors. II. New perspectives on efferent signaling between brain, neuroendocrine cells, and gut epithelial cells, *Am J Physiol Gastrointest Liver Physiol* 289:G377, 2005.

Heitzmann D, Warth R: Physiology and pathophysiology of potassium channels in gastrointestinal epithelia, *Physiol Rev* 88:1119, 2008.

Hocker M: Molecular mechanisms of gastrin-dependent gene regulation, *Ann N Y Acad Sci* 1014:97, 2004.

Hylemon PB, Zhou H, Pandak WM, Ren S, Gil G, Dent P: Bile acids as regulatory molecules, *J Lipid Res* 50:1509, 2009.

Jain RN, Samuelson LC: Differentiation of the gastric mucosa. II. Role of gastrin in gastric epithelial cell proliferation and maturation, *Am J Physiol Gastrointest Liver Physiol* 291:G762, 2006.

Laine L, Takeuchi K, Tarnawski A: Gastric mucosal defense and cytoprotection: bench to bedside, *Gastroenterology* 135:41, 2008.

Lefebvre P, Cariou B, Lien F, et al: Role of bile acids and bile acid receptors in metabolic regulation, *Physiol Rev* 89:147, 2009.

Portincasa P, Di Ciaula A, Wang HH, et al: Coordinate regulation of gallbladder motor function in the gut-liver axis, *Hepatology* 47:2112, 2008.

Portincasa P, Moschetta A, Palasciano G: Cholesterol gallstone disease, *Lancet* 368:230, 2006.

Russell DW: Fifty years of advances in bile acid synthesis and metabolism, *J Lipid Res* 50(Suppl):S120, 2009.

Trauner M, Boyer JL: Bile salt transporters: molecular characterization, function, and regulation, *Physiol Rev* 83:633, 2003.

Wallace JL: Prostaglandins, NSAIDs, and gastric mucosal protection: why doesn't the stomach digest itself? *Physiol Rev* 88:1547, 2008.

Williams JA, Chen X, Sabbatini ME: Small G proteins as key regulators of pancreatic digestive enzyme secretion, *Am J Physiol Endocrinol Metab* 296:E405, 2009.

Zanner R, Gratzl M, Prinz C: Circle of life of secretory vesicles in gastric enterochromaffin-like cells, *Ann N Y Acad Sci* 971:389, 2002.

Digestion and Absorption in the Gastrointestinal Tract

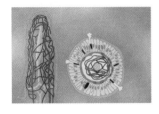

The major foods on which the body lives (with the exception of small quantities of substances such as vitamins and minerals) can be classified as *carbohydrates, fats,* and *proteins.* They generally cannot be absorbed in their natural forms through the gastrointestinal mucosa and, for this reason, are useless as nutrients without preliminary digestion. Therefore, this chapter discusses the processes by which carbohydrates, fats, and proteins are digested into small enough compounds for absorption and the mechanisms by which the digestive end products, as well as water, electrolytes, and other substances, are absorbed.

Digestion of the Various Foods by Hydrolysis

Hydrolysis of Carbohydrates. Almost all the carbohydrates of the diet are either large *polysaccharides* or *disaccharides,* which are combinations of *monosaccharides* bound to one another by *condensation.* This means that a hydrogen ion (H^+) has been removed from one of the monosaccharides, and a hydroxyl ion (−OH) has been removed from the next one. The two monosaccharides then combine with each other at these sites of removal, and the hydrogen and hydroxyl ions combine to form water (H_2O).

When carbohydrates are digested, the above process is reversed and the carbohydrates are converted into monosaccharides. Specific enzymes in the digestive juices of the gastrointestinal tract return the hydrogen and hydroxyl ions from water to the polysaccharides and thereby separate the monosaccharides from each other. This process, called *hydrolysis,* is the following (in which R″-R′ is a disaccharide):

$$R''\text{-}R' + H_2O \xrightarrow[\text{enzyme}]{\text{digestive}} R''OH + R'H$$

Hydrolysis of Fats. Almost the entire fat portion of the diet consists of triglycerides (neutral fats), which are combinations of three *fatty acid* molecules condensed with a single *glycerol* molecule. During condensation, three molecules of water are removed.

Digestion of the triglycerides consists of the reverse process: the fat-digesting enzymes return three molecules of water to the triglyceride molecule and thereby split the fatty acid molecules away from the glycerol. Here again, the digestive process is one of *hydrolysis.*

Hydrolysis of Proteins. Proteins are formed from multiple *amino acids* that are bound together by *peptide linkages.* At each linkage, a hydroxyl ion has been removed from one amino acid and a hydrogen ion has been removed from the succeeding one; thus, the successive amino acids in the protein chain are also bound together by condensation, and digestion occurs by the reverse effect: hydrolysis. That is, the proteolytic enzymes return hydrogen and hydroxyl ions from water molecules to the protein molecules to split them into their constituent amino acids.

Therefore, the chemistry of digestion is simple because, in the case of all three major types of food, the same basic process of *hydrolysis* is involved. The only difference lies in the types of enzymes required to promote the hydrolysis reactions for each type of food.

All the digestive enzymes are proteins. Their secretion by the different gastrointestinal glands was discussed in Chapter 64.

Digestion of Carbohydrates

Carbohydrate Foods of the Diet. Only three major sources of carbohydrates exist in the normal human diet. They are *sucrose,* which is the disaccharide known popularly as cane sugar; *lactose,* which is a disaccharide

789

found in milk; and *starches,* which are large polysaccharides present in almost all nonanimal foods, particularly in potatoes and different types of grains. Other carbohydrates ingested to a slight extent are *amylose, glycogen, alcohol, lactic acid, pyruvic acid, pectins, dextrins,* and minor quantities of *carbohydrate derivatives in meats.*

The diet also contains a large amount of cellulose, which is a carbohydrate. However, no enzymes capable of hydrolyzing cellulose are secreted in the human digestive tract. Consequently, cellulose cannot be considered a food for humans.

Digestion of Carbohydrates in the Mouth and Stomach.

When food is chewed, it is mixed with saliva, which contains the digestive enzyme *ptyalin* (an α-amylase) secreted mainly by the parotid glands. This enzyme hydrolyzes starch into the disaccharide *maltose* and other small polymers of glucose that contain three to nine glucose molecules, as shown in Figure 65-1. However, the food remains in the mouth only a short time, so probably not more than 5 percent of all the starches will have become hydrolyzed by the time the food is swallowed.

However, starch digestion sometimes continues in the body and fundus of the stomach for as long as 1 hour before the food becomes mixed with the stomach secretions. Then activity of the salivary amylase is blocked by acid of the gastric secretions because the amylase is essentially nonactive as an enzyme once the pH of the medium falls below about 4.0. Nevertheless, on the average, before food and its accompanying saliva do become completely mixed with the gastric secretions, as much as 30 to 40 percent of the starches will have been hydrolyzed mainly to form *maltose.*

Digestion of Carbohydrates in the Small Intestine

Digestion by Pancreatic Amylase. Pancreatic secretion, like saliva, contains a large quantity of α-amylase that is almost identical in its function with the α-amylase of saliva but is several times as powerful. Therefore, within 15 to 30 minutes after the chyme empties from the stomach into the duodenum and mixes with pancreatic juice, virtually all the carbohydrates will have become digested.

In general, the carbohydrates are almost totally converted into *maltose* and/or *other small glucose polymers* before passing beyond the duodenum or upper jejunum.

Hydrolysis of Disaccharides and Small Glucose Polymers into Monosaccharides by Intestinal Epithelial Enzymes. The enterocytes lining the villi of the small intestine contain four enzymes (*lactase, sucrase, maltase,* and *α-dextrinase*), which are capable of splitting the disaccharides lactose, sucrose, and maltose, plus other small glucose polymers, into their constituent monosaccharides. These enzymes are located *in the enterocytes* covering *the intestinal microvilli brush border,* so the disaccharides are digested as they come in contact with these enterocytes.

Lactose splits into a molecule of *galactose* and a molecule of *glucose.* Sucrose splits into a molecule of *fructose* and a molecule of *glucose.* Maltose and other small glucose polymers all split into *multiple molecules of glucose.* Thus, the final products of carbohydrate digestion are all monosaccharides. They are all water soluble and are absorbed immediately into the portal blood.

In the ordinary diet, which contains far more starches than all other carbohydrates combined, glucose represents more than 80 percent of the final products of carbohydrate digestion, and galactose and fructose each represent seldom more than 10 percent.

The major steps in carbohydrate digestion are summarized in Figure 65-1.

Digestion of Proteins

Proteins of the Diet. The dietary proteins are chemically long chains of amino acids bound together by *peptide linkages.* A typical linkage is the following:

$$R - CH - C \overbrace{(OH + H)}\ N - CH - COOH \rightarrow$$

with NH_2 on the first CH, O double-bonded to C, H on N, R on the second CH.

$$R - CH - C - N - CH - COOH + H_2O$$

with NH_2 on the first CH, O double-bonded to C, H on N, R on the second CH.

The characteristics of each protein are determined by the types of amino acids in the protein molecule and by the sequential arrangements of these amino acids. The physical and chemical characteristics of different proteins important in human tissues are discussed in Chapter 69.

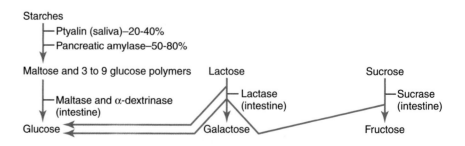

Figure 65-1 Digestion of carbohydrates.

Starches
— Ptyalin (saliva)–20-40%
— Pancreatic amylase–50-80%

Maltose and 3 to 9 glucose polymers   Lactose   Sucrose

— Maltase and α-dextrinase   — Lactase   — Sucrase
  (intestine)   (intestine)   (intestine)

Glucose   Galactose   Fructose

Digestion of Proteins in the Stomach. *Pepsin,* the important peptic enzyme of the stomach, is most active at a pH of 2.0 to 3.0 and is inactive at a pH above about 5.0. Consequently, for this enzyme to cause digestion of protein, the stomach juices must be acidic. As explained in Chapter 64, the gastric glands secrete a large quantity of hydrochloric acid. This hydrochloric acid is secreted by the parietal (oxyntic) cells in the glands at a pH of about 0.8, but by the time it is mixed with the stomach contents and with secretions from the nonoxyntic glandular cells of the stomach, the pH then averages around 2.0 to 3.0, a highly favorable range of acidity for pepsin activity.

One of the important features of pepsin digestion is its ability to digest the protein *collagen,* an albuminoid type of protein that is affected little by other digestive enzymes. Collagen is a major constituent of the intercellular connective tissue of meats; therefore, for the digestive enzymes of the digestive tract to penetrate meats and digest the other meat proteins, it is necessary that the collagen fibers be digested. Consequently, in persons who lack pepsin in the stomach juices, the ingested meats are less well penetrated by the other digestive enzymes and, therefore, may be poorly digested.

As shown in Figure 65-2, pepsin only initiates the process of protein digestion, usually providing only 10 to 20 percent of the total protein digestion to convert the protein to proteoses, peptones, and a few polypeptides. This splitting of proteins occurs as a result of hydrolysis at the peptide linkages between amino acids.

Most Protein Digestion Results from Actions of Pancreatic Proteolytic Enzymes.

Most protein digestion occurs in the upper small intestine, in the duodenum and jejunum, under the influence of proteolytic enzymes from pancreatic secretion. Immediately on entering the small intestine from the stomach, the partial breakdown products of the protein foods are attacked by major proteolytic pancreatic enzymes: *trypsin, chymotrypsin, carboxypolypeptidase,* and *proelastase,* as shown in Figure 65-2.

Both trypsin and chymotrypsin split protein molecules into small polypeptides; carboxypolypeptidase then cleaves individual amino acids from the carboxyl ends of the polypeptides. *Proelastase,* in turn, is converted into *elastase,* which then digests elastin fibers that partially hold meats together.

Only a small percentage of the proteins are digested all the way to their constituent amino acids by the pancreatic juices. Most remain as dipeptides and tripeptides.

Digestion of Peptides by Peptidases in the Enterocytes That Line the Small Intestinal Villi.

The last digestive stage of the proteins in the intestinal lumen is achieved by the enterocytes that line the villi of the small intestine, mainly in the duodenum and jejunum. These cells have a *brush border* that consists of hundreds of *microvilli* projecting from the surface of each cell. In the membrane of each of these microvilli are multiple *peptidases* that protrude through the membranes to the exterior, where they come in contact with the intestinal fluids.

Two types of peptidase enzymes are especially important, *aminopolypeptidase* and several *dipeptidases.* They succeed in splitting the remaining larger polypeptides into tripeptides and dipeptides and a few into amino acids. Both the amino acids plus the dipeptides and tripeptides are easily transported through the microvillar membrane to the interior of the enterocyte.

Finally, inside the cytosol of the enterocyte are multiple other peptidases that are specific for the remaining types of linkages between amino acids. Within minutes, virtually all the last dipeptides and tripeptides are digested to the final stage to form single amino acids; these then pass on through to the other side of the enterocyte and thence into the blood.

More than 99 percent of the final protein digestive products that are absorbed are individual amino acids, with only rare absorption of peptides and very, very rare absorption of whole protein molecules. Even these few absorbed molecules of whole protein can sometimes cause serious allergic or immunologic disturbances, as discussed in Chapter 34.

Digestion of Fats

Fats of the Diet. By far the most abundant fats of the diet are the neutral fats, also known as *triglycerides,* each molecule of which is composed of a glycerol nucleus and three fatty acid side chains, as shown in Figure 65-3.

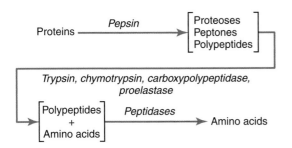

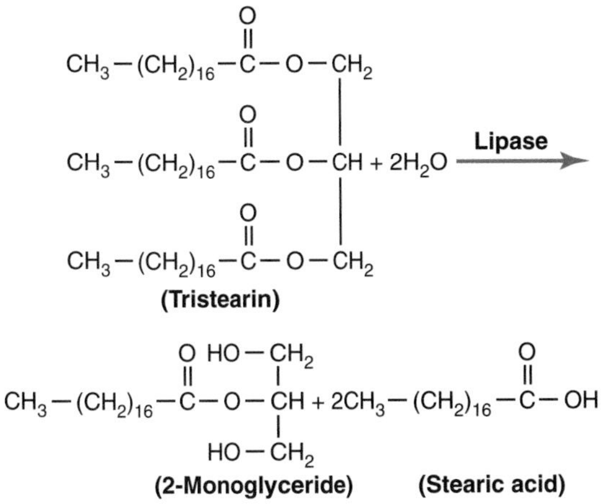

Figure 65-2 Digestion of proteins.

$$CH_3-(CH_2)_{16}-\overset{\overset{O}{\|}}{C}-O-CH_2$$

$$CH_3-(CH_2)_{16}-\overset{\overset{O}{\|}}{C}-O-CH + 2H_2O \quad \xrightarrow{\textbf{Lipase}}$$

$$CH_3-(CH_2)_{16}-\overset{\overset{O}{\|}}{C}-O-CH_2$$

(Tristearin)

$$CH_3-(CH_2)_{16}-\overset{\overset{O}{\|}}{C}-O-\overset{\overset{HO-CH_2}{|}}{CH} + 2CH_3-(CH_2)_{16}-\overset{\overset{O}{\|}}{C}-OH$$

$$HO-CH_2$$

(2-Monoglyceride)   (Stearic acid)

Figure 65-3 Hydrolysis of neutral fat catalyzed by lipase.

Neutral fat is a major constituent in food of animal origin but much, much less so in food of plant origin.

In the usual diet are also small quantities of phospholipids, cholesterol, and cholesterol esters. The phospholipids and cholesterol esters contain fatty acid and therefore can be considered fats. Cholesterol, however, is a sterol compound that contains no fatty acid, but it does exhibit some of the physical and chemical characteristics of fats; plus, it is derived from fats and is metabolized similarly to fats. Therefore, cholesterol is considered, from a dietary point of view, a fat.

Digestion of Fats in the Intestine. A small amount of triglycerides is digested *in the stomach* by *lingual lipase* that is secreted by lingual glands in the mouth and swallowed with the saliva. This amount of digestion is less than 10 percent and generally unimportant. Instead, essentially all fat digestion occurs in the small intestine as follows.

The First Step in Fat Digestion Is Emulsification by Bile Acids and Lecithin. The first step in fat digestion is physically to break the fat globules into small sizes so that the water-soluble digestive enzymes can act on the globule surfaces. This process is called *emulsification of the fat,* and it begins by agitation in the stomach to mix the fat with the products of stomach digestion.

Then, most of the emulsification occurs in the duodenum under the influence of *bile,* the secretion from the liver that does not contain any digestive enzymes. However, bile does contain a large quantity of *bile salts,* as well as the phospholipid *lecithin.* Both of these, *but especially the lecithin,* are extremely important for emulsification of the fat. The polar parts (the points where ionization occurs in water) of the bile salts and lecithin molecules are highly soluble in water, whereas most of the remaining portions of their molecules are highly soluble in fat. Therefore, the fat-soluble portions of these liver secretions dissolve in the surface layer of the fat globules, with the polar portions projecting. The polar projections, in turn, are soluble in the surrounding watery fluids, which greatly decreases the interfacial tension of the fat and makes it soluble as well.

When the interfacial tension of a globule of nonmiscible fluid is low, this nonmiscible fluid, on agitation, can be broken up into many tiny particles far more easily than it can when the interfacial tension is great. Consequently, a major function of the bile salts and lecithin, especially the lecithin, in the bile is to make the fat globules readily fragmentable by agitation with the water in the small bowel. This action is the same as that of many detergents that are widely used in household cleaners for removing grease.

Each time the diameters of the fat globules are significantly decreased as a result of agitation in the small intestine, the total surface area of the fat increases manyfold. Because the average diameter of the fat particles in the intestine after emulsification has occurred is less than 1 micrometer, this represents an increase of as much as 1000-fold in total surface areas of the fats caused by the emulsification process.

The lipase enzymes are water-soluble compounds and can attack the fat globules only on their surfaces. Consequently, this detergent function of bile salts and lecithin is very important for digestion of fats.

Triglycerides Are Digested by Pancreatic Lipase. By far the most important enzyme for digestion of the triglycerides is *pancreatic lipase,* present in enormous quantities in pancreatic juice, enough to digest within 1 minute all triglycerides that it can reach. In addition, the enterocytes of the small intestine contain additional lipase, known as *enteric lipase,* but this is usually not needed.

End Products of Fat Digestion Are Free Fatty Acids. Most of the triglycerides of the diet are split by pancreatic lipase into *free fatty acids* and *2-monoglycerides,* as shown in Figure 65-4.

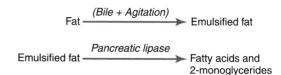

Figure 65-4 Digestion of fats.

Bile Salts Form Micelles That Accelerate Fat Digestion. The hydrolysis of triglycerides is a highly reversible process; therefore, accumulation of monoglycerides and free fatty acids in the vicinity of digesting fats quickly blocks further digestion. But the bile salts play the additional important role of removing the monoglycerides and free fatty acids from the vicinity of the digesting fat globules almost as rapidly as these end products of digestion are formed. This occurs in the following way.

Bile salts, when in high enough concentration in water, have the propensity to form *micelles,* which are small spherical, cylindrical globules 3 to 6 nanometers in diameter composed of 20 to 40 molecules of bile salt. These develop because each bile salt molecule is composed of a sterol nucleus that is highly fat-soluble and a polar group that is highly water-soluble. The sterol nucleus encompasses the fat digestate, forming a small fat globule in the middle of a resulting micelle, with polar groups of bile salts projecting outward to cover the surface of the micelle. Because these polar groups are negatively charged, they allow the entire micelle globule to dissolve in the water of the digestive fluids and to remain in stable solution until the fat is absorbed into the blood.

The bile salt micelles also act as a transport medium to carry the monoglycerides and free fatty acids, both of which would otherwise be relatively insoluble, to the brush borders of the intestinal epithelial cells. There the monoglycerides and free fatty acids are absorbed into the blood, as discussed later, but the bile salts themselves are released back into the chyme to be used again and again for this "ferrying" process.

Digestion of Cholesterol Esters and Phospholipids. Most cholesterol in the diet is in the form of cholesterol esters, which are combinations of free cholesterol and one molecule of fatty acid. Phospholipids also contain fatty acid within their molecules. Both the cholesterol esters and the phospholipids are hydrolyzed by two other lipases in the pancreatic secretion that free the fatty acids—the enzyme *cholesterol ester hydrolase* to hydrolyze the cholesterol ester, and *phospholipase A$_2$* to hydrolyze the phospholipid.

The bile salt micelles play the same role in "ferrying" free cholesterol and phospholipid molecule digestates that they play in "ferrying" monoglycerides and free fatty acids. Indeed, essentially no cholesterol is absorbed without this function of the micelles.

Basic Principles of Gastrointestinal Absorption

It is suggested that the reader review the basic principles of transport of substances through cell membranes discussed in Chapter 4. The following paragraphs present specialized applications of these transport processes during gastrointestinal absorption.

Anatomical Basis of Absorption

The total quantity of fluid that must be absorbed each day by the intestines is equal to the ingested fluid (about 1.5 liters) plus that secreted in the various gastrointestinal secretions (about 7 liters). This comes to a total of 8 to 9 liters. All but about 1.5 liters of this is absorbed in the small intestine, leaving only 1.5 liters to pass through the ileocecal valve into the colon each day.

The stomach is a poor absorptive area of the gastrointestinal tract because it lacks the typical villus type of absorptive membrane, and also because the junctions between the epithelial cells are tight junctions. Only a few highly lipid-soluble substances, such as alcohol and some drugs like aspirin, can be absorbed in small quantities.

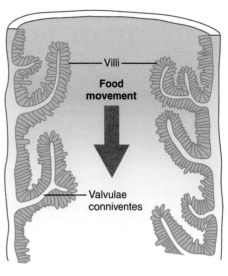

Figure 65-5 Longitudinal section of the small intestine, showing the valvulae conniventes covered by villi.

Folds of Kerckring, Villi, and Microvilli Increase the Mucosal Absorptive Area by Nearly 1000-Fold. Figure 65-5 demonstrates the absorptive surface of the small intestinal mucosa, showing many folds called *valvulae conniventes* (or *folds of Kerckring*), which increase the surface area of the absorptive mucosa about threefold. These folds extend circularly most of the way around the intestine and are especially well developed in the duodenum and jejunum, where they often protrude up to 8 millimeters into the lumen.

Also located on the epithelial surface of the small intestine all the way down to the ileocecal valve are millions of small *villi*. These project about 1 millimeter from the surface of the mucosa, as shown on the surfaces of the valvulae conniventes in Figure 65-5 and in individual detail in Figure 65-6. The villi lie so close to one another in the upper small intestine that they touch in most areas,

Figure 65-6 Functional organization of the villus. *A,* Longitudinal section. *B,* Cross section showing a basement membrane beneath the epithelial cells and a brush border at the other ends of these cells.

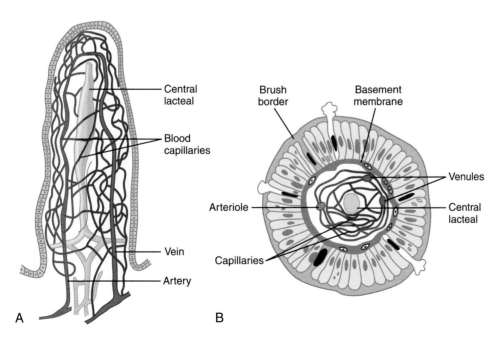

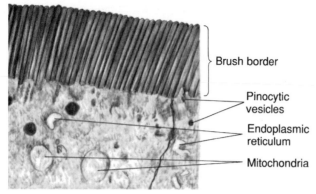

Figure 65-7 Brush border of a gastrointestinal epithelial cell, showing also absorbed pinocytic vesicles, mitochondria, and endoplasmic reticulum lying immediately beneath the brush border. (Courtesy Dr. William Lockwood.)

but their distribution is less profuse in the distal small intestine. The presence of villi on the mucosal surface enhances the total absorptive area another 10-fold.

Finally, each intestinal epithelial cell on each villus is characterized by a *brush border,* consisting of as many as 1000 *microvilli* 1 micrometer in length and 0.1 micrometer in diameter protruding into the intestinal chyme; these microvilli are shown in the electron micrograph in Figure 65-7. This increases the surface area exposed to the intestinal materials at least another 20-fold.

Thus, the combination of the folds of Kerckring, the villi, and the microvilli increases the total absorptive area of the mucosa perhaps 1000-fold, making a tremendous total area of 250 or more square meters for the entire small intestine—about the surface area of a tennis court.

Figure 65-6*A* shows in longitudinal section the general organization of the villus, emphasizing (1) the advantageous arrangement of the vascular system for absorption of fluid and dissolved material into the portal blood and (2) the arrangement of the *"central lacteal"* lymph vessel for absorption into the lymph. Figure 65-6*B* shows a cross section of the villus, and Figure 65-7 shows many small *pinocytic vesicles,* which are pinched-off portions of infolded enterocyte membrane forming vesicles of absorbed fluids that have been entrapped. Small amounts of substances are absorbed by this physical process of *pinocytosis.*

Extending from the epithelial cell body into each microvillus of the brush border are multiple actin filaments that contract rhythmically to cause continual movement of the microvilli, keeping them constantly exposed to new quantities of intestinal fluid.

Absorption in the Small Intestine

Absorption from the small intestine each day consists of several hundred grams of carbohydrates, 100 or more grams of fat, 50 to 100 grams of amino acids, 50 to 100 grams of ions, and 7 to 8 liters of water. The absorptive *capacity* of the normal small intestine is far greater than

this: as much as several kilograms of carbohydrates per day, 500 grams of fat per day, 500 to 700 grams of proteins per day, and 20 or more liters of water per day. The *large* intestine can absorb still additional water and ions, although very few nutrients.

Absorption of Water by Osmosis

Isosmotic Absorption. Water is transported through the intestinal membrane entirely by *diffusion.* Furthermore, this diffusion obeys the usual laws of osmosis. Therefore, when the chyme is dilute enough, water is absorbed through the intestinal mucosa into the blood of the villi almost entirely by osmosis.

Conversely, water can also be transported in the opposite direction—from plasma into the chyme. This occurs especially when hyperosmotic solutions are discharged from the stomach into the duodenum. Within minutes, sufficient water usually will be transferred by osmosis to make the chyme isosmotic with the plasma.

Absorption of Ions

Sodium Is Actively Transported Through the Intestinal Membrane. Twenty to 30 grams of sodium are secreted in the intestinal secretions each day. In addition, the average person eats 5 to 8 grams of sodium each day. Therefore, to prevent net loss of sodium into the feces, the intestines must absorb 25 to 35 grams of sodium each day, which is equal to about one seventh of all the sodium present in the body.

Whenever significant amounts of intestinal secretions are lost to the exterior, as in extreme diarrhea, the sodium reserves of the body can sometimes be depleted to lethal levels within hours. Normally, however, less than 0.5 percent of the intestinal sodium is lost in the feces each day because it is rapidly absorbed through the intestinal mucosa. Sodium also plays an important role in helping to absorb sugars and amino acids, as subsequent discussions reveal.

The basic mechanism of sodium absorption from the intestine is shown in Figure 65-8. The principles of this mechanism, discussed in Chapter 4, are also essentially the same as for absorption of sodium from the gallbladder and renal tubules as discussed in Chapter 27.

The motive power for sodium absorption is provided by active transport of sodium from inside the epithelial cells through the basal and lateral walls of these cells into paracellular spaces. This active transport obeys the usual laws of active transport: It requires energy, and the energy process is catalyzed by appropriate adenosine triphosphatase (ATP) enzymes in the cell membrane (see Chapter 4). Part of the sodium is absorbed along with chloride ions; in fact, the negatively charged chloride ions are mainly passively "dragged" by the positive electrical charges of the sodium ions.

Active transport of sodium through the basolateral membranes of the cell reduces the sodium concentration inside the cell to a low value ($\approx 50\,\text{mEq/L}$), as shown

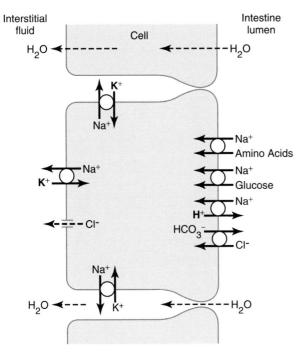

Figure 65-8 Absorption of sodium, chloride, glucose, and amino acids through the intestinal epithelium. Note also osmotic absorption of water (i.e., water "follows" sodium through the epithelial membrane).

in Figure 65-8. Because the sodium concentration in the chyme is normally about 142 mEq/L (i.e., about equal to that in plasma), sodium moves down this steep electrochemical gradient from the chyme through the brush border of the epithelial cell into the epithelial cell cytoplasm. Sodium is also co-transported through the brush border membrane by several specific carrier proteins, including (1) sodium-glucose co-transporter, (2) sodium-amino acid co-transporters, and (3) sodium-hydrogen exchanger. These transporters function similarly as in the renal tubules, described in Chapter 27, and provide still more sodium ions to be transported by the epithelial cells into the paracellular spaces. At the same time they also provide secondary active absorption of glucose and amino acids, powered by the active Na^+-K^+ ATPase pump on the basolateral membrane.

Osmosis of the Water. The next step in the transport process is osmosis of water by transcellular and paracellular pathways. This occurs because a large osmotic gradient has been created by the elevated concentration of ions in the paracellular space. Much of this osmosis occurs through the tight junctions between the apical borders of the epithelial cells (paracellular pathway), but much also occurs through the cells themselves (transcellular pathway). And osmotic movement of water creates flow of fluid into and through the paracellular spaces and, finally, into the circulating blood of the villus.

Aldosterone Greatly Enhances Sodium Absorption. When a person becomes dehydrated, large amounts of aldosterone almost always are secreted by the cortices of the adrenal glands. Within 1 to 3 hours this aldosterone causes increased activation of the enzyme and transport mechanisms for all aspects of sodium absorption by the intestinal epithelium. And the increased sodium absorption in turn causes secondary increases in absorption of chloride ions, water, and some other substances.

This effect of aldosterone is especially important in the colon because it allows virtually no loss of sodium chloride in the feces and also little water loss. Thus, the function of aldosterone in the intestinal tract is the same as that achieved by aldosterone in the renal tubules, which also serves to conserve sodium chloride and water in the body when a person becomes dehydrated.

Absorption of Chloride Ions in the Small Intestine. In the upper part of the small intestine, chloride ion absorption is rapid and occurs mainly by diffusion (i.e., absorption of sodium ions through the epithelium creates electronegativity in the chyme and electropositivity in the paracellular spaces between the epithelial cells). Then chloride ions move along this electrical gradient to "follow" the sodium ions. Chloride is also absorbed across the brush border membrane of parts of the ileum and large intestine by a brush border membrane chloride-bicarbonate exchanger; chloride exits the cell on the basolateral membrane through chloride channels.

Absorption of Bicarbonate Ions in the Duodenum and Jejunum. Often large quantities of bicarbonate ions must be reabsorbed from the upper small intestine because large amounts of bicarbonate ions have been secreted into the duodenum in both pancreatic secretion and bile. The bicarbonate ion is absorbed in an indirect way as follows: When sodium ions are absorbed, moderate amounts of hydrogen ions are secreted into the lumen of the gut in exchange for some of the sodium. These hydrogen ions in turn combine with the bicarbonate ions to form carbonic acid (H_2CO_3), which then dissociates to form water and carbon dioxide. The water remains as part of the chyme in the intestines, but the carbon dioxide is readily absorbed into the blood and subsequently expired through the lungs. Thus, this is so-called "active absorption of bicarbonate ions." It is the same mechanism that occurs in the tubules of the kidneys.

Secretion of Bicarbonate Ions in the Ileum and Large Intestine—Simultaneous Absorption of Chloride Ions

The epithelial cells on the surfaces of the villi in the ileum, as well as on all surfaces of the large intestine, have a special capability of secreting bicarbonate ions in exchange for absorption of chloride ions (see Figure 65-8). This is important because it provides alkaline bicarbonate ions that neutralize acid products formed by bacteria in the large intestine.

Extreme Secretion of Chloride Ions, Sodium Ions, and Water from the Large Intestine Epithelium in Some Types of Diarrhea. Deep in the spaces between the intestinal epithelial folds are immature epithelial cells that continually divide to form new epithelial cells. These in turn spread outward over the luminal surfaces of the intestines. While still in the deep folds, the epithelial cells secrete sodium chloride and water into the intestinal lumen. This secretion in turn is reabsorbed by the older epithelial cells outside the folds, thus providing flow of water for absorbing intestinal digestates.

The toxins of cholera and of some other types of diarrheal bacteria can stimulate the epithelial fold secretion so greatly that this secretion often becomes much greater than can be reabsorbed, thus sometimes causing loss of 5 to 10 liters of water and sodium chloride as *diarrhea* each day. Within 1 to 5 days, many severely affected patients die from this loss of fluid alone.

Extreme diarrheal secretion is initiated by entry of a subunit of cholera toxin into the epithelial cells. This stimulates formation of excess cyclic adenosine monophosphate, which opens tremendous numbers of chloride channels, allowing chloride ions to flow rapidly from inside the cell into the intestinal crypts. In turn, this is believed to activate a sodium pump that pumps sodium ions into the crypts to go along with the chloride ions. Finally, all this extra sodium chloride causes extreme osmosis of water from the blood, thus providing rapid flow of fluid along with the salt. All this excess fluid washes away most of the bacteria and is of value in combating the disease, but too much of a good thing can be lethal because of serious dehydration of the whole body that might ensue. In most instances, the life of a cholera victim can be saved by administration of tremendous amounts of sodium chloride solution to make up for the loss.

Active Absorption of Calcium, Iron, Potassium, Magnesium, and Phosphate. *Calcium ions* are actively absorbed into the blood, especially from the duodenum, and the amount of calcium ion absorption is exactly controlled to supply the daily need of the body for calcium. One important factor controlling calcium absorption is *parathyroid hormone* secreted by the parathyroid glands, and another is *vitamin D.* Parathyroid hormone activates vitamin D, and the activated vitamin D in turn greatly enhances calcium absorption. These effects are discussed in Chapter 79.

Iron ions are also actively absorbed from the small intestine. The principles of iron absorption and regulation of its absorption in proportion to the body's need for iron, especially for the formation of hemoglobin, are discussed in Chapter 32.

Potassium, magnesium, phosphate, and probably *still other ions* can also be actively absorbed through the intestinal mucosa. In general, the monovalent ions are absorbed with ease and in great quantities. Conversely, bivalent ions are normally absorbed in only small amounts; for example, maximum absorption of calcium ions is only 1/50 as great as the normal absorption of sodium ions. Fortunately, only small quantities of the bivalent ions are normally required daily by the body.

Absorption of Nutrients

Carbohydrates Are Mainly Absorbed as Monosaccharides

Essentially all the carbohydrates in the food are absorbed in the form of monosaccharides; only a small fraction is absorbed as disaccharides and almost none as larger carbohydrate compounds. By far the most abundant of the absorbed monosaccharides is *glucose,* usually accounting for more than 80 percent of carbohydrate calories absorbed. The reason for this is that glucose is the final digestion product of our most abundant carbohydrate food, the starches. The remaining 20 percent of absorbed monosaccharides is composed almost entirely of *galactose* and *fructose,* the galactose derived from milk and the fructose as one of the monosaccharides digested from cane sugar.

Virtually all the monosaccharides are absorbed by an active transport process. Let us first discuss the absorption of glucose.

Glucose Is Transported by a Sodium Co-Transport Mechanism. In the absence of sodium transport through the intestinal membrane, virtually no glucose can be absorbed. The reason is that glucose absorption occurs in a co-transport mode with active transport of sodium (see Figure 65-8).

There are two stages in the transport of sodium through the intestinal membrane. First is active transport of sodium ions through the basolateral membranes of the intestinal epithelial cells into the blood, thereby depleting sodium inside the epithelial cells. Second, decrease of sodium inside the cells causes sodium from the intestinal lumen to move through the brush border of the epithelial cells to the cell interiors by a process of *secondary active transport.* That is, a sodium ion combines with a *transport protein,* but the transport protein will not transport the sodium to the interior of the cell until the protein also combines with some other appropriate substance such as glucose. Intestinal glucose also combines simultaneously with the same transport protein and then both the sodium ion and glucose molecule are transported together to the interior of the cell. Thus, the low concentration of sodium inside the cell literally "drags" sodium to the interior of the cell and along with it the glucose at the same time. Once inside the epithelial cell, other transport proteins and enzymes cause facilitated diffusion of the glucose through the cell's basolateral membrane into the paracellular space and from there into the blood.

To summarize, it is the initial active transport of sodium through the basolateral membranes of the intestinal epithelial cells that provides the eventual motive force for moving glucose also through the membranes.

Absorption of Other Monosaccharides. Galactose is transported by almost exactly the same mechanism as glucose. Conversely, fructose transport does not occur by the sodium co-transport mechanism. Instead, fructose is transported by facilitated diffusion all the way through the intestinal epithelium but not coupled with sodium transport.

Much of the fructose, on entering the cell, becomes phosphorylated, then converted to glucose, and finally transported in the form of glucose the rest of the way into the blood. Because fructose is not co-transported with sodium, its overall rate of transport is only about one half that of glucose or galactose.

Absorption of Proteins as Dipeptides, Tripeptides, or Amino Acids

As explained earlier in the chapter, most proteins, after digestion, are absorbed through the luminal membranes of the intestinal epithelial cells in the form of dipeptides, tripeptides, and a few free amino acids. The energy for most of this transport is supplied by a sodium co-transport mechanism in the same way that sodium co-transport of glucose occurs. That is, most peptide or amino acid molecules bind in the cell's microvillus membrane with a specific transport protein that requires sodium binding before transport can occur. After binding, the sodium ion then moves down its electrochemical gradient to the interior of the cell and pulls the amino acid or peptide along with it. This is called *co-transport* (or *secondary active transport*) *of the amino acids and peptides* (see Figure 65-8). A few amino acids do not require this sodium co-transport mechanism but instead are transported by special membrane transport proteins in the same way that fructose is transported, by facilitated diffusion.

At least five types of transport proteins for transporting amino acids and peptides have been found in the luminal membranes of intestinal epithelial cells. This multiplicity of transport proteins is required because of the diverse binding properties of different amino acids and peptides.

Absorption of Fats

Earlier in this chapter, it was pointed out that when fats are digested to form monoglycerides and free fatty acids, both of these digestive end products first become dissolved in the central lipid portions of *bile micelles.* Because the molecular dimensions of these micelles are only 3 to 6 nanometers in diameter, and because of their highly charged exterior, they are soluble in chyme. In this form, the monoglycerides and free fatty acids are carried to the surfaces of the microvilli of the intestinal cell brush border and then penetrate into the recesses among the moving, agitating microvilli. Here, both the monoglycerides and fatty acids diffuse immediately out of the micelles and into the interior of the epithelial cells, which is possible because the lipids are also soluble in the epithelial cell membrane. This leaves the bile micelles still in the chyme, where they function again and again to help absorb still more monoglycerides and fatty acids.

Thus, the micelles perform a "ferrying" function that is highly important for fat absorption. In the presence of an abundance of bile micelles, about 97 percent of the fat is absorbed; in the absence of the bile micelles, only 40 to 50 percent can be absorbed.

After entering the epithelial cell, the fatty acids and monoglycerides are taken up by the cell's smooth endoplasmic reticulum; here, they are mainly used to form new triglycerides that are subsequently released in the form of *chylomicrons* through the base of the epithelial cell, to flow upward through the thoracic lymph duct and empty into the circulating blood.

Direct Absorption of Fatty Acids into the Portal Blood. Small quantities of short- and medium-chain fatty acids, such as those from butterfat, are absorbed directly into the portal blood rather than being converted into triglycerides and absorbed by way of the lymphatics. The cause of this difference between short- and long-chain fatty acid absorption is that the short-chain fatty acids are more water-soluble and mostly are not reconverted into triglycerides by the endoplasmic reticulum. This allows direct diffusion of these short-chain fatty acids from the intestinal epithelial cells directly into the capillary blood of the intestinal villi.

Absorption in the Large Intestine: Formation of Feces

About 1500 milliliters of chyme normally pass through the ileocecal valve into the large intestine each day. Most of the water and electrolytes in this chyme are absorbed in the colon, usually leaving less than 100 milliliters of fluid to be excreted in the feces. Also, essentially all the ions are absorbed, leaving only 1 to 5 mEq each of sodium and chloride ions to be lost in the feces.

Most of the absorption in the large intestine occurs in the proximal one half of the colon, giving this portion the name *absorbing colon*, whereas the distal colon functions principally for feces storage until a propitious time for feces excretion and is therefore called the *storage colon.*

Absorption and Secretion of Electrolytes and Water. The mucosa of the large intestine, like that of the small intestine, has a high capability for active absorption of sodium, and the electrical potential gradient created by absorption of the sodium causes chloride absorption as well. The tight junctions between the epithelial cells of the large intestinal epithelium are much tighter than those of the small intestine. This prevents significant amounts of back-diffusion of ions through these junctions, thus allowing the large intestinal mucosa to absorb sodium ions far more completely—that is, against a much higher concentration gradient—than can occur in the small intestine. This is especially true when large quantities of aldosterone are available because aldosterone greatly enhances sodium transport capability.

In addition, as occurs in the distal portion of the small intestine, the mucosa of the large intestine secretes *bicarbonate ions* while it simultaneously absorbs an equal number of chloride ions in an exchange transport process that has already been described. The bicarbonate helps neutralize the acidic end products of bacterial action in the large intestine.

Absorption of sodium and chloride ions creates an osmotic gradient across the large intestinal mucosa, which in turn causes absorption of water.

Maximum Absorption Capacity of the Large Intestine. The large intestine can absorb a maximum of 5 to 8 liters of fluid and electrolytes each day. When the total quantity entering the large intestine through the ileocecal valve or by way of large intestine secretion exceeds this amount, the excess appears in the feces as diarrhea. As noted earlier in the chapter, toxins from cholera or certain other bacterial infections often cause the crypts in the terminal ileum and in the large intestine to secrete 10 or more liters of fluid each day, leading to severe and sometimes lethal diarrhea.

Bacterial Action in the Colon. *Numerous bacteria, especially colon bacilli, are present even normally in the absorbing colon.* They are capable of digesting small amounts of cellulose, in this way providing a few calories of extra nutrition for the body. In herbivorous animals, this source of energy is significant, although it is of negligible importance in human beings.

Other substances formed as a result of bacterial activity are vitamin K, vitamin B_{12}, thiamine, riboflavin, and various gases that contribute to *flatus* in the colon, especially carbon dioxide, hydrogen gas, and methane. The bacteria-formed vitamin K is especially important because the amount of this vitamin in the daily ingested foods is normally insufficient to maintain adequate blood coagulation.

Composition of the Feces. The feces normally are about three-fourths *water* and one-fourth *solid matter* that is composed of about 30 percent *dead bacteria,* 10 to 20 percent *fat,* 10 to 20 percent *inorganic matter,* 2 to 3 percent *protein,* and 30 percent *undigested roughage* from the food and dried constituents of digestive juices, such as bile pigment and sloughed epithelial cells. The brown color of feces is caused by *stercobilin* and *urobilin,* derivatives of bilirubin. The odor is caused principally by products of bacterial action; these products vary from one person to another, depending on each person's colonic bacterial flora and on the type of food eaten. The actual odoriferous products include *indole, skatole, mercaptans,* and *hydrogen sulfide.*

Bibliography

Barrett KE: New ways of thinking about (and teaching about) intestinal epithelial function, *Adv Physiol Educ* 32:25, 2008.

Barrett KE, Keely SJ: Chloride secretion by the intestinal epithelium: molecular basis and regulatory aspects, *Annu Rev Physiol* 62:535, 2000.

Black DD: Development and physiological regulation of intestinal lipid absorption. I. Development of intestinal lipid absorption: cellular events in chylomicron assembly and secretion, *Am J Physiol Gastrointest Liver Physiol* 293:G519, 2007.

Bröer S: Amino acid transport across mammalian intestinal and renal epithelia, *Physiol Rev* 88:249, 2008.

Bröer S: Apical transporters for neutral amino acids: physiology and pathophysiology, *Physiology (Bethesda)* 23:95, 2008.

Bronner F: Recent developments in intestinal calcium absorption, *Nutr Rev* 67:109, 2009.

Daniel H: Molecular and integrative physiology of intestinal peptide transport, *Annu Rev Physiol* 66:361, 2004.

Field M: Intestinal ion transport and the pathophysiology of diarrhea, *J Clin Invest* 111:931, 2003.

Hui DY, Labonté ED, Howles PN: Development and physiological regulation of intestinal lipid absorption. III. Intestinal transporters and cholesterol absorption, *Am J Physiol Gastrointest Liver Physiol* 294:G839, 2008.

Iqbal J, Hussain MM: Intestinal lipid absorption, *Am J Physiol Endocrinol Metab* 296:E1183, 2009.

Kullak-Ublick GA, Stieger B, Meier PJ: Enterohepatic bile salt transporters in normal physiology and liver disease, *Gastroenterology* 126:322, 2004.

Kunzelmann K, Mall M: Electrolyte transport in the mammalian colon: mechanisms and implications for disease, *Physiol Rev* 82:245, 2002.

Leturque A, Brot-Laroche E, Le Gall M: GLUT2 mutations, translocation, and receptor function in diet sugar managing, *Am J Physiol Endocrinol Metab* 296:E985, 2009.

Mansbach CM 2nd, Gorelick F: Development and physiological regulation of intestinal lipid absorption. II. Dietary lipid absorption, complex lipid synthesis, and the intracellular packaging and secretion of chylomicrons, *Am J Physiol Gastrointest Liver Physiol* 293:G645, 2007.

Pacha J: Development of intestinal transport function in mammals, *Physiol Rev* 80:1633, 2000.

Rothman S, Liebow C, Isenman L: Conservation of digestive enzymes, *Physiol Rev* 82:1, 2002.

Schulzke JD, Ploeger S, Amasheh M, et al: Epithelial tight junctions in intestinal inflammation, *Ann N Y Acad Sci* 1165:294, 2009.

Stevens CE, Hume ID: Contributions of microbes in vertebrate gastrointestinal tract to production and conservation of nutrients, *Physiol Rev* 78:393, 1998.

West AR, Oates PS: Mechanisms of heme iron absorption: current questions and controversies, *World J Gastroenterol* 14:4101, 2008.

Williams KJ: Molecular processes that handle—and mishandle—dietary lipids, *J Clin Invest* 118:3247, 2008.

Zachos NC, Kovbasnjuk O, Donowitz M: Regulation of intestinal electroneutral sodium absorption and the brush border Na^+/H^+ exchanger by intracellular calcium, *Ann N Y Acad Sci* 1165:240, 2009.

Physiology of Gastrointestinal Disorders

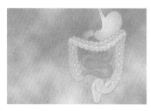

Effective therapy for most gastrointestinal disorders depends on a basic knowledge of gastrointestinal physiology. The purpose of this chapter is to discuss a few representative types of gastrointestinal malfunction that have special physiologic bases or consequences.

Disorders of Swallowing and of the Esophagus

Paralysis of the Swallowing Mechanism. Damage to the fifth, ninth, or tenth cerebral nerve can cause paralysis of significant portions of the swallowing mechanism. Also, a few diseases, such as *poliomyelitis* or *encephalitis,* can prevent normal swallowing by damaging the swallowing center in the brain stem. Finally, paralysis of the swallowing muscles, as occurs in *muscle dystrophy* or in failure of neuromuscular transmission in *myasthenia gravis* or *botulism,* can also prevent normal swallowing.

When the swallowing mechanism is partially or totally paralyzed, the abnormalities that can occur include (1) complete abrogation of the swallowing act so that swallowing cannot occur, (2) failure of the glottis to close so that food passes into the lungs instead of the esophagus, and (3) failure of the soft palate and uvula to close the posterior nares so that food refluxes into the nose during swallowing.

One of the most serious instances of paralysis of the swallowing mechanism occurs when patients are under deep anesthesia. Often, while on the operating table, they vomit large quantities of materials from the stomach into the pharynx; then, instead of swallowing the materials again, they simply suck them into the trachea because the anesthetic has blocked the reflex mechanism of swallowing. As a result, such patients occasionally choke to death on their own vomitus.

Achalasia and Megaesophagus. *Achalasia* is a condition in which the lower esophageal sphincter fails to relax during swallowing. As a result, food swallowed into the esophagus then fails to pass from the esophagus into the stomach. Pathological studies have shown damage in the neural network of the myenteric plexus in the lower two thirds of the esophagus. As a result, the musculature of the lower esophagus

remains spastically contracted and the myenteric plexus has lost its ability to transmit a signal to cause "receptive relaxation" of the gastroesophageal sphincter as food approaches this sphincter during swallowing.

When achalasia becomes severe, the esophagus often cannot empty the swallowed food into the stomach for many hours, instead of the few seconds that is the normal time. Over months and years, the esophagus becomes tremendously enlarged until it often can hold as much as 1 liter of food, which often becomes putridly infected during the long periods of esophageal stasis. The infection may also cause ulceration of the esophageal mucosa, sometimes leading to severe substernal pain or even rupture and death. Considerable benefit can be achieved by stretching the lower end of the esophagus by means of a balloon inflated on the end of a swallowed esophageal tube. Antispasmotic drugs (drugs that relax smooth muscle) can also be helpful.

Disorders of the Stomach

Gastritis—Inflammation of the Gastric Mucosa. Mild to moderate chronic gastritis is exceedingly common in the population as a whole, especially in the middle to later years of adult life.

The inflammation of gastritis may be only superficial and therefore not very harmful, or it can penetrate deeply into the gastric mucosa, in many long-standing cases causing almost complete atrophy of the gastric mucosa. In a few cases, gastritis can be acute and severe, with ulcerative excoriation of the stomach mucosa by the stomach's own peptic secretions.

Research suggests that much gastritis is caused by chronic bacterial infection of the gastric mucosa. This often can be treated successfully by an intensive regimen of antibacterial therapy.

In addition, certain ingested irritant substances can be especially damaging to the protective gastric mucosal barrier—that is, to the mucous glands and to the tight epithelial junctions between the gastric lining cells—often leading to severe acute or chronic gastritis. Two of the most common of these substances are excesses of *alcohol* or *aspirin.*

Gastric Barrier and Its Penetration in Gastritis. Absorption of food from the stomach directly into the blood is normally slight. This low level of absorption is mainly due to two specific features of the gastric mucosa: (1) It is lined with highly resistant mucous cells that secrete viscid and adherent mucus and (2) it has tight junctions between the adjacent epithelial cells. These two together plus other impediments to gastric absorption are called the "gastric barrier."

The gastric barrier normally is resistant enough to diffusion so that even the highly concentrated hydrogen ions of the gastric juice, averaging about 100,000 times the concentration of hydrogen ions in plasma, seldom diffuse even to the slightest extent through the lining mucus as far as the epithelial membrane itself. In gastritis, the permeability of the barrier is greatly increased. The hydrogen ions do then diffuse into the stomach epithelium, creating additional havoc and leading to a vicious circle of progressive stomach mucosal damage and atrophy. It also makes the mucosa susceptible to digestion by the peptic digestive enzymes, thus frequently resulting in a *gastric ulcer*.

Chronic Gastritis Can Lead to Gastric Atrophy and Loss of Stomach Secretions. In many people who have chronic gastritis, the mucosa gradually becomes more and more atrophic until little or no gastric gland digestive secretion remains. It is also believed that some people develop autoimmunity against the gastric mucosa, which also leads eventually to gastric atrophy. Loss of the stomach secretions in gastric atrophy leads to *achlorhydria* and, occasionally, to *pernicious anemia*.

Achlorhydria (and Hypochlorhydria). *Achlorhydria* means simply that the stomach fails to secrete hydrochloric acid; it is diagnosed when the pH of the gastric secretions fails to decrease below 6.5 after maximal stimulation. *Hypochlorhydria* means diminished acid secretion. When acid is not secreted, pepsin also usually is not secreted; even when it is, the lack of acid prevents it from functioning because pepsin requires an acid medium for activity.

Gastric Atrophy May Cause Pernicious Anemia. Pernicious anemia is a common accompaniment of gastric atrophy and achlorhydria. Normal gastric secretions contain a glycoprotein called *intrinsic factor*, secreted by the same parietal cells that secrete hydrochloric acid. Intrinsic factor must be present for adequate absorption of vitamin B_{12} from the ileum. That is, intrinsic factor combines with vitamin B_{12} in the stomach and protects it from being digested and destroyed as it passes into the small intestine. Then, when the intrinsic factor–vitamin B_{12} complex reaches the terminal ileum, the intrinsic factor binds with receptors on the ileal epithelial surface. This in turn makes it possible for the vitamin B_{12} to be absorbed.

In the absence of intrinsic factor, only about 1/50 of the vitamin B_{12} is absorbed. And, without intrinsic factor, an adequate amount of vitamin B_{12} is not made available from the foods to cause young, newly forming red blood cells to mature in the bone marrow. The result is *pernicious anemia*. This is discussed in more detail in Chapter 32.

Peptic Ulcer

A peptic ulcer is an excoriated area of stomach or intestinal mucosa caused principally by the digestive action of gastric juice or upper small intestinal secretions. Figure 66-1 shows the points in the gastrointestinal tract at which peptic ulcers most frequently occur, demonstrating that the most frequent site is within a few centimeters of the pylorus. In addition, peptic ulcers frequently occur along the lesser curvature of the antral end of the stomach or, more rarely, in the lower end of the esophagus where stomach juices frequently reflux.

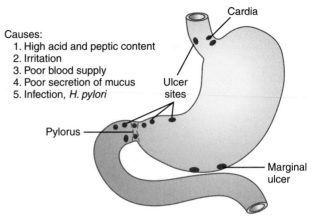

Causes:
1. High acid and peptic content
2. Irritation
3. Poor blood supply
4. Poor secretion of mucus
5. Infection, *H. pylori*

Figure 66-1 Peptic ulcer. *H. pylori, Helicobacter pylori.*

A type of peptic ulcer called a *marginal ulcer* also often occurs wherever a surgical opening such as a gastrojejunostomy has been made between the stomach and the jejunum of the small intestine.

Basic Cause of Peptic Ulceration. The usual cause of peptic ulceration is an *imbalance* between the rate of secretion of gastric juice and the degree of protection afforded by (1) the gastroduodenal mucosal barrier and (2) the neutralization of the gastric acid by duodenal juices. It will be recalled that all areas normally exposed to gastric juice are well supplied with mucous glands, beginning with compound mucous glands in the lower esophagus plus the mucous cell coating of the stomach mucosa, the mucous neck cells of the gastric glands, the deep pyloric glands that secrete mainly mucus, and, finally, the glands of Brunner's of the upper duodenum, which secrete a highly alkaline mucus.

In addition to the mucus protection of the mucosa, the duodenum is protected by the *alkalinity of the small intestinal secretions*. Especially important is *pancreatic secretion*, which contains large quantities of sodium bicarbonate that neutralize the hydrochloric acid of the gastric juice, thus also inactivating pepsin and preventing digestion of the mucosa. In addition, large amounts of bicarbonate ions are provided in (1) the secretions of the large Brunner's glands in the first few centimeters of the duodenal wall and (2) in bile coming from the liver.

Finally, two feedback control mechanisms normally ensure that this neutralization of gastric juices is complete, as follows:

1. When excess acid enters the duodenum, it inhibits gastric secretion and peristalsis in the stomach, both by nervous reflexes and by hormonal feedback from the duodenum, thereby decreasing the rate of gastric emptying.

2. The presence of acid in the small intestine liberates *secretin* from the intestinal mucosa, which then passes by way of the blood to the pancreas to promote rapid secretion of pancreatic juice. This juice also contains a high concentration of sodium bicarbonate, thus making still more sodium bicarbonate available for neutralization of the acid.

Therefore, a peptic ulcer can be caused in either of two ways: (1) excess secretion of acid and pepsin by the gastric mucosa or (2) diminished ability of the gastroduodenal mucosal barrier to protect against the digestive properties of the stomach acid–pepsin secretion.

Specific Causes of Peptic Ulcer in the Human Being

Bacterial Infection by *Helicobacter pylori* Breaks Down the Gastroduodenal Mucosal Barrier and Stimulates Gastric Acid Secretion. At least 75 percent of peptic ulcer patients have been found to have chronic infection of the terminal portions of the gastric mucosa and initial portions of the duodenal mucosa, most often caused by the bacterium *Helicobacter pylori*. Once this infection begins, it can last a lifetime unless it is eradicated by antibacterial therapy. Furthermore, the bacterium is capable of penetrating the mucosal barrier both by virtue of its physical capability to burrow through the barrier and by releasing ammonium that liquefies the barrier and stimulates the secretion of hydrochloric acid. As a result, the strong acidic digestive juices of the stomach secretions can then penetrate into the underlying epithelium and literally digest the gastrointestinal wall, thus leading to peptic ulceration.

Other Causes of Ulceration. In many people who have peptic ulcers in the initial portion of the duodenum, the rate of gastric acid secretion is greater than normal, sometimes as much as twice normal. Although part of this increased secretion may be stimulated by bacterial infection, studies in both animals and human beings have shown that excess secretion of gastric juices for any reason (for instance, even in psychic disturbances) may cause peptic ulceration.

Other factors that predispose to ulcers include (1) *smoking*, presumably because of increased nervous stimulation of the stomach secretory glands; (2) *alcohol*, because it tends to break down the mucosal barrier; and (3) *aspirin* and other nonsteroidal anti-inflammatory drugs that also have a strong propensity for breaking down this barrier.

Treatment of Peptic Ulcers. Since discovery of the bacterial infectious basis for much peptic ulceration, therapy has changed immensely. Initial reports are that almost all patients with peptic ulceration can be treated effectively by two measures: (1) use of *antibiotics* along with other agents to kill infectious bacteria and (2) administration of an acid-suppressant drug, especially *ranitidine*, an antihistaminic that blocks the stimulatory effect of histamine on gastric gland histamine$_2$ receptors, thus reducing gastric acid secretion by 70 to 80 percent.

In the past, before these approaches to peptic ulcer therapy were developed, it was often necessary to remove as much as four fifths of the stomach, thus reducing stomach acid–peptic juices enough to cure most patients. Another therapy was to cut the two vagus nerves that supply parasympathetic stimulation to the gastric glands. This blocked almost all secretion of acid and pepsin and often cured the ulcer or ulcers within 1 week after the operation. However, much of the basal stomach secretion returned after a few months and in many patients the ulcer also returned.

The newer physiologic approaches to therapy may prove to be miraculous. Even so, in a few instances, the patient's condition is so severe, including massive bleeding from the ulcer, that heroic operative procedures often must still be used.

Disorders of the Small Intestine

Abnormal Digestion of Food in the Small Intestine—Pancreatic Failure

A serious cause of abnormal digestion is failure of the pancreas to secrete pancreatic juice into the small intestine. Lack of pancreatic secretion frequently occurs (1) in *pancreatitis* (which is discussed later), (2) when the *pancreatic duct is blocked* by a gallstone at the papilla of Vater, or (3) after the *head of the pancreas has been removed* because of malignancy.

Loss of pancreatic juice means loss of trypsin, chymotrypsin, carboxypolypeptidase, pancreatic amylase, pancreatic lipase, and still a few other digestive enzymes. Without these enzymes, up to 60 percent of the fat entering the small intestine may be unabsorbed, as well as one third to one half of the proteins and carbohydrates. As a result, large portions of the ingested food cannot be used for nutrition and copious, fatty feces are excreted.

Pancreatitis—Inflammation of the Pancreas. Pancreatitis can occur in the form of either *acute pancreatitis* or *chronic pancreatitis*.

The most common cause of pancreatitis is *drinking excess alcohol*, and the second most common cause is *blockage of the papilla of Vater* by a gallstone; the two together account for more than 90 percent of all cases. When a gallstone blocks the papilla of Vater, this blocks the main secretory duct from the pancreas and the common bile duct. The pancreatic enzymes are then dammed up in the ducts and acini of the pancreas. Eventually, so much trypsinogen accumulates that it *overcomes the trypsin inhibitor* in the secretions and a small quantity of trypsinogen becomes activated to form trypsin. Once this happens, the trypsin activates still more trypsinogen, as well as chymotrypsinogen and carboxypolypeptidase, resulting in a vicious circle until most of the proteolytic enzymes in the pancreatic ducts and acini become activated. These enzymes rapidly digest large portions of the pancreas, sometimes completely and permanently destroying the ability of the pancreas to secrete digestive enzymes.

Malabsorption by the Small Intestinal Mucosa—Sprue

Occasionally, nutrients are not adequately absorbed from the small intestine even though the food has become well digested. Several diseases can cause decreased absorption by the mucosa; they are often classified together under the general term *"sprue."* Malabsorption also can occur when large portions of the small intestine have been removed.

Nontropical Sprue. One type of sprue, called variously *idiopathic sprue, celiac disease* (in children), or *gluten enteropathy*, results from the toxic effects of *gluten* present in certain types of grains, especially wheat and rye. Only some people are susceptible to this effect, but in those who are susceptible, gluten has a direct destructive effect on intestinal enterocytes. In milder forms of the disease, only the microvilli of the absorbing enterocytes on the villi are destroyed, thus decreasing the absorptive surface area as much as twofold. In the more severe forms, the villi themselves become blunted or disappear altogether, thus still further reducing the absorptive area of the gut. Removal of wheat and rye flour from the diet frequently results in cure within weeks, especially in children with this disease.

Tropical Sprue. A different type of sprue called *tropical sprue* frequently occurs in the tropics and can often be treated with antibacterial agents. Even though no specific bacterium has been implicated as the cause, it is believed that this variety of sprue is usually caused by inflammation of the intestinal mucosa resulting from unidentified infectious agents.

Malabsorption in Sprue. In the early stages of sprue, intestinal absorption of fat is more impaired than absorption of other digestive products. The fat that appears in the stools is almost entirely in the form of salts of fatty acids rather than undigested fat, demonstrating that the problem is one of absorption, not of digestion. In fact, the condition is frequently called *steatorrhea*, which means simply excess fats in the stools.

In severe cases of sprue, in addition to malabsorption of fats there is also impaired absorption of proteins, carbohydrates, calcium, vitamin K, folic acid, and vitamin B$_{12}$. As a result, the person suffers (1) severe nutritional deficiency, often developing wasting of the body; (2) osteomalacia (demineralization of the bones because of lack of calcium); (3) inadequate blood coagulation caused by lack of vitamin K; and (4) macrocytic anemia of the pernicious anemia type, owing to diminished vitamin B$_{12}$ and folic acid absorption.

Disorders of the Large Intestine

Constipation

Constipation means *slow movement of feces through the large intestine;* it is often associated with large quantities of dry, hard feces in the descending colon that accumulate because of overabsorption of fluid. Any pathology of the intestines that obstructs movement of intestinal contents, such as tumors, adhesions that constrict the intestines, or ulcers, can cause constipation. A frequent functional cause of constipation is irregular bowel habits that have developed through a lifetime of inhibition of the normal defecation reflexes.

Infants are seldom constipated, but part of their training in the early years of life requires that they learn to control defecation; this control is effected by inhibiting the natural defecation reflexes. Clinical experience shows that if one does not allow defecation to occur when the defecation reflexes are excited or if one overuses laxatives to take the place of natural bowel function, the reflexes themselves become progressively less strong over months or years, and the colon becomes *atonic.* For this reason, if a person establishes regular bowel habits early in life, defecating when the gastrocolic and duodenocolic reflexes cause mass movements in the large intestine, the development of constipation in later life is much less likely.

Constipation can also result from spasm of a small segment of the sigmoid colon. It should be recalled that motility normally is weak in the large intestine, so even a slight degree of spasm is often capable of causing serious constipation. After the constipation has continued for several days and excess feces have accumulated above a spastic sigmoid colon, excessive colonic secretions often then lead to a day or so of diarrhea. After this, the cycle begins again, with repeated bouts of alternating constipation and diarrhea.

Megacolon (Hirschsprung's Disease). Occasionally, constipation is so severe that bowel movements occur only once every several days or sometimes only once a week. This allows tremendous quantities of fecal matter to accumulate in the colon, causing the colon sometimes to distend to a diameter of 3 to 4 inches. The condition is called *megacolon,* or *Hirschsprung's disease.*

A frequent cause of megacolon is lack of or deficiency *of ganglion cells in the myenteric plexus in a segment of the sigmoid colon.* As a consequence, neither defecation reflexes nor strong peristaltic motility can occur in this area of the large intestine. The sigmoid itself becomes small and almost spastic while feces accumulate proximal to this area, causing megacolon in the ascending, transverse, and descending colons.

Diarrhea

Diarrhea results from rapid movement of fecal matter through the large intestine. Several causes of diarrhea with important physiologic sequelae are the following.

Enteritis—Inflammation of the Intestinal Tract. Enteritis means inflammation usually caused either by a virus or by bacteria in the intestinal tract. In usual *infectious diarrhea,* the infection is most extensive in the large intestine and the distal end of the ileum. Everywhere the infection is present, the mucosa becomes irritated and its rate of secretion becomes greatly enhanced. In addition, motility of the intestinal wall usually increases manifold. As a result, large quantities of fluid are made available for washing the infectious agent toward the anus, and at the same time strong propulsive movements propel this fluid forward. This is an important mechanism for ridding the intestinal tract of a debilitating infection.

Of special interest is diarrhea caused by *cholera* (and less often by other bacteria such as some pathogenic colon bacilli). As explained in Chapter 65, cholera toxin directly stimulates excessive secretion of electrolytes and fluid from the crypts of Lieberkühn in the distal ileum and colon. The amount can be 10 to 12 liters per day, although the colon can usually reabsorb a maximum of only 6 to 8 liters per day. Therefore, loss of fluid and electrolytes can be so debilitating within several days that death can ensue.

The most important physiologic basis of therapy in cholera is to replace the fluid and electrolytes as rapidly as they are lost, mainly by giving the patient intravenous solutions. With proper therapy, along with the use of antibiotics, almost no cholera patients die but without therapy up to 50 percent do.

Psychogenic Diarrhea. Everyone is familiar with the diarrhea that accompanies periods of nervous tension, such as during examination time or when a soldier is about to go into battle. This type of diarrhea, called *psychogenic* emotional diarrhea, is caused by excessive stimulation of the parasympathetic nervous system, which greatly excites both (1) motility and (2) excess secretion of mucus in the distal colon. These two effects added together can cause marked diarrhea.

Ulcerative Colitis. Ulcerative colitis is a disease in which extensive areas of the walls of the large intestine become inflamed and ulcerated. The motility of the ulcerated colon is often so great that *mass movements* occur much of the day rather than for the usual 10 to 30 minutes. Also, the colon's secretions are greatly enhanced. As a result, the patient has repeated diarrheal bowel movements.

The cause of ulcerative colitis is unknown. Some clinicians believe that it results from an allergic or immune destructive effect, but it also could result from chronic bacterial infection not yet understood. Whatever the cause, there is a strong hereditary tendency for susceptibility to ulcerative colitis. Once the condition has progressed far, the ulcers seldom will heal until an ileostomy is performed to allow the small intestinal contents to drain to the exterior rather than to pass through the colon. Even then the ulcers sometimes fail to heal, and the only solution might be surgical removal of the entire colon.

Paralysis of Defecation in Spinal Cord Injuries

From Chapter 63 it will be recalled that defecation is normally initiated by accumulating feces in the rectum, which causes a spinal cord–mediated *defecation reflex* passing from the rectum to the *conus medullaris* of the spinal cord and then back to the descending colon, sigmoid, rectum, and anus.

When the spinal cord is injured somewhere between the conus medullaris and the brain, the voluntary portion of the defecation act is blocked while the basic cord reflex for defecation is still intact. Nevertheless, loss of the voluntary aid to defecation—that is, loss of the increased abdominal pressure and relaxation of the voluntary anal sphincter—often makes defecation a difficult process in the person with this type of upper cord injury. But because the cord defecation reflex can still occur, a small enema to excite action of this cord reflex, usually given in the morning shortly after a meal, can often cause adequate defecation. In this way, people with spinal cord injuries that do not destroy the conus medullaris of the spinal cord can usually control their bowel movements each day.

General Disorders of the Gastrointestinal Tract

Vomiting

Vomiting is the means by which the upper gastrointestinal tract rids itself of its contents when almost any part of the upper tract becomes excessively irritated, overdistended, or even overexcitable. Excessive distention or irritation of the duodenum provides an especially strong stimulus for vomiting.

The sensory signals that initiate vomiting originate mainly from the pharynx, esophagus, stomach, and upper portions of the small intestines. And the nerve impulses are transmitted, as shown in Figure 66-2, by both vagal and sympathetic afferent nerve fibers to multiple distributed nuclei in the brain stem that all together are called the "vomiting center." From here, *motor impulses* that cause the actual vomiting are transmitted from the vomiting center by way of the fifth, seventh, ninth, tenth, and twelfth cranial nerves to the upper gastrointestinal tract, through vagal and sympathetic nerves to the lower tract, and through spinal nerves to the diaphragm and abdominal muscles.

Antiperistalsis, the Prelude to Vomiting. In the early stages of excessive gastrointestinal irritation or overdistention, *antiperistalsis* begins to occur often many minutes before vomiting appears. Antiperistalsis means peristalsis *up* the digestive tract rather than downward. This may begin as far down in the intestinal tract as the ileum, and the antiperistaltic wave travels backward up the intestine at a rate of 2 to 3 cm/sec; this process can actually push a large share of the lower small intestine contents all the way back to the duodenum and stomach within 3 to 5 minutes. Then, as these upper portions of the gastrointestinal tract, especially the duodenum, become overly

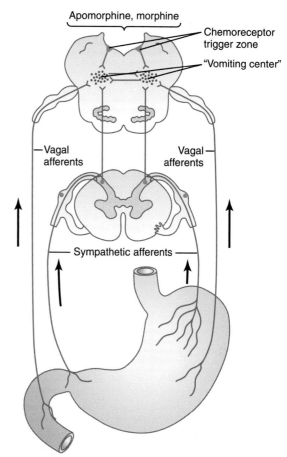

Figure 66-2 Neutral connections of the "vomiting center." This so-called vomiting center includes multiple sensory, motor, and control nuclei mainly in the medullary and pontile reticular formation but also extending into the spinal cord.

distended, this distention becomes the exciting factor that initiates the actual vomiting act.

At the onset of vomiting, strong intrinsic contractions occur in both the duodenum and the stomach, along with partial relaxation of the esophageal-stomach sphincter, thus allowing vomitus to begin moving from the stomach into the esophagus. From here, a specific vomiting act involving the abdominal muscles takes over and expels the vomitus to the exterior, as explained in the next paragraph.

Vomiting Act. Once the vomiting center has been sufficiently stimulated and the vomiting act instituted, the first effects are (1) a deep breath, (2) raising of the hyoid bone and larynx to pull the upper esophageal sphincter open, (3) closing of the glottis to prevent vomitus flow into the lungs, and (4) lifting of the soft palate to close the posterior nares. Next comes a strong downward contraction of the diaphragm along with simultaneous contraction of all the abdominal wall muscles. This squeezes the stomach between the diaphragm and the abdominal muscles, building the intragastric pressure to a high level. Finally, the lower esophageal sphincter relaxes completely, allowing expulsion of the gastric contents upward through the esophagus.

Thus, the vomiting act results from a squeezing action of the muscles of the abdomen associated with simultaneous contraction of the stomach wall and opening of the esophageal sphincters so that the gastric contents can be expelled.

"Chemoreceptor Trigger Zone" in the Brain Medulla for Initiation of Vomiting by Drugs or by Motion Sickness. Aside from the vomiting initiated by irritative stimuli in the gastrointestinal tract, vomiting can also be caused by nervous signals arising in areas of the brain. This is particularly true for a small area located bilaterally on the floor of the fourth ventricle called the *chemoreceptor trigger zone for vomiting.* Electrical stimulation of this area can initiate vomiting; but, more important, administration of certain drugs, including apomorphine, morphine, and some digitalis derivatives, can directly stimulate this chemoreceptor trigger zone and initiate vomiting. Destruction of this area blocks this type of vomiting but does not block vomiting resulting from irritative stimuli in the gastrointestinal tract itself.

Also, it is well known that rapidly changing direction or rhythm of motion of the body can cause certain people to vomit. The mechanism for this is the following: The motion stimulates receptors in the vestibular labyrinth of the inner ear, and from here impulses are transmitted mainly by way of the brain stem *vestibular nuclei into the cerebellum,* then to the *chemoreceptor trigger zone,* and finally to the *vomiting center* to cause vomiting.

Nausea

Everyone has experienced the sensation of nausea and knows that it is often a prodrome of vomiting. Nausea is the conscious recognition of subconscious excitation in an area of the medulla closely associated with or part of the vomiting center, and it can be caused by (1) irritative impulses coming from the gastrointestinal tract, (2) impulses that originate in the lower brain associated with motion sickness, or (3) impulses from the cerebral cortex to initiate vomiting. Vomiting occasionally occurs without the prodromal sensation of nausea, indicating that only certain portions of the vomiting center are associated with the sensation of nausea.

Gastrointestinal Obstruction

The gastrointestinal tract can become obstructed at almost any point along its course, as shown in Figure 66-3. Some common causes of obstruction are (1) *cancer,* (2) *fibrotic constriction resulting from ulceration or from peritoneal adhesions,* (3) *spasm of a segment of the gut,* and (4) *paralysis of a segment of the gut.*

The abnormal consequences of obstruction depend on the point in the gastrointestinal tract that becomes obstructed. If the obstruction occurs at the pylorus, which results often from fibrotic constriction after peptic ulceration, persistent vomiting of stomach contents occurs. This depresses bodily nutrition; it also causes excessive loss of hydrogen ions from the stomach and can result in various degrees of *whole-body metabolic alkalosis.*

If the obstruction is beyond the stomach, antiperistaltic reflux from the small intestine causes intestinal juices to flow backward into the stomach, and these juices are vomited along with the stomach secretions. In this instance, the person loses large amounts of water and electrolytes. He or she becomes severely dehydrated, but the loss of acid from the stomach and base from the small intestine may be approximately equal, so little change in acid-base balance occurs.

If the obstruction is near the distal end of the large intestine, feces can accumulate in the colon for a week or more.

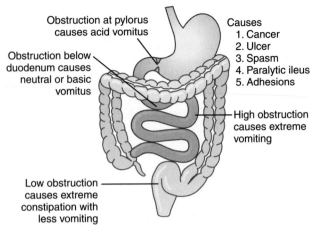

Obstruction at pylorus causes acid vomitus

Obstruction below duodenum causes neutral or basic vomitus

Causes
1. Cancer
2. Ulcer
3. Spasm
4. Paralytic ileus
5. Adhesions

High obstruction causes extreme vomiting

Low obstruction causes extreme constipation with less vomiting

Figure 66-3 Obstruction in different parts of the gastrointestinal tract.

The patient develops an intense feeling of constipation, but at first vomiting is not severe. After the large intestine has become completely filled and it finally becomes impossible for additional chyme to move from the small intestine into the large intestine, severe vomiting does then occur. Prolonged obstruction of the large intestine can finally cause rupture of the intestine itself or dehydration and circulatory shock resulting from the severe vomiting.

Gases in the Gastrointestinal Tract; "Flatus"

Gases, called *flatus,* can enter the gastrointestinal tract from three sources: (1) swallowed air, (2) gases formed in the gut as a result of bacterial action, or (3) gases that diffuse from the blood into the gastrointestinal tract. Most gases in the stomach are mixtures of nitrogen and oxygen derived from swallowed air. In the typical person these gases are expelled by belching. Only small amounts of gas normally occur in the small intestine, and much of this gas is air that passes from the stomach into the intestinal tract.

In the large intestine, most of the gases are derived from bacterial action, including especially *carbon dioxide, methane,* and *hydrogen.* When methane and hydrogen become suitably mixed with oxygen, an actual explosive mixture is sometimes formed. Use of the electric cautery during sigmoidoscopy has been known to cause a mild explosion.

Certain foods are known to cause greater expulsion of flatus through the anus than others—beans, cabbage, onion, cauliflower, corn, and certain irritant foods such as vinegar. Some of these foods serve as a suitable medium for gas-forming bacteria, especially unabsorbed fermentable types of carbohydrates. For instance, beans contain an indigestible carbohydrate that passes into the colon and becomes a superior food for colonic bacteria. But in other instances, excess expulsion of gas results from irritation of the large intestine, which promotes rapid peristaltic expulsion of gases through the anus before they can be absorbed.

The amount of gases entering or forming in the large intestine each day averages 7 to 10 liters, whereas the average amount expelled through the anus is usually only about 0.6 liter. The remainder is normally absorbed into the blood through the intestinal mucosa and expelled through the lungs.

Bibliography

Andoh A, Yagi Y, Shioya M, et al: Mucosal cytokine network in inflammatory bowel disease, *World J Gastroenterol* 14:5154, 2008.

Binder HJ: Mechanisms of diarrhea in inflammatory bowel diseases, *Ann N Y Acad Sci* 1165:285, 2009.

Bjarnason I, Takeuchi K: Intestinal permeability in the pathogenesis of NSAID-induced enteropathy, *J Gastroenterol* 44(Suppl 19):23, 2009.

Blaser MJ, Atherton JC: *Helicobacter pylori* persistence: biology and disease, *J Clin Invest* 113:321, 2004.

Casanova JL, Abel L: Revisiting Crohn's disease as a primary immunodeficiency of macrophages, *J Exp Med* 206:1839, 2009.

Cover TL, Blaser MJ: *Helicobacter pylori* in health and disease, *Gastroenterology* 136:1863, 2009.

Elson CO: Genes, microbes, and T cells—new therapeutic targets in Crohn's disease, *N Engl J Med* 346:614, 2002.

Fox JG, Wang TC: Inflammation, atrophy, and gastric cancer, *J Clin Invest* 117:60, 2007.

Hunt KA, van Heel DA: Recent advances in coeliac disease genetics, *Gut* 58:473, 2009.

Kahrilas PJ: Clinical practice. Gastroesophageal reflux disease, *N Engl J Med* 359:1700, 2008.

Korzenik JR, Podolsky DK: Evolving knowledge and therapy of inflammatory bowel disease, *Nat Rev Drug Discov* 5:197, 2006.

Kozuch PL, Hanauer SB: Treatment of inflammatory bowel disease: a review of medical therapy, *World J Gastroenterol* 14:354, 2008.

Kunzelmann K, Mall M: Electrolyte transport in the mammalian colon: mechanisms and implications for disease, *Physiol Rev* 82:245, 2002.

Laine L, Takeuchi K, Tarnawski A: Gastric mucosal defense and cytoprotection: bench to bedside, *Gastroenterology* 135:41, 2008.

Laroux FS, Pavlick KP, Wolf RE, Grisham MB: Dysregulation of intestinal mucosal immunity: implications in inflammatory bowel disease, *News Physiol Sci* 16:272, 2001.

McMahon BP, Jobe BA, Pandolfino JE, Gregersen H: Do we really understand the role of the oesophagogastric junction in disease? *World J Gastroenterol* 15:144, 2009.

Podolsky DK: Inflammatory bowel disease, *N Engl J Med* 347:417, 2002.

Schulzke JD, Ploeger S, Amasheh M, et al: Epithelial tight junctions in intestinal inflammation, *Ann N Y Acad Sci* 1165:294, 2009.

Singh S, Graff LA, Bernstein CN: Do NSAIDs, antibiotics, infections, or stress trigger flares in IBD? *Am J Gastroenterol* 104:1298, 2009.

Suerbaum S, Michetti P: *Helicobacter pylori* infection, *N Engl J Med* 347(15):1175, 2002.

Tonsi AF, Bacchion M, Crippa S, et al: Acute pancreatitis at the beginning of the 21st century: the state of the art, *World J Gastroenterol* 15:2945, 2009.

Wolfe MM, Lichtenstein DR, Singh G: Gastrointestinal toxicity of nonsteroidal antiinflammatory drugs, *N Engl J Med* 340(24):1888, 1999.

Xavier RJ, Podolsky DK: Unravelling the pathogenesis of inflammatory bowel disease, *Nature* 448:427, 2007.

XIII

Metabolism and Temperature Regulation

67. Metabolism of Carbohydrates, and Formation of Adenosine Triphosphate

68. Lipid Metabolism

69. Protein Metabolism

70. The Liver as an Organ

71. Dietary Balances; Regulation of Feeding; Obesity and Starvation; Vitamins and Minerals

72. Energetics and Metabolic Rate

73. Body Temperature Regulation, and Fever

Metabolism of Carbohydrates, and Formation of Adenosine Triphosphate

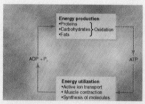

The next few chapters deal with metabolism in the body—the chemical processes that make it possible for the cells to continue living. It is not the purpose of this textbook to present the chemical details of all the various cellular reactions, because this lies in the discipline of biochemistry. Instead, these chapters are devoted to (1) a review of the principal chemical processes of the cell and (2) an analysis of their physiologic implications, especially the manner in which they fit into the overall body homeostasis.

Release of Energy from Foods, and the Concept of "Free Energy"

Most of the chemical reactions in the cells are aimed at making the energy in foods available to the various physiologic systems of the cell. For instance, energy is required for muscle activity, secretion by the glands, maintenance of membrane potentials by the nerve and muscle fibers, synthesis of substances in the cells, absorption of foods from the gastrointestinal tract, and many other functions.

Coupled Reactions. All the energy foods—carbohydrates, fats, and proteins—can be oxidized in the cells, and during this process, large amounts of energy are released. These same foods can also be burned with pure oxygen outside the body in an actual fire, also releasing large amounts of energy; in this case, however, the energy is released suddenly, all in the form of heat. The energy needed by the physiologic processes of the cells is not heat but energy to cause mechanical movement in the case of muscle function, to concentrate solutes in the case of glandular secretion, and to effect other cell functions. To provide this energy, the chemical reactions must be "coupled" with the systems responsible for these physiologic functions. This coupling is accomplished by special cellular enzyme and energy transfer systems, some of which are explained in this and subsequent chapters.

"Free Energy." The amount of energy liberated by complete oxidation of a food is called the *free energy of oxidation of the food*, and this is generally represented by the symbol ΔG. Free energy is usually expressed in terms of calories per mole of substance. For instance, the amount of free energy liberated by complete oxidation of 1 mole (180 grams) of glucose is 686,000 calories.

Adenosine Triphosphate Is the "Energy Currency" of the Body

Adenosine triphosphate (ATP) is an essential link between energy-utilizing and energy-producing functions of the body (Figure 67-1). For this reason, ATP has been called the energy currency of the body, and it can be gained and spent repeatedly.

Energy derived from the oxidation of carbohydrates, proteins, and fats is used to convert adenosine diphosphate (ADP) to ATP, which is then consumed by the various reactions of the body that are necessary for (1) active transport of molecules across cell membranes; (2) contraction of muscles and performance of mechanical work; (3) various synthetic reactions that create hormones, cell membranes, and many other essential molecules of the body; (4) conduction of nerve impulses; (5) cell division and growth; and (6) many other physiologic functions that are necessary to maintain and propagate life.

ATP is a labile chemical compound that is present in all cells. ATP is a combination of adenine, ribose, and three phosphate radicals as shown in Figure 67-2. The last two phosphate radicals are connected with the remainder of the molecule by high-energy bonds, which are indicated by the symbol ~.

The amount of free energy in each of these high-energy bonds per mole of ATP is about 7300 calories under standard conditions and about 12,000 calories under the usual

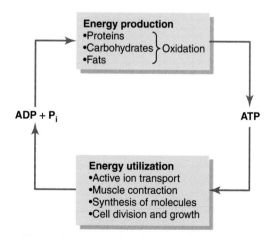

Figure 67-1 Adenosine triphosphate (ATP) as the central link between energy-producing and energy-utilizing systems of the body. ADP, adenosine diphosphate; P_i, inorganic phosphate.

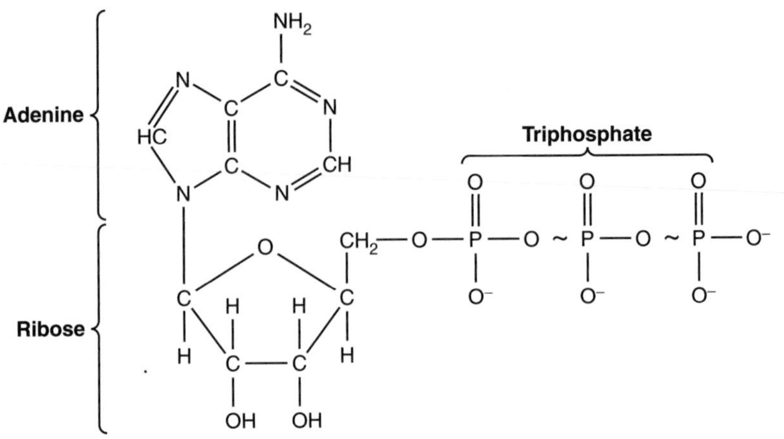

Figure 67-2 Chemical structure of adenosine triphosphate (ATP).

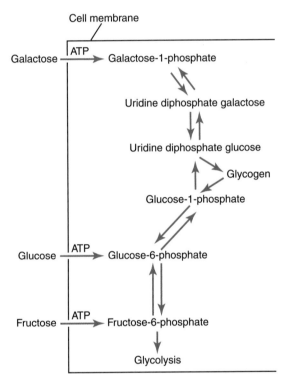

conditions of temperature and concentrations of the reactants in the body. Therefore, in the body, removal of each of the last two phosphate radicals liberates about 12,000 calories of energy. After loss of one phosphate radical from ATP, the compound becomes ADP, and after loss of the second phosphate radical, it becomes *adenosine monophosphate* (AMP). The interconversions among ATP, ADP, and AMP are the following:

$$\text{ATP} \underset{+12,000\ cal}{\overset{-12,000\ cal}{\rightleftarrows}} \left\{ \begin{array}{c} \text{ADP} \\ + \\ \text{PO}_3 \end{array} \right\} \underset{+12,000\ cal}{\overset{-12,000\ cal}{\rightleftarrows}} \left\{ \begin{array}{c} \text{AMP} \\ + \\ \text{2PO}_3 \end{array} \right\}$$

ATP is present everywhere in the cytoplasm and nucleoplasm of all cells, and essentially all the physiologic mechanisms that require energy for operation obtain it directly from ATP (or another similar high-energy compound, guanosine triphosphate [GTP]). In turn, the food in the cells is gradually oxidized, and the released energy is used to form new ATP, thus always maintaining a supply of this substance. All these energy transfers take place by means of coupled reactions.

The principal purpose of this chapter is to explain how the energy from carbohydrates can be used to form ATP in the cells. Normally, 90 percent or more of all the carbohydrates utilized by the body are used for this purpose.

Central Role of Glucose in Carbohydrate Metabolism

As explained in Chapter 65, the final products of carbohydrate digestion in the alimentary tract are almost entirely glucose, fructose, and galactose—with glucose representing, on average, about 80 percent of these. After absorption from the intestinal tract, much of the fructose and almost all the galactose are rapidly converted into glucose in the liver. Therefore, little fructose and galactose are present in the circulating blood. *Glucose thus becomes the final common pathway for the transport of almost all carbohydrates to the tissue cells.*

In liver cells, appropriate enzymes are available to promote interconversions among the monosaccharides—glucose, fructose, and galactose—as shown in Figure 67-3. Furthermore, the dynamics of the reactions are such that when the liver releases the monosaccharides back into the blood, the final product is almost entirely glucose. The reason for this is that the liver cells contain large amounts of *glucose phosphatase*. Therefore, glucose-6-phosphate can be degraded to glucose

Figure 67-3 Interconversions of the three major monosaccharides—glucose, fructose, and galactose—in liver cells.

and phosphate, and the glucose can then be transported through the liver cell membrane back into the blood.

Once again, it should be emphasized that usually more than 95 percent of all the monosaccharides that circulate in the blood are the final conversion product, glucose.

Transport of Glucose Through the Cell Membrane

Before glucose can be used by the body's tissue cells, it must be transported through the tissue cell membrane into the cellular cytoplasm. However, glucose *cannot easily diffuse through the pores* of the cell membrane because the maximum molecular weight of particles that can diffuse readily is about 100, and glucose has a molecular weight of 180. Yet glucose does pass to the interior of the cells with a reasonable degree of freedom by the mechanism of *facilitated diffusion*. The principles of this type of transport are discussed in Chapter 4. Basically, they are the following. Penetrating through the lipid matrix of the cell membrane are large numbers of protein *carrier* molecules that can bind with glucose. In this bound form, the glucose can be transported by the carrier from one side of the membrane to the other side and then released. Therefore, if the concentration of glucose is greater on one side of the membrane than on the other side, more glucose will be transported from the high-concentration area to the low-concentration area than in the opposite direction.

The transport of glucose through the membranes of most tissue cells is quite different from that which occurs through the gastrointestinal membrane or through the epithelium of the renal tubules. In both cases, the glucose is transported by the mechanism of *active sodium-glucose co-transport*, in which active transport of sodium provides energy for absorbing glucose *against a concentration difference*. This sodium-glucose co-transport mechanism functions only in certain special epithelial cells that are specifically adapted for active absorption of glucose. At other cell membranes, glucose is transported only from higher concentration toward lower concentration by *facilitated diffusion*, made possible by the special binding properties of membrane *glucose carrier protein*. The details of *facilitated diffusion* for cell membrane transport are presented in Chapter 4.

Insulin Increases Facilitated Diffusion of Glucose

The rate of glucose transport, as well as transport of some other monosaccharides, is greatly increased by insulin. When large amounts of insulin are secreted by the pancreas, the rate of glucose transport into most cells increases to 10 or more times the rate of transport when no insulin is secreted. Conversely, the amounts of glucose that can diffuse to the insides of most cells of the body in the absence of insulin, with the exception of liver and brain cells, are far too little to supply the amount of glucose normally required for energy metabolism.

In effect, the rate of carbohydrate utilization by most cells is controlled by the rate of insulin secretion from the pancreas. The functions of insulin and its control of carbohydrate metabolism are discussed in detail in Chapter 78.

Phosphorylation of Glucose

Immediately on entry into the cells, glucose combines with a phosphate radical in accordance with the following reaction:

$$\text{Glucose} \xrightarrow[\text{+ATP}]{\text{glucokinase or hexokinase}} \text{Glucose-6-phosphate}$$

This phosphorylation is promoted mainly by the enzyme *glucokinase* in the liver and by *hexokinase* in most other cells. The phosphorylation of glucose is almost completely irreversible except in the liver cells, the renal tubular epithelial cells, and the intestinal epithelial cells; in these cells, another enzyme, *glucose phosphatase*, is also available, and when this is activated, it can reverse the reaction. In most tissues of the body, phosphorylation serves to *capture* the glucose in the cell. That is, because of its almost instantaneous binding with phosphate, the glucose will not diffuse back out, except from those special cells, especially liver cells, that have phosphatase.

Glycogen Is Stored in Liver and Muscle

After absorption into a cell, glucose can be used immediately for release of energy to the cell, or it can be stored in the form of *glycogen*, which is a large polymer of glucose.

All cells of the body are capable of storing at least some glycogen, but certain cells can store large amounts, especially *liver cells*, which can store up to 5 to 8 percent of their weight as glycogen, and *muscle cells*, which can store up to 1 to 3 percent glycogen. The glycogen molecules can be polymerized to almost any molecular weight, with the average molecular weight being 5 million or greater; most of the glycogen precipitates in the form of solid granules.

This conversion of the monosaccharides into a high-molecular-weight precipitated compound (glycogen) makes it possible to store large quantities of carbohydrates without significantly altering the osmotic pressure of the intracellular fluids. High concentrations of low-molecular-weight soluble monosaccharides would play havoc with the osmotic relations between intracellular and extracellular fluids.

Glycogenesis—Formation of Glycogen

The chemical reactions for glycogenesis are shown in Figure 67-4. From this figure, it can be seen that *glucose-6-phosphate* can become *glucose-1-phosphate*; this is converted to *uridine diphosphate glucose*, which is finally converted into glycogen. Several specific enzymes are required to cause these conversions, and any monosaccharide that can be converted into glucose can enter into the reactions. Certain smaller compounds, including *lactic acid, glycerol, pyruvic acid,* and some *deaminated amino acids,* can also be converted into glucose or closely allied compounds and then converted into glycogen.

Glycogenolysis—Breakdown of Stored Glycogen

Glycogenolysis means the breakdown of the cell's stored glycogen to re-form glucose in the cells. The glucose can then be used to provide energy. Glycogenolysis does not occur by reversal of the same chemical reactions that form glycogen; instead, each succeeding glucose molecule on each branch of the glycogen polymer is split away by *phosphorylation*, catalyzed by the enzyme *phosphorylase*.

Under resting conditions, the phosphorylase is in an inactive form, so that glycogen will remain stored. When it is necessary to re-form glucose from glycogen, the phosphorylase must first be activated. This can be accomplished in several ways, including the following two.

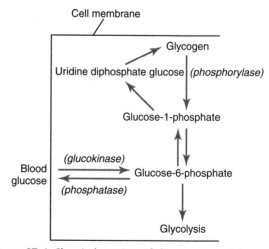

Figure 67-4 Chemical reactions of glycogenesis and glycogenolysis, showing also interconversions between blood glucose and liver glycogen. (The phosphatase required for the release of glucose from the cell is present in liver cells but not in most other cells.)

Activation of Phosphorylase by Epinephrine or by Glucagon. Two hormones, *epinephrine* and *glucagon*, can activate phosphorylase and thereby cause rapid glycogenolysis. The initial effect of each of these hormones is to promote the formation of *cyclic AMP* in the cells, which then initiates a cascade of chemical reactions that activates the phosphorylase. This is discussed in detail in Chapter 78.

Epinephrine is released by the adrenal medullae when the sympathetic nervous system is stimulated. Therefore, one of the functions of the sympathetic nervous system is to increase the availability of glucose for rapid energy metabolism. This function of epinephrine occurs markedly in both liver cells and muscle, thereby contributing, along with other effects of sympathetic stimulation, to preparing the body for action, as discussed fully in Chapter 60.

Glucagon is a hormone secreted by the *alpha cells* of the pancreas when the blood glucose concentration falls too low. It stimulates formation of cyclic AMP mainly in the liver cells, and this in turn promotes conversion of liver glycogen into glucose and its release into the blood, thereby elevating the blood glucose concentration. The function of glucagon in blood glucose regulation is discussed more fully in Chapter 78.

Release of Energy from Glucose by the Glycolytic Pathway

Because complete oxidation of 1 gram-mole of glucose releases 686,000 calories of energy and only 12,000 calories of energy are required to form 1 gram-mole of ATP, energy would be wasted if glucose were decomposed all at once into water and carbon dioxide while forming only a single ATP molecule. Fortunately, cells of the body contain special protein enzymes that cause the glucose molecule to split a little at a time in many successive steps, so that its energy is released in small packets to form one molecule of ATP at a time, forming a total of 38 moles of ATP for each mole of glucose metabolized by the cells.

The next sections describe the basic principles of the processes by which the glucose molecule is progressively dissected and its energy released to form ATP.

Glycolysis—Splitting Glucose to Form Pyruvic Acid

By far the most important means of releasing energy from the glucose molecule is initiated by *glycolysis*. The end products of glycolysis are then oxidized to provide energy. Glycolysis means splitting of the glucose molecule to form *two molecules of pyruvic acid*.

Glycolysis occurs by 10 successive chemical reactions, shown in Figure 67-5. Each step is catalyzed by at least one specific protein enzyme. Note that glucose is first converted into fructose-1,6-diphosphate and then split into two three-carbon-atom molecules, glyceraldehyde-3-phosphate, each of which is then converted through five additional steps into pyruvic acid.

Formation of ATP During Glycolysis. Despite the many chemical reactions in the glycolytic series, only a small portion of the free energy in the glucose molecule is released at most steps. However, between the 1,3-diphosphoglyceric acid and the 3-phosphoglyceric acid stages, and again between the phosphoenolpyruvic acid and the pyruvic acid stages, the packets of energy released are greater than 12,000 calories per mole, the amount required to form ATP, and

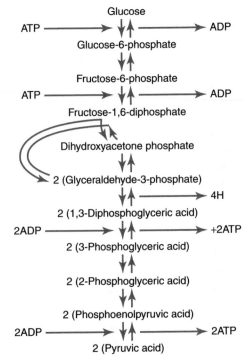

Figure 67-5 Sequence of chemical reactions responsible for glycolysis.

the reactions are coupled in such a way that ATP is formed. Thus, a total of 4 moles of ATP are formed for each mole of fructose-1,6-diphosphate that is split into pyruvic acid.

Yet, 2 moles of ATP are required to phosphorylate the original glucose to form fructose-1,6-diphosphate before glycolysis could begin. Therefore, *the net gain in ATP molecules by the entire glycolytic process is only 2 moles for each mole of glucose utilized*. This amounts to 24,000 calories of energy that becomes transferred to ATP, but during glycolysis, a total of 56,000 calories of energy were lost from the original glucose, giving an overall *efficiency* for ATP formation of only 43 percent. The remaining 57 percent of the energy is lost in the form of heat.

Conversion of Pyruvic Acid to Acetyl Coenzyme A

The next stage in the degradation of glucose is a two-step conversion of the two pyruvic acid molecules from Figure 67-5 into two molecules of *acetyl coenzyme A* (acetyl-CoA), in accordance with the following reaction:

$$2CH_3 - \overset{\overset{\textstyle O}{\|}}{C} - COOH + 2CoA - SH \rightarrow$$
(Pyruvic acid)   (Coenzyme A)

$$2CH_3 - \overset{\overset{\textstyle O}{\|}}{C} - S - CoA + 2CO_2 + 4H$$
(Acetyl-CoA)

Two carbon dioxide molecules and four hydrogen atoms are released from this reaction, while the remaining portions of the two pyruvic acid molecules combine with coenzyme A, a derivative of the vitamin pantothenic acid, to form two molecules of acetyl-CoA. In this conversion, no ATP is formed, but up to six molecules of ATP are formed when the four released hydrogen atoms are later oxidized, as discussed later.

Citric Acid Cycle (Krebs Cycle)

The next stage in the degradation of the glucose molecule is called the *citric acid cycle* (also called the *tricarboxylic acid cycle* or the *Krebs cycle* in honor of Hans Krebs for his discovery of the citric acid cycle). This is a sequence of chemical reactions in which the acetyl portion of acetyl-CoA is degraded to carbon dioxide and hydrogen atoms. These reactions all occur in the *matrix of the mitochondrion*. The released hydrogen atoms add to the number of these atoms that will subsequently be oxidized (as discussed later), releasing tremendous amounts of energy to form ATP.

Figure 67-6 shows the different stages of the chemical reactions in the citric acid cycle. The substances to the left are added during the chemical reactions, and the products of the chemical reactions are shown to the right. Note at the top of the column that the cycle begins with *oxaloacetic acid*, and at the bottom of the chain of reactions, *oxaloacetic acid* is formed again. Thus, the cycle can continue over and over.

In the initial stage of the citric acid cycle, *acetyl-CoA* combines with *oxaloacetic acid* to form *citric acid*. The coenzyme A portion of the acetyl-CoA is released and can be used again and again for the formation of still more quantities of acetyl-CoA from pyruvic acid. The acetyl portion, however, becomes an integral part of the citric acid molecule. During the successive stages of the citric acid cycle, several molecules of water are added, as shown on the left in the figure, and *carbon dioxide* and *hydrogen atoms* are released at other stages in the cycle, as shown on the right in the figure.

The net results of the entire citric acid cycle are given in the explanation at the bottom of Figure 67-6, demonstrating that for each molecule of glucose originally metabolized, two acetyl-CoA molecules enter into the citric acid cycle, along with six molecules of water. These are then degraded into 4 carbon dioxide molecules, 16 hydrogen atoms, and 2 molecules of coenzyme A. Two molecules of ATP are formed, as follows.

Formation of ATP in the Citric Acid Cycle. The citric acid cycle itself does not cause a great amount of energy to be released; in only one of the chemical reactions—during the change from α-ketoglutaric acid to succinic acid—is a molecule of ATP formed. Thus, for each molecule of glucose metabolized, two acetyl-CoA molecules pass through the citric acid cycle, each forming a molecule of ATP, or a total of two molecules of ATP formed.

Function of Dehydrogenases and Nicotinamide Adenine Dinucleotide in Causing Release of Hydrogen Atoms in the Citric Acid Cycle. As already noted at several points in this discussion, hydrogen atoms are released during different chemical reactions of the citric acid cycle—4 hydrogen atoms during glycolysis, 4 during formation of acetyl-CoA from pyruvic acid and 16 in the citric acid cycle; *this makes a total of 24 hydrogen atoms released for each original molecule of glucose*. However, the hydrogen atoms are not simply turned loose in the intracellular fluid. Instead, they are released in packets of two, and in each instance, the release is catalyzed by a specific protein enzyme called a *dehydrogenase*. Twenty of the 24 hydrogen atoms immediately combine with nicotinamide adenine dinucleotide (NAD$^+$), a derivative of the vitamin niacin, in accordance with the following reaction:

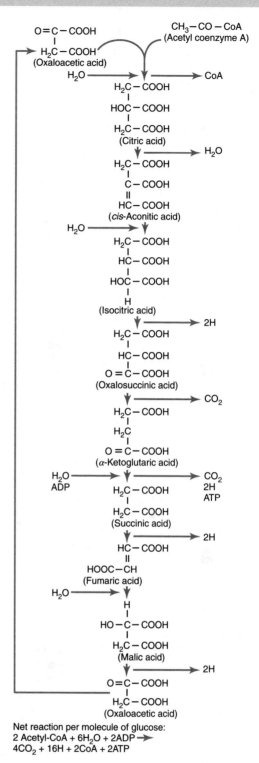

Figure 67-6 Chemical reactions of the citric acid cycle, showing the release of carbon dioxide and a number of hydrogen atoms during the cycle.

$$\text{Substrate} \overset{\displaystyle H}{\underset{\displaystyle H}{\diagdown}} + \text{NAD}^+ \xrightarrow{\textit{dehydrogenase}}$$

$$\text{NADH} + \text{H}^+ + \text{Substrate}$$

This reaction will not occur without intermediation of the specific dehydrogenase or without the availability of NAD$^+$ to act as a hydrogen carrier. Both the free hydrogen ion and the hydrogen bound with NAD$^+$ subsequently enter into multiple oxidative chemical reactions that form tremendous quantities of ATP, as discussed later.

The remaining four hydrogen atoms released during the breakdown of glucose—the four released during the citric acid cycle between the succinic and fumaric acid stages—combine with a specific dehydrogenase but are not subsequently released to NAD$^+$. Instead, they pass directly from the dehydrogenase into the oxidative process.

Function of Decarboxylases in Causing Release of Carbon Dioxide.
Referring again to the chemical reactions of the citric acid cycle, as well as to those for the formation of acetyl-CoA from pyruvic acid, we find that there are three stages in which carbon dioxide is released. To cause the release of carbon dioxide, other specific protein enzymes, called *decarboxylases*, split the carbon dioxide away from the substrate. The carbon dioxide is then dissolved in the body fluids and transported to the lungs, where it is expired from the body (see Chapter 40).

Formation of Large Quantities of ATP by Oxidation of Hydrogen—the Process of Oxidative Phosphorylation
Despite all the complexities of (1) glycolysis, (2) the citric acid cycle, (3) dehydrogenation, and (4) decarboxylation, pitifully small amounts of ATP are formed during all these processes—only two ATP molecules in the glycolysis scheme and another two in the citric acid cycle for each molecule of glucose metabolized. Instead, almost 90 percent of the total ATP created through glucose metabolism is formed during subsequent oxidation of the hydrogen atoms that were released at early stages of glucose degradation. Indeed, the principal function of all these earlier stages is to make the hydrogen of the glucose molecule available in forms that can be oxidized.

Oxidation of hydrogen is accomplished, as illustrated in Figure 67-7, by a series of enzymatically catalyzed reactions *in the mitochondria*. These reactions (1) split each hydrogen atom into a hydrogen ion and an electron and (2) use the electrons eventually to combine dissolved oxygen of the fluids with water molecules to form hydroxyl ions. Then the hydrogen and hydroxyl ions combine with each other to form water. During this sequence of oxidative reactions, tremendous quantities of energy are released to form ATP. Formation of ATP in this manner is called *oxidative phosphorylation*. This occurs entirely in the mitochondria by a highly specialized process called the *chemiosmotic mechanism*.

Chemiosmotic Mechanism of the Mitochondria to Form ATP
Ionization of Hydrogen, the Electron Transport Chain, and Formation of Water. The first step in oxidative phosphorylation in the mitochondria is to ionize the hydrogen atoms that

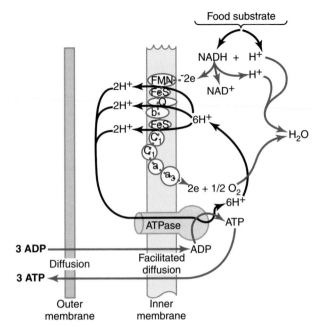

Figure 67-7 Mitochondrial chemiosmotic mechanism of oxidative phosphorylation for forming large quantities of ATP. This figure shows the relationship of the oxidative and phosphorylation steps at the outer and inner membranes of the mitochondrion.

have been removed from the food substrates. As described earlier, these hydrogen atoms are removed in pairs: one immediately becomes a hydrogen ion, H$^+$; the other combines with NAD$^+$ to form NADH. The upper portion of Figure 67-7 shows the subsequent fate of the NADH and H$^+$. The initial effect is to release the other hydrogen atom from the NADH to form another hydrogen ion, H$^+$; this process also reconstitutes NAD$^+$ that will be reused again and again.

The electrons that are removed from the hydrogen atoms to cause the hydrogen ionization immediately enter an *electron transport chain of electron acceptors* that are an integral part of the inner membrane (the shelf membrane) of the mitochondrion. The electron acceptors can be reversibly reduced or oxidized by accepting or giving up electrons. The important members of this electron transport chain include *flavoprotein*, several *iron sulfide proteins, ubiquinone,* and *cytochromes B, C1, C, A,* and *A3*. Each electron is shuttled from one of these acceptors to the next until it finally reaches cytochrome A3, which is called *cytochrome oxidase* because it is capable of giving up two electrons and thus reducing elemental oxygen to form ionic oxygen, which then combines with hydrogen ions to form water.

Thus, Figure 67-7 shows the transport of electrons through the electron chain and then their ultimate use by cytochrome oxidase to cause the formation of water molecules. During the transport of these electrons through the electron transport chain, energy is released that is used to cause the synthesis of ATP, as follows.

Pumping of Hydrogen Ions into the Outer Chamber of the Mitochondrion, Caused by the Electron Transport Chain. As the electrons pass through the electron transport chain, large amounts of energy are released. This energy is used to pump hydrogen ions from the inner matrix of the mitochondrion (to the right in Figure 67-7) into the outer chamber between the inner and outer mitochondrial membranes (to the left). This creates a high concentration of positively charged hydrogen ions in this chamber; it also creates a strong negative electrical potential in the inner matrix.

Formation of ATP. The next step in oxidative phosphorylation is to convert ADP into ATP. This occurs in conjunction with a large protein molecule that protrudes all the way through the inner mitochondrial membrane and projects with a knoblike head into the inner mitochondrial matrix. This molecule is an ATPase, the physical nature of which is shown in Figure 67-7. It is called *ATP synthetase*.

The high concentration of positively charged hydrogen ions in the outer chamber and the large electrical potential difference across the inner membrane cause the hydrogen ions to flow into the inner mitochondrial matrix *through the substance of the ATPase molecule*. In doing so, energy derived from this hydrogen ion flow is used by ATPase to convert ADP into ATP by combining ADP with a free ionic phosphate radical (Pi), thus adding another high-energy phosphate bond to the molecule.

The final step in the process is transfer of ATP from the inside of the mitochondrion back to the cell cytoplasm. This occurs by facilitated diffusion outward through the inner membrane and then by simple diffusion through the permeable outer mitochondrial membrane. In turn, ADP is continually transferred in the other direction for continual conversion into ATP. *For each two electrons that pass through the entire electron transport chain (representing the ionization of two hydrogen atoms), up to three ATP molecules are synthesized.*

Summary of ATP Formation During the Breakdown of Glucose

We can now determine the total number of ATP molecules that, under optimal conditions, can be formed by the energy from one molecule of glucose.

1. During glycolysis, four molecules of ATP are formed and two are expended to cause the initial phosphorylation of glucose to get the process going. This gives a net gain of *two molecules of ATP*.

2. During each revolution of the citric acid cycle, one molecule of ATP is formed. However, because each glucose molecule splits into two pyruvic acid molecules, there are two revolutions of the cycle for each molecule of glucose metabolized, giving a net production of *two more molecules of ATP*.

3. During the entire schema of glucose breakdown, a total of 24 hydrogen atoms are released during glycolysis and during the citric acid cycle. Twenty of these atoms are oxidized in conjunction with the chemiosmotic mechanism shown in Figure 67-7, with the release of three ATP molecules per two atoms of hydrogen metabolized. This gives an additional *30 ATP molecules*.

4. The remaining four hydrogen atoms are released by their dehydrogenase into the chemiosmotic oxidative schema in the mitochondrion beyond the first stage of Figure 67-7. Two ATP molecules are usually released for every two hydrogen atoms oxidized, thus giving a total of *four more ATP molecules*.

Now, adding all the ATP molecules formed, we find a maximum of *38 ATP molecules* formed for each molecule of glucose degraded to carbon dioxide and water. Thus, 456,000 calories of energy can be stored in the form of ATP, whereas 686,000 calories are released during the complete oxidation of each gram-molecule of glucose. This represents an overall maximum *efficiency* of energy transfer of 66 percent. The remaining 34 percent of the energy becomes heat and, therefore, cannot be used by the cells to perform specific functions.

Control of Energy Release from Stored Glycogen When the Body Needs Additional Energy: Effect of ATP and ADP Cell Concentrations in Controlling the Rate of Glycolysis

Continual release of energy from glucose when the cells do not need energy would be an extremely wasteful process. Instead, glycolysis and the subsequent oxidation of hydrogen atoms are continually controlled in accordance with the cells' need for ATP. This control is accomplished by multiple feedback control mechanisms within the chemical schemata. Among the more important of these are the effects of cell concentrations of both ADP and ATP in controlling the rates of chemical reactions in the energy metabolism sequence.

One important way in which ATP helps control energy metabolism is to inhibit the enzyme *phosphofructokinase*. Because this enzyme promotes the formation of fructose-1,6-diphosphate, one of the initial steps in the glycolytic series of reactions, the net effect of excess cellular ATP is to slow or even stop glycolysis, which in turn stops most carbohydrate metabolism. Conversely, ADP (and AMP as well) causes the opposite change in this enzyme, greatly increasing its activity. Whenever ATP is used by the tissues for energizing a major fraction of almost all intracellular chemical reactions, this reduces the ATP inhibition of the enzyme phosphofructokinase and at the same time increases its activity as a result of the excess ADP formed. Thus, the glycolytic process is set in motion, and the total cellular store of ATP is replenished.

Another control linkage is the *citrate ion* formed in the citric acid cycle. An excess of this ion also *strongly inhibits phosphofructokinase*, thus preventing the glycolytic process from getting ahead of the citric acid cycle's ability to use the pyruvic acid formed during glycolysis.

A third way by which the ATP-ADP-AMP system controls carbohydrate metabolism, as well as controlling energy release from fats and proteins, is the following: Referring to the various chemical reactions for energy release, we see that if all the ADP in the cell has already been converted into ATP, additional ATP simply cannot be formed. As a result, the entire sequence involved in the use of foodstuffs—glucose, fats, and proteins—to form ATP is stopped. Then, when ATP is used by the cell to energize the different physiologic functions in the cell, the newly formed ADP and AMP turn on the energy processes again, and ADP and AMP are almost instantly returned to the ATP state. In this way, essentially a full store of ATP is automatically maintained, except during extreme cellular activity, such as very strenuous exercise.

Anaerobic Release of Energy—"Anaerobic Glycolysis"

Occasionally, oxygen becomes either unavailable or insufficient, so oxidative phosphorylation cannot take place. Yet even under these conditions, a small amount of energy can still be released to the cells by the glycolysis stage of carbohydrate degradation, because the chemical reactions for the breakdown of glucose to pyruvic acid do not require oxygen.

This process is extremely wasteful of glucose because only 24,000 calories of energy are used to form ATP for each molecule of glucose metabolized, which represents only a little over 3 percent of the total energy in the glucose molecule. Nevertheless, this release of glycolytic energy to the cells, which is called *anaerobic energy*, can be a lifesaving measure for up to a few minutes when oxygen becomes unavailable.

Formation of Lactic Acid During Anaerobic Glycolysis Allows Release of Extra Anaerobic Energy. The *law of mass action* states that as the end products of a chemical reaction build up in a reacting medium, the rate of the reaction decreases, approaching zero. The two end products of the glycolytic reactions (see Figure 67-5) are (1) pyruvic acid and (2) hydrogen atoms combined with NAD$^+$ to form NADH and H$^+$. The buildup of either or both of these would stop the glycolytic process and prevent further formation of ATP. When their quantities begin to be excessive, these two end products react with each other to form lactic acid, in accordance with the following equation:

$$CH_3-\underset{\underset{\text{(Pyruvic acid)}}{}}{\overset{\overset{\text{OH}}{||}}{C}}-COOH + NADH + H^+ \underset{}{\overset{lactic\ dehydrogenase}{\rightleftharpoons}}$$

$$CH_3-\underset{\underset{\underset{\text{(Lactic acid)}}{}}{|}}{\overset{\overset{\text{OH}}{|}}{\underset{H}{C}}}-COOH + NAD^+$$

Thus, under anaerobic conditions, the major portion of the pyruvic acid is converted into lactic acid, which diffuses readily out of the cells into the extracellular fluids and even into the intracellular fluids of other less active cells. Therefore, lactic acid represents a type of "sinkhole" into which the glycolytic end products can disappear, thus allowing glycolysis to proceed far longer than would otherwise be possible. Indeed, glycolysis could proceed for only a few seconds without this conversion. Instead, it can proceed for several minutes, supplying the body with considerable extra quantities of ATP, even in the absence of respiratory oxygen.

Reconversion of Lactic Acid to Pyruvic Acid When Oxygen Becomes Available Again. When a person begins to breathe oxygen again after a period of anaerobic metabolism, the lactic acid is rapidly reconverted to pyruvic acid and NADH plus H$^+$. Large portions of these are immediately oxidized to form large quantities of ATP. This excess ATP then causes as much as three fourths of the remaining excess pyruvic acid to be converted back into glucose.

Thus, the large amount of lactic acid that forms during anaerobic glycolysis is not lost from the body because, when oxygen is available again, the lactic acid can be either reconverted to glucose or used directly for energy. By far the greatest portion of this reconversion occurs in the liver, but a small amount can also occur in other tissues.

Use of Lactic Acid by the Heart for Energy. Heart muscle is especially capable of converting lactic acid to pyruvic acid and then using the pyruvic acid for energy. This occurs to a great extent during heavy exercise, when large amounts of lactic acid are released into the blood from the skeletal muscles and consumed as an extra energy source by the heart.

Release of Energy from Glucose by the Pentose Phosphate Pathway

In almost all the body's muscles, essentially all the carbohydrates utilized for energy are degraded to pyruvic acid by glycolysis and then oxidized. However, this glycolytic scheme is not the only means by which glucose can be degraded and used to provide energy. A second important mechanism for the breakdown and oxidation of glucose is called the *pentose phosphate pathway* (or *phosphogluconate pathway*), which is responsible for as much as 30 percent of the glucose breakdown *in the liver and even more than this in fat cells.*

This pathway is especially important because it can provide energy independently of all the enzymes of the citric acid cycle and therefore is an alternative pathway for energy metabolism when certain enzymatic abnormalities occur in cells. It has a special capacity for providing energy to multiple cellular synthetic processes.

Release of Carbon Dioxide and Hydrogen by the Pentose Phosphate Pathway. Figure 67-8 shows most of the basic chemical reactions in the pentose phosphate pathway. It demonstrates that glucose, during several stages of conversion, can release one molecule of carbon dioxide and four atoms of hydrogen, with the resultant formation of a five-carbon sugar, D-ribulose. This substance can change progressively into several other five-, four-, seven-, and three-carbon sugars. Finally, various combinations of these sugars can resynthesize glucose. However, *only five molecules of glucose are resynthesized for every six molecules of glucose that initially enter into the reactions.* That is, the pentose phosphate pathway is a cyclical process in which one molecule of glucose is metabolized for each revolution of the cycle. Thus, by repeating the cycle again and again, all the glucose can

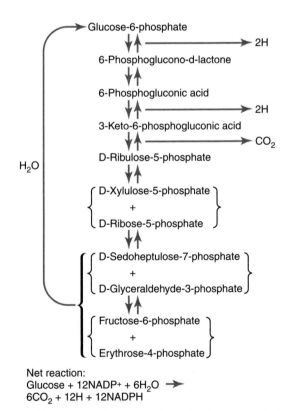

Net reaction:
Glucose + 12NADP$^+$ + 6H$_2$O $\longrightarrow$
6CO$_2$ + 12H + 12NADPH

Figure 67-8 Pentose phosphate pathway for glucose metabolism.

eventually be converted into carbon dioxide and hydrogen, and the hydrogen can enter the oxidative phosphorylation pathway to form ATP; more often, however, it is used for the synthesis of fat or other substances, as follows.

Use of Hydrogen to Synthesize Fat; the Function of Nicotinamide Adenine Dinucleotide Phosphate. The hydrogen released during the pentose phosphate cycle does not combine with NAD^+ as in the glycolytic pathway but combines with nicotinamide adenine dinucleotide phosphate ($NADP^+$), which is almost identical to NAD^+ except for an extra phosphate radical, P. This difference is extremely significant because only hydrogen bound with $NADP^+$ in the form of NADPH can be used for the synthesis of fats from carbohydrates (as discussed in Chapter 68) and for the synthesis of some other substances.

When the glycolytic pathway for using glucose becomes slowed because of cellular inactivity, the pentose phosphate pathway remains operative (mainly in the liver) to break down any excess glucose that continues to be transported into the cells, and NADPH becomes abundant to help convert acetyl-CoA, also derived from glucose, into long fatty acid chains. This is another way in which energy in the glucose molecule is used other than for the formation of ATP—in this instance, *for the formation and storage of fat in the body.*

Glucose Conversion to Glycogen or Fat

When glucose is not immediately required for energy, the extra glucose that continually enters the cells is either stored as glycogen or converted into fat. Glucose is preferentially stored as glycogen until the cells have stored as much glycogen as they can—an amount sufficient to supply the energy needs of the body for only 12 to 24 hours.

When the glycogen-storing cells (primarily liver and muscle cells) approach saturation with glycogen, the additional glucose is converted into fat in liver and fat cells and is stored as fat in the fat cells. Other steps in the chemistry of this conversion are discussed in Chapter 68.

Formation of Carbohydrates from Proteins and Fats—"Gluconeogenesis"

When the body's stores of carbohydrates decrease below normal, moderate quantities of glucose can be formed from *amino acids* and the *glycerol* portion of fat. This process is called *gluconeogenesis.*

Gluconeogenesis is especially important in preventing an excessive reduction in the blood glucose concentration during fasting. Glucose is the primary substrate for energy in tissues such as the brain and the red blood cells, and adequate amounts of glucose must be present in the blood for several hours between meals. The liver plays a key role in maintaining blood glucose levels during fasting by converting its stored glycogen to glucose (glycogenolysis) and by synthesizing glucose, mainly from lactate and amino acids (gluconeogenesis). Approximately 25 percent of the liver's glucose production during fasting is from gluconeogenesis, helping to provide a steady supply of glucose to the brain. During prolonged fasting, the kidneys also synthesize considerable amounts of glucose from amino acids and other precursors.

About 60 percent of the amino acids in the body proteins can be converted easily into carbohydrates; the remaining 40 percent have chemical configurations that make this difficult or impossible. Each amino acid is converted into glucose by a slightly different chemical process. For instance, alanine can be converted directly into pyruvic acid simply by deamination; the pyruvic acid is then converted into glucose or stored glycogen. Several of the more complicated amino acids can be converted into different sugars that contain three-, four-, five-, or seven-carbon atoms; they can then enter the phosphogluconate pathway and eventually form glucose. Thus, by means of deamination plus several simple interconversions, many of the amino acids can become glucose. Similar interconversions can change glycerol into glucose or glycogen.

Regulation of Gluconeogenesis. Diminished carbohydrates in the cells and decreased blood sugar are the basic stimuli that increase the rate of gluconeogenesis. Diminished carbohydrates can directly reverse many of the glycolytic and phosphogluconate reactions, thus allowing the conversion of deaminated amino acids and glycerol into carbohydrates. In addition, the hormone *cortisol* is especially important in this regulation, as follows.

Effect of Corticotropin and Glucocorticoids on Gluconeogenesis. When normal quantities of carbohydrates are not available to the cells, the adenohypophysis, for reasons not completely understood, begins to secrete increased quantities of the hormone *corticotropin*. This stimulates the adrenal cortex to produce large quantities of *glucocorticoid hormones*, especially *cortisol*. In turn, cortisol mobilizes proteins from essentially all cells of the body, making these available in the form of amino acids in the body fluids. A high proportion of these immediately become deaminated in the liver and provide ideal substrates for conversion into glucose. Thus, one of the most important means by which gluconeogenesis is promoted is through the release of glucocorticoids from the adrenal cortex.

Blood Glucose

The normal blood glucose concentration in a person who has not eaten a meal within the past 3 to 4 hours is about 90 mg/dl. After a meal containing large amounts of carbohydrates, this level seldom rises above 140 mg/dl unless the person has diabetes mellitus, which is discussed in Chapter 78.

The regulation of blood glucose concentration is intimately related to the pancreatic hormones insulin and glucagon; this subject is discussed in detail in Chapter 78 in relation to the functions of these hormones.

Bibliography

Barthel A, Schmoll D: Novel concepts in insulin regulation of hepatic gluconeogenesis, *Am J Physiol Endocrinol Metab* 285:E685, 2003.

Ceulemans H, Bollen M: Functional diversity of protein phosphatase-1, a cellular economizer and reset button, *Physiol Rev* 84:1, 2004.

Ferrer JC, Favre C, Gomis RR, et al: Control of glycogen deposition, *FEBS Lett* 546:127, 2003.

Gunter TE, Yule DI, Gunter KK, et al: Calcium and mitochondria, *FEBS Lett* 567:96, 2004.

Jackson JB: Proton translocation by transhydrogenase, *FEBS Lett* 545:18, 2003.

Jiang G, Zhang BB: Glucagon and regulation of glucose metabolism, *Am J Physiol Endocrinol Metab* 284:E671, 2003.

Krebs HA: The tricarboxylic acid cycle, *Harvey Lect* 44:165, 1948–1949.

Kunji ER: The role and structure of mitochondrial carriers, *FEBS Lett* 564:239, 2004.

Lam TK, Carpentier A, Lewis GF, et al: Mechanisms of the free fatty acid-induced increase in hepatic glucose production, *Am J Physiol Endocrinol Metab* 284:E863, 2003.

Mills DA, Ferguson-Miller S: Understanding the mechanism of proton movement linked to oxygen reduction in cytochrome c oxidase: lessons from other proteins, *FEBS Lett* 545:47, 2003.

Murphy MP: How mitochondria produce reactive oxygen species, *Biochem J* 417:1, 2009.

Navarro A, Boveris A: The mitochondrial energy transduction system and the aging process, *Am J Physiol Cell Physiol* 292:C670, 2007.

Pilkis SJ, Granner DK: Molecular physiology of the regulation of hepatic gluconeogenesis and glycolysis, *Annu Rev Physiol* 54:885, 1992.

Riddell MC: The endocrine response and substrate utilization during exercise in children and adolescents, *J Appl Physiol* 105:725, 2008.

Roden M, Bernroider E: Hepatic glucose metabolism in humans—its role in health and disease, *Best Pract Res Clin Endocrinol Metab* 17:365, 2003.

Starkov AA: The role of mitochondria in reactive oxygen species metabolism and signaling, *Ann N Y Acad Sci* 1147:37, 2008.

Wahren J, Ekberg K: Splanchnic regulation of glucose production, *Annu Rev Nutr* 27:329, 2007.

Lipid Metabolism

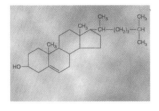

Several chemical compounds in food and in the body are classified as *lipids*. They include (1) *neutral fat*, also known as *triglycerides;* (2) *phospholipids;* (3) *cholesterol;* and (4) a few others of less importance. Chemically, the basic lipid moiety of the triglycerides and the phospholipids is *fatty acids*, which are long-chain hydrocarbon organic acids. A typical fatty acid, palmitic acid, is the following: $CH_3(CH_2)_{14}COOH$.

Although cholesterol does not contain fatty acid, its sterol nucleus is synthesized from portions of fatty acid molecules, thus giving it many of the physical and chemical properties of other lipid substances.

The triglycerides are used in the body mainly to provide energy for the different metabolic processes, a function they share almost equally with the carbohydrates. However, some lipids, especially cholesterol, the phospholipids, and small amounts of triglycerides, are used to form the membranes of all cells of the body and to perform other cellular functions.

Basic Chemical Structure of Triglycerides (Neutral Fat). Because most of this chapter deals with the utilization of triglycerides for energy, the following typical structure of the triglyceride molecule should be understood.

$$CH_3-(CH_2)_{16}-COO-CH_2$$
$$|$$
$$CH_3-(CH_2)_{16}-COO-CH$$
$$|$$
$$CH_3-(CH_2)_{16}-COO-CH_2$$

Tristearin

Note that three long-chain fatty acid molecules are bound with one molecule of glycerol. The three fatty acids most commonly present in the triglycerides of the human body are (1) *stearic acid* (shown in the tristearin example), which has an 18-carbon chain and is fully saturated with hydrogen atoms; (2) *oleic acid*, which also has an 18-carbon chain but has one double bond in the middle of the chain; and (3) *palmitic acid*, which has 16 carbon atoms and is fully saturated.

Transport of Lipids in the Body Fluids

Transport of Triglycerides and Other Lipids from the Gastrointestinal Tract by Lymph—the Chylomicrons

As explained in Chapter 65, almost all the fats in the diet, with the principal exception of a few short-chain fatty acids, are absorbed from the intestines into the intestinal lymph. During digestion, most triglycerides are split into monoglycerides and fatty acids. Then, while passing through the intestinal epithelial cells, the monoglycerides and fatty acids are resynthesized into new molecules of triglycerides that enter the lymph as minute, dispersed droplets called *chylomicrons* (Figure 68-1), whose diameters are between 0.08 and 0.6 micron. A small amount of *apoprotein B* is adsorbed to the outer surfaces of the chylomicrons. This leaves the remainder of the protein molecules projecting into the surrounding water and thereby increases the suspension stability of the chylomicrons in the lymph fluid and prevents their adherence to the lymphatic vessel walls.

Most of the cholesterol and phospholipids absorbed from the gastrointestinal tract enter the chylomicrons. Thus, although the chylomicrons are composed principally of triglycerides, they also contain about 9 percent phospholipids, 3 percent cholesterol, and 1 percent apoprotein B. The chylomicrons are then transported upward through the thoracic duct and emptied into the circulating venous blood at the juncture of the jugular and subclavian veins.

Removal of the Chylomicrons from the Blood

About 1 hour after a meal that contains large quantities of fat, the chylomicron concentration in the plasma may rise to 1 to 2 percent of the total plasma, and because of the large size of the chylomicrons, the plasma appears turbid and sometimes yellow. However, the chylomicrons have a half-life of less than 1 hour, so the plasma becomes clear again within a few hours. The fat of the chylomicrons is removed mainly in the following way.

Chylomicron Triglycerides Are Hydrolyzed by Lipoprotein Lipase, and Fat Is Stored in Adipose Tissue. Most of the chylomicrons are removed from the circulating blood as they pass through the capillaries of

819

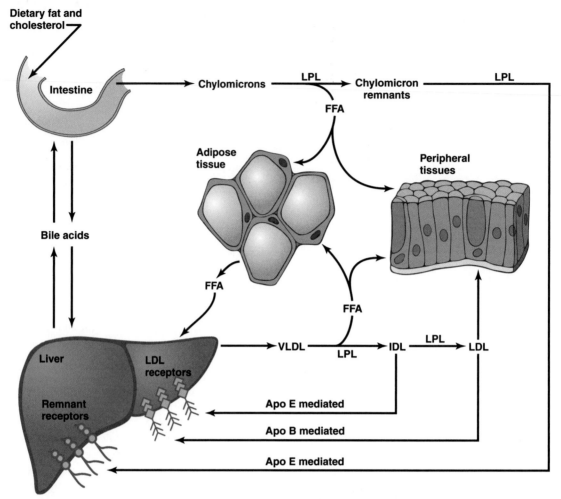

Figure 68-1 Summary of major pathways for metabolism of chylomicrons synthesized in the intestine and very low density lipoprotein (*VLDL*) synthesized in the liver. Apo B, apolipoprotein B; Apo E, apolipoprotein E; FFA, free fatty acids; HDL, high-density lipoprotein; IDL, intermediate-density lipoprotein; LDL, low-density lipoprotein; LPL, lipoprotein lipase.

various tissues, especially adipose tissue, skeletal muscle, and heart. These tissues synthesize the enzyme *lipoprotein lipase*, which is transported to the surface of capillary endothelial cells, where it hydrolyzes the triglycerides of chylomicrons as they come in contact with the endothelial wall, thus releasing fatty acids and glycerol (see Figure 68-1).

The fatty acids released from the chylomicrons, being highly miscible with the membranes of the cells, diffuse into the fat cells of the adipose tissue and muscle cells. Once inside these cells, the fatty acids can be used for fuel or again synthesized into triglycerides, with new glycerol being supplied by the metabolic processes of the storage cells, as discussed later in the chapter. The lipase also causes hydrolysis of phospholipids; this, too, releases fatty acids to be stored in the cells in the same way.

After the triglycerides are removed from the chylomicrons, the cholesterol-enriched *chylomicron remnants* are rapidly cleared from the plasma. The chylomicron remnants bind to receptors on endothelial cells in the liver sinusoids. *Apolipoprotein-E* on the surface of the chylomicron remnants and secreted by liver cells also plays an important role in initiating clearance of these plasma lipoproteins.

"Free Fatty Acids" Are Transported in the Blood in Combination with Albumin

When fat that has been stored in the adipose tissue is to be used elsewhere in the body to provide energy, it must first be transported from the adipose tissue to the other tissue. It is transported mainly in the form of *free fatty acids*. This is achieved by hydrolysis of the triglycerides back into fatty acids and glycerol.

At least two classes of stimuli play important roles in promoting this hydrolysis. First, when the amount of glucose available to the fat cell is inadequate, one of the glucose breakdown products, *α-glycerophosphate*, is also available in insufficient quantities. Because this substance is required to maintain the glycerol portion of triglycerides, the result is hydrolysis of triglycerides. Second, a *hormone-sensitive cellular lipase* can be activated by several hormones from the endocrine glands, and this also promotes rapid hydrolysis of triglycerides. This is discussed later in the chapter.

On leaving fat cells, fatty acids ionize strongly in the plasma and the ionic portion combines immediately with albumin molecules of the plasma proteins. Fatty acids bound in this manner are called *free fatty acids* or *nonesterified fatty acids*, to distinguish them from other fatty acids in the plasma that exist in the form of (1) esters of glycerol, (2) cholesterol, or (3) other substances.

The concentration of free fatty acids in the plasma under resting conditions is about 15 mg/dl, which is a total of only 0.45 gram of fatty acids in the entire circulatory system. Even this small amount accounts for almost all the transport of fatty acids from one part of the body to another for the following reasons:

1. Despite the minute amount of free fatty acid in the blood, its rate of "turnover" is extremely rapid: *half the plasma fatty acid is replaced by new fatty acid every 2 to 3 minutes*. One can calculate that at this rate, almost all the normal energy requirements of the body can be provided by the oxidation of transported free fatty acids, without using any carbohydrates or proteins for energy.

2. Conditions that increase the rate of utilization of fat for cellular energy also increase the free fatty acid concentration in the blood; in fact, the concentration sometimes increases fivefold to eightfold. Such a large increase occurs especially in cases of *starvation* and in *diabetes mellitus;* in both these conditions, the person derives little or no metabolic energy from carbohydrates.

Under normal conditions, only about 3 molecules of fatty acid combine with each molecule of albumin, but as many as 30 fatty acid molecules can combine with a single albumin molecule when the need for fatty acid transport is extreme. This shows how variable the rate of lipid transport can be under different physiologic conditions.

Lipoproteins—Their Special Function in Transporting Cholesterol and Phospholipids

In the postabsorptive state, after all the chylomicrons have been removed from the blood, more than 95 percent of all the lipids in the plasma are in the form of *lipoprotein.* These are small particles—much smaller than chylomicrons, but qualitatively similar in composition—containing *triglycerides, cholesterol, phospholipids*, and *protein.* The total concentration of lipoproteins in the plasma averages about 700 milligrams per 100 milliliters of plasma—that is, 700 mg/dl. This can be broken down into the following individual lipoprotein constituents:

	mg/dl of Plasma
Cholesterol	180
Phospholipids	160
Triglycerides	160
Protein	200

Types of Lipoproteins. Aside from the chylomicrons, which are themselves very large lipoproteins, there are four major types of lipoproteins, classified by their densities as measured in the ultracentrifuge: (1) *very low density lipoproteins (VLDLs),* which contain high concentrations of triglycerides and moderate concentrations of both cholesterol and phospholipids; (2) *intermediate-density lipoproteins (IDLs),* which are very low density lipoproteins from which a share of the triglycerides has been removed, so the concentrations of cholesterol and phospholipids are increased; (3) *low-density lipoproteins (LDLs),* which are derived from intermediate-density lipoproteins by the removal of almost all the triglycerides, leaving an especially high concentration of cholesterol and a moderately high concentration of phospholipids; and (4) *high-density lipoproteins (HDLs),* which contain a high concentration of protein (about

50 percent) but much smaller concentrations of cholesterol and phospholipids.

Formation and Function of Lipoproteins. Almost all the lipoproteins are formed in the liver, which is also where most of the plasma cholesterol, phospholipids, and triglycerides are synthesized. In addition, small quantities of HDLs are synthesized in the intestinal epithelium during the absorption of fatty acids from the intestines.

The primary function of the lipoproteins is to transport their lipid components in the blood. The VLDLs transport triglycerides synthesized in the liver mainly to the adipose tissue, whereas the other lipoproteins are especially important in the different stages of phospholipid and cholesterol transport from the liver to the peripheral tissues or from the periphery back to the liver. Later in the chapter, we discuss in more detail special problems of cholesterol transport in relation to the disease *atherosclerosis,* which is associated with the development of fatty lesions on the insides of arterial walls.

Fat Deposits

Adipose Tissue

Large quantities of fat are stored in two major tissues of the body, the *adipose tissue* and the *liver.* The adipose tissue is usually called *fat deposits*, or simply tissue fat.

The major function of adipose tissue is storage of triglycerides until they are needed to provide energy elsewhere in the body. A subsidiary function is to provide heat insulation for the body, as discussed in Chapter 73.

Fat Cells (Adipocytes). The fat cells (adipocytes) of adipose tissue are modified fibroblasts that store almost pure triglycerides in quantities as great as 80 to 95 percent of the entire cell volume. Triglycerides inside the fat cells are generally in a liquid form. When the tissues are exposed to prolonged cold, the fatty acid chains of the cell triglycerides, over a period of weeks, become either shorter or more unsaturated to decrease their melting point, thereby always allowing the fat to remain in a liquid state. This is particularly important because only liquid fat can be hydrolyzed and transported from the cells.

Fat cells can synthesize very small amounts of fatty acids and triglycerides from carbohydrates; this function supplements the synthesis of fat in the liver, as discussed later in the chapter.

Exchange of Fat Between the Adipose Tissue and the Blood—Tissue Lipases. As discussed earlier, large quantities of lipases are present in adipose tissue. Some of these enzymes catalyze the deposition of cell triglycerides from the chylomicrons and lipoproteins. Others, when activated by hormones, cause splitting of the triglycerides of the fat cells to release free fatty acids. Because of the rapid exchange of fatty acids, the triglycerides in fat cells are renewed about once every 2 to 3 weeks, which means that the fat stored in the tissues today is not the same fat that was stored last month, thus emphasizing the dynamic state of storage fat.

Liver Lipids

The principal functions of the liver in lipid metabolism are to (1) degrade fatty acids into small compounds that can be used for energy; (2) synthesize triglycerides, mainly from carbohydrates, but to a lesser extent from proteins as well; and

(3) synthesize other lipids from fatty acids, especially cholesterol and phospholipids.

Large quantities of triglycerides appear in the liver (1) during the early stages of starvation, (2) in diabetes mellitus, and (3) in any other condition in which fat instead of carbohydrates is being used for energy. In these conditions, large quantities of triglycerides are mobilized from the adipose tissue, transported as free fatty acids in the blood, and redeposited as triglycerides in the liver, where the initial stages of much of fat degradation begin. Thus, under normal physiological conditions, the total amount of triglycerides in the liver is determined to a great extent by the overall rate at which lipids are being used for energy.

The liver may also store large amounts of lipids in *lipodystrophy*, a condition characterized by atrophy or genetic deficiency of adipocytes.

The liver cells, in addition to containing triglycerides, contain large quantities of phospholipids and cholesterol, which are continually synthesized by the liver. Also, the liver cells are much more capable than other tissues of desaturating fatty acids, so liver triglycerides normally are much more unsaturated than the triglycerides of adipose tissue. This capability of the liver to desaturate fatty acids is functionally important to all tissues of the body because many structural elements of all cells contain reasonable quantities of unsaturated fats and their principal source is the liver. This desaturation is accomplished by a dehydrogenase in the liver cells.

Use of Triglycerides for Energy: Formation of Adenosine Triphosphate

The dietary intake of fat varies considerably in persons of different cultures, averaging as little as 10 to 15 percent of caloric intake in some Asian populations to as much as 35 to 50 percent of the calories in many Western populations. For many persons the use of fats for energy is therefore as important as the use of carbohydrates is. In addition, many of the carbohydrates ingested with each meal are converted into triglycerides, then stored, and used later in the form of fatty acids released from the triglycerides for energy.

Hydrolysis of Triglycerides. The first stage in using triglycerides for energy is their hydrolysis into fatty acids and glycerol. Then, both the fatty acids and the glycerol are transported in the blood to the active tissues, where they will be oxidized to give energy. Almost all cells—with some exceptions, such as brain tissue and red blood cells—can use fatty acids for energy.

Glycerol, on entering the active tissue, is immediately changed by intracellular enzymes into *glycerol-3-phosphate*, which enters the glycolytic pathway for glucose breakdown and is thus used for energy. Before the fatty acids can be used for energy, they must be processed further in the following way.

Entry of Fatty Acids into Mitochondria. Degradation and oxidation of fatty acids occur only in the mitochondria. Therefore, the first step for the use of fatty acids is their transport into the mitochondria. This is a carrier-mediated process that uses *carnitine* as the carrier substance. Once inside the mitochondria, fatty acids split away from carnitine and are degraded and oxidized.

Degradation of Fatty Acids to Acetyl Coenzyme A by Beta-Oxidation. The fatty acid molecule is degraded in the mitochondria by progressive release of two-carbon segments in the form of *acetyl coenzyme A (acetyl-CoA)*. This process, which is shown in Figure 68-2, is called the *beta-oxidation* process for degradation of fatty acids.

To understand the essential steps in the beta-oxidation process, note that in equation 1 the first step is combination of the fatty acid molecule with coenzyme A (CoA) to form fatty acyl-CoA. In equations 2, 3, and 4, the *beta carbon* (the second carbon from the right) of the fatty acyl-CoA binds with an oxygen molecule—that is, the beta carbon becomes oxidized.

Then, in equation 5, the right-hand two-carbon portion of the molecule is split off to release acetyl-CoA into the cell fluid. At the same time, another CoA molecule binds at the end of the remaining portion of the fatty acid molecule, and this forms a new fatty acyl-CoA molecule; this time, however, the molecule is two carbon atoms shorter because of the loss of the first acetyl-CoA from its terminal end.

Next, this shorter fatty acyl-CoA enters into equation 2 and progresses through equations 3, 4, and 5 to release still another acetyl-CoA molecule, thus shortening the original fatty acid molecule by another two carbons. In addition to the released acetyl-CoA molecules, four atoms of hydrogen are released from the fatty acid molecule at the same time, entirely separate from the acetyl-CoA.

Oxidation of Acetyl-CoA. The acetyl-CoA molecules formed by beta-oxidation of fatty acids in the mitochondria enter immediately into the *citric acid cycle* (see

$$\text{(1) } RCH_2CH_2CH_2COOH + CoA + ATP \xrightleftharpoons{\text{Thiokinase}} RCH_2CH_2CH_2COCoA + AMP + Pyrophosphate$$
$$\text{(Fatty acid)} \qquad\qquad \text{(Fatty acyl-CoA)}$$

$$\text{(2) } RCH_2CH_2CH_2COCoA + FAD \xrightarrow{\text{Acyl dehydrogenase}} RCH_2CH=CHCOCoA + FADH_2$$
$$\text{(Fatty acyl-CoA)}$$

$$\text{(3) } RCH_2CH=CHCOCoA + H_2O \xrightleftharpoons{\text{Enoyl hydrase}} RCH_2CHOHCH_2COCoA$$

$$\text{(4) } RCH_2CHOHCH_2COCoA + NAD^+ \xrightleftharpoons[\text{dehydrogenase}]{\beta\text{-Hydroxyacyl}} RCH_2COCH_2COCoA + NADH + H^+$$

$$\text{(5) } RCH_2COCH_2COCoA + CoA \xrightleftharpoons{\text{Thiolase}} RCH_2COCoA + CH_3COCoA$$
$$\text{(Fatty acyl-CoA) (Acetyl-CoA)}$$

Figure 68-2 Beta-oxidation of fatty acids to yield acetyl coenzyme A.

Chapter 67), combining first with oxaloacetic acid to form citric acid, which then is degraded into carbon dioxide and hydrogen atoms. The hydrogen is subsequently oxidized by the *chemiosmotic oxidative system of the mitochondria*, which was also explained in Chapter 67. The net reaction in the citric acid cycle for each molecule of acetyl-CoA is the following:

$$CH_3COCoA + \text{Oxaloacetic acid} + 3H_2O + ADP$$

$$\xrightarrow{\text{Citric acid cycle}}$$

$$2CO_2 + 8H + HCoA + ATP + \text{Oxaloacetic acid}$$

Thus, after initial degradation of fatty acids to acetyl-CoA, their final breakdown is precisely the same as that of the acetyl-CoA formed from pyruvic acid during the metabolism of glucose. And the extra hydrogen atoms are also oxidized by the same *chemiosmotic oxidative system of the mitochondria* that is used in carbohydrate oxidation, liberating large amounts of adenosine triphosphate (ATP).

Large Amounts of ATP Are Formed by Oxidation of Fatty Acids. In Figure 68-2, note that the four separate hydrogen atoms released each time a molecule of acetyl-CoA is split from the fatty acid chain are released in the forms $FADH_2$, NADH, and H^+. Therefore, for every stearic fatty acid molecule that is split to form 9 acetyl-CoA molecules, 32 extra hydrogen atoms are removed. In addition, for each of the 9 molecules of acetyl-CoA that are subsequently degraded by the citric acid cycle, 8 more hydrogen atoms are removed, making another 72 hydrogens. This makes a total of 104 hydrogen atoms eventually released by the degradation of each stearic acid molecule. Of this group, 34 are removed from the degrading fatty acids by flavoproteins, and 70 are removed by nicotinamide adenine dinucleotide (NAD^+) as NADH and H^+.

These two groups of hydrogen atoms are oxidized in the mitochondria, as discussed in Chapter 67, but they enter the oxidative system at different points. Therefore, 1 molecule of ATP is synthesized for each of the 34 flavoprotein hydrogens, and 1.5 molecules of ATP are synthesized for each of the 70 NADH and H^+ hydrogens. This makes 34 plus 105, or a total of 139 molecules of ATP formed by the oxidation of hydrogen derived from each molecule of stearic acid. Another nine molecules of ATP are formed in the citric acid cycle itself (separate from the ATP released by the oxidation of hydrogen), one for each of the nine acetyl-CoA molecules metabolized. Thus, a total of 148 molecules of ATP are formed during the complete oxidation of 1 molecule of stearic acid. However, two high-energy bonds are consumed in the initial combination of CoA with the stearic acid molecule, making a *net gain* of 146 molecules of ATP.

Formation of Acetoacetic Acid in the Liver and Its Transport in the Blood

A large share of the initial degradation of fatty acids occurs in the liver, especially when excessive amounts of lipids are being used for energy. However, the liver uses only a small proportion of the fatty acids for its own intrinsic metabolic processes. Instead, when the fatty acid chains have been split into acetyl-CoA, two molecules of acetyl-CoA condense to form one molecule of acetoacetic acid, which is then transported in the blood to the other cells throughout the body, where it is used for energy. The chemical processes are the following:

$$2CH_3COCoA + H_2O \underset{\text{other cells}}{\overset{\text{liver cells}}{\rightleftharpoons}}$$

Acetyl-CoA

$$CH_3COCH_2COOH + 2HCoA$$

Acetoacetic acid

Part of the acetoacetic acid is also converted into *β-hydroxybutyric acid*, and minute quantities are converted into *acetone* in accord with the following reactions:

The acetoacetic acid, β-hydroxybutyric acid, and acetone diffuse freely through the liver cell membranes and are transported by the blood to the peripheral tissues. Here they again diffuse into the cells, where reverse reactions occur and acetyl-CoA molecules are formed. These in turn enter the citric acid cycle and are oxidized for energy, as already explained.

Normally, the acetoacetic acid and β-hydroxybutyric acid that enter the blood are transported so rapidly to the tissues that their combined concentration in the plasma seldom rises above 3 mg/dl. Yet, despite this small *concentration* in the blood, large *quantities* are actually transported, as is also true for free fatty acid transport. The rapid transport of both these substances results from their high solubility in the membranes of the target cells, which allows almost instantaneous diffusion into the cells.

Ketosis in Starvation, Diabetes, and Other Diseases. The concentrations of acetoacetic acid, β-hydroxybutyric acid, and acetone occasionally rise to levels many times normal in the blood and interstitial fluids; this condition is called *ketosis* because acetoacetic acid is a keto acid. The three compounds are called *ketone bodies*. Ketosis occurs especially in starvation, in diabetes mellitus, and sometimes even when a person's diet is composed almost entirely of fat. In all these states, essentially no carbohydrates are metabolized—in starvation and with a high-fat diet because carbohydrates are not available, and in diabetes because insulin is not available to cause glucose transport into the cells.

When carbohydrates are not used for energy, almost all the energy of the body must come from metabolism of fats. We shall see later in the chapter that the unavailability of carbohydrates automatically increases the rate of removal of fatty acids from adipose tissues; in addition, several hormonal factors—such as increased secretion of glucocorticoids by the adrenal cortex, increased secretion of glucagon by the pancreas, and decreased secretion of insulin by the pancreas—further enhance the removal of fatty acids from the fat tissues. As a result, tremendous quantities of fatty acids become available (1) to the peripheral tissue cells to be used for energy and (2) to the liver cells, where much of the fatty acid is converted to ketone bodies.

823

The ketone bodies pour out of the liver to be carried to the cells. For several reasons, the cells are limited in the amount of ketone bodies that can be oxidized; the most important reason is the following: One of the products of carbohydrate metabolism is the *oxaloacetate* that is required to bind with acetyl-CoA before it can be processed in the citric acid cycle. Therefore, deficiency of oxaloacetate derived from carbohydrates limits the entry of acetyl-CoA into the citric acid cycle, and when there is a simultaneous outpouring of large quantities of acetoacetic acid and other ketone bodies from the liver, the blood concentrations of acetoacetic acid and β-hydroxybutyric acid sometimes rise to as high as 20 times normal, thus leading to extreme acidosis, as explained in Chapter 30.

The acetone that is formed during ketosis is a volatile substance, some of which is blown off in small quantities in the expired air of the lungs. This gives the breath an acetone smell that is frequently used as a diagnostic criterion of ketosis.

Adaptation to a High-Fat Diet. When changing slowly from a carbohydrate diet to an almost completely fat diet, a person's body adapts to use far more acetoacetic acid than usual, and in this instance, ketosis normally does not occur. For instance, the Inuit (Eskimos), who sometimes live mainly on a fat diet, do not develop ketosis. Undoubtedly, several factors, none of which is clear, enhance the rate of acetoacetic acid metabolism by the cells. After a few weeks, even the brain cells, which normally derive almost all their energy from glucose, can derive 50 to 75 percent of their energy from fats.

Synthesis of Triglycerides from Carbohydrates

Whenever a greater quantity of carbohydrates enters the body than can be used immediately for energy or can be stored in the form of glycogen, the excess is rapidly converted into triglycerides and stored in this form in the adipose tissue.

In human beings, most triglyceride synthesis occurs in the liver, but minute quantities are also synthesized in the adipose tissue itself. The triglycerides formed in the liver are transported mainly in VLDLs to the adipose tissue, where they are stored.

Conversion of Acetyl-CoA into Fatty Acids. The first step in the synthesis of triglycerides is conversion of carbohydrates into acetyl-CoA. As explained in Chapter 67, this occurs during the normal degradation of glucose by the glycolytic system. Because fatty acids are actually large polymers of acetic acid, it is easy to understand how acetyl-CoA can be converted into fatty acids. However, the synthesis of fatty acids from acetyl-CoA is not achieved by simply reversing the oxidative degradation described earlier. Instead, this occurs by the two-step process shown in Figure 68-3, using *malonyl-CoA* and NADPH as the principal intermediates in the polymerization process.

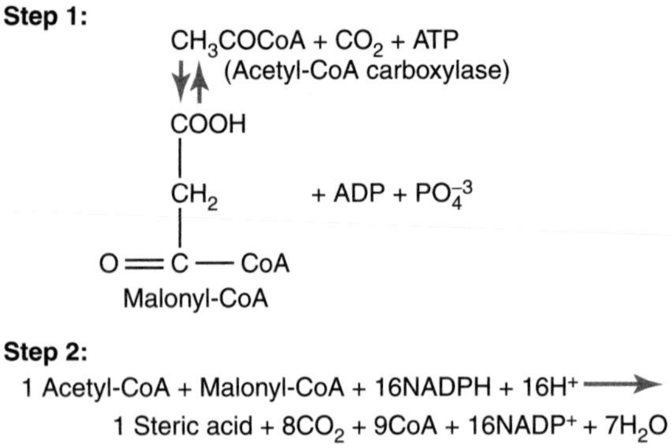

Step 1:

$$CH_3COCoA + CO_2 + ATP$$
(Acetyl-CoA carboxylase)

$$\begin{array}{c} COOH \\ | \\ CH_2 \qquad + ADP + PO_4^{-3} \\ | \\ O{=}C{-}CoA \end{array}$$
Malonyl-CoA

Step 2:

1 Acetyl-CoA + Malonyl-CoA + 16NADPH + 16H$^+$ $\longrightarrow$
1 Steric acid + 8CO$_2$ + 9CoA + 16NADP$^+$ + 7H$_2$O

Figure 68-3 Synthesis of fatty acids.

Combination of Fatty Acids with α-Glycerophosphate to Form Triglycerides. Once the synthesized fatty acid chains have grown to contain 14 to 18 carbon atoms, they bind with glycerol to form triglycerides. The enzymes that cause this conversion are highly specific for fatty acids with chain lengths of 14 carbon atoms or greater, a factor that controls the physical quality of the triglycerides stored in the body.

As shown in Figure 68-4, the glycerol portion of triglycerides is furnished by α-glycerophosphate, which is another product derived from the glycolytic scheme of glucose degradation. This mechanism is discussed in Chapter 67.

Efficiency of Carbohydrate Conversion into Fat.

During triglyceride synthesis, only about 15 percent of the original energy in the glucose is lost in the form of heat; the remaining 85 percent is transferred to the stored triglycerides.

Importance of Fat Synthesis and Storage. Fat synthesis from carbohydrates is especially important for two reasons:

1. The ability of the different cells of the body to store carbohydrates in the form of glycogen is generally slight; a maximum of only a few hundred grams of glycogen can be stored in the liver, the skeletal muscles, and all other tissues of the body put together. In contrast, many kilograms of fat can be stored in adipose tissue. Therefore, fat synthesis provides a means by which the energy of excess ingested carbohydrates (and proteins) can be stored for later use. Indeed, the average person has almost 150 times as much energy stored in the form of fat as stored in the form of carbohydrate.

2. Each gram of fat contains almost two and a half times the calories of energy contained by each gram of glycogen. Therefore, for a given weight gain, a person can store several times as much energy in the form of fat as in the form

Figure 68-4 Overall schema for synthesis of triglycerides from glucose.

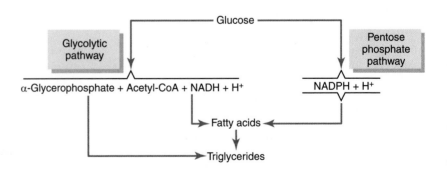

of carbohydrate, which is exceedingly important when an animal must be highly motile to survive.

Failure to Synthesize Fats from Carbohydrates in the Absence of Insulin. When insufficient insulin is available, as occurs in serious diabetes mellitus, fats are poorly synthesized, if at all, for the following reasons: First, when insulin is not available, glucose does not enter the fat and liver cells satisfactorily, so little of the acetyl-CoA and NADPH needed for fat synthesis can be derived from glucose. Second, lack of glucose in the fat cells greatly reduces the availability of α-glycerophosphate, which also makes it difficult for the tissues to form triglycerides.

Synthesis of Triglycerides from Proteins

Many amino acids can be converted into acetyl-CoA, as discussed in Chapter 69. The acetyl-CoA can then be synthesized into triglycerides. Therefore, when people have more proteins in their diets than their tissues can use as proteins, a large share of the excess is stored as fat.

Regulation of Energy Release from Triglycerides

Carbohydrates Are Preferred over Fats for Energy When Excess Carbohydrates Are Available. When excess quantities of carbohydrates are available in the body, carbohydrates are used preferentially over triglycerides for energy. There are several reasons for this "fat-sparing" effect of carbohydrates. One of the most important is the following: The fats in adipose tissue cells are present in two forms: stored triglycerides and small quantities of free fatty acids. They are in constant equilibrium with each other. When excess quantities of α-*glycerophosphate* are present (which occurs when excess carbohydrates are available), the excess α-glycerophosphate binds the free fatty acids in the form of stored triglycerides. As a result, the equilibrium between free fatty acids and triglycerides shifts toward the stored triglycerides; consequently, only minute quantities of fatty acids are available to be used for energy. Because α-glycerophosphate is an important product of glucose metabolism, the availability of large amounts of glucose automatically inhibits the use of fatty acids for energy.

Second, when carbohydrates are available in excess, fatty acids are synthesized more rapidly than they are degraded. This effect is caused partially by the large quantities of acetyl-CoA formed from the carbohydrates and by the low concentration of free fatty acids in the adipose tissue, thus creating conditions appropriate for the conversion of acetyl-CoA into fatty acids.

An even more important effect that promotes the conversion of carbohydrates to fats is the following: The first step, which is the rate-limiting step, in the synthesis of fatty acids is carboxylation of acetyl-CoA to form malonyl-CoA. The rate of this reaction is controlled primarily by the enzyme *acetyl-CoA carboxylase*, the activity of which is accelerated in the presence of intermediates of the citric acid cycle. When excess carbohydrates are being used, these intermediates increase, automatically causing increased synthesis of fatty acids.

Thus, an excess of carbohydrates in the diet not only acts as a fat-sparer but also increases fat stores. In fact, all the excess carbohydrates not used for energy or stored in the small glycogen deposits of the body are converted to fat for storage.

Acceleration of Fat Utilization for Energy in the Absence of Carbohydrates. All the fat-sparing effects of carbohydrates are lost and actually reversed when carbohydrates are not available. The equilibrium shifts in the opposite direction, and fat is mobilized from the adipose cells and used for energy in place of carbohydrates.

Also important are several hormonal changes that take place to promote rapid fatty acid mobilization from adipose tissue. Among the most important of these is a marked decrease in pancreatic secretion of insulin caused by the absence of carbohydrates. This not only reduces the rate of glucose utilization by the tissues but also decreases fat storage, which further shifts the equilibrium in favor of fat metabolism in place of carbohydrates.

Hormonal Regulation of Fat Utilization. At least seven of the hormones secreted by the endocrine glands have significant effects on fat utilization. Some important hormonal effects on fat metabolism—in addition to *insulin lack*, discussed in the previous paragraph—are noted here.

Probably the most dramatic increase that occurs in fat utilization is that observed during heavy exercise. This results almost entirely from release of *epinephrine* and *norepinephrine* by the adrenal medullae during exercise, as a result of sympathetic stimulation. These two hormones directly activate *hormone-sensitive triglyceride lipase*, which is present in abundance in the fat cells, and this causes rapid breakdown of triglycerides and mobilization of fatty acids. Sometimes the free fatty acid concentration in the blood of an exercising person rises as much as eightfold, and the use of these fatty acids by the muscles for energy is correspondingly increased. Other types of stress that activate the sympathetic nervous system can also increase fatty acid mobilization and utilization in a similar manner.

Stress also causes large quantities of *corticotropin* to be released by the anterior pituitary gland, and this causes the adrenal cortex to secrete extra quantities of *glucocorticoids*. Both corticotropin and glucocorticoids activate either the same hormone-sensitive triglyceride lipase as that activated by epinephrine and norepinephrine or a similar lipase. When corticotropin and glucocorticoids are secreted in excessive amounts for long periods, as occurs in the endocrine condition called Cushing's syndrome, fats are frequently mobilized to such a great extent that ketosis results. Corticotropin and glucocorticoids are then said to have a *ketogenic effect*. *Growth hormone* has an effect similar to but weaker than that of corticotropin and glucocorticoids in activating hormone-sensitive lipase. Therefore, growth hormone can also have a mild ketogenic effect.

Finally, *thyroid hormone* causes rapid mobilization of fat, which is believed to result indirectly from an increased overall rate of energy metabolism in all cells of the body under the influence of this hormone. The resulting reduction in acetyl-CoA and other intermediates of both fat and carbohydrate metabolism in the cells is a stimulus to fat mobilization.

The effects of the different hormones on metabolism are discussed further in the chapters dealing with each hormone.

Obesity

Obesity means deposition of excess fat in the body. This subject is discussed in Chapter 71 in relation to dietary balances, but briefly, it is caused by the ingestion of greater amounts of food than can be used by the body for energy. The excess food, whether fats, carbohydrates, or proteins, is then stored almost entirely as fat in the adipose tissue, to be used later for energy.

Several strains of rodents have been found in which *hereditary obesity* occurs. In at least one of these, the obesity is caused by ineffective mobilization of fat from the adipose tissue by tissue lipase, while synthesis and storage of fat continue normally. Such a one-way process causes progressive enhancement of the fat stores, resulting in severe obesity.

Phospholipids and Cholesterol

Phospholipids

The major types of body phospholipids are *lecithins, cephalins,* and *sphingomyelin;* their typical chemical formulas are shown in Figure 68-5. Phospholipids always contain one or more fatty acid molecules and one phosphoric acid radical, and they usually contain a nitrogenous base. Although the chemical structures of phospholipids are somewhat variant, their physical properties are similar because they are all lipid soluble, transported in lipoproteins, and used throughout the body for various structural purposes, such as in cell membranes and intracellular membranes.

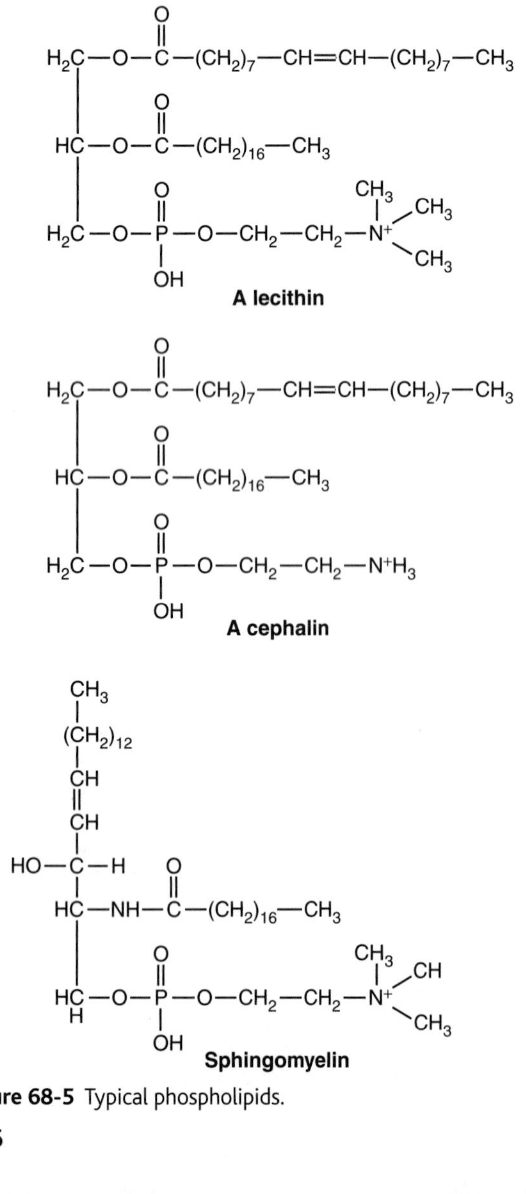

Formation of Phospholipids. Phospholipids are synthesized in essentially all cells of the body, although certain cells have a special ability to form great quantities of them. Probably 90 percent are formed in the liver cells; substantial quantities are also formed by the intestinal epithelial cells during lipid absorption from the gut.

The rate of phospholipid formation is governed to some extent by the usual factors that control the overall rate of fat metabolism because, when triglycerides are deposited in the liver, the rate of phospholipid formation increases. Also, certain specific chemical substances are needed for the formation of some phospholipids. For instance, *choline,* either obtained in the diet or synthesized in the body, is necessary for the formation of lecithin, because choline is the nitrogenous base of the lecithin molecule. Also, *inositol* is necessary for the formation of some cephalins.

Specific Uses of Phospholipids. Several functions of the phospholipids are the following: (1) Phospholipids are an important constituent of lipoproteins in the blood and are essential for the formation and function of most of these; in their absence, serious abnormalities of transport of cholesterol and other lipids can occur. (2) Thromboplastin, which is necessary to initiate the clotting process, is composed mainly of one of the cephalins. (3) Large quantities of sphingomyelin are present in the nervous system; this substance acts as an electrical insulator in the myelin sheath around nerve fibers. (4) Phospholipids are donors of phosphate radicals when these radicals are necessary for different chemical reactions in the tissues. (5) Perhaps the most important of all the functions of phospholipids is participation in the formation of structural elements—mainly membranes—in cells throughout the body, as discussed in the next section of this chapter in connection with a similar function for cholesterol.

Cholesterol

Cholesterol, the formula of which is shown in Figure 68-6, is present in the diets of all people, and it can be absorbed slowly from the gastrointestinal tract into the intestinal lymph. It is highly fat soluble but only slightly soluble in water. It is specifically capable of forming esters with fatty acids. Indeed, about 70 percent of the cholesterol in the lipoproteins of the plasma is in the form of cholesterol esters.

Formation of Cholesterol. Besides the cholesterol absorbed each day from the gastrointestinal tract, which is called *exogenous cholesterol,* an even greater quantity is formed in the cells of the body, called *endogenous cholesterol.* Essentially all the endogenous cholesterol that circulates in the lipoproteins of the plasma is formed by the liver, but all other cells of the body form at least some cholesterol, which is consistent with the fact that many of the membranous structures of all cells are partially composed of this substance.

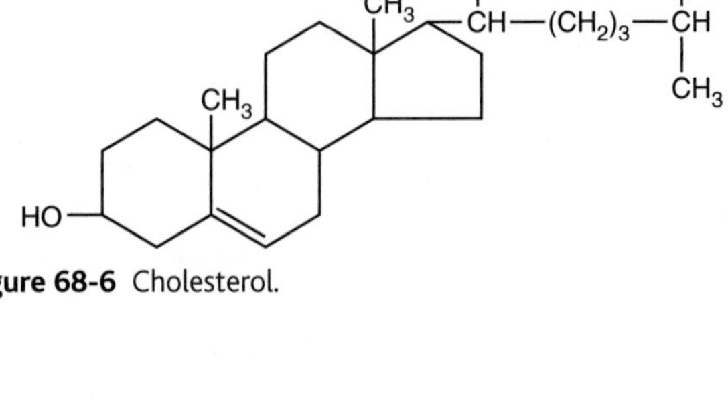

Figure 68-5 Typical phospholipids.

Figure 68-6 Cholesterol.

The basic structure of cholesterol is a sterol nucleus. This is synthesized entirely from multiple molecules of acetyl-CoA. In turn, the sterol nucleus can be modified by means of various side chains to form (1) cholesterol; (2) cholic acid, which is the basis of the bile acids formed in the liver; and (3) many important steroid hormones secreted by the adrenal cortex, the ovaries, and the testes (these hormones are discussed in later chapters).

Factors That Affect Plasma Cholesterol Concentration—Feedback Control of Body Cholesterol. Among the important factors that affect plasma cholesterol concentration are the following:

1. An increase in the *amount of cholesterol ingested each day* increases the plasma concentration slightly. However, when cholesterol is ingested, the rising concentration of cholesterol inhibits the most essential enzyme for endogenous synthesis of cholesterol, 3-hydroxy-3-methylglutaryl CoA reductase, thus providing an intrinsic feedback control system to prevent an excessive increase in plasma cholesterol concentration. As a result, plasma cholesterol concentration *usually* is not changed upward or downward more than ±15 percent by altering the amount of cholesterol in the diet, although the response of individuals differs markedly.

2. A *highly saturated fat* diet increases blood cholesterol concentration 15 to 25 percent, especially when this is associated with excess weight gain and obesity. This results from increased fat deposition in the liver, which then provides increased quantities of acetyl-CoA in the liver cells for the production of cholesterol. Therefore, to decrease the blood cholesterol concentration, it is usually just as important, if not more important, to maintain a diet low in saturated fat as to maintain a diet low in cholesterol.

3. Ingestion of fat containing highly *unsaturated fatty acids* usually depresses the blood cholesterol concentration a slight to moderate amount. The mechanism of this effect is unknown, despite the fact that this observation is the basis of much present-day dietary strategy.

4. *Lack of insulin* or *thyroid hormone* increases the blood cholesterol concentration, whereas excess thyroid hormone decreases the concentration. These effects are probably caused mainly by changes in the degree of activation of specific enzymes responsible for the metabolism of lipid substances.

5. *Genetic disorders* of cholesterol metabolism may greatly increase plasma cholesterol levels. For example, mutations of the *LDL receptor* gene prevent the liver from adequately removing the cholesterol-rich LDLs from the plasma. As discussed later, this causes the liver to produce excessive amounts of cholesterol. Mutations of the gene that encodes *apolipoprotein B*, the part of the LDL that binds to the receptor, also cause excessive cholesterol production by the liver.

Specific Uses of Cholesterol in the Body. By far the most abundant nonmembranous use of cholesterol in the body is to form cholic acid in the liver. As much as 80 percent of cholesterol is converted into cholic acid. As explained in Chapter 70, this is conjugated with other substances to form bile salts, which promote digestion and absorption of fats.

A small quantity of cholesterol is used by (1) the adrenal glands to form *adrenocortical hormones*, (2) the ovaries to form *progesterone* and *estrogen*, and (3) the testes to form *testosterone*. These glands can also synthesize their own sterols and then form hormones from them, as discussed in the chapters on endocrinology.

A large amount of cholesterol is precipitated in the corneum of the skin. This, along with other lipids, makes the skin highly resistant to the absorption of water-soluble substances and to the action of many chemical agents because cholesterol and the other skin lipids are highly inert to acids and to many solvents that might otherwise easily penetrate the body. Also, these lipid substances help prevent water evaporation from the skin; without this protection, the amount of evaporation can be 5 to 10 liters per day (as occurs in burn patients who have lost their skin) instead of the usual 300 to 400 milliliters.

Cellular Structural Functions of Phospholipids and Cholesterol—Especially for Membranes

The previously mentioned uses of phospholipids and cholesterol are of only minor importance in comparison with their function of forming specialized structures, mainly membranes, in all cells of the body. In Chapter 2, it was pointed out that large quantities of phospholipids and cholesterol are present in both the cell membrane and the membranes of the internal organelles of all cells. It is also known that the *ratio* of membrane cholesterol to phospholipids is especially important in determining the fluidity of the cell membranes.

For membranes to be formed, substances that are not soluble in water must be available. In general, the only substances in the body that are not soluble in water (besides the inorganic substances of bone) are the lipids and some proteins. Thus, the physical integrity of cells everywhere in the body is based mainly on phospholipids, cholesterol, and certain insoluble proteins. The polar charges on the phospholipids also reduce the interfacial tension between the cell membranes and the surrounding fluids.

Another fact that indicates the importance of phospholipids and cholesterol for the formation of structural elements of the cells is the slow turnover rates of these substances in most nonhepatic tissues—turnover rates measured in months or years. For instance, their function in brain cells to provide memory processes is related mainly to their indestructible physical properties.

Atherosclerosis

Atherosclerosis is a disease of the large and intermediate-sized arteries in which fatty lesions called *atheromatous plaques* develop on the inside surfaces of the arterial walls. *Arteriosclerosis*, in contrast, is a general term that refers to thickened and stiffened blood vessels of all sizes.

One abnormality that can be measured very early in blood vessels that later become atherosclerotic is *damage to the vascular endothelium*. This, in turn, increases the expression of adhesion molecules on endothelial cells and decreases their ability to release nitric oxide and other substances that help prevent adhesion of macromolecules, platelets, and monocytes to the endothelium. After damage to the vascular endothelium occurs, circulating monocytes and lipids (mostly LDLs) begin to accumulate at the site of injury (Figure 68-7A). The monocytes cross the endothelium, enter the *intima* of the vessel wall, and differentiate to become *macrophages*, which then ingest and oxidize the accumulated lipoproteins, giving the macrophages a foamlike appearance.

Figure 68-7 Development of atherosclerotic plaque. *A,* Attachment of a monocyte to an adhesion molecule on a damaged endothelial cell of an artery. The monocyte then migrates through the endothelium into the intimal layer of the arterial wall and is transformed into a macrophage. The macrophage then ingests and oxidizes lipoprotein molecules, becoming a macrophage foam cell. The foam cells release substances that cause inflammation and growth of the intimal layer. *B,* Additional accumulation of macrophages and growth of the intima cause the plaque to grow larger and accumulate lipids. Eventually, the plaque could occlude the vessel or rupture, causing the blood in the artery to coagulate and form a thrombus. (Modified from Libby P: Inflammation in atherosclerosis. Nature 420:868, 2002.)

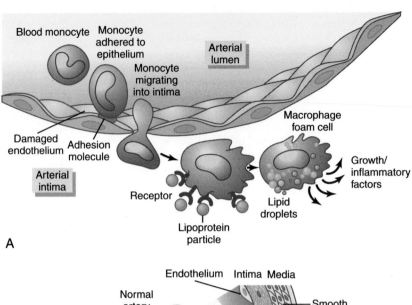

A

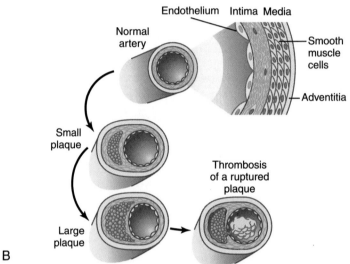

B

These *macrophage foam cells* then aggregate on the blood vessel and form a visible *fatty streak.*

With time, the fatty streaks grow larger and coalesce, and the surrounding fibrous and smooth muscle tissues proliferate to form larger and larger plaques (see Figure 68-7*B*). Also, the macrophages release substances that cause *inflammation* and further proliferation of smooth muscle and fibrous tissue on the inside surfaces of the arterial wall. The lipid deposits plus the cellular proliferation can become so large that the plaque bulges into the lumen of the artery and greatly reduces blood flow, sometimes completely occluding the vessel. Even without occlusion, the fibroblasts of the plaque eventually deposit extensive amounts of dense connective tissue; *sclerosis* (fibrosis) becomes so great that the arteries become stiff and unyielding. Still later, calcium salts often precipitate with the cholesterol and other lipids of the plaques, leading to bony-hard calcifications that can make the arteries rigid tubes. Both of these later stages of the disease are called "hardening of the arteries."

Atherosclerotic arteries lose most of their distensibility, and because of the degenerative areas in their walls, they are easily ruptured. Also, where the plaques protrude into the flowing blood, their rough surfaces can cause blood clots to develop, with resultant thrombus or embolus formation (see Chapter 36), leading to a sudden blockage of all blood flow in the artery.

Almost half of all deaths in the United States and Europe are due to vascular disease. About two thirds of these deaths are caused by thrombosis of one or more coronary arteries. The remaining one third are caused by thrombosis or hemorrhage of vessels in other organs of the body, especially the brain (causing strokes), but also the kidneys, liver, gastrointestinal tract, limbs, and so forth.

Basic Causes of Atherosclerosis—the Roles of Cholesterol and Lipoproteins

Increased Low-Density Lipoproteins. An important factor in causing atherosclerosis is a high blood plasma concentration of cholesterol in the form of low-density lipoproteins. The plasma concentration of these high-cholesterol LDLs is increased by several factors, including eating highly saturated fat in the daily diet, obesity, and physical inactivity. To a lesser extent, eating excess cholesterol may also raise plasma levels of LDLs.

An interesting example occurs in rabbits, which normally have low plasma cholesterol concentrations because of their vegetarian diet. Simply feeding these animals large quantities of cholesterol as part of their daily diet leads to serious atherosclerotic plaques throughout their arterial systems.

Familial Hypercholesterolemia. This is a disease in which the person inherits defective genes for the formation of LDL receptors on the membrane surfaces of the body's cells. In the absence of these receptors, the liver cannot absorb either intermediate-density or low-density lipoprotein. Without this absorption, the cholesterol machinery of the liver cells goes on a rampage, producing new cholesterol; it is no longer responsive to the feedback inhibition of too much plasma cholesterol. As a result, the number of VLDLs released by the liver into the plasma increases immensely.

Patients with full-blown familial hypercholesterolemia may have blood cholesterol concentrations of 600 to 1000 mg/dl, levels that are four to six times normal. Many of these people die before age 20 because of myocardial infarction or other sequelae of atherosclerotic blockage of blood vessels throughout the body.

Heterozygous familial hypercholesterolemia is relatively common and occurs in about one in 500 people. The more severe form of this disorder caused by homozygous mutations is much rarer, occurring in only about one of every million births on average.

Role of High-Density Lipoproteins in Preventing Atherosclerosis. Much less is known about the function of HDLs compared with that of LDLs. It is believed that HDLs can actually absorb cholesterol crystals that are beginning to be deposited in arterial walls. Whether this mechanism is true or not, HDLs do help protect against the development of atherosclerosis. Consequently, when a person has a high *ratio* of high-density to low-density lipoproteins, the likelihood of developing atherosclerosis is greatly reduced.

Other Major Risk Factors for Atherosclerosis

In some people with perfectly normal levels of cholesterol and lipoproteins, atherosclerosis still develops. Some of the factors that are known to predispose to atherosclerosis are (1) *physical inactivity* and *obesity*, (2) *diabetes mellitus*, (3) *hypertension*, (4) *hyperlipidemia*, and (5) *cigarette smoking*.

Hypertension, for example, increases the risk for atherosclerotic coronary artery disease by at least twofold. Likewise, a person with diabetes mellitus has, on average, more than a twofold increased risk of developing coronary artery disease. When hypertension and diabetes mellitus occur together, the risk for coronary artery disease is increased by more than eightfold. And when hypertension, diabetes mellitus, and hyperlipidemia are all present, the risk for atherosclerotic coronary artery disease is increased almost 20-fold, suggesting that these factors interact in a synergistic manner to increase the risk of developing atherosclerosis. In many overweight and obese patients, these three risk factors do occur together, greatly increasing their risk for atherosclerosis, which in turn may lead to heart attack, stroke, and kidney disease.

In early and middle adulthood, men are more likely to develop atherosclerosis than are women of comparable age, suggesting that male sex hormones might be atherogenic or, conversely, that female sex hormones might be protective.

Some of these factors cause atherosclerosis by increasing the concentration of LDLs in the plasma. Others, such as hypertension, lead to atherosclerosis by causing damage to the vascular endothelium and other changes in the vascular tissues that predispose to cholesterol deposition.

To add to the complexity of atherosclerosis, experimental studies suggest that *excess blood levels of iron* can lead to atherosclerosis, perhaps by forming free radicals in the blood that damage the vessel walls. About one quarter of all people have a special type of LDL called lipoprotein(a), containing an additional protein, *apolipoprotein(a)*, that almost doubles

the incidence of atherosclerosis. The precise mechanisms of these atherogenic effects have yet to be discovered.

Prevention of Atherosclerosis

The most important measures to protect against the development of atherosclerosis and its progression to serious vascular disease are (1) maintaining a healthy weight, being physically active, and eating a diet that contains mainly unsaturated fat with a low cholesterol content; (2) preventing hypertension by maintaining a healthy diet and being physically active, or effectively controlling blood pressure with antihypertensive drugs if hypertension does develop; (3) effectively controlling blood glucose with insulin treatment or other drugs if diabetes develops; and (4) avoiding cigarette smoking.

Several types of drugs that lower plasma lipids and cholesterol have proved to be valuable in preventing atherosclerosis. Most of the cholesterol formed in the liver is converted into bile acids and secreted in this form into the duodenum; then, more than 90 percent of these same bile acids is reabsorbed in the terminal ileum and used over and over again in the bile. Therefore, any agent that combines with the bile acids in the gastrointestinal tract and prevents their reabsorption into the circulation can decrease the total bile acid pool in the circulating blood. This causes far more of the liver cholesterol to be converted into new bile acids. Thus, simply eating *oat bran*, which binds bile acids and is a constituent of many breakfast cereals, increases the proportion of liver cholesterol that forms new bile acids rather than forming new LDLs and atherogenic plaques. *Resin agents* can also be used to bind bile acids in the gut and increase their fecal excretion, thereby reducing cholesterol synthesis by the liver.

Another group of drugs called *statins* competitively inhibits *hydroxymethylglutaryl-coenzyme A (HMG-CoA) reductase*, a rate-limiting enzyme in the synthesis of cholesterol. This inhibition decreases cholesterol synthesis and increases LDL receptors in the liver, usually causing a 25 to 50 percent reduction in plasma levels of LDLs. The statins may also have other beneficial effects that help prevent atherosclerosis, such as attenuating vascular inflammation. These drugs are now widely used to treat patients who have increased plasma cholesterol levels.

In general, studies show that for each 1 mg/dl decrease in LDL cholesterol in the plasma, there is about a 2 percent decrease in mortality from atherosclerotic heart disease. Therefore, appropriate preventive measures are valuable in decreasing heart attacks.

Bibliography

Adiels M, Olofsson SO, Taskinen MR, Borén J: Overproduction of very low-density lipoproteins is the hallmark of the dyslipidemia in the metabolic syndrome, *Arterioscler Thromb Vasc Biol* 28:1225, 2008.

Black DD: Development and Physiological Regulation of Intestinal Lipid Absorption. I. Development of intestinal lipid absorption: cellular events in chylomicron assembly and secretion, *Am J Physiol Gastrointest Liver Physiol* 293:G519, 2007.

Brown MS, Goldstein JL: A proteolytic pathway that controls the cholesterol content of membranes, cells, and blood, *Proc Natl Acad Sci U S A* 96:11041, 1999.

Bugger H, Abel ED: Molecular mechanisms for myocardial mitochondrial dysfunction in the metabolic syndrome, *Clin Sci (Lond)* 114:195, 2008.

Hahn C, Schwartz MA: The role of cellular adaptation to mechanical forces in atherosclerosis, *Arterioscler Thromb Vasc Biol* 28:2101, 2008.

Jaworski K, Sarkadi-Nagy E, Duncan RE, et al: Regulation of triglyceride metabolism IV. Hormonal regulation of lipolysis in adipose tissue, *Am J Physiol Gastrointest Liver Physiol* 293:G1, 2007.

Mansbach CM 2nd, Gorelick F: Development and physiological regulation of intestinal lipid absorption. II. Dietary lipid absorption, complex lipid synthesis, and the intracellular packaging and secretion of chylomicrons, *Am J Physiol Gastrointest Liver Physiol* 293:G645, 2008.

Mooradian AD, Haas MJ, Wehmeier KR, Wong NC: Obesity-related changes in high-density lipoprotein metabolism, *Obesity (Silver Spring)* 16:1152, 2008.

Roden M: How free fatty acids inhibit glucose utilization in human skeletal muscle, *News Physiol Sci* 19:92, 2004.

Tabet F, Rye KA: High-density lipoproteins, inflammation and oxidative stress, *Clin Sci (Lond)* 116:87, 2009.

Williams KJ: Molecular processes that handle—and mishandle—dietary lipids, *J Clin Invest* 118:3247, 2008.

Zernecke A, Shagdarsuren E, Weber C: Chemokines in atherosclerosis: an update, *Arterioscler Thromb Vasc Biol* 28:1897, 2008.

Protein Metabolism

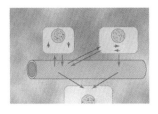

About three quarters of the body solids are proteins. These include structural proteins, enzymes, nucleoproteins, proteins that transport oxygen, proteins of the muscle that cause muscle contraction, and many other types that perform specific intracellular and extracellular functions throughout the body.

The basic chemical properties that explain proteins' diverse functions are so extensive that they constitute a major portion of the entire discipline of biochemistry. For this reason, the current discussion is confined to a few specific aspects of protein metabolism that are important as background for other discussions in this text.

Basic Properties

Amino Acids

The principal constituents of proteins are amino acids, 20 of which are present in the body proteins in significant quantities. Figure 69-1 shows the chemical formulas of these 20 amino acids, demonstrating that they all have two features in common: each amino acid has an acidic group ($-COOH$) and a nitrogen atom attached to the molecule, usually represented by the amino group ($-NH_2$).

Peptide Linkages and Peptide Chains. The amino acids of proteins are aggregated into long chains by means of *peptide linkages*. The chemical nature of this linkage is demonstrated by the following reaction:

$$R-CH-CO(OH)+R'-CH-COOH \rightarrow$$
$$\overset{|}{NH_2} \qquad \overset{|}{H)NH}$$

$$R-CH-CO$$
$$\overset{|}{NH_2}$$
$$|$$
$$NH + H_2O$$
$$|$$
$$R'-CH-COOH$$

Note in this reaction that the nitrogen of the amino radical of one amino acid bonds with the carbon of the carboxyl radical of the other amino acid. A hydrogen ion is released from the amino radical, and a hydroxyl ion is released from the carboxyl radical; these two combine to form a molecule of water. After the peptide linkage has been formed, an amino radical and a carboxyl radical are still at opposite ends of the new, longer molecule. Each of these radicals is capable of combining with additional amino acids to form a *peptide chain*. Some complicated protein molecules have many thousand amino acids combined by peptide linkages, and even the smallest protein molecule usually has more than 20 amino acids combined by peptide linkages. The average is about 400 amino acids.

Other Linkages in Protein Molecules. Some protein molecules are composed of several peptide chains rather than a single chain, and these chains are bound to one another by other linkages, often by *hydrogen bonding* between the CO and NH radicals of the peptides, as follows:

$$
\begin{array}{ccc}
& C = O \cdots\cdots H-N & \\
R-HC & & CH-R' \\
& N-H \cdots\cdots O = C &
\end{array}
$$

Many peptide chains are coiled or folded, and the successive coils or folds are held in a tight spiral or in other shapes by similar hydrogen bonding and other forces.

Transport and Storage of Amino Acids

Blood Amino Acids

The normal concentration of amino acids in the blood is between 35 and 65 mg/dl. This is an average of about 2 mg/dl for each of the 20 amino acids, although some are present in far greater amounts than others. Because the amino acids are relatively strong acids, they exist in the blood principally in the ionized state, resulting from the removal of one hydrogen atom from the NH_2 radical. They actually account for 2 to 3 milliequivalents of the negative ions in the blood. The precise distribution of the different amino acids in the blood depends to some extent on the types of proteins eaten, but the concentrations of at least some individual amino acids are regulated by selective synthesis in the different cells.

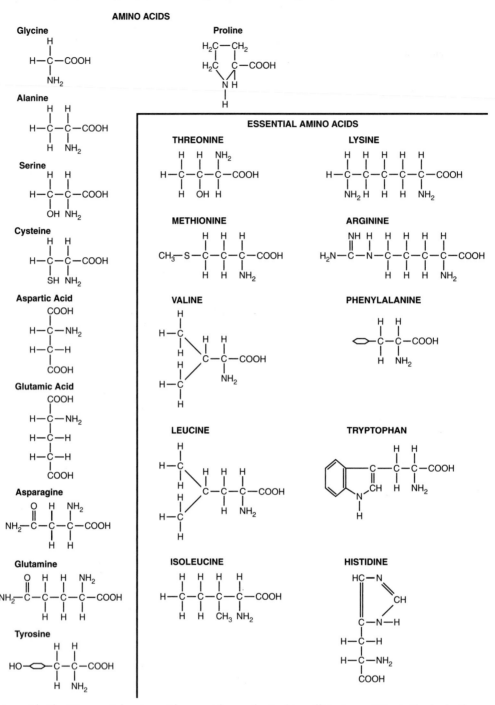

Figure 69-1 Amino acids. The 10 *essential* amino acids cannot be synthesized in sufficient quantities in the body; these essential amino acids must be obtained, already formed, from food.

Fate of Amino Acids Absorbed from the Gastrointestinal Tract. The products of protein digestion and absorption in the gastrointestinal tract are almost entirely amino acids; only rarely are polypeptides or whole protein molecules absorbed from the digestive tract into the blood. Soon after a meal, the amino acid concentration in a person's blood rises, but the increase is usually only a few milligrams per deciliter, for two reasons: First, protein digestion and absorption are usually extended over 2 to 3 hours, which allows only small quantities of amino acids to be absorbed at a time. Second, after entering the blood, the excess amino acids are absorbed within 5 to 10 minutes by cells throughout the body, especially by the liver. Therefore, almost never do large concentrations of amino acids accumulate in the blood and tissue fluids. Nevertheless, the turnover rate of the amino acids is so rapid that many grams of proteins can be carried from one part of the body to another in the form of amino acids each hour.

Active Transport of Amino Acids into the Cells. The molecules of all the amino acids are much too large to diffuse readily through the pores of the cell membranes. Therefore, significant quantities of amino acids can move either inward or outward through the membranes only by facilitated transport or active transport using carrier mechanisms. The nature of some of the carrier mechanisms is still poorly understood, but a few are discussed in Chapter 4.

Renal Threshold for Amino Acids. In the kidneys, the different amino acids can be *actively reabsorbed* through the proximal tubular epithelium, which removes them from the glomerular filtrate and returns them to the blood if they should filter into the renal tubules through the glomerular membranes. However, as is true of other active transport mechanisms in the renal tubules, there is an upper limit to the rate at which each type of amino acid can be transported. For this reason, when the concentration of a particular type of amino acid becomes too high in the plasma and glomerular filtrate, the excess that cannot be actively reabsorbed is lost into the urine.

Storage of Amino Acids as Proteins in the Cells

Almost immediately after entry into tissue cells, amino acids combine with one another by peptide linkages, under the direction of the cell's messenger RNA and ribosomal system, to form cellular proteins. Therefore, the concentration of free amino acids inside the cells usually remains low. Thus, storage of large quantities of free amino acids does not occur in the cells; instead, they are stored mainly in the form of actual proteins. But many of these intracellular proteins can be rapidly decomposed again into amino acids under the influence of intracellular lysosomal digestive enzymes; these amino acids can then be transported back out of the cell into the blood. Special exceptions to this reversal process are the proteins in the chromosomes of the nucleus and the structural proteins such as collagen and muscle contractile proteins; these proteins do not participate significantly in this reverse digestion and transport back out of the cells.

Some tissues of the body participate in the storage of amino acids to a greater extent than others. For instance, the liver, which is a large organ and has special systems for processing amino acids, can store large quantities of rapidly exchangeable proteins; this is also true to a lesser extent of the kidneys and the intestinal mucosa.

Release of Amino Acids from the Cells as a Means of Regulating Plasma Amino Acid Concentration. Whenever plasma amino acid concentrations fall below normal levels, the required amino acids are transported out of the cells to replenish their supply in the plasma. In this way, the plasma concentration of each type of amino acid is maintained at a reasonably constant value. Later, it is noted that some of the hormones secreted by the endocrine glands are able to alter the balance between tissue proteins and circulating amino acids. For instance, growth hormone and insulin increase the formation of tissue proteins, whereas adrenocortical glucocorticoid hormones increase the concentration of plasma amino acids.

Reversible Equilibrium Between the Proteins in Different Parts of the Body. Because cellular proteins in the liver (and, to a much less extent, in other tissues) can be synthesized rapidly from plasma amino acids, and because many of these proteins can be degraded and returned to the plasma almost as rapidly, there is constant interchange and equilibrium between the plasma amino acids and labile proteins in virtually all cells of the body. For instance, if any particular tissue requires proteins, it can synthesize new proteins from the amino acids of the blood; in turn, the blood amino acids are replenished by degradation of proteins from other cells of the body, especially from the liver cells. These effects are particularly noticeable in relation to protein synthesis in cancer cells. Cancer cells are often prolific users of amino acids; therefore, the proteins of the other cells can become markedly depleted.

Upper Limit for the Storage of Proteins. Each particular type of cell has an upper limit with regard to the amount of proteins it can store. After all the cells have reached their limits, the excess amino acids still in the circulation are degraded into other products and used for energy, as discussed subsequently, or they are converted to fat or glycogen and stored in these forms.

Functional Roles of the Plasma Proteins

The major types of protein present in the plasma are *albumin, globulin*, and *fibrinogen*.

A major function of *albumin* is to provide *colloid osmotic pressure* in the plasma, which prevents plasma loss from the capillaries, as discussed in Chapter 16.

The *globulins* perform a number of *enzymatic functions* in the plasma, but equally important, they are principally responsible for the body's both natural and acquired *immunity* against invading organisms, discussed in Chapter 34.

Fibrinogen polymerizes into long fibrin threads during blood coagulation, thereby *forming blood clots* that help repair leaks in the circulatory system, discussed in Chapter 36.

Formation of the Plasma Proteins. Essentially all the albumin and fibrinogen of the plasma proteins, as well as 50 to 80 percent of the globulins, are formed in the liver. The remaining globulins are formed almost entirely in the lymphoid tissues. They are mainly the gamma globulins that constitute the antibodies used in the immune system.

The rate of plasma protein formation by the liver can be extremely high, as much as 30 g/day. Certain disease conditions cause rapid loss of plasma proteins; severe burns that denude large surface areas of the skin can cause the loss of several liters of plasma through the denuded areas each day. The rapid production of plasma proteins by the liver is valuable in preventing death in such states. Occasionally, a person with severe renal disease loses as much as 20 grams of plasma protein in the urine each day for months, and it is continually replaced mainly by liver production of the required proteins.

In *cirrhosis of the liver*, large amounts of fibrous tissue develop among the liver parenchymal cells, causing a reduction in their ability to synthesize plasma proteins. As discussed in Chapter 25, this leads to decreased plasma colloid osmotic pressure, which causes generalized edema.

Plasma Proteins as a Source of Amino Acids for the Tissues. When the tissues become depleted of proteins, the plasma proteins can act as a source of rapid replacement. Indeed, whole plasma proteins can be imbibed in toto by tissue macrophages through the process of pinocytosis; once in these cells, they are split into amino acids that are transported back into the blood and used throughout the body to build cellular proteins wherever needed. In this way, the plasma proteins function as a labile protein storage medium and represent a readily available source of amino acids whenever a particular tissue requires them.

Reversible Equilibrium Between the Plasma Proteins and the Tissue Proteins. There is a constant state of equilibrium, as shown in Figure 69-2, among the plasma proteins, the amino acids of the plasma, and the tissue proteins. It has been estimated from radioactive tracer studies that normally about

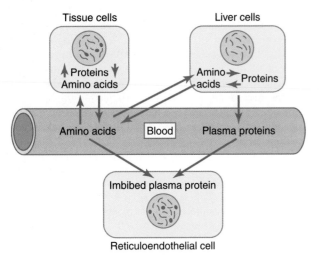

Figure 69-2 Reversible equilibrium among the tissue proteins, plasma proteins, and plasma amino acids.

400 grams of body protein are synthesized and degraded each day as part of the continual state of flux of amino acids. This demonstrates the general principle of reversible exchange of amino acids among the different proteins of the body. Even during starvation or severe debilitating diseases, the ratio of total tissue proteins to total plasma proteins in the body remains relatively constant at about 33:1.

Because of this reversible equilibrium between plasma proteins and the other proteins of the body, one of the most effective therapies for severe, acute whole-body protein deficiency is intravenous transfusion of plasma protein. Within a few days, or sometimes within hours, the amino acids of the administered protein are distributed throughout the cells of the body to form new proteins as needed.

Essential and Nonessential Amino Acids

Ten of the amino acids normally present in animal proteins can be synthesized in the cells, whereas the other 10 either cannot be synthesized or are synthesized in quantities too small to supply the body's needs. This second group of amino acids that cannot be synthesized is called the *essential amino acids*. Use of the word "essential" does not mean that the other 10 "nonessential" amino acids are not required for the formation of proteins, but only that the others are *not essential in the diet* because they can be synthesized in the body.

Synthesis of the nonessential amino acids depends mainly on the formation of appropriate α-keto acids, which are the precursors of the respective amino acids. For instance, *pyruvic acid*, which is formed in large quantities during the glycolytic breakdown of glucose, is the keto acid precursor of the amino acid *alanine*. Then, by the process of *transamination*, an amino radical is transferred to the α-keto acid, and the keto

oxygen is transferred to the donor of the amino radical. This reaction is shown in Figure 69-3. Note in this figure that the amino radical is transferred to the pyruvic acid from another chemical that is closely allied to the amino acids—*glutamine*. Glutamine is present in the tissues in large quantities, and one of its principal functions is to serve as an amino radical storehouse. In addition, amino radicals can be transferred from *asparagine, glutamic acid*, and *aspartic acid*.

Transamination is promoted by several enzymes, among which are the *aminotransferases*, which are derivatives of pyridoxine, one of the B vitamins (B_6). Without this vitamin, the amino acids are synthesized only poorly and protein formation cannot proceed normally.

Use of Proteins for Energy

Once the cells are filled to their limits with stored protein, any additional amino acids in the body fluids are degraded and used for energy or are stored mainly as fat or secondarily as glycogen. This degradation occurs almost entirely in the liver, and it begins with *deamination*, which is explained in the following section.

Deamination. Deamination means removal of the amino groups from the amino acids. This occurs mainly by *transamination*, which means transfer of the amino group to some acceptor substance, which is the reverse of the transamination explained earlier in relation to the synthesis of amino acids.

The greatest amount of deamination occurs by the following transamination schema:

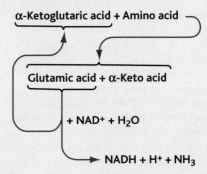

Note from this schema that the amino group from the amino acid is transferred to α-ketoglutaric acid, which then becomes glutamic acid. The glutamic acid can then transfer the amino group to still other substances or release it in the form of ammonia (NH_3). In the process of losing the amino group, the glutamic acid once again becomes α-ketoglutaric acid, so the cycle can be repeated again and again. To initiate this process, the excess amino acids in the cells, especially in the liver, induce the activation of large quantities of *aminotransferases*, the enzymes responsible for initiating most deamination.

Figure 69-3 Synthesis of alanine from pyruvic acid by transamination.

$$NH_2-\underset{\underset{O}{\|}}{C}-CH_2-CH_2-\underset{\underset{NH_2}{|}}{CH}-COOH \quad + \quad CH_3-\underset{\underset{O}{\|}}{C}-COOH \xrightarrow{\textit{Transaminase}}$$

(Glutamine) (Pyruvic acid)

$$NH_2-\underset{\underset{O}{\|}}{C}-CH_2-CH_2-\underset{\underset{O}{\|}}{C}-COOH \quad + \quad CH_3-\underset{\underset{NH}{|}}{C}-COOH$$

(α-Ketoglutamic acid) (Alanine)

Urea Formation by the Liver. The ammonia released during deamination of amino acids is removed from the blood almost entirely by conversion into urea; two molecules of ammonia and one molecule of carbon dioxide combine in accordance with the following net reaction:

$$2\ NH_3 + CO_2 \rightarrow H_2N\!-\!\underset{\underset{O}{\|}}{C}\!-\!NH_2 + H_2O$$

Essentially all urea formed in the human body is synthesized in the liver. In the absence of the liver or in serious liver disease, ammonia accumulates in the blood. This is extremely toxic, especially to the brain, often leading to a state called *hepatic coma*.

The stages in the formation of urea are essentially the following:

After its formation, the urea diffuses from the liver cells into the body fluids and is excreted by the kidneys.

Oxidation of Deaminated Amino Acids. Once amino acids have been deaminated, the resulting keto acids can, in most instances, be oxidized to release energy for metabolic purposes. This usually involves two successive processes: (1) The keto acid is changed into an appropriate chemical substance that can enter the citric acid cycle, and (2) this substance is degraded by the cycle and used for energy in the same manner that acetyl coenzyme A (acetyl-CoA) derived from carbohydrate and lipid metabolism is used, as explained in Chapters 67 and 68. In general, the amount of adenosine triphosphate (ATP) formed for each gram of protein that is oxidized is slightly less than that formed for each gram of glucose oxidized.

Gluconeogenesis and Ketogenesis. Certain deaminated amino acids are similar to the substrates normally used by the cells, mainly the liver cells, to synthesize glucose or fatty acids. For instance, deaminated alanine is pyruvic acid. This can be converted into either glucose or glycogen. Alternatively, it can be converted into acetyl-CoA, which can then be polymerized into fatty acids. Also, two molecules of acetyl-CoA can condense to form acetoacetic acid, which is one of the ketone bodies, as explained in Chapter 68.

The conversion of amino acids into glucose or glycogen is called *gluconeogenesis*, and the conversion of amino acids into keto acids or fatty acids is called *ketogenesis*. Of the 20 deaminated amino acids, 18 have chemical structures that allow them to be converted into glucose, and 19 of them can be converted into fatty acids.

Obligatory Degradation of Proteins

When a person eats no proteins, a certain proportion of body proteins is degraded into amino acids and then deaminated and oxidized. This involves 20 to 30 grams of protein each day, which is called the *obligatory loss* of proteins. Therefore, to prevent net loss of protein from the body, one must ingest a minimum of 20 to 30 grams of protein each day; to be on the safe side, a minimum of 60 to 75 grams is usually recommended.

The ratios of the different amino acids in the dietary protein must be about the same as the ratios in the body tissues if the entire dietary protein is to be fully usable to form new proteins in the tissues. If one particular type of essential amino acid is low in concentration, the others become unusable because cells synthesize either whole proteins or none at all, as explained in Chapter 3 in relation to protein synthesis. The unusable amino acids are deaminated and oxidized. A protein that has a ratio of amino acids different from that of the average body protein is called a *partial protein* or *incomplete protein*, and such a protein is less valuable for nutrition than is a *complete protein*.

Effect of Starvation on Protein Degradation. Except for the 20 to 30 grams of obligatory protein degradation each day, the body uses almost entirely carbohydrates or fats for energy, as long as they are available. However, after several weeks of starvation, when the quantities of stored carbohydrates and fats begin to run out, the amino acids of the blood are rapidly deaminated and oxidized for energy. From this point on, the proteins of the tissues degrade rapidly—as much as 125 grams daily—and, as a result, cellular functions deteriorate precipitously. Because carbohydrate and fat utilization for energy normally occurs in preference to protein utilization, carbohydrates and fats are called *protein sparers*.

Hormonal Regulation of Protein Metabolism

Growth Hormone Increases the Synthesis of Cellular Proteins. Growth hormone causes the tissue proteins to increase. The precise mechanism by which this occurs is not known, but it is believed to result mainly from increased transport of amino acids through the cell membranes, acceleration of the DNA and RNA transcription and translation processes for protein synthesis, and decreased oxidation of tissue proteins.

Insulin Is Necessary for Protein Synthesis. Total lack of insulin reduces protein synthesis to almost zero. Insulin accelerates the transport of some amino acids into cells, which could be the stimulus to protein synthesis. Also, insulin reduces protein degradation and increases the availability of glucose to the cells, so the need for amino acids for energy is correspondingly reduced.

Glucocorticoids Increase Breakdown of Most Tissue Proteins. The glucocorticoids secreted by the adrenal cortex *decrease* the quantity of protein in *most* tissues while increasing the amino acid concentration in the plasma, as well as increasing *both liver proteins and plasma proteins*. It is believed that the glucocorticoids act by increasing the rate of breakdown of extrahepatic proteins, thereby making increased quantities of amino acids available in the body fluids. This allows the liver to synthesize increased quantities of hepatic cellular proteins and plasma proteins.

Testosterone Increases Protein Deposition in Tissues. Testosterone, the male sex hormone, causes increased deposition of protein in tissues throughout the body, especially the contractile proteins of the muscles (30 to 50 percent increase). The mechanism of this effect is unknown, but it is definitely different from the effect of growth hormone, in the following way: Growth hormone causes tissues to continue growing almost indefinitely, whereas testosterone causes the muscles and, to a much lesser extent, some other protein tissues to enlarge for only several months. Once the muscles and other protein tissues have reached a maximum, despite continued administration of testosterone, further protein deposition ceases.

Estrogen. Estrogen, the principal female sex hormone, also causes some deposition of protein, but its effect is relatively insignificant in comparison with that of testosterone.

Thyroxine. Thyroxine increases the rate of metabolism of all cells and, as a result, indirectly affects protein metabolism. If insufficient carbohydrates and fats are available for energy, thyroxine causes rapid degradation of proteins and uses them for energy. Conversely, if adequate quantities of carbohydrates and fats are available and excess amino acids are also available in the extracellular fluid, thyroxine can actually increase the rate of protein synthesis. In growing animals or human beings, deficiency of thyroxine causes growth to be greatly inhibited because of lack of protein synthesis. In essence, it is believed that thyroxine has little specific effect on protein metabolism but does have an important general effect by increasing the rates of both normal anabolic and normal catabolic protein reactions.

Bibliography

Altenberg GA: The engine of ABC proteins, *News Physiol Sci* 18:191, 2003.

Bröer S: Apical transporters for neutral amino acids: physiology and pathophysiology, *Physiology (Bethesda)* 23:95, 2008.

Bröer S: Amino acid transport across mammalian intestinal and renal epithelia, *Physiol Rev* 88:249, 2008.

Daniel H: Molecular and integrative physiology of intestinal peptide transport, *Annu Rev Physiol* 66:361, 2004.

Finn PF, Dice JF: Proteolytic and lipolytic responses to starvation, *Nutrition* 22:830, 2006.

Jans DA, Hubner S: Regulation of protein transport to the nucleus: central role of phosphorylation, *Physiol Rev* 76:651, 1996.

Kuhn CM: Anabolic steroids, *Recent Prog Horm Res* 57:411, 2002.

Moriwaki H, Miwa Y, Tajika M, et al: Branched-chain amino acids as a protein- and energy-source in liver cirrhosis, *Biochem Biophys Res Commun* 313:405, 2004.

Phillips SM: Dietary protein for athletes: from requirements to metabolic advantage, *Appl Physiol Nutr Metab* 31:647, 2006.

Tang JE, Phillips SM: Maximizing muscle protein anabolism: the role of protein quality, *Curr Opin Clin Nutr Metab Care* 12:66, 2009.

Tavernarakis N: Ageing and the regulation of protein synthesis: a balancing act? *Trends Cell Biol* 18:228, 2008.

Wolfe RR, Miller SL, Miller KB: Optimal protein intake in the elderly, *Clin Nutr* 27:675, 2008.

The Liver as an Organ

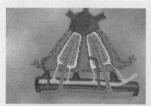

Although the liver is a discrete organ, it performs many different functions that interrelate with one another. This becomes especially evident in abnormalities of the liver because many of its functions are disturbed simultaneously. This chapter summarizes the liver's different functions, including (1) filtration and storage of blood; (2) metabolism of carbohydrates, proteins, fats, hormones, and foreign chemicals; (3) formation of bile; (4) storage of vitamins and iron; and (5) formation of coagulation factors.

Physiologic Anatomy of the Liver

The liver is the largest organ in the body, contributing about 2 percent of the total body weight, or about 1.5 kilograms (3.3 pounds) in the average adult human. The basic functional unit of the liver is the *liver lobule*, which is a cylindrical structure several millimeters in length and 0.8 to 2 millimeters in diameter. The human liver contains 50,000 to 100,000 individual lobules.

The liver lobule, shown in cut-away format in Figure 70-1, is constructed around a *central vein* that empties into the hepatic veins and then into the vena cava. The lobule itself is composed principally of many liver *cellular plates* (two of which are shown in Figure 70-1) that radiate from the central vein like spokes in a wheel. Each hepatic plate is usually two cells thick, and between the adjacent cells lie small *bile canaliculi* that empty into *bile ducts* in the fibrous septa separating the adjacent liver lobules.

In the septa are small *portal venules* that receive their blood mainly from the venous outflow of the gastrointestinal tract by way of the portal vein. From these venules blood flows into flat, branching *hepatic sinusoids* that lie between the hepatic plates and then into the central vein. Thus, the hepatic cells are exposed continuously to portal venous blood.

Hepatic arterioles are also present in the interlobular septa. These arterioles supply arterial blood to the septal tissues between the adjacent lobules, and many of the small arterioles also empty directly into the hepatic sinusoids, most frequently emptying into those located about one-third the distance from the interlobular septa, as shown in Figure 70-1.

In addition to the hepatic cells, the venous sinusoids are lined by two other cell types: (1) typical *endothelial cells* and (2) large *Kupffer cells* (also called *reticuloendothelial cells*), which are resident macrophages that line the sinusoids and are capable of phagocytizing bacteria and other foreign matter in the hepatic sinus blood.

The endothelial lining of the sinusoids has extremely large pores, some of which are almost 1 micrometer in diameter. Beneath this lining, lying between the endothelial cells and the hepatic cells, are narrow tissue spaces called the *spaces of Disse*, also known as the *perisinusoidal spaces*. The millions of spaces of Disse connect with lymphatic vessels in the interlobular septa. Therefore, excess fluid in these spaces is removed through the lymphatics. Because of the large pores in the endothelium, substances in the plasma move freely into the spaces of Disse. Even large portions of the plasma proteins diffuse freely into these spaces.

Hepatic Vascular and Lymph Systems

The function of the hepatic vascular system is discussed in Chapter 15 in connection with the portal veins and can be summarized as follows.

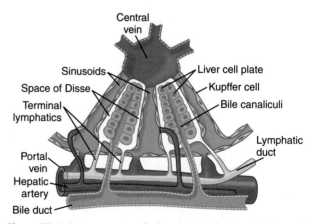

Figure 70-1 Basic structure of a liver lobule, showing the liver cellular plates, the blood vessels, the bile-collecting system, and the lymph flow system composed of the spaces of Disse and the interlobular lymphatics. (Modified from Guyton AC, Taylor AE, Granger HJ: Circulatory Physiology. Vol 2: Dynamics and Control of the Body Fluids. Philadelphia: WB Saunders, 1975.)

Blood Flows Through the Liver from the Portal Vein and Hepatic Artery

The Liver Has High Blood Flow and Low Vascular Resistance. About 1050 milliliters of blood flows from the portal vein into the liver sinusoids each minute, and an additional 300 milliliters flows into the sinusoids from the hepatic artery, the total averaging about 1350 ml/min. This amounts to 27 percent of the resting cardiac output.

The pressure in the portal vein leading into the liver averages about 9 mm Hg and the pressure in the hepatic vein leading from the liver into the vena cava normally averages almost exactly 0 mm Hg. This small pressure difference, only 9 mm Hg, shows that the resistance to blood flow through the hepatic sinusoids is normally very low, especially when one considers that about 1350 milliliters of blood flows by this route each minute.

Cirrhosis of the Liver Greatly Increases Resistance to Blood Flow. When liver parenchymal cells are destroyed, they are replaced with fibrous tissue that eventually contracts around the blood vessels, thereby greatly impeding the flow of portal blood through the liver. This disease process is known as *cirrhosis of the liver*. It results most commonly from chronic alcoholism or from excess fat accumulation in the liver and subsequent liver inflammation, a condition called *nonalcoholic steatohepatitis, or NASH*. A less severe form of fat accumulation and inflammation of the liver, *nonalcoholic fatty liver disease* (NAFLD), is the most common cause of liver disease in many industrialized countries, including the United States, and is usually associated with obesity and type II diabetes.

Cirrhosis can also follow ingestion of poisons such as carbon tetrachloride, viral diseases such as infectious hepatitis, obstruction of the bile ducts, and infectious processes in the bile ducts.

The portal system is also occasionally blocked by a large clot that develops in the portal vein or its major branches. When the portal system is suddenly blocked, the return of blood from the intestines and spleen through the liver portal blood flow system to the systemic circulation is tremendously impeded, resulting in *portal hypertension* and increasing the capillary pressure in the intestinal wall to 15 to 20 mm Hg above normal. The patient often dies within a few hours because of excessive loss of fluid from the capillaries into the lumens and walls of the intestines.

The Liver Functions as a Blood Reservoir

Because the liver is an expandable organ, large quantities of blood can be stored in its blood vessels. Its normal blood volume, including both that in the hepatic veins and that in the hepatic sinuses, is about 450 milliliters, or almost 10 percent of the body's total blood volume. When high pressure in the right atrium causes backpressure in the liver, the liver expands, and 0.5 to 1 liter of extra blood is occasionally stored in the hepatic veins and sinuses. This occurs especially in cardiac failure with peripheral congestion, which is discussed in Chapter 22. Thus, in effect, the liver is a large, expandable, venous organ capable of acting as a valuable blood reservoir in times of excess blood volume and capable of supplying extra blood in times of diminished blood volume.

The Liver Has Very High Lymph Flow

Because the pores in the hepatic sinusoids are very permeable and allow ready passage of both fluid and proteins into the spaces of Disse, the lymph draining from the liver usually has a protein concentration of about 6 g/dl, which is only slightly less than the protein concentration of plasma. Also, the high permeability of the liver sinusoid epithelium allows large quantities of lymph to form. Therefore, about half of all the lymph formed in the body under resting conditions arises in the liver.

High Hepatic Vascular Pressures Can Cause Fluid Transudation into the Abdominal Cavity from the Liver and Portal Capillaries—Ascites. When the pressure in the hepatic veins rises only 3 to 7 mm Hg above normal, excessive amounts of fluid begin to transude into the lymph and leak through the outer surface of the liver capsule directly into the abdominal cavity. This fluid is almost pure plasma, containing 80 to 90 percent as much protein as normal plasma. At vena caval pressures of 10 to 15 mm Hg, hepatic lymph flow increases to as much as 20 times normal, and the "sweating" from the surface of the liver can be so great that it causes large amounts of free fluid in the abdominal cavity, which is called *ascites*. Blockage of portal flow through the liver also causes high capillary pressures in the entire portal vascular system of the gastrointestinal tract, resulting in edema of the gut wall and transudation of fluid through the serosa of the gut into the abdominal cavity. This, too, can cause ascites.

Regulation of Liver Mass—Regeneration

The liver possesses a remarkable ability to restore itself after significant hepatic tissue loss from either partial hepatectomy or acute liver injury, as long as the injury is uncomplicated by viral infection or inflammation. Partial hepatectomy, in which up to 70 percent of the liver is removed, causes the remaining lobes to enlarge and restore the liver to its original size. This regeneration is remarkably rapid and requires only 5 to 7 days in rats. During liver regeneration, hepatocytes are estimated to replicate once or twice, and after the original size and volume of the liver are achieved, the hepatocytes revert to their usual quiescent state.

Control of this rapid regeneration of the liver is still poorly understood, but *hepatocyte growth factor (HGF)* appears to be important in causing liver cell division and growth. HGF is produced by mesenchymal cells in the liver and in other tissues, but not by hepatocytes. Blood levels of HGF rise more than 20-fold after partial hepatectomy, but mitogenic responses are usually found only in the liver after these operations, suggesting that HGF may be activated only in the affected organ. Other growth factors, especially *epidermal growth factor*, and cytokines such as *tumor necrosis factor* and *interleukin-6* may also be involved in stimulating regeneration of liver cells.

After the liver has returned to its original size, the process of hepatic cell division is terminated. Again, the factors involved are not well understood, although *transforming growth factor-β*, a cytokine secreted by hepatic cells, is a potent inhibitor of liver cell proliferation and has been suggested as the main terminator of liver regeneration.

Physiologic experiments indicate that liver growth is closely regulated by some unknown signal related to body size, so an optimal liver-to-body weight ratio is maintained for optimal metabolic function. In liver diseases associated with fibrosis, inflammation, or viral infections, however, the regenerative process of the liver is severely impaired and liver function deteriorates.

Hepatic Macrophage System Serves a Blood-Cleansing Function

Blood flowing through the intestinal capillaries picks up many bacteria from the intestines. Indeed, a sample of blood taken from the portal veins before it enters the liver almost always grows colon bacilli when cultured, whereas growth of colon bacilli from blood in the systemic circulation is extremely rare.

Special high-speed motion pictures of the action of Kupffer cells, the large phagocytic macrophages that line the hepatic venous sinuses, have demonstrated that these cells efficiently cleanse blood as it passes through the sinuses; when a bacterium comes into momentary contact with a Kupffer cell, in less than 0.01 second the bacterium passes inward through the wall of the Kupffer cell to become permanently lodged therein until it is digested. Probably less than 1 percent of the bacteria entering the portal blood from the intestines succeeds in passing through the liver into the systemic circulation.

Metabolic Functions of the Liver

The liver is a large, chemically reactant pool of cells that have a high rate of metabolism, sharing substrates and energy from one metabolic system to another, processing and synthesizing multiple substances that are transported to other areas of the body, and performing myriad other metabolic functions. For these reasons, a major share of the entire discipline of biochemistry is devoted to the metabolic reactions in the liver. But here, let us summarize those metabolic functions that are especially important in understanding the integrated physiology of the body.

Carbohydrate Metabolism

In carbohydrate metabolism, the liver performs the following functions, as summarized in Chapter 67:

1. Storage of large amounts of glycogen
2. Conversion of galactose and fructose to glucose
3. Gluconeogenesis
4. Formation of many chemical compounds from intermediate products of carbohydrate metabolism

The liver is especially important for maintaining a normal blood glucose concentration. Storage of glycogen allows the liver to remove excess glucose from the blood, store it, and then return it to the blood when the blood glucose concentration begins to fall too low. This is called the *glucose buffer function* of the liver. In a person with poor liver function, blood glucose concentration after a meal rich in carbohydrates may rise two to three times as much as in a person with normal liver function.

Gluconeogenesis in the liver is also important in maintaining a normal blood glucose concentration because gluconeogenesis occurs to a significant extent only when the glucose concentration falls below normal. Then large amounts of amino acids and glycerol from triglycerides are converted into glucose, thereby helping to maintain a relatively normal blood glucose concentration.

Fat Metabolism

Although most cells of the body metabolize fat, certain aspects of fat metabolism occur mainly in the liver. Specific functions of the liver in fat metabolism, as summarized from Chapter 68, are the following:

1. Oxidation of fatty acids to supply energy for other body functions
2. Synthesis of large quantities of cholesterol, phospholipids, and most lipoproteins
3. Synthesis of fat from proteins and carbohydrates

To derive energy from neutral fats, the fat is first split into glycerol and fatty acids; then the fatty acids are split by *beta-oxidation* into two-carbon acetyl radicals that form *acetyl coenzyme A* (acetyl-CoA). This can enter the citric acid cycle and be oxidized to liberate tremendous amounts of energy. Beta-oxidation can take place in all cells of the body, but it occurs especially rapidly in the hepatic cells. The liver cannot use all the acetyl-CoA that is formed; instead, it is converted by the condensation of two molecules of acetyl-CoA into *acetoacetic acid*, a highly soluble acid that passes from the hepatic cells into the extracellular fluid and is then transported throughout the body to be absorbed by other tissues. These tissues reconvert the acetoacetic acid into acetyl-CoA and then oxidize it in the usual manner. Thus, the liver is responsible for a major part of the metabolism of fats.

About 80 percent of the cholesterol synthesized in the liver is converted into bile salts, which are secreted into the bile; the remainder is transported in the lipoproteins and carried by the blood to the tissue cells everywhere in the body. Phospholipids are likewise synthesized in the liver and transported principally in the lipoproteins. Both cholesterol and phospholipids are used by the cells to form membranes, intracellular structures, and multiple chemical substances that are important to cellular function.

Almost all the fat synthesis in the body from carbohydrates and proteins also occurs in the liver. After fat is synthesized in the liver, it is transported in the lipoproteins to the adipose tissue to be stored.

Protein Metabolism

The body cannot dispense with the liver's contribution to protein metabolism for more than a few days without death ensuing. The most important functions of the liver in protein metabolism, as summarized from Chapter 69, are the following:

1. Deamination of amino acids
2. Formation of urea for removal of ammonia from the body fluids
3. Formation of plasma proteins
4. Interconversions of the various amino acids and synthesis of other compounds from amino acids

Deamination of amino acids is required before they can be used for energy or converted into carbohydrates or fats. A small amount of deamination can occur in the other tissues of the body, especially in the kidneys, but this is much less important than the deamination of amino acids by the liver.

Formation of urea by the liver removes ammonia from the body fluids. Large amounts of ammonia are formed by the deamination process, and additional amounts are continually formed in the gut by bacteria and then absorbed into the blood. Therefore, if the liver does not form urea, the plasma ammonia concentration rises rapidly and results in *hepatic coma* and death. Indeed, even greatly decreased blood flow through the liver—as occurs occasionally when a shunt develops between the portal vein and the vena cava—can cause excessive ammonia in the blood, an extremely toxic condition.

Essentially all the plasma proteins, with the exception of part of the gamma globulins, are formed by the hepatic cells. This accounts for about 90 percent of all the plasma proteins. The remaining gamma globulins are the antibodies formed mainly by plasma cells in the lymph tissue of the body. The liver can form plasma proteins at a maximum rate of 15 to 50 g/day. Therefore, even if as much as half the plasma proteins are lost from the body, they can be replenished in 1 or 2 weeks.

It is particularly interesting that plasma protein depletion causes rapid mitosis of the hepatic cells and growth of the liver to a larger size; these effects are coupled with rapid output of plasma proteins until the plasma concentration returns to normal. With chronic liver disease (e.g., cirrhosis), plasma proteins, such as albumin, may fall to very low levels, causing generalized edema and ascites, as explained in Chapter 29.

Among the most important functions of the liver is its ability to synthesize certain amino acids and to synthesize other important chemical compounds from amino acids. For instance, the so-called nonessential amino acids can all be synthesized in the liver. To do this, a keto acid having the same chemical composition (except at the keto oxygen) as that of the amino acid to be formed is synthesized. Then an amino radical is transferred through several stages of *transamination* from an available amino acid to the keto acid to take the place of the keto oxygen.

Other Metabolic Functions of the Liver

The Liver Is a Storage Site for Vitamins. The liver has a particular propensity for storing vitamins and has long been known as an excellent source of certain vitamins in the treatment of patients. The vitamin stored in greatest quantity in the liver is vitamin A, but large quantities of vitamin D and vitamin B_{12} are normally stored as well. Sufficient quantities of vitamin A can be stored to prevent vitamin A deficiency for as long as 10 months. Sufficient vitamin D can be stored to prevent deficiency for 3 to 4 months, and enough vitamin B_{12} can be stored to last for at least 1 year and maybe several years.

The Liver Stores Iron as Ferritin. Except for the iron in the hemoglobin of the blood, by far the greatest proportion of iron in the body is stored in the liver in the form of *ferritin*. The hepatic cells contain large amounts of a protein called *apoferritin*, which is capable of combining reversibly with iron. Therefore, when iron is available in the body fluids in extra quantities, it combines with apoferritin to form ferritin and is stored in this form in the hepatic cells until needed elsewhere. When the iron in the circulating body fluids reaches a low level, the ferritin releases the iron. Thus, the apoferritin-ferritin system of the liver acts as a *blood iron buffer*, as well as an iron storage medium. Other functions of the liver in relation to iron metabolism and red blood cell formation are considered in Chapter 32.

The Liver Forms the Blood Substances Used in Coagulation. Substances formed in the liver that are used in the coagulation process include *fibrinogen, prothrombin, accelerator globulin, Factor VII*, and several other important factors. Vitamin K is required by the metabolic processes of the liver for the formation of several of these substances, especially prothrombin and Factors VII, IX, and X. In the absence of vitamin K, the concentrations of all these decrease markedly and this almost prevents blood coagulation.

The Liver Removes or Excretes Drugs, Hormones, and Other Substances. The active chemical medium of the liver is well known for its ability to detoxify or excrete into the bile many drugs, including sulfonamides, penicillin, ampicillin, and erythromycin.

In a similar manner, several of the hormones secreted by the endocrine glands are either chemically altered or excreted by the liver, including thyroxine and essentially all the steroid hormones, such as estrogen, cortisol, and aldosterone. Liver damage can lead to excess accumulation of one or more of these hormones in the body fluids and therefore cause overactivity of the hormonal systems.

Finally, one of the major routes for excreting calcium from the body is secretion by the liver into the bile, which then passes into the gut and is lost in the feces.

Measurement of Bilirubin in the Bile as a Clinical Diagnostic Tool

The formation of bile by the liver and the function of the bile salts in the digestive and absorptive processes of the intestinal tract are discussed in Chapters 64 and 65. In addition, many substances are excreted in the bile and then eliminated in the feces. One of these is the greenish yellow pigment *bilirubin*. This is a major end product of hemoglobin degradation, as pointed out in Chapter 32. However, it also provides *an exceedingly valuable tool for diagnosing both hemolytic blood diseases and various types of liver diseases*. Therefore, while referring to Figure 70-2, let us explain this.

Briefly, when the red blood cells have lived out their life span (on average, 120 days) and have become too fragile to exist in the circulatory system, their cell membranes rupture, and the released hemoglobin is phagocytized by tissue macrophages (also called the *reticuloendothelial system*) throughout the body. The hemoglobin is first split into *globin* and *heme*, and the heme ring is opened to give (1) free iron, which is transported in the blood by transferrin, and (2) a straight chain of four pyrrole nuclei, which is the substrate from which bilirubin will eventually be formed. The first substance formed is *biliverdin*, but this is rapidly reduced to *free bilirubin*, also called *unconjugated bilirubin*, which is gradually released from the macrophages into the plasma. This form of bilirubin immediately combines strongly with plasma albumin and is transported in this combination throughout the blood and interstitial fluids.

Within hours, the unconjugated bilirubin is absorbed through the hepatic cell membrane. In passing to the inside of the liver cells, it is released from the plasma albumin and soon thereafter conjugated about 80 percent with glucuronic acid to form *bilirubin glucuronide*, about 10 percent with sulfate to form *bilirubin sulfate*, and about 10 percent with a multitude of other substances. In these forms, the bilirubin is excreted from the hepatocytes by an active transport process into the bile canaliculi and then into the intestines.

Formation and Fate of Urobilinogen. Once in the intestine, about half of the "conjugated" bilirubin is converted by bacterial action into the substance *urobilinogen*, which is highly soluble. Some of the urobilinogen is reabsorbed through the intestinal mucosa back into the blood. Most of

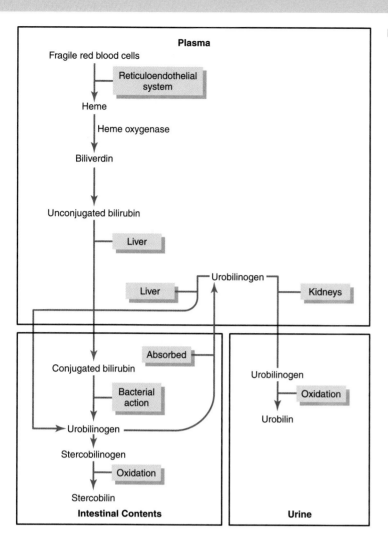

Figure 70-2 Bilirubin formation and excretion.

this is re-excreted by the liver back into the gut, but about 5 percent is excreted by the kidneys into the urine. After exposure to air in the urine, the urobilinogen becomes oxidized to *urobilin*; alternatively, in the feces, it becomes altered and oxidized to form *stercobilin*. These interrelations of bilirubin and the other bilirubin products are shown in Figure 70-2.

Jaundice—Excess Bilirubin in the Extracellular Fluid

Jaundice refers to a yellowish tint to the body tissues, including a yellowness of the skin and deep tissues. The usual cause of jaundice is large quantities of bilirubin in the extracellular fluids, either unconjugated or conjugated bilirubin. The normal plasma concentration of bilirubin, which is almost entirely the unconjugated form, averages 0.5 mg/dl of plasma. In certain abnormal conditions, this can rise to as high as 40 mg/dl, and much of it can become the conjugated type. The skin usually begins to appear jaundiced when the concentration rises to about three times normal—that is, above 1.5 mg/dl.

The common causes of jaundice are (1) increased destruction of red blood cells, with rapid release of bilirubin into the blood, and (2) obstruction of the bile ducts or damage to the liver cells so that even the usual amounts of bilirubin cannot be excreted into the gastrointestinal tract. These two types of jaundice are called, respectively, *hemolytic jaundice* and *obstructive jaundice*. They differ from each other in the following ways.

Hemolytic Jaundice Is Caused by Hemolysis of Red Blood Cells. In hemolytic jaundice, the excretory function of the liver is not impaired, but red blood cells are hemolyzed so rapidly that the hepatic cells simply cannot excrete the bilirubin as quickly as it is formed. Therefore, the plasma concentration of free bilirubin rises to above-normal levels. Likewise, the rate of formation of *urobilinogen* in the intestine is greatly increased, and much of this is absorbed into the blood and later excreted in the urine.

Obstructive Jaundice Is Caused by Obstruction of Bile Ducts or Liver Disease. In obstructive jaundice, caused either by obstruction of the bile ducts (which most often occurs when a gallstone or cancer blocks the common bile duct) or by damage to the hepatic cells (which occurs in *hepatitis*), the rate of bilirubin formation is normal, but the bilirubin formed cannot pass from the blood into the intestines. The unconjugated bilirubin still enters the liver cells and becomes conjugated in the usual way. This conjugated bilirubin is then returned to the blood, probably by rupture of the congested bile canaliculi and direct emptying of the bile into the lymph leaving the liver. Thus, *most of the bilirubin in the plasma becomes the conjugated type* rather than the unconjugated type.

Diagnostic Differences Between Hemolytic and Obstructive Jaundice. Chemical laboratory tests can be used to differentiate between unconjugated and conjugated bilirubin in the plasma. In hemolytic jaundice, almost all the bilirubin is in the "unconjugated" form; in obstructive jaundice, it is mainly in the "conjugated" form. A test called the *van den Bergh reaction* can be used to differentiate between the two.

When there is total obstruction of bile flow, no bilirubin can reach the intestines to be converted into urobilinogen by bacteria. Therefore, no urobilinogen is reabsorbed into the blood, and none can be excreted by the kidneys into the urine. Consequently, in *total* obstructive jaundice, tests for urobilinogen in the urine are completely negative. Also, the stools become clay colored owing to a lack of stercobilin and other bile pigments.

Another major difference between unconjugated and conjugated bilirubin is that the kidneys can excrete small quantities of the highly soluble conjugated bilirubin but not the albumin-bound unconjugated bilirubin. Therefore, in severe obstructive jaundice, significant quantities of conjugated bilirubin appear in the urine. This can be demonstrated simply by shaking the urine and observing the foam, which turns an intense yellow. Thus, by understanding the physiology of bilirubin excretion by the liver and by the use of a few simple tests, it is often possible to differentiate among multiple types of hemolytic diseases and liver diseases, as well as to determine the severity of the disease.

Bibliography

Anderson N, Borlak J: Molecular mechanisms and therapeutic targets in steatosis and steatohepatitis, *Pharmacol Rev* 60:31, 2008.

Ankoma-Sey V: Hepatic regeneration—revisiting the myth of Prometheus, *News Physiol Sci* 14:149, 1999.

Bhutani VK, Maisels MJ, Stark AR, Buonocore G: Expert Committee for Severe Neonatal Hyperbilirubinemia; European Society for Pediatric Research; American Academy of Pediatrics. Management of jaundice and prevention of severe neonatal hyperbilirubinemia in infants >or=35 weeks gestation, *Neonatology* 94:63, 2008.

Fevery J: Bilirubin in clinical practice: a review, *Liver Int* 28:592, 2008.

Friedman SL: Hepatic stellate cells: protean, multifunctional, and enigmatic cells of the liver, *Physiol Rev* 88:125, 2008.

Lefebvre P, Cariou B, Lien F, et al: Role of bile acids and bile acid receptors in metabolic regulation, *Physiol Rev* 89:147, 2009.

Maisels MJ, McDonagh AF: Phototherapy for neonatal jaundice, *N Engl J Med* 358:920, 2008.

Marchesini G, Moscatiello S, Di Domizio S, Forlani G: Obesity-associated liver disease, *J Clin Endocrinol Metab* 93(11 Suppl 1):S74, 2008.

Postic C, Girard J: Contribution of de novo fatty acid synthesis to hepatic steatosis and insulin resistance: lessons from genetically engineered mice, *J Clin Invest* 118:829, 2008.

Preiss D, Sattar N: Non-alcoholic fatty liver disease: an overview of prevalence, diagnosis, pathogenesis and treatment considerations, *Clin Sci (Lond)* 115:141, 2008.

Reichen J: The role of the sinusoidal endothelium in liver function, *News Physiol Sci* 14:117, 1999.

Roma MG, Crocenzi FA, Sánchez Pozzi EA: Hepatocellular transport in acquired cholestasis: new insights into functional, regulatory and therapeutic aspects, *Clin Sci (Lond)* 114:567, 2008.

Ryter SW, Alam J, Choi AM: Heme oxygenase-1/carbon monoxide: from basic science to therapeutic applications, *Physiol Rev* 86(2):583–650, 2006.

Sanyal AJ, Bosch J, Blei A, Arroyo V: Portal hypertension and its complications, *Gastroenterology* 134:1715, 2008.

Sozio M, Crabb DW: Alcohol and lipid metabolism, *Am J Physiol Endocrinol Metab* 295:E10, 2008.

Dietary Balances; Regulation of Feeding; Obesity and Starvation; Vitamins and Minerals

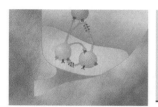

Energy Intake and Output Are Balanced Under Steady-State Conditions

Intake of carbohydrates, fats, and proteins provides energy that can be used to perform various body functions or stored for later use. Stability of body weight and composition over long periods requires that a person's energy intake and energy expenditure be balanced. When a person is overfed and energy intake persistently exceeds expenditure, most of the excess energy is stored as fat, and body weight increases; conversely, loss of body mass and starvation occur when energy intake is insufficient to meet the body's metabolic needs.

Because different foods contain different proportions of proteins, carbohydrates, fats, minerals, and vitamins, appropriate balances must also be maintained among these constituents so that all segments of the body's metabolic systems can be supplied with the requisite materials. This chapter discusses the mechanisms by which food intake is regulated in accordance with the body's metabolic needs and some of the problems of maintaining balance among the different types of foods.

Dietary Balances

Energy Available in Foods

The energy liberated from each gram of carbohydrate as it is oxidized to carbon dioxide and water is 4.1 Calories (1 Calorie equals 1 kilocalorie), and that liberated from fat is 9.3 Calories. The energy liberated from metabolism of the average dietary protein as each gram is oxidized to carbon dioxide, water, and urea is 4.35 Calories. Also, these substances vary in the average percentages that are absorbed from the gastrointestinal tract: about 98 percent of carbohydrate, 95 percent of fat, and 92 percent of protein. Therefore, the average *physiologically available energy* in each gram of these three foodstuffs is as follows:

	Calories
Carbohydrate	4
Fat	9
Protein	4

Average Americans receive about 15 percent of their energy from protein, 40 percent from fat, and 45 percent from carbohydrate. In most non-Western countries, the quantity of energy derived from carbohydrates far exceeds that derived from both proteins and fats. Indeed, in some parts of the world where meat is scarce, the energy received from fats and proteins combined may be no greater than 15 to 20 percent.

Table 71-1 gives the compositions of selected foods, demonstrating especially the high proportions of fat and protein in meat products and the high proportion of carbohydrate in most vegetable and grain products. Fat is deceptive in the diet because it usually exists as nearly 100 percent fat, whereas both proteins and carbohydrates are mixed in watery media so that each of these normally represents less than 25 percent of the weight. Therefore, the fat of one pat of butter mixed with an entire helping of potato sometimes contains as much energy as the potato itself.

Average Daily Requirement for Protein Is 30 to 50 Grams. Twenty to 30 grams of the body proteins are degraded and used to produce other body chemicals daily. Therefore, all cells must continue to form new proteins to take the place of those that are being destroyed, and a supply of protein is necessary in the diet for this purpose. An average person can maintain normal stores of protein, provided the *daily intake is above 30 to 50 grams.*

Some proteins have inadequate quantities of certain essential amino acids and therefore cannot be used to replace the degraded proteins. Such proteins are called *partial proteins*, and when they are present in large quantities in the diet, the daily protein requirement is much greater than normal. In general, proteins derived from animal foodstuffs are more complete than are proteins derived from vegetable and grain sources. For example, the protein of corn has almost no tryptophan, one of the essential amino acids. Therefore, individuals in low-income countries who consume cornmeal as the principal source of protein sometimes develop the protein-deficiency syndrome called *kwashiorkor*, which consists of failure to grow, lethargy, depressed mentality, and edema caused by low plasma protein concentration.

Carbohydrates and Fats Act as "Protein Sparers." When the diet contains an abundance of carbohydrates and fats, almost all the body's energy is derived from these two substances, and little is derived from proteins.

Therefore, both carbohydrates and fats are said to be *protein sparers*. Conversely, in starvation, after the carbohydrates and fats have been depleted, the body's protein

Table 71-1 Protein, Fat, and Carbohydrate Content of Different Foods

Food	% Protein	% Fat	% Carbohydrate	Fuel Value per 100 Grams (Calories)
Apples	0.3	0.4	14.9	64
Asparagus	2.2	0.2	3.9	26
Bacon, fat	6.2	76.0	0.7	712
broiled	25.0	55.0	1.0	599
Beef (average)	17.5	22.0	1.0	268
Beets, fresh	1.6	0.1	9.6	46
Bread, white	9.0	3.6	49.8	268
Butter	0.6	81.0	0.4	733
Cabbage	1.4	0.2	5.3	29
Carrots	1.2	0.3	9.3	45
Cashew nuts	19.6	47.2	26.4	609
Cheese, cheddar, American	23.9	32.3	1.7	393
Chicken, total edible	21.6	2.7	1.0	111
Chocolate	5.5	52.9	18.0	570
Corn (maize)	10.0	4.3	73.4	372
Haddock	17.2	0.3	0.5	72
Lamb, leg (average)	18.0	17.5	1.0	230
Milk, fresh whole	3.5	3.9	4.9	69
Molasses	0.0	0.0	60.0	240
Oatmeal, dry, uncooked	14.2	7.4	68.2	396
Oranges	0.9	0.2	11.2	50
Peanuts	26.9	44.2	23.6	600
Peas, fresh	6.7	0.4	17.7	101
Pork, ham	15.2	31.0	1.0	340
Potatoes	2.0	0.1	19.1	85
Spinach	2.3	0.3	3.2	25
Strawberries	0.8	0.6	8.1	41
Tomatoes	1.0	0.3	4.0	23
Tuna, canned	24.2	10.8	0.5	194
Walnuts, English	15.0	64.4	15.6	702

stores are consumed rapidly for energy, sometimes at rates approaching several hundred grams per day rather than the normal daily rate of 30 to 50 grams.

Methods for Determining Metabolic Utilization of Carbohydrates, Fats, and Proteins

"Respiratory Quotient" Is the Ratio of CO_2 Production to O_2 Utilization and Can Be Used to Estimate Fat and Carbohydrate Utilization. When carbohydrates are metabolized with oxygen, exactly one carbon dioxide molecule is formed for each molecule of oxygen consumed. This ratio of carbon dioxide output to oxygen usage is called the *respiratory quotient*, so the respiratory quotient for carbohydrates is 1.0.

When fat is oxidized in the body's cells, an average of 70 carbon dioxide molecules are formed for each 100 molecules of oxygen consumed. The respiratory quotient for the metabolism of fat therefore averages 0.70. When proteins are oxidized by the cells, the average respiratory quotient is 0.80. The reason that the respiratory quotients for fats and proteins are lower than those for carbohydrates is that a portion of the oxygen metabolized with these foods is required to combine with the excess hydrogen atoms present in their molecules, so less carbon dioxide is formed in relation to the oxygen used.

Now let us see how one can make use of the respiratory quotient to determine the relative utilization of different foods by the body. First, it will be recalled from Chapter 39 that the output of carbon dioxide by the lungs divided by the uptake of oxygen during the same period is called the *respiratory exchange ratio*. Over a period of 1 hour or more, the respiratory exchange ratio exactly equals the average respiratory quotient of the metabolic reactions throughout the body. If a person has a respiratory quotient of 1.0, he or she is metabolizing almost entirely carbohydrates, because the respiratory quotients for both fat and protein metabolism are considerably less than 1.0. Likewise, when the respiratory quotient is about 0.70, the body is metabolizing almost entirely fats, to the exclusion of carbohydrates and proteins. And, finally, if we ignore the normally small amount of protein metabolism, respiratory quotients between 0.70 and 1.0 describe the approximate ratios of carbohydrate to fat metabolism. To be more exact, one can first determine the protein utilization by measuring nitrogen excretion as discussed in the next section. Then, using the appropriate mathematical formula, one can calculate almost exactly the utilization of the three foodstuffs.

Some of the important findings from studies of respiratory quotients are the following:

1. Immediately after a meal, almost all the food that is metabolized is carbohydrates, so the respiratory quotient at that time approaches 1.0.

2. About 8 to 10 hours after a meal, the body has already used up most of its readily available carbohydrates, and the respiratory quotient approaches that for fat metabolism, about 0.70.

3. In untreated diabetes mellitus, little carbohydrate can be used by the body's cells under any conditions because insulin is required for this. Therefore, when diabetes is severe, most of the time the respiratory quotient remains near that for fat metabolism, 0.70.

Nitrogen Excretion Can Be Used to Assess Protein Metabolism. The average protein contains about 16 percent nitrogen. During metabolism of the protein, about 90 percent of this nitrogen is excreted in the urine in the form of urea, uric acid, creatinine, and other nitrogen products. The remaining 10 percent is excreted in the feces. Therefore, the rate of protein breakdown in the body can be estimated by measuring the amount of nitrogen in the urine, then adding 10 percent for the nitrogen excreted in the feces, and multiplying by 6.25 (i.e., 100/16) to determine the total amount of protein metabolism in grams per day. Thus, excretion of 8 grams of nitrogen in the urine each day means that there has been about 55 grams of protein breakdown. If the daily intake of protein is less than the daily breakdown of protein, the person is said to have a *negative nitrogen balance*, which means that his or her body stores of protein are decreasing daily.

Regulation of Food Intake and Energy Storage

Stability of the body's total mass and composition over long periods requires that energy intake match energy expenditure. As discussed in Chapter 72, only about 27 percent of the energy ingested normally reaches the functional systems of the cells, and much of this is eventually converted to heat, which is generated as a result of protein metabolism, muscle activity, and activities of the various organs and tissues of the body. Excess energy intake is stored mainly as fat, whereas a deficit of energy intake causes loss of total body mass until energy expenditure eventually equals energy intake or death occurs.

Although there is considerable variability in the amount of energy storage (i.e., fat mass) in different individuals, maintenance of an adequate energy supply is necessary for survival. Therefore, the body is endowed with powerful physiologic control systems that help maintain adequate energy intake. Deficits of energy stores, for example, rapidly activate multiple mechanisms that cause hunger and drive a person to seek food. In athletes and laborers, energy expenditure for the high level of muscle activity may be as high as 6000 to 7000 Calories per day, compared with only about 2000 Calories per day for sedentary individuals. Thus, a large energy expenditure associated with physical work usually stimulates equally large increases in caloric intake.

What are the physiological mechanisms that sense changes in energy balance and influence the quest for food? Maintenance of adequate energy supply in the body is so critical that there are multiple short-term and long-term control systems that regulate not only food intake but also energy expenditure and energy stores. In the next few sections we describe some of these control systems and their operation in physiological conditions, as well as in obesity and starvation.

Neural Centers Regulate Food Intake

The sensation of *hunger* is associated with a craving for food and several other physiological effects, such as rhythmical contractions of the stomach and restlessness, which cause the person to seek an adequate food supply. A person's *appetite is a desire for food*, often of a particular type, and is useful in helping to choose the quality of the food to be eaten. If the quest for food is successful, the feeling of *satiety* occurs. Each of these feelings is influenced by environmental and cultural factors, as well as by physiologic controls that influence specific centers of the brain, especially the hypothalamus.

The Hypothalamus Contains Hunger and Satiety Centers. Several neuronal centers of the hypothalamus participate in the control of food intake. The *lateral nuclei of the hypothalamus serve as a feeding center*, and stimulation of this area causes an animal to eat voraciously *(hyperphagia)*. Conversely, destruction of the lateral hypothalamus causes lack of desire for food and progressive *inanition*, a condition characterized by marked weight loss, muscle weakness, and decreased metabolism. The lateral hypothalamic feeding center operates by exciting the motor drives to search for food.

The *ventromedial nuclei of the hypothalamus serve as the satiety center*. This center is believed to give a sense of nutritional satisfaction that inhibits the feeding center. Electrical stimulation of this region can cause complete satiety, and even in the presence of highly appetizing food, the animal refuses to eat *(aphagia)*. Conversely, destruction of the ventromedial nuclei causes voracious and continued eating until the animal becomes extremely obese, sometimes weighing as much as four times normal.

845

The *paraventricular, dorsomedial,* and *arcuate nuclei* of the hypothalamus also play a major role in regulating food intake. For example, lesions of the paraventricular nuclei often cause excessive eating, whereas lesions of the dorsomedial nuclei usually depress eating behavior. As discussed later, the arcuate nuclei are the sites in the hypothalamus where multiple hormones released from the gastrointestinal tract and adipose tissue converge to regulate food intake, as well as energy expenditure.

There is much chemical cross-talk among the neurons on the hypothalamus, and together, these centers coordinate the processes that control eating behavior and the perception of satiety. These hypothalamic nuclei also influence the secretion of several hormones that are important in regulating energy balance and metabolism, including those from the thyroid and adrenal glands, as well as the pancreatic islet cells.

The hypothalamus receives neural signals from the gastrointestinal tract that provide sensory information about stomach filling; chemical signals from nutrients in the blood (glucose, amino acids, and fatty acids) that signify satiety; signals from gastrointestinal hormones; signals from hormones released by adipose tissue; and signals from the cerebral cortex (sight, smell, and taste) that influence feeding behavior. Some of these inputs to the hypothalamus are shown in Figure 71-1.

The hypothalamic feeding and satiety centers have a high density of receptors for neurotransmitters and hormones that influence feeding behavior. A few of the many substances that have been shown to alter appetite and feeding behavior in experimental studies are listed in Table 71-2 and are generally categorized as (1) *orexigenic* substances that stimulate feeding or (2) *anorexigenic* substances that inhibit feeding.

Neurons and Neurotransmitters in the Hypothalamus That Stimulate or Inhibit Feeding.

There are two distinct types of neurons in the arcuate nuclei of the hypothalamus that are especially important as controllers of both appetite and energy expenditure (Figure 71-2): (1) *pro-opiomelanocortin (POMC) neurons* that produce α-melanocyte-stimulating hormone (α-MSH) together with cocaine- and amphetamine-related transcript (CART) and (2) *neurons that produce the orexigenic substances neuropeptide Y (NPY) and agouti-related protein (AGRP).* Activation of the POMC neurons decreases food intake and increases energy expenditure, whereas activation of the NPY-AGRP neurons increases food intake and reduces energy expenditure. As discussed later, these neurons appear to be the major targets for several hormones that regulate appetite, including *leptin, insulin, cholecystokinin (CCK),* and *ghrelin.* In fact, the neurons of the arcuate nuclei appear to be a site of convergence of many of the nervous and peripheral signals that regulate energy stores.

The POMC neurons release α-MSH, which then acts on *melanocortin receptors* found especially in neurons of the *paraventricular nuclei.* Although there are at least

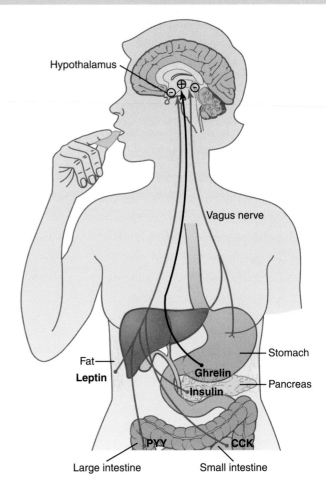

Figure 71-1 Feedback mechanisms for control of food intake. Stretch receptors in the stomach activate sensory afferent pathways in the vagus nerve and inhibit food intake. Peptide YY (*PYY*), cholecystokinin (*CCK*), and insulin are gastrointestinal hormones that are released by the ingestion of food and suppress further feeding. Ghrelin is released by the stomach, especially during fasting, and stimulates appetite. Leptin is a hormone produced in increasing amounts by fat cells as they increase in size; it inhibits food intake.

five subtypes of melanocortin receptors (MCR), *MCR-3* and *MCR-4* are especially important in regulating food intake and energy balance. Activation of these receptors reduces food intake while increasing energy expenditure. Conversely, inhibition of MCR-3 and MCR-4 greatly increases food intake and decreases energy expenditure. The effect of MCR activation to increase energy expenditure appears to be mediated, at least in part, by activation of neuronal pathways that project from the paraventricular nuclei to the *nucleus tractus solitarius* and stimulate sympathetic nervous system activity.

The hypothalamic melanocortin system plays a powerful role in regulating energy stores of the body, and defective signaling of the melanocortin pathway is associated with extreme obesity. In fact, mutations of MCR-4 represent the most common known monogenic (single-gene) cause of human obesity, and some studies suggest that MCR-4 mutations may account for as much as 5 to 6 percent of early-onset severe obesity in children. In contrast, excessive activation of the melanocortin system reduces appetite. Some studies suggest that this activation may

Table 71-2 Neurotransmitters and Hormones That Influence Feeding and Satiety Centers in the Hypothalamus

Decrease Feeding (Anorexigenic)	Increase Feeding (Orexigenic)
α-Melanocyte-stimulating hormone (α-MSH)	Neuropeptide Y (NPY)
Leptin	Agouti-related protein (AGRP)
Serotonin	Melanin-concentrating hormone (MCH)
Norepinephrine	Orexins A and B
Corticotropin-releasing hormone	Endorphins
Insulin	Galanin (GAL)
Cholecystokinin (CCK)	Amino acids (glutamate and γ-aminobutyric acid)
Glucagon-like peptide (GLP)	Cortisol
Cocaine- and amphetamine-regulated transcript (CART)	Ghrelin
Peptide YY (PYY)	Endocannabinoids

play a role in causing the anorexia associated with severe infections, cancer tumors, or uremia.

AGRP released from the orexigenic neurons of the hypothalamus is a natural antagonist of MCR-3 and MCR-4 and probably increases feeding by inhibiting the effects of α-MSH to stimulate melanocortin receptors (see Figure 71-2). Although the role of AGRP in normal physiologic control of food intake is unclear, excessive formation of AGRP in mice and humans, due to gene mutations, is associated with increased food intake and obesity.

NPY is also released from orexigenic neurons of the arcuate nuclei. When energy stores of the body are low, orexigenic neurons are activated to release NPY, which stimulates appetite. At the same time, firing of the POMC neurons is reduced, thereby decreasing the activity of the melanocortin pathway and further stimulating appetite.

Neural Centers That Influence the Mechanical Process of Feeding. Another aspect of feeding is the mechanical act of the feeding process itself. If the brain is sectioned below the hypothalamus but above the mesencephalon, the animal can still perform the basic mechanical features of the feeding process. It can salivate, lick its lips,

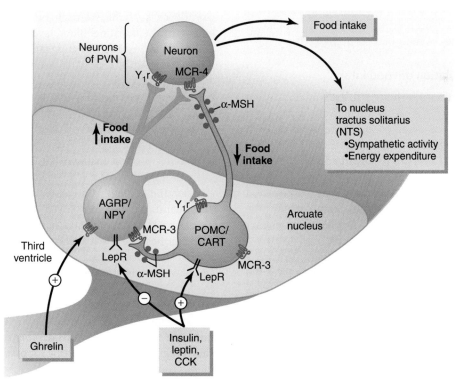

Figure 71-2 Control of energy balance by two types of neurons of the arcuate nuclei: (1) pro-opiomelanocortin (*POMC*) neurons that release α-melanocyte-stimulating hormone (*α-MSH*) and cocaine- and amphetamine-regulated transcript (*CART*), decreasing food intake and increasing energy expenditure and (2) neurons that produce agouti-related protein (*AGRP*) and neuropeptide Y (*NPY*), increasing food intake and reducing energy expenditure. α-MSH released by POMC neurons stimulates melanocortin receptors (*MCR-3* and *MCR-4*) in the paraventricular nuclei (*PVN*), which then activate neuronal pathways that project to the nucleus tractus solitarius (*NTS*) and increase sympathetic activity and energy expenditure. AGRP acts as an antagonist of MCR-4. Insulin, leptin, and cholecystokinin (*CCK*) are hormones that inhibit AGRP-NPY neurons and stimulate adjacent POMC-CART neurons, thereby reducing food intake. Ghrelin, a hormone secreted from the stomach, activates AGRP-NPY neurons and stimulates food intake. LepR, leptin receptor; Y₁R, neuropeptide Y1 receptor. (Redrawn from Barsh GS, Schwartz MW: Nature Rev Genetics 3:589, 2002.)

chew food, and swallow. Therefore, *the actual mechanics of feeding are controlled by centers in the brain stem*. The function of the other centers in feeding, then, is to control the quantity of food intake and to excite these centers of feeding mechanics to activity.

Neural centers higher than the hypothalamus also play important roles in the control of feeding, particularly in the control of appetite. These centers include the *amygdala* and the *prefrontal cortex*, which are closely coupled with the hypothalamus. It will be recalled from the discussion of the sense of smell in Chapter 53 that portions of the amygdala are a major part of the olfactory nervous system. Destructive lesions in the amygdala have demonstrated that some of its areas increase feeding, whereas others inhibit feeding. In addition, stimulation of some areas of the amygdala elicits the mechanical act of feeding. An important effect of destruction of the amygdala on both sides of the brain is a "psychic blindness" in the choice of foods. In other words, the animal (and presumably the human being as well) loses or at least partially loses the appetite control that determines the type and quality of food it eats.

Factors That Regulate Quantity of Food Intake

Regulation of the quantity of food intake can be divided into *short-term regulation*, which is concerned primarily with preventing overeating at each meal, and *long-term regulation*, which is concerned primarily with maintenance of normal quantities of energy stores in the body.

Short-Term Regulation of Food Intake

When a person is driven by hunger to eat voraciously and rapidly, what turns off the eating when he or she has eaten enough? There has not been enough time for changes in the body's energy stores to occur, and it takes hours for enough nutritional factors to be absorbed into the blood to cause the necessary inhibition of eating. Yet it is important that the person not overeat and that he or she eat an amount of food that approximates nutritional needs. The following are several types of rapid feedback signals that are important for these purposes.

Gastrointestinal Filling Inhibits Feeding. When the gastrointestinal tract becomes distended, especially the stomach and the duodenum, stretch inhibitory signals are transmitted mainly by way of the vagi to suppress the feeding center, thereby reducing the desire for food (see Figure 71-1).

Gastrointestinal Hormonal Factors Suppress Feeding. *Cholecystokinin (CCK)*, released mainly in response to fat and proteins entering the duodenum, enters the blood and acts as a hormone to influence several gastrointestinal functions such as gallbladder contraction, gastric emptying, gut motility, and gastric acid secretion as discussed in Chapters 62, 63, and 64. However, CCK also activates receptors on local sensory nerves in the duodenum, sending messages to the brain via the vagus nerve that contribute to satiation and meal cessation. The effect of CCK is short-lived and chronic administration of CCK by itself has no major effect on body weight. Therefore, CCK functions mainly to prevent overeating during meals but may not play a major role in the frequency of meals or the total energy consumed.

Peptide YY (PYY) is secreted from the entire gastrointestinal tract, but especially from the ileum and colon. Food intake stimulates release of PYY, with blood concentrations rising to peak levels 1 to 2 hours after ingesting a meal. These peak levels of PYY are influenced by the number of calories ingested and the composition of the food, with higher levels of PYY observed after meals with a high fat content. Although injections of PYY into mice have been shown to decrease food intake for 12 hours or more, the importance of this gastrointestinal hormone in regulating appetite in humans is still unclear.

For reasons that are not entirely understood, the presence of food in the intestines stimulates them to secrete *glucagon-like peptide (GLP)*, which in turn enhances glucose-dependent *insulin* production and secretion from the pancreas. Glucagon-like peptide and insulin both tend to suppress appetite. Thus, eating a meal stimulates the release of several gastrointestinal hormones that may induce satiety and reduce further intake of food (see Figure 71-1).

Ghrelin—a Gastrointestinal Hormone—Increases Feeding. *Ghrelin* is a hormone released mainly by the oxyntic cells of the stomach but also, to a much less extent, by the intestine. Blood levels of ghrelin rise during fasting, peak just before eating, and then fall rapidly after a meal, suggesting a possible role in stimulating feeding. Also, administration of ghrelin increases food intake in experimental animals, further supporting the possibility that it may be an orexigenic hormone. However, its physiologic role in humans is still uncertain.

Oral Receptors Meter Food Intake. When an animal with an esophageal fistula is fed large quantities of food, even though this food is immediately lost again to the exterior, the degree of hunger is decreased after a reasonable quantity of food has passed through the mouth. This effect occurs despite the fact that the gastrointestinal tract does not become the least bit filled. Therefore, it is postulated that various "oral factors" related to feeding, such as chewing, salivation, swallowing, and tasting, "meter" the food as it passes through the mouth, and after a certain amount has passed, the hypothalamic feeding center becomes inhibited. However, the inhibition caused by this metering mechanism is considerably less intense and of shorter duration, usually lasting for only 20 to 40 minutes, than is the inhibition caused by gastrointestinal filling.

Intermediate and Long-Term Regulation of Food Intake

An animal that has been starved for a long time and is then presented with unlimited food eats a far greater quantity than does an animal that has been on a regular diet. Conversely, an animal that has been force-fed for several weeks eats very little when allowed to eat according to its own desires. Thus, the feeding control mechanism of the body is geared to the nutritional status of the body.

Effect of Blood Concentrations of Glucose, Amino Acids, and Lipids on Hunger and Feeding. It has long been known that a decrease in blood glucose concentration causes hunger, which has led to the so-called *glucostatic theory of hunger and feeding regulation*. Similar studies have demonstrated the same effect for blood amino acid concentration and blood concentration of breakdown products of lipids such as the keto acids and some fatty acids, leading to the *aminostatic* and *lipostatic* theories of regulation. That is, when the availability of any of the three major types of food decreases, the desire for feeding is increased, eventually returning the blood metabolite concentrations back toward normal.

Neurophysiological studies of function in specific areas of the brain also support the glucostatic, aminostatic, and lipostatic theories, by the following observations: (1) A rise in blood *glucose* level *increases the rate of firing of glucoreceptor neurons in the satiety center in the ventromedial and paraventricular nuclei of the hypothalamus.* (2) The same increase in blood glucose level simultaneously *decreases* the firing of *glucosensitive neurons* in the *hunger center of the lateral hypothalamus.* In addition, some amino acids and lipid substances affect the rates of firing of these same neurons or other closely associated neurons.

Temperature Regulation and Food Intake. When an animal is exposed to cold, it tends to increase feeding; when it is exposed to heat, it tends to decrease its caloric intake. This is caused by interaction within the hypothalamus between the temperature-regulating system (see Chapter 73) and the food intake–regulating system. This is important because increased food intake in a cold animal (1) increases its metabolic rate and (2) provides increased fat for insulation, both of which tend to correct the cold state.

Feedback Signals from Adipose Tissue Regulate Food Intake. Most of the stored energy in the body consists of fat, the amount of which can vary considerably in different individuals. What regulates this energy reserve, and why is there so much variability among individuals?

Studies in humans and in experimental animals indicate that the hypothalamus senses energy storage through the actions of *leptin*, a peptide hormone released from adipocytes. When the amount of adipose tissue increases (signaling excess energy storage), the adipocytes produce increased amounts of leptin, which is released into the blood. Leptin then circulates to the brain, where it moves across the blood-brain barrier by facilitated diffusion and occupies leptin receptors at multiple sites in the hypothalamus, especially the POMC neurons of the arcuate nuclei and neurons of the paraventricular nuclei.

Stimulation of leptin receptors in these hypothalamic nuclei initiates multiple actions that decrease fat storage, including (1) decreased production in the hypothalamus of appetite stimulators, such as *NPY* and *AGRP*; (2) *activation of POMC neurons*, causing release of α-MSH and activation of melanocortin receptors; (3) increased production in the hypothalamus of substances, such as *corticotropin-releasing hormone*, that decrease food intake; (4) *increased sympathetic nerve activity* (through neural projections from the hypothalamus to the vasomotor centers), which increases metabolic rate and energy expenditure; and (5) *decreased insulin secretion* by the pancreatic beta cells, which decreases energy storage. Thus, leptin is an important means by which the adipose tissue signals the brain that enough energy has been stored and that intake of food is no longer necessary.

In mice or humans with mutations that render their fat cells unable to produce leptin or mutations that cause defective leptin receptors in the hypothalamus, marked hyperphagia and morbid obesity occur. In most obese humans, however, there does not appear to be a deficiency of leptin production because plasma leptin levels increase in proportion with increasing adiposity. Therefore, some physiologists believe that obesity may be associated with *leptin resistance*; that is, leptin receptors or postreceptor signaling pathways normally activated by leptin may be defective in obese people, who continue to eat despite very high levels of leptin.

Another explanation for the failure of leptin to prevent increasing adiposity in obese individuals is that there are many redundant systems that control feeding behavior, as well as social and cultural factors that can cause continued excess food intake even in the presence of high levels of leptin.

Summary of Long-Term Regulation. Even though our information on the different feedback factors in long-term feeding regulation is imprecise, we can make the following general statement: When the energy stores of the body fall below normal, the feeding centers of the hypothalamus and other areas of the brain become highly active, and the person exhibits increased hunger, as well as searching for food. Conversely, when the energy stores (mainly the fat stores) are already abundant, the person usually loses the sensation of hunger and develops a state of satiety.

Importance of Having Both Long- and Short-Term Regulatory Systems for Feeding

The long-term regulatory system for feeding, which includes all the nutritional energy feedback mechanisms, helps maintain constant stores of nutrients in the tissues, preventing them from becoming too low or too high. The short-term regulatory stimuli serve two other purposes. First, they tend to make the person eat smaller quantities at each eating session, thus allowing food to pass through the gastrointestinal tract at a steadier pace so that its digestive and absorptive mechanisms can work at optimal rates rather than becoming periodically overburdened. Second, they help prevent the person from eating amounts at each meal that would be too much for the metabolic storage systems once all the food has been absorbed.

Obesity

Obesity can be defined as an excess of body fat. A surrogate marker for body fat content is the body mass index (BMI), which is calculated as:

$$BMI = Weight\ in\ kg/Height\ in\ m^2$$

In clinical terms, a BMI between 25 and 29.9 kg/m^2 is called overweight, and a BMI greater than 30 kg/m^2 is called obese. BMI is not a direct estimate of adiposity and does not take into account the fact that some individuals have a high BMI due to a large muscle mass. A better way to define obesity is to actually measure the percentage of total body fat. Obesity is usually defined as 25 percent or greater total body fat in men and 35 percent or greater in women. Although percentage of body fat can be estimated with various methods, such as measuring skin-fold thickness, bioelectrical impedance, or underwater weighing, these methods are rarely used in clinical practice, where BMI is commonly used to assess obesity.

The prevalence of obesity in children and adults in the United States and in many other industrialized countries is rapidly increasing, rising by more than 30 percent over the past decade. Approximately 65 percent of adults in the United States are overweight, and nearly 33 percent of adults are obese.

Obesity Results from Greater Energy Intake Than Energy Expenditure. When greater quantities of energy (in the form of food) enter the body than are expended, the body weight increases, and most of the excess energy is stored as fat. Therefore, excessive adiposity (obesity) is caused by energy intake in excess of energy output. For each 9.3 Calories of excess energy that enter the body, approximately 1 gram of fat is stored.

Fat is stored mainly in adipocytes in subcutaneous tissue and in the intraperitoneal cavity, although the liver and other tissues of the body often accumulate significant amounts of lipids in obese persons. The metabolic processes involved in fat storage were discussed in Chapter 68.

It was previously believed that the number of adipocytes could increase substantially only during infancy and childhood and that excess energy intake in children led to *hyperplastic obesity*, associated with increased numbers of adipocytes and only small increases in adipocyte size. In contrast, obesity developing in adults was thought to increase only adipocyte size, resulting in *hypertrophic obesity*. Recent studies, however, have shown that new adipocytes can differentiate from fibroblast-like preadipocytes at any period of life and that the development of obesity in adults is accompanied by increased numbers, as well as increased size, of adipocytes. An extremely obese person may have as many as four times as many adipocytes, each containing twice as much lipid, as a lean person.

Once a person has become obese and a stable weight is obtained, energy intake once again equals energy output. For a person to lose weight, energy intake must be *less* than energy expenditure.

Decreased Physical Activity and Abnormal Feeding Regulation as Causes of Obesity

The causes of obesity are complex. Although genes play an important role in programming the powerful physiological mechanisms that regulate food intake and energy metabolism, lifestyle and environmental factors may play the dominant role in many obese people. The rapid increase in the prevalence of obesity in the past 20 to 30 years emphasizes the important role of lifestyle and environmental factors because genetic changes could not have occurred so rapidly.

Sedentary Lifestyle Is a Major Cause of Obesity. Regular physical activity and physical training are known to increase muscle mass and decrease body fat mass, whereas inadequate physical activity is typically associated with decreased muscle mass and increased adiposity. For example, studies have shown a close association between sedentary behaviors, such as prolonged television watching, and obesity.

About 25 to 30 percent of the energy used each day by the average person goes into muscular activity, and in a laborer, as much as 60 to 70 percent is used in this way. In obese people, increased physical activity usually increases energy expenditure more than food intake, resulting in significant weight loss. Even a single episode of strenuous exercise may increase basal energy expenditure for several hours after the physical activity is stopped. Because muscular activity is by far the most important means by which energy is expended in the body, increased physical activity is often an effective means of reducing fat stores.

Abnormal Feeding Behavior Is an Important Cause of Obesity. Although powerful physiological mechanisms regulate food intake, there are also important environmental and psychological factors that can cause abnormal feeding behavior, excessive energy intake, and obesity.

Environmental, Social, and Psychological Factors Contribute to Abnormal Feeding. As discussed previously, the importance of environmental factors is evident from the rapid increase in the prevalence of obesity in most industrialized countries, which has coincided with an abundance of high-energy foods (especially fatty foods) and sedentary lifestyles.

Psychological factors may contribute to obesity in some people. For example, people often gain large amounts of weight during or after stressful situations, such as the death of a parent, a severe illness, or even mental depression. It seems that eating can be a means of releasing tension.

Childhood Overnutrition as a Possible Cause of Obesity. One factor that may contribute to obesity is the prevalent idea that healthy eating habits require three meals a day and that each meal must be filling. Many young children are forced into this habit by overly solicitous parents, and the children continue to practice it throughout life.

The rate of formation of new fat cells is especially rapid in the first few years of life, and the greater the rate of fat storage, the greater the number of fat cells. The number of fat cells in obese children is often as much as three times that in normal children. Therefore, it has been suggested that overnutrition of children—especially in infancy and, to a lesser extent, during the later years of childhood—can lead to a lifetime of obesity.

Neurogenic Abnormalities as a Cause of Obesity. We previously pointed out that lesions in the ventromedial nuclei of the hypothalamus cause an animal to eat excessively and become obese. People with hypophysial tumors that encroach on the hypothalamus often develop progressive obesity, demonstrating that obesity in human beings, too, can result from damage to the hypothalamus.

Although hypothalamic damage is almost never found in obese people, it is possible that the functional organization of the hypothalamic or other neurogenic feeding centers in obese individuals is different from that in nonobese persons. Also, there may be abnormalities of neurotransmitters or receptor mechanisms in the neural pathways of the hypothalamus that control feeding. In support of this theory, an obese person who has reduced to normal weight by strict dietary measures usually develops intense hunger that is demonstrably far greater than that of a normal person. This indicates that the "set-point" of an obese person's feeding control system is at a much higher level of nutrient storage than that of a nonobese person.

Studies in experimental animals also indicate that when food intake is restricted in obese animals, there are marked neurotransmitter changes in the hypothalamus that greatly increase hunger and oppose weight loss. Some of these changes include increased formation of orexigenic neurotransmitters such as NPY and decreased formation of anorexic substances such as leptin and α-MSH.

Genetic Factors as a Cause of Obesity. Obesity definitely runs in families. Yet it has been difficult to determine the precise role of genetics in contributing to obesity because family members generally share many of the same eating habits and physical activity patterns. Current evidence, however, suggests that 20 to 25 percent of cases of obesity may be caused by genetic factors.

Genes can contribute to obesity by causing abnormalities of (1) one or more of the pathways that regulate the feeding centers and (2) energy expenditure and fat storage. Three of the monogenic (single-gene) causes of obesity are (1) *mutations of MCR-4*, the most common monogenic form of obesity discovered thus far; (2) *congenital leptin deficiency* caused by mutations of the leptin gene, which are very rare; and (3) *mutations of the leptin receptor*, also very rare. All these monogenic forms of obesity account for only a very small percentage of obesity. It is likely that many gene variations interact with environmental factors to influence the amount and distribution of body fat.

Treatment of Obesity

Treatment of obesity depends on decreasing energy input below energy expenditure and creating a sustained negative energy balance until the desired weight loss is achieved. In other words, this means either reducing energy intake or increasing energy expenditure. The current National Institutes of Health (NIH) guidelines recommend a decrease in caloric intake of 500 kilocalories per day for overweight and moderately obese persons (BMI > 25 but < 35 kg/m²) to achieve a weight loss of approximately 1 pound each week. A more aggressive energy deficit of 500 to 1000 kilocalories per day is recommended for persons with BMIs greater than 35 kg/m². Typically, such an energy deficit, if it can be achieved and sustained, will cause a weight loss of about 1 to 2 pounds per week, or about a 10 percent weight loss after 6 months. For most people attempting to lose weight, increasing physical activity is also an important component of successful long-term weight loss.

To decrease energy intake, most reducing diets are designed to contain large quantities of "bulk," which is generally made up of non-nutritive cellulose substances. This bulk distends the stomach and thereby partially appeases hunger. In experimental animals, such a procedure simply makes the animal increase its food intake even more, but human beings can often fool themselves because their food intake is sometimes controlled as much by habit as by hunger. As pointed out later in connection with starvation, it is important to prevent vitamin deficiencies during the dieting period.

Various *drugs for decreasing the degree of hunger* have been used in the treatment of obesity. The most widely used drugs are *amphetamines* (or amphetamine derivatives), which directly inhibit the feeding centers in the brain. One drug for treating obesity is *sibutramine*, a sympathomimetic that reduces food intake and increases energy expenditure. The danger in using these drugs is that they simultaneously overexcite the sympathetic nervous system and raise the blood pressure. Also, a person soon adapts to the drug, so weight reduction is usually no greater than 5 to 10 percent.

Another group of drugs works by altering lipid metabolism. For example, *orlistat, a lipase inhibitor, reduces the intestinal digestion of fat.* This causes a portion of the ingested fat to be lost in the feces and therefore reduces energy absorption. However, fecal fat loss may cause unpleasant gastrointestinal side effects, as well as loss of fat-soluble vitamins in the feces.

Significant weight loss can be achieved in many obese persons with increased physical activity. The more exercise one gets, the greater the daily energy expenditure and the more rapidly the obesity disappears. Therefore, forced exercise is often an essential part of treatment. The current clinical guidelines for the treatment of obesity recommend that the first step be lifestyle modifications that include increased physical activity combined with a reduction in caloric intake. For morbidly obese patients with BMIs greater than 40, or for patients with BMIs greater than 35 and conditions such as hypertension or type II diabetes that predispose them to other serious diseases, various surgical procedures can be used to decrease the fat mass of the body or to decrease the amount of food that can be eaten at each meal.

Two of the most common surgical procedures used in the United States to treat morbid obesity are gastric bypass surgery and gastric banding surgery. *Gastric bypass surgery* involves construction of a small pouch in the proximal part of the stomach that is then connected to the jejunum with a section of small bowel of varying lengths; the pouch is separated from the remaining part of the stomach with staples. *Gastric banding surgery* involves placing an adjustable band around the stomach near its upper end; this also creates a small stomach pouch that restricts the amount of food that can be eaten at each meal. Although these surgical procedures generally produce substantial weight loss in obese patients, they are major operations, and their long-term effects on overall health and mortality are still uncertain.

Inanition, Anorexia, and Cachexia

Inanition is the opposite of obesity and is characterized by extreme weight loss. It can be caused by inadequate availability of food or by pathophysiological conditions that greatly decrease the desire for food, including psychogenic disturbances, hypothalamic abnormalities, and factors released from peripheral tissues. In many instances, especially in those with serious diseases such as cancer, the reduced desire for food may be associated with increased energy expenditure, causing serious weight loss.

Anorexia can be defined as *a reduction in food intake caused primarily by diminished appetite*, as opposed to the literal definition of "not eating." This definition emphasizes the important role of central neural mechanisms in the pathophysiology of anorexia in diseases such as cancer, when other common problems, such as pain and nausea, may also cause a person to consume less food. *Anorexia nervosa* is an abnormal psychic state in which a person loses all desire for food and even becomes nauseated by food; as a result, severe inanition occurs.

Cachexia is a metabolic disorder of increased energy expenditure leading to weight loss greater than that caused by reduced food intake alone. Anorexia and cachexia often occur together in many types of cancer or in the "wasting syndrome" observed in patients with acquired immunodeficiency syndrome (AIDS) and chronic inflammatory disorders. Almost all types of cancer cause both anorexia and cachexia, and more than half of cancer patients develop anorexia-cachexia syndrome during the course of their disease.

Central neural and peripheral factors are believed to contribute to cancer-induced anorexia and cachexia. Several inflammatory cytokines, including *tumor necrosis factor-α, interleukin-6, interleukin-1β,* and a *proteolysis-inducing factor,* have been shown to cause anorexia and cachexia. Most of these inflammatory cytokines appear to mediate anorexia by activation of the *melanocortin system* in the hypothalamus. The precise mechanisms by which cytokines or tumor products interact with the melanocortin pathway to decrease food intake are still unclear, but blockade of the hypothalamic melanocortin receptors appears to almost completely prevent their anorexic and cachectic effects in experimental animals. Additional research, however, is necessary to better understand the pathophysiological mechanisms of anorexia and cachexia in cancer patients and to develop therapeutic agents to improve their nutritional status and survival.

Starvation

Depletion of Food Stores in the Body Tissues During Starvation. Even though the tissues preferentially use carbohydrate for energy over both fat and protein, the quantity of carbohydrate normally stored in the entire body is only a few hundred grams (mainly glycogen in the liver and muscles), and it can supply the energy required for body functions for perhaps half a day. Therefore, except for the first few hours of starvation, the major effects are progressive depletion of tissue fat and protein. Because fat is the prime source of energy (100 times as much fat energy is stored in the normal person as carbohydrate energy), the rate of fat depletion continues unabated, as shown in Figure 71-3, until most of the fat stores in the body are gone.

Protein undergoes three phases of depletion: rapid depletion at first, then greatly slowed depletion, and, finally, rapid depletion again shortly before death. The initial rapid depletion is caused by the use of easily mobilized protein for direct metabolism or for conversion to glucose and then metabolism of glucose mainly by the brain. After the readily mobilized protein stores have been depleted during the early phase of starvation, the remaining protein is not so easily removed. At this time, the rate of gluconeogenesis decreases to one-third to one-fifth its previous rate, and the rate of depletion of protein becomes greatly decreased. The lessened availability of glucose then initiates a series of events that leads to excessive fat utilization and conversion of some of the fat

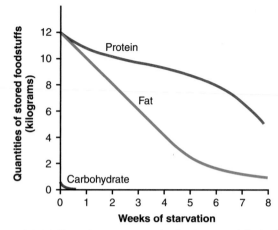

Figure 71-3 Effect of starvation on the food stores of the body.

breakdown products to ketone bodies, producing the state of *ketosis,* which is discussed in Chapter 68. The ketone bodies, like glucose, can cross the blood-brain barrier and can be used by the brain cells for energy. Therefore, about two thirds of the brain's energy is now derived from these ketone bodies, principally from beta-hydroxybutyrate. This sequence of events leads to at least partial preservation of the protein stores of the body.

There finally comes a time when the fat stores are almost depleted, and the only remaining source of energy is protein. At that time, the protein stores once again enter a stage of rapid depletion. Because proteins are also essential for the maintenance of cellular function, death ordinarily ensues when the proteins of the body have been depleted to about half their normal level.

Vitamin Deficiencies in Starvation. The stores of some of the vitamins, especially the water-soluble vitamins—the vitamin B group and vitamin C—do not last long during starvation. Consequently, after a week or more of starvation, mild vitamin deficiencies usually begin to appear, and after several weeks, severe vitamin deficiencies can occur. These deficiencies can add to the debility that leads to death.

Vitamins

Daily Requirements of Vitamins. A vitamin is an organic compound needed in small quantities for normal metabolism that cannot be manufactured in the cells of the body. Lack of vitamins in the diet can cause important metabolic deficits. Table 71-3 lists the amounts of important vitamins required daily by the average person. These requirements vary considerably, depending on such factors as body size, rate of growth, amount of exercise, and pregnancy.

Storage of Vitamins in the Body. Vitamins are stored to a slight extent in all cells. Some vitamins are stored to a major extent in the liver. For instance, the quantity of vitamin A stored in the liver may be sufficient to maintain a person for 5 to 10 months without any intake of vitamin A. The quantity of vitamin D stored in the liver is usually sufficient to maintain a person for 2 to 4 months without any additional intake of vitamin D.

The storage of most water-soluble vitamins is relatively slight. This applies especially to most vitamin B compounds. When a person's diet is deficient in vitamin B compounds,

Table 71-3 Required Daily Amounts of Vitamins

Vitamin	Amount
A	5000 IU
Thiamine	1.5 mg
Riboflavin	1.8 mg
Niacin	20 mg
Ascorbic acid	45 mg
D	400 IU
E	15 IU
K	70 μg
Folic acid	0.4 mg
B_{12}	3 μg
Pyridoxine	2 mg
Pantothenic acid	Unknown

clinical symptoms of the deficiency can sometimes be recognized within a few days (except for vitamin B_{12}, which can last in the liver in a bound form for a year or longer). Absence of vitamin C, another water-soluble vitamin, can cause symptoms within a few weeks and can cause death from scurvy in 20 to 30 weeks.

Vitamin A

Vitamin A occurs in animal tissues as *retinol*. This vitamin does not occur in foods of vegetable origin, but *provitamins* for the formation of vitamin A do occur in abundance in many vegetable foods. These are the yellow and red *carotenoid pigments*, which, because their chemical structures are similar to that of vitamin A, can be changed into vitamin A in the liver.

Vitamin A Deficiency Causes "Night Blindness" and Abnormal Epithelial Cell Growth. One basic function of vitamin A is its use in the formation of the retinal pigments of the eye, which is discussed in Chapter 50. Vitamin A is needed to form the visual pigments and, therefore, to prevent night blindness.

Vitamin A is also necessary for normal growth of most cells of the body and especially for normal growth and proliferation of the different types of epithelial cells. When vitamin A is lacking, the epithelial structures of the body tend to become stratified and keratinized. Vitamin A deficiency manifests itself by (1) scaliness of the skin and sometimes acne; (2) failure of growth of young animals, including cessation of skeletal growth; (3) failure of reproduction, associated especially with atrophy of the germinal epithelium of the testes and sometimes with interruption of the female sexual cycle; and (4) keratinization of the cornea, with resultant corneal opacity and blindness.

In vitamin A deficiency, the damaged epithelial structures often become infected (e.g., conjunctivae of the eyes, linings of the urinary tract, and respiratory passages). Vitamin A has been called an "anti-infection" vitamin.

Thiamine (Vitamin B_1)

Thiamine operates in the metabolic systems of the body principally as *thiamine pyrophosphate*; this compound functions as a *cocarboxylase*, operating mainly in conjunction with a protein decarboxylase for decarboxylation of pyruvic acid and other α-keto acids, as discussed in Chapter 67.

Thiamine deficiency *(beriberi)* causes decreased utilization of pyruvic acid and some amino acids by the tissues, but increased utilization of fats. Thus, thiamine is specifically needed for the final metabolism of carbohydrates and many amino acids. The decreased utilization of these nutrients is responsible for many debilities associated with thiamine deficiency.

Thiamine Deficiency Causes Lesions of the Central and Peripheral Nervous Systems. The central nervous system normally depends almost entirely on the metabolism of carbohydrates for its energy. In thiamine deficiency, the utilization of glucose by nervous tissue may be decreased 50 to 60 percent and is replaced by the utilization of ketone bodies derived from fat metabolism. The neuronal cells of the central nervous system frequently show chromatolysis and swelling during thiamine deficiency, changes that are characteristic of neuronal cells with poor nutrition. These changes can disrupt communication in many portions of the central nervous system.

Thiamine deficiency can cause *degeneration of myelin sheaths* of nerve fibers in both the peripheral nerves and the central nervous system. Lesions in the peripheral nerves frequently cause them to become extremely irritable, resulting in "polyneuritis," characterized by pain radiating along the course of one or many peripheral nerves. Also, fiber tracts in the cord can degenerate to such an extent that *paralysis* occasionally results; even in the absence of paralysis, the muscles atrophy, resulting in severe weakness.

Thiamine Deficiency Weakens the Heart and Causes Peripheral Vasodilation. A person with severe thiamine deficiency eventually develops *cardiac failure* because of weakened cardiac muscle. Further, the venous return of blood to the heart may be increased to as much as two times normal. This occurs because thiamine deficiency causes *peripheral vasodilation* throughout the circulatory system, presumably as a result of decreased release of metabolic energy in the tissues, leading to local vascular dilation. The cardiac effects of thiamine deficiency are due partly to high blood flow into the heart and partly to primary weakness of the cardiac muscle. *Peripheral edema* and *ascites* also occur to a major extent in some people with thiamine deficiency, mainly because of cardiac failure.

Thiamine Deficiency Causes Gastrointestinal Tract Disturbances. Among the gastrointestinal symptoms of thiamine deficiency are indigestion, severe constipation, anorexia, gastric atony, and hypochlorhydria. All these effects presumably result from failure of the smooth muscle and glands of the gastrointestinal tract to derive sufficient energy from carbohydrate metabolism.

The overall picture of thiamine deficiency, including polyneuritis, cardiovascular symptoms, and gastrointestinal disorders, is frequently referred to as *beriberi*—especially when the cardiovascular symptoms predominate.

Niacin

Niacin, also called *nicotinic acid*, functions in the body as coenzymes in the form of nicotinamide adenine dinucleotide (NAD) and nicotinamide adenine dinucleotide phosphate (NADP). These coenzymes are hydrogen acceptors; they combine with hydrogen atoms as they are removed from food substrates by many types of dehydrogenases. The typical operation of both these coenzymes is presented in Chapter 67. When a deficiency of niacin exists, the normal rate of dehydrogenation cannot be maintained; therefore, oxidative delivery of energy from the foodstuffs to the functioning elements of all cells cannot occur at normal rates.

In the early stages of niacin deficiency, simple physiological changes such as muscle weakness and poor glandular secretion may occur, but in severe niacin deficiency, actual tissue death ensues. Pathological lesions appear in many parts of the central nervous system, and permanent dementia or many types of psychoses may result. Also, the skin develops a cracked, pigmented scaliness in areas that are exposed to mechanical irritation or sun irradiation; thus, it appears that in persons with niacin deficiency, the skin is unable to repair irritative damage.

Niacin deficiency causes intense irritation and inflammation of the mucous membranes of the mouth and other portions of the gastrointestinal tract, resulting in many digestive abnormalities that can lead to widespread gastrointestinal hemorrhage in severe cases. It is possible that this results from generalized depression of metabolism in the gastrointestinal epithelium and failure of appropriate epithelial repair.

The clinical entity called *pellagra* and the canine disease called *black tongue* are caused mainly by niacin deficiency. Pellagra is greatly exacerbated in people on a corn diet because corn is deficient in the amino acid tryptophan, which can be converted in limited quantities to niacin in the body.

Riboflavin (Vitamin B$_2$)

Riboflavin normally combines in the tissues with phosphoric acid to form two coenzymes, *flavin mononucleotide (FMN)* and *flavin adenine dinucleotide (FAD)*. They operate as hydrogen carriers in important oxidative systems of the mitochondria. NAD, operating in association with specific dehydrogenases, usually accepts hydrogen removed from various food substrates and then passes the hydrogen to FMN or FAD; finally, the hydrogen is released as an ion into the mitochondrial matrix to become oxidized by oxygen (described in Chapter 67).

Deficiency of riboflavin in experimental animals causes severe dermatitis, vomiting, diarrhea, muscle spasticity that finally becomes muscle weakness, coma and decline in body temperature, and then death. Thus, severe riboflavin deficiency can cause many of the same effects as a lack of niacin in the diet; presumably, the debilities that result in each instance are due to generally depressed oxidative processes within the cells.

In the human being, there are no known cases of riboflavin deficiency severe enough to cause the marked debilities noted in experimental animals, but mild riboflavin deficiency is probably common. Such deficiency causes digestive disturbances, burning sensations of the skin and eyes, cracking at the corners of the mouth, headaches, mental depression, forgetfulness, and so on.

Although the manifestations of riboflavin deficiency are usually relatively mild, this deficiency frequently occurs in association with deficiency of thiamine, niacin, or both. Many deficiency syndromes, including *pellagra, beriberi, sprue,* and *kwashiorkor,* are probably due to a combined deficiency of a number of vitamins, as well as other aspects of malnutrition.

Vitamin B$_{12}$

Several *cobalamin* compounds that possess the common prosthetic group shown next exhibit so-called vitamin B$_{12}$ activity. Note that this prosthetic group contains cobalt, which has bonds similar to those of iron in the hemoglobin molecule. It is likely that the cobalt atom functions in much the same way that the iron atom functions to combine reversibly with other substances.

Vitamin B$_{12}$ Deficiency Causes Pernicious Anemia. Vitamin B$_{12}$ performs several metabolic functions, acting as a hydrogen acceptor coenzyme. Its most important function is to act as a coenzyme for reducing ribonucleotides to deoxyribonucleotides, a step that is necessary in the replication of genes. This could explain the major functions of vitamin B$_{12}$: (1) promotion of growth and (2) promotion of red blood cell formation and maturation. This red cell function is described in detail in Chapter 32 in relation to pernicious anemia, a type of anemia caused by failure of red blood cell maturation when vitamin B$_{12}$ is deficient.

Vitamin B$_{12}$ Deficiency Causes Demyelination of the Large Nerve Fibers of the Spinal Cord. The demyelination of nerve fibers in people with vitamin B$_{12}$ deficiency occurs especially in the posterior columns, and occasionally the lateral columns, of the spinal cord. As a result, many people with pernicious anemia have loss of peripheral sensation and, in severe cases, even become paralyzed.

The usual cause of vitamin B$_{12}$ deficiency is not lack of this vitamin in the food but deficiency of formation of *intrinsic factor*, which is normally secreted by the parietal cells of the gastric glands and is essential for absorption of vitamin B$_{12}$ by the ileal mucosa. This is discussed in Chapters 32 and 66.

Folic Acid (Pteroylglutamic Acid)

Several pteroylglutamic acids exhibit the "folic acid effect." Folic acid functions as a carrier of hydroxymethyl and formyl groups. *Perhaps its most important use in the body is in the synthesis of purines and thymine, which are required for formation of DNA.* Therefore, folic acid, like vitamin B$_{12}$, is required for replication of the cellular genes. This may explain one of the most important functions of folic acid—to promote growth. Indeed, when it is absent from the diet, an animal grows very little.

Folic acid is an even more potent growth promoter than vitamin B$_{12}$ and, like vitamin B$_{12}$, is important for the maturation of red blood cells, as discussed in Chapter 32. However, vitamin B$_{12}$ and folic acid each perform specific and different chemical functions in promoting growth and maturation of red blood cells. One of the significant effects of folic acid deficiency is the development of *macrocytic anemia*, almost identical to that which occurs in pernicious anemia. This often can be treated effectively with folic acid alone.

Pyridoxine (Vitamin B$_6$)

Pyridoxine exists in the form of *pyridoxal phosphate* in the cells and functions as a coenzyme for many chemical reactions related to amino acid and protein metabolism. *Its most important role is that of coenzyme in the transamination process for the synthesis of amino acids.* As a result, pyridoxine plays many key roles in metabolism, especially protein metabolism. Also, it is believed to act in the transport of some amino acids across cell membranes.

Dietary lack of pyridoxine in lower animals can cause dermatitis, decreased rate of growth, development of fatty liver, anemia, and evidence of mental deterioration. Rarely, in children, pyridoxine deficiency has been known to cause seizures, dermatitis, and gastrointestinal disturbances such as nausea and vomiting.

Pantothenic Acid

Pantothenic acid is mainly incorporated in the body into *coenzyme A (CoA)*, which has many metabolic roles in the cells. Two of these discussed at length in Chapters 67 and 68 are (1) conversion of decarboxylated pyruvic acid into acetyl-CoA before its entry into the citric acid cycle and (2) degradation of fatty acid molecules into multiple molecules of acetyl-CoA. *Thus, lack of pantothenic acid can lead to depressed metabolism of both carbohydrates and fats.*

Deficiency of pantothenic acid in lower animals can cause retarded growth, failure of reproduction, graying of the hair, dermatitis, fatty liver, and hemorrhagic adrenocortical necrosis. In the human being, no definite deficiency syndrome has been proved, presumably because of the wide occurrence of this vitamin in almost all foods and because small amounts can probably be synthesized in the body. This does not mean that pantothenic acid is not of value in the metabolic systems of the body; indeed, it is perhaps as necessary as any other vitamin.

Ascorbic Acid (Vitamin C)

Ascorbic Acid Deficiency Weakens Collagen Fibers Throughout the Body. Ascorbic acid is essential for activating the enzyme *prolyl hydroxylase*, which promotes the hydroxylation step in the formation of hydroxyproline, an integral constituent of collagen. Without ascorbic acid, the collagen fibers that are formed in virtually all tissues of the body are defective and weak. Therefore, this vitamin is essential for the growth and strength of the fibers in subcutaneous tissue, cartilage, bone, and teeth.

Ascorbic Acid Deficiency Causes Scurvy. Deficiency of ascorbic acid for 20 to 30 weeks, which occurred frequently during long ship voyages in the past, causes *scurvy*. One of the most important effects of scurvy is *failure of wounds to heal*. This is caused by failure of the cells to deposit collagen fibrils and intercellular cement substances. As a result, healing of a wound may require several months instead of the several days ordinarily necessary.

Lack of ascorbic acid also causes *cessation of bone growth*. The cells of the growing epiphyses continue to proliferate, but no new collagen is laid down between the cells, and the bones fracture easily at the point of growth because of failure to ossify. Also, when an already ossified bone fractures in a person with ascorbic acid deficiency, the osteoblasts cannot form new bone matrix. Consequently, the fractured bone does not heal.

The *blood vessel walls become extremely fragile* in scurvy because of (1) failure of the endothelial cells to be cemented together properly and (2) failure to form the collagen fibrils normally present in vessel walls. The capillaries are especially likely to rupture, and as a result, many small petechial hemorrhages occur throughout the body. The hemorrhages beneath the skin cause purpuric blotches, sometimes over the entire body. To test for ascorbic acid deficiency, one can produce such petechial hemorrhages by inflating a blood pressure cuff over the upper arm; this occludes the venous return of blood, the capillary pressure rises, and red blotches occur on the forearm if the ascorbic acid deficiency is sufficiently severe.

In extreme scurvy, the muscle cells sometimes fragment; lesions of the gums occur, with loosening of the teeth; infections of the mouth develop; and vomiting of blood, bloody stools, and cerebral hemorrhage can all occur. Finally, high fever often develops before death.

Vitamin D

Vitamin D increases calcium absorption from the gastrointestinal tract and helps control calcium deposition in the bone. The mechanism by which vitamin D increases calcium absorption is mainly to promote active transport of calcium through the epithelium of the ileum. In particular, it increases the formation of a calcium-binding protein in the intestinal epithelial cells that aids in calcium absorption. The specific functions of vitamin D in relation to overall body calcium metabolism and bone formation are presented in Chapter 79.

Vitamin E

Several related compounds exhibit so-called vitamin E activity. Only rare instances of proved vitamin E deficiency have occurred in human beings. In experimental animals, lack of vitamin E can cause degeneration of the germinal epithelium in the testis and, therefore, can cause male sterility. Lack of vitamin E can also cause resorption of a fetus after conception in the female. Because of these effects of vitamin E deficiency, vitamin E is sometimes called the "antisterility vitamin." Deficiency of vitamin E prevents normal growth and sometimes causes degeneration of the renal tubular cells and the muscle cells.

Vitamin E is believed to play a protective role in the prevention of oxidation of unsaturated fats. In the absence of vitamin E, the quantity of unsaturated fats in the cells becomes diminished, causing abnormal structure and function of such cellular organelles as the mitochondria, the lysosomes, and even the cell membrane.

Vitamin K

Vitamin K is an essential co-factor to a liver enzyme that adds a carboxyl group to factors II (prothrombin), VII (proconvertin), IX, and X, all of which are important in blood coagulation. Without this carboxylation these coagulation factors are inactive. Therefore, when vitamin K deficiency occurs, blood clotting is retarded. The function of this vitamin and its relation to some of the anticoagulants, such as dicumarol, are presented in greater detail in Chapter 36.

Several compounds, both natural and synthetic, exhibit vitamin K activity. Because vitamin K is synthesized by bacteria in the colon, it is rare for a person to have a bleeding tendency because of vitamin K deficiency in the diet. However, when the bacteria of the colon are destroyed by the administration of large quantities of antibiotic drugs, vitamin K deficiency occurs rapidly because of the paucity of this compound in the normal diet.

Mineral Metabolism

The functions of many of the minerals, such as sodium, potassium, and chloride, are presented at appropriate points in the text. Only specific functions of minerals not covered elsewhere are mentioned here. The body content of the most important minerals is listed in Table 71-4, and the daily requirements of these are given in Table 71-5.

Table 71-4 Average Content of a 70-Kilogram Man

Constituent	Amount (grams)
Water	41,400
Fat	12,600
Protein	12,600
Carbohydrate	300
Sodium	63
Potassium	150
Calcium	1,160
Magnesium	21
Chloride	85
Phosphorus	670
Sulfur	112
Iron	3
Iodine	0.014

Table 71-5 Average Required Daily Amounts of Minerals for Adults

Mineral	Amount
Sodium	3.0 g
Potassium	1.0 g
Chloride	3.5 g
Calcium	1.2 g
Phosphorus	1.2 g
Iron	18.0 mg
Iodine	150.0 µg
Magnesium	0.4 g
Cobalt	Unknown
Copper	Unknown
Manganese	Unknown
Zinc	15 mg

Magnesium. Magnesium is about one sixth as plentiful in cells as potassium. Magnesium is required as a catalyst for many intracellular enzymatic reactions, particularly those related to carbohydrate metabolism.

The extracellular fluid magnesium concentration is slight, only 1.8 to 2.5 mEq/L. Increased extracellular concentration of magnesium depresses nervous system activity, as well as skeletal muscle contraction. This latter effect can be blocked by the administration of calcium. Low magnesium concentration causes increased irritability of the nervous system, peripheral vasodilation, and cardiac arrhythmias, especially after acute myocardial infarction.

Calcium. Calcium is present in the body mainly in the form of calcium phosphate in the bone. This subject is discussed in detail in Chapter 79, as is the calcium content of extracellular fluid. Excess quantities of calcium ions in extracellular fluid can cause the heart to stop in systole and can act as a mental depressant. At the other extreme, low levels

of calcium can cause spontaneous discharge of nerve fibers, resulting in tetany, as discussed in Chapter 79.

Phosphorus. *Phosphate is the major anion of intracellular fluid.* Phosphates have the ability to combine reversibly with many coenzyme systems and with multiple other compounds that are necessary for the operation of metabolic processes. Many important reactions of phosphates have been catalogued at other points in this text, especially in relation to the functions of adenosine triphosphate, adenosine diphosphate, phosphocreatine, and so forth. Also, bone contains a tremendous amount of calcium phosphate, which is discussed in Chapter 79.

Iron. The function of iron in the body, especially in relation to the formation of hemoglobin, is discussed in Chapter 32. *Two thirds of the iron in the body is in the form of hemoglobin,* although smaller quantities are present in other forms, especially in the liver and the bone marrow. Electron carriers containing iron (especially the cytochromes) are present in the mitochondria of all cells of the body and are essential for most of the oxidation that occurs in the cells. Therefore, iron is absolutely essential for both the transport of oxygen to the tissues and the operation of oxidative systems within the tissue cells, without which life would cease within a few seconds.

Important Trace Elements in the Body. A few elements are present in the body in such small quantities that they are called *trace elements.* The amounts of these elements in foods are also usually minute. Yet without any one of them, a specific deficiency syndrome is likely to develop. Three of the most important are iodine, zinc, and fluorine.

Iodine. The best known of the trace elements is iodine. This element is discussed in Chapter 76 in connection with the formation and function of thyroid hormone; as shown in Table 71-4, the entire body contains an average of only 14 milligrams. Iodine is essential for the formation of *thyroxine* and *triiodothyronine,* the two thyroid hormones that are essential for maintenance of normal metabolic rates in all cells of the body.

Zinc. Zinc is an integral part of many enzymes, one of the most important of which is *carbonic anhydrase,* present in especially high concentration in the red blood cells. This enzyme is responsible for rapid combination of carbon dioxide with water in the red blood cells of the peripheral capillary blood and for rapid release of carbon dioxide from the pulmonary capillary blood into the alveoli. Carbonic anhydrase is also present to a major extent in the gastrointestinal mucosa, the tubules of the kidney, and the epithelial cells of many glands of the body. Consequently, zinc in small quantities is essential for the performance of many reactions related to carbon dioxide metabolism.

Zinc is also a component of *lactic dehydrogenase* and is therefore important for the interconversions between pyruvic acid and lactic acid. Finally, zinc is a component of some *peptidases* and is important for the digestion of proteins in the gastrointestinal tract.

Fluorine. Fluorine does not seem to be a necessary element for metabolism, but the presence of a small quantity of fluorine in the body during the period of life when the teeth are being formed subsequently protects against caries. Fluorine does not make the teeth stronger but has a poorly understood effect in suppressing the cariogenic process. It has been suggested that fluorine is deposited in the hydroxyapatite crystals of the tooth enamel and combines with and therefore blocks the functions of various trace metals that are necessary for activation of the bacterial enzymes that cause caries. Therefore, when fluorine is present, the enzymes remain inactive and cause no caries.

Excessive intake of fluorine causes *fluorosis*, which manifests in its mild state by mottled teeth and in its more severe state by enlarged bones. It has been postulated that in this condition, fluorine combines with trace metals in some of the metabolic enzymes, including the phosphatases, so that various metabolic systems become partially inactivated. According to this theory, the mottled teeth and enlarged bones are due to abnormal enzyme systems in the odontoblasts and osteoblasts. Even though the mottled teeth are highly resistant to the development of caries, the structural strength of these teeth may be considerably lessened by the mottling process.

Bibliography

Bray GA: Lifestyle and pharmacological approaches to weight loss: efficacy and safety, *J Clin Endocrinol Metab* 93(11 Suppl 1):S81, 2008.

Coll AP: Effects of pro-opiomelanocortin (POMC) on food intake and body weight: mechanisms and therapeutic potential?, *Clin Sci (Lond)* 113:171, 2007.

Cone RD: Studies on the physiological functions of the melanocortin system, *Endocr Rev* 27:736, 2006.

da Silva AA, Kuo JJ, Hall JE: Role of hypothalamic melanocortin 3/4-receptors in mediating chronic cardiovascular, renal, and metabolic actions of leptin, *Hypertension* 43:1312, 2004.

Davy KP, Hall JE: Obesity and hypertension: two epidemics or one?, *Am J Physiol Regul Integr Comp Physiol* 286:R803, 2004.

Farooqi IS, O'Rahilly S: Mutations in ligands and receptors of the leptin-melanocortin pathway that lead to obesity, *Nat Clin Pract Endocrinol Metab* 4:569, 2008.

Friedman JM, Halaas JL: Leptin and the regulation of body weight in mammals, *Nature* 395:763, 1998.

Gao Q, Horvath TL: Cross-talk between estrogen and leptin signaling in the hypothalamus, *Am J Physiol Endocrinol Metab* 294(5):E817, 2008.

Hall JE: The kidney, hypertension, and obesity, *Hypertension* 4:625, 2003.

Hall JE, Henegar JR, Dwyer TM, et al: Is obesity a major cause of chronic kidney disease? *Adv Ren Replace Ther* 11:41, 2004.

Hall JE, Jones DW: What can we do about the "epidemic" of obesity, *Am J Hypertens* 15:657, 2002.

Holst JJ: The physiology of glucagon-like peptide 1, *Physiol Rev* 87:1409, 2007.

Jones G, Strugnell SA, DeLuca HF: Current understanding of the molecular actions of vitamin D, *Physiol Rev* 78:1193, 1998.

Laviano A, Inui A, Marks DL, et al: Neural control of the anorexia-cachexia syndrome, *Am J Physiol Endocrinol Metab* 295:E1000, 2008.

Lucock M: Is folic acid the ultimate functional food component for disease prevention?, *BMJ* 328:211, 2004.

Marty N, Dallaporta M, Thorens B: Brain glucose sensing, counterregulation, and energy homeostasis, *Physiology (Bethesda)* 22:241, 2007.

Morton GJ, Cummings DE, Baskin DG, et al: Central nervous system control of food intake and body weight, *Nature* 443:289, 2006.

National Institutes of Health: *Clinical Guidelines on the Identification, Evaluation, and Treatment of Overweight and Obesity in Adults: The Evidence Report*, Bethesda MD, 1998, National Heart, Lung, and Blood Institute and National Institute of Diabetes and Digestive and Kidney Diseases. Available at: http://www.nhlbi.nih.gov/guidelines/index.htm.

Powers HJ: Riboflavin (vitamin B$_2$) and health, *Am J Clin Nutr* 77:1352, 2003.

Tallam LS, da Silva AA, Hall JE: Melanocortin-4 receptor mediates chronic cardiovascular and metabolic actions of leptin, *Hypertension* 48:58, 2006.

Woods SC, D'Alessio DA: Central control of body weight and appetite, *J Clin Endocrinol Metab* 93(11 Suppl 1):S37, 2008.

Energetics and Metabolic Rate

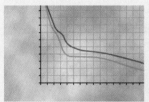

Adenosine Triphosphate (ATP) Functions as an "Energy Currency" in Metabolism

Carbohydrates, fats, and proteins can all be used by cells to synthesize large quantities of adenosine triphosphate (ATP), which can be used as an energy source for almost all other cellular functions. For this reason, ATP has been called an energy "currency" in cell metabolism. Indeed, the transfer of energy from foodstuffs to most functional systems of the cells can be done only through this medium of ATP (or the similar nucleotide guanosine triphosphate, GTP). Many of the attributes of ATP are presented in Chapter 2.

An attribute of ATP that makes it highly valuable as an energy currency is the large quantity of free energy (about 7300 calories, or 7.3 Calories [kilocalories], per mole under standard conditions, but as much as 12,000 calories under physiological conditions) vested in each of its two high-energy phosphate bonds. The amount of energy in each bond, when liberated by decomposition of ATP, is enough to cause almost any step of any chemical reaction in the body to take place if appropriate energy transfer is achieved. Some chemical reactions that require ATP energy use only a few hundred of the available 12,000 calories, and the remainder of this energy is lost in the form of heat.

ATP Is Generated by Combustion of Carbohydrates, Fats, and Proteins. In previous chapters, we discussed the transfer of energy from various foods to ATP. To summarize, ATP is produced from the following processes:

1. *Combustion of carbohydrates*—mainly glucose, but also smaller amounts of other sugars such as fructose; this occurs in the cytoplasm of the cell through the anaerobic process of *glycolysis* and in the cell mitochondria through the aerobic *citric acid (Krebs) cycle*.

2. *Combustion of fatty acids* in the cell mitochondria by *beta-oxidation*.

3. *Combustion of proteins*, which requires hydrolysis to their component amino acids and degradation of the amino acids to intermediate compounds of the citric acid cycle and then to acetyl coenzyme A and carbon dioxide.

ATP Energizes the Synthesis of Cellular Components. Among the most important intracellular processes that require ATP energy is the formation of peptide linkages between amino acids during the synthesis of proteins. The different peptide linkages, depending on which types of amino acids are linked, require from 500 to 5000 calories of energy per mole. From the discussion of protein synthesis in Chapter 3 recall that four high-energy phosphate bonds are expended during the cascade of reactions required to form each peptide linkage. This provides a total of 48,000 calories of energy, which is far more than the 500 to 5000 calories eventually stored in each of the peptide linkages.

ATP energy is also used in the synthesis of glucose from lactic acid and in the synthesis of fatty acids from acetyl coenzyme A. In addition, ATP energy is used for the synthesis of cholesterol, phospholipids, the hormones, and almost all other substances of the body. Even the urea excreted by the kidneys requires ATP for its formation from ammonia. One might wonder why energy is expended to form urea, which is simply discarded by the body. However, remembering the extreme toxicity of ammonia in the body fluids, one can see the value of this reaction, which keeps the ammonia concentration of the body fluids at a low level.

ATP Energizes Muscle Contraction. Muscle contraction will not occur without energy from ATP. Myosin, one of the important contractile proteins of the muscle fiber, acts as an enzyme to cause breakdown of ATP into adenosine diphosphate (ADP), thus releasing the energy required to cause contraction. Only a small amount of ATP is normally degraded in muscles when muscle contraction is not occurring, but this rate of ATP usage can rise to at least 150 times the resting level during short bursts of maximal contraction. The mechanism by which ATP energy is used to cause muscle contraction is discussed in Chapter 6.

ATP Energizes Active Transport Across Membranes. In Chapters 4, 27, and 65, active transport of electrolytes and various nutrients across cell membranes and from the renal tubules and gastrointestinal tract into the blood is discussed. We noted that active transport of most electrolytes and substances such as glucose, amino acids, and acetoacetate can occur against an electrochemical gradient, even though the natural diffusion of the substances would be in the opposite direction. To oppose the electrochemical gradient requires energy, which is provided by ATP.

ATP Energizes Glandular Secretion. The same principles apply to glandular secretion as to the absorption of substances against concentration gradients because energy is required to concentrate substances as they are secreted by the glandular cells. In addition, energy is required to synthesize the organic compounds to be secreted.

ATP Energizes Nerve Conduction. The energy used during propagation of a nerve impulse is derived from the potential energy stored in the form of concentration differences of ions across the membranes. That is, a high concentration of potassium inside the fiber and a low concentration outside the fiber constitute a type of energy storage. Likewise, a high concentration of sodium on the outside of the membrane and a low concentration on the inside represent another store of energy. The energy needed to pass each action potential along the fiber membrane is derived from this energy storage, with small amounts of potassium transferring out of the cell and sodium into the cell during each of the action potentials. However, active transport systems energized by ATP then retransport the ions back through the membrane to their former positions.

Phosphocreatine Functions as an Accessory Storage Depot for Energy and as an "ATP Buffer"

Despite the paramount importance of ATP as a coupling agent for energy transfer, this substance is not the most abundant store of high-energy phosphate bonds in the cells. *Phosphocreatine*, which also contains high-energy phosphate bonds, is three to eight times more abundant than ATP. Also, the high-energy bond (~) of phosphocreatine contains about 8500 calories per mole under standard conditions and as many as 13,000 calories per mole under conditions in the body (37 °C and low concentrations of the reactants). This is slightly greater than the 12,000 calories per mole in each of the two high-energy phosphate bonds of ATP. The formula for creatinine phosphate is the following:

$$\underset{\substack{|\\ \text{HOOC}-\text{CH}_2}}{} - \overset{\substack{\text{CH}_3 \quad \text{NH} \; \text{H} \quad \text{O}\\ |\qquad \| \quad | \qquad \|}}{\text{N}-\text{C}-\text{N}\sim\overset{\substack{|\\ \text{O}\\ |\\ \text{H}}}{\text{P}}-\text{OH}}$$

Unlike ATP, phosphocreatine cannot act as a direct coupling agent for energy transfer between the foods and the functional cellular systems, but it can transfer energy interchangeably with ATP. When extra amounts of ATP are available in the cell, much of its energy is used to synthesize phosphocreatine, thus building up this storehouse of energy. Then, when the ATP begins to be used up, the energy in the phosphocreatine is transferred rapidly back to ATP and then to the functional systems of the cells. This reversible interrelation between ATP and phosphocreatine is demonstrated by the following equation:

Phosphocreatine + ADP
↓↑
ATP + Creatine

Note that the higher energy level of the high-energy phosphate bond in phosphocreatine (1000 to 1500 calories per mole greater than that in ATP) causes the reaction between phosphocreatine and ADP to proceed rapidly toward the formation of new ATP every time even the slightest amount of ATP expends its energy elsewhere. Therefore, the slightest usage of ATP by the cells calls forth the energy from the phosphocreatine to synthesize new ATP. This effect keeps the concentration of ATP at an almost constant high level as long as any phosphocreatine remains. For this reason, we can call the ATP-phosphocreatine system an ATP "buffer" system. One can readily understand the importance of keeping the concentration of ATP nearly constant because the rates of almost all the metabolic reactions in the body depend on this constancy.

Anaerobic Versus Aerobic Energy

Anaerobic energy means energy that can be derived from foods without the simultaneous utilization of oxygen; *aerobic energy* means energy that can be derived from foods only by oxidative metabolism. In the discussions in Chapters 67 through 69, we noted that carbohydrates, fats, and proteins can all be oxidized to cause synthesis of ATP. However, *carbohydrates are the only significant foods that can be used to provide energy without the utilization of oxygen*; this energy release occurs during glycolytic breakdown of glucose or glycogen to pyruvic acid. For each mole of glucose that is split into pyruvic acid, 2 moles of ATP are formed. However, when stored glycogen in a cell is split to pyruvic acid, each mole of glucose in the glycogen gives rise to 3 moles of ATP. The reason for this difference is that free glucose entering the cell must be phosphorylated by using 1 mole of ATP before it can begin to be split; this is not true of glucose derived from glycogen because it comes from the glycogen already in the phosphorylated state, without the additional expenditure of ATP. *Thus, the best source of energy under anaerobic conditions is the stored glycogen of the cells.*

Anaerobic Energy Utilization During Hypoxia. One of the prime examples of anaerobic energy utilization occurs in acute hypoxia. When a person stops breathing, there is already a small amount of oxygen stored in the lungs and an additional amount stored in the hemoglobin of the blood. This oxygen is sufficient to keep the metabolic processes functioning for only about 2 minutes. Continued life beyond this time requires an additional source of energy. This can be derived for another minute or so from glycolysis—that is, the glycogen of the cells splitting into pyruvic acid, and the pyruvic acid becoming lactic acid, which diffuses out of the cells, as described in Chapter 67.

Anaerobic Energy Utilization During Strenuous Bursts of Activity Is Derived Mainly from Glycolysis. Skeletal muscles can perform extreme feats of strength for a few seconds but are much less capable during prolonged activity. Most of the extra energy required during these bursts of activity cannot come from the oxidative processes because they are too slow to respond. Instead, the extra energy comes from anaerobic sources: (1) ATP already present in the muscle cells, (2) phosphocreatine in the cells, and (3) anaerobic energy released by glycolytic breakdown of glycogen to lactic acid.

The maximum amount of ATP in muscle is only about 5 mmol/L of intracellular fluid, and this amount can maintain maximum muscle contraction for no more than a second or so. The amount of phosphocreatine in the cells is three to eight times this amount, but even by using all the phosphocreatine, maximum contraction can be maintained for only 5 to 10 seconds.

Release of energy by glycolysis can occur much more rapidly than can oxidative release of energy. Consequently, most of the extra energy required during strenuous activity that lasts for more than 5 to 10 seconds but less than 1 to 2 minutes is derived from anaerobic glycolysis. As a result, the glycogen content of muscles during strenuous bouts of exercise is reduced, whereas the lactic acid concentration of the blood rises. After the exercise is over, oxidative metabolism is used to reconvert about four fifths of the lactic acid into glucose;

the remainder becomes pyruvic acid and is degraded and oxidized in the citric acid cycle. The reconversion to glucose occurs principally in the liver cells, and the glucose is then transported in the blood back to the muscles, where it is stored once more in the form of glycogen.

Extra Consumption of Oxygen Repays the Oxygen Debt After Completion of Strenuous Exercise. After a period of strenuous exercise, a person continues to breathe hard and to consume large amounts of oxygen for at least a few minutes and sometimes for as long as 1 hour thereafter. This additional oxygen is used (1) to reconvert the lactic acid that has accumulated during exercise back into glucose, (2) to reconvert adenosine monophosphate and ADP to ATP, (3) to reconvert creatine and phosphate to phosphocreatine, (4) to re-establish normal concentrations of oxygen bound with hemoglobin and myoglobin, and (5) to raise the concentration of oxygen in the lungs to its normal level. This extra consumption of oxygen after exercise is called *repaying the oxygen debt*.

The principle of oxygen debt is discussed further in Chapter 84 in relation to sports physiology; the ability of a person to build up an oxygen debt is especially important in many types of athletics.

Summary of Energy Utilization by the Cells

With the background of the past few chapters and of the preceding discussion, we can now synthesize a composite picture of overall energy utilization by the cells, as shown in Figure 72-1. This figure demonstrates the anaerobic utilization of glycogen and glucose to form ATP and the aerobic utilization of compounds derived from carbohydrates, fats, proteins, and other substances to form additional ATP. In turn, ATP is in reversible equilibrium with phosphocreatine in the cells, and because larger quantities of phosphocreatine are present in the cells than ATP, much of the cells' stored energy is in this energy storehouse.

Energy from ATP can be used by the different functioning systems of the cells to provide for synthesis and growth, muscle contraction, glandular secretion, nerve impulse conduction, active absorption, and other cellular activities. If greater amounts of energy are demanded for cellular activities than can be provided by oxidative metabolism, the phosphocreatine storehouse is used first, and then anaerobic breakdown of glycogen follows rapidly. Thus, oxidative metabolism cannot deliver bursts of extreme energy to the

cells nearly as rapidly as the anaerobic processes can, but at slower rates of usage, the oxidative processes can continue as long as energy stores (mainly fat) exist.

Control of Energy Release in the Cell

Rate Control of Enzyme-Catalyzed Reactions. Before discussing the control of energy release in the cell, it is necessary to consider the basic principles of *rate control* of enzymatically catalyzed chemical reactions, which are the types of reactions that occur almost universally throughout the body.

The mechanism by which an enzyme catalyzes a chemical reaction is for the enzyme first to combine loosely with one of the substrates of the reaction. This alters the bonding forces on the substrate sufficiently so that it can react with other substances. Therefore, the rate of the overall chemical reaction is determined by both the concentration of the enzyme and the concentration of the substrate that binds with the enzyme. The basic equation expressing this concept is as follows:

$$\text{Rate of reaction} = \frac{K_1 \times [\text{Enzyme}] \times [\text{Substrate}]}{K_2 + [\text{Substrate}]}$$

This is called the *Michaelis-Menten equation*. Figure 72-2 shows the application of this equation.

Role of Enzyme Concentration in Regulation of Metabolic Reactions. Figure 72-2 shows that *when the substrate concentration is high*, as shown in the right half of the figure, the rate of a chemical reaction is determined almost entirely by the concentration of the enzyme. Thus, as the enzyme concentration increases from an arbitrary value of 1 up to 2, 4, or 8, the rate of the reaction increases proportionately, as demonstrated by the rising levels of the curves. As an example, when large quantities of glucose enter the renal tubules in a person with diabetes mellitus—that is, the substrate glucose is in great excess in the tubules—further increases in tubular glucose have little effect on glucose reabsorption, because the transport enzymes are saturated. Under these conditions, the rate of reabsorption of the glucose is limited by the concentration of the transport enzymes in the proximal tubular cells, not by the concentration of the glucose itself.

Role of Substrate Concentration in Regulation of Metabolic Reactions. Note also in Figure 72-2 that when the substrate

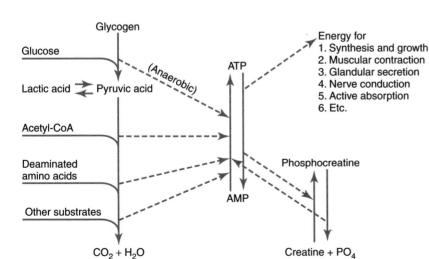

Figure 72-1 Overall schema of energy transfer from foods to the adenylic acid system and then to the functional elements of the cells. (Modified from Soskin S, Levine R: Carbohydrate Metabolism. Chicago: University of Chicago Press, 1952.)

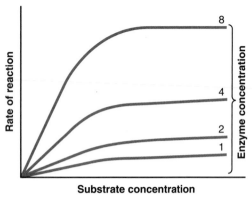

Figure 72-2 Effect of substrate and enzyme concentrations on the rate of enzyme-catalyzed reaction.

concentration becomes low enough that only a small portion of the enzyme is required in the reaction, the rate of the reaction becomes directly proportional to the substrate concentration, as well as the enzyme concentration. This is the relationship seen in the absorption of substances from the intestinal tract and renal tubules when their concentrations are low.

Rate Limitation in a Series of Reactions. Almost all chemical reactions of the body occur in series, with the product of one reaction acting as a substrate for the next reaction, and so on. Therefore, the overall rate of a complex series of chemical reactions is determined mainly by the rate of reaction of the slowest step in the series. This is called the *rate-limiting step* in the entire series.

ADP Concentration as a Rate-Controlling Factor in Energy Release. Under *resting* conditions, the concentration of ADP in the cells is extremely slight, so the chemical reactions that depend on ADP as one of the substrates are quite slow. They include all the oxidative metabolic pathways that release energy from food, as well as essentially all other pathways for the release of energy in the body. Thus, *ADP is a major rate-limiting factor* for almost all energy metabolism of the body.

When the cells become active, regardless of the type of activity, ATP is converted into ADP, increasing the concentration of ADP in direct proportion to the degree of activity of the cell. This ADP then automatically increases the rates of all the reactions for the metabolic release of energy from food. Thus, by this simple process, the amount of energy released in the cell is controlled by the degree of activity of the cell. In the absence of cellular activity, the release of energy stops because all the ADP soon becomes ATP.

Metabolic Rate

The *metabolism* of the body simply means all the chemical reactions in all the cells of the body, and the *metabolic rate* is normally expressed in terms of the rate of heat liberation during chemical reactions.

Heat Is the End Product of Almost All the Energy Released in the Body. In discussing many of the metabolic reactions in the preceding chapters, we noted that not all the energy in foods is transferred to ATP; instead, a large portion of this energy becomes heat. On average, 35 percent of the energy in foods becomes heat during ATP formation. Then, still more energy becomes heat as it is transferred from ATP

to the functional systems of the cells, so even under optimal conditions, no more than 27 percent of all the energy from food is finally used by the functional systems.

Even when 27 percent of the energy reaches the functional systems of the cells, most of this eventually becomes heat. For example, when proteins are synthesized, large portions of ATP are used to form the peptide linkages and this stores energy in these linkages. But there is also continuous turnover of proteins—some being degraded while others are being formed. When proteins are degraded, the energy stored in the peptide linkages is released in the form of heat into the body.

Another example is the energy used for muscle activity. Much of this energy simply overcomes the viscosity of the muscles themselves or of the tissues so that the limbs can move. This viscous movement causes friction within the tissues, which generates heat.

Consider also the energy expended by the heart in pumping blood. The blood distends the arterial system, and this distention itself represents a reservoir of potential energy. As the blood flows through the peripheral vessels, the friction of the different layers of blood flowing over one another and the friction of the blood against the walls of the vessels turn all this energy into heat.

Essentially all the energy expended by the body is eventually converted into heat. The only significant exception occurs when the muscles are used to perform some form of work outside the body. For instance, when the muscles elevate an object to a height or propel the body up steps, a type of potential energy is created by raising a mass against gravity. But when external expenditure of energy is not taking place, all the energy released by the metabolic processes eventually becomes body heat.

The Calorie. To discuss the metabolic rate of the body and related subjects quantitatively, it is necessary to use some unit for expressing the quantity of energy released from the different foods or expended by the different functional processes of the body. Most often, the *Calorie* is the unit used for this purpose. It will be recalled that 1 *calorie*—spelled with a small "c" and often called a *gram calorie*—is the quantity of heat required to raise the temperature of 1 gram of water 1°C. The calorie is much too small a unit when referring to energy in the body. Consequently, the Calorie—sometimes spelled with a capital "C" and often called a *kilocalorie*, which is equivalent to 1000 calories—is the unit ordinarily used in discussing energy metabolism.

Measurement of the Whole-Body Metabolic Rate

Direct Calorimetry Measures Heat Liberated from the Body. Because a person ordinarily is not performing any external work, the whole-body metabolic rate can be determined by simply measuring the total quantity of heat liberated from the body in a given time.

In determining the metabolic rate by direct calorimetry, one measures the quantity of heat liberated from the body in a large, specially constructed *calorimeter*. The subject is placed in an air chamber that is so well insulated that no heat can leak through the walls of the chamber. Heat formed by the subject's body warms the air of the chamber. However, the air temperature within the chamber is maintained at a constant level by forcing the air through pipes in a cool water bath. The rate of heat gain by the water bath, which can be measured with an accurate thermometer, is equal to the rate at which heat is liberated by the subject's body.

Direct calorimetry is physically difficult to perform and is used only for research purposes.

Indirect Calorimetry—The "Energy Equivalent" of Oxygen. Because more than 95 percent of the energy expended in the body is derived from reactions of oxygen with the different foods, the whole-body metabolic rate can also be calculated with a high degree of accuracy from the rate of oxygen utilization. When 1 liter of oxygen is metabolized with glucose, 5.01 Calories of energy are released; when metabolized with starches, 5.06 Calories are released; with fat, 4.70 Calories; and with protein, 4.60 Calories.

Using these figures, it is striking how nearly equivalent are the quantities of energy liberated per liter of oxygen, regardless of the type of food being metabolized. For the average diet, the *quantity of energy liberated per liter of oxygen used in the body averages about 4.825 Calories.* This is called the *energy equivalent* of oxygen; using this energy equivalent, one can calculate with a high degree of precision the rate of heat liberation in the body from the quantity of oxygen used in a given period of time.

If a person metabolizes only carbohydrates during the period of the metabolic rate determination, the calculated quantity of energy liberated, based on the value for the average energy equivalent of oxygen (4.825 Calories/L), would be about 4 percent too little. Conversely, if the person obtains most energy from fat, the calculated value would be about 4 percent too great.

Energy Metabolism—Factors That Influence Energy Output

As discussed in Chapter 71, energy intake is balanced with energy output in healthy adults who maintain a stable body weight. About 45 percent of daily energy intake is derived from carbohydrates, 40 percent from fats, and 15 percent from proteins in the average American diet. Energy output can also be partitioned into several measurable components, including energy used for (1) performing essential metabolic functions of the body (the "basal" metabolic rate); (2) performing various physical activities; (3) digesting, absorbing, and processing food; and (4) maintaining body temperature.

Overall Energy Requirements for Daily Activities

An average man who weighs 70 kilograms and lies in bed all day uses about 1650 Calories of energy. The process of eating and digesting food increases the amount of energy used each day by an additional 200 or more Calories, so the same man lying in bed and eating a reasonable diet requires a dietary intake of about 1850 Calories per day. If he sits in a chair all day without exercising, his total energy requirement reaches 2000 to 2250 Calories. Therefore, the daily energy requirement for a very sedentary man performing only essential functions is about 2000 Calories.

The amount of energy used to perform daily physical activities is normally about 25 percent of the total energy expenditure, but it can vary markedly in different individuals, depending on the type and amount of physical activity. For example, walking up stairs requires about 17 times as much energy as lying in bed asleep. In general, over a 24-hour period, a person performing heavy labor can achieve a maximal rate of energy utilization as great as 6000 to 7000 Calories, or as much as 3.5 times the energy used under conditions of no physical activity.

Basal Metabolic Rate (BMR)—The Minimum Energy Expenditure for the Body to Exist

Even when a person is at complete rest, considerable energy is required to perform all the chemical reactions of the body. This minimum level of energy required to exist is called the *basal metabolic rate* (BMR) and accounts for about 50 to 70 percent of the daily energy expenditure in most sedentary individuals (Figure 72-3).

Because the level of physical activity is highly variable among different individuals, measurement of the BMR provides a useful means of comparing one person's metabolic rate with that of another. The usual method for determining BMR is to measure the rate of oxygen utilization over a given period of time under the following conditions:

1. The person must not have eaten food for at least 12 hours.
2. The BMR is determined after a night of restful sleep.
3. No strenuous activity is performed for at least 1 hour before the test.
4. All psychic and physical factors that cause excitement must be eliminated.
5. The temperature of the air must be comfortable and between 68° and 80°F.
6. No physical activity is permitted during the test.

The BMR normally averages about 65 to 70 Calories per hour in an average 70-kilogram man. Although much of the BMR is accounted for by essential activities of the central nervous system, heart, kidneys, and other organs, the *variations* in BMR among different individuals are related mainly to differences in the amount of skeletal muscle and body size.

Skeletal muscle, even under resting conditions, accounts for 20 to 30 percent of the BMR. For this reason, BMR is usually corrected for differences in body size by expressing it as Calories per hour per square meter of body surface area, calculated from height and weight. The average values for males and females of different ages are shown in Figure 72-4.

Much of the decline in BMR with increasing age is probably related to loss of muscle mass and replacement of muscle with adipose tissue, which has a lower rate of metabolism. Likewise, slightly lower BMRs in women, compared with men, are due partly to their lower percentage of muscle mass

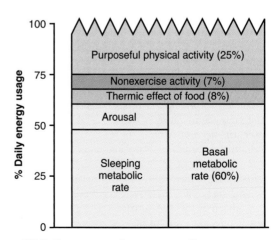

Figure 72-3 Components of energy expenditure.

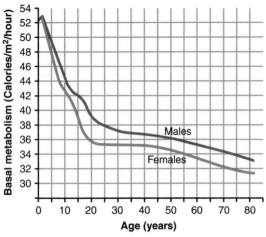

Figure 72-4 Normal basal metabolic rates at different ages for each sex.

and higher percentage of adipose tissue. However, other factors can influence the BMR, as discussed next.

Thyroid Hormone Increases Metabolic Rate. When the thyroid gland secretes maximal amounts of thyroxine, the metabolic rate sometimes rises 50 to 100 percent above normal. Conversely, total loss of thyroid secretion decreases the metabolic rate to 40 to 60 percent of normal. As discussed in Chapter 76, thyroxine increases the rates of the chemical reactions of many cells in the body and therefore increases metabolic rate. Adaptation of the thyroid gland— with increased secretion in cold climates and decreased secretion in hot climates—contributes to the differences in BMRs among people living in different geographical zones; for example, people living in arctic regions have BMRs 10 to 20 percent higher than those of persons living in tropical regions.

Male Sex Hormone Increases Metabolic Rate. The male sex hormone testosterone can increase the metabolic rate about 10 to 15 percent. The female sex hormones may increase the BMR a small amount, but usually not enough to be significant. Much of this effect of the male sex hormone is related to its anabolic effect to increase skeletal muscle mass.

Growth Hormone Increases Metabolic Rate. Growth hormone can increase the metabolic rate by stimulating cellular metabolism and by increasing skeletal muscle mass. In adults with growth hormone deficiency, replacement therapy with recombinant growth hormone increases basal metabolic rate by about 20 percent.

Fever Increases Metabolic Rate. Fever, regardless of its cause, increases the chemical reactions of the body by an average of about 120 percent for every 10 °C rise in temperature. This is discussed in more detail in Chapter 73.

Sleep Decreases Metabolic Rate. The metabolic rate decreases 10 to 15 percent below normal during sleep. This fall is due to two principal factors: (1) decreased tone of the skeletal musculature during sleep and (2) decreased activity of the central nervous system.

Malnutrition Decreases Metabolic Rate. Prolonged malnutrition can decrease the metabolic rate 20 to 30 percent, presumably due to the paucity of food substances in the cells. In the final stages of many disease conditions, the inanition that accompanies the disease causes a marked decrease in metabolic rate, to the extent that the body temperature may fall several degrees shortly before death.

Energy Used for Physical Activities

The factor that most dramatically increases metabolic rate is strenuous exercise. Short bursts of maximal muscle contraction in a single muscle can liberate as much as 100 times its normal resting amount of heat for a few seconds. For the entire body, maximal muscle exercise can increase the overall heat production of the body for a few seconds to about 50 times normal, or to about 20 times normal for more sustained exercise in a well-trained individual.

Table 72-1 shows the energy expenditure during different types of physical activity for a 70-kilogram man. Because of the great variation in the amount of physical activity among individuals, this component of energy expenditure is the most important reason for the differences in caloric intake required to maintain energy balance. However, in industrialized countries where food supplies are plentiful, such as the United States, caloric intake often periodically exceeds energy expenditure, and the excess energy is stored mainly as fat. This underscores the importance of maintaining a proper level of physical activity to prevent excess fat stores and obesity.

Even in sedentary individuals who perform little or no daily exercise or physical work, significant energy is spent on spontaneous physical activity required to maintain muscle tone and body posture and on other nonexercise activities such as "fidgeting." Together, these nonexercise activities account for about 7 percent of a person's daily energy usage.

Energy Used for Processing Food—Thermogenic Effect of Food

After a meal is ingested, the metabolic rate increases as a result of the different chemical reactions associated with digestion, absorption, and storage of food in the body. This is called the *thermogenic effect of food* because these processes require energy and generate heat.

After a meal that contains a large quantity of carbohydrates or fats, the metabolic rate usually increases about 4 percent.

Table 72-1 Energy Expenditure During Different Types of Activity for a 70-Kilogram Man

Form of Activity	Calories per Hour
Sleeping	65
Awake lying still	77
Sitting at rest	100
Standing relaxed	105
Dressing and undressing	118
Typewriting rapidly	140
Walking slowly (2.6 miles per hour)	200
Carpentry, metalworking, industrial painting	240
Sawing wood	480
Swimming	500
Running (5.3 miles per hour)	570
Walking up stairs rapidly	1100

Extracted from data compiled by Professor M.S. Rose.

However, after a high-protein meal, the metabolic rate usually begins rising within an hour, reaching a maximum of about 30 percent above normal, and this lasts for 3 to 12 hours. This effect of protein on the metabolic rate is called the *specific dynamic action of protein*. The thermogenic effect of food accounts for about 8 percent of the total daily energy expenditure in many persons.

Energy Used for Nonshivering Thermogenesis—Role of Sympathetic Stimulation

Although physical work and the thermogenic effect of food cause liberation of heat, these mechanisms are not aimed primarily at regulation of body temperature. Shivering provides a regulated means of producing heat by increasing muscle activity in response to cold stress, as discussed in Chapter 73. Another mechanism, *nonshivering thermogenesis*, can also produce heat in response to cold stress. This type of thermogenesis is stimulated by sympathetic nervous system activation, which releases norepinephrine and epinephrine, which in turn increase metabolic activity and heat generation.

In certain types of fat tissue, called *brown fat*, sympathetic nervous stimulation causes liberation of large amounts of heat. This type of fat contains large numbers of mitochondria and many small globules of fat instead of one large fat globule. In these cells, the process of oxidative phosphorylation in the mitochondria is mainly "uncoupled." That is, when the cells are stimulated by the sympathetic nerves, the mitochondria produce a large amount of heat but almost no ATP, so almost all the released oxidative energy immediately becomes heat.

A neonate has a considerable number of brown fat cells, and maximal sympathetic stimulation can increase the child's metabolism more than 100 percent. The magnitude of this type of thermogenesis in an adult human, who has virtually no brown fat, is probably less than 15 percent, although this might increase significantly after cold adaptation.

Nonshivering thermogenesis may also serve as a buffer against obesity. Recent studies indicate that sympathetic nervous system activity is increased in obese persons who have a persistent excess caloric intake. The mechanism responsible for sympathetic activation in obese persons is uncertain, but it may be mediated partly through the effects of increased leptin, which activates pro-opiomelanocortin neurons in the hypothalamus. Sympathetic stimulation, by increasing thermogenesis, helps to limit excess weight gain.

Bibliography

Argyropoulos G, Harper ME: Uncoupling proteins and thermoregulation, *J Appl Physiol* 92:2187, 2002.

Cahill GF Jr: Fuel metabolism in starvation, *Annu Rev Nutr* 26:1, 2006.

Cannon B, Nedergaard J: Brown adipose tissue: function and physiological significance, *Physiol Rev* 84:277, 2004.

Harper ME, Green K, Brand MD: The efficiency of cellular energy transduction and its implications for obesity, *Annu Rev Nutr* 28:13, 2008.

Harper ME, Seifert EL: Thyroid hormone effects on mitochondrial energetics, *Thyroid* 18:145, 2008.

Kim B: Thyroid hormone as a determinant of energy expenditure and the basal metabolic rate, *Thyroid* 18:141, 2008.

Levine JA: Measurement of energy expenditure, *Public Health Nutr* 8:1123, 2005.

Levine JA, Vander Weg MW, Hill JO, Klesges RC: Non-exercise activity thermogenesis: the crouching tiger, hidden dragon of societal weight gain, *Arterioscler Thromb Vasc Biol* 26:729, 2006.

Lowell BB, Bachman ES: Beta-adrenergic receptors, diet-induced thermogenesis, and obesity, *J Biol Chem* 278:29385, 2003.

Morrison SF, Nakamura K, Madden CJ: Central control of thermogenesis in mammals, *Exp Physiol* 93:773, 2008.

Murphy E, Steenbergen C: Mechanisms underlying acute protection from cardiac ischemia-reperfusion injury, *Physiol Rev* 88:581, 2008.

National Institutes of Health: *Clinical Guidelines on the Identification, Evaluation, and Treatment of Overweight and Obesity in Adults: The Evidence Report*, Bethesda, MD, 1998, National Heart, Lung, and Blood Institute and National Institute of Diabetes and Digestive and Kidney Diseases. Available at: http://www.nhlbi.nih.gov/guidelines/index.htm.

Saks V, Favier R, Guzun R, Schlattner U, Wallimann T: Molecular system bioenergetics: regulation of substrate supply in response to heart energy demands, *J Physiol* 15:577, 769, 2006.

Silva JE: Thermogenic mechanisms and their hormonal regulation, *Physiol Rev* 86:435, 2006.

van Baak MA: Meal-induced activation of the sympathetic nervous system and its cardiovascular and thermogenic effects in man, *Physiol Behav* 94:178, 2008.

Westerterp KR: Limits to sustainable human metabolic rate, *J Exp Biol* 204:3183, 2001.

Westerterp KR: Impacts of vigorous and non-vigorous activity on daily energy expenditure, *Proc Nutr Soc* 62:645, 2003.

Body Temperature Regulation, and Fever

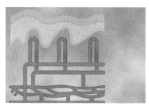

Normal Body Temperatures

Body Core Temperature and Skin Temperature. The temperature of the deep tissues of the body—the "core" of the body—remains very constant, within ±1°F (±0.6°C), except when a person develops a febrile illness. Indeed, a nude person can be exposed to temperatures as low as 55°F or as high as 130°F in *dry* air and still maintain an almost constant core temperature. The mechanisms for regulating body temperature represent a beautifully designed control system. In this chapter we discuss this system as it operates in health and in disease.

The *skin temperature*, in contrast to the *core temperature*, rises and falls with the temperature of the surroundings. The skin temperature is important when we refer to the skin's ability to lose heat to the surroundings.

Normal Core Temperature. No single core temperature can be considered normal because measurements in many healthy people have shown a *range* of normal temperatures measured orally, as shown in Figure 73-1, from less than 97°F (36°C) to over 99.5°F (37.5°C). The average normal core temperature is generally considered to be between 98.0° and 98.6°F when measured orally and about 1°F higher when measured rectally.

The body temperature increases during exercise and varies with temperature extremes of the surroundings because the temperature regulatory mechanisms are not perfect. When excessive heat is produced in the body by strenuous exercise, the temperature can rise temporarily to as high as 101°F to 104°F. Conversely, when the body is exposed to extreme cold, the temperature can fall below 96°F.

Body Temperature Is Controlled by Balancing Heat Production and Heat Loss

When the rate of heat production in the body is greater than the rate at which heat is being lost, heat builds up in the body and the body temperature rises. Conversely,

when heat loss is greater, both body heat and body temperature decrease. Most of the remainder of this chapter is concerned with this balance between heat production and heat loss and the mechanisms by which the body controls each of these.

Heat Production

Heat production is a principal by-product of metabolism. In Chapter 72, which summarizes body energetics, we discuss the different factors that determine the rate of heat production, called the *metabolic rate of the body*. The most important of these factors are listed again here: (1) basal rate of metabolism of all the cells of the body; (2) extra rate of metabolism caused by muscle activity, including muscle contractions caused by shivering; (3) extra metabolism caused by the effect of thyroxine (and, to a less extent, other hormones, such as growth hormone and testosterone) on the cells; (4) extra metabolism caused by the effect of epinephrine, norepinephrine, and sympathetic stimulation on the cells; (5) extra metabolism caused by increased chemical activity in the cells themselves, especially when the cell temperature increases; and (6) extra metabolism needed for digestion, absorption, and storage of food (thermogenic effect of food).

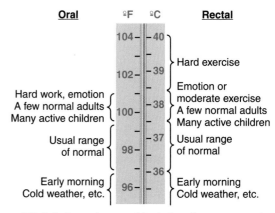

Figure 73-1 Estimated range of body "core" temperature in normal people. (Redrawn from DuBois EF: Fever. Springfield, Ill: Charles C Thomas, 1948.)

Heat Loss

Most of the heat produced in the body is generated in the deep organs, especially in the liver, brain, and heart, and in the skeletal muscles during exercise. Then this heat is transferred from the deeper organs and tissues to the skin, where it is lost to the air and other surroundings. Therefore, the rate at which heat is lost is determined almost entirely by two factors: (1) how rapidly heat can be conducted from where it is produced in the body core to the skin and (2) how rapidly heat can then be transferred from the skin to the surroundings. Let us begin by discussing the system that insulates the core from the skin surface.

Insulator System of the Body

The skin, the subcutaneous tissues, and especially the fat of the subcutaneous tissues act together as a heat insulator for the body. The fat is important because it conducts heat only *one third* as readily as other tissues. When no blood is flowing from the heated internal organs to the skin, the insulating properties of the normal male body are about equal to three-quarters the insulating properties of a usual suit of clothes. In women, this insulation is even better.

The insulation beneath the skin is an effective means of maintaining normal internal core temperature, even though it allows the temperature of the skin to approach the temperature of the surroundings.

Blood Flow to the Skin from the Body Core Provides Heat Transfer

Blood vessels are distributed profusely beneath the skin. Especially important is a continuous venous plexus that is supplied by inflow of blood from the skin capillaries, shown in Figure 73-2. In the most exposed areas of the body—the hands, feet, and ears—blood is also supplied to the plexus directly from the small arteries through highly muscular *arteriovenous anastomoses*.

The rate of blood flow into the skin venous plexus can vary tremendously—from barely above zero to as great as 30 percent of the total cardiac output. A high rate of skin flow causes heat to be conducted from the core of the body to the skin with great efficiency, whereas reduction in the rate of skin flow can decrease the heat conduction from the core to very little.

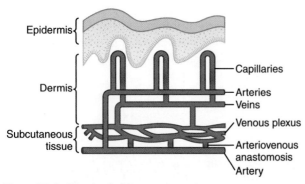

Figure 73-2 Skin circulation.

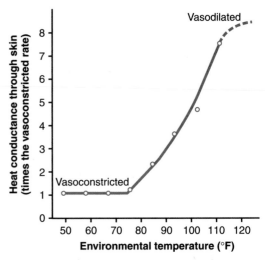

Figure 73-3 Effect of changes in the environmental temperature on heat conductance from the body core to the skin surface. (Modified from Benzinger TH: Heat and Temperature Fundamentals of Medical Physiology. New York: Dowden, Hutchinson & Ross, 1980.)

Figure 73-3 shows quantitatively the effect of environmental air temperature on conductance of heat from the core to the skin surface and then conductance into the air, demonstrating an approximate eightfold increase in heat conductance between the fully vasoconstricted state and the fully vasodilated state.

Therefore, the skin is an effective controlled *"heat radiator" system*, and the flow of blood to the skin is a most effective mechanism for heat transfer from the body core to the skin.

Control of Heat Conduction to the Skin by the Sympathetic Nervous System. Heat conduction to the skin by the blood is controlled by the degree of vasoconstriction of the arterioles and the arteriovenous anastomoses that supply blood to the venous plexus of the skin. This vasoconstriction is controlled almost entirely by the sympathetic nervous system in response to changes in body core temperature and changes in environmental temperature. This is discussed later in the chapter in connection with control of body temperature by the hypothalamus.

Basic Physics of How Heat Is Lost from the Skin Surface

The various methods by which heat is lost from the skin to the surroundings are shown in Figure 73-4. They include *radiation, conduction*, and *evaporation*, which are explained next.

Radiation. As shown in Figure 73-4, in a nude person sitting inside at normal room temperature, about 60 percent of total heat loss is by radiation.

Loss of heat by radiation means loss in the form of infrared heat rays, a type of electromagnetic wave. Most infrared heat rays that radiate from the body have wavelengths of 5 to 20 micrometers, 10 to 30 times the wavelengths of light rays. All objects that are not at absolute zero temperature radiate such rays. The human body

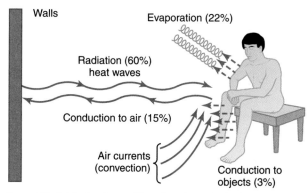

Figure 73-4 Mechanisms of heat loss from the body.

radiates heat rays in all directions. Heat rays are also being radiated from the walls of rooms and other objects toward the body. If the temperature of the body is greater than the temperature of the surroundings, a greater quantity of heat is radiated from the body than is radiated to the body.

Conduction. As shown in Figure 73-4, only minute quantities of heat, about 3 percent, are normally lost from the body by direct conduction from the surface of the body to *solid objects*, such as a chair or a bed. Loss of heat by *conduction to air*, however, represents a sizable proportion of the body's heat loss (about 15 percent) even under normal conditions.

It will be recalled that heat is actually the kinetic energy of molecular motion, and the molecules of the skin are continually undergoing vibratory motion. Much of the energy of this motion can be transferred to the air if the air is colder than the skin, thus increasing the velocity of the air molecules' motion. Once the temperature of the air adjacent to the skin equals the temperature of the skin, no further loss of heat occurs in this way because now an equal amount of heat is conducted from the air to the body. Therefore, conduction of heat from the body to the air is self-limited *unless the heated air moves away from the skin*, so new, unheated air is continually brought in contact with the skin, a phenomenon called *air convection*.

Convection. The removal of heat from the body by convection air currents is commonly called *heat loss by convection*. Actually, the heat must first be *conducted* to the air and then carried away by the convection air currents.

A small amount of convection almost always occurs around the body because of the tendency for air adjacent to the skin to rise as it becomes heated. Therefore, in a nude person seated in a comfortable room without gross air movement, about 15 percent of his or her total heat loss occurs by conduction to the air and then by air convection away from the body.

Cooling Effect of Wind. When the body is exposed to wind, the layer of air immediately adjacent to the skin is replaced by new air much more rapidly than normally, and heat loss by convection increases accordingly. The cooling effect of wind at low velocities is about proportional to the *square root of the wind velocity*. For instance,

a wind of 4 miles per hour is about twice as effective for cooling as a wind of 1 mile per hour.

Conduction and Convection of Heat from a Person Suspended in Water. Water has a specific heat several thousand times as great as that of air, so each unit portion of water adjacent to the skin can absorb far greater quantities of heat than air can. Also, heat conductivity in water is very great in comparison with that in air. Consequently, it is impossible for the body to heat a thin layer of water next to the body to form an "insulator zone" as occurs in air. Therefore, the rate of heat loss to water is usually many times greater than the rate of heat loss to air.

Evaporation. When water evaporates from the body surface, 0.58 Calorie (kilocalorie) of heat is lost for each gram of water that evaporates. Even when a person is not sweating, water still evaporates *insensibly* from the skin and lungs at a rate of about 600 to 700 ml/day. This causes continual heat loss at a rate of 16 to 19 Calories per hour. This insensible evaporation through the skin and lungs cannot be controlled for purposes of temperature regulation because it results from continual diffusion of water molecules through the skin and respiratory surfaces. However, loss of heat by *evaporation of sweat* can be controlled by regulating the rate of sweating, which is discussed later in the chapter.

Evaporation Is a Necessary Cooling Mechanism at Very High Air Temperatures. As long as skin temperature is greater than the temperature of the surroundings, heat can be lost by radiation and conduction. But when the temperature of the surroundings becomes greater than that of the skin, instead of losing heat, the body gains heat by both radiation and conduction. Under these conditions, *the only means by which the body can rid itself of heat is by evaporation*.

Therefore, anything that prevents adequate evaporation when the surrounding temperature is higher than the skin temperature will cause the internal body temperature to rise. This occurs occasionally in human beings who are born with congenital absence of sweat glands. These people can tolerate cold temperatures as well as normal people can, but they are likely to die of heatstroke in tropical zones because without the evaporative refrigeration system, they cannot prevent a rise in body temperature when the air temperature is above that of the body.

Effect of Clothing on Conductive Heat Loss. Clothing entraps air next to the skin in the weave of the cloth, thereby increasing the thickness of the so-called *private zone* of air adjacent to the skin and also decreasing the flow of convection air currents. Consequently, the rate of heat loss from the body by conduction and convection is greatly depressed. A usual suit of clothes decreases the rate of heat loss to about half that from the nude body, but arctic-type clothing can decrease this heat loss to as little as one sixth.

About half the heat transmitted from the skin to the clothing is radiated to the clothing instead of being conducted across the small intervening space. Therefore, coating the inside of clothing with a thin layer of gold, which reflects radiant heat back to the body, makes the insulating properties of clothing far more effective than otherwise. Using this technique, clothing for use in the arctic can be decreased in weight by about half.

The effectiveness of clothing in maintaining body temperature is almost completely lost when the clothing becomes wet because the high conductivity of water increases the rate of heat transmission through cloth 20-fold or more. Therefore, one of the most important factors for protecting the body against cold in arctic regions is extreme caution against allowing the clothing to become wet. Indeed, one must be careful not to become overheated even temporarily because sweating in one's clothes makes them much less effective thereafter as an insulator.

Sweating and Its Regulation by the Autonomic Nervous System

Stimulation of the anterior hypothalamus-preoptic area in the brain either electrically or by excess heat causes sweating. The nerve impulses from this area that cause sweating are transmitted in the autonomic pathways to the spinal cord and then through sympathetic outflow to the skin everywhere in the body.

It should be recalled from the discussion of the autonomic nervous system in Chapter 60 that the sweat glands are innervated by *cholinergic* nerve fibers (fibers that secrete acetylcholine but that run in the sympathetic nerves along with the adrenergic fibers). These glands can also be stimulated to some extent by epinephrine or norepinephrine circulating in the blood, even though the glands themselves do not have adrenergic innervation. This is important during exercise, when these hormones are secreted by the adrenal medullae and the body needs to lose excessive amounts of heat produced by the active muscles.

Mechanism of Sweat Secretion. In Figure 73-5, the sweat gland is shown to be a tubular structure consisting of two parts: (1) a deep subdermal *coiled portion* that secretes the sweat, and (2) a *duct portion* that passes outward through the dermis and epidermis of the skin. As is true of so many other glands, the secretory portion of the sweat gland secretes a fluid called the *primary secretion* or *precursor secretion*; the concentrations of constituents in the fluid are then modified as the fluid flows through the duct.

The precursor secretion is an active secretory product of the epithelial cells lining the coiled portion of the sweat gland. Cholinergic sympathetic nerve fibers ending on or near the glandular cells elicit the secretion.

The composition of the precursor secretion is similar to that of plasma, except that it does not contain plasma proteins. The concentration of sodium is about 142 mEq/L and that of chloride is about 104 mEq/L, with much smaller concentrations of the other solutes of plasma. As this precursor solution flows through the duct portion of the gland, it is modified by reabsorption of most of the sodium and chloride ions. The degree of this reabsorption depends on the rate of sweating, as follows.

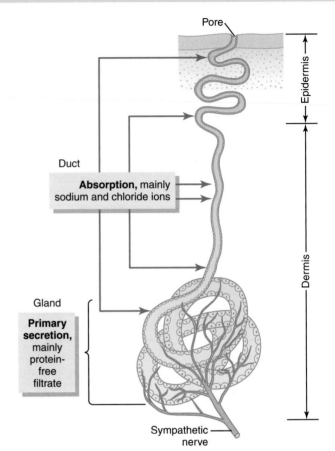

Figure 73-5 Sweat gland innervated by an acetylcholine-secreting sympathetic nerve. A *primary protein-free secretion* is formed by the glandular portion, but most of the electrolytes are reabsorbed in the duct, leaving a dilute, watery secretion.

When the sweat glands are stimulated only slightly, the precursor fluid passes through the duct slowly. In this instance, essentially all the sodium and chloride ions are reabsorbed, and the concentration of each falls to as low as 5 mEq/L. This reduces the osmotic pressure of the sweat fluid to such a low level that most of the water is also reabsorbed, which concentrates most of the other constituents. Therefore, at low rates of sweating, such constituents as urea, lactic acid, and potassium ions are usually very concentrated.

Conversely, when the sweat glands are strongly stimulated by the sympathetic nervous system, large amounts of precursor secretion are formed, and the duct may reabsorb only slightly more than half the sodium chloride; the concentrations of sodium and chloride ions are then (in an *unacclimatized* person) a maximum of about 50 to 60 mEq/L, slightly less than half the concentrations in plasma. Furthermore, the sweat flows through the glandular tubules so rapidly that little of the water is reabsorbed. Therefore, the other dissolved constituents of sweat are only moderately increased in concentration—urea is about twice that in the plasma, lactic acid about 4 times, and potassium about 1.2 times.

There is a significant loss of sodium chloride in the sweat when a person is unacclimatized to heat. There is much less electrolyte loss, despite increased sweating capacity, once a person has become acclimatized, as follows.

Acclimatization of the Sweating Mechanism to Heat—Role of Aldosterone. Although a normal, unacclimatized person seldom produces more than about 1 liter of sweat per hour, when this person is exposed to hot weather for 1 to 6 weeks, he or she begins to sweat more profusely, often increasing maximum sweat production to as much as 2 to 3 L/hour. Evaporation of this much sweat can remove heat from the body at a rate *more than 10 times* the normal basal rate of heat production. This increased effectiveness of the sweating mechanism is caused by a change in the internal sweat gland cells themselves to increase their sweating capability.

Also associated with acclimatization is a further decrease in the concentration of sodium chloride in the sweat, which allows progressively better conservation of body salt. Most of this effect is caused by *increased secretion of aldosterone* by the adrenocortical glands, which results from a slight decrease in sodium chloride concentration in the extracellular fluid and plasma. An *unacclimatized* person who sweats profusely often loses 15 to 30 grams of salt each day for the first few days. After 4 to 6 weeks of acclimatization, the loss is usually 3 to 5 g/day.

Loss of Heat by Panting

Many lower animals have little ability to lose heat from the surfaces of their bodies, for two reasons: (1) the surfaces are often covered with fur, and (2) the skin of most lower animals is not supplied with sweat glands, which prevents most of the evaporative loss of heat from the skin. A substitute mechanism, the *panting* mechanism, is used by many lower animals as a means of dissipating heat.

The phenomenon of panting is "turned on" by the thermoregulator centers of the brain. That is, when the blood becomes overheated, the hypothalamus initiates neurogenic signals to decrease the body temperature. One of these signals initiates panting. The actual panting process is controlled by a *panting center* that is associated with the pneumotaxic respiratory center located in the pons.

When an animal pants, it breathes in and out rapidly, so large quantities of new air from the exterior come in contact with the upper portions of the respiratory passages; this cools the blood in the respiratory passage mucosa as a result of water evaporation from the mucosal surfaces, especially evaporation of saliva from the tongue. Yet panting does not increase the alveolar ventilation more than is required for proper control of the blood gases because each breath is extremely shallow; therefore, most of the air that enters the alveoli is dead-space air mainly from the trachea and not from the atmosphere.

Regulation of Body Temperature—Role of the Hypothalamus

Figure 73-6 shows what happens to the body "core" temperature of a nude person after a few hours' exposure to *dry* air ranging from 30° to 160°F. The precise dimensions of this curve depend on the wind movement of the air, the

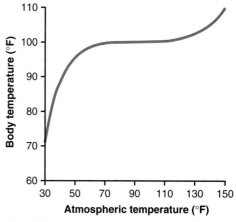

Figure 73-6 Effect of high and low atmospheric temperatures of several hours' duration, under dry conditions, on the internal body "core" temperature. Note that the internal body temperature remains stable despite wide changes in atmospheric temperature.

amount of moisture in the air, and even the nature of the surroundings. In general, a nude person in dry air between 55° and 130° F is capable of maintaining a normal body core temperature somewhere between 97° and 100°F.

The temperature of the body is regulated almost entirely by nervous feedback mechanisms, and almost all these operate through *temperature-regulating centers* located in the *hypothalamus*. For these feedback mechanisms to operate, there must also be temperature detectors to determine when the body temperature becomes either too high or too low.

Role of the Anterior Hypothalamic-Preoptic Area in Thermostatic Detection of Temperature

Experiments have been performed in which minute areas in the brain of an animal have been either heated or cooled by use of a *thermode*. This small, needle-like device is heated by electrical means or by passing hot water through it, or it is cooled by cold water. The principal areas in the brain where heat or cold from a thermode affects body temperature control are the preoptic and anterior hypothalamic nuclei of the hypothalamus.

Using the thermode, the anterior hypothalamic-preoptic area has been found to contain large numbers of heat-sensitive neurons, as well as about one-third as many cold-sensitive neurons. These neurons are believed to function as temperature sensors for controlling body temperature. The heat-sensitive neurons increase their firing rate 2- to 10-fold in response to a 10°C increase in body temperature. The cold-sensitive neurons, by contrast, increase their firing rate when the body temperature falls.

When the preoptic area is heated, the skin all over the body immediately breaks out in a profuse sweat, whereas the skin blood vessels over the entire body become greatly dilated. This is an immediate reaction to cause the body to lose heat, thereby helping to return the body temperature toward the normal level. In addition, any excess body heat production is inhibited. Therefore, it is clear that the hypothalamic-preoptic area has the capability to serve as a thermostatic body temperature control center.

Detection of Temperature by Receptors in the Skin and Deep Body Tissues

Although the signals generated by the temperature receptors of the hypothalamus are extremely powerful in controlling body temperature, receptors in other parts of the body play additional roles in temperature regulation. This is especially true of temperature receptors in the skin and in a few specific deep tissues of the body.

It will be recalled from the discussion of sensory receptors in Chapter 48 that the skin is endowed with both *cold* and *warmth* receptors. There are far more cold receptors than warmth receptors—in fact, 10 times as many in many parts of the skin. Therefore, peripheral detection of temperature mainly concerns detecting cool and cold instead of warm temperatures.

When the skin is chilled over the entire body, immediate reflex effects are invoked and begin to increase the temperature of the body in several ways: (1) by providing a strong stimulus to cause shivering, with a resultant increase in the rate of body heat production; (2) by inhibiting the process of sweating, if this is already occurring; and (3) by promoting skin vasoconstriction to diminish loss of body heat from the skin.

Deep body temperature receptors are found mainly in the *spinal cord*, in the *abdominal viscera*, and in or around the *great veins* in the upper abdomen and thorax. These deep receptors function differently from the skin receptors because they are exposed to the body core temperature rather than the body surface temperature. Yet, like the skin temperature receptors, they detect mainly cold rather than warmth. It is probable that both the skin and the deep body receptors are concerned with preventing *hypothermia*—that is, preventing low body temperature.

Posterior Hypothalamus Integrates the Central and Peripheral Temperature Sensory Signals

Even though many temperature sensory signals arise in peripheral receptors, these signals contribute to body temperature control mainly through the hypothalamus. The area of the hypothalamus that they stimulate is located bilaterally in the posterior hypothalamus approximately at the level of the mammillary bodies. The temperature sensory signals from the anterior hypothalamic-preoptic area are also transmitted into this posterior hypothalamic area. Here the signals from the preoptic area and the signals from elsewhere in the body are combined and integrated to control the heat-producing and heat-conserving reactions of the body.

Neuronal Effector Mechanisms That Decrease or Increase Body Temperature

When the hypothalamic temperature centers detect that the body temperature is either too high or too low, they institute appropriate temperature-decreasing or temperature-increasing procedures. The reader is probably familiar with most of these from personal experience, but special features are the following.

Temperature-Decreasing Mechanisms When the Body Is Too Hot

The temperature control system uses three important mechanisms to reduce body heat when the body temperature becomes too great:

1. *Vasodilation of skin blood vessels*. In almost all areas of the body, the skin blood vessels become intensely dilated. This is caused by inhibition of the sympathetic centers in the posterior hypothalamus that cause vasoconstriction. Full vasodilation can increase the rate of heat transfer to the skin as much as eightfold.

2. *Sweating*. The effect of increased body temperature to cause sweating is demonstrated by the blue curve in Figure 73-7, which shows a sharp increase in the rate of evaporative heat loss resulting from sweating when the body core temperature rises above the critical level of 37°C (98.6°F). An additional 1°C increase in body temperature causes enough sweating to remove 10 times the basal rate of body heat production.

3. *Decrease in heat production*. The mechanisms that cause excess heat production, such as shivering and chemical thermogenesis, are strongly inhibited.

Temperature-Increasing Mechanisms When the Body Is Too Cold

When the body is too cold, the temperature control system institutes exactly opposite procedures. They are:

1. *Skin vasoconstriction throughout the body*. This is caused by stimulation of the posterior hypothalamic sympathetic centers.

2. *Piloerection*. Piloerection means hairs "standing on end." Sympathetic stimulation causes the arrector pili

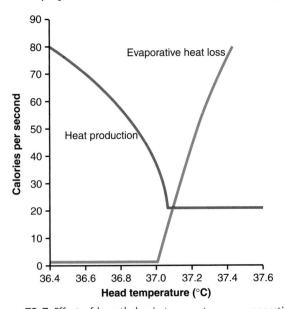

Figure 73-7 Effect of hypothalamic temperature on evaporative heat loss from the body and on heat production caused primarily by muscle activity and shivering. This figure demonstrates the extremely critical temperature level at which increased heat loss begins and heat production reaches a minimum stable level.

muscles attached to the hair follicles to contract, which brings the hairs to an upright stance. This is not important in human beings, but in lower animals, upright projection of the hairs allows them to entrap a thick layer of "insulator air" next to the skin, so transfer of heat to the surroundings is greatly depressed.

3. *Increase in thermogenesis (heat production).* Heat production by the metabolic systems is increased by promoting shivering, sympathetic excitation of heat production, and thyroxine secretion. These methods of increasing heat require additional explanation, which follows.

Hypothalamic Stimulation of Shivering. Located in the dorsomedial portion of the posterior hypothalamus near the wall of the third ventricle is an area called the *primary motor center for shivering.* This area is normally inhibited by signals from the heat center in the anterior hypothalamic-preoptic area but is excited by cold signals from the skin and spinal cord. Therefore, as shown by the sudden increase in "heat production" (see the red curve in Figure 73-7), this center becomes activated when the body temperature falls even a fraction of a degree below a critical temperature level. It then transmits signals that cause shivering through bilateral tracts down the brain stem, into the lateral columns of the spinal cord, and finally to the anterior motor neurons. These signals are nonrhythmical and do not cause the actual muscle shaking. Instead, they increase the tone of the skeletal muscles throughout the body by facilitating the activity of the anterior motor neurons. When the tone rises above a certain critical level, shivering begins. This probably results from feedback oscillation of the muscle spindle stretch reflex mechanism, which is discussed in Chapter 54. *During maximum shivering, body heat production can rise to four to five times normal.*

Sympathetic "Chemical" Excitation of Heat Production. As pointed out in Chapter 72, an increase in either sympathetic stimulation or circulating norepinephrine and epinephrine in the blood can cause an immediate increase in the rate of cellular metabolism. This effect is called *chemical thermogenesis,* or *nonshivering thermogenesis.* It results at least partially from the ability of norepinephrine and epinephrine to *uncouple* oxidative phosphorylation, which means that excess foodstuffs are oxidized and thereby release energy in the form of heat but do not cause ATP to be formed.

The degree of chemical thermogenesis that occurs in an animal is almost directly proportional to the amount of *brown fat* in the animal's tissues. This is a type of fat that contains large numbers of special mitochondria where uncoupled oxidation occurs, as described in Chapter 72. Brown fat is richly supplied with sympathetic nerves that release norepinephrine, which stimulates tissue expression of *mitochondrial uncoupling protein* (also called *thermogenin*) and increases thermogenesis.

Acclimatization greatly affects the intensity of chemical thermogenesis; some animals, such as rats, that have been exposed to a cold environment for several weeks exhibit a 100 to 500 percent increase in heat production when acutely exposed to cold, in contrast to the unacclimatized animal, which responds with an increase of perhaps one third as much. This increased thermogenesis also leads to a corresponding increase in food intake.

In adult human beings, who have almost no brown fat, it is rare for chemical thermogenesis to increase the rate of heat production more than 10 to 15 percent. However, in infants, who *do* have a small amount of brown fat in the interscapular space, chemical thermogenesis can increase the rate of heat production 100 percent, which is probably an important factor in maintaining normal body temperature in neonates.

Increased Thyroxine Output as a Long-Term Cause of Increased Heat Production. Cooling the anterior hypothalamic-preoptic area also increases production of the neurosecretory hormone *thyrotropin-releasing hormone* by the hypothalamus. This hormone is carried by way of the hypothalamic portal veins to the anterior pituitary gland, where it stimulates secretion of *thyroid-stimulating hormone.*

Thyroid-stimulating hormone in turn stimulates increased output of *thyroxine* by the thyroid gland, as explained in Chapter 76. The increased thyroxine activates uncoupling protein and increases the rate of cellular metabolism throughout the body, which is yet another mechanism of *chemical thermogenesis.* This increase in metabolism does not occur immediately but requires several weeks' exposure to cold to make the thyroid gland hypertrophy and reach its new level of thyroxine secretion.

Exposure of animals to extreme cold for several weeks can cause their thyroid glands to increase in size 20 to 40 percent. However, human beings seldom allow themselves to be exposed to the same degree of cold as that to which animals are often subjected. Therefore, we still do not know, quantitatively, how important the thyroid mechanism of adaptation to cold is in the human being.

Isolated measurements have shown that military personnel residing for several months in the arctic develop increased metabolic rates; some Inuit (Eskimos) also have abnormally high basal metabolic rates. Further, the continuous stimulatory effect of cold on the thyroid gland may explain the much higher incidence of toxic thyroid goiters in people who live in cold climates than in those who live in warm climates.

Concept of a "Set-Point" for Temperature Control

In the example of Figure 73-7, it is clear that at a critical body core temperature of about 37.1°C (98.8°F), drastic changes occur in the rates of both heat loss and heat production. At temperatures above this level, the rate of heat loss is greater than that of heat production, so the body temperature falls and approaches the 37.1°C level. At temperatures below this level, the rate of heat production is greater than that of heat loss, so the body temperature rises and again approaches the 37.1°C level. This crucial temperature level is called the "set-point" of the temperature control mechanism. That is, all the temperature control mechanisms continually attempt to bring the body temperature back to this set-point level.

Feedback Gain for Body Temperature Control. Let us recall the discussion of feedback gain of control systems presented in Chapter 1. Feedback gain is a measure of the effectiveness of a control system. In the case of body temperature control, it is important for the internal core temperature to change as little as possible, even though the environmental temperature might change greatly from day to day or even hour to hour. The *feedback gain* of the temperature control system is equal to the ratio of the change in environmental temperature to the change in body core temperature minus 1.0 (see Chapter 1 for this formula). Experiments have shown that the body temperature of humans changes about 1°C for each 25° to 30°C change in environmental temperature. Therefore, the feedback gain of the total mechanism for body temperature control averages about 27 (28/1.0 − 1.0 = 27), which is an extremely high gain for a biological control system (the baroreceptor arterial pressure control system, by comparison, has a feedback gain of <2).

Skin Temperature Can Slightly Alter the Set-Point for Core Temperature Control

The critical temperature set-point in the hypothalamus above which sweating begins and below which shivering begins is determined mainly by the degree of activity of the heat temperature receptors in the anterior hypothalamic-preoptic area. However, temperature signals from the peripheral areas of the body, especially from the skin and certain deep body tissues (spinal cord and abdominal viscera), also contribute slightly to body temperature regulation. But how do they contribute? The answer is that they alter the set-point of the hypothalamic temperature control center. This effect is shown in Figures 73-8 and 73-9.

Figure 73-8 demonstrates the effect of different skin temperatures on the set-point for sweating, showing that the set-point increases as the skin temperature decreases. Thus, for the person represented in this figure, the hypothalamic set-point increased from 36.7°C when the skin temperature was higher than 33°C to a set-point of 37.4°C when the skin temperature had fallen to 29°C. Therefore, when the skin temperature was high, sweating began at a lower hypothalamic temperature than when the skin temperature was low. One can readily understand the value of such a system because it is important that sweating be inhibited when the skin temperature is low; otherwise, the combined effect of low skin temperature and sweating could cause far too much loss of body heat.

A similar effect occurs in shivering, as shown in Figure 73-9. That is, when the skin becomes cold, it drives the

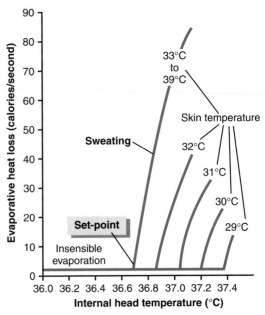

Figure 73-8 Effect of changes in the internal head temperature on the rate of evaporative heat loss from the body. Note that the skin temperature determines the set-point level at which sweating begins. (Courtesy Dr. T. H. Benzinger.)

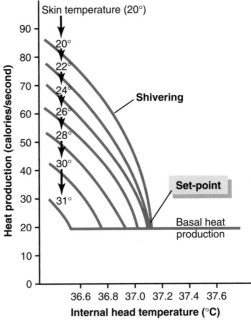

Figure 73-9 Effect of changes in the internal head temperature on the rate of heat production by the body. Note that the skin temperature determines the set-point level at which shivering begins. (Courtesy Dr. T. H. Benzinger.)

hypothalamic centers to the shivering threshold even when the hypothalamic temperature itself is still on the hot side of normal. Here again, one can understand the value of the control system because a cold skin temperature would soon lead to a deeply depressed body temperature unless heat production were increased. Thus, a cold skin temperature actually "anticipates" a fall in internal body temperature and prevents this.

Behavioral Control of Body Temperature

Aside from the subconscious mechanisms for body temperature control, the body has another temperature-control mechanism that is even more potent. This is *behavioral control of temperature*, which can be explained as follows: Whenever the internal body temperature becomes too high, signals from the temperature-controlling areas in the brain give the person a psychic sensation of being overheated. Conversely, whenever the body becomes too cold, signals from the skin and probably also from some deep body receptors elicit the feeling of cold discomfort. Therefore, the person makes appropriate environmental adjustments to re-establish comfort, such as moving into a heated room or wearing well-insulated clothing in freezing weather. This is a much more powerful system of body temperature control than most physiologists have acknowledged in the past. Indeed, this is the only really effective mechanism to maintain body heat control in severely cold environments.

Local Skin Temperature Reflexes

When a person places a foot under a hot lamp and leaves it there for a short time, *local vasodilation* and mild *local sweating* occur. Conversely, placing the foot in cold water causes local vasoconstriction and local cessation of sweating. These reactions are caused by local effects of temperature directly on the blood vessels and also by local cord reflexes conducted from skin receptors to the spinal cord and back to the same skin area and the sweat glands. The *intensity* of these local effects is, in addition, controlled by the central brain temperature controller, so their overall effect is proportional to the hypothalamic heat control signal *times* the local signal. Such reflexes can help prevent excessive heat exchange from locally cooled or heated portions of the body.

Regulation of Internal Body Temperature Is Impaired by Cutting the Spinal Cord. After cutting the spinal cord in the neck above the sympathetic outflow from the cord, regulation of body temperature becomes extremely poor because the hypothalamus can no longer control either skin blood flow or the degree of sweating anywhere in the body. This is true even though the local temperature reflexes originating in the skin, spinal cord, and intra-abdominal receptors still exist. These reflexes are extremely weak in comparison with hypothalamic control of body temperature.

In people with this condition, body temperature must be regulated principally by the patient's psychic response to cold and hot sensations in the head region—that is, by behavioral control of clothing and by moving into an appropriate warm or cold environment.

Abnormalities of Body Temperature Regulation

Fever

Fever, which means a body temperature above the usual range of normal, can be caused by abnormalities in the brain itself or by toxic substances that affect the temperature-regulating centers. Some causes of fever (and also of subnormal body temperatures) are presented in Figure 73-10.

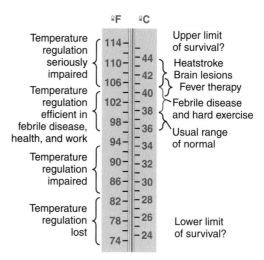

Figure 73-10 Body temperatures under different conditions. (Redrawn from DuBois EF: Fever. Springfield, Ill: Charles C Thomas, 1948.)

They include bacterial diseases, brain tumors, and environmental conditions that may terminate in heatstroke.

Resetting the Hypothalamic Temperature-Regulating Center in Febrile Diseases—Effect of Pyrogens

Many proteins, breakdown products of proteins, and certain other substances, especially lipopolysaccharide toxins released from bacterial cell membranes, can cause the set-point of the hypothalamic thermostat to rise. Substances that cause this effect are called *pyrogens*. Pyrogens released from toxic bacteria or those released from degenerating body tissues cause fever during disease conditions. When the set-point of the hypothalamic temperature-regulating center becomes higher than normal, all the mechanisms for raising the body temperature are brought into play, including heat conservation and increased heat production. Within a few hours after the set-point has been increased, the body temperature also approaches this level, as shown in Figure 73-11.

Mechanism of Action of Pyrogens in Causing Fever— Role of Cytokines. Experiments in animals have shown that some pyrogens, when injected into the hypothalamus, can act directly and immediately on the hypothalamic temperature-regulating center to increase its set-point. Other pyrogens function indirectly and may require several hours of latency before causing their effects. This is true of many of the bacterial pyrogens, especially the *endotoxins* from gram-negative bacteria.

When bacteria or breakdown products of bacteria are present in the tissues or in the blood, they are *phagocytized by the blood leukocytes, by tissue macrophages*, and *by large granular killer lymphocytes*. All these cells digest the bacterial products and then release cytokines, a diverse group of peptide signaling molecules involved in the innate and adaptive immune responses. One of the most important of these cytokines in causing fever is *interleukin-1 (IL-1)*, also called *leukocyte pyrogen* or

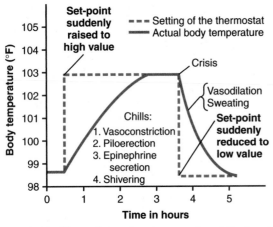

Figure 73-11 Effects of changing the set-point of the hypothalamic temperature controller.

endogenous pyrogen. Interleukin-1 is released from macrophages into the body fluids and, on reaching the hypothalamus, almost immediately activates the processes to produce fever, sometimes increasing the body temperature a noticeable amount in only 8 to 10 minutes. *As little as one ten millionth of a gram of endotoxin lipopolysaccharide* from bacteria, acting in concert with the blood leukocytes, tissue macrophages, and killer lymphocytes, can cause fever. The amount of interleukin-1 that is formed in response to lipopolysaccharide to cause fever is only a few nanograms.

Several experiments have suggested that interleukin-1 causes fever by first inducing the formation of one of the prostaglandins, mainly prostaglandin E$_2$, or a similar substance, which acts in the hypothalamus to elicit the fever reaction. When prostaglandin formation is blocked by drugs, the fever is either completely abrogated or at least reduced. In fact, this may be the explanation for the manner in which aspirin reduces fever because aspirin impedes the formation of prostaglandins from arachidonic acid. Drugs such as aspirin that reduce fever are called *antipyretics*.

Fever Caused by Brain Lesions. When a brain surgeon operates in the region of the hypothalamus, severe fever almost always occurs; rarely, the opposite effect, hypothermia, occurs, demonstrating both the potency of the hypothalamic mechanisms for body temperature control and the ease with which abnormalities of the hypothalamus can alter the set-point of temperature control. Another condition that frequently causes prolonged high temperature is compression of the hypothalamus by a brain tumor.

Characteristics of Febrile Conditions

Chills. When the set-point of the hypothalamic temperature-control center is suddenly changed from the normal level to higher than normal (as a result of tissue destruction, pyrogenic substances, or dehydration), the body temperature usually takes several hours to reach the new temperature set-point.

Figure 73-11 demonstrates the effect of suddenly increasing the temperature set-point to a level of 103°F.

Because the blood temperature is now less than the set-point of the hypothalamic temperature controller, the usual responses that cause elevation of body temperature occur. During this period, the person experiences chills and feels extremely cold, even though his or her body temperature may already be above normal. Also, the skin becomes cold because of vasoconstriction and the person shivers. Chills can continue until the body temperature reaches the hypothalamic set-point of 103°F. Then the person no longer experiences chills but instead feels neither cold nor hot. As long as the factor that is causing the higher set-point of the hypothalamic temperature controller is present, the body temperature is regulated more or less in the normal manner, but at the high temperature set-point level.

Crisis, or "Flush". If the factor that is causing the high temperature is removed, the set-point of the hypothalamic temperature controller will be reduced to a lower value—perhaps even back to the normal level, as shown in Figure 73-11. In this instance, the body temperature is still 103°F, but the hypothalamus is attempting to regulate the temperature to 98.6°F. This situation is analogous to excessive heating of the anterior hypothalamic-preoptic area, which causes intense sweating and the sudden development of hot skin because of vasodilation everywhere. This sudden change of events in a febrile state is known as the "crisis" or, more appropriately, the "flush." In the days before the advent of antibiotics, the crisis was always anxiously awaited because once this occurred, the doctor assumed that the patient's temperature would soon begin falling.

Heatstroke

The upper limit of air temperature that one can stand depends to a great extent on whether the air is dry or wet. If the air is dry and sufficient convection air currents are flowing to promote rapid evaporation from the body, a person can withstand several hours of air temperature at 130°F. Conversely, if the air is 100 percent humidified or if the body is in water, the body temperature begins to rise whenever the environmental temperature rises above about 94°F. If the person is performing heavy work, the critical *environmental temperature* above which heatstroke is likely to occur may be as low as 85° to 90°F.

When the body temperature rises beyond a critical temperature, into the range of 105° to 108°F, the person is likely to develop *heatstroke*. The symptoms include dizziness, abdominal distress sometimes accompanied by vomiting, sometimes delirium, and eventually loss of consciousness if the body temperature is not soon decreased. These symptoms are often exacerbated by a degree of *circulatory shock* brought on by excessive loss of fluid and electrolytes in the sweat.

The hyperpyrexia itself is also exceedingly damaging to the body tissues, especially the brain, and is responsible for many of the effects. In fact, even a few minutes of very high body temperature can sometimes be fatal. For this reason, many authorities recommend immediate treatment of heatstroke by placing the person in a cold water bath. Because this often induces uncontrollable shivering, with a considerable increase in the rate of heat production, others have suggested that sponge or spray cooling of the skin is likely to be more effective for rapidly decreasing the body core temperature.

Harmful Effects of High Temperature. The pathological findings in a person who dies of hyperpyrexia are local hemorrhages and parenchymatous degeneration of cells throughout the entire body, but especially in the brain. Once neuronal cells are destroyed, they can never be replaced. Also, damage to the liver, kidneys, and other organs can often be severe enough that failure of one or more of these organs eventually causes death, but sometimes not until several days after the heatstroke.

Acclimatization to Heat. It can be extremely important to acclimatize people to extreme heat. Examples of people requiring acclimatization are soldiers on duty in the tropics and miners working in the 2-mile-deep gold mines of South Africa, where the temperature approaches body temperature and the humidity approaches 100 percent. A person exposed to heat for several hours each day while performing a reasonably heavy workload will develop increased tolerance to hot and humid conditions in 1 to 3 weeks.

Among the most important physiological changes that occur during this acclimatization process are an approximately twofold increase in the maximum rate of sweating, an increase in plasma volume, and diminished loss of salt in the sweat and urine to almost none; the last two effects result from increased secretion of aldosterone by the adrenal glands.

Exposure of the Body to Extreme Cold

Unless treated immediately, a person exposed to ice water for 20 to 30 minutes ordinarily dies because of heart standstill or heart fibrillation. By that time, the internal body temperature will have fallen to about 77°F. If warmed rapidly by the application of external heat, the person's life can often be saved.

Loss of Temperature Regulation at Low Temperatures. As noted in Figure 73-10, once the body temperature has fallen below about 85°F, the ability of the hypothalamus to regulate temperature is lost; it is greatly impaired even when the body temperature falls below about 94°F. Part of the reason for this diminished temperature regulation is that the rate of chemical heat production in each cell is depressed almost twofold for each 10°F decrease in body temperature. Also, sleepiness develops (later followed by coma), which depresses the activity of the central nervous system heat control mechanisms and prevents shivering.

Frostbite. When the body is exposed to extremely low temperatures, surface areas can freeze; the freezing is called *frostbite*. This occurs especially in the lobes of the ears and in the digits of the hands and feet. If the freeze has been sufficient to cause extensive formation of ice crystals in the cells, permanent damage usually results, such as permanent circulatory impairment and local tissue damage. Often gangrene follows thawing, and the frostbitten areas must be removed surgically.

Cold-Induced Vasodilation Is a Final Protection Against Frostbite at Almost Freezing Temperatures. When the temperature of tissues falls almost to freezing, the smooth muscle in the vascular wall becomes paralyzed because of the cold itself, and sudden vasodilation occurs, often manifested by a flush of the skin. This mechanism helps prevent frostbite by delivering warm blood to the skin. This mechanism is far less developed in humans than in most lower animals that live in the cold all the time.

Artificial Hypothermia. It is easy to decrease the temperature of a person by first administering a strong sedative to depress the reactivity of the hypothalamic temperature controller and then cooling the person with ice or cooling blankets until the temperature falls. The temperature can then be maintained below 90°F for several days to a week or more by continual sprinkling of cool water or alcohol on the body. Such artificial cooling has been used during heart surgery so that the heart can be stopped artificially for many minutes at a time. Cooling to this extent does not cause tissue damage, but it does slow the heart and greatly depresses cell metabolism so that the body's cells can survive 30 minutes to more than 1 hour without blood flow during the surgical procedure.

Bibliography

Aronoff DM, Neilson EG: Antipyretics: mechanisms of action and clinical use in fever suppression, *Am J Med* 111:304, 2001.

Benarroch EE: Thermoregulation: recent concepts and remaining questions, *Neurology* 69:1293, 2007.

Blatteis CM: Endotoxic fever: new concepts of its regulation suggest new approaches to its management, *Pharmacol Ther* 111:194, 2006.

Blatteis CM: The onset of fever: new insights into its mechanism, *Prog Brain Res* 162:3, 2007.

Conti B, Tabarean I, Andrei C, Bartfai T: Cytokines and fever, *Front Biosci* 9:1433, 2004.

Florez-Duquet M, McDonald RB: Cold-induced thermoregulation and biological aging, *Physiol Rev* 78:339, 1998.

González-Alonso J, Crandall CG, Johnson JM: The cardiovascular challenge of exercising in the heat, *J Physiol* 586:45, 2008.

Horowitz M: Matching the heart to heat-induced circulatory load: heat-acclimatory responses, *News Physiol Sci* 18:215, 2003.

Katschinski DM: On heat and cells and proteins, *News Physiol Sci* 19:11, 2004.

Kenney WL, Munce TA: Aging and human temperature regulation, *J Appl Physiol* 95:2598, 2003.

Kozak W, Kluger MJ, Tesfaigzi J, et al: Molecular mechanisms of fever and endogenous antipyresis, *Ann N Y Acad Sci* 917:121, 2000.

Morrison SF: Central pathways controlling brown adipose tissue thermogenesis, *News Physiol Sci* 19:67, 2004.

Morrison SF, Nakamura K, Madden CJ: Central control of thermogenesis in mammals, *Exp Physiol* 93:773, 2008.

Olsen TS, Weber UJ, Kammersgaard LP: Therapeutic hypothermia for acute stroke, *Lancet Neurol* 2:410, 2003.

Romanovsky AA: Thermoregulation: some concepts have changed. Functional architecture of the thermoregulatory system, *Am J Physiol Regul Integr Comp Physiol* 292:R37, 2007.

Rowland T: Thermoregulation during exercise in the heat in children: old concepts revisited, *J Appl Physiol* 105:718, 2008.

Saper CB: Neurobiological basis of fever, *Ann N Y Acad Sci* 856:90, 1998.

Simon A, van der Meer JW: Pathogenesis of familial periodic fever syndromes or hereditary autoinflammatory syndromes, *Am J Physiol Regul Integr Comp Physiol* 292:R86, 2007.

Steinman L: Nuanced roles of cytokines in three major human brain disorders, *J Clin Invest* 118:3557, 2008.

UNIT XIV

Endocrinology and Reproduction

74. Introduction to Endocrinology

75. Pituitary Hormones and Their Control by the Hypothalamus

76. Thyroid Metabolic Hormones

77. Adrenocortical Hormones

78. Insulin, Glucagon, and Diabetes Mellitus

79. Parathyroid Hormone, Calcitonin, Calcium and Phosphate Metabolism, Vitamin D, Bone, and Teeth

80. Reproductive and Hormonal Functions of the Male (and Function of the Pineal Gland)

81. Female Physiology Before Pregnancy and Female Hormones

82. Pregnancy and Lactation

83. Fetal and Neonatal Physiology

Introduction to Endocrinology

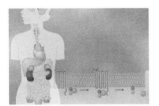

Coordination of Body Functions by Chemical Messengers

The multiple activities of the cells, tissues, and organs of the body are coordinated by the interplay of several types of chemical messenger systems:

1. *Neurotransmitters* are released by axon terminals of neurons into the synaptic junctions and act locally to control nerve cell functions.

2. *Endocrine hormones* are released by glands or specialized cells into the circulating blood and influence the function of target cells at another location in the body.

3. *Neuroendocrine hormones* are secreted by neurons into the circulating blood and influence the function of target cells at another location in the body.

4. *Paracrines* are secreted by cells into the extracellular fluid and affect neighboring target cells of a different type.

5. *Autocrines* are secreted by cells into the extracellular fluid and affect the function of the same cells that produced them.

6. *Cytokines* are peptides secreted by cells into the extracellular fluid and can function as autocrines, paracrines, or endocrine hormones. Examples of cytokines include the *interleukins* and other *lymphokines* that are secreted by helper cells and act on other cells of the immune system (see Chapter 34). Cytokine hormones (e.g., *leptin*) produced by adipocytes are sometimes called *adipokines*.

In the next few chapters, we discuss mainly the endocrine and neuroendocrine hormone systems, keeping in mind that many of the body's chemical messenger systems interact with one another to maintain homeostasis. For example, the adrenal medullae and the pituitary gland secrete their hormones primarily in response to neural stimuli. The neuroendocrine cells, located in the hypothalamus, have axons that terminate in the posterior pituitary gland and median eminence and secrete several neurohormones, including *antidiuretic hormone* (ADH), *oxytocin,* and *hypophysiotropic hormones,* which control the secretion of anterior pituitary hormones.

The *endocrine hormones* are carried by the circulatory system to cells throughout the body, including the nervous system in some cases, where they bind with receptors and initiate many cell reactions. Some endocrine hormones affect many different types of cells of the body; for example, *growth hormone* (from the anterior pituitary gland) causes growth in most parts of the body, and *thyroxine* (from the thyroid gland) increases the rate of many chemical reactions in almost all the body's cells.

Other hormones affect mainly specific *target tissues* because these tissues have abundant receptors for the hormone. For example, *adrenocorticotropic hormone* (ACTH) from the anterior pituitary gland specifically stimulates the adrenal cortex, causing it to secrete adrenocortical hormones, and the *ovarian hormones* have their main effects on the female sex organs and the secondary sexual characteristics of the female body.

Figure 74-1 shows the anatomical loci of the major endocrine glands and endocrine tissues of the body, except for the placenta, which is an additional source of the sex hormones. Table 74-1 provides an overview of the different hormone systems and their most important actions.

The multiple hormone systems play a key role in regulating almost all body functions, including metabolism, growth and development, water and electrolyte balance, reproduction, and behavior. For instance, without growth hormone, a person would be a dwarf. Without thyroxine and triiodothyronine from the thyroid gland, almost all the chemical reactions of the body would become sluggish and the person would become sluggish as well. Without insulin from the pancreas, the body's cells could use little of the food carbohydrates for energy. And without the sex hormones, sexual development and sexual functions would be absent.

Chemical Structure and Synthesis of Hormones

Three general classes of hormones exist:

1. *Proteins and polypeptides,* including hormones secreted by the anterior and posterior pituitary gland, the pancreas (insulin and glucagon), the parathyroid gland (parathyroid hormone), and many others (see Table 74-1).

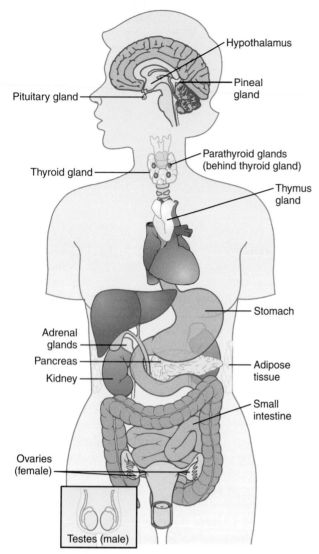

Figure 74-1 Anatomical loci of the principal endocrine glands and tissues of the body.

2. *Steroids* secreted by the adrenal cortex (cortisol and aldosterone), the ovaries (estrogen and progesterone), the testes (testosterone), and the placenta (estrogen and progesterone).

3. *Derivatives of the amino acid tyrosine,* secreted by the thyroid (thyroxine and triiodothyronine) and the adrenal medullae (epinephrine and norepinephrine). There are no known polysaccharides or nucleic acid hormones.

Polypeptide and Protein Hormones Are Stored in Secretory Vesicles Until Needed. Most of the hormones in the body are polypeptides and proteins. These hormones range in size from small peptides with as few as 3 amino acids (thyrotropin-releasing hormone) to proteins with almost 200 amino acids (growth hormone and prolactin). In general, polypeptides with 100 or more amino acids are called *proteins,* and those with fewer than 100 amino acids are referred to as *peptides.*

Protein and peptide hormones are synthesized on the rough end of the endoplasmic reticulum of the different endocrine cells, in the same fashion as most other proteins (Figure 74-2). They are usually synthesized first as larger proteins that are not biologically active *(preprohormones)* and are cleaved to form smaller *prohormones* in the endoplasmic reticulum. These are then transferred to the Golgi apparatus for packaging into secretory vesicles. In this process, enzymes in the vesicles cleave the prohormones to produce smaller, biologically active hormones and inactive fragments. The vesicles are stored within the cytoplasm, and many are bound to the cell membrane until their secretion is needed. Secretion of the hormones (as well as the inactive fragments) occurs when the secretory vesicles fuse with the cell membrane and the granular contents are extruded into the interstitial fluid or directly into the blood stream by *exocytosis.*

In many cases, the stimulus for exocytosis is an increase in cytosolic calcium concentration caused by depolarization of the plasma membrane. In other instances, stimulation of an endocrine cell surface receptor causes increased cyclic adenosine monophosphate (cAMP) and subsequently activation of protein kinases that initiate secretion of the hormone. The peptide hormones are water soluble, allowing them to enter the circulatory system easily, where they are carried to their target tissues.

Steroid Hormones Are Usually Synthesized from Cholesterol and Are Not Stored. The chemical structure of steroid hormones is similar to that of cholesterol, and in most instances hormones are synthesized from cholesterol itself. They are lipid soluble and consist of three cyclohexyl rings and one cyclopentyl ring combined into a single structure (Figure 74-3).

Although there is usually very little hormone storage in steroid-producing endocrine cells, large stores of cholesterol esters in cytoplasm vacuoles can be rapidly mobilized for steroid synthesis after a stimulus. Much of the cholesterol in steroid-producing cells comes from the plasma, but there is also de novo synthesis of cholesterol in steroid-producing cells. Because the steroids are highly lipid soluble, once they are synthesized, they simply diffuse across the cell membrane and enter the interstitial fluid and then the blood.

Amine Hormones Are Derived from Tyrosine. The two groups of hormones derived from tyrosine, the thyroid and the adrenal medullary hormones, are formed by the actions of enzymes in the cytoplasmic compartments of the glandular cells. The thyroid hormones are synthesized and stored in the thyroid gland and incorporated into macromolecules of the protein *thyroglobulin,* which is stored in large follicles within the thyroid gland. Hormone secretion occurs when the amines are split from thyroglobulin, and the free hormones are then released into the blood stream. After entering the blood, most of the thyroid hormones combine with plasma proteins, especially *thyroxine-binding globulin,* which slowly releases the hormones to the target tissues.

Table 74-1 Endocrine Glands, Hormones, and Their Functions and Structure

Gland/Tissue	Hormones	Major Functions	Chemical Structure
Hypothalamus (Chapter 75)	Thyrotropin-releasing hormone (TRH)	Stimulates secretion of thyroid-stimulating hormone (TSH) and prolactin	Peptide
	Corticotropin-releasing hormone (CRH)	Causes release of adrenocorticotropic hormone (ACTH)	Peptide
	Growth hormone–releasing hormone (GHRH)	Causes release of growth hormone	Peptide
	Growth hormone inhibitory hormone (GHIH) (somatostatin)	Inhibits release of growth hormone	Peptide
	Gonadotropin-releasing hormone (GnRH)	Causes release of luteinizing hormone (LH) and follicle-stimulating hormone (FSH)	
	Dopamine or prolactin-inhibiting factor (PIF)	Inhibits release of prolactin	Amine
Anterior pituitary (Chapter 75)	Growth hormone	Stimulates protein synthesis and overall growth of most cells and tissues	Peptide
	TSH	Stimulates synthesis and secretion of thyroid hormones (thyroxine and triiodothyronine)	Peptide
	ACTH	Stimulates synthesis and secretion of adrenocortical hormones (cortisol, androgens, and aldosterone)	Peptide
	Prolactin	Promotes development of the female breasts and secretion of milk	Peptide
	FSH	Causes growth of follicles in the ovaries and sperm maturation in Sertoli cells of testes	Peptide
	LH	Stimulates testosterone synthesis in Leydig cells of testes; stimulates ovulation, formation of corpus luteum, and estrogen and progesterone synthesis in ovaries	Peptide
Posterior pituitary (Chapter 75)	Antidiuretic hormone (ADH) (also called *vasopressin*)	Increases water reabsorption by the kidneys and causes vasoconstriction and increased blood pressure	Peptide
	Oxytocin	Stimulates milk ejection from breasts and uterine contractions	Peptide
Thyroid (Chapter 76)	Thyroxine (T_4) and triiodothyronine (T_3)	Increases the rates of chemical reactions in most cells, thus increasing body metabolic rate	Amine
	Calcitonin	Promotes deposition of calcium in the bones and decreases extracellular fluid calcium ion concentration	Peptide
Adrenal cortex (Chapter 77)	Cortisol	Has multiple metabolic functions for controlling metabolism of proteins, carbohydrates, and fats; also has anti-inflammatory effects	Steroid
	Aldosterone	Increases renal sodium reabsorption, potassium secretion, and hydrogen ion secretion	Steroid
Adrenal medulla (Chapter 60)	Norepinephrine, epinephrine	Same effects as sympathetic stimulation	Amine
Pancreas (Chapter 78)	Insulin (β cells)	Promotes glucose entry in many cells, and in this way controls carbohydrate metabolism	Peptide

(Continued)

Table 74-1 Endocrine Glands, Hormones, and Their Functions and Structure—Cont'd

Gland/Tissue	Hormones	Major Functions	Chemical Structure
	Glucagon (α cells)	Increases synthesis and release of glucose from the liver into the body fluids	Peptide
Parathyroid (Chapter 79)	Parathyroid hormone (PTH)	Controls serum calcium ion concentration by increasing calcium absorption by the gut and kidneys and releasing calcium from bones	Peptide
Testes (Chapter 80)	Testosterone	Promotes development of male reproductive system and male secondary sexual characteristics	Steroid
Ovaries (Chapter 81)	Estrogens	Promotes growth and development of female reproductive system, female breasts, and female secondary sexual characteristics	Steroid
	Progesterone	Stimulates secretion of "uterine milk" by the uterine endometrial glands and promotes development of secretory apparatus of breasts	Steroid
Placenta (Chapter 82)	Human chorionic gonadotropin (HCG)	Promotes growth of corpus luteum and secretion of estrogens and progesterone by corpus luteum	Peptide
	Human somatomammotropin	Probably helps promote development of some fetal tissues as well as the mother's breasts	Peptide
	Estrogens	See actions of estrogens from ovaries	Steroid
	Progesterone	See actions of progesterone from ovaries	Steroid
Kidney (Chapter 26)	Renin	Catalyzes conversion of angiotensinogen to angiotensin I (acts as an enzyme)	Peptide
	1,25-Dihydroxycholecalciferol	Increases intestinal absorption of calcium and bone mineralization	Steroid
	Erythropoietin	Increases erythrocyte production	Peptide
Heart (Chapter 22)	Atrial natriuretic peptide (ANP)	Increases sodium excretion by kidneys, reduces blood pressure	Peptide
Stomach (Chapter 64)	Gastrin	Stimulates HCl secretion by parietal cells	Peptide
Small intestine (Chapter 64)	Secretin	Stimulates pancreatic acinar cells to release bicarbonate and water	Peptide
	Cholecystokinin (CCK)	Stimulates gallbladder contraction and release of pancreatic enzymes	Peptide
Adipocytes (Chapter 71)	Leptin	Inhibits appetite, stimulates thermogenesis	Peptide

Epinephrine and norepinephrine are formed in the adrenal medulla, which normally secretes about four times more epinephrine than norepinephrine. Catecholamines are taken up into preformed vesicles and stored until secreted. Similar to the protein hormones stored in secretory granules, catecholamines are also released from adrenal medullary cells by exocytosis. Once the catecholamines enter the circulation, they can exist in the plasma in free form or in conjugation with other substances.

Hormone Secretion, Transport, and Clearance from the Blood

Onset of Hormone Secretion After a Stimulus, and Duration of Action of Different Hormones. Some hormones, such as norepinephrine and epinephrine, are secreted within seconds after the gland is stimulated, and they may develop full action within another few seconds to minutes; the actions of other hormones, such as thyroxine or growth hormone, may require months for full effect. Thus, each of the different hormones has its own characteristic onset and duration of action—each tailored to perform its specific control function.

Concentrations of Hormones in the Circulating Blood, and Hormonal Secretion Rates. The concentrations of hormones required to control most metabolic and endocrine functions are incredibly small. Their concentrations in the blood range from as little as 1 picogram (which is one millionth of one millionth of a gram) in each milliliter of blood up to at most a few micrograms (a few millionths of a gram) per milliliter of blood. Similarly, the rates of secretion of the various hormones are extremely small, usually measured in micrograms or milligrams per day. We shall see later in this

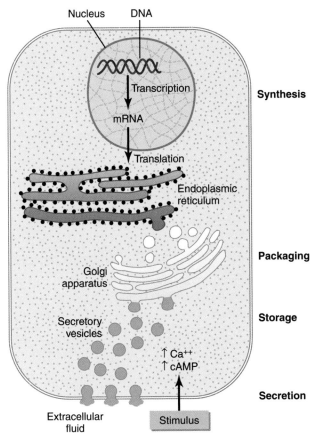

Figure 74-2 Synthesis and secretion of peptide hormones. The stimulus for hormone secretion often involves changes in intracellular calcium or changes in cyclic adenosine monophosphate (cAMP) in the cell.

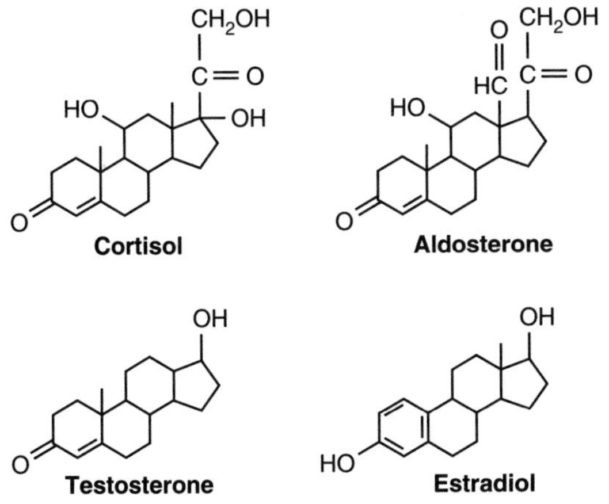

Figure 74-3 Chemical structures of several steroid hormones.

chapter that highly specialized mechanisms are available in the target tissues that allow even these minute quantities of hormones to exert powerful control over the physiological systems.

Feedback Control of Hormone Secretion

Negative Feedback Prevents Overactivity of Hormone Systems. Although the plasma concentrations of many hormones fluctuate in response to vari-

ous stimuli that occur throughout the day, all hormones studied thus far appear to be closely controlled. In most instances, this control is exerted through *negative feedback mechanisms* that ensure a proper level of hormone activity at the target tissue. After a stimulus causes release of the hormone, conditions or products resulting from the action of the hormone tend to suppress its further release. In other words, the hormone (or one of its products) has a negative feedback effect to prevent oversecretion of the hormone or overactivity at the target tissue.

The controlled variable is sometimes not the secretory rate of the hormone itself but the degree of activity of the target tissue. Therefore, only when the target tissue activity rises to an appropriate level will feedback signals to the endocrine gland become powerful enough to slow further secretion of the hormone. Feedback regulation of hormones can occur at all levels, including gene transcription and translation steps involved in the synthesis of hormones and steps involved in processing hormones or releasing stored hormones.

Surges of Hormones Can Occur with Positive Feedback. In a few instances, *positive feedback* occurs when the biological action of the hormone causes additional secretion of the hormone. One example of this is the surge of *luteinizing hormone* (LH) that occurs as a result of the stimulatory effect of estrogen on the anterior pituitary before ovulation. The secreted LH then acts on the ovaries to stimulate additional secretion of estrogen, which in turn causes more secretion of LH. Eventually, LH reaches an appropriate concentration and typical negative feedback control of hormone secretion is then exerted.

Cyclical Variations Occur in Hormone Release. Superimposed on the negative and positive feedback control of hormone secretion are periodic variations in hormone release that are influenced by seasonal changes, various stages of development and aging, the diurnal (daily) cycle, and sleep. For example, the secretion of growth hormone is markedly increased during the early period of sleep but is reduced during the later stages of sleep. In many cases, these cyclical variations in hormone secretion are due to changes in activity of neural pathways involved in controlling hormone release.

Transport of Hormones in the Blood

Water-soluble hormones (peptides and catecholamines) are dissolved in the plasma and transported from their sites of synthesis to target tissues, where they diffuse out of the capillaries, into the interstitial fluid, and ultimately to target cells.

Steroid and thyroid hormones, in contrast, circulate in the blood mainly bound to plasma proteins. Usually less than 10 percent of steroid or thyroid hormones in the plasma exist free in solution. For example, more than 99 percent of the thyroxine in the blood is bound to plasma proteins. However, protein-bound hormones cannot easily diffuse across the capillaries and gain access to their target cells and are therefore biologically inactive until they dissociate from plasma proteins.

The relatively large amounts of hormones bound to proteins serve as reservoirs, replenishing the concentration of free hormones when they are bound to target receptors or lost from the circulation. Binding of hormones to plasma proteins greatly slows their clearance from the plasma.

"Clearance" of Hormones from the Blood

Two factors can increase or decrease the concentration of a hormone in the blood. One of these is the rate of hormone secretion into the blood. The second is the rate of removal of the hormone from the blood, which is called the *metabolic clearance rate.* This is usually expressed in terms of the number of milliliters of plasma cleared of the hormone per minute. To calculate this clearance rate, one measures (1) the rate of disappearance of the hormone from the plasma (e.g., nanograms per minute) and (2) the plasma concentration of the hormone (e.g., nanograms per milliliter of plasma). Then, the metabolic clearance rate is calculated by the following formula:

Metabolic clearance rate = Rate of disappearance of hormone from the plasma / Concentration of hormone

The usual procedure for making this measurement is the following: A purified solution of the hormone to be measured is tagged with a radioactive substance. Then the radioactive hormone is infused at a constant rate into the blood stream until the radioactive concentration in the plasma becomes steady. At this time, the rate of disappearance of the radioactive hormone from the plasma equals the rate at which it is infused, which gives one the rate of disappearance. At the same time, the plasma concentration of the radioactive hormone is measured using a standard radioactive counting procedure. Then, using the formula just cited, the metabolic clearance rate is calculated.

Hormones are "cleared" from the plasma in several ways, including (1) metabolic destruction by the tissues, (2) binding with the tissues, (3) excretion by the liver into the bile, and (4) excretion by the kidneys into the urine. For certain hormones, a decreased metabolic clearance rate may cause an excessively high concentration of the hormone in the circulating body fluids. For instance, this occurs for several of the steroid hormones when the liver is diseased because these hormones are conjugated mainly in the liver and then "cleared" into the bile.

Hormones are sometimes degraded at their target cells by enzymatic processes that cause endocytosis of the cell membrane hormone-receptor complex; the hormone is then metabolized in the cell, and the receptors are usually recycled back to the cell membrane.

Most of the peptide hormones and catecholamines are water soluble and circulate freely in the blood. They are usually degraded by enzymes in the blood and tissues and rapidly excreted by the kidneys and liver, thus remaining in the blood for only a short time. For example, the half-life of angiotensin II circulating in the blood is less than a minute.

Hormones that are bound to plasma proteins are cleared from the blood at much slower rates and may remain in the circulation for several hours or even days. The half-life of adrenal steroids in the circulation, for example, ranges between 20 and 100 minutes, whereas the half-life of the protein-bound thyroid hormones may be as long as 1 to 6 days.

Mechanisms of Action of Hormones

Hormone Receptors and Their Activation

The first step of a hormone's action is to bind to specific *receptors* at the target cell. Cells that lack receptors for the hormones do not respond. Receptors for some hormones are located on the target cell membrane, whereas other hormone receptors are located in the cytoplasm or the nucleus. When the hormone combines with its receptor, this usually initiates a cascade of reactions in the cell, with each stage becoming more powerfully activated so that even small concentrations of the hormone can have a large effect.

Hormonal receptors are large proteins, and each cell that is to be stimulated usually has some 2000 to 100,000 receptors. Also, each receptor is usually highly specific for a single hormone; this determines the type of hormone that will act on a particular tissue. The target tissues that are affected by a hormone are those that contain its specific receptors.

The locations for the different types of hormone receptors are generally the following:

1. *In or on the surface of the cell membrane.* The membrane receptors are specific mostly for the protein, peptide, and catecholamine hormones.

2. *In the cell cytoplasm.* The primary receptors for the different steroid hormones are found mainly in the cytoplasm.

3. *In the cell nucleus.* The receptors for the thyroid hormones are found in the nucleus and are believed to be located in direct association with one or more of the chromosomes.

The Number and Sensitivity of Hormone Receptors Are Regulated. The number of receptors in a target cell usually does not remain constant from day to day, or even from minute to minute. The receptor proteins themselves are often inactivated or destroyed during the course of their function, and at other times they are reactivated or new ones are manufactured by the protein-manufacturing mechanism of the cell. For instance, increased hormone concentration and increased binding with its target cell receptors sometimes cause the number of active receptors to decrease. This *down-regulation* of the receptors can occur as a result of (1) inactivation of some of the receptor molecules; (2) inactivation of some of the intracellular protein signaling molecules; (3) temporary sequestration of the receptor to the inside of the cell, away from the site of action of hormones that interact with cell membrane receptors; (4) destruction of the receptors by lysosomes after they are internalized; or (5) decreased production of the receptors. In each case, receptor down-regulation decreases the target tissue's responsiveness to the hormone.

Some hormones cause *up-regulation* of receptors and intracellular signaling proteins; that is, the stimulating hormone induces greater than normal formation of receptor or intracellular signaling molecules by the protein-manufacturing machinery of the target cell, or greater availability of the receptor for interaction with the hormone. When this occurs, the target tissue becomes progressively more sensitive to the stimulating effects of the hormone.

Intracellular Signaling After Hormone Receptor Activation

Almost without exception, a hormone affects its target tissues by first forming a hormone-receptor complex. This alters the function of the receptor itself, and the activated receptor initiates the hormonal effects. To explain this, let us give a few examples of the different types of interactions.

Ion Channel–Linked Receptors. Virtually all the neurotransmitter substances, such as acetylcholine and norepinephrine, combine with receptors in the postsynaptic membrane. This almost always causes a change in the structure of the receptor, usually opening or closing a channel for one or more ions. Some of these *ion channel–linked receptors* open (or close) channels for sodium ions, others for potassium ions, others for calcium ions, and so forth. The altered movement of these ions through the channels causes the subsequent effects on the postsynaptic cells. Although a few hormones may exert some of their actions through activation of ion channel receptors, most hormones that open or close ions channels

do this indirectly by coupling with G protein–linked or enzyme-linked receptors, as discussed next.

G Protein–Linked Hormone Receptors. Many hormones activate receptors that indirectly regulate the activity of target proteins (e.g., enzymes or ion channels) by coupling with groups of cell membrane proteins called *heterotrimeric GTP-binding proteins (G proteins)* (Figure 74-4). Of more than 1000 known G protein–coupled receptors, all have seven transmembrane segments that loop in and out of the cell membrane. Some parts of the receptor that protrude into the cell cytoplasm (especially the cytoplasmic tail of the receptor) are coupled to G proteins that include three (i.e., trimeric) parts—the α, β, and γ subunits. When the ligand (hormone) binds to the extracellular part of the receptor, a conformational change occurs in the receptor that activates the G proteins and induces intracellular signals that either (1) open or close cell membrane ion channels or (2) change the activity of an enzyme in the cytoplasm of the cell.

The trimeric G proteins are named for their ability to bind *guanosine nucleotides*. In their inactive state, the α, β, and γ subunits of G proteins form a complex that binds *guanosine diphosphate* (GDP) on the α subunit. When the receptor is activated, it undergoes a conformational change that causes the GDP-bound trimeric G protein to associate with the cytoplasmic part of the receptor and to exchange GDP for *guanosine triphosphate* (GTP). Displacement of GDP by GTP causes the α subunit to dissociate from the trimeric complex and to associate with other intracellular signaling proteins; these proteins, in turn, alter the activity of ion channels or intracellular enzymes such as *adenylyl cyclase* or *phospholipase C*, which alters cell function.

The signaling event is terminated when the hormone is removed and the α subunit inactivates itself by converting its bound GTP to GDP; then the α subunit once again combines with the β and γ subunits to form an inactive, membrane-bound trimeric G protein.

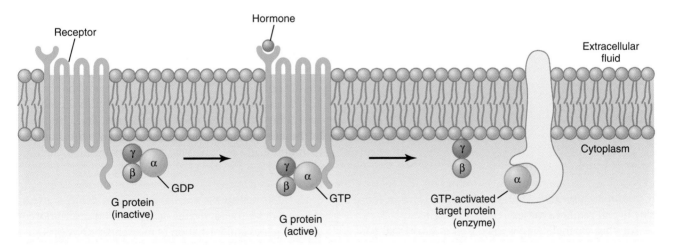

Figure 74-4 Mechanism of activation of a G protein–coupled receptor. When the hormone activates the receptor, the inactive α, β, and γ G protein complex associates with the receptor and is activated, with an exchange of guanosine triphosphate (GTP) for guanosine diphosphate (GDP). This causes the α subunit (to which the GTP is bound) to dissociate from the β and γ subunits of the G protein and to interact with membrane-bound target proteins (enzymes) that initiate intracellular signals.

Some hormones are coupled to *inhibitory G proteins* (denoted G_i proteins), whereas others are coupled to *stimulatory G proteins* (denoted G_s proteins). Thus, depending on the coupling of a hormone receptor to an inhibitory or stimulatory G protein, a hormone can either increase or decrease the activity of intracellular enzymes. This complex system of cell membrane G proteins provides a vast array of potential cell responses to different hormones in the various target tissues of the body.

Enzyme-Linked Hormone Receptors. Some receptors, when activated, function directly as enzymes or are closely associated with enzymes that they activate. These *enzyme-linked receptors* are proteins that pass through the membrane only once, in contrast to the seven-transmembrane G protein–coupled receptors. Enzyme-linked receptors have their hormone-binding site on the outside of the cell membrane and their catalytic or enzyme-binding site on the inside. When the hormone binds to the extracellular part of the receptor, an enzyme immediately inside the cell membrane is activated (or occasionally inactivated). Although many enzyme-linked receptors have intrinsic enzyme activity, others rely on enzymes that are closely associated with the receptor to produce changes in cell function.

One example of an enzyme-linked receptor is the *leptin receptor* (Figure 74-5). Leptin is a hormone secreted by fat cells and has many physiological effects, but it is especially important in regulating appetite and energy balance, as discussed in Chapter 71. The leptin receptor is a member of a large family of *cytokine receptors* that do not themselves contain enzymatic activity but signal through associated enzymes. In the case of the leptin receptor, one of the signaling pathways occurs through a *tyrosine kinase* of the *janus kinase* (JAK) family, *JAK2*. The leptin receptor exists as a dimer (i.e., in two parts), and binding of leptin to the extracellular part of the receptor alters its conformation, enabling phosphorylation and activation of the intracellular associated JAK2 molecules. The activated JAK2 molecules then phosphorylate other tyrosine residues within the leptin receptor–JAK2 complex to mediate intracellular signaling. The intracellular signals include phosphorylation of *signal transducer and activator of transcription* (STAT) proteins, which activates transcription by leptin target genes to initiate protein synthesis. Phosphorylation of JAK2 also leads to activation of other intracellular enzyme pathways such as *mitogen-activated protein kinases* (MAPK) and *phosphatidylinositol 3-kinase* (PI3K). Some of the effects of leptin occur rapidly as a result of activation of these intracellular enzymes, whereas other actions occur more slowly and require synthesis of new proteins.

Another example, one widely used in hormonal control of cell function, is for the hormone to bind with a special transmembrane receptor, which then becomes the activated enzyme *adenylyl cyclase* at the end that protrudes to the interior of the cell. This cyclase catalyzes

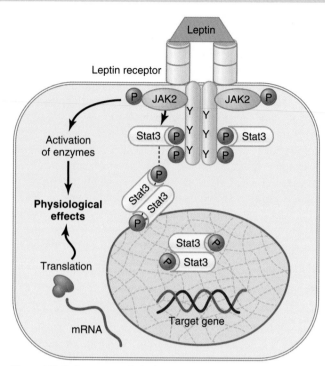

Figure 74-5 An enzyme-linked receptor—the leptin receptor. The receptor exists as a homodimer (two identical parts), and leptin binds to the extracellular part of the receptor, causing phosphorylation and activation of the intracellular associated janus kinase 2 (JAK2). This causes phosphorylation of signal transducer and activator of transcription (STAT) proteins, which then activates the transcription of target genes and the synthesis of proteins. JAK2 phosphorylation also activates several other enzyme systems that mediate some of the more rapid effects of leptin.

the formation of cAMP, which has a multitude of effects inside the cell to control cell activity, as discussed later. cAMP is called a *second messenger* because it is not the hormone itself that directly institutes the intracellular changes; instead, the cAMP serves as a second messenger to cause these effects.

For a few peptide hormones, such as atrial natriuretic peptide (ANP), *cyclic guanosine monophosphate* (cGMP), which is only slightly different from cAMP, serves in a similar manner as a second messenger.

Intracellular Hormone Receptors and Activation of Genes. Several hormones, including adrenal and gonadal steroid hormones, thyroid hormones, retinoid hormones, and vitamin D, bind with protein receptors inside the cell rather than in the cell membrane. Because these hormones are lipid soluble, they readily cross the cell membrane and interact with receptors in the cytoplasm or nucleus. The activated hormone-receptor complex then binds with a specific regulatory (promoter) sequence of the DNA called the *hormone response element,* and in this manner either activates or represses transcription of specific genes and formation of messenger RNA (mRNA) (Figure 74-6). Therefore, minutes, hours, or even days after the hormone has entered the cell, newly formed proteins appear in the cell and become the controllers of new or altered cellular functions.

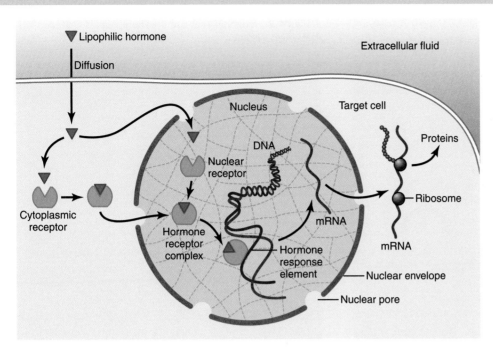

Figure 74-6 Mechanisms of interaction of lipophilic hormones, such as steroids, with intracellular receptors in target cells. After the hormone binds to the receptor in the cytoplasm or in the nucleus, the hormone-receptor complex binds to the hormone response element (promoter) on the DNA. This either activates or inhibits gene transcription, formation of messenger RNA (mRNA), and protein synthesis.

Many different tissues have identical intracellular hormone receptors, but the genes that the receptors regulate are different in the various tissues. An intracellular receptor can activate a gene response only if the appropriate combination of gene regulatory proteins is present, and many of these regulatory proteins are tissue specific. Thus, the responses of different tissues to a hormone are determined not only by the specificity of the receptors but also by the expression of genes that the receptor regulates.

Second Messenger Mechanisms for Mediating Intracellular Hormonal Functions

We noted earlier that one of the means by which hormones exert intracellular actions is to stimulate formation of the second messenger cAMP inside the cell membrane. The cAMP then causes subsequent intracellular effects of the hormone. Thus, the only direct effect that the hormone has on the cell is to activate a single type of membrane receptor. The second messenger does the rest.

cAMP is not the only second messenger used by the different hormones. Two other especially important ones are (1) calcium ions and associated *calmodulin* and (2) products of membrane phospholipid breakdown.

Adenylyl Cyclase–cAMP Second Messenger System

Table 74-2 shows a few of the many hormones that use the adenylyl cyclase-cAMP mechanism to stimulate their target tissues, and Figure 74-7 shows the adenylyl cyclase–cAMP second messenger system. Binding of the hormones with the receptor allows coupling of the receptor to a *G protein*. If the G protein stimulates the adenylyl cyclase–cAMP system, it is called a G_s *protein*, denoting a stimulatory G protein. Stimulation of adenylyl cyclase, a membrane-bound enzyme, by the G_s protein then

Table 74-2 Hormones That Use the Adenylyl Cyclase–cAMP Second Messenger System

Adrenocorticotropic hormone (ACTH)
Angiotensin II (epithelial cells)
Calcitonin
Catecholamines (β receptors)
Corticotropin-releasing hormone (CRH)
Follicle-stimulating hormone (FSH)
Glucagon
Human chorionic gonadotropin (HCG)
Luteinizing hormone (LH)
Parathyroid hormone (PTH)
Secretin
Somatostatin
Thyroid-stimulating hormone (TSH)
Vasopressin (V_2 receptor, epithelial cells)

catalyzes the conversion of a small amount of cytoplasmic *adenosine triphosphate* (ATP) into cAMP inside the cell. This then activates *cAMP-dependent protein kinase*, which phosphorylates specific proteins in the cell, triggering biochemical reactions that ultimately lead to the cell's response to the hormone.

Once cAMP is formed inside the cell, it usually activates a *cascade of enzymes*. That is, first one enzyme is activated, which activates a second enzyme, which activates a third, and so forth. The importance of this mechanism is that only a few molecules of activated adenylyl cyclase immediately inside the cell membrane can cause many more molecules of the next enzyme to be activated, which can cause still more molecules of the third enzyme to be activated, and so forth. In this way, even the slightest amount of hormone acting on the cell surface can initiate a powerful cascading activating force for the entire cell.

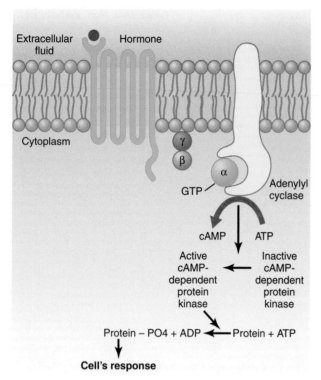

Figure 74-7 Cyclic adenosine monophosphate (cAMP) mechanism by which many hormones exert their control of cell function. ADP, adenosine diphosphate; ATP, adenosine triphosphate.

Table 74-3 Hormones That Use the Phospholipase C Second Messenger System

Angiotensin II (vascular smooth muscle)
Catecholamines (α receptors)
Gonadotropin-releasing hormone (GnRH)
Growth hormone–releasing hormone (GHRH)
Oxytocin
Thyrotropin releasing hormone (TRH)
Vasopressin (V1 receptor, vascular smooth muscle)

phosphate (PIP_2), into two different second messenger products: *inositol triphosphate* (IP_3) and *diacylglycerol* (DAG). The IP_3 mobilizes calcium ions from mitochondria and the endoplasmic reticulum, and the calcium ions then have their own second messenger effects, such as smooth muscle contraction and changes in cell secretion.

DAG, the other lipid second messenger, activates the enzyme *protein kinase C* (PKC), which then phosphorylates a large number of proteins, leading to the cell's response (Figure 74-8). In addition to these effects, the lipid portion of DAG is *arachidonic acid*, which is the precursor for the *prostaglandins* and other local hormones that cause multiple effects in tissues throughout the body.

If binding of the hormone to its receptors is coupled to an inhibitory G protein (denoted G_i protein), adenylyl cyclase will be inhibited, reducing the formation of cAMP and ultimately leading to an inhibitory action in the cell. Thus, depending on the coupling of the hormone receptor to an inhibitory or a stimulatory G protein, a hormone can either increase or decrease the concentration of cAMP and phosphorylation of key proteins inside the cell.

The specific action that occurs in response to increases or decreases of cAMP in each type of target cell depends on the nature of the intracellular machinery—some cells have one set of enzymes, and other cells have other enzymes. Therefore, different functions are elicited in different target cells, such as initiating synthesis of specific intracellular chemicals, causing muscle contraction or relaxation, initiating secretion by the cells, and altering cell permeability.

Thus, a thyroid cell stimulated by cAMP forms the metabolic hormones thyroxine and triiodothyronine, whereas the same cAMP in an adrenocortical cell causes secretion of the adrenocortical steroid hormones. In epithelial cells of the renal tubules, cAMP increases their permeability to water.

Cell Membrane Phospholipid Second Messenger System

Some hormones activate transmembrane receptors that activate the enzyme *phospholipase C* attached to the inside projections of the receptors (Table 74-3). This enzyme catalyzes the breakdown of some phospholipids in the cell membrane, especially *phosphatidylinositol bi-*

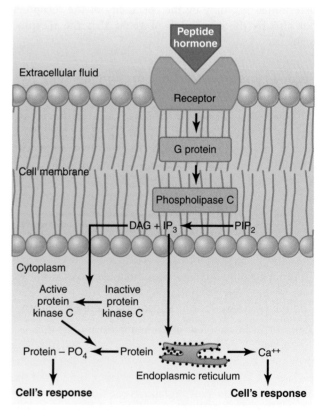

Figure 74-8 The cell membrane phospholipid second messenger system by which some hormones exert their control of cell function. DAG, diacylglycerol; IP_3, inositol triphosphate; PIP_2, phosphatidylinositol biphosphate.

Calcium-Calmodulin Second Messenger System

Another second messenger system operates in response to the entry of calcium into the cells. Calcium entry may be initiated by (1) changes in membrane potential that open calcium channels or (2) a hormone interacting with membrane receptors that open calcium channels.

On entering a cell, calcium ions bind with the protein *calmodulin.* This protein has four calcium sites, and when three or four of these sites have bound with calcium, the calmodulin changes its shape and initiates multiple effects inside the cell, including activation or inhibition of protein kinases. Activation of calmodulin-dependent protein kinases causes, via phosphorylation, activation or inhibition of proteins involved in the cell's response to the hormone. For example, one specific function of calmodulin is to activate *myosin light chain kinase,* which acts directly on the myosin of smooth muscle to cause smooth muscle contraction.

The normal calcium ion concentration in most cells of the body is 10^{-8} to 10^{-7} mol/L, which is not enough to activate the calmodulin system. But when the calcium ion concentration rises to 10^{-6} to 10^{-5} mol/L, enough binding occurs to cause all the intracellular actions of calmodulin. This is almost exactly the same amount of calcium ion change that is required in skeletal muscle to activate troponin C, which causes skeletal muscle contraction, as explained in Chapter 7. It is interesting that troponin C is similar to calmodulin in both function and protein structure.

Hormones That Act Mainly on the Genetic Machinery of the Cell

Steroid Hormones Increase Protein Synthesis

Another means by which hormones act—specifically, the steroid hormones secreted by the adrenal cortex, ovaries, and testes—is to cause synthesis of proteins in the target cells. These proteins then function as enzymes, transport proteins, or structural proteins, which in turn provide other functions of the cells.

The sequence of events in steroid function is essentially the following:

1. The steroid hormone diffuses across the cell membrane and enters the cytoplasm of the cell, where it binds with a specific *receptor protein.*

2. The combined receptor protein–hormone then diffuses into or is transported into the nucleus.

3. The combination binds at specific points on the DNA strands in the chromosomes, which activates the transcription process of specific genes to form mRNA.

4. The mRNA diffuses into the cytoplasm, where it promotes the translation process at the ribosomes to form new proteins.

To give an example, *aldosterone,* one of the hormones secreted by the adrenal cortex, enters the cytoplasm of renal tubular cells, which contain a specific receptor protein

often called the *mineralocorticoid receptor.* Therefore, in these cells, the sequence of events cited earlier ensues. After about 45 minutes, proteins begin to appear in the renal tubular cells and promote sodium reabsorption from the tubules and potassium secretion into the tubules. Thus, the full action of the steroid hormone is characteristically delayed for at least 45 minutes—up to several hours or even days. This is in marked contrast to the almost instantaneous action of some of the peptide and amino acid–derived hormones, such as vasopressin and norepinephrine.

Thyroid Hormones Increase Gene Transcription in the Cell Nucleus

The thyroid hormones *thyroxine* and *triiodothyronine* cause increased transcription by specific genes in the nucleus. To accomplish this, these hormones first bind directly with receptor proteins in the nucleus; these receptors are *activated transcription factors* located within the chromosomal complex, and they control the function of the gene promoters, as explained in Chapter 3.

Two important features of thyroid hormone function in the nucleus are the following:

1. They activate the genetic mechanisms for the formation of many types of intracellular proteins—probably 100 or more. Many of these are enzymes that promote enhanced intracellular metabolic activity in virtually all cells of the body.

2. Once bound to the intranuclear receptors, the thyroid hormones can continue to express their control functions for days or even weeks.

Measurement of Hormone Concentrations in the Blood

Most hormones are present in the blood in extremely minute quantities; some concentrations are as low as one billionth of a milligram (1 picogram) per milliliter. Therefore, it was difficult to measure these concentrations by the usual chemical means. An extremely sensitive method, however, was developed about 45 years ago that revolutionized the measurement of hormones, their precursors, and their metabolic end products. This method is called *radioimmunoassay.*

Radioimmunoassay

The method of performing radioimmunoassay is as follows. First, an antibody that is highly specific for the hormone to be measured is produced.

Second, a small quantity of this antibody is (1) mixed with a quantity of fluid from the animal containing the hormone to be measured and (2) mixed simultaneously with an appropriate amount of purified standard hormone that has been tagged with a radioactive isotope. However, one specific condition must be met: There must be too little antibody to bind completely both the radioactively tagged hormone and the hormone in the fluid to be assayed. Therefore, the natural hormone in the assay fluid and the radioactive standard hormone *compete for the binding sites* of the antibody. In the process of competing, the quantity of each of the two hormones, the natural and the radioactive, that binds is proportional to its concentration in the assay fluid.

Third, after binding has reached equilibrium, the antibody-hormone complex is separated from the remainder of the solution, and the quantity of radioactive hormone bound in this complex is measured by radioactive counting techniques. If a large amount of radioactive hormone has bound with the antibody, it is clear that there was only a small amount of natural hormone to compete with the radioactive hormone, and therefore the concentration of the natural hormone in the assayed fluid was small. Conversely, if only a small amount of radioactive hormone has bound, it is clear that there was a large amount of natural hormone to compete for the binding sites.

Fourth, to make the assay highly quantitative, the radioimmunoassay procedure is also performed for "standard" solutions of untagged hormone at several concentration levels. Then a "standard curve" is plotted, as shown in Figure 74-9. By comparing the radioactive counts recorded from the "unknown" assay procedures with the standard curve, one can determine within an error of 10 to 15 percent the concentration of the hormone in the "unknown" assayed fluid. As little as billionths or even trillionths of a gram of hormone can often be assayed in this way.

Enzyme-Linked Immunosorbent Assay

Enzyme-linked immunosorbent assays (ELISAs) can be used to measure almost any protein, including hormones. This test combines the specificity of antibodies with the sensitivity of simple enzyme assays. Figure 74-10 shows the basic elements of this method, which is often

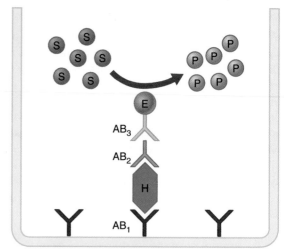

Figure 74-10 Basic principles of the enzyme-linked immunosorbent assay (ELISA) for measuring the concentration of a hormone (H). AB_1 and AB_2 are antibodies that recognize the hormone at different binding sites, and AB_3 is an antibody that recognizes AB_2. E is an enzyme linked to AB_3 that catalyzes the formation of a colored fluorescent product (P) from a substrate (S). The amount of the product is measured using optical methods and is proportional to the amount of hormone in the well if there are excess antibodies in the well.

performed on plastic plates that each have 96 small wells. Each well is coated with an antibody (AB_1) that is specific for the hormone being assayed. Samples or standards are added to each of the wells, followed by a second antibody (AB_2) that is also specific for the hormone but binds to a different site of the hormone molecule. A third antibody (AB_3) that is added recognizes AB_2 and is coupled to an enzyme that converts a suitable substrate to a product that can be easily detected by colorimetric or fluorescent optical methods.

Because each molecule of enzyme catalyzes the formation of many thousands of product molecules, even small amounts of hormone molecules can be detected. In contrast to competitive radioimmunoassay methods, ELISA methods use excess antibodies so that all hormone molecules are captured in antibody-hormone complexes. Therefore, the amount of hormone present in the sample or in the standard is proportional to the amount of product formed.

The ELISA method has become widely used in clinical laboratories because (1) it does not employ radioactive isotopes, (2) much of the assay can be automated using 96-well plates, and (3) it has proved to be a cost-effective and accurate method for assessing hormone levels.

Bibliography

Alberts B, Johnson A, Lewis J, et al: *Molecular Biology of the Cell*, ed 5, New York, 2008, Garland Science.

Antunes-Rodrigues J, de Castro M, Elias LL, et al: Neuroendocrine control of body fluid metabolism, *Physiol Rev* 84:169, 2004.

Aranda A, Pascual A: Nuclear hormone receptors and gene expression, *Physiol Rev* 81:1269, 2001.

Bezbradica JS, Medzhitov R: Integration of cytokine and heterologous receptor signaling pathways, *Nat Immunol* 10:333, 2009.

Dayan CM, Panicker V: Novel insights into thyroid hormones from the study of common genetic variation, *Nat Rev Endocrinol* 5:211, 2009.

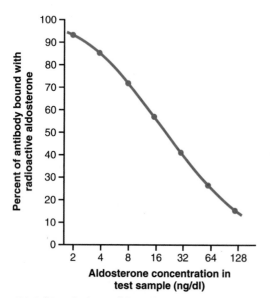

Figure 74-9 "Standard curve" for radioimmunoassay of aldosterone. (Courtesy Dr. Manis Smith.)

Funder JW: Reconsidering the roles of the mineralocorticoid receptor, *Hypertension* 53:286, 2009.

Gao Q, Horvath TL: Cross-talk between estrogen and leptin signaling in the hypothalamus, *Am J Physiol Endocrinol Metab* 294:E817, 2008.

Heldring N, Pike A, Andersson S, et al: Estrogen receptors: how do they signal and what are their targets? *Physiol Rev* 87:905, 2007.

Kuhn M: Structure, regulation, and function of mammalian membrane guanylyl cyclase receptors, with a focus on guanylyl cyclase-A, *Circ Res* 93:700, 2003.

Mogi M, Iwai M, Horiuchi M: Emerging concepts of regulation of angiotensin II receptors: new players and targets for traditional receptors, *Arterioscler Thromb Vasc Biol* 27:2532, 2007.

Morris AJ, Malbon CC: Physiological regulation of G protein-linked signaling, *Physiol Rev* 79:1373, 1999.

Pires-daSilva A, Sommer RJ: The evolution of signaling pathways in animal development, *Nat Rev Genet* 4:39, 2003.

Psarra AM, Sekeris CE: Glucocorticoid receptors and other nuclear transcription factors in mitochondria and possible functions, *Biochim Biophys Acta* 1787:431, 2009.

Spat A, Hunyady L: Control of aldosterone secretion: a model for convergence in cellular signaling pathways, *Physiol Rev* 84:489, 2004.

Tasken K, Aandahl EM: Localized effects of cAMP mediated by distinct routes of protein kinase A, *Physiol Rev* 84:137, 2004.

Wettschureck N, Offermanns S: Mammalian G proteins and their cell type specific functions, *Physiol Rev* 85:1159, 2005.

Yang J, Young MJ: The mineralocorticoid receptor and its coregulators, *J Mol Endocrinol* 43:53, 2009.

Yen PM: Physiological and molecular basis of thyroid hormone action, *Physiol Rev* 81:1097, 2001.

Pituitary Hormones and Their Control by the Hypothalamus

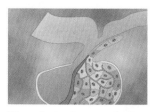

Pituitary Gland and Its Relation to the Hypothalamus

The Pituitary Gland Has Two Distinct Parts— The Anterior and Posterior Lobes. The *pituitary gland* (Figure 75-1), also called the *hypophysis,* is a small gland—about 1 centimeter in diameter and 0.5 to 1 gram in weight—that lies in the *sella turcica,* a bony cavity at the base of the brain, and is connected to the hypothalamus by the *pituitary* (or *hypophysial*) stalk. Physiologically, the pituitary gland is divisible into two distinct portions: the *anterior pituitary,* also known as the *adenohypophysis,* and the *posterior pituitary,* also known as the *neurohypophysis.* Between these is a small, relatively avascular zone called the *pars intermedia,* which is much less developed in the human being but is larger and much more functional in some lower animals.

Embryologically, the two portions of the pituitary originate from different sources—the anterior pituitary from *Rathke's pouch,* which is an embryonic invagination of the pharyngeal epithelium, and the posterior pituitary from a neural tissue outgrowth from the hypothalamus. The origin of the anterior pituitary from the pharyngeal epithelium explains the epithelioid nature of its cells, and the origin of the posterior pituitary from neural tissue explains the presence of large numbers of glial-type cells in this gland.

Six important peptide hormones plus several hormones of lesser importance are secreted by the *anterior* pituitary, and two important peptide hormones are secreted by the *posterior* pituitary. The hormones of the anterior pituitary play major roles in the control of metabolic functions throughout the body, as shown in Figure 75-2.

• *Growth hormone* promotes growth of the entire body by affecting protein formation, cell multiplication, and cell differentiation.

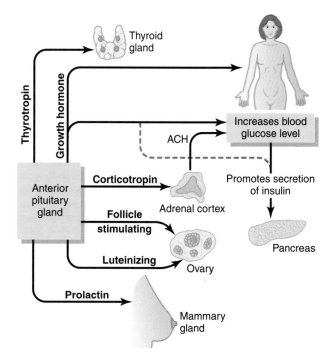

Figure 75-2 Metabolic functions of the anterior pituitary hormones. ACH, adrenal corticosteroid hormones.

Figure 75-1 Pituitary gland.

- *Adrenocorticotropin (corticotropin)* controls the secretion of some of the adrenocortical hormones, which affect the metabolism of glucose, proteins, and fats.
- *Thyroid-stimulating hormone (thyrotropin)* controls the rate of secretion of thyroxine and triiodothyronine by the thyroid gland, and these hormones control the rates of most intracellular chemical reactions in the body.
- *Prolactin* promotes mammary gland development and milk production.
- Two separate gonadotropic hormones, *follicle-stimulating hormone* and *luteinizing hormone,* control growth of the ovaries and testes, as well as their hormonal and reproductive activities.

The two hormones secreted by the posterior pituitary play other roles.

- *Antidiuretic hormone* (also called *vasopressin*) controls the rate of water excretion into the urine, thus helping to control the concentration of water in the body fluids.
- *Oxytocin* helps express milk from the glands of the breast to the nipples during suckling and helps in the delivery of the baby at the end of gestation.

Anterior Pituitary Gland Contains Several Different Cell Types That Synthesize and Secrete Hormones.

Usually, there is one cell type for each major hormone formed in the anterior pituitary gland. With special stains attached to high-affinity antibodies that bind with the distinctive hormones, at least five cell types can be differentiated (Figure 75-3). Table 75-1 provides

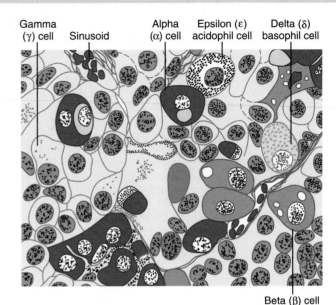

Figure 75-3 Cellular structure of the anterior pituitary gland. (Redrawn from Guyton AC: Physiology of the Human Body, 6th ed. Philadelphia: Saunders College Publishing, 1984.)

a summary of these cell types, the hormones they produce, and their physiological actions. These five cell types are:

1. *Somatotropes*—human growth hormone (hGH)
2. *Corticotropes*—adrenocorticotropin (ACTH)
3. *Thyrotropes*—thyroid-stimulating hormone (TSH)
4. *Gonadotropes*—gonadotropic hormones, which include both luteinizing hormone (LH) and follicle-stimulating hormone (FSH)
5. *Lactotropes*—prolactin (PRL)

Table 75-1 Cells and Hormones of the Anterior Pituitary Gland and Their Physiological Functions

Cell	Hormone	Chemistry	Physiological Action
Somatotropes	Growth hormone (GH; somatotropin)	Single chain of 191 amino acids	Stimulates body growth; stimulates secretion of IGF-1; stimulates lipolysis; inhibits actions of insulin on carbohydrate and lipid metabolism
Corticotropes	Adrenocorticotropic hormone (ACTH; corticotropin)	Single chain of 39 amino acids	Stimulates production of glucocorticoids and androgens by the adrenal cortex; maintains size of zona fasciculata and zona reticularis of cortex
Thyrotropes	Thyroid-stimulating hormone (TSH; thyrotropin)	Glycoprotein of two subunits, α (89 amino acids) and β (112 amino acids)	Stimulates production of thyroid hormones by thyroid follicular cells; maintains size of follicular cells
Gonadotropes	Follicle-stimulating hormone (FSH)	Glycoprotein of two subunits, α (89 amino acids) and β (112 amino acids)	Stimulates development of ovarian follicles; regulates spermatogenesis in the testis
	Luteinizing hormone (LH)	Glycoprotein of two subunits, α (89 amino acids) and β (115 amino acids)	Causes ovulation and formation of the corpus luteum in the ovary; stimulates production of estrogen and progesterone by the ovary; stimulates testosterone production by the testis
Lactotropes Mammotropes	Prolactin (PRL)	Single chain of 198 amino acids	Stimulates milk secretion and production

IGF, insulin-like growth factor.

About 30 to 40 percent of the anterior pituitary cells are somatotropes that secrete growth hormone, and about 20 percent are corticotropes that secrete ACTH. Each of the other cell types accounts for only 3 to 5 percent of the total; nevertheless, they secrete powerful hormones for controlling thyroid function, sexual functions, and milk secretion by the breasts.

Somatotropes stain strongly with acid dyes and are therefore called *acidophils*. Thus, pituitary tumors that secrete large quantities of human growth hormone are called *acidophilic tumors.*

Posterior Pituitary Hormones Are Synthesized by Cell Bodies in the Hypothalamus. The bodies of the cells that secrete the *posterior* pituitary hormones are not located in the pituitary gland itself but are large neurons, called *magnocellular neurons*, located in the *supraoptic* and *paraventricular nuclei* of the hypothalamus. The hormones are then transported in the axoplasm of the neurons' nerve fibers passing from the hypothalamus to the posterior pituitary gland. This is discussed later in the chapter.

Hypothalamus Controls Pituitary Secretion

Almost all secretion by the pituitary is controlled by either hormonal or nervous signals from the hypothalamus. Indeed, when the pituitary gland is removed from its normal position beneath the hypothalamus and transplanted to some other part of the body, its rates of secretion of the different hormones (except for prolactin) fall to very low levels.

Secretion from the posterior pituitary is controlled by nerve signals that originate in the hypothalamus and terminate in the posterior pituitary. In contrast, secretion by the anterior pituitary is controlled by hormones called *hypothalamic releasing* and *hypothalamic inhibitory hormones* (or *factors*) secreted within the hypothalamus and then conducted, as shown in Figure 75-4, to the anterior pituitary through minute blood vessels called *hypothalamic-hypophysial portal vessels*. In the anterior pituitary, these releasing and inhibitory hormones act on the glandular cells to control their secretion. This system of control is discussed in the next section of this chapter.

The hypothalamus receives signals from many sources in the nervous system. Thus, when a person is exposed to pain, a portion of the pain signal is transmitted into the hypothalamus. Likewise, when a person experiences some powerful depressing or exciting thought, a portion of the signal is transmitted into the hypothalamus. Olfactory stimuli denoting pleasant or unpleasant smells transmit strong signal components directly and through the amygdaloid nuclei into the hypothalamus. Even the concentrations of nutrients, electrolytes, water, and various hormones in the blood excite or inhibit various portions of the hypothalamus. Thus, the hypothalamus is a collecting center for information concerning the internal well-being

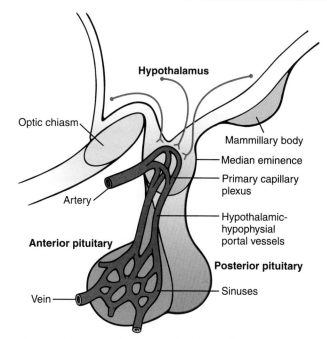

Figure 75-4 Hypothalamic-hypophysial portal system.

of the body, and much of this information is used to control secretions of the many globally important pituitary hormones.

Hypothalamic-Hypophysial Portal Blood Vessels of the Anterior Pituitary Gland

The anterior pituitary is a highly vascular gland with extensive capillary sinuses among the glandular cells. Almost all the blood that enters these sinuses passes first through another capillary bed in the lower hypothalamus. The blood then flows through small *hypothalamic-hypophysial portal blood vessels* into the anterior pituitary sinuses. Figure 75-4 shows the lowermost portion of the hypothalamus, called the *median eminence*, which connects inferiorly with the pituitary stalk. Small arteries penetrate into the median eminence and then additional small vessels return to its surface, coalescing to form the hypothalamic-hypophysial portal blood vessels. These pass downward along the pituitary stalk to supply blood to the anterior pituitary sinuses.

Hypothalamic Releasing and Inhibitory Hormones Are Secreted into the Median Eminence. Special neurons in the hypothalamus synthesize and secrete the *hypothalamic releasing* and *inhibitory hormones* that control secretion of the anterior pituitary hormones. These neurons originate in various parts of the hypothalamus and send their nerve fibers to the median eminence and *tuber cinereum*, an extension of hypothalamic tissue into the pituitary stalk.

The endings of these fibers are different from most endings in the central nervous system, in that their function is not to transmit signals from one neuron to another but rather to secrete the hypothalamic releasing and inhibitory hormones into the tissue fluids. These hormones are immediately absorbed into the hypothalamic-hypophysial portal system and carried directly to the sinuses of the anterior pituitary gland.

Hypothalamic Releasing and Inhibitory Hormones Control Anterior Pituitary Secretion. The function of the releasing and inhibitory hormones is to control secretion of the anterior pituitary hormones. For most of the anterior pituitary hormones, it is the releasing hormones that are important, but for prolactin, a hypothalamic inhibitory hormone probably exerts more control. The major hypothalamic releasing and inhibitory hormones are summarized in Table 75-2 and are the following:

1. *Thyrotropin-releasing hormone* (TRH), which causes release of thyroid-stimulating hormone
2. *Corticotropin-releasing hormone* (CRH), which causes release of adrenocorticotropin
3. *Growth hormone–releasing hormone* (GHRH), which causes release of growth hormone, and *growth hormone inhibitory hormone* (GHIH), also called *somatostatin,* which inhibits release of growth hormone
4. *Gonadotropin-releasing hormone* (GnRH), which causes release of the two gonadotropic hormones, luteinizing hormone and follicle-stimulating hormone
5. *Prolactin inhibitory hormone* (PIH), which causes inhibition of prolactin secretion

Additional hypothalamic hormones include one that stimulates prolactin secretion and perhaps others that inhibit release of the anterior pituitary hormones. Each of the more important hypothalamic hormones is discussed in detail as the specific hormonal systems controlled by them are presented in this and subsequent chapters.

Specific Areas in the Hypothalamus Control Secretion of Specific Hypothalamic Releasing and Inhibitory Hormones. All or most of the hypothalamic hormones are secreted at nerve endings in the median eminence before being transported to the anterior pituitary gland. Electrical stimulation of this region excites these nerve endings and, therefore, causes release of essentially all the hypothalamic hormones. However, the neuronal cell bodies that give rise to these median eminence nerve endings are located in other discrete areas of the hypothalamus or in closely related areas of the basal brain. The specific loci of the neuronal cell bodies that form the different hypothalamic releasing or inhibitory hormones are still poorly known, so it would be misleading to attempt delineation here.

Physiological Functions of Growth Hormone

All the major anterior pituitary hormones, except for growth hormone, exert their principal effects by stimulating target glands, including thyroid gland, adrenal cortex, ovaries, testicles, and mammary glands. The functions of each of these pituitary hormones are so intimately concerned with the functions of the respective target glands that, except for growth hormone, their functions are discussed in subsequent chapters along with the target glands. Growth hormone, in contrast to other hormones, does not function through a target gland but exerts its effects directly on all or almost all tissues of the body.

Growth Hormone Promotes Growth of Many Body Tissues

Growth hormone, also called *somatotropic hormone* or *somatotropin,* is a small protein molecule that contains 191 amino acids in a single chain and has a molecular weight of 22,005. It causes growth of almost all tissues of the body that are capable of growing. It promotes increased sizes of the cells and increased mitosis, with development of greater numbers of cells and specific differentiation of certain types of cells such as bone growth cells and early muscle cells.

Figure 75-5 shows typical weight charts of two growing littermate rats, one of which received daily injections of growth hormone and the other of which did not receive

Table 75-2 Hypothalamic Releasing and Inhibitory Hormones That Control Secretion of the Anterior Pituitary Gland

Hormone	Structure	Primary Action on Anterior Pituitary
Thyrotropin-releasing hormone (TRH)	Peptide of 3 amino acids	Stimulates secretion of TSH by thyrotropes
Gonadotropin-releasing hormone (GnRH)	Single chain of 10 amino acids	Stimulates secretion of FSH and LH by gonadotropes
Corticotropin-releasing hormone (CRH)	Single chain of 41 amino acids	Stimulates secretion of ACTH by corticotropes
Growth hormone-releasing hormone (GHRH)	Single chain of 44 amino acids	Stimulates secretion of growth hormone by somatotropes
Growth hormone inhibitory hormone (somatostatin)	Single chain of 14 amino acids	Inhibits secretion of growth hormone by somatotropes
Prolactin-inhibiting hormone (PIH)	Dopamine (a catecholamine)	Inhibits synthesis and secretion of prolactin by lactotropes

ACTH, adrenocorticotropic hormone; FSH, follicle-stimulating hormone; LH, luteinizing hormone; TSH, thyroid-stimulating hormone.

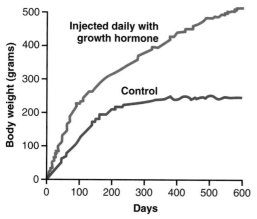

Figure 75-5 Comparison of weight gain of a rat injected daily with growth hormone with that of a normal littermate.

growth hormone. This figure shows marked enhancement of growth in the rat given growth hormone, in the early days of life and even after the two rats reached adulthood. In the early stages of development, all organs of the treated rat increased proportionately in size; after adulthood was reached, most of the bones stopped lengthening, but many of the soft tissues continued to grow. This results from the fact that once the epiphyses of the long bones have united with the shafts, further lengthening of bone cannot occur, even though most other tissues of the body can continue to grow throughout life.

Growth Hormone Has Several Metabolic Effects

Aside from its general effect in causing growth, growth hormone has multiple specific metabolic effects, including (1) increased rate of protein synthesis in most cells of the body; (2) increased mobilization of fatty acids from adipose tissue, increased free fatty acids in the blood, and increased use of fatty acids for energy; and (3) decreased rate of glucose utilization throughout the body. Thus, in effect, growth hormone enhances body protein, uses up fat stores, and conserves carbohydrates.

Growth Hormone Promotes Protein Deposition in Tissues

Although the precise mechanisms by which growth hormone increases protein deposition are not known, a series of different effects are known, all of which could lead to enhanced protein deposition.

Enhancement of Amino Acid Transport Through the Cell Membranes. Growth hormone directly enhances transport of most amino acids through the cell membranes to the interior of the cells. This increases the amino acid concentrations in the cells and is presumed to be at least partly responsible for the increased protein synthesis. This control of amino acid transport is similar to the effect of insulin in controlling glucose transport through the membrane, as discussed in Chapters 67 and 78.

Enhancement of RNA Translation to Cause Protein Synthesis by the Ribosomes. Even when the amino acid concentrations are not increased in the cells, growth hormone still increases RNA translation, causing protein to be synthesized in greater amounts by the ribosomes in the cytoplasm.

Increased Nuclear Transcription of DNA to Form RNA. Over more prolonged periods (24 to 48 hours), growth hormone also stimulates the transcription of DNA in the nucleus, causing the formation of increased quantities of RNA. This promotes more protein synthesis and promotes growth if sufficient energy, amino acids, vitamins, and other requisites for growth are available. In the long run, this may be the most important function of growth hormone.

Decreased Catabolism of Protein and Amino Acids. In addition to the increase in protein synthesis, there is a decrease in the breakdown of cell protein. A probable reason for this is that growth hormone also mobilizes large quantities of free fatty acids from the adipose tissue, and these are used to supply most of the energy for the body's cells, thus acting as a potent "protein sparer."

Summary. Growth hormone enhances almost all facets of amino acid uptake and protein synthesis by cells, while at the same time reducing the breakdown of proteins.

Growth Hormone Enhances Fat Utilization for Energy

Growth hormone has a specific effect in causing the release of fatty acids from adipose tissue and, therefore, increasing the concentration of fatty acids in the body fluids. In addition, in tissues throughout the body, growth hormone enhances the conversion of fatty acids to acetyl coenzyme A (acetyl-CoA) and its subsequent utilization for energy. Therefore, under the influence of growth hormone, fat is used for energy in preference to the use of carbohydrates and proteins.

Growth hormone's ability to promote fat utilization, together with its protein anabolic effect, causes an increase in lean body mass. However, mobilization of fat by growth hormone requires several hours to occur, whereas enhancement of protein synthesis can begin in minutes under the influence of growth hormone.

"Ketogenic" Effect of Excessive Growth Hormone. Under the influence of excessive amounts of growth hormone, fat mobilization from adipose tissue sometimes becomes so great that large quantities of acetoacetic acid are formed by the liver and released into the body fluids, thus causing *ketosis*. This excessive mobilization of fat from the adipose tissue also frequently causes a fatty liver.

Growth Hormone Decreases Carbohydrate Utilization

Growth hormone causes multiple effects that influence carbohydrate metabolism, including (1) decreased glucose uptake in tissues such as skeletal muscle and fat, (2) increased glucose production by the liver, and (3) increased insulin secretion.

Each of these changes results from growth hormone–induced "insulin resistance," which attenuates insulin's actions to stimulate the uptake and utilization of glucose in skeletal muscle and adipose tissue and to inhibit gluconeogenesis (glucose production) by the liver; this leads to increased blood glucose concentration and a compensatory increase in insulin secretion. For these reasons, growth hormone's effects are called *diabetogenic,* and excess secretion of growth hormone can produce metabolic disturbances similar to those found in patients with type II (non-insulin-dependent) diabetes, who are also resistant to the metabolic effects of insulin.

We do not know the precise mechanism by which growth hormone causes insulin resistance and decreased glucose utilization by the cells. However, growth hormone–induced increases in blood concentrations of fatty acids likely contribute to impairment of insulin's actions on tissue glucose utilization. Experimental studies indicate that raising blood levels of fatty acids above normal rapidly decreases the sensitivity of the liver and skeletal muscle to insulin's effects on carbohydrate metabolism.

Necessity of Insulin and Carbohydrate for the Growth-Promoting Action of Growth Hormone. Growth hormone fails to cause growth in animals that lack a pancreas; it also fails to cause growth if carbohydrates are excluded from the diet. This shows that adequate insulin activity and adequate availability of carbohydrates are necessary for growth hormone to be effective. Part of this requirement for carbohydrates and insulin is to provide the energy needed for the metabolism of growth, but there seem to be other effects as well. Especially important is insulin's ability to enhance the transport of some amino acids into cells, in the same way that it stimulates glucose transport.

Growth Hormone Stimulates Cartilage and Bone Growth

Although growth hormone stimulates increased deposition of protein and increased growth in almost all tissues of the body, its most obvious effect is to increase growth of the skeletal frame. This results from multiple effects of growth hormone on bone, including (1) increased deposition of protein by the chondrocytic and osteogenic cells that cause bone growth, (2) increased rate of reproduction of these cells, and (3) a specific effect of converting chondrocytes into osteogenic cells, thus causing deposition of new bone.

There are two principal mechanisms of bone growth. First, in response to growth hormone stimulation, the long bones grow in length at the epiphyseal cartilages, where the epiphyses at the ends of the bone are separated from the shaft. This growth first causes deposition of new cartilage, followed by its conversion into new bone, thus elongating the shaft and pushing the epiphyses farther and farther apart. At the same time, the epiphyseal cartilage itself is progressively used up, so by late adolescence, no additional epiphyseal cartilage remains to provide for further long bone growth. At this time, bony fusion occurs between the shaft and the epiphysis at each end, so no further lengthening of the long bone can occur.

Second, *osteoblasts* in the bone periosteum and in some bone cavities deposit new bone on the surfaces of older bone. Simultaneously, *osteoclasts* in the bone (discussed in detail in Chapter 79) remove old bone. When the rate of deposition is greater than that of resorption, the thickness of the bone increases. *Growth hormone strongly stimulates osteoblasts.* Therefore, the bones can continue to become thicker throughout life under the influence of growth hormone; this is especially true for the membranous bones. For instance, the jaw bones can be stimulated to grow even after adolescence, causing forward protrusion of the chin and lower teeth. Likewise, the bones of the skull can grow in thickness and give rise to bony protrusions over the eyes.

Growth Hormone Exerts Much of Its Effect Through Intermediate Substances Called "Somatomedins" (Also Called "Insulin-Like Growth Factors")

When growth hormone is supplied directly to cartilage chondrocytes cultured outside the body, proliferation or enlargement of the chondrocytes usually fails to occur. Yet growth hormone injected into the intact animal does cause proliferation and growth of the same cells.

In brief, it has been found that growth hormone causes the liver (and, to a much less extent, other tissues) to form several small proteins called *somatomedins* that have the potent effect of increasing all aspects of bone growth. Many of the somatomedin effects on growth are similar to the effects of insulin on growth. Therefore, the somatomedins are also called insulin-like growth factors (IGFs).

At least four somatomedins have been isolated, but by far the most important of these is *somatomedin C* (also called insulin-like growth factor-1, or IGF-I). The molecular weight of somatomedin C is about 7500, and its concentration in the plasma closely follows the rate of growth hormone secretion.

The pygmies of Africa have a congenital inability to synthesize significant amounts of somatomedin C. Therefore, even though their plasma concentration of growth hormone is either normal or high, they have diminished amounts of somatomedin C in the plasma; this apparently accounts for the small stature of these people. Some other dwarfs (e.g., the Lévi-Lorain dwarf) also have this problem.

It has been postulated that most, if not all, of the growth effects of growth hormone result from somatomedin C and other somatomedins, rather than from direct effects of growth hormone on the bones and other peripheral tissues. Even so, experiments have demonstrated that injection of growth hormone directly into the epiphyseal cartilages of bones of living animals causes the specific growth of these cartilage areas, and the amount of growth hormone required for this is minute. Some aspects of the somatomedin hypothesis are still questionable.

One possibility is that growth hormone can cause the formation of enough somatomedin C in the local tissue to cause local growth. It is also possible that growth hormone itself is directly responsible for increased growth in some tissues and that the somatomedin mechanism is an alternative means of increasing growth but not always a necessary one.

Short Duration of Action of Growth Hormone but Prolonged Action of Somatomedin C.

Growth hormone attaches only weakly to the plasma proteins in the blood. Therefore, it is released from the blood into the tissues rapidly, having a half-time in the blood of less than 20 minutes. By contrast, somatomedin C attaches strongly to a carrier protein in the blood that, like somatomedin C, is produced in response to growth hormone. As a result, somatomedin C is released only slowly from the blood to the tissues, with a half-time of about 20 hours. This greatly prolongs the growth-promoting effects of the bursts of growth hormone secretion shown in Figure 75-6.

Regulation of Growth Hormone Secretion

For many years it was believed that growth hormone was secreted primarily during the period of growth but then disappeared from the blood at adolescence. This has proved to be untrue. After adolescence, secretion decreases slowly with aging, finally falling to about 25 percent of the adolescent level in very old age.

Growth hormone is secreted in a pulsatile pattern, increasing and decreasing. The precise mechanisms that control secretion of growth hormone are not fully understood, but several factors related to a person's state of nutrition or stress are known to stimulate secretion: (1) *starvation*, especially with severe *protein deficiency*; (2) *hypoglycemia* or *low concentration of fatty acids in the blood*; (3) *exercise*; (4) *excitement*; (5) *trauma*; and (6) *ghrelin*, a hormone secreted by the stomach before meals. Growth hormone also characteristically increases during the first 2 hours of *deep sleep*, as shown in Figure 75-6. Table 75-3 summarizes some of the factors that are known to influence growth hormone secretion.

Table 75-3 Factors That Stimulate or Inhibit Secretion of Growth Hormone

Stimulate Growth Hormone Secretion	Inhibit Growth Hormone Secretion
Decreased blood glucose	Increased blood glucose
Decreased blood free fatty acids	Increased blood free fatty acids
Increased blood amino acids (arginine)	Aging
Starvation or fasting, protein deficiency	Obesity
Trauma, stress, excitement	Growth hormone inhibitory hormone (somatostatin)
Exercise	Growth hormone (exogenous)
Testosterone, estrogen	Somatomedins (insulin-like growth factors)
Deep sleep (stages II and IV)	
Growth hormone–releasing hormone	
Ghrelin	

The normal concentration of growth hormone in the plasma of an adult is between 1.6 and 3 ng/ml; in a child or adolescent, it is about 6 ng/ml. These values often increase to as high as 50 ng/ml after depletion of the body stores of proteins or carbohydrates during prolonged starvation.

Under acute conditions, hypoglycemia is a far more potent stimulator of growth hormone secretion than is an acute decrease in protein intake. Conversely, in chronic conditions, growth hormone secretion seems to correlate more with the degree of cellular protein depletion than with the degree of glucose insufficiency. For instance, the extremely high levels of growth hormone that occur during starvation are closely related to the amount of protein depletion.

Figure 75-7 demonstrates the effect of protein deficiency on plasma growth hormone and then the effect of adding protein to the diet. The first column shows very high levels of growth hormone in children with extreme protein deficiency during the protein malnutrition condition called *kwashiorkor*; the second column shows the levels in the same children after 3 days of treatment with more than adequate quantities of carbohydrates in their diets, demonstrating that the carbohydrates did not lower the plasma growth hormone concentration. The third and fourth columns show the levels after treatment with protein supplements for 3 and 25 days, respectively, with a concomitant decrease in the hormone.

These results demonstrate that under severe conditions of protein malnutrition, adequate calories alone are not sufficient to correct the excess production of growth hormone. The protein deficiency must also be corrected before the growth hormone concentration will return to normal.

Role of the Hypothalamus, Growth Hormone-Releasing Hormone, and Somatostatin in the Control of Growth Hormone Secretion

From the preceding description of the many factors that can affect growth hormone secretion, one can readily understand the perplexity of physiologists as they attempted

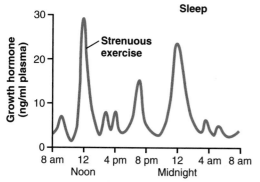

Figure 75-6 Typical variations in growth hormone secretion throughout the day, demonstrating the especially powerful effect of strenuous exercise and also the high rate of growth hormone secretion that occurs during the first few hours of deep sleep.

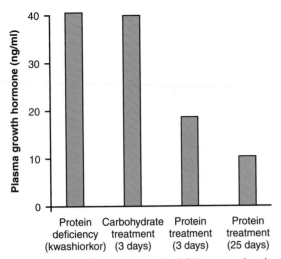

Figure 75-7 Effect of extreme protein deficiency on the plasma concentration of growth hormone in the disease kwashiorkor. Also shown is the failure of carbohydrate treatment but the effectiveness of protein treatment in lowering growth hormone concentration. (Drawn from data in Pimstone BL, Barbezat G, Hansen JD, et al: Studies on growth hormone secretion in protein-calorie malnutrition. Am J Clin Nutr 21:482, 1968.)

to unravel the mysteries of regulation of growth hormone secretion. It is known that growth hormone secretion is controlled by two factors secreted in the hypothalamus and then transported to the anterior pituitary gland through the hypothalamic-hypophysial portal vessels. They are *growth hormone–releasing hormone* and *growth hormone inhibitory hormone* (also called *somatostatin*). Both of these are polypeptides; GHRH is composed of 44 amino acids, and somatostatin is composed of 14 amino acids.

The part of the hypothalamus that causes secretion of GHRH is the ventromedial nucleus; this is the same area of the hypothalamus that is sensitive to blood glucose concentration, causing satiety in hyperglycemic states and hunger in hypoglycemic states. The secretion of somatostatin is controlled by other nearby areas of the hypothalamus. Therefore, it is reasonable to believe that some of the same signals that modify a person's behavioral feeding instincts also alter the rate of growth hormone secretion.

In a similar manner, hypothalamic signals depicting emotions, stress, and trauma can all affect hypothalamic control of growth hormone secretion. In fact, experiments have shown that catecholamines, dopamine, and serotonin, each of which is released by a different neuronal system in the hypothalamus, all increase the rate of growth hormone secretion.

Most of the control of growth hormone secretion is probably mediated through GHRH rather than through the inhibitory hormone somatostatin. GHRH stimulates growth hormone secretion by attaching to specific cell membrane receptors on the outer surfaces of the growth hormone cells in the pituitary gland. The receptors activate the adenylyl cyclase system inside the cell membrane, increasing the intracellular level of cyclic adenosine monophosphate (cAMP). This has both short-term and

long-term effects. The short-term effect is to increase calcium ion transport into the cell; within minutes, this causes fusion of the growth hormone secretory vesicles with the cell membrane and release of the hormone into the blood. The long-term effect is to increase transcription in the nucleus by the genes to stimulate the synthesis of new growth hormone.

When growth hormone is administered directly into the blood of an animal over a period of hours, the rate of endogenous growth hormone secretion decreases. This demonstrates that growth hormone secretion is subject to typical negative feedback control, as is true for essentially all hormones. The nature of this feedback mechanism and whether it is mediated mainly through inhibition of GHRH or enhancement of somatostatin, which inhibits growth hormone secretion, are uncertain.

In summary, our knowledge of the regulation of growth hormone secretion is not sufficient to describe a composite picture. Yet because of the extreme secretion of growth hormone during starvation and its important long-term effect to promote protein synthesis and tissue growth, we can propose the following: the major long-term controller of growth hormone secretion is the long-term state of nutrition of the tissues themselves, especially their level of protein nutrition. That is, nutritional deficiency or excess tissue need for cellular proteins—for instance, after a severe bout of exercise when the muscles' nutritional status has been taxed—in some way increases the rate of growth hormone secretion. Growth hormone, in turn, promotes synthesis of new proteins while at the same time conserving the proteins already present in the cells.

Abnormalities of Growth Hormone Secretion

Panhypopituitarism. This term means decreased secretion of all the anterior pituitary hormones. The decrease in secretion may be congenital (present from birth), or it may occur suddenly or slowly at any time during life, most often resulting from a pituitary tumor that destroys the pituitary gland.

Dwarfism. Most instances of dwarfism result from generalized deficiency of anterior pituitary secretion (panhypopituitarism) during childhood. In general, all the physical parts of the body develop in appropriate proportion to one another, but the rate of development is greatly decreased. A child who has reached the age of 10 years may have the bodily development of a child aged 4 to 5 years, and the same person at age 20 years may have the bodily development of a child aged 7 to 10 years.

A person with panhypopituitary dwarfism does not pass through puberty and never secretes sufficient quantities of gonadotropic hormones to develop adult sexual functions. In one third of such dwarfs, however, only growth hormone is deficient; these persons do mature sexually and occasionally reproduce. In one type of dwarfism (the African pygmy and the Lévi-Lorain dwarf), the rate of growth hormone secretion is normal or high, but there is a hereditary inability to form somatomedin C, which is a key step for the promotion of growth by growth hormone.

Treatment with Human Growth Hormone. Growth hormones from different species of animals are sufficiently different from one another that they will cause growth only in the one species or, at most, closely related species. For this reason, growth hormone prepared from lower animals (except, to some extent, from primates) is not effective in human beings. Therefore, the growth hormone of the human being is called *human growth hormone* to distinguish it from the others.

In the past, because growth hormone had to be prepared from human pituitary glands, it was difficult to obtain sufficient quantities to treat patients with growth hormone deficiency, except on an experimental basis. However, human growth hormone can now be synthesized by *Escherichia coli* bacteria as a result of successful application of recombinant DNA technology. Therefore, this hormone is now available in sufficient quantities for treatment purposes. Dwarfs who have pure growth hormone deficiency can be completely cured if treated early in life. Human growth hormone may also prove to be beneficial in other metabolic disorders because of its widespread metabolic functions.

Panhypopituitarism in the Adult. Panhypopituitarism first occurring in adulthood frequently results from one of three common abnormalities. Two tumorous conditions, craniopharyngiomas or chromophobe tumors, may compress the pituitary gland until the functioning anterior pituitary cells are totally or almost totally destroyed. The third cause is thrombosis of the pituitary blood vessels. This abnormality occasionally occurs when a new mother develops circulatory shock after the birth of her baby.

The general effects of adult panhypopituitarism are (1) hypothyroidism, (2) depressed production of glucocorticoids by the adrenal glands, and (3) suppressed secretion of the gonadotropic hormones so that sexual functions are lost. Thus, the picture is that of a lethargic person (from lack of thyroid hormones) who is gaining weight (because of lack of fat mobilization by growth, adrenocorticotropic, adrenocortical, and thyroid hormones) and has lost all sexual functions. Except for the abnormal sexual functions, the patient can usually be treated satisfactorily by administering adrenocortical and thyroid hormones.

Gigantism. Occasionally, the acidophilic, growth hormone–producing cells of the anterior pituitary gland become excessively active, and sometimes even acidophilic tumors occur in the gland. As a result, large quantities of growth hormone are produced. All body tissues grow rapidly, including the bones. If the condition occurs before adolescence, before the epiphyses of the long bones have become fused with the shafts, height increases so that the person becomes a giant— up to 8 feet tall.

The giant ordinarily has *hyperglycemia*, and the beta cells of the islets of Langerhans in the pancreas are prone to degenerate because they become overactive owing to the hyperglycemia. Consequently, in about 10 percent of giants, full-blown *diabetes mellitus* eventually develops.

In most giants, panhypopituitarism eventually develops if they remain untreated because the gigantism is usually caused by a tumor of the pituitary gland that grows until the gland itself is destroyed. This eventual general deficiency of pituitary hormones usually causes death in early adulthood. However, once gigantism is diagnosed, further effects can often be blocked by microsurgical removal of the tumor or by irradiation of the pituitary gland.

Acromegaly. If an acidophilic tumor occurs after adolescence—that is, after the epiphyses of the long bones have fused with the shafts—the person cannot grow taller, but the bones can become thicker and the soft tissues can continue to grow. This condition, shown in Figure 75-8, is known as *acromegaly*. Enlargement is especially marked in the bones of the hands and feet and in the *membranous bones*, including the cranium, nose, bosses on the forehead, supraorbital ridges, lower jawbone, and portions of the vertebrae, because their growth does not cease at adolescence. Consequently, the lower jaw protrudes forward, sometimes as much as half an inch, the forehead slants forward because of excess development of the supraorbital ridges, the nose increases to as much as twice normal size, the feet require size 14 or larger shoes, and the fingers become extremely thickened so that the hands are almost twice normal size. In addition to these effects, changes in the vertebrae ordinarily cause a hunched

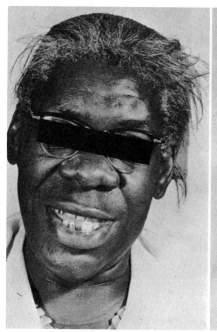 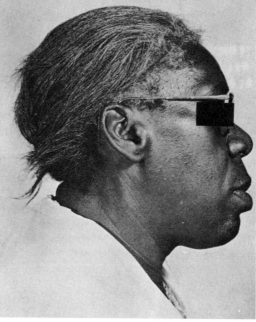

Figure 75-8 Acromegalic patient

back, which is known clinically as *kyphosis*. Finally, many soft tissue organs, such as the tongue, the liver, and especially the kidneys, become greatly enlarged.

Possible Role of Decreased Growth Hormone Secretion in Causing Changes Associated with Aging

In people who have lost the ability to secrete growth hormone, some features of the aging process accelerate. For instance, a 50-year-old person who has been without growth hormone for many years may have the appearance of a person aged 65. The aged appearance seems to result mainly from decreased protein deposition in most tissues of the body and increased fat deposition in its place. The physical and physiological effects are increased wrinkling of the skin, diminished rates of function of some of the organs, and diminished muscle mass and strength.

As one ages, the average plasma concentration of growth hormone in an otherwise normal person changes approximately as follows:

	ng/ml
5 to 20 years	6
20 to 40 years	3
40 to 70 years	1.6

Thus, it is possible that some of the normal aging effects result from diminished growth hormone secretion. In fact, some studies of growth hormone therapy in older people have demonstrated three important beneficial effects: (1) increased protein deposition in the body, especially in the muscles; (2) decreased fat deposits; and (3) a feeling of increased energy. Other studies, however, have shown that treatment of elderly patients with recombinant growth hormone may produce several undesirable side effects including insulin resistance and diabetes, edema, carpal tunnel syndrome, and arthralgias (joint pain). Therefore, recombinant growth hormone therapy is generally not recommended for use in healthy elderly patients with normal endocrine function.

Posterior Pituitary Gland and Its Relation to the Hypothalamus

The *posterior pituitary gland,* also called the *neurohypophysis,* is composed mainly of glial-like cells called *pituicytes.* The pituicytes do not secrete hormones; they act simply as a supporting structure for large numbers of *terminal nerve fibers* and *terminal nerve endings* from nerve tracts that originate in the *supraoptic* and *paraventricular nuclei* of the hypothalamus, as shown in Figure 75-9. These tracts pass to the neurohypophysis through the *pituitary stalk* (hypophysial stalk). The nerve endings are bulbous knobs that contain many secretory granules. These endings lie on the surfaces of capillaries, where they secrete two posterior pituitary hormones: (1) *antidiuretic hormone* (ADH), also called *vasopressin,* and (2) *oxytocin.*

If the pituitary stalk is cut above the pituitary gland but the entire hypothalamus is left intact, the posterior pituitary hormones continue to be secreted normally, after a transient decrease for a few days; they are then secreted by the cut ends of the fibers within the hypothalamus and not by the

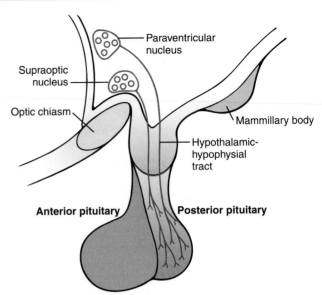

Figure 75-9 Hypothalamic control of the posterior pituitary.

nerve endings in the posterior pituitary. The reason for this is that the hormones are initially synthesized in the cell bodies of the supraoptic and paraventricular nuclei and are then transported in combination with "carrier" proteins called *neurophysins* down to the nerve endings in the posterior pituitary gland, requiring several days to reach the gland.

ADH is formed primarily in the supraoptic nuclei, whereas oxytocin is formed primarily in the paraventricular nuclei. Each of these nuclei can synthesize about one sixth as much of the second hormone as of its primary hormone.

When nerve impulses are transmitted downward along the fibers from the supraoptic or paraventricular nuclei, the hormone is immediately released from the secretory granules in the nerve endings by the usual secretory mechanism of *exocytosis* and is absorbed into adjacent capillaries. Both the neurophysin and the hormone are secreted together, but because they are only loosely bound to each other, the hormone separates almost immediately. The neurophysin has no known function after leaving the nerve terminals.

Chemical Structures of Antidiuretic Hormone and Oxytocin
Both oxytocin and ADH (vasopressin) are polypeptides, each containing nine amino acids. Their amino acid sequences are the following:

Vasopressin: Cys-Tyr-Phe-Gln-Asn-Cys-Pro-Arg-GlyNH$_2$
Oxytocin: Cys-Tyr-Ile-Gln-Asn-Cys-Pro-Leu-GlyNH$_2$

Note that these two hormones are almost identical except that in vasopressin, phenylalanine and arginine replace isoleucine and leucine of the oxytocin molecule. The similarity of the molecules explains their partial functional similarities.

Physiological Functions of Antidiuretic Hormone

The injection of extremely minute quantities of ADH—as small as 2 nanograms—can cause decreased excretion of water by the kidneys (antidiuresis). This antidiuretic effect is discussed in detail in Chapter 28. Briefly, in the absence of ADH, the collecting tubules and ducts become almost impermeable to water, which prevents significant reabsorption of water and therefore allows extreme loss of water into the urine, also causing extreme dilution of the urine. Conversely, in the presence of ADH, the permeability of the collecting ducts and tubules to water increases greatly and allows most of the water to be reabsorbed as the tubular fluid passes through these ducts, thereby conserving water in the body and producing very concentrated urine.

The precise mechanism by which ADH acts on the collecting ducts to increase their permeability is only partially known. Without ADH, the luminal membranes of the tubular epithelial cells of the collecting ducts are almost impermeable to water. However, immediately inside the cell membrane are a large number of special vesicles that have highly water-permeable pores called *aquaporins*. When ADH acts on the cell, it first combines with membrane receptors that activate adenylyl cyclase and cause the formation of cAMP inside the tubular cell cytoplasm. This causes phosphorylation of elements in the special vesicles, which then causes the vesicles to insert into the apical cell membranes, thus providing many areas of high water permeability. All this occurs within 5 to 10 minutes. Then, in the absence of ADH, the entire process reverses in another 5 to 10 minutes. Thus, this process temporarily provides many new pores that allow free diffusion of water from the tubular fluid through the tubular epithelial cells and into the renal interstitial fluid. Water is then absorbed from the collecting tubules and ducts by osmosis, as explained in Chapter 28 in relation to the urine-concentrating mechanism of the kidneys.

Regulation of Antidiuretic Hormone Production

Increased Extracellular Fluid Osmolarity Stimulates Antidiuretic Hormone Secretion. When a concentrated electrolyte solution is injected into the artery that supplies the hypothalamus, the ADH neurons in the supraoptic and paraventricular nuclei immediately transmit impulses into the posterior pituitary to release large quantities of ADH into the circulating blood, sometimes increasing the ADH secretion to as high as 20 times normal. Conversely, injection of a dilute solution into this artery causes cessation of the impulses and therefore almost total cessation of ADH secretion. Thus, the concentration of ADH in the body fluids can change from small amounts to large amounts, or vice versa, in only a few minutes.

Somewhere in or near the hypothalamus are modified neuron receptors called *osmoreceptors.* When the extracellular fluid becomes too concentrated, fluid is pulled by osmosis out of the osmoreceptor cell, decreasing its size and initiating appropriate nerve signals in the hypothalamus to cause additional ADH secretion. Conversely, when the extracellular fluid becomes too dilute, water moves by osmosis in the opposite direction, into the cell, and this decreases the signal for ADH secretion. Although some researchers place these osmoreceptors in the hypothalamus itself (possibly even in the supraoptic nuclei), others believe that they are located in the *organum vasculosum,*

a highly vascular structure in the anteroventral wall of the third ventricle.

Regardless of the mechanism, concentrated body fluids stimulate the supraoptic nuclei, whereas dilute body fluids inhibit them. A feedback control system is available to control the total osmotic pressure of the body fluids.

Further details on the control of ADH secretion and the role of ADH in controlling renal function and body fluid osmolality are presented in Chapter 28.

Low Blood Volume and Low Blood Pressure Stimulate ADH Secretion—Vasoconstrictor Effects of ADH

Whereas minute concentrations of ADH cause increased water conservation by the kidneys, higher concentrations of ADH have a potent effect of constricting the arterioles throughout the body and therefore increasing the arterial pressure. For this reason, ADH has another name, *vasopressin.*

One of the stimuli for causing intense ADH secretion is decreased blood volume. This occurs strongly when the blood volume decreases 15 to 25 percent or more; the secretory rate then sometimes rises to as high as 50 times normal. The cause of this is the following.

The atria have stretch receptors that are excited by overfilling. When excited, they send signals to the brain to inhibit ADH secretion. Conversely, when the receptors are unexcited as a result of underfilling, the opposite occurs, with greatly increased ADH secretion. Decreased stretch of the baroreceptors of the carotid, aortic, and pulmonary regions also stimulates ADH secretion. For further details about this blood volume-pressure feedback mechanism, refer to Chapter 28.

Oxytocic Hormone

Oxytocin Causes Contraction of the Pregnant Uterus. The hormone *oxytocin*, in accordance with its name, powerfully stimulates contraction of the pregnant uterus, especially toward the end of gestation. Therefore, many obstetricians believe that this hormone is at least partially responsible for causing birth of the baby. This is supported by the following facts: (1) In a hypophysectomized animal, the duration of labor is prolonged, indicating a possible effect of oxytocin during delivery. (2) The amount of oxytocin in the plasma increases during labor, especially during the last stage. (3) Stimulation of the cervix in a pregnant animal elicits nervous signals that pass to the hypothalamus and cause increased secretion of oxytocin. These effects and this possible mechanism for aiding in the birth process are discussed in more detail in Chapter 82.

Oxytocin Aids in Milk Ejection by the Breasts. Oxytocin also plays an especially important role in lactation—a role that is far better understood than its role in delivery. In lactation, oxytocin causes milk to be expressed from the alveoli into the ducts of the breast so that the baby can obtain it by suckling.

This mechanism works as follows: The suckling stimulus on the nipple of the breast causes signals to be transmitted through sensory nerves to the oxytocin neurons in the paraventricular and supraoptic nuclei in the hypothalamus, which causes release of oxytocin by the posterior pituitary gland. The oxytocin is then carried by the blood to the breasts, where it causes contraction of *myoepithelial cells* that lie outside of and form a latticework surrounding the alveoli of the mammary glands. In less than a minute after the beginning of suckling, milk begins to flow. This mechanism is called *milk letdown* or *milk ejection.* It is discussed further in Chapter 82 in relation to the physiology of lactation.

Bibliography

Antunes-Rodrigues J, de Castro M, Elias LL, et al: Neuroendocrine control of body fluid metabolism, *Physiol Rev* 84:169, 2004.

Boone M, Deen PM: Physiology and pathophysiology of the vasopressin-regulated renal water reabsorption, *Pflugers Arch* 456:1005, 2008.

Burbach JP, Luckman SM, Murphy D, et al: Gene regulation in the magnocellular hypothalamo-neurohypophysial system, *Physiol Rev* 81:1197, 2001.

Chiamolera MI, Wondisford FE: Thyrotropin-releasing hormone and the thyroid hormone feedback mechanism, *Endocrinology* 150:1091, 2009.

Dattani M, Preece M: Growth hormone deficiency and related disorders: insights into causation, diagnosis, and treatment, *Lancet* 363:1977, 2004.

Donaldson ZR, Young LJ: Oxytocin, vasopressin, and the neurogenetics of sociality, *Science* 322:900, 2008.

Dunger DB: Determinants of short stature and the response to growth hormone therapy, *Horm Res* 71(Suppl 2):2, 2009.

Eugster EA, Pescovitz OH: Gigantism, *J Clin Endocrinol Metab* 84:4379, 1999.

Freeman ME, Kanyicska B, Lerant A, et al: Prolactin: structure, function, and regulation of secretion, *Physiol Rev* 80:1523, 2000.

Gimpl G, Fahrenholz F: The oxytocin receptor system: structure, function, and regulation, *Physiol Rev* 81:629, 2001.

Lohmeier TE: Neurohypophysial hormones, *Am J Physiol Regul Integr Comp Physiol* 285:R715, 2003.

McEwen BS: Physiology and neurobiology of stress and adaptation: central role of the brain, *Physiol Rev* 87:873, 2007.

Melmed S: Acromegaly pathogenesis and treatment, *J Clin Invest* 119:3189, 2009.

Møller N, Jørgensen JO: Effects of growth hormone on glucose, lipid, and protein metabolism in human subjects, *Endocr Rev* 30:152, 2009.

Nielsen S, Frokiaer J, Marples D, et al: Aquaporins in the kidney: from molecules to medicine, *Physiol Rev* 82:205, 2002.

Ohlsson C, Mohan S, Sjögren K, et al: The role of liver-derived insulin-like growth factor-I, *Endocr Rev* 30:494, 2009.

Rosenfeld RG: The future of research into growth hormone responsiveness, *Horm Res* 71(Suppl 2):71, 2009.

Rosenfeld RG, Hwa V: The growth hormone cascade and its role in mammalian growth, *Horm Res* 71(Suppl 2):36, 2009.

Schrier RW: Vasopressin and aquaporin 2 in clinical disorders of water homeostasis, *Semin Nephrol* 28:289, 2008.

Stricker EM, Sved AF: Controls of vasopressin secretion and thirst: similarities and dissimilarities in signals, *Physiol Behav* 77:731, 2002.

Zhu X, Gleiberman AS, Rosenfeld MG: Molecular physiology of pituitary development: signaling and transcriptional networks, *Physiol Rev* 87:933, 2007.

Thyroid Metabolic Hormones

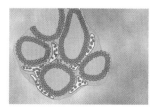

The thyroid gland, located immediately below the larynx on each side of and anterior to the trachea, is one of the largest of the endocrine glands, normally weighing 15 to 20 grams in adults. The thyroid secretes two major hormones, *thyroxine* and *triiodothyronine*, commonly called T_4 and T_3, respectively. Both of these hormones profoundly increase the metabolic rate of the body. Complete lack of thyroid secretion usually causes the basal metabolic rate to fall 40 to 50 percent below normal, and extreme excesses of thyroid secretion can increase the basal metabolic rate to 60 to 100 percent above normal. Thyroid secretion is controlled primarily by *thyroid-stimulating hormone* (TSH) secreted by the anterior pituitary gland.

The thyroid gland also secretes *calcitonin*, an important hormone for calcium metabolism that is considered in detail in Chapter 79.

The purpose of this chapter is to discuss the formation and secretion of the thyroid hormones, their metabolic functions, and regulation of their secretion.

Synthesis and Secretion of the Thyroid Metabolic Hormones

About 93 percent of the metabolically active hormones secreted by the thyroid gland is *thyroxine*, and 7 percent *triiodothyronine*. However, almost all the thyroxine is eventually converted to triiodothyronine in the tissues, so both are functionally important. The functions of these two hormones are qualitatively the same, but they differ in rapidity and intensity of action. Triiodothyronine is about four times as potent as thyroxine, but it is present in the blood in much smaller quantities and persists for a much shorter time than does thyroxine.

Physiologic Anatomy of the Thyroid Gland. The thyroid gland is composed, as shown in Figure 76-1, of large numbers of closed *follicles* (100 to 300 micrometers in diameter) filled with a secretory substance called

colloid and lined with *cuboidal epithelial cells* that secrete into the interior of the follicles. The major constituent of colloid is the large glycoprotein *thyroglobulin*, which contains the thyroid hormones. Once the secretion has entered the follicles, it must be absorbed back through the follicular epithelium into the blood before it can function in the body. The thyroid gland has a blood flow about five times the weight of the gland each minute, which is a blood supply as great as that of any other area of the body, with the possible exception of the adrenal cortex.

Iodine Is Required for Formation of Thyroxine

To form normal quantities of thyroxine, about 50 milligrams of ingested iodine in the form of iodides are required *each year*, or about *1 mg/week*. To prevent iodine deficiency, common table salt is iodized with about 1 part sodium iodide to every 100,000 parts sodium chloride.

Fate of Ingested Iodides. Iodides ingested orally are absorbed from the gastrointestinal tract into the blood in about the same manner as chlorides. Normally, most of the iodides are rapidly excreted by the kidneys, but only after about one fifth are selectively removed from the circulating blood by the cells of the thyroid gland and used for synthesis of the thyroid hormones.

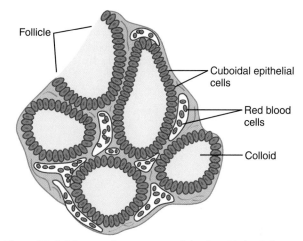

Figure 76-1 Microscopic appearance of the thyroid gland, showing secretion of thyroglobulin into the follicles.

907

Iodide Pump—the Sodium-Iodide Symporter (Iodide Trapping)

The first stage in the formation of thyroid hormones, shown in Figure 76-2, is transport of iodides from the blood into the thyroid glandular cells and follicles. The basal membrane of the thyroid cell has the specific ability to pump the iodide actively to the interior of the cell. This is achieved by the action of a *sodium-iodide symporter* (NIS), which co-transports one iodide ion along with two sodium ions across the basolateral (plasma) membrane into the cell. The energy for transporting iodide against a concentration gradient comes from the sodium-potassium ATPase pump, which pumps sodium out of the cell, thereby establishing a low intracellular sodium concentration and a gradient for facilitated diffusion of sodium into the cell.

This process of concentrating the iodide in the cell is called *iodide trapping*. In a normal gland, the iodide pump concentrates the iodide to about 30 times its concentration in the blood. When the thyroid gland becomes maximally active, this concentration ratio can rise to as high as 250 times. The rate of iodide trapping by the thyroid is influenced by several factors, the most important being the concentration of TSH; TSH stimulates and hypophysectomy greatly diminishes the activity of the iodide pump in thyroid cells.

Iodide is transported out of the thyroid cells across the apical membrane into the follicle by a chloride-iodide ion counter-transporter molecule called *pendrin*. The thyroid epithelial cells also secrete into the follicle thyroglobulin that contains tyrosine amino acids to which the iodide ions will bind, as discussed in the next section.

Thyroglobulin and Chemistry of Thyroxine and Triiodothyronine Formation

Formation and Secretion of Thyroglobulin by the Thyroid Cells.

The thyroid cells are typical protein-secreting glandular cells, as shown in Figure 76-2. The endoplasmic reticulum and Golgi apparatus synthesize and secrete into the follicles a large glycoprotein molecule called *thyroglobulin,* with a molecular weight of about 335,000.

Each molecule of thyroglobulin contains about 70 tyrosine amino acids, and they are the major substrates that combine with iodine to form the thyroid hormones. Thus, the thyroid hormones form *within* the thyroglobulin molecule. That is, the thyroxine and triiodothyronine hormones formed from the tyrosine amino acids remain part of the thyroglobulin molecule during synthesis of the thyroid hormones and even afterward as stored hormones in the follicular colloid.

Oxidation of the Iodide Ion.

The first essential step in the formation of the thyroid hormones is conversion of the iodide ions to an *oxidized form of iodine*, either nascent iodine (I^0) or I_3^-, that is then capable of combining directly with the amino acid tyrosine. This oxidation of iodine is promoted by the enzyme *peroxidase* and its accompanying *hydrogen peroxide*, which provide a potent system capable of oxidizing iodides. The peroxidase is either located in the apical membrane of the cell or attached to it, thus providing the oxidized iodine at exactly the point in the cell where the thyroglobulin molecule issues forth from the Golgi apparatus and through the cell membrane into the stored thyroid gland colloid. When the peroxidase system is blocked or when it is hereditarily absent from the cells, the rate of formation of thyroid hormones falls to zero.

Iodination of Tyrosine and Formation of the Thyroid Hormones—"Organification" of Thyroglobulin.

The binding of iodine with the thyroglobulin molecule is called *organification* of the thyroglobulin. Oxidized iodine even in the molecular form will bind directly but slowly with the amino acid tyrosine. In the thyroid cells, however, the oxidized iodine is associated with thyroid

Figure 76-2 Thyroid cellular mechanisms for iodine transport, thyroxine and triiodothyronine formation, and thyroxine and triiodothyronine release into the blood. DIT, diiodotyrosine; MIT, monoiodotyrosine; NIS, sodium-iodide symporter; RT_3, reverse triiodothyronine; T_3, triiodothyronine; T_4, thyroxine; T_G, thyroglobulin.

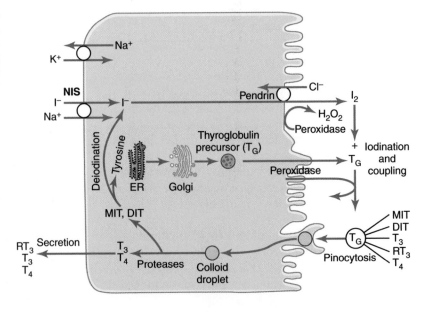

peroxidase enzyme (Figure 76-2) that causes the process to occur within seconds or minutes. Therefore, almost as rapidly as the thyroglobulin molecule is released from the Golgi apparatus or as it is secreted through the apical cell membrane into the follicle, iodine binds with about one sixth of the tyrosine amino acids within the thyroglobulin molecule.

Figure 76-3 shows the successive stages of iodination of tyrosine and final formation of the two important thyroid hormones, thyroxine and triiodothyronine. Tyrosine is first iodized to *monoiodotyrosine* and then to *diiodotyrosine*. Then, during the next few minutes, hours, and even days, more and more of the iodotyrosine residues become *coupled* with one another.

The major hormonal product of the coupling reaction is the molecule *thyroxine (T_4)*, which is formed when two molecules of diiodotyrosine are joined together; the thyroxine then remains part of the thyroglobulin molecule. Or one molecule of monoiodotyrosine couples with one molecule of diiodotyrosine to form *triiodothyronine (T_3)*, which represents about one fifteenth of the final hormones. Small amounts of *reverse T_3 (RT_3)* are formed by coupling of diiodotyrosine with monoiodotyrosine, but RT_3 does not appear to be of functional significance in humans.

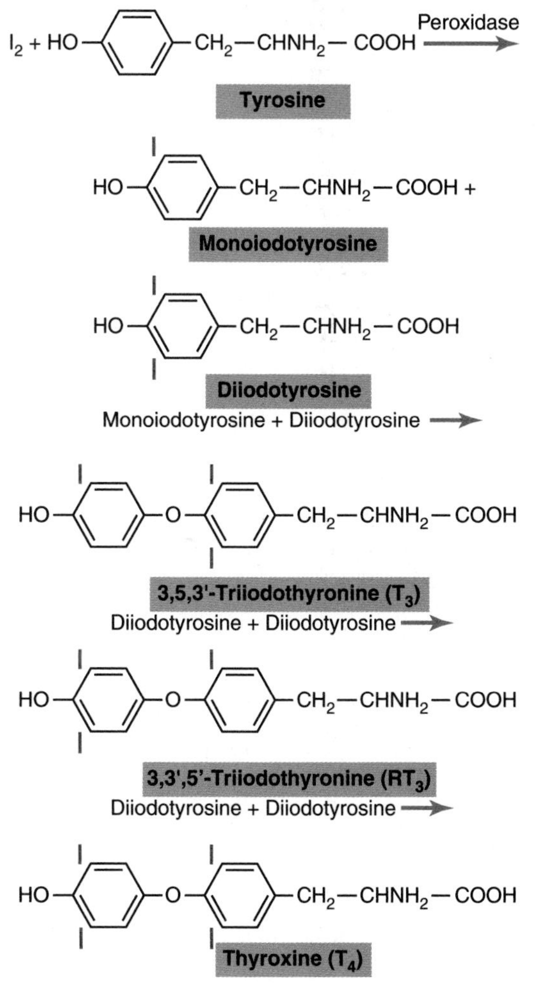

Figure 76-3 Chemistry of thyroxine and triiodothyronine formation.

Storage of Thyroglobulin.

The thyroid gland is unusual among the endocrine glands in its ability to store large amounts of hormone. After synthesis of the thyroid hormones has run its course, each thyroglobulin molecule contains up to 30 thyroxine molecules and a few triiodothyronine molecules. In this form, the thyroid hormones are stored in the follicles in an amount sufficient to supply the body with its normal requirements of thyroid hormones for 2 to 3 months. Therefore, when synthesis of thyroid hormone ceases, the physiologic effects of deficiency are not observed for several months.

Release of Thyroxine and Triiodothyronine from the Thyroid Gland

Thyroglobulin itself is not released into the circulating blood in measurable amounts; instead, thyroxine and triiodothyronine must first be cleaved from the thyroglobulin molecule, and then these free hormones are released. This process occurs as follows: The apical surface of the thyroid cells sends out pseudopod extensions that close around small portions of the colloid to form *pinocytic vesicles* that enter the apex of the thyroid cell. Then *lysosomes* in the cell cytoplasm immediately fuse with these vesicles to form digestive vesicles containing digestive enzymes from the lysosomes mixed with the colloid. Multiple *proteases* among the enzymes digest the thyroglobulin molecules and release thyroxine and triiodothyronine in free form. These then diffuse through the base of the thyroid cell into the surrounding capillaries. Thus, the thyroid hormones are released into the blood.

About three quarters of the iodinated tyrosine in the thyroglobulin never become thyroid hormones but remain monoiodotyrosine and diiodotyrosine. During the digestion of the thyroglobulin molecule to cause release of thyroxine and triiodothyronine, these iodinated tyrosines also are freed from the thyroglobulin molecules. However, they are not secreted into the blood. Instead, their iodine is cleaved from them by a *deiodinase enzyme* that makes virtually all this iodine available again for recycling within the gland for forming additional thyroid hormones. In the congenital absence of this deiodinase enzyme, many persons become iodine deficient because of failure of this recycling process.

Daily Rate of Secretion of Thyroxine and Triiodothyronine.

About 93 percent of the thyroid hormone released from the thyroid gland is normally thyroxine and only 7 percent is triiodothyronine. However, during the ensuing few days, about one half of the thyroxine is slowly deiodinated to form additional triiodothyronine. Therefore, the hormone finally delivered to and used by the tissues is mainly triiodothyronine, a total of about 35 micrograms of triiodothyronine per day.

Transport of Thyroxine and Triiodothyronine to Tissues

Thyroxine and Triiodothyronine Are Bound to Plasma Proteins. On entering the blood, more than

909

99 percent of the thyroxine and triiodothyronine combines immediately with several of the plasma proteins, all of which are synthesized by the liver. They combine mainly with *thyroxine-binding globulin* and much less so with *thyroxine-binding prealbumin* and *albumin*.

Thyroxine and Triiodothyronine Are Released Slowly to Tissue Cells. Because of high affinity of the plasma-binding proteins for the thyroid hormones, these substances—in particular, thyroxine—are released to the tissue cells slowly. Half the thyroxine in the blood is released to the tissue cells about every 6 days, whereas half the triiodothyronine—because of its lower affinity—is released to the cells in about 1 day.

On entering the tissue cells, both thyroxine and triiodothyronine again bind with intracellular proteins, the thyroxine binding more strongly than the triiodothyronine. Therefore, they are again stored, but this time in the target cells themselves, and they are used slowly over a period of days or weeks.

Thyroid Hormones Have Slow Onset and Long Duration of Action. After injection of a large quantity of thyroxine into a human being, essentially no effect on the metabolic rate can be discerned for 2 to 3 days, thereby demonstrating that there is a *long latent* period before thyroxine activity begins. Once activity does begin, it increases progressively and reaches a maximum in 10 to 12 days, as shown in Figure 76-4. Thereafter, it decreases with a half-life of about 15 days. Some of the activity persists for as long as 6 weeks to 2 months.

The actions of triiodothyronine occur about four times as rapidly as those of thyroxine, with a latent period as short as 6 to 12 hours and maximal cellular activity occurring within 2 to 3 days.

Most of the latency and prolonged period of action of these hormones are probably caused by their binding with proteins both in the plasma and in the tissue cells, followed by their slow release. However, we shall see in subsequent discussions that part of the latent period also results from the manner in which these hormones perform their functions in the cells themselves.

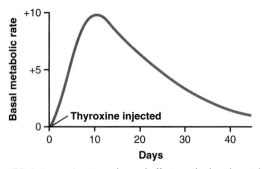

Figure 76-4 Approximate prolonged effect on the basal metabolic rate caused by administering a single large dose of thyroxine.

Physiological Functions of the Thyroid Hormones

Thyroid Hormones Increase the Transcription of Large Numbers of Genes

The general effect of thyroid hormone is to activate nuclear transcription of large numbers of genes (Figure 76-5). Therefore, in virtually all cells of the body, great numbers of protein enzymes, structural proteins, transport proteins, and other substances are synthesized. The net result is generalized increase in functional activity throughout the body.

Most of the Thyroxine Secreted by the Thyroid Is Converted to Triiodothyronine. Before acting on the genes to increase genetic transcription, one iodide is removed from almost all the thyroxine, thus forming triiodothyronine. Intracellular thyroid hormone receptors have a high affinity for triiodothyronine. Consequently, more than 90 percent of the thyroid hormone molecules that bind with the receptors is triiodothyronine.

Thyroid Hormones Activate Nuclear Receptors. The thyroid hormone receptors are either attached to the DNA genetic strands or located in proximity to them. The thyroid hormone receptor usually forms a heterodimer with *retinoid X receptor* (RXR) at specific *thyroid hormone response elements* on the DNA. On binding with thyroid hormone, the receptors become activated and initiate the transcription process. Then large numbers of different types of messenger RNA are formed, followed within another few minutes or hours by RNA translation on the cytoplasmic ribosomes to form hundreds of new intracellular proteins. However, not all the proteins are increased by similar percentages—some only slightly, and others at least as much as sixfold. It is believed that most of the actions of thyroid hormone result from the subsequent enzymatic and other functions of these new proteins.

Thyroid hormones also appear to have *nongenomic* cellular effects that are independent of their effects on gene transcription. For example, some effects of thyroid hormones occur within minutes, too rapidly to be explained by changes in protein synthesis, and are not affected by inhibitors of gene transcription and translation. Such actions have been described in several tissues, including the heart and pituitary, as well as adipose tissue. The site of nongenomic thyroid hormone action appears to be the plasma membrane, cytoplasm, and perhaps some cell organelles such as mitochondria. Nongenomic actions of thyroid hormone include the regulation of ion channels and oxidative phosphorylation and appear to involve the activation of intracellular secondary messengers such as cyclic AMP or protein kinase signaling cascades.

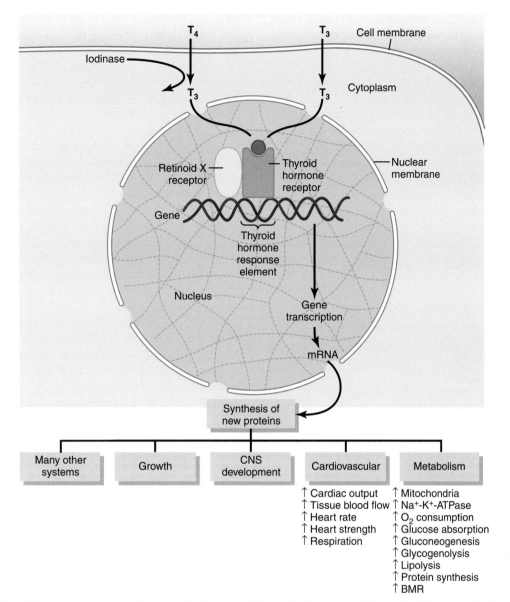

Figure 76-5 Thyroid hormone activation of target cells. Thyroxine (T₄) and triiodothyronine (T₃) readily diffuse through the cell membrane. Much of the T₄ is deiodinated to form T₃, which interacts with the thyroid hormone receptor, bound as a heterodimer with a retinoid X receptor, of the thyroid hormone response element of the gene. This causes either increases or decreases in transcription of genes that lead to formation of proteins, thus producing the thyroid hormone response of the cell. The actions of thyroid hormone on cells of several different systems are shown. mRNA, messenger ribonucleic acid.

Thyroid Hormones Increase Cellular Metabolic Activity

The thyroid hormones increase the metabolic activities of almost all the tissues of the body. The basal metabolic rate can increase to 60 to 100 percent above normal when large quantities of the hormones are secreted. The rate of utilization of foods for energy is greatly accelerated. Although the rate of protein synthesis is increased, at the same time the rate of protein catabolism is also increased. The growth rate of young people is greatly accelerated. The mental processes are excited, and the activities of most of the other endocrine glands are increased.

Thyroid Hormones Increase the Number and Activity of Mitochondria. When thyroxine or triiodothyronine is given to an animal, the mitochondria in most cells of the animal's body increase in size and number. Furthermore, the total membrane surface area of the mitochondria increases almost directly in proportion to the increased metabolic rate of the whole animal. Therefore, one of the principal functions of thyroxine might be simply to increase the number and activity of mitochondria, which in turn increases the rate of formation of adenosine triphosphate (ATP) to energize cellular function. However, the increase in the number and activity of mitochondria could be the *result* of increased activity of the cells as well as the cause of the increase.

Thyroid Hormones Increase Active Transport of Ions through Cell Membranes. One of the enzymes that increases its activity in response to thyroid hormone is *Na-K-ATPase*. This in turn increases the rate of transport of both sodium and potassium ions through the cell membranes of some tissues. Because this process uses energy and increases the amount of heat produced in the body, it has been suggested that this might be one of the mechanisms by which thyroid hormone increases the body's metabolic rate. In fact, thyroid hormone also causes the cell membranes of most cells to become leaky to sodium ions, which further activates the sodium pump and further increases heat production.

Effect of Thyroid Hormone on Growth

Thyroid hormone has both general and specific effects on growth. For instance, it has long been known that thyroid hormone is essential for the metamorphic change of the tadpole into the frog.

In humans, the effect of thyroid hormone on growth is manifest mainly in growing children. In those who are hypothyroid, the rate of growth is greatly retarded. In those who are hyperthyroid, excessive skeletal growth often occurs, causing the child to become considerably taller at an earlier age. However, the bones also mature more rapidly and the epiphyses close at an early age, so the duration of growth and the eventual height of the adult may actually be shortened.

An important effect of thyroid hormone is to promote growth and development of the brain during fetal life and for the first few years of postnatal life. If the fetus does not secrete sufficient quantities of thyroid hormone, growth and maturation of the brain both before birth and afterward are greatly retarded and the brain remains smaller than normal. Without specific thyroid therapy within days or weeks after birth, the child without a thyroid gland will remain mentally deficient throughout life. This is discussed more fully later in the chapter.

Effects of Thyroid Hormone on Specific Bodily Mechanisms

Stimulation of Carbohydrate Metabolism. Thyroid hormone stimulates almost all aspects of carbohydrate metabolism, including rapid uptake of glucose by the cells, enhanced glycolysis, enhanced gluconeogenesis, increased rate of absorption from the gastrointestinal tract, and even increased insulin secretion with its resultant secondary effects on carbohydrate metabolism. All these effects probably result from the overall increase in cellular metabolic enzymes caused by thyroid hormone.

Stimulation of Fat Metabolism. Essentially all aspects of fat metabolism are also enhanced under the influence of thyroid hormone. In particular, lipids are mobilized rapidly from the fat tissue, which decreases the fat stores of the body to a greater extent than almost any other tissue element. This also increases the free fatty acid concentration in the plasma and greatly accelerates the oxidation of free fatty acids by the cells.

Effect on Plasma and Liver Fats. *Increased* thyroid hormone *decreases* the concentrations of cholesterol, phospholipids, and triglycerides in the plasma, even though it *increases* the free fatty acids. Conversely, *decreased* thyroid secretion greatly *increases* the plasma concentrations of cholesterol, phospholipids, and triglycerides and almost always causes excessive deposition of fat in the liver as well. The large increase in circulating plasma cholesterol in prolonged hypothyroidism is often associated with severe atherosclerosis, discussed in Chapter 68.

One of the mechanisms by which thyroid hormone decreases the plasma cholesterol concentration is to increase significantly the rate of cholesterol secretion in the bile and consequent loss in the feces. A possible mechanism for the increased cholesterol secretion is that thyroid hormone induces increased numbers of low-density lipoprotein receptors on the liver cells, leading to rapid removal of low-density lipoproteins from the plasma by the liver and subsequent secretion of cholesterol in these lipoproteins by the liver cells.

Increased Requirement for Vitamins. Because thyroid hormone increases the quantities of many bodily enzymes and because vitamins are essential parts of some of the enzymes or coenzymes, thyroid hormone increases the need for vitamins. Therefore, a relative vitamin deficiency can occur when excess thyroid hormone is secreted, unless at the same time increased quantities of vitamins are made available.

Increased Basal Metabolic Rate. Because thyroid hormone increases metabolism in almost all cells of the body, excessive quantities of the hormone can occasionally increase the basal metabolic rate 60 to 100 percent above normal. Conversely, when no thyroid hormone is produced, the basal metabolic rate falls to almost one-half normal. Figure 76-6 shows the approximate relation between the daily supply of thyroid hormones and the basal metabolic rate. Extreme amounts of the hormones are required to cause high basal metabolic rates.

Decreased Body Weight. Greatly increased thyroid hormone almost always decreases the body weight, and greatly decreased thyroid hormone almost always increases the body weight; these effects do not always occur because thyroid hormone also increases the appetite, and this may counterbalance the change in the metabolic rate.

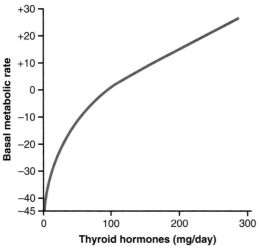

Figure 76-6 Approximate relation of daily rate of thyroid hormone (T_4 and T_3) secretion to the basal metabolic rate.

Effect of Thyroid Hormones on the Cardiovascular System

Increased Blood Flow and Cardiac Output. Increased metabolism in the tissues causes more rapid utilization of oxygen than normal and release of greater than normal quantities of metabolic end products from the tissues. These effects cause vasodilation in most body tissues, thus increasing blood flow. The rate of blood flow in the skin especially increases because of the increased need for heat elimination from the body. As a consequence of the increased blood flow, cardiac output also increases, sometimes rising to 60 percent or more above normal when excessive thyroid hormone is present and falling to only 50 percent of normal in severe hypothyroidism.

Increased Heart Rate. The heart rate increases considerably more under the influence of thyroid hormone than would be expected from the increase in cardiac output. Therefore, thyroid hormone seems to have a direct effect on the excitability of the heart, which in turn increases the heart rate. This effect is of particular importance because the heart rate is one of the sensitive physical signs that the clinician uses in determining whether a patient has excessive or diminished thyroid hormone production.

Increased Heart Strength. The increased enzymatic activity caused by increased thyroid hormone production apparently increases the strength of the heart when only a slight excess of thyroid hormone is secreted. This is analogous to the increase in heart strength that occurs in mild fevers and during exercise. However, when thyroid hormone is increased markedly, the heart muscle strength becomes depressed because of long-term excessive protein catabolism. Indeed, some severely thyrotoxic patients die of cardiac decompensation secondary to myocardial failure and to increased cardiac load imposed by the increase in cardiac output.

Normal Arterial Pressure. The *mean* arterial pressure usually remains about normal after administration of thyroid hormone. Because of increased blood flow through the tissues between heartbeats, the pulse pressure is often increased, with the systolic pressure elevated in hyperthyroidism 10 to 15 mm Hg and the diastolic pressure reduced a corresponding amount.

Increased Respiration. The increased rate of metabolism increases the utilization of oxygen and formation of carbon dioxide; these effects activate all the mechanisms that increase the rate and depth of respiration.

Increased Gastrointestinal Motility. In addition to increased appetite and food intake, which has been discussed, thyroid hormone increases both the rates of secretion of the digestive juices and the motility of the gastrointestinal tract. Hyperthyroidism therefore often results in diarrhea, whereas lack of thyroid hormone can cause constipation.

Excitatory Effects on the Central Nervous System. In general, thyroid hormone increases the rapidity of cerebration but also often dissociates this; conversely, lack of thyroid hormone decreases this function. The hyperthyroid individual is likely to have extreme nervousness and many psychoneurotic tendencies, such as anxiety complexes, extreme worry, and paranoia.

Effect on the Function of the Muscles. Slight increase in thyroid hormone usually makes the muscles react with vigor, but when the quantity of hormone becomes excessive, the muscles become weakened because of excess protein catabolism. Conversely, lack of thyroid hormone causes the muscles to become sluggish and they relax slowly after a contraction.

Muscle Tremor. One of the most characteristic signs of hyperthyroidism is a fine muscle tremor. This is not the coarse tremor that occurs in Parkinson disease or in shivering because it occurs at the rapid frequency of 10 to 15 times per second. The tremor can be observed easily by placing a sheet of paper on the extended fingers and noting the degree of vibration of the paper. This tremor is believed to be caused by increased reactivity of the neuronal synapses in the areas of the spinal cord that control muscle tone. The tremor is an important means for assessing the degree of thyroid hormone effect on the central nervous system.

Effect on Sleep. Because of the exhausting effect of thyroid hormone on the musculature and on the central nervous system, the hyperthyroid subject often has a feeling of constant tiredness, but because of the excitable effects of thyroid hormone on the synapses, it is difficult to sleep. Conversely, extreme somnolence is characteristic of hypothyroidism, with sleep sometimes lasting 12 to 14 hours a day.

Effect on Other Endocrine Glands. Increased thyroid hormone increases the rates of secretion of several other endocrine glands, but it also increases the need of the tissues for the hormones. For instance, increased thyroxine secretion increases the rate of glucose metabolism everywhere in the body and therefore causes a corresponding need for increased insulin secretion by the pancreas. Also, thyroid hormone increases many metabolic activities related to bone formation and, as a consequence, increases the need for parathyroid hormone. Thyroid hormone also increases the rate at which adrenal glucocorticoids are inactivated by the liver. This leads to feedback increase in adrenocorticotropic hormone (ACTH) production by the anterior pituitary and, therefore, increased rate of glucocorticoid secretion by the adrenal glands.

Effect of Thyroid Hormone on Sexual Function. For normal sexual function, thyroid secretion needs to be approximately normal. In men, lack of thyroid hormone is likely to cause loss of libido; great excesses of the hormone, however, sometimes cause impotence.

In women, lack of thyroid hormone often causes *menorrhagia* and *polymenorrhea*—that is, respectively, excessive and frequent menstrual bleeding. Yet, strangely enough, in other women thyroid lack may cause irregular periods and occasionally even *amenorrhea*.

A hypothyroid woman, like a man, is likely to have greatly decreased libido. To make the picture still more confusing, in the hyperthyroid woman, *oligomenorrhea*, which means greatly reduced bleeding, is common, and occasionally amenorrhea results.

The action of thyroid hormone on the gonads cannot be pinpointed to a specific function but probably results from a combination of direct metabolic effects on the gonads, as well as excitatory and inhibitory feedback effects operating through the anterior pituitary hormones that control the sexual functions.

Regulation of Thyroid Hormone Secretion

To maintain normal levels of metabolic activity in the body, precisely the right amount of thyroid hormone must be secreted at all times; to achieve this, specific feedback mechanisms operate through the hypothalamus and anterior pituitary gland to control the rate of thyroid secretion. These mechanisms are as follows.

TSH (from the Anterior Pituitary Gland) Increases Thyroid Secretion. TSH, also known as *thyrotropin*, is an anterior pituitary hormone, a glycoprotein with a molecular weight of about 28,000. This hormone, also discussed in Chapter 74, increases the secretion of thyroxine and triiodothyronine by the thyroid gland. Its specific effects on the thyroid gland are as follows:

1. *Increased proteolysis of the thyroglobulin* that has already been stored in the follicles, with resultant release of the thyroid hormones into the circulating blood and diminishment of the follicular substance itself

2. *Increased activity of the iodide pump*, which increases the rate of "iodide trapping" in the glandular cells, sometimes increasing the ratio of intracellular to extracellular iodide concentration in the glandular substance to as much as eight times normal

3. *Increased iodination of tyrosine* to form the thyroid hormones

4. *Increased size and increased secretory activity of the thyroid cells*

5. *Increased number of thyroid cells* plus a change from cuboidal to columnar cells and much infolding of the thyroid epithelium into the follicles

In summary, TSH increases all the known secretory activities of the thyroid glandular cells.

The most important early effect after administration of TSH is to initiate proteolysis of the thyroglobulin, which causes release of thyroxine and triiodothyronine into the blood within 30 minutes. The other effects require hours or even days and weeks to develop fully.

Cyclic Adenosine Monophosphate Mediates the Stimulatory Effect of TSH. In the past, it was difficult to explain the many and varied effects of TSH on the thyroid cell. It is now clear that most of these effects result from activation of the "second messenger" *cyclic adenosine monophosphate* (cAMP) system of the cell.

The first event in this activation is binding of TSH with specific TSH receptors on the basal membrane surfaces of the thyroid cell. This then activates *adenylyl cyclase* in the membrane, which increases the formation of cAMP inside the cell. Finally, the cAMP acts as a *second messenger* to activate protein kinase, which causes multiple phosphorylations throughout the cell. The result is both an immediate increase in secretion of thyroid hormones and prolonged growth of the thyroid glandular tissue itself.

This method for control of thyroid cell activity is similar to the function of cAMP as a "second messenger" in many other target tissues of the body, as discussed in Chapter 74.

Anterior Pituitary Secretion of TSH Is Regulated by Thyrotropin-Releasing Hormone from the Hypothalamus

Anterior pituitary secretion of TSH is controlled by a hypothalamic hormone, *thyrotropin-releasing hormone* (TRH), which is secreted by nerve endings in the median eminence of the hypothalamus. From the median eminence, the TRH is then transported to the anterior pituitary by way of the hypothalamic-hypophysial portal blood, as explained in Chapter 74.

TRH has been obtained in pure form. It is a simple substance, a tripeptide amide—*pyroglutamyl-histidyl-proline-amide*. TRH directly affects the anterior pituitary gland cells to increase their output of TSH. When the blood portal system from the hypothalamus to the anterior pituitary gland becomes blocked, the rate of secretion of TSH by the anterior pituitary decreases greatly but is not reduced to zero.

The molecular mechanism by which TRH causes the TSH-secreting cells of the anterior pituitary to produce TSH is first to bind with TRH receptors in the pituitary cell membrane. This in turn *activates the phospholipase second messenger system* inside the pituitary cells to produce large amounts of phospholipase C, followed by a cascade of other second messengers, including calcium ions and diacyl glycerol, which eventually leads to TSH release.

Effects of Cold and Other Neurogenic Stimuli on TRH and TSH Secretion.

One of the best-known stimuli for increasing the rate of TRH secretion by the hypothalamus, and therefore TSH secretion by the anterior pituitary gland, is exposure of an animal to cold. This effect almost certainly results from excitation of the hypothalamic centers for body temperature control. Exposure of rats for several weeks to severe cold increases the output of thyroid hormones sometimes to more than 100 percent of normal and can increase the basal metabolic rate as much as 50 percent. Indeed, persons moving to arctic regions have been known to develop basal metabolic rates 15 to 20 percent above normal.

Various emotional reactions can also affect the output of TRH and TSH and therefore indirectly affect the secretion of thyroid hormones. Excitement and anxiety—conditions that greatly stimulate the sympathetic nervous system—cause an acute decrease in secretion of TSH, perhaps because these states increase the metabolic rate and body heat and therefore exert an inverse effect on the heat control center.

Neither these emotional effects nor the effect of cold is observed after the hypophysial stalk has been cut, demonstrating that both of these effects are mediated by way of the hypothalamus.

Feedback Effect of Thyroid Hormone to Decrease Anterior Pituitary Secretion of TSH

Increased thyroid hormone in the body fluids decreases secretion of TSH by the anterior pituitary. When the rate of thyroid hormone secretion rises to about 1.75 times normal, the rate of TSH secretion falls essentially to zero. Almost all this feedback depressant effect occurs even when the anterior pituitary has been separated from the hypothalamus. Therefore, as shown in Figure 76-7, it is probable that increased thyroid hormone inhibits anterior pituitary secretion of TSH mainly by a direct effect on the anterior pituitary gland itself. Regardless of the mechanism of the feedback, its effect is to maintain an almost constant concentration of free thyroid hormones in the circulating body fluids.

Antithyroid Substances Suppress Thyroid Secretion

The best known antithyroid drugs are *thiocyanate, propylthiouracil,* and high concentrations of *inorganic iodides.* The mechanism by which each of these drugs blocks thyroid secretion is different from the others, and can be explained as follows.

Thiocyanate Ions Decrease Iodide Trapping.

The same active pump that transports iodide ions into the thyroid cells can also pump thiocyanate ions, perchlorate ions, and nitrate ions. Therefore, the administration of thiocyanate (or one of the other ions as well) in high enough concentration can cause competitive inhibition of iodide transport into the cell—that is, inhibition of the iodide-trapping mechanism.

The decreased availability of iodide in the glandular cells does not stop the formation of thyroglobulin; it merely prevents the thyroglobulin that is formed from becoming iodinated and therefore from forming the thyroid hormones. This deficiency of the thyroid hormones in turn leads to increased secretion of TSH by the anterior pituitary gland, which causes overgrowth of the thyroid gland even though the gland still does not form adequate quantities of thyroid hormones. Therefore, the use of thiocyanates and some other ions to block thyroid secretion can lead to development of a greatly enlarged thyroid gland, which is called a *goiter.*

Propylthiouracil Decreases Thyroid Hormone Formation.

Propylthiouracil (and other, similar compounds, such as methimazole and carbimazole) prevents formation of thyroid hormone from iodides and tyrosine. The mechanism of this is partly to block the peroxidase enzyme that is required for iodination of tyrosine and partly to block the coupling of two iodinated tyrosines to form thyroxine or triiodothyronine.

Propylthiouracil, like thiocyanate, does not prevent formation of thyroglobulin. The absence of thyroxine and triiodothyronine in the thyroglobulin can lead to tremendous feedback enhancement of TSH secretion by the anterior pituitary gland, thus promoting growth of the glandular tissue and forming a goiter.

Iodides in High Concentrations Decrease Thyroid Activity and Thyroid Gland Size.

When iodides are present in the blood in *high concentration* (100 times the normal plasma level), most activities of the thyroid gland are decreased, but often they remain decreased for only a few weeks. The effect is to reduce the rate of iodide trapping so that the rate of iodination of tyrosine to form thyroid hormones is also decreased. Even more important, the normal endocytosis of colloid from the follicles by the thyroid glandular cells is paralyzed by the high iodide concentrations. Because this is the first step in release of the thyroid hormones from the storage colloid, there is almost immediate shutdown of thyroid hormone secretion into the blood.

Because iodides in high concentrations decrease all phases of thyroid activity, they slightly decrease the size of the thyroid gland and especially decrease its blood supply, in contradistinction to the opposite effects caused by most of the other antithyroid agents. For this reason, iodides are frequently administered to patients for 2 to 3 weeks before surgical removal of the thyroid gland to decrease the necessary amount of surgery, especially to decrease the amount of bleeding.

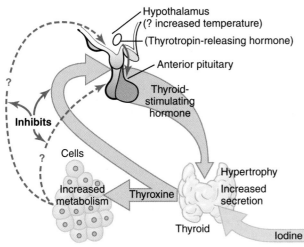

Figure 76-7 Regulation of thyroid secretion.

Diseases of the Thyroid

Hyperthyroidism

Most effects of hyperthyroidism are obvious from the preceding discussion of the various physiologic effects of thyroid hormone. However, some specific effects should be mentioned in connection especially with the development, diagnosis, and treatment of hyperthyroidism.

Causes of Hyperthyroidism (Toxic Goiter, Thyrotoxicosis, Graves' Disease). In most patients with hyperthyroidism, the thyroid gland is increased to two to three times' normal size, with tremendous hyperplasia and infolding of the follicular cell lining into the follicles, so the number of cells is increased greatly. Also, each cell increases its rate of secretion severalfold; radioactive iodine uptake studies indicate that some of these hyperplastic glands secrete thyroid hormone at rates 5 to 15 times normal.

Graves' disease, the most common form of hyperthyroidism, is an autoimmune disease in which antibodies called *thyroid-stimulating immunoglobulins* (TSIs) form against the TSH receptor in the thyroid gland. These antibodies bind with the same membrane receptors that bind TSH and induce continual activation of the cAMP system of the cells, with resultant development of hyperthyroidism. The TSI antibodies have a prolonged stimulating effect on the thyroid gland, lasting for as long as 12 hours, in contrast to a little over 1 hour for TSH. The high level of thyroid hormone secretion caused by TSI in turn suppresses anterior pituitary formation of TSH. Therefore, TSH concentrations are less than normal (often essentially zero) rather than enhanced in almost all patients with Graves' disease.

The antibodies that cause hyperthyroidism almost certainly occur as the result of autoimmunity that has developed against thyroid tissue. Presumably, at some time in the history of the person, an excess of thyroid cell antigens was released from the thyroid cells and this has resulted in the formation of antibodies against the thyroid gland itself.

Thyroid Adenoma. Hyperthyroidism occasionally results from a localized adenoma (a tumor) that develops in the thyroid tissue and secretes large quantities of thyroid hormone. This is different from the more usual type of hyperthyroidism in that it is usually not associated with evidence of any autoimmune disease. An interesting effect of the adenoma is that as long as it continues to secrete large quantities of thyroid hormone, secretory function in the remainder of the thyroid gland is almost totally inhibited because the thyroid hormone from the adenoma depresses the production of TSH by the pituitary gland.

Symptoms of Hyperthyroidism

The symptoms of hyperthyroidism are obvious from the preceding discussion of the physiology of the thyroid hormones: (1) a high state of excitability, (2) intolerance to heat, (3) increased sweating, (4) mild to extreme weight loss (sometimes as much as 100 pounds), (5) varying degrees of diarrhea, (6) muscle weakness, (7) nervousness or other psychic disorders, (8) extreme fatigue but inability to sleep, and (9) tremor of the hands.

Exophthalmos. Most people with hyperthyroidism develop some degree of protrusion of the eyeballs, as shown in Figure 76-8. This condition is called *exophthalmos.* A major degree of exophthalmos occurs in about one third of

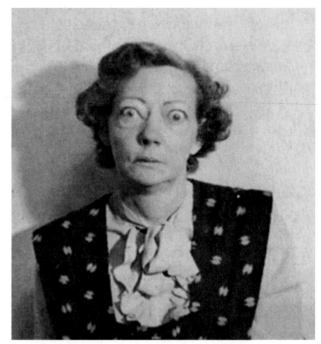

Figure 76-8 Patient with exophthalmic hyperthyroidism. Note protrusion of the eyes and retraction of the superior eyelids. The basal metabolic rate was +40. (Courtesy Dr. Leonard Posey.)

hyperthyroid patients, and the condition sometimes becomes so severe that the eyeball protrusion stretches the optic nerve enough to damage vision. Much more often, the eyes are damaged because the eyelids do not close completely when the person blinks or is asleep. As a result, the epithelial surfaces of the eyes become dry and irritated and often infected, resulting in ulceration of the cornea.

The cause of the protruding eyes is edematous swelling of the retro-orbital tissues and degenerative changes in the extraocular muscles. In most patients, immunoglobulins that react with the eye muscles can be found in the blood. Furthermore, the concentration of these immunoglobulins is usually highest in patients who have high concentrations of TSIs. Therefore, there is much reason to believe that exophthalmos, like hyperthyroidism itself, is an autoimmune process. The exophthalmos is usually greatly ameliorated with treatment of the hyperthyroidism.

Diagnostic Tests for Hyperthyroidism. For the usual case of hyperthyroidism, the most accurate diagnostic test is direct measurement of the concentration of "free" thyroxine (and sometimes triiodothyronine) in the plasma, using appropriate radioimmunoassay procedures.

Other tests that are sometimes used are as follows:

1. The basal metabolic rate is usually increased to +30 to +60 in severe hyperthyroidism.

2. The concentration of TSH in the plasma is measured by radioimmunoassay. In the usual type of thyrotoxicosis, anterior pituitary secretion of TSH is so completely suppressed by the large amounts of circulating thyroxine and triiodothyronine that there is almost no plasma TSH.

3. The concentration of TSI is measured by radioimmunoassay. This is usually high in thyrotoxicosis but low in thyroid adenoma.

Physiology of Treatment in Hyperthyroidism. The most direct treatment for hyperthyroidism is surgical removal of most of the thyroid gland. In general, it is desirable to prepare the patient for surgical removal of the gland before the operation. This is done by administering propylthiouracil, usually for several weeks, until the basal metabolic rate of the patient has returned to normal. Then, administration of high concentrations of iodides for 1 to 2 weeks immediately before operation causes the gland itself to recede in size and its blood supply to diminish. By using these preoperative procedures, the operative mortality is less than 1 in 1000 in the better hospitals, whereas before development of modern procedures, operative mortality was 1 in 25.

Treatment of the Hyperplastic Thyroid Gland with Radioactive Iodine

Eighty to 90 percent of an injected dose of iodide is absorbed by the hyperplastic, toxic thyroid gland within 1 day after injection. If this injected iodine is radioactive, it can destroy most of the secretory cells of the thyroid gland. Usually 5 millicuries of radioactive iodine is given to the patient, whose condition is reassessed several weeks later. If the patient is still hyperthyroid, additional doses are administered until normal thyroid status is reached.

Hypothyroidism

The effects of hypothyroidism, in general, are opposite to those of hyperthyroidism, but there are a few physiological mechanisms peculiar to hypothyroidism. Hypothyroidism, like hyperthyroidism, is often initiated by autoimmunity against the thyroid gland (*Hashimoto disease*), but immunity that destroys the gland rather than stimulates it. The thyroid glands of most of these patients first have autoimmune "thyroiditis," which means thyroid inflammation. This causes progressive deterioration and finally fibrosis of the gland, with resultant diminished or absent secretion of thyroid hormone. Several other types of hypothyroidism also occur, often associated with development of enlarged thyroid glands, called *thyroid goiter*, as follows.

Endemic Colloid Goiter Caused by Dietary Iodide Deficiency. The term "goiter" means a greatly enlarged thyroid gland. As pointed out in the discussion of iodine metabolism, about 50 milligrams of iodine are required *each year* for the formation of adequate quantities of thyroid hormone. In certain areas of the world, notably in the Swiss Alps, the Andes, and the Great Lakes region of the United States, insufficient iodine is present in the soil for the foodstuffs to contain even this minute quantity. Therefore, in the days before iodized table salt, many people who lived in these areas developed extremely large thyroid glands, called *endemic goiters.*

The mechanism for development of large endemic goiters is the following: Lack of iodine prevents production of both thyroxine and triiodothyronine. As a result, no hormone is available to inhibit production of TSH by the anterior pituitary; this causes the pituitary to secrete excessively large quantities of TSH. The TSH then stimulates the thyroid cells to secrete tremendous amounts of thyroglobulin colloid into the follicles, and the gland grows larger and larger. But because of lack of iodine, thyroxine and triiodothyronine production does not occur in the thyroglobulin molecule and therefore does not cause the normal suppression of TSH production by the anterior pituitary. The follicles become tremendous in size, and the thyroid gland may increase to 10 to 20 times' normal size.

Idiopathic Nontoxic Colloid Goiter. Enlarged thyroid glands similar to those of endemic colloid goiter can also occur in people who do not have iodine deficiency. These goitrous glands may secrete normal quantities of thyroid hormones, but more frequently, the secretion of hormone is depressed, as in endemic colloid goiter.

The exact cause of the enlarged thyroid gland in patients with idiopathic colloid goiter is not known, but most of these patients show signs of mild thyroiditis; therefore, it has been suggested that the thyroiditis causes slight hypothyroidism, which then leads to increased TSH secretion and progressive growth of the noninflamed portions of the gland. This could explain why these glands are usually nodular, with some portions of the gland growing while other portions are being destroyed by thyroiditis.

In some persons with colloid goiter, the thyroid gland has an abnormality of the enzyme system required for formation of the thyroid hormones. Among the abnormalities often encountered are the following:

1. *Deficient iodide-trapping mechanism,* in which iodine is not pumped adequately into the thyroid cells

2. *Deficient peroxidase system,* in which the iodides are not oxidized to the iodine state

3. *Deficient coupling of iodinated tyrosines in the thyroglobulin molecule* so that the final thyroid hormones cannot be formed

4. *Deficiency of the deiodinase enzyme,* which prevents recovery of iodine from the iodinated tyrosines that are not coupled to form the thyroid hormones (this is about two thirds of the iodine), thus leading to iodine deficiency

Finally, some foods contain *goitrogenic substances* that have a propylthiouracil-type of antithyroid activity, thus also leading to TSH-stimulated enlargement of the thyroid gland. Such goitrogenic substances are found especially in some varieties of turnips and cabbages.

Physiological Characteristics of Hypothyroidism. Whether hypothyroidism is due to thyroiditis, endemic colloid goiter, idiopathic colloid goiter, destruction of the thyroid gland by irradiation, or surgical removal of the thyroid gland, the physiological effects are the same. They include fatigue and extreme somnolence with sleeping up to 12 to 14 hours a day, extreme muscular sluggishness, slowed heart rate, decreased cardiac output, decreased blood volume, sometimes increased body weight, constipation, mental sluggishness, failure of many trophic functions in the body evidenced by depressed growth of hair and scaliness of the skin, development of a froglike husky voice, and, in severe cases, development of an edematous appearance throughout the body called myxedema.

Myxedema. *Myxedema* develops in the patient with almost total lack of thyroid hormone function. Figure 76-9 shows such a patient, demonstrating bagginess under the eyes and swelling of the face. In this condition, for reasons not explained, greatly increased quantities of hyaluronic acid and chondroitin sulfate bound with protein form excessive tissue gel in the interstitial spaces, and this causes the total quantity of interstitial fluid to increase. Because of the

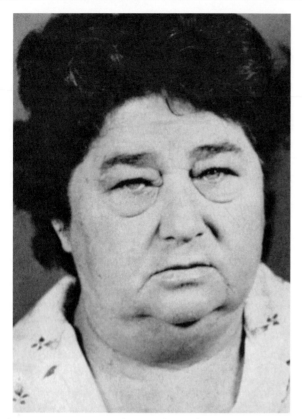

Figure 76-9 Patient with myxedema. (Courtesy Dr. Herbert Langford.)

gel nature of the excess fluid, it is mainly immobile and the edema is the nonpitting type.

Atherosclerosis in Hypothyroidism. As pointed out earlier, lack of thyroid hormone increases the quantity of blood cholesterol because of altered fat and cholesterol metabolism and diminished liver excretion of cholesterol in the bile. The increase in blood cholesterol is usually associated with increased atherosclerosis. Therefore, many hypothyroid patients, particularly those with myxedema, develop atherosclerosis, which in turn results in peripheral vascular disease, deafness, and coronary artery disease with consequent early death.

Diagnostic Tests in Hypothyroidism. The tests already described for diagnosis of hyperthyroidism give opposite results in hypothyroidism. The free thyroxine in the blood is low. The basal metabolic rate in myxedema ranges between −30 and −50. And the secretion of TSH by the anterior pituitary when a test dose of TRH is administered is usually greatly increased (except in those rare instances of hypothyroidism caused by depressed response of the pituitary gland to TRH).

Treatment of Hypothyroidism. Figure 76-4 shows the effect of thyroxine on the basal metabolic rate, demonstrating that the hormone normally has a duration of action of more than 1 month. Consequently, it is easy to maintain a steady level of thyroid hormone activity in the body by daily oral ingestion of a tablet or more containing thyroxine. Furthermore, proper treatment of the hypothyroid patient results in such complete normality that formerly myxedematous patients have lived into their 90s after treatment for more than 50 years.

Cretinism

Cretinism is caused by extreme hypothyroidism during fetal life, infancy, or childhood. This condition is characterized especially by failure of body growth and by mental retardation. It results from congenital lack of a thyroid gland (*congenital cretinism*), from failure of the thyroid gland to produce thyroid hormone because of a genetic defect of the gland, or from iodine lack in the diet *(endemic cretinism)*. The severity of endemic cretinism varies greatly, depending on the amount of iodine in the diet, and whole populaces of an endemic geographic iodine-deficient soil area have been known to have cretinoid tendencies.

A neonate without a thyroid gland may have normal appearance and function because it was supplied with some (but usually not enough) thyroid hormone by the mother while in utero. A few weeks after birth, however, the neonate's movements become sluggish and both physical and mental growth begin to be greatly retarded. Treatment of the neonate with cretinism at any time with adequate iodine or thyroxine usually causes normal return of physical growth, but unless the cretinism is treated within a few weeks after birth, mental growth remains permanently retarded. This results from retardation of the growth, branching, and myelination of the neuronal cells of the central nervous system at this critical time in the normal development of the mental powers.

Skeletal growth in the child with cretinism is characteristically more inhibited than is soft tissue growth. As a result of this disproportionate rate of growth, the soft tissues are likely to enlarge excessively, giving the child with cretinism an obese, stocky, and short appearance. Occasionally the tongue becomes so large in relation to the skeletal growth that it obstructs swallowing and breathing, inducing a characteristic guttural breathing that sometimes chokes the child.

Bibliography

Bizhanova A, Kopp P: The sodium-iodide symporter NIS and pendrin in iodide homeostasis of the thyroid, *Endocrinology* 150:1084, 2009.

Brent GA: Clinical practice. Graves' disease, *N Engl J Med* 358:2594, 2008.

Chiamolera MI, Wondisford FE: Thyrotropin-releasing hormone and the thyroid hormone feedback mechanism, *Endocrinology* 150:1091, 2009.

De La Vieja A, Dohan O, Levy O, et al: Molecular analysis of the sodium/iodide symporter: impact on thyroid and extrathyroid pathophysiology, *Physiol Rev* 80:1083, 2000.

Dayan CM: Interpretation of thyroid function tests, *Lancet* 357:619, 2001.

Dayan CM, Panicker V: Novel insights into thyroid hormones from the study of common genetic variation, *Nat Rev Endocrinol* 5:211, 2009.

Dohan O, De La Vieja A, Paroder V, et al: The sodium/iodide Symporter (NIS): characterization, regulation, and medical significance, *Endocr Rev* 24:48, 2003.

Gereben B, Zavacki AM, Ribich S, et al: Cellular and molecular basis of deiodinase-regulated thyroid hormone signaling, *Endocr Rev* 29:898, 2008.

Heuer H, Visser TJ: Pathophysiological importance of thyroid hormone transporters, *Endocrinology* 150:1078, 2009.

Kharlip J, Cooper DS: Recent developments in hyperthyroidism, *Lancet* 373:1930, 2009.

Klein I, Danzi S: Thyroid disease and the heart, *Circulation* 116:1725, 2007.

O'Reilly DS: Thyroid function tests—time for a reassessment, *BMJ* 320:1332, 2000.

Pearce EN, Farwell AP, Braverman LE: Thyroiditis, *N Engl J Med* 348:2646, 2003.

St Germain DL, Galton VA, Hernandez A: Defining the roles of the iodothyronine deiodinases: current concepts and challenges, *Endocrinology* 150:1097, 2009.

Szkudlinski MW, Fremont V, Ronin C, et al: Thyroid-stimulating hormone and thyroid-stimulating hormone receptor structure-function relationships, *Physiol Rev* 82:473, 2002.

Vasudevan N, Ogawa S, Pfaff D: Estrogen and thyroid hormone receptor interactions: physiological flexibility by molecular specificity, *Physiol Rev* 82:923, 2002.

Yen PM: Physiological and molecular basis of thyroid hormone action, *Physiol Rev* 81:1097, 2001.

Zimmermann MB: Iodine deficiency, *Endocr Rev* 30:376, 2009.

UNIT XIV

Adrenocortical Hormones

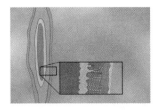

The two *adrenal glands,* each of which weighs about 4 grams, lie at the superior poles of the two kidneys. As shown in Figure 77-1, each gland is composed of two distinct parts, the *adrenal medulla* and the *adrenal cortex.* The adrenal medulla, the central 20 percent of the gland, is functionally related to the sympathetic nervous system; it secretes the hormones *epinephrine* and *norepinephrine* in response to sympathetic stimulation. In turn, these hormones cause almost the same effects as direct stimulation of the sympathetic nerves in all parts of the body. These hormones and their effects are discussed in detail in Chapter 60 in relation to the sympathetic nervous system.

The adrenal cortex secretes an entirely different group of hormones, called *corticosteroids.* These hormones are all synthesized from the steroid cholesterol, and they all have similar chemical formulas. However, slight differences in their molecular structures give them several different but very important functions.

Corticosteroids: Mineralocorticoids, Glucocorticoids, and Androgens. Two major types of adrenocortical hormones, the *mineralocorticoids* and the *glucocorticoids,* are secreted by the adrenal cortex. In addition to these, small amounts of sex hormones are secreted, especially *androgenic hormones,* which exhibit about the same effects in the body as the male sex hormone testosterone. They are normally of only slight importance, although in certain abnormalities of the adrenal cortices, extreme quantities can be secreted (which is discussed later in the chapter) and can result in masculinizing effects.

The *mineralocorticoids* have gained this name because they especially affect the electrolytes (the "minerals") of the extracellular fluids, especially sodium and potassium. The *glucocorticoids* have gained their name because they exhibit important effects that increase blood glucose concentration. They have additional effects on both protein and fat metabolism that are equally as important to body function as their effects on carbohydrate metabolism.

More than 30 steroids have been isolated from the adrenal cortex, but two are of exceptional importance to the normal endocrine function of the human body: *aldosterone,* which is the principal mineralocorticoid, and *cortisol,* which is the principal glucocorticoid.

Synthesis and Secretion of Adrenocortical Hormones

The Adrenal Cortex Has Three Distinct Layers. Figure 77-1 shows that the adrenal cortex is composed of three relatively distinct layers:

1. The *zona glomerulosa,* a thin layer of cells that lies just underneath the capsule, constitutes about 15 percent of the adrenal cortex. These cells are the only ones in the adrenal gland capable of secreting significant amounts of *aldosterone* because they contain the enzyme *aldosterone synthase,* which is necessary for

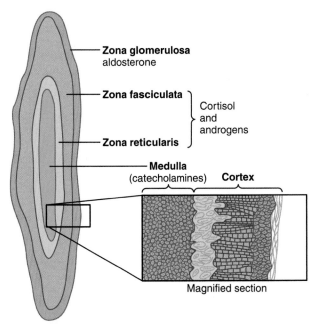

Figure 77-1 Secretion of adrenocortical hormones by the different zones of the adrenal cortex and secretion of catecholamines by the adrenal medulla.

synthesis of aldosterone. The secretion of these cells is controlled mainly by the extracellular fluid concentrations of *angiotensin II* and *potassium,* both of which stimulate aldosterone secretion.

2. The *zona fasciculata,* the middle and widest layer, constitutes about 75 percent of the adrenal cortex and secretes the glucocorticoids *cortisol* and *corticosterone,* as well as small amounts of *adrenal androgens* and *estrogens.* The secretion of these cells is controlled in large part by the hypothalamic-pituitary axis via *adrenocorticotropic hormone* (ACTH).

3. The *zona reticularis,* the deep layer of the cortex, secretes the adrenal androgens *dehydroepiandrosterone* (DHEA) and *androstenedione,* as well as small amounts of estrogens and some glucocorticoids. ACTH also regulates secretion of these cells, although other factors such as *cortical androgen-stimulating hormone,* released from the pituitary, may also be involved. The mechanisms for controlling adrenal androgen production, however, are not nearly as well understood as those for glucocorticoids and mineralocorticoids.

Aldosterone and cortisol secretion are regulated by independent mechanisms. Factors such as angiotensin II that specifically increase the output of aldosterone and cause hypertrophy of the zona glomerulosa have no effect on the other two zones. Similarly, factors such as ACTH that increase secretion of cortisol and adrenal androgens and cause hypertrophy of the zona fasciculata and zona reticularis have little effect on the zona glomerulosa.

Adrenocortical Hormones Are Steroids Derived from Cholesterol. All human steroid hormones, including those produced by the adrenal cortex, are synthesized from cholesterol. Although the cells of the adrenal cortex can synthesize de novo small amounts of cholesterol from acetate, approximately 80 percent of the cholesterol used for steroid synthesis is provided by low-density lipoproteins (LDL) in the circulating plasma. The LDLs, which have high concentrations of cholesterol, diffuse from the plasma into the interstitial fluid and attach to specific receptors contained in structures called *coated pits* on the adrenocortical cell membranes. The coated pits are then internalized by *endocytosis,* forming vesicles that eventually fuse with cell lysosomes and release cholesterol that can be used to synthesize adrenal steroid hormones.

Transport of cholesterol into the adrenal cells is regulated by feedback mechanisms that can markedly alter the amount available for steroid synthesis. For example, ACTH, which stimulates adrenal steroid synthesis, increases the number of adrenocortical cell receptors for LDL, as well as the activity of enzymes that liberate cholesterol from LDL.

Once the cholesterol enters the cell, it is delivered to the mitochondria, where it is cleaved by the enzyme *cholesterol desmolase* to form *pregnenolone;* this is the rate-limiting step in the eventual formation of adrenal steroids (Figure 77-2). In all three zones of the adrenal cortex, this initial step in steroid synthesis is stimulated by the different factors that control secretion of the major hormone products aldosterone and cortisol. For example, both ACTH, which stimulates cortisol secretion, and angiotensin II, which stimulates

aldosterone secretion, increase the conversion of cholesterol to pregnenolone.

Synthetic Pathways for Adrenal Steroids. Figure 77-2 gives the principal steps in the formation of the important steroid products of the adrenal cortex: aldosterone, cortisol, and the androgens. Essentially all these steps occur in two of the organelles of the cell, the *mitochondria* and the *endoplasmic reticulum,* some steps occurring in one of these organelles and some in the other. Each step is catalyzed by a specific enzyme system. A change in even a single enzyme in the schema can cause vastly different types and relative proportions of hormones to be formed. For example, very large quantities of masculinizing sex hormones or other steroid compounds not normally present in the blood can occur with altered activity of only one of the enzymes in this pathway.

The chemical formulas of aldosterone and cortisol, which are the most important mineralocorticoid and glucocorticoid hormones, respectively, are shown in Figure 77-2. Cortisol has a keto-oxygen on carbon number 3 and is hydroxylated at carbon numbers 11 and 21. The mineralocorticoid aldosterone has an oxygen atom bound at the number 18 carbon.

In addition to aldosterone and cortisol, other steroids having glucocorticoid or mineralocorticoid activities, or both, are normally secreted in small amounts by the adrenal cortex. And several additional potent steroid hormones not normally formed in the adrenal glands have been synthesized and are used in various forms of therapy. Some of the more important of the corticosteroid hormones, including the synthetic ones, are the following, as summarized in Table 77-1.

Mineralocorticoids

- Aldosterone (very potent, accounts for about 90 percent of all mineralocorticoid activity)
- Deoxycorticosterone (1/30 as potent as aldosterone, but very small quantities secreted)
- Corticosterone (slight mineralocorticoid activity)
- 9α-Fluorocortisol (synthetic, slightly more potent than aldosterone)
- Cortisol (very slight mineralocorticoid activity, but large quantity secreted)
- Cortisone (slight mineralocorticoid activity)

Glucocorticoids

- Cortisol (very potent, accounts for about 95 percent of all glucocorticoid activity)
- Corticosterone (provides about 4 percent of total glucocorticoid activity, but much less potent than cortisol)
- Cortisone (almost as potent as cortisol)
- Prednisone (synthetic, four times as potent as cortisol)
- Methylprednisone (synthetic, five times as potent as cortisol)
- Dexamethasone (synthetic, 30 times as potent as cortisol)

It is clear from this list that some of these hormones have both glucocorticoid and mineralocorticoid activities. It is especially significant that cortisol normally has some mineralocorticoid activity, because some syndromes of excess cortisol secretion can cause significant mineralocorticoid effects, along with its much more potent glucocorticoid effects.

The intense glucocorticoid activity of the synthetic hormone dexamethasone, which has almost zero

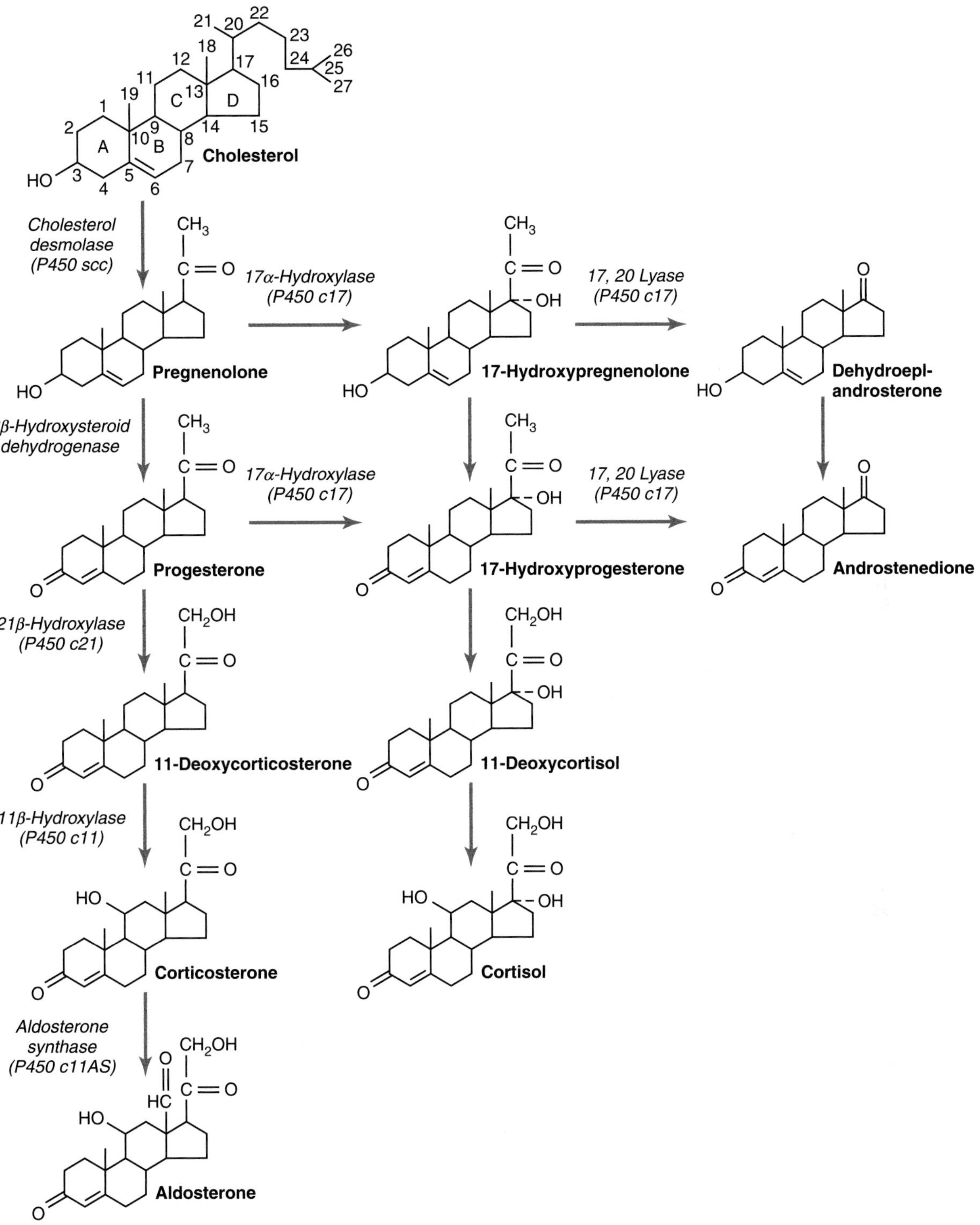

Figure 77-2 Pathways for synthesis of steroid hormones by the adrenal cortex. The enzymes are shown in italics.

mineralocorticoid activity, makes this an especially important drug for stimulating specific glucocorticoid activity.

Adrenocortical Hormones Are Bound to Plasma Proteins. Approximately 90 to 95 percent of the cortisol in the plasma binds to plasma proteins, especially a globulin called *cortisol-binding globulin* or *transcortin* and, to a lesser extent, to albumin. This high degree of binding to plasma proteins slows the elimination of cortisol from the plasma; therefore, cortisol has a relatively long half-life of 60 to 90 minutes. Only about 60 percent of circulating aldosterone

combines with the plasma proteins, so about 40 percent is in the free form; as a result, aldosterone has a relatively short half-life of about 20 minutes. These hormones are transported throughout the extracellular fluid compartment in both the combined and free forms.

Binding of adrenal steroids to the plasma proteins may serve as a reservoir to lessen rapid fluctuations in free hormone concentrations, as would occur, for example, with cortisol during brief periods of stress and episodic secretion of ACTH. This reservoir function may also help to ensure a

Table 77-1 Adrenal Steroid Hormones in Adults; Synthetic Steroids and Their Relative Glucocorticoid and Mineralocorticoid Activities

Steroids	Average Plasma Concentration (free and bound, µg/100 ml)	Average Amount Secreted (mg/24 hr)	Glucocorticoid Activity	Mineralocorticoid Activity
Adrenal Steroids				
Cortisol	12	15	1.0	1.0
Corticosterone	0.4	3	0.3	15.0
Aldosterone	0.006	0.15	0.3	3000
Deoxycorticosterone	0.006	0.2	0.2	100
Dehydroepiandrosterone	175	20	—	—
Synthetic Steroids				
Cortisone	—	—	0.8	1.0
Prednisolone	—	—	4	0.8
Methylprednisone	—	—	5	—
Dexamethasone	—	—	30	—
9α-fluorocortisol	—	—	10	125

Glucocorticoid and mineralocorticoid activities of the steroids are relative to cortisol, with cortisol being 1.0.

relatively uniform distribution of the adrenal hormones to the tissues.

Adrenocortical Hormones Are Metabolized in the Liver. The adrenal steroids are degraded mainly in the liver and conjugated especially to *glucuronic acid* and, to a lesser extent, sulfates. These substances are inactive and do not have mineralocorticoid or glucocorticoid activity. About 25 percent of these conjugates are excreted in the bile and then in the feces. The remaining conjugates formed by the liver enter the circulation but are not bound to plasma proteins, are highly soluble in the plasma, and are therefore filtered readily by the kidneys and excreted in the urine. Diseases of the liver markedly depress the rate of inactivation of adrenocortical hormones, and kidney diseases reduce the excretion of the inactive conjugates.

The normal concentration of aldosterone in blood is about 6 nanograms (6 billionths of a gram) per 100 milliliters, and the average secretory rate is approximately 150 µg/day (0.15 mg/day). The blood concentration of aldosterone, however, depends greatly on several factors including dietary intake of sodium and potassium.

The concentration of cortisol in the blood averages 12 µg/100 ml, and the secretory rate averages 15 to 20 mg/day. However, blood concentration and secretion rate of cortisol fluctuate throughout the day, rising in the early morning and declining in the evening, as discussed later.

Functions of the Mineralocorticoids—Aldosterone

Mineralocorticoid Deficiency Causes Severe Renal Sodium Chloride Wasting and Hyperkalemia. Total loss of adrenocortical secretion usually causes death within 3 days to 2 weeks unless the person receives extensive salt therapy or injection of mineralocorticoids.

Without mineralocorticoids, potassium ion concentration of the extracellular fluid rises markedly, sodium and chloride are rapidly lost from the body, and the total extracellular fluid volume and blood volume become greatly reduced. The person soon develops diminished cardiac output, which progresses to a shocklike state, followed by death. This entire sequence can be prevented by the administration of aldosterone or some other mineralocorticoid. Therefore, the mineralocorticoids are said to be the acute "lifesaving" portion of the adrenocortical hormones. The glucocorticoids are equally necessary, however, allowing the person to resist the destructive effects of life's intermittent physical and mental "stresses," as discussed later in the chapter.

Aldosterone Is the Major Mineralocorticoid Secreted by the Adrenals. Aldosterone exerts nearly 90 percent of the mineralocorticoid activity of the adrenocortical secretions, but cortisol, the major glucocorticoid secreted by the adrenal cortex, also provides a significant amount of mineralocorticoid activity. Aldosterone's mineralocorticoid activity is about 3000 times greater than that of cortisol, but the plasma concentration of cortisol is nearly 2000 times that of aldosterone.

Cortisol can also bind to mineralocorticoid receptors with high affinity. However, the renal epithelial cells also contain the enzyme 11β-hydroxysteroid dehydrogenase type 2, which converts cortisol to cortisone. Because cortisone does not avidly bind mineralocorticoid receptors, cortisol does not normally exert significant mineralocorticoid effects. However, in patients with genetic deficiency of 11β-hydroxysteroid dehydrogenase type 2 activity, cortisol may have substantial mineralocorticoid effects. This condition is called *apparent mineralocorticoid excess syndrome* (AME) because the patient has essentially the same pathophysiological changes as a patient with excess aldosterone secretion, except that plasma aldosterone levels are very low. Ingestion of large amounts of licorice, which contains glycyrrhetinic acid, may also cause AME due to its ability to block 11β-hydroxysteroid dehydrogenase type 2 enzyme activity.

Renal and Circulatory Effects of Aldosterone

Aldosterone Increases Renal Tubular Reabsorption of Sodium and Secretion of Potassium. It will be recalled from Chapter 27 that aldosterone increases reabsorption of sodium and simultaneously increases secretion of potassium by the renal tubular epithelial cells, especially in the *principal cells of the collecting tubules* and, to a lesser extent, in the distal tubules and collecting ducts. Therefore, aldosterone causes sodium to be conserved in the extracellular fluid while increasing potassium excretion in the urine.

A high concentration of aldosterone in the plasma can transiently decrease the sodium loss into the urine to as little as a few milliequivalents a day. At the same time, potassium loss into the urine transiently increases severalfold. Therefore, the net effect of excess aldosterone in the plasma is to increase the total quantity of sodium in the extracellular fluid while decreasing the potassium.

Conversely, total lack of aldosterone secretion can cause transient loss of 10 to 20 grams of sodium in the urine a day, an amount equal to one tenth to one fifth of all the sodium in the body. At the same time, potassium is conserved tenaciously in the extracellular fluid.

Excess Aldosterone Increases Extracellular Fluid Volume and Arterial Pressure but Has Only a Small Effect on Plasma Sodium Concentration. Although aldosterone has a potent effect in decreasing the rate of sodium ion excretion by the kidneys, the concentration of sodium in the extracellular fluid often rises only a few milliequivalents. The reason for this is that when sodium is reabsorbed by the tubules, there is simultaneous osmotic absorption of almost equivalent amounts of water. Also, small increases in extracellular fluid sodium concentration stimulate thirst and increased water intake, if water is available. Therefore, the extracellular fluid volume increases almost as much as the retained sodium, but without much change in sodium concentration.

Even though aldosterone is one of the body's most powerful sodium-retaining hormones, only transient sodium retention occurs when excess amounts are secreted. An aldosterone-mediated increase in extracellular fluid volume lasting more than 1 to 2 days also leads to an increase in arterial pressure, as explained in Chapter 19. The rise in arterial pressure then increases kidney excretion of both salt and water, called *pressure natriuresis* and *pressure diuresis*, respectively. Thus, after the extracellular fluid volume increases 5 to 15 percent above normal, arterial pressure also increases 15 to 25 mm Hg, and this elevated blood pressure returns the renal output of salt and water to normal despite the excess aldosterone (Figure 77-3).

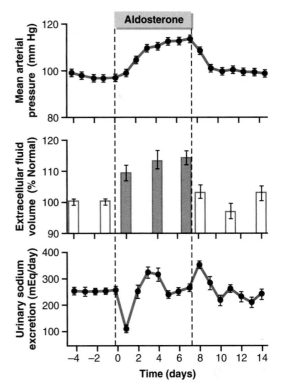

Figure 77-3 Effect of aldosterone infusion on arterial pressure, extracellular fluid volume, and sodium excretion in dogs. Although aldosterone was infused at a rate that raised plasma concentrations to about 20 times normal, note the "escape" from sodium retention on the second day of infusion as arterial pressure increased and urinary sodium excretion returned to normal. (Drawn from data in Hall JE, Granger JP, Smith MJ Jr, et al: Role of hemodynamics and arterial pressure in aldosterone "escape." Hypertension 6 (suppl I):I183-192, 1984.)

This return to normal of salt and water excretion by the kidneys as a result of pressure natriuresis and diuresis is called *aldosterone escape.* Thereafter, the rate of gain of salt and water by the body is zero, and balance is maintained between salt and water intake and output by the kidneys despite continued excess aldosterone. In the meantime, however, the person has developed hypertension, which lasts as long as the person remains exposed to high levels of aldosterone.

Conversely, when aldosterone secretion becomes zero, large amounts of salt are lost in the urine, not only diminishing the amount of sodium chloride in the extracellular fluid but also decreasing the extracellular fluid volume. The result is severe extracellular fluid dehydration and low blood volume, leading to *circulatory shock.* Without therapy, this usually causes death within a few days after the adrenal glands suddenly stop secreting aldosterone.

Excess Aldosterone Causes Hypokalemia and Muscle Weakness; Too Little Aldosterone Causes Hyperkalemia and Cardiac Toxicity. Excess aldosterone not only causes loss of potassium ions from the extracellular fluid into the urine but also stimulates transport of potassium from the extracellular fluid into most cells of the body. Therefore, excessive secretion of aldosterone, as occurs with some types of adrenal tumors, may cause a serious decrease in the plasma potassium concentration, sometimes from the normal value of 4.5 mEq/L to as low as 2 mEq/L. This condition is called *hypokalemia.* When the potassium ion concentration falls below about one-half normal, severe muscle weakness often develops. This is caused by alteration of the electrical excitability of the nerve and muscle fiber membranes (see Chapter 5), which prevents transmission of normal action potentials.

Conversely, when aldosterone is deficient, the extracellular fluid potassium ion concentration can rise far above normal. When it rises to 60 to 100 percent above normal, serious cardiac toxicity, including weakness of heart contraction and development of arrhythmia, becomes evident; progressively higher concentrations of potassium lead inevitably to heart failure.

Excess Aldosterone Increases Tubular Hydrogen Ion Secretion and Causes Alkalosis. Aldosterone not only causes potassium to be secreted into the tubules in exchange for sodium reabsorption in the principal cells of the renal collecting tubules but also causes secretion of hydrogen ions in exchange for sodium in the *intercalated cells* of the cortical collecting tubules. This decreases the hydrogen ion concentration in the extracellular fluid, causing a metabolic alkalosis.

Aldosterone Stimulates Sodium and Potassium Transport in Sweat Glands, Salivary Glands, and Intestinal Epithelial Cells

Aldosterone has almost the same effects on sweat glands and salivary glands as it has on the renal tubules. Both these glands form a primary secretion that contains large quantities of sodium chloride, but much of the sodium chloride, on passing through the excretory ducts, is reabsorbed, whereas potassium and bicarbonate ions are secreted. Aldosterone greatly increases the reabsorption of sodium chloride and the secretion of potassium by the ducts. The effect on the sweat glands is important to conserve body salt in hot environments, and the effect on the salivary glands is necessary to conserve salt when excessive quantities of saliva are lost.

Aldosterone also greatly enhances sodium absorption by the intestines, especially in the colon, which prevents loss of sodium in the stools. Conversely, in the absence of aldosterone, sodium absorption can be poor, leading to failure to absorb chloride and other anions and water as well. The unabsorbed sodium chloride and water then lead to diarrhea, with further loss of salt from the body.

Cellular Mechanism of Aldosterone Action

Although for many years we have known the overall effects of mineralocorticoids on the body, the molecular mechanisms of aldosterone's actions on the tubular cells to increase transport of sodium are still not fully understood. However, the cellular sequence of events that leads to increased sodium reabsorption seems to be the following.

First, because of its lipid solubility in the cellular membranes, aldosterone diffuses readily to the interior of the tubular epithelial cells.

Second, in the cytoplasm of the tubular cells, aldosterone combines with a highly specific cytoplasmic *mineralocorticoid receptor* (MR) protein (Figure 77-4), a protein that has a stereomolecular configuration that allows only aldosterone or similar compounds to combine with it. Although renal tubular epithelial cell MR receptors also have a high affinity for cortisol, the enzyme 11β-hydroxysteroid dehydrogenase type 2 normally converts most of the cortisol to cortisone, which does not readily bind to MR receptors, as discussed previously.

Third, the aldosterone-receptor complex or a product of this complex diffuses into the nucleus, where it may undergo further alterations, finally inducing one or more specific portions of the DNA to form one or more types of messenger RNA related to the process of sodium and potassium transport.

Fourth, the messenger RNA diffuses back into the cytoplasm, where, operating in conjunction with the ribosomes, it causes protein formation. The proteins formed are a mixture of (1) one or more enzymes and (2) membrane transport proteins that, all acting together, are required for sodium, potassium, and hydrogen transport through the cell membrane (see Figure 77-4). One of the enzymes especially increased is *sodium-potassium adenosine triphosphatase,* which serves as the principal part of the pump for sodium and potassium exchange at the *basolateral membranes* of the renal tubular cells.

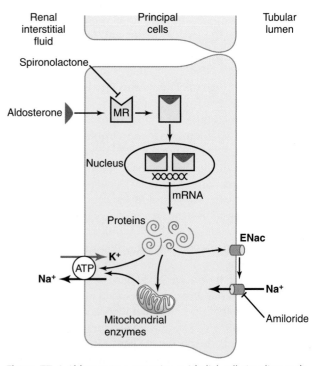

Figure 77-4 Aldosterone-responsive epithelial cell signaling pathways. ENaC, epithelial sodium channel proteins; MR, mineralocorticoid receptor. Activation of the MR by aldosterone can be antagonized with spironolactone. Amiloride is a drug that can be used to block ENaC.

Additional proteins, perhaps equally important, are *epithelial sodium channel* (ENaC) proteins inserted into the *luminal membrane* of the same tubular cells that allow rapid diffusion of sodium ions from the tubular lumen into the cell; then the sodium is pumped the rest of the way by the sodium-potassium pump located in the basolateral membranes of the cell.

Thus, aldosterone does not have a major immediate effect on sodium transport; rather, this effect must await the sequence of events that leads to the formation of the specific intracellular substances required for sodium transport. About 30 minutes is required before new RNA appears in the cells, and about 45 minutes is required before the rate of sodium transport begins to increase; the effect reaches maximum only after several hours.

Possible Nongenomic Actions of Aldosterone and Other Steroid Hormones

Recent studies suggest that many steroids, including aldosterone, elicit not only slowly developing *genomic* effects that have a latency of 60 to 90 minutes and require gene transcription and synthesis of new proteins, but also more rapid *nongenomic* effects that take place in a few seconds or minutes.

These nongenomic actions are believed to be mediated by binding of steroids to cell membrane receptors that are coupled to second messenger systems, similar to those used for peptide hormone signal transduction. For example, aldosterone has been shown to increase formation of cAMP in vascular smooth muscle cells and in epithelial cells of the renal collecting tubules in less than 2 minutes, a time period that is far too short for gene transcription and synthesis of new proteins. In other cell types, aldosterone has been shown to rapidly stimulate the phosphatidylinositol second messenger system. However, the precise structure of receptors responsible for the rapid effects of aldosterone has not been determined, nor is the physiological significance of these nongenomic actions of steroids well understood.

Regulation of Aldosterone Secretion

The regulation of aldosterone secretion is so deeply intertwined with the regulation of extracellular fluid electrolyte concentrations, extracellular fluid volume, blood volume, arterial pressure, and many special aspects of renal function that it is difficult to discuss the regulation of aldosterone secretion independently of all these other factors. This subject is presented in detail in Chapters 28 and 29, to which the reader is referred. However, it is important to list here some of the more important points of aldosterone secretion control.

The regulation of aldosterone secretion by the zona glomerulosa cells is almost entirely independent of the regulation of cortisol and androgens by the zona fasciculata and zona reticularis.

Four factors are known to play essential roles in the regulation of aldosterone. In the probable order of their importance, they are as follows:

1. Increased potassium ion concentration in the extracellular fluid greatly *increases* aldosterone secretion.

2. Increased angiotensin II concentration in the extracellular fluid also greatly *increases* aldosterone secretion.

3. Increased sodium ion concentration in the extracellular fluid *very slightly decreases* aldosterone secretion.

4. ACTH from the anterior pituitary gland is necessary for aldosterone secretion but has little effect in controlling the rate of secretion in most physiological conditions.

Of these factors, *potassium ion concentration* and the *renin-angiotensin system* are by far the most potent in regulating aldosterone secretion. A small percentage increase in potassium concentration can cause a severalfold increase in aldosterone secretion. Likewise, activation of the renin-angiotensin system, usually in response to diminished blood flow to the kidneys or to sodium loss, can increase in aldosterone secretion severalfold. In turn, the aldosterone acts on the kidneys (1) to help them excrete the excess potassium ions and (2) to increase the blood volume and arterial pressure, thus returning the renin-angiotensin system toward its normal level of activity. These feedback control mechanisms are essential for maintaining life, and the reader is referred again to Chapters 27 and 29 for a more complete description of their functions.

Figure 77-5 shows the effects on plasma aldosterone concentration caused by blocking the formation of angiotensin

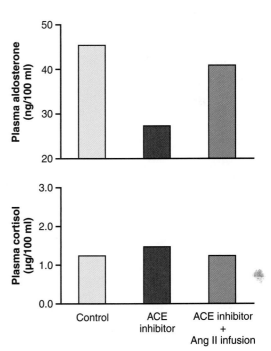

Figure 77-5 Effects of treating sodium-depleted dogs with an angiotensin-converting enzyme (ACE) inhibitor for 7 days to block formation of angiotensin II (Ang II) and of infusing exogenous Ang II to restore plasma Ang II levels after ACE inhibition. Note that blocking Ang II formation reduced plasma aldosterone concentration with little effect on cortisol, demonstrating the important role of Ang II in stimulating aldosterone secretion during sodium depletion. (Drawn from data in Hall JE, Guyton AC, Smith MJ Jr, et al: Chronic blockade of angiotensin II formation during sodium deprivation. Am J Physiol 237:F424, 1979.)

II with an angiotensin-converting enzyme inhibitor after several weeks of a low-sodium diet that increases plasma aldosterone concentration. Note that blocking angiotensin II formation markedly decreases plasma aldosterone concentration without significantly changing cortisol concentration; this indicates the important role of angiotensin II in stimulating aldosterone secretion when sodium intake and extracellular fluid volume are reduced.

By contrast, the effects of sodium ion concentration per se and of ACTH in controlling aldosterone secretion are usually minor. Nevertheless, a 10 to 20 percent decrease in extracellular fluid sodium ion concentration, which occurs on rare occasions, can perhaps increase aldosterone secretion by about 50 percent. In the case of ACTH, if there is even a small amount of ACTH secreted by the anterior pituitary gland, it is usually enough to permit the adrenal glands to secrete whatever amount of aldosterone is required, but total absence of ACTH can significantly reduce aldosterone secretion. Therefore, ACTH appears to play a "permissive" role in regulation of aldosterone secretion.

Functions of the Glucocorticoids

Even though mineralocorticoids can save the life of an acutely adrenalectomized animal, the animal still is far from normal. Instead, its metabolic systems for utilization of proteins, carbohydrates, and fats remain considerably deranged. Furthermore, the animal cannot resist different types of physical or even mental stress, and minor illnesses such as respiratory tract infections can lead to death. Therefore, the glucocorticoids have functions just as important to the long-continued life of the animal as those of the mineralocorticoids. They are explained in the following sections.

At least 95 percent of the glucocorticoid activity of the adrenocortical secretions results from the secretion of *cortisol*, known also as *hydrocortisone*. In addition to this, a small but significant amount of glucocorticoid activity is provided by *corticosterone*.

Effects of Cortisol on Carbohydrate Metabolism

Stimulation of Gluconeogenesis. By far the best-known metabolic effect of cortisol and other glucocorticoids on metabolism is the ability to stimulate gluconeogenesis (formation of carbohydrate from proteins and some other substances) by the liver, often increasing the rate of gluconeogenesis as much as 6- to 10-fold. This results mainly from two effects of cortisol.

1. *Cortisol increases the enzymes required to convert amino acids into glucose in the liver cells.* This results from the effect of the glucocorticoids to activate DNA transcription in the liver cell nuclei in the same way that aldosterone functions in the renal tubular cells, with formation of messenger RNAs that in turn lead to the array of enzymes required for gluconeogenesis.

2. *Cortisol causes mobilization of amino acids from the extrahepatic tissues mainly from muscle.* As a result, more amino acids become available in the plasma to enter into the gluconeogenesis process of the liver and thereby to promote the formation of glucose.

One of the effects of increased gluconeogenesis is a marked increase in glycogen storage in the liver cells. This effect of cortisol allows other glycolytic hormones, such as epinephrine and glucagon, to mobilize glucose in times of need, such as between meals.

Decreased Glucose Utilization by Cells. Cortisol also causes a moderate decrease in the rate of glucose utilization by most cells in the body. Although the cause of this decrease is unknown, most physiologists believe that somewhere between the point of entry of glucose into the cells and its final degradation, cortisol directly delays the rate of glucose utilization. A suggested mechanism is based on the observation that glucocorticoids depress the oxidation of nicotinamide-adenine dinucleotide (NADH) to form NAD^+. Because NADH must be oxidized to allow glycolysis, this effect could account for the diminished utilization of glucose by the cells.

Elevated Blood Glucose Concentration and "Adrenal Diabetes." Both the increased rate of gluconeogenesis and the moderate reduction in the rate of glucose utilization by the cells cause the blood glucose concentrations to rise. The rise in blood glucose in turn stimulates secretion of insulin. The increased plasma levels of insulin, however, are not as effective in maintaining plasma glucose as they are under normal conditions. For reasons that are not entirely clear, high levels of glucocorticoid reduce the sensitivity of many tissues, especially skeletal muscle and adipose tissue, to the stimulatory effects of insulin on glucose uptake and utilization. One possible explanation is that high levels of fatty acids, caused by the effect of glucocorticoids to mobilize lipids from fat depots, may impair insulin's actions on the tissues. In this way, excess secretion of glucocorticoids may produce disturbances of carbohydrate metabolism similar to those found in patients with excess levels of growth hormone.

The increase in blood glucose concentration is occasionally great enough (50 percent or more above normal) that the condition is called *adrenal diabetes*. Administration of insulin lowers the blood glucose concentration only a moderate amount in adrenal diabetes—not nearly as much as it does in pancreatic diabetes—because the tissues are resistant to the effects of insulin.

Effects of Cortisol on Protein Metabolism

Reduction in Cellular Protein. One of the principal effects of cortisol on the metabolic systems of the body is reduction of the protein stores in essentially all body cells except those of the liver. This is caused by both decreased protein synthesis and increased catabolism of protein already in the cells. Both these effects may result partly from decreased amino acid transport into extrahepatic tissues, as discussed later; this is probably not the major cause because cortisol also depresses the formation of RNA and subsequent protein synthesis in many extrahepatic tissues, especially in muscle and lymphoid tissue.

In the presence of great excesses of cortisol, the muscles can become so weak that the person cannot rise from the squatting position. And the immunity functions of the lymphoid tissue can be decreased to a small fraction of normal.

Cortisol Increases Liver and Plasma Proteins. Coincidentally with the reduced proteins elsewhere in the body, the liver proteins become enhanced. Furthermore, the plasma proteins (which are produced by the liver and then released into the blood) are also increased. These increases are exceptions to the protein depletion that occurs elsewhere in the body. It is believed that this difference results from a possible effect of cortisol to enhance amino acid transport into liver cells (but not into most other cells) and to enhance the liver enzymes required for protein synthesis.

Increased Blood Amino Acids, Diminished Transport of Amino Acids into Extrahepatic Cells, and Enhanced Transport into Hepatic Cells. Studies in isolated tissues have demonstrated that cortisol depresses amino acid transport into muscle cells and perhaps into other extrahepatic cells.

The decreased transport of amino acids into extrahepatic cells decreases their intracellular amino acid concentrations and consequently decreases the synthesis of protein. Yet catabolism of proteins in the cells continues to release amino acids from the already existing proteins, and these diffuse out of the cells to increase the plasma amino acid concentration. Therefore, *cortisol mobilizes amino acids from the nonhepatic tissues* and in doing so diminishes the tissue stores of protein.

The increased plasma concentration of amino acids and enhanced transport of amino acids into the hepatic cells by cortisol could also account for enhanced utilization of amino acids by the liver to cause such effects as (1) increased rate of deamination of amino acids by the liver, (2) increased protein synthesis in the liver, (3) increased formation of plasma proteins by the liver, and (4) increased conversion of amino acids to glucose—that is, enhanced gluconeogenesis. Thus, it is possible that many of the effects of cortisol on the metabolic systems of the body result mainly from this ability of cortisol to mobilize amino acids from the peripheral tissues while at the same time increasing the liver enzymes required for the hepatic effects.

Effects of Cortisol on Fat Metabolism

Mobilization of Fatty Acids. In much the same manner that cortisol promotes amino acid mobilization from muscle, it also promotes mobilization of fatty acids from adipose tissue. This increases the concentration of free fatty acids in the plasma, which also increases their utilization for energy. Cortisol also seems to have a direct effect to enhance the oxidation of fatty acids in the cells.

The mechanism by which cortisol promotes fatty acid mobilization is not completely understood. However, part of the effect probably results from diminished transport of glucose into the fat cells. Recall that α-glycerophosphate, which is derived from glucose, is required for both deposition and maintenance of triglycerides in these cells. In its absence the fat cells begin to release fatty acids.

The increased mobilization of fats by cortisol, combined with increased oxidation of fatty acids in the cells, helps shift the metabolic systems of the cells from utilization of glucose for energy to utilization of fatty acids in times of starvation or other stresses. This cortisol mechanism, however, requires several hours to become fully developed—not nearly so rapid or so powerful an effect as a similar shift elicited by a decrease in insulin, as we discuss in Chapter 78. Nevertheless, the increased use of fatty acids for metabolic energy is an important factor for long-term conservation of body glucose and glycogen.

Obesity Caused by Excess Cortisol. Despite the fact that cortisol can cause a moderate degree of fatty acid mobilization from adipose tissue, many people with excess cortisol secretion develop a peculiar type of obesity, with excess deposition of fat in the chest and head regions of the body, giving a buffalo-like torso and a rounded "moon face." Although the cause is unknown, it has been suggested that this obesity results from excess stimulation of food intake, with fat being generated in some tissues of the body more rapidly than it is mobilized and oxidized.

Cortisol Is Important in Resisting Stress and Inflammation

Almost any type of stress, whether physical or neurogenic, causes an immediate and marked increase in ACTH secretion by the anterior pituitary gland, followed within minutes by greatly increased adrenocortical secretion of cortisol. This is demonstrated dramatically by the experiment shown in Figure 77-6, in which corticosteroid formation and secretion increased sixfold in a rat within 4 to 20 minutes after fracture of two leg bones.

Some of the different types of stress that increase cortisol release are the following:

1. Trauma of almost any type
2. Infection
3. Intense heat or cold
4. Injection of norepinephrine and other sympathomimetic drugs
5. Surgery
6. Injection of necrotizing substances beneath the skin
7. Restraining an animal so that it cannot move
8. Almost any debilitating disease

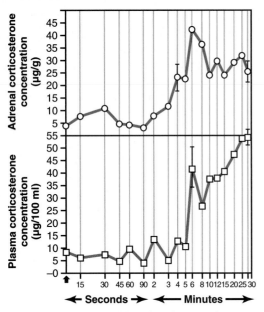

Figure 77-6 Rapid reaction of the adrenal cortex of a rat to stress caused by fracture of the tibia and fibula at time zero. (In the rat, corticosterone is secreted in place of cortisol.) (Courtesy Drs. Guillemin, Dear, and Lipscomb.)

Even though we know that cortisol secretion often increases greatly in stressful situations, we are not sure why this is of significant benefit to the animal. One possibility is that the glucocorticoids cause rapid mobilization of amino acids and fats from their cellular stores, making them immediately available both for energy and for synthesis of other compounds, including glucose, needed by the different tissues of the body. Indeed, it has been shown in a few instances that damaged tissues that are momentarily depleted of proteins can use the newly available amino acids to form new proteins that are essential to the lives of the cells. Also, the amino acids are perhaps used to synthesize other essential intracellular substances, such as purines, pyrimidines, and creatine phosphate, which are necessary for maintenance of cellular life and reproduction of new cells.

But all this is mainly supposition. It is supported only by the fact that cortisol usually does not mobilize the basic functional proteins of the cells, such as the muscle contractile proteins and the proteins of neurons, until almost all other proteins have been released. This preferential effect of cortisol in mobilizing labile proteins could make amino acids available to needy cells to synthesize substances essential to life.

Anti-Inflammatory Effects of High Levels of Cortisol

When tissues are damaged by trauma, by infection with bacteria, or in other ways, they almost always become "inflamed." In some conditions, such as in rheumatoid arthritis, the inflammation is more damaging than the trauma or disease itself. The administration of large amounts of cortisol can usually block this inflammation or even reverse many of its effects once it has begun. Before attempting to explain the way in which cortisol

functions to block inflammation, let us review the basic steps in the inflammation process, discussed in more detail in Chapter 33.

Five main stages of inflammation occur: (1) release from the damaged tissue cells of chemical substances that activate the inflammation process—chemicals such as histamine, bradykinin, proteolytic enzymes, prostaglandins, and leukotrienes; (2) an increase in blood flow in the inflamed area caused by some of the released products from the tissues, an effect called *erythema*; (3) leakage of large quantities of almost pure plasma out of the capillaries into the damaged areas because of increased capillary permeability, followed by clotting of the tissue fluid, thus causing a *nonpitting type of edema*; (4) infiltration of the area by leukocytes; and (5) after days or weeks, ingrowth of fibrous tissue that often helps in the healing process.

When large amounts of cortisol are secreted or injected into a person, the cortisol has two basic *anti-inflammatory effects:* (1) it can block the early stages of the inflammation process before inflammation even begins, or (2) if inflammation has already begun, it causes rapid resolution of the inflammation and increased rapidity of healing. These effects are explained further as follows.

Cortisol Prevents the Development of Inflammation by Stabilizing Lysosomes and by Other Effects. Cortisol has the following effects in preventing inflammation:

1. *Cortisol stabilizes the lysosomal membranes.* This is one of its most important anti-inflammatory effects because it is much more difficult than normal for the membranes of the intracellular lysosomes to rupture. Therefore, most of the proteolytic enzymes that are released by damaged cells to cause inflammation, which are mainly stored in the lysosomes, are released in greatly decreased quantity.

2. *Cortisol decreases the permeability of the capillaries,* probably as a secondary effect of the reduced release of proteolytic enzymes. This prevents loss of plasma into the tissues.

3. *Cortisol decreases both migration of white blood cells into the inflamed area and phagocytosis of the damaged cells.* These effects probably result from the fact that cortisol diminishes the formation of prostaglandins and leukotrienes that otherwise would increase vasodilation, capillary permeability, and mobility of white blood cells.

4. *Cortisol suppresses the immune system, causing lymphocyte reproduction to decrease markedly.* The T lymphocytes are especially suppressed. In turn, reduced amounts of T cells and antibodies in the inflamed area lessen the tissue reactions that would otherwise promote the inflammation process.

5. *Cortisol attenuates fever mainly because it reduces the release of interleukin-1 from the white blood cells,* which is one of the principal excitants to the hypothalamic temperature control system. The decreased temperature in turn reduces the degree of vasodilation.

Thus, cortisol has an almost global effect in reducing all aspects of the inflammatory process. How much of this results from the simple effect of cortisol in stabilizing lysosomal and cell membranes versus its effect to reduce the formation of prostaglandins and leukotrienes from arachidonic acid in damaged cell membranes and other effects of cortisol is unclear.

Cortisol Causes Resolution of Inflammation. Even after inflammation has become well established, the administration of cortisol can often reduce inflammation within hours to a few days. The immediate effect is to block most of the factors that promote the inflammation. But in addition, the rate of healing is enhanced. This probably results from the same, mainly undefined, factors that allow the body to resist many other types of physical stress when large quantities of cortisol are secreted. Perhaps this results from the mobilization of amino acids and use of these to repair the damaged tissues; perhaps it results from the increased glucogenesis that makes extra glucose available in critical metabolic systems; perhaps it results from increased amounts of fatty acids available for cellular energy; or perhaps it depends on some effect of cortisol for inactivating or removing inflammatory products.

Regardless of the precise mechanisms by which the anti-inflammatory effect occurs, this effect of cortisol plays a major role in combating certain types of diseases, such as rheumatoid arthritis, rheumatic fever, and acute glomerulonephritis. All these diseases are characterized by severe local inflammation, and the harmful effects on the body are caused mainly by the inflammation itself and not by other aspects of the disease.

When cortisol or other glucocorticoids are administered to patients with these diseases, almost invariably the inflammation begins to subside within 24 hours. And even though the cortisol does not correct the basic disease condition, merely preventing the damaging effects of the inflammatory response, this alone can often be a lifesaving measure.

Other Effects of Cortisol

Cortisol Blocks the Inflammatory Response to Allergic Reactions. The basic allergic reaction between antigen and antibody is not affected by cortisol, and even some of the secondary effects of the allergic reaction still occur. However, because the inflammatory response is responsible for many of the serious and sometimes lethal effects of allergic reactions, administration of cortisol, followed by its effect in reducing inflammation and the release of inflammatory products, can be lifesaving. For instance, cortisol effectively prevents shock or death in anaphylaxis, which otherwise kills many people, as explained in Chapter 34.

Effect on Blood Cells and on Immunity in Infectious Diseases. Cortisol decreases the number of eosinophils and lymphocytes in the blood; this effect begins within a few minutes after the injection of cortisol and becomes marked within a few hours. Indeed, a finding of lymphocytopenia or eosinopenia is an important diagnostic criterion for overproduction of cortisol by the adrenal gland.

Likewise, the administration of large doses of cortisol causes significant atrophy of all the lymphoid tissue throughout the body, which in turn decreases the output of both T cells and antibodies from the lymphoid tissue. As a result, the level of immunity for almost all foreign invaders of the body is decreased. This occasionally can lead to fulminating infection and death from diseases that would otherwise not be lethal, such as fulminating tuberculosis in a person whose disease had previously been arrested. Conversely, this ability of cortisol and other glucocorticoids to suppress immunity makes them useful drugs in preventing immunological rejection of transplanted hearts, kidneys, and other tissues.

Cortisol increases the production of red blood cells by mechanisms that are unclear. When excess cortisol is secreted by the adrenal glands, polycythemia often results, and conversely, when the adrenal glands secrete no cortisol, anemia often results.

Cellular Mechanism of Cortisol Action

Cortisol, like other steroid hormones, exerts its effects by first interacting with intracellular receptors in target cells. Because cortisol is lipid soluble, it can easily diffuse through the cell membrane. Once inside the cell, cortisol binds with its protein receptor in the cytoplasm, and the hormone-receptor complex then interacts with specific regulatory DNA sequences, called *glucocorticoid response elements*, to induce or repress gene transcription. Other proteins in the cell, called *transcription factors*, are also necessary for the hormone-receptor complex to interact appropriately with the glucocorticoid response elements.

Glucocorticoids increase or decrease transcription of many genes to alter synthesis of mRNA for the proteins that mediate their multiple physiological effects. Thus, most of the metabolic effects of cortisol are not immediate but require 45 to 60 minutes for proteins to be synthesized, and up to several hours or days to fully develop. Recent evidence suggests that glucocorticoids, especially at high concentrations, may also have some rapid *nongenomic effects* on cell membrane ion transport that may contribute to their therapeutic benefits.

Regulation of Cortisol Secretion by Adrenocorticotropic Hormone from the Pituitary Gland

ACTH Stimulates Cortisol Secretion. Unlike aldosterone secretion by the zona glomerulosa, which is controlled mainly by potassium and angiotensin acting directly on the adrenocortical cells, secretion of cortisol is controlled almost entirely by ACTH secreted by the anterior pituitary gland. This hormone, also called *corticotropin* or *adrenocorticotropin*, also enhances the production of adrenal androgens.

Chemistry of ACTH. ACTH has been isolated in pure form from the anterior pituitary. It is a large polypeptide, having a chain length of 39 amino acids. A smaller polypeptide, a digested product of ACTH having a chain length of 24 amino acids, has all the effects of the total molecule.

ACTH Secretion Is Controlled by Corticotropin-Releasing Factor from the Hypothalamus. In the same way that other pituitary hormones are controlled by releasing factors from the hypothalamus, an important releasing factor also controls ACTH secretion. This is called *corticotropin-releasing factor* (CRF). It is secreted into the primary capillary plexus of the hypophysial portal system in the median eminence of the hypothalamus and then carried to the anterior pituitary gland, where it induces ACTH secretion. CRF is a peptide composed of 41 amino acids. The cell bodies of the neurons that secrete CRF are located mainly in the paraventricular nucleus of the hypothalamus. This nucleus in turn receives many nervous connections from the limbic system and lower brain stem.

The anterior pituitary gland can secrete only minute quantities of ACTH in the absence of CRF. Instead, most conditions that cause high ACTH secretory rates initiate this secretion by signals that begin in the basal regions of the brain, including the hypothalamus, and are then transmitted by CRF to the anterior pituitary gland.

ACTH Activates Adrenocortical Cells to Produce Steroids by Increasing Cyclic Adenosine Monophosphate (cAMP). The principal effect of ACTH on the adrenocortical cells is to activate *adenylyl cyclase* in the cell membrane. This then induces the formation of *cAMP* in the cell cytoplasm, reaching its maximal effect in about 3 minutes. The cAMP in turn activates the intracellular enzymes that cause formation of the adrenocortical hormones. This is another example of cAMP as a *second messenger* signal system.

The most important of all the ACTH-stimulated steps for controlling adrenocortical secretion is activation of the enzyme *protein kinase A*, which *causes initial conversion of cholesterol to pregnenolone.* This initial conversion is the "rate-limiting" step for all the adrenocortical hormones, which explains why ACTH is normally necessary for any

adrenocortical hormones to be formed. Long-term stimulation of the adrenal cortex by ACTH not only increases secretory activity but also causes hypertrophy and proliferation of the adrenocortical cells, especially in the zona fasciculata and zona reticularis, where cortisol and the androgens are secreted.

Physiological Stress Increases ACTH and Adrenocortical Secretion

As pointed out earlier in the chapter, almost any type of physical or mental stress can lead within minutes to greatly enhanced secretion of ACTH and consequently cortisol as well, often increasing cortisol secretion as much as 20-fold. This effect was demonstrated by the rapid and strong adrenocortical secretory responses after trauma shown in Figure 77-6.

Pain stimuli caused by physical stress or tissue damage are transmitted first upward through the brain stem and eventually to the median eminence of the hypothalamus, as shown in Figure 77-7. Here CRF is secreted into the hypophysial portal system. Within minutes the entire control sequence leads to large quantities of cortisol in the blood.

Mental stress can cause an equally rapid increase in ACTH secretion. This is believed to result from increased activity in the limbic system, especially in the region of the amygdala and hippocampus, both of which then transmit signals to the posterior medial hypothalamus.

Inhibitory Effect of Cortisol on the Hypothalamus and on the Anterior Pituitary to Decrease ACTH Secretion. Cortisol has direct negative feedback effects on (1) the hypothalamus to decrease the formation of CRF and (2) the anterior pituitary gland to decrease the formation of ACTH. Both of these feedbacks help regulate

Figure 77-7 Mechanism for regulation of glucocorticoid secretion. ACTH, adrenocorticotropic hormone; CRF, corticotropin-releasing factor.

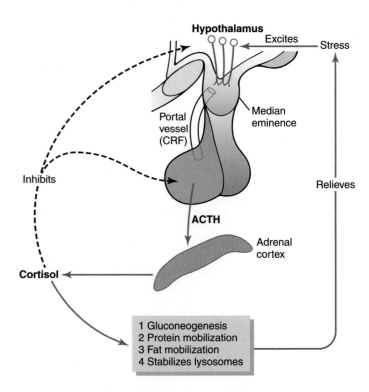

the plasma concentration of cortisol. That is, whenever the cortisol concentration becomes too great, the feedbacks automatically reduce the ACTH toward a normal control level.

Summary of the Cortisol Control System

Figure 77-7 shows the overall system for control of cortisol secretion. The key to this control is the excitation of the hypothalamus by different types of stress. Stress stimuli activate the entire system to cause rapid release of cortisol, and the cortisol in turn initiates a series of metabolic effects directed toward relieving the damaging nature of the stressful state.

There is also direct feedback of the cortisol to both the hypothalamus and the anterior pituitary gland to decrease the concentration of cortisol in the plasma at times when the body is not experiencing stress. However, the stress stimuli are the prepotent ones; they can always break through this direct inhibitory feedback of cortisol, causing either periodic exacerbations of cortisol secretion at multiple times during the day (Figure 77-8) or prolonged cortisol secretion in times of chronic stress.

Circadian Rhythm of Glucocorticoid Secretion. The secretory rates of CRF, ACTH, and cortisol are high in the early morning but low in the late evening, as shown in Figure 77-8; the plasma cortisol level ranges between a high of about 20 µg/dl an hour before arising in the morning and a low of about 5 µg/dl around midnight. This effect results from a 24-hour cyclical alteration in the signals from the hypothalamus that cause cortisol secretion. When a person changes daily sleeping habits, the cycle changes correspondingly. Therefore, measurements of blood cortisol levels are meaningful only when expressed in terms of the time in the cycle at which the measurements are made.

Synthesis and Secretion of ACTH in Association with Melanocyte-Stimulating Hormone, Lipotropin, and Endorphin

When ACTH is secreted by the anterior pituitary gland, several other hormones that have similar chemical structures are secreted simultaneously. The reason for this is that the gene that is transcribed to form the RNA molecule that causes ACTH synthesis initially causes the formation of a considerably larger protein, a preprohormone called *proopiomelanocortin* (POMC), which is the precursor of ACTH and several other peptides, including *melanocyte-stimulating hormone* (MSH), *β-lipotropin*, *β-endorphin*, and a few others (Figure 77-9). Under normal conditions, none of these hormones is secreted in enough quantity by the pituitary to have a significant effect on the human body, but when the rate of secretion of ACTH is high, as may occur in Addison's disease, formation of some of the other POMC-derived hormones may also be increased.

The POMC gene is actively transcribed in several tissues, including the corticotroph cells of the anterior pituitary, POMC neurons in the arcuate nucleus of the hypothalamus, cells of the dermis, and lymphoid tissue. In all of these cell types, POMC is processed to form a series of smaller peptides. The precise type of POMC-derived products from a particular tissue depends on the type of processing enzymes present in the tissue. Thus, pituitary corticotroph cells express *prohormone convertase 1* (PC1),

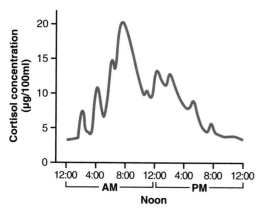

Figure 77-8 Typical pattern of cortisol concentration during the day. Note the oscillations in secretion as well as a daily secretory surge an hour or so after awaking in the morning.

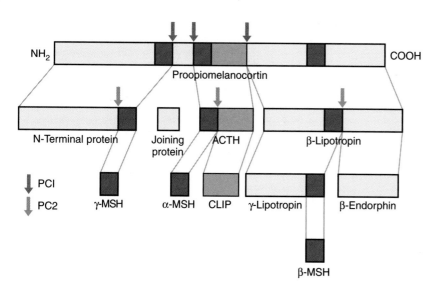

Figure 77-9 Proopiomelanocortin (POMC) processing by prohormone convertase 1 (PC1, *red arrows*) and PC 2 (*blue arrows*). Tissue-specific expression of these two enzymes results in different peptides produced in various tissues. The anterior pituitary expresses PC1, resulting in formation of N-terminal peptide, joining peptide, ACTH, and β-lipotropin. Expression of PC2 within the hypothalamus leads to the production of α-, β-, and γ-melanocyte stimulating hormone (MSH), but not ACTH. CLIP, corticotropin-like intermediate peptide.

but not PC2, resulting in the production of N-terminal peptide, joining peptide, ACTH, and β-lipotropin. In the hypothalamus, the expression of PC2 leads to the production of α-, β-, and γ-MSH and β-endorphin but not ACTH. As discussed in Chapter 71, α-MSH formed by neurons of the hypothalamus plays a major role in appetite regulation.

In *melanocytes* located in abundance between the dermis and epidermis of the skin, MSH stimulates formation of the black pigment *melanin* and disperses it to the epidermis. Injection of MSH into a person over 8 to 10 days can greatly increase darkening of the skin. The effect is much greater in people who have genetically dark skins than in light-skinned people.

In some lower animals, an intermediate "lobe" of the pituitary gland, called the *pars intermedia,* is highly developed, lying between the anterior and posterior pituitary lobes. This lobe secretes an especially large amount of MSH. Furthermore, this secretion is independently controlled by the hypothalamus in response to the amount of light to which the animal is exposed or in response to other environmental factors. For instance, some arctic animals develop darkened fur in the summer and yet have entirely white fur in the winter.

ACTH, because it contains an MSH sequence, has about 1/30 as much melanocyte-stimulating effect as MSH. Furthermore, because the quantities of pure MSH secreted in the human being are extremely small, whereas those of ACTH are large, it is likely that ACTH is normally more important than MSH in determining the amount of melanin in the skin.

Adrenal Androgens

Several moderately active male sex hormones called *adrenal androgens* (the most important of which is *dehydroepiandrosterone*) are continually secreted by the adrenal cortex, especially during fetal life, as discussed more fully in Chapter 83. Also, progesterone and estrogens, which are female sex hormones, are secreted in minute quantities.

Normally, the adrenal androgens have only weak effects in humans. It is possible that part of the early development of the male sex organs results from childhood secretion of adrenal androgens. The adrenal androgens also exert mild effects in the female, not only before puberty but also throughout life. Much of the growth of the pubic and axillary hair in the female results from the action of these hormones.

In extra-adrenal tissues, some of the adrenal androgens are converted to testosterone, the primary male sex hormone, which probably accounts for much of their androgenic activity. The physiological effects of androgens are discussed in Chapter 80 in relation to male sexual function.

Abnormalities of Adrenocortical Secretion

Hypoadrenalism (Adrenal Insufficiency)—Addison's Disease

Addison's disease results from an inability of the adrenal cortices to produce sufficient adrenocortical hormones, and this in turn is most frequently caused by *primary atrophy or injury* of the adrenal cortices. In about 80 percent of the cases, the atrophy is caused by autoimmunity against the cortices. Adrenal gland hypofunction is also frequently caused by tuberculous destruction of the adrenal glands or invasion of the adrenal cortices by cancer.

In some cases, adrenal insufficiency is secondary to impaired function of the pituitary gland, which fails to produce sufficient ACTH. When ACTH output is too low, cortisol and aldosterone production decrease and eventually, the adrenal glands may atrophy due to lack of ACTH stimulation. Secondary adrenal insufficiency is much more common than Addison's disease, which is sometimes called *primary adrenal insufficiency*. Disturbances in severe adrenal insufficiency are as follows.

Mineralocorticoid Deficiency. Lack of aldosterone secretion greatly decreases renal tubular sodium reabsorption and consequently allows sodium ions, chloride ions, and water to be lost into urine in great profusion. The net result is a greatly decreased extracellular fluid volume. Furthermore, hyponatremia, hyperkalemia, and mild acidosis develop because of failure of potassium and hydrogen ions to be secreted in exchange for sodium reabsorption.

As the extracellular fluid becomes depleted, plasma volume falls, red blood cell concentration rises markedly, cardiac output and blood pressure decrease, and the patient dies in shock, death usually occurring in the untreated patient 4 days to 2 weeks after complete cessation of mineralocorticoid secretion.

Glucocorticoid Deficiency. Loss of cortisol secretion makes it impossible for a person with Addison's disease to maintain normal blood glucose concentration between meals because he or she cannot synthesize significant quantities of glucose by gluconeogenesis. Furthermore, lack of cortisol reduces the mobilization of both proteins and fats from the tissues, thereby depressing many other metabolic functions of the body. This sluggishness of energy mobilization when cortisol is not available is one of the major detrimental effects of glucocorticoid lack. Even when excess quantities of glucose and other nutrients are available, the person's muscles are weak, indicating that glucocorticoids are necessary to maintain other metabolic functions of the tissues in addition to energy metabolism.

Lack of adequate glucocorticoid secretion also makes a person with Addison's disease highly susceptible to the deteriorating effects of different types of stress, and even a mild respiratory infection can cause death.

Melanin Pigmentation. Another characteristic of most people with Addison's disease is melanin pigmentation of the mucous membranes and skin. This melanin is not always deposited evenly but occasionally is deposited in blotches, and it is deposited especially in the thin skin areas, such as the mucous membranes of the lips and the thin skin of the nipples.

The cause of the melanin deposition is believed to be the following: When cortisol secretion is depressed, the normal negative feedback to the hypothalamus and anterior pituitary gland is also depressed, therefore allowing tremendous rates of ACTH secretion, as well as simultaneous secretion of increased amounts of MSH. Probably the tremendous amounts of ACTH cause most of the pigmenting effect because they can stimulate formation of melanin by the melanocytes in the same way that MSH does.

Treatment of People with Addison's Disease. An untreated person with total adrenal destruction dies within a few days to a few weeks because of weakness and usually circulatory shock. Yet such a person can live for years if small quantities of mineralocorticoids and glucocorticoids are administered daily.

Addisonian Crisis. As noted earlier in the chapter, great quantities of glucocorticoids are occasionally secreted in response to different types of physical or mental stress. In a person with Addison's disease, the output of glucocorticoids does not increase during stress. Yet whenever different types of trauma, disease, or other stresses, such as surgical operations, supervene, a person is likely to have an acute need for excessive amounts of glucocorticoids and often must be given 10 or more times the normal quantities of glucocorticoids to prevent death.

This critical need for extra glucocorticoids and the associated severe debility in times of stress is called an *addisonian crisis*.

Hyperadrenalism—Cushing's Syndrome

Hypersecretion by the adrenal cortex causes a complex cascade of hormone effects called *Cushing's syndrome.* Many of the abnormalities of Cushing's syndrome are ascribable to abnormal amounts of cortisol, but excess secretion of androgens may also cause important effects. Hypercortisolism can occur from multiple causes, including (1) adenomas of the anterior pituitary that secrete large amounts of ACTH, which then causes adrenal hyperplasia and excess cortisol secretion; (2) abnormal function of the hypothalamus that causes high levels of corticotropin-releasing hormone (CRH), which stimulates excess ACTH release; (3) "ectopic secretion" of ACTH by a tumor elsewhere in the body, such as an abdominal carcinoma; and (4) adenomas of the adrenal cortex. When Cushing's syndrome is secondary to excess secretion of ACTH by the anterior pituitary, this is referred to as *Cushing's disease.*

Excess ACTH secretion is the most common cause of Cushing's syndrome and is characterized by high plasma levels of ACTH and cortisol. Primary overproduction of cortisol by the adrenal glands accounts for about 20 to 25 percent of clinical cases of Cushing's syndrome and is usually associated with reduced ACTH levels due to cortisol feedback inhibition of ACTH secretion by the anterior pituitary gland.

Administration of large doses of dexamethasone, a synthetic glucocorticoid, can be used to distinguish between *ACTH-dependent* and *ACTH-independent* Cushing's syndrome. In patients who have overproduction of ACTH due to an ACTH-secreting pituitary adenoma or to hypothalamic-pituitary dysfunction, even large doses of dexamethasone usually do not suppress ACTH secretion. In contrast, patients with primary adrenal overproduction of cortisol (ACTH-independent) usually have low or undetectable levels of ACTH. The dexamethasone test, although widely used, can sometimes give an incorrect diagnosis because some ACTH-secreting pituitary tumors respond to dexamethasone with suppressed ACTH secretion. Therefore, it is usually considered to be a first step in the differential diagnosis of Cushing's syndrome.

Cushing's syndrome can also occur when large amounts of glucocorticoids are administered over prolonged periods for therapeutic purposes. For example, patients with chronic inflammation associated with diseases such as rheumatoid arthritis are often treated with glucocorticoids and may develop some of the clinical symptoms of Cushing's syndrome.

A special characteristic of Cushing's syndrome is mobilization of fat from the lower part of the body, with concomitant extra deposition of fat in the thoracic and upper abdominal regions, giving rise to a buffalo torso. The excess secretion of steroids also leads to an edematous appearance of the face, and the androgenic potency of some of the hormones sometimes causes acne and hirsutism (excess growth of facial hair). The appearance of the face is frequently described as a "moon face," as demonstrated in the untreated patient with Cushing's syndrome to the left in Figure 77-10. About 80 percent of patients have hypertension, presumably because of the mineralocorticoid effects of cortisol.

Effects on Carbohydrate and Protein Metabolism. The abundance of cortisol secreted in Cushing's syndrome can cause increased blood glucose concentration, sometimes to

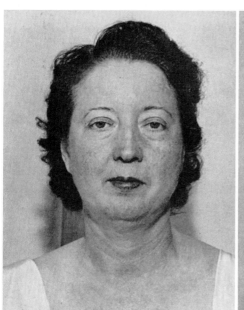 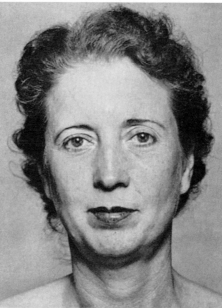

Figure 77-10 A person with Cushing's syndrome before (*left*) and after (*right*) subtotal adrenalectomy. (Courtesy Dr. Leonard Posey.)

values as high as 200 mg/dl after meals—as much as twice normal. This results mainly from enhanced gluconeogenesis and decreased glucose utilization by the tissues.

The effects of glucocorticoids on protein catabolism are often profound in Cushing's syndrome, causing greatly decreased tissue proteins almost everywhere in the body with the exception of the liver; the plasma proteins also remain unaffected. The loss of protein from the muscles in particular causes severe weakness. The loss of protein synthesis in the lymphoid tissues leads to a suppressed immune system, so many of these patients die of infections. Even the protein collagen fibers in the subcutaneous tissue are diminished so that the subcutaneous tissues tear easily, resulting in development of large *purplish striae* where they have torn apart. In addition, severely diminished protein deposition in the bones often causes severe *osteoporosis* with consequent weakness of the bones.

Treatment of Cushing's Syndrome. Treatment of Cushing's syndrome consists of removing an adrenal tumor if this is the cause or decreasing the secretion of ACTH, if this is possible. Hypertrophied pituitary glands or even small tumors in the pituitary that oversecrete ACTH can sometimes be surgically removed or destroyed by radiation. Drugs that block steroidogenesis, such as *metyrapone, ketoconazole,* and *aminoglutethimide,* or that inhibit ACTH secretion, such as *serotonin antagonists* and *GABA-transaminase inhibitors,* can also be used when surgery is not feasible. If ACTH secretion cannot easily be decreased, the only satisfactory treatment is usually bilateral partial (or even total) adrenalectomy, followed by administration of adrenal steroids to make up for any insufficiency that develops.

Primary Aldosteronism (Conn's Syndrome)

Occasionally a small tumor of the zona glomerulosa cells occurs and secretes large amounts of aldosterone; the resulting condition is called "primary aldosteronism" or "Conn's syndrome." Also, in a few instances, hyperplastic adrenal cortices secrete aldosterone rather than cortisol. The effects of the excess aldosterone are discussed in detail earlier in the chapter. The most important effects are hypokalemia, mild metabolic alkalosis, slight increase in extracellular fluid volume and blood volume, very slight increase in plasma sodium concentration (usually > 4 to 6 mEq/L increase), and, almost always, hypertension. Especially interesting in primary aldosteronism are occasional periods of muscle paralysis caused by the hypokalemia. The paralysis is caused by a depressant effect of low extracellular potassium concentration on action potential transmission by the nerve fibers, as explained in Chapter 5.

One of the diagnostic criteria of primary aldosteronism is a decreased plasma renin concentration. This results from feedback suppression of renin secretion caused by the excess aldosterone or by the excess extracellular fluid volume and arterial pressure resulting from the aldosteronism. Treatment of primary aldosteronism may include surgical removal of the tumor or of most of the adrenal tissue when hyperplasia is the cause. Another option for treatment is pharmacological antagonism of the mineralocorticoid receptor with spironolactone or eplerenone.

Adrenogenital Syndrome

An occasional adrenocortical tumor secretes excessive quantities of androgens that cause intense masculinizing effects

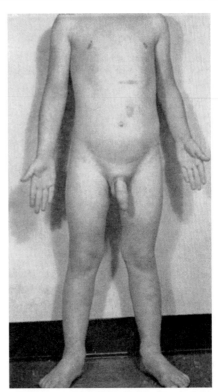

Figure 77-11 Adrenogenital syndrome in a 4-year-old boy. (Courtesy Dr. Leonard Posey.)

throughout the body. If this occurs in a female, she develops virile characteristics, including growth of a beard, a much deeper voice, occasionally baldness if she also has the genetic trait for baldness, masculine distribution of hair on the body and the pubis, growth of the clitoris to resemble a penis, and deposition of proteins in the skin and especially in the muscles to give typical masculine characteristics.

In the prepubertal male, a virilizing adrenal tumor causes the same characteristics as in the female plus rapid development of the male sexual organs, as shown in Figure 77-11, which depicts a 4-year-old boy with adrenogenital syndrome. In the adult male, the virilizing characteristics of adrenogenital syndrome are usually obscured by the normal virilizing characteristics of the testosterone secreted by the testes. It is often difficult to make a diagnosis of adrenogenital syndrome in the adult male. In adrenogenital syndrome, the excretion of 17-ketosteroids (which are derived from androgens) in the urine may be 10 to 15 times normal. This finding can be used in diagnosing the disease.

Bibliography

Adcock IM, Barnes PJ: Molecular mechanisms of corticosteroid resistance, *Chest* 134:394, 2008.

Biller BM, Grossman AB, Stewart PM, et al: Treatment of adrenocorticotropin-dependent Cushing's syndrome: a consensus statement, *J Clin Endocrinol Metab* 93:2454, 2008.

Boldyreff B, Wehling M: Aldosterone: refreshing a slow hormone by swift action, *News Physiol Sci* 19:97, 2004.

Bornstein SR: Predisposing factors for adrenal insufficiency, *N Engl J Med* 360:2328, 2009.

Boscaro M, Arnaldi G: Approach to the patient with possible Cushing's syndrome, *J Clin Endocrinol Metab.* 94:3121, 2009.

Boscaro M, Barzon L, Fallo F, et al: Cushing's syndrome, *Lancet* 357:783, 2001.

de Paula RB, da Silva AA, Hall JE: Aldosterone antagonism attenuates obesity-induced hypertension and glomerular hyperfiltration, *Hypertension* 43:41, 2004.

Fuller PJ, Young MJ: Mechanisms of mineralocorticoid action, *Hypertension* 46:1227, 2005.

Funder JW: Reconsidering the roles of the mineralocorticoid receptor, *Hypertension* 53:286, 2009.

Funder JW: Aldosterone and the cardiovascular system: genomic and nongenomic effects, *Endocrinology* 147:5564, 2006.

Hall JE, Granger JP, Smith MJ Jr, et al: Role of renal hemodynamics and arterial pressure in aldosterone "escape", *Hypertension* 6:I183, 1984.

Larsen PR, Kronenberg HM, Melmed S, et al: *Williams Textbook of Endocrinology*, ed 10, Philadelphia, 2003, WB Saunders Co.

Levin ER: Rapid signaling by steroid receptors, *Am J Physiol Regul Integr Comp Physiol* 295:R1425, 2008.

Lösel RM, Falkenstein E, Feuring M, et al: Nongenomic steroid action: Controversies, questions, and answers, *Physiol Rev* 83:965, 2003.

Oberleithner H: Unorthodox sites and modes of aldosterone action, *News Physiol Sci* 19:51, 2004.

O'shaughnessy KM, Karet FE: Salt handling and hypertension, *J Clin Invest* 113:1075, 2004.

Pippal JB, Fuller PJ: Structure-function relationships in the mineralocorticoid receptor, *J Mol Endocrinol* 41:405, 2008.

Raff H: Utility of salivary cortisol measurements in Cushing's syndrome and adrenal insufficiency, *J Clin Endocrinol Metab* 94:3647, 2009.

Rickard AJ, Young MJ: Corticosteroid receptors, macrophages and cardiovascular disease, *J Mol Endocrinol* 42:449, 2009.

Spat A, Hunyady L: Control of aldosterone secretion: a model for convergence in cellular signaling pathways, *Physiol Rev* 84:489, 2004.

Speiser PW, White PC: Congenital adrenal hyperplasia, *N Engl J Med* 349:776, 2003.

Sowers JR, Whaley-Connell A, Epstein M: Narrative review: the emerging clinical implications of the role of aldosterone in the metabolic syndrome and resistant hypertension, *Ann Intern Med* 150:776, 2009.

Stockand JD: New ideas about aldosterone signaling in epithelia, *Am J Physiol Renal Physiol* 282:F559, 2002.

Vinson GP: The adrenal cortex and life, *Mol Cell Endocrinol* 300:2, 2009.

Insulin, Glucagon, and Diabetes Mellitus

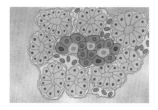

The pancreas, in addition to its digestive functions, secretes two important hormones, *insulin* and *glucagon*, that are crucial for normal regulation of glucose, lipid, and protein metabolism. Although the pancreas secretes other hormones, such as *amylin, somatostatin,* and *pancreatic polypeptide*, their functions are not as well established. The main purpose of this chapter is to discuss the physiological roles of insulin and glucagon and the pathophysiology of diseases, especially *diabetes mellitus*, caused by abnormal secretion or activity of these hormones.

Physiologic Anatomy of the Pancreas. The pancreas is composed of two major types of tissues, as shown in Figure 78-1: (1) the *acini,* which secrete digestive juices into the duodenum, and (2) the *islets of Langerhans,* which secrete insulin and glucagon directly into the blood. The digestive secretions of the pancreas are discussed in Chapter 64.

The human pancreas has 1 to 2 million islets of Langerhans, each only about 0.3 millimeter in diameter and organized around small capillaries into which its cells secrete their hormones. The islets contain three major types of cells, *alpha, beta,* and *delta* cells, which are distinguished from one another by their morphological and staining characteristics.

The beta cells, constituting about 60 percent of all the cells of the islets, lie mainly in the middle of each islet and secrete *insulin* and *amylin,* a hormone that is often secreted in parallel with insulin, although its function is unclear. The alpha cells, about 25 percent of the total, secrete *glucagon.* And the delta cells, about 10 percent of the total, secrete *somatostatin.* In addition, at least one other type of cell, the *PP cell,* is present in small numbers in the islets and secretes a hormone of uncertain function called *pancreatic polypeptide.*

The close interrelations among these cell types in the islets of Langerhans allow cell-to-cell communication and direct control of secretion of some of the hormones by the other hormones. For instance, insulin inhibits glucagon secretion, amylin inhibits insulin secretion, and somatostatin inhibits the secretion of both insulin and glucagon.

Insulin and Its Metabolic Effects

Insulin was first isolated from the pancreas in 1922 by Banting and Best, and almost overnight the outlook for the severely diabetic patient changed from one of rapid decline and death to that of a nearly normal person. Historically, insulin has been associated with "blood sugar," and true enough, insulin has profound effects on carbohydrate metabolism. Yet it is abnormalities of fat metabolism, causing such conditions as acidosis and arteriosclerosis, that are the usual causes of death in diabetic patients. Also, in patients with prolonged diabetes, diminished ability to synthesize proteins leads to wasting of the tissues and many cellular functional disorders. Therefore, it is clear that insulin affects fat and protein metabolism almost as much as it does carbohydrate metabolism.

Insulin Is a Hormone Associated with Energy Abundance

As we discuss insulin in the next few pages, it will become apparent that insulin secretion is associated with energy abundance. That is, when there is great abundance of energy-giving foods in the diet, especially excess amounts of carbohydrates, insulin secretion increases. In turn, the insulin plays an important role in storing the excess

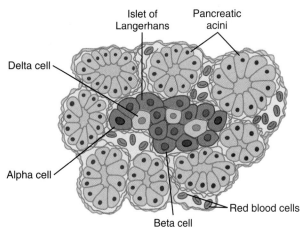

Figure 78-1 Physiologic anatomy of an islet of Langerhans in the pancreas.

energy. In the case of excess carbohydrates, it causes them to be stored as glycogen mainly in the liver and muscles. Also, all the excess carbohydrates that cannot be stored as glycogen are converted under the stimulus of insulin into fats and stored in the adipose tissue. In the case of proteins, insulin has a direct effect in promoting amino acid uptake by cells and conversion of these amino acids into protein. In addition, it inhibits the breakdown of the proteins that are already in the cells.

Insulin Chemistry and Synthesis

Insulin is a small protein; human insulin has a molecular weight of 5808. It is composed of two amino acid chains, shown in Figure 78-2, connected to each other by disulfide linkages. When the two amino acid chains are split apart, the functional activity of the insulin molecule is lost.

Insulin is synthesized in the beta cells by the usual cell machinery for protein synthesis, as explained in Chapter 3, beginning with translation of the insulin RNA by ribosomes attached to the endoplasmic reticulum to form *preproinsulin*. This initial preproinsulin has a molecular weight of about 11,500, but it is then cleaved in the endoplasmic reticulum to form a *proinsulin* with a molecular weight of about 9000 and consisting of three

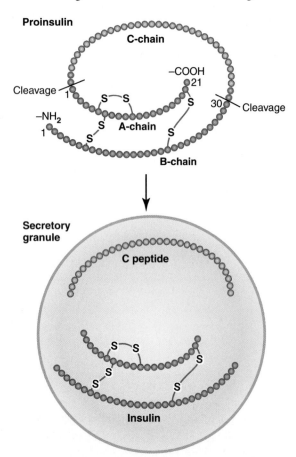

Figure 78-2 Schematic of the human proinsulin molecule, which is cleaved in the Golgi apparatus of the pancreatic beta cells to form connecting peptide (C peptide), and insulin, which is composed of the A and B chains connected by disulfide bonds. The C peptide and insulin are packaged in granules and secreted in equimolar amounts, along with a small amount of proinsulin.

chains of peptides, A, B, and C. Most of the proinsulin is further cleaved in the Golgi apparatus to form insulin, composed of the A and B chain connected by disulfide linkages, and the C chain peptide, called *connecting peptide* (*C peptide*). The insulin and C peptide are packaged in the secretory granules and secreted in equimolar amounts. About 5 to 10 percent of the final secreted product is still in the form of proinsulin.

The proinsulin and C peptide have virtually no insulin activity. However, C peptide binds to a membrane structure, most likely a G protein–coupled membrane receptor, and elicits activation of at least two enzyme systems, sodium-potassium ATPase and endothelial nitric oxide synthase. Although both of these enzymes have multiple physiological functions, the importance of C peptide in regulating these enzymes is still uncertain.

Measurement of C peptide levels by radioimmunoassay can be used in insulin-treated diabetic patients to determine how much of their own natural insulin they are still producing. Patients with type 1 diabetes who are unable to produce insulin will usually have greatly decreased levels of C peptide.

When insulin is secreted into the blood, it circulates almost entirely in an unbound form; it has a plasma half-life that averages only about 6 minutes, so it is mainly cleared from the circulation within 10 to 15 minutes. Except for that portion of the insulin that combines with receptors in the target cells, the remainder is degraded by the enzyme *insulinase* mainly in the liver, to a lesser extent in the kidneys and muscles, and slightly in most other tissues. This rapid removal from the plasma is important because, at times, it is as important to turn off rapidly as to turn on the control functions of insulin.

Activation of Target Cell Receptors by Insulin and the Resulting Cellular Effects

To initiate its effects on target cells, insulin first binds with and activates a membrane receptor protein that has a molecular weight of about 300,000 (Figure 78-3). It is the activated receptor that causes the subsequent effects.

The insulin receptor is a combination of four subunits held together by disulfide linkages: *two alpha subunits* that lie entirely outside the cell membrane and *two beta subunits* that penetrate through the membrane, protruding into the cell cytoplasm. The insulin binds with the alpha subunits on the outside of the cell, but because of the linkages with the beta subunits, the portions of the beta subunits protruding into the cell become autophosphorylated. Thus, the insulin receptor is an example of an *enzyme-linked receptor*, discussed in Chapter 74. Autophosphorylation of the beta subunits of the receptor activates a local *tyrosine kinase*, which in turn causes phosphorylation of multiple other intracellular enzymes including a group called *insulin-receptor substrates (IRS)*. Different types of IRS (e.g., IRS-1, IRS-2, IRS-3) are expressed in different tissues. The net effect is to activate some of these enzymes while inactivating others. In this

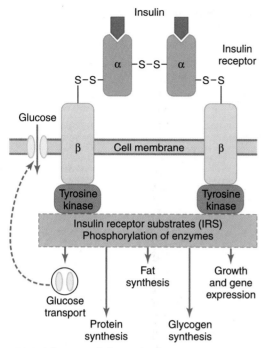

Figure 78-3 Schematic of the insulin receptor. Insulin binds to the α-subunit of its receptor, which causes autophosphorylation of the β-subunit receptor, which in turn induces tyrosine kinase activity. The receptor tyrosine kinase activity begins a cascade of cell phosphorylation that increases or decreases the activity of enzymes, including insulin receptor substrates, that mediate the effects on glucose, fat, and protein metabolism. For example, glucose transporters are moved to the cell membrane to assist glucose entry into the cell.

way, insulin directs the intracellular metabolic machinery to produce the desired effects on carbohydrate, fat, and protein metabolism. The end effects of insulin stimulation are the following:

1. Within seconds after insulin binds with its membrane receptors, the membranes of about 80 percent of the body's cells markedly increase their uptake of glucose. This is especially true of muscle cells and adipose cells but *is not true of most neurons in the brain.* The increased glucose transported into the cells is immediately phosphorylated and becomes a substrate for all the usual carbohydrate metabolic functions. The increased glucose transport is believed to result from translocation of multiple intracellular vesicles to the cell membranes; these vesicles carry multiple molecules of glucose transport proteins, which bind with the cell membrane and facilitate glucose uptake into the cells. When insulin is no longer available, these vesicles separate from the cell membrane within about 3 to 5 minutes and move back to the cell interior to be used again and again as needed.

2. The cell membrane becomes more permeable to many of the amino acids, potassium ions, and phosphate ions, causing increased transport of these substances into the cell.

3. Slower effects occur during the next 10 to 15 minutes to change the activity levels of many more intracellular metabolic enzymes. These effects result mainly from the changed states of phosphorylation of the enzymes.

4. Much slower effects continue to occur for hours and even several days. They result from changed rates of translation of messenger RNAs at the ribosomes to form new proteins and still slower effects from changed rates of transcription of DNA in the cell nucleus. In this way, insulin remolds much of the cellular enzymatic machinery to achieve its metabolic goals.

Effect of Insulin on Carbohydrate Metabolism

Immediately after a high-carbohydrate meal, the glucose that is absorbed into the blood causes rapid secretion of insulin, which is discussed in detail later in the chapter. The insulin in turn causes rapid uptake, storage, and use of glucose by almost all tissues of the body, but especially by the muscles, adipose tissue, and liver.

Insulin Promotes Muscle Glucose Uptake and Metabolism

During much of the day, muscle tissue depends not on glucose for its energy but on fatty acids. The principal reason for this is that the normal *resting muscle* membrane is only slightly permeable to glucose, except when the muscle fiber is stimulated by insulin; between meals, the amount of insulin that is secreted is too small to promote significant amounts of glucose entry into the muscle cells.

However, under two conditions the muscles do use large amounts of glucose. One of these is during moderate or heavy exercise. This usage of glucose does not require large amounts of insulin because exercising muscle fibers become more permeable to glucose even in the absence of insulin because of the contraction process itself.

The second condition for muscle usage of large amounts of glucose is during the few hours after a meal. At this time the blood glucose concentration is high and the pancreas is secreting large quantities of insulin. The extra insulin causes rapid transport of glucose into the muscle cells. This causes the muscle cell during this period to use glucose preferentially over fatty acids, as discussed later.

Storage of Glycogen in Muscle. If the muscles are not exercising after a meal and yet glucose is transported into the muscle cells in abundance, then most of the glucose is stored in the form of muscle glycogen instead of being used for energy, up to a limit of 2 to 3 percent concentration. The glycogen can later be used for energy by the muscle. It is especially useful for short periods of extreme energy use by the muscles and even to provide spurts of anaerobic energy for a few minutes at a time by glycolytic breakdown of the glycogen to lactic acid, which can occur even in the absence of oxygen.

Quantitative Effect of Insulin to Assist Glucose Transport through the Muscle Cell Membrane. The quantitative effect of insulin to facilitate glucose transport through the muscle cell membrane is demonstrated by the experimental results shown in Figure 78-4. The lower curve labeled "control" shows the concentration of free glucose measured inside the cell, demonstrating that the glucose concentration remained almost zero despite

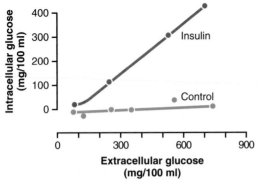

Figure 78-4 Effect of insulin in enhancing the concentration of glucose inside muscle cells. Note that in the absence of insulin (control), the intracellular glucose concentration remains near zero, despite high extracellular glucose concentrations. (Data from Eisenstein AB: The Biochemical Aspects of Hormone Action. Boston: Little, Brown, 1964.)

increased extracellular glucose concentration up to as high as 750 mg/100 ml. In contrast, the curve labeled "insulin" demonstrates that the intracellular glucose concentration rose to as high as 400 mg/100 ml when insulin was added. Thus, it is clear that insulin can increase the rate of transport of glucose into the resting muscle cell by at least 15-fold.

Insulin Promotes Liver Uptake, Storage, and Use of Glucose

One of the most important of all the effects of insulin is to cause most of the glucose absorbed after a meal to be stored almost immediately in the liver in the form of glycogen. Then, between meals, when food is not available and the blood glucose concentration begins to fall, insulin secretion decreases rapidly and the liver glycogen is split back into glucose, which is released back into the blood to keep the glucose concentration from falling too low.

The mechanism by which insulin causes glucose uptake and storage in the liver includes several almost simultaneous steps:

1. Insulin *inactivates liver phosphorylase,* the principal enzyme that causes liver glycogen to split into glucose. This prevents breakdown of the glycogen that has been stored in the liver cells.

2. Insulin causes *enhanced uptake of glucose* from the blood by the liver cells. It does this by *increasing the activity of the enzyme glucokinase,* which is one of the enzymes that causes the initial phosphorylation of glucose after it diffuses into the liver cells. Once phosphorylated, the glucose is *temporarily* trapped inside the liver cells because phosphorylated glucose cannot diffuse back through the cell membrane.

3. Insulin also increases the activities of the enzymes that promote glycogen synthesis, including especially *glycogen synthase,* which is responsible for polymerization of the monosaccharide units to form the glycogen molecules.

The net effect of all these actions is to increase the amount of glycogen in the liver. The glycogen can increase to a total of about 5 to 6 percent of the liver mass, which is equivalent to almost 100 grams of stored glycogen in the whole liver.

Glucose Is Released from the Liver Between Meals. When the blood glucose level begins to fall to a low level between meals, several events transpire that cause the liver to release glucose back into the circulating blood:

1. The decreasing blood glucose causes the pancreas to decrease its insulin secretion.

2. The lack of insulin then reverses all the effects listed earlier for glycogen storage, essentially stopping further synthesis of glycogen in the liver and preventing further uptake of glucose by the liver from the blood.

3. The lack of insulin (along with increase of glucagon, which is discussed later) activates the enzyme *phosphorylase,* which causes the splitting of glycogen into *glucose phosphate.*

4. The enzyme *glucose phosphatase,* which had been inhibited by insulin, now becomes activated by the insulin lack and causes the phosphate radical to split away from the glucose; this allows the free glucose to diffuse back into the blood.

Thus, the liver removes glucose from the blood when it is present in excess after a meal and returns it to the blood when the blood glucose concentration falls between meals. Ordinarily, about 60 percent of the glucose in the meal is stored in this way in the liver and then returned later.

Insulin Promotes Conversion of Excess Glucose into Fatty Acids and Inhibits Gluconeogenesis in the Liver. When the quantity of glucose entering the liver cells is more than can be stored as glycogen or can be used for local hepatocyte metabolism, *insulin promotes the conversion of all this excess glucose into fatty acids.* These fatty acids are subsequently packaged as triglycerides in very-low-density lipoproteins and transported in this form by way of the blood to the adipose tissue and deposited as fat.

Insulin also *inhibits gluconeogenesis.* It does this mainly by decreasing the quantities and activities of the liver enzymes required for gluconeogenesis. However, part of the effect is caused by an action of insulin that decreases the release of amino acids from muscle and other extrahepatic tissues and in turn the availability of these necessary precursors required for gluconeogenesis. This is discussed further in relation to the effect of insulin on protein metabolism.

Lack of Effect of Insulin on Glucose Uptake and Usage by the Brain

The brain is quite different from most other tissues of the body in that insulin has little effect on uptake or use of glucose. Instead, *most of the brain cells are permeable to glucose and can use glucose without the intermediation of insulin.*

The brain cells are also quite different from most other cells of the body in that they normally use only glucose for energy and can use other energy substrates, such as fats, only with difficulty. Therefore, it is essential that the blood glucose level always be maintained above a critical level, which is one of the most important functions of the blood glucose control system. When the blood glucose falls too low, into the range of 20 to 50 mg/100 ml, symptoms of *hypoglycemic shock* develop, characterized by progressive nervous irritability that leads to fainting, seizures, and even coma.

Effect of Insulin on Carbohydrate Metabolism in Other Cells

Insulin increases glucose transport into and glucose usage by most other cells of the body (with the exception of the brain cells, as noted) in the same way that it affects glucose transport and usage in muscle cells. The transport of glucose into adipose cells mainly provides substrate for the glycerol portion of the fat molecule. Therefore, in this indirect way, insulin promotes deposition of fat in these cells.

Effect of Insulin on Fat Metabolism

Although not quite as visible as the acute effects of insulin on carbohydrate metabolism, insulin's effects on fat metabolism are, in the long run, equally important. Especially dramatic is the long-term effect of *insulin lack* in causing extreme atherosclerosis, often leading to heart attacks, cerebral strokes, and other vascular accidents. But first, let us discuss the acute effects of insulin on fat metabolism.

Insulin Promotes Fat Synthesis and Storage

Insulin has several effects that lead to fat storage in adipose tissue. First, insulin increases the utilization of glucose by most of the body's tissues, which automatically decreases the utilization of fat, thus functioning as a fat sparer. However, insulin also promotes fatty acid synthesis. This is especially true when more carbohydrates are ingested than can be used for immediate energy, thus providing the substrate for fat synthesis. Almost all this synthesis occurs in the liver cells, and the fatty acids are then transported from the liver by way of the blood lipoproteins to the adipose cells to be stored. The different factors that lead to increased fatty acid synthesis in the liver include the following:

1. *Insulin increases the transport of glucose into the liver cells.* After the liver glycogen concentration reaches 5 to 6 percent, this in itself inhibits further glycogen synthesis. Then all the additional glucose entering the liver cells becomes available to form fat. The glucose is first split to pyruvate in the glycolytic pathway, and the pyruvate subsequently is converted to acetyl coenzyme A (acetyl-CoA), the substrate from which fatty acids are synthesized.

2. *An excess of citrate and isocitrate ions is formed by the citric acid cycle when excess amounts of glucose are being used for energy.* These ions then have a direct effect in activating *acetyl-CoA carboxylase,* the enzyme required to carboxylate acetyl-CoA to form *malonyl-CoA,* the first stage of fatty acid synthesis.

3. *Most of the fatty acids are then synthesized within the liver and used to form triglycerides,* the usual form of storage fat. They are released from the liver cells to the blood in the lipoproteins. Insulin activates *lipoprotein lipase* in the capillary walls of the adipose tissue, which splits the triglycerides again into fatty acids, a requirement for them to be absorbed into the adipose cells, where they are again converted to triglycerides and stored.

Role of Insulin in Storage of Fat in the Adipose Cells. Insulin has two other essential effects that are required for fat storage in adipose cells:

1. *Insulin inhibits the action of hormone-sensitive lipase.* This is the enzyme that causes hydrolysis of the triglycerides already stored in the fat cells. Therefore, the release of fatty acids from the adipose tissue into the circulating blood is inhibited.

2. *Insulin promotes glucose transport through the cell membrane into the fat cells* in the same way that it promotes glucose transport into muscle cells. Some of this glucose is then used to synthesize minute amounts of fatty acids, but more important, it also forms large quantities of α-glycerol phosphate. This substance supplies the *glycerol* that combines with fatty acids to form the triglycerides that are the storage form of fat in adipose cells. Therefore, when insulin is not available, even storage of the large amounts of fatty acids transported from the liver in the lipoproteins is almost blocked.

Insulin Deficiency Increases Use of Fat for Energy

All aspects of fat breakdown and use for providing energy are greatly enhanced in the absence of insulin. This occurs even normally between meals when secretion of insulin is minimal, but it becomes extreme in diabetes mellitus when secretion of insulin is almost zero. The resulting effects are as follows.

Insulin Deficiency Causes Lipolysis of Storage Fat and Release of Free Fatty Acids. In the absence of insulin, all the effects of insulin noted earlier that cause storage of fat are reversed. The most important effect is that the enzyme *hormone-sensitive lipase* in the fat cells becomes strongly activated. This causes hydrolysis of the stored triglycerides, releasing large quantities of fatty acids and glycerol into the circulating blood. Consequently, the plasma concentration of free fatty acids begins to rise within minutes. These free fatty acids then become the main energy substrate used by essentially all tissues of the body except the brain.

Figure 78-5 shows the effect of insulin lack on the plasma concentrations of free fatty acids, glucose, and

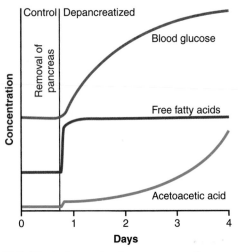

Figure 78-5 Effect of removing the pancreas on the approximate concentrations of blood glucose, plasma free fatty acids, and acetoacetic acid.

acetoacetic acid. Note that almost immediately after removal of the pancreas, the free fatty acid concentration in the plasma begins to rise, more rapidly even than the concentration of glucose.

Insulin Deficiency Increases Plasma Cholesterol and Phospholipid Concentrations. The excess of fatty acids in the plasma associated with insulin deficiency also promotes liver conversion of some of the fatty acids into phospholipids and cholesterol, two of the major products of fat metabolism. These two substances, along with excess triglycerides formed at the same time in the liver, are then discharged into the blood in the lipoproteins. Occasionally the plasma lipoproteins increase as much as threefold in the absence of insulin, giving a total concentration of plasma lipids of several percent rather than the normal 0.6 percent. This high lipid concentration—especially the high concentration of cholesterol—promotes the development of atherosclerosis in people with serious diabetes.

Excess Usage of Fats During Insulin Lack Causes Ketosis and Acidosis. Insulin lack also causes excessive amounts of *acetoacetic acid* to be formed in the liver cells due to the following effect: In the absence of insulin but in the presence of excess fatty acids in the liver cells, the carnitine transport mechanism for transporting fatty acids into the mitochondria becomes increasingly activated. In the mitochondria, beta oxidation of the fatty acids then proceeds rapidly, releasing extreme amounts of acetyl-CoA. A large part of this excess acetyl-CoA is then condensed to form acetoacetic acid, which is then released into the circulating blood. Most of this passes to the peripheral cells, where it is again converted into acetyl-CoA and used for energy in the usual manner.

At the same time, the absence of insulin also depresses the utilization of acetoacetic acid in the peripheral tissues. Thus, so much acetoacetic acid is released from the liver that it cannot all be metabolized by the tissues. As shown in Figure 78-5, the concentration of acetoacetic acid rises during the days after cessation of insulin secretion, sometimes reaching concentrations of 10 mEq/L or more, which is a severe state of body fluid acidosis.

As explained in Chapter 68, some of the acetoacetic acid is also converted into β-hydroxybutyric acid and *acetone*. These two substances, along with the acetoacetic acid, are called *ketone bodies,* and their presence in large quantities in the body fluids is called *ketosis.* We see later that in severe diabetes the acetoacetic acid and the β-hydroxybutyric acid can cause severe *acidosis* and *coma,* which may lead to death.

Effect of Insulin on Protein Metabolism and on Growth

Insulin Promotes Protein Synthesis and Storage. During the few hours after a meal when excess quantities of nutrients are available in the circulating blood, proteins, carbohydrates, and fats are stored in the tissues; insulin is required for this to occur. The manner in which insulin causes protein storage is not as well understood as the mechanisms for both glucose and fat storage. Some of the facts follow.

1. *Insulin stimulates transport of many of the amino acids into the cells.* Among the amino acids most strongly transported are *valine, leucine, isoleucine, tyrosine,* and *phenylalanine.* Thus, insulin shares with growth hormone the capability of increasing the uptake of amino acids into cells. However, the amino acids affected are not necessarily the same ones.

2. *Insulin increases the translation of messenger RNA,* thus forming new proteins. In some unexplained way, insulin "turns on" the ribosomal machinery. In the absence of insulin, the ribosomes simply stop working, almost as if insulin operates an "on-off" mechanism.

3. Over a longer period of time, *insulin also increases the rate of transcription of selected DNA genetic sequences* in the cell nuclei, thus forming increased quantities of RNA and still more protein synthesis—especially promoting a vast array of enzymes for storage of carbohydrates, fats, and proteins.

4. *Insulin inhibits the catabolism of proteins,* thus decreasing the rate of amino acid release from the cells, especially from the muscle cells. Presumably this results from the ability of insulin to diminish the normal degradation of proteins by the cellular lysosomes.

5. *In the liver, insulin depresses the rate of gluconeogenesis.* It does this by decreasing the activity of the enzymes that promote gluconeogenesis. Because the substrates most used for synthesis of glucose by gluconeogenesis are the plasma amino acids, this suppression of gluconeogenesis conserves the amino acids in the protein stores of the body.

In summary, insulin promotes protein formation and prevents the degradation of proteins.

Insulin Deficiency Causes Protein Depletion and Increased Plasma Amino Acids. Virtually all protein storage comes to a halt when insulin is not available. The catabolism of proteins increases, protein synthesis stops, and large quantities of amino acids are dumped into the plasma. The plasma amino acid concentration rises considerably, and most of the excess amino acids are used either directly for energy or as substrates for gluconeogenesis. This degradation of the amino acids also leads to enhanced urea excretion in the urine. The resulting protein wasting is one of the most serious of all the effects of severe diabetes mellitus. It can lead to extreme weakness and many deranged functions of the organs.

Insulin and Growth Hormone Interact Synergistically to Promote Growth. Because insulin is required for the synthesis of proteins, it is as essential for growth of an animal as growth hormone is. This is demonstrated in Figure 78-6, which shows that a depancreatized, hypophysectomized rat without therapy hardly grows at all. Furthermore, the administration of either growth hormone or insulin one at a time causes almost no growth. Yet a combination of these hormones causes dramatic growth. Thus, it appears that the two hormones function synergistically to promote growth, each performing a specific function that is separate from that of the other. Perhaps a small part of this necessity for both hormones results from the fact that each promotes cellular uptake of a different selection of amino acids, all of which are required if growth is to be achieved.

Mechanisms of Insulin Secretion

Figure 78-7 shows the basic cellular mechanisms for insulin secretion by the pancreatic beta cells in response to increased blood glucose concentration, the primary controller of insulin secretion. The beta cells have a large number of *glucose transporters* (GLUT 2) that permit a rate of glucose influx that is proportional to the blood concentration in the physiological range. Once inside the cells, glucose is phosphorylated to glucose-6-phosphate by

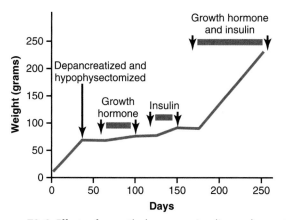

Figure 78-6 Effect of growth hormone, insulin, and growth hormone plus insulin on growth in a depancreatized and hypophysectomized rat.

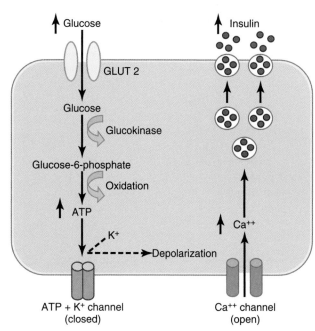

Figure 78-7 Basic mechanisms of glucose stimulation of insulin secretion by beta cells of the pancreas. GLUT, glucose transporter.

glucokinase. This appears to be the rate limiting step for glucose metabolism in the beta cell and is considered the major mechanism for glucose sensing and adjustment of the amount of secreted insulin to the blood glucose levels.

The glucose-6-phosphate is subsequently oxidized to form adenosine triphosphate (ATP), which inhibits the *ATP-sensitive potassium channels* of the cell. Closure of the potassium channels depolarizes the cell membrane, thereby opening *voltage-gated calcium channels*, which are sensitive to changes in membrane voltage. This produces an influx of calcium that stimulates fusion of the docked insulin-containing vesicles with the cell membrane and secretion of insulin into the extracellular fluid by *exocytosis.*

Other nutrients, such as certain amino acids, can also be metabolized by the beta cells to increase intracellular ATP levels and stimulate insulin secretion. Some hormones, such as glucagon, glucose-dependent insulinotropic peptide (gastric inhibitory peptide), and acetylcholine, increase intracellular calcium levels through other signaling pathways and enhance the effect of glucose, although they do not have major effects on insulin secretion in the absence of glucose. Other hormones, including somatostatin and norepinephrine (by activating α-adrenergic receptors), inhibit exocytosis of insulin.

Sulfonylurea drugs stimulate insulin secretion by binding to the ATP-sensitive potassium channels and blocking their activity. This results in a depolarizing effect that triggers insulin secretion, making these drugs useful in stimulating insulin secretion in patients with type II diabetes, as we discuss later. Table 78-1 summarizes some of the factors that can increase or decrease insulin secretion.

Control of Insulin Secretion

Formerly, it was believed that insulin secretion was controlled almost entirely by the blood glucose concentration.

Table 78-1 Factors and Conditions That Increase or Decrease Insulin Secretion

Increase Insulin Secretion	Decrease Insulin Secretion
Increased blood glucose	Decreased blood glucose
Increased blood free fatty acids	Fasting
Increased blood amino acids	Somatostatin
Gastrointestinal hormones (gastrin, cholecystokinin, secretin, gastric inhibitory peptide)	α-Adrenergic activity
	Leptin
Glucagon, growth hormone, cortisol	
Parasympathetic stimulation; acetylcholine	
β-Adrenergic stimulation	
Insulin resistance; obesity	
Sulfonylurea drugs (glyburide, tolbutamide)	

However, as more has been learned about the metabolic functions of insulin for protein and fat metabolism, it has become apparent that blood amino acids and other factors also play important roles in controlling insulin secretion (see Table 78-1).

Increased Blood Glucose Stimulates Insulin Secretion. At the normal *fasting* level of blood glucose of 80 to 90 mg/100 ml, the rate of insulin secretion is minimal—on the order of 25 ng/min/kg of body weight, a level that has only slight physiological activity. If the blood glucose concentration is suddenly increased to a level two to three times normal and kept at this high level thereafter, insulin secretion increases markedly in two stages, as shown by the changes in plasma insulin concentration seen in Figure 78-8.

1. Plasma insulin concentration increases almost 10-fold within 3 to 5 minutes after the acute elevation of the blood glucose; this results from immediate dumping of preformed insulin from the beta cells of the islets

of Langerhans. However, the initial high rate of secretion is not maintained; instead, the insulin concentration decreases about halfway back toward normal in another 5 to 10 minutes.

2. Beginning at about 15 minutes, insulin secretion rises a second time and reaches a new plateau in 2 to 3 hours, this time usually at a rate of secretion even greater than that in the initial phase. This secretion results both from additional release of preformed insulin and from activation of the enzyme system that synthesizes and releases new insulin from the cells.

Feedback Relation between Blood Glucose Concentration and Insulin Secretion Rate. As the concentration of blood glucose rises above 100 mg/100 ml of blood, the rate of insulin secretion rises rapidly, reaching a peak some 10 to 25 times the basal level at blood glucose concentrations between 400 and 600 mg/100 ml, as shown in Figure 78-9. Thus, the increase in insulin secretion under a glucose stimulus is dramatic both in its rapidity and in the tremendous level of secretion achieved. Furthermore, the turn-off of insulin secretion is almost equally as rapid, occurring within 3 to 5 minutes after reduction in blood glucose concentration back to the fasting level.

This response of insulin secretion to an elevated blood glucose concentration provides an extremely important feedback mechanism for regulating blood glucose concentration. That is, any rise in blood glucose increases insulin secretion and the insulin in turn increases transport of glucose into liver, muscle, and other cells, thereby reducing the blood glucose concentration back toward the normal value.

Other Factors That Stimulate Insulin Secretion

Amino Acids. In addition to the stimulation of insulin secretion by excess blood glucose, some of the amino acids have a similar effect. The most potent of these are *arginine* and *lysine*. This effect differs from glucose stimulation of insulin secretion in the following way: Amino acids administered in the absence of a rise in blood glucose cause only a small increase in insulin secretion. However, when administered at the same time that the blood glucose concentration

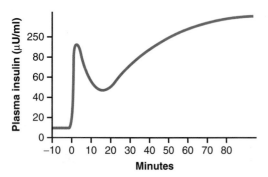

Figure 78-8 Increase in plasma insulin concentration after a sudden increase in blood glucose to two to three times the normal range. Note an initial rapid surge in insulin concentration and then a delayed but higher and continuing increase in concentration beginning 15 to 20 minutes later.

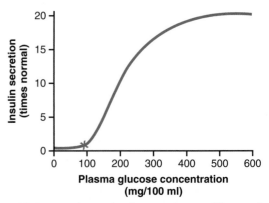

Figure 78-9 Approximate insulin secretion at different plasma glucose levels.

is elevated, the glucose-induced secretion of insulin may be as much as doubled in the presence of the excess amino acids. Thus, the *amino acids strongly potentiate the glucose stimulus for insulin secretion.*

The stimulation of insulin secretion by amino acids is important because the insulin in turn promotes transport of amino acids into the tissue cells, as well as intracellular formation of protein. That is, insulin is important for proper utilization of excess amino acids in the same way that it is important for the utilization of carbohydrates.

Gastrointestinal Hormones. A mixture of several important gastrointestinal hormones—*gastrin, secretin, cholecystokinin,* and *glucose-dependent insulinotrophic peptide* (which seems to be the most potent)—causes a moderate increase in insulin secretion. These hormones are released in the gastrointestinal tract after a person eats a meal. They then cause an "anticipatory" increase in blood insulin in preparation for the glucose and amino acids to be absorbed from the meal. These gastrointestinal hormones generally act the same way as amino acids to increase the sensitivity of insulin response to increased blood glucose, almost doubling the rate of insulin secretion as the blood glucose level rises.

Other Hormones and the Autonomic Nervous System. Other hormones that either directly increase insulin secretion or potentiate the glucose stimulus for insulin secretion include *glucagon, growth hormone, cortisol,* and, to a lesser extent, *progesterone* and *estrogen*. The importance of the stimulatory effects of these hormones is that prolonged secretion of any one of them in large quantities can occasionally lead to exhaustion of the beta cells of the islets of Langerhans and thereby increase the risk for developing diabetes mellitus. Indeed, diabetes often occurs in people who are maintained on high pharmacological doses of some of these hormones. Diabetes is particularly common in giants or acromegalic people with growth hormone–secreting tumors, or in people whose adrenal glands secrete excess glucocorticoids.

Under some conditions, stimulation of the parasympathetic nerves to the pancreas can increase insulin secretion, whereas sympathetic nerve stimulation may decrease insulin secretion. However, it is doubtful that these effects play a major role in physiological regulation of insulin secretion.

Role of Insulin (and Other Hormones) in "Switching" Between Carbohydrate and Lipid Metabolism

From the preceding discussions, it should be clear that insulin promotes the utilization of carbohydrates for energy, whereas it depresses the utilization of fats. Conversely, lack of insulin causes fat utilization mainly to the exclusion of glucose utilization, except by brain tissue. Furthermore, the signal that controls this switching mechanism is principally the blood glucose concentration. When the glucose concentration is low, insulin secretion is suppressed and fat is used almost exclusively for energy everywhere except in the brain. When the glucose concentration is high, insulin secretion is stimulated and carbohydrate is used instead of fat. The excess blood glucose is stored in the form of liver glycogen, liver fat, and muscle glycogen. Therefore, one of the most important functional roles of insulin in the body is to control which of

these two foods from moment to moment will be used by the cells for energy.

At least four other known hormones also play important roles in this switching mechanism: *growth hormone* from the anterior pituitary gland, *cortisol* from the adrenal cortex, *epinephrine* from the adrenal medulla, and *glucagon* from the alpha cells of the islets of Langerhans in the pancreas. Glucagon is discussed in the next section of this chapter. Both growth hormone and cortisol are secreted in response to hypoglycemia, and both inhibit cellular utilization of glucose while promoting fat utilization. However, the effects of both of these hormones develop slowly, usually requiring many hours for maximal expression.

Epinephrine is especially important in increasing plasma glucose concentration during periods of stress when the sympathetic nervous system is excited. However, epinephrine acts differently from the other hormones in that it increases the plasma fatty acid concentration at the same time. The reasons for these effects are as follows: (1) epinephrine has the potent effect of causing glycogenolysis in the liver, thus releasing within minutes large quantities of glucose into the blood; (2) it also has a direct lipolytic effect on the adipose cells because it activates adipose tissue hormone-sensitive lipase, thus greatly enhancing the blood concentration of fatty acids as well. Quantitatively, the enhancement of fatty acids is far greater than the enhancement of blood glucose. Therefore, epinephrine especially enhances the utilization of fat in such stressful states as exercise, circulatory shock, and anxiety.

Glucagon and Its Functions

Glucagon, a hormone secreted by the *alpha cells* of the islets of Langerhans when the blood glucose concentration falls, has several functions that are diametrically opposed to those of insulin. Most important of these functions is to increase the blood glucose concentration, an effect that is exactly the opposite that of insulin.

Like insulin, glucagon is a large polypeptide. It has a molecular weight of 3485 and is composed of a chain of 29 amino acids. On injection of purified glucagon into an animal, a profound *hyperglycemic* effect occurs. Only 1 µg/kg of glucagon can elevate the blood glucose concentration about 20 mg/100 ml of blood (a 25 percent increase) in about 20 minutes. For this reason, glucagon is also called the *hyperglycemic hormone*.

Effects on Glucose Metabolism

The major effects of glucagon on glucose metabolism are (1) breakdown of liver glycogen (*glycogenolysis*) and (2) increased *gluconeogenesis* in the liver. Both of these effects greatly enhance the availability of glucose to the other organs of the body.

Glucagon Causes Glycogenolysis and Increased Blood Glucose Concentration. The most dramatic effect of glucagon is its ability to cause glycogenolysis in the liver, which in turn increases the blood glucose concentration within minutes.

It does this by the following complex cascade of events:

1. Glucagon activates *adenylyl cyclase* in the hepatic cell membrane,
2. Which causes the formation of *cyclic adenosine monophosphate*,
3. Which activates *protein kinase regulator protein*,
4. Which activates *protein kinase*,
5. Which activates *phosphorylase b kinase*,
6. Which converts *phosphorylase b* into *phosphorylase a*,
7. Which promotes the degradation of glycogen into glucose-1-phosphate,
8. Which is then dephosphorylated; and the glucose is released from the liver cells.

This sequence of events is exceedingly important for several reasons. First, it is one of the most thoroughly studied of all the *second messenger* functions of cyclic adenosine monophosphate. Second, it demonstrates a cascade system in which *each succeeding product is produced in greater quantity than the preceding product*. Therefore, it represents a potent *amplifying* mechanism; this type of amplifying mechanism is widely used throughout the body for controlling many, if not most, cellular metabolic systems, often causing as much as a millionfold amplification in response. This explains how *only a few micrograms of glucagon can cause the blood glucose level to double or increase even more within a few minutes*.

Infusion of glucagon for about 4 hours can cause such intensive liver glycogenolysis that all the liver stores of glycogen become depleted.

Glucagon Increases Gluconeogenesis

Even after all the glycogen in the liver has been exhausted under the influence of glucagon, continued infusion of this hormone still causes continued hyperglycemia. This results from the effect of glucagon to increase the rate of amino acid uptake by the liver cells and then the conversion of many of the amino acids to glucose by gluconeogenesis. This is achieved by activating multiple enzymes that are required for amino acid transport and gluconeogenesis, especially activation of the enzyme system for converting pyruvate to phosphoenolpyruvate, a rate-limiting step in gluconeogenesis.

Other Effects of Glucagon

Most other effects of glucagon occur only when its concentration rises well above the maximum normally found in the blood. Perhaps the most important effect is that *glucagon activates adipose cell lipase,* making increased quantities of fatty acids available to the energy systems of the body. Glucagon also inhibits the storage of triglycerides in the liver, which prevents the liver from removing fatty acids from the blood; this also helps make additional

amounts of fatty acids available for the other tissues of the body.

Glucagon in high concentrations also (1) enhances the strength of the heart; (2) increases blood flow in some tissues, especially the kidneys; (3) enhances bile secretion; and (4) inhibits gastric acid secretion. All these effects are probably of minimal importance in the normal function of the body.

Regulation of Glucagon Secretion

Increased Blood Glucose Inhibits Glucagon Secretion. The blood glucose concentration is by far the most potent factor that controls glucagon secretion. Note specifically, however, that *the effect of blood glucose concentration on glucagon secretion is in exactly the opposite direction from the effect of glucose on insulin secretion.*

This is demonstrated in Figure 78-10, showing that a *decrease* in the blood glucose concentration from its normal fasting level of about 90 mg/100 ml of blood down to hypoglycemic levels can increase the plasma concentration of glucagon severalfold. Conversely, increasing the blood glucose to hyperglycemic levels decreases plasma glucagon. Thus, in hypoglycemia, glucagon is secreted in large amounts; it then greatly increases the output of glucose from the liver and thereby serves the important function of correcting the hypoglycemia.

Increased Blood Amino Acids Stimulate Glucagon Secretion. High concentrations of amino acids, as occur in the blood after a protein meal (especially the amino acids *alanine* and *arginine*), *stimulate* the secretion of glucagon. This is the same effect that amino acids have in stimulating insulin secretion. Thus, in this instance, the glucagon and insulin responses are not opposites. The importance of amino acid stimulation of glucagon secretion is that the glucagon then promotes rapid conversion of the amino acids to glucose, thus making even more glucose available to the tissues.

Exercise Stimulates Glucagon Secretion. In exhaustive exercise, the blood concentration of glucagon often increases fourfold to fivefold. What causes this is not understood because the blood glucose concentration

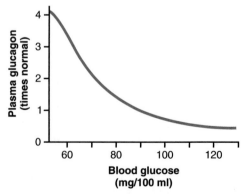

Figure 78-10 Approximate plasma glucagon concentration at different blood glucose levels.

does not necessarily fall. A beneficial effect of the glucagon is that it prevents a decrease in blood glucose.

One of the factors that might increase glucagon secretion in exercise is increased circulating amino acids. Other factors, such as β-adrenergic stimulation of the islets of Langerhans, may also play a role.

Somatostatin Inhibits Glucagon and Insulin Secretion

The *delta cells* of the islets of Langerhans secrete the hormone *somatostatin,* a 14 amino acid polypeptide that has an extremely short half-life of only 3 minutes in the circulating blood. Almost all factors related to the ingestion of food stimulate somatostatin secretion. They include (1) increased blood glucose, (2) increased amino acids, (3) increased fatty acids, and (4) increased concentrations of several of the gastrointestinal hormones released from the upper gastrointestinal tract in response to food intake.

In turn, somatostatin has multiple inhibitory effects as follows:

1. Somatostatin acts locally within the islets of Langerhans themselves to depress the secretion of both insulin and glucagon.
2. Somatostatin decreases the motility of the stomach, duodenum, and gallbladder.
3. Somatostatin decreases both secretion and absorption in the gastrointestinal tract.

Putting all this information together, it has been suggested that the principal role of somatostatin is to extend the period of time over which the food nutrients are assimilated into the blood. At the same time, the effect of somatostatin to depress insulin and glucagon secretion decreases the utilization of the absorbed nutrients by the tissues, thus preventing rapid exhaustion of the food and therefore making it available over a longer period of time.

It should also be recalled that somatostatin is the same chemical substance as *growth hormone inhibitory hormone,* which is secreted in the hypothalamus and suppresses anterior pituitary gland growth hormone secretion.

Summary of Blood Glucose Regulation

In a normal person, the blood glucose concentration is narrowly controlled, usually between 80 and 90 mg/100 ml of blood in the fasting person each morning before breakfast. This concentration increases to 120 to 140 mg/100 ml during the first hour or so after a meal, but the feedback systems for control of blood glucose return the glucose concentration rapidly back to the control level, usually within 2 hours after the last absorption of carbohydrates. Conversely, in starvation, the gluconeogenesis function of the liver provides the glucose that is required to maintain the fasting blood glucose level.

The mechanisms for achieving this high degree of control have been presented in this chapter. Let us summarize them.

1. *The liver functions as an important blood glucose buffer system.* That is, when the blood glucose rises to a high concentration after a meal and the rate of insulin secretion also increases, as much as two thirds of the glucose absorbed from the gut is almost immediately stored in the liver in the form of glycogen. Then, during the succeeding hours, when both the blood glucose concentration and the rate of insulin secretion fall, the liver releases the glucose back into the blood. In this way, the liver decreases the fluctuations in blood glucose concentration to about one third of what they would otherwise be. In fact, in patients with severe liver disease, it becomes almost impossible to maintain a narrow range of blood glucose concentration.

2. *Both insulin and glucagon function as important feedback control systems for maintaining a normal blood glucose concentration.* When the glucose concentration rises too high, increased insulin secretion causes the blood glucose concentration to decrease toward normal. Conversely, a decrease in blood glucose stimulates glucagon secretion; the glucagon then functions in the opposite direction to increase the glucose toward normal. Under most normal conditions, the insulin feedback mechanism is much more important than the glucagon mechanism, but in instances of starvation or excessive utilization of glucose during exercise and other stressful situations, the glucagon mechanism also becomes valuable.

3. Also, in severe hypoglycemia, a direct effect of low blood glucose on the hypothalamus stimulates the sympathetic nervous system. The epinephrine secreted by the adrenal glands further increases release of glucose from the liver. This also helps protect against severe hypoglycemia.

4. And finally, over a period of hours and days, both growth hormone and cortisol are secreted in response to prolonged hypoglycemia. They both decrease the rate of glucose utilization by most cells of the body, converting instead to greater amounts of fat utilization. This, too, helps return the blood glucose concentration toward normal.

Importance of Blood Glucose Regulation. One might ask the question: Why is it so important to maintain a constant blood glucose concentration, particularly because most tissues can shift to utilization of fats and proteins for energy in the absence of glucose? The answer is that glucose is the only nutrient that normally can be used by the *brain, retina,* and *germinal epithelium of the gonads* in sufficient quantities to supply them optimally with their required energy. Therefore, it is important to maintain the blood glucose concentration at a sufficiently high level to provide this necessary nutrition.

Most of the glucose formed by gluconeogenesis during the interdigestive period is used for metabolism in the brain. Indeed, it is important that the pancreas not secrete any insulin during this time; otherwise, the scant supplies of glucose that are available would all go into the muscles and other peripheral tissues, leaving the brain without a nutritive source.

It is also important that the blood glucose concentration not rise too high for four reasons: (1) Glucose can exert a large amount of osmotic pressure in the extracellular fluid, and if the glucose concentration rises to excessive values, this can cause considerable cellular dehydration. (2) An excessively high level of blood glucose concentration causes loss of glucose in the urine. (3) Loss of glucose in the urine also causes osmotic diuresis by the kidneys, which can deplete the body of its fluids and electrolytes. (4) Long-term increases in blood glucose may cause damage to many tissues, especially to blood vessels. Vascular injury associated with uncontrolled diabetes mellitus leads to increased risk for heart attack, stroke, end-stage renal disease, and blindness.

Diabetes Mellitus

Diabetes mellitus is a syndrome of impaired carbohydrate, fat, and protein metabolism caused by either lack of insulin secretion or decreased sensitivity of the tissues to insulin. There are two general types of diabetes mellitus:

1. *Type I diabetes*, also called *insulin-dependent diabetes mellitus* (IDDM), is caused by lack of insulin secretion.

2. *Type II diabetes*, also called *non-insulin-dependent diabetes mellitus* (NIDDM), is initially caused by decreased sensitivity of target tissues to the metabolic effect of insulin. This reduced sensitivity to insulin is often called *insulin resistance.*

In both types of diabetes mellitus, metabolism of all the main foodstuffs is altered. The basic effect of insulin lack or insulin resistance on glucose metabolism is to prevent the efficient uptake and utilization of glucose by most cells of the body, except those of the brain. As a result, blood glucose concentration increases, cell utilization of glucose falls increasingly lower, and utilization of fats and proteins increases.

Type I Diabetes—Deficiency of Insulin Production by Beta Cells of the Pancreas

Injury to the beta cells of the pancreas or diseases that impair insulin production can lead to type I diabetes. *Viral infections* or *autoimmune disorders* may be involved in the destruction of beta cells in many patients with type I diabetes, although heredity also plays a major role in determining the susceptibility of the beta cells to destruction by these insults. In some instances, there may be a hereditary tendency for beta cell degeneration even without viral infections or autoimmune disorders.

The usual onset of type I diabetes occurs at about 14 years of age in the United States, and for this reason it is often called *juvenile diabetes mellitus.* However, type I diabetes can occur at any age, including adulthood, following disorders that lead to destruction of pancreatic beta cells. Type I diabetes may develop abruptly, over a period of a few days or weeks, with three principal sequelae: (1) increased blood glucose, (2) increased utilization of fats for energy and

for formation of cholesterol by the liver, and (3) depletion of the body's proteins. Approximately 5 to 10 percent of people with diabetes mellitus have the type I form of the disease.

Blood Glucose Concentration Rises to High Levels in Diabetes Mellitus. The lack of insulin decreases the efficiency of peripheral glucose utilization and augments glucose production, raising plasma glucose to 300 to 1200 mg/100 ml. The increased plasma glucose then has multiple effects throughout the body.

Increased Blood Glucose Causes Loss of Glucose in the Urine. The high blood glucose causes more glucose to filter into the renal tubules than can be reabsorbed, and the excess glucose spills into the urine. This normally occurs when the blood glucose concentration rises above 180 mg/100 ml, a level that is called the blood "threshold" for the appearance of glucose in the urine. When the blood glucose level rises to 300 to 500 mg/100 ml—common values in people with severe untreated diabetes—100 or more grams of glucose can be lost into the urine each day.

Increased Blood Glucose Causes Dehydration. The very high levels of blood glucose (sometimes as high as 8 to 10 times normal in severe untreated diabetes) can cause severe cell dehydration throughout the body. This occurs partly because glucose does not diffuse easily through the pores of the cell membrane, and the increased osmotic pressure in the extracellular fluids causes osmotic transfer of water out of the cells.

In addition to the direct cellular dehydrating effect of excessive glucose, the loss of glucose in the urine causes *osmotic diuresis.* That is, the osmotic effect of glucose in the renal tubules greatly decreases tubular reabsorption of fluid. The overall effect is massive loss of fluid in the urine, causing dehydration of the extracellular fluid, which in turn causes compensatory dehydration of the intracellular fluid, for reasons discussed in Chapter 26. Thus, *polyuria* (excessive urine excretion), *intracellular and extracellular dehydration*, and *increased thirst* are classic symptoms of diabetes.

Chronic High Glucose Concentration Causes Tissue Injury. When blood glucose is poorly controlled over long periods in diabetes mellitus, blood vessels in multiple tissues throughout the body begin to function abnormally and undergo structural changes that result in inadequate blood supply to the tissues. This in turn leads to increased risk for heart attack, stroke, end-stage kidney disease, retinopathy and blindness, and ischemia and gangrene of the limbs.

Chronic high glucose concentration also causes damage to many other tissues. For example, *peripheral neuropathy*, which is abnormal function of peripheral nerves, and *autonomic nervous system dysfunction* are frequent complications of chronic, uncontrolled diabetes mellitus. These abnormalities can result in impaired cardiovascular reflexes, impaired bladder control, decreased sensation in the extremities, and other symptoms of peripheral nerve damage.

The precise mechanisms that cause tissue injury in diabetes are not well understood but probably involve multiple effects of high glucose concentrations and other metabolic abnormalities on proteins of endothelial and vascular smooth muscle cells, as well as other tissues. In addition, *hypertension*, secondary to renal injury, and *atherosclerosis*, secondary to abnormal lipid metabolism, often develop in patients with diabetes and amplify the tissue damage caused by the elevated glucose.

Diabetes Mellitus Causes Increased Utilization of Fats and Metabolic Acidosis. The shift from carbohydrate to fat metabolism in diabetes increases the release of keto acids, such as acetoacetic acid and β-hydroxybutyric acid, into the plasma more rapidly than they can be taken up and oxidized by the tissue cells. As a result, the patient develops severe *metabolic acidosis* from the excess keto acids, which, in association with dehydration due to the excessive urine formation, can cause severe acidosis. This leads rapidly to *diabetic coma* and death unless the condition is treated immediately with large amounts of insulin.

All the usual physiological compensations that occur in metabolic acidosis take place in diabetic acidosis. They include *rapid and deep breathing,* which causes increased expiration of carbon dioxide; this buffers the acidosis but also depletes extracellular fluid bicarbonate stores. The kidneys compensate by decreasing bicarbonate excretion and generating new bicarbonate that is added back to the extracellular fluid.

Although extreme acidosis occurs only in the most severe instances of uncontrolled diabetes, when the pH of the blood falls below about 7.0, *acidotic coma* and death can occur within hours. The overall changes in the electrolytes of the blood as a result of severe diabetic acidosis are shown in Figure 78-11.

Excess fat utilization in the liver occurring over a long time causes large amounts of cholesterol in the circulating blood and increased deposition of cholesterol in the arterial walls. This leads to severe *arteriosclerosis* and other vascular lesions, as discussed earlier.

Diabetes Causes Depletion of the Body's Proteins. Failure to use glucose for energy leads to increased utilization and decreased storage of proteins and fat. Therefore, a person with severe untreated diabetes mellitus suffers rapid weight loss and *asthenia* (lack of energy) despite eating large amounts of food *(polyphagia).* Without treatment, these metabolic abnormalities can cause severe wasting of the body tissues and death within a few weeks.

Type II Diabetes—Resistance to the Metabolic Effects of Insulin

Type II diabetes is far more common than type I, accounting for about 90 to 95 percent of all cases of diabetes mellitus. In most cases, the onset of type II diabetes occurs after age 30, often between the ages of 50 and 60 years, and the disease develops gradually. Therefore, this syndrome is often referred to as *adult-onset diabetes.* In recent years, however, there has been a steady increase in the number of younger individuals, some younger than 20 years old, with type II diabetes. This trend appears to be related mainly to the increasing prevalence of *obesity, the most important risk factor for type II diabetes* in children and adults.

Obesity, Insulin Resistance, and "Metabolic Syndrome" Usually Precede Development of Type II Diabetes. Type II diabetes, in contrast to type I, is associated with *increased* plasma insulin concentration *(hyperinsulinemia).* This occurs as a compensatory response by the pancreatic beta cells for diminished sensitivity of target tissues to the metabolic effects of insulin, a condition referred to as *insulin resistance.* The decrease in insulin sensitivity impairs carbohydrate utilization and storage, raising blood glucose and stimulating a compensatory increase in insulin secretion.

Development of insulin resistance and impaired glucose metabolism is usually a gradual process, beginning with excess weight gain and obesity. The mechanisms that link obesity with insulin resistance, however, are still uncertain. Some studies suggest that there are fewer insulin receptors, especially in the skeletal muscle, liver, and adipose tissue, in obese than in lean subjects. However, most of the insulin resistance appears to be caused by abnormalities of the signaling pathways that link receptor activation with multiple cellular effects. Impaired insulin signaling appears to be closely related to toxic effects of lipid accumulation in tissues such as skeletal muscle and liver secondary to excess weight gain.

Insulin resistance is part of a cascade of disorders that is often called the *"metabolic syndrome."* Some of the features of the metabolic syndrome include (1) obesity, especially accumulation of abdominal fat; (2) insulin resistance; (3) fasting hyperglycemia; (4) lipid abnormalities, such as increased blood triglycerides and decreased blood high-density lipoprotein-cholesterol; and (5) hypertension. All of the features of the metabolic syndrome are closely related to accumulation of excess adipose tissue in the abdominal cavity around the visceral organs.

The role of insulin resistance in contributing to some of the components of the metabolic syndrome is uncertain, although it is clear that insulin resistance is the primary cause of increased blood glucose concentration. The major adverse consequence of the metabolic syndrome is cardiovascular disease including atherosclerosis and injury to various organs throughout the body. Several of the metabolic abnormalities associated with the syndrome increase the risk for cardiovascular disease, and insulin resistance predisposes to the development of type II diabetes mellitus, also a major cause of cardiovascular disease.

Other Factors That Can Cause Insulin Resistance and Type II Diabetes. Although most patients with type II diabetes are overweight or have substantial accumulation of visceral fat, severe insulin resistance and type II diabetes can also occur as a result of other acquired or genetic conditions that impair insulin signaling in peripheral tissues (Table 78-2).

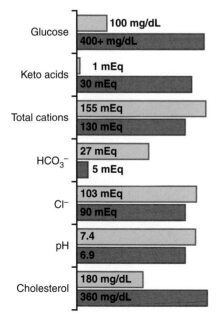

Figure 78-11 Changes in blood constituents in diabetic coma, showing normal values (*lavender bars*) and diabetic coma values (*red bars*).

Table 78-2 Some Causes of Insulin Resistance

- Obesity/overweight (especially excess visceral adiposity)
- Excess glucocorticoids (Cushing's syndrome or steroid therapy)
- Excess growth hormone (acromegaly)
- Pregnancy, gestational diabetes
- Polycystic ovary disease
- Lipodystrophy (acquired or genetic; associated with lipid accumulation in liver)
- Autoantibodies to the insulin receptor
- Mutations of insulin receptor
- Mutations of the peroxisome proliferators' activator receptor γ (PPARγ)
- Mutations that cause genetic obesity (e.g., melanocortin receptor mutations)
- Hemochromatosis (a hereditary disease that causes tissue iron accumulation)

Polycystic ovary syndrome (PCOS), for example, is associated with marked increases in ovarian androgen production and insulin resistance and is one of the most common endocrine disorders in women, affecting approximately 6 percent of all women during their reproductive life. Although the pathogenesis of PCOS remains uncertain, insulin resistance and hyperinsulinemia are found in approximately 80 percent of affected women. The long-term consequences include increased risk for diabetes mellitus, increased blood lipids, and cardiovascular disease.

Excess formation of *glucocorticoids (Cushing's syndrome)* or *growth hormone (acromegaly)* also decreases the sensitivity of various tissues to the metabolic effects of insulin and can lead to development of diabetes mellitus. Genetic causes of obesity and insulin resistance, if severe enough, also can lead to type II diabetes and many other features of the metabolic syndrome including cardiovascular disease.

Development of Type II Diabetes During Prolonged Insulin Resistance. With prolonged and severe insulin resistance, even the increased levels of insulin are not sufficient to maintain normal glucose regulation. As a result, moderate hyperglycemia occurs after ingestion of carbohydrates in the early stages of the disease.

In the later stages of type II diabetes, the pancreatic beta cells become "exhausted" or damaged and are unable to produce enough insulin to prevent more severe hyperglycemia, especially after the person ingests a carbohydrate-rich meal.

Some obese people, although having marked insulin resistance and greater than normal increases in blood glucose after a meal, never develop clinically significant diabetes mellitus; apparently, the pancreas in these people produces enough insulin to prevent severe abnormalities of glucose metabolism. In others, however, the pancreas gradually becomes exhausted from secreting large amounts of insulin or damaged by factors associated with lipid accumulation in the pancreas, and full-blown diabetes mellitus occurs. Some studies suggest that genetic factors play an important role in determining whether an individual's pancreas can sustain the high output of insulin over many years that is necessary to avoid the severe abnormalities of glucose metabolism in type II diabetes.

In many instances, type II diabetes can be effectively treated, at least in the early stages, with exercise, caloric restriction, and weight reduction, and no exogenous insulin administration is required. Drugs that increase insulin sensitivity, such as *thiazolidinediones*, drugs that suppress liver glucose production, such as *metformin*, or drugs that cause additional release of insulin by the pancreas, such as *sulfonylureas*, may also be used. However, in the later stages of type II diabetes, insulin administration is usually required to control plasma glucose.

Physiology of Diagnosis of Diabetes Mellitus

Table 78-3 compares some of clinical features of type I and type II diabetes mellitus. The usual methods for diagnosing diabetes are based on various chemical tests of the urine and the blood.

Urinary Glucose. Simple office tests or more complicated quantitative laboratory tests may be used to determine the quantity of glucose lost in the urine. In general, a normal person loses undetectable amounts of glucose, whereas a person with diabetes loses glucose in small to large amounts, in proportion to the severity of disease and the intake of carbohydrates.

Fasting Blood Glucose and Insulin Levels. The fasting blood glucose level in the early morning is normally 80 to 90 mg/100 ml, and 110 mg/100 ml is considered to be the upper limit of normal. A fasting blood glucose level above this value often indicates diabetes mellitus or at least marked insulin resistance.

In type I diabetes, plasma insulin levels are very low or undetectable during fasting and even after a meal. In type II diabetes, plasma insulin concentration may be severalfold higher than normal and usually increases to a greater extent after ingestion of a standard glucose load during a glucose tolerance test (see the next paragraph).

Glucose Tolerance Test. As demonstrated by the bottom curve in Figure 78-12, called a "glucose tolerance curve," when a normal, fasting person ingests 1 gram of glucose per kilogram of body weight, the blood glucose level rises from about 90 mg/100 ml to 120 to 140 mg/100 ml and falls back to below normal in about 2 hours.

In a person with diabetes, the fasting blood glucose concentration is almost always above 110 mg/100 ml and often

Table 78-3 Clinical Characteristics of Patients with Type I and Type II Diabetes Mellitus

Feature	Type I	Type II
Age at onset	Usually <20 yr	Usually >30 yr
Body mass	Low (wasted) to Normal	Obese
Plasma insulin	Low or absent	Normal to high initially
Plasma glucagon	High, can be suppressed	High, resistant to suppression
Plasma glucose	Increased	Increased
Insulin sensitivity	Normal	Reduced
Therapy	Insulin	Weight loss, thiazolidinediones, metformin, sulfonylureas, insulin

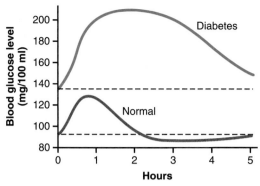

Figure 78-12 Glucose tolerance curve in a normal person and in a person with diabetes.

above 140 mg/100 ml. Also, the glucose tolerance test is almost always abnormal. On ingestion of glucose, these people exhibit a much greater than normal rise in blood glucose level, as demonstrated by the upper curve in Figure 78-12, and the glucose level falls back to the control value only after 4 to 6 hours; furthermore, it fails to fall *below* the control level. The slow fall of this curve and its failure to fall below the control level demonstrate that either (1) the normal increase in insulin secretion after glucose ingestion does not occur or (2) there is decreased sensitivity to insulin. A diagnosis of diabetes mellitus can usually be established on the basis of such a curve, and type I and type II diabetes can be distinguished from each other by measurements of plasma insulin, with plasma insulin being low or undetectable in type I diabetes and increased in type II diabetes.

Acetone Breath. As pointed out in Chapter 68, small quantities of acetoacetic acid in the blood, which increase greatly in severe diabetes, are converted to acetone. This is volatile and vaporized into the expired air. Consequently, one can frequently make a diagnosis of type I diabetes mellitus simply by smelling acetone on the breath of a patient. Also, keto acids can be detected by chemical means in the urine and their quantitation aids in determining the severity of the diabetes. In the early stages of type II diabetes, however, keto acids are usually not produced in excess amounts. However, when insulin resistance becomes severe and there is greatly increased utilization of fats for energy, keto acids are then produced in persons with type II diabetes.

Treatment of Diabetes

Effective treatment of type I diabetes mellitus requires administration of enough insulin so that the patient will have carbohydrate, fat, and protein metabolism that is as normal as possible. Insulin is available in several forms. "Regular" insulin has a duration of action that lasts from 3 to 8 hours, whereas other forms of insulin (precipitated with zinc or with various protein derivatives) are absorbed slowly from the injection site and therefore have effects that last as long as 10 to 48 hours. Ordinarily, a patient with severe type I diabetes is given a single dose of one of the longer-acting insulins each day to increase overall carbohydrate metabolism throughout the day. Then additional quantities of regular insulin are given during the day at those times when the blood glucose level tends to rise too high, such as at mealtimes. Thus, each patient is provided with an individualized pattern of treatment.

In persons with type II diabetes, dieting and exercise are usually recommended in an attempt to induce weight loss

and to reverse the insulin resistance. If this fails, drugs may be administered to increase insulin sensitivity or to stimulate increased production of insulin by the pancreas. In many persons, however, exogenous insulin must be used to regulate blood glucose.

In the past, the insulin used for treatment was derived from animal pancreata. However, human insulin produced by the recombinant DNA process has become more widely used because some patients develop immunity and sensitization against animal insulin, thus limiting its effectiveness.

Relation of Treatment to Arteriosclerosis. Diabetic patients, mainly because of their high levels of circulating cholesterol and other lipids, develop atherosclerosis, arteriosclerosis, severe coronary heart disease, and multiple microcirculatory lesions far more easily than do normal people. Indeed, those who have poorly controlled diabetes throughout childhood are likely to die of heart disease in early adulthood.

In the early days of treating diabetes, the tendency was to severely reduce the carbohydrates in the diet so that the insulin requirements would be minimized. This procedure kept the blood glucose from increasing too high and attenuated loss of glucose in the urine, but it did not prevent many of the abnormalities of fat metabolism. Consequently, the current tendency is to allow the patient an almost normal carbohydrate diet and to give enough insulin to metabolize the carbohydrates. This decreases the rate of fat metabolism and depresses the high level of blood cholesterol.

Because the complications of diabetes, such as atherosclerosis, increased susceptibility to infection, diabetic retinopathy, cataracts, hypertension, and chronic renal disease, are closely associated with the levels of blood lipids and blood glucose, most physicians also use lipid-lowering drugs to help prevent these disturbances.

Insulinoma—Hyperinsulinism

Although much rarer than diabetes, excessive insulin production occasionally occurs from an adenoma of an islet of Langerhans. About 10 to 15 percent of these adenomas are malignant, and occasionally metastases from the islets of Langerhans spread throughout the body, causing tremendous production of insulin by both the primary and metastatic cancers. Indeed, more than 1000 grams of glucose have had to be administered every 24 hours to prevent hypoglycemia in some of these patients.

Insulin Shock and Hypoglycemia. As already emphasized, the central nervous system normally derives essentially all its energy from glucose metabolism, and insulin is not necessary for this use of glucose. However, if high levels of insulin cause blood glucose to fall to low values, the metabolism of the central nervous system becomes depressed. Consequently, in patients with insulin-secreting tumors or in patients with diabetes who administer too much insulin to themselves, the syndrome called *insulin shock* may occur as follows.

As the blood glucose level falls into the range of 50 to 70 mg/100 ml, the central nervous system usually becomes excitable because this degree of hypoglycemia sensitizes neuronal activity. Sometimes various forms of hallucinations result, but more often the patient simply experiences extreme nervousness, trembles all over, and breaks out in a sweat. As the blood glucose level falls to 20 to 50 mg/100 ml, clonic seizures and loss of consciousness are likely to occur. As the glucose level falls still lower, the seizures cease and only a state of coma remains. Indeed, at times it is difficult by simple clinical observation to distinguish between diabetic coma as a result of insulin-lack acidosis and coma due to hypoglycemia caused by excess insulin. The acetone breath and the rapid, deep breathing of diabetic coma are not present in hypoglycemic coma.

Proper treatment for a patient who has hypoglycemic shock or coma is immediate intravenous administration of large quantities of glucose. This usually brings the patient out of shock within a minute or more. Also, the administration of glucagon (or, less effectively, epinephrine) can cause glycogenolysis in the liver and thereby increase the blood glucose level extremely rapidly. If treatment is not administered immediately, permanent damage to the neuronal cells of the central nervous system often occurs.

Bibliography

Ahrén B: Islet G protein-coupled receptors as potential targets for treatment of type 2 diabetes, *Nat Rev Drug Discov* 8:369, 2009.

Bansal P, Wang Q: Insulin as a physiological modulator of glucagon secretion, *Am J Physiol Endocrinol Metab* 295:E751, 2008.

Barthel A, Schmoll D: Novel concepts in insulin regulation of hepatic gluconeogenesis, *Am J Physiol Endocrinol Metab* 285:E685, 2003.

Bashan N, Kovsan J, Kachko I, et al: Positive and negative regulation of insulin signaling by reactive oxygen and nitrogen species, *Physiol Rev* 89:27, 2009.

Bryant NJ, Govers R, James DE: Regulated transport of the glucose transporter GLUT4, *Nat Rev Mol Cell Biol* 3:267, 2002.

Civitarese AE, Ravussin E: Mitochondrial energetics and insulin resistance, *Endocrinology* 149:950, 2008.

Concannon P, Rich SS, Nepom GT: Genetics of type 1A diabetes, *N Engl J Med* 360:1646, 2009.

Cornier MA, Dabelea D, Hernandez TL, et al: The metabolic syndrome, *Endocr Rev* 29:777, 2008.

Dunne MJ, Cosgrove KE, Shepherd RM, et al: Hyperinsulinism in infancy: from basic science to clinical disease, *Physiol Rev* 84:239, 2004.

Hall JE, Summers RL, Brands MW, et al: Resistance to the metabolic actions of insulin and its role in hypertension, *Am J Hypertens* 7:772, 1994.

Hattersley AT: Unlocking the secrets of the pancreatic beta cell: man and mouse provide the key, *J Clin Invest* 114:314, 2004.

Holst JJ: The physiology of glucagon-like peptide 1, *Physiol Rev* 87:1409, 2007.

Hussain MA, Theise ND: Stem-cell therapy for diabetes mellitus, *Lancet* 364:203, 2004.

Ishiki M, Klip A: Recent developments in the regulation of glucose transporter-4 traffic: new signals, locations, and partners, *Endocrinology* 146:5071, 2005.

Kowluru A: Regulatory roles for small G proteins in the pancreatic beta-cell: lessons from models of impaired insulin secretion, *Am J Physiol Endocrinol Metab* 285:E669, 2003.

MacDonald PE, Rorsman P: The ins and outs of secretion from pancreatic beta-cells: control of single-vesicle exo- and endocytosis, *Physiology (Bethesda)* 22:113, 2007.

Møller N, Jørgensen JO: Effects of growth hormone on glucose, lipid, and protein metabolism in human subjects, *Endocr Rev* 30:152, 2009.

Reece EA, Leguizamón G, Wiznitzer A: Gestational diabetes: the need for a common ground, *Lancet* 373:1789, 2009.

Roden M: How free fatty acids inhibit glucose utilization in human skeletal muscle, *News Physiol Sci* 19:92, 2004.

Salehi M, Aulinger BA, D'Alessio DA: Targeting beta-cell mass in type 2 diabetes: promise and limitations of new drugs based on incretins, *Endocr Rev* 29:367, 2008.

Saltiel AR: Putting the brakes on insulin signaling, *N Engl J Med* 349:2560, 2003.

Savage DB, Petersen KF, Shulman GI: Disordered lipid metabolism and the pathogenesis of insulin resistance, *Physiol Rev* 87:507, 2007.

Scheuner D, Kaufman RJ: The unfolded protein response: a pathway that links insulin demand with beta-cell failure and diabetes, *Endocr Rev* 29:317, 2008.

Stefan N, Kantartzis K, Häring HU: Causes and metabolic consequences of fatty liver, *Endocr Rev* 29:939, 2008.

Thaler JP, Cummings DE: Hormonal and metabolic mechanisms of diabetes remission after gastrointestinal surgery, *Endocrinology* 150:2518, 2009.

Williams DL: Finding the sweet spot: peripheral versus central glucagon-like peptide 1 action in feeding and glucose homeostasis, *Endocrinology* 150:2997, 2009.

Wang H, Eckel RH: Lipoprotein lipase: from gene to obesity, *Am J Physiol Endocrinol Metab* 297:E271, 2009.

Parathyroid Hormone, Calcitonin, Calcium and Phosphate Metabolism, Vitamin D, Bone, and Teeth

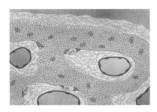

The physiology of calcium and phosphate metabolism, formation of bone and teeth, and regulation of *vitamin D, parathyroid hormone* (PTH), and *calcitonin* are all closely intertwined. Extracellular calcium ion concentration, for example, is determined by the interplay of calcium absorption from the intestine, renal excretion of calcium, and bone uptake and release of calcium, each of which is regulated by the hormones just noted. Because phosphate homeostasis and calcium homeostasis are closely associated, they are discussed together in this chapter.

Overview of Calcium and Phosphate Regulation in the Extracellular Fluid and Plasma

Extracellular fluid calcium concentration is normally regulated precisely, seldom rising or falling more than a few percent from the normal value of about 9.4 mg/dl, which is equivalent to 2.4 mmol calcium per liter. This precise control is essential because calcium plays a key role in many physiologic processes, including contraction of skeletal, cardiac, and smooth muscles; blood clotting; and transmission of nerve impulses, to name just a few. Excitable cells, such as neurons, are sensitive to changes in calcium ion concentrations, and increases in calcium ion concentration above normal *(hypercalcemia)* cause progressive depression of the nervous system; conversely, decreases in calcium concentration *(hypocalcemia)* cause the nervous system to become more excited.

An important feature of extracellular calcium regulation is that only about 0.1 percent of the total body calcium is in the extracellular fluid, about 1 percent is in the cells and its organelles, and the rest is stored in bones. Therefore, the bones can serve as large reservoirs, releasing calcium when extracellular fluid concentration decreases and storing excess calcium.

Approximately 85 percent of the body's phosphate is stored in bones, 14 to 15 percent is in the cells, and less than 1 percent is in the extracellular fluid. Although extracellular fluid phosphate concentration is not nearly as well regulated as calcium concentration, phosphate serves several important functions and is controlled by many of the same factors that regulate calcium.

Calcium in the Plasma and Interstitial Fluid

The calcium in the plasma is present in three forms, as shown in Figure 79-1: (1) About 41 percent (1 mmol/L) of the calcium is combined with the plasma proteins and in this form is nondiffusible through the capillary membrane; (2) about 9 percent of the calcium (0.2 mmol/L) is diffusible through the capillary membrane but is combined with anionic substances of the plasma and interstitial fluids (citrate and phosphate, for instance) in such a manner that it is not ionized; and (3) the remaining 50 percent of the calcium in the plasma is both diffusible through the capillary membrane and ionized.

Thus, the plasma and interstitial fluids have a normal calcium *ion* concentration of about 1.2 mmol/L (or 2.4 mEq/L, because it is a divalent ion), a level only one-half the total plasma calcium concentration. This ionic calcium is the form that is important for most functions of calcium in the body, including the effect of calcium on the heart, the nervous system, and bone formation.

Inorganic Phosphate in the Extracellular Fluids

Inorganic phosphate in the plasma is mainly in two forms: $HPO_4^=$ and $H_2PO_4^-$. The concentration of $HPO_4^=$ is about 1.05 mmol/L, and the concentration of $H_2PO_4^-$ is about 0.26 mmol/L. When the total quantity of phosphate in the extracellular fluid rises, so does the quantity of each of these two types of phosphate ions. Furthermore, when the pH of the extracellular fluid becomes more acidic, there is a relative increase in $H_2PO_4^-$ and a decrease in $HPO_4^=$, whereas the opposite occurs when the extracellular fluid becomes alkaline. These relations were presented in the discussion of acid-base balance in Chapter 30.

Because it is difficult to determine chemically the exact quantities of $HPO_4^=$ and $H_2PO_4^-$ in the blood, ordinarily the total quantity of phosphate is expressed in terms of milligrams of *phosphorus* per deciliter (100 ml) of blood. The average total quantity of inorganic phosphorus

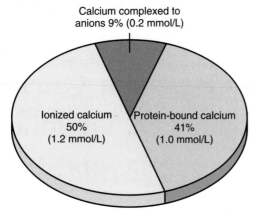

Figure 79-1 Distribution of ionized calcium (Ca⁺⁺), diffusible but un-ionized calcium complexed to anions, and nondiffusible protein-bound calcium in blood plasma.

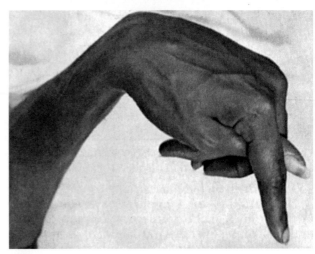

Figure 79-2 Hypocalcemic tetany in the hand, called *carpopedal spasm.*

represented by both phosphate ions is about 4 mg/dl, varying between normal limits of 3 to 4 mg/dl in adults and 4 to 5 mg/dl in children.

Nonbone Physiologic Effects of Altered Calcium and Phosphate Concentrations in the Body Fluids

Changing the level of phosphate in the extracellular fluid from far below normal to two to three times normal does not cause major immediate effects on the body. In contrast, even slight increases or decreases of calcium ion in the extracellular fluid can cause extreme immediate physiological effects. In addition, chronic hypocalcemia or hypophosphatemia greatly decreases bone mineralization, as explained later in the chapter.

Hypocalcemia Causes Nervous System Excitement and Tetany. When the extracellular fluid concentration of calcium ions falls below normal, the nervous system becomes progressively more excitable because this causes increased neuronal membrane permeability to sodium ions, allowing easy initiation of action potentials. At plasma calcium ion concentrations about 50 percent below normal, the peripheral nerve fibers become so excitable that they begin to discharge spontaneously, initiating trains of nerve impulses that pass to the peripheral skeletal muscles to elicit tetanic muscle contraction. Consequently, hypocalcemia causes tetany. It also occasionally causes seizures because of its action of increasing excitability in the brain.

Figure 79-2 shows tetany in the hand, which usually occurs before tetany develops in most other parts of the body. This is called "carpopedal spasm."

Tetany ordinarily occurs when the blood concentration of calcium falls from its normal level of 9.4 mg/dl to about 6 mg/dl, which is only 35 percent below the normal calcium concentration, and it is usually lethal at about 4 mg/dl.

In laboratory animals, in which calcium can gradually be reduced beyond the usual lethal levels, very extreme hypocalcemia can cause other effects that are seldom evident in patients, such as marked dilatation of the heart, changes in cellular enzyme activities, increased membrane permeability in some cells (in addition to nerve cells), and impaired blood clotting.

Hypercalcemia Depresses Nervous System and Muscle Activity. When the level of calcium in the body fluids rises above normal, the nervous system becomes depressed and reflex activities of the central nervous system are sluggish. Also, increased calcium ion concentration decreases the QT interval of the heart and causes lack of appetite and constipation, probably because of depressed contractility of the muscle walls of the gastrointestinal tract.

These depressive effects begin to appear when the blood level of calcium rises above about 12 mg/dl, and they can become marked as the calcium level rises above 15 mg/dl. When the level of calcium rises above about 17 mg/dl in the blood, calcium phosphate crystals are likely to precipitate throughout the body; this condition is discussed later in connection with parathyroid poisoning.

Absorption and Excretion of Calcium and Phosphate

Intestinal Absorption and Fecal Excretion of Calcium and Phosphate. The usual rates of intake are about 1000 mg/day each for calcium and phosphorus, about the amounts in 1 liter of milk. Normally, divalent cations such as calcium ions are poorly absorbed from the intestines. However, as discussed later, *vitamin D* promotes calcium absorption by the intestines, and about 35 percent (350 mg/day) of the ingested calcium is usually absorbed; the calcium remaining in the intestine is excreted in the feces. An additional 250 mg/day of calcium enters the intestines via secreted gastrointestinal juices and sloughed mucosal cells. Thus, about 90 percent (900 mg/day) of the daily intake of calcium is excreted in the feces (Figure 79-3).

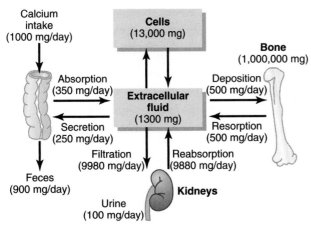

Calcium
intake
(1000 mg/day)

Cells
(13,000 mg)

Bone
(1,000,000 mg)

Absorption
(350 mg/day)

Extracellular
fluid
(1300 mg)

Deposition
(500 mg/day)

Secretion
(250 mg/day)

Resorption
(500 mg/day)

Filtration
(9980 mg/day)

Reabsorption
(9880 mg/day)

Feces
(900 mg/day)

Kidneys

Urine
(100 mg/day)

Figure 79-3 Overview of calcium exchange between different tissue compartments in a person ingesting 1000 mg of calcium per day. Note that most of the ingested calcium is normally eliminated in the feces, although the kidneys have the capacity to excrete large amounts by reducing tubular reabsorption of calcium.

Intestinal absorption of phosphate occurs easily. Except for the portion of phosphate that is excreted in the feces in combination with nonabsorbed calcium, almost all the dietary phosphate is absorbed into the blood from the gut and later excreted in the urine.

Renal Excretion of Calcium and Phosphate. Approximately 10 percent (100 mg/day) of the ingested calcium is excreted in the urine. About 41 percent of the plasma calcium is bound to plasma proteins and is therefore not filtered by the glomerular capillaries. The rest is combined with anions such as phosphate (9 percent) or ionized (50 percent) and is filtered through the glomeruli into the renal tubules.

Normally, the renal tubules reabsorb 99 percent of the filtered calcium and about 100 mg/day are excreted in the urine. Approximately 90 percent of the calcium in the glomerular filtrate is reabsorbed in the proximal tubules, loops of Henle, and early distal tubules.

Then in the late distal tubules and early collecting ducts, reabsorption of the remaining 10 percent is selective, depending on the calcium ion concentration in the blood.

When calcium concentration is low, this reabsorption is great, so almost no calcium is lost in the urine. Conversely, even a minute increase in blood calcium ion concentration above normal increases calcium excretion markedly. We shall see later in the chapter that the most important factor controlling this reabsorption of calcium in the distal portions of the nephron, and therefore controlling the rate of calcium excretion, is PTH.

Renal phosphate excretion is controlled by an *overflow mechanism*, as explained in Chapter 29. That is, when phosphate concentration in the plasma is below the critical value of about 1 mmol/L, all the phosphate in the glomerular filtrate is reabsorbed and no phosphate is lost in the urine. But above this critical concentration, the rate of phosphate loss is directly proportional to the additional

increase. Thus, the kidneys regulate the phosphate concentration in the extracellular fluid by altering the rate of phosphate excretion in accordance with the plasma phosphate concentration and the rate of phosphate filtration by the kidneys.

However, as discussed later in the chapter, PTH can greatly increase phosphate excretion by the kidneys, thereby playing an important role in the control of plasma phosphate concentration and calcium concentration.

Bone and Its Relation to Extracellular Calcium and Phosphate

Bone is composed of a tough *organic matrix* that is greatly strengthened by deposits of *calcium salts*. Average *compact bone* contains by weight about 30 percent matrix and 70 percent salts. *Newly formed bone* may have a considerably higher percentage of matrix in relation to salts.

Organic Matrix of Bone. The organic matrix of bone is 90 to 95 percent *collagen fibers*, and the remainder is a homogeneous gelatinous medium called *ground substance*. The collagen fibers extend primarily along the lines of tensional force and give bone its powerful tensile strength.

The ground substance is composed of extracellular fluid plus *proteoglycans*, especially *chondroitin sulfate* and *hyaluronic acid*. The precise function of each of these is not known, although they do help to control the deposition of calcium salts.

Bone Salts. The crystalline salts deposited in the organic matrix of bone are composed principally of *calcium* and *phosphate*. The formula for the major crystalline salt, known as *hydroxyapatite*, is the following:

$$Ca_{10}(PO_4)_6(OH)_2$$

Each crystal—about 400 angstroms long, 10 to 30 angstroms thick, and 100 angstroms wide—is shaped like a long, flat plate. The relative ratio of calcium to phosphorus can vary markedly under different nutritional conditions, the Ca/P ratio on a weight basis varying between 1.3 and 2.0.

Magnesium, sodium, potassium, and *carbonate* ions are also present among the bone salts, although x-ray diffraction studies fail to show definite crystals formed by them. Therefore, they are believed to be conjugated to the hydroxyapatite crystals rather than organized into distinct crystals of their own. This ability of many types of ions to conjugate to bone crystals extends to many ions normally foreign to bone, such as *strontium, uranium, plutonium, the other transuranic elements, lead, gold, other heavy metals,* and *at least 9 of 14 of the major radioactive products released by explosion of the hydrogen bomb.* Deposition of radioactive substances in the bone can cause prolonged irradiation of the bone tissues, and if a sufficient amount is deposited, an osteogenic sarcoma (bone cancer) eventually develops in most cases.

Tensile and Compressional Strength of Bone.

Each collagen fiber of *compact* bone is composed of repeating periodic segments every 640 angstroms along its length; hydroxyapatite crystals lie adjacent to each segment of the fiber, bound tightly to it. This intimate bonding prevents "shear" in the bone; that is, it prevents the crystals and collagen fibers from slipping out of place, which is essential in providing strength to the bone. In addition, the segments of adjacent collagen fibers overlap one another, also causing hydroxyapatite crystals to be overlapped like bricks keyed to one another in a brick wall.

The collagen fibers of bone, like those of tendons, have great tensile strength, whereas the calcium salts have great compressional strength. These combined properties plus the degree of bondage between the collagen fibers and the crystals provide a bony structure that has both extreme tensile strength and compressional strength.

Precipitation and Absorption of Calcium and Phosphate in Bone—Equilibrium with the Extracellular Fluids

Hydroxyapatite Does Not Precipitate in Extracellular Fluid Despite Supersaturation of Calcium and Phosphate Ions.

The concentrations of calcium and phosphate ions in extracellular fluid are considerably greater than those required to cause precipitation of hydroxyapatite. However, inhibitors are present in almost all tissues of the body, as well as in plasma, to prevent such precipitation; one such inhibitor is *pyrophosphate*. Therefore, hydroxyapatite crystals fail to precipitate in normal tissues except in bone despite the state of supersaturation of the ions.

Mechanism of Bone Calcification.

The initial stage in bone production is the secretion of *collagen molecules* (called collagen monomers) and *ground substance* (mainly proteoglycans) by *osteoblasts*. The collagen monomers polymerize rapidly to form collagen fibers; the resultant tissue becomes *osteoid*, a cartilage-like material differing from cartilage in that calcium salts readily precipitate in it. As the osteoid is formed, some of the osteoblasts become entrapped in the osteoid and become quiescent. At this stage they are called *osteocytes*.

Within a few days after the osteoid is formed, calcium salts begin to precipitate on the surfaces of the collagen fibers. The precipitates first appear at intervals along each collagen fiber, forming minute nidi that rapidly multiply and grow over a period of days and weeks into the finished product, *hydroxyapatite crystals.*

The initial calcium salts to be deposited are not hydroxyapatite crystals but amorphous compounds (noncrystalline), a mixture of salts such as $CaHPO_4 \cdot 2H_2O$, $Ca_3(PO_4)_2 \cdot 3H_2O$, and others. Then by a process of substitution and addition of atoms, or reabsorption and reprecipitation, these salts are converted into the hydroxyapatite crystals over a period of weeks or months. A few percent may remain permanently in the amorphous form. This is important because these amorphous salts can be absorbed rapidly when there is need for extra calcium in the extracellular fluid.

The mechanism that causes calcium salts to be deposited in osteoid is not fully understood. One theory holds that at the time of formation, the collagen fibers are specially constituted in advance for causing precipitation of calcium salts. The osteoblasts supposedly also secrete a substance into the osteoid to neutralize an inhibitor (believed to be pyrophosphate) that normally prevents hydroxyapatite crystallization. Once the pyrophosphate has been neutralized, the natural affinity of the collagen fibers for calcium salts causes the precipitation.

Precipitation of Calcium in Nonosseous Tissues Under Abnormal Conditions.

Although calcium salts almost never precipitate in normal tissues besides bone, under abnormal conditions, they do precipitate. For instance, they precipitate in arterial walls in *arteriosclerosis* and cause the arteries to become bonelike tubes. Likewise, calcium salts frequently deposit in degenerating tissues or in old blood clots. Presumably, in these instances, the inhibitor factors that normally prevent deposition of calcium salts disappear from the tissues, thereby allowing precipitation.

Calcium Exchange Between Bone and Extracellular Fluid

If soluble calcium salts are injected intravenously, the calcium ion concentration may increase immediately to high levels. However, within 30 to 60 minutes, the calcium ion concentration returns to normal. Likewise, if large quantities of calcium ions are removed from the circulating body fluids, the calcium ion concentration again returns to normal within 30 minutes to about 1 hour. These effects result in great part from the fact that the bone contains a type of *exchangeable* calcium that is always in equilibrium with the calcium ions in the extracellular fluids.

A small portion of this exchangeable calcium is also the calcium found in all tissue cells, especially in highly permeable types of cells such as those of the liver and the gastrointestinal tract. However, most of the exchangeable calcium is in the bone. It normally amounts to about 0.4 to 1 percent of the total bone calcium. This calcium is deposited in the bones in a form of readily mobilizable salt such as $CaHPO_4$ and other amorphous calcium salts.

The importance of exchangeable calcium is that it provides a rapid *buffering* mechanism to keep the calcium ion concentration in the extracellular fluids from rising to excessive levels or falling to low levels under transient conditions of excess or decreased availability of calcium.

Deposition and Absorption of Bone—Remodeling of Bone

Deposition of Bone by the Osteoblasts. Bone is continually being deposited by *osteoblasts,* and it is continually being absorbed where *osteoclasts* are active (Figure 79-4). Osteoblasts are found on the outer surfaces of the bones and in the bone cavities. A small amount of osteoblastic activity occurs continually in all living bones (on about 4 percent of all surfaces at any given time in an adult), so at least some new bone is being formed constantly.

Absorption of Bone—Function of the Osteoclasts. Bone is also being continually absorbed in the presence of osteoclasts, which are large, phagocytic, multinucleated cells (as many as 50 nuclei), derivatives of monocytes or monocyte-like cells formed in the bone marrow. The osteoclasts are normally active on less than 1 percent of the bone surfaces of an adult. Later in the chapter we see that PTH controls the bone absorptive activity of osteoclasts.

Histologically, bone absorption occurs immediately adjacent to the osteoclasts. The mechanism of this absorption is believed to be the following: The osteoclasts send out villus-like projections toward the bone, forming a ruffled border adjacent to the bone (Figure 79-5). The villi secrete two types of substances: (1) proteolytic enzymes, released from the lysosomes of the osteoclasts, and (2) several acids, including citric acid and lactic acid, released from the mitochondria and secretory vesicles. The enzymes digest or dissolve the organic matrix of the bone, and the acids cause dissolution of the bone salts. The osteoclastic cells also imbibe by phagocytosis minute particles of bone matrix and crystals, eventually also dissoluting these and releasing the products into the blood.

As discussed later, parathyroid hormone (PTH) stimulates osteoclast activity and bone resorption, but this occurs through an indirect mechanism. PTH binds to receptors on the adjacent osteoblasts, causing them to release cytokines, including *osteoprotegerin ligand* (OPGL), which is also called *RANK ligand.* OPGL activates receptors on preosteoclast cells, causing them to differentiate into mature multinucleated osteoclasts. The mature osteoclasts then develop

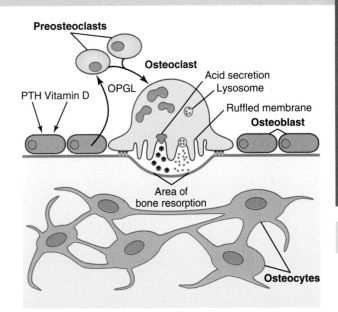

Figure 79-5 Bone resorption by osteoclasts. Parathyroid hormone (PTH) binds to receptors on osteoblasts, causing them to release osteoprotegerin ligand (OPGL), which binds to receptors on preosteoclast cells. This causes the cells to differentiate into mature osteoclasts. The osteoclasts then develop a ruffled border and release enzymes from lysosomes, as well as acids that promote bone resorption. Osteocytes are osteoblasts that have become encased in bone matrix during bone tissue production; the osteocytes form a system of interconnected cells that spreads all through the bone.

a ruffled border and release enzymes and acids that promote bone resorption.

Osteoblasts also produce osteoprotegerin (OPG), sometimes called *osteoclastogenesis inhibitory factor* (OCIF), a cytokine which inhibits bone resorption. OPG acts as a "decoy" receptor, binding to OPGL and preventing OPGL from interacting with its receptor, thereby inhibiting differentiation of preosteoclasts into mature osteoclasts that resorb bone. OPG opposes the bone resorptive activity of PTH and mice with genetic deficiency of OPG have severe decreases in bone mass compared with mice with normal OPG formation. Although the factors that regulate OPG are not well understood, vitamin D and PTH appear to stimulate production of mature osteoclasts through the dual action of inhibiting OPG production and stimulating OPGL formation. On the other hand, the hormone estrogen stimulates OPG production.

The therapeutic importance of the OPG-OPGL pathway is currently being exploited. Novel drugs that mimic the action of OPG by blocking the interaction of OPGL with its receptor appear to be useful for treating bone loss in postmenopausal women and in some patients with bone cancer.

Bone Deposition and Absorption Are Normally in Equilibrium. Normally, except in growing bones, the rates of bone deposition and absorption are equal to each other, so the total mass of bone remains constant. Osteoclasts usually exist in small but concentrated masses, and once a mass of osteoclasts begins to develop, it usually eats away at the bone for about 3 weeks, creating a tunnel that ranges in diameter from 0.2 to 1 millimeter and is several millimeters long. At the end of this time, the osteoclasts disappear and the tunnel

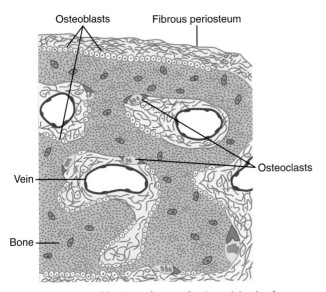

Figure 79-4 Osteoblastic and osteoclastic activity in the same bone.

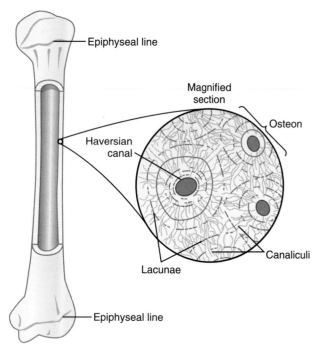

Figure 79-6 Structure of bone.

is invaded by osteoblasts instead; then new bone begins to develop. Bone deposition then continues for several months, the new bone being laid down in successive layers of concentric circles *(lamellae)* on the inner surfaces of the cavity until the tunnel is filled. Deposition of new bone ceases when the bone begins to encroach on the blood vessels supplying the area. The canal through which these vessels run, called the *haversian canal,* is all that remains of the original cavity. Each new area of bone deposited in this way is called an *osteon,* as shown in Figure 79-6.

Value of Continual Bone Remodeling. The continual deposition and absorption of bone have several physiologically important functions. First, bone ordinarily adjusts its strength in proportion to the degree of bone stress. Consequently, bones thicken when subjected to heavy loads. Second, even the shape of the bone can be rearranged for proper support of mechanical forces by deposition and absorption of bone in accordance with stress patterns. Third, because old bone becomes relatively brittle and weak, new organic matrix is needed as the old organic matrix degenerates. In this manner, the normal toughness of bone is maintained. Indeed, the bones of children, in whom the rates of deposition and absorption are rapid, show little brittleness in comparison with the bones of the elderly, in whom the rates of deposition and absorption are slow.

Control of the Rate of Bone Deposition by Bone "Stress." Bone is deposited in proportion to the compressional load that the bone must carry. For instance, the bones of athletes become considerably heavier than those of nonathletes. Also, if a person has one leg in a cast but continues to walk on the opposite leg, the bone of the leg in the cast becomes thin and as much as 30 percent decalcified within a few weeks, whereas the opposite bone remains thick and normally calcified. Therefore, continual physical stress stimulates osteoblastic deposition and calcification of bone.

Bone stress also determines the shape of bones under certain circumstances. For instance, if a long bone of the leg

breaks in its center and then heals at an angle, the compression stress on the inside of the angle causes increased deposition of bone. Increased absorption occurs on the outer side of the angle where the bone is not compressed. After many years of increased deposition on the inner side of the angulated bone and absorption on the outer side, the bone can become almost straight, especially in children because of the rapid remodeling of bone at younger ages.

Repair of a Fracture Activates Osteoblasts. Fracture of a bone in some way maximally activates all the periosteal and intraosseous osteoblasts involved in the break. Also, immense numbers of new osteoblasts are formed almost immediately from *osteoprogenitor cells,* which are bone stem cells in the surface tissue lining bone, called the *"bone membrane."* Therefore, within a short time, a large bulge of osteoblastic tissue and new organic bone matrix, followed shortly by the deposition of calcium salts, develops between the two broken ends of the bone. This is called a *callus.*

Many orthopedic surgeons use the phenomenon of bone stress to accelerate the rate of fracture healing. This is done by use of special mechanical fixation apparatuses for holding the ends of the broken bone together so that the patient can continue to use the bone immediately. This causes stress on the opposed ends of the broken bones, which accelerates osteoblastic activity at the break and often shortens convalescence.

Vitamin D

Vitamin D has a potent effect to increase calcium absorption from the intestinal tract; it also has important effects on bone deposition and bone absorption, as discussed later. However, vitamin D itself is not the active substance that actually causes these effects. Instead, vitamin D must first be converted through a succession of reactions in the liver and the kidneys to the final active product, *1,25-dihydroxycholecalciferol,* also called $1,25(OH)_2D_3$. Figure 79-7 shows the succession of steps that lead to the formation of this substance from vitamin D. Let us discuss these steps.

Cholecalciferol (Vitamin D_3) Is Formed in the Skin. Several compounds derived from sterols belong to the vitamin D family, and they all perform more or less the same functions. Vitamin D_3 (also called *cholecalciferol*) is the most important of these and is formed in the skin as a result of irradiation of *7-dehydrocholesterol,* a substance normally in the skin, by ultraviolet rays from the sun. Consequently, appropriate exposure to the sun prevents vitamin D deficiency. The additional vitamin D compounds that we ingest in food are identical to the cholecalciferol formed in the skin, except for the substitution of one or more atoms that do not affect their function.

Cholecalciferol Is Converted to 25-Hydroxycholecalciferol in the Liver. The first step in the activation of cholecalciferol is to convert it to 25-hydroxycholecalciferol; this occurs in the liver. The process is limited because the 25-hydroxycholecalciferol has a feedback inhibitory

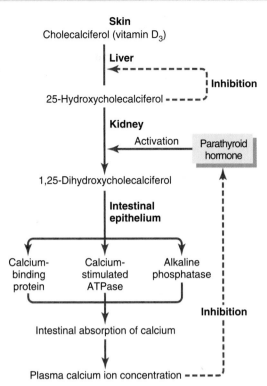

Figure 79-7 Activation of vitamin D₃ to form 1,25-dihydroxy-cholecalciferol and the role of vitamin D in controlling the plasma calcium concentration.

effect on the conversion reactions. This feedback effect is extremely important for two reasons.

First, the feedback mechanism precisely regulates the concentration of 25-hydroxycholecalciferol in the plasma, an effect that is shown in Figure 79-8. Note that the intake of vitamin D₃ can increase many times and yet the concentration of 25-hydroxycholecalciferol remains nearly normal. This high degree of feedback control prevents excessive action of vitamin D when intake of vitamin D₃ is altered over a wide range.

Second, this controlled conversion of vitamin D₃ to 25-hydroxycholecalciferol conserves the vitamin D

stored in the liver for future use. Once it is converted, it persists in the body for only a few weeks, whereas in the vitamin D form, it can be stored in the liver for many months.

Formation of 1,25-Dihydroxycholecalciferol in the Kidneys and Its Control by Parathyroid Hormone. Figure 79-7 also shows the conversion in the proximal tubules of the kidneys of 25-hydroxycholecalciferol to *1,25-dihydroxycholecalciferol*. This latter substance is by far the most active form of vitamin D because the previous products in the scheme of Figure 79-7 have less than 1/1000 of the vitamin D effect. Therefore, in the absence of the kidneys, vitamin D loses almost all its effectiveness.

Note also in Figure 79-7 that the conversion of 25-hydroxycholecalciferol to 1,25-dihydroxycholecalciferol requires PTH. In the absence of PTH, almost none of the 1,25-dihydroxycholecalciferol is formed. Therefore, PTH exerts a potent influence in determining the functional effects of vitamin D in the body.

Calcium Ion Concentration Controls the Formation of 1,25-Dihydroxycholecalciferol. Figure 79-9 demonstrates that the plasma concentration of 1,25-dihydroxycholecalciferol is inversely affected by the concentration of calcium in the plasma. There are two reasons for this. First, the calcium ion itself has a slight effect in preventing the conversion of 25-hydroxycholecalciferol to 1,25-dihydroxycholecalciferol. Second, and even more important, as we shall see later in the chapter, the rate of secretion of PTH is greatly suppressed when the plasma calcium ion concentration rises above 9 to 10 mg/100 ml. Therefore, at calcium concentrations below this level, PTH promotes the conversion of 25-hydroxycholecalciferol to 1,25-dihydroxycholecalciferol in the kidneys. At higher calcium concentrations, when PTH is suppressed, the 25-hydroxycholecalciferol is converted to a different

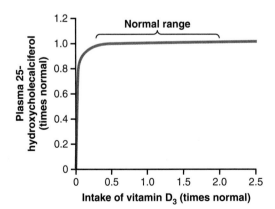

Figure 79-8 Effect of increasing vitamin D₃ intake on the plasma concentration of 25-hydroxycholecalciferol. This figure shows that increases in vitamin D intake, up to 2.5 times normal, have little effect on the final quantity of activated vitamin D that is formed. Deficiency of activated vitamin D occurs only at very low levels of vitamin D intake.

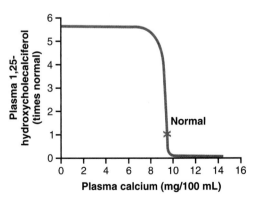

Figure 79-9 Effect of plasma calcium concentration on the plasma concentration of 1,25-dihydroxycholecalciferol. This figure shows that a slight decrease in calcium concentration below normal causes increased formation of activated vitamin D, which in turn leads to greatly increased absorption of calcium from the intestine.

compound—24,25-dihydroxycholecalciferol—that has almost no vitamin D effect.

When the plasma calcium concentration is already too high, the formation of 1,25-dihydroxycholecalciferol is greatly depressed. Lack of this in turn decreases the absorption of calcium from the intestines, the bones, and the renal tubules, thus causing the calcium ion concentration to fall back toward its normal level.

Actions of Vitamin D

The active form of vitamin D, 1,25-dihydroxycholecalciferol, has several effects on the intestines, kidneys, and bones that increase absorption of calcium and phosphate into the extracellular fluid and contribute to feedback regulation of these substances.

Vitamin D receptors are present in most cells in the body and are located mainly in the nuclei of target cells. Similar to receptors for steroids and thyroid hormone, the vitamin D receptor has hormone-binding and DNA-binding domains. The vitamin D receptor forms a complex with another intracellular receptor, the *retinoid-X receptor*, and this complex binds to DNA and activates transcription in most instances. In some cases, however, vitamin D suppresses transcription. Although the vitamin D receptor binds several forms of cholecalciferol, its affinity for 1,25-dihydroxycholecalciferol is roughly 1000 times that for 25-hydroxycholecalciferol, which explains their relative biological potencies.

"Hormonal" Effect of Vitamin D to Promote Intestinal Calcium Absorption.

1,25-Dihydroxycholecalciferol itself functions as a type of "hormone" to promote intestinal absorption of calcium. It does this principally by increasing, over a period of about 2 days, formation of *calbindin*, a *calcium-binding protein*, in the intestinal epithelial cells. This protein functions in the brush border of these cells to transport calcium into the cell cytoplasm. Then the calcium moves through the basolateral membrane of the cell by facilitated diffusion. The rate of calcium absorption is directly proportional to the quantity of this calcium-binding protein. Furthermore, this protein remains in the cells for several weeks after the 1,25-dihydroxycholecalciferol has been removed from the body, thus causing a prolonged effect on calcium absorption.

Other effects of 1,25-dihydroxycholecalciferol that might play a role in promoting calcium absorption are the formation of (1) a calcium-stimulated ATPase in the brush border of the epithelial cells and (2) an alkaline phosphatase in the epithelial cells. The precise details of all these effects are unclear.

Vitamin D Promotes Phosphate Absorption by the Intestines.

Although phosphate is usually absorbed easily, phosphate flux through the gastrointestinal epithelium is enhanced by vitamin D. It is believed that this results from a direct effect of 1,25-dihydroxycholecalciferol, but it is possible that it results secondarily from this hormone's action on calcium absorption, the calcium in turn acting as a transport mediator for the phosphate.

Vitamin D Decreases Renal Calcium and Phosphate Excretion.

Vitamin D also increases calcium and phosphate reabsorption by the epithelial cells of the renal tubules, thereby tending to decrease excretion of these substances in the urine. However, this is a weak effect and probably not of major importance in regulating the extracellular fluid concentration of these substances.

Effect of Vitamin D on Bone and Its Relation to Parathyroid Hormone Activity.

Vitamin D plays important roles in both bone absorption and bone deposition. The administration of *extreme quantities of vitamin D causes absorption of bone.* In the absence of vitamin D, the effect of PTH in causing bone absorption (discussed in the next section) is greatly reduced or even prevented. The mechanism of this action of vitamin D is not known, but it is believed to result from the effect of 1,25-dihydroxycholecalciferol to increase calcium transport through cellular membranes.

Vitamin D in smaller quantities promotes bone calcification. One of the ways in which it does this is to increase calcium and phosphate absorption from the intestines. However, even in the absence of such increase, it enhances the mineralization of bone. Here again, the mechanism of the effect is unknown, but it probably also results from the ability of 1,25-dihydroxycholecalciferol to cause transport of calcium ions through cell membranes—but in this instance, perhaps in the opposite direction through the osteoblastic or osteocytic cell membranes.

Parathyroid Hormone

Parathyroid hormone provides a powerful mechanism for controlling extracellular calcium and phosphate concentrations by regulating intestinal reabsorption, renal excretion, and exchange between the extracellular fluid and bone of these ions. Excess activity of the parathyroid gland causes rapid absorption of calcium salts from the bones, with resultant *hypercalcemia* in the extracellular fluid; conversely, hypofunction of the parathyroid glands causes *hypocalcemia*, often with resultant tetany.

Physiologic Anatomy of the Parathyroid Glands.

Normally there are four parathyroid glands in humans; they are located immediately behind the thyroid gland—one behind each of the upper and each of the lower poles of the thyroid. Each parathyroid gland is about 6 millimeters long, 3 millimeters wide, and 2 millimeters thick and has a macroscopic appearance of dark brown fat. The parathyroid glands are difficult to locate during thyroid operations because they often look like just another lobule of the thyroid gland. For this reason, before the importance of these glands was generally recognized, total or subtotal thyroidectomy frequently resulted in removal of the parathyroid glands as well.

Removal of half the parathyroid glands usually causes no major physiologic abnormalities. However, removal of three of the four normal glands causes transient hypoparathyroidism. But even a small quantity of remaining parathyroid tissue is usually capable of hypertrophying to satisfactorily perform the function of all the glands.

The parathyroid gland of the adult human being, shown in Figure 79-10, contains mainly *chief cells* and a small to moderate number of *oxyphil cells,* but oxyphil cells are absent in many animals and in young humans. The chief cells are believed to secrete most, if not all, of the PTH. The function of the oxyphil cells is not certain, but the cells are believed to be modified or depleted chief cells that no longer secrete hormone.

Chemistry of Parathyroid Hormone. PTH has been isolated in a pure form. It is first synthesized on the ribosomes in the form of a preprohormone, a polypeptide chain of 110 amino acids. This is cleaved first to a prohormone with 90 amino acids, then to the hormone itself with 84 amino acids by the endoplasmic reticulum and Golgi apparatus, and finally packaged in secretory granules in the cytoplasm of the cells. The final hormone has a molecular weight of about 9500. Smaller compounds with as few as 34 amino acids adjacent to the N terminus of the molecule have also been isolated from the parathyroid glands that exhibit full PTH activity. In fact, because the kidneys rapidly remove the whole 84-amino acid hormone within minutes but fail to remove many of the fragments

for hours, a large share of the hormonal activity is caused by the fragments.

Effect of Parathyroid Hormone on Calcium and Phosphate Concentrations in the Extracellular Fluid

Figure 79-11 shows the approximate effects on the blood calcium and phosphate concentrations caused by suddenly infusing PTH into an animal and continuing this for several hours. Note that at the onset of infusion the calcium ion concentration begins to rise and reaches a plateau in about 4 hours. The phosphate concentration, however, falls more rapidly than the calcium rises and reaches a depressed level within 1 or 2 hours. The rise in calcium concentration is caused principally by two effects: (1) an effect of PTH to increase calcium and phosphate absorption from the bone and (2) a rapid effect of PTH to decrease the excretion of calcium by the kidneys. The decline in phosphate concentration is caused by a strong effect of PTH to increase renal phosphate excretion, an effect that is usually great enough to override increased phosphate absorption from the bone.

Parathyroid Hormone Increases Calcium and Phosphate Absorption from the Bone

PTH has two effects on bone in causing absorption of calcium and phosphate. One is a rapid phase that begins in minutes and increases progressively for several hours. This phase results from activation of the already existing bone cells (mainly the osteocytes) to promote calcium and phosphate absorption. The second phase is a much slower one, requiring several days or even weeks to become fully developed; it results from proliferation of the osteoclasts, followed by greatly increased osteoclastic reabsorption of the bone itself, not merely absorption of the calcium phosphate salts from the bone.

Rapid Phase of Calcium and Phosphate Absorption from Bone—Osteolysis. When large quantities of PTH are injected, the calcium ion concentration in the blood begins to rise within minutes, long before any new bone cells can be developed. Histological and physiological studies have shown that PTH causes removal of bone salts from two areas in the bone: (1) from the bone matrix in

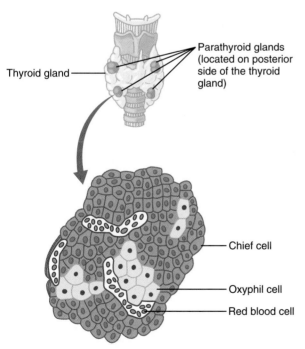

Figure 79-10 The four parathyroid glands lie immediately behind the thyroid gland. Almost all of the parathyroid hormone (PTH) is synthesized and secreted by the chief cells. The function of the oxyphil cells is uncertain, but they may be modified or depleted chief cells that no longer secrete PTH.

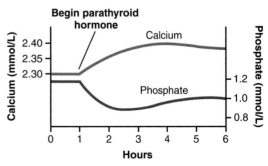

Figure 79-11 Approximate changes in calcium and phosphate concentrations during the first 5 hours of parathyroid hormone infusion at a moderate rate.

the vicinity of the osteocytes lying within the bone itself and (2) in the vicinity of the osteoblasts along the bone surface.

One does not usually think of either osteoblasts or osteocytes functioning to cause bone salt absorption, because both these types of cells are osteoblastic in nature and normally associated with bone deposition and its calcification. However, studies have shown that the osteoblasts and osteocytes form a system of interconnected cells that spreads all through the bone and over all the bone surfaces except the small surface areas adjacent to the osteoclasts (see Figure 79-5). In fact, long, filmy processes extend from osteocyte to osteocyte throughout the bone structure, and these processes also connect with the surface osteocytes and osteoblasts. This extensive system is called the *osteocytic membrane system,* and it is believed to provide a membrane that separates the bone itself from the extracellular fluid.

Between the osteocytic membrane and the bone is a small amount of *bone fluid.* Experiments suggest that the osteocytic membrane pumps calcium ions from the bone fluid into the extracellular fluid, creating a calcium ion concentration in the bone fluid only one-third that in the extracellular fluid. When the osteocytic pump becomes excessively activated, the bone fluid calcium concentration falls even lower, and calcium phosphate salts are then absorbed from the bone. This effect is called *osteolysis,* and it occurs without absorption of the bone's fibrous and gel matrix. When the pump is inactivated, the bone fluid calcium concentration rises to a higher level and calcium phosphate salts are redeposited in the matrix.

But where does PTH fit into this picture? First, the cell membranes of both the osteoblasts and the osteocytes have receptor proteins for binding PTH. PTH can activate the calcium pump strongly, thereby causing rapid removal of calcium phosphate salts from those amorphous bone crystals that lie near the cells. PTH is believed to stimulate this pump by increasing the calcium permeability of the bone fluid side of the osteocytic membrane, thus allowing calcium ions to diffuse into the membrane cells from the bone fluid. Then the calcium pump on the other side of the cell membrane transfers the calcium ions the rest of the way into the extracellular fluid.

Slow Phase of Bone Absorption and Calcium Phosphate Release—Activation of the Osteoclasts. A much better known effect of PTH and one for which the evidence is much clearer is its activation of the osteoclasts. Yet the osteoclasts do not themselves have membrane receptor proteins for PTH. Instead, it is believed that the activated osteoblasts and osteocytes send secondary "signals" to the osteoclasts. As discussed previously, a major secondary signal is *osteoprotegerin ligand,* which activates receptors on preosteoclast cells and transforms them into mature osteoclasts that set about their usual task of gobbling up the bone over a period of weeks or months.

Activation of the osteoclastic system occurs in two stages: (1) immediate activation of the osteoclasts that are already formed and (2) formation of new osteoclasts.

Several days of excess PTH usually cause the osteoclastic system to become well developed, but it can continue to grow for months under the influence of strong PTH stimulation.

After a few months of excess PTH, osteoclastic resorption of bone can lead to weakened bones and secondary stimulation of the osteoblasts that attempt to correct the weakened state. Therefore, the late effect is actually to enhance both osteoblastic and osteoclastic activity. Still, even in the late stages, there is more bone absorption than bone deposition in the presence of continued excess PTH.

Bone contains such great amounts of calcium in comparison with the total amount in all the extracellular fluids (about 1000 times as much) that even when PTH causes a great rise in calcium concentration in the fluids, it is impossible to discern any immediate effect on the bones. Prolonged administration or secretion of PTH—over a period of many months or years—finally results in very evident absorption in all the bones and even development of large cavities filled with large, multinucleated osteoclasts.

Parathyroid Hormone Decreases Calcium Excretion and Increases Phosphate Excretion by the Kidneys

Administration of PTH causes rapid loss of phosphate in the urine owing to the effect of the hormone to diminish proximal tubular reabsorption of phosphate ions.

PTH also increases renal tubular reabsorption of calcium at the same time that it diminishes phosphate reabsorption. Moreover, it increases the rate of reabsorption of magnesium ions and hydrogen ions while it decreases the reabsorption of sodium, potassium, and amino acid ions in much the same way that it affects phosphate. The increased calcium absorption occurs mainly in the *late distal tubules,* the *collecting tubules,* the early collecting ducts, and possibly the ascending loop of Henle to a lesser extent.

Were it not for the effect of PTH on the kidneys to increase calcium reabsorption, continual loss of calcium into the urine would eventually deplete both the extracellular fluid and the bones of this mineral.

Parathyroid Hormone Increases Intestinal Absorption of Calcium and Phosphate

At this point, we should be reminded again that PTH greatly enhances both calcium and phosphate absorption from the intestines by increasing the formation in the kidneys of 1,25-dihydroxycholecalciferol from vitamin D, as discussed earlier in the chapter.

Cyclic Adenosine Monophosphate Mediates the Effects of Parathyroid Hormone. A large share of the effect of PTH on its target organs is mediated by the cyclic adenosine monophosphate (cAMP) *second messenger* mechanism. Within a few minutes after PTH administration, the concentration of cAMP increases in the osteocytes, osteoclasts, and other target cells. This cAMP in turn is probably responsible for such functions as osteoclastic secretion of enzymes and acids to cause bone reabsorption and formation of 1,25-dihydroxy-cholecalciferol in the kidneys. Other direct effects of PTH probably function independently of the second messenger mechanism.

Control of Parathyroid Secretion by Calcium Ion Concentration

Even the slightest decrease in calcium ion concentration in the extracellular fluid causes the parathyroid glands to increase their rate of secretion within minutes; if the decreased calcium concentration persists, the glands will hypertrophy, sometimes fivefold or more. For instance, the parathyroid glands become greatly enlarged in *rickets,* in which the level of calcium is usually depressed only a small amount. They also become greatly enlarged in *pregnancy,* even though the decrease in calcium ion concentration in the mother's extracellular fluid is hardly measurable, and they are greatly enlarged during *lactation* because calcium is used for milk formation.

Conversely, conditions that increase the calcium ion concentration above normal cause decreased activity and reduced size of the parathyroid glands. Such conditions include (1) excess quantities of calcium in the diet, (2) increased vitamin D in the diet, and (3) bone absorption caused by factors other than PTH (e.g., bone absorption caused by disuse of the bones).

Changes in extracellular fluid calcium ion concentration are detected by a *calcium-sensing receptor* (CaSR) in parathyroid cell membranes. The CaSR is a G protein–coupled receptor that, when stimulated by calcium ions, activates phospholipase C and increases intracellular inositol 1,4,5-triphosphate and diacylglycerol formation. This stimulates release of calcium from intracellular stores, which, in turn, *decreases* PTH secretion. Conversely, decreased extracellular fluid calcium ion concentration inhibits these pathways and stimulates PTH secretion. This contrasts with many endocrine tissues in which hormone secretion is stimulated when these pathways are activated.

Figure 79-12 shows the approximate relation between plasma calcium concentration and plasma PTH concentration. The solid red curve shows the acute effect when the calcium concentration is changed over a period of a few hours. This shows that even small decreases in calcium concentration from the normal value can double or triple the plasma PTH. The approximate chronic effect that one finds when the calcium ion concentration changes over a period of many weeks, thus allowing time for the glands to hypertrophy greatly, is shown by the dashed red line; this demonstrates that a decrease of only a fraction of a milligram per deciliter in plasma calcium concentration can double PTH secretion. This is the basis of the body's extremely potent feedback system for long-term control of plasma calcium ion concentration.

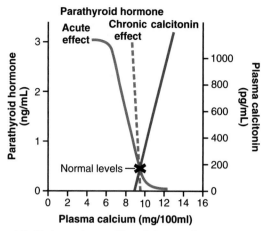

Figure 79-12 Approximate effect of plasma calcium concentration on the plasma concentrations of parathyroid hormone and calcitonin. Note especially that long-term, chronic changes in calcium concentration of only a few percentage points can cause as much as 100 percent change in parathyroid hormone concentration.

Summary of Effects of Parathyroid Hormone. Figure 79-13 summarizes the main effects of increased PTH secretion in response to decreased extracellular fluid calcium ion concentration: (1) PTH stimulates bone resorption, causing release of calcium into the extracellular fluid; (2) PTH increases reabsorption of calcium and decreases phosphate reabsorption by the renal tubules, leading to decreased excretion of calcium and increased excretion of phosphate; and (3) PTH is

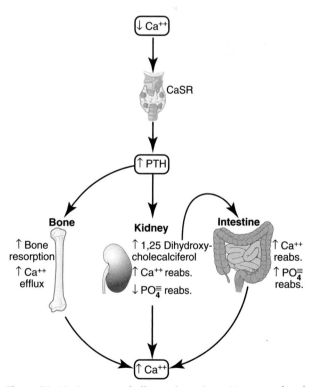

Figure 79-13 Summary of effects of parathyroid hormone (PTH) on bone, the kidneys, and the intestine in response to decreased extracellular fluid calcium ion concentration. CaSR, calcium sensing receptor.

necessary for conversion of 25-hydroxycholecalciferol to 1,25-dihydroxycholecalciferol, which, in turn, increases calcium absorption by the intestines. These actions together provide a powerful means of regulating extracellular fluid calcium concentration.

Calcitonin

Calcitonin, a peptide hormone secreted by the thyroid gland, tends to *decrease* plasma calcium concentration and, in general, has effects opposite to those of PTH. However, the quantitative role of calcitonin in humans is far less than that of PTH in regulating calcium ion concentration.

Synthesis and secretion of calcitonin occur in the *parafollicular cells*, or *C cells*, lying in the interstitial fluid between the follicles of the thyroid gland. These cells constitute only about 0.1 percent of the human thyroid gland and are the remnants of the *ultimobranchial glands* of lower animals, such as fish, amphibians, reptiles, and birds. Calcitonin is a 32-amino acid peptide with a molecular weight of about 3400.

Increased Plasma Calcium Concentration Stimulates Calcitonin Secretion. The primary stimulus for calcitonin secretion is increased extracellular fluid calcium ion concentration. This contrasts with PTH secretion, which is stimulated by decreased calcium concentration.

In young animals, but much less so in older animals and in humans, an increase in plasma calcium concentration of about 10 percent causes an immediate twofold or more increase in the rate of secretion of calcitonin, which is shown by the blue line in Figure 79-12. This provides a second hormonal feedback mechanism for controlling the plasma calcium ion concentration, but one that is relatively weak and works in a way opposite that of the PTH system.

Calcitonin Decreases Plasma Calcium Concentration. In some young animals, calcitonin decreases blood calcium ion concentration rapidly, beginning within minutes after injection of the calcitonin, in at least two ways.

1. The immediate effect is to decrease the absorptive activities of the osteoclasts and possibly the osteolytic effect of the osteocytic membrane throughout the bone, thus shifting the balance in favor of deposition of calcium in the exchangeable bone calcium salts. This effect is especially significant in young animals because of the rapid interchange of absorbed and deposited calcium.

2. The second and more prolonged effect of calcitonin is to decrease the formation of new osteoclasts. Also, because osteoclastic resorption of bone leads secondarily to osteoblastic activity, decreased numbers of osteoclasts are followed by decreased numbers of osteoblasts. Therefore, over a long period, the net result is reduced osteoclastic and osteoblastic activity and, consequently, little prolonged effect on plasma calcium ion concentration. That is, the effect on plasma calcium is mainly a transient one, lasting for a few hours to a few days at most.

Calcitonin also has minor effects on calcium handling in the kidney tubules and the intestines. Again, the effects are opposite those of PTH, but they appear to be of such little importance that they are seldom considered.

Calcitonin Has a Weak Effect on Plasma Calcium Concentration in the Adult Human. The reason for the weak effect of calcitonin on plasma calcium is twofold. First, any initial reduction of the calcium ion concentration caused by calcitonin leads within hours to a powerful stimulation of PTH secretion, which almost overrides the calcitonin effect. When the thyroid gland is removed and calcitonin is no longer secreted, the long-term blood calcium ion concentration is not measurably altered, which again demonstrates the overriding effect of the PTH system of control.

Second, in the adult, the daily rates of absorption and deposition of calcium are small, and even after the rate of absorption is slowed by calcitonin, this still has only a small effect on plasma calcium ion concentration. The effect of calcitonin in children is much greater because bone remodeling occurs rapidly in children, with absorption and deposition of calcium as great as 5 grams or more per day—equal to 5 to 10 times the total calcium in all the extracellular fluid. Also, in certain bone diseases, such as *Paget disease*, in which osteoclastic activity is greatly accelerated, calcitonin has a much more potent effect of reducing the calcium absorption.

Summary of Control of Calcium Ion Concentration

At times, the amount of calcium absorbed into or lost from the body fluids is as much as 0.3 gram in 1 hour. For instance, in cases of diarrhea, several grams of calcium can be secreted in the intestinal juices, passed into the intestinal tract, and lost into the feces each day.

Conversely, after ingestion of large quantities of calcium, particularly when there is also an excess of vitamin D activity, a person may absorb as much as 0.3 gram in 1 hour. This figure compares with a *total quantity of calcium in all the extracellular fluid of about 1 gram.* The addition or subtraction of 0.3 gram to or from such a small amount of calcium in the extracellular fluid would cause serious hypercalcemia or hypocalcemia. However, there is a first line of defense to prevent this from occurring even before the parathyroid and calcitonin hormonal feedback systems have a chance to act.

Buffer Function of the Exchangeable Calcium in Bones—The First Line of Defense. The exchangeable calcium salts in the bones, discussed earlier in this chapter, are amorphous calcium phosphate compounds, probably mainly $CaHPO_4$ or some similar compound loosely bound in the bone and in reversible equilibrium with the calcium and phosphate ions in the extracellular fluid.

The quantity of these salts that is available for exchange is about 0.5 to 1 percent of the total calcium salts of the bone, a total of 5 to 10 grams of calcium. Because of the ease of deposition of these exchangeable salts and their ease of resolubility, an increase in the concentrations of extracellular fluid calcium and phosphate ions above normal causes immediate deposition of exchangeable salt. Conversely, a decrease in these concentrations causes immediate absorption of exchangeable salt. This reaction is rapid because the amorphous bone crystals are extremely small and their total surface area exposed to the fluids of the bone is perhaps 1 acre or more.

Also, about 5 percent of all the blood flows through the bones each minute—that is, about 1 percent of all the extracellular fluid each minute. Therefore, about one half of any excess calcium that appears in the extracellular fluid is removed by this buffer function of the bones in about 70 minutes.

In addition to the buffer function of the bones, the *mitochondria* of many of the tissues of the body, especially of the liver and intestine, contain a significant amount of exchangeable calcium (a total of about 10 grams in the whole body) that provides an additional buffer system for helping to maintain constancy of the extracellular fluid calcium ion concentration.

Hormonal Control of Calcium Ion Concentration—The Second Line of Defense. At the same time that the exchangeable calcium mechanism in the bones is "buffering" the calcium in the extracellular fluid, both the parathyroid and the calcitonin hormonal systems are beginning to act. Within 3 to 5 minutes after an acute increase in the calcium ion concentration, the rate of PTH secretion decreases. As already explained, this sets into play multiple mechanisms for reducing the calcium ion concentration back toward normal.

At the same time that PTH decreases, calcitonin increases. In young animals and possibly in young children (but probably to a smaller extent in adults), the calcitonin causes rapid deposition of calcium in the bones, and perhaps in some cells of other tissues. Therefore, in very young animals, excess calcitonin can cause a high calcium ion concentration to return to normal perhaps considerably more rapidly than can be achieved by the exchangeable calcium-buffering mechanism alone.

In prolonged calcium excess or prolonged calcium deficiency, only the PTH mechanism seems to be really important in maintaining a normal plasma calcium ion concentration. When a person has a continuing deficiency of calcium in the diet, PTH can often stimulate enough calcium absorption from the bones to maintain a normal

plasma calcium ion concentration for 1 year or more, but eventually, even the bones will run out of calcium. Thus, in effect, the bones are a large buffer-reservoir of calcium that can be manipulated by PTH. Yet when the bone reservoir either runs out of calcium or, oppositely, becomes saturated with calcium, the long-term control of extracellular calcium ion concentration resides almost entirely in the roles of PTH and vitamin D in controlling calcium absorption from the gut and calcium excretion in the urine.

Pathophysiology of Parathyroid Hormone, Vitamin D, and Bone Disease

Hypoparathyroidism

When the parathyroid glands do not secrete sufficient PTH, the osteocytic resorption of exchangeable calcium decreases and the osteoclasts become almost totally inactive. As a result, calcium reabsorption from the bones is so depressed that the level of calcium in the body fluids decreases. Yet because calcium and phosphates are not being absorbed from the bone, the bone usually remains strong.

When the parathyroid glands are suddenly removed, the calcium level in the blood falls from the normal of 9.4 mg/dl to 6 to 7 mg/dl within 2 to 3 days and the blood phosphate concentration may double. When this low calcium level is reached, the usual signs of tetany develop. Among the muscles of the body especially sensitive to tetanic spasm are the laryngeal muscles. Spasm of these muscles obstructs respiration, which is the usual cause of death in tetany unless appropriate treatment is applied.

Treatment of Hypoparathyroidism with PTH and Vitamin D. PTH is occasionally used for treating hypoparathyroidism. However, because of the expense of this hormone, because its effect lasts for a few hours at most, and because the tendency of the body to develop antibodies against it makes it progressively less and less effective, hypoparathyroidism is usually not treated with PTH administration.

In most patients with hypoparathyroidism, the administration of extremely large quantities of vitamin D, to as high as 100,000 units per day, along with intake of 1 to 2 grams of calcium, keeps the calcium ion concentration in a normal range. At times, it might be necessary to administer 1,25-dihydroxycholecalciferol instead of the nonactivated form of vitamin D because of its much more potent and much more rapid action. This can also cause unwanted effects because it is sometimes difficult to prevent overactivity by this activated form of vitamin D.

Primary Hyperparathyroidism

In primary hyperparathyroidism, an abnormality of the parathyroid glands causes inappropriate, excess PTH secretion. The cause of primary hyperparathyroidism ordinarily is a tumor of one of the parathyroid glands; such tumors occur much more frequently in women than in men or children, mainly because pregnancy and lactation stimulate the parathyroid glands and therefore predispose to the development of such a tumor.

Hyperparathyroidism causes extreme osteoclastic activity in the bones. This elevates the calcium ion concentration in the extracellular fluid while usually depressing the concentration of phosphate ions because of increased renal excretion of phosphate.

Bone Disease in Hyperparathyroidism. Although in mild hyperparathyroidism new bone can be deposited rapidly enough to compensate for the increased osteoclastic resorption of bone, in severe hyperparathyroidism the osteoclastic absorption soon far outstrips osteoblastic deposition, and the bone may be eaten away almost entirely. Indeed, the reason a hyperparathyroid person seeks medical attention is often a broken bone. Radiographs of the bone typically show extensive decalcification and, occasionally, large punched-out cystic areas of the bone that are filled with osteoclasts in the form of so-called giant cell osteoclast "tumors." Multiple fractures of the weakened bones can result from only slight trauma, especially where cysts develop. The cystic bone disease of hyperparathyroidism is called *osteitis fibrosa cystica.*

Osteoblastic activity in the bones also increases greatly in a vain attempt to form enough new bone to make up for the old bone absorbed by the osteoclastic activity. When the osteoblasts become active, they secrete large quantities of *alkaline phosphatase.* Therefore, one of the important diagnostic findings in hyperparathyroidism is a high level of plasma alkaline phosphatase.

Effects of Hypercalcemia in Hyperparathyroidism. Hyperparathyroidism can at times cause the plasma calcium level to rise to 12 to 15 mg/dl and, rarely, even higher. The effects of such elevated calcium levels, as detailed earlier in the chapter, are depression of the central and peripheral nervous systems, muscle weakness, constipation, abdominal pain, peptic ulcer, lack of appetite, and depressed relaxation of the heart during diastole.

Parathyroid Poisoning and Metastatic Calcification. When, on rare occasions, extreme quantities of PTH are secreted, the level of calcium in the body fluids rises rapidly to high values. Even the extracellular fluid phosphate concentration often rises markedly instead of falling, as is usually the case, probably because the kidneys cannot excrete rapidly enough all the phosphate being absorbed from the bone. Therefore, the calcium and phosphate in the body fluids become greatly supersaturated, so calcium phosphate ($CaHPO_4$) crystals begin to deposit in the alveoli of the lungs, the tubules of the kidneys, the thyroid gland, the acid-producing area of the stomach mucosa, and the walls of the arteries throughout the body. This extensive *metastatic* deposition of calcium phosphate can develop within a few days.

Ordinarily, the level of calcium in the blood must rise above 17 mg/dl before there is danger of parathyroid poisoning, but once such elevation develops along with concurrent elevation of phosphate, death can occur in only a few days.

Formation of Kidney Stones in Hyperparathyroidism. Most patients with mild hyperparathyroidism show few signs of bone disease and few general abnormalities as a result of elevated calcium, but they do have an extreme tendency to form kidney stones. The reason is that the excess calcium and phosphate absorbed from the intestines or mobilized from the bones in hyperparathyroidism must eventually be excreted by the kidneys, causing a proportionate increase in the concentrations of these substances in the urine. As a result, crystals of calcium phosphate tend to precipitate in the kidney, forming calcium phosphate stones. Also, calcium oxalate stones develop because even normal levels of oxalate cause calcium precipitation at high calcium levels.

Because the solubility of most renal stones is slight in alkaline media, the tendency for formation of renal calculi is considerably greater in alkaline urine than in acid urine. For this reason, acidotic diets and acidic drugs are frequently used for treating renal calculi.

Secondary Hyperparathyroidism

In secondary hyperparathyroidism, high levels of PTH occur as a compensation for *hypocalcemia* rather than as a primary abnormality of the parathyroid glands. This contrasts with primary hyperparathyroidism, which is associated with hypercalcemia.

Secondary hyperparathyroidism can be caused by vitamin D deficiency or chronic renal disease in which the damaged kidneys are unable to produce sufficient amounts of the active form of vitamin D, 1,25-dihydroxycholecalciferol. As discussed in more detail in the next section, the vitamin D deficiency leads to *osteomalacia* (inadequate mineralization of the bones) and high levels of PTH cause absorption of the bones.

Rickets Caused by Vitamin D Deficiency

Rickets occurs mainly in children. It results from calcium or phosphate deficiency in the extracellular fluid, usually caused by lack of vitamin D. If the child is adequately exposed to sunlight, the 7-dehydrocholesterol in the skin becomes activated by the ultraviolet rays and forms vitamin D_3, which prevents rickets by promoting calcium and phosphate absorption from the intestines, as discussed earlier in the chapter.

Children who remain indoors through the winter in general do not receive adequate quantities of vitamin D without some supplementation in the diet. Rickets tends to occur especially in the spring months because vitamin D formed during the preceding summer is stored in the liver and available for use during the early winter months. Also, calcium and phosphate absorption from the bones can prevent clinical signs of rickets for the first few months of vitamin D deficiency.

Plasma Concentrations of Calcium and Phosphate Decrease in Rickets. The plasma calcium concentration in rickets is only slightly depressed, but the level of phosphate is greatly depressed. This is because the parathyroid glands prevent the calcium level from falling by promoting bone absorption every time the calcium level begins to fall. However, there is no good regulatory system for preventing a falling level of phosphate, and the increased parathyroid activity actually increases the excretion of phosphates in the urine.

Rickets Weakens the Bones. During prolonged rickets, the marked compensatory increase in PTH secretion causes extreme osteoclastic absorption of the bone; this in turn causes the bone to become progressively weaker and imposes marked physical stress on the bone, resulting in rapid osteoblastic activity as well. The osteoblasts lay down large quantities of osteoid, which does not become calcified because of insufficient calcium and phosphate ions. Consequently, the newly formed, uncalcified, and weak osteoid gradually takes the place of the older bone that is being reabsorbed.

Tetany in Rickets. In the early stages of rickets, tetany almost never occurs because the parathyroid glands continually stimulate osteoclastic absorption of bone and, therefore, maintain an almost normal level of calcium in the extracellular fluid. However, when the bones finally become exhausted of calcium, the level of calcium may fall rapidly. As the blood level of calcium falls below 7 mg/dl, the usual signs of tetany develop and the child may die of tetanic respiratory spasm unless intravenous calcium is administered, which relieves the tetany immediately.

Treatment of Rickets. The treatment of rickets depends on supplying adequate calcium and phosphate in the diet and, equally important, on administering large amounts of vitamin D. If vitamin D is not administered, little calcium and phosphate are absorbed from the gut.

Osteomalacia—"Adult Rickets." Adults seldom have a serious *dietary* deficiency of vitamin D or calcium because large quantities of calcium are not needed for bone growth as in children. However, serious deficiencies of both vitamin D and calcium occasionally occur as a result of *steatorrhea* (failure to absorb fat) because vitamin D is fat-soluble and calcium tends to form insoluble soaps with fat; consequently, in steatorrhea, both vitamin D and calcium tend to pass into the feces. Under these conditions, an adult occasionally has such poor calcium and phosphate absorption that adult rickets can occur, although this almost never proceeds to the stage of tetany but often is a cause of severe bone disability.

Osteomalacia and Rickets Caused by Renal Disease. "Renal rickets" is a type of osteomalacia that results from prolonged kidney damage. The cause of this condition is mainly failure of the damaged kidneys to form 1,25-dihydroxycholecalciferol, the active form of vitamin D. In patients whose kidneys have been removed or destroyed and who are being treated by hemodialysis, the problem of renal rickets is often a severe one.

Another type of renal disease that leads to rickets and osteomalacia is *congenital hypophosphatemia*, resulting from congenitally reduced reabsorption of phosphates by the renal tubules. This type of rickets must be treated with phosphate compounds instead of calcium and vitamin D, and it is called *vitamin D–resistant rickets.*

Osteoporosis—Decreased Bone Matrix

Osteoporosis is the most common of all bone diseases in adults, especially in old age. It is different from osteomalacia and rickets because it results from diminished organic bone matrix rather than from poor bone calcification. In osteoporosis the osteoblastic activity in the bone is usually less than normal, and consequently the rate of bone osteoid deposition is depressed. But occasionally, as in hyperparathyroidism, the cause of the diminished bone is excess osteoclastic activity.

The many common causes of osteoporosis are (1) *lack of physical stress on the bones* because of inactivity; (2) *malnutrition* to the extent that sufficient protein matrix cannot be formed; (3) *lack of vitamin C,* which is necessary for the secretion of intercellular substances by all cells, including formation of osteoid by the osteoblasts; (4) *postmenopausal lack of estrogen secretion* because estrogens decrease the number and activity of osteoclasts; (5) *old age,* in which growth hormone and other growth factors diminish greatly, plus the fact that many of the protein anabolic functions also deteriorate with age, so bone matrix cannot be deposited satisfactorily; and (6) *Cushing's syndrome,* because massive quantities of glucocorticoids secreted in this disease cause decreased deposition of protein throughout the body and increased catabolism of protein and have the specific effect of depressing osteoblastic activity. Thus, many diseases of deficiency of protein metabolism can cause osteoporosis.

Physiology of the Teeth

The teeth cut, grind, and mix the food eaten. To perform these functions, the jaws have powerful muscles capable of providing an occlusive force between the front teeth of 50 to 100 pounds and for the jaw teeth, 150 to 200 pounds. Also, the upper and lower teeth are provided with projections and facets that interdigitate, so the upper set of teeth fits with the lower. This fitting is called *occlusion,* and it allows even small particles of food to be caught and ground between the tooth surfaces.

Function of the Different Parts of the Teeth

Figure 79-14 shows a sagittal section of a tooth, demonstrating its major functional parts: the *enamel, dentin, cementum,* and *pulp.* The tooth can also be divided into the *crown,* which is the portion that protrudes out from the gum into the mouth, and the *root,* which is the portion within the bony socket of the jaw. The collar between the crown and the root where the tooth is surrounded by the gum is called the *neck.*

Enamel. The outer surface of the tooth is covered by a layer of enamel that is formed before eruption of the tooth by special epithelial cells called *ameloblasts.* Once the tooth has erupted, no more enamel is formed. Enamel is composed of large and dense crystals of hydroxyapatite with adsorbed carbonate, magnesium, sodium, potassium, and other ions embedded in a fine meshwork of strong and almost insoluble protein fibers that are similar in physical characteristics (but not chemically identical) to the keratin of hair.

The crystalline structure of the salts makes the enamel extremely hard, much harder than the dentin. Also, the special protein fiber meshwork, although constituting

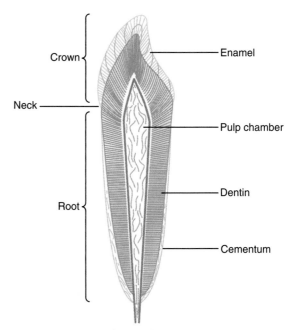

Figure 79-14 Functional parts of a tooth.

only about 1 percent of the enamel mass, makes enamel resistant to acids, enzymes, and other corrosive agents because this protein is one of the most insoluble and resistant proteins known.

Dentin. The main body of the tooth is composed of dentin, which has a strong, bony structure. Dentin is made up principally of hydroxyapatite crystals similar to those in bone but much denser. These crystals are embedded in a strong meshwork of collagen fibers. In other words, the principal constituents of dentin are much the same as those of bone. The major difference is its histological organization because dentin does not contain any osteoblasts, osteocytes, osteoclasts, or spaces for blood vessels or nerves. Instead, it is deposited and nourished by a layer of cells called *odontoblasts,* which line its inner surface along the wall of the pulp cavity.

The calcium salts in dentin make it extremely resistant to compressional forces, and the collagen fibers make it tough and resistant to tensional forces that might result when the teeth are struck by solid objects.

Cementum. Cementum is a bony substance secreted by cells of the *periodontal membrane,* which lines the tooth socket. Many collagen fibers pass directly from the bone of the jaw, through the periodontal membrane, and then into the cementum. These collagen fibers and the cementum hold the tooth in place. When the teeth are exposed to excessive strain, the layer of cementum becomes thicker and stronger. Also, it increases in thickness and strength with age, causing the teeth to become more firmly seated in the jaws by adulthood and later.

Pulp. The pulp cavity of each tooth is filled with *pulp,* which is composed of connective tissue with an abundant supply of nerve fibers, blood vessels, and lymphatics. The cells lining the surface of the pulp cavity are the odontoblasts, which, during the formative years of the tooth, lay down the dentin but at the same time encroach more and more on the pulp cavity, making it smaller. In later life, the dentin stops growing and the pulp cavity remains essentially constant in size. However, the odontoblasts are still viable and send projections into small *dentinal tubules* that penetrate all the way through the dentin; they are of importance for exchange of calcium, phosphate, and other minerals with the dentin.

Dentition

Humans and most other mammals develop two sets of teeth during a lifetime. The first teeth are called the deciduous teeth, or milk teeth, and they number 20 in humans. They erupt between the seventh month and the second year of life, and they last until the sixth to the 13th year. After each deciduous tooth is lost, a permanent tooth replaces it and an additional 8 to 12 molars appear posteriorly in the jaws, making the total number of permanent teeth 28 to 32, depending on whether the four wisdom teeth finally appear, which does not occur in everyone.

Formation of the Teeth. Figure 79-15 shows the formation and eruption of teeth. Figure 79-15*A* shows invagination of the oral epithelium into the *dental lamina;* this is followed by the development of a tooth-producing organ. The epithelial cells above form ameloblasts, which form the enamel on the outside of the tooth. The epithelial cells below invaginate upward into the middle of the tooth to form the pulp cavity and the odontoblasts that secrete dentin. Thus, enamel is formed on the outside of the tooth, and dentin is formed on the inside, giving rise to an early tooth, as shown in Figure 79-15*B.*

Eruption of Teeth. During early childhood, the teeth begin to protrude outward from the bone through the oral epithelium into the mouth. The cause of "eruption" is unknown, although several theories have been offered in an attempt to explain this phenomenon. The most likely theory is that growth of the tooth root and the bone underneath the tooth progressively shoves the tooth forward.

Development of the Permanent Teeth. During embryonic life, a tooth-forming organ also develops in the deeper dental lamina for each permanent tooth that will be needed after the deciduous teeth are gone. These tooth-producing organs slowly form the permanent teeth throughout the first 6 to 20 years of life. When each permanent tooth becomes fully formed, it, like the deciduous tooth, pushes outward through the bone. In so doing, it erodes the root of the deciduous tooth and

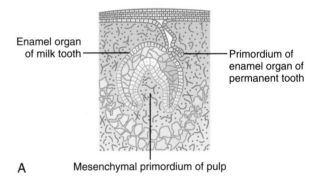

Enamel organ of milk tooth

Primordium of enamel organ of permanent tooth

A   Mesenchymal primordium of pulp

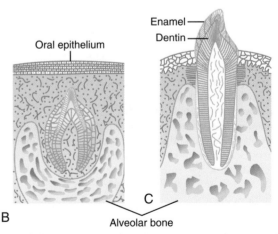

Oral epithelium

Enamel

Dentin

B

C

Alveolar bone

Figure 79-15 *A,* Primordial tooth organ. *B,* Developing tooth. *C,* Erupting tooth.

eventually causes it to loosen and fall out. Soon thereafter, the permanent tooth erupts to take the place of the original one.

Metabolic Factors Influence Development of the Teeth. The rate of development and the speed of eruption of teeth can be accelerated by both thyroid and growth hormones. Also, the deposition of salts in the early-forming teeth is affected considerably by various factors of metabolism, such as the availability of calcium and phosphate in the diet, the amount of vitamin D present, and the rate of PTH secretion. When all these factors are normal, the dentin and enamel will be correspondingly healthy, but when they are deficient, the calcification of the teeth also may be defective and the teeth will be abnormal throughout life.

Mineral Exchange in Teeth

The salts of teeth, like those of bone, are composed of hydroxyapatite with adsorbed carbonates and various cations bound together in a hard crystalline substance. Also, new salts are constantly being deposited while old salts are being reabsorbed from the teeth, as occurs in bone. Deposition and reabsorption occur mainly in the dentin and cementum and to a limited extent in the enamel. In the enamel, these processes occur mostly by diffusional exchange of minerals with the saliva instead of with the fluids of the pulp cavity.

The rate of absorption and deposition of minerals in the cementum is about equal to that in the surrounding bone of the jaw, whereas the rate of deposition and absorption of minerals in the dentin is only one-third that of bone. The cementum has characteristics almost identical to those of usual bone, including the presence of osteoblasts and osteoclasts, whereas dentin does not have these characteristics, as explained earlier. This difference undoubtedly explains the different rates of mineral exchange.

In summary, continual mineral exchange occurs in the dentin and cementum of teeth, although the mechanism of this exchange in dentin is unclear. However, enamel exhibits extremely slow mineral exchange, so it maintains most of its original mineral complement throughout life.

Dental Abnormalities

The two most common dental abnormalities are *caries* and *malocclusion*. Caries refers to erosion of the teeth, whereas malocclusion is failure of the projections of the upper and lower teeth to interdigitate properly.

Caries and the Role of Bacteria and Ingested Carbohydrates. It is generally agreed that caries result from the action of bacteria on the teeth, the most common of which is *Streptococcus mutans*. The first event in the development of caries is the deposit of *plaque*, a film of precipitated products of saliva and food, on the teeth. Large numbers of bacteria inhabit this plaque and are readily available to cause caries. These bacteria depend to a great extent on carbohydrates for their food. When carbohydrates are available, their metabolic systems are strongly activated and they multiply. In addition, they form acids (particularly lactic acid) and proteolytic enzymes. The acids are the major culprit in causing caries because the calcium salts of teeth are slowly dissolved in a highly acidic medium. And once the salts have become absorbed, the remaining organic matrix is rapidly digested by the proteolytic enzymes.

The enamel of the tooth is the primary barrier to the development of caries. Enamel is far more resistant to demineralization by acids than is dentin, primarily because the crystals of enamel are dense, but also because each enamel crystal is about 200 times as large in volume as each dentin crystal. Once the carious process has penetrated through the enamel to the dentin, it proceeds many times as rapidly because of the high degree of solubility of the dentin salts.

Because of the dependence of the caries bacteria on carbohydrates for their nutrition, it has frequently been taught that eating a diet high in carbohydrate content will lead to excessive development of caries. However, it is not the quantity of carbohydrate ingested but the frequency with which it is eaten that is important. If carbohydrates are eaten in many small parcels throughout the day, such as in the form of candy, the bacteria are supplied with their preferential metabolic substrate for many hours of the day and the development of caries is greatly increased.

Role of Fluorine in Preventing Caries. Teeth formed in children who drink water that contains small amounts of fluorine develop enamel that is more resistant to caries than the enamel in children who drink water that does not contain fluorine. Fluorine does not make the enamel harder than usual, but fluorine ions replace many of the hydroxyl ions in the hydroxyapatite crystals, which in turn makes the enamel several times less soluble. Fluorine may also be toxic to the bacteria. Finally, when small pits do develop in the enamel, fluorine is believed to promote deposition of calcium phosphate to "heal" the enamel surface. Regardless of the precise means by which fluorine protects the teeth, it is known that small amounts of fluorine deposited in enamel make teeth about three times as resistant to caries as teeth without fluorine.

Malocclusion. Malocclusion is usually caused by a hereditary abnormality that causes the teeth of one jaw to grow to abnormal positions. In malocclusion, the teeth do not interdigitate properly and therefore cannot perform their normal grinding or cutting action adequately. Malocclusion occasionally also results in abnormal displacement of the lower jaw in relation to the upper jaw, causing such undesirable effects as pain in the mandibular joint and deterioration of the teeth.

The orthodontist can usually correct malocclusion by applying prolonged gentle pressure against the teeth with appropriate braces. The gentle pressure causes absorption of alveolar jaw bone on the compressed side of the tooth and deposition of new bone on the tensional side of the tooth. In this way, the tooth gradually moves to a new position as directed by the applied pressure.

Bibliography

Berndt T, Kumar R: Novel mechanisms in the regulation of phosphorus homeostasis, *Physiology (Bethesda)* 24:17, 2009.

Bilezikian JP, Silverberg SJ: Clinical practice. Asymptomatic primary hyperparathyroidism, *N Engl J Med* 350:1746, 2004.

Canalis E, Giustina A, Bilezikian JP: Mechanisms of anabolic therapies for osteoporosis, *N Engl J Med* 357:905, 2007.

Chen RA, Goodman WG: Role of the calcium-sensing receptor in parathyroid gland physiology, *Am J Physiol Renal Physiol* 286:F1005, 2004.

Compston JE: Sex steroids and bone, *Physiol Rev* 81:419, 2001.

Delmas PD: Treatment of postmenopausal osteoporosis, *Lancet* 359:2018, 2002.

Fraser WD: Hyperparathyroidism, *Lancet* 374:145, 2009.

Goodman WG, Quarles LD: Development and progression of secondary hyperparathyroidism in chronic kidney disease: lessons from molecular genetics, *Kidney Int* 74:276, 2008.

Hoenderop JG, Nilius B, Bindels RJ: Calcium absorption across epithelia, *Physiol Rev* 85:373, 2005.

Holick MF: Vitamin D deficiency, *N Engl J Med* 357:266, 2007.

Hofer AM, Brown EM: Extracellular calcium sensing and signalling, *Nat Rev Mol Cell Biol* 4:530, 2003.

Jones G, Strugnell SA, DeLuca HF: Current understanding of the molecular actions of vitamin D, *Physiol Rev* 78:1193, 1998.

Kearns AE, Khosla S, Kostenuik PJ: Receptor activator of nuclear factor kappaB ligand and osteoprotegerin regulation of bone remodeling in health and disease, *Endocr Rev* 29:155, 2008.

Khosla S, Amin S, Orwoll E: Osteoporosis in men, *Endocr Rev* 29:441, 2008.

Khosla S, Westendorf JJ, Oursler MJ: Building bone to reverse osteoporosis and repair fractures, *J Clin Invest* 118:421, 2008.

Marx SJ: Hyperparathyroid and hypoparathyroid disorders, *N Engl J Med* 343:1863, 2000.

Peng JB, Brown EM, Hediger MA: Apical entry channels in calcium-transporting epithelia, *News Physiol Sci* 18:158, 2003.

Quarles LD: Endocrine functions of bone in mineral metabolism regulation, *J Clin Invest* 118:3820, 2008.

Seeman E, Delmas PD: Bone quality—the material and structural basis of bone strength and fragility, *N Engl J Med* 354:2250, 2006.

Shoback D: Clinical practice. Hypoparathyroidism, *N Engl J Med* 359:391, 2008.

Silver J, Naveh-Many T: Phosphate and the parathyroid, *Kidney Int* 75:898, 2009.

Silver J, Kilav R, Naveh-Many T: Mechanisms of secondary hyperparathyroidism, *Am J Physiol Renal Physiol* 283:F367, 2002.

Smajilovic S, Tfelt-Hansen J: Novel role of the calcium-sensing receptor in blood pressure modulation, *Hypertension* 52:994, 2008.

Tordoff MG: Calcium: taste, intake, and appetite, *Physiol Rev* 81:1567, 2001.

Wharton B, Bishop N: Rickets, *Lancet* 362:1389, 2003.

Zaidi M: Skeletal remodeling in health and disease, *Nat Med* 13:791, 2007.

Reproductive and Hormonal Functions of the Male (and Function of the Pineal Gland)

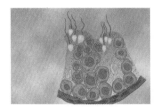

The reproductive functions of the male can be divided into three major subdivisions: (1) spermatogenesis, which means the formation of sperm; (2) performance of the male sexual act; and (3) regulation of male reproductive functions by the various hormones. Associated with these reproductive functions are the effects of the male sex hormones on the accessory sexual organs, cellular metabolism, growth, and other functions of the body.

Physiologic Anatomy of the Male Sexual Organs

Figure 80-1A shows the various portions of the male reproductive system, and Figure 80-1B gives a more detailed structure of the testis and epididymis. The testis is composed of up to 900 coiled *seminiferous tubules,* each averaging more than one-half meter long, in which the sperm are formed. The sperm then empty into the *epididymis,* another coiled tube about 6 meters long. The epididymis leads into the *vas deferens,* which enlarges into the *ampulla of the vas deferens* immediately before the vas enters the body of the *prostate gland.*

Two *seminal vesicles,* one located on each side of the prostate, empty into the prostatic end of the ampulla, and the contents from both the ampulla and the seminal vesicles pass into an *ejaculatory duct* leading through the body of the prostate gland and then emptying into the *internal urethra.* *Prostatic ducts* also empty from the prostate gland into the ejaculatory duct and from there into the prostatic urethra.

Finally, the *urethra* is the last connecting link from the testis to the exterior. The urethra is supplied with mucus derived from a large number of minute *urethral glands* located along its entire extent and even more so from bilateral *bulbourethral glands* (Cowper glands) located near the origin of the urethra.

Spermatogenesis

During formation of the embryo, the *primordial germ cells* migrate into the testes and become immature germ cells called *spermatogonia,* which lie in two or

three layers of the inner surfaces of the *seminiferous tubules* (a cross section of one is shown in Figure 80-2A). The spermatogonia begin to undergo mitotic division, beginning at puberty, and continually proliferate and differentiate through definite stages of development to form sperm, as shown in Figure 80-2B.

Steps of Spermatogenesis

Spermatogenesis occurs in the seminiferous tubules during active sexual life as the result of stimulation by anterior

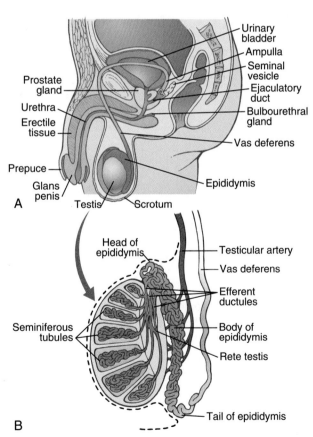

Figure 80-1 *A,* Male reproduction system. (Modified from Bloom V, Fawcett DW: Textbook of Histology, 10th ed. Philadelphia: WB Saunders, 1975.) *B,* Internal structure of the testis and relation of the testis to the epididymis. (Redrawn from Guyton AC: Anatomy and Physiology. Philadelphia: Saunders College Publishing, 1985.)

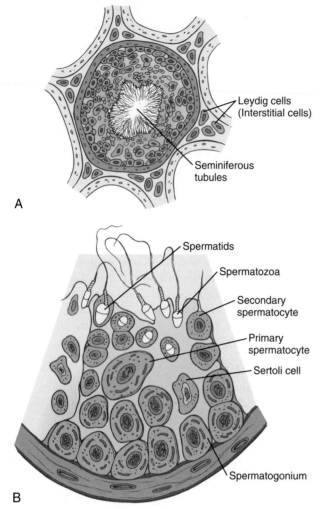

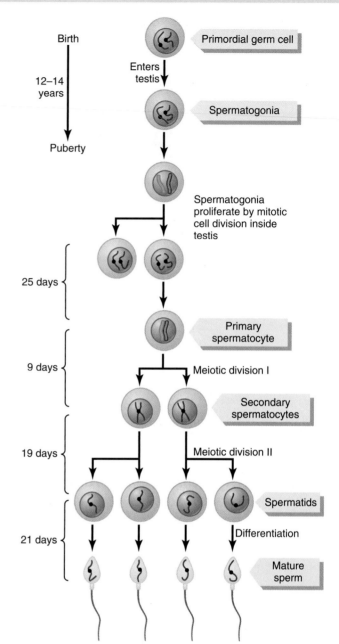

Figure 80-2 *A*, Cross section of a seminiferous tubule. *B*, Stages in the development of sperm from spermatogonia.

Figure 80-3 Cell divisions during spermatogenesis. During embryonic development the primordial germ cells migrate to the testis, where they become spermatogonia. At puberty (usually 12 to 14 years after birth), the spermatogonia proliferate rapidly by mitosis. Some begin meiosis to become primary spermatocytes and continue through meiotic division I to become secondary spermatocytes. After completion of meiotic division II, the secondary spermatocytes produce spermatids, which differentiate to form spermatozoa.

pituitary gonadotropic hormones, beginning at an average age of 13 years and continuing throughout most of the remainder of life but decreasing markedly in old age.

In the first stage of spermatogenesis, the spermatogonia migrate among *Sertoli cells* toward the central lumen of the seminiferous tubule. The Sertoli cells are large, with overflowing cytoplasmic envelopes that surround the developing spermatogonia all the way to the central lumen of the tubule.

Meiosis. Spermatogonia that cross the barrier into the Sertoli cell layer become progressively modified and enlarged to form large *primary spermatocytes* (Figure 80-3). Each of these, in turn, undergoes meiotic division to form two *secondary spermatocytes*. After another few days, these too divide to form *spermatids* that are eventually modified to become *spermatozoa* (sperm).

During the change from the spermatocyte stage to the spermatid stage, the 46 chromosomes (23 pairs of chromosomes) of the spermatocyte are divided, so 23 chromosomes go to one spermatid and the other 23 to the second spermatid. This also divides the chromosomal genes so that only one half of the genetic characteristics of the eventual fetus are provided by the father, whereas the other half are derived from the oocyte provided by the mother.

The entire period of spermatogenesis, from spermatogonia to spermatozoa, takes about 74 days.

Sex Chromosomes. In each spermatogonium, one of the 23 pairs of chromosomes carries the genetic information that determines the sex of each eventual offspring. This pair is composed of one X chromosome, which is called the *female chromosome,* and one Y chromosome, the *male chromosome.* During meiotic division, the male Y chromosome goes to one spermatid that then becomes a *male sperm,* and the female X chromosome goes to another spermatid that becomes a *female sperm.* The sex of the eventual offspring is determined by which of these two types of sperm fertilizes the ovum. This is discussed further in Chapter 82.

Formation of Sperm. When the spermatids are first formed, they still have the usual characteristics of epithelioid cells, but soon they begin to differentiate and elongate into spermatozoa. As shown in Figure 80-4, each spermatozoon is composed of a *head* and a *tail.* The head comprises the condensed nucleus of the cell with only a thin cytoplasmic and cell membrane layer around its surface. On the outside of the anterior two thirds of the head is a thick cap called the *acrosome* that is formed mainly from the Golgi apparatus. This contains a number of enzymes similar to those found in lysosomes of the typical cell, including *hyaluronidase* (which can digest proteoglycan filaments of tissues) and powerful *proteolytic enzymes* (which can digest proteins). These enzymes play important roles in allowing the sperm to enter the ovum and fertilize it.

The tail of the sperm, called the *flagellum,* has three major components: (1) a central skeleton constructed of 11 microtubules, collectively called the *axoneme*—the structure of this is similar to that of cilia found on the surfaces of other types of cells described in Chapter 2; (2) a thin cell membrane covering the axoneme; and (3) a collection of

mitochondria surrounding the axoneme in the proximal portion of the tail (called the *body of the tail*).

Back-and-forth movement of the tail (flagellar movement) provides motility for the sperm. This movement results from a rhythmical longitudinal sliding motion between the anterior and posterior tubules that make up the axoneme. The energy for this process is supplied in the form of adenosine triphosphate, which is synthesized by the mitochondria in the body of the tail.

Normal sperm move in a fluid medium at a velocity of 1 to 4 mm/min. This allows them to move through the female genital tract in quest of the ovum.

Hormonal Factors That Stimulate Spermatogenesis

The role of hormones in reproduction is discussed later, but at this point, let us note that several hormones play essential roles in spermatogenesis. Some of these are as follows:

1. *Testosterone,* secreted by the *Leydig cells* located in the interstitium of the testis (see Figure 80-2), is essential for growth and division of the testicular germinal cells, which is the first stage in forming sperm.

2. *Luteinizing hormone,* secreted by the anterior pituitary gland, stimulates the Leydig cells to secrete testosterone.

3. *Follicle-stimulating hormone,* also secreted by the anterior pituitary gland, stimulates the *Sertoli cells;* without this stimulation, the conversion of the spermatids to sperm (the process of spermiogenesis) will not occur.

4. *Estrogens,* formed from testosterone by the Sertoli cells when they are stimulated by follicle-stimulating hormone, are probably also essential for spermiogenesis.

5. *Growth hormone* (as well as most of the other body hormones) is necessary for controlling background metabolic functions of the testes. Growth hormone specifically promotes early division of the spermatogonia themselves; in its absence, as in pituitary dwarfs, spermatogenesis is severely deficient or absent, thus causing infertility.

Maturation of Sperm in the Epididymis

After formation in the seminiferous tubules, the sperm require several days to pass through the 6-meter-long tubule of the *epididymis.* Sperm removed from the seminiferous tubules and from the early portions of the epididymis are nonmotile, and they cannot fertilize an ovum. However, after the sperm have been in the epididymis for 18 to 24 hours, they develop the *capability of motility,* even though several inhibitory proteins in the epididymal fluid still prevent final motility until after ejaculation.

Storage of Sperm in the Testes. The two testes of the human adult form up to 120 million sperm each day. A small quantity of these can be stored in the epididymis,

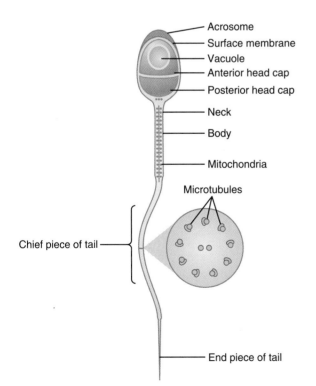

Figure 80-4 Structure of the human spermatozoon.

Labels for Figure 80-4:
- Acrosome
- Surface membrane
- Vacuole
- Anterior head cap
- Posterior head cap
- Neck
- Body
- Mitochondria
- Microtubules
- Chief piece of tail
- End piece of tail

but most are stored in the vas deferens. They can remain stored, maintaining their fertility, for at least a month. During this time, they are kept in a deeply suppressed, inactive state by multiple inhibitory substances in the secretions of the ducts. Conversely, with a high level of sexual activity and ejaculations, storage may be no longer than a few days.

After ejaculation, the sperm become motile, and they also become capable of fertilizing the ovum, a process called *maturation*. The Sertoli cells and the epithelium of the epididymis secrete a special nutrient fluid that is ejaculated along with the sperm. This fluid contains hormones (including both testosterone and estrogens), enzymes, and special nutrients that are essential for sperm maturation.

Physiology of the Mature Sperm. The normal motile, fertile sperm are capable of flagellated movement through the fluid medium at velocities of 1 to 4 mm/min. The activity of sperm is greatly enhanced in a neutral and slightly alkaline medium, as exists in the ejaculated semen, but it is greatly depressed in a mildly acidic medium. A strong acidic medium can cause rapid death of sperm.

The activity of sperm increases markedly with increasing temperature, but so does the rate of metabolism, causing the life of the sperm to be considerably shortened. Although sperm can live for many weeks in the suppressed state in the genital ducts of the testes, life expectancy of ejaculated sperm in the female genital tract is only 1 to 2 days.

Function of the Seminal Vesicles

Each seminal vesicle is a tortuous, loculated tube lined with a secretory epithelium that secretes a mucoid material containing an abundance of *fructose, citric acid,* and other nutrient substances, as well as large quantities of *prostaglandins* and *fibrinogen.* During the process of emission and ejaculation, each seminal vesicle empties its contents into the ejaculatory duct shortly after the vas deferens empties the sperm. This adds greatly to the bulk of the ejaculated semen, and the fructose and other substances in the seminal fluid are of considerable nutrient value for the ejaculated sperm until one of the sperm fertilizes the ovum.

Prostaglandins are believed to aid fertilization in two ways: (1) by reacting with the female cervical mucus to make it more receptive to sperm movement and (2) by possibly causing backward, reverse peristaltic contractions in the uterus and fallopian tubes to move the ejaculated sperm toward the ovaries (a few sperm reach the upper ends of the fallopian tubes within 5 minutes).

Function of the Prostate Gland

The prostate gland secretes a thin, milky fluid that contains calcium, citrate ion, phosphate ion, a clotting enzyme, and a profibrinolysin. During emission, the capsule of the prostate gland contracts simultaneously with the contractions of the vas deferens so that the thin, milky

fluid of the prostate gland adds further to the bulk of the semen. A slightly alkaline characteristic of the prostatic fluid may be quite important for successful fertilization of the ovum because the fluid of the vas deferens is relatively acidic owing to the presence of citric acid and metabolic end products of the sperm and, consequently, helps to inhibit sperm fertility. Also, the vaginal secretions of the female are acidic (pH of 3.5 to 4.0). Sperm do not become optimally motile until the pH of the surrounding fluids rises to about 6.0 to 6.5. Consequently, it is probable that the slightly alkaline prostatic fluid helps to neutralize the acidity of the other seminal fluids during ejaculation and thus enhances the motility and fertility of the sperm.

Semen

Semen, which is ejaculated during the male sexual act, is composed of the fluid and sperm from the vas deferens (about 10 percent of the total), fluid from the seminal vesicles (almost 60 percent), fluid from the prostate gland (about 30 percent), and small amounts from the mucous glands, especially the bulbourethral glands. Thus, the bulk of the semen is seminal vesicle fluid, which is the last to be ejaculated and serves to wash the sperm through the ejaculatory duct and urethra.

The average pH of the combined semen is about 7.5, the alkaline prostatic fluid having more than neutralized the mild acidity of the other portions of the semen. The prostatic fluid gives the semen a milky appearance, and fluid from the seminal vesicles and mucous glands gives the semen a mucoid consistency. Also, a clotting enzyme from the prostatic fluid causes the fibrinogen of the seminal vesicle fluid to form a weak fibrin coagulum that holds the semen in the deeper regions of the vagina where the uterine cervix lies. The coagulum then dissolves during the next 15 to 30 minutes because of lysis by fibrinolysin formed from the prostatic profibrinolysin. In the early minutes after ejaculation, the sperm remain relatively immobile, possibly because of the viscosity of the coagulum. As the coagulum dissolves, the sperm simultaneously become highly motile.

Although sperm can live for many weeks in the male genital ducts, once they are ejaculated in the semen, their maximal life span is only 24 to 48 hours at body temperature. At lowered temperatures, however, semen can be stored for several weeks, and when frozen at temperatures below –100°C, sperm have been preserved for years.

"Capacitation" of Spermatozoa Is Required for Fertilization of the Ovum

Although spermatozoa are said to be "mature" when they leave the epididymis, their activity is held in check by multiple inhibitory factors secreted by the genital duct epithelia. Therefore, when they are first expelled in the semen, they are unable to fertilize the ovum. However, on coming in contact with the fluids of the female genital tract, multiple changes occur that activate the sperm for the final processes of fertilization. These collective changes are called *capacitation of the spermatozoa*. This normally requires from 1 to 10 hours. Some changes that are believed to occur are the following:

1. The uterine and fallopian tube fluids wash away the various inhibitory factors that suppress sperm activity in the male genital ducts.

2. While the spermatozoa remain in the fluid of the male genital ducts, they are continually exposed to many floating vesicles from the seminiferous tubules containing large amounts of cholesterol. This cholesterol is continually added to the cellular membrane covering the sperm acrosome, toughening this membrane and preventing release of its enzymes. After ejaculation, the sperm deposited in the vagina swim away from the cholesterol vesicles upward into the uterine cavity, and they gradually lose much of their other excess cholesterol over the next few hours. In so doing, the membrane at the head of the sperm (the acrosome) becomes much weaker.

3. The membrane of the sperm also becomes much more permeable to calcium ions, so calcium now enters the sperm in abundance and changes the activity of the flagellum, giving it a powerful whiplash motion in contrast to its previously weak undulating motion. In addition, the calcium ions cause changes in the cellular membrane that cover the leading edge of the acrosome, making it possible for the acrosome to release its enzymes rapidly and easily as the sperm penetrates the granulosa cell mass surrounding the ovum, and even more so as it attempts to penetrate the zona pellucida of the ovum itself.

Thus, multiple changes occur during the process of capacitation. Without these, the sperm cannot make its way to the interior of the ovum to cause fertilization.

Acrosome Enzymes, the "Acrosome Reaction," and Penetration of the Ovum

Stored in the acrosome of the sperm are large quantities of *hyaluronidase* and *proteolytic enzymes*. Hyaluronidase depolymerizes the hyaluronic acid polymers in the intercellular cement that holds the ovarian granulosa cells together. The proteolytic enzymes digest proteins in the structural elements of tissue cells that still adhere to the ovum.

When the ovum is expelled from the ovarian follicle into the fallopian tube, it still carries with it multiple layers of granulosa cells. Before a sperm can fertilize the ovum, it must dissolute these granulosa cell layers, and then it must penetrate though the thick covering of the ovum itself, the *zona pellucida*. To achieve this, the stored enzymes in the acrosome begin to be released. It is believed that the hyaluronidase among these enzymes is especially important in opening pathways between the granulosa cells so that the sperm can reach the ovum.

When the sperm reaches the zona pellucida of the ovum, the anterior membrane of the sperm binds spe-

cifically with receptor proteins in the zona pellucida. Next, the entire acrosome rapidly dissolves and all the acrosomal enzymes are released. Within minutes, these enzymes open a penetrating pathway for passage of the sperm head through the zona pellucida to the inside of the ovum. Within another 30 minutes, the cell membranes of the sperm head and of the oocyte fuse with each other to form a single cell. At the same time, the genetic material of the sperm and the oocyte combine to form a completely new cell genome, containing equal numbers of chromosomes and genes from mother and father. This is the process of *fertilization;* then the embryo begins to develop, as discussed in Chapter 82.

Why Does Only One Sperm Enter the Oocyte? With as many sperm as there are, why does only one enter the oocyte? The reason is not entirely known, but within a few minutes after the first sperm penetrates the zona pellucida of the ovum, calcium ions diffuse inward through the oocyte membrane and cause multiple cortical granules to be released by exocytosis from the oocyte into the perivitelline space. These granules contain substances that permeate all portions of the zona pellucida and prevent binding of additional sperm, and they even cause any sperm that have already begun to bind to fall off. Thus, almost never does more than one sperm enter the oocyte during fertilization.

Abnormal Spermatogenesis and Male Fertility

The seminiferous tubular epithelium can be destroyed by a number of diseases. For instance, bilateral *orchitis* (inflammation) of the testes resulting from *mumps* causes sterility in some affected males. Also, some male infants are born with degenerate tubular epithelia as a result of strictures in the genital ducts or other abnormalities. Finally, another cause of sterility, usually temporary, is *excessive temperature of the testes.*

Effect of Temperature on Spermatogenesis. Increasing the temperature of the testes can prevent spermatogenesis by causing degeneration of most cells of the seminiferous tubules besides the spermatogonia. It has often been stated that the reason the testes are located in the dangling scrotum is to maintain the temperature of these glands below the internal temperature of the body, although usually only about 2°C below the internal temperature. On cold days, scrotal reflexes cause the musculature of the scrotum to contract, pulling the testes close to the body to maintain this 2° differential. Thus, the scrotum acts as a cooling mechanism for the testes (but a *controlled* cooling), without which spermatogenesis might be deficient during hot weather.

Cryptorchidism

Cryptorchidism means failure of a testis to descend from the abdomen into the scrotum at or near the time of birth of a fetus. During development of the male fetus, the testes are derived from the genital ridges in the abdomen. However, at about 3 weeks to 1 month before birth of the baby, the testes normally descend through the inguinal canals into the scrotum. Occasionally this descent does not occur or occurs incompletely, so one or both testes remain in the abdomen, in the inguinal canal, or elsewhere along the route of descent.

A testis that remains throughout life in the abdominal cavity is incapable of forming sperm. The tubular epithelium becomes degenerate, leaving only the interstitial structures of the testis. It has been claimed that even the few degrees' higher temperature in the abdomen than in the scrotum is sufficient to cause this degeneration of the tubular epithelium and, consequently, to cause sterility, although this is not certain. Nevertheless, for this reason, operations to relocate the cryptorchid testes from the abdominal cavity into the scrotum before the beginning of adult sexual life can be performed on boys who have undescended testes.

Testosterone secretion by the fetal testes is the normal stimulus that causes the testes to descend into the scrotum from the abdomen. Therefore, many, if not most, instances of cryptorchidism are caused by abnormally formed testes that are unable to secrete enough testosterone. The surgical operation for cryptorchidism in these patients is unlikely to be successful.

Effect of Sperm Count on Fertility. The usual quantity of semen ejaculated during each coitus averages about 3.5 milliliters, and in each milliliter of semen is an average of about 120 million sperm, although even in "normal" males this can vary from 35 million to 200 million. This means an average total of 400 million sperm are usually present in the several milliliters of each ejaculate. When the number of sperm in each milliliter falls below about 20 million, the person is likely to be infertile. Thus, even though only a single sperm is necessary to fertilize the ovum, for reasons not understood, the ejaculate usually must contain a tremendous number of sperm for only one sperm to fertilize the ovum.

Effect of Sperm Morphology and Motility on Fertility. Occasionally a man has a normal number of sperm but is still infertile. When this occurs, sometimes as many as one-half the sperm are found to be abnormal physically, having two heads, abnormally shaped heads, or abnormal tails, as shown in Figure 80-5. At other times, the sperm appear to be structurally normal, but for reasons not understood, they are either entirely nonmotile or relatively nonmotile. Whenever the majority of the sperm are morphologically abnormal or are nonmotile, the person is likely to be infertile, even though the remainder of the sperm appear to be normal.

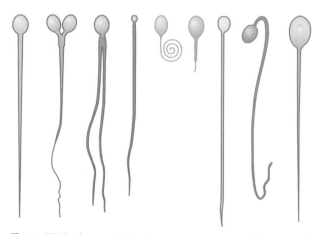

Figure 80-5 Abnormal infertile sperm, compared with a normal sperm on the right.

Male Sexual Act

Neuronal Stimulus for Performance of the Male Sexual Act

The most important source of sensory nerve signals for initiating the male sexual act is the *glans penis*. The glans contains an especially sensitive sensory end-organ system that transmits into the central nervous system that special modality of sensation called *sexual sensation*. The slippery massaging action of intercourse on the glans stimulates the sensory end-organs, and the sexual signals in turn pass through the pudendal nerve, then through the sacral plexus into the sacral portion of the spinal cord, and finally up the cord to undefined areas of the brain.

Impulses may also enter the spinal cord from areas adjacent to the penis to aid in stimulating the sexual act. For instance, stimulation of the anal epithelium, the scrotum, and perineal structures in general can send signals into the cord that add to the sexual sensation. Sexual sensations can even originate in internal structures, such as in areas of the urethra, bladder, prostate, seminal vesicles, testes, and vas deferens. Indeed, one of the causes of "sexual drive" is filling of the sexual organs with secretions. Mild infection and inflammation of these sexual organs sometimes cause almost continual sexual desire, and some "aphrodisiac" drugs, such as cantharidin, irritate the bladder and urethral mucosa, inducing inflammation and vascular congestion.

Psychic Element of Male Sexual Stimulation. Appropriate psychic stimuli can greatly enhance the ability of a person to perform the sexual act. Simply thinking sexual thoughts or even dreaming that the act of intercourse is being performed can initiate the male act, culminating in ejaculation. Indeed, *nocturnal emissions* during dreams occur in many males during some stages of sexual life, especially during the teens.

Integration of the Male Sexual Act in the Spinal Cord. Although psychic factors usually play an important part in the male sexual act and can initiate or inhibit it, brain function is probably not necessary for its performance because appropriate genital stimulation can cause ejaculation in some animals and occasionally in humans after their spinal cords have been cut above the lumbar region. The male sexual act results from inherent reflex mechanisms integrated in the sacral and lumbar spinal cord, and these mechanisms can be initiated by either psychic stimulation from the brain or actual sexual stimulation from the sex organs, but usually it is a combination of both.

Stages of the Male Sexual Act

Penile Erection—Role of the Parasympathetic Nerves. Penile erection is the first effect of male sexual stimulation, and the degree of erection is proportional to the degree of stimulation, whether psychic or physical. Erection is caused by parasympathetic impulses that pass from the sacral portion of the spinal cord through the pelvic nerves to the penis. These parasympathetic nerve fibers, in contrast to most other parasympathetic fibers, are believed to release *nitric oxide* and/or *vasoactive intestinal peptide* in addition to acetylcholine. Nitric oxide activates the enzyme *guanylyl cyclase,* causing increased formation of *cyclic guanosine monophosphate* (GMP). The cyclic GMP especially relaxes the arteries of the penis and the trabecular meshwork of smooth muscle fibers in the *erectile tissue* of the *corpora cavernosa* and *corpus spongiosum* in the shaft of the penis, shown in Figure 80-6. As the vascular smooth muscles relax, blood flow into the penis increases, causing release of nitric oxide from the vascular endothelial cells and further vasodilation.

The erectile tissue of the penis consists of large cavernous sinusoids, which are normally relatively empty of blood but become dilated tremendously when arterial blood flows rapidly into them under pressure while the venous outflow is partially occluded. Also, the erectile bodies, especially the two corpora cavernosa, are surrounded by strong fibrous coats; therefore, high pressure within the sinusoids causes ballooning of the erectile tissue to such an extent that the penis becomes hard and elongated. This is the phenomenon of *erection.*

Lubrication Is a Parasympathetic Function. During sexual stimulation, the parasympathetic impulses, in addition to promoting erection, cause the urethral glands and the bulbourethral glands to secrete mucus. This mucus flows through the urethra during intercourse to aid in the lubrication during coitus. However, most of the lubrication of coitus is provided by the female sexual organs rather than by the male. Without satisfactory lubrication, the male sexual act is seldom successful because unlubricated intercourse causes grating, painful sensations that inhibit rather than excite sexual sensations.

Emission and Ejaculation Are Functions of the Sympathetic Nerves. Emission and ejaculation are the culmination of the male sexual act. When the sexual stimulus becomes extremely intense, the reflex centers of the spinal cord begin to emit *sympathetic impulses* that leave the cord at T-12 to L-2 and pass to the genital organs through the hypogastric and pelvic sympathetic nerve plexuses to initiate *emission,* the forerunner of ejaculation.

Emission begins with contraction of the vas deferens and the ampulla to cause expulsion of sperm into the internal urethra. Then, contractions of the muscular coat of the prostate gland followed by contraction of the seminal vesicles expel prostatic and seminal fluid also into the urethra, forcing the sperm forward. All these fluids mix in the internal urethra with mucus already secreted by the bulbourethral glands to form the semen. The process to this point is *emission.*

The filling of the internal urethra with semen elicits sensory signals that are transmitted through the pudendal nerves to the sacral regions of the cord, giving the feeling of sudden fullness in the internal genital organs. Also, these sensory signals further excite rhythmical contraction of the internal genital organs and cause contraction of the ischiocavernosus and bulbocavernosus muscles that compress the bases of the penile erectile tissue. These effects together cause rhythmical, wavelike increases in pressure in both the erectile tissue of the penis and the genital ducts and urethra, which "ejaculate" the semen from the urethra to the exterior. This final process is called *ejaculation.* At the same time, rhythmical contractions of the pelvic muscles and even of some of the muscles of the body trunk cause thrusting movements of the pelvis and penis, which also help propel the semen into the deepest recesses of the vagina and perhaps even slightly into the cervix of the uterus.

This entire period of emission and ejaculation is called the *male orgasm.* At its termination, the male sexual excitement disappears almost entirely within 1 to 2 minutes and erection ceases, a process called *resolution.*

Testosterone and Other Male Sex Hormones

Secretion, Metabolism, and Chemistry of the Male Sex Hormone

Secretion of Testosterone by the Interstitial Cells of Leydig in the Testes. The testes secrete several male sex hormones, which are collectively called *androgens,* including *testosterone, dihydrotestosterone,* and *androstenedione.* Testosterone is so much more abundant than the others that one can consider it to be the primary testicular hormone, although as we shall see, much, if not most, of the testosterone is eventually converted into the more active hormone dihydrotestosterone in the target tissues.

Testosterone is formed by the *interstitial cells of Leydig,* which lie in the interstices between the seminiferous tubules and constitute about 20 percent of the mass of the adult testes, as shown in Figure 80-7. Leydig cells

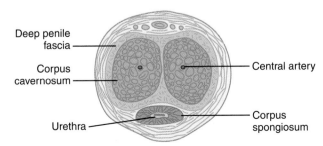

Deep penile fascia

Corpus cavernosum

Urethra

Central artery

Corpus spongiosum

Figure 80-6 Erectile tissue of the penis.

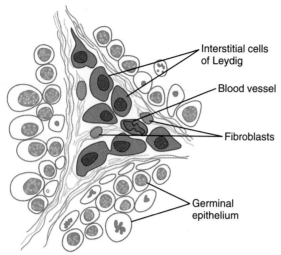

Figure 80-7 Interstitial cells of Leydig, the cells that secrete testosterone, located in the interstices between the seminiferous tubules.

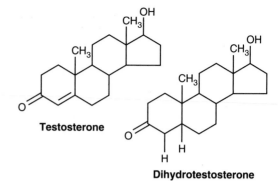

Figure 80-8 Testosterone and dihydrotestosterone.

are almost nonexistent in the testes during childhood when the testes secrete almost no testosterone, but they *are* numerous in the newborn male infant for the first few months of life and in the adult male after puberty; at both these times the testes secrete large quantities of testosterone. Furthermore, when tumors develop from the interstitial cells of Leydig, great quantities of testosterone are secreted. Finally, when the germinal epithelium of the testes is destroyed by x-ray treatment or excessive heat, the Leydig cells, which are less easily destroyed, often continue to produce testosterone.

Secretion of Androgens Elsewhere in the Body. The term "androgen" means any steroid hormone that has masculinizing effects, including testosterone; it also includes male sex hormones produced elsewhere in the body besides the testes. For instance, the adrenal glands secrete at least five androgens, although the total masculinizing activity of all these is normally so slight (<5 percent of the total in the adult male) that even in women they do not cause significant masculine characteristics, except for causing growth of pubic and axillary hair. But when an adrenal tumor of the adrenal androgen-producing cells occurs, the quantity of androgenic hormones may then become great enough to cause all the usual male secondary sexual characteristics to occur even in the female. These effects are described in connection with the adrenogenital syndrome in Chapter 77.

Rarely, embryonic rest cells in the ovary can develop into a tumor that produces excessive quantities of androgens in women; one such tumor is the *arrhenoblastoma*. The normal ovary also produces minute quantities of androgens, but they are not significant.

Chemistry of the Androgens. All androgens are steroid compounds, as shown by the formulas in Figure 80-8 for *testosterone* and *dihydrotestosterone*. Both in the testes and in the adrenals, the androgens can be synthesized either from cholesterol or directly from acetyl coenzyme A.

Metabolism of Testosterone. After secretion by the testes, about 97 percent of the testosterone becomes either loosely bound with plasma albumin or more tightly bound with a beta globulin called *sex hormone-binding globulin*

and circulates in the blood in these states for 30 minutes to several hours. By that time, the testosterone is either transferred to the tissues or degraded into inactive products that are subsequently excreted.

Much of the testosterone that becomes fixed to the tissues is converted within the tissue cells to *dihydrotestosterone*, especially in certain target organs such as the prostate gland in the adult and the external genitalia of the male fetus. Some actions of testosterone are dependent on this conversion, whereas other actions are not. The intracellular functions are discussed later in the chapter.

Degradation and Excretion of Testosterone. The testosterone that does not become fixed to the tissues is rapidly converted, mainly by the liver, into *androsterone* and *dehydroepiandrosterone* and simultaneously conjugated as either glucuronides or sulfates (glucuronides, particularly). These are excreted either into the gut by way of the liver bile or into the urine through the kidneys.

Production of Estrogen in the Male. In addition to testosterone, small amounts of estrogens are formed in the male (about one-fifth the amount in the nonpregnant female) and a reasonable quantity of estrogens can be recovered from a man's urine. The exact source of estrogens in the male is unclear, but the following are known: (1) the concentration of estrogens in the fluid of the seminiferous tubules is quite high and probably plays an important role in spermiogenesis. This estrogen is believed to be formed by the Sertoli cells by converting testosterone to estradiol. (2) Much larger amounts of estrogens are formed from testosterone and androstanediol in other tissues of the body, especially the liver, probably accounting for as much as 80 percent of the total male estrogen production.

Functions of Testosterone

In general, testosterone is responsible for the distinguishing characteristics of the masculine body. Even during fetal life, the testes are stimulated by chorionic gonadotropin from the placenta to produce moderate quantities of testosterone throughout the entire period of fetal development and for 10 or more weeks after birth; thereafter, essentially no testosterone is produced during childhood until about the ages of 10 to 13 years. Then testosterone production increases rapidly under the stimulus of anterior pituitary gonadotropic hormones at the onset of puberty and lasts throughout most of the remainder of life, as shown in Figure 80-9, dwindling rapidly beyond age 50 to become 20 to 50 percent of the peak value by age 80.

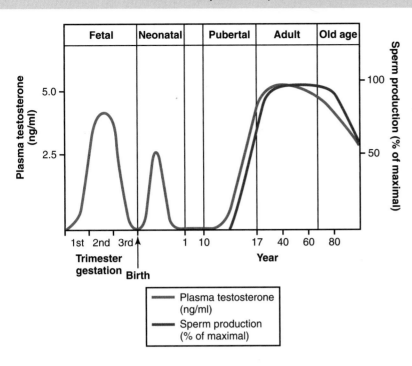

Figure 80-9 The different stages of male sexual function as reflected by average plasma testosterone concentrations (*red line*) and sperm production (*blue line*) at different ages. (Modified from Griffin JF, Wilson JD: The testis. In: Bondy PK, Rosenberg LE [eds]: Metabolic Control and Disease, 8th ed. Philadelphia: WB Saunders, 1980.)

Functions of Testosterone During Fetal Development

Testosterone begins to be elaborated by the male fetal testes at about the seventh week of embryonic life. Indeed, one of the major functional differences between the female and the male sex chromosome is that the male chromosome has the *SRY (sex-determining region Y) gene* that encodes a protein called the *testis determining factor* (also called the *SRY protein*). The SRY protein initiates a cascade of gene activations that cause the genital ridge cells to differentiate into cells that secrete testosterone and eventually become the testes, whereas the female chromosome causes this ridge to differentiate into cells that secrete estrogens.

Injection of large quantities of male sex hormone into pregnant animals causes development of male sexual organs even though the fetus is female. Also, removal of the testes in the early male fetus causes development of female sexual organs.

Thus, testosterone secreted first by the genital ridges and later by the fetal testes is responsible for the development of the male body characteristics, including the formation of a penis and a scrotum rather than formation of a clitoris and a vagina. Also, it causes formation of the prostate gland, seminal vesicles, and male genital ducts, while at the same time suppressing the formation of female genital organs.

Effect of Testosterone to Cause Descent of the Testes. The testes usually descend into the scrotum during the last 2 to 3 months of gestation when the testes begin secreting reasonable quantities of testosterone. If a male child is born with undescended but otherwise normal testes, administration of testosterone usually causes the testes to descend in the usual manner if the inguinal canals are large enough to allow the testes to pass.

Administration of gonadotropic hormones, which stimulate the Leydig cells of the newborn child's testes to produce testosterone, can also cause the testes to descend. Thus, the stimulus for descent of the testes is testosterone, indicating again that testosterone is an important hormone for male sexual development during fetal life.

Effect of Testosterone on Development of Adult Primary and Secondary Sexual Characteristics

After puberty, increasing amounts of testosterone secretion cause the penis, scrotum, and testes to enlarge about eightfold before the age of 20 years. In addition, testosterone causes the secondary sexual characteristics of the male to develop, beginning at puberty and ending at maturity. These secondary sexual characteristics, in addition to the sexual organs themselves, distinguish the male from the female as follows.

Effect on the Distribution of Body Hair. Testosterone causes growth of hair (1) over the pubis, (2) upward along the linea alba of the abdomen sometimes to the umbilicus and above, (3) on the face, (4) usually on the chest, and (5) less often on other regions of the body, such as the back. It also causes the hair on most other portions of the body to become more prolific.

Baldness. Testosterone decreases the growth of hair on the top of the head; a man who does not have functional testes does not become bald. However, many virile men never become bald because baldness is a result of two factors: first, a *genetic background* for the development of baldness and, second, superimposed on this genetic background, *large quantities of androgenic hormones*. A woman who has the appropriate genetic background and who develops a long-sustained androgenic tumor becomes bald in the same manner as does a man.

Effect on the Voice. Testosterone secreted by the testes or injected into the body causes hypertrophy of the laryngeal mucosa and enlargement of the larynx. The effects cause at first a relatively discordant, "cracking" voice, but this gradually changes into the typical adult masculine voice.

Testosterone Increases Thickness of the Skin and Can Contribute to Development of Acne. Testosterone increases the thickness of the skin over the entire body and increases the ruggedness of the subcutaneous tissues. Testosterone also increases the rate of secretion by some or perhaps all the body's sebaceous glands. Especially important is excessive secretion by the sebaceous glands of the face because this can result in *acne.* Therefore, acne is one of the most common features of male adolescence when the body is first becoming introduced to increased testosterone. After several years of testosterone secretion, the skin normally adapts to the testosterone in a way that allows it to overcome the acne.

Testosterone Increases Protein Formation and Muscle Development. One of the most important male characteristics is development of increasing musculature after puberty, averaging about a 50 percent increase in muscle mass over that in the female. This is associated with increased protein in the nonmuscle parts of the body as well. Many of the changes in the skin are due to deposition of proteins in the skin, and the changes in the voice also result partly from this protein anabolic function of testosterone.

Because of the great effect that testosterone and other androgens have on the body musculature, synthetic androgens are widely used by athletes to improve their muscular performance. This practice is to be severely deprecated because of prolonged harmful effects of excess androgens, as we discuss in Chapter 84 in relation to sports physiology. Testosterone or synthetic androgens are also occasionally used in old age as a "youth hormone" to improve muscle strength and vigor, but with questionable results.

Testosterone Increases Bone Matrix and Causes Calcium Retention. After the great increase in circulating testosterone that occurs at puberty (or after prolonged injection of testosterone), the bones grow considerably thicker and deposit considerable additional calcium salts. Thus, testosterone increases the total quantity of bone matrix and causes calcium retention. The increase in bone matrix is believed to result from the general protein anabolic function of testosterone plus deposition of calcium salts in response to the increased protein.

Testosterone has a specific effect on the pelvis to (1) narrow the pelvic outlet, (2) lengthen it, (3) cause a funnel-like shape instead of the broad ovoid shape of the female pelvis, and (4) greatly increase the strength of the entire pelvis for load-bearing. In the absence of testosterone, the male pelvis develops into a pelvis that is similar to that of the female.

Because of the ability of testosterone to increase the size and strength of bones, it is sometimes used in older men to treat osteoporosis.

When great quantities of testosterone (or any other androgen) are secreted abnormally in the still-growing child, the rate of bone growth increases markedly, causing a spurt in total body height. However, the testosterone also causes the epiphyses of the long bones to unite with the shafts of the bones at an early age. Therefore, despite the rapidity of growth, this early uniting of the epiphyses prevents the person from growing as tall as he would have grown had testosterone not been secreted at all. Even in normal men, the final adult height is slightly less than that which occurs in males castrated before puberty.

Testosterone Increases Basal Metabolic Rate. Injection of large quantities of testosterone can increase the basal metabolic rate by as much as 15 percent. Also, even the usual quantity of testosterone secreted by the testes during adolescence and early adult life increases the rate of metabolism some 5 to 10 percent above the value that it would be were the testes not active. This increased rate of metabolism is possibly an indirect result of the effect of testosterone on protein anabolism, the increased quantity of proteins—the enzymes especially—increasing the activities of all cells.

Testosterone Increases Red Blood Cells. When normal quantities of testosterone are injected into a castrated adult, the number of red blood cells per cubic millimeter of blood increases 15 to 20 percent. Also, the average man has about 700,000 more red blood cells per cubic millimeter than the average woman. Despite the strong association of testosterone and increased hematocrit, testosterone does not appear to directly increase erythropoietin levels or have a direct effect on red blood cell production. The effect of testosterone to increase red blood cell production may be at least partly indirect due to the increased metabolic rate that occurs after testosterone administration.

Effect on Electrolyte and Water Balance. As pointed out in Chapter 77, many steroid hormones can increase the reabsorption of sodium in the distal tubules of the kidneys. Testosterone also has such an effect, but only to a minor degree in comparison with the adrenal mineralocorticoids. Nevertheless, after puberty, the blood and extracellular fluid volumes of the male in relation to body weight increase as much as 5 to 10 percent.

Basic Intracellular Mechanism of Action of Testosterone

Most of the effects of testosterone result basically from increased rate of protein formation in the target cells. This has been studied extensively in the prostate gland, one of the organs that is most affected by testosterone. In this gland, testosterone enters the prostatic cells within a few minutes after secretion. Then it is most often converted, under the influence of the intracellular enzyme 5α-reductase, to *dihydrotestosterone,* and this in turn binds with a cytoplasmic "receptor protein." This combination migrates to the cell nucleus, where it binds with a nuclear protein and induces DNA-RNA transcription.

Within 30 minutes, RNA polymerase has become activated and the concentration of RNA begins to increase in the prostatic cells; this is followed by progressive increase in cellular protein. After several days, the quantity of DNA in the prostate gland has also increased and there has been a simultaneous increase in the number of prostatic cells.

Testosterone stimulates production of proteins virtually everywhere in the body, although more specifically affecting those proteins in "target" organs or tissues responsible for the development of both primary and secondary male sexual characteristics.

Recent studies suggest that testosterone, like other steroidal hormones, may also exert some rapid, *nongenomic effects* that do not require synthesis of new proteins. The physiological role of these nongenomic actions of testosterone, however, has yet to be determined.

Control of Male Sexual Functions by Hormones from the Hypothalamus and Anterior Pituitary Gland

A major share of the control of sexual functions in both the male and the female begins with secretion of *gonadotropin-releasing hormone* (GnRH) by the hypothalamus (Figure 80-10). This hormone in turn stimulates the anterior pituitary gland to secrete two other hormones called *gonadotropic hormones*: (1) *luteinizing hormone* (LH) and (2) *follicle-stimulating hormone* (FSH). In turn, LH is the primary stimulus for the secretion of testosterone by the testes, and FSH mainly stimulates spermatogenesis.

GnRH and Its Effect in Increasing the Secretion of LH and FSH

GnRH is a 10-amino acid peptide secreted by neurons whose cell bodies are located in the *arcuate nuclei of the hypothalamus*. The endings of these neurons terminate mainly in the median eminence of the hypothalamus, where they release GnRH into the hypothalamic-hypophysial portal vascular system. Then the GnRH is transported to the anterior pituitary gland in the hypophysial portal blood and stimulates the release of the two gonadotropins, LH and FSH.

GnRH is secreted intermittently a few minutes at a time once every 1 to 3 hours. The intensity of this hormone's stimulus is determined in two ways: (1) by the frequency of these cycles of secretion and (2) by the quantity of GnRH released with each cycle.

The secretion of LH by the anterior pituitary gland is also cyclical, with LH following fairly faithfully the pulsatile release of GnRH. Conversely, FSH secretion increases and decreases only slightly with each fluctuation of GnRH secretion; instead, it changes more slowly over a period of many hours in response to longer-term changes in GnRH. Because of the much closer relation between GnRH secretion and LH secretion, GnRH is also widely known as *LH-releasing hormone.*

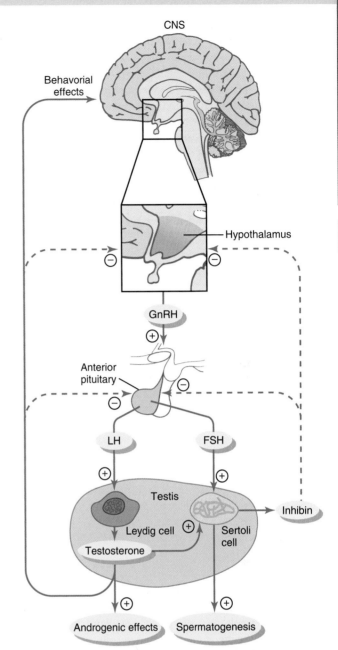

Figure 80-10 Feedback regulation of the hypothalamic-pituitary-testicular axis in males. Stimulatory effects are shown by ⊕ and negative feedback inhibitory effects are shown by ⊖. FSH, follicle-stimulating hormone; GnRH, gonadotropin-releasing hormone; LH, luteinizing hormone.

Gonadotropic Hormones: LH and FSH

Both of the gonadotropic hormones, LH and FSH, are secreted by the same cells, called *gonadotropes*, in the anterior pituitary gland. In the absence of GnRH secretion from the hypothalamus, the gonadotropes in the pituitary gland secrete almost no LH or FSH.

LH and FSH are *glycoproteins*. They exert their effects on their target tissues in the testes mainly by *activating the cyclic adenosine monophosphate second messenger system,* which in turn activates specific enzyme systems in the respective target cells.

Regulation of Testosterone Production by LH.

Testosterone is secreted by the *interstitial cells of Leydig* in the testes, but only when they are stimulated by LH from the anterior pituitary gland. Furthermore, the quantity of testosterone secreted increases approximately in direct proportion to the amount of LH available.

Mature Leydig cells are normally found in a child's testes for a few weeks after birth but then disappear until after the age of about 10 years. However, injection of purified LH into a child at any age or secretion of LH at puberty causes testicular interstitial cells that look like fibroblasts to evolve into functioning Leydig cells.

Inhibition of Anterior Pituitary Secretion of LH and FSH by Testosterone-Negative Feedback Control of Testosterone Secretion.

The testosterone secreted by the testes in response to LH has the reciprocal effect of inhibiting anterior pituitary secretion of LH (see Figure 80-10). Most of this inhibition probably results from a direct effect of testosterone on the hypothalamus to decrease the secretion of GnRH. This in turn causes a corresponding decrease in secretion of both LH and FSH by the anterior pituitary, and the decrease in LH reduces the secretion of testosterone by the testes. Thus, whenever secretion of testosterone becomes too great, this automatic negative feedback effect, operating through the hypothalamus and anterior pituitary gland, reduces the testosterone secretion back toward the desired operating level. Conversely, too little testosterone allows the hypothalamus to secrete large amounts of GnRH, with a corresponding increase in anterior pituitary LH and FSH secretion and consequent increase in testicular testosterone secretion.

Regulation of Spermatogenesis by FSH and Testosterone

FSH binds with specific FSH receptors attached to the Sertoli cells in the seminiferous tubules. This causes the Sertoli cells to grow and secrete various spermatogenic substances. Simultaneously, testosterone (and dihydrotestosterone) diffusing into the seminiferous tubules from the Leydig cells in the interstitial spaces also has a strong tropic effect on spermatogenesis. Thus, to initiate spermatogenesis, both FSH and testosterone are necessary.

Role of Inhibin in Negative Feedback Control of Seminiferous Tubule Activity.

When the seminiferous tubules fail to produce sperm, secretion of FSH by the anterior pituitary gland increases markedly. Conversely, when spermatogenesis proceeds too rapidly, pituitary secretion of FSH diminishes. The cause of this negative feedback effect on the anterior pituitary is believed to be secretion by the Sertoli cells of still another hormone called *inhibin* (see Figure 80-10). This hormone has a strong direct effect on the anterior pituitary gland to inhibit the secretion of FSH and possibly a slight effect on the hypothalamus to inhibit secretion of GnRH.

Inhibin is a glycoprotein, like both LH and FSH, having a molecular weight between 10,000 and 30,000. It has been isolated from cultured Sertoli cells. Its potent inhibitory feedback effect on the anterior pituitary gland

provides an important negative feedback mechanism for control of spermatogenesis, operating simultaneously with and in parallel to the negative feedback mechanism for control of testosterone secretion.

Human Chorionic Gonadotropin Secreted by the Placenta During Pregnancy Stimulates Testosterone Secretion by the Fetal Testes

During pregnancy the hormone *human chorionic gonadotropin* (hCG) is secreted by the placenta, and it circulates both in the mother and in the fetus. This hormone has almost the same effects on the sexual organs as LH.

During pregnancy, if the fetus is a male, hCG from the placenta causes the testes of the fetus to secrete testosterone. This testosterone is critical for promoting formation of the male sexual organs, as pointed out earlier. We discuss hCG and its functions during pregnancy in greater detail in Chapter 82.

Puberty and Regulation of Its Onset

Initiation of the onset of puberty has long been a mystery. But it has now been determined that *during childhood the hypothalamus simply does not secrete significant amounts of GnRH.* One of the reasons for this is that, during childhood, the slightest secretion of any sex steroid hormones exerts a strong inhibitory effect on hypothalamic secretion of GnRH. Yet for reasons still not understood, at the time of puberty, the secretion of hypothalamic GnRH breaks through the childhood inhibition and adult sexual life begins.

Male Adult Sexual Life and Male Climacteric. After puberty, gonadotropic hormones are produced by the male pituitary gland for the remainder of life, and at least some spermatogenesis usually continues until death. Most men, however, begin to exhibit slowly decreasing sexual functions in their late 50s or 60s, and one study showed that the average age for terminating intersexual relations was 68, although the variation was great. This decline in sexual function is related to decrease in testosterone secretion, as shown in Figure 80-9. The decrease in male sexual function is called the *male climacteric.* Occasionally the male climacteric is associated with symptoms of hot flashes, suffocation, and psychic disorders similar to the menopausal symptoms of the female. These symptoms can be abrogated by administration of testosterone, synthetic androgens, or even estrogens that are used for treatment of menopausal symptoms in the female.

Abnormalities of Male Sexual Function

Prostate Gland and Its Abnormalities

The prostate gland remains relatively small throughout childhood and begins to grow at puberty under the stimulus of testosterone. This gland reaches an almost stationary size by the age of 20 years and remains at this size up to the age of about 50 years. At that time, in some men it begins to involute, along with decreased production of testosterone by the testes.

A benign prostatic fibroadenoma frequently develops in the prostate in many older men and can cause urinary obstruction. This hypertrophy is caused not by testosterone but instead by abnormal overgrowth of prostate tissue itself.

Cancer of the prostate gland is a different problem and accounts for about 2 to 3 percent of all male deaths. Once cancer of the prostate gland does occur, the cancerous cells are usually stimulated to more rapid growth by testosterone and are inhibited by removal of both testes so that testosterone cannot be formed. Prostatic cancer usually can be inhibited by administration of estrogens. Even some patients who have prostatic cancer that has already metastasized to almost all the bones of the body can be successfully treated for a few months to years by removal of the testes, by estrogen therapy, or by both; after this therapy the metastases usually diminish in size and the bones partially heal. This treatment does not stop the cancer but does slow it and sometimes greatly diminishes the severe bone pain.

Hypogonadism in the Male

When the testes of a male fetus are nonfunctional during fetal life, none of the male sexual characteristics develop in the fetus. Instead, female organs are formed. The reason for this is that the basic genetic characteristic of the fetus, whether male or female, is to form female sexual organs if there are no sex hormones. But in the presence of testosterone, formation of female sexual organs is suppressed, and instead, male organs are induced.

When a boy loses his testes before puberty, a state of eunuchism ensues in which he continues to have infantile sex organs and other infantile sexual characteristics throughout life. The height of an adult eunuch is slightly greater than that of a normal man because the bone epiphyses are slow to unite, although the bones are quite thin and the muscles are considerably weaker than those of a normal man. The voice is childlike, there is no loss of hair on the head, and the normal adult masculine hair distribution on the face and elsewhere does not occur.

When a man is castrated after puberty, some of his male secondary sexual characteristics revert to those of a child and others remain of adult masculine character. The sexual organs regress slightly in size but not to a childlike state, and the voice regresses from the bass quality only slightly. However, there is loss of masculine hair production, loss of the thick masculine bones, and loss of the musculature of the virile male.

Also in a castrated adult male, sexual desires are decreased but not lost, provided sexual activities have been practiced previously. Erection can still occur as before, although with less ease, but it is rare that ejaculation can take place, primarily because the semen-forming organs degenerate and there has been a loss of the testosterone-driven psychic desire.

Some instances of hypogonadism are caused by a genetic inability of the hypothalamus to secrete normal amounts of GnRH. This is often associated with a simultaneous abnormality of the feeding center of the hypothalamus, causing the person to greatly overeat. Consequently, obesity occurs along with eunuchism. A patient with this condition is shown in Figure 80-11; the condition is called *adiposogenital syndrome, Fröhlich syndrome,* or *hypothalamic eunuchism.*

Testicular Tumors and Hypergonadism in the Male

Interstitial Leydig cell tumors develop in rare instances in the testes, but when they do develop, they sometimes produce as much as 100 times the normal quantities of testosterone. When such tumors develop in young children, they cause

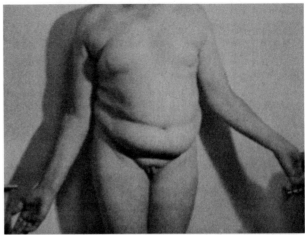
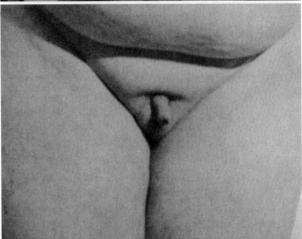

Figure 80-11 Adiposogenital syndrome in an adolescent male. Note the obesity and childlike sexual organs. (Courtesy Dr. Leonard Posey.)

rapid growth of the musculature and bones but also cause early uniting of the epiphyses, so that the eventual adult height is actually considerably less than that which would have been achieved otherwise. Such interstitial cell tumors also cause excessive development of the male sexual organs, all skeletal muscles, and other male sexual characteristics. In the adult male, small interstitial cell tumors are difficult to diagnose because masculine features are already present.

Much more common than the interstitial Leydig cell tumors are tumors of the germinal epithelium. Because germinal cells are capable of differentiating into almost any type of cell, many of these tumors contain multiple tissues, such as placental tissue, hair, teeth, bone, skin, and so forth, all found together in the same tumorous mass called a *teratoma*. These tumors often secrete few hormones, but if a significant quantity of placental tissue develops in the tumor, it may secrete large quantities of hCG with functions similar to those of LH. Also, estrogenic hormones are sometimes secreted by these tumors and cause the condition called *gynecomastia* (overgrowth of the breasts).

Erectile Dysfunction in the Male

Erectile dysfunction, also called "impotence," is characterized by an inability of the man to develop or maintain an *erection* of sufficient rigidity for satisfactory sexual intercourse.

Neurological problems, such as trauma to the parasympathetic nerves from prostate surgery, deficient levels of testosterone, and some *drugs (nicotine, alcohol, antidepressants)* can also contribute to erectile dysfunction.

In men older than age 40, erectile dysfunction is most often caused by underlying vascular disease. As discussed previously, adequate blood flow and nitric oxide formation are essential for penile erection. Vascular disease, which can occur as a result of uncontrolled *hypertension, diabetes,* and *atherosclerosis,* reduces the ability of the body's blood vessels, including those in the penis, to dilate. Part of this impaired vasodilation is due to decreased release of nitric oxide.

Erectile dysfunction caused by vascular disease can often be successfully treated with *phosphodiesterase-5 (PDE-5) inhibitors* such as sildenafil (Viagra), vardenafil (Levitra) or tadalafil (Cialis). These drugs increase cyclic GMP levels in the erectile tissue by inhibiting the enzyme *phosphodiesterase-5,* which rapidly degrades cyclic GMP. Thus, by inhibiting the degradation of cyclic GMP, the PDE-5 inhibitors enhance and prolong the effect of cyclic GMP to cause erection.

Pineal Gland—Its Function in Controlling Seasonal Fertility in Some Animals

For as long as the pineal gland has been known to exist, myriad functions have been ascribed to it, including its (1) enhancing sex, (2) staving off infection, (3) promoting sleep, (4) enhancing mood, and (5) increasing longevity (as much as 10 to 25 percent). It is known from comparative anatomy that the pineal gland is a vestigial remnant of what was a third eye located high in the back of the head in some lower animals. Many physiologists have been content with the idea that this gland is a nonfunctional remnant, but others have claimed for many years that it plays important roles in the control of sexual activities and reproduction.

But now, after years of research, it appears that the pineal gland does indeed play a regulatory role in sexual and reproductive function. In lower animals that bear their young at certain seasons of the year and in which the pineal gland has been removed or the nervous circuits to the pineal gland have been sectioned, the normal periods of seasonal fertility are lost. To these animals, such seasonal fertility is important because it allows birth of the offspring at the time of year, usually springtime or early summer, when survival is most likely. The mechanism of this effect is not entirely clear, but it seems to be the following.

First, the pineal gland is controlled by the amount of light or "time pattern" of light seen by the eyes each day. For instance, in the hamster, greater than 13 hours of *darkness* each day activates the pineal gland, whereas less than that amount of darkness fails to activate it, with a critical balance between activation and nonactivation. The nervous pathway involves the passage of light signals from the eyes to the suprachiasmal nucleus of the hypothalamus and then to the pineal gland, activating pineal secretion.

Second, the pineal gland secretes *melatonin* and several other, similar substances. Either melatonin or one of the other substances is believed to pass either by way of the blood or through the fluid of the third ventricle to the anterior pituitary gland to *decrease* gonadotropic hormone secretion.

Thus, in the presence of pineal gland secretion, gonadotropic hormone secretion is suppressed in some species of animals, and the gonads become inhibited and even partly involuted. This is what presumably occurs during the early winter months when there is increasing darkness. But after about 4 months of dysfunction, gonadotropic hormone secretion breaks through the inhibitory effect of the pineal gland and the gonads become functional once more, ready for a full springtime of activity.

But does the pineal gland have a similar function for control of reproduction in humans? The answer to this question is unknown. However, tumors often occur in the region of the pineal gland. Some of these secrete excessive quantities of pineal hormones, whereas others are tumors of surrounding tissue and press on the pineal gland to destroy it. Both types of tumors are often associated with hypogonadal or hypergonadal function. So perhaps the pineal gland does play at least some role in controlling sexual drive and reproduction in humans.

Bibliography

Brennan J, Capel B: One tissue, two fates: molecular genetic events that underlie testis versus ovary development, *Nat Rev Genet* 5:509, 2004.

Compston JE: Sex steroids and bone, *Physiol Rev* 81:419, 2001.

Foradori CD, Weiser MJ, Handa RJ: Non-genomic actions of androgens, *Front Neuroendocrinol* 29:169, 2008.

Foresta C, Zuccarello D, Garolla A, et al: Role of hormones, genes, and environment in human cryptorchidism, *Endocr Rev* 29:560, 2008.

Kocer A, Reichmann J, Best D, et al: Germ cell sex determination in mammals, *Mol Hum Reprod* 15:205, 2009.

Lahn BT, Pearson NM, Jegalian K: The human Y chromosome, in the light of evolution, *Nat Rev Genet* 2:207, 2001.

Lanfranco F, Kamischke A, Zitzmann M, et al: Klinefelter's syndrome, *Lancet* 364:273, 2004.

Matzuk M, Lamb D: The biology of infertility: research advances and clinical challenges, *Nat Med* 14:1197, 2008.

McVary KT: Clinical practice. Erectile dysfunction, *N Engl J Med* 357:2472, 2007.

Michels G, Hoppe UC: Rapid actions of androgens, *Front Neuroendocrinol* 29:182, 2008.

Nelson WG, De Marzo AM, Isaacs WB: Prostate cancer, *N Engl J Med* 349:366, 2003.

Park SY, Jameson JL: Transcriptional regulation of gonadal development and differentiation, *Endocrinology* 146:1035, 2005.

Plant TM, Marshall GR: The functional significance of FSH in spermatogenesis and the control of its secretion in male primates, *Endocr Rev* 22:764, 2001.

Reckelhoff JF, Yanes LL, Iliescu R, et al: Testosterone supplementation in aging men and women: possible impact on cardiovascular-renal disease, *Am J Physiol Renal Physiol* 289:F941, 2005.

Rhoden EL, Morgentaler A: Risks of testosterone-replacement therapy and recommendations for monitoring, *N Engl J Med* 350:482, 2004.

Simonneaux V, Ribelayga C: Generation of the melatonin endocrine message in mammals: a review of the complex regulation of melatonin synthesis by norepinephrine, peptides, and other pineal transmitters, *Pharmacol Rev* 55:325, 2003.

Walker WH: Molecular mechanisms of testosterone action in spermatogenesis, *Steroids* 74:602, 2009.

Wang RS, Yeh S, Tzeng CR, et al: Androgen receptor roles in spermatogenesis and fertility: lessons from testicular cell-specific androgen receptor knockout mice, *Endocr Rev* 30:119, 2009.

Wilhelm D, Palmer S, Koopman P: Sex determination and gonadal development in mammals, *Physiol Rev* 87:1, 2007.

Yan W: Male infertility caused by spermiogenic defects: lessons from gene knockouts, *Mol Cell Endocrinol* 306:24, 2009.

Female Physiology Before Pregnancy and Female Hormones

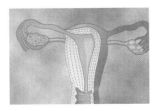

Female reproductive functions can be divided into two major phases: (1) preparation of the female body for conception and pregnancy and (2) the period of pregnancy itself. This chapter is concerned with preparation of the female body for pregnancy, and Chapter 82 presents the physiology of pregnancy and childbirth.

Physiologic Anatomy of the Female Sexual Organs

Figures 81-1 and 81-2 show the principal organs of the human female reproductive tract, including the *ovaries*, *fallopian tubes* (also called *uterine tubes*), *uterus*, and *vagina*. Reproduction begins with the development of ova in the ovaries. In the middle of each monthly sexual cycle, a single ovum is expelled from an ovarian follicle into the abdominal cavity near the open fimbriated ends of the two fallopian tubes. This ovum then passes through one of the fallopian tubes into the uterus; if it has been fertilized by a sperm, it implants in the uterus, where it develops into a fetus, a placenta, and fetal membranes—and eventually into a baby.

During fetal life, the outer surface of the ovary is covered by a *germinal epithelium*, which embryologically is derived from the epithelium of the germinal ridges. As the female fetus develops, *primordial ova* differentiate from this germinal epithelium and migrate into the substance of the ovarian cortex. Each ovum then collects around it a layer of spindle cells from the ovarian *stroma* (the supporting tissue of the ovary) and causes them to take on epithelioid characteristics; they are then called *granulosa cells*. The ovum surrounded by a single layer of granulosa cells is called a *primordial follicle*. The ovum at this stage is still immature, requiring two more cell divisions before it can be fertilized by a sperm. At this time, the ovum is called a *primary oocyte*.

During all the reproductive years of adult life, between about 13 and 46 years of age, 400 to 500 of the primordial follicles develop enough to expel their ova—one each month; the remainder degenerate (become *atretic*). At the end of reproductive capability (at *menopause*), only a few primordial follicles remain in the ovaries and even these degenerate soon thereafter.

Female Hormonal System

The female hormonal system, like that of the male, consists of three hierarchies of hormones, as follows:

1. A hypothalamic releasing hormone, *gonadotropin-releasing hormone* (GnRH)

2. The anterior pituitary sex hormones, *follicle-stimulating hormone* (FSH) and *luteinizing hormone* (LH), both of which are secreted in response to the release of GnRH from the hypothalamus

3. The ovarian hormones, *estrogen* and *progesterone*, which are secreted by the ovaries in response to the two female sex hormones from the anterior pituitary gland

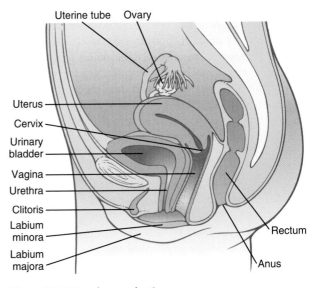

Figure 81-1 Female reproductive organs.

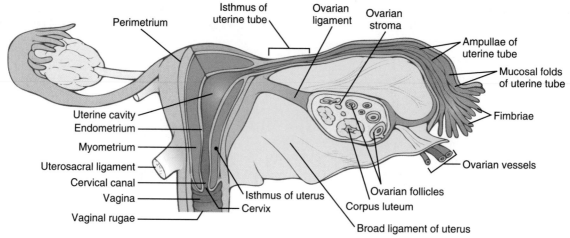

Figure 81-2 Internal structures of the uterus, ovary, and a uterine tube. (Redrawn from Guyton AC: Physiology of the Human Body, 6th ed. Philadelphia: Saunders College Publishing, 1984.)

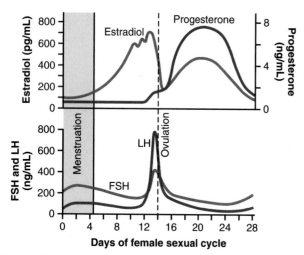

Figure 81-3 Approximate plasma concentrations of the gonadotropins and ovarian hormones during the normal female sexual cycle. FSH, follicle-stimulating hormone; LH, luteinizing hormone.

These various hormones are secreted at drastically differing rates during different parts of the female monthly sexual cycle. Figure 81-3 shows the approximate changing concentrations of the anterior pituitary gonadotropic hormones FSH and LH (bottom two curves) and of the ovarian hormones estradiol (estrogen) and progesterone (top two curves).

The amount of GnRH released from the hypothalamus increases and decreases much less drastically during the monthly sexual cycle. It is secreted in short pulses averaging once every 90 minutes, as occurs in the male.

Monthly Ovarian Cycle; Function of the Gonadotropic Hormones

The normal reproductive years of the female are characterized by monthly rhythmical changes in the rates of secretion of the female hormones and corresponding physical changes in the ovaries and other sexual organs. This rhythmical pattern is called the *female monthly*

sexual cycle (or, less accurately, the *menstrual cycle*). The duration of the cycle averages 28 days. It may be as short as 20 days or as long as 45 days in some women, although abnormal cycle length is frequently associated with decreased fertility.

There are two significant results of the female sexual cycle. First, only a *single* ovum is normally released from the ovaries each month, so normally only a single fetus will begin to grow at a time. Second, the uterine endometrium is prepared in advance for implantation of the fertilized ovum at the required time of the month.

Gonadotropic Hormones and Their Effects on the Ovaries

The ovarian changes that occur during the sexual cycle depend completely on the gonadotropic hormones *FSH* and *LH*, secreted by the anterior pituitary gland. In the absence of these hormones, the ovaries remain inactive, which is the case throughout childhood, when almost no pituitary gonadotropic hormones are secreted. At age 9 to 12 years, the pituitary begins to secrete progressively more FSH and LH, which leads to onset of normal monthly sexual cycles beginning between the ages of 11 and 15 years. This period of change is called *puberty*, and the time of the first menstrual cycle is called *menarche*. Both FSH and LH are small glycoproteins having molecular weights of about 30,000.

During each month of the female sexual cycle, there is a cyclical increase and decrease of both FSH and LH, as shown in the bottom of Figure 81-3. These cyclical variations cause cyclical ovarian changes, which are explained in the following sections.

Both FSH and LH stimulate their ovarian target cells by combining with highly specific FSH and LH receptors in the ovarian target cell membranes. In turn, the activated receptors increase the cells' rates of secretion and usually the growth and proliferation of the cells as well. Almost all these stimulatory effects result from *activation of the cyclic adenosine monophosphate second messenger*

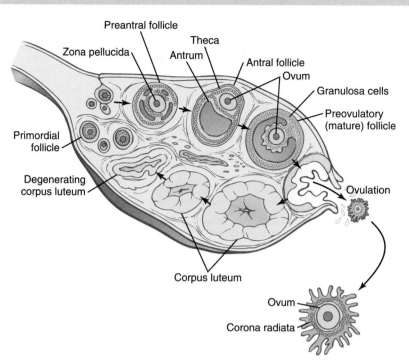

Figure 81-4 Stages of follicular growth in the ovary, also showing formation of the corpus luteum.

system in the cell cytoplasm, which causes the formation of *protein kinase* and multiple *phosphorylations of key enzymes* that stimulate sex hormone synthesis, as explained in Chapter 74.

Ovarian Follicle Growth—"Follicular" Phase of the Ovarian Cycle

Figure 81-4 shows the progressive stages of follicular growth in the ovaries. When a female child is born, each ovum is surrounded by a single layer of granulosa cells; the ovum, with this granulosa cell sheath, is called a *primordial follicle*, as shown in the figure. Throughout childhood, the granulosa cells are believed to provide nourishment for the ovum and to secrete an *oocyte maturation-inhibiting factor* that keeps the ovum suspended in its primordial state in the prophase stage of meiotic division. Then, after puberty, when FSH and LH from the anterior pituitary gland begin to be secreted in significant quantities, the ovaries, together with some of the follicles within them, begin to grow.

The first stage of follicular growth is moderate enlargement of the ovum itself, which increases in diameter twofold to threefold. Then follows growth of additional layers of granulosa cells in some of the follicles; these follicles are known as *primary follicles.*

Development of Antral and Vesicular Follicles.
During the first few days of each monthly female sexual cycle, the concentrations of both FSH and LH secreted by the anterior pituitary gland increase slightly to moderately, with the increase in FSH slightly greater than that of LH and preceding it by a few days. These hormones, especially FSH, cause accelerated growth of 6 to 12 primary follicles each month. The initial effect is rapid proliferation of the granulosa cells, giving rise to many more layers of these cells. In addition, spindle cells derived from the ovary interstitium collect in several layers outside the granulosa cells, giving rise to a second mass of cells called the *theca.* This is divided into two layers. In the *theca interna,* the cells take on epithelioid characteristics similar to those of the granulosa cells and develop the ability to secrete additional steroid sex hormones (estrogen and progesterone). The outer layer, the *theca externa,* develops into a highly vascular connective tissue capsule that becomes the capsule of the developing follicle.

After the early proliferative phase of growth, lasting for a few days, the mass of granulosa cells secretes a *follicular fluid* that contains a high concentration of estrogen, one of the important female sex hormones (discussed later). Accumulation of this fluid causes an *antrum* to appear within the mass of granulosa cells, as shown in Figure 81-4.

The early growth of the primary follicle up to the antral stage is stimulated mainly by FSH alone. Then greatly accelerated growth occurs, leading to still larger follicles called *vesicular follicles.* This accelerated growth is caused by the following: (1) Estrogen is secreted into the follicle and causes the granulosa cells to form increasing numbers of FSH receptors; this causes a positive feedback effect because it makes the granulosa cells even more sensitive to FSH. (2) The pituitary FSH and the estrogens combine to promote LH receptors on the original granulosa cells, thus allowing LH stimulation to occur in addition to FSH stimulation and creating an even more rapid increase in follicular secretion. (3) The increasing estrogens from the follicle plus the increasing LH from the anterior pituitary gland act together to cause proliferation of the follicular thecal cells and increase their secretion as well.

Once the antral follicles begin to grow, their growth occurs almost explosively. The ovum itself also enlarges in diameter another threefold to fourfold, giving a total ovum diameter increase up to 10-fold, or a mass increase of 1000-fold. As the follicle enlarges, the ovum remains embedded in a mass of granulosa cells located at one pole of the follicle.

Only One Follicle Fully Matures Each Month, and the Remainder Undergo Atresia.

After a week or more of growth—but before ovulation occurs—one of the follicles begins to outgrow all the others; the remaining 5 to 11 developing follicles involute (a process called *atresia*), and these follicles are said to become *atretic*.

The cause of the atresia is unknown, but it has been postulated to be the following: The large amounts of estrogen from the most rapidly growing follicle act on the hypothalamus to depress further enhancement of FSH secretion by the anterior pituitary gland, in this way blocking further growth of the less well developed follicles. Therefore, the largest follicle continues to grow because of its intrinsic positive feedback effects, while all the other follicles stop growing and actually involute.

This process of atresia is important because it normally allows only one of the follicles to grow large enough each month to ovulate; this usually prevents more than one child from developing with each pregnancy. The single follicle reaches a diameter of 1 to 1.5 centimeters at the time of ovulation and is called the *mature follicle*.

Ovulation

Ovulation in a woman who has a normal 28-day female sexual cycle occurs 14 days after the onset of menstruation. Shortly before ovulation the protruding outer wall of the follicle swells rapidly, and a small area in the center of the follicular capsule, called the *stigma*, protrudes like a nipple. In another 30 minutes or so, fluid begins to ooze from the follicle through the stigma, and about 2 minutes later, the stigma ruptures widely, allowing a more viscous fluid, which has occupied the central portion of the follicle, to evaginate outward. This viscous fluid carries with it the ovum surrounded by a mass of several thousand small granulosa cells, called the *corona radiata*.

Surge of LH Is Necessary for Ovulation. LH is necessary for final follicular growth and ovulation. Without this hormone, even when large quantities of FSH are available, the follicle will not progress to the stage of ovulation.

About 2 days before ovulation (for reasons that are not completely understood but are discussed in more detail later in the chapter), the rate of secretion of LH by the anterior pituitary gland increases markedly, rising 6- to 10-fold and peaking about 16 hours before ovulation. FSH also increases about twofold to threefold at the same time, and the FSH and LH act synergistically to cause rapid swelling of the follicle during the last few days before ovulation. The LH also has a specific effect on the granulosa and theca cells, converting them mainly to progesterone-secreting cells. Therefore, the rate of secretion of estrogen begins to fall about 1 day before ovulation, while increasing amounts of progesterone begin to be secreted.

It is in this environment of (1) rapid growth of the follicle, (2) diminishing estrogen secretion after a prolonged phase of excessive estrogen secretion, and (3) initiation of secretion of progesterone that ovulation occurs. Without the initial preovulatory surge of LH, ovulation will not take place.

Initiation of Ovulation. Figure 81-5 gives a schema for the initiation of ovulation, showing the role of the large quantity of LH secreted by the anterior pituitary gland. This LH causes rapid secretion of follicular steroid hormones that contain progesterone. Within a few hours, two events occur, both of which are necessary for ovulation: (1) The *theca externa* (the capsule of the follicle) begins to release proteolytic enzymes from lysosomes, and these cause dissolution of the follicular capsular wall and consequent weakening of the wall, resulting in further swelling of the entire follicle and degeneration of the stigma. (2) Simultaneously there is rapid growth of new blood vessels into the follicle wall, and at the same time, prostaglandins (local hormones that cause vasodilation) are secreted into the follicular tissues. These two effects cause plasma transudation into the follicle, which contributes to follicle swelling. Finally, the combination of follicle swelling and simultaneous degeneration of the stigma causes follicle rupture, with discharge of the ovum.

Corpus Luteum—"Luteal" Phase of the Ovarian Cycle

During the first few hours after expulsion of the ovum from the follicle, the remaining granulosa and theca interna cells change rapidly into *lutein cells.* They enlarge in diameter two or more times and become filled with lipid inclusions that give them a yellowish appearance.

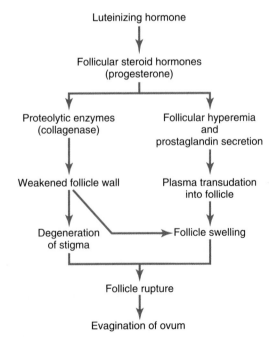

Figure 81-5 Postulated mechanism of ovulation.

This process is called *luteinization,* and the total mass of cells together is called the *corpus luteum,* which is shown in Figure 81-4. A well-developed vascular supply also grows into the corpus luteum.

The *granulosa cells* in the corpus luteum develop extensive intracellular smooth endoplasmic reticula that form large amounts of the female sex hormones *progesterone* and *estrogen* (more progesterone than estrogen during the luteal phase). The *theca cells* form mainly the androgens *androstenedione* and *testosterone* rather than female sex hormones. However, most of these hormones are also converted by the enzyme *aromatase* in the granulosa cells into estrogens, the female hormones.

The corpus luteum normally grows to about 1.5 centimeters in diameter, reaching this stage of development 7 to 8 days after ovulation. Then it begins to involute and eventually loses its secretory function and its yellowish, lipid characteristic about 12 days after ovulation, becoming the *corpus albicans;* during the ensuing few weeks, this is replaced by connective tissue and over months is absorbed.

Luteinizing Function of LH.
The change of granulosa and theca interna cells into lutein cells is dependent mainly on LH secreted by the anterior pituitary gland. In fact, this function gives LH its name—"luteinizing," for "yellowing." Luteinization also depends on extrusion of the ovum from the follicle. A yet uncharacterized local hormone in the follicular fluid, called *luteinization-inhibiting factor,* seems to hold the luteinization process in check until after ovulation.

Secretion by the Corpus Luteum: An Additional Function of LH.
The corpus luteum is a highly secretory organ, secreting large amounts of both *progesterone* and *estrogen.* Once LH (mainly that secreted during the ovulatory surge) has acted on the granulosa and theca cells to cause luteinization, the newly formed lutein cells seem to be programmed to go through a preordained sequence of (1) proliferation, (2) enlargement, and (3) secretion, followed by (4) degeneration. All this occurs in about 12 days. We shall see in the discussion of pregnancy in Chapter 82 that another hormone with almost exactly the same properties as LH, *chorionic gonadotropin,* which is secreted by the placenta, can act on the corpus luteum to prolong its life—usually maintaining it for at least the first 2 to 4 months of pregnancy.

Involution of the Corpus Luteum and Onset of the Next Ovarian Cycle.
Estrogen in particular and progesterone to a lesser extent, secreted by the corpus luteum during the luteal phase of the ovarian cycle, have strong feedback effects on the anterior pituitary gland to maintain low secretory rates of both FSH and LH.

In addition, the lutein cells secrete small amounts of the hormone *inhibin,* the same as the inhibin secreted by the Sertoli cells of the male testes. This hormone inhibits secretion by the anterior pituitary gland, especially FSH secretion. Low blood concentrations of both FSH and LH result, and loss of these hormones finally causes the corpus luteum to degenerate completely, a process called *involution* of the corpus luteum.

Final involution normally occurs at the end of almost exactly 12 days of corpus luteum life, which is around the 26th day of the normal female sexual cycle, 2 days before menstruation begins. At this time, the sudden cessation of secretion of estrogen, progesterone, and inhibin by the corpus luteum removes the feedback inhibition of the anterior pituitary gland, allowing it to begin secreting increasing amounts of FSH and LH again. FSH and LH initiate the growth of new follicles, beginning a new ovarian cycle. The paucity of secretion of progesterone and estrogen at this time also leads to menstruation by the uterus, as explained later.

Summary

About every 28 days, gonadotropic hormones from the anterior pituitary gland cause about 8 to 12 new follicles to begin to grow in the ovaries. One of these follicles finally becomes "mature" and ovulates on the 14th day of the cycle. During growth of the follicles, mainly estrogen is secreted.

After ovulation, the secretory cells of the ovulating follicle develop into a corpus luteum that secretes large quantities of both the major female hormones, progesterone and estrogen. After another 2 weeks, the corpus luteum degenerates, whereupon the ovarian hormones estrogen and progesterone decrease greatly and menstruation begins. A new ovarian cycle then follows.

Functions of the Ovarian Hormones— Estradiol and Progesterone

The two types of ovarian sex hormones are the *estrogens* and the *progestins.* By far the most important of the estrogens is the hormone *estradiol,* and by far the most important progestin is *progesterone.* The estrogens mainly promote proliferation and growth of specific cells in the body that are responsible for the development of most secondary sexual characteristics of the female. The progestins function mainly to prepare the uterus for pregnancy and the breasts for lactation.

Chemistry of the Sex Hormones

Estrogens.
In the normal *nonpregnant* female, estrogens are secreted in significant quantities only by the ovaries, although minute amounts are also secreted by the adrenal cortices. During *pregnancy,* tremendous quantities of estrogens are also secreted by the placenta, as discussed in Chapter 82.

Only three estrogens are present in significant quantities in the plasma of the human female: β-estradiol, estrone, and *estriol,* the formulas for which are shown in Figure 81-6. The principal estrogen secreted by the ovaries is β-estradiol. Small amounts of estrone are also secreted,

Figure 81-6 Synthesis of the principal female hormones. The chemical structures of the precursor hormones, including progesterone, are shown in Figure 77-2.

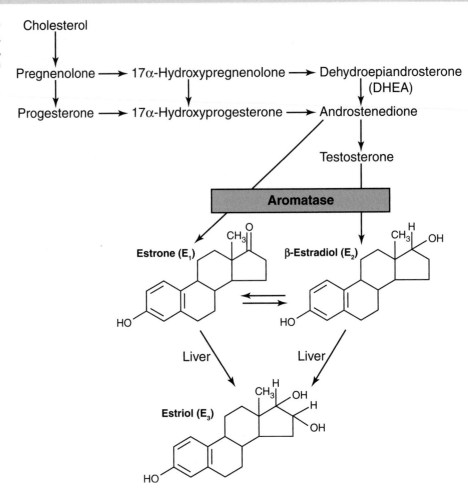

Synthesis of the Estrogens and Progestins. Note from the chemical formulas of the estrogens and progesterone in Figure 81-6 that they are all steroids. They are synthesized in the ovaries mainly from cholesterol derived from the blood but also to a slight extent from acetyl coenzyme A, multiple molecules of which can combine to form the appropriate steroid nucleus.

During synthesis, mainly progesterone and androgens (testosterone and androstenedione) are synthesized first; then, during the follicular phase of the ovarian cycle, before these two initial hormones can leave the ovaries, almost all the androgens and much of the progesterone are converted into estrogens by the enzyme aromatase in the granulosa cells. Because the theca cells lack the aromatase, they cannot convert androgens to estrogens. However, androgens diffuse out of the theca cells into the adjacent granulosa cells, where they are converted to estrogens by aromatase, the activity of which is stimulated by FSH (Figure 81-7).

During the luteal phase of the cycle, far too much progesterone is formed for all of it to be converted, which accounts for the large secretion of progesterone into the circulating blood at this time. Also, about one-fifteenth as much testosterone is secreted into the plasma of the female by the ovaries as is secreted into the plasma of the male by the testes.

but most of this is formed in the peripheral tissues from androgens secreted by the adrenal cortices and by ovarian thecal cells. Estriol is a weak estrogen; it is an oxidative product derived from both estradiol and estrone, with the conversion occurring mainly in the liver.

The estrogenic potency of β-estradiol is 12 times that of estrone and 80 times that of estriol. Considering these relative potencies, one can see that the total estrogenic effect of β-estradiol is usually many times that of the other two together. For this reason, β-estradiol is considered the major estrogen, although the estrogenic effects of estrone are not negligible.

Progestins. By far the most important of the progestins is progesterone. However, small amounts of another progestin, 17-α-hydroxyprogesterone, are secreted along with progesterone and have essentially the same effects. Yet for practical purposes, it is usually reasonable to consider progesterone the only important progestin.

In the normal nonpregnant female, progesterone is secreted in significant amounts only during the latter half of each ovarian cycle, when it is secreted by the corpus luteum.

As we shall see in Chapter 82, large amounts of progesterone are also secreted by the placenta during pregnancy, especially after the fourth month of gestation.

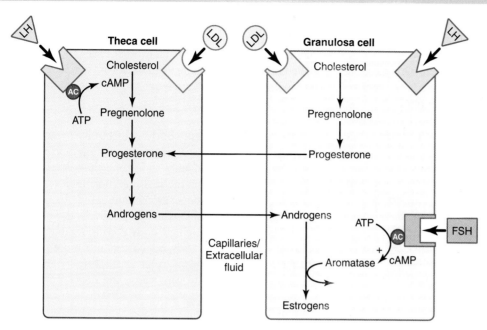

Figure 81-7 Interaction of follicular theca and granulosa cells for production of estrogens. The theca cells, under the control of luteinizing hormone (LH), produce androgens that diffuse into the granulosa cells. In mature follicles, follicle stimulating hormone (FSH) acts on granulosa cells to stimulate aromatase activity, which converts the androgens to estrogens. AC, adenylate cyclase; ATP, adenosine triphosphate; cAMP, cyclic adenosine monophosphate; LDL, low-density lipoproteins.

Estrogens and Progesterone Are Transported in the Blood Bound to Plasma Proteins. Both estrogens and progesterone are transported in the blood bound mainly with plasma albumin and with specific estrogen- and progesterone-binding globulins. The binding between these hormones and the plasma proteins is loose enough that they are rapidly released to the tissues over a period of 30 minutes or so.

Functions of the Liver in Estrogen Degradation. The liver conjugates the estrogens to form glucuronides and sulfates, and about one fifth of these conjugated products is excreted in the bile; most of the remainder is excreted in the urine. Also, the liver converts the potent estrogens estradiol and estrone into the almost totally impotent estrogen estriol. Therefore, diminished liver function actually *increases* the activity of estrogens in the body, sometimes causing *hyperestrinism*.

Fate of Progesterone. Within a few minutes after secretion, almost all the progesterone is degraded to other steroids that have no progestational effect. As with the estrogens, the liver is especially important for this metabolic degradation.

The major end product of progesterone degradation is *pregnanediol.* About 10 percent of the original progesterone is excreted in the urine in this form. Therefore, one can estimate the rate of progesterone formation in the body from the rate of this excretion.

Functions of the Estrogens—Their Effects on the Primary and Secondary Female Sex Characteristics

A primary function of the estrogens is to cause cellular proliferation and growth of the tissues of the sex organs and other tissues related to reproduction.

Effect of Estrogens on the Uterus and External Female Sex Organs. During childhood, estrogens are secreted only in minute quantities, but at puberty, the quantity secreted in the female under the influence of the pituitary gonadotropic hormones increases 20-fold or more. At this time, the female sex organs change from those of a child to those of an adult. The ovaries, fallopian tubes, uterus, and vagina all increase several times in size. Also, the external genitalia enlarge, with deposition of fat in the mons pubis and labia majora and enlargement of the labia minora.

In addition, estrogens change the vaginal epithelium from a cuboidal into a stratified type, which is considerably more resistant to trauma and infection than is the prepubertal cuboidal cell epithelium. Vaginal infections in children can often be cured by the administration of estrogens simply because of the resulting increased resistance of the vaginal epithelium.

During the first few years after puberty, the size of the uterus increases twofold to threefold, but more important than the increase in uterus size are the changes that take place in the uterine endometrium under the influence of estrogens. Estrogens cause marked proliferation of the endometrial stroma and greatly increased development of the endometrial glands, which will later aid in providing nutrition to the implanted ovum. These effects are discussed later in the chapter in connection with the endometrial cycle.

Effect of Estrogens on the Fallopian Tubes. The estrogens' effect on the mucosal lining of the fallopian tubes is similar to that on the uterine endometrium. They cause the glandular tissues of this lining to proliferate; especially important, they cause the number of ciliated epithelial cells that line the fallopian tubes to increase. Also, activity of the cilia is considerably enhanced. These cilia always beat toward the uterus, which helps propel the fertilized ovum in that direction.

Effect of Estrogens on the Breasts. The primordial breasts of females and males are exactly alike. In fact, under the influence of appropriate hormones, the masculine breast during the first 2 decades of life can develop sufficiently to produce milk in the same manner as the female breast.

Estrogens cause (1) development of the stromal tissues of the breasts, (2) growth of an extensive ductile system, and (3) deposition of fat in the breasts. The lobules and alveoli of the breast develop to a slight extent under the influence of estrogens alone, but it is progesterone and prolactin that cause the ultimate determinative growth and function of these structures.

In summary, the estrogens initiate growth of the breasts and of the milk-producing apparatus. They are also responsible for the characteristic growth and external appearance of the mature female breast. However, they do not complete the job of converting the breasts into milk-producing organs.

Effect of Estrogens on the Skeleton. Estrogens inhibit osteoclastic activity in the bones and therefore stimulate bone growth. As discussed in Chapter 79, at least part of this effect is due to stimulation of *osteoprotegerin,* also called *osteoclastogenesis inhibitory factor,* a cytokine that inhibits bone resorption.

At puberty, when the female enters her reproductive years, her growth in height becomes rapid for several years. However, estrogens have another potent effect on skeletal growth: They cause uniting of the epiphyses with the shafts of the long bones. This effect of estrogen in the female is much stronger than the similar effect of testosterone in the male. As a result, growth of the female usually ceases several years earlier than growth of the male. A female eunuch who is devoid of estrogen production usually grows several inches taller than a normal mature female because her epiphyses do not unite at the normal time.

Osteoporosis of the Bones Caused by Estrogen Deficiency in Old Age. After menopause, almost no estrogens are secreted by the ovaries. This estrogen deficiency leads to (1) increased osteoclastic activity in the bones, (2) decreased bone matrix, and (3) decreased deposition of bone calcium and phosphate. In some women this effect is extremely severe, and the resulting condition is *osteoporosis,* described in Chapter 79. Because this can greatly weaken the bones and lead to bone fracture, especially fracture of the vertebrae, many postmenopausal women are treated prophylactically with estrogen replacement to prevent the osteoporotic effects.

Estrogens Slightly Increase Protein Deposition. Estrogens cause a slight increase in total body protein, which is evidenced by a slight positive nitrogen balance when estrogens are administered. This mainly results from the growth-promoting effect of estrogen on the sexual organs, the bones, and a few other tissues of the body. The enhanced protein deposition caused by testosterone is much more general and much more powerful than that caused by estrogens.

Estrogens Increase Body Metabolism and Fat Deposition. Estrogens increase the whole-body metabolic rate slightly, but only about one third as much as the increase caused by the male sex hormone testosterone. They also cause deposition of increased quantities of fat in the subcutaneous tissues. As a result, the percentage of body fat in the female body is considerably greater than that in the male body, which contains more protein. In addition to deposition of fat in the breasts and subcutaneous tissues, estrogens cause the deposition of fat in the buttocks and thighs, which is characteristic of the feminine figure.

Estrogens Have Little Effect on Hair Distribution. Estrogens do not greatly affect hair distribution. However, hair does develop in the pubic region and in the axillae after puberty. Androgens formed in increased quantities by the female adrenal glands after puberty are mainly responsible for this.

Effect of Estrogens on the Skin. Estrogens cause the skin to develop a texture that is soft and usually smooth, but even so, the skin of a woman is thicker than that of a child or a castrated female. Also, estrogens cause the skin to become more vascular; this is often associated with increased warmth of the skin and also promotes greater bleeding of cut surfaces than is observed in men.

Effect of Estrogens on Electrolyte Balance. The chemical similarity of estrogenic hormones to adrenocortical hormones has been pointed out. Estrogens, like aldosterone and some other adrenocortical hormones, cause sodium and water retention by the kidney tubules. This effect of estrogens is normally slight and rarely of significance, but during pregnancy, the tremendous formation of estrogens by the placenta may contribute to body fluid retention, as discussed in Chapter 82.

Functions of Progesterone

Progesterone Promotes Secretory Changes in the Uterus. By far the most important function of progesterone is *to promote secretory changes in the uterine endometrium* during the latter half of the monthly female sexual cycle, thus preparing the uterus for implantation of the fertilized ovum. This function is discussed later in connection with the endometrial cycle of the uterus.

In addition to this effect on the endometrium, progesterone decreases the frequency and intensity of uterine contractions, thereby helping to prevent expulsion of the implanted ovum.

Effect of Progesterone on the Fallopian Tubes.
Progesterone also promotes increased secretion by the mucosal lining of the fallopian tubes. These secretions are necessary for nutrition of the fertilized, dividing ovum as it traverses the fallopian tube before implantation.

Progesterone Promotes Development of the Breasts.
Progesterone promotes development of the lobules and alveoli of the breasts, causing the alveolar cells to proliferate, enlarge, and become secretory in nature. However, progesterone does not cause the alveoli to secrete milk; as discussed in Chapter 82, milk is secreted only after the prepared breast is further stimulated by *prolactin* from the anterior pituitary gland.

Progesterone also causes the breasts to swell. Part of this swelling is due to the secretory development in the lobules and alveoli, but part also results from increased fluid in the tissue.

Monthly Endometrial Cycle and Menstruation

Associated with the monthly cyclical production of estrogens and progesterone by the ovaries is an endometrial cycle in the lining of the uterus that operates through the following stages: (1) proliferation of the uterine endometrium; (2) development of secretory changes in the endometrium; and (3) desquamation of the endometrium, which is known as *menstruation*. The various phases of this endometrial cycle are shown in Figure 81-8.

Proliferative Phase (Estrogen Phase) of the Endometrial Cycle, Occurring Before Ovulation.
At the beginning of each monthly cycle, most of the endometrium has been desquamated by menstruation. After menstruation, only a thin layer of endometrial stroma remains and the only epithelial cells that are left are those located in the remaining deeper portions of the glands and crypts of the endometrium. *Under the influence of estrogens,* secreted in increasing quantities by the ovary during the first part of the monthly ovarian cycle, the stromal cells and the epithelial cells proliferate rapidly. The endometrial surface is re-epithelialized within 4 to 7 days after the beginning of menstruation.

Then, during the next week and a half, before ovulation occurs, the endometrium increases greatly in thickness, owing to increasing numbers of stromal cells and to progressive growth of the endometrial glands and new blood vessels into the endometrium. At the time of ovulation, the endometrium is 3 to 5 millimeters thick.

The endometrial glands, especially those of the cervical region, secrete a thin, stringy mucus. The mucus strings actually align themselves along the length of the cervical canal, forming channels that help guide sperm in the proper direction from the vagina into the uterus.

Secretory Phase (Progestational Phase) of the Endometrial Cycle, Occurring After Ovulation.
During most of the latter half of the monthly cycle, after ovulation has occurred, progesterone and estrogen together are secreted in large quantities by the corpus luteum. The estrogens cause slight additional cellular proliferation in the endometrium during this phase of the cycle, whereas progesterone causes marked swelling and secretory development of the endometrium. The glands increase in tortuosity; an excess of secretory substances accumulates in the glandular epithelial cells. Also, the cytoplasm of the stromal cells increases; lipid and glycogen deposits increase greatly in the stromal cells; and the blood supply to the endometrium further increases in proportion to the developing secretory activity, with the blood vessels becoming highly tortuous. At the peak of the secretory phase, about 1 week after ovulation, the endometrium has a thickness of 5 to 6 millimeters.

The whole purpose of all these endometrial changes is to produce a highly secretory endometrium that contains large amounts of stored nutrients to provide appropriate conditions for implantation of a *fertilized* ovum during the latter half of the monthly cycle. From the time a fertilized ovum enters the uterine cavity from the fallopian tube (which occurs 3 to 4 days after ovulation) until the time the ovum implants (7 to 9 days after ovulation), the uterine secretions, called "uterine milk," provide nutrition for the early dividing ovum. Then, once the ovum implants in the endometrium, the trophoblastic cells on the surface of the implanting ovum (in the blastocyst stage) begin to digest the endometrium and absorb the endometrial stored substances, thus making great quantities of nutrients available to the early implanting embryo.

Menstruation.
If the ovum is not fertilized, about 2 days before the end of the monthly cycle, the corpus luteum in the ovary suddenly involutes and the ovarian hormones (estrogens and progesterone) decrease to low levels of secretion, as shown in Figure 81-3. Menstruation follows.

Menstruation is caused by the reduction of estrogens and progesterone, especially progesterone, at the end of the monthly ovarian cycle. The first effect is decreased stimulation of the endometrial cells by these two hormones, followed rapidly by involution of the endometrium itself to about 65 percent of its previous thickness. Then, during the 24 hours preceding the onset of menstruation, the tortuous blood vessels leading to the mucosal layers of the endometrium become vasospastic, presumably

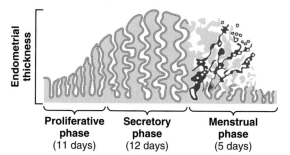

Figure 81-8 Phases of endometrial growth and menstruation during each monthly female sexual cycle.

because of some effect of involution, such as release of a vasoconstrictor material—possibly one of the vasoconstrictor types of prostaglandins that are present in abundance at this time.

The vasospasm, the decrease in nutrients to the endometrium, and the loss of hormonal stimulation initiate necrosis in the endometrium, especially of the blood vessels. As a result, blood at first seeps into the vascular layer of the endometrium and the hemorrhagic areas grow rapidly over a period of 24 to 36 hours. Gradually, the necrotic outer layers of the endometrium separate from the uterus at the sites of the hemorrhages until, about 48 hours after the onset of menstruation, all the superficial layers of the endometrium have desquamated. The mass of desquamated tissue and blood in the uterine cavity, plus contractile effects of prostaglandins or other substances in the decaying desquamate, all acting together, initiate uterine contractions that expel the uterine contents.

During normal menstruation, approximately 40 milliliters of blood and an additional 35 milliliters of serous fluid are lost. The menstrual fluid is normally nonclotting because a *fibrinolysin* is released along with the necrotic endometrial material. If excessive bleeding occurs from the uterine surface, the quantity of fibrinolysin may not be sufficient to prevent clotting. The presence of clots during menstruation is often clinical evidence of uterine pathology.

Within 4 to 7 days after menstruation starts, the loss of blood ceases because, by this time, the endometrium has become re-epithelialized.

Leukorrhea During Menstruation. During menstruation, tremendous numbers of leukocytes are released along with the necrotic material and blood. It is probable that some substance liberated by the endometrial necrosis causes this outflow of leukocytes. As a result of these leukocytes and possibly other factors, the uterus is highly resistant to infection during menstruation, even though the endometrial surfaces are denuded. This is of extreme protective value.

Regulation of the Female Monthly Rhythm—Interplay Between the Ovarian and Hypothalamic-Pituitary Hormones

Now that we have presented the major cyclical changes that occur during the monthly female sexual cycle, we can attempt to explain the basic rhythmical mechanism that causes the cyclical variations.

The Hypothalamus Secretes GnRH, Which Causes the Anterior Pituitary Gland to Secrete LH and FSH

As pointed out in Chapter 74, secretion of most of the anterior pituitary hormones is controlled by "releasing hormones" formed in the hypothalamus and then transported to the anterior pituitary gland by way of the hypothalamic-hypophysial portal system. In the case of the gonadotropins, one releasing hormone, *GnRH*, is important. This hormone has been purified and has been found to be a decapeptide with the following formula:

Glu‑His‑Trp‑Ser‑Tyr‑Gly‑Leu‑Arg‑Pro‑Gly‑NH$_2$

Intermittent, Pulsatile Secretion of GnRH by the Hypothalamus Stimulates Pulsatile Release of LH from the Anterior Pituitary Gland. The hypothalamus does not secrete GnRH continuously but instead secretes it in pulses lasting 5 to 25 minutes that occur every 1 to 2 hours. The lower curve in Figure 81-9 shows the electrical pulsatile signals in the hypothalamus that cause the hypothalamic pulsatile output of GnRH.

It is intriguing that when GnRH is infused continuously so that it is available all the time rather than in pulses, its ability to cause the release of LH and FSH by the anterior pituitary gland is lost. Therefore, for reasons unknown, the pulsatile nature of GnRH release is essential to its function.

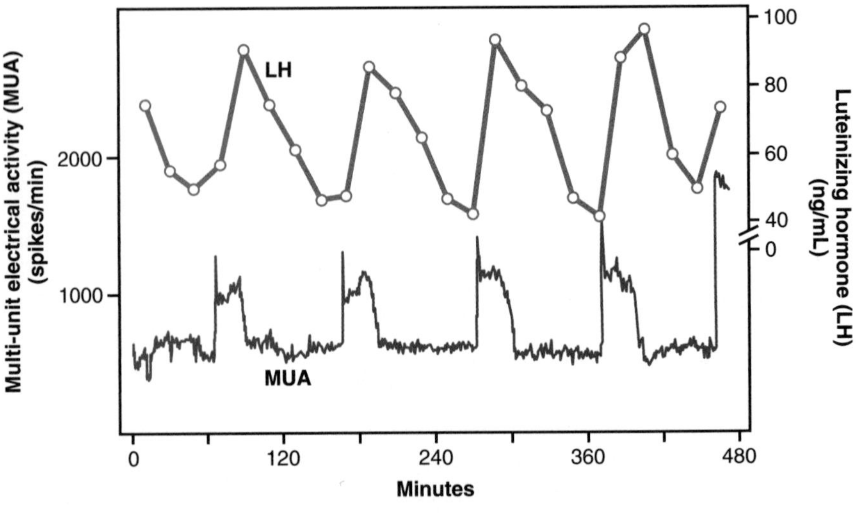

Figure 81-9 *Upper curve:* Pulsatile change in luteinizing hormone (LH) in the peripheral circulation of a pentobarbital-anesthetized ovariectomized rhesus monkey. *Lower curve:* Minute-by-minute recording of multi-unit electrical activity (MUA) in the mediobasal hypothalamus. (Data from Wilson RC, Kesner JS, Kaufman JM, et al: Central electrophysiologic correlates of pulsatile luteinizing hormone secretion. Neuroendocrinology 39:256, 1984.)

The pulsatile release of GnRH also causes intermittent output of LH secretion about every 90 minutes. This is shown by the upper curve in Figure 81-9.

Hypothalamic Centers for Release of GnRH. The neuronal activity that causes pulsatile release of GnRH occurs primarily in the mediobasal hypothalamus, especially in the arcuate nuclei of this area. Therefore, it is believed that these arcuate nuclei control most female sexual activity, although neurons located in the preoptic area of the anterior hypothalamus also secrete GnRH in moderate amounts. Multiple neuronal centers in the higher brain's "limbic" system (the system for psychic control) transmit signals into the arcuate nuclei to modify both the intensity of GnRH release and the frequency of the pulses, thus providing a partial explanation of why psychic factors often modify female sexual function.

Negative Feedback Effects of Estrogen and Progesterone to Decrease LH and FSH Secretion

Estrogen in small amounts has a strong effect to inhibit the production of both LH and FSH. Also, when progesterone is available, the inhibitory effect of estrogen is multiplied, even though progesterone by itself has little effect (Figure 81-10).

These feedback effects seem to operate mainly on the anterior pituitary gland directly, but they also operate to a lesser extent on the hypothalamus to decrease secretion of GnRH, especially by altering the frequency of the GnRH pulses.

Inhibin from the Corpus Luteum Inhibits FSH and LH Secretion. In addition to the feedback effects of estrogen and progesterone, other hormones seem to be involved, especially *inhibin*, which is secreted along with the steroid sex hormones by the granulosa cells of the ovarian corpus luteum in the same way that Sertoli cells secrete inhibin in the male testes (see Figure 81-10). This hormone has the same effect in the female as in the male—inhibiting the secretion of FSH and, to a lesser extent, LH by the anterior pituitary gland. Therefore, it is believed that inhibin might be especially important in causing the decrease in secretion of FSH and LH at the end of the monthly female sexual cycle.

Positive Feedback Effect of Estrogen Before Ovulation—The Preovulatory LH Surge

For reasons not completely understood, the anterior pituitary gland secretes greatly increased amounts of LH for 1 to 2 days beginning 24 to 48 hours before ovulation. This effect is demonstrated in Figure 81-3. The figure shows a much smaller preovulatory surge of FSH as well.

Experiments have shown that infusion of estrogen into a female above a critical rate for 2 to 3 days during the latter part of the first half of the ovarian cycle will cause rapidly accelerating growth of the ovarian follicles, as well as rapidly accelerating secretion of ovarian estrogens. During

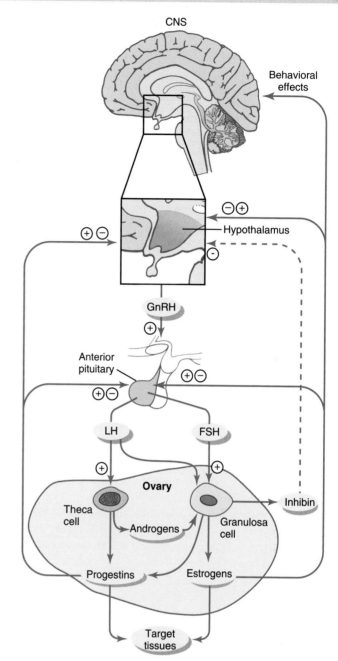

Figure 81-10 Feedback regulation of the hypothalamic-pituitary-ovarian axis in females. Stimulatory effects are shown by ⊕ and negative feedback inhibitory effects are shown by ⊖. Estrogens and progestins exert both negative and positive feedback effects on the anterior pituitary and hypothalamus depending on the stage of the ovarian cycle. Inhibin has a negative feedback effect on the anterior pituitary. FSH, follicle-stimulating hormone; GnRH, gonadotropin-releasing hormone; LH, luteinizing hormone.

this period, secretions of both FSH and LH by the anterior pituitary gland are at first slightly suppressed. Then secretion of LH increases abruptly sixfold to eightfold, and secretion of FSH increases about twofold. The greatly increased secretion of LH causes ovulation to occur.

The cause of this abrupt surge in LH secretion is not known. However, several possible explanations are as follows: (1) It has been suggested that estrogen at this point in the cycle has a peculiar *positive feedback effect* of stimulating pituitary secretion of LH and, to a lesser extent, FSH (see Figure 81-10); this is in sharp contrast to its normal negative feedback effect that occurs during the remainder of the female monthly cycle. (2) The granulosa cells of the follicles begin to secrete small but increasing quantities of progesterone a day or so before the preovulatory LH surge, and it has been suggested that this might be the factor that stimulates the excess LH secretion.

Without this normal preovulatory surge of LH, ovulation will not occur.

Feedback Oscillation of the Hypothalamic-Pituitary-Ovarian System

Now, after discussing much of the known information about the interrelations of the different components of the female hormonal system, we can explain the feedback oscillation that controls the rhythm of the female sexual cycle. It seems to operate in approximately the following sequence of three events.

1. **Postovulatory Secretion of the Ovarian Hormones, and Depression of the Pituitary Gonadotropins.** The easiest part of the cycle to explain is the events that occur during the postovulatory phase—between ovulation and the beginning of menstruation. During this time, the corpus luteum secretes large quantities of progesterone and estrogen, as well as the hormone inhibin. All these hormones together have a combined negative feedback effect on the anterior pituitary gland and hypothalamus, causing the suppression of both FSH and LH secretion and decreasing them to their lowest levels about 3 to 4 days before the onset of menstruation. These effects are shown in Figure 81-3.

2. **Follicular Growth Phase.** Two to 3 days before menstruation, the corpus luteum has regressed to almost total involution and the secretion of estrogen, progesterone, and inhibin from the corpus luteum decreases to a low ebb. This releases the hypothalamus and anterior pituitary from the negative feedback effect of these hormones. Therefore, a day or so later, at about the time that menstruation begins, pituitary secretion of FSH begins to increase again, as much as twofold; then, several days after menstruation begins, LH secretion increases slightly as well. These hormones initiate new ovarian follicle growth and a progressive increase in the secretion of estrogen, reaching a peak estrogen secretion at about 12.5 to 13 days after the onset of the new female monthly sexual cycle.

   During the first 11 to 12 days of this follicle growth, the rates of pituitary secretion of the gonadotropins FSH and LH decrease slightly because of the negative feedback effect, mainly of estrogen, on the anterior pituitary gland. Then there is a sudden, marked increase in the secretion of LH and, to a lesser extent, FSH. This is the preovulatory surge of LH and FSH, which is followed by ovulation.

3. **Preovulatory Surge of LH and FSH Causes Ovulation.** About 11½ to 12 days after the onset of the monthly cycle, the decline in secretion of FSH and LH comes to an abrupt halt. It is believed that the high level of estrogens at this time (or the beginning of progesterone secretion by the follicles) causes a positive feedback stimulatory effect on the anterior pituitary, as explained earlier, which leads to a terrific surge in the secretion of LH and, to a lesser extent, FSH. Whatever the cause of this preovulatory LH and FSH surge, the great excess of LH leads to both ovulation and subsequent development of and secretion by the corpus luteum. Thus, the hormonal system begins its new round of secretions until the next ovulation.

Anovulatory Cycles—Sexual Cycles at Puberty

If the preovulatory surge of LH is not of sufficient magnitude, ovulation will not occur and the cycle is said to be "anovulatory." The phases of the sexual cycle continue, but they are altered in the following ways: First, lack of ovulation causes failure of development of the corpus luteum, so there is almost no secretion of progesterone during the latter portion of the cycle. Second, the cycle is shortened by several days but the rhythm continues. Therefore, it is likely that progesterone is not required for maintenance of the cycle itself, although it can alter its rhythm.

The first few cycles after the onset of puberty are usually anovulatory, as are the cycles occurring several months to years before menopause, presumably because the LH surge is not potent enough at these times to cause ovulation.

Puberty and Menarche

Puberty means the onset of adult sexual life, and *menarche* means the beginning of the cycle of menstruation. The period of puberty is caused by a gradual increase in gonadotropic hormone secretion by the pituitary, beginning in about the eighth year of life, as shown in Figure 81-11,

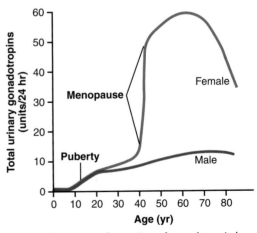

Figure 81-11 Total rates of secretion of gonadotropic hormones throughout the sexual lives of female and male human beings, showing an especially abrupt increase in gonadotropic hormones at menopause in the female.

and usually culminating in the onset of puberty and menstruation between ages 11 and 16 years in girls (average, 13 years).

In the female, as in the male, the infantile pituitary gland and ovaries are capable of full function if appropriately stimulated. However, as is also true in the male, and for reasons not understood, the hypothalamus does not secrete significant quantities of GnRH during childhood. Experiments have shown that the hypothalamus is capable of secreting this hormone, but the appropriate signal from some other area of brain to cause the secretion is lacking. Therefore, it is now believed that the onset of puberty is initiated by some maturation process that occurs elsewhere in the brain, perhaps somewhere in the limbic system.

Figure 81-12 shows (1) the increasing levels of estrogen secretion at puberty, (2) the cyclical variation during the monthly sexual cycle, (3) the further increase in estrogen secretion during the first few years of reproductive life, (4) the progressive decrease in estrogen secretion toward the end of reproductive life, and, finally, (5) almost no estrogen or progesterone secretion beyond menopause.

Menopause

At age 40 to 50 years, the sexual cycle usually becomes irregular and ovulation often fails to occur. After a few months to a few years, the cycle ceases altogether, as shown in Figure 81-12. The period during which the cycle ceases and the female sex hormones diminish to almost none is called *menopause.*

The cause of menopause is "burning out" of the ovaries. Throughout a woman's reproductive life, about 400 of the primordial follicles grow into mature follicles and ovulate, and hundreds of thousands of ova degenerate. At about age 45 years, only a few primordial follicles remain to be stimulated by FSH and LH, and, as shown in Figure 81-12, the production of estrogens by the ovaries decreases as the number of primordial follicles approaches zero. When estrogen production falls below a critical value, the estrogens can no longer inhibit the production of the gonadotropins FSH and LH. Instead, as shown in Figure 81-11, the gonadotropins FSH and LH (mainly FSH) are produced

after menopause in large and continuous quantities, but as the remaining primordial follicles become atretic, the production of estrogens by the ovaries falls virtually to zero.

At the time of menopause, a woman must readjust her life from one that has been physiologically stimulated by estrogen and progesterone production to one devoid of these hormones. The loss of estrogens often causes marked physiological changes in the function of the body, including (1) "hot flushes" characterized by extreme flushing of the skin, (2) psychic sensations of dyspnea, (3) irritability, (4) fatigue, (5) anxiety, and (6) decreased strength and calcification of bones throughout the body. These symptoms are of sufficient magnitude in about 15 percent of women to warrant treatment. If counseling fails, daily administration of estrogen in small quantities usually reverses the symptoms, and by gradually decreasing the dose, postmenopausal women can likely avoid severe symptoms.

Abnormalities of Secretion by the Ovaries

Hypogonadism-Reduced Secretion by the Ovaries. Less than normal secretion by the ovaries can result from poorly formed ovaries, lack of ovaries, or genetically abnormal ovaries that secrete the wrong hormones because of missing enzymes in the secretory cells. When ovaries are absent from birth or when they become nonfunctional before puberty, *female eunuchism* occurs. In this condition the usual secondary sexual characteristics do not appear, and the sexual organs remain infantile. Especially characteristic of this condition is prolonged growth of the long bones because the epiphyses do not unite with the shafts as early as they do in a normal woman. Consequently, the female eunuch is essentially as tall as or perhaps even slightly taller than her male counterpart of similar genetic background.

When the ovaries of a fully developed woman are removed, the sexual organs regress to some extent so that the uterus becomes almost infantile in size, the vagina becomes smaller, and the vaginal epithelium becomes thin and easily damaged. The breasts atrophy and become pendulous, and the pubic hair becomes thinner. The same changes occur in women after menopause.

Irregularity of Menses, and Amenorrhea Caused by Hypogonadism. As pointed out in the preceding discussion of menopause, the quantity of estrogens produced by the ovaries must rise above a critical value in order to cause rhythmical sexual cycles. Consequently, in hypogonadism or when the gonads are secreting small quantities of estrogens as a result of other factors, such as *hypothyroidism,* the ovarian cycle often does not occur normally. Instead, several months may elapse between menstrual periods or menstruation may cease altogether (amenorrhea). Prolonged ovarian cycles are frequently associated with failure of ovulation, presumably because of insufficient secretion of LH at the time of the preovulatory surge of LH, which is necessary for ovulation.

Hypersecretion by the Ovaries. Extreme hypersecretion of ovarian hormones by the ovaries is a rare clinical entity because excessive secretion of estrogens automatically decreases the production of gonadotropins by the pituitary, and this limits

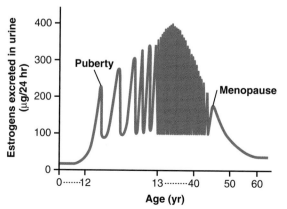

Figure 81-12   Estrogen secretion throughout the sexual life of the female human being.

the production of ovarian hormones. Consequently, hypersecretion of feminizing hormones is usually recognized clinically only when a feminizing tumor develops.

A rare *granulosa cell tumor* can develop in an ovary, occurring more often after menopause than before. These tumors secrete large quantities of estrogens, which exert the usual estrogenic effects, including hypertrophy of the uterine endometrium and irregular bleeding from this endometrium. In fact, bleeding is often the first and only indication that such a tumor exists.

Female Sexual Act

Stimulation of the Female Sexual Act. As is true in the male sexual act, successful performance of the female sexual act depends on both psychic stimulation and local sexual stimulation.

Thinking sexual thoughts can lead to female sexual desire, and this aids greatly in the performance of the female sexual act. Such desire is based on psychological and physiological drive, although sexual desire does increase in proportion to the level of sex hormones secreted. Desire also changes during the monthly sexual cycle, reaching a peak near the time of ovulation, probably because of the high levels of estrogen secretion during the preovulatory period.

Local sexual stimulation in women occurs in more or less the same manner as in men because massage and other types of stimulation of the vulva, vagina, and other perineal regions can create sexual sensations. The glans of the *clitoris* is especially sensitive for initiating sexual sensations.

As in the male, the sexual sensory signals are transmitted to the sacral segments of the spinal cord through the pudendal nerve and sacral plexus. Once these signals have entered the spinal cord, they are transmitted to the cerebrum. Also, local reflexes integrated in the sacral and lumbar spinal cord are at least partly responsible for some of the reactions in the female sexual organs.

Female Erection and Lubrication. Located around the introitus and extending into the clitoris is erectile tissue almost identical to the erectile tissue of the penis. This erectile tissue, like that of the penis, is controlled by the parasympathetic nerves that pass through the nervi erigentes from the sacral plexus to the external genitalia. In the early phases of sexual stimulation, parasympathetic signals dilate the arteries of the erectile tissue, probably resulting from release of acetylcholine, nitric oxide, and vasoactive intestinal polypeptide (VIP) at the nerve endings. This allows rapid accumulation of blood in the erectile tissue so that the introitus tightens around the penis; this aids the male greatly in his attainment of sufficient sexual stimulation for ejaculation to occur.

Parasympathetic signals also pass to the bilateral Bartholin glands located beneath the labia minora and cause them to secrete mucus immediately inside the introitus. This mucus is responsible for much of the lubrication during sexual intercourse, although much is also provided by mucus secreted by the vaginal epithelium and a small amount from the male urethral glands. This lubrication is necessary during intercourse to establish a satisfactory massaging sensation rather than an irritative sensation, which may be provoked by a dry vagina. A massaging sensation constitutes the optimal stimulus for evoking the appropriate reflexes that culminate in both the male and female climaxes.

Female Orgasm. When local sexual stimulation reaches maximum intensity, and especially when the local sensations are supported by appropriate psychic conditioning signals from the cerebrum, reflexes are initiated that cause the female orgasm, also called the *female climax*. The female orgasm is analogous to emission and ejaculation in the male, and it may help promote fertilization of the ovum. Indeed, the human female is known to be somewhat more fertile when inseminated by normal sexual intercourse rather than by artificial methods, thus indicating an important function of the female orgasm. Possible reasons for this are as follows.

First, during the orgasm, the perineal muscles of the female contract rhythmically, which results from spinal cord reflexes similar to those that cause ejaculation in the male. It is possible that these reflexes increase uterine and fallopian tube motility during the orgasm, thus helping to transport the sperm upward through the uterus toward the ovum; information on this subject is scanty, however. Also, the orgasm seems to cause dilation of the cervical canal for up to 30 minutes, thus allowing easy transport of the sperm.

Second, in many lower animals, copulation causes the posterior pituitary gland to secrete oxytocin; this effect is probably mediated through the brain amygdaloid nuclei and then through the hypothalamus to the pituitary. The oxytocin causes increased rhythmical contractions of the uterus, which have been postulated to cause increased transport of the sperm. A few sperm have been shown to traverse the entire length of the fallopian tube in the cow in about 5 minutes, a rate at least 10 times as fast as that which the swimming motions of the sperm themselves could possibly achieve. Whether this occurs in the human female is unknown.

In addition to the possible effects of the orgasm on fertilization, the intense sexual sensations that develop during the orgasm also pass to the cerebrum and cause intense muscle tension throughout the body. But after culmination of the sexual act, this gives way during the succeeding minutes to a sense of satisfaction characterized by relaxed peacefulness, an effect called *resolution*.

Female Fertility

Fertile Period of Each Sexual Cycle. The ovum remains viable and capable of being fertilized after it is expelled from the ovary probably no longer than 24 hours. Therefore, sperm must be available soon after ovulation if fertilization is to take place. A few sperm can remain fertile in the female reproductive tract for up to 5 days. Therefore, for fertilization to take place, intercourse must occur sometime between 4 and 5 days before ovulation up to a few hours after ovulation. Thus, the period of female fertility during each month is short, about 4 to 5 days.

Rhythm Method of Contraception. One of the commonly practiced methods of contraception is to avoid intercourse near the time of ovulation. The difficulty with this method of contraception is predicting the exact time of ovulation. Yet the interval from ovulation until the next succeeding onset of menstruation is almost always between 13 and 15 days. Therefore, if the menstrual cycle is regular, with an exact periodicity of 28 days, ovulation usually occurs within 1 day of the 14th day of the cycle. If, in contrast, the periodicity of the cycle is 40 days, ovulation usually occurs within 1 day of the 26th day of the cycle. Finally, if the periodicity of the cycle is 21 days, ovulation usually occurs within 1 day of the seventh day of the cycle. Therefore, it is usually stated that avoidance of intercourse for 4 days before the calculated day of ovulation and 3 days afterward prevents conception. But such a method of contraception can be used only when the periodicity of the menstrual cycle is regular. The failure rate of this method of contraception, resulting in an unintentional pregnancy, may be as high as 20 to 25 percent per year.

Hormonal Suppression of Fertility—"The Pill." It has long been known that administration of either estrogen or progesterone, if given in appropriate quantities during the first half of the monthly cycle, can inhibit ovulation. The reason for this is that appropriate administration of either of these hormones can prevent the preovulatory surge of LH secretion by the pituitary gland, which is essential in causing ovulation.

Why the administration of estrogen or progesterone prevents the preovulatory surge of LH secretion is not fully understood. However, experimental work has suggested that immediately before the surge occurs, there is probably a sudden depression of estrogen secretion by the ovarian follicles, and this might be the necessary signal that causes the subsequent feedback effect on the anterior pituitary that leads to the LH surge. The administration of sex hormones (estrogens or progesterone) could prevent the initial ovarian hormonal depression that might be the initiating signal for ovulation.

The challenge in devising methods for the hormonal suppression of ovulation has been in developing appropriate combinations of estrogens and progestins that suppress ovulation but do not cause other, unwanted effects. For instance, too much of either hormone can cause abnormal menstrual bleeding patterns. However, use of certain synthetic progestins in place of progesterone, especially the 19-norsteroids, along with small amounts of estrogens usually prevents ovulation yet allows an almost normal pattern of menstruation. Therefore, almost all "pills" used for the control of fertility consist of some combination of synthetic estrogens and synthetic progestins. The main reason for using synthetic estrogens and progestins is that the *natural* hormones are almost entirely destroyed by the liver within a short time after they are absorbed from the gastrointestinal tract into the portal circulation. However, many of the *synthetic* hormones can resist this destructive propensity of the liver, thus allowing oral administration.

Two of the most commonly used synthetic estrogens are *ethinyl estradiol* and *mestranol*. Among the most commonly used progestins are *norethindrone, norethynodrel, ethynodiol,* and *norgestrel*. The drug is usually begun in the early stages of the monthly cycle and continued beyond the time that ovulation would normally occur. Then the drug is stopped, allowing menstruation to occur and a new cycle to begin.

The failure rate, resulting in an unintentional pregnancy, for hormonal suppression of fertility using various forms of the "pill" is about 8 to 9 percent per year.

Abnormal Conditions That Cause Female Sterility. About 5 to 10 percent of women are infertile. Occasionally, no abnormality can be discovered in the female genital organs, in which case it must be assumed that the infertility is due to either abnormal physiological function of the genital system or abnormal genetic development of the ova themselves.

The most common cause of female sterility is failure to ovulate. This can result from hyposecretion of gonadotropic hormones, in which case the intensity of the hormonal stimuli is simply insufficient to cause ovulation, or it can result from abnormal ovaries that do not allow ovulation. For instance, thick ovarian capsules occasionally exist on the outsides of the ovaries, making ovulation difficult.

Because of the high incidence of anovulation in sterile women, special methods are often used to determine whether ovulation occurs. These methods are based mainly on the effects of progesterone on the body because the normal increase in progesterone secretion usually does not occur during the latter half of anovulatory cycles. In the absence of progestational effects, the cycle can be assumed to be anovulatory.

One of these tests is simply to analyze the urine for a surge in pregnanediol, the end product of progesterone metabolism, during the latter half of the sexual cycle; the lack of this substance indicates failure of ovulation. Another common test is for the woman to chart her body temperature throughout the cycle. Secretion of progesterone during the latter half of the cycle raises the body temperature about 0.5°F, with the temperature rise coming abruptly at the time of ovulation. Such a temperature chart, showing the point of ovulation, is illustrated in Figure 81-13.

Lack of ovulation caused by hyposecretion of the pituitary gonadotropic hormones can sometimes be treated by appropriately timed administration of *human chorionic gonadotropin*, a hormone (discussed in Chapter 82) that is extracted from the human placenta. This hormone, although secreted by the placenta, has almost the same effects as LH and is therefore a powerful stimulator of ovulation. However, excess use of this hormone can cause ovulation from many follicles simultaneously; this results in multiple births, an effect that has caused as many as eight babies (stillborn in many cases) to be born to mothers treated for infertility with this hormone.

One of the most common causes of female sterility is *endometriosis,* a common condition in which endometrial tissue almost identical to that of the normal uterine endometrium grows and even menstruates in the pelvic cavity surrounding the uterus, fallopian tubes, and ovaries. Endometriosis causes fibrosis throughout the pelvis, and this fibrosis sometimes so enshrouds the ovaries that an ovum cannot be released into the abdominal cavity. Often, endometriosis occludes the fallopian tubes, either at the fimbriated ends or elsewhere along their extent.

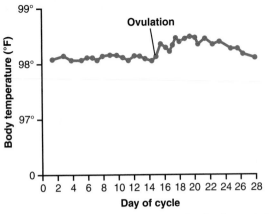

Figure 81-13 Elevation in body temperature shortly after ovulation.

Another common cause of female infertility is *salpingitis*, that is, *inflammation of the fallopian tubes;* this causes fibrosis in the tubes, thereby occluding them. In the past, such inflammation occurred mainly as a result of gonococcal infection. But with modern therapy, this is becoming a less prevalent cause of female infertility.

Still another cause of infertility is secretion of abnormal mucus by the uterine cervix. Ordinarily, at the time of ovulation, the hormonal environment of estrogen causes the secretion of mucus with special characteristics that allow rapid mobility of sperm into the uterus and actually guide the sperm up along mucous "threads." Abnormalities of the cervix itself, such as low-grade infection or inflammation, or abnormal hormonal stimulation of the cervix, can lead to a viscous mucous plug that prevents fertilization.

Bibliography

Barton M, Meyer MR: Postmenopausal hypertension: mechanisms and therapy, *Hypertension* 54:11, 2009.

Beral V, Banks E, Reeves G: Evidence from randomised trials on the long-term effects of hormone replacement therapy, *Lancet* 360:942, 2002.

Blaustein JD: Progesterone and progestin receptors in the brain: the neglected ones, *Endocrinology* 149:2737, 2008.

Bulun SE: Endometriosis, *N Engl J Med* 360:268, 2009.

Compston JE: Sex steroids and bone, *Physiol Rev* 81:419, 2001.

de la Iglesia HO, Schwartz WJ: Minireview: timely ovulation: circadian regulation of the female hypothalamo-pituitary-gonadal axis, *Endocrinology* 147:1148, 2006.

Federman DD: The biology of human sex differences, *N Engl J Med* 354:1507, 2006.

Grady D: Clinical practice. Management of menopausal symptoms, *N Engl J Med* 355:2338, 2006.

Gruber CJ, Tschugguel W, Schneeberger C, et al: Production and actions of estrogens, *N Engl J Med* 346:340, 2002.

Hamilton-Fairley D, Taylor A: Anovulation, *BMJ* 327:546, 2003.

Heldring N, Pike A, Andersson S, et al: Estrogen receptors: how do they signal and what are their targets, *Physiol Rev* 87:905, 2007.

Jabbour HN, Kelly RW, Fraser HM, et al: Endocrine regulation of menstruation, *Endocr Rev* 27:17, 2006.

Moriarty K, Kim KH, Bender JR: Minireview: estrogen receptor-mediated rapid signaling, *Endocrinology* 147:5557, 2006.

Nadal A, Diaz M, Valverde MA: The estrogen trinity: membrane, cytosolic, and nuclear effects, *News Physiol Sci* 16:251, 2001.

Nelson HD: Menopause, *Lancet* 371:760, 2008.

Nilsson S, Makela S, Treuter E, et al: Mechanisms of estrogen action, *Physiol Rev* 81:1535, 2001.

Niswender GD, Juengel JL, Silva PJ, et al: Mechanisms controlling the function and life span of the corpus luteum, *Physiol Rev* 80:1, 2000.

Petitti DB: Combination estrogen-progestin oral contraceptives, *N Engl J Med* 349:1443, 2003.

Riggs BL: The mechanisms of estrogen regulation of bone resorption, *J Clin Invest* 106:1203, 2000.

Santen RJ, Brodie H, Simpson ER, et al: History of aromatase: saga of an important biological mediator and therapeutic target, *Endocr Rev* 30:343, 2009.

Smith S, Pfeifer SM, Collins JA: Diagnosis and management of female infertility, *JAMA* 290:1767, 2003.

Stocco C, Telleria C, Gibori G: The molecular control of corpus luteum formation, function, and regression, *Endocr Rev* 28:117, 2007.

Toran-Allerand CD: A plethora of estrogen receptors in the brain: where will it end? *Endocrinology* 145:1069, 2004.

Vasudevan N, Ogawa S, Pfaff D: Estrogen and thyroid hormone receptor interactions: physiological flexibility by molecular specificity, *Physiol Rev* 82:923, 2002.

Xing D, Nozell S, Chen YF, et al: Estrogen and mechanisms of vascular protection, *Arterioscler Thromb Vasc Biol* 29:289, 2009.

Pregnancy and Lactation

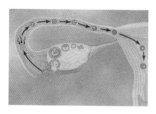

In Chapters 80 and 81, the sexual functions of the male and female are described to the point of fertilization of the ovum. If the ovum becomes fertilized, a new sequence of events called *gestation*, or *pregnancy*, takes place, and the fertilized ovum eventually develops into a full-term fetus. The purpose of this chapter is to discuss the early stages of ovum development after fertilization and then to discuss the physiology of pregnancy. In Chapter 83, some special aspects of fetal and early childhood physiology are discussed.

Maturation and Fertilization of the Ovum

While still in the ovary, the ovum is in the *primary oocyte* stage. Shortly before it is released from the ovarian follicle, its nucleus divides by meiosis and a *first polar body* is expelled from the nucleus of the oocyte. The primary oocyte then becomes the *secondary oocyte*. In this process, each of the 23 pairs of chromosomes loses one of its partners, which becomes incorporated in a *polar body* that is expelled. This leaves 23 *unpaired* chromosomes in the secondary oocyte. It is at this time that the ovum, still in the secondary oocyte stage, is ovulated into the abdominal cavity. Then, almost immediately, it enters the fimbriated end of one of the fallopian tubes.

Entry of the Ovum into the Fallopian Tube (Uterine Tube). When ovulation occurs, the ovum, along with a hundred or more attached granulosa cells that constitute the *corona radiata*, is expelled directly into the peritoneal cavity and must then enter one of the fallopian tubes (also called uterine tubes) to reach the cavity of the uterus. The fimbriated ends of each fallopian tube fall naturally around the ovaries. The inner surfaces of the fimbriated tentacles are lined with ciliated epithelium, and the *cilia* are activated by estrogen from the ovaries, which causes the cilia to beat toward the opening, or *ostium*, of the involved fallopian tube. One can actually see a slow fluid current flowing toward the ostium. By this means, the ovum enters one of the fallopian tubes.

Although one might suspect that many ova fail to enter the fallopian tubes, conception studies suggest that up to 98 percent succeed in this task. Indeed, in some recorded cases, women with one ovary removed and the opposite fallopian tube removed have had several children with relative ease of conception, thus demonstrating that ova can even enter the opposite fallopian tube.

Fertilization of the Ovum. After the male ejaculates semen into the vagina during intercourse, a few sperm are transported within 5 to 10 minutes upward from the vagina and through the uterus and fallopian tubes to the *ampullae* of the fallopian tubes near the ovarian ends of the tubes. This transport of the sperm is aided by contractions of the uterus and fallopian tubes stimulated by prostaglandins in the male seminal fluid and also by oxytocin released from the posterior pituitary gland of the female during her orgasm. Of the almost half a billion sperm deposited in the vagina, a few thousand succeed in reaching each ampulla.

Fertilization of the ovum normally takes place in the ampulla of one of the fallopian tubes soon after both the sperm and the ovum enter the ampulla. But before a sperm can enter the ovum, it must first penetrate the multiple layers of granulosa cells attached to the outside of the ovum (the *corona radiata*) and then bind to and penetrate the *zona pellucida* surrounding the ovum. The mechanisms used by the sperm for these purposes are presented in Chapter 80.

Once a sperm has entered the ovum (which is still in the secondary oocyte stage of development), the oocyte divides again to form the *mature ovum* plus a *second polar body* that is expelled. The mature ovum still carries in its nucleus (now called the *female pronucleus*) 23 chromosomes. One of these chromosomes is the female chromosome, known as the *X chromosome*.

In the meantime, the fertilizing sperm has also changed. On entering the ovum, its head swells to form a *male pronucleus*, shown in Figure 82-1*D*. Later, the 23 unpaired chromosomes of the male pronucleus and the 23 unpaired chromosomes of the female pronucleus align themselves

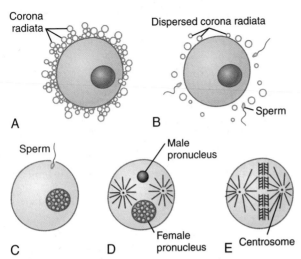

A

B

Sperm

Male pronucleus

Female pronucleus

Centrosome

C   D   E

Figure 82-1 Fertilization of the ovum. *A,* The mature ovum surrounded by the corona radiata. *B,* Dispersal of the corona radiata. *C,* Entry of the sperm. *D,* Formation of the male and female pronuclei. *E,* Reorganization of a full complement of chromosomes and beginning division of the ovum. (Modified from Arey LB: Developmental Anatomy: A Textbook and Laboratory Manual of Embryology, 7th ed. Philadelphia: WB Saunders, 1974.)

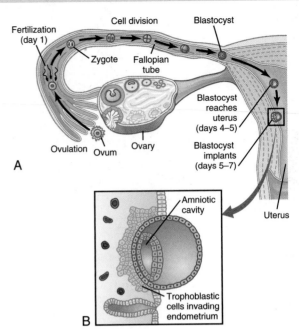

Figure 82-2 *A,* Ovulation, fertilization of the ovum in the fallopian tube, and implantation of the blastocyst in the uterus. *B,* Action of trophoblast cells in implantation of the blastocyst in the uterine endometrium.

to re-form a complete complement of 46 chromosomes (23 pairs) in the *fertilized ovum* (Figure 82-1*E*).

What Determines the Sex of the Fetus That Is Created?

After formation of the mature sperm, half of these carry in their genome an X chromosome (the female chromosome) and half carry a Y chromosome (the male chromosome). Therefore, if an X chromosome from a sperm combines with an X chromosome from an ovum, giving an XX combination, a female child will be born, as explained in Chapter 80. But if a Y chromosome from a sperm is paired with an X chromosome from an ovum, giving an XY combination, a male child will be born.

Transport of the Fertilized Ovum in the Fallopian Tube

After fertilization has occurred, an additional 3 to 5 days is normally required for transport of the fertilized ovum through the remainder of the fallopian tube into the cavity of the uterus (Figure 82-2). This transport is effected mainly by a feeble fluid current in the tube resulting from epithelial secretion plus action of the ciliated epithelium that lines the tube; the cilia always beat toward the uterus. Weak contractions of the fallopian tube may also aid the ovum passage.

The fallopian tubes are lined with a rugged, cryptoid surface that impedes passage of the ovum despite the fluid current. Also, the *isthmus* of the fallopian tube (the last 2 centimeters before the tube enters the uterus) remains spastically contracted for about the first 3 days after ovulation. After this time, the rapidly increasing progesterone secreted by the ovarian corpus luteum first promotes

increasing progesterone receptors on the fallopian tube smooth muscle cells; then the progesterone activates the receptors, exerting a tubular relaxing effect that allows entry of the ovum into the uterus.

This delayed transport of the fertilized ovum through the fallopian tube allows several stages of cell division to occur before the dividing ovum—now called a *blastocyst,* with about 100 cells—enters the uterus. During this time, the fallopian tube secretory cells produce large quantities of secretions used for the nutrition of the developing blastocyst.

Implantation of the Blastocyst in the Uterus

After reaching the uterus, the developing blastocyst usually remains in the uterine cavity an additional 1 to 3 days before it implants in the endometrium; thus, implantation ordinarily occurs on about the fifth to seventh day after ovulation. Before implantation, the blastocyst obtains its nutrition from the uterine endometrial secretions, called "uterine milk."

Implantation results from the action of *trophoblast cells* that develop over the surface of the blastocyst. These cells secrete proteolytic enzymes that digest and liquefy the adjacent cells of the uterine endometrium. Some of the fluid and nutrients released are actively transported by the same trophoblast cells into the blastocyst, adding more sustenance for growth. Figure 82-3 shows an early implanted human blastocyst, with a small embryo. Once implantation has taken place, the trophoblast cells and other adjacent cells (from the blastocyst and the uterine endometrium) proliferate rapidly, forming the placenta and the various membranes of pregnancy.

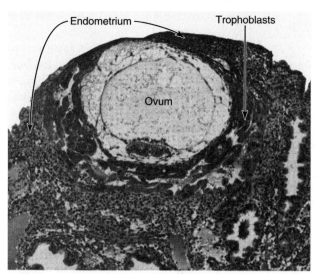

Figure 82-3 Implantation of the early human embryo, showing trophoblastic digestion and invasion of the endometrium. (Courtesy Dr. Arthur Hertig.)

Early Nutrition of the Embryo

In Chapter 81, we pointed out that the progesterone secreted by the ovarian corpus luteum during the latter half of each monthly sexual cycle has an effect on the uterine endometrium, converting the endometrial stromal cells into large swollen cells containing extra quantities of glycogen, proteins, lipids, and even some minerals necessary for development of the *conceptus* (the embryo and its adjacent parts or associated membranes). Then, when the conceptus implants in the endometrium, the continued secretion of progesterone causes the endometrial cells to swell further and to store even more nutrients. These cells are now called *decidual cells,* and the total mass of cells is called the *decidua.*

As the trophoblast cells invade the decidua, digesting and imbibing it, the stored nutrients in the decidua are used by the embryo for growth and development. During the first week after implantation, this is the only means by which the embryo can obtain nutrients; the embryo continues to obtain at least some of its nutrition in this way for up to 8 weeks, although the placenta also begins to provide nutrition after about the 16th day beyond fertilization (a little more than 1 week after implantation). Figure 82-4 shows this trophoblastic period of nutrition, which gradually gives way to placental nutrition.

Function of the Placenta

Developmental and Physiologic Anatomy of the Placenta
While the trophoblastic cords from the blastocyst are attaching to the uterus, blood capillaries grow into the cords from the vascular system of the newly forming embryo. About 21 days after fertilization, blood also begins to be pumped by the heart of the human embryo. Simultaneously, *blood sinuses* supplied with blood from the mother develop around

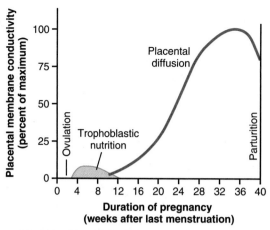

Figure 82-4 Nutrition of the fetus. Most of the early nutrition is due to trophoblastic digestion and absorption of nutrients from the endometrial decidua, and essentially all the later nutrition results from diffusion through the placental membrane.

the outsides of the trophoblastic cords. The trophoblast cells send out more and more projections, which become *placental villi* into which fetal capillaries grow. Thus, the villi, carrying fetal blood, are surrounded by sinuses that contain maternal blood.

The final structure of the placenta is shown in Figure 82-5. Note that the fetus's blood flows through two *umbilical arteries,* then into the capillaries of the villi, and finally back through a single *umbilical vein* into the fetus. At the same time, the mother's blood flows from her *uterine arteries* into large *maternal sinuses* that surround the villi and then back into the *uterine veins* of the mother. The lower part of Figure 82-5 shows the relation between the fetal blood of each fetal placental villus and the blood of the mother surrounding the outsides of the villus in the fully developed placenta.

The total surface area of all the villi of the mature placenta is only a few square meters—many times less than the area of the pulmonary membrane in the lungs. Nevertheless, nutrients and other substances pass through this placental membrane mainly by diffusion in much the same manner that diffusion occurs through the alveolar membranes of the lungs and the capillary membranes elsewhere in the body.

Placental Permeability and Membrane Diffusion Conductance

The major function of the placenta is to provide for diffusion of foodstuffs and oxygen from the mother's blood into the fetus's blood and diffusion of excretory products from the fetus back into the mother.

In the early months of pregnancy, the placental membrane is still thick because it is not fully developed. Therefore, its permeability is low. Further, the surface area is small because the placenta has not grown significantly. Therefore, the total diffusion conductance is minuscule at first. Conversely, in later pregnancy, the permeability increases because of thinning of the membrane diffusion layers and because the surface area expands many times over, thus giving the tremendous increase in placental diffusion shown in Figure 82-4.

Rarely, "breaks" occur in the placental membrane, which allows fetal blood cells to pass into the mother or,

PLACENTA

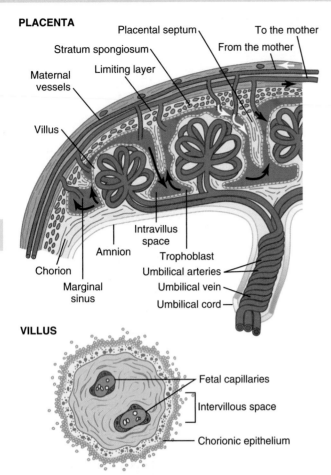

Figure 82-5 *Above,* Organization of the mature placenta. *Below,* Relation of the fetal blood in the villus capillaries to the mother's blood in the intervillous spaces. (Modified from Gray H, Goss CM: Anatomy of the Human Body, 25th ed. Philadelphia: Lea & Febiger, 1948; and from Arey LB: Developmental Anatomy: A Textbook and Laboratory Manual of Embryology, 7th ed. Philadelphia: WB Saunders, 1974.)

even less commonly, the mother's cells to pass into the fetus. Fortunately, it is rare for the fetus to bleed severely into the mother's circulation because of a ruptured placental membrane.

Diffusion of Oxygen Through the Placental Membrane. Almost the same principles for diffusion of oxygen through the pulmonary membrane (discussed in detail in Chapter 39) are applicable for diffusion of oxygen through the placental membrane. The dissolved oxygen in the blood of the large maternal sinuses passes into the fetal blood by *simple diffusion,* driven by an oxygen pressure gradient from the mother's blood to the fetus's blood. Near the end of pregnancy, the mean P_{O_2} of the mother's blood in the placental sinuses is about 50 mm Hg, and the mean P_{O_2} in the fetal blood after it becomes oxygenated in the placenta is about 30 mm Hg. Therefore, the mean pressure gradient for diffusion of oxygen through the placental membrane is about 20 mm Hg.

One might wonder how it is possible for a fetus to obtain sufficient oxygen when the fetal blood leaving the placenta has a P_{O_2} of only 30 mm Hg. There are three reasons why even this low P_{O_2} is capable of allowing the fetal blood to

transport almost as much oxygen to the fetal tissues as is transported by the mother's blood to her tissues.

First, the hemoglobin of the fetus is mainly *fetal hemoglobin,* a type of hemoglobin synthesized in the fetus before birth. Figure 82-6 shows the comparative oxygen dissociation curves for maternal hemoglobin and fetal hemoglobin, demonstrating that the curve for fetal hemoglobin is shifted to the left of that for maternal hemoglobin. This means that at the low P_{O_2} levels in fetal blood, the fetal hemoglobin can carry 20 to 50 percent more oxygen than maternal hemoglobin can.

Second, the *hemoglobin concentration of fetal blood is about 50 percent greater than that of the mother;* this is an even more important factor in enhancing the amount of oxygen transported to the fetal tissues.

Third, the *Bohr effect,* which is explained in relation to the exchange of carbon dioxide and oxygen in the lung in Chapter 40, provides another mechanism to enhance the transport of oxygen by fetal blood. That is, hemoglobin can carry more oxygen at a low P_{CO_2} than it can at a high P_{CO_2}. The fetal blood entering the placenta carries large amounts of carbon dioxide, but much of this carbon dioxide diffuses from the fetal blood into the maternal blood. Loss of the carbon dioxide makes the fetal blood more alkaline, whereas the increased carbon dioxide in the maternal blood makes it more acidic.

These changes cause the capacity of fetal blood to combine with oxygen to increase and that of maternal blood to decrease. This forces still more oxygen from the maternal blood, while enhancing oxygen uptake by the fetal blood. Thus, the Bohr shift operates in one direction in the maternal blood and in the other direction in the fetal blood. These two effects make the Bohr shift twice as important here as it is for oxygen exchange in the lungs; therefore, it is called the *double Bohr effect.*

By these three means, the fetus is capable of receiving more than adequate oxygen through the placental

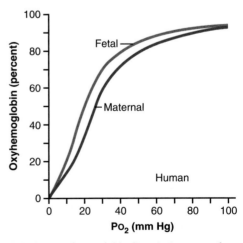

Figure 82-6 Oxygen-hemoglobin dissociation curves for maternal and fetal blood, showing that fetal blood can carry a greater quantity of oxygen than can maternal blood for a given blood P_{O_2}. (Data from Metcalfe J, Moll W, Bartels H: Gas exchange across the placenta. Fed Proc 23:775, 1964.)

membrane, despite the fact that the fetal blood leaving the placenta has a Po$_2$ of only 30 mm Hg.

The total *diffusing capacity* of the entire placenta for oxygen at term is about 1.2 milliliters of oxygen per minute per millimeter of mercury oxygen pressure difference across the membrane. This compares favorably with that of the lungs of the newborn baby.

Diffusion of Carbon Dioxide Through the Placental Membrane. Carbon dioxide is continually formed in the tissues of the fetus in the same way that it is formed in maternal tissues, and the only means for excreting the carbon dioxide from the fetus is through the placenta into the mother's blood. The Pco$_2$ of the fetal blood is 2 to 3 mm Hg higher than that of the maternal blood. This small pressure gradient for carbon dioxide across the membrane is more than sufficient to allow adequate diffusion of carbon dioxide because the extreme solubility of carbon dioxide in the placental membrane allows carbon dioxide to diffuse about 20 times as rapidly as oxygen.

Diffusion of Foodstuffs Through the Placental Membrane. Other metabolic substrates needed by the fetus diffuse into the fetal blood in the same manner as oxygen does. For instance, in the late stages of pregnancy, the fetus often uses as much glucose as the entire body of the mother uses. To provide this much glucose, the trophoblast cells lining the placental villi provide for *facilitated diffusion* of glucose through the placental membrane. That is, the glucose is transported by carrier molecules in the trophoblast cells of the membrane. Even so, the glucose level in fetal blood is 20 to 30 percent lower than that in maternal blood.

Because of the high solubility of fatty acids in cell membranes, these also diffuse from the maternal blood into the fetal blood, but more slowly than glucose, so that glucose is used more easily by the fetus for nutrition. Also, such substances as ketone bodies and potassium, sodium, and chloride ions diffuse with relative ease from the maternal blood into the fetal blood.

Excretion of Waste Products Through the Placental Membrane. In the same manner that carbon dioxide diffuses from the fetal blood into the maternal blood, other excretory products formed in the fetus also diffuse through the placental membrane into the maternal blood and are then excreted along with the excretory products of the mother. These include especially the *nonprotein nitrogens* such as *urea, uric acid,* and *creatinine.* The level of urea in fetal blood is only slightly greater than that in maternal blood because urea diffuses through the placental membrane with great ease. However, creatinine, which does not diffuse as easily, has a fetal blood concentration considerably higher than that in the mother's blood. Therefore, excretion from the fetus depends mainly, if not entirely, on the diffusion gradients across the placental membrane and its permeability. Because there are higher concentrations of the excretory products in the fetal blood than in the maternal blood, there is continual diffusion of these substances from the fetal blood to the maternal blood.

Hormonal Factors in Pregnancy

In pregnancy, the placenta forms especially large quantities of *human chorionic gonadotropin, estrogens, progesterone,* and *human chorionic somatomammotropin,* the first three of which, and probably the fourth as well, are all essential to a normal pregnancy.

Human Chorionic Gonadotropin Causes Persistence of the Corpus Luteum and Prevents Menstruation

Menstruation normally occurs in a nonpregnant woman about 14 days after ovulation, at which time most of the endometrium of the uterus sloughs away from the uterine wall and is expelled to the exterior. If this should happen after an ovum has implanted, the pregnancy would terminate. However, this is prevented by the secretion of human chorionic gonadotropin by the newly developing embryonic tissues in the following manner.

Coincidental with the development of the trophoblast cells from the early fertilized ovum, the hormone *human chorionic gonadotropin* is secreted by the syncytial trophoblast cells into the fluids of the mother, as shown in Figure 82-7. The secretion of this hormone can first be

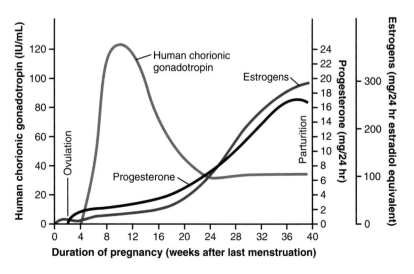

Figure 82-7 Rates of secretion of estrogens and progesterone, and concentration of human chorionic gonadotropin at different stages of pregnancy.

measured in the blood 8 to 9 days after ovulation, shortly after the blastocyst implants in the endometrium. Then the rate of secretion rises rapidly to reach a maximum at about 10 to 12 weeks of pregnancy and decreases back to a lower value by 16 to 20 weeks. It continues at this elevated level for the remainder of pregnancy.

Function of Human Chorionic Gonadotropin. Human chorionic gonadotropin is a glycoprotein having a molecular weight of about 39,000 and much the same molecular structure and function as luteinizing hormone secreted by the pituitary gland. By far, its most important function is to prevent involution of the corpus luteum at the end of the monthly female sexual cycle. Instead, it causes the corpus luteum to secrete even larger quantities of its sex hormones—progesterone and estrogens—for the next few months. These sex hormones prevent menstruation and cause the endometrium to continue to grow and store large amounts of nutrients rather than being shed in the menstruum. As a result, the *decidua-like cells* that develop in the endometrium during the normal female sexual cycle become actual *decidual cells—* greatly swollen and nutritious—at about the time that the blastocyst implants.

Under the influence of human chorionic gonadotropin, the corpus luteum in the mother's ovary grows to about twice its initial size by a month or so after pregnancy begins. Its continued secretion of estrogens and progesterone maintains the decidual nature of the uterine endometrium, which is necessary for the early development of the fetus.

If the corpus luteum is removed before approximately the seventh week of pregnancy, spontaneous abortion almost always occurs, sometimes even up to the 12th week. After that time, the placenta secretes sufficient quantities of progesterone and estrogens to maintain pregnancy for the remainder of the gestation period. The corpus luteum involutes slowly after the 13th to 17th week of gestation.

Effect of Human Chorionic Gonadotropin on the Fetal Testes. Human chorionic gonadotropin also exerts an *interstitial cell*–stimulating effect on the testes of the male fetus, resulting in the production of testosterone in male fetuses until the time of birth. This small secretion of testosterone during gestation is what causes the fetus to grow male sex organs instead of female organs. Near the end of pregnancy, the testosterone secreted by the fetal testes also causes the testes to descend into the scrotum.

Secretion of Estrogens by the Placenta

The placenta, like the corpus luteum, secretes both estrogens and progesterone. Histochemical and physiological studies show that these two hormones, like most other placental hormones, are secreted by the *syncytial trophoblast* cells of the placenta.

Figure 82-7 shows that toward the end of pregnancy, the daily production of placental estrogens increases to about 30 times the mother's normal level of production. However, the secretion of estrogens by the placenta is quite different from secretion by the ovaries. Most important, the estrogens secreted by the placenta are not synthesized de novo from basic substrates in the placenta. Instead, they are formed almost entirely from androgenic steroid compounds, *dehydroepiandrosterone* and *16-hydroxy-dehydroepiandrosterone,* which are formed both in the mother's adrenal glands and in the adrenal glands of the fetus. These weak androgens are transported by the blood to the placenta and converted by the trophoblast cells into estradiol, estrone, and estriol. (The cortices of the fetal adrenal glands are extremely large, and about 80 percent consists of a so-called *fetal zone,* the primary function of which seems to be to secrete dehydroepiandrosterone during pregnancy.)

Function of Estrogen in Pregnancy. In the discussions of estrogens in Chapter 81, we pointed out that these hormones exert mainly a proliferative function on most reproductive and associated organs of the mother. During pregnancy, the extreme quantities of estrogens cause (1) enlargement of the mother's uterus, (2) enlargement of the mother's breasts and growth of the breast ductal structure, and (3) enlargement of the mother's female external genitalia.

The estrogens also relax the pelvic ligaments of the mother, so the sacroiliac joints become relatively limber and the symphysis pubis becomes elastic. These changes allow easier passage of the fetus through the birth canal. There is much reason to believe that estrogens also affect many general aspects of fetal development during pregnancy, for example, by affecting the rate of cell reproduction in the early embryo.

Secretion of Progesterone by the Placenta

Progesterone is also essential for a successful pregnancy— in fact, it is just as important as estrogen. In addition to being secreted in moderate quantities by the corpus luteum at the beginning of pregnancy, it is secreted later in tremendous quantities by the placenta, averaging about a 10-fold increase during the course of pregnancy, as shown in Figure 82-7.

The special effects of progesterone that are essential for the normal progression of pregnancy are as follows:

1. Progesterone causes decidual cells to develop in the uterine endometrium, and these cells play an important role in the nutrition of the early embryo.

2. Progesterone decreases the contractility of the pregnant uterus, thus preventing uterine contractions from causing spontaneous abortion.

3. Progesterone contributes to the development of the conceptus even before implantation because it specifically increases the secretions of the mother's fallopian tubes and uterus to provide appropriate nutritive matter for the developing *morula* (the spherical mass of 16 to 32 blastomeres formed before the blastula) and *blastocyst.* There is also reason to believe that

progesterone affects cell cleavage in the early developing embryo.

4. The progesterone secreted during pregnancy helps the estrogen prepare the mother's breasts for lactation, which is discussed later in this chapter.

Human Chorionic Somatomammotropin

A more recently discovered placental hormone is called *human chorionic somatomammotropin.* It is a protein with a molecular weight of about 22,000, and it begins to be secreted by the placenta at about the fifth week of pregnancy. Secretion of this hormone increases progressively throughout the remainder of pregnancy in direct proportion to the weight of the placenta. Although the functions of chorionic somatomammotropin are uncertain, it is secreted in quantities several times greater than all the other pregnancy hormones combined. It has several possible important effects.

First, when administered to several types of lower animals, human chorionic somatomammotropin causes at least partial development of the animal's breasts and in some instances causes lactation. Because this was the first function of the hormone discovered, it was first named *human placental lactogen* and was believed to have functions similar to those of prolactin. However, attempts to promote lactation in humans with its use have not been successful.

Second, this hormone has weak actions similar to those of growth hormone, causing the formation of protein tissues in the same way that growth hormone does. It also has a chemical structure similar to that of growth hormone, but 100 times as much human chorionic somatomammotropin as growth hormone is required to promote growth.

Third, human chorionic somatomammotropin causes decreased insulin sensitivity and decreased utilization of glucose in the mother, thereby making larger quantities of glucose available to the fetus. Because glucose is the major substrate used by the fetus to energize its growth, the possible importance of such a hormonal effect is obvious. Further, the hormone promotes the release of free fatty acids from the fat stores of the mother, thus providing this alternative source of energy for the mother's metabolism during pregnancy. Therefore, it appears that human chorionic somatomammotropin is a general metabolic hormone that has specific nutritional implications for both the mother and the fetus.

Other Hormonal Factors in Pregnancy

Almost all the nonsexual endocrine glands of the mother also react markedly to pregnancy. This results mainly from the increased metabolic load on the mother but also, to some extent, from the effects of placental hormones on the pituitary and other glands. Some of the most notable effects are the following.

Pituitary Secretion. The anterior pituitary gland of the mother enlarges at least 50 percent during pregnancy and increases its production of *corticotropin, thyrotropin,* and *prolactin.* Conversely, pituitary secretion of follicle-stimulating hormone and luteinizing hormone is almost totally suppressed as a result of the inhibitory effects of estrogens and progesterone from the placenta.

Increased Corticosteroid Secretion. The rate of adrenocortical secretion of the *glucocorticoids* is moderately increased throughout pregnancy. It is possible that these glucocorticoids help mobilize amino acids from the mother's tissues so that these can be used for synthesis of tissues in the fetus.

Pregnant women usually have about a twofold increase in the secretion of *aldosterone,* reaching a peak at the end of gestation. This, along with the actions of estrogens, causes a tendency for even a normal pregnant woman to reabsorb excess sodium from her renal tubules and, therefore, to retain fluid, occasionally leading to *pregnancy-induced hypertension.*

Increased Thyroid Gland Secretion. The mother's thyroid gland ordinarily enlarges up to 50 percent during pregnancy and increases its production of thyroxine a corresponding amount. The increased thyroxine production is caused at least partly by a thyrotropic effect of *human chorionic gonadotropin* secreted by the placenta and by small quantities of a specific thyroid-stimulating hormone, *human chorionic thyrotropin,* also secreted by the placenta.

Increased Parathyroid Gland Secretion. The mother's parathyroid glands usually enlarge during pregnancy; this is especially true if the mother is on a calcium-deficient diet. Enlargement of these glands causes calcium absorption from the mother's bones, thereby maintaining normal calcium ion concentration in the mother's extracellular fluid even while the fetus removes calcium to ossify its own bones. This secretion of parathyroid hormone is even more intensified during lactation after the baby's birth because the growing baby requires many times more calcium than the fetus does.

Secretion of "Relaxin" by the Ovaries and Placenta. Another substance besides the estrogens and progesterone, a hormone called *relaxin,* is secreted by the corpus luteum of the ovary and by placental tissues. Its secretion is increased by a stimulating effect of human chorionic gonadotropin at the same time that the corpus luteum and the placenta secrete large quantities of estrogens and progesterone.

Relaxin is a 48-amino acid polypeptide having a molecular weight of about 9000. This hormone, when injected, causes relaxation of the ligaments of the symphysis pubis in the estrous rat and guinea pig. This effect is weak or possibly even absent in pregnant women. Instead, this role is probably played mainly by the estrogens, which also cause relaxation of the pelvic ligaments. It has also been claimed that relaxin softens the cervix of the pregnant woman at the time of delivery.

Response of the Mother's Body to Pregnancy

Most apparent among the many reactions of the mother to the fetus and to the excessive hormones of pregnancy is the increased size of the various sexual organs. For instance, the uterus increases from about 50 grams to 1100 grams, and the breasts approximately double in size. At the same time, the vagina enlarges and the introitus opens more widely.

Also, the various hormones can cause marked changes in a pregnant woman's appearance, sometimes resulting in the development of edema, acne, and masculine or acromegalic features.

Weight Gain in the Pregnant Woman

The average weight gain during pregnancy is about 25 to 35 pounds, with most of this gain occurring during the last two trimesters. Of this, about 8 pounds is fetus and 4 pounds is amniotic fluid, placenta, and fetal membranes. The uterus increases about 3 pounds and the breasts another 2 pounds, still leaving an average weight increase of 8 to 18 pounds. About 5 pounds of this is extra fluid in the blood and extracellular fluid, and the remaining 3 to 13 pounds is generally fat accumulation. The extra fluid is excreted in the urine during the first few days after birth, that is, after loss of the fluid-retaining hormones from the placenta.

During pregnancy, a woman often has a greatly increased desire for food, partly as a result of removal of food substrates from the mother's blood by the fetus and partly because of hormonal factors. Without appropriate prenatal control of diet, the mother's weight gain can be as great as 75 pounds instead of the usual 25 to 35 pounds.

Metabolism During Pregnancy

As a consequence of the increased secretion of many hormones during pregnancy, including thyroxine, adrenocortical hormones, and the sex hormones, the basal metabolic rate of the pregnant woman increases about 15 percent during the latter half of pregnancy. As a result, she frequently has sensations of becoming overheated. Also, owing to the extra load that she is carrying, greater amounts of energy than normal must be expended for muscle activity.

Nutrition During Pregnancy

By far the greatest growth of the fetus occurs during the last trimester of pregnancy; its weight almost doubles during the last 2 months of pregnancy. Ordinarily, the mother does not absorb sufficient protein, calcium, phosphates, and iron from her diet during the last months of pregnancy to supply these extra needs of the fetus. However, anticipating these extra needs, the mother's body has already been storing these substances—some in the placenta, but most in the normal storage depots of the mother.

If appropriate nutritional elements are not present in a pregnant woman's diet, a number of maternal deficiencies can occur, especially in calcium, phosphates, iron, and the vitamins. For example, the fetus needs about 375 milligrams of iron to form its blood, and the mother needs an additional 600 milligrams to form her own extra blood. The normal store of nonhemoglobin iron in the mother at the outset of pregnancy is often only 100 milligrams and almost never more than 700 milligrams. Therefore, without sufficient iron in her food, a pregnant woman usually develops *hypochromic anemia*. Also, it is especially important that she receive vitamin D, because although the total quantity of calcium used by the fetus is small, calcium is normally poorly absorbed by the mother's gastrointestinal tract without vitamin D. Finally, shortly before birth of the baby, vitamin K is often added to the mother's diet so that the baby will have sufficient prothrombin to prevent hemorrhage, particularly brain hemorrhage, caused by the birth process.

Changes in the Maternal Circulatory System During Pregnancy

Blood Flow Through the Placenta, and Maternal Cardiac Output Increases During Pregnancy. About 625 milliliters of blood flows through the maternal circulation of the placenta each minute during the last month of pregnancy. This, plus the general increase in the mother's metabolism, increases the mother's cardiac output to 30 to 40 percent above normal by the 27th week of pregnancy; then, for reasons unexplained, the cardiac output falls to only a little above normal during the last 8 weeks of pregnancy, despite the high uterine blood flow.

Maternal Blood Volume Increases During Pregnancy. The maternal blood volume shortly before term is about 30 percent above normal. This increase occurs mainly during the latter half of pregnancy, as shown by the curve of Figure 82-8. The cause of the increased volume is likely due, at least in part, to aldosterone and estrogens, which are greatly increased in pregnancy, and to increased fluid retention by the kidneys. Also, the bone marrow becomes increasingly active and produces extra red blood cells to go with the excess fluid volume. Therefore, at the time of birth of the baby, the mother has about 1 to 2 liters of extra blood in her circulatory system. Only about one fourth of this amount is normally lost through bleeding during delivery of the baby, thereby allowing a considerable safety factor for the mother.

Maternal Respiration Increases During Pregnancy

Because of the increased basal metabolic rate of a pregnant woman and because of her greater size, the total amount of oxygen used by the mother shortly before birth of the baby is about 20 percent above normal and a commensurate amount of carbon dioxide is formed. These effects cause the mother's minute ventilation to increase. It is also believed that the high levels of progesterone during pregnancy increase the minute ventilation even more, because progesterone increases the respiratory center's sensitivity to carbon dioxide. The net result is an increase in minute ventilation of about 50 percent and a decrease in arterial P_{CO_2} to several millimeters of mercury below that in a nonpregnant woman. Simultaneously, the growing uterus presses upward against the abdominal contents, which press upward against the diaphragm, so the total excursion of the diaphragm is decreased. Consequently, the respiratory rate is increased to maintain the extra ventilation.

Maternal Kidney Function During Pregnancy

The rate of urine formation by a pregnant woman is usually slightly increased because of increased fluid intake and increased load of excretory products. But in addition, several special alterations of kidney function occur.

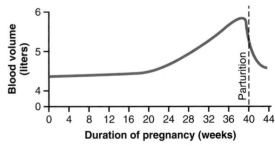

Figure 82-8 Effect of pregnancy to increase the mother's blood volume.

First, the renal tubules' reabsorptive capacity for sodium, chloride, and water is increased as much as 50 percent as a consequence of increased production of salt and water retaining hormones, especially steroid hormones by the placenta and adrenal cortex.

Second, the renal blood flow and glomerular filtration rate increase up to 50 percent during normal pregnancy due to renal vasodilation. Although the mechanisms that cause renal vasodilation in pregnancy are still unclear, some studies suggest that increased levels of nitric oxide or the ovarian hormone relaxin may contribute to these changes. The increased glomerular filtration rate likely occurs, at least in part, as a compensation for increased tubular reabsorption of salt and water. Thus, the *normal* pregnant woman ordinarily accumulates only about 5 pounds of extra water and salt.

Amniotic Fluid and Its Formation

Normally, the volume of *amniotic fluid* (the fluid inside the uterus in which the fetus floats) is between 500 milliliters and 1 liter, but it can be only a few milliliters or as much as several liters. Isotope studies of the rate of formation of amniotic fluid show that, on average, the water in amniotic fluid is replaced once every 3 hours and the electrolytes sodium and potassium are replaced an average of once every 15 hours. A large portion of the fluid is derived from renal excretion by the fetus. Likewise, a certain amount of absorption occurs by way of the gastrointestinal tract and lungs of the fetus. However, even after in utero death of a fetus, some turnover of the amniotic fluid is still present, which indicates that some of the fluid is formed and absorbed directly through the amniotic membranes.

Preeclampsia and Eclampsia

About 5 percent of all pregnant women experience a rapid rise in arterial blood pressure to hypertensive levels during the last few months of pregnancy. This is also associated with leakage of large amounts of protein into the urine. This condition is called *preeclampsia* or *toxemia of pregnancy*. It is often characterized by excess salt and water retention by the mother's kidneys and by weight gain and development of edema and hypertension in the mother. In addition, there is impaired function of the vascular endothelium and arterial spasm occurs in many parts of the mother's body, most significantly in the kidneys, brain, and liver. Both the renal blood flow and the glomerular filtration rate are decreased, which is exactly opposite to the changes that occur in the normal pregnant woman. The renal effects also include thickened glomerular tufts that contain a protein deposit in the basement membranes.

Various attempts have been made to prove that preeclampsia is caused by excessive secretion of placental or adrenal hormones, but proof of a hormonal basis is still lacking. Another theory is that preeclampsia results from some type of autoimmunity or allergy in the mother caused by the presence of the fetus. In support of this, the acute symptoms usually disappear within a few days after birth of the baby.

There is also evidence that preeclampsia is initiated by *insufficient blood supply to the placenta*, resulting in the placenta's release of substances that cause widespread dysfunction of the maternal vascular endothelium. During normal placental development, the trophoblasts invade the arterioles of the uterine endometrium and completely remodel the maternal arterioles into large blood vessels with low resistance to blood flow. In patients with preeclampsia, the maternal arterioles fail to undergo these adaptive changes, for reasons that are still unclear, and there is insuf-

ficient blood supply to the placenta. This, in turn, causes the placenta to release various substances that enter the mother's circulation and cause impaired vascular endothelial function, decreased blood flow to the kidneys, excess salt and water retention, and increased blood pressure.

Although the factors that link reduced placental blood supply with maternal endothelial dysfunction are still uncertain, some experimental studies suggest a role for increased levels of *inflammatory cytokines* such as *tumor necrosis factor-α and interleukin-6*. Placental factors that impede angiogenesis (blood vessel growth) have also been shown to contribute to increased inflammatory cytokines and preeclampsia. For example, the antiangiogenic proteins *soluble fms-related tyrosine kinase 1* (s-Flt1) and *soluble endoglin* are increased in the blood of women with preeclampsia. These substances are released by the placenta into the maternal circulation in response to ischemia and hypoxia of the placenta. Soluble endoglin and s-Flt1 have multiple effects that may impair function of the maternal vascular endothelium and result in hypertension, proteinuria, and the other systemic manifestations of preeclampsia. However, the precise role of the various factors released from the ischemic placenta in causing the multiple cardiovascular and renal abnormalities in women with preeclampsia is still uncertain.

Eclampsia is an extreme degree of preeclampsia, characterized by vascular spasm throughout the body; clonic seizures in the mother, sometimes followed by coma; greatly decreased kidney output; malfunction of the liver; often extreme hypertension; and a generalized toxic condition of the body. It usually occurs shortly before birth of the baby. Without treatment, a high percentage of eclamptic mothers die. However, with optimal and immediate use of rapidly acting vasodilating drugs to reduce the arterial pressure to normal, followed by immediate termination of pregnancy—by cesarean section if necessary—the mortality even in eclamptic mothers has been reduced to 1 percent or less.

Parturition

Increased Uterine Excitability Near Term

Parturition means birth of the baby. Toward the end of pregnancy, the uterus becomes progressively more excitable, until finally it develops such strong rhythmical contractions that the baby is expelled. The exact cause of the increased activity of the uterus is not known, but at least two major categories of effects lead up to the intense contractions responsible for parturition: (1) progressive hormonal changes that cause increased excitability of the uterine musculature and (2) progressive mechanical changes.

Hormonal Factors That Increase Uterine Contractility

Increased Ratio of Estrogens to Progesterone. Progesterone inhibits uterine contractility during pregnancy, thereby helping to prevent expulsion of the fetus. Conversely, estrogens have a definite tendency to increase the degree of uterine contractility, partly because estrogens increase the number of gap junctions between the adjacent uterine smooth muscle cells, but also because of other poorly understood effects. Both progesterone and estrogen are secreted in progressively greater quantities throughout most of pregnancy, but from the seventh month onward, estrogen secretion continues to increase while progesterone secretion remains constant or perhaps even decreases slightly. Therefore, it has been postulated that the *estrogen-to-progesterone ratio* increases sufficiently toward the end of pregnancy to be at least partly responsible for the increased contractility of the uterus.

Oxytocin Causes Contraction of the Uterus. Oxytocin is a hormone secreted by the neurohypophysis that specifically causes uterine contraction (see Chapter 75). There are four reasons to believe that oxytocin might be important in increasing the contractility of the uterus near term: (1) The uterine muscle increases its oxytocin receptors and, therefore, increases its responsiveness to a given dose of oxytocin during the latter few months of pregnancy. (2) The rate of oxytocin secretion by the neurohypophysis is considerably increased at the time of labor. (3) Although hypophysectomized animals can still deliver their young at term, labor is prolonged. (4) Experiments in animals indicate that irritation or stretching of the uterine cervix, as occurs during labor, can cause a neurogenic reflex through the paraventricular and supraoptic nuclei of the hypothalamus that causes the posterior pituitary gland (the neurohypophysis) to increase its secretion of oxytocin.

Effect of Fetal Hormones on the Uterus. The fetus's pituitary gland secretes increasing quantities of oxytocin, which might play a role in exciting the uterus. Also, the fetus's adrenal glands secrete large quantities of cortisol, another possible uterine stimulant. In addition, the fetal membranes release prostaglandins in high concentration at the time of labor. These, too, can increase the intensity of uterine contractions.

Mechanical Factors That Increase Uterine Contractility

Stretch of the Uterine Musculature. Simply stretching smooth muscle organs usually increases their contractility. Further, intermittent stretch, as occurs repeatedly in the uterus because of fetal movements, can also elicit smooth muscle contraction. Note especially that twins are born, on average, *19 days* earlier than a single child, which emphasizes the importance of mechanical stretch in eliciting uterine contractions.

Stretch or Irritation of the Cervix. There is reason to believe that stretching or irritating the uterine cervix is particularly important in eliciting uterine contractions. For instance, the obstetrician frequently induces labor by rupturing the membranes so that the head of the baby stretches the cervix more forcefully than usual or irritates it in other ways.

The mechanism by which cervical irritation excites the body of the uterus is not known. It has been suggested that stretching or irritation of nerves in the cervix initiates reflexes to the body of the uterus, but the effect could also result simply from myogenic transmission of signals from the cervix to the body of the uterus.

Onset of Labor—A Positive Feedback Mechanism for Its Initiation

During most of the months of pregnancy, the uterus undergoes periodic episodes of weak and slow rhythmical contractions called *Braxton Hicks contractions.* These contractions become progressively stronger toward the end of pregnancy; then they change suddenly, within hours, to become exceptionally strong contractions that start stretching the cervix and later force the baby through the birth canal, thereby causing parturition. This process is called *labor,* and the strong contractions that result in final parturition are called *labor contractions.*

We do not know what suddenly changes the slow, weak rhythmicity of the uterus into strong labor contractions. However, on the basis of experience with other types of physiological control systems, a theory has been proposed for explaining the onset of labor. The *positive feedback* theory suggests that stretching of the cervix by the fetus's head finally becomes great enough to elicit a strong reflex increase in contractility of the uterine body. This pushes the baby forward, which stretches the cervix more and initiates more positive feedback to the uterine body. Thus, the process repeats until the baby is expelled. This theory is shown in Figure 82-9, and the observations supporting it are the following.

First, labor contractions obey all the principles of positive feedback. That is, once the strength of uterine contraction becomes greater than a critical value, each contraction leads to subsequent contractions that become stronger and stronger until maximum effect is achieved. Referring to the discussion in Chapter 1 of positive

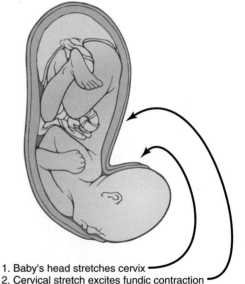

1. Baby's head stretches cervix
2. Cervical stretch excites fundic contraction
3. Fundic contraction pushes baby down and stretches cervix some more
4. Cycle repeats over and over again

Figure 82-9 Theory for the onset of intensely strong contractions during labor.

feedback in control systems, one can see that this is the precise nature of all positive feedback mechanisms when the feedback gain becomes greater than a critical value.

Second, two known types of positive feedback increase uterine contractions during labor: (1) Stretching of the cervix causes the entire body of the uterus to contract, and this contraction stretches the cervix even more because of the downward thrust of the baby's head. (2) Cervical stretching also causes the pituitary gland to secrete oxytocin, which is another means for increasing uterine contractility.

To summarize, we can assume that multiple factors increase the contractility of the uterus toward the end of pregnancy. Eventually a uterine contraction becomes strong enough to irritate the uterus, especially at the cervix, and this increases uterine contractility still more because of positive feedback, resulting in a second uterine contraction stronger than the first, a third stronger than the second, and so forth. Once these contractions become strong enough to cause this type of feedback, with each succeeding contraction greater than the preceding one, the process proceeds to completion—all *because positive feedback initiates a vicious circle when the gain of the feedback is greater than a critical level.*

One might ask about the many instances of false labor, in which the contractions become stronger and stronger and then fade away. Remember that for a vicious circle to continue, *each* new cycle of the positive feedback must be stronger than the previous one. If at any time after labor starts some contractions fail to re-excite the uterus sufficiently, the positive feedback could go into a retrograde decline and the labor contractions would fade away.

Abdominal Muscle Contractions During Labor

Once uterine contractions become strong during labor, pain signals originate both from the uterus and from the birth canal. These signals, in addition to causing suffering, elicit neurogenic reflexes in the spinal cord to the abdominal muscles, causing intense contractions of these muscles. The abdominal contractions add greatly to the force that causes expulsion of the baby.

Mechanics of Parturition

The uterine contractions during labor begin mainly at the top of the uterine fundus and spread downward over the body of the uterus. Also, the intensity of contraction is great in the top and body of the uterus but weak in the lower segment of the uterus adjacent to the cervix. Therefore, each uterine contraction tends to force the baby downward toward the cervix.

In the early part of labor, the contractions might occur only once every 30 minutes. As labor progresses, the contractions finally appear as often as once every 1 to 3 minutes and the intensity of contraction increases greatly, with only a short period of relaxation between contractions. The combined contractions of the uterine and abdominal musculature during delivery of the baby cause a downward force on the fetus of about 25 pounds during each strong contraction.

It is fortunate that the contractions of labor occur intermittently, because strong contractions impede or sometimes even stop blood flow through the placenta and would cause death of the fetus if the contractions were continuous. Indeed, overuse of various uterine stimulants, such as oxytocin, can cause uterine spasm rather than rhythmical contractions and can lead to death of the fetus.

In more than 95 percent of births, the head is the first part of the baby to be expelled, and in most of the remaining instances, the buttocks are presented first. When the baby enters the birth canal with the buttocks or feet first, this is called a *breech* presentation.

The head acts as a wedge to open the structures of the birth canal as the fetus is forced downward. The first major obstruction to expulsion of the fetus is the uterine cervix. Toward the end of pregnancy, the cervix becomes soft, which allows it to stretch when labor contractions begin in the uterus. The so-called *first stage of labor* is a period of progressive cervical dilation, lasting until the cervical opening is as large as the head of the fetus. This stage usually lasts for 8 to 24 hours in the first pregnancy but often only a few minutes after many pregnancies.

Once the cervix has dilated fully, the fetal membranes usually rupture and the amniotic fluid is lost suddenly through the vagina. Then the fetus's head moves rapidly into the birth canal, and with additional force from above, it continues to wedge its way through the canal until delivery is effected. This is called the *second stage of labor,* and it may last from as little as 1 minute after many pregnancies to 30 minutes or more in the first pregnancy.

Separation and Delivery of the Placenta

For 10 to 45 minutes after birth of the baby, the uterus continues to contract to a smaller and smaller size, which causes a *shearing* effect between the walls of the uterus and the placenta, thus separating the placenta from its implantation site. Separation of the placenta opens the placental sinuses and causes bleeding. The amount of bleeding is limited to an average of 350 milliliters by the following mechanism: The smooth muscle fibers of the uterine musculature are arranged in figures of eight around the blood vessels as the vessels pass through the uterine wall. Therefore, contraction of the uterus after delivery of the baby constricts the vessels that had previously supplied blood to the placenta. In addition, it is believed that vasoconstrictor prostaglandins formed at the placental separation site cause additional blood vessel spasm.

Labor Pains

With each uterine contraction, the mother experiences considerable pain. The cramping pain in early labor is probably caused mainly by hypoxia of the uterine muscle resulting from compression of the blood vessels in the uterus. This pain is not felt when the visceral sensory *hypogastric nerves,* which carry the visceral sensory fibers leading from the uterus, have been sectioned.

However, during the second stage of labor, when the fetus is being expelled through the birth canal, much more severe pain is caused by cervical stretching, perineal stretching, and stretching or tearing of structures in the vaginal canal itself. This pain is conducted to the mother's spinal cord and brain by somatic nerves instead of by the visceral sensory nerves.

Involution of the Uterus After Parturition

During the first 4 to 5 weeks after parturition, the uterus involutes. Its weight becomes less than half its immediate postpartum weight within 1 week, and in 4 weeks, if the mother lactates, the uterus may become as small as it was before pregnancy. This effect of lactation results from the suppression of pituitary gonadotropin and ovarian hormone secretion during the first few months of lactation, as discussed later. During early involution of the uterus, the placental site on the endometrial surface autolyzes, causing a vaginal discharge known as "lochia," which is first bloody and then serous in nature, continuing for a total of about 10 days. After this time, the endometrial surface becomes re-epithelialized and ready for normal, nongravid sex life again.

Lactation

Development of the Breasts

The breasts, shown in Figure 82-10, begin to develop at puberty. This development is stimulated by the estrogens of the monthly female sexual cycle; estrogens stimulate

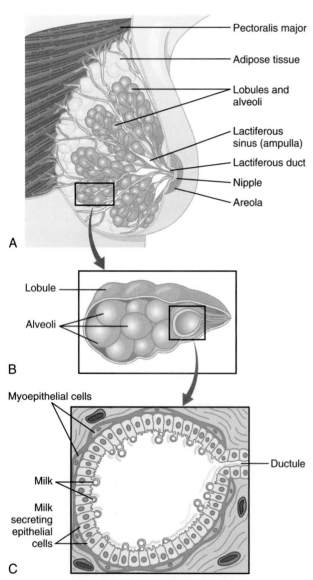

A

Lobule

Alveoli

B

Myoepithelial cells

Milk

Milk secreting epithelial cells

Ductule

C

Figure 82-10 The breast and its secretory lobules, alveoli, and lactiferous ducts (milk ducts) that constitute its mammary gland (*A*). The enlargements show a lobule (*B*) and milk-secreting cells of an alveolus (*C*).

Pectoralis major

Adipose tissue

Lobules and alveoli

Lactiferous sinus (ampulla)

Lactiferous duct

Nipple

Areola

growth of the breasts' *mammary glands* plus the deposition of fat to give the breasts mass. In addition, far greater growth occurs during the high-estrogen state of pregnancy, and only then does the glandular tissue become completely developed for the production of milk.

Estrogens Stimulate Growth of the Ductal System of the Breasts. All through pregnancy, the large quantities of estrogens secreted by the placenta cause the ductal system of the breasts to grow and branch. Simultaneously, the stroma of the breasts increases in quantity, and large quantities of fat are laid down in the stroma.

Also important for growth of the ductal system are at least four other hormones: *growth hormone, prolactin, the adrenal glucocorticoids,* and *insulin.* Each of these is known to play at least some role in protein metabolism, which presumably explains their function in the development of the breasts.

Progesterone Is Required for Full Development of the Lobule-Alveolar System. Final development of the breasts into milk-secreting organs also requires *progesterone.* Once the ductal system has developed, progesterone—acting synergistically with estrogen, as well as with the other hormones just mentioned—causes additional growth of the breast lobules, with budding of alveoli and development of secretory characteristics in the cells of the alveoli. These changes are analogous to the secretory effects of progesterone on the endometrium of the uterus during the latter half of the female menstrual cycle.

Prolactin Promotes Lactation

Although estrogen and progesterone are essential for the physical development of the breasts during pregnancy, a specific effect of both these hormones is to inhibit *the actual secretion of milk.* Conversely, the hormone *prolactin* has exactly the opposite effect on milk secretion—promoting it. This hormone is secreted by the mother's anterior pituitary gland, and its concentration in her blood rises steadily from the fifth week of pregnancy until birth of the baby, at which time it has risen to 10 to 20 times the normal nonpregnant level. This high level of prolactin at the end of pregnancy is shown in Figure 82-11.

In addition, the placenta secretes large quantities of *human chorionic somatomammotropin,* which probably has lactogenic properties, thus supporting the prolactin from the mother's pituitary during pregnancy. Even so, because of the suppressive effects of estrogen and progesterone, no more than a few milliliters of fluid are secreted each day until after the baby is born. The fluid secreted during the last few days before and the first few days after parturition is called *colostrum;* it contains essentially the same concentrations of proteins and lactose as milk, but it has almost no fat and its maximum rate of production is about 1/100 the subsequent rate of milk production.

Immediately after the baby is born, the sudden loss of both estrogen and progesterone secretion from the

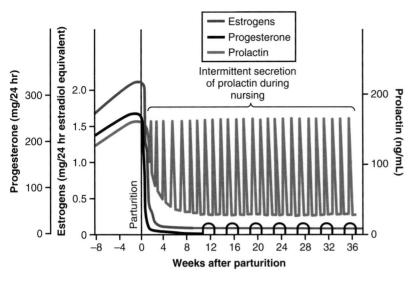

Figure 82-11 Changes in rates of secretion of estrogens, progesterone, and prolactin for 8 weeks before parturition and 36 weeks thereafter. Note especially the decrease of prolactin secretion back to basal levels within a few weeks after parturition, but also the intermittent periods of marked prolactin secretion (for about 1 hour at a time) during and after periods of nursing.

placenta allows the lactogenic effect of prolactin from the mother's pituitary gland to assume its natural milk-promoting role, and over the next 1 to 7 days, the breasts begin to secrete copious quantities of milk instead of colostrum. This secretion of milk requires an adequate background secretion of most of the mother's other hormones as well, but most important are *growth hormone, cortisol, parathyroid hormone,* and *insulin.* These hormones are necessary to provide the amino acids, fatty acids, glucose, and calcium required for milk formation.

After birth of the baby, the *basal level* of prolactin secretion returns to the nonpregnant level over the next few weeks, as shown in Figure 82-11. However, each time the mother nurses her baby, nervous signals from the nipples to the hypothalamus cause a 10- to 20-fold surge in prolactin secretion that lasts for about 1 hour, which is also shown in Figure 82-11. This prolactin acts on the mother's breasts to keep the mammary glands secreting milk into the alveoli for the subsequent nursing periods. If this prolactin surge is absent or blocked as a result of hypothalamic or pituitary damage or if nursing does not continue, the breasts lose their ability to produce milk within 1 week or so. However, milk production can continue for several years if the child continues to suckle, although the rate of milk formation normally decreases considerably after 7 to 9 months.

Hypothalamus Secretes Prolactin Inhibitory Hormone. The hypothalamus plays an essential role in controlling prolactin secretion, as it does for almost all the other anterior pituitary hormones. However, this control is different in one aspect: The hypothalamus mainly *stimulates* production of all the other hormones, but it mainly *inhibits* prolactin production. Consequently, damage to the hypothalamus or blockage of the hypothalamic-hypophysial portal system often increases prolactin secretion while it depresses secretion of the other anterior pituitary hormones.

Therefore, it is believed that anterior pituitary secretion of prolactin is controlled either entirely or almost entirely by an inhibitory factor formed in the hypothalamus and transported through the hypothalamic-hypophysial portal system to the anterior pituitary gland. This factor is called *prolactin inhibitory hormone.* It is almost certainly the same as the catecholamine *dopamine,* which is known to be secreted by the arcuate nuclei of the hypothalamus and can decrease prolactin secretion as much as 10-fold.

Suppression of the Female Ovarian Cycles in Nursing Mothers for Many Months After Delivery. In most nursing mothers, the ovarian cycle (and ovulation) does not resume until a few weeks after cessation of nursing. The reason seems to be that the same nervous signals from the breasts to the hypothalamus that cause prolactin secretion during suckling—either because of the nervous signals themselves or because of a subsequent effect of increased prolactin—inhibit secretion of gonadotropin-releasing hormone by the hypothalamus. This, in turn, suppresses formation of the pituitary gonadotropic hormones—luteinizing hormone and follicle-stimulating hormone. However, after several months of lactation, in some mothers, especially in those who nurse their babies only some of the time, the pituitary begins to secrete sufficient gonadotropic hormones to reinstate the monthly sexual cycle, even though nursing continues.

Ejection (or "Let-Down") Process in Milk Secretion—Function of Oxytocin

Milk is secreted continuously into the alveoli of the breasts, but it does not flow easily from the alveoli into the ductal system and, therefore, does not continually leak from the breast nipples. Instead, the milk must be *ejected* from the alveoli into the ducts before the baby can obtain it. This is caused by a combined neurogenic and hormonal reflex that involves the posterior pituitary hormone *oxytocin,* as follows.

When the baby suckles, it receives virtually no milk for the first half minute or so. Sensory impulses must first be transmitted through somatic nerves from the nipples to the mother's spinal cord and then to her hypothalamus, where they cause nerve signals that promote *oxytocin* secretion at the same time that they cause prolactin secretion. The oxytocin is carried in the blood to the breasts, where it causes *myoepithelial cells* (which surround the outer walls of the alveoli) to contract, thereby expressing the milk from the alveoli into the ducts at a pressure of +10 to 20 mm Hg. Then the baby's suckling becomes effective in removing the milk. Thus, within 30 seconds to 1 minute after a baby begins to suckle, milk begins to flow. This process is called *milk ejection* or *milk let-down*.

Suckling on one breast causes milk flow not only in that breast but also in the opposite breast. It is especially interesting that fondling of the baby by the mother or hearing the baby crying often gives enough of an emotional signal to the hypothalamus to cause milk ejection.

Inhibition of Milk Ejection.

A particular problem in nursing a baby comes from the fact that many psychogenic factors or even generalized sympathetic nervous system stimulation throughout the mother's body can inhibit oxytocin secretion and consequently depress milk ejection. For this reason, many mothers must have an undisturbed period of adjustment after childbirth if they are to be successful in nursing their babies.

Milk Composition and the Metabolic Drain on the Mother Caused by Lactation

Table 82-1 lists the contents of human milk and cow's milk. The concentration of lactose in human milk is about 50 percent greater than in cow's milk, but the concentration of protein in cow's milk is ordinarily two or more times greater than in human milk. Finally, only one third as much ash, which contains calcium and other minerals, is found in human milk compared with cow's milk.

At the height of lactation in the human mother, 1.5 liters of milk may be formed each day (and even more if the mother has twins). With this degree of lactation, great quantities of energy are drained from the mother; approximately 650 to 750 kilocalories per liter (or 19 to 22 kilocalories per ounce) are contained in breast milk, although the composition and caloric content of the milk depends on the mother's diet and other factors such as the fullness of the breasts. Large amounts of metabolic sub-strates are also lost from the mother. For instance, about 50 grams of fat enter the milk each day, as well as about 100 grams of lactose, which must be derived by conversion from the mother's glucose. Also, 2 to 3 grams of calcium phosphate may be lost each day; unless the mother is drinking large quantities of milk and has an adequate intake of vitamin D, the output of calcium and phosphate by the lactating mammae will often be much greater than the intake of these substances. To supply the needed calcium and phosphate, the parathyroid glands enlarge greatly and the bones become progressively decalcified. The mother's bone decalcification is usually not a big problem during pregnancy, but it can become more important during lactation.

Antibodies and Other Anti-infectious Agents in Milk.

Not only does milk provide the newborn baby with needed nutrients, but it also provides important protection against infection. For instance, multiple types of *antibodies* and other anti-infectious agents are secreted in milk along with the nutrients. Also, several different types of white blood cells are secreted, including both *neutrophils* and *macrophages,* some of which are especially lethal to bacteria that could cause deadly infections in newborn babies. Particularly important are antibodies and macrophages that destroy *Escherichia coli* bacteria, which often cause lethal diarrhea in newborns.

When cow's milk is used to supply nutrition for the baby in place of mother's milk, the protective agents in it are usually of little value because they are normally destroyed within minutes in the internal environment of the human being.

Bibliography

Alexander BT, Bennett WA, Khalil RA, et al: Preeclampsia: linking placental ischemia with cardiovascular-renal dysfunction, *News Physiol Sci* 16:282, 2001.

Augustine RA, Ladyman SR, Grattan DR: From feeding one to feeding many: hormone-induced changes in bodyweight homeostasis during pregnancy, *J Physiol* 586:387, 2008.

Barnhart KT: Clinical practice. Ectopic pregnancy, *N Engl J Med* 361:379, 2009.

Ben-Jonathan N, Hnasko R: Dopamine as a prolactin (PRL) inhibitor, *Endocr Rev* 22:724, 2001.

Freeman ME, Kanyicska B, Lerant A, et al: Prolactin: structure, function, and regulation of secretion, *Physiol Rev* 80:1523, 2000.

Gimpl G, Fahrenholz F: The oxytocin receptor system: structure, function, and regulation, *Physiol Rev* 81:629, 2001.

Goldenberg RL, Culhane JF, Iams JD, Romero R: Epidemiology and causes of preterm birth, *Lancet* 371:75, 2008.

Khalaf Y: ABC of subfertility: tubal subfertility, *BMJ* 327:610, 2003.

Labbok MH, Clark D, Goldman AS: Breastfeeding: maintaining an irreplaceable immunological resource, *Nat Rev Immunol* 4:565, 2004.

LaMarca HL, Rosen JM: Hormones and mammary cell fate—what will I become when I grow up? *Endocrinology* 149:4317, 2008.

Murphy VE, Smith R, Giles WB, et al: Endocrine regulation of human fetal growth: the role of the mother, placenta, and fetus, *Endocr Rev* 27:141, 2006.

Osol G, Mandala M: Maternal uterine vascular remodeling during pregnancy, *Physiology (Bethesda)* 24:58, 2009.

Roberts JM, Gammill HS: Preeclampsia: recent insights, *Hypertension* 46:1243, 2005.

Table 82-1 Composition of Milk

Constituent	Human Milk (%)	Cow's Milk (%)
Water	88.5	87.0
Fat	3.3	3.5
Lactose	6.8	4.8
Casein	0.9	2.7
Lactalbumin and other proteins	0.4	0.7
Ash	0.2	0.7

Shennan DB, Peaker M: Transport of milk constituents by the mammary gland, *Physiol Rev* 80:925, 2000.

Sherwood OD: Relaxin's physiological roles and other diverse actions, *Endocr Rev* 25:205, 2004.

Simhan HN, Caritis SN: Prevention of preterm delivery, *N Engl J Med* 357:477, 2–7.

Smith R: Parturition, *N Engl J Med* 356:271, 2007.

Wang A, Rana S, Karumanchi SA: Preeclampsia: the role of angiogenic factors in its pathogenesis, *Physiology (Bethesda)* 24:147, 2009.

Wu G, Bazer FW, Cudd TA, et al: Maternal nutrition and fetal development, *J Nutr* 134:2169, 2004.

UNIT XIV

CHAPTER 83

Fetal and Neonatal Physiology

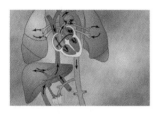

A complete discussion of fetal development, functioning of the child immediately after birth, and growth and development through the early years of life lies within the province of formal courses in obstetrics and pediatrics. However, many physiologic principles are peculiar to the infant and this chapter discusses the more important of these.

Growth and Functional Development of the Fetus

Initial development of the placenta and fetal membranes occurs far more rapidly than development of the fetus. In fact, during the first 2 to 3 weeks after implantation of the blastocyst, the fetus remains almost microscopic, but thereafter, as shown in Figure 83-1, the length of the fetus increases almost in proportion to age. At 12 weeks, the length is about 10 centimeters; at 20 weeks, 25 centimeters; and at term (40 weeks), 53 centimeters (about 21 inches). Because the weight of the fetus is approximately proportional to the cube of length, the weight increases almost in proportion to the cube of the age of the fetus.

Note in Figure 83-1 that the weight remains minuscule during the first 12 weeks and reaches 1 pound only at 23 weeks (5½ months) of gestation. Then, during the last trimester of pregnancy, the fetus gains rapidly, so 2 months before birth, the weight averages 3 pounds, 1 month before birth 4.5 pounds, and at birth 7 pounds—the final birth weight varying from as low as 4.5 pounds to as high as 11 pounds in normal infants with normal gestational periods.

Development of the Organ Systems

Within 1 month after fertilization of the ovum, the gross characteristics of all the different organs of the fetus have already begun to develop, and during the next 2 to 3 months, most of the details of the different organs are established. Beyond month 4, the organs of the fetus are grossly the same as those of the neonate. However, cellular development in each organ is usually far from complete and requires the full remaining 5 months of pregnancy for complete development. Even at birth, certain structures, particularly in the nervous system,

the kidneys, and the liver, lack full development, as discussed in more detail later in the chapter.

Circulatory System. The human heart begins beating during the fourth week after fertilization, contracting at a rate of about 65 beats/min. This increases steadily to about 140 beats/min immediately before birth.

Formation of Blood Cells. Nucleated red blood cells begin to be formed in the yolk sac and mesothelial layers of the placenta at about the third week of fetal development. This is followed 1 week later (at 4 to 5 weeks) by formation of non-nucleated red blood cells by the fetal mesenchyme and also by the endothelium of the fetal blood vessels. Then, at 6 weeks, the liver begins to form blood cells, and in the third month, the spleen and other lymphoid tissues of the body begin forming blood cells. Finally, from the third month on, the bone marrow gradually becomes the principal source of the red blood cells, as well as most of the white blood cells, except for continued lymphocyte and plasma cell production in lymphoid tissue.

Respiratory System. Respiration cannot occur during fetal life because there is no air to breathe in the amniotic cavity. However, attempted respiratory movements do take place beginning at the end of the first trimester of pregnancy. Tactile stimuli and fetal asphyxia especially cause these attempted respiratory movements.

During the last 3 to 4 months of pregnancy, the respiratory movements of the fetus are mainly inhibited, for reasons unknown, and the lungs remain almost completely deflated. The inhibition of respiration during the later months of fetal life prevents filling of the lungs with fluid and debris from the

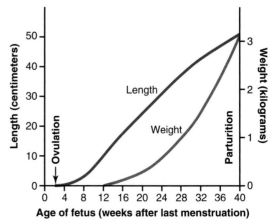

Figure 83-1 Growth of the fetus.

meconium excreted by the fetus's gastrointestinal tract into the amniotic fluid. Also, small amounts of fluid are secreted into the lungs by the alveolar epithelium up until the moment of birth, thus keeping only clean fluid in the lungs.

Nervous System. Most of the reflexes of the fetus that involve the spinal cord and even the brain stem are present by the third to fourth months of pregnancy. However, those nervous system functions that involve the cerebral cortex are still only in the early stages of development even at birth. Indeed, myelinization of some major tracts of the brain becomes complete only after about 1 year of postnatal life.

Gastrointestinal Tract. By midpregnancy the fetus begins to ingest and absorb large quantities of amniotic fluid, and during the last 2 to 3 months, gastrointestinal function approaches that of the normal neonate. By that time, small quantities of *meconium* are continually formed in the gastrointestinal tract and excreted from the anus into the amniotic fluid. Meconium is composed partly of residue from swallowed amniotic fluid and partly of *mucus,* epithelial cells, and other residues of excretory products from the gastrointestinal mucosa and glands.

Kidneys. The fetal kidneys begin to excrete urine during the second trimester pregnancy, and fetal urine accounts for about 70 to 80 percent of the amniotic fluid. Abnormal kidney development or severe impairment of kidney function in the fetus greatly reduces the formation of amniotic fluid *(oligohydramnios)* and can lead to fetal death.

Although the fetal kidneys form urine, the renal control systems for regulating fetal extracellular fluid volume and electrolyte balances, and especially acid-base balance, are almost nonexistent until late fetal life and do not reach full development until a few months after birth.

Fetal Metabolism. The fetus uses mainly glucose for energy, and the fetus has a high capability to store fat and protein, much if not most of the fat being synthesized from glucose rather than being absorbed directly from the mother's blood. In addition to these generalities, there are special problems of fetal metabolism in relation to calcium, phosphate, iron, and some vitamins.

Metabolism of Calcium and Phosphate. Figure 83-2 shows the rates of calcium and phosphate accumulation in the fetus, demonstrating that about 22.5 grams of calcium and 13.5 grams of phosphorus are accumulated in the average fetus during gestation. About one half of these accumulate during the last 4 weeks of gestation, which is coincident with the period of rapid ossification of the fetal bones and with the period of rapid weight gain of the fetus.

During the earlier part of fetal life, the bones are relatively unossified and have mainly a cartilaginous matrix. Indeed, x-ray films ordinarily do not show any ossification until after the fourth month of pregnancy.

Note especially that the total amounts of calcium and phosphate needed by the fetus during gestation represent only about 2 percent of the quantities of these substances in the mother's bones. Therefore, this is a minimal drain from the mother. Much greater drain occurs after birth during lactation.

Accumulation of Iron. Figure 83-2 also shows that iron accumulates in the fetus even more rapidly than calcium and phosphate. Most of the iron is in the form of hemoglobin, which begins to be formed as early as the third week after fertilization of the ovum.

Small amounts of iron are concentrated in the mother's uterine progestational endometrium even before implantation of the ovum; this iron is ingested into the embryo by the trophoblastic cells and is used to form the very early red blood cells. About one third of the iron in a fully developed fetus is normally stored in the liver. This iron can then be used for several months after birth by the neonate for formation of additional hemoglobin.

Utilization and Storage of Vitamins. The fetus needs vitamins equally as much as the adult and in some instances to a far greater extent. In general, the vitamins function the same in the fetus as in the adult, as discussed in Chapter 71. Special functions of several vitamins should be mentioned, however.

The B vitamins, especially vitamin B_{12} and folic acid, are necessary for formation of red blood cells and nervous tissue, as well as for overall growth of the fetus.

Vitamin C is necessary for appropriate formation of intercellular substances, especially the bone matrix and fibers of connective tissue.

Vitamin D is necessary for normal bone growth in the fetus, but even more important, the mother needs it for adequate absorption of calcium from her gastrointestinal tract. If the mother has plenty of vitamin D in her body fluids, large quantities of the vitamin will be stored by the fetal liver to be used by the neonate for several months after birth.

Vitamin E, although the mechanisms of its functions are not entirely clear, is necessary for normal development of the early embryo. In its absence in laboratory animals, spontaneous abortion usually occurs at an early stage of pregnancy.

Vitamin K is used by the fetal liver for formation of Factor VII, prothrombin, and several other blood coagulation factors. When vitamin K is insufficient in the mother, Factor VII and prothrombin become deficient in the fetus and the mother. Because most vitamin K is formed by bacterial action in the mother's colon, the neonate has no adequate source of vitamin K for the first week or so of life after birth until normal colonic bacterial flora become established in the newborn infant. Therefore, prenatal storage in the fetal liver of at least small amounts of vitamin K derived from the mother is helpful in preventing fetal hemorrhage, particularly hemorrhage in the brain when the head is traumatized by squeezing through the birth canal.

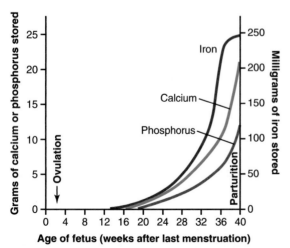

Figure 83-2 Iron, calcium, and phosphorus storage in the fetus at different stages of gestation.

Adjustments of the Infant to Extrauterine Life

Onset of Breathing

The most obvious effect of birth on the baby is loss of the placental connection with the mother and, therefore, loss of this means of metabolic support. One of the most important immediate adjustments required of the infant is to begin breathing.

Cause of Breathing at Birth. After normal delivery from a mother who has not been depressed by anesthetics, the child ordinarily begins to breathe within seconds and has a normal respiratory rhythm within less than 1 minute after birth. The promptness with which the fetus begins to breathe indicates that breathing is initiated by sudden exposure to the exterior world, probably resulting from (1) a slightly asphyxiated state incident to the birth process, but also from (2) sensory impulses that originate in the suddenly cooled skin. In an infant who does not breathe immediately, the body becomes progressively more hypoxic and hypercapnic, which provides additional stimulus to the respiratory center and usually causes breathing within an additional minute after birth.

Delayed or Abnormal Breathing at Birth—Danger of Hypoxia. If the mother has been depressed by a general anesthetic during delivery, which at least partially anesthetizes the fetus as well, the onset of respiration is likely to be delayed for several minutes, thus demonstrating the importance of using as little anesthesia as feasible. Also, many infants who have had head trauma during delivery or who undergo prolonged delivery are slow to breathe or sometimes do not breathe at all. This can result from two possible effects: First, in a few infants, intracranial hemorrhage or brain contusion causes a concussion syndrome with a greatly depressed respiratory center. Second, and probably much more important, prolonged fetal hypoxia during delivery can cause serious depression of the respiratory center.

Hypoxia frequently occurs during delivery because of (1) compression of the umbilical cord; (2) premature separation of the placenta; (3) excessive contraction of the uterus, which can cut off the mother's blood flow to the placenta; or (4) excessive anesthesia of the mother, which depresses oxygenation even of her blood.

Degree of Hypoxia That an Infant Can Tolerate. In an adult, failure to breathe for only 4 minutes often causes death, but a neonate often survives as long as 10 minutes of failure to breathe after birth. Permanent and serious brain impairment often ensues if breathing is delayed more than 8 to 10 minutes. Indeed, actual lesions develop mainly in the thalamus, in the inferior colliculi, and in other brain stem areas, thus permanently affecting many of the motor functions of the body.

Expansion of the Lungs at Birth. At birth, the walls of the alveoli are at first collapsed because of the surface tension of the viscid fluid that fills them. More than 25 mm Hg of negative inspiratory pressure in the lungs is usually required to oppose the effects of this surface tension and to open the alveoli for the first time. But once the alveoli do open, further respiration can be effected with relatively weak respiratory movements. Fortunately, the first inspirations of the normal neonate are extremely powerful, usually capable of creating as much as 60 mm Hg negative pressure in the intrapleural space.

Figure 83-3 shows the tremendous negative intrapleural pressures required to open the lungs at the onset of breathing. At the top is shown the pressure-volume curve ("compliance" curve) for the first breath after birth. Observe, first, the lower part of the curve *beginning at the zero pressure point* and moving to the right. The curve shows that the volume of air in the lungs remains almost exactly zero until the negative pressure has reached −40 centimeters water (−30 mm Hg). Then, as the negative pressure increases to −60 centimeters of water, about 40 milliliters of air enters the lungs. To deflate the lungs, considerable positive pressure, about +40 centimeters of water, is required because of viscous resistance offered by the fluid in the bronchioles.

Note that the second breath is much easier, with far less negative and positive pressures required. Breathing does not become completely normal until about 40 minutes after birth, as shown by the third compliance curve, the shape of which compares favorably with that for the normal adult, as shown in Chapter 38.

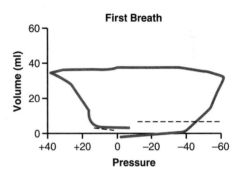

First Breath

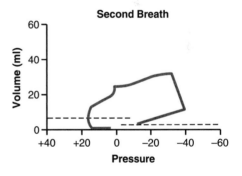

Second Breath

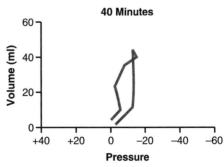

40 Minutes

Figure 83-3 Pressure-volume curves of the lungs ("compliance" curves) of a neonate immediately after birth, showing the extreme forces required for breathing during the first two breaths of life and development of a nearly normal compliance curve within 40 minutes after birth. (Redrawn from Smith CA: The first breath. Sci Am 209:32, 1963, © 1963 by Scientific American, Inc. All rights reserved.)

Respiratory Distress Syndrome Caused When Surfactant Secretion Is Deficient. A small number of infants, especially premature infants and infants born of diabetic mothers, develop severe respiratory distress in the early hours to the first several days after birth, and some die within the next day or so. The alveoli of these infants at death contain large quantities of proteinaceous fluid, almost as if pure plasma had leaked out of the capillaries into the alveoli. The fluid also contains desquamated alveolar epithelial cells. This condition is called *hyaline membrane disease* because microscopic slides of the lung show the material filling the alveoli to look like a hyaline membrane.

A characteristic finding in respiratory distress syndrome is failure of the respiratory epithelium to secrete adequate quantities of *surfactant*, a substance normally secreted into the alveoli that decreases the surface tension of the alveolar fluid, therefore allowing the alveoli to open easily during inspiration. The surfactant-secreting cells (type II alveolar epithelial cells) do not begin to secrete surfactant until the last 1 to 3 months of gestation. Therefore, many premature babies and a few full-term babies are born without the capability to secrete sufficient surfactant, which causes both a collapse tendency of the alveoli and development of pulmonary edema. The role of surfactant in preventing these effects is discussed in Chapter 37.

Circulatory Readjustments at Birth

Equally as essential as the onset of breathing at birth are immediate circulatory adjustments that allow adequate blood flow through the lungs. Also, circulatory adjustments during the first few hours of life cause more and more blood flow through the baby's liver, which up to this point has had little blood flow. To describe these readjustments, we must first consider the anatomical structure of the fetal circulation.

Specific Anatomical Structure of the Fetal Circulation. Because the lungs are mainly nonfunctional during fetal life and because the liver is only partially functional, it is not necessary for the fetal heart to pump much blood through either the lungs or the liver. However, the fetal heart must pump large quantities of blood through the placenta. Therefore, special anatomical arrangements cause the fetal circulatory system to operate much differently from that of the newborn baby.

First, as shown in Figure 83-4, blood returning from the placenta through the umbilical vein passes through the *ductus venosus*, mainly bypassing the liver. Then most of the blood entering the right atrium from the inferior vena cava is directed in a straight pathway across the posterior aspect of the right atrium and through the *foramen ovale* directly into the left atrium. Thus, the well-oxygenated blood from the placenta enters mainly the left side of the heart, rather than the right side, and is pumped by the left ventricle mainly into the arteries of the head and forelimbs.

The blood entering the right atrium from the superior vena cava is directed downward through the tricuspid valve into the right ventricle. This blood is mainly deoxygenated blood from the head region of the fetus. It is pumped by the right ventricle into the pulmonary artery and then mainly through the *ductus arteriosus* into the descending aorta, then through the two umbilical arteries into the placenta, where the deoxygenated blood becomes oxygenated.

Figure 83-5 gives the relative percentages of the total blood pumped by the heart that pass through the different vascular

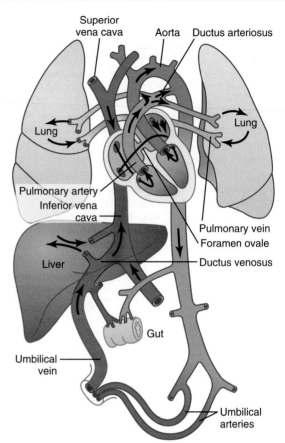

Figure 83-4 Organization of the fetal circulation. (Modified from Arey LB: Developmental Anatomy: A Textbook and Laboratory Manual of Embryology, 7th ed. Philadelphia: WB Saunders, 1974.)

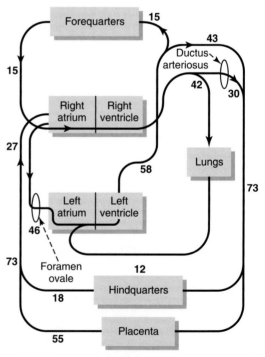

Figure 83-5 Diagram of the fetal circulatory system, showing relative distribution of blood flow to the different vascular areas. The numerals represent the percentage of the total output from both sides of the heart flowing through each particular area.

circuits of the fetus. This figure shows that 55 percent of all the blood goes through the placenta, leaving only 45 percent to pass through all the tissues of the fetus. Furthermore, during fetal life, only 12 percent of the blood flows through the lungs; immediately after birth, virtually all the blood flows through the lungs.

Changes in the Fetal Circulation at Birth. The basic changes in the fetal circulation at birth are discussed in Chapter 23 in relation to congenital anomalies of the ductus arteriosus and foramen ovale that persist throughout life in a few persons. Briefly, these changes are the following.

Decreased Pulmonary and Increased Systemic Vascular Resistances at Birth. The primary changes in the circulation at birth are, first, loss of the tremendous blood flow through the placenta, which approximately doubles the systemic vascular resistance at birth. This increases the aortic pressure, as well as the pressures in the left ventricle and left atrium.

Second, the *pulmonary vascular resistance greatly decreases* as a result of expansion of the lungs. In the unexpanded fetal lungs, the blood vessels are compressed because of the small volume of the lungs. Immediately on expansion, these vessels are no longer compressed and the resistance to blood flow decreases severalfold. Also, in fetal life, the hypoxia of the lungs causes considerable tonic vasoconstriction of the lung blood vessels, but vasodilation takes place when aeration of the lungs eliminates the hypoxia. All these changes together reduce the resistance to blood flow through the lungs as much as fivefold, which *reduces the pulmonary arterial pressure, right ventricular pressure,* and *right atrial pressure.*

Closure of the Foramen Ovale. The *low right atrial pressure* and the *high left atrial pressure* that occur secondarily to the changes in pulmonary and systemic resistances at birth cause blood now to attempt to flow backward through the foramen ovale; that is, from the left atrium into the right atrium, rather than in the other direction, as occurred during fetal life. Consequently, the small valve that lies over the foramen ovale on the left side of the atrial septum closes over this opening, thereby preventing further flow through the foramen ovale.

In two thirds of all people, the valve becomes adherent over the foramen ovale within a few months to a few years and forms a permanent closure. But even if permanent closure does not occur, the left atrial pressure throughout life normally remains 2 to 4 mm Hg greater than the right atrial pressure and the backpressure keeps the valve closed.

Closure of the Ductus Arteriosus. The ductus arteriosus also closes, but for different reasons. First, the increased systemic resistance elevates the aortic pressure while the decreased pulmonary resistance reduces the pulmonary arterial pressure. As a consequence, after birth, blood begins to flow backward from the aorta into the pulmonary artery through the ductus arteriosus, rather than in the other direction, as in fetal life. However, after only a few hours, the muscle wall of the ductus arteriosus constricts markedly and within 1 to 8 days, the constriction is usually sufficient to stop all blood flow. This is called *functional closure* of the ductus arteriosus. Then, during the next 1 to 4 months, the ductus arteriosus ordinarily becomes anatomically occluded by growth of fibrous tissue into its lumen.

The cause of ductus arteriosus closure relates to the increased oxygenation of the blood flowing through the ductus. In fetal life the Po_2 of the ductus blood is only 15 to 20 mm Hg, but it increases to about 100 mm Hg within a few hours after birth. Furthermore, many experiments have shown that the degree of contraction of the smooth muscle in the ductus wall is highly related to this availability of oxygen.

In one of several thousand infants, the ductus fails to close, resulting in a *patent ductus arteriosus,* the consequences of which are discussed in Chapter 23. The failure of closure has been postulated to result from excessive ductus dilation caused by vasodilating prostaglandins in the ductus wall. In fact, administration of the drug *indomethacin,* which blocks synthesis of prostaglandins, often leads to closure.

Closure of the Ductus Venosus. In fetal life the portal blood from the fetus's abdomen joins the blood from the umbilical vein, and these together pass by way of the *ductus venosus* directly into the vena cava immediately below the heart but above the liver, thus bypassing the liver.

Immediately after birth, blood flow through the umbilical vein ceases, but most of the portal blood still flows through the ductus venosus, with only a small amount passing through the channels of the liver. However, within 1 to 3 hours the muscle wall of the ductus venosus contracts strongly and closes this avenue of flow. As a consequence, the portal venous pressure rises from near 0 to 6 to 10 mm Hg, which is enough to force portal venous blood flow through the liver sinuses. Although the ductus venosus rarely fails to close, we know almost nothing about what causes the closure.

Nutrition of the Neonate

Before birth, the fetus derives almost all its energy from glucose obtained from the mother's blood. After birth, the amount of glucose stored in the infant's body in the form of liver and muscle glycogen is sufficient to supply the infant's needs for only a few hours. The liver of the neonate is still far from functionally adequate at birth, which prevents significant gluconeogenesis. Therefore, the infant's blood glucose concentration frequently falls the first day to as low as 30 to 40 mg/dl of plasma, less than half the normal value. Fortunately, however, appropriate mechanisms are available for the infant to use its stored fats and proteins for metabolism until mother's milk can be provided 2 to 3 days later.

Special problems are also frequently associated with getting an adequate fluid supply to the neonate because the infant's rate of body fluid turnover averages seven times that of an adult, and the mother's milk supply requires several days to develop. Ordinarily, the infant's weight decreases 5 to 10 percent and sometimes as much as 20 percent within the first 2 to 3 days of life. Most of this weight loss is loss of fluid rather than of body solids.

Special Functional Problems in the Neonate

An important characteristic of the neonate is instability of the various hormonal and neurogenic control systems. This results partly from immature development of the different organs of the body and partly from the fact that the control systems simply have not become adjusted to the new way of life.

Respiratory System

The normal rate of respiration in a neonate is about 40 breaths per minute, and tidal air with each breath averages 16 milliliters. This gives a total minute respiratory volume of 640 ml/min, which is about twice as great in relation to the body weight as that of an adult. *The functional residual capacity of the infant's lungs is only one-half that of an adult in relation to body weight.* This difference causes excessive cyclical increases and decreases in the newborn baby's blood gas concentrations if the respiratory rate becomes slowed because it is the residual air in the lungs that smoothes out the blood gas variations.

Circulation

Blood Volume. The blood volume of a neonate immediately after birth averages about 300 milliliters, but if the infant is left attached to the placenta for a few minutes after birth or if the umbilical cord is stripped to force blood out of its vessels into the baby, an additional 75 milliliters of blood enters the infant, to make a total of 375 milliliters. Then, during the ensuing few hours, fluid is lost into the neonate's tissue spaces from this blood, which increases the hematocrit but returns the blood volume once again to the normal value of about 300 milliliters. Some pediatricians believe that this extra blood volume caused by stripping the umbilical cord can lead to mild pulmonary edema with some degree of respiratory distress, but the extra red blood cells are often valuable to the infant.

Cardiac Output. The cardiac output of the neonate averages 500 ml/min, which, like respiration and body metabolism, is about twice as much in relation to body weight as in the adult. Occasionally a child is born with an especially low cardiac output caused by hemorrhage of much of its blood volume from the placenta at birth.

Arterial Pressure. The arterial pressure during the first day after birth averages about 70 mm Hg systolic and 50 mm Hg diastolic; this increases slowly during the next several months to about 90/60. Then there is a much slower rise during the subsequent years until the adult pressure of 115/70 is attained at adolescence.

Blood Characteristics. The red blood cell count in the neonate averages about 4 million per cubic millimeter. If blood is stripped from the cord into the infant, the red blood cell count rises an additional 0.5 to 0.75 million during the first few hours of life, giving a red blood cell count of about 4.75 million per cubic millimeter, as shown in Figure 83-6. Subsequent to this, however, few new red blood cells are formed in the infant during the first few weeks of life, presumably because the hypoxic stimulus of fetal life is no longer present to stimulate red cell production. Thus, as shown in Figure 83-6, the average red blood cell count falls to less than 4 million per cubic millimeter by about 6 to 8 weeks of age. From that time on, increasing activity by the baby provides the appropriate stimulus for returning the red blood cell count to normal within another 2 to 3 months. Immediately after birth, the white blood cell count of the neonate is about 45,000 per cubic millimeter, which is about five times as great as that of the normal adult.

Neonatal Jaundice and Erythroblastosis Fetalis. Bilirubin formed in the fetus can cross the placenta into the mother and be excreted through the liver of the mother, but immediately after birth, the only means for ridding the neonate of bilirubin is through the neonate's own liver, which

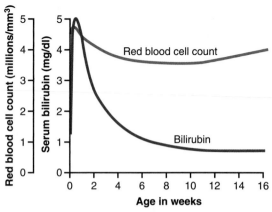

Figure 83-6 Changes in the red blood cell count and in serum bilirubin concentration during the first 16 weeks of life, showing physiological anemia at 6 to 12 weeks of life and physiological hyperbilirubinemia during the first 2 weeks of life.

for the first week or so of life functions poorly and is incapable of conjugating significant quantities of bilirubin with glucuronic acid for excretion into the bile. Consequently, the plasma bilirubin concentration rises from a normal value of less than 1 mg/dl to an average of 5 mg/dl during the first 3 days of life and then gradually falls back to normal as the liver becomes functional. This effect, called *physiological hyperbilirubinemia*, is shown in Figure 83-6, and it is associated with mild *jaundice* (yellowness) of the infant's skin and especially of the sclerae of its eyes for a week or two.

However, by far the most important abnormal cause of serious neonatal jaundice is *erythroblastosis fetalis*, which is discussed in detail in Chapter 32 in relation to Rh factor incompatibility between the fetus and mother. Briefly, the *erythroblastotic baby* inherits Rh-positive red cells from the father, while the mother is Rh negative. The mother then becomes immunized against the Rh-positive factor (a protein) in the fetus's blood cells, and her antibodies destroy fetal red cells, releasing extreme quantities of bilirubin into the fetus's plasma and often causing fetal death for lack of adequate red cells. Before the advent of modern obstetrical therapeutics, this condition occurred either mildly or seriously in 1 of every 50 to 100 neonates.

Fluid Balance, Acid-Base Balance, and Renal Function

The rate of fluid intake and fluid excretion in the newborn infant is seven times as great in relation to weight as in the adult, which means that even a slight percentage alteration of fluid intake or fluid output can cause rapidly developing abnormalities.

The rate of metabolism in the infant is also twice as great in relation to body mass as in the adult, which means that twice as much acid is normally formed, creating a tendency toward acidosis in the infant. Functional development of the kidneys is not complete until the end of about the first month of life. For instance, the kidneys of the neonate can concentrate urine to only 1.5 times the osmolality of the plasma, whereas the adult can concentrate the urine to three to four times the plasma osmolarity. Therefore, considering the immaturity of the kidneys, together with the marked fluid turnover in the infant and rapid formation of acid, one can readily understand that among the most important problems of infancy are acidosis, dehydration, and, more rarely, overhydration.

Liver Function

During the first few days of life, liver function in the neonate may be quite deficient, as evidenced by the following effects:

1. The liver of the neonate conjugates bilirubin with glucuronic acid poorly and therefore excretes bilirubin only slightly during the first few days of life.

2. The liver of the neonate is deficient in forming plasma proteins, so the plasma protein concentration falls during the first weeks of life to 15 to 20 percent less than that for older children. Occasionally the protein concentration falls so low that the infant develops hypoproteinemic edema.

3. The gluconeogenesis function of the liver is particularly deficient. As a result, the blood glucose level of the unfed neonate falls to about 30 to 40 mg/dl (about 40 percent of normal) and the infant must depend mainly on its stored fats for energy until sufficient feeding can occur.

4. The liver of the neonate usually also forms too little of the blood factors needed for normal blood coagulation.

Digestion, Absorption, and Metabolism of Energy Foods; and Nutrition

In general, the ability of the neonate to digest, absorb, and metabolize foods is no different from that of the older child, with the following three exceptions.

First, *secretion of pancreatic amylase in the neonate is deficient*, so the neonate uses starches less adequately than do older children.

Second, *absorption of fats from the gastrointestinal tract is somewhat less than that in the older child.* Consequently, milk with a high fat content, such as cow's milk, is frequently inadequately absorbed.

Third, because the liver functions imperfectly during at least the first week of life, *the glucose concentration in the blood is unstable and low.*

The neonate is especially capable of synthesizing and storing proteins. Indeed, with an adequate diet, up to 90 percent of the ingested amino acids is used for formation of body proteins. This is a much higher percentage than in adults.

Increased Metabolic Rate and Poor Body Temperature Regulation. The normal metabolic rate of the neonate in relation to body weight is about twice that of the adult, which accounts also for the twice as great cardiac output and twice as great minute respiratory volume in relation to body weight in the infant.

Because the body surface area is large in relation to body mass, heat is readily lost from the body. As a result, the body temperature of the neonate, particularly of premature infants, falls easily. Figure 83-7 shows that the body temperature of even a normal infant often falls several degrees during the first few hours after birth but returns to normal in 7 to 10 hours. Still, the body temperature regulatory mechanisms remain poor during the early days of life, allowing marked deviations in temperature, which are also shown in Figure 83-7.

Nutritional Needs During the Early Weeks of Life. At birth, a neonate is usually in complete nutritional balance, provided the mother has had an adequate diet. Furthermore, function of the gastrointestinal system is usually more than adequate to digest and assimilate all the nutritional needs of the infant if appropriate nutrients are provided in the diet.

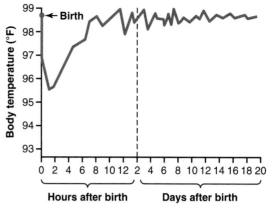

Figure 83-7 Fall in body temperature of the neonate immediately after birth, and instability of body temperature during the first few days of life.

However, three specific problems do occur in the early nutrition of the infant.

Need for Calcium and Vitamin D. The neonate is in a stage of rapid ossification of its bones at birth, so a ready supply of calcium throughout infancy is necessary. This is ordinarily supplied adequately by the usual diet of milk. Yet absorption of calcium by the gastrointestinal tract is poor in the absence of vitamin D. Therefore, the vitamin D–deficient infant can develop severe rickets in only a few weeks. This is particularly true in premature babies because their gastrointestinal tracts absorb calcium even less effectively than those of normal infants.

Necessity for Iron in the Diet. If the mother has had adequate amounts of iron in her diet, the liver of the infant usually has stored enough iron to keep forming blood cells for 4 to 6 months after birth. But if the mother has had insufficient iron in her diet, severe anemia is likely to occur in the infant after about 3 months of life. To prevent this possibility, early feeding of the infant with egg yolk, which contains reasonably large quantities of iron, or the administration of iron in some other form is desirable by the second or third month of life.

Vitamin C Deficiency in Infants. Ascorbic acid (vitamin C) is not stored in significant quantities in the fetal tissues, yet it is required for proper formation of cartilage, bone, and other intercellular structures of the infant. Furthermore, milk provides only small supplies of ascorbic acid, especially cow's milk, which has only one fourth as much as human milk. For this reason, orange juice or other sources of ascorbic acid are often prescribed by the third week of life.

Immunity

The neonate inherits much immunity from the mother because many protein antibodies diffuse from the mother's blood through the placenta into the fetus. However, the neonate does not form antibodies of its own to a significant extent. By the end of the first month, the baby's gamma globulins, which contain the antibodies, have decreased to less than half the original level, with a corresponding decrease in immunity. Thereafter, the baby's own immunity system begins to form antibodies and the gamma globulin concentration returns essentially to normal by the age of 12 to 20 months.

Despite the decrease in gamma globulins soon after birth, the antibodies inherited from the mother protect the infant for about 6 months against most major childhood infectious diseases, including diphtheria, measles, and polio. Therefore, immunization against these diseases before 6 months is usually unnecessary. Conversely, the inherited antibodies against whooping cough are normally insufficient to protect the neonate; therefore, for full safety, the infant requires immunization against this disease within the first month or so of life.

Allergy. The newborn infant is seldom subject to allergy. Several months later, however, when the infant's own antibodies first begin to form, extreme allergic states can develop, often resulting in serious eczema, gastrointestinal abnormalities, and even anaphylaxis. As the child grows older and still higher degrees of immunity develop, these allergic manifestations usually disappear. This relation of immunity to allergy is discussed in Chapter 34.

Endocrine Problems

Ordinarily, the endocrine system of the infant is highly developed at birth, and the infant seldom exhibits any immediate endocrine abnormalities. However, there are special instances in which the endocrinology of infancy is important:

1. If a pregnant mother bearing a female child is treated with an androgenic hormone or if an androgenic tumor develops during pregnancy, the child will be born with a high degree of masculinization of her sexual organs, thus resulting in a type of *hermaphroditism.*

2. The sex hormones secreted by the placenta and by the mother's glands during pregnancy occasionally cause the neonate's breasts to form milk during the first days of life. Sometimes the breasts then become inflamed, or infectious mastitis develops.

3. An infant born of an untreated diabetic mother will have considerable hypertrophy and hyperfunction of the islets of Langerhans in the pancreas. As a consequence, the infant's blood glucose concentration may fall to lower than 20 mg/dl shortly after birth. Fortunately, however, in the neonate, unlike in the adult, insulin shock or coma from this low level of blood glucose concentration only rarely develops.

   Maternal type II diabetes is the most common cause of large babies. Type II diabetes in the mother is associated with resistance to the metabolic effects of insulin and compensatory increases in plasma insulin concentration. The high levels of insulin are believed to stimulate fetal growth and contribute to increased birth weight. Increased supply of glucose and other nutrients to the fetus may also contribute to increased fetal growth. However, most of the increased fetal weight is due to increased body fat; there is usually little increase in body length, although the size of some organs may be increased *(organomegaly).*

   In the mother with uncontrolled type I diabetes (caused by lack of insulin secretion), fetal growth may be stunted because of metabolic deficits in the mother and growth and tissue maturation of the neonate are often impaired. Also, there is a high rate of intrauterine mortality. Among the fetuses that do come to term, there is still a high mortality rate. Two thirds of the infants who die succumb to *respiratory distress syndrome,* described earlier in the chapter.

4. Occasionally a child is born with hypofunctional adrenal cortices, often resulting from *agenesis* of the adrenal glands or *exhaustion atrophy*, which can occur when the adrenal glands have been vastly overstimulated.

5. If a pregnant woman has hyperthyroidism or is treated with excess thyroid hormone, the infant is likely to be born with a temporarily hyposecreting thyroid gland. Conversely, if before pregnancy a woman had had her thyroid gland removed, her pituitary gland may secrete great quantities of thyrotropin during gestation and the child might be born with temporary hyperthyroidism.

6. In a fetus lacking thyroid hormone secretion, the bones grow poorly and there is mental retardation. This causes the condition called *cretin dwarfism*, discussed in Chapter 76.

Special Problems of Prematurity

All the problems in neonatal life just noted are severely exacerbated in prematurity. They can be categorized under the following two headings: (1) immaturity of certain organ systems and (2) instability of the different homeostatic control systems. Because of these effects, a premature baby seldom lives if it is born more than 3 months before term.

Immature Development of the Premature Infant

Almost all the organ systems of the body are immature in the premature infant and require particular attention if the life of the premature baby is to be saved.

Respiration. The respiratory system is especially likely to be underdeveloped in the premature infant. The vital capacity and the functional residual capacity of the lungs are especially small in relation to the size of the infant. Also, surfactant secretion is depressed or absent. As a consequence, *respiratory distress syndrome* is a common cause of death. Also, the low functional residual capacity in the premature infant is often associated with periodic breathing of the Cheyne-Stokes type.

Gastrointestinal Function. Another major problem of the premature infant is to ingest and absorb adequate food. If the infant is more than 2 months premature, the digestive and absorptive systems are almost always inadequate. The absorption of fat is so poor that the premature infant must have a low-fat diet. Furthermore, the premature infant has unusual difficulty in absorbing calcium and, therefore, can develop severe rickets before the difficulty is recognized. For this reason, special attention must be paid to adequate calcium and vitamin D intake.

Function of Other Organs. Immaturity of other organ systems that frequently causes serious difficulties in the premature infant includes (1) immaturity of the liver, which results in poor intermediary metabolism and often a bleeding tendency as a result of poor formation of coagulation factors; (2) immaturity of the kidneys, which are particularly deficient in their ability to rid the body of acids, thereby predisposing to acidosis and to serious fluid balance abnormalities; (3) immaturity of the blood-forming mechanism of the bone marrow, which allows rapid development of anemia; and (4) depressed formation of gamma globulin by the lymphoid system, which often leads to serious infection.

Instability of the Homeostatic Control Systems in the Premature Infant

Immaturity of the different organ systems in the premature infant creates a high degree of instability in the homeostatic mechanisms of the body. For instance, the acid-base balance can vary tremendously, particularly when the rate of food intake varies from time to time. Likewise, the blood protein concentration is usually low because of immature liver development, often leading to *hypoproteinemic edema*. And inability of the infant to regulate its calcium ion concentration may bring on hypocalcemic tetany. Also, the blood glucose concentration can vary between the extremely wide limits of 20 to more than 100 mg/dl, depending principally on the regularity of feeding. It is no wonder, then, with these extreme variations in the internal environment of the premature infant, that mortality is high if a baby is born 3 or more months prematurely.

Instability of Body Temperature. One of the particular problems of the premature infant is inability to maintain normal body temperature. Its temperature tends to approach that of its surroundings. At normal room temperature, the infant's temperature may stabilize in the low 90°s or even in the 80°sF. Statistical studies show that a body temperature maintained below 96°F (35.5°C) is associated with a particularly high incidence of death, which explains the almost mandatory use of the incubator in treatment of prematurity.

Danger of Blindness Caused by Excess Oxygen Therapy in the Premature Infant

Because premature infants frequently develop respiratory distress, oxygen therapy has often been used in treating prematurity. However, it has been discovered that use of excess oxygen in treating premature infants, especially in early prematurity, can lead to blindness. The reason is that too much oxygen stops the growth of new blood vessels in the retina. Then when oxygen therapy is stopped, the blood vessels try to make up for lost time and burst forth with a great mass of vessels growing all through the vitreous humor, blocking light from the pupil to the retina. And later, the vessels are replaced with a mass of fibrous tissue where the eye's clear vitreous humor should be.

This condition is known as *retrolental fibroplasias* and causes permanent blindness. For this reason, it is particularly important to avoid treatment of premature infants with high concentrations of respiratory oxygen. Physiologic studies indicate that the premature infant is usually safe with up to 40 percent oxygen in the air breathed, but some child physiologists believe that complete safety can be achieved only at normal oxygen concentration in the air that is breathed.

Growth and Development of the Child

The major physiologic problems of the child beyond the neonatal period are related to special metabolic needs for growth, which have been fully covered in the sections of this book on metabolism and endocrinology.

Figure 83-8 shows the changes in heights of boys and girls from the time of birth until the age of 20 years. Note especially that these parallel each other almost exactly until the end of the first decade of life. Between the ages of 11 and 13 years, the female estrogens begin to be formed and cause rapid growth in height but early uniting of the epiphyses

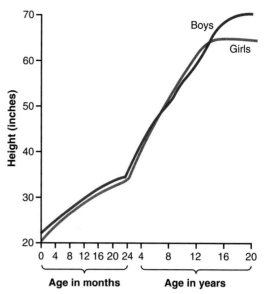

Figure 83-8 Average height of boys and girls from infancy to 20 years of age.

of the long bones at about the 14th to 16th year of life, so growth in height then ceases. This contrasts with the effect of testosterone in the male, which causes extra growth at a slightly later age—mainly between ages 13 and 17 years. The male, however, undergoes more prolonged growth because of delayed uniting of the epiphyses, so his final height is considerably greater than that of the female.

Behavioral Growth

Behavioral growth is principally a problem of maturity of the nervous system. It is difficult to dissociate maturity of the anatomical structures of the nervous system from maturity caused by training. Anatomical studies show that certain major tracts in the central nervous system are not completely myelinated until the end of the first year of life. For this reason, it is frequently stated that the nervous system is not

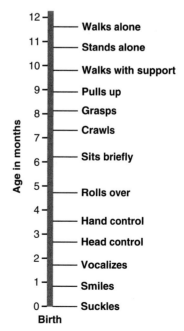

Figure 83-9 Behavioral development of the infant during the first year of life.

fully functional at birth. The brain cortex and its associated functions, such as vision, seem to require several months after birth for final functional development to occur.

At birth, the infant brain mass is only 26 percent of the adult brain mass and 55 percent at 1 year, but it reaches almost adult proportions by the end of the second year. This is also associated with closure of the fontanels and sutures of the skull, which allows only 20 percent additional growth of the brain beyond the first 2 years of life. Figure 83-9 shows a normal progress chart for the infant during the first year of life. Comparison of this chart with the baby's actual development is used for clinical assessment of mental and behavioral growth.

Bibliography

Baraldi E, Filippone M: Chronic lung disease after premature birth, *N Engl J Med* 357:1946, 2007.

Bissonnette JM: Mechanisms regulating hypoxic respiratory depression during fetal and postnatal life, *Am J Physiol Regul Integr Comp Physiol* 278:R1391, 2000.

Cannon B, Nedergaard J: Brown adipose tissue: function and physiological significance, *Physiol Rev* 84:277, 2004.

Cetin I, Alvino G, Cardellicchio M: Long chain fatty acids and dietary fats in fetal nutrition, *J Physiol* 587:3441, 2009.

Challis JRG, Matthews SG, Gibb W, et al: Endocrine and paracrine regulation of birth at term and preterm, *Endocr Rev* 21:514, 2000.

Fowden AL, Giussani DA, Forhead AJ: Intrauterine programming of physiological systems: causes and consequences, *Physiology (Bethesda)* 21:29, 2006.

Goldenberg RL, Culhane JF, Iams JD, et al: Epidemiology and causes of preterm birth, *Lancet* 371:75, 2008.

Gluckman PD, Hanson MA, Cooper C, et al: Effect of in utero and early-life conditions on adult health and disease, *N Engl J Med* 359:61, 2008.

Hilaire G, Duron B: Maturation of the mammalian respiratory system, *Physiol Rev* 79:325, 1999.

Johnson MH: Functional brain development in humans, *Nat Rev Neurosci* 2:475, 2001.

Kinney HC, Thach BT: The sudden infant death syndrome, *N Engl J Med* 361:795, 2009.

Kovacs CS, Kronenberg HM: Maternal-fetal calcium and bone metabolism during pregnancy, puerperium, and lactation, *Endocr Rev* 18:832, 1997.

Labbok MH, Clark D, Goldman AS: Breastfeeding: maintaining an irreplaceable immunological resource, *Nat Rev Immunol* 4:565, 2004.

Maisels MJ, McDonagh AF: Phototherapy for neonatal jaundice, *N Engl J Med* 358:920, 2008.

McMurtry IF: Pre- and postnatal lung development, maturation, and plasticity, *Am J Physiol Lung Cell Mol Physiol* 282:L341, 2002.

Ojeda NB, Grigore D, Alexander BT: Developmental programming of hypertension: insight from animal models of nutritional manipulation, *Hypertension* 52:44, 2008.

Osol G, Mandala M: Maternal uterine vascular remodeling during pregnancy, *Physiology (Bethesda)* 24:58, 2009.

Ross MG, Nijland MJ: Development of ingestive behavior, *Am J Physiol* 274:R879, 1998.

Saigal S, Doyle LW: An overview of mortality and sequelae of preterm birth from infancy to adulthood, *Lancet* 371:261, 2008.

Sports Physiology

84. Sports Physiology

Sports Physiology

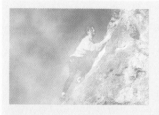

There are few stresses to which the body is exposed that approach the extreme stresses of heavy exercise. In fact, if some of the extremes of exercise were continued for even moderately prolonged periods, they might be lethal. Therefore, sports physiology is mainly a discussion of the ultimate limits to which several of the bodily mechanisms can be stressed. To give one simple example: In a person who has extremely high fever approaching the level of lethality, the body metabolism increases to about 100 percent above normal. By comparison, the metabolism of the body during a marathon race may increase to 2000 percent above normal.

Female and Male Athletes

Most of the quantitative data that are given in this chapter are for the young male athlete, not because it is desirable to know only these values but because it is only in male athletes that relatively complete measurements have been made. However, for those measurements that have been made in the female athlete, similar basic physiologic principles apply, except for quantitative differences caused by differences in body size, body composition, and the presence or absence of the male sex hormone testosterone.

In general, most quantitative values for women—such as muscle strength, pulmonary ventilation, and cardiac output, all of which are related mainly to the muscle mass—vary between two thirds and three quarters of the values recorded in men. When measured in terms of strength per square centimeter of cross-sectional area, the female muscle can achieve almost exactly the same maximal force of contraction as that of the male—between 3 and 4 kg/cm². Therefore, most of the difference in total muscle performance lies in the extra percentage of the male body that is muscle, caused by endocrine differences that we discuss later.

The performance capabilities of the female versus male athlete are illustrated by the relative running speeds for a marathon race. In a comparison, the top female performer had a running speed that was 11 percent less than that of the top male performer. For other events, however, women have at times held records faster than men—for instance, for the two-way swim across the English Channel, where the availability of extra fat seems to be an advantage for heat insulation, buoyancy, and extra long-term energy.

Testosterone secreted by the male testes has a powerful *anabolic effect* in causing greatly increased deposition of protein everywhere in the body, but especially in the muscles. In fact, even a male who participates in very little sports activity but who nevertheless has a normal level of testosterone will have muscles that grow about 40 percent larger than those of a comparable female without the testosterone.

The female sex hormone *estrogen* probably also accounts for some of the difference between female and male performance, although not nearly so much as testosterone. Estrogen increases the deposition of fat in the female, especially in the breasts, hips, and subcutaneous tissue. At least partly for this reason, the average nonathletic female has about 27 percent body fat composition, in contrast to the nonathletic male, who has about 15 percent. This is a detriment to the highest levels of athletic performance in those events in which performance depends on speed or on ratio of total body muscle strength to body weight.

Muscles in Exercise

Strength, Power, and Endurance of Muscles

The final common determinant of success in athletic events is what the muscles can do for you—what strength they can give when it is needed, what power they can achieve in the performance of work, and how long they can continue their activity.

The strength of a muscle is determined mainly by its size, with a *maximal contractile force between 3 and 4 kg/cm²* of muscle cross-sectional area. Thus, a man who is well supplied with testosterone or who has enlarged his muscles through an exercise training program will have correspondingly increased muscle strength.

To give an example of muscle strength, a world-class weight lifter might have a quadriceps muscle with a cross-sectional area as great as 150 square centimeters. This would translate into a maximal contractile strength of 525 kilograms (or 1155 pounds), with all this force applied to the patellar tendon. Therefore, one can readily understand how it is possible for this tendon at times to be ruptured or actually to be avulsed from its insertion into the tibia below the knee. Also, when such forces occur in tendons that span a joint, similar forces are applied to the surfaces of the joint or sometimes to ligaments spanning the joints, thus accounting for such happenings as displaced cartilages, compression fractures about the joint, and torn ligaments.

The *holding strength* of muscles is about 40 percent greater than the contractile strength. That is, if a muscle is already contracted and a force then attempts to stretch out the muscle, as occurs when landing after a jump, this requires about 40 percent more force than can be achieved by a shortening contraction. Therefore, the force of 525 kilograms calculated above for the patellar tendon during muscle contraction becomes 735 kilograms (1617 pounds) during holding contractions. This further compounds the problems of the tendons, joints, and ligaments. It can also lead to internal tearing in the muscle itself. In fact, forceful stretching of a maximally contracted muscle is one of the surest ways to create the highest degree of muscle soreness.

Mechanical work performed by a muscle is the amount of force applied by the muscle multiplied by the distance over which the force is applied. The *power* of muscle contraction is different from muscle strength because power is a measure of the total amount of work that the muscle performs in a unit period of time. Power is therefore determined not only by the strength of muscle contraction but also by its *distance of contraction* and the *number of times that it contracts each minute*. Muscle power is generally measured in *kilogram meters (kg-m) per minute*. That is, a muscle that can lift 1 kilogram weight to a height of 1 meter or that can move some object laterally against a force of 1 kilogram for a distance of 1 meter in 1 minute is said to have a power of 1 kg-m/min. The maximal power achievable by all the muscles in the body of a highly trained athlete with all the muscles working together is approximately the following:

	kg-m/min
First 8 to 10 seconds	7000
Next 1 minute	4000
Next 30 minutes	1700

Thus, it is clear that a person has the capability of extreme power surges for short periods of time, such as during a 100-meter dash that is completed entirely within 10 seconds, whereas for long-term endurance events, the power output of the muscles is only one fourth as great as during the initial power surge.

This does not mean that one's athletic performance is four times as great during the initial power surge as it is for the next 30 minutes, because the *efficiency* for translation of muscle power output into athletic performance is often much less during rapid activity than during less rapid but sustained activity. Thus, the velocity of the 100-meter dash is only 1.75 times as great as the velocity of a 30-minute race, despite the fourfold difference in short-term versus long-term muscle power capability.

Another measure of muscle performance is *endurance*. This, to a great extent, depends on the nutritive support for the muscle—more than anything else on the amount of glycogen that has been stored in the muscle before the period of exercise. A person on a high-carbohydrate diet stores far more glycogen in muscles than a person on either a mixed diet or a high-fat diet. Therefore, endurance is greatly enhanced by a high-carbohydrate diet. When athletes run at speeds typical for the marathon race, their endurance (as measured by the time that they can sustain the race until complete exhaustion) is approximately the following:

	Minutes
High-carbohydrate diet	240
Mixed diet	120
High-fat diet	85

The corresponding amounts of glycogen stored in the muscle before the race started explain these differences. The amounts stored are approximately the following:

	g/kg Muscle
High-carbohydrate diet	40
Mixed diet	20
High-fat diet	6

Muscle Metabolic Systems in Exercise

The same basic metabolic systems are present in muscle as in other parts of the body; these are discussed in detail in Chapters 67 through 73. However, special quantitative measures of the activities of three metabolic systems are exceedingly important in understanding the limits of physical activity. These systems are (1) *the phosphocreatine-creatine system,* (2) *the glycogen-lactic acid system,* and (3) *the aerobic system.*

Adenosine Triphosphate. The source of energy actually used to cause muscle contraction is adenosine triphosphate (ATP), which has the following basic formula:

$$\text{Adenosine-PO}_3 \sim \text{PO}_3 \sim \text{PO}_3^-$$

The bonds attaching the last two phosphate radicals to the molecule, designated by the symbol ~, are *high-energy phosphate bonds.* Each of these bonds stores 7300 calories of energy per mole of ATP under standard conditions (and even slightly more than this under the physical conditions in the body, which is discussed in detail in Chapter 67). Therefore, when one phosphate radical is removed, more than 7300 calories of energy are released to energize the muscle contractile process. Then, when the second phosphate radical is removed, still another 7300 calories become available. Removal of the first phosphate converts the ATP into *adenosine diphosphate* (ADP), and removal of the second converts this ADP into *adenosine monophosphate* (AMP).

The amount of ATP present in the muscles, even in a well-trained athlete, is sufficient to sustain maximal muscle power for only about 3 seconds, maybe enough for one half of a 50-meter dash. Therefore, except for a few seconds at a time, it is essential that new ATP be formed continuously, even during the performance of short athletic events. Figure 84-1 shows the overall metabolic system, demonstrating the breakdown of ATP first to ADP and then to AMP, with the release of energy to the muscles for contraction. The left-hand side of the figure shows the three metabolic systems that provide a continuous supply of ATP in the muscle fibers.

Phosphocreatine-Creatine System

Phosphocreatine (also called *creatine phosphate*) is another chemical compound that has a high-energy phosphate bond, with the following formula:

$$\text{Creatine} \sim \text{PO}_3^-$$

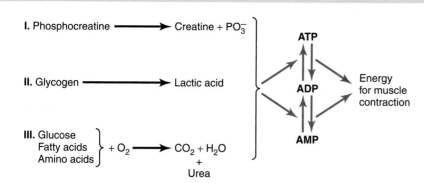

Figure 84-1 Important metabolic systems that supply energy for muscle contraction.

I. Phosphocreatine $\longrightarrow$ Creatine + PO_3^-

II. Glycogen $\longrightarrow$ Lactic acid

III. Glucose
Fatty acids } + O_2 $\longrightarrow$ CO_2 + H_2O
Amino acids   +
                                            Urea

ATP

ADP   Energy
                       for muscle
AMP   contraction

This can decompose to *creatine* and *phosphate ion,* as shown in Figure 84-1, and in doing so releases large amounts of energy. In fact, the high-energy phosphate bond of phosphocreatine has more energy than the bond of ATP, 10,300 calories per mole compared with 7300 for the ATP bond. Therefore, phosphocreatine can easily provide enough energy to reconstitute the high-energy bond of ATP. Furthermore, most muscle cells have two to four times as much phosphocreatine as ATP.

A special characteristic of energy transfer from phosphocreatine to ATP is that it occurs within a small fraction of a second. Therefore, all the energy stored in the muscle phosphocreatine is almost instantaneously available for muscle contraction, just as is the energy stored in ATP.

The combined amounts of cell ATP and cell phosphocreatine are called the *phosphagen energy system.* These together can provide maximal muscle power for 8 to 10 seconds, almost enough for the 100-meter run. *Thus, the energy from the phosphagen system is used for maximal short bursts of muscle power.*

Glycogen-Lactic Acid System. The stored glycogen in muscle can be split into glucose and the glucose then used for energy. The initial stage of this process, called *glycolysis,* occurs without use of oxygen and, therefore, is said to be *anaerobic metabolism* (see Chapter 67). During glycolysis, each glucose molecule is split into two *pyruvic acid molecules,* and energy is released to form four ATP molecules for each original glucose molecule, as explained in Chapter 67. Ordinarily, the pyruvic acid then enters the mitochondria of the muscle cells and reacts with oxygen to form still many more ATP molecules. However, when there is insufficient oxygen for this second stage (the oxidative stage) of glucose metabolism to occur, most of the pyruvic acid then is converted into *lactic acid,* which diffuses out of the muscle cells into the interstitial fluid and blood. Therefore, much of the muscle glycogen is transformed to lactic acid, but in doing so, considerable amounts of ATP are formed entirely without the consumption of oxygen.

Another characteristic of the glycogen-lactic acid system is that it can form ATP molecules about 2.5 times as rapidly as can the oxidative mechanism of the mitochondria. Therefore, when large amounts of ATP are required for short to moderate periods of muscle contraction, this anaerobic glycolysis mechanism can be used as a rapid source of energy. It is, however, only about one half as rapid as the phosphagen system. Under optimal conditions, the glycogen-lactic acid system can provide 1.3 to 1.6 minutes of maximal muscle activity in addition to the 8 to 10 seconds provided by the phosphagen system, although at somewhat reduced muscle power.

Aerobic System. The aerobic system is the oxidation of foodstuffs in the mitochondria to provide energy. That is, as shown to the left in Figure 84-1, glucose, fatty acids, and amino acids from the foodstuffs—after some intermediate processing—combine with oxygen to release tremendous amounts of energy that are used to convert AMP and ADP into ATP, as discussed in Chapter 67.

In comparing this aerobic mechanism of energy supply with the glycogen-lactic acid system and the phosphagen system, the relative *maximal rates of power generation* in terms of moles of ATP generation per minute are the following:

	Moles of ATP/min
Phosphagen system	4
Glycogen-lactic acid system	2.5
Aerobic system	1

When comparing the same systems for endurance, the relative values are the following:

	Time
Phosphagen system	8-10 seconds
Glycogen-lactic acid system	1.3-1.6 minutes
Aerobic system	Unlimited time (as long as nutrients last)

Thus, one can readily see that the phosphagen system is the one used by the muscle for power surges of a few seconds, and the aerobic system is required for prolonged athletic activity. In between is the glycogen-lactic acid system, which is especially important for giving extra power during such intermediate races as the 200- to 800-meter runs.

What Types of Sports Use Which Energy Systems? By considering the vigor of a sports activity and its duration, one can estimate closely which of the energy systems is used for each activity. Various approximations are presented in Table 84-1.

Recovery of the Muscle Metabolic Systems After Exercise. In the same way that the energy from phosphocreatine can be used to reconstitute ATP, energy from the glycogen-lactic acid system can be used to reconstitute both phosphocreatine and ATP. And then energy from the oxidative metabolism of the aerobic system can be used to reconstitute all the other systems—the ATP, the phosphocreatine, and the glycogen-lactic acid system.

Table 84-1 Energy Systems Used in Various Sports

Phosphagen System, Almost Entirely

100-meter dash
Jumping
Weight lifting
Diving
Football dashes
Baseball triple

Phosphagen and Glycogen-Lactic Acid Systems

200-meter dash
Basketball
Ice hockey dashes
Glycogen-Lactic Acid System, Mainly
400-meter dash
100-meter swim
Tennis
Soccer

Glycogen-Lactic Acid and Aerobic Systems

800-meter dash
200-meter swim
1500-meter skating
Boxing
2000-meter rowing
1500-meter run
1-mile run
400-meter swim

Aerobic System

10,000-meter skating
Cross-country skiing
Marathon run (26.2 miles, 42.2km)
Jogging

Reconstitution of the lactic acid system means mainly the removal of the excess lactic acid that has accumulated in all the fluids of the body. This is especially important because *lactic acid causes extreme fatigue.* When adequate amounts of energy are available from oxidative metabolism, removal of lactic acid is achieved in two ways: (1) A small portion of it is converted back into pyruvic acid and then metabolized oxidatively by all the body tissues. (2) The remaining lactic acid is reconverted into glucose mainly in the liver, and the glucose in turn is used to replenish the glycogen stores of the muscles.

Recovery of the Aerobic System After Exercise. Even during the early stages of heavy exercise, a portion of one's aerobic energy capability is depleted. This results from two effects: (1) the so-called *oxygen debt* and (2) *depletion of the glycogen stores* of the muscles.

Oxygen Debt. The body normally contains about 2 liters of stored oxygen that can be used for aerobic metabolism even without breathing any new oxygen. This stored oxygen consists of the following: (1) 0.5 liter in the air of the lungs, (2) 0.25 liter dissolved in the body fluids, (3) 1 liter combined with the hemoglobin of the blood, and (4) 0.3 liter

stored in the muscle fibers themselves, combined mainly with myoglobin, an oxygen-binding chemical similar to hemoglobin.

In heavy exercise, almost all this stored oxygen is used within a minute or so for aerobic metabolism. Then, after the exercise is over, this stored oxygen must be replenished by breathing extra amounts of oxygen over and above the normal requirements. In addition, about 9 liters more oxygen must be consumed to provide for reconstituting both the phosphagen system and the lactic acid system. All this extra oxygen that must be "repaid," about 11.5 liters, is called the oxygen debt.

Figure 84-2 shows this principle of oxygen debt. During the first 4 minutes of the figure, the person exercises heavily, and the rate of oxygen uptake increases more than 15-fold. Then, even after the exercise is over, the oxygen uptake still remains above normal, at first very high while the body is reconstituting the phosphagen system and repaying the stored oxygen portion of the oxygen debt, and then for another 40 minutes at a lower level while the lactic acid is removed. The early portion of the oxygen debt is called the *alactacid oxygen debt* and amounts to about 3.5 liters. The latter portion is called the *lactic acid oxygen debt* and amounts to about 8 liters.

Recovery of Muscle Glycogen. Recovery from exhaustive muscle glycogen depletion is not a simple matter. This often requires days, rather than the seconds, minutes, or hours required for recovery of the phosphagen and lactic acid metabolic systems. Figure 84-3 shows this recovery process under three conditions: first, in people on a high-carbohydrate diet; second, in people on a high-fat, high-protein diet; and third, in people with no food. Note that on a high-carbohydrate diet, full recovery occurs in about 2 days. Conversely, people on a high-fat, high-protein diet or on no food at all show very little recovery even after as long as 5 days. The messages of this comparison are (1) that it is important for an athlete to have a high-carbohydrate diet before a grueling athletic event and (2) not to participate in exhaustive exercise during the 48 hours preceding the event.

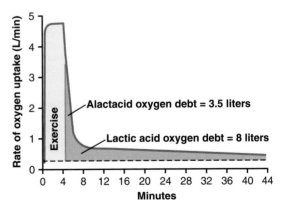

Figure 84-2 Rate of oxygen uptake by the lungs during maximal exercise for 4 minutes and then for about 40 minutes after the exercise is over. This figure demonstrates the principle of *oxygen debt.*

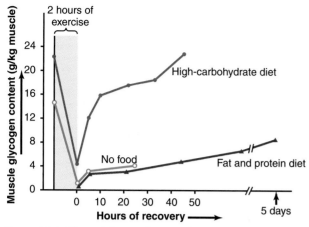

Figure 84-3 Effect of diet on the rate of muscle glycogen replenishment after prolonged exercise. (Redrawn from Fox EL: Sports Physiology. Philadelphia: Saunders College Publishing, 1979.)

Nutrients Used During Muscle Activity

In addition to the large usage of carbohydrates by the muscles during exercise, especially during the early stages of exercise, muscles use large amounts of fat for energy in the form of *fatty acids* and *acetoacetic acid* (see Chapter 68), and they use to a much less extent proteins in the form of *amino acids*. In fact, even under the best conditions, in endurance athletic events that last longer than 4 to 5 hours, the glycogen stores of the muscle become almost totally depleted and are of little further use for energizing muscle contraction. Instead, the muscle now depends on energy from other sources, mainly from fats.

Figure 84-4 shows the approximate relative usage of carbohydrates and fat for energy during prolonged exhaustive exercise under three dietary conditions: high-carbohydrate diet, mixed diet, and high-fat diet. Note that most of the energy is derived from carbohydrates during the first few seconds or minutes of the exercise, but at the time of exhaustion, as much as 60 to 85 percent of the energy is being derived from fats, rather than carbohydrates.

Not all the energy from carbohydrates comes from the stored *muscle* glycogen. In fact, almost as much glycogen is

stored in the *liver* as in the muscles, and this can be released into the blood in the form of glucose and then taken up by the muscles as an energy source. In addition, glucose solutions given to an athlete to drink during the course of an athletic event can provide as much as 30 to 40 percent of the energy required during prolonged events such as marathon races.

Therefore, if muscle glycogen and blood glucose are available, they are the energy nutrients of choice for intense muscle activity. Even so, for a long-term endurance event, one can expect fat to supply more than 50 percent of the required energy after about the first 3 to 4 hours.

Effect of Athletic Training on Muscles and Muscle Performance

Importance of Maximal Resistance Training. One of the cardinal principles of muscle development during athletic training is the following: Muscles that function under no load, even if they are exercised for hours on end, increase little in strength. At the other extreme, muscles that contract at more than 50 percent maximal force of contraction will develop strength rapidly even if the contractions are performed only a few times each day. Using this principle, experiments on muscle building have shown that *six nearly maximal muscle contractions performed in three sets 3 days a week give approximately optimal increase in muscle strength, without producing chronic muscle fatigue.*

The upper curve in Figure 84-5 shows the approximate percentage increase in strength that can be achieved in a previously untrained young person by this resistive training program, demonstrating that the muscle strength increases about 30 percent during the first 6 to 8 weeks but almost plateaus after that time. Along with this increase in strength is an approximately equal percentage increase in muscle mass, which is called *muscle hypertrophy.*

In old age, many people become so sedentary that their muscles atrophy tremendously. In these instances, muscle training often increases muscle strength more than 100 percent.

Muscle Hypertrophy. The average size of a person's muscles is determined to a great extent by heredity plus the level of testosterone secretion, which, in men, causes considerably larger muscles than in women. With training, however, the muscles can become hypertrophied perhaps an additional 30 to 60 percent. Most of this hypertrophy results from

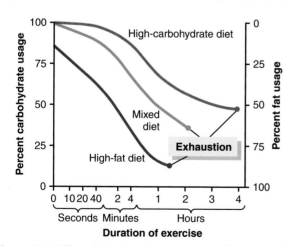

Figure 84-4 Effect of duration of exercise, as well as type of diet on relative percentages of carbohydrate or fat used for energy by muscles. (Based partly on data in Fox EL: Sports Physiology. Philadelphia: Saunders College Publishing, 1979.)

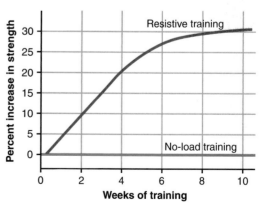

Figure 84-5 Approximate effect of optimal resistive exercise training on increase in muscle strength over a training period of 10 weeks.

increased diameter of the muscle fibers rather than increased numbers of fibers. However, a very few greatly enlarged muscle fibers are believed to split down the middle along their entire length to form entirely new fibers, thus increasing the number of fibers slightly.

The changes that occur inside the hypertrophied muscle fibers themselves include (1) increased numbers of myofibrils, proportionate to the degree of hypertrophy; (2) up to 120 percent increase in mitochondrial enzymes; (3) as much as 60 to 80 percent increase in the components of the phosphagen metabolic system, including both ATP and phosphocreatine; (4) as much as 50 percent increase in stored glycogen; and (5) as much as 75 to 100 percent increase in stored triglyceride (fat). Because of all these changes, the capabilities of both the anaerobic and the aerobic metabolic systems are increased, increasing especially the maximum oxidation rate and efficiency of the oxidative metabolic system as much as 45 percent.

Fast-Twitch and Slow-Twitch Muscle Fibers. In the human being, all muscles have varying percentages of *fast-twitch* and *slow-twitch muscle fibers.* For instance, the gastrocnemius muscle has a higher preponderance of fast-twitch fibers, which gives it the capability of forceful and rapid contraction of the type used in jumping. In contrast, the soleus muscle has a higher preponderance of slow-twitch muscle fibers and therefore is used to a greater extent for prolonged lower leg muscle activity.

The basic differences between the fast-twitch and the slow-twitch fibers are the following:

1. Fast-twitch fibers are about twice as large in diameter.

2. The enzymes that promote rapid release of energy from the phosphagen and glycogen-lactic acid energy systems are two to three times as active in fast-twitch fibers as in slow-twitch fibers, thus making the maximal power that can be achieved for very short periods of time by fast-twitch fibers about twice as great as that of slow-twitch fibers.

3. Slow-twitch fibers are mainly organized for endurance, especially for generation of aerobic energy. They have far more mitochondria than the fast-twitch fibers. In addition, they contain considerably more myoglobin, a hemoglobin-like protein that combines with oxygen within the muscle fiber; the extra myoglobin increases the rate of diffusion of oxygen throughout the fiber by shuttling oxygen from one molecule of myoglobin to the next. In addition, the enzymes of the aerobic metabolic system are considerably more active in slow-twitch fibers than in fast-twitch fibers.

4. The number of capillaries is greater in the vicinity of slow-twitch fibers than in the vicinity of fast-twitch fibers.

In summary, fast-twitch fibers can deliver extreme amounts of power for a few seconds to a minute or so. Conversely, slow-twitch fibers provide endurance, delivering prolonged strength of contraction over many minutes to hours.

Hereditary Differences Among Athletes for Fast-Twitch Versus Slow-Twitch Muscle Fibers. Some people have considerably more fast-twitch than slow-twitch fibers, and others have more slow-twitch fibers; this could determine to some extent the athletic capabilities of different individuals. Athletic training has not been shown to change the relative proportions of fast-twitch and slow-twitch fibers however much an athlete might want to develop one type of athletic prowess over another. Instead, this seems to be determined almost entirely by genetic inheritance, and this in turn helps determine which area of athletics is most suited to each person: some people appear to be born to be marathoners; others are born to be sprinters and jumpers. For example, the following are recorded percentages of fast-twitch versus slow-twitch fiber in the quadriceps muscles of different types of athletes:

	Fast-Twitch	Slow-Twitch
Marathoners	18	82
Swimmers	26	74
Average male	55	45
Weight lifters	55	45
Sprinters	63	37
Jumpers	63	37

Respiration in Exercise

Although one's respiratory ability is of relatively little concern in the performance of sprint types of athletics, it is critical for maximal performance in endurance athletics.

Oxygen Consumption and Pulmonary Ventilation in Exercise. Normal oxygen consumption for a young man at rest is about 250 ml/min. However, under maximal conditions, this can be increased to approximately the following average levels:

	ml/min
Untrained average male	3600
Athletically trained average male	4000
Male marathon runner	5100

Figure 84-6 shows the relation between *oxygen consumption* and *total pulmonary ventilation* at different levels of exercise. It is clear from this figure, as would be expected, that there is a linear relation. Both oxygen consumption and total pulmonary ventilation increase about 20-fold between the resting state and maximal intensity of exercise *in the well-trained athlete.*

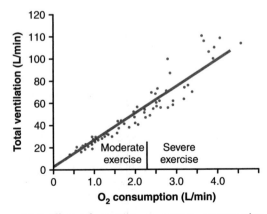

Figure 84-6 Effect of exercise on oxygen consumption and ventilatory rate. (Redrawn from Gray JS: Pulmonary Ventilation and Its Physiological Regulation. Springfield, Ill: Charles C Thomas, 1950.)

Limits of Pulmonary Ventilation. How severely do we stress our respiratory systems during exercise? This can be answered by the following comparison for a normal young man:

	L/min
Pulmonary ventilation at maximal exercise	100-110
Maximal breathing capacity	150-170

Thus, the maximal breathing capacity is about 50 percent greater than the actual pulmonary ventilation during maximal exercise. This provides an element of safety for athletes, giving them extra ventilation that can be called on in such conditions as (1) exercise at high altitudes, (2) exercise under very hot conditions, and (3) abnormalities in the respiratory system.

The important point is that the respiratory system is not normally the most limiting factor in the delivery of oxygen to the muscles during maximal muscle aerobic metabolism. We shall see shortly that the ability of the heart to pump blood to the muscles is usually a greater limiting factor.

Effect of Training on $\dot{V}o_2$ Max. The abbreviation for the rate of oxygen usage under maximal aerobic metabolism is $\dot{V}o_2$ Max. Figure 84-7 shows the progressive effect of athletic training on $\dot{V}o_2$ Max recorded in a group of subjects beginning at the level of no training and then pursuing the training program for 7 to 13 weeks. In this study, it is surprising that the $\dot{V}o_2$ Max increased only about 10 percent. Furthermore, the frequency of training, whether two times or five times per week, had little effect on the increase in $\dot{V}o_2$ Max. Yet, as pointed out earlier, the $\dot{V}o_2$ Max of a marathoner is about 45 percent greater than that of an untrained person. Part of this greater $\dot{V}o_2$ Max of the marathoner probably is genetically determined; that is, those people who have greater chest sizes in relation to body size and stronger respiratory muscles select themselves to become marathoners. However, it is also likely that many years of training increase the marathoner's $\dot{V}o_2$ Max by values considerably greater than the 10 percent that has been recorded in short-term experiments such as that in Figure 84-7.

Oxygen-Diffusing Capacity of Athletes. The *oxygen-diffusing capacity* is a measure of the rate at which oxygen can diffuse from the pulmonary alveoli into the blood. This is expressed in terms of *milliliters of oxygen that will diffuse each minute for each millimeter of mercury difference between alveolar partial pressure of oxygen and pulmonary blood oxygen pressure.* That is, if the partial pressure of oxygen in the alveoli is 91 mm Hg and the oxygen pressure in the blood is 90 mm Hg, the amount of oxygen that diffuses through the respiratory membrane each minute is equal to the diffusing capacity. The following are measured values for different diffusing capacities:

	ml/min
Nonathlete at rest	23
Nonathlete during maximal exercise	48
Speed skaters during maximal exercise	64
Swimmers during maximal exercise	71
Oarsman during maximal exercise	80

The most startling fact about these results is the several-fold increase in diffusing capacity between the resting state and the state of maximal exercise. This results mainly from the fact that blood flow through many of the pulmonary capillaries is sluggish or even dormant in the resting state, whereas in maximal exercise, increased blood flow through the lungs causes all the pulmonary capillaries to be perfused at their maximal rates, thus providing a far greater surface area through which oxygen can diffuse into the pulmonary capillary blood.

It is also clear from these values that those athletes who require greater amounts of oxygen per minute have higher diffusing capacities. Is this because people with naturally greater diffusing capacities choose these types of sports, or is it because something about the training procedures increases the diffusing capacity? The answer is not known, but it is very likely that training, particularly endurance training, does play an important role.

Blood Gases During Exercise. Because of the great usage of oxygen by the muscles in exercise, one would expect the oxygen pressure of the arterial blood to decrease markedly during strenuous athletics and the carbon dioxide pressure of the venous blood to increase far above normal. However, this normally is not the case. Both of these values remain nearly normal, demonstrating the extreme ability of the respiratory system to provide adequate aeration of the blood even during heavy exercise.

This demonstrates another important point: *The blood gases do not always have to become abnormal for respiration to be stimulated in exercise.* Instead, respiration is stimulated mainly by neurogenic mechanisms during exercise, as discussed in Chapter 41. Part of this stimulation results from direct stimulation of the respiratory center by the same nervous signals that are transmitted from the brain to the muscles to cause the exercise. An additional part is believed to result from sensory signals transmitted into the respiratory center from the contracting muscles and moving joints. All this extra nervous stimulation of respiration is normally sufficient to provide almost exactly the necessary increase in pulmonary ventilation required to keep the blood respiratory gases—the oxygen and the carbon dioxide—very near to normal.

Effect of Smoking on Pulmonary Ventilation in Exercise. It is widely known that smoking can decrease an athlete's "wind." This is true for many reasons. First, one effect of nicotine is constriction of the terminal bronchioles of the lungs, which increases the resistance of airflow into and out of the lungs. Second, the irritating effects of the smoke itself

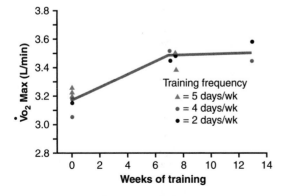

Figure 84-7 Increase in $\dot{V}o_2$ Max over a period of 7 to 13 weeks of athletic training. (Redrawn from Fox EL: Sports Physiology. Philadelphia: Saunders College Publishing, 1979.)

cause increased fluid secretion into the bronchial tree, as well as some swelling of the epithelial linings. Third, nicotine paralyzes the cilia on the surfaces of the respiratory epithelial cells that normally beat continuously to remove excess fluids and foreign particles from the respiratory passageways. As a result, much debris accumulates in the passageways and adds further to the difficulty of breathing. Putting all these factors together, even a light smoker often feels respiratory strain during maximal exercise, and the level of performance may be reduced.

Much more severe are the effects of chronic smoking. There are few chronic smokers in whom some degree of emphysema does not develop. In this disease, the following occur: (1) chronic bronchitis, (2) obstruction of many of the terminal bronchioles, and (3) destruction of many alveolar walls. In severe emphysema, as much as four fifths of the respiratory membrane can be destroyed; then even the slightest exercise can cause respiratory distress. In fact, many such patients cannot even perform the simple feat of walking across the floor of a single room without gasping for breath.

Cardiovascular System in Exercise

Muscle Blood Flow. A key requirement of cardiovascular function in exercise is to deliver the required oxygen and other nutrients to the exercising muscles. For this purpose, the muscle blood flow increases drastically during exercise. Figure 84-8 shows a recording of muscle blood flow in the calf of a person for a period of 6 minutes during moderately strong intermittent contractions. Note not only the great increase in flow—about 13-fold—but also the flow decrease during each muscle contraction. Two points can be made from this study: (1) The actual contractile process itself temporarily decreases muscle blood flow because the contracting skeletal muscle compresses the intramuscular blood vessels; therefore, strong *tonic* muscle contractions can cause rapid muscle fatigue because of lack of delivery of enough oxygen and other nutrients during the continuous contraction. (2) The blood flow to muscles during exercise increases markedly. The following comparison shows the maximal increase in blood flow that can occur in a well-trained athlete.

	ml/100 g Muscle/min
Resting blood flow	3.6
Blood flow during maximal exercise	90

Thus, muscle blood flow can increase a maximum of about 25-fold during the most strenuous exercise. Almost one-half this increase in flow results from intramuscular vasodilation caused by the direct effects of increased muscle metabolism, as explained in Chapter 21. The remaining increase results from multiple factors, the most important of which is probably the moderate increase in arterial blood pressure that occurs in exercise, usually about a 30 percent increase. The increase in pressure not only forces more blood through the blood vessels but also stretches the walls of the arterioles and further reduces the vascular resistance. Therefore, a 30 percent increase in blood pressure can often more than double the blood flow; this multiplies the great increase in flow already caused by the metabolic vasodilation at least another twofold.

Work Output, Oxygen Consumption, and Cardiac Output During Exercise. Figure 84-9 shows the interrelations among work output, oxygen consumption, and cardiac output during exercise. It is not surprising that all these are directly related to one another, as shown by the linear functions, because the muscle work output increases oxygen consumption, and increased oxygen consumption in turn dilates the muscle blood vessels, thus increasing venous return and cardiac output. Typical cardiac outputs at several levels of exercise are the following:

	L/min
Cardiac output in young man at rest	5.5
Maximal cardiac output during exercise in young untrained man	23
Maximal cardiac output during exercise in average male marathoner	30

Thus, the normal untrained person can increase cardiac output a little over fourfold, and the well-trained athlete can increase output about sixfold. (Individual marathoners have been clocked at cardiac outputs as great as 35 to 40 L/min, seven to eight times normal resting output.)

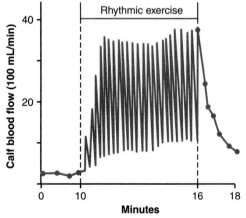

Figure 84-8 Effects of muscle exercise on blood flow in the calf of a leg during strong rhythmical contraction. The blood flow was much less during contraction than between contractions. (Redrawn from Barcroft H, Dornhors AC: Blood flow through human calf during rhythmic exercise. J Physiol 109:402, 1949.)

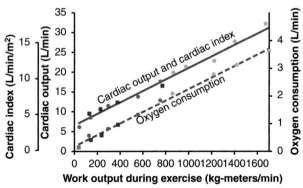

Figure 84-9 Relation between cardiac output and work output (*solid line*) and between oxygen consumption and work output (*dashed line*) during different levels of exercise. (Redrawn from Guyton AC, Jones CE, Coleman TB: Circulatory Physiology: Cardiac Output and Its Regulation. Philadelphia: WB Saunders, 1973.)

Effect of Training on Heart Hypertrophy and on Cardiac Output. From the foregoing data, it is clear that marathoners can achieve maximal cardiac outputs about 40 percent greater than those achieved by untrained persons. This results mainly from the fact that the heart chambers of marathoners enlarge about 40 percent; along with this enlargement of the chambers, the heart mass also increases 40 percent or more. Therefore, not only do the skeletal muscles hypertrophy during athletic training, but so does the heart. However, heart enlargement and increased pumping capacity occur almost entirely in the endurance types, not in the sprint types, of athletic training.

Even though the heart of the marathoner is considerably larger than that of the normal person, resting cardiac output is almost exactly the same as that in the normal person. However, this normal cardiac output is achieved by a large stroke volume at a reduced heart rate. Table 84-2 compares stroke volume and heart rate in the untrained person and the marathoner.

Thus, the heart-pumping effectiveness of each heartbeat is 40 to 50 percent greater in the highly trained athlete than in the untrained person, but there is a corresponding decrease in heart rate at rest.

Role of Stroke Volume and Heart Rate in Increasing the Cardiac Output. Figure 84-10 shows the approximate changes in stroke volume and heart rate as the cardiac output increases from its resting level of about 5.5 L/min to 30 L/min in the marathon runner. The *stroke volume* increases from 105 to 162 milliliters, an increase of about 50 percent, whereas the heart rate increases from 50 to 185 beats/min,

an increase of 270 percent. Therefore, the heart rate increase accounts by far for a greater proportion of the increase in cardiac output than does the increase in stroke volume during strenuous exercise. The stroke volume normally reaches its maximum by the time the cardiac output has increased only halfway to its maximum. Any further increase in cardiac output must occur by increasing the heart rate.

Relation of Cardiovascular Performance to V̇o₂ Max. During maximal exercise, both the heart rate and stroke volume are increased to about 95 percent of their maximal levels. Because the cardiac output is equal to stroke volume *times* heart rate, one finds that the cardiac output is about 90 percent of the maximum that the person can achieve. This is in contrast to about 65 percent of maximum for pulmonary ventilation. Therefore, one can readily see that the cardiovascular system is normally much more limiting on V̇o₂ Max than is the respiratory system, because oxygen utilization by the body can never be more than the rate at which the cardiovascular system can transport oxygen to the tissues.

For this reason, it is frequently stated that the level of athletic performance that can be achieved by the marathoner mainly depends on the performance capability of his or her heart, because this is the most limiting link in the delivery of adequate oxygen to the exercising muscles. Therefore, the 40 percent greater cardiac output that the marathoner can achieve over the average untrained male is probably the single most important physiologic benefit of the marathoner's training program.

Effect of Heart Disease and Old Age on Athletic Performance. Because of the critical limitation that the cardiovascular system places on maximal performance in endurance athletics, one can readily understand that any type of heart disease that reduces maximal cardiac output will cause an almost corresponding decrease in achievable total body muscle power. Therefore, a person with congestive heart failure frequently has difficulty achieving even the muscle power required to climb out of bed, much less to walk across the floor.

The maximal cardiac output of older people also decreases considerably—there is as much as a 50 percent decrease between ages 18 and 80. Also, there is even more decrease in maximal breathing capacity. For these reasons, as well as reduced skeletal muscle mass, the maximal achievable muscle power is greatly reduced in old age.

Body Heat in Exercise

Almost all the energy released by the body's metabolism of nutrients is eventually converted into body heat. This applies even to the energy that causes muscle contraction for the following reasons: First, the maximal efficiency for conversion of nutrient energy into muscle work, even under the best of conditions, is only 20 to 25 percent; the remainder of the nutrient energy is converted into heat during the course of the intracellular chemical reactions. Second, almost all the energy that does go into creating muscle work still becomes body heat because all but a small portion of this energy is used for (1) overcoming viscous resistance to the movement of the muscles and joints, (2) overcoming the friction of the blood flowing through the blood vessels, and (3) other, similar effects—all of which convert the muscle contractile energy into heat.

Table 84-2 Comparison of Cardiac Function Between Marathoner and Nonathlete

	Stroke Volume (ml)	Heart Rate (beats/min)
Resting		
Nonathlete	75	75
Marathoner	105	50
Maximum		
Nonathlete	110	195
Marathoner	162	185

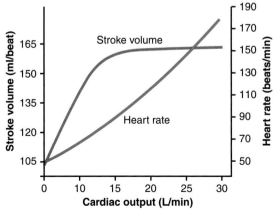

Figure 84-10 Approximate stroke volume output and heart rate at different levels of cardiac output in a marathon athlete.

Now, recognizing that the oxygen consumption by the body can increase as much as 20-fold in the well-trained athlete and that the amount of heat liberated in the body is almost exactly proportional to the oxygen consumption (as discussed in Chapter 72), one quickly realizes that tremendous amounts of heat are injected into the internal body tissues when performing endurance athletic events. Next, with a vast rate of heat flow into the body, on a very hot and humid day so that the sweating mechanism cannot eliminate the heat, an intolerable and even lethal condition called *heatstroke* can easily develop in the athlete.

Heatstroke. During endurance athletics, even under normal environmental conditions, the body temperature often rises from its normal level of 98.6° to 102° or 103°F (37° to 40°C). With very hot and humid conditions or excess clothing, the body temperature can easily rise to 106° to 108°F (41° to 42°C). At this level, the elevated temperature itself becomes destructive to tissue cells, especially the brain cells. When this happens, multiple symptoms begin to appear, including extreme weakness, exhaustion, headache, dizziness, nausea, profuse sweating, confusion, staggering gait, collapse, and unconsciousness.

This whole complex is called *heatstroke,* and failure to treat it immediately can lead to death. In fact, even though the person has stopped exercising, the temperature does not easily decrease by itself. One of the reasons for this is that at these high temperatures, the temperature-regulating mechanism itself often fails (see Chapter 73). A second reason is that in heatstroke, the very high body temperature approximately doubles the rates of all intracellular chemical reactions, thus liberating still more heat.

The treatment of heatstroke is to reduce the body temperature as rapidly as possible. The most practical way to do this is to remove all clothing, maintain a spray of cool water on all surfaces of the body or continually sponge the body, and blow air over the body with a fan. Experiments have shown that this treatment can reduce the temperature either as rapidly or almost as rapidly as any other procedure, although some physicians prefer total immersion of the body in water containing a mush of crushed ice if available.

Body Fluids and Salt in Exercise

As much as a 5- to 10-pound weight loss has been recorded in athletes in a period of 1 hour during endurance athletic events under hot and humid conditions. Essentially all this weight loss results from loss of sweat. Loss of enough sweat to decrease body weight only 3 percent can significantly diminish a person's performance, and a 5 to 10 percent rapid decrease in weight can often be serious, leading to muscle cramps, nausea, and other effects. Therefore, it is essential to replace fluid as it is lost.

Replacement of Sodium Chloride and Potassium. Sweat contains a large amount of sodium chloride, for which reason it has long been stated that all athletes should take salt (sodium chloride) tablets when performing exercise on hot and humid days. However, overuse of salt tablets has often done as much harm as good. Furthermore, if an athlete becomes acclimatized to the heat by progressive increase in athletic exposure over a period of 1 to 2 weeks rather than

performing maximal athletic feats on the first day, the sweat glands also become acclimatized, so the amount of salt lost in the sweat becomes only a small fraction of that lost before acclimatization. This sweat gland acclimatization results mainly from increased aldosterone secretion by the adrenal cortex. The aldosterone in turn has a direct effect on the sweat glands, increasing reabsorption of sodium chloride from the sweat before the sweat itself issues forth from the sweat gland tubules onto the surface of the skin. Once the athlete is acclimatized, only rarely do salt supplements need to be considered during athletic events.

Experience by military units exposed to heavy exercise in the desert has demonstrated still another electrolyte problem—the loss of potassium. Potassium loss results partly from the increased secretion of aldosterone during heat acclimatization, which increases the loss of potassium in the urine, as well as in the sweat. As a consequence of these findings, some of the supplemental fluids for athletics contain properly proportioned amounts of potassium along with sodium, usually in the form of fruit juices.

Drugs and Athletes

Without belaboring this issue, let us list some of the effects of drugs in athletics.

First, *caffeine* is believed by some to increase athletic performance. In one experiment on a marathon runner, running time for the marathon was improved by 7 percent by judicious use of caffeine in amounts similar to those found in one to three cups of coffee. Yet experiments by others have failed to confirm any advantage, thus leaving this issue in doubt.

Second, use of *male sex hormones (androgens)* or other anabolic steroids to increase muscle strength undoubtedly can increase athletic performance under some conditions, especially in women and even in men. However, anabolic steroids also greatly increase the risk of cardiovascular damage because they often cause hypertension, decreased high-density blood lipoproteins, and increased low-density lipoproteins, all of which promote heart attacks and strokes.

In men, any type of male sex hormone preparation also leads to decreased testicular function, including both decreased formation of sperm and decreased secretion of the person's own natural testosterone, with residual effects sometimes lasting at least for many months and perhaps indefinitely. In a woman, even more dire effects can occur because she is not normally adapted to the male sex hormone—hair on the face, a bass voice, ruddy skin, and cessation of menses.

Other drugs, such as *amphetamines* and *cocaine,* have been reputed to increase one's athletic performance. It is equally true that overuse of these drugs can lead to deterioration of performance. Furthermore, experiments have failed to prove the value of these drugs except as a psychic stimulant. Some athletes have been known to die during athletic events because of interaction between such drugs and the norepinephrine and epinephrine released by the sympathetic nervous system during exercise. One of the possible causes of death under these conditions is overexcitability of the heart, leading to ventricular fibrillation, which is lethal within seconds.

Body Fitness Prolongs Life

Multiple studies have now shown that people who maintain appropriate body fitness, using judicious regimens of exercise and weight control, have the additional benefit of prolonged life. Especially between the ages of 50 and 70, studies have shown mortality to be three times less in the most fit people than in the least fit.

But why does body fitness prolong life? The following are some of the most important reasons.

Body fitness and weight control greatly reduce cardiovascular disease. This results from (1) maintenance of moderately lower blood pressure and (2) reduced blood cholesterol and low-density lipoprotein along with increased high-density lipoprotein. As pointed out earlier, these changes all work together to reduce the number of heart attacks, brain strokes, and kidney disease.

The athletically fit person has more bodily reserves to call on when he or she does become sick. For instance, an 80-year-old nonfit person may have a respiratory system that limits oxygen delivery to the tissues to no more than 1 L/min; this means a *respiratory reserve of no more than threefold to fourfold.* However, an athletically fit old person may have twice as much reserve. This is especially important in preserving life when the older person develops conditions such as pneumonia that can rapidly require all available respiratory reserve. In addition, the ability to increase cardiac output in times of need (the "cardiac reserve") is often 50 percent greater in the athletically fit old person than in the nonfit person.

Exercise and overall body fitness also reduce the risk for several chronic metabolic disorders associated with obesity such as insulin resistance and type II diabetes. Moderate exercise, even in the absence of significant weight loss, has been shown to improve insulin sensitivity and reduce, or in some cases eliminate, the need for insulin treatment in patients with type II diabetes.

Improved body fitness also reduces the risk for several types of cancers, including breast, prostate, and colon cancer. Much of the beneficial effects of exercise may be related to reduction in obesity. However, studies in experimental animals and in humans have also shown that regular exercise reduces the risk for many chronic diseases through mechanisms that are incompletely understood but are, at least to some extent, independent of weight loss or decreased adiposity.

Bibliography

Allen DG, Lamb GD, Westerblad H: Skeletal muscle fatigue: cellular mechanisms, *Physiol Rev* 88:287, 2008.

Blair SN, LaMonte MJ, Nichaman MZ: The evolution of physical activity recommendations. How much is enough, *Am J Clin Nutr* 79:913S, 2004.

Cairns SP, Lindinger MI: Do multiple ionic interactions contribute to skeletal muscle fatigue? *J Physiol* 586:4039, 2008.

Favier FB, Benoit H, Freyssenet D: Cellular and molecular events controlling skeletal muscle mass in response to altered use, *Pflugers Arch* 456:587, 2008.

Fitts RH: The cross-bridge cycle and skeletal muscle fatigue, *J Appl Physiol* 104:551, 2008.

Glass JD: Signalling pathways that mediate skeletal muscle hypertrophy and atrophy, *Nat Cell Biol* 5:87, 2003.

González-Alonso J, Crandall CG, Johnson JM: The cardiovascular challenge of exercising in the heat, *J Physiol* 586:45, 2008.

Guyton AC, Jones CE, Coleman TB: *Circulatory Physiology: Cardiac Output and Its Regulation*, ed 2, Philadelphia, 1973, WB Saunders Co.

Levine BD: $\dot{V}o_2$ Max: what do we know, and what do we still need to know?, *J Physiol* 586:25, 2008.

Powers SK, Jackson MJ: Exercise-induced oxidative stress: cellular mechanisms and impact on muscle force production, *Physiol Rev* 88:1243, 2008.

Rennie MJ, Wackerhage H, Spangenburg EE, et al: Control of the size of the human muscle mass, *Annu Rev Physiol* 66:799, 2004.

Romer LM, Polkey MI: Exercise-induced respiratory muscle fatigue: implications for performance, *J Appl Physiol* 104:879, 2008.

Sandri M: Signaling in muscle atrophy and hypertrophy, *Physiology (Bethesda)* 23:160, 2008.

Schiaffino S, Sandri M, Murgia M: Activity-dependent signaling pathways controlling muscle diversity and plasticity, *Physiology (Bethesda)* 22:269, 2007.

Seals DR, Desouza CA, Donato AJ, et al: Habitual exercise and arterial aging, *J Appl Physiol* 105:1323, 2008.

Sjöqvist F, Garle M, Rane A: Use of doping agents, particularly anabolic steroids, in sports and society, *Lancet* 371:1872, 2008.

Tschakovsky ME, Hughson RL: Interaction of factors determining oxygen uptake at the onset of exercise, *J Appl Physiol* 86:1101, 1999.

Note: Page numbers followed by *b* indicate boxes; *f*, figures; *t*, tables.

A

A bands, of skeletal muscle, 71, 72*f*
A fibers, 563–564, 563*f*
  Aδ cold fibers, 592
  Aδ fast pain fibers, 584, 585, 587
  Aα motor fibers, 656, 659
  Aγ motor fibers, 656, 659
Abdominal compression reflex, 209
Abdominal muscles
  in expiration, 465, 466*f*
  in labor, 1013
  spasm of, in peritonitis, 665
Absence syndrome, 726
Absolute refractory period, 69
Absorbing colon, 797, 798
Absorption. *See* Kidney(s), reabsorption by;
    Large intestine, absorption in; Small
    intestine, absorption in.
Acceleration of head
  angular, 677, 677*f*
  linear, 676–677
Acceleratory forces, in aviation and
    spacecraft, 531–533, 531*f*, 532*f*
Acclimatization to altitude, 510
  alveolar P$_{O_2}$ and, 527, 528–530
  work capacity and, 530, 530*t*
Acclimatization to cold, chemical
    thermogenesis and, 873
Acclimatization to heat, 877
  sweating and, 871, 877
Accommodation
  of eye, 601, 601*f*
    autonomic control of, 631–632, 735
    pupillary reaction to, 632
  of mechanoreceptors, 562
ACE (angiotensin-converting enzyme)
    inhibitors
  adverse effects of, 320–321
  antihypertensive effects of, 374
Acetate, vasodilation caused by, 200
Acetazolamide, 398, 503
Acetoacetic acid, 823–824, 839
  in diabetes mellitus, 393, 953
  insulin lack and, 944
Acetone, 823
  on breath, 953–954
  ketosis and, 823, 824
Acetyl coenzyme A (acetyl-CoA), 22
  acetoacetic acid produced from, 823
  in acetylcholine synthesis, 732
  amino acids converted to, 825
  cholesterol synthesis from, 827
  in citric acid cycle, 813–814, 813*f*
    after fatty acid oxidation, 822–823
  from fatty acid beta-oxidation, 822,
    822*f*, 823
  fatty acid synthesis from, 824, 824*f*, 825

Acetyl coenzyme A (acetyl-CoA) (*Continued*)
  pantothenic acid and, 855
  pyruvic acid conversion to, 812–813
  steroid synthesis from, 992
Acetylcholine
  in basal ganglia, 692–693, 692*f*
  of brain stem reticular neurons, 711
    sleep and, 722
  cardiac effects of, 119, 120
    bradycardia as, 144
  as central nervous system transmitter, 551
  of cholinergic nerve endings, 731–732
    drugs with potentiating effect on, 740
  coronary blood flow and, 247
  gastric secretions and, 778, 779
  gastrointestinal smooth muscle and, 755, 756
  Huntington's disease and, 694
  molecular structure of, 731
  at neuromuscular junction
    secretion of, 73, 83–86, 84*f*
    synthesis of, 83, 86
  pancreatic secretions and, 782
  pharmacologic actions of, 740
  as smooth muscle neurotransmitter, 95, 96
  synthesis of, 732
Acetylcholine receptors. *See also*
    Acetylcholine-gated ion channels.
  in myasthenia gravis, 86
  principal types of, 733
Acetylcholine system, in brain, 712, 713, 713*f*
Acetylcholine-gated ion channels, 48,
    73–74, 83–84, 84*f*, 85, 85*f*. *See also*
    Acetylcholine receptors.
Acetylcholinesterase
  at neuromuscular junction, 83, 84*f*, 85, 86
  at parasympathetic nerve endings, 732
Acetylcholinesterase inhibitors, 86, 740
  for myasthenia gravis, 86–87
Acetyl-CoA. *See* Acetyl coenzyme
    A (acetyl-CoA).
Acetyl-CoA carboxylase, 825
Acetylsalicylic acid. *See* Aspirin
    (acetylsalicylic acid).
Achalasia, 765, 799
Achlorhydria, 778, 800
Acid(s)
  definition of, 379
  nonvolatile, 385, 387, 388, 390
    anion gap and, 395
  sour taste of, 645, 646*t*
  strong and weak, 379–380
Acid hydrolases, of lysosomes, 19, 20
Acid-base disorders. *See also* Acidosis; Alkalosis.
  clinical causes of, 392–393
  diagnosis of, 393–395, 394*f*
  mixed, 394–395, 394*f*
  treatment of, 393

Acid-base nomogram, 394–395, 394*f*
Acid-base regulation. *See also* Hydrogen ions.
  buffer systems in, 380–381
    ammonia, 388–389, 389*f*
    bicarbonate, 381–383, 382*f*
    gastrointestinal mucus and, 775
    isohydric principle and, 383–384
    phosphate, 383, 388, 388*f*
    protein, 383–384, 413
    respiratory, 385
  fundamental definitions for, 379–380
  kidneys in, 380, 385–388, 386*f*, 387*f*
    correction of acidosis by, 387, 391
    correction of alkalosis by, 387,
      391–392
    phosphate and ammonia buffers in,
      388–389, 388*f*, 389*f*
    quantification of, 389–391, 390*t*
  overview of, 379, 380
  precision of, 379, 380
  respiratory system in, 380, 384–385, 384*f*
Acidophil cells, 896*f*, 897
Acidophilic tumors, 897, 903–904
Acidosis. *See also* Acid-base disorders.
  bicarbonate reabsorption in, 386, 387, 390
  calcium and
    protein-bound, 367
    reabsorption of, 369
  characteristics of, 391*t*
  chronic, ammonium excretion in,
    389, 391
  definition of, 379, 380
  metabolic, 391, 391*t*
    anion gap in, 395, 395*t*
    clinical causes of, 392–393
    definition of, 382
    in diabetes mellitus, 951
    diagnosis of, 394
    hydrogen ion secretion in, 390
    hyperchloremic, 395, 395*t*
    potassium homeostasis and, 362
    renal correction of, 391
  in neonate, 1024
  neuronal depression in, 557
  potassium homeostasis and, 364, 367
  renal correction of, 391
  in renal failure, 406
  respiratory, 382, 385, 391, 391*t*
    clinical causes of, 392
    diagnosis of, 393–394
    hydrogen ion secretion in, 390
    renal correction of, 391
  in shock, 278
  treatment of, 393
Acini
  of pancreas, 773, 780–781, 939, 939*f*
  of salivary glands, 773, 774*f*, 775, 776

Acquired (adaptive) immunity, 433–442.
  See also Antibodies; Antigen(s);
  Lymphocytes.
  basic types of, 433, 434
  passive, 442
  tolerance to own tissues in, 442
Acquired immunodeficiency syndrome (AIDS)
  helper T cells in, 440–441
  wasting syndrome in, 852
Acromegaly, 903–904, 903*f*
  diabetes mellitus in, 952
Acrosome, 975, 975*f*, 977
Acrosome reaction, 977
ACTH. *See* Adrenocorticotropic hormone
  (ACTH; corticotropin).
Actin
  in ameboid movement, 23
  of cardiac muscle, 101, 103
    Frank-Starling mechanism and, 110
    ventricular volume and, 108
  in cell membrane support, 16
  coated pits and, 18–19, 18*f*
  in intestinal microvilli, 794
  in mitosis, 39
  in phagocytosis, 19
  of platelets, 451, 454
  of skeletal muscle
    contraction mechanism and, 74, 74*f*,
      75–76, 75*f*, 76*f*
    hypertrophy and, 81
    muscle tension and, 77, 77*f*
    structural features of, 71, 72*f*, 73*f*, 74*f*,
      75, 75*f*
  of smooth muscle, 92, 92*f*, 93–94
Action potential(s). *See also* Membrane
    potential(s).
  calcium ions in, 64
    in gastrointestinal smooth muscle,
      754–755
  cardiac, 102–104, 102*f*
    atrial, 117
    duration of contraction and, 104
    electrocardiogram and, 122, 122*f*
    excitation-contraction coupling
      and, 103, 104
    plateau in, 66, 66*f*
    prolonged ventricular, 147, 148*f*
    in Purkinje fibers, 102*f*, 103, 117
    sinus nodal, 115–116, 116*f*, 117
    spontaneous rhythmicity in, 66–67, 66*f*
    ventricular, 102, 102*f*, 122, 122*f*
  nerve, 60–63, 61*f*
    anions and, 64
    energy expenditure by, 65, 66*f*, 68
    energy of ATP for, 860
    excitation of, 68–69, 68*f*
    initiation of, 64
    inspiratory, 505
    on motor nerve, 73
    olfactory, 649, 650
    as positive feedback, 8–9, 64
    propagation of, 64–65, 65*f*
    re-establishing ionic gradients
      after, 65
    refractory period after, 69
    stages of, 61
    summary of, 63, 63*f*
    threshold for, 64–65, 68–69, 68*f*
    velocity of, 68
  neuronal
    of brain stem reticular area, 711
    in cerebellum, 684, 685
    facilitation and, 708
    generation in axon, 553–554
    postganglionic, 732
    at presynaptic terminal, 547–548
    of retinal ganglion cells, 617, 619

Action potential(s), neuronal (*Continued*)
    summation and, 554*f*, 555
    threshold for, 555, 556–557, 556*f*
  plateau in
    with cardiac muscle, 66, 66*f*
    with smooth muscle, 95*f*, 96
  receptor potentials and, 561–562, 561*f*
  recording with oscilloscope, 69, 69*f*
  rhythmical, 66–67, 66*f*
  skeletal muscle, 74, 83, 87, 88, 88*f*, 89*f*
    end plate potential and, 84, 85, 85*f*
    energy for, 78
  smooth muscle, 95–96, 95*f*
    of bladder, 306–308
    excited by stretch, 96
    gastrointestinal, 754–755, 754*f*
    plateau in, 95*f*, 96
    slow wave, 95*f*, 96
    of stomach, 766
Action tremor, 687–688, 689
Active hyperemia, 194
Active transport, 14, 18, 52–56
  of amino acids into cells, 832–833
  through cellular sheets, 55–56, 55*f*
  vs. diffusion, 45–46, 46*f*
  energy from ATP for, 859
  primary, 52–54, 53*f*
  in renal tubular reabsorption, 324–328,
    325*f*, 326*f*, 327*f*
  in salivary ducts, 775
  secondary, 52–53, 54–55, 55*f*. *See also*
    Co-transport.
  thyroid hormones and, 912
Acupuncture, 588
Acute local potentials, 68, 69
Acute subthreshold potentials, 68, 68*f*
Acute tubular necrosis, 400–401
Adaptation
  of olfactory sensations, 650
  of sensory receptors, 562–563, 562*f*
  of taste, 648
Adaptive control systems, 9
Adaptive immunity. *See* Acquired (adaptive)
    immunity.
Addison disease, 934–935
  hyperkalemia in, 361, 365
  hyponatremia in, 294–295, 360
    salt appetite and, 360
  volume depletion in, 375
Addisonian crisis, 935
Adenine, 27, 28, 28*f*, 30, 31*t*
Adenohypophysis. *See* Pituitary gland, anterior.
Adenosine
  blood flow control and, 192–193
    in cardiac muscle, 247
    in gut wall, 761
    in skeletal muscle, 243–244
  coronary ischemia and, 248
  irreversible shock and, 278–279
Adenosine diphosphate (ADP)
  control of glycolysis by, 815
  conversion to ATP, 809–810
    in mitochondria, 814*f*, 815
  metabolic rate and, 862
  oxygen usage and, 500, 501, 501*f*
  platelet aggregation and, 452
Adenosine monophosphate (AMP),
    809–810. *See also* Cyclic adenosine
    monophosphate (cAMP).
Adenosine triphosphate (ATP), 21–23
  in active transport, 52–53
    by calcium pump, 54
    renal tubular, 324–325, 325*f*, 326, 326*f*
    by sodium-potassium pump, 53, 53*f*
  in cardiac muscle, 248
  chemical structure of, 809, 810*f*
  ciliary movement and, 25

Adenosine triphosphate (ATP) (*Continued*)
  control of glycolysis by, 815
  conversion into cAMP, 889
  depleted in irreversible shock, 278–279
  as energy currency, 809–810, 809*f*, 859–861
    anaerobic vs. aerobic, 860–861
    functions energized by, 859, 860
    nutrients degraded for, 859
    phosphocreatine buffer of, 860
    summary of, 861, 861*f*
  energy released per mole of, 809–810
  from fatty acid oxidation, 823
  flagellar movement and, 975
  gastrointestinal secretions and, 774
  glycogen-lactic acid system and, 1033, 1033*f*
  high-energy bonds of, 21, 809, 859
  mitochondrial synthesis of, 16, 22, 22*f*
  nerve fiber ionic gradients and, 65
  in olfactory cilium, 649, 649*f*
  phosphocreatine and, 1033, 1033*f*
  in postganglionic nerve endings, 732
  production of, 812
    acetyl-CoA and, 812–813
    citric acid cycle and, 813–814, 813*f*
    glycolysis and, 812, 812*f*
    oxidative phosphorylation and,
      814–815, 814*f*
    summary of, 815
  in protein synthesis, 34, 34*f*
  in RNA synthesis, 30
  in skeletal muscle, 73, 74, 75, 76, 78–79
    of athletes, 1032–1034, 1033*f*, 1033*t*
  in smooth muscle, 93, 94
  structure of, 21
  uses of, 22–23, 22*f*
  as vasodilator, in skeletal muscle, 243–244
Adenylyl cyclase. *See also* Cyclic adenosine
    monophosphate (cAMP).
  ACTH and, 932
  adrenergic or cholinergic receptors and, 733
  antidiuretic hormone and, 905
  glucagon and, 948
  growth hormone secretion and, 902
  hormonal activity and, 889–890, 889*b*, 890*f*
  hormone receptors and, 888
  memory and, 707–708
  in olfactory cilium, 649, 649*f*
  in smooth muscle, 97
  thyroid hormone secretion and, 914
ADH. *See* Antidiuretic hormone (ADH;
    vasopressin).
Adhesion molecules
  in inflammation, 428, 429*f*
  in T-cell activation, 440, 440*f*
Adipocytes (fat cells), 12, 821
  cytokine hormones produced by, 881
  deficiency of, 822
  obesity and, 850
Adipokines, 881
Adipose tissue, 821
  fatty acid diffusion into, 820, 820*f*
  fatty acid mobilization from, 823, 825
    cortisol and, 929
  fatty acid storage in, 825
    insulin and, 943
  food intake and feedback from, 849
  lipase in, 821, 826
  triglyceride storage in, 824, 825
  triglyceride synthesis in, 824, 825
Adiposogenital syndrome, 985, 985*f*
ADP. *See* Adenosine diphosphate (ADP).
Adrenal cortex. *See also* Adrenocortical
    hormones.
  anatomy of, 921, 921*f*
  cholesterol used by, 827
  fetal, 1008
  neonatal hypofunction of, 1026

Adrenal diabetes, 928
Adrenal glands
    adenoma of, 935
    anatomy of, 921, 921f
Adrenal insufficiency. *See* Addison disease.
Adrenal medulla. *See also* Epinephrine;
        Norepinephrine.
    anatomy of, 921, 921f
    exercise and, fat utilization in, 825
    function of, 736
        basal secretion in, 737
        duration of action in, 732, 736
        receptors and, 733
    hypovolemic shock and, 275
    sympathetic nerve fibers and, 730
    sympathetic vasoconstrictor system and, 204
Adrenergic drugs, 739–740
Adrenergic fibers, 731–732
Adrenergic receptors, 733, 733t. *See also* Alpha
        adrenergic receptors; Beta adrenergic
        receptors.
    drugs causing block of, 740
Adrenocortical hormones, 921–937. *See also*
        Androgens, adrenal; Glucocorticoids;
        Mineralocorticoids.
    abnormalities of, 934–936, 935f, 936f
    classification of, 921
    excretion of, 924
    metabolism of, in liver, 924
    plasma protein binding of, 923–924
    pregnancy and, 1009
    properties of, 922–923, 924t
    synthesis and secretion of, 921–924, 921f,
        923f, 924t
Adrenocorticotropic hormone (ACTH;
        corticotropin), 896, 896t
    adrenocortical hormone synthesis and, 922
    aldosterone secretion and, 927, 928
    chemistry of, 931
    cortisol secretion and, 931–934, 932f
    deficiency of, 934
    excess of, 935, 936
    gluconeogenesis and, 817
    ketogenic effect of, 825
    pregnancy and, 1009
    regulation of, by hypothalamus, 931–932
    synthesis and secretion of, 933–934
    thyroid hormones and, 913–914
Adrenogenital syndrome, 936, 936f
Aerobic energy, 860. *See also* Oxidative
        metabolism.
    for exercise, 1033, 1033f, 1033t, 1034b
    recovery after, 1034, 1034f, 1035f
Afferent arteriole(s), renal, 304–305, 305f,
        307f, 311f
    glomerular filtration rate and, 315, 316, 316f
    myogenic mechanism and, 321
    physiologic control of, 317–318, 319
    reabsorption rate and, 336
    tubuloglomerular feedback and, 320, 320f
Affinity constant, 438
Afterdischarge, 567–568
    crossed extensor reflex and, 663, 663f
    flexor reflex and, 662, 662f
Afterload, 109
Agglutination
    by antibodies, 438
    by complement system, 439
    of red blood cells, 446
        in blood typing, 447, 447t
Agglutinins, 446, 446f, 446t
    anti-Rh, 447
    in blood typing, 447, 447t
Agglutinogens, 445, 446t, 447
Agonist and antagonist muscles, 81
    neuronal circuits and, 566
Agouti-related protein, 846, 847, 847f, 849

AIDS. *See* Acquired immunodeficiency
        syndrome (AIDS).
Air hunger, 522
Airflow resistance, in bronchial tree, 473
Airplane. *See* Aviation.
Airway obstruction
    atelectasis secondary to, 519, 519f
    in emphysema, 517, 518
    forced expiratory volume in 1 second
        and, 517, 517f
    maximum expiratory flow and,
        516–517, 516f
    sleep apnea caused by, 513
Airway resistance
    in asthma, 520
    hypoxia and, 520
Akinesia, 693
Alactacid oxygen debt, 1034, 1034f
Alarm reaction
    arterial pressure elevation in, 205
    sympathetic nervous system in, 738–739
Albinos, visual acuity of, 611
Albumin, 833. *See also* Plasma proteins.
    bilirubin transport by, 840, 842
    cortisol bound to, 923
    fatty acid transport by, 820, 821
    glomerular filtration of, 313–314, 313t
    plasma colloid osmotic pressure and,
        184, 184t, 833
    for plasma volume measurement, 290
    thyroid hormones bound to, 909–910
Alcohol
    cirrhosis and, 838
    gastric absorption of, 793
    gastritis caused by, 799
    pancreatitis caused by, 801
    peptic ulcer and, 801
Alcoholic headache, 591
Aldosterone, 924–928
    angiotensin II and, 221–222
    arterial pressure control and, 221–222,
        227f, 228
    in cardiac failure, 260
    chemical formula of, 922, 923f
    circulatory effects of, 925–926, 925f
    concentration of, in blood, 924
    cortisol and, 924–925
    deficiency of, 924, 934
    excess of, 925–926, 925f
        alkalosis caused by, 390
        hypernatremia caused by, 296
        hypertension caused by, 407
        metabolic alkalosis caused by, 393
    extracellular fluid osmolarity and, 359–360
    extracellular fluid sodium and,
        359–360, 359f
    intestinal sodium absorption and,
        795, 797, 926
    mechanism of action, 891, 926–927, 926f
    nongenomic actions of, 927
    obesity and, 225
    plasma protein binding of, 923
    potassium homeostasis and, 361
        renal secretion in, 337–338, 364–366,
        364f, 365f, 366f, 925
    pregnancy and, 1009
    properties of, 922, 924t
    regulation of secretion of, 927–928, 927f
    renal effects of, 925–926, 925f
    salivary glands and, 926
    sodium reabsorption and, 328, 337–338,
        375, 925
    sweat glands and, 926
    sweating and, acclimatization of, 871, 877
    synthesis of, 921–922, 923f
    tubular reabsorption and, 328,
        337–338, 338t

Aldosterone antagonists, 332, 333f, 398t, 399
Aldosterone escape, 925
Aldosteronism, primary, 936
    alkalosis in, 390
    hypertension caused by, 219–220
    hypokalemia in, 361, 365
Alimentary tract. *See* Gastrointestinal tract.
Alkali, definition of, 379
Alkaline phosphatase, in hyperparathyroidism,
        968
Alkalosis. *See also* Acid-base disorders.
    in aldosterone excess, 390
    bicarbonate excretion in, 385, 390
    calcium and
        protein-bound, 367
        reabsorption of, 369
    characteristics of, 391t
    definition of, 379, 380
    grand mal attack and, 726
    metabolic, 391t, 392
        aldosterone excess with, 926
        bicarbonate excretion in, 387
        clinical causes of, 393
        definition of, 382
        diagnosis of, 394
        hydrogen ion secretion and, 390
        potassium homeostasis and, 362
        vomiting as cause of, 393, 804
    neuronal excitability in, 557
    renal correction of, 391–392
    respiratory, 391t, 392
        clinical causes of, 392
        diagnosis of, 394
        at high altitude, 529
        hydrogen ion secretion and, 390
    treatment of, 393
Allergic reactions
    in asthma, 520
    cortisol and, 931
    eosinophils in, 430
    mast cells and basophils in, 431
Allergy, 443–444
    in infant, 1026
Allografts, 449
All-or-nothing principle, of action
        potential, 65
Alpha adrenergic receptors, 733, 733t
    in coronary vessels, 248
    drugs acting on, 739
    drugs blocking, 740
    of vascular smooth muscle, norepinephrine
        and, 204
Alpha waves, 723f, 724–725, 724f, 725f
Altitude. *See* High altitude.
Alveolar air, 487–489, 487t
    expired air and, 487t, 489, 489f
    rate of replacement of, 487–488, 488f
Alveolar ducts, 489, 489f
Alveolar macrophages, 427, 428, 474
Alveolar membrane, 5. *See also* Respiratory
        membrane.
Alveolar pressure, 466–467, 466f
Alveolar ventilation, 471–472
    acid-base balance and, 384–385, 384f
    carbon dioxide partial pressure and
        alveolar, 488–489, 489f
        blood, 508, 508f, 510, 510f
    during exercise, 510–511, 511f
    at high altitude, 529
    oxygen partial pressure and
        alveolar, 488, 488f
        blood, 509, 509f, 510, 510f
    pH of blood and, 508, 508f, 510, 510f
    ventilation-perfusion ratio and, 492–494
Alveolus(i), pulmonary, 489, 489f, 490f
    fluid balance with interstitium, 482, 482f
Alzheimer's disease, 727–728

Amacrine cells, 610*f*, 617, 617*f*
  action potentials of, 617
  functions of, 618–619
  neurotransmitters released by, 617
  visual contrast and, 618
  visual pathway and, 617, 617*f*
Ameboid movement, 23–24, 23*f*, 425
Ameloblasts, 969, 970
Amiloride, 332, 333*f*, 399
  Liddle's syndrome and, 408–409
Amino acids
  active transport into cells, 832–833
  in blood, 831–833
    equilibrium between proteins and, 833–834, 834*f*
    glucagon secretion and, 948
    glucocorticoids and, 835, 929
    regulation of levels of, 833
  deamination of, 834–835, 839
  as energy source, 834–835
    in starvation, 835
  essential, 832*f*, 834
    deficiency of, 843
  facilitated diffusion of, 50
  glucose synthesis from, 817
    cortisol and, 928
  growth hormone and, 899, 900
  insulin and metabolism of, 944–945
  insulin secretion and, 946–947
  nonessential, 832*f*
    synthesis of, 834, 834*f*, 840
  plasma proteins as source of, 833
  as protein digestion products, 791
  in protein synthesis
    RNA codons for, 29*f*, 30, 31–32, 31*t*, 32*f*
    transfer RNA and, 31, 32, 32*f*, 34, 34*f*
  renal reabsorption of, 311–312, 325, 326*f*
    upper limit of, 833
  sodium co-transport of, 54–55, 794–795, 795*f*, 797
  storage of, 833
  structures of, 831, 832*f*
  tyrosine, hormones derived from, 882–884
Aminoaciduria, 408
Aminopolypeptidase, 791
Aminostatic theory of hunger and feeding, 849
Aminotransferases, 834
Amitriptyline, 727
Ammonia
  from amino acid deamination, 834, 835
  hepatic coma and, 835
  urea derived from, 835, 839–840, 859
Ammonia buffer system, 388–389, 389*f*
Ammonium chloride, for alkalosis, 393
Ammonium ion
  buffering by, 388–389, 389*f*
  excretion of, 389, 389*f*, 390, 391
Amnesia
  anterograde, 709, 719
  retrograde, 709
Amniotic fluid, 1011
  fetal urine in, 1020
  ingestion of, 1020
Amorphosynthesis, 577
AMP (adenosine monophosphate), 809–810. *See also* Cyclic adenosine monophosphate (cAMP).
Amphetamines
  athletic performance and, 1040
  for weight loss, 851
Ampulla, of semicircular duct, 675*f*, 676, 676*f*
Amygdala, 719–720
  anterior commissure and, 705
  feeding and, 848

α-Amylase(s)
  pancreatic, 781, 790
    in neonate, 1025
  salivary. *See* Ptyalin.
Amylin, 939
Amyloid plaques, in Alzheimer's disease, 728
Amyloidosis, nephrotic syndrome associated with, 404
Anaerobic energy, 860–861
Anaerobic glycolysis, 815–816, 860–861
  in muscle, 1033
Anaerobic metabolism, brain's lack of, 749
Anal sphincters, 771, 771*f*, 772
Analgesia system of brain and spinal cord, 586–588, 587*f*
Anaphase, 38*f*, 39
Anaphylactic shock, 280, 443
  sympathomimetic drugs for, 281
Anaphylaxis, 443
Anchoring filaments, of lymphatic capillaries, 187, 187*f*, 188
Androgens. *See also* Testosterone.
  adrenal, 921, 934, 980
    excess of, tumor-produced, 936
    in pregnancy, 1008
    synthesis of, 922, 923*f*
  athletic performance and, 1040
  ovarian production of, 980, 991, 992, 992*f*, 993*f*
  testicular production of, 979–980, 980*f*
Androstenedione
  adrenal synthesis of, 922, 923*f*
  ovarian synthesis of, 991
  testicular synthesis of, 979
Androsterone, 980
Anemia, 420–421
  aplastic, 420
  in chronic renal failure, 406
  circulatory effects of, 233, 420–421
  cyanosis and, 521–522
  hematocrit in, 287
  hemolytic, 420
  hypoxia in, 420–421, 521
  macrocytic, in folic acid deficiency, 854
  megaloblastic, 415*f*, 420
  microcytic, hypochromic, 415*f*, 420
  in neonate, 1025
  pernicious, 417, 420, 778, 800, 854
  in pregnancy, 1010
  red blood cell characteristics in, 415*f*
Anesthesia
  cardiac arrest during, 153
  general
    cardiac arrest caused by, 279, 281
    neurogenic shock caused by, 279
  paralysis of swallowing in, 799
  respiratory depression caused by, 512
  spinal
    cardiac output and, 239, 239*f*
    neurogenic shock caused by, 279
Anesthetics
  local, as membrane stabilizers, 69
  synaptic transmission and, 557
Angina pectoris, 252. *See also* Myocardial ischemia.
  bypass surgery for, 252
  cardiac hypertrophy leading to, 272
  current of injury in, 141
  drug treatment for, 252
    nitrates in, 196
Angiogenesis, 197, 198
  cancer growth and, 41
  at high altitude, 529
  inhibitors of, 198
Angiogenin, 198
Angioplasty, coronary artery, 253

Angiostatin, 198
Angiotensin I, 220–221
Angiotensin II, 220–221, 220*f*
  aldosterone secretion and, 921–922, 927–928
  endothelial cell receptors for, nitric oxide and, 196
  extracellular fluid osmolarity and, 359–360
  extracellular fluid sodium and, 359–360
  glomerular filtration rate and, 318, 320–321
  hypertension involving, 223–224, 223*f*
  in hypovolemic shock, 275
  obesity and, 225
  renal effects of, 221–222, 222*f*
  renal reabsorption and, 337, 338–339, 338*f*, 338*t*, 376
  renal sodium and water excretion and, 374–375, 374*f*
  thirst and, 358
  as vasoconstrictor, 199
    limited long-term effect of, 200
    nitric oxide and, 196
Angiotensin II receptor antagonists, 374
Angiotensinases, 221
Angiotensin-converting enzyme (ACE) inhibitors
  adverse effects of, 320–321
  antihypertensive effects of, 374
Angiotensinogen, 220
Angular acceleration, of head, 677, 677*f*
Angular gyrus area, 700, 701, 702, 704*f*, 705
Anion gap, 395, 395*t*
Anorexia, 851–852
Anorexia nervosa, 851–852
Anorexigenic substances, 846–847, 847*t*, 851
Anovulatory cycles, 998, 1001
ANP. *See* Atrial natriuretic peptide (ANP).
Anterior commissure, 705
Anterior motor neurons. *See* Motor neurons, anterior.
Anterograde amnesia, 709, 719
Anterolateral system, 573, 580–581, 581*f*
  thermal signals in, 593
  types of sensations in, 573
Antibodies, 437–438, 437*f*. *See also* Immunoglobulin(s).
  autoantibodies, hyperthyroidism caused by, 916
  classes of, 438
  infusion of, 442
  mechanisms of action of, 438, 438*f*, 439*f*
  in milk, 1016
  in neonate, 1025–1026
  opsonization and, 425
  in saliva, 776
Anticholinesterases. *See* Acetylcholinesterase inhibitors.
Anticoagulants
  in blood, 457
  for clinical use, 459–460
  in tissues, 453
Anticodons, 32
Antidiuretic hormone (ADH; vasopressin), 896, 904–905. *See also* Diabetes insipidus.
  arterial blood pressure and, 357, 905
  atrial stretch reflex and, 208
  blood volume and, 357, 357*f*, 905
  in cardiac failure, 260
  chemical structure of, 904
  disorders associated with, 354–355
  extracellular fluid osmolarity and, 905
  extracellular fluid volume and, 375–376
  factors affecting level of, 357, 357*t*
  hypernatremia caused by deficit of, 295
  hyponatremia caused by excess of, 295
  hypothalamus and, 356, 356*f*, 716, 904
  in hypovolemic shock, 275, 279

Antidiuretic hormone (ADH; vasopressin)
(*Continued*)
osmoreceptor feedback and, 355–357, 355*f*,
356*f*, 357*f*, 905
salt intake and, 217
synthesis and release of, 355, 356, 356*f*
urine concentration and, 345, 346, 346*f*,
347–348, 348*t*, 350, 350*f*
urea and, 350–351, 353
as vasoconstrictor, 199, 905
water reabsorption and, 339, 339*f*, 904–905
Antigen(s), 434
antibody binding of, 438
in blood cells, 445
released by macrophages, 436, 437
self-antigens, 434–435
Antigen-presenting cells, 440, 440*f*
Antioncogenes, 40
Antiperistalsis, 803, 804
Antipyretics, 876
Antipyrine, 289
Antithrombin III, 457
heparin and, 457
Antithyroid substances, 915
in foods, 917
Antral follicles, 989–990
Antrum, gastric, 766, 766*f*
Anuria, 399, 401
Aortic baroreceptors, 205–206, 206*f*
Aortic bodies, 208, 507, 508, 508*f*, 509
high altitude and, 529
Aortic coarctation, 224, 269
Aortic pressure, 158, 159*f*
cardiac cycle and, 105, 105*f*, 107
cardiac output and, 112, 112*f*
pulsations in, 168, 169*f*
abnormal contours of, 169, 169*f*
transmission to peripheral arteries,
169–170, 169*f*, 170*f*
Aortic regurgitation
circulatory dynamics in, 268
murmur of, 267, 267*f*, 268
pressure pulse associated with, 169, 169*f*
Aortic stenosis
aortic pressure pulse in, 169, 169*f*
circulatory dynamics in, 268
congenital, 269
murmur of, 267, 267*f*, 268
work output associated with, 108
Aortic valve, 105*f*, 106–107, 107*f*
aortic pressure curve and, 107
second heart sound and, 107, 266, 266*f*
Aphasia, 703–704
Aplastic anemia, 420
Aplysia, 707, 707*f*, 708
Apocrine glands, autonomic control of, 735
Apoferritin, 840
Apolipoprotein(a), 829
Apolipoprotein B, mutations of, 827
Apolipoprotein E
Alzheimer's disease and, 728
chylomicron removal from blood
and, 820, 820*f*
Apoprotein B, 819
Apoptosis, 40
Apparent mineralocorticoid excess syndrome,
924–925
Appendix, pain pathways from, 589–590, 589*f*
Appetite, 845. *See also* Hunger.
diminished level of, 851–852
gastric secretion and, 779
higher brain centers and, 848
hypothalamus and, 846–847
Appetite area of brain, 776
Aquaporins, 47, 905
aquaporin-2, antidiuretic hormone
and, 339, 339*f*

Aqueous humor, 606, 606*f*
formation of, 606, 606*f*
outflow of, 607, 607*f*
Aqueous veins, 607, 607*f*
Arachidonic acid, 890
Arachnoidal villi, 746*f*, 747
cerebrospinal fluid pressure and, 747–748
Arcuate fasciculus, 704–705, 704*f*
Arcuate nuclei
food intake and, 846–847, 847*f*, 847*t*
leptin and, 849
gonadotropin-releasing hormone and, 997
Area postrema, blood-brain barrier and,
748–749
Arginine, nitric oxide synthesis from, 195, 196*f*
Argyll Robertson pupil, 632
Aromatase, 991, 992, 992*f*, 993*f*
Arousal, pain signals and, 586
Arrhythmias, cardiac, 143–153
atrial fibrillation, 151–152, 152*f*
in mitral valvular disease, 269
atrial flutter, 152–153, 152*f*, 153*f*
atrioventricular block, 144–145, 144*f*, 145*f*
cardiac arrest, 153
circulatory arrest and, 281
cardiac hypertrophy leading to, 272
causes of, 143
hyperkalemia and, 926
in long QT syndromes, 147, 148*f*
paroxysmal tachycardia, 148–149
atrial, 148, 148*f*
ventricular, 148–149, 149*f*
partial intraventricular block, 145–146, 145*f*
as premature contractions. *See* Premature
contractions.
sinoatrial block, 144, 144*f*
sinus rhythm abnormalities, 143–144,
143*f*, 144*f*. *See also* Bradycardia;
Tachycardia(s).
supraventricular tachycardias, 148
torsades de pointes, 147, 148*f*
ventricular fibrillation as. *See* Ventricular
fibrillation.
Arterial blood pressure. *See also* Blood pressure.
acceleratory forces and, 531, 531*f*
age-related increase in, 171, 171*f*
blood flow and, 165–166, 165*f*, 166*f*
autoregulation of, 165–166, 165*f*,
194–195, 194*f*, 200, 217, 744–745, 745*f*
cerebral, 744–745, 745*f*
cardiac output and, 112, 112*f*, 216*f*,
217, 217*f*
in cardiogenic shock, 259
in different parts of circulation, 158, 159*f*
exercise-related increase in, 244–245
extracellular fluid volume and, 217, 217*f*
gravitational effect on, 173, 174
mean value of, 171, 171*f*
measurement of, clinical, 170–171, 170*f*
of neonate, 1024
reference level for, 174–175, 174*f*
regulation of. *See* Arterial blood pressure
control.
renal blood flow and, 319, 319*f*, 320, 321
renal reabsorption rate and, 336
respiratory waves in, 210
shock and, 273
hypovolemic, 274–275, 274*f*
thyroid hormones and, 913
urine output and, 337
vascular resistance and, 165
Arterial blood pressure control, 159
aldosterone and, 925, 925*f*
as homeostatic mechanism, 6, 7–8
integrated system for, 226–228, 227*f*
nervous, 204–209, 373–374
antidiuretic hormone and, 357

Arterial blood pressure control, nervous
(*Continued*)
brain stem in, 739
cardiac output and, 232, 232*f*
in CNS ischemic response, 209,
210–211, 210*f*
hypothalamus and, 715
parasympathetic, 736
reflex mechanisms in, 205–209,
206*f*, 207*f*
respiratory waves and, 210
skeletal nerves and muscles in, 209–210
sympathetic, 735–736
thirst and, 358
vasomotor waves and, 210–211, 210*f*
by renal–body fluid system, 213–220,
227–228, 227*f*, 371–373, 371*f*, 372*f*
chronic hypertension and, 218–220,
218*f*, 220*f*
pressure diuresis in, 213–218, 214*f*, 215*f*
salt in, 217–218, 376. *See also* Pressure
natriuresis.
total peripheral resistance and,
216–217, 216*f*, 217*f*
by renin-angiotensin system, 220–222,
220*f*, 221*f*, 222*f*
hypertension and, 223–224, 223*f*
Arterial pressure pulses, 168–171. *See also*
Pulse pressure.
abnormal contours of, 169, 169*f*
compliance and, 168, 169–170
damping of, 170
transmission to peripheral arteries,
169–170, 169*f*, 170*f*
typical record of, 168, 169*f*
Arterial system, volume-pressure curve of,
167–168, 168*f*
Arteries
blood volume in, 157
distensibility of, 167–168, 168*f*
function of, 157
sympathetic innervation of, 201, 202*f*
Arterioles, 177, 178*f*. *See also*
Metarterioles.
blood volume in, 157
of brain, 743, 743*f*, 744, 745
function of, 157
hepatic, 837
in nervous control of arterial pressure, 205
renal. *See* Afferent arteriole(s), renal;
Efferent arteriole(s), renal.
resistance of, fourth power of radius
and, 164
sympathetic innervation of, 201, 202*f*
sympathetic tone of, 737
vasodilator agents and, 193
bradykinin as, 199
histamine as, 199–200
Arteriosclerosis. *See also* Atherosclerosis.
atherosclerosis-induced, 828
calcium deposition in, 958
definition of, 827
diabetes mellitus and, 953
pulse pressure in, 168–169, 169*f*
stroke associated with, 745
Arteriovenous anastomoses, cutaneous,
868, 868*f*
heat conduction and, 868
Arteriovenous fistula
cardiac failure associated with,
263–264, 264*f*
cardiac output with, 232, 239, 239*f*, 240
circulatory changes associated with,
239–240, 239*f*
Articulation, of speech, 704
Artificial kidney. *See* Dialysis, renal.
Ascites, 298, 300, 838

Ascorbic acid. *See* Vitamin C.
Aspirin (acetylsalicylic acid)
  acidosis caused by, 393
  fever and, 876
  gastric absorption of, 793
  gastritis caused by, 799
  peptic ulcer and, 801
Association areas, 699–701, 699f
  caudate nucleus and, 691, 692
  granular neurons in, 697
  limbic, 699f, 700
  parieto-occipitotemporal, 699–700,
    699f, 702
  prefrontal, 699f, 700, 702–703
  Wernicke area and, 701
Aster, mitotic, 38–39, 38f
Astereognosis, 577
Asthma, 444, 473, 520
  airway obstruction in, 517, 520
Astigmatism, 603, 603f, 604f
Astrocytes, in cerebral blood flow regulation,
  743, 743f, 744
Astronauts. *See* Spacecraft.
Ataxia, 689
Atelectasis, 519, 519f
  in oxygen toxicity, 537
Atheromatous plaques, 827, 828, 828f
Atherosclerosis, 827–829. *See also*
    Arteriosclerosis.
  Alzheimer's disease and, 728
  cholesterol and, 828, 829
  coronary, 248
    acute occlusion caused by,
      248–249
    bypass surgery for, 252
    collateral circulation and, 249
    risk factors for, 829
  diabetes mellitus, 953
  in hypothyroidism, 918
  prevention of, 829
  renal artery, 403
  risk factors for, 828–829
  systolic pressure increase in, 171
Athetosis, 691
Athletes, bradycardia in, 143–144. *See also*
    Sports physiology.
Atmospheric hypoxia, 520, 521, 522.
    See also High altitude.
Atopic allergies, 443
ATP. *See* Adenosine triphosphate (ATP).
ATP synthetase, 22, 815
ATPase(s). *See also* Calcium ATPase;
    Hydrogen ATPase; Hydrogen-
    potassium ATPase pump; Sodium-
    potassium ATPase pump.
  in active transport, 53, 53f, 54
  in kidneys, 324–325, 325f
  mitochondrial, 814f, 815
  of myosin head, 75, 76
ATP-sensitive potassium channels, of
    pancreatic beta cells, 945, 945f
Atria
  action potential in, 117
  cardiac impulse in, 118, 118f
  electrocardiogram and, 133–134, 133f
  as primer pumps, 104–106
Atrial fibrillation, 151–152, 152f
  in mitral valvular disease, 269
Atrial flutter, 152–153, 152f, 153f
Atrial heart sound, 266, 267f
Atrial natriuretic peptide (ANP)
  blood volume and, 376
  in cardiac failure, 260–261
  renal reabsorption and, 339
  sodium excretion and, 376
Atrial paroxysmal tachycardia, 148, 148f
Atrial premature contractions, 146, 146f

Atrial pressure
  cardiac cycle and, 105, 105f, 106
  ventricular function curves and, 110–111,
    110f
Atrial stretch receptors, 208–209
  antidiuretic hormone and, 905
  respiratory waves and, 210
  sodium excretion and, 376
Atrial syncytium, 102
Atrial T wave, 122
  vectorial analysis of, 133–134, 133f
Atrial tachycardia, paroxysmal, 148, 148f
Atrioventricular (A-V) block
  causes of, 144
  ectopic pacemaker associated with, 119
  first-degree, 144–145, 144f
  second-degree, 145, 145f
  third-degree (complete), 145, 145f
Atrioventricular (A-V) bundle, 102, 115, 116f,
    117, 117f
  blocking of impulses in, 144. *See also*
    Atrioventricular (A-V) block.
  ectopic pacemaker in, 119–120
  ischemia of, 144
  one-way conduction through, 117–118
  premature contractions originating in, 146
  sympathetic effects on, 120
  timing of impulse in, 117f, 118
Atrioventricular (A-V) nodal paroxysmal
    tachycardia, 148
Atrioventricular (A-V) nodal premature
    contractions, 146, 146f
Atrioventricular (A-V) node, 115, 116f,
    117, 117f
  as ectopic pacemaker, 119
  inflammation of, 144
  intrinsic rhythmicity of, 119
  ischemia of, 144
  parasympathetic effects on, 119–120
    blocking of conduction by, 144
  premature contractions originating in,
    146, 146f
  sympathetic effects on, 120
Atrioventricular (A-V) valves, 105f, 106–107,
    107f. *See also* Mitral valve; Tricuspid
    valve.
  first heart sound and, 107, 265
Atrophy, of skeletal muscle, 81, 82
Audiogram, 642, 642f
Audiometer, 642
Auditory cortex, 639, 639f, 640–641, 640f
  speech and, 704–705, 704f
Auditory receptive aphasia, 703
Auerbach's plexus. *See* Myenteric plexus.
Augmented unipolar limb leads. *See* Unipolar
    limb leads, augmented.
Auscultation, of heart sounds, 266, 266f
Auscultatory method, for blood pressure
    measurement, 170–171, 170f
Autocrines, 881
Autograft, 449
Autoimmune diseases, 442
Autolysis, 19–20
Autonomic ganglia
  drugs blocking transmission through, 740
  nicotinic receptors in, 733
  peripheral sympathetic, 729
  prevertebral, 729
  sympathetic chains of, 729, 730f
Autonomic nervous system, 729–741. *See*
    also Parasympathetic nervous system;
    Sympathetic nervous system.
  in arterial pressure control, acute, 205
  brain stem control of, 739, 739f
  circulatory control by, 201–204, 202f,
    204f, 205
  eye control by, 631–632, 631f

Autonomic nervous system (*Continued*)
  functional characteristics of, 731–737
    cholinergic and adrenergic fibers
      in, 731–732
    excitation and inhibition in, 733–735, 734t
    receptors on organs and, 732–733, 733t
    specific organs and, 734t, 735–736
    stimulus frequency required in, 736
    tone in, 737
  gastrointestinal tract and. *See* Gastrointestinal
    tract, autonomic control of.
  hypothalamic influence on, 739, 739f
  insulin secretion and, 947
  organization of, 729–731, 730f, 731f
  pharmacology of, 739–740
  rapidity and intensity of effects, 729
  smooth muscle and, 94–95, 94f
Autonomic reflexes, 665, 729, 738
  bowel activity and, 772
  local, 738
Autoregulation of blood flow, 165–166, 165f,
    194–195, 194f, 200, 217
  cerebral, 744–745, 745f
  renal, 317, 319–321, 319f, 320f
Autoregulatory escape, gastrointestinal blood
    flow and, 762
A-V block. *See* Atrioventricular (A-V) block.
Aviation. *See also* High altitude; Spacecraft.
  acceleratory forces in, 531–533, 531f
  acute hypoxia in, 528
  breathing air vs. breathing oxygen in, 528
  deceleratory forces in parachuting in,
    532–533
Axis deviation, 135–137, 135f, 136f, 137f
Axon, 543, 544f, 547, 547f
Axonal streaming, 551
Axoneme, 25, 975
Azathioprine, for immunosuppression, in
    transplantation, 449
Azotemia. *See* Uremia.

B
B lymphocytes, 433, 434. *See also* Antibodies;
    Lymphocytes.
  as antigen-presenting cells, 440
  helper T cells and, 436, 437, 441, 441f
  interleukins and, 441
  memory cells of, 437
  plasma cells formed by. *See* Plasma cells.
  preprocessing of, 435, 435f, 442
  specificity of, 435–436, 436f
Bacteria
  in colon, 798, 855
  dental caries and, 971
  evolution of, 17–18, 18f
  in feces, 798
  fever and, 875–876
  lysosomal killing of, 20
  phagocytosis of, 19, 20. *See also*
    Phagocytosis.
Bainbridge reflex, 208–209, 229–230
Balance. *See* Equilibrium.
Baldness, 981
Ballistic movements, cerebellar control of, 688
Barometric pressure, at different altitudes,
    527, 528t
Baroreceptor reflexes, 205–209, 206f, 207f, 738
  acute neurogenic hypertension and,
    224–225
  adaptation and, 562
  in cardiac failure, acute stage, 255–256, 256f
  as homeostatic mechanism, 6, 7–8
  in hypovolemic shock, 275
  in integrated pressure response, 227, 227f
  oscillation of, 210, 210f
  renal sodium and water excretion and,
    373–374

Bartholin glands, 1000
Bartter's syndrome, 408
Basal ganglia, 689–694
  as accessory motor system, 689
  anatomical relations of, 690, 690*f*
  clinical syndromes associated with, 693–694
    Huntington's disease, 694
    Parkinson's disease, 691, 693–694
  dopamine system and, 712, 713, 713*f*
  gamma efferents and, 659
  in integrated motor control, 695
  neglect syndrome and, 692, 692*f*
  neuronal circuitry of, 690, 690*f*
    caudate circuit, 690*f*, 691–692, 691*f*
    putamen circuit, 690–691, 690*f*, 691*f*
  neurotransmitters in, 692–693, 692*f*
  overall motor control by, 681
  patterns of motor activity and, 690–691, 695
  scaling of movements and, 692
  timing of movements and, 692
Basal metabolic rate (BMR), 863–864, 864*f*, 867
  in pregnancy, 1010
  testosterone and, 982
  thyroid hormones and, 907, 911, 912, 913*f*
    in hyperthyroidism, 916
    in hypothyroidism, 918
Base(s)
  as components of DNA, 27, 28, 28*f*, 29
  definition of, 379
  strong and weak, 379–380
Basement membrane, of capillaries, 177, 178*f*
Basilar fibers, of cochlea, 635
  hair cells and, 636*f*, 637, 637*f*
  traveling wave and, 635, 636
Basilar membrane, of cochlea, 634–635, 634*f*, 635*f*
  hair cells and, 637
  loudness and, 638
  sound frequency and, 638
  traveling wave along, 635, 635*f*, 636*f*
Basket cells, 685
Basophil erythroblasts, 415, 415*f*
Basophils, 423, 423*t*, 424*f*, 431
  allergies and, 443
  complement fragments and, 439, 439*f*
  eosinophil chemotactic factor of, 430
  heparin produced by, 431, 439, 457
Bathorhodopsin, 611–612, 611*f*
Bends. *See* Decompression sickness.
Beriberi, 853, 854
  cardiac failure associated with, 263, 264, 264*f*, 853
  cardiac output in, 232
  hypoxia in, 521
  peripheral vasodilation in, 194, 853
Beta adrenergic receptors, 733, 733*t*
  of bronchiolar smooth muscle, 473
  of cardiac muscle, sympathetic stimulation and, 120
  in coronary vessels, 248
  drugs acting on, 739
  potassium homeostasis and, 361–362
Beta blockers, 740
  for angina pectoris, 252
  hyperkalemia caused by, 361–362
Beta waves, 723*f*, 724–725, 724*f*, 725*f*
Beta-aminoisobutyricaciduria, 408
Beta-amyloid peptide, in Alzheimer's disease, 728
Beta-oxidation of fatty acids, 822, 822*f*, 839
Betz cells, 669–670. *See also* Pyramidal cells.
Bicarbonate. *See also* Sodium bicarbonate.
  in bile, 784, 785
  carbon dioxide transported as, 502–503, 502*f*
  in cerebrospinal fluid, at high altitude, 529
  diarrhea-related loss of, 392

Bicarbonate (*Continued*)
  gastric acid secretion and, 777–778, 778*f*
  in gastrointestinal mucus, 775
    duodenal, 786
  intestinal absorption of, 795
  intestinal secretion of
    in large intestine, 787, 795, 797
    in small intestine, 787, 795
  pancreatic secretion of, 780–782, 782*f*
    mucosal protection and, 800
    regulation of, 782–783, 783*f*
  in plasma
    carbon dioxide transport and, 413
    measurement of, 393–395, 394*f*
  renal excretion of, 389, 390
    in alkalosis, 392
  renal reabsorption of, 332–333, 332*f*, 385, 386–388, 386*f*, 387*f*
    carbonic anhydrase inhibitors and, 398
    factors affecting, 390–391, 390*t*
  in saliva, 774*f*, 775
  vomiting-related loss of, 393
Bicarbonate buffer system, 381–383, 382*f*
  intracellular fluid and, 383
Bicarbonate-chloride carrier protein, 502–503
Bile, 783–786
  composition of, 784–785, 784*t*
  excretion of calcium in, 840
  excretion of hormones in, 886
  functions of, 783, 785
  release into duodenum, 784*f*, 785
  secretion of, 783–784, 785
    secretin and, 784, 784*f*, 785
  storage and concentration of, 784, 784*f*, 785
Bile acids. *See also* Bile salts.
  cholesterol and, 827, 829
  functions of, 783
Bile canaliculi, 783–784, 837, 837*f*
Bile ducts, 783–784, 837, 837*f*
  obstruction of, 841–842
Bile salts. *See also* Bile acids.
  cholesterol and, 839
  cholic acid for, 827
  concentration in bile, 784, 784*t*
  enterohepatic circulation of, 785
  in fat digestion and absorption, 785, 792
Bilirubin, 419–420, 783, 840–842
  concentration in bile, 784, 784*t*
  concentration in plasma, 841
  conjugated, 840, 841–842, 841*f*
  fecal color and, 798
  formation and transformations of, 840–841, 841*f*
  jaundice and, 841–842
    in neonate, 1024
  in neonate, 1024, 1024*f*
  from transfusion reactions, 1025
  unconjugated, 840, 841–842, 841*f*
Biliverdin, 840
Binocular vision, 605, 605*f*. *See also* Stereopsis.
2,3-Biphosphoglycerate (BPG), 500, 500*f*
Bipolar cells, 609, 610*f*, 616–617, 617*f*
  transmitters at synapses of, 617
  two types of, 618, 619–620
  visual pathway and, 617, 617*f*
Bipolar disorder, 727
Bipolar limb leads, 124–126, 125*f*, 126*f*
  vectorial analysis of potentials in, 131, 131*f*
    atrial T wave, 133–134, 133*f*
    axes for, 130, 130*f*
    increased voltage in, 136*f*, 137
    mean electrical axis, 134–135, 135*f*
    P wave, 133, 133*f*
    QRS complex, 131–132, 132*f*
    T wave, 133, 133*f*
Bitemporal hemianopsia, 627
Bitter taste, 645–646, 646*t*, 647

Bladder. *See also* Micturition; Micturition reflex.
  anatomy of, physiologic, 306–308, 307*f*
  atonic, 310
  external sphincter of, 308, 308*f*, 310
  innervation of, 308, 308*f*
  internal sphincter of. *See* Urethra, posterior.
  irritation of, intestinal activity and, 772
  pressure changes in, 309, 309*f*
Blastocyst, 1004, 1004*f*, 1005*f*
  progesterone and, 1008–1009
Bleeding tendencies. *See also* Hemorrhage.
  in factor deficiencies, 457–458
  in thrombocytopenia, 458
Bleeding time, 460
Blind spot, 627
Blindness, in premature infant, 197–198, 1027
Blood. *See also* Extracellular fluid.
  cleansing of, by spleen, 175
  reservoirs of, 175, 175*f*
  viscosity of, 161–162, 163, 164
    anemia and, 420–421
    hematocrit and, 165, 165*f*
    mountain sickness and, 531
    plasma loss and, 279
    in polycythemia, 421
Blood cells, genesis of, 414–415, 414*f*. *See also* Leukocytes (white blood cells); Red blood cells (erythrocytes)
Blood coagulation. *See also* Clot *entries*; Hemostasis.
  abnormalities of
    with bleeding, 457–458
    with thromboembolism, 459
  clotting factors in, 452*t*, 453
    hepatic synthesis of, 840
  initiation of, 454–456, 455*f*, 456*f*
  mechanism of, 453–454
  in neonate, 1025
  outside the body, 460
  positive feedback in, 8, 9
  prevention of, in normal vascular system, 456–457
  in ruptured vessel, 452, 452*f*
  tests of, 460–461, 460*f*
Blood flow, 160–162. *See also* Circulation.
  arterial pressure and, 165–166, 165*f*, 166*f*
  cardiac output and, 159
  cerebral. *See* Cerebral blood flow.
  definition of, 160
  diameter of vessel and, 163–164, 163*f*
  in different tissues and organs, 191, 192*t*
  gastrointestinal. *See* Gastrointestinal tract, blood flow in.
  interstitial fluid P_{CO_2} and, 497, 498*f*
  interstitial fluid P_{O_2} and, 496–497, 496*f*
  laminar, 161, 161*f*
  in liver, 838
  metabolic oxygen use and, 501
  methods for measuring, 160–161, 160*f*, 161*f*
  in muscle. *See* Skeletal muscle, blood flow in.
  needs of tissues for, 191, 192–193
  pressure difference and, 159, 160
  pulmonary. *See* Pulmonary circulation.
  regulation of. *See* Blood flow control.
  renal. *See* Renal blood flow.
  resistance to. *See* Vascular resistance.
  in skin, heat loss and, 868, 868*f*
  in thyroid gland, 907
  thyroid hormones and, 913
  in total circulation, 160
  turbulent, 161–162, 161*f*
  units of, 160
  velocity of
    cross-sectional area and, 158
    parabolic profile for, 161, 161*f*
    turbulence and, 161–162

Blood flow control
  humoral, 199–200
  local, 191
    acute, 191, 192–196, 192f, 193f
    autoregulation in, 165–166, 165f,
      194–195, 194f, 200, 217
    cardiac output and, 230–231
    long-term, 191–192, 196–198, 197f
    tissue factors affecting, 97
    tissue needs and, 158–159
Blood gases. See also Carbon dioxide partial
    pressure (Pco$_2$); Oxygen partial
    pressure (Po$_2$).
  during exercise, 1037
  measurement of, 515–516
Blood glucose
  cortisol and, 928
    in Cushing syndrome, 935–936
  diagnosis of diabetes and, 952–953, 953f
  glucagon and, 947–948, 948f
  gluconeogenesis and, 839
  hepatic buffering of, 839
  hunger and, 766, 849
  importance of regulation of, 949–950
  insulin secretion and, 946, 946f, 947
  in neonate, 1023, 1025
    of diabetic mother, 1026
    premature, 1027
  normal level of, 817
  renal blood flow and, 321
  summary of regulation of, 949–950
  urinary excretion and, 327
Blood pressure. See also Arterial blood
    pressure; Capillary pressure; Venous
    pressures.
  definition of, 162
  measurement of, high-fidelity, 162, 162f
  in parts of circulation, 158, 159f
  standard units of, 162
Blood transfusion, 280–281. See also
    Transfusion; Transfusion reactions.
  blood types in, 445, 446t
Blood types
  O-A-B, 445–447, 446f, 446t
  Rh, 447–449
Blood typing, 446–447, 447t
Blood vessels. See also Arteries; Arterioles;
    Capillaries; Veins.
  autonomic control of, 729–730, 730f, 731,
    734t, 735
    adrenal medullae in, 736
    intrinsic tone of, 737
Blood volume, 287. See also Extracellular fluid
    volume.
  antidiuretic hormone and, 357, 357f, 905
  aortic valve disease and, 268
  atrial natriuretic peptide and, 376
  atrial reflexes and, 208
  cardiac output and, 233, 238, 238f
  conditions causing large increases in,
    376–377
  vs. extracellular fluid volume, 373, 373f
  hemorrhage and. See also Hypovolemic
    shock.
    compensatory mechanisms, 275–276
  at high altitude, 529
  in lungs, 157, 478–479
  mean circulatory filling pressure and,
    236, 236f
  measurement of, 290
  mitral valve disease and, 269
  of neonate, 1024
  in pregnancy, 1010, 1010f
  regulation of, 371–373, 372f
  testosterone and, 982
  venous return and, 238, 238f
Blood-brain barrier, 748–749

Blood–cerebrospinal fluid barrier, 748–749
Blue weakness, 616
BMR. See Basal metabolic rate (BMR).
Body mass index (BMI), 850
Bohr effect, 500, 500f
  double, 1006
  fetal blood and, 1006
Bone, 957–960. See also Fractures.
  calcification of, 958
    vitamin D and, 962
  calcium exchange with, 958, 967
    in pregnancy, 1009
  deposition and absorption of, 959–960,
    959f
  estrogenic effects on, 994
  in fetus, 1020
  growth hormone and, 900
    somatomedins and, 900–901
  growth mechanisms of, 900
  hydroxyapatite in, 957, 958
  organic matrix of, 957
  parathyroid hormone and, 963–964
  phosphate in extracellular fluid and, 958
  radioactive substances in, 957–958
  rickets and, 968
  salts of, 957–958
  strength of, 958, 960
  structure of, 959–960, 960f
  testosterone and, 982
  thyroid hormones and, 912
    in cretinism, 918
  vitamin D and, 962
Bone fluid, 964
Bone marrow
  B lymphocyte processing in, 435, 442
  leukopenia and, 431
  macrophages of, 427–428
  response of, to inflammation, 429, 430, 430f
Bone marrow aplasia, 420
Bony labyrinth, 634, 674
Botulinum toxin, 85
Bowman's capsule, 305–306, 305f, 310–311,
    311f, 312, 313f
  pressure in, 314–315, 314f
Boyle's law, 535
BPG (2,3-biphosphoglycerate), 500, 500f
Bradycardia, sinus, 143–144, 143f
Bradykinin, 199, 200
  in asthma, 520
  glomerular filtration rate and, 319
  in gut wall, 761
  from mast cells and basophils, 431
  as pain stimulus, 583, 584
  in salivary glands, 776
Brain. See also Basal ganglia; Cerebellum;
    Cerebral cortex; Nervous system.
  acceleration injury to, 746
  activating systems of, 711–713
    neurohormonal systems, 711,
      712–713, 713f
    reticular excitatory area, 711–712, 712f
  blood flow in. See Cerebral blood flow.
  capillaries of, tight junctions of, 178
  carbon dioxide in blood and, 200
  childhood development of, 1027–1028
  glucose for, 949
    insulin and, 942–943
  growth of, thyroid hormones and, 912
  interstitial fluid pressure in, 183
  metabolism of, 749–750
  reticular inhibitory area and, 712, 712f
  vegetative functions of, 714,
    715–717, 716f
Brain damage
  Cheyne-Stokes breathing in, 512
  circulatory arrest causing, 282
  neurogenic shock caused by, 279–280

Brain edema, 749
  in acute mountain sickness, 530
  hyponatremia with, 295, 296f
  negative acceleratory forces causing,
    531–532
  respiratory depression in, 512
  treatment of, 749
Brain stem. See also Medulla; Pons.
  autonomic control centers of, 739, 739f
  basal ganglia input from, 692–693, 692f
  cerebellar functions and, 686–687, 694
  cerebellar input from, 683, 683f
  cerebellar signals to, 684
  cerebral activation by, 711–713
    continuous excitatory signals in,
      711–712, 712f
    neurohormonal systems in, 711,
      712–713, 713f
  cerebral inhibition by, 712
  chewing and, 763
  feeding and, 847–848
  functions of, 673
  gastrointestinal reflexes and, 757
  hypothalamus and, 715
  limbic system and, 715
  motor functions and, 673–674, 673f, 674f
    anencephaly and, 678–679
    gamma efferents in, 659, 660
    stretch reflexes and, 660
  pain pathways to, 586
  salivatory nuclei in, 776, 776f
  swallowing and, 764, 765
  vestibular nuclei in, 678, 678f
  vomiting center in, 803, 803f, 804
Brain waves. See Electroencephalogram
    (EEG).
Braxton Hicks contractions, 1012
Breasts
  anatomy of, 1014f
  development of, 1014
  estrogens and, 994, 1014
  of neonate, 1026
  progesterone and, 995, 1014
Breathing. See also Respiration.
  cardiac output curve and, 234, 234f
  work of, 468
Broca's area, 668–669, 669f, 699f,
    700, 704–705
Brodmann's areas, 574–575, 575f
Bronchi, 472–473
Bronchial circulation, 477
  shunt blood and, 496, 496f
Bronchioles, 472–473
  particles entrapped in, 474
Bronchospasm
  in anaphylaxis, 443
  in asthma, 444
Brown fat, 865, 873
Brown-Séquard syndrome, 590
Brunner glands, 786, 800
Brush border, intestinal, 790, 791, 794, 794f
Buccal glands, 775
Buffer nerves, from baroreceptors, 207
Buffer systems, 380–381
  ammonia, 388–389, 389f
  bicarbonate, 381–383, 382f
    intracellular fluid and, 383
  gastrointestinal mucus and, 775
  isohydric principle and, 383–384
  phosphate, 383, 388, 388f
  proteins, 383–384
    hemoglobin, 383, 413
  respiratory, 385
Bulboreticular facilitatory region, 711
  gamma efferents and, 659–660
  stretch reflexes and, 660
Bulbourethral glands, 307f, 973, 973f, 979

Bulk flow
in artificial kidney, 409
into peritubular capillary, 323–324, 324*f*
Bumetanide, 331, 331*f*, 397
Bundle branch block
axis deviation in, 136–137, 136*f*, 137*f*
QRS prolongation in, 138, 142
T wave and, 142
Bundle branches, 115, 116*f*, 118. *See also*
Purkinje fibers.
Bundle of His. *See* Atrioventricular (A-V)
bundle.
Burns
plasma loss in, 279
water loss caused by, 285

C
C cells, thyroid, 966
C fibers, 563–564, 563*f*
analgesia system and, 587
cold receptors and, 592
pain sensation and, 584, 585, 586
visceral, 588
sympathetic, 729–730
warmth receptors and, 592
C peptide, 940, 940*f*
Cachexia, 852
Caffeine, 557
athletic performance and, 1040
Caisson disease. *See* Decompression sickness.
Cajal, interstitial cells of, 754
Calbindin, 962
Calcarine fissure, 623, 624, 624*f*
Calcitonin, 965*f*, 966
renal calcium reabsorption and, 368–369
Calcitriol, 304
Calcium, 856
action potential and, 64
in gastrointestinal smooth muscle,
754–755
blood coagulation and, 453, 453*f*, 454, 455,
455*f*, 456, 456*f*
prevention of, 460
in bone, 957
deposition of, 958
exchange with extracellular fluid,
958, 967
parathyroid hormone and, 963–964
in cardiac muscle
excitation-contraction coupling and,
103–104, 104*f*
sympathetic stimulation and, 120
exchangeable, 958, 967
excretion of, in bile, 840
exocytosis and, 21
of gastrointestinal secretions, 774
in extracellular fluid and plasma,
955–957, 957*f*
calcitonin and, 965*f*, 966
cardiac muscle contraction and,
103–104, 104*f*, 112
excess or deficiency of, 367, 856, 956, 956*f*
forms of, 955, 956*f*
as nerve membrane stabilizer, 69
normal range of, 7, 7*t*
parathyroid hormone and, 963–966, 963*f*,
965*f*, 967
regulation of, 367–368, 368*f*
in rickets, 968
of smooth muscle, 97–98
summary of, 966–967
vitamin D activation and, 961–962, 961*f*
fecal excretion of, 367, 368, 956–957, 957*f*
fetal accumulation of, 1020, 1020*f*
in gastrointestinal smooth muscle
action potential and, 754–755
tonic contraction and, 755

Calcium (*Continued*)
intestinal absorption of, 796, 956–957, 957*f*
parathyroid hormone and, 796, 964–965
vitamin D and, 796, 855, 962, 964–965
neonatal need for, 1025, 1026, 1027
in nonosseous tissues, 958
peptide hormone secretion and, 882
plasma protein binding of, 312
at postganglionic nerve endings, 732
renal excretion of, 368, 369*t*, 957, 957*f*
renal reabsorption of, 339, 368–369, 368*f*
parathyroid hormone and, 964
as second messenger, in hormone action,
890, 891
in skeletal muscle contraction, 75–76,
88–89, 88*f*, 89*f*
in smooth muscle, 93–94, 94*f*, 97–98
sodium channels and, 64, 69
sodium counter-transport of, 55, 55*f*
vasoconstriction induced by, 200
Calcium ATPase, 324–325
of cardiac muscle, 104, 104*f*
Calcium carbonate, of vestibular system, 675
Calcium ion channels. *See also* Calcium-
sodium channels
of cardiac muscle, 102–103, 104*f*
hormone receptors and, 891
memory system of *Aplysia* and, 707, 708
of smooth muscle, 97
voltage-gated, 64
at neuromuscular junction, 83, 84*f*, 86
of pancreatic beta cells, 945, 945*f*
at presynaptic terminal, 548
of smooth muscle, 96
Calcium pumps, 54
of cardiac muscle, 104, 104*f*
renal, 368–369, 368*f*
of skeletal muscle, 74, 88–89, 88*f*, 89*f*
of smooth muscle, 97, 98
Calcium release channels, 88, 88*f*, 103
Calcium-sensing receptor (CaSR), 965
Calcium-sodium channels.
in cardiac muscle, 102–103
in gastrointestinal smooth muscle, 754–755
Calmodulin, 93–94, 94*f*
hormone action and, 891
Calorie, 862
Calorimeter, 862, 863
Calsequestrin, 88, 88*f*
cAMP. *See* Cyclic adenosine monophosphate
(cAMP).
cAMP-dependent protein kinase, 889
Cancer
anorexia-cachexia in, 852
genetic mechanisms of, 40–41
Capacitance, vascular, 167. *See also* Vascular
compliance.
sympathetic control of, 168
Capillaries
blood flow in
average, 179
intermittent character of, 178–179
velocity of, 158
blood volume in, 157
cerebral, 743, 743*f*, 745
barriers at, 748–749
edema and, 749
diffusion across walls of, 4–5, 4*f*,
179–180, 179*f*
concentration difference and, 180
molecular size and, 179–180, 180*t*
distance from any single cell, 4–5, 177
fluid filtration across, 181–186, 181*f*
excess, causing edema, 297
into potential spaces, 300
function of, 157
in gastrointestinal tract, pores of, 178

Capillaries (*Continued*)
glomerular. *See* Glomerular capillaries.
increase in number of, 197, 197*f*
at high altitude, 529
intercellular clefts of, 177–178, 178*f*
diffusion through, 179–180
lymphatic, 186*f*, 187, 187*f*, 188, 188*f*
pumping by, 188–189
organization of, 177, 178*f*
peritubular. *See* Peritubular capillaries
permeability decrease in, cortisol-
induced, 930
permeability increase in
bradykinin-induced, 199
in circulatory shock, 277
edema caused by, 297
histamine-induced, 199–200
pores in, 157, 158, 177–178, 178*f*
diffusion through, 4–5, 179–180
fluid filtration and, 181
permeabilities for various molecules,
179–180, 180*t*
pressures in
gravity and, 173–174
hydrostatic. *See* Capillary pressure.
pulmonary, 158
systemic, 158
pulmonary. *See* Pulmonary capillaries.
of skeletal muscle, blood flow during
exercise, 243
surface area of, 177
wall structure of, 177, 178*f*
Capillary filtration coefficient, 181, 185
Capillary fluid shift, for arterial pressure
regulation, 227, 227*f*
Capillary pressure, 181, 181*f*, 184*t*, 185*t*
edema caused by increased in, 297
increased blood volume and, 238
lymph flow and, 188
measurement of, 181–182, 182*f*
Carbachol, 86
Carbaminohemoglobin, 503
Carbohydrates
absence of, fat utilization in, 823, 825
absorption of, 796
in athlete's diet, 1034, 1035, 1035*f*
in cell, 12, 13
of cell membrane, 14
dental caries and, 971
dietary sources of, 789–790
digestion of, 789–790, 790*f*
pancreatic enzyme for, 781, 790
as energy source. *See* Glucose, energy
production from.
excess of, fat metabolism and, 825
in foods
energy available in, 843–844
metabolic utilization of, 844–845
growth hormone and, 899–900
metabolism of. *See also* Glucose.
insulin and, 941–943, 942*f*, 947
liver's functions in, 839
thyroid hormones and, 912
storage of. *See* Glycogen.
synthesis of, in Golgi apparatus, 20
triglycerides synthesized from, 824–825, 824*f*
Carbon dioxide
diffusing capacity for, 491–492, 492*f*
diffusion coefficient of, 487*t*
diffusion of. *See also* Diffusion, of gases.
through capillary membrane, 179
from cells to capillaries to alveoli,
497–498, 497*f*, 498*f*, 502
in extracellular fluid
acid-base balance and, 384
normal range of, 7*t*
regulation of, 6, 7

Carbon dioxide (*Continued*)
in large intestine, 804
lipid solubility of, 46
from metabolism
of carbohydrates, 812–813, 813*f*, 814, 816–817, 816*f*
mitochondrial, 22
placental diffusion of, 1007
removal by lungs, 5
respiratory control by, 507–508, 507*f*, 508*f*
transport in blood, 495, 502–504, 502*f*, 503*f*, 504*f*
pH change caused by, 504
in urea synthesis, 835
as vasoconstrictor, 200
as vasodilator, 97, 200
in skeletal muscle, 243–244
Carbon dioxide dissociation curve, 503, 503*f*
Carbon dioxide partial pressure (PCO_2). *See also* Hypercapnia.
alveolar, 488–489, 489*f*
in deep-sea diving, 537
ventilation-perfusion ratio and, 492–494, 493*f*
blood
cerebral blood flow and, 743–744, 744*f*
chemoreceptors and, 208, 509
exercise and, 511, 511*f*, 1037
measurement of, 515–516
respiratory control and, 507–508, 508*f*, 510, 510*f*, 512–513, 512*f*
in extracellular fluid, 382, 384, 385
in acidosis, 390, 391, 392
in alkalosis, 390, 392
high levels of, 537
in interstitial fluid, 497–498, 498*f*
oxygen-hemoglobin dissociation curve and, 500, 500*f*
plasma measurement of, 393–395, 394*f*
solubility coefficient and, 486
Carbon monoxide
diffusing capacity for, 492, 492*f*
hemoglobin combination with, 501–502, 501*f*
Carbonate ions, in bone, 957–958
Carbonic acid
in bicarbonate buffer system, 32, 381
cerebral blood flow and, 744
intestinal bicarbonate absorption and, 795
pancreatic secretions and, 781, 782–783, 782*f*
in red blood cells, 502–503
Carbonic anhydrase
gastric acid secretion and, 777–778
in kidney, 381
bicarbonate reabsorption and, 386–387, 386*f*, 389*f*
pancreatic secretions and, 781, 782*f*
in red blood cells, 413, 502, 502*f*, 503
zinc in, 856
Carbonic anhydrase inhibitors, 398, 398*t*, 503
Carboxypolypeptidase, 781, 791
Carcinogens, 41
Cardiac. *See also* Heart.
Cardiac arrest, 153
circulatory arrest and, 281
Cardiac catheterization, premature contractions caused by, 146
Cardiac cycle, 104–107, 105*f*
current flows around heart in, 123–124, 124*f*
volume-pressure diagram during, 108–109, 108*f*, 109*f*
Cardiac failure, 255–264
acute, in anemia, 421
aortic valve lesions with, 268, 269
blood volume in, 376–377

Cardiac failure (*Continued*)
causes of, 255
chemical energy expended in, 109, 110
Cheyne-Stokes breathing in, 512
circulatory dynamics in, 255–258
acute stage, 255–256, 256*f*, 262, 262*f*
chronic stage, 256–257, 256*f*
compensated, 256*f*, 257, 262, 262*f*
decompensated, 257–258, 257*f*, 262–263, 263*f*
graphical analysis of, 262–264, 262*f*, 263*f*, 264*f*
definition of, 255
edema caused by, 298
efficiency of heart in, 110
extracellular fluid volume in, 375, 376–377
high-output, graphical analysis of, 263–264, 264*f*
hypertension and, 218
hypertrophy leading to, 272
left-sided
pulmonary circulation in, 478–479, 481
pulmonary edema in, 259, 482, 483
unilateral, 259
low-output, 259
peripheral edema in, 259–261, 260*f*
pulmonary edema in, 256
as acute edema, 259, 261
decompensated, 258
left-sided, 259
quantitative graphical analysis of, 262–264, 262*f*
in acute stage, 262, 262*f*
during compensation, 262, 262*f*
with decompensation, 262–263, 263*f*
in high-output failure, 263–264, 264*f*
red blood cell production in, 416
right-sided, emphysema leading to, 518
in thiamine deficiency, 263, 264, 264*f*, 853
unilateral, 259
Cardiac hypertrophy, 272. *See also* Ventricular hypertrophy.
athletic training and, 1039
cardiac output and, 231
in congenital heart disease, 272
after myocardial infarction, 256
in valvular heart disease, 272
Cardiac index, 229
age and, 229, 230*f*
Cardiac muscle, 101–104
action potentials in. *See* Action potential(s), cardiac.
contractile strength of
body temperature and, 112
exercise and, 245
sympathetic stimulation of, 111, 120, 203, 231
thyroid hormones and, 913
vagal stimulation and, 111, 203
contraction of
chemical energy for, 109–110
duration of, 104
efficiency of, 110
coronary artery arrangement in, 247, 247*f*
coronary blood flow control and, 247
excitation-contraction coupling in, 103–104, 104*f*
Frank-Starling mechanism and, 110, 111
histology of, 101, 102*f*
hypertrophy of, 272. *See also* Cardiac hypertrophy.
infarcted, 249–250
metabolism of, 248
recording electrical potentials from, 123–124, 124*f*
refractory period of, 103, 103*f*
shock-related lesions in, 277–278

Cardiac muscle (*Continued*)
vs. skeletal muscle, 102–104
spiraling layers of, 118
as syncytium, 101–102, 102*f*
three types of, 101
velocity of signal conduction in, 103
in atria, 117
by Purkinje fibers, 117
Cardiac output, 229
anemia and, 233, 420–421
arterial pressure and, 112, 112*f*, 216*f*, 217, 217*f*
with arteriovenous fistula, 232, 239, 239*f*, 240
blood volume and, 238, 238*f*
definition of, 160
during exercise, 210, 230, 230*f*, 232, 244, 245, 245*f*
athletic training and, 1038, 1038*f*, 1039, 1039*f*
at high altitude, 529
limits achievable, 231, 231*f*
measurement methods for, 240–241, 240*f*, 241*f*
after myocardial infarction, 250
of neonate, 1024
normal values of, 160, 229
pathologically high, 232–233, 233*f*
pathologically low, 232, 233–234, 233*f*
in pregnancy, 1010
regulation of
by local tissue flows, 159, 230–231, 234
by nervous system, 111, 111*f*, 232, 232*f*
quantitative analysis of, 234. *See also* Cardiac output curves; Venous return curves.
by venous return. *See* Venous return, cardiac output and.
shock and, 273
hypovolemic, 274–275, 274*f*
septic, 280
skeletal muscle contraction and, 209–210
sympathetic inhibition and, 239, 239*f*
sympathetic stimulation and, 238–239, 239*f*
thyroid hormones and, 913
total peripheral resistance and, 230–231, 230*f*
reduced, 232–233
volume-loading hypertension and, 219, 220*f*
Cardiac output curves, 231, 231*f*, 234–235
combinations of patterns of, 235, 235*f*
exercise and, 245, 245*f*
external pressure on heart and, 234, 234*f*, 235
in heart failure. *See* Cardiac failure, circulatory dynamics in.
in hypovolemic shock, 276, 276*f*
with simultaneous venous return curves, 238–240, 238*f*
Cardiac reserve, 257, 261–262, 261*f*
patent ductus arteriosus and, 270
in valvular disease, 269
Cardiac surgery, extracorporeal circulation during, 271–272
Cardiogenic shock, 233, 250, 259, 273. *See also* Circulatory shock.
Cardiopulmonary resuscitation (CPR), 151, 153
Cardiotachometer, 144
in sinus arrhythmia, 144, 144*f*
Cardiotonic drugs, 258, 261
Caries, dental, 971
fluorine and, 971
Carnitine, 822
Carotenoids, 853
Carotid bodies, 208, 507, 508, 508*f*, 509, 509*f*
high altitude and, 529
rhythmical output signal and, 568, 569*f*

Carotid sinus baroreceptors, 205–206, 206*f*, 207
Carotid sinus syndrome, 144
Carrier proteins, 14, 45, 46
   active transport and, 46, 46*f*, 52–53
   facilitated diffusion and, 46, 46*f*, 49–50, 49*f*
Carrier-mediated diffusion. *See* Facilitated diffusion.
Cartilage, growth hormone and, 900–901
Caspases, 40
CaSR (calcium-sensing receptor), 965
Catalases, 536–537
Cataracts, 604
Catecholamines. *See* Epinephrine; Norepinephrine.
Catechol-*O*-methyl transferase
   epinephrine degradation by, 732
   norepinephrine degradation by, 732
Caudate circuit, 690*f*, 691–692, 691*f*
Caudate nucleus, 670, 690, 690*f*, 691, 691*f*
   dopamine system and, 713, 713*f*
   Huntington's disease and, 694
   neurotransmitters in, 692–693, 692*f*
   Parkinson's disease and, 693
Caveolae
   of capillary endothelial cells, 178, 178*f*
   of smooth muscle fibers, 98, 98*f*
Caveolins, 178, 178*f*
CCK. *See* Cholecystokinin (CCK).
Cecum, ileocecal sphincter and, 770
Celiac disease, 801
Celiac ganglion, 729, 730*f*, 757
Cell(s), 3, 11–25, 11*f*, 12*f*
   basic characteristics common to, 3
   basic substances of, 11, 12
   compared to precellular life, 17–18, 18*f*
   cytoplasm of, 11, 11*f*, 14
   cytoskeleton of, 11, 16–17, 17*f*
   damaged, lysosomal removal of, 19–20
   functional systems of, 18–23
      for digestion, 19–20, 19*f*. *See also* Lysosomes.
      for energy extraction, 21–23, 22*f*
      for ingestion, 18–19, 18*f*
      for synthesis, 20–21, 20*f*
   life cycle of, 37
   locomotion of, 23–25, 23*f*, 24*f*
   membranous structures of, 13–14, 13*f*
   nuclear membrane of, 11, 11*f*, 13, 17, 17*f*
   nucleoli of, 12*f*, 17, 17*f*, 32
   nucleus of, 11, 11*f*, 17, 17*f*
      evolution of, 18
   number of, in human body, 3
   organelles of, 12, 12*f*, 14–17. *See also* Endoplasmic reticulum; Golgi apparatus; Lysosomes; Mitochondria; Peroxisomes.
   overall structure of, 11, 11*f*, 12, 12*f*
   secretory vesicles of, 16, 16*f*, 21
Cell death, apoptotic, 40
Cell differentiation, 39–40
Cell growth, 39
   of cancer cells, 41
Cell membrane, 11, 11*f*, 13–14, 13*f*, 45, 46*f*
   cholesterol in, 13, 14, 827
   diffusion through. *See* Diffusion through cell membrane.
   oxygen toxicity to, 537
   phospholipids in, 826, 827
   replenishment of, 21
Cell reproduction, 37–39, 38*f*
   control of, 39
Cell volume
   hypernatremia-related changes in, 296
   hyponatremia-related changes in, 295, 296*f*
   in intracellular edema, 296
   osmotic equilibrium and, 291–292, 292*f*
   sodium-potassium pump and, 53

Cell-mediated immunity, 433, 434, 435*f*, 439–440, 440*f*. *See also* T lymphocytes.
Cellulose, 790, 798
Cementum, 969, 969*f*, 970
   mineral exchange in, 971
Central fissure, of cerebral cortex, 575, 575*f*
Central nervous system (CNS). *See also* Brain; Spinal cord.
   childhood development of, 1027–1028
   fetal development of, 1020
   major levels of function in, 545–546
   thyroid hormones and, 913
      muscle tremor and, 913
Central nervous system ischemic response, 209, 210–211, 210*f*, 227, 227*f*
   in cardiac failure, acute stage, 255–256, 256*f*
   in hypovolemic shock, 274, 275
Central venous catheter, 174
Central venous pressure, 172. *See also* Right atrial pressure.
Centrifugal acceleratory forces, 531–532
Centrioles, 12*f*, 17, 38–39, 38*f*
Centromere, 38, 38*f*, 39
Centrosome, 38
Cephalic phase
   of gastric secretion, 779, 780*f*
   of pancreatic secretion, 782
Cephalins
   chemical structure of, 826, 826*f*
   thromboplastin and, 826
Cerebellum, 681–689
   anatomical folds of, 682, 682*f*
   anatomical functional areas of, 681–682, 682*f*
   auditory pathways and, 639
   ballistic movements and, 688
   basal ganglia and, 690*f*
   clinical abnormalities of, 689
      smooth progression of movements and, 688
   correction of motor errors by, 686
   damping function of, 687–688, 689
   deep nuclei of, 683–684, 684*f*, 685
   functional unit of, 684–685, 684*f*
   gamma efferents and, 659
   inhibitory cells in, 685, 686
   input pathways to, 682–683, 683*f*
   in integrated motor control, 694
   motor cortex fibers leading to, 670
   output signals from, 683–684, 684*f*
   overall motor control by, 681, 686–689, 687*f*
   representation of body in, 682, 682*f*
   turn-on and turn-off signals from, 685–686, 694
   vestibular system and, 677, 678, 678*f*
Cerebral blood flow, 743–746
   autoregulation of, 744–745, 745*f*
   blockage of, 745–746. *See also* Stroke.
   cessation of, 743
   in hypovolemic shock, 274–275
   local neuronal activity and, 744, 745*f*
   measurement of, 744
   microcirculation in, 745
   normal rate of, 743
   regulation of, 195, 743–745, 744*f*, 745*f*
   vessel architecture for, 743, 743*f*
Cerebral cortex, 545–546
   anatomic divisions of, 574–575, 575*f*
   brain stem excitatory signals and, 711–712, 712*f*
   connections between hemispheres of, 702, 705
   corticofugal signals from
      from primary visual cortex, 624
      sensory input and, 581–582
   dimensions of, 697
   equilibrium status and, 678

Cerebral cortex (*Continued*)
   functional areas of, 667, 668*f*, 698, 698*f*, 699*f*. *See also* Association areas.
      for facial recognition, 700–701, 700*f*
      in nondominant hemisphere, 702
   hearing and. *See* Auditory cortex.
   histologic structure of, 697, 698*f*
   language and, 699–700, 699*f*, 703–705, 704*f*. *See also* Speech.
   layers of, 697
   limbic, 714–715, 714*f*, 720
   motor control by. *See* Motor cortex.
   pain perception and, 586
   somatosensory. *See* Somatosensory cortex.
   thalamus and, 697–698, 698*f*
   thought and, 705–706
   vasomotor center controlled by, 204
   vision and. *See* Visual cortex.
Cerebral ischemia
   arterial pressure response to, 209
   vasomotor paralysis caused by, 279–280
Cerebrocerebellum, 686, 688–689
Cerebrospinal fluid (CSF), 746–749
   absorption of, 747
   barrier between blood and, 748–749
   bicarbonate in, at high altitude, 529
   cushioning function of, 746
   flow of, 746, 746*f*, 747
   formation of, 746, 747
   obstruction to flow of, 748
   osmolarity of, 747
      thirst and, 358
   perivascular spaces and, 746, 747, 747*f*
   spaces occupied by, 746, 746*f*
Cerebrospinal fluid pressure, 747–748
   decreased, headache caused by, 591
   elevated
      blood pressure response to, 209, 210–211, 210*f*
      papilledema secondary to, 748
      in pathological conditions, 748
      respiratory depression secondary to, 512
   measurement of, 748
   normal level of, 747
Cerebrovascular disease, dementia in, 728
CFU (colony-forming unit), 414*f*, 415
cGMP. *See* Cyclic guanosine monophosphate (cGMP).
Channels. *See* Ion channels; Protein channels.
Chemical gating. *See* Ligand-gated channels.
Chemical messengers, 881
Chemical pain stimuli, 583
   tissue damage and, 584
   visceral, 588
Chemical synapses, 546–547
Chemical thermogenesis, 873
Chemiosmotic mechanism, of ATP formation, 22, 814–815, 814*f*
   starting with fatty acids, 823
Chemoreceptor reflexes, 208
   in cardiac failure, acute stage, 255–256, 256*f*
   in integrated pressure response, 227, 227*f*
   oscillation of, 210
Chemoreceptor trigger zone, 803*f*, 804
Chemoreceptors, 208, 508–510, 508*f*, 509*f*, 559, 560*b*
   at high altitude, 529
Chemosensitive area, of respiratory center, 507–508, 507*f*
Chemotaxis
   ameboid movement and, 24
   complement protein C5a and, 439, 439*f*
   of eosinophils, 430
   of neutrophils and macrophages, 424*f*, 425, 428
Chenodeoxycholic acid, 785

Chest leads, 126, 126f
Chewing, 763
Chewing reflex, 763
Cheyne-Stokes breathing, 512–513, 512f
Chief cells
   gastric. See Peptic (chief) cells.
   parathyroid, 963, 963f
Child, growth and development of, 1027–1028,
   1027f. See also Infant.
Chills, and fever, 876, 876f
Chloride. See also Sodium chloride.
   absorption of
      in large intestine, 795, 797
      in small intestine, 795
   anion gap and, 395
   in cerebrospinal fluid, 747
   diffusion through capillary pores, 179, 180t
   gastric acid secretion and, 777–778, 778f
   intestinal absorption of, 794, 795, 795f, 797
   intestinal water secretion and, 787
   neuronal somal membrane and, 552,
      552f, 553
   plasma concentration of, with reduced GFR,
      404, 405f
   in red blood cells, 502–503
   renal reabsorption of, 328
   in saliva, 774f, 775, 776
   in sweat gland secretions, 870–871
Chloride ion channels
   intestinal, 795
      diarrhea and, 796
   of postsynaptic neuronal membrane, 548,
      550, 554
   presynaptic inhibition and, 554
Chloride shift, 502–503
Chloride-bicarbonate exchanger, 795
Chloride-iodide counter-transporter, 908
Cholecalciferol. See Vitamin D.
Cholecystokinin (CCK), 758, 758t
   food intake and, 846, 846f, 847f, 848
   gallbladder emptying and, 768,
      785, 784f
   molecular structure of, 780
   pancreatic secretions and, 782, 783
   small intestine peristalsis and, 769
   stomach emptying and, 768
Cholera, 796, 802
Cholesterol, 826–827
   absorption of, bile salts and, 785
   adrenocortical hormone synthesis from,
      922, 923f
   in bile, 783, 784, 784t, 786
      gallstones and, 786, 786f
   bile salts synthesized from, 785
   blood level of
      atherosclerosis and, 828, 829
      control of, 827
      insulin and, 944
      thyroid hormones and, 912, 918
   of capillary membrane, 178, 178f
   of cell membranes, 13, 14, 827
   in chylomicron remnants, 820
   in chylomicrons, 819
   dietary, 792
   endogenous, 826, 827
   genetic disorders affecting, 827
   intestinal absorption of, 793
   as lipid, 819
   in lipoproteins, 821, 821t
   in seminiferous tubules, 977
   steroid hormone synthesis from, 827, 882
   structure of, 826f, 827
   synthesis of, 826–827
      in endoplasmic reticulum, 20
      in liver, 822, 826, 839
   uses of, 827
Cholesterol desmolase, 922, 923f

Cholesterol ester hydrolase, 792–793
Cholesterol esterase, 781
Cholesterol esters, 826
   dietary, 792
   digestion of, 792–793
   steroid synthesis from, 882
Cholic acid, 785, 827
Choline, in lecithin synthesis, 826
Choline acetyltransferase, 551, 732
Cholinergic drugs, 740
Cholinergic fibers, 731–732
   to sweat glands, 870
Cholinesterase, 551
Chondroitin sulfate, 20
Chorda tympani, 647, 648f
Chordae tendineae, 107, 107f
Chorea, 691
Choroid, 611
Choroid plexus, 746, 747, 747f
   barriers at, 748–749
Chromatic aberration, 631
Chromatids, 38–39
Chromatin material, 17, 17f
Chromosomes, 17, 38
   transcriptional regulation and, 36, 38
Chronic obstructive pulmonary disease
      (COPD), ventilation-perfusion
      abnormalities in, 494
Chylomicron remnants, 820, 820f
Chylomicrons
   formation of, 797, 819
   pathways involving, 820f
   removal from blood, 819–820
   transport of, 819
Chyme
   in colon, 770, 797
   in small intestine, 768, 769, 770, 781, 782
      cholecystokinin and, 783
      water absorption and, 794
   in stomach, 765, 766, 767–768
Chymotrypsin, 781, 791
Chymotrypsinogen, 781
Cilia, 24–25, 24f. See also Stereocilia.
   of fallopian tubes, 993–994, 1003, 1004
   of respiratory epithelium, 473
   of vestibular hair cells, 675, 675f, 676
Ciliary body, aqueous humor formed by,
      606, 606f
Ciliary ganglion, 631, 631f
Ciliary muscle
   control of, 601, 631–632, 734t, 735
   innervation of, 631
Ciliary processes, 606, 606f
Circle of Willis, 743
Circulation. See also Blood flow; Systemic
      circulation.
   basic principles of, 4, 4f, 158–159
   fetal, 1022–1023, 1022f
   microcirculation, 177–178, 178f
   neonatal
      readjustments in, 1022–1023
      special problems in, 1024, 1024f
   nervous regulation of, 201–204, 202f,
      204f. See also Arterial blood pressure
      control, nervous.
   parts of, 157, 158f
      cross-sectional areas of, 157, 158, 158t
      pressures in, 158, 159f
      volumes of blood in, 157, 158f
Circulatory arrest, 281–282
   vasomotor failure in, 277
Circulatory shock, 234, 273–282. See also
      Cardiogenic shock.
   in aldosterone deficiency, 925
   anaphylactic, 280
      sympathomimetic drugs for, 281
   arterial pressure in, 273

Circulatory shock (Continued)
   causes of, 273
   circulatory arrest and, 281
   definition of, 273
   gastrointestinal vasoconstriction during, 762
   heatstroke with, 876
   hemorrhagic. See Hypovolemic shock.
   histamine-induced, 280
   hypovolemic. See Hypovolemic shock
   neurogenic, 279–280
      sympathomimetic drugs for, 281
   renal ischemia in, 401
   septic, 280
   stages of, 274
   tissue deterioration in, 273–274, 277–278,
      278f
   treatment of, 280–281
Circulatory system, 4–5, 4f
Circus movement, 149–150, 149f, 152
   after myocardial infarction, 251
Cirrhosis, 838
   edema in, 298, 377–378, 833
Citrate
   as anticoagulant, 456, 460
   phosphofructokinase inhibition by, 815
   vasodilation caused by, 200
Citric acid, in seminal vesicles, 976
Citric acid cycle, 22, 813–814, 813f, 815
   acetoacetic acid and, 823
   amino acid degradation products in, 835
   fatty acid oxidation and, 822–823
   fatty acid synthesis and, 825
      with excess glucose, 943
Clathrin, 18–19, 18f
   at neuromuscular junction, 86
Clearance methods, renal, 340–343, 340t,
      341f, 342f, 343t
Climacteric, male, 984
Climbing fibers, 684, 684f, 685, 686
Clonus, 660, 660f
Clostridial infections, hyperbaric oxygen
      therapy for, 540
Clot dissolution or fibrous organization, 453
Clot formation, 452, 452f, 454. See also Blood
      coagulation.
   outside the body, 460
Clot lysis, 457
Clot retraction, 452, 452f, 454
   thrombocytopenia and, 458
Clotting factors, 452, 452t, 453
   deficiencies of, 457–458
   initiation of coagulation and, 454–456,
      455f, 456f
Clotting time, 460
CNS. See Central nervous system (CNS).
Coagulation. See Blood coagulation.
Coated pits, 18–19, 18f
   adrenocortical hormone synthesis and, 922
   at neuromuscular junction, 86
Cobalamin. See Vitamin B$_{12}$.
Cocaine- and amphetamine-related transcript,
      846, 847f
Cochlea. See Hearing, cochlea in.
Cochlear nerve, 634f, 636–637, 636f, 638
Cochlear nuclei, 639, 639f
Codons, 29f, 30, 31–32, 31t, 32f
Coenzyme A. See Acetyl coenzyme
      A (acetyl-CoA).
Colchicine, 39
Cold environment, 877. See also Temperature,
      body.
   acclimatization to, 873
   thyroid-stimulating hormone and, 915
Cold receptors, 592–593, 592f. See also
      Thermoreceptive senses.
Cold-sensitive neurons, 871
Colitis, ulcerative, 771, 802–803

Collagen
  ascorbic acid and, 855
  of bone, 957, 958
  digestion of, 791
  of lungs, 467
  of sarcolemma, 71
  of teeth, 970
Collagen fiber bundles, 180, 180*f*, 181
Collateral circulation, 198
  in heart, 249, 249*f*
Collecting duct, 306, 306*f*, 307*f*
  transport properties of, 333–334, 333*f*
  urine concentration and, 348*t*, 350,
    350*f*, 352*f*, 353
Collecting tubule, 306, 306*f*, 332–333,
    332*f*, 333*f*
  aldosterone and, 337
  urine concentration and, 346, 346*f*, 348*t*,
    352*f*, 353
Colloid, of thyroid gland, 907, 907*f*, 908, 909
Colloid goiter, 917
Colloid osmotic pressure. *See also* Osmotic
    pressure
  interstitial fluid, 181, 181*f*, 184, 184*t*, 185*t*
    in lungs, 481, 482*t*
    lymph flow and, 188, 189
  plasma, 181, 181*f*, 184, 184*t*, 185*t*
    albumin and, 184, 184*t*, 833
    lymph flow and, 188
  plasma substitutes and, 281
  reabsorption in kidney and, 335–337, 335*f*,
    336*t*, 337*f*
Colon. *See* Large intestine (colon).
Colonoileal reflex, 757
Colony-forming unit (CFU), 414*f*, 415
Color blindness, 616, 616*f*
Color blobs, 625, 625*f*
Color vision, 615–616, 615*f*, 616*f*
  dorsal lateral geniculate nucleus and, 624
  ganglion cells in, 619, 620–621
  pigments in, 609, 614, 614*f*
  visual cortex and, 624*f*, 625, 625*f*, 626, 627
  white light and, 616
Colostrum, 1014
Coma
  hepatic, 835
  vs. sleep, 721
Committed stem cells, 414, 415, 423–424
Compensatory pause, 146
Complement system, 433, 438–439, 439*f*
  opsonization and, 425
Complete atrioventricular block, 145, 145*f*
Complete protein, 835
Complex cells, of visual cortex, 626, 627
Complex spike, 684
Compliance, pulmonary
  of lungs, 467, 467*f*
  of lungs plus thorax, 468
Compliance, vascular. *See* Vascular compliance.
Conceptus, 1005
Concussion, brain edema secondary to, 749
Conductance of blood vessels, 163
  in parallel circuit, 164
Conduction system. *See* Heart, excitatory and
    conductive system of
Conductive heat loss, 869, 869*f*
  clothing and, 869–870
  in water, 869
Cones, 609
  of central fovea, 619
  color blindness and, 616
  dark adaptation by, 614–615
  electrotonic conduction in, 617–618
  neural circuitry and, 616–617, 617*f*
    pathway to ganglion cells, 617, 617*f*
  neurotransmitter released by, 617
  number of, 619

Cones (*Continued*)
  photochemistry of, 611, 613, 613*f*,
    614, 614*f*
  spectral sensitivities of, 615, 615*f*
  structure of, 609, 610*f*
Congenital heart disease. *See also* Patent ductus
    arteriosus
  axis deviation in, 135–136, 136*f*
  cardiac hypertrophy in, 272
  causes of, 271
  circulatory dynamics in, 269–271, 270*f*, 271*f*
  valvular, 267
Conn syndrome. *See* Aldosteronism, primary
Connecting tubule, 306, 306*f*
Consciousness, 706
Constipation, 802
Constricted lung diseases, 516, 516*f*
Constrictor waves, gastric, 766
Contact junctions, of smooth muscle, 95
Contact lenses, 604
Contraception
  hormonal, 1001
  rhythm method of, 1001
Contractility, cardiac. *See* Cardiac muscle,
    contractile strength of.
Contrecoup injury, 746
Control systems of body, 6–9. *See also*
    Feedback; Homeostasis.
  adaptive, 9
  for arterial blood pressure, 6, 7–8. *See also*
    Arterial blood pressure control.
  for extracellular fluid characteristics, 7
    carbon dioxide concentration, 6, 7
    oxygen concentration, 6
  gain of, 7–8
Convective heat loss, 869, 869*f*
  clothing and, 869–870
  in water, 869
  wind and, 869
Convergence, in neuronal pathways, 566, 566*f*
Converting enzyme, 220–221, 220*f*
COPD (chronic obstructive pulmonary
    disease), ventilation-perfusion
    abnormalities in, 494
Cord righting reflex, 664
Cordotomy, 586
Corona radiata, 989*f*, 990, 1003, 1004*f*
Coronary arteries, 246, 246*f*
  acute occlusion of, 248–249. *See also*
    Myocardial infarction.
    causes of death after, 250–251
    collateral circulation and, 249, 251, 256
  arrangement within cardiac muscle,
    247, 247*f*
  collateral circulation involving, 249, 249*f*
Coronary artery bypass surgery, 252, 259
Coronary artery disease, 246, 248–250
  catheter-based treatment of, 253, 259
  pain in, 252. *See also* Angina pectoris.
Coronary artery spasm, 249
Coronary blood flow
  control of, 247–248
    adenosine in, 193
  epicardial vs. subendocardial, 247, 247*f*
  during exercise, 246
  in hypovolemic shock, 274–275, 276
  phasic changes in, 246, 246*f*
  at rest, 246
Coronary blood supply, 246, 246*f*
Coronary embolus, 248–249
Coronary steal, 251–252
Coronary thrombosis, 248–249
  collateral development following, 198
  spasm leading to, 249
Coronary venous blood flow, 246
Corpus albicans, 991
Corpus callosum, 702, 705

Corpus luteum, 989*f*, 990–991
  inhibin secreted by, 991, 997
  in pregnancy, 1008
  relaxin secreted by, 1009
Cortical level of nervous system, 545–546
Cortical nephrons, 306, 307*f*
Corticofugal signals, 581–582
  from primary visual cortex, 624
Corticopontocerebellar tract, 682, 687
Corticorubral tract, 670–671, 671*f*
Corticospinal (pyramidal) tract, 655*f*, 656,
    669–670, 670*f*
  cerebellum and, 687, 687*f*
  corticorubrospinal pathway and, 670–671
  lesions in, 673
Corticosteroids. *See* Adrenocortical hormones.
Corticosterone
  activity of, 928
  properties of, 922, 924*t*
  synthesis of, 922, 923*f*
Corticotropes, 896, 896*t*, 897, 933–934
Corticotropin. *See* Adrenocorticotropic
    hormone (ACTH; corticotropin)
Corticotropin-releasing factor (CRF). *See*
    Corticotropin-releasing hormone
    (CRH).
Corticotropin-releasing hormone (CRH),
    898, 898*t*, 931–932
  appetite suppression by, 849
Cortisol, 921
  anti-inflammatory effects of, 930–931
    in allergic reactions, 931
  carbohydrate metabolism and, 928
  chemical formula of, 922, 923*f*
  circadian rhythm of secretion, 933, 933*f*
  concentration in blood, 924
  deficiency of, 934
  excess of, 935–936
  fat metabolism and, 929
  gluconeogenesis and, 817
  insulin secretion and, 947
  lymphocytopenia caused by, 931
  mechanism of action, 931
  mineralocorticoid activity of, 924–925
  plasma protein binding of, 923
  properties of, 922, 924*t*
  protein metabolism and, 928–929
  regulation of, by ACTH, 931–934, 932*f*
  stress and, 929, 930, 930*f*
  synthesis of, 922, 923*f*
Cortisol-binding globulin, 923
Cortisone, 922, 924*t*
Co-transport, 54–55, 55*f*. *See also* Sodium
    co-transport.
  renal tubular, 325–326, 326*f*
Cough reflex, 473, 512
Coumarins, 459–460
Counter-transport, 54, 55, 55*f*
  renal tubular, 326, 326*f*
Coup injury, 746
Coupled chemical reactions, 809
Cowper glands. *See* Bulbourethral glands.
CPR (cardiopulmonary resuscitation), 151, 153
Cramp, muscle, 665
Cramping pain, visceral, 588–589
Creatine phosphate. *See* Phosphocreatine.
Creatinine
  chronic renal failure and, 406
  excretion of, 329
    with reduced GFR, 404, 405*f*
  placental diffusion of, 1007
  plasma concentration of, 341, 341*f*, 342*f*
    with reduced GFR, 404, 405*f*
Creatinine clearance, 341
Cretinism, 918, 1026
CRF (corticotropin-releasing factor). *See*
    Corticotropin-releasing hormone (CRH).

CRH (corticotropin-releasing hormone), 898, 898*t*, 931–932
  appetite suppression by, 849
Cribriform plate, 651
Crisis, febrile, 876, 876*f*
Crista ampullaris, 675*f*, 676, 676*f*, 677
Critical closing pressure, 166, 166*f*
Crossed extensor reflex, 663, 663*f*
Crown, of tooth, 969, 969*f*
Cryptorchidism, 977–978
Crypts of Lieberkühn, 773, 786–787, 786*f*
  of large intestine, 787
    extreme diarrhea and, 796, 802
CSF. *See* Cerebrospinal fluid (CSF).
Cupula, 676, 676*f*, 677
Curare, 85
Curariform drugs, 86
Current of injury, 138–141
  fibrillation tendency and, 250–251
  J point and, 138–140, 139*f*
  myocardial ischemia or infarction and, 138, 140–141, 140*f*, 141*f*
  QRS complex and, 138, 139*f*
Cushing disease, 935
Cushing reaction, 209
Cushing syndrome, 935–936, 935*f*
  diabetes mellitus in, 952
  ketosis in, 825
  osteoporosis in, 969
Cyanide poisoning, 521
Cyanosis, 521–522
Cyclic adenosine monophosphate (cAMP).
    See also Adenylyl cyclase.
  ACTH and, 932
  adrenergic or cholinergic receptors and, 733
  aldosterone and, 927
  antidiuretic hormone and, 905
  chloride channels and, 796
  glucagon and, 948
  gonadotropic hormones and, 983, 988–989
  growth hormone and, 902
  hormonal activity and, 889–890, 889*b*, 890*f*
  hormone secretion and, 882
  memory and, 707–708
  in olfactory cilium, 649, 649*f*
  parathyroid hormone and, 964–965
  phosphorylase activation and, 36, 812
  in postsynaptic neuron, 549, 549*f*
  as second messenger, 888
  in smooth muscle, 97
  thyroid hormone and, 914
Cyclic guanosine monophosphate (cGMP)
  nitric oxide and, 195, 196
  penile erection and, 978–979
  phosphodiesterase-5 inhibitors and, 196, 986
  photoreceptor sodium channels and, 612–613, 612*f*, 613–614, 613*f*
  in postsynaptic neuron, 549, 549*f*
  in smooth muscle, 97
Cyclosporine, for immunosuppression, in transplantation, 449
Cystic duct, 783–784
Cystinuria, essential, 408
Cystitis, 403–404
Cystometrogram, 309, 309*f*
Cytochrome oxidase, 814
  cyanide poisoning and, 521
Cytochromes, of electron transport chain, 814
Cytokines, 881
  enzyme-linked receptors for, 888
  fever and, 875–876
Cytosine, 27, 28, 28*f*, 30, 31*t*
Cytoskeleton, 11, 16–17, 17*f*
Cytosol, 14
Cytotoxic T cells, 440, 441, 441*f*

D
DAG (diacylglycerol), 890
Dark adaptation curve, 614–615, 614*f*
Dead space
  anatomic, 471–472
  physiologic, 471–472, 493, 494
Dead space air, expired air and, 489, 489*f*
Dead space volume, 471, 471*f*
Deafness, 642, 642*f*
Deamination of amino acids, 834–835, 839
Decarboxylases, 814
Decerebrate rigidity, 674
Decibel unit, 638–639, 638*f*
Decidua, 1005
Decidual cells, 1005, 1008
Declarative memory, 706
Decompression sickness, 537, 538–539, 538*f*
Decremental conduction, 556, 556*f*
Deep cerebellar nuclei, 683–684, 684*f*, 685, 688
  lesions of, 689
Deep nuclear cells, 684–685, 684*f*, 687
Deep receptors, 560*b*, 580
Deep sensations, 571
Deep-sea diving, 535–540
  decompression after, 537–539
  depth of
    gas volume vs., 535
    pressure vs., 535, 536*f*
  high partial pressures in, 535–539
    of carbon dioxide, 537
    of nitrogen, 535
    of oxygen, 499, 535–537, 536*f*
  with SCUBA apparatus, 539, 539*f*
Defecation, 771–772
  parasympathetic stimulation and, 787
Defecation reflexes, 771–772, 771*f*, 803
  parasympathetic, 738, 757, 771, 771*f*
  spinal, 757
Defibrillation
  atrial, 152
  ventricular, 151, 151*f*
    in cardiopulmonary resuscitation, 151
Deglutition. *See* Swallowing.
Dehydration
  aldosterone secretion in, 795
  in diabetes mellitus, 950
  diarrhea with, 796
  hypernatremia caused by, 295, 295*t*
  in hyponatremia, 294–295, 295*t*
  hypovolemic shock in, 279
    fluid therapy for, 280
  in neonate, 1024
Dehydroepiandrosterone (DHEA), 922, 923*f*, 924*t*, 934, 980
  placental estrogen synthesis from, 1008
Dehydrogenases, 813, 814, 815
Deiodinase, 909
  deficiency of, 917
Delayed compliance of vessels, 168, 168*f*
Delayed-reaction allergy, 443
Delta waves, 723*f*, 724–725, 725*f*
Dementia, 726
  in Alzheimer's disease, 727–728
  cerebrovascular disease and, 728
  in Huntington's disease, 694
Demyelination
  osmotic-mediated, 295
  in vitamin B$_{12}$ deficiency, 854
Dendrites, 543, 544*f*, 547, 547*f*
  excitation and inhibition transmitted by, 555–556, 556*f*
Dendritic cells, 440
Denervation, of skeletal muscle, 82
Denervation supersensitivity, 737, 737*f*
Dense bars, of neuromuscular junction, 83, 84*f*
Dense bodies, of smooth muscle, 92, 92*f*
Dental lamina, 970–971

Dentate nucleus, 683, 684, 684*f*, 688
  lesions of, 689
Dentin, 969, 969*f*, 970
  caries and, 971
  development of, 970, 970*f*
  mineral exchange in, 971
Dentinal tubules, 970
Deoxycorticosterone, 922, 923*f*, 924*t*
Deoxyribonucleic acid. *See* DNA (deoxyribonucleic acid).
Deoxyribose, 27, 28*f*
Depolarization, of action potential, 61, 61*f*, 64–65
  calcium channels and, 64
Depolarization waves, 121–123, 122*f*. *See also* P wave; QRS complex.
  current flow in chest and, 124, 124*f*
  slow conduction of, T wave and, 142
L-Deprenyl, 693
Depression, mental, 726–727
Depth of focus, 602, 602*f*
Depth perception, 605, 605*f*, 630
Dermatomes, 582, 582*f*
Desmopressin, 354–355
Detoxification, enzymes for, 20
Detrusor muscle, 306–308, 307*f*, 309
  micturition reflex and, 309
  parasympathetic fibers to, 308
Deuteranope, 616
Dexamethasone, 922–923, 924*t*
Dexamethasone suppression test, 935
Dextran solution, 281
α-Dextrinase, 790
DHEA. *See* Dehydroepiandrosterone (DHEA).
Diabetes insipidus, 295
  central, 354
  nephrogenic, 354–355, 408
Diabetes mellitus, 939, 950–954
  acidosis in, 393
  arteriosclerosis and, 953
  atherosclerosis and, 829
  brain metabolism in, 749–750
  diagnosis of, 952–953, 953*f*
  end-stage renal disease caused by, 402, 403
  fatty acids in blood in, 821
  gigantism with, 903
  glomerular filtration rate in, 321
  hyperkalemia in, 361
  ketosis in, 823
  maternal, 1026
  metabolic utilization of nutrients in, 845
  triglycerides in liver in, 822
  type I, 950–951
    C peptide in, 940
    clinical characteristics of, 952*t*
    fetal morbidity in mothers with, 1026
    treatment of, 953
  type II, 950, 951–952
    clinical characteristics of, 952*t*
    large babies of mothers with, 1026
    treatment of, 953
  urinary glucose excretion in, 327
  urine output in, 397
Diacylglycerol (DAG), 890
Dialysis, renal, 409–410, 409*f*
  hypertension associated with, 219
Dialyzing fluid, 409–410, 410*t*
Diapedesis, 415
  by lymphocytes, 425
  by monocytes, 425
  by neutrophils, 424*f*, 425, 428, 429*f*
Diarrhea, 802–803
  calcium loss in, 966
  hyponatremia caused by, 294–295
  intestinal absorption capacity and, 797–798

Diarrhea (*Continued*)
  metabolic acidosis caused by, 392
  psychogenic, 802
  as response to irritation, 787
  severe, 796, 797–798
Diastole, 105, 105*f*
  duration of, heart rate and, 105
  filling of ventricles during, 105*f*, 106
Diastolic blood pressure, 158, 168
  age-related increase in, 171, 171*f*
  measurement of, 170–171, 170*f*
Diastolic pressure curve, 108, 108*f*
Dicer enzyme, 32–33, 33*f*
Diet. *See* Food intake.
Differentiation, cellular, 39–40
Differentiation inducers, of hematopoietic
    stem cells, 415
Diffuse junctions, of smooth muscle, 94–95
Diffusing capacity, 491–492, 492*f*
  at high altitude, 529
Diffusion
  of gases. *See also* Carbon dioxide, diffusion
      of; Oxygen, diffusion of.
    physics of, 485–487, 486*f*
    through respiratory membrane,
        485, 486, 487, 489–492, 492*f*
  as molecular and ionic motion, 46
  osmosis and, 290
Diffusion across capillary walls, 4–5, 4*f*,
    179–180, 179*f*
  concentration difference and, 180
  molecular size and, 179–180, 180*t*
Diffusion coefficient of a gas, 487, 487*t*
  respiratory membrane and, 490–491
Diffusion potential, 57–58, 57*f*
  resting membrane potential and,
    60, 60*f*
Diffusion through cell membrane, 18, 45,
    46–47, 46*f*. *See also* Ion channels;
    Protein channels.
  vs. active transport, 45–46
  facilitated, 46, 46*f*, 49–50, 49*f*
    in glucose reabsorption, 326, 326*f*
    in sodium reabsorption, 325
  in pores and channels, 46–48, 46*f*, 47*f*,
    48*f*, 49*f*
  rate of, 49, 49*f*
    factors affecting, 50–51, 50*f*
  simple, 46, 46*f*
    vs. facilitated diffusion, 49, 49*f*
  of water, 46, 47, 51–52, 51*f*
Diffusion through interstitium, 180–181
Diffusion through respiratory membrane, 485,
    486, 487, 489–492, 492*f*.
    See also Carbon dioxide, diffusion of;
    Oxygen, diffusion of.
Digestion, 789–793
  of carbohydrates, 789–790, 790*f*
    pancreatic enzyme for, 781, 790
  of fats, 789, 791–793, 791*f*
  of proteins, 789, 790–791, 791*f*
    enterogastric reflexes and, 767, 768
    pancreatic enzymes in, 781, 791
Digestive enzymes, 773
  gastric. *See* Pepsin.
  intestinal, 787, 790
  pancreatic, 780–781
    carbohydrates and, 781, 790
    cholecystokinin and, 783
    fats and, 781, 792–793, 792*f*
    loss of, 801
    optimal pH for, 783
    phases of secretion, 782
    proteins and, 781, 791, 791*f*
    regulation of, 782–783, 783*f*
  salivary, 774*f*, 775, 790
Digestive vesicle, 19, 19*f*, 426

Digitalis
  in cardiogenic shock, 259
  diuresis caused by, 263
  in heart failure, 258
    with acute pulmonary edema, 261
    decompensated, 263, 263*f*
  ventricular tachycardia caused by, 149
Digitalis toxicity, T-wave changes in, 142, 142*f*
Dihydropyridine receptors, 88, 88*f*
Dihydrotestosterone, 979, 980, 982–983
  chemical structure of, 980*f*
Diisopropyl fluorophosphate, 86
Diopters, 600, 600*f*
Dipeptidases, 791
Disaccharides
  dietary sources of, 789–790
  digestion of, 787, 789, 790, 790*f*
Discharge zone, 565–566, 565*f*
Disse, spaces of, 837, 837*f*, 838
Disseminated intravascular coagulation, 459
  in septic shock, 280
Dissociation constant, 381
Distal tubule, 306, 306*f*. *See also* Macula densa.
  calcium reabsorption in, 368–369
  diluting segment of, 331
  potassium secretion by, 364, 366, 366*f*
  transport properties of, 331–333, 332*f*, 333*f*
  urine concentration and, 346, 346*f*, 348*t*,
    350, 350*f*, 352*f*, 353
Distensibility, vascular, 167–168, 168*f*. *See also*
    Vascular compliance.
Diuretics, 397–399, 398*f*, 398*t*
  for essential hypertension, 226
  in heart failure, 258
    with acute pulmonary edema, 261
  hyponatremia caused by, 294–295
  metabolic alkalosis caused by, 393
Divergence, in neuronal pathways, 566, 566*f*
Diving. *See* Deep-sea diving.
DNA (deoxyribonucleic acid), 27, 27*f*. *See also*
    Transcription.
  methylation of, 36
  mitochondrial, 16
  nuclear location of, 17, 17*f*
  replication of, 37–38
  structure of, 27–29, 28*f*, 29*f*
  viral, 18
DNA ligase, 37–38
DNA polymerase, 37–38
DNA proofreading, 37–38
DNA repair, 37–38
Dominant hemisphere, 701–702
  corpus callosum and, 705
Donnan effect, 184, 287
L-Dopa, 693, 727
Dopamine
  in basal ganglia, 692–693, 692*f*
    Parkinson's disease and, 693
  as central nervous system transmitter, 551
  in norepinephrine synthesis, 732
  prolactin secretion and, 1015
  schizophrenia and, 727
Dopamine system, in brain, 712, 713, 713*f*
Doppler flowmeter, 160–161, 161*f*
Dorsal column–medial lemniscal system,
    573–580
  anatomy of, 573–574, 573*f*, 574*f*, 575*f*
  overview of, 573
  position sense and, 580
  rapidly changing sensations in, 579
  signal transmission and analysis in, 577–579,
    578*f*
  spatial orientation of fibers in, 574
  types of sensations in, 573
Dorsal lateral geniculate nucleus,
    623–624, 623*f*
Dorsal respiratory group, 505–506, 506*f*

Down syndrome, Alzheimer's disease
    characteristics in, 728
Dreaming, 712–713, 721
Drinking, threshold for, 358
Dropped beats, 145, 145*f*
Ductus arteriosus, 269–270, 270*f*, 1022, 1022*f*.
    See also Patent ductus arteriosus.
  closure of, 270, 1023
Ductus venosus, 1022, 1022*f*, 1023
Duodenocolic reflex, 771
Duodenum. *See also* Small intestine.
  mucus secreted in, 786
  peptic ulcer of, 800, 800*f*, 801
  stomach emptying and, 767–768
Dural sinuses, negative pressure in, 173
Dwarfism, 902–903
Dynamic proprioception, 580
Dynein, of cilia, 25
Dynorphin, 587
Dysarthria, 689
Dysbarism. *See* Decompression sickness.
Dysdiadochokinesia, 689
Dyslexia, 701, 703
Dysmetria, 689
Dyspnea, 522

E
Ear. *See* Hearing.
ECG. *See* Electrocardiogram (ECG).
Echocardiography, cardiac output estimated
    by, 240
Eclampsia, 1011
Ectopic beat. *See* Premature contractions.
Ectopic foci, causes of, 146
Ectoplasm, 16
Eddy currents, 161
Edema, 296–300
  capillary filtration and, 185–186
  cerebral. *See* Brain edema.
  extracellular, 297
    in cirrhosis, 298
    excess fluid and, 373, 373*f*
    general causes of, 297
    in heart failure, 298
    in kidney disease, 298
    plasma protein decrease with, 298
    safety factors preventing, 298–300,
        299*f*, 373
    specific causes of, 297–298
  generalized, in renal failure, 406
  histamine-induced, 199–200
  hypoproteinemic, in neonate, 1027
  hypoxia associated with, 521
  interstitial fluid pressure and, 189
  interstitial free fluid in, 181, 299
  intracellular, 296
  myxedema, 917–918, 918*f*
  in nephrotic syndrome, 377
  nonpitting, 299
  of optic disc, 748
  pitting, 299
  in potential spaces, 300
Edinger-Westphal nucleus, 631, 631*f*, 632
EEG. *See* Electroencephalogram (EEG).
Effectors, 543
Efference copy, 683, 687
Efferent arteriole(s), renal, 304–305, 305*f*, 306,
    307*f*, 311*f*
  angiotensin II and, 338, 339
  glomerular filtration rate and, 315, 316, 316*f*
  physiologic control of, 317–318
  reabsorption rate and, 336
  tubuloglomerular feedback and, 320, 320*f*
Efficiency, of cardiac contraction, 110
Effusion, 300
Einthoven's law, 125
Einthoven's triangle, 125, 125*f*

Ejaculation, 979
   as sympathetic function, 738, 979
Ejaculatory duct, 973, 973f, 976
Ejection, period of, 105f, 106, 108, 108f, 109f
Ejection fraction, 106
Elastase, 791
Elastic recoil, 465
Elastin, of lungs, 467
Electric shock
   defibrillation with
      atrial, 152
      ventricular, 151, 151f
   fibrillation caused by, 150, 150f
Electrical alternans, 145–146, 145f
Electrical synapses, 546
Electrocardiogram (ECG)
   in angina pectoris, 141
   atrial contraction and, 122
   in atrial fibrillation, 152, 152f
   in atrial flutter, 152–153, 153f
   in atrioventricular block
      first-degree, 144–145, 144f
      second-degree, 145, 145f
      third-degree (complete), 145, 145f
   in bundle branch block, 136–137, 136f,
      137f, 138
      T wave and, 142
   cardiac cycle and, 105, 105f
   current flows and, 123–124, 124f
   in electrical alternans, 145–146, 145f
   high-voltage, 135f, 136f, 137
      premature ventricular contractions with,
         146–147
   leads used for, 124–127, 125f, 126f. See also
         Bipolar limb leads.
      axes of, 130, 130f
   in long QT syndrome, 147, 148f
   low-voltage, 137, 137f
   in myocardial ischemia or infarction
      current of injury in, 140–141, 140f, 141f
      in mild ischemia, 142, 142f
   normal, 121–123, 121f
      vectorial analysis of, 131–134, 132f, 133f
   normal voltages in, 123
   in paroxysmal tachycardia
      atrial, 148, 148f
      ventricular, 148–149, 149f
   in partial intraventricular block,
      145–146, 145f
   position of heart in chest and, 135
   with premature contractions
      atrial, 146, 146f
      A-V nodal or A-V bundle, 146, 146f
      ventricular, 146–147, 147f
   QRS prolongation in, 137–138, 141
   QRS with bizarre patterns in, 138, 141
   recording methods for, 123
   in sinoatrial nodal block, 144, 144f
   in sinus bradycardia, 143f
   in sinus tachycardia, 143, 143f
   torsades de pointes in, 147, 148f
   vectorial analysis of, 129–142
      atrial T wave in, 133–134, 133f
      axes in, 130, 130f
      axis deviation in, 135–137
      current of injury in, 138–141, 139f,
         140f, 141f
      direction of vector in, 129, 130f
      instantaneous mean vector in, 129, 129f
      mean electrical axis in, 134–137, 135f
      of normal ECG, 131–134, 132f, 133f
      P wave in, 133–134, 133f
      of potentials in each lead, 130–131,
         130f, 131f
      with premature ventricular contractions,
         147, 147f
      principles of, 129–131

Electrocardiogram (ECG), vectorial analysis
         of (Continued)
      projected vector in, 130, 130f, 131, 131f
      QRS complex in, 131–132, 132f
      T wave in, 133, 133f
      vectorcardiogram in, 134, 134f
   ventricular contraction and, 122–123
   in ventricular fibrillation, 150–151, 151f
   in ventricular hypertrophy, 135–136, 135f,
      136f, 137–138
   voltage abnormalities in, 136f, 137, 137f
   voltage and time calibration of, 123
Electroconvulsive therapy, 727
Electroencephalogram (EEG), 723, 724
   epilepsy and, 725, 725f, 726
   frequencies of waves in, 723, 724–725, 724f
   normal types of waves in, 723f, 724
   in sleep and wakefulness, 723, 724, 725, 725f
   voltages in, 723, 724–725
Electrolytes. See also specific electrolytes.
   in gastrointestinal secretions, 774–775
   in large intestine, 797–798
      diarrhea and, 797, 802
   renal regulation of, 303, 304f, 311–312
   in stomach contents, 768
Electromagnetic flowmeter, 160, 160f
   for cardiac output measurement, 240, 240f
Electromagnetic receptors, 559, 560b
Electron transport chain, 814–815, 814f
Electrotonic conduction, 555, 556, 556f
   in retinal neurons, 617–618
ELISA (enzyme-linked immunosorbent
      assay), 892, 892f
Emboli, 459
Embryo. See also Fetus; Implantation.
   ameboid movement by cells of, 24
   cell differentiation in, 40
   early nutrition of, 995, 1005, 1008
Emission, 979
Emmetropia, 602, 602f
Emotional arousal, thyroid-stimulating
      hormone and, 915
Emotions. See Limbic system.
Emphysema, pulmonary, 517–518, 518f
   low-voltage ECG associated with, 137
   respiratory surface area in, 491
   ventilation-perfusion abnormalities in,
      494, 518
Enamel, of teeth, 969–970, 969f
   development of, 970, 970f
   mineral exchange in, 971
   resistance to caries, 971
End plate potential, 84, 85–86, 85f
End-diastolic pressure, 108
   as preload, 109
End-diastolic volume, 106, 108, 109f
Endocochlear potential, 637–638
Endocrine glands
   anatomical loci of, 881, 882f
   autonomic control of, 734t, 735
   energy from ATP for, 859
   in infancy, problems of, 1026
   overview of, 883t
   regulatory functions of, 5–6
Endocrine hormones, 881. See also Hormones.
Endocytosis, 18–19, 18f
   adrenocortical hormone synthesis and, 922
   in ameboid movement, 23, 23f
   in capillary endothelium, 178
Endogenous pyrogen, 875–876
Endolymph, 637–638, 676, 677
Endometrial cycle, 995–996, 995f
Endometriosis, infertility secondary to, 1001
Endometrium
   estrogen and, 993
   implantation in. See Implantation.
   progesterone and, 994

Endoplasmic reticulum, 12f, 14–15, 15f
   gastrointestinal secretions and, 774, 774f
   Golgi apparatus and, 15, 15f, 20–21
   of muscle fiber. See Sarcoplasmic reticulum.
   nuclear membrane and, 17, 17f
   platelets and, 451, 454
   ribosomes and, 14, 20, 20f, 33–34, 34f
   secretory vesicles and, 16
   specific functions of, 20, 20f
Endoplasmic reticulum vesicles, 15, 15f,
      20–21, 20f
Endorphins, 587
   β-endorphin, 933–934, 933f
Endostatin, 198
Endothelial cells
   of arteries and arterioles
      nitric oxide and, 195–196, 196f
      shear stress on, 195–196
   of capillaries, 177–178, 178f
      diffusion through, 179–180
   clotting and, 452, 457, 459
   of hepatic sinusoids, 837
   of lymphatic capillaries, 187, 187f, 188–189
   platelet fusion with, 452
Endothelial damage
   atherosclerosis and, 827–828, 828f, 829
   endothelin release in, 196
Endothelial-derived relaxing or constricting
      factors, 195–196, 196f
Endothelin, 196
   glomerular filtration rate and, 318
Endotoxin
   in circulatory shock, 277
   clotting activated by, 459
   fever and, 875–876
End-stage renal disease (ESRD), 401–402, 402f,
      402t. See also Renal failure, chronic.
   dialysis for, 409–410, 409f, 410t
      hypertension associated with, 219
   transplantation for, 409
End-systolic volume, 106, 108, 109f
Energy abundance, insulin and, 939–940
Energy equivalent of oxygen, 863
Energy expenditure, 863–865. See also
      Metabolic rate.
   in cachexia, 852
   components of, 863, 863f
   for daily activities, 863
   for essential metabolic functions,
      863–864, 864f
   hypothalamus and, 846, 849
   for nonshivering thermogenesis, 865
   for physical activities, 864, 864t
   for processing food, 864–865
   of pulmonary ventilation, 468
   for skeletal muscle contraction, 73, 74, 75,
      76, 78–79
Energy release
   heat as end product of, 862
   rate of, 861–862. See also Metabolic rate.
Energy sources. See Adenosine triphosphate
      (ATP), as energy currency; Fats, as
      energy source; Food(s), energy
      available in; Glucose, energy
      production from; Protein(s), as
      energy source; Triglycerides, energy
      production from.
Enhancers, 35f, 36
Enkephalins, 587, 587f
   in basal ganglia, 692–693, 692f
Enteric lipase, 792
Enteric nervous system, 755, 756, 756f
   autonomic influences on, 735, 755, 756–757
   defecation reflex and, 771
   gallbladder emptying and, 785
   gastric pepsinogen secretion and, 779
   glandular secretions and, 773

Enteric nervous system (*Continued*)
neurotransmitters of, 756–757
pancreatic secretions and, 782
peristalsis and, 759
reflexes in, 757
sensory fibers and, 755, 757
small intestine and, 769
stomach emptying and, 767
Enteritis, 802
Enterochromaffin-like cells, 779
Enterocytes. *See also* Villi, intestinal.
of crypts, secretions of, 786–787
digestive enzymes of, 787, 790, 791, 792
replacement of, 787
Enterogastric reflexes, 757, 767–768
reverse, 780
Enterohepatic circulation, of bile salts, 785
Enterokinase, 781
Enzyme-linked immunosorbent assay
(ELISA), 892, 892f
Enzymes, 11, 27
G-protein activation of, 887, 887f
hormone receptors linked to, 888, 888f
membrane proteins as, 13, 14
reaction rates and, 861–862, 862f
regulation of, 35, 36–37
synthetic functions of, 35
Eosinophilic chemotactic factor, in asthma, 520
Eosinophils, 423, 423t, 424f, 430
Epididymis, 973, 973f
spermatozoal maturation in, 975, 976
Epidural space, negative pressure in, 183
Epilepsy, 725–726, 725f. *See also* Seizures.
neuronal circuits in, 569
Epinephrine
adrenal medullar secretion of, 730, 732,
736, 884, 921
basal level of, 737
in hypovolemic shock, 275
adrenergic receptors and, 733
bronchiolar dilation and, 473
coronary blood flow and, 247, 248
fatty acid mobilization caused by, 825
gastrointestinal smooth muscle and, 755,
756, 757
glomerular filtration rate and, 318
glucose availability and, 812
insulin secretion and, 947
metabolic rate and, 867
phosphorylase activation by, 812
for shock, 281
sweat glands and, 870
as sympathomimetic drug, 739
synthesis of, 732, 884
thermogenesis and, 873
as vasoconstrictor, 199, 204
in skeletal muscle, 244
vasodilation in skeletal muscles and, 204, 244
Eplerenone, 332, 333f, 399
Equilibrium. *See also* Posture; Vestibular
apparatus.
cerebellum and, 686–687
exteroceptive information and, 678
footpad pressure and, 678
neck proprioceptors and, 678
sensation of, 571
static, 676–677
visual information and, 678
Erectile dysfunction, 985–986
phosphodiesterase-5 inhibitors for, 196
Erection
female, 1000
penile, 196, 738, 978–979, 979f
Erythroblastosis fetalis, 415f, 420, 447–448,
1024
Erythroblasts, 415f, 420. *See also*
Proerythroblasts.

Erythrocytes. *See* Red blood cells (erythrocytes).
Erythropoietin, 304, 416–417, 416f
kidney disease and, 304, 406, 416
Esophageal reflux, 765
Esophageal secretions, 776–777
Esophageal sphincter
lower, 765
upper, 764
Esophagus
achalasia of, 799
ulcer of, 800
ESRD. *See* End-stage renal disease (ESRD).
β-Estradiol, 991–992, 992f
hepatic degradation of, 993
Estriol, 991–992, 992f, 993
Estrogen(s), 987, 988f, 991
breast development and, 994, 1014
chemistry of, 991–992, 992f, 993f
in contraceptive drugs, 1001
excretion of, 993
fat deposition and, 994, 1031
functions of, 993–994
gonadotropin inhibition by, 997, 998
hepatic degradation of, 993
hypersecretion of, 999–1000
life cycle variations in, 999, 999f
in luteal phase, 991
in male, 980
menstrual cycle and, 995
osteoporosis and, 969
in ovarian follicles, 989, 990
plasma protein binding of, 993
in pregnancy, 1007f, 1008
preovulatory surge of luteinizing hormone
and, 997–998
protein deposition in tissues and, 836
spermatogenesis and, 975
synthesis of
in adrenal cortex, 922
in ovaries, 992, 992f, 993f
uterine contractility and, 1011–1012
Estrone, 991–992, 992f, 993
Ethacrynic acid, 397
Eunuchism, 985
female, 999
Evans blue dye, 290
Evaporative heat loss, 869, 869f. *See also*
Sweating.
hypothalamic control of, 872, 872f
by panting, 871
at very high air temperatures, 869
Excitation-contraction coupling
in cardiac muscle, 103–104, 104f
in skeletal muscle, 87, 88–89, 88f, 89f
Excitatory postsynaptic potential, 553, 553f,
554, 554f
dendrites and, 556
summation of, 553, 554f, 555
Excitatory presynaptic terminals, 547
Excitatory receptors, 547, 549–550
Excitatory stimulus, 565
reciprocal inhibition and, 566–567, 567f
Excitatory transmitter, 548
Excited zone, 565–566, 565f
Excretion rate, calculation of, 340t
Exercise. *See also* Sports physiology.
anaerobic glycolysis in, 860–861
arterial pressure increase in, 205, 210,
232, 232f
blood flow control to skeletal muscle and,
191, 195, 196–197, 198, 243–244
cardiac output during, 210, 230, 230f, 232,
244, 245, 245f
athletic training and, 1038, 1038f,
1039, 1039f
circulatory readjustments in, 244–245
coronary blood flow during, 246

Exercise (*Continued*)
energy expenditure in, 864, 864t
fat utilization in, 825
gastrointestinal vasoconstriction during, 762
glucagon secretion and, 948–949
growth hormone secretion and, 901, 902
hyperkalemia caused by, 362
lactic acid produced in, for cardiac
energy, 816
life-prolonging effect of, 1041
lymphatic pump during, 188
obesity and, 850, 851
oxygen debt in, 861
oxygen diffusing capacity during, 491
oxygen transport during, 498–499, 499f
oxygen uptake by blood during, 495–496
oxygen-hemoglobin dissociation curve
and, 500
pulmonary circulation and, 480, 481f
respiratory regulation during, 510–511,
510f, 511f
sweat glands and, 870
valvular heart lesions and, 269
Exercise testing, of cardiac reserve, 261–262
Exocytosis, 19, 21
in ameboid movement, 23, 23f
of catecholamines, 884
of gastrointestinal secretions, 774
of peptide hormones, 882
of protein hormones, 882
Exophthalmos, in hyperthyroidism, 916, 916f
Expanded tip tactile receptors, 560f, 572
Expiratory compliance curve, 467, 467f
Expiratory reserve volume, 469, 469f
Expired air, 487t, 489, 489f
External work, cardiac, 108–109, 108f, 109f
Exteroreceptive sensations, 571, 678
Extracellular fluid, 3–4, 286, 286f, 287. *See also*
Interstitial fluid; Plasma.
calcium in. *See* Calcium, in extracellular
fluid and plasma.
in chronic renal failure, 406, 406f
composition of, 7, 7t, 45, 45f, 287, 288f, 288t
distribution between interstitium and blood,
373, 373f
as internal environment, 3, 9
intracellular fluid and, 3–4
exchange between compartments, 290
osmotic equilibrium of, 291–292, 292f
mixing of, 4–5
nutrients in, origins of, 5
osmolality of, 52
osmolarity of. *See* Extracellular fluid
osmolarity.
pH of, 7, 7t, 380t. *See also* Acid-base
regulation.
potassium concentration in, 364, 364f,
365f, 366f
regulation of, 7
carbon dioxide concentration, 6, 7
oxygen concentration, 6
sodium in. *See* Sodium, extracellular fluid.
transport through body, 4–5, 4f
volume of. *See* Extracellular fluid volume.
Extracellular fluid osmolarity. *See also* Plasma,
osmolarity of.
in abnormal states, 292–294, 293f,
293t, 294t
glucose and, 950
potassium distribution and, 362
regulation of, 345, 355
angiotensin II and aldosterone in,
359–360, 359f
by osmoreceptor-ADH system, 345,
355–357, 355f, 356f, 357f, 358–359,
360, 905
by thirst, 357–360, 358t, 359f

Extracellular fluid volume. *See also* Blood volume.
in abnormal states, 292–294, 293*f*, 293*t*, 294*t*
aldosterone and, 925, 925*f*
antidiuretic hormone and, 375–376
arterial blood pressure and, 217, 217*f*
angiotensin II and, 221, 374–375
conditions causing large increases in, 376–378
depletion of, alkalosis secondary to, 390
diuretics and, 397, 398*f*
hypertension and, 218, 219, 220*f*
measurement of, 289, 289*t*
regulation of, 370–371
by renal–body fluid system, 371–373, 372*f*
salt and, 217–218
salt appetite and, 360
testosterone and, 982
thirst and, 358
Extracorporeal circulation, in cardiac surgery, 271–272
Extrafusal muscle fibers, 656*f*, 657, 659
Extrapyramidal system, 671
Extrasystole. *See* Premature contractions.
Extrinsic pathway of coagulation, 454–455, 455*f*, 456
Eye movements, 627
fixation movements, 628–630, 629*f*, 678
muscular control of, 627–628, 628*f*
neural pathways for, 628, 628*f*
vestibular apparatus and, 677
voluntary, premotor cortex and, 669
Eyes. *See also* Visual *entries.*
accommodation of, 601, 601*f*
autonomic control of, 631–632, 735
pupillary reaction to, 632
autonomic control of, 631–632, 631*f*, 734*t*, 735
equilibrium maintenance and, 678
fluid system of, 606–608, 606*f*, 607*f*
focusing of. *See* Accommodation.
headache associated with, 592
lens of. *See* Lens, of eye.
ophthalmoscopic examination of, 605–606, 605*f*
optics of, 600–605
accommodation in, 601, 601*f*
camera analogy in, 600, 600*f*
depth of focus in, 602, 602*f*
depth perception in, 605, 605*f*, 630
pupillary diameter in, 601–602, 602*f*
refractive errors in, 602–604, 602*f*, 603*f*, 604*f*
visual acuity in, 604–605, 604*f*
protruding, in hyperthyroidism, 916, 916*f*
pupillary diameter of, 601–602, 602*f*
autonomic control of, 632
dark adaptation by, 615

F
Facial recognition areas, 700–701, 700*f*
Facilitated diffusion, 46, 46*f*, 49–50, 49*f*
in glucose reabsorption, 326, 326*f*
in sodium reabsorption, 325
Facilitated zone, 565–566, 565*f*
Facilitation of neurons, 545, 555, 565–566
memory and, 707–708, 707*f*
F-actin, 75, 75*f*
FAD (flavin adenine dinucleotide), 854
Fainting
acute venous dilation in, 233
emotional, 204
in long QT syndromes, 147
in Stokes-Adams syndrome, 119, 145
Fallopian tubes
anatomy of, 987, 987*f*, 988*f*
entry of ovum into, 1003, 1004*f*

Fallopian tubes (*Continued*)
estrogenic effects on, 993–994
infertility associated with, 1002
progesterone and, 995
transport of fertilized ovum in, 1004, 1004*f*
transport of sperm in, 1000, 1003
Familial hypercholesterolemia, 828–829
Fanconi's syndrome, 408
Farsightedness, 602, 602*f*, 603, 603*f*
Fasciculus, 72*f*
Fast muscle fibers, 79
Fast pain, 583
Fast sodium channels, 64
in cardiac muscle, 66, 102, 115
sinus nodal action potential and, 116
ventricular action potential and, 115–116
Fastigial nucleus, 683, 684, 684*f*
lesions of, 689
Fasting blood glucose, 952
Fast-sharp pain pathway, 584–585, 585*f*
Fast-twitch muscle fibers, 1036, 1036*t*
Fat cells. *See* Adipocytes (fat cells).
Fatigue
of neuromuscular junction, 85–86
of skeletal muscle, 80–81
of synapses, 557
in reverberatory circuit, 567–568
stabilizing effect of, 569–570, 569*f*
Fats. *See also* Lipids; Triglycerides.
absorption of, 797
bile salts and, 785
deposits of, 821–822. *See also* Adipose tissue.
estrogen and, 994, 1031
dietary
gallstones and, 786
types of, 791–792
digestion of, 789, 791–793, 791*f*
bile acids and, 783
bile salts and, 785
gallbladder emptying and, 785
pancreatic enzymes for, 781, 783*f*
in stomach, 792
emulsification of, 792, 792*f*
as energy source. *See also* Triglycerides, energy production from.
for athletes, 1035, 1035*f*
in diabetes mellitus, 951
growth hormone and, 899
with high-fat diet, 824
hormonal regulation of, 825
insulin and, 943–944, 944*f*, 947
liver and, 821–822
in feces, 798
in foods
energy available in, 843–844
metabolic utilization of, 844–845
glucose storage as, 817
glucose synthesis from, 817
malabsorption of, 802
metabolism of, in liver, 839
neonatal utilization of, 1025, 1026
stomach emptying and, 768
storage of, 850. *See also* Adipose tissue.
depleted in starvation, 852, 852*f*
insulin and, 943
as thermal insulation, 868
Fatty acids
absorption of, 797
bile salts and, 785
amino acid conversion to, 835
beta-oxidation of, 822, 822*f*, 839
chemical structures of, 819
cholecystokinin release and, 783
chylomicron release of, 819–820, 820*f*
as energy source, 822–825, 822*f*
in absence of carbohydrates, 823, 825
for cardiac muscle, 248

Fatty acids, as energy source (*Continued*)
cortisol and, 929
regulation of, 825–826
unavailability of carbohydrates and, 824
free. *See* Free fatty acids.
glucagon and, 948
glucose conversion to, 817
insulin and, 942
hepatic degradation of, 821–822
nonesterified, 820
placental diffusion of, 1007
in plasma
cortisol and, 929
forms of, 820
growth hormone and, 899, 900, 901
protein binding of, 312, 820, 821
transport of, 820–821, 822
synthesis of
from carbohydrate excess, 825
insulin and, 943
in liver, 824, 824*f*
three most common, 819
transport into mitochondria, 822
from triglyceride hydrolysis, 789, 792
triglyceride synthesis from, in intestinal epithelium, 797, 819
Fatty liver disease, nonalcoholic, 838
Fatty streaks, 827–828
Feces
bile in, 840
clay-colored, 842
composition of, 798
fat in, 802
formation of, 797–798
intestinal mucus and, 787
nitrogen in, 845
water loss in, 285, 286*t*
Feedback
enzyme regulation and, 37
genetic regulation and, 37
negative, 7–8, 8*f*, 9
delayed, 9
in hormone systems, 885
positive, 8–9, 8*f*
in hormone systems, 885
Feedback gain, 7–8
body temperature and, 874
Feed-forward control, 9
Feeding center, hypothalamic, 845
Female fertility, 1000–1002
Female hormones, 987–988. *See also* Ovarian cycle; Ovarian hormones.
plasma concentrations of, 988, 988*f*
Female sexual act, 1000
Female sexual organs, 987, 987*f*, 988*f*
in pregnancy, 1009–1010
Fenestrated capillaries, glomerular, 312
Fenn effect, 76
Ferritin, 418*f*, 419–420, 840
Fertility, female, 1000–1002
Fertilization, 977, 1003–1004, 1004*f*
cervical mucus and, 1002
female orgasm and, 1000
limitation to one sperm, 977
prostaglandins and, 976
time during cycle and, 1000–1001
Fetal cells, transplantation of, for Parkinson's disease, 693
Fetal zone, of adrenal cortex, 1008
Fetus. *See also* Embryo.
circulation in, 1022–1023, 1022*f*
growth of, 1019, 1019*f*
hemoglobin of, 1006
hormones of, uterine contraction and, 1012
nutrition of, 1005, 1005*f*. *See also* Placenta.
human chorionic somatomammotropin and, 1009

Fetus (*Continued*)
  organ system development, 1019–1020
  respiratory movements of, 1019–1020
  testosterone in, 980, 981, 981*f*, 984
FEV_1 (forced expiratory volume in 1 second), 517, 517*f*
Fever, 875–877, 875*f*
  brain lesions or surgery and, 876
  chills associated with, 876, 876*f*
  cortisol and, 930
  crisis of, 876, 876*f*
  heart rate and, 143
  hypothalamic set-point and, 875–876, 876*f*
  metabolic rate and, 864
  pyrogens and, 875–876
  in septic shock, 280
Fibrillar proteins, 11, 16–17
Fibrin, 453–454, 453*f*
  in platelet plug formation, 452, 452*f*
Fibrinogen, 453–454, 453*f*, 833
  in seminal vesicle fluid, 976
Fibrinolysin, in menstrual fluid, 996
Fibrin-stabilizing factor, 451, 454
Fibroblast growth factor, angiogenesis and, 198
Fibroblasts, ameboid movement by, 24
Fibromuscular hyperplasia, 403
Fick principle, 240–241, 240*f*
Fields of vision, 627, 627*f*
Fifth cranial nerve, reticular excitatory signals and, 711–712, 712*f*
Fight or flight reaction, 739
Filaments, of cytoskeleton, 16
Filariasis, lymphatic, 297
Filling pressure. *See* Mean circulatory filling pressure; Mean systemic filling pressure.
Filtration coefficient, capillary, 181, 185
  glomerular, 312, 314
  peritubular, 336
Filtration fraction, glomerular, 312, 315
  calculation of, 342
  reabsorption rate and, 336
Filtration pressure, mean, at pulmonary capillary, 482, 482*t*
Filtration pressure, net, 181, 184, 185–186
  abnormal, edema and, 185–186
First heart sound, 265–266, 267*f*
First-degree incomplete heart block, 144–145, 144*f*
Fitness, life-prolonging effect of, 1041. *See also* Exercise.
Fixation movements of eyes, 628–630, 629*f*, 678
Flagellum of sperm, 24, 975, 975*f*, 977
Flatus, 798, 804
Flavin adenine dinucleotide (FAD), 854
Flavin mononucleotide (FMN), 854
Flavoprotein, 814, 823
Flexor reflex, 661–663, 662*f*, 663*f*
Flocculonodular lobe, 678, 678*f*, 681, 682*f*
  equilibrium and, 686
  inputs to, 683, 683*f*
  lesions of, 689
  vestibular nuclei and, 682*f*, 683
Flowmeters, 160–161, 160*f*, 161*f*
  electromagnetic, for cardiac output measurement, 240, 240*f*
Fluid absorption into capillaries, 181, 186. *See also* Net reabsorption pressure.
Fluid balance
  of intake and output, 285–286, 286*t*
  in neonate, 1024
Fluid compartments, 286, 286*f*. *See also* Extracellular fluid; Intracellular fluid; Potential spaces.
  measurement of volumes in, 287–290, 289*f*, 289*t*

Fluid filtration across capillaries, 181–186, 181*f*. *See also* Net filtration pressure.
Fluid retention, renal, in cardiac failure, 256, 257, 262
  decompensated, 257–258, 263
  high-output, 264
  peripheral edema and, 260–261
Fluid therapy, calculations for, 292–294, 293*f*, 293*t*, 294*t*
Fluorine, 856–857
  dental caries and, 971
9α-Fluorocortisol, 922, 924*t*
Fluorosis, 857
Flush, febrile, 876, 876*f*
FMN (flavin mononucleotide), 854
Foam cells, 827–828, 828*f*
Focal epilepsy, 725, 726
Focal length, 597*f*, 598–599, 599*f*
Focal line, 598, 598*f*, 599*f*
Focal point, 597–598, 597*f*
Folds of Kerckring, 793, 793*f*
Folic acid, 854
  in fetus, 1020
  impaired absorption of, 802
  red blood cell production and, 417, 420, 854
Follicle(s)
  ovarian. *See* Ovarian follicle(s).
  thyroid, 907, 907*f*
    thyroglobulin storage in, 909
Follicle-stimulating hormone (FSH), 896, 896*t*
  in female, 987, 988–989, 988*f*
    follicular phase and, 989–990, 998
    luteal phase and, 991
    after menopause, 999
    in pregnancy, 1009
    preovulatory surge of, 988*f*, 997, 998
    regulation of cycle and, 996, 997–998, 997*f*
  in male, 983–984, 983*f*
    spermatogenesis and, 975, 983, 983*f*, 984
Follicular phase, 989–990, 989*f*, 990*f*, 998
Food(s)
  compositions of, 843, 844*t*
  energy available in, 809–810, 843–844, 844*t*
    regulation of intake and, 843, 845–849, 846*f*, 847*f*, 847*t*
  metabolic utilization of, 844–845
  thermogenic effect of, 864–865, 867
Food intake, regulation of, 843, 845–849
  factors affecting quantity, 848–849
  neural centers for, 845–848, 846*f*, 847*f*, 847*t*
Foot processes, of astrocytes, 743*f*, 744
Foramen ovale, 1022, 1022*f*, 1023
Forced expiratory vital capacity (FVC), 517, 517*f*
Forced expiratory volume in 1 second (FEV_1), 517, 517*f*
Foreign chemicals, renal excretion of, 303, 311–312, 330
Fornix, 714*f*, 718–719
Fourth (atrial) heart sound, 266, 267*f*
Fovea, 609, 610*f*, 616, 617, 617*f*, 619
  accommodation and, 631
  involuntary visual fixation and, 629, 629*f*
  visual cortex representation of, 624
Fractures
  in hypoparathyroidism, 968
  muscle spasm associated with, 664–665
  repair of, 960
  vertebral, acceleratory forces causing, 532–533
Frank-Starling mechanism, 110–111, 229
FRC. *See* Functional residual capacity (FRC).
Free energy, 809
Free fatty acids. *See also* Fatty acids.
  in adipose tissue, 825
  in blood, 820–821, 822
    during exercise, 825
    insulin and, 943–944, 944*f*

Free nerve endings, 560*f*, 571
  fiber types leading from, 572
  as pain receptors, 583
  spatial summation and, 564, 564*f*
  tickle and itch detection by, 572–573
  as warmth receptors, 592
Free radicals
  high alveolar P_{O_2} and, 536–537
  oxygen-derived, high alveolar P_{O_2} and, 536–537
Free-water clearance, 354
Frequency principle, 638
Frequency summation, of skeletal muscle contractions, 80, 80*f*
Frostbite, 877
Fructose, 790
  intestinal absorption of, 796
  in liver, 810, 810*f*
  in seminal vesicles, 976
FSH. *See* Follicle-stimulating hormone (FSH).
Functional residual capacity (FRC), 469, 469*f*
  in asthma, 520
  determination of, 470–471
  in neonate, 1024
Furosemide, 331, 331*f*, 397
Fusiform cells, of cerebral cortex, 697, 698*f*
FVC (forced expiratory vital capacity), 517, 517*f*

G
G cells, gastric acid secretion and, 779
G proteins
  calcium-sensing receptor coupled to, 965
  hormone receptors linked to, 887–888, 887*f*
    adenylyl cyclase-cAMP and, 889, 890, 890*f*
  inhibitory, 888
  in olfactory cilium, 649, 649*f*
  in postsynaptic neuron, 548–549, 549*f*
  stimulatory, 888
GABA (gamma-aminobutyric acid), 551
  in basal ganglia, 692–693, 692*f*
    Huntington's disease and, 692–693, 692*f*, 694
  of granular neurons, 697
  presynaptic inhibition and, 554
G-actin, 75
Gain, of control system, 7–8
  for body temperature, 874
Galactose, 790
  absorption of, 796
  in liver, 810, 810*f*
Gallbladder, 783–784, 784*f*, 785
  emptying of, 784*f*, 785
Galloping reflex, 664
Gallstones, 786, 786*f*
  blocking pancreatic duct, 801
  obstructive jaundice and, 841
Gamma globulins, 833, 840. *See also* Antibodies.
  in neonate, 1025
Gamma-aminobutyric acid. *See* GABA (gamma-aminobutyric acid).
Ganglia, autonomic. *See* Autonomic ganglia.
Ganglion cells, of retina, 610*f*, 617, 617*f*
  cortical input from, 625, 626
  excitation of, 617, 619–621, 620*f*
  number of, 619
  thalamic input from, 624
  three types of, 619
  visual pathway and, 617, 617*f*
Gap junctions, 546
  in cardiac muscle, 101–102, 117
  in gastrointestinal smooth muscle, 753
  in unitary smooth muscle, 91
Gas, gastrointestinal, 798, 804

Gas exchange. *See* Respiratory membrane; Ventilation-perfusion ratio.
Gas gangrene, hyperbaric oxygen therapy for, 540
Gases
  diffusion coefficients of, 487, 487*t*
  diffusion of
    physics of, 485–487, 486*f*
    through respiratory membrane, 485, 486, 487, 489–492, 492*f*
  solubility coefficients of, 485–486, 486*t*
  volume-pressure relationship, 535
Gastric. *See also* Stomach.
Gastric acid. *See* Hydrochloric acid, gastric.
Gastric atrophy, 800
Gastric banding surgery, 851
Gastric barrier, 778, 799–800
Gastric bypass surgery, 851
Gastric glands. *See* Oxyntic (gastric) glands.
Gastric inhibitory peptide (GIP), 758, 758*t*
  gastric secretion and, 780
  stomach emptying and, 768
Gastric phase
  of gastric secretion, 779, 780*f*
  of pancreatic secretion, 782
Gastric secretion, 777–780
  gastric glands and. *See* Oxyntic (gastric) glands.
  inhibition by intestinal factors, 780
  in interdigestive period, 780
  phases of, 779, 780*f*
  pyloric glands and, 777, 778, 779
  surface mucous cells and, 777, 779
Gastric ulcer, 800. *See also* Peptic ulcer.
Gastrin, 758, 758*t*
  gastric acid secretion and, 778, 779
  molecular structure of, 779, 780
  secretion of, 777, 778
    duodenal, 779
  small intestine peristalsis and, 769
  stomach emptying and, 767, 768
Gastrin cells, 779
Gastritis, 799–800
Gastrocolic reflex, 757, 771
Gastroenteric reflex, 769
Gastroesophageal sphincter, 765
Gastroileal reflex, 769–770
Gastrointestinal hormones, 757–759, 758*t*, 761
  glandular secretions and, 774
  insulin secretion and, 947
  small intestine peristalsis and, 769
  stomach emptying and, 768
Gastrointestinal motility
  autonomic influences on, 735
  of colon, 770–772, 770*f*, 771*f*. *See also* Defecation.
  enteric nervous system and. *See* Myenteric plexus.
  hormonal control of, 757–759, 758*t*
  movements in. *See* Mixing movements, gastrointestinal; Peristalsis; Propulsive movements.
  muscle properties and. *See* Gastrointestinal smooth muscle.
  parasympathetic tone and, 737
  reflexes affecting, 757
  sensory nerve fibers and, 757
  of small intestine, 768–770, 768*f*, 770*f*
  of stomach
    mixing function of, 765, 766
    peristalsis in, 766, 767
  swallowing and, 763–765, 764*f*
  thyroid hormones and, 913
Gastrointestinal obstruction, 804, 804*f*
  plasma loss in, 279

Gastrointestinal secretion(s), 773–788. *See also* Digestive enzymes.
  autonomic control of, 734*t*, 735, 773–774
  autonomic reflexes and, 738
  daily volume of, 775*t*
  esophageal, 776–777
  functions of, 773
  gastric, 777–780, 777*f*, 778*f*, 780*f*. *See also* Oxyntic (gastric) glands.
  glands providing
    complex, 773, 774*f*
    secretion mechanism of, 774–775
    stimulation of, 773–774
    types of, 773
    typical cell of, 774*f*
  of large intestine, 787
  of liver. *See* Bile.
  pancreatic. *See* Pancreatic secretions.
  pH of, 775*t*
  saliva as, 775–776. *See also* Salivary glands.
  of small intestine, 786–787, 786*f*
Gastrointestinal smooth muscle
  electrical activity of, 753–755, 754*f*
  sympathetic nervous system and, 757
  as syncytium, 753
  tonic contraction of, 755
  wall structure and, 753, 754*f*
Gastrointestinal tract. *See also* Enteric nervous system.
  anatomy of, 753, 754*f*
  autonomic control of, 755, 756–757
    glands and, 734*t*, 735, 738, 773–774
  autonomic reflexes affecting
    bowel activity and, 772
    glands and, 738
  blood flow in, 759–762
    arterial blood supply, 760–761, 760*f*
    during exercise or shock, 762
    gut activity and, 761
    through intestinal villi, 761–762, 761*f*
    nervous control of, 762
    splanchnic circulation and, 759–760, 760*f*
  functional aspects of, 753
  glands in. *See* Gastrointestinal secretion(s).
  homeostatic functions of, 5
  reflexes affecting, 757
  sensory nerve fibers from, 755, 756*f*, 757
  wall structure of, 753, 754*f*. *See also* Gastrointestinal smooth muscle.
Gated channels, 47, 48, 48*f*, 49*f*
G-CSF (granulocyte colony-stimulating factor), in inflammation, 430, 430*f*
GDP. *See* Guanosine diphosphate (GDP).
Gene(s), 27–29
  nuclear location of, 17
  schema of control by, 27, 27*f*
  silencing of, 33
Gene expression, 27
  cell differentiation and, 40
  regulation of, 35–36, 35*f*
    microRNA in, 32–33, 33*f*
Gene transcription. *See* Transcription.
Genetic code, 29, 29*f*
Geniculocalcarine tract, 623, 623*f*, 625
Germ cells, primordial, 973, 974*f*
Germinal epithelium, 987
GFR. *See* Glomerular filtration rate (GFR).
GH. *See* Growth hormone (GH; somatotropin).
Ghrelin, 846, 846*f*, 847*f*, 848
  growth hormone secretion and, 901
GHRH (growth hormone–releasing hormone), 898, 898*t*, 901–902
Giant pyramidal cells, 669–670
Gigantism, 903
Gigantocellular neurons, 713, 713*f*
GIP. *See* Gastric inhibitory peptide (GIP).
Gitelman's syndrome, 408

Glands. *See* Endocrine glands.
Glans penis, 978
Glaucoma, 607–608
Glial feet, 745. *See also* Foot processes.
Global aphasia, 703, 704
Globin, 840
Globulins, 833. *See also* Immunoglobulin(s).
Globus pallidus, 690, 690*f*, 691–692, 691*f*
  Huntington's disease and, 694
  lesions in, 691
  neurotransmitters in, 692–693, 692*f*
Glomerular capillaries, 304–306, 311, 311*f*, 312–314, 313*f*
  colloid osmotic pressure in, 314, 314*f*, 315, 315*f*, 316
  fenestrae of, 178, 312
  hydrostatic pressure in, 182, 312, 314, 314*f*, 315–316
  selective permeability of, 178, 179–180, 313–314, 313*f*, 313*t*
Glomerular filtrate, composition of, 312
Glomerular filtration, 310–314, 311*f*
  of representative substances, 323, 324*t*
Glomerular filtration rate (GFR)
  advantages of normal high level, 312
  aging and, 403, 403*f*
  autoregulation of, 319–321, 319*f*, 320*f*
  in cardiac failure, 260
  in chronic renal failure, 404–405, 405*f*, 405*t*
  determinants of, 312, 314–316, 314*f*, 315*f*, 316*f*, 316*t*
  estimation of
    with creatinine concentration, 341, 341*f*, 342*f*
    with inulin clearance, 340–341, 340*t*, 341*f*
  as fraction of plasma flow, 312
  physiologic control of, 317–319, 318*t*
  in pregnancy, 1011
Glomerulonephritis
  acute, 400
  autoimmune, 442
  chronic, 403
    hypertension in, 407
    nephrotic syndrome in, 404
  end-stage renal disease caused by, 402
Glomerulosclerosis, 403
Glomerulotubular balance, 319, 334–335
Glomerulus(i), in olfactory bulb, 649*f*, 651
Glomerulus(i), of kidney, 305–306
  age-related loss of, 403, 403*f*
Glomus cells, 509
Glossopharyngeal nerve
  carotid baroreceptors and, 205, 206*f*
  carotid bodies and, 508*f*, 509
  in circulatory control, 203
  swallowing and, 764*f*, 765
  taste signals and, 647, 648*f*
Glossopharyngeal neuralgia, 590
Glucagon, 947–949
  chemistry of, 947
  fat metabolism and, 948
  glucose metabolism and, 947–948
  for hypoglycemic shock, 954
  insulin and, 947, 949
  phosphorylase activation by, 812, 948
  regulation of secretion of, 948–949, 948*f*
  secretion of, by alpha cells, 939, 947
  small intestine motility and, 769
  somatostatin and, 949
Glucagon-like peptide, appetite and, 848
Glucocorticoids, 921, 928. *See also* Cortisol.
  deficiency of, 934, 935
  excess of, 935–936
  gluconeogenesis and, 817
  for immunosuppression, in transplantation, 449
  ketogenic effect of, 825

Glucocorticoids (*Continued*)
  nongenomic effects of, 931
  pregnancy and, 1009
  properties of, 922–923, 924*t*
  protein metabolism and, 835
  for shock, 281
  synthesis of, 922
Glucokinase, 811, 811*f*, 942, 945, 945*f*
Gluconeogenesis, 817
  from amino acids, 835
  blood glucose concentration and, 839
  cortisol and, 928
  glucagon and, 947, 948
  insulin and, 942, 944
  in kidneys, 304
  in neonate, 1025
Glucose
  absorption of, 796
  for athletes, 1035
  for brain cells, 749–750
  from carbohydrate digestion, 790, 790*f*
  central role of, in carbohydrate metabolism, 810, 810*f*
  in cerebrospinal fluid, 747
  circulatory shock and, 277, 281
  cortisol and utilization of, 928
  diffusion through capillary pores, 179, 180*t*
  energy production from, 812
    acetyl-CoA and, 812–813
    citric acid cycle and, 813–814, 813*f*
    efficiency of, 815
    glycolysis and, 812, 812*f*
    oxidative phosphorylation and, 814–815, 814*f*
    by pentose phosphate pathway, 816–817, 816*f*
    as preferred source, 825
    summary of, 815
  in extracellular fluid, normal range of, 7, 7*t*
  facilitated diffusion of, 50, 810–811
    insulin and, 811
    placental, 1007
    in renal reabsorption, 326, 326*f*
  fatty acids derived from, 817
  in fetal metabolism, 1007, 1020
  for gonads, 949
  insulin and, 941–943, 942*f*
  phosphorylation of, 811
  placental diffusion of, 1007
  plasma level of. *See* Blood glucose.
  renal reabsorption of, 311–312, 325–326, 326*f*
    transport maximum for, 326–327, 327*f*
  sodium co-transport of, 54–55, 55*f*, 325–326, 326*f*, 794–795, 795*f*, 796, 811
  solutions of, 294
    isotonic, 291–292
  storage of. *See* Glycogen.
  transport through cell membrane, 810–811. *See also* Facilitated diffusion; Sodium co-transport.
    insulin and, 811, 941–942, 942*f*, 943
  urinary, 950, 952
  vasodilation caused by lack of, 194
Glucose phosphatase, 810, 811
Glucose tolerance test, 952–953, 953*f*
Glucose transporters, 50, 325–326, 326*f*. *See also* Sodium co-transport.
  of pancreatic beta cells, 945, 945*f*
Glucose-dependent insulinotropic peptide, 758
  gastric secretion and, 780
  stomach emptying and, 768
Glucose-6-phosphate, 810, 811
  glycogen synthesis from, 811, 811*f*
Glucostatic theory of hunger and feeding, 849
Glucuronic acid, steroids conjugated to, 924

Glutamate
  at Aδ pain fiber endings, 585
  in basal ganglia, 692–693
  at C pain fiber endings, 586
  as central nervous system transmitter, 551
  cochlear hair cells and, 637
  of granular neurons, 697
  as photoreceptor transmitter, 617
  schizophrenia and, 727
  umami taste and, 646
Glutamic acid, 834
Glutamine
  as amino radical donor, 834
  ammonium ion produced from, 388–389, 389*f*
Gluten enteropathy, 801
Glycerol, 789, 819
  as energy source, 822
  glucose synthesis from, 817
  triglyceride hydrolysis and, 820
Glycerol esters, in plasma, 820
Glycerol-3-phosphate, 822
α-Glycerophosphate, 820, 824, 824*f*, 825
Glycine, as central nervous system transmitter, 551
Glycinuria, simple, 408
Glycocalyx, 14
  endothelial, clotting activation and, 456–457
Glycogen, 12, 14, 20, 811–812
  glucose storage as, 811, 817
    as anaerobic energy source, 860–861
    compared to fat storage, 824–825
    depleted in starvation, 852
    insulin and, 941, 942
    in muscle, 941
  in skeletal muscle, 78, 80–81, 811, 941
    during exercise, 1032, 1032*t*, 1035
    recovery of, 1034, 1035*f*
Glycogenesis, 811, 811*f*
Glycogen-lactic acid system, 1033–1034, 1033*f*, 1034*b*, 1036
Glycogenolysis, 811–812, 811*f*
  glucagon and, 947–948
Glycolipids, of cell membrane, 14
Glycolysis, 22, 812, 812*f*, 815
  anaerobic, 815–816, 860–861, 1033
  in cardiac muscle, 248
  feedback control of, 815
  glycerol used in, 822
  in shocked tissue, 278
  in skeletal muscle, 78, 79, 1033
    hypertrophy and, 81
Glycoproteins, of cell membrane, 14
Glycosuria, renal, 408–409
GM-CSF (granulocyte-monocyte colony-stimulating factor), in inflammation, 430, 430*f*
GMP (guanosine monophosphate). *See* Cyclic guanosine monophosphate (cGMP).
GnRH. *See* Gonadotropin-releasing hormone (GnRH).
Goblet cells, of gastrointestinal tract, 773
  in crypts of Lieberkühn, 786, 786*f*
Goiter
  antithyroid substances and, 915, 917
  endemic, 917
  hypothyroidism with, 917
  idiopathic nontoxic, 917
  toxic. *See* Hyperthyroidism.
Goitrogenic substances, 917
Goldblatt hypertension, 223–224, 223*f*, 403
Goldman equation, 58
Goldman-Hodgkin-Katz equation, 58
Golgi apparatus, 12*f*, 15, 15*f*, 16
  gastrointestinal secretions and, 774, 774*f*
  platelets and, 451, 454
  specific functions of, 20–21, 20*f*

Golgi tendon organs, 560*f*, 657, 661, 661*f*
  cerebellar input from, 661
  feedback to motor cortex, 672
  nerve fibers from, 564, 656*f*
Gonadotropes, 896, 896*t*
Gonadotropic hormones. *See also*
    Follicle-stimulating hormone (FSH);
    Luteinizing hormone (LH).
  female infertility and, 1001
  female sexual cycle and, 988–991, 990*f*
  life cycle variation in, 998*f*
  in male, 983–984, 983*f*
  pineal gland and, 986
Gonadotropin-releasing hormone (GnRH), 898, 898*t*
  in childhood, 999
  in female, 987, 988, 996–997, 997*f*
  in male, 983, 983*f*
    genetic deficiency of, 985, 985*f*
  puberty and, 984
Gradient-time transport, 327–328
Grand mal epilepsy, 725–726, 725*f*
Granular cells, of cerebral cortex, 697, 698*f*
Granular endoplasmic reticulum, 14, 15*f*, 20, 20*f*
Granule cell layer, of cerebellum, 684–685, 684*f*
Granule cells, in olfactory bulb, 650, 652
Granulocyte colony-stimulating factor (G-CSF), in inflammation, 430, 430*f*
Granulocyte-monocyte colony-stimulating factor (GM-CSF), in inflammation, 430, 430*f*
Granulocytes, 423, 423*t*, 424, 424*f*. *See also* Basophils; Eosinophils; Neutrophils.
  produced in inflammation, 429, 430, 430*f*
Granulosa cell tumor, 1000
Granulosa cells, 987, 989, 989*f*, 990. *See also* Corona radiata.
  of corpus luteum, 991
  estrogen synthesis in, 992, 993*f*
  inhibin secreted by, 991, 997
Graves disease, 916
Gravitational pressure
  arterial pressure and, 174
  reference level and, 174–175, 174*f*
  venous pressure and, 172–173, 173*f*, 174
Gravity. *See also* Vestibular apparatus.
  acceleratory forces and, 531–533, 531*f*, 532*f*
  brain stem nuclei and, 673–674
  weightlessness and, 533–534
Gray ramus(i), 729–730, 730*f*
Greater circulation, 157
Ground substance, 20
  of bone, 957, 958
Growth, thyroid hormones and, 912
Growth factors, 39
Growth hormone (GH; somatotropin), 895, 896*t*, 898–904
  abnormalities of secretion of, 902–904, 903*f*
  aging and, 901, 904
  carbohydrate utilization and, 899–900
  cartilage and bone growth and, 900
  cells secreting, 896, 896*t*, 897
  daily variations in secretion, 901, 901*f*
  diabetogenic effect of, 900
  fat utilization and, 899
  general growth-promoting effect of, 898–899, 899*f*
  in hypoglycemia, 901, 949
  insulin and, 900, 945, 945*f*, 947
  ketogenic effect of, 825
  metabolic effects of, 899
  metabolic rate and, 864
  plasma concentration of, 901
  protein deposition in tissues and, 899, 904
  protein synthesis and, 835, 899

Growth hormone (GH; somatotropin)
(*Continued*)
regulation of secretion of, 901–902, 901*t*, 902*f*
short duration of action, 901
somatomedins and, 900–901
spermatogenesis and, 975
therapy with
for dwarfism, 902–903
in older people, 904
Growth hormone–inhibitory hormone, 898, 898*t*, 901–902, 949
Growth hormone–releasing hormone (GHRH), 898, 898*t*, 901–902
Growth inducers, of hematopoietic stem cells, 415
GTP. *See* Guanosine triphosphate (GTP).
GTP-binding proteins. *See* G proteins.
Guanine, 27, 28, 28*f*, 30, 31*t*
Guanosine diphosphate (GDP), hormone receptors and, 887, 887*f*
Guanosine monophosphate (GMP). *See* Cyclic guanosine monophosphate (cGMP).
Guanosine triphosphate (GTP), 810, 859
hormone receptors and, 887, 887*f*
Guanylyl cyclase
penile erection and, 978–979
in smooth muscle, 97
Gynecomastia, tumor-induced, 985

H
H band, 72*f*
Habituation, 706, 707, 718
Hagfish, 213
Hair(s)
estrogens and, 994
olfactory, 649
testosterone and, 981
Hair cells
of cochlea, 634–635, 636–638, 636*f*, 637*f*
loudness and, 638
retrograde pathways to, 641–642
of vestibular apparatus, 675–676, 675*f*, 676*f*, 677, 677*f*
Hair end-organ, 560*f*, 572
adaptation of, 562, 562*f*
Haldane effect, 503–504, 504*f*
Hallucinations, hippocampal seizures with, 719
Hand skills, cortical control of, 669
Hashimoto disease, 917
Haustrations, 770
Haversian canal, 959–960, 960*f*
Hay fever, 443
HDLs. *See* High-density lipoproteins (HDLs).
Head orientation, maculae and, 674–676
Head rotation
cortical control of, 669
vestibular system and, 676, 677, 677*f*, 678
Headache, 590–592, 591*f*
Head-down position, for shock, 281
Hearing, 633–643
abnormalities of, 642, 642*f*
attenuation reflex in, 634
bone conduction and, 634, 642, 642*f*
central mechanisms in, 639–642, 639*f*, 640*f*
retrograde pathways in, 641–642
cochlea in, 634–639
functional anatomy and, 634–635, 634*f*, 635*f*
organ of Corti and, 634–635, 634*f*, 636–638, 636*f*, 637*f*, 641–642
ossicular system and, 633–634, 633*f*
traveling wave and, 635, 635*f*, 636*f*
direction of sound and, 641
frequency of sound and, 638–639, 638*f*
auditory cortex and, 640
auditory pathways and, 639–640
loudness and, 638–639, 638*f*

Hearing, loudness and (*Continued*)
attenuation reflex and, 634
auditory pathways and, 639
ossicular system in, 633–634, 633*f*
of sound patterns, 640–641
speech and, 703, 704–705, 704*f*
tympanic membrane in, 633–634, 633*f*
Heart. *See also* Cardiac *entries.*
athletic training and, 1038, 1038*f*, 1038*t*, 1039, 1039*f*, 1039*t*
autonomic regulation of, 110, 111, 111*f*, 119–120, 734*t*, 735
blood flow through, 101, 101*f*
as blood reservoir, 175
electrical currents in region of, 124, 124*f*
enlargement of. *See* Cardiac hypertrophy.
excitatory and conductive system of, 115–118, 116*f. See also* Bundle branches; Purkinje fibers.
cardiac cycle and, 104–105
control of, 118–120
muscle fibers of, 101
spread and timing of impulse, 118, 118*f*
velocity of conduction in, 103, 117
fetal, 1019
Frank-Starling mechanism and, 110–111, 229
lactic acid as energy for, 816
oxygen consumption by, 109
regulation of pumping by, 110–112, 231
rupture of, 251
structure of, 101*f*
work output of, 107–109, 108*f*, 109*f*, 110
during exercise, 1038, 1038*f*
Heart failure. *See* Cardiac failure.
Heart rate
arterial pressure regulation and, 205
atrial reflex control of, 208–209
body temperature and, 112, 143
duration of cardiac cycle and, 105
duration of contraction and, 104
from electrocardiogram, 123
exercise and, 244, 245
athletic training and, 1039, 1039*f*
hypothalamus and, 715
in hypovolemic shock, 274
irregular, 144, 144*f*
in atrial fibrillation, 152
parasympathetic regulation of, 201
right atrial wall stretch and, 110, 229–230
slow, 143–144, 143*f*
sympathetic stimulation of, 111, 120, 143
cardiac output and, 231
vasomotor center and, 203
thyroid hormones and, 913
vagal stimulation and, 111, 119–120
Heart sounds, 107, 265–268
auscultation of, 266, 266*f*
frequencies of, 265, 266*f*
normal, 265–266
with patent ductus arteriosus, 267*f*, 270
with valvular lesions, 267–268, 267*f*
Heart-lung machines, 271–272
Heat. *See also* Warmth receptors.
as metabolic end product, 862
metabolic rate measurement and, 862–863
from nonshivering thermogenesis, 865
Heat loss, 868–871
blood flow to skin and, 868, 868*f*
evaporative. *See* Evaporative heat loss; Sweating.
insulator system of body and, 868
mechanisms of, 868–870, 869*f*
panting in, 871
at very high air temperatures, 869
to water vs. air, 869, 876

Heat production. *See* Thermogenesis (heat production).
Heat-sensitive neurons, 871
Heatstroke, 876–877, 1040
Helicobacter pylori, 801
Helicotrema, 635, 635*f*
traveling wave toward, 635, 636
Helium, in deep diving, 539
Helium dilution method, 470–471
Helper T cells, 436, 437, 440–441, 441*f*
cyclosporine and, 449
Hematocrit, 165, 165*f*, 287
in blood volume calculation, 290
at high altitude, 529, 530
splenic reservoir of red cells and, 175
viscosity of blood and, 165, 165*f*
Hematopoietic stem cells, pluripotential, 414–415, 414*f*, 423–424
Heme, 840
Hemiballismus, 691
Hemoglobin. *See also* Oxygen-hemoglobin dissociation curve.
acid-base buffering by, 383, 413
combination with carbon monoxide, 501–502, 501*f*
combination with oxygen, 418, 498–499, 498*f*, 499*f*
degradation of, 419–420, 840
deoxygenated, in cyanosis, 521–522
fetal, 1006
oxygen transport by, vs. dissolved state, 498, 501
oxygen transport capacity of, 413
oxygen-buffering function of, 6, 499
high alveolar P_{O_2} and, 536, 537
quantity in red blood cells, 413
quantity in whole blood, 413
at high altitude, 529
red blood cells and, 413
structure of, 418, 418*f*
synthesis of, 417, 417*f*
Hemoglobin S, 420
Hemolysins, 446
Hemolysis, in transfusion reactions, 446
Hemolytic anemia, 420
Hemolytic jaundice, 841–842
Hemophilia, 458
Hemorrhage. *See also* Bleeding tendencies.
adjustment to
blood volume and, 373–374
delayed compliance in, 168
renin-angiotensin system in, 221, 221*f*
sympathetic control in, 168
vasopressin in, 199
venous constriction in, 175
anemia secondary to, 420
Hemorrhagic shock. *See* Hypovolemic shock.
Hemosiderin, 418*f*, 419
Hemostasis. *See also* Blood coagulation.
definition of, 451
events in, 451
clot dissolution or fibrosis, 453
clot formation, 452, 452*f*
platelet plug formation, 451–452
vascular constriction, 451
Henderson-Hasselbalch equation, 382
blood CO_2 measurement and, 515
Henry's law, 485–486
Heparin, 457
clinical use of, 459, 460
from mast cells and basophils, 431, 439, 457
Hepatic arterioles, 837
Hepatic artery, 837*f*, 838
Hepatic coma, 835
Hepatic vein, 837*f*, 838
elevated pressure in, 838
Hepatitis, jaundice in, 841

Hepatocyte growth factor, 838
Hepatocytes, bile secretion by, 783
Hereditary spherocytosis, 420
Hering-Breuer inflation reflex, 506
Hering's nerves
  baroreceptors and, 205–206, 206*f*
  chemoreceptors and, 208
Hermaphroditism, 1026
Herpes zoster, 590
Hexagonal reference system, 130
Hexokinase, 811
High altitude
  acclimatization to, 510
    alveolar Po$_2$ and, 527, 528–530
    work capacity and, 530, 530*t*
  acute hypoxia at, 528
  alveolar Pco$_2$ at, 527, 528*t*, 529
  alveolar Po$_2$ at, 499, 527, 528*t*
    acclimatization of natives, 529–530, 530*f*
    acclimatization over time, 528–529
    breathing pure oxygen, 528, 528*t*
  alveolar ventilation at, 510
  arterial oxygen saturation at, 527, 528*f*, 528*t*
  barometric pressures at, 527, 528*t*
  mountain sickness at
    acute, 530
    chronic, 530–531
  polycythemia at, 421
  red blood cell production at, 416
  tissue vascularity increase at, 197–198
  work capacity at, 530, 530*t*
High-density lipoproteins (HDLs), 821
  atherosclerosis and, 829
High-energy phosphate compounds. *See*
    Adenosine triphosphate (ATP);
    Phosphocreatine.
High-fat diet, adaptation to, 824
Hindbrain, motor control and, 694
Hippocampus, 714, 714*f*, 718–719
  learning and, 719
  memory storage and, 709, 719
  olfaction and, 651
  schizophrenia and, 727
Hirschsprung disease, 802
His bundle. *See* Atrioventricular (A-V) bundle.
Histamine
  anaphylaxis and, 443
  in asthma, 520
  bronchiolar constriction caused by, 473
  gastric acid secretion and, 778, 779, 801
  hay fever and, 443
  from mast cells and basophils, 431, 439
  shock induced by, 280
  urticaria and, 443
  as vasodilator, 199–200
Histiocytes, 426, 428
Histones, 36, 38, 40
Hives, 443
HLA (human leukocyte antigen
    complex), 449
HMG-CoA reductase, 827
  statins and, 829
Homeostasis, 4. *See also* Control systems
    of body.
  automaticity of body and, 9
  circulatory system and, 4–5, 4*f*
  nutrients and, 5
  in premature infant, 1027
  protection of body and, 6
  regulatory systems and, 5–6
  removal of metabolic products and, 5
  reproduction and, 6
Homonymous hemianopsia, 627
Horizontal cells, 609, 610*f*, 617, 617*f*
  function of, 618
  inhibitory, 620, 620*f*
  neurotransmitters released by, 617

Hormone response element, 888, 889*f*
  for cortisol, 931
  for thyroid hormones, 910, 911*f*, 913*f*
Hormone-gated receptors, of smooth
    muscle, 97
Hormones, 881–893. *See also* Endocrine glands.
  anatomical loci of sources of, 881, 882*f*
  chemical messenger systems and, 881
  clearance from blood, 886
  concentrations of, in blood, 884–885
    measurement of, 891–892, 892*f*
  general classes of, 881–884
  insulin secretion stimulated by, 947
  mechanisms of action, 886–891
    genetic machinery and, 888–889, 891
    intracellular signaling in, 887–889, 887*f*,
        888*f*, 889*f*
    receptors in, 886–889
    second messengers in, 888, 889–891,
        889*b*, 890*b*, 890*f*
  overview of, 883*t*
  regulatory functions of, 5–6
  secretion of, 884–885, 885*f*
    cyclical variations in, 885
    feedback control of, 885
  structures of, 881–884
  synthesis of, 881–884
  transport of, in blood, 885–886
Hormone-sensitive lipase, 820, 825
  insulin and, 943
Horner's syndrome, 632
Human chorionic gonadotropin
  for female infertility, 1001
  fetal testes and, 984, 1008
  in pregnancy, 1007–1008, 1007*f*
Human chorionic somatomammotropin,
    1009, 1014
Human chorionic thyrotropin, 1009
Human growth hormone, 902–903. *See also*
    Growth hormone (GH; somatotropin).
Human leukocyte antigen (HLA) complex, 449
Human placental lactogen, 1009
Humidification of air, 487, 487*t*
Humoral immunity, 433, 434, 435*f*,
    437–439, 437*f*. *See also* Antibodies;
    B lymphocytes.
Hunger, 845. *See also* Appetite.
  hypothalamus and, 716
Hunger contractions, 766
Hunger pangs, 766
Huntington's disease, 694
Hyaline membrane disease, 1022. *See also*
    Neonatal respiratory distress syndrome.
Hyaluronic acid, 20
  in proteoglycan filaments, 180
Hyaluronidase, in acrosome, 975, 977
Hydrocephalus, 748
Hydrochloric acid, gastric
  deficiency of, 778, 800
  emotional stimuli and, 780
  organisms destroyed by, 433
  pepsinogen secretion and, 778, 779
  peptic ulcer and, 800, 801
    treatment and, 801
  pH of, 380, 380*t*, 777
    pepsin activity and, 791
  protein digestion and, 791
  secretin release caused by, 782
  secretion of, 777–778, 777*f*, 778*f*
    stimulation of, 778, 779
Hydrocortisone. *See* Cortisol.
Hydrogen atoms
  from fatty acid oxidation, 823
  oxidation of, 814–815
  from pentose phosphate pathway,
    816–817, 816*f*
Hydrogen ATPase, 324–325, 387–388, 387*f*

Hydrogen bonding
  in DNA, 28, 29
  in DNA replication, 37
  in protein synthesis, 32
  in proteins, 831
  in transcription, 30
Hydrogen gas, in large intestine, 804
Hydrogen ions. *See also* Acid-base disorders;
    Acid-base regulation; pH.
  acids and, 379–380
  arterial blood, chemoreceptors and, 208
  arteriolar dilation or constriction and, 200
  cerebral blood flow and, 744
  concentration in body fluids, 380, 380*t*
    precise regulation of, 379
  in oxidative phosphorylation, 814–815, 814*f*
  primary active transport of, 54
  renal excretion of, with reduced GFR,
    404, 405*f*
  renal secretion of, 311–312, 326, 326*f*,
    332–333, 334
    aldosterone excess and, 926
    bicarbonate reabsorption and, 385,
        386–388, 386*f*, 387*f*, 390–391, 390*t*
    factors affecting, 390–391, 390*t*
  respiratory control by, 507, 507*f*, 508, 508*f*
    chemoreceptors and, 509
    high altitude and, 529
  sodium counter-transport of, 55, 55*f*,
    326, 326*f*
    intestinal, 794–795
  sour taste and, 645
  vasodilation associated with, 97
Hydrogen peroxide, oxidation by, 15–16
  high alveolar Po$_2$ and, 536–537
  of iodide, 908
  in leukocytes, 426
Hydrogen-potassium ATPase pump, 324–325
  gastric acid secretion and, 777–778, 778*f*
  potassium reabsorption and, 364.
Hydrolase enzymes, in lysosomes, 15, 19–20
Hydrolysis, 789
Hydronephrosis, 315
Hydrostatic pressure
  in capillaries. *See* Capillary pressure.
  in interstitium. *See* Interstitial fluid
      hydrostatic pressure.
  reabsorption in kidney and, 335–337, 335*f*,
      336*t*, 337*f*
  venous pressure and, 172–173
Hydroxyapatite
  of bone, 957, 958
  of teeth, 969, 970, 971
β-Hydroxybutyric acid, 823
  ketosis and, 823, 852
Hydroxyl ions, of neutrophils and
    macrophages, 426
Hydroxymethylglutaryl CoA (HMG-CoA)
    reductase, 827
  statins and, 829
17α-Hydroxyprogesterone, 992
Hyperalgesia, 583–584, 590
Hyperbaric oxygen therapy, 540
Hyperbarism, 535
Hyperbilirubinemia, physiologic, 1024, 1024*f*
Hypercalcemia, 367, 956. *See also* Calcium, in
    extracellular fluid and plasma.
  in hyperparathyroidism, 968
Hypercapnia, 522
  dyspnea secondary to, 522
Hyperchloremic metabolic acidosis, 395, 395*t*
Hypercholesterolemia, familial, 828–829
Hypereffective heart, 231, 231*f*
Hyperemia
  active, 194
  reactive, 194
Hyperglycemia, gigantism with, 903

Hyperinsulinemia, 951, 952
Hyperinsulinism, 953
Hyperkalemia, 361
    acidosis secondary to, 391
    aldosterone deficiency and, 926
    in mineralocorticoid deficiency, 924
Hyperlipidemia, coronary artery disease
        and, 829
Hypernatremia, 294, 295–296, 295t
Hyperopia, 602, 602f, 603, 603f
Hyperosmotic dehydration, 295, 295t
Hyperosmotic overhydration, 295t, 296
Hyperosmotic solution, 292
Hyperparathyroidism
    primary, 967–968
    secondary, 968
        in chronic renal failure, 407
Hyperpolarization
    of cardiac fibers, 66f, 67, 120
        atrioventricular nodal, 120
        sinus nodal, 116, 120
    of photoreceptor membrane, 612–613,
        617–618
    of postsynaptic membrane, 554
    of smooth muscle, 97
        gastrointestinal, 755
Hypersensitivity, 443–444
Hypertension
    acute neurogenic, 224–225
    in aldosteronism, primary, 219–220
    Alzheimer's disease and, 728
    in aortic coarctation, 224
    atherosclerosis and, 829
    cerebral blood flow and, 744–745, 745f
    chronic
        definition of, 218
        impaired renal fluid excretion and,
            218–220, 218f, 220f
        lethal effects of, 218
    coronary artery disease and, 829
    endothelial damage in, 196
    essential (primary), 225–226, 226f
        treatment of, 226
    genetic causes of, 225
    Goldblatt types of, 223–224, 223f
    kidney disease and, 406, 407
        dialysis and, 219
        as end-stage renal disease, 402
        as nephrosclerosis, 403
    left ventricular hypertrophy in, 135–136,
        135f, 137
    in preeclampsia, 224, 1011
    pregnancy-induced, 1009
    renal artery stenosis and, 223–224, 223f
    renal ischemia and, 224
    renin-angiotensin system and, 223–224,
        223f
    stroke secondary to, 745
    volume-loading, 218–219, 218f, 220f
        combined with vasoconstriction,
            224–225
Hyperthyroidism, 916, 916f
    cardiac output in, 233
    in neonate, 1026
Hypertonic solutions, 292, 292f
    fluid shifts and osmolarities caused
        by, 293, 293f
Hyperventilation, alkalosis secondary to, 392
Hypocalcemia, 367, 956, 956f. See also Calcium,
        in extracellular fluid and plasma.
    hyperparathyroidism secondary to, 968
Hypochlorhydria, 800
Hypochromic anemia, 419
    microcytic, 415f, 420
Hypoeffective heart, 231, 231f
Hypogastric plexus, 729, 730f
    bladder and, 308

Hypoglycemia
    cortisol secretion in, 949
    epinephrine and, 949
    growth hormone secretion in, 901, 949
Hypoglycemic shock, 943
Hypogonadism
    female, 999
    male, 985, 985f
Hypokalemia, 361
    aldosterone excess and, 925–926
    alkalosis secondary to, 391
Hyponatremia, 294–295, 295t, 296f
Hypo-osmotic dehydration, 294–295, 295t
Hypo-osmotic overhydration, 295, 295t
Hypo-osmotic solution, 292
Hypoparathyroidism, 967
Hypophosphatemia
    congenital, 969
    renal, 408
Hypotension, antidiuretic hormone and, 905
Hypothalamic inhibitory hormones,
        897–898, 898t
Hypothalamic releasing hormones,
        897–898, 898t
Hypothalamic-hypophysial portal vessels,
        897–898, 897f
Hypothalamus, 714, 714f, 715–718, 716f
    amygdala and, 719
    autonomic control by, 739, 739f
    behavioral functions of, 717
    blood-brain barrier and, 748–749
    hunger and satiety centers of, 845–846, 846f
        anorexia and, 852
        leptin and, 849
        neurons and neurotransmitters in,
            846–847, 847f, 847t, 849
        obesity and, 850–851
    lesions in, 717
    osmoreceptors in, 355, 356f, 905
    pain signals and, 587
    pineal gland and, 986
    pituitary and
        anterior, 716–717, 897–898, 897f, 898t,
            901–902
        posterior, 895, 897, 904, 904f, 905, 906
    reward and punishment functions of,
        717–718
    sleep and, 722
    temperature regulation and. See
        Temperature, body, hypothalamic
        regulation of.
    vasodilator system and, 204
    vasomotor center controlled by, 204
    vegetative and endocrine control functions
        of, 715–717
    visual fibers to, 623
Hypothermia, 877
    artificial, 877
    deep body temperature receptors
        and, 872
Hypothyroidism, 917–918, 918f
    cardiac output in, 234
    in fetal life, infancy, or childhood, 918
    menstrual irregularities in, 999
    in neonate, 1026
Hypotonia
    deep cerebellar nuclei and, 689
    motor cortex lesions with, 673
Hypotonic solutions, 292, 292f
    fluid shifts and osmolarities caused
        by, 293, 293f
Hypoventilation, hypoxia secondary to, 520
    hypercapnia and, 522
    oxygen therapy in, 521
Hypovolemic shock, 274–279
    arterial pressure and, 274–275, 274f
    bleeding volume and, 274–275, 274f

Hypovolemic shock (Continued)
    cardiac output and, 274–275, 274f
    in dehydration, 279
        fluid therapy for, 280
    gastrointestinal vasoconstriction in, 762
    irreversible, 278–279, 278f
    nonprogressive (compensated), 275–276
    in plasma loss, 279
    progressive, 275, 275f, 276–278, 276f
    in trauma, 279
    treatment of, 280–281
Hypoxia
    acute, at high altitude, 528
    anaerobic energy during, 860
    in anemia, 420–421, 521
    causes of, 520, 521
    dyspnea secondary to, 522
    effects on the body, 521
    erythropoietin secretion in, 304, 416
    in neonate, 1021
    neuronal depression in, 557
    polycythemia secondary to, 421

I
I bands, of skeletal muscle, 71, 72f
I cells, intestinal, 783
IDLs (intermediate-density lipoproteins), 821
Ig. See Immunoglobulin entries.
Iggo dome receptor, 572, 572f
IL. See Interleukin entries.
Ileocecal sphincter, 756, 769–770, 770f
Ileocecal valve
    feedback control of, 770
    function of, 769–770, 770f
    ileal peristalsis and, 769, 770f
Image formation. See also Visual image(s).
    by lenses, 599–600, 599f
    on retina, 601
Imipramine, 727
Immune system, homeostatic functions of, 6
Immunity. See Acquired (adaptive) immunity;
        Innate immunity.
Immunization, 433, 437, 442.
Immunoglobulin(s), 437–438, 437f. See also
        Antibodies.
Immunoglobulin E (IgE), 431, 438
    allergy and, 443–444
Immunoglobulin G (IgG), 438
Immunoglobulin M (IgM), 438
    transfusion reaction caused by, 446
Immunosuppression
    by cortisol, 930, 931
    for transplantation, 449–450
Impedance matching, by ossicular system,
        633–634
Impermeant solutes, 291, 292
Implantation, 1004, 1004f, 1005f
    endometrial nutrients and, 995, 1004, 1008
Inanition, 851
    hypothalamic feeding center and, 845
Incisura, in aortic pressure curve, 107,
        169f, 170f
    aortic regurgitation and, 169
Incomplete intraventricular block,
        145–146, 145f
Incontinence, overflow, 310
Incus, 633, 633f
Indicator-dilution method, 241, 241f, 287–290,
        289f, 289t
Indifferent electrode, 126
Infant. See also Child; Neonate.
    allergy in, 1026
    endocrine problems in, 1026
    premature, 1026–1027
        retrolental fibroplasia in, 197–198, 1027
Inferior colliculus, 639–640, 639f
Inferior olivary nuclei, 670, 683

Inferior olive
  basal ganglia and, 690*f*
  cerebellum and, 683, 684, 684*f*, 686, 687
Inferior salivatory nucleus, 648
Infertility
  female, 1001–1002
  male, 977, 978
Inflammation, 428
  atherosclerosis and, 828, 829
  chemotaxis of leukocytes in, 424*f*, 425
  complement system in, 439
  cortisol and, 930–931
    in allergic reactions, 931
  intracellular edema secondary to, 296
  macrophages and neutrophils in, 428–430,
    429*f*, 430*f*
  mast cells in, 431
  stages of, 930
  walling-off effect of, 428
Inflammatory cytokines, anorexia-cachexia
    and, 852
Infrared radiation, 868–869
Ingestion of food, 763
  mastication in, 763
  swallowing in, 763–765, 764*f*
Inhibin
  in female, 991, 997, 998
  in male, 984
Inhibition circuit, reciprocal, 566–567, 567*f*
Inhibitory neuronal circuits, 569
Inhibitory postsynaptic potential, 553*f*,
    554–555
  dendrites and, 556
  summation and, 555
Inhibitory presynaptic terminals, 547
Inhibitory receptors, 547, 549, 550
Inhibitory transmitter, 548
Inhibitory zone, 566
Injury potential. *See* Current of injury.
Innate immunity, 433. *See also* Complement
    system; Natural killer lymphocytes;
    Phagocytosis.
Inositol, in cephalin synthesis, 826
Inositol triphosphate (IP$_3$), 890
INR (international normalized ratio), 461
Insensible water loss, 285, 286*t*
  heat loss caused by, 869
Inspiratory capacity, 469, 469*f*
Inspiratory compliance curve, 467, 467*f*
Inspiratory reserve volume, 469, 469*f*
Insulin, 939–947
  appetite and, 846, 846*f*, 847*f*, 848
  blood cholesterol and, 827
  carbohydrate absence and, 825
  carbohydrate metabolism and, 941–943,
    942*f*, 947
  chemistry of, 940, 940*f*
  circulatory shock and, 277
  control of secretion of, 945–947, 946*f*
  cortisol and, 928
  energy abundance and, 939–940
  energy storage and, 849
  factors affecting secretion of, 946*t*
  fat storage and, 943
  fat synthesis and, 825
  fat utilization and, 943–944, 944*f*, 947
  glucagon and, 949
  glucose transport into cells and, 811, 941
  growth hormone and, 900, 945, 945*f*, 947
  mechanisms of secretion of, 945, 945*f*
  overtreatment with, brain metabolism
    and, 749–750
  plasma half-life of, 940
  plasma level of, 952
  potassium homeostasis and, 361
  protein storage and, 835, 945
  protein synthesis and, 835, 944

Insulin (*Continued*)
  receptor activation by, 940–941, 941*f*
  small intestine peristalsis and, 769
  somatostatin and, 949
  in switching between carbohydrates
    and lipids, 947
  synthesis of, 940, 940*f*
  treatment of diabetes with, 953
Insulin receptors, 940–941, 941*f*
Insulin resistance, 950, 951–952, 952*b*, 953
  growth hormone–induced, 900
Insulin shock, 953–954
Insulinase, 940
Insulin-like growth factor 1 (somatomedin C),
    900–901
Insulin-like growth factors (somatomedins),
    900–901
Insulinoma, 953
Insulin-receptor substrates, 940–941, 941*f*
Integral membrane proteins, 13*f*, 14
Integrins, on neutrophils, 428
Intelligence, 701
Intention tremor, 687–688, 689
Intercalated cells, renal, 332–333, 332*f*
  hydrogen ion secretion by, 54, 333,
    387–388, 387*f*
  potassium reabsorption by, 364
Intercalated disks, 101–102, 102*f*
  of Purkinje fibers, 117
Interleukin(s), 881
Interleukin-1 (IL-1)
  fever and, 875–876, 930
  in inflammation, 430, 430*f*
  in lymphocyte activation, 436, 441*f*
Interleukin-2 (IL-2), from helper T cells,
    440, 441
Interleukin-3 (IL-3), hematopoietic stem cells
    and, 415
Intermediate-density lipoproteins
    (IDLs), 821
Intermediolateral horn, 729, 730*f*
Internal capsule, of brain, 690, 690*f*
International normalized ratio (INR), 461
Interneurons, in motor control, spinal,
    655*f*, 656
Internodal pathways, cardiac, 115, 116*f*,
    117, 117*f*
Interphase, 37, 38
Interphase nucleus, 17, 17*f*
Interplexiform cells, 617
Interposed nucleus, 683, 684, 687
  lesions of, 689
Interstitial cells of Cajal, 754
Interstitial fluid, 180–181, 180*f*, 286, 286*f*, 287.
    See also Lymphatic system.
  carbon dioxide partial pressure (Pco_2) in,
    497–498, 498*f*
  composition of, 287, 288*t*
  fibrinogen leaking into, 453–454
  osmolarity of, 288*t*, 291
  oxygen partial pressure (Po_2) in,
    496–497, 496*f*
  pH of, 380, 380*t*
  plasma proteins in, 184, 185, 189
  protein concentration in, 185, 187, 189
  renal, physical forces and, 335–337, 335*f*,
    336*t*, 337*f*
  renal medullary, hyperosmotic, 347–349,
    349*f*, 350–352, 350*f*, 351*f*, 352*f*, 353
    impaired formation of, 354
  transport between plasma and, 4–5, 4*f*
  volume of, 189
    calculation of, 290
Interstitial fluid colloid osmotic pressure,
    181, 181*f*, 184, 184*t*, 185*t*
  in lungs, 481, 482*t*
  lymph flow and, 188, 189

Interstitial fluid hydrostatic pressure,
    181, 181*f*, 182–184, 184*t*, 185*t*
  lymph flow and, 187–188, 187*f*, 189
  negative, 182, 183–184, 189
    edema and, 298–299, 299*f*, 300
    in lungs, 481, 482, 482*t*
    in potential spaces, 300
Interstitial nephritis, 403
Interstitium, 180–181, 180*f*
  excess extracellular fluid in, 373, 373*f*
  free fluid in, 180*f*, 181, 183, 299
  ground substance in, 20
Intestinal obstruction, plasma loss in, 279.
    See also Gastrointestinal
    obstruction.
Intestinal phase
  of gastric secretion, 779, 780, 780*f*
  of pancreatic secretion, 782
Intestine. *See* Large intestine (colon);
    Small intestine.
Intra-abdominal pressure, venous pressure
    in legs and, 172
Intracellular edema, 296
Intracellular fluid, 3, 286, 286*f*
  buffers in
    phosphate as, 383
    proteins as, 383–384
  composition of, 45, 45*f*, 287, 288*f*, 288*t*
  extracellular fluid and, 3–4
    exchange between compartments, 290
    osmotic equilibrium of, 291–292, 292*f*
  of neuronal somal, 553
  osmolality of, 52
  osmolarity of, 288*t*, 291
    in abnormal states, 292–294, 293*f*,
      293*t*, 294*t*
  pH of, 380, 380*t*
  volume calculation of, 290
    in abnormal states, 292–294, 293*f*,
      293*t*, 294*t*
Intracranial pressure. *See* Cerebrospinal fluid
    pressure.
Intrafusal muscle fibers, 656, 656*f*, 657–658,
    657*f*, 659, 660
Intramural plexus. *See* Enteric nervous
    system.
Intraocular pressure, 607–608, 607*f*
Intrapleural pressure, cardiac output curve
    and, 234, 234*f*, 235, 235*f*
Intrapleural space, negative pressure
    in, 183
Intravenous solutions, nutritive, 294. *See also*
    Saline solutions.
Intraventricular block, partial, 145–146, 145*f*
Intrinsic factor, 417, 420, 800
  secretion of, 777, 778
Intrinsic pathway of coagulation,
    454–456, 456*f*
Inulin, water reabsorption and, 334
Inulin clearance, 340–341, 340*t*, 341*f*, 343
Inulin space, 289
Iodide
  antithyroid activity of, 915, 917
  dietary
    absorption of, 907
    deficiency of, 917, 918
    requirement for, 856, 907
  oxidation of, 908, 908*f*
  radioactive, for hyperthyroidism, 917
  in thyroid hormone synthesis, 908–909,
    908*f*, 909*f*, 914
Iodide trapping, 908, 914
  deficient mechanism of, 917
  high iodide concentration and, 915
  thiocyanate and, 915
Iodinase, 908–909
Iodine, 856. *See also* Iodide.

Ion channels, 14. *See also* Acetylcholine-gated ion channels; Calcium ion channels; Chloride ion channels; Potassium ion channels; Protein channels; Sodium ion channels; Voltage-gated channels.
  of adrenergic or cholinergic receptors, 732–733
  G-protein–activated
    hormones and, 887
    in postsynaptic membrane, 549, 549*f*
  of interstitial cells of Cajal, 754
  in postsynaptic membrane, 548, 550
    G-protein–activated, 549, 549*f*
    receptors linked to, 887
Ionizing radiation, cancer caused by, 41
Ionophore component, of postsynaptic receptor, 548
Ions, in cell, 11
IP$_3$ (inositol triphosphate), 890
Iris, innervation of, 631, 631*f*, 632
Iron, 418–419, 856
  absorption of, 419, 796
  atherosclerosis and, 829
  daily loss of, 419
  fetal accumulation of, 1020, 1020*f*
  functions of, 418
  from hemoglobin degradation, 840
  neonatal need for, 1025
  in pregnancy, 1010
  transport, storage and metabolism of, 418–419, 418*f*, 840
Iron lung, 522*f*, 523
Iron sulfide proteins, 814
Irritant receptors, in airways, 512
Ischemia. *See also* Cerebral ischemia; Myocardial ischemia; Renal ischemia.
  intracellular edema secondary to, 296
  as pain stimulus, 584
    visceral, 588
Ischemic heart disease, 246, 248–250. *See also* Myocardial ischemia.
Islets of Langerhans, 939, 939*f*
  adenoma of, 953
Isograft, 449
Isogravimetric method, for capillary pressure measurement, 182, 182*f*
Isohydric principle, 383–384
Isomaltase, 787
Isometric contraction
  of skeletal muscle, 79, 79*f*
  of ventricle, 106
Isometric relaxation, of ventricle, 106
Isopropyl norepinephrine, 733
Isosmotic solutions, 292
Isosthenuria, 405, 406*f*
Isotonic contraction, of skeletal muscle, 79, 79*f*
Isotonic solutions, 291–292, 292*f*
Isovolumic contraction, 105*f*, 106, 108, 108*f*, 109*f*
Isovolumic relaxation, 105*f*, 106, 108, 108*f*, 109*f*
Itch detection, 572–573
  anterolateral system and, 573
  scratch reflex and, 664

J

J point, 138–140, 139*f*
J receptors, in lung, 512
Jacksonian epilepsy, 726
Janus kinases (JAKs), leptin receptor and, 888, 888*f*
Jaundice, 841–842
  neonatal, 1024, 1024*f*
  in transfusion reactions, 448
Joint angulation, position receptors and, 580
Joint receptors
  adaptation of, 562, 562*f*
  of neck, 678
  predictive function of, 563
  Ruffini's endings as, 572

Joint spaces, effusion in, 300
Junctional potential, 96
Juxtaglomerular apparatus, 195, 320, 320*f*, 331
Juxtaglomerular cells, 220, 320, 320*f*
Juxtamedullary nephrons, 306, 307*f*
  countercurrent mechanism and, 306, 307*f*, 348

K

Kallidin, 199, 761
Kallikrein, 199
  in salivary glands, 776
Keratoconus, 604
Kernicterus, 448
Keto acids
  amino acid synthesis from, 834, 834*f*, 840
  conversion of amino acids to, 834, 835
  in diabetes mellitus, 953
  oxidation of, 835
Ketogenesis, 835
α-Ketoglutaric acid, 834
Ketone bodies, 823, 824
  insulin lack and, 944
  in starvation, 852
Ketosis, 823–824
  hormonally induced, 825
    by growth hormone, 899
  insulin lack and, 944
  in starvation, 852
Kidney(s). *See also* Renal *entries.*
  acid-base balance and. *See* Acid-base regulation, kidneys in.
  anatomy of, physiologic, 304–306, 305*f*, 306*f*, 307*f*
  arterioles of. *See* Afferent arteriole(s), renal; Efferent arteriole(s), renal.
  blood flow control in, 195
  blood pressure and. *See* Arterial blood pressure control, by renal–body fluid system; Renin-angiotensin system.
  blood supply of, 304–305, 305*f*
  drugs and, 330
  fetal, 1020
  functions of, 303–304
  gluconeogenesis in, 817
  homeostatic functions of, 5
  interstitial fluid pressure in, 183
  irritation of, intestinal activity and, 772
  in neonate, 1024
  oxygen consumption by, 316, 317*f*
  reabsorption by, 311*f*, 312, 323, 324*f*
    arterial pressure and, 337
    calculation from renal clearance, 340*t*, 342–343, 343*f*
    in different parts of nephron, 329–334
    glomerulotubular balance and, 334–335
    hormonal control of, 337–339, 338*f*, 338*t*, 339*f*
    hydrostatic and osmotic forces in, 335–337, 335*f*, 336*t*, 337*f*
    mechanisms of, 323–329
    regulation of, 334–339
    of representative substances, 323, 324*t*. *See also specific substances.*
    summary of, 334, 334*f*
    transport maximum for, 326–327, 327*f*, 327*t*
  secretion by, 311*f*, 312, 323, 334
    calculation from renal clearance, 340*t*, 342–343
    counter-transport in, 326, 326*f*
    of hydrogen ions, 311–312, 326, 326*f*, 332–333, 334
    of organic acids and bases, 329*f*, 330
    of potassium, 311–312, 332, 333, 333*f*, 337–338
    transport maximum for, 326, 327, 327*t*
  shock-related lesions in, 277–278

Kidney disease, 399. *See also* Renal failure.
  anemia in, 304
  edema in, 298
  hypertension and, 406, 407
    in end-stage renal disease, 402
    in nephrosclerosis, 403
    nephrotic syndrome in, 404
    osteomalacia and rickets in, 969
    tubular disorders, 408–409
Kidney function testing, clearance methods for, 341*f*, 342*f*
Kidney stones, in hypoparathyroidism, 968
Kidney transplantation, 409
Kilocalorie, 862
Kinesiology, 81
Kinesthesia, 580
Kinetic energy, of blood flow, cardiac work and, 108
Kininogen, high-molecular-weight, 455
Kinins, 199
Kinocilium, 675–676, 675*f*
Klüver-Bucy syndrome, 720
Knee jerk, 660, 660*f*
Korotkoff sounds, 170–171
Krause's corpuscle, 560*f*
Krebs cycle. *See* Citric acid cycle.
Kupffer cells, 427, 427*f*, 837, 839
Kwashiorkor, 843, 854
  growth hormone in, 901, 902*f*
Kyphosis, in acromegaly, 903–904

L

Labeled line principle, 559
Labor, 1012–1013, 1012*f*
Labor pains, 1013
Lacrimal glands, autonomic control of, 734*t*, 735
Lactase, 787, 790
Lactation, 1014–1016
  metabolic drain on mother from, 1016
  oxytocin and, 716, 905–906
  parathyroid enlargement in, 965
Lactic acid
  from anaerobic glycolysis, 816, 860–861
  as energy source for heart, 816
  ischemic pain and, 584
  from muscle glycogen, 1033–1034, 1033*f*
  reconversion to pyruvic acid, 816
  removal of, 1033–1034
  shock and, 278
  in skeletal muscle, 78
    as vasodilator, 243–244
  in sweat, 870
Lactic acid oxygen debt, 1034, 1034*f*
Lactic dehydrogenase, zinc in, 856
Lactose, 789–790
Lactotropes, 896, 896*t*
Laminar flow, of blood, 161, 161*f*, 162
Language, 699–700, 699*f*, 702, 703–705, 704*f*. *See also* Speech.
Large intestine (colon)
  absorption in, 797–798
    active transport in, 55–56, 55*f*
    of chloride, 795, 797, 926
    of sodium, 795, 797, 926
  bacterial action in, 798, 804
  disorders of, 802–803. *See also* Diarrhea.
  functions of, 770
  gas in, 798, 804
  movements of, 770–772, 770*f*, 771*f*. *See also* Defecation.
  obstruction of, 804, 804*f*
  secretions of, 787
    bicarbonate in, 795
  storage function of, 797
Larynx, 474–475, 474*f*
Lateral geniculate body, 623–624, 623*f*

Lateral inhibition, 578–579, 578f
  in auditory system, 640
  in cerebellum, 685
  in motor system, 656
  in retina, 618, 618f, 620, 620f
Lateral lemniscus, 639, 639f
Lateral motor system of the cord, 671
Law of the gut, 759
LDLs. *See* Low-density lipoproteins (LDLs).
Learned patterns of movement, 690, 695
Learning
  hippocampus in, 719
  neuronal connectivity and, 708
  reflexive, 709
  reward or punishment and, 718
Lecithin
  in bile, 784, 784t, 786, 792
  chemical structure of, 826, 826f
Left atrial pressure, 478, 478f
  in left-sided heart failure, 481
  pulmonary edema and, 482–483, 482f
Left bundle branch block
  left axis deviation in, 136, 136f
  T wave and, 142
Left ventricle
  volume-pressure curves of, 108–109,
    108f, 109f
  work done by, 107–109, 108f, 109f
Left ventricular dilatation, QRS prolongation
  in, 137–138
Left ventricular hypertrophy. *See also* Cardiac
  hypertrophy; Ventricular hypertrophy.
  aortic valve lesions and, 268
  electrocardiogram with, 135–136, 135f, 137
    QRS prolongation in, 137–138
Left-to-right shunt, 269. *See also* Patent ductus
  arteriosus.
Lengthening reaction, 661
Lens, of eye
  accommodation of, 601, 601f
    autonomic control of, 631–632, 735
    pupillary reaction to, 632
  in analogy to camera, 600, 600f
  cataracts in, 604
Lenses, physical principles of
  concave, 598, 598f
  convex, 597–598, 597f
  cylindrical, 598, 598f, 599f
  focal length of, 597f, 598–599, 599f
  focal point of, 597–598, 597f
  image formation by, 599–600, 599f
  refractive power of, 599f, 600, 600f
Leptin, 846, 846f, 847f
  as cytokine hormone, 881
  fat storage and, 849
  obesity and, 851, 865
Leptin receptor, 888, 888f
Leukemias, 431–432
Leukocyte pyrogen, 875–876
Leukocytes (white blood cells), 423–425.
    See also specific cell types.
  ameboid movement by, 24
  concentration of, in blood, 423
  genesis of, 423–424, 424f
  life span of, 424–425
  types of, 423
    as percentages, 423, 423t
Leukopenia, 431
Leukorrhea, during menstruation, 996
Leukotrienes, bronchoconstriction caused
  by, 443
Lever systems, in skeletal muscle function,
  81, 81f
Leydig cell tumors, 985
Leydig cells, 974f, 975, 979–980, 980f
LH. *See* Luteinizing hormone (LH).
Licorice, 924–925

Liddle's syndrome, 408–409
Lidocaine, for paroxysmal tachycardia, 148
Ligand-gated channels, 47, 48
Ligands, 14, 19
Light and dark adaptation, 614–615, 614f
Limb leads. *See* Bipolar limb leads.
Limbic association area, 699f, 700
Limbic cortex, 714–715, 714f, 720
Limbic system, 714–715, 714f. *See also*
    Amygdala; Hippocampus;
    Hypothalamus.
  Alzheimer's disease and, 727
  gonadotropin-releasing hormone and, 997
  manic-depressive illness and, 727
  motivation and, 695
  olfaction and, 651
  Parkinson's disease and, 693
  psychomotor seizure and, 726
  reward and punishment functions
    of, 717–718
  schizophrenia and, 727
Liminal zone, 565–566, 565f
Linear acceleration, of head, 676–677
Linear acceleratory forces, 532–533, 532f
Lingual glands, 792
Lingual lipase, 792
Lipase(s)
  in adipose tissue, 821, 826, 943
    glucagon and, 948
  enteric, 792
  hormone-sensitive, 820, 821, 825
    insulin and, 943
  intestinal, 787
  lingual, 792
  in macrophages, 426
  pancreatic, 781, 792–793, 792f
Lipase inhibitor, for weight loss, 851
Lipid bilayer, 13–14, 13f, 45, 46, 46f. *See also*
    Cell membrane.
Lipids. *See also* Cholesterol; Fats; Phospholipids.
  absorption of, bile salts and, 785
  of cell membranes, 12, 13
    glycolipids, 14
  in cells, 12
  classification of, 819
  synthesis of, in endoplasmic reticulum,
    20, 20f
  transport of, in body fluids, 819–821
Lipodystrophy, 822
Lipopolysaccharide. *See* Endotoxin.
Lipoprotein(a), 829
Lipoprotein lipase, 819–820, 820f
  insulin and, 943
Lipoproteins, 821. *See also* High-density
    lipoproteins (HDLs); Low-density
    lipoproteins (LDLs).
  insulin and, 944
  phospholipids in, 826
Lipostatic theory of hunger and feeding, 849
β-Lipotropin, 933–934, 933f
Lissauer, tract of
  pain signals in, 585f
  thermal signals in, 593
Liver, 837–842. *See also* Hepatic *entries.*
  acetoacetic acid formed in, 823–824
  adrenocortical hormones metabolized
    in, 924
  amino acid storage by, 833
  anatomic organization of, 837, 837f
  B lymphocyte processing in, 435
  bile salt synthesis by, 785
  bile secretion by, 783–784, 784f, 785
  as blood reservoir, 175, 838
  capillaries of, permeability of, 178,
    179–180
  coagulation factors formed in, 840
  detoxifying function of, 840

Liver (*Continued*)
  excretory functions of, 840
  fatty acid degradation in, 823
  glucose buffer function of, 839, 949
  glycogen in, 811, 811f
  homeostatic functions of, 5
  insulin action on, 942
  iron storage in, 840
  lipids in, 821–822
  lymphatic system in, 837, 837f, 838
  macrophages in, 427
  metabolic functions of, 839–840
  monosaccharides in, 810, 810f
  neonatal function of, 1025
  protein synthesis in
    cortisol and, 929
    of plasma proteins, 833
  regeneration of, 838
  shock-related injury to, 277, 278f
  sinusoids of, 837, 837f
    blood flow in, 838
    phagocytosis of bacteria in, 839
    reticuloendothelial cells of, 759–760, 837
  vascular system of, 837f, 838
  vitamin storage in, 840
Liver disease, 838. *See also* Cirrhosis.
  bilirubin and, 840, 841–842
  clotting factor deficiencies in, 457–458
Local sign principle, 662–663
Lochia, 1013–1014
Locomotive reflexes, 663–664
Locus ceruleus, and norepinephrine system,
  551, 712–713, 713f
Long QT syndromes, 147, 148f
Loop diuretics, 331, 331f, 397–398, 398t
Loop of Henle, 306, 306f
  calcium reabsorption in, 368–369
  glomerulotubular balance of, 335
  magnesium reabsorption in, 370
  transport properties of, 330–331, 330f, 331f
  urine concentration and, 346, 346f,
    352–353, 352f
    hyperosmotic medulla and, 348–349,
      348t, 349f
Loudness, 638–639, 638f
  attenuation reflex and, 634
  auditory pathways and, 639
Low-density lipoproteins (LDLs), 821
  adrenocortical hormone synthesis and, 922
  atherosclerosis and, 828–829
  receptors for
    mutations affecting, 827, 828–829
    statins and, 829
Low-pressure receptors, 208
Lumirhodopsin, 611–612, 611f
Lung(s). *See also* Pulmonary *entries.*
  as blood reservoir, 175, 478
  blood volume in, 157, 478–479
  circulation of. *See* Pulmonary circulation.
  compliance of, 467, 467f
    hypoxia and, 520
    thoracic cage and, 468
  consolidation of, 518
  elastic forces of, 465, 467
    surface tension and, 467–468
    work and, 468
  macrophages in, 427
  massive collapse of, 519, 519f
  neonatal expansion of, 1021, 1021f
  recoil pressure of, 467
  shock-related injury to, 277–278
Lupus erythematosus, 442
  chronic glomerulonephritis in, 403
Luteal phase, 989f, 990–991
Lutein cells, 990–991
Luteinization, 990–991
Luteinization-inhibiting factor, 991

Luteinizing hormone (LH), 896, 896*t*
 in female, 987, 988–989, 988*f*
  follicular phase and, 989–990
  luteal phase and, 991
  after menopause, 999
  ovulation and, 990, 990*f*
  in pregnancy, 1009
  preovulatory surge of, 885, 988*f*,
   997–998, 1001
  regulation of cycle and, 996, 996*f*,
   997–998, 997*f*
 in male, 983–984, 983*f*
  spermatogenesis and, 975
Lymph
 formation of, 187
  in liver, 838
 intestinal absorption into, 187
 rate of flow, 187–189, 187*f*
Lymph nodes
 macrophages in, 426–427
 structure of, 426–427, 427*f*
Lymphatic capillaries, 186*f*, 187, 187*f*,
  188, 188*f*
 pumping by, 188–189
Lymphatic pump, 188, 189
Lymphatic system, 181, 186–189, 186*f*
 cerebral substitute for, 747
 chylomicrons in, 797, 819
 edema and, 297, 300
 interstitial fluid pressure and, 183–184, 189
 interstitial fluid protein concentration
  and, 187, 189
 interstitial fluid volume and, 189
 intestinal villi and, 769, 793*f*, 794
 in liver, 837, 837*f*, 838
 net filtration and, 185
 potential spaces drained by, 300
 pulmonary, 477, 481, 482, 482*f*
 valves in, 187, 187*f*, 188, 188*f*
Lymphedema, 297
Lymphoblast, 423–424, 424*f*
Lymphocytes, 423, 423*t*, 424, 434, 435*f*.
   See also B lymphocytes;
   T lymphocytes.
 activation of clones of, 436
 life span of, 425
 preprocessing of, 434–435
  tolerance and, 442
 specificity of, 435–436, 436*f*
Lymphocytic leukemias, 431
Lymphocytic lineage, 423–424, 424*f*
Lymphocytopenia, cortisol-induced, 931
Lymphoid tissues, 434
 cortisol-induced atrophy of, 931
Lymphokines, 436, 440–441, 441*f*, 881
Lysine monohydrochloride, for alkalosis, 393
Lysis
 by antibodies, 438
 by complement system, 439, 439*f*
  in transfusion reaction, 446
Lysoferrin, 20
Lysosomes, 12*f*, 15, 19–20, 19*f*
 amino acids released by, 833
 circulatory shock and, 277
  glucocorticoids and, 281
 inflammation and, 930
 of leukocytes, 426
 in thyroid hormone release, 909
Lysozyme, 20, 433
 in saliva, 776
Lytic complex, 439, 446

M
M line, 73*f*
Machinery murmur, 270
Macrocytes, 417
Macromotor units, 82

Macrophages, 425–426
 alveolar, 427, 428, 474
 ameboid movement by, 24, 425
 as antigen-presenting cells, 440
 atherosclerosis and, 827–828, 828*f*
 chemotaxis by, 439
 helper T cells and, 441
 hemoglobin uptake by, 419–420
 hepatic (Kupffer cells), 427, 427*f*, 837, 839
 in inflammation, 428–430, 430*f*
 in lymphocyte activation, 436, 437
 in milk, 1016
 in monocyte-macrophage system, 426–428,
  427*f*
 opsonization and, 439
 pinocytosis in, 18
 pyrogens released by, 875–876
 tissue, 426–428
  development from monocytes, 429
  hemoglobin incorporated by, 840
  platelet removal by, 451–452
  response to infection, 428
Macula densa, 195, 306, 306*f*, 320, 320*f*, 331
 glomerular filtration rate and, 319–320,
  320*f*
Maculae, 674–675, 675*f*, 676–677
 hair cells of, 675–676, 675*f*
 linear acceleration and, 676–677
Magnesium, 856
 in bone, 957–958
 extracellular fluid concentration of, 369,
  370, 856
 intestinal absorption of, 796
 renal excretion of, 369–370
Magnet reaction, 663
Magnocellular neurons, 356, 897
Major basic protein, 430
Major histocompatibility complex (MHC)
  proteins, 440, 440*f*, 441*f*
Malabsorption, 801–802
Male climacteric, 984
Male hormones
 androgenic. *See* Androgens; Testosterone.
 hypothalamic-pituitary axis and,
  983–984, 983*f*
Male hypogonadism, 985, 985*f*
Male sexual act, 978–979
Male sexual organs, 973, 973*f*
Malleus, 633, 633*f*
Malnutrition, and metabolic rate, 864. *See also*
  Starvation.
Malocclusion, 971–972
Malonyl-CoA, 824, 824*f*, 825
Maltase, 787, 790
Maltose, 790
Manic-depressive psychosis, 727
Mannitol, for brain edema, 749
Marginal ulcer, 800
Margination, 424*f*, 428, 429*f*
Mark time reflex, 664
Mass discharge, 738
Mass movements, in colon, 770–771
Mass reflex, 665
Mast cells, 431
 allergies and, 443
 asthma and, 520
 complement fragments and, 439, 439*f*
 eosinophil chemotactic factor of, 430
 heparin produced by, 431, 439, 457
Mastication, 763
Maximum expiratory flow, 516–517, 516*f*
Mayer waves, 210–211
M-CSF (monocyte colony-stimulating factor),
  in inflammation, 430, 430*f*
Mean circulatory filling pressure, 236, 236*f*
Mean electrical axis of ventricles, 134–137, 135*f*
 conditions causing deviation of, 135–137

Mean filtration pressure, at pulmonary
  capillary, 482, 482*t*
Mean pulmonary filling pressure, in left-sided
  heart failure, 259
Mean QRS vector, 129, 135, 135*f*
Mean systemic filling pressure, 235, 235*f*,
  236–237, 236*f*, 238–239, 238*f*
 in decompensated cardiac failure, 262–263
 exercise and, 244–245
 after myocardial infarction, 255–256
  fluid retention and, 256, 258
 in neurogenic shock, 279
Meat, digestion of
 collagen in, 791
 elastin in, 791
Mechanical pain stimuli, 583
Mechanical ventilation, 522–523, 522*f*
Mechanical work, energy of ATP for, 22, 23
Mechanoreceptive senses, 571
Mechanoreceptors, 559, 560*b*. *See also specific*
  receptor types.
 adaptation of, 562–563, 562*f*
 of skin and deep tissues, 559, 560*b*, 560*f*
Meconium, 1020
Medial forebrain bundle, 715, 717
Medial geniculate nucleus, 639, 639*f*, 640
Medial lemniscus(i), 573, 574, 574*f*, 575*f*
Medial longitudinal fasciculus, 628, 628*f*, 630
 vestibular signals in, 678
Medial motor system of the cord, 671
Median eminence, 897, 897*f*, 898
Medulla. *See also* Brain stem.
 chemoreceptor trigger zone in, 804
 circulatory control by, 202, 202*f*, 203, 204*f*
  baroreceptor signals and, 206
 pyramids of, 669, 670*f*
 respiratory control by, 505–508, 506*f*, 507*f*,
  508*f*, 509. *See also* Respiratory center.
 reticular inhibitory area in, 712, 712*f*
 swallowing and, 764, 765
Medullary collecting duct, 333–334, 333*f*
Medullary reticular nuclei, 673, 673*f*, 674
 decerebrate rigidity and, 674
Medullary reticulospinal tract, 674, 674*f*
Megacolon, 802
Megaesophagus, 799
Megakaryocytes, 423, 424, 451
Megaloblastic anemia, 415*f*, 420
Meiosis
 in ovary, 1003
 in testis, 974, 974*f*
Meissner's corpuscles, 560*f*, 571, 572
 vibrations detected by, 572, 579
Meissner's plexus. *See* Submucosal plexus.
Melanin
 Addison disease and, 934
 of retina, 609–611
 of skin, 934
Melanocortin receptors, 846–847, 847*f*,
  849, 851
 anorexia and, 852
Melanocyte-stimulating hormone, 933–934,
  933*f*
 α form of, 846, 847, 847*f*, 849, 933–934, 933*f*
  obesity and, 851
 β form of, 933–934, 933*f*
 γ form of, 933–934, 933*f*
Melatonin, pineal gland secretion of, 986
Membrane. *See* Cell membrane.
Membrane potential(s). *See also* Action
  potential(s); Receptor potentials;
  Resting membrane potential.
 diffusion potential, 57–58, 57*f*
  resting membrane potential and, 60, 60*f*
 measurement of, 58–59, 58*f*, 59*f*
  oscilloscope in, 69, 69*f*
 of olfactory cells, 650

Membrane transport, 45–56. *See also* Active transport; Diffusion.
  basic mechanisms of, 45–46, 46f
  energy of ATP for, 22–23, 22f
Membranous labyrinth, 674, 675f
Memory, 545, 706–707
  Alzheimer's disease and, 727–728
  classification of, 706–707
  hippocampus and, 709, 719
  intermediate long-term, 706, 707–708
  long-term, 706, 708
    thalamus and, 712
  reward or punishment and, 718
  short-term, 706, 707
    consolidation of, 708–709
  Wernicke area and, 701
  working, 703, 706
Memory B cells, 437
Memory T cells, 440
Memory traces, 706
Menarche, 988, 998–999
Meningitis, headache of, 591
Menopause, 987, 998f, 999, 999f
  osteoporosis secondary to, 969, 994
Menstrual cycle, 988, 995–996, 995f. *See also* Ovarian cycle.
  absent, 999
  anovulatory, 998, 1001
  irregular, 999
  thyroid hormones and, 914, 999
Menstruation, 995–996
  leukorrhea during, 996
  prevented by human chorionic gonadotropin, 1007, 1008
Merkel's discs, 572, 572f
Meromyosin, 72f
Mesencephalon
  motor function and, 670f, 673
  reticular substance of, 711
Mesenteric ganglia, 757
Mesolimbic dopaminergic system, 727
Messenger RNA (mRNA), 29f, 31–32, 32f. *See also* Transcription; Translation.
  microRNA and, 32–33, 33f
Metabolic clearance rate, of hormone, 886
Metabolic end products, removal of, 5
Metabolic rate, 862–863. *See also* Energy expenditure.
  ADP in control of, 862
  basal. *See* Basal metabolic rate (BMR).
  blood flow to tissue and, 192, 192f
    cardiac output and, 234
  epinephrine and, 736
  estrogens and, 994
  factors determining, 867
  interstitial fluid P_{CO_2} and, 498, 498f
  after a meal, 864–865
  measurement of, 862–863
  in neonate, 1025
  thermogenesis and, 873
Metabolic syndrome, 951
Metabolism
  blood flow and, cerebral, 743
  of cardiac muscle, 248
  definition of, 862
Metaphase, 38f, 39
Metarhodopsin, 611–612, 611f, 613, 614
Metarterioles, 177, 178f
  in local blood flow control, 193, 193f
  sympathetic innervation of, 201
  vasomotion of, 178–179, 193
Metastatic calcification, in hyperparathyroidism, 968
Methacholine, 86
Methane, in large intestine, 804
Methoxamine, as sympathomimetic drug, 739
Methyl alcohol, acidosis caused by, 393

Methylmercaptan, 650
Methylprednisone, 922, 924t
MHC (major histocompatibility complex) proteins, 440, 440f, 441f
Micelles, 785, 786, 792, 793, 797
Michaelis-Menten equation, 861
Microcirculation, 177–178, 178f. *See also* Capillaries.
Microcytic, hypochromic anemia, 415f, 420
Microglia, 428
Microgravity, 533–534
Microprocessor complex, 32–33
MicroRNA (miRNA), 31, 32–33, 33f
Microtubules, 11, 16, 17, 17f
  of cilia, 24, 25
  of flagellum, 975, 975f
  of mitotic apparatus, 17, 38–39
Microvilli
  of intestinal epithelium, 790, 791, 794, 794f
    gluten and, 801
  of taste bud, 646, 647f
Micturition, 306
  abnormalities of, 310
Micturition reflex, 306, 309–310, 738
  neurologic injury and, 310
Micturition waves, 309, 309f
Middle cerebral artery, blockage of, 745
Migraine headache, 591
Milk
  composition of, 1016, 1016t
  ejection of, 906, 1015–1016
Mineral(s), 855–857. *See also specific minerals.*
  body content of, 856t
  daily requirements of, 856t
Mineralocorticoid receptor, 891, 926, 926f
Mineralocorticoid receptor antagonists, 399
Mineralocorticoids, 921. *See also* Aldosterone.
  deficiency of, 924, 934
  properties of, 922–923, 924t
  synthesis of, 921–922
Minimal change nephropathy, 313–314, 404
Minute respiratory volume, 471
Minute work output, cardiac, 107–108
Miosis, 632
miRNA. *See* MicroRNA (miRNA).
Mirror neurons, 668
Mitochondria, 12f, 16, 16f, 21–23, 22f
  citric acid cycle in, 813
  exchangeable calcium in, 967
  fatty acid metabolism in, 822–823
  fatty acid transport into, 822
  high altitude and, 529
  oxidative phosphorylation in, 814–815, 814f
  of photoreceptors, 609, 610f
  of platelets, 451, 454
  of presynaptic terminals, 547, 547f
  of skeletal muscle, 73, 73f
    in fast vs. slow fibers, 79
  of sperm, 975, 975f
  thyroid hormones and, 911–912
Mitochondrial uncoupling protein, 873
Mitosis, 17, 37, 38–39, 38f
  prevention of, with colchicine, 39
Mitral cells, 651, 651f, 652
Mitral regurgitation
  circulatory dynamics in, 268–269
  murmur of, 267–268, 267f
Mitral stenosis
  circulatory dynamics in, 268–269
  murmur of, 267f, 268
  pulmonary capillary pressure in, 483
Mitral valve, 106–107, 107f
  first heart sound and, 265, 266, 266f
Mixed acid-base disorders, 394–395, 394f
Mixing movements, gastrointestinal, 759
  of colon, 770
  of small intestine, 768–769, 768f

Mixing waves, gastric, 766
Modality of sensation, 559
Modiolus, 635, 636–637, 637f
Molecular layer, of cerebellum, 684–685, 684f
Monoamine oxidase, of adrenergic nerve endings, 732
Monoamine oxidase inhibitors, 727
Monocyte colony-stimulating factor (M-CSF), in inflammation, 430, 430f
Monocyte-macrophage system, 426–428, 427f
Monocytes, 423, 423t, 424, 425
  atherosclerosis and, 827–828, 828f
  diapedesis by, 425
  in inflammation, 429
    increased production of, 429, 430, 430f
Monoglycerides, 791f, 792, 792f
  absorption of, 797
    bile salts and, 785, 792
  resynthesis of triglycerides from, 797, 819
Monosaccharides, 789, 790
  absorption of, 796
  in liver cells, 810, 810f
Morphine, respiratory depression caused by, 512
Morula, 1008–1009
Mossy fibers, 684–685, 684f
Motilin, 758–759, 758t
  small intestine peristalsis and, 769
Motion sickness
  nausea in, 804
  in spacecraft, 533
  vomiting in, 804
Motivation, 695. *See also* Limbic system; Punishment centers; Reward centers.
Motor aphasia, 704
Motor apraxia, 669
Motor cortex, 667–673. *See also* Premotor area; Supplementary motor area.
  basal ganglia and, 689, 690f, 691
  cerebellar input from, 682, 683, 686, 687, 687f
  cerebrocerebellum and, 688
  columnar arrangement of neurons in, 671–672
  lesions in, 673
  pathways from, 669–670, 670f
    red nucleus and, 670–671, 671f
  prefrontal association area and, 700
  representations of body in, 667, 668f
  role of, 694–695
  sensory pathways to, 670
  somatosensory feedback to, 672
  somatosensory input to, 575, 575f, 577, 670
  specialized areas of, 668–669, 669f
  speech and, 704–705
  spinal cord excitation by, 671–673, 672f
  subareas of, 667–668, 668f
  vasomotor center excitation by, 204
  voluntary movements and, 667, 673, 686
Motor end plate, 83, 84f. *See also* Neuromuscular junction.
Motor functions, 543–544, 544f
  basal ganglia in. *See* Basal ganglia.
  brain stem in, 673–674, 673f, 674f
    anencephaly and, 678–679
    gamma efferents in, 659, 660
    stretch reflexes and, 660
  cerebellum in. *See* Cerebellum.
  cerebral cortex in. *See* Motor cortex.
  cognitive control of, 691–692, 695
  integrated control of, 694–695
  spinal cord in, 655
    excitation by cortex for, 671–673, 672f
    organization of, 655–657, 655f, 656f
    pathways from cortex for, 669–671, 670f, 671f
    reflexes and. *See* Spinal cord reflexes.
    sensory receptors and. *See* Golgi tendon organs; Muscle spindles.

Motor imagery, 686
Motor nerve fibers, classification of, 563*f*, 655, 656
Motor neurons, anterior, 547, 547*f*, 552, 655, 655*f*. *See also* Spinal cord reflexes.
  alpha, 655, 656, 656*f*, 659
  corticospinal tract and, 669, 672, 672*f*
  gamma, 655, 656, 656*f*, 657, 657*f*, 658, 659, 660
  inhibition of, Golgi tendon organ and, 661
  pathways converging on, 672, 672*f*
  pontine reticulospinal tract and, 673–674
  Renshaw cells and, 656
  rubrospinal tract and, 671, 672, 672*f*
Motor units, 80, 656
  after poliomyelitis, 82
Mountain sickness
  acute, 530
  chronic, 530–531
Movement receptors, 563
mRNA. *See* Messenger RNA (mRNA).
Mucin, salivary, 775
Mucopolysaccharides, in cardiac T tubules, 103
Mucous cells
  of gastric surface, 777, 779
  of gastrointestinal tract, 773
  of pyloric glands, 778
Mucous glands, 773
  esophageal, 776–777
Mucous neck cells, gastric, 777, 777*f*, 778
Mucus
  gastrointestinal tract, 773, 775
    in large intestine, 787
    in saliva, 774*f*, 775, 776
    in small intestine, 786
    in stomach, 777, 778, 779, 780, 799–800
  in respiratory passages, 473
Multiple fiber summation, 80
Mumps orchitis, 977
Murmurs, cardiac
  with patent ductus arteriosus, 267*f*, 270
  in valvular heart disease, 267–268
Muscarinic receptors, 733
  drugs acting on, 740
  drugs blocking, 740
Muscle. *See* Cardiac muscle; Skeletal muscle; Smooth muscle.
Muscle contraction
  energy of ATP for, 22, 22*f*, 23, 859
  heat dissipated in, 862
Muscle cramps, 665
Muscle impulse, 64–65
Muscle spasm
  headache caused by, 591
  pain caused by, 584
  spinal cord reflexes causing, 664–665
Muscle spasticity, stroke leading to, 673
Muscle spindles, 560*f*, 656*f*, 657
  adaptation of, 562, 562*f*
  cerebellar input from, 661, 683, 683*f*
  feedback to motor cortex, 672
  joint angulation and, 580
  nerve fibers from, 564, 656, 656*f*
  receptor function of, 657–658, 657*f*
  stretch reflex and, 658–659, 658*f*, 659*f*, 672
    clinical applications of, 660, 660*f*
Muscle stretch reflex, 658–659, 658*f*, 659*f*, 672, 694
  clinical applications of, 660, 660*f*
Muscle tone
  central control of, 694
  of skeletal muscle, 80
Muscle weakness
  aldosterone excess and, 925–926
  cortisol excess and, 929
Muscularis mucosae, contractions of, 769

Musculoskeletal system, homeostatic functions of, 5
Mutations, 38
  cancer caused by, 40–41
Myasthenia gravis, 86–87, 442
Mydriasis, 632
Myelin sheath, 67, 67*f*, 68, 68*f*. *See also* Demyelination.
  sphingomyelin of, 826
  thiamine deficiency and, 853
Myelinated nerve fibers, 67, 67*f*
  absolute refractory period of, 69
  classification of, 563, 563*f*
  saltatory conduction in, 68, 68*f*
  velocity of conduction in, 68, 563
Myeloblasts, 423–424, 424*f*
Myelocytic lineage, 423–424, 424*f*
Myelogenous leukemias, 431
Myenteric plexus, 755, 756, 756*f*
  of colon, deficient in megacolon, 802
  of esophagus, 765
  gastroenteric reflex and, 769
  parasympathetic neurons in, 757
  peristalsis and, 759
  reflexes of, from cecum to ileum, 770
  of small intestine, 769, 780
Myenteric reflexes, 759
  defecation and, 771
  peristaltic rush and, 769
  stomach emptying and, 767
Myocardial infarction, 249–250
  acute anterior wall, 140, 140*f*
    recovery from, 141, 141*f*
  acute posterior wall, 140–141, 140*f*
    recovery from, 141, 141*f*
  cardiogenic shock secondary to, 259
  causes of death after, 250–251
  circulatory effects of. *See* Cardiac failure, circulatory dynamics in.
  current of injury in, 140–141, 140*f*, 141*f*
  low-voltage ECG after series of, 137, 137*f*
  recovery from
    function of heart after, 252, 256–257, 256*f*
    rest during, 251–252
    stages of, 251–252, 251*f*
  subendocardial, 249–250
Myocardial ischemia. *See also* Angina pectoris.
  ectopic foci caused by, 146
  electrocardiogram in
    current of injury and, 138, 140–141, 140*f*, 141*f*
    in mild ischemia, 142, 142*f*
  metabolism of cardiac muscle in, 248
  pain in, 252
  vasospastic, 248
Myofibrils, of skeletal muscle, 71, 72*f*, 73*f*, 74*f*
  T tubules and, 87, 87*f*, 88
Myogenic mechanism, 321
  renal blood flow and, 321
Myoglobin, 79, 1036
Myopia, 602–603, 602*f*, 603*f*
Myosin
  in ameboid movement, 23
  as ATP-degrading enzyme, 859
  of cardiac muscle, 101, 103
    Frank-Starling mechanism and, 110
    ventricular volume and, 108
  coated pits and, 18–19, 18*f*
  in mitosis, 39
  of platelets, 451, 454
  of skeletal muscle
    contraction mechanism and, 74, 74*f*, 75–76, 76*f*
    hypertrophy and, 81
    muscle tension and, 77, 77*f*
    structural features of, 71, 72*f*, 73*f*, 74–75, 74*f*
  of smooth muscle, 92–94, 92*f*

Myosin light chain kinase, 93–94, 94*f*
  calmodulin and, 891
Myosin phosphatase, 94, 94*f*
Myxedema, 917–918, 918*f*

N
NAD⁺. *See* Nicotinamide adenine dinucleotide (NAD⁺).
Naming objects, cortical area for, 699*f*, 700
Nasal cavity, 472*f*, 474
Nasal field of vision, 627
Nasal glands, autonomic control of, 735
Nasal sinuses, headache associated with, 591–592, 591*f*
NASH (nonalcoholic steatohepatitis), 838
Natriuretic drugs, for essential hypertension, 226
Natural killer lymphocytes, 433
Nausea, 804
Nearsightedness, 602–603, 602*f*, 603*f*
Neck proprioceptors, 678
Necrosis
  cellular, 40
  in hypovolemic shock, 277–278, 278*f*
Negative feedback, 7–8, 8*f*, 9
  delayed, 9
  in hormone systems, 885
Neglect syndrome, 692, 692*f*
Neocortex, 715
Neonatal respiratory distress syndrome, 468, 519, 1022, 1026
Neonate. *See also* Infant.
  circulation of
    readjustments in, 1022–1023
    special problems in, 1024, 1024*f*
  immunity in, 1025–1026
  jaundice in, 1024, 1024*f*
  liver function in, 1025
  nutrition of, 1023, 1025, 1026
  renal function in, 1024
  respiration in, 1021–1022, 1021*f*, 1024, 1026
  special functional problems in, 1023–1026
  temperature regulation in, 873, 1025, 1025*f*
    prematurity and, 1027
  weight loss in, 1023
Neospinothalamic tract, 585
Neostigmine, 86
  for myasthenia gravis, 86–87
Nephritis, interstitial, 403
Nephrogenic diabetes insipidus, 295
Nephron(s), 305–306, 306*f*, 307*f*. *See also* Distal tubule; Loop of Henle; Proximal tubule.
  age-related loss of, 403
  transport and permeability properties of, 348*t*
Nephrosclerosis, 403
  benign, 403
  malignant, 403
Nephrotic syndrome, 404
  edema in, 298, 377
Nernst equation, 50, 57–58
Nernst potential, of neuron membrane, 552–553
Nerve fibers, physiologic classification of, 563–564, 563*f*
Nerve impulse, 64–65. *See also* Action potential(s), nerve.
Nerve trunks
  myelinated fibers in, 67, 67*f*
    saltatory conduction in, 68, 68*f*
    velocity of conduction in, 68
  unmyelinated fibers in, 67, 67*f*
Nervous system. *See also* Central nervous system (CNS); Enteric nervous system; Synapses.
  compared with computer, 546, 546*f*
  general design of, 543–545, 544*f*
  integrative function of, 544–545
  regulatory functions of, 5

Net acid excretion, 390
Net filtration, 185
Net filtration pressure, 181, 184, 185–186
  abnormal, edema and, 185–186
  glomerular, 314, 314*f*
Net reabsorption pressure, 185, 186
Neuroendocrine hormones, 881
Neurogenic bladder, 310
Neurogenic shock, 279–280
  sympathomimetic drugs for, 281
Neurohormonal systems, in brain, 711,
    712–713, 713*f*
Neurohypophysis. *See* Pituitary gland, posterior.
Neuromuscular junction
  of skeletal muscle, 83
    acetylcholine action at, 73, 83–86, 84*f*
    acetylcholine synthesis at, 83, 86
    drugs acting at, 85, 86
    fatigue of, 85–86
    myasthenia gravis and, 86–87
    structure of, 83, 84*f*
  of smooth muscle, 94–95, 94*f*
Neuron(s). *See also* Axon; Dendrites; Soma of
    neuron; Synapses.
  central nervous system, 543, 544*f*
  continuously discharging, 568
  excitation of, 552–555, 552*f*, 553*f*, 554*f*.
      See also Action potential(s), neuronal.
    dendrite functions in, 555–556, 556*f*
    drug effects on, 557
    rate of firing and, 556–557, 556*f*
    excitatory state of, 556–557, 556*f*
  facilitation of, 545, 555
  inhibition of, 553*f*, 554–555
  inhibitory state of, 556–557
  metabolism of, 749
  morphologic variations in, 547
    motor. *See* Motor neurons, anterior.
  rate of firing of, for different neuron types,
      556–557, 556*f*
  resting membrane potential of soma, 552, 552*f*
Neuronal circuits
  inhibitory, 569
  instability and stability of, 569–570, 569*f*
Neuronal pools, 564–568
  grossly inhibitory, 569
  prolongation of signal by, 567–568
  relaying of signals through, 565–567, 565*f*,
      566*f*, 567*f*
Neuropeptide Y, 846, 847, 847*f*, 849, 851
Neuropeptides, 550, 550*b*, 551–552
Neurophysins, 904
Neurotransmitters, 546, 547, 550–552, 550*b*, 881
  in basal ganglia, 692–693, 692*f*
  in enteric nervous system, 756–757
  in hypothalamus, feeding and, 847*f*, 847*t*
  neurohormonal control of brain activity by,
      712–713, 713*f*
  release from presynaptic terminal, 548
  of retinal neurons, 617
Neutral fats. *See* Triglycerides.
Neutrophilia, 428–429
Neutrophils, 423, 423*t*, 424*f*
  chemotaxis by, 439
  diapedesis by, 424*f*, 425, 428, 429*f*
  in infection, 425–426
  in inflammation, 428–430, 429*f*
  in milk, 1016
  opsonization and, 439
Niacin, 853–854
Nicotinamide adenine dinucleotide (NAD⁺),
    813, 814
  in deamination, 834
  in fatty acid oxidation, 822*f*, 823
  glucocorticoids and, 928
  lactic acid formation and, 816
  niacin requirement and, 853–854

Nicotinamide adenine dinucleotide phosphate
    (NADP⁺)
  in fatty acid synthesis, 824, 824*f*
  niacin requirement and, 853–854
  pentose phosphate pathway and, 816*f*, 817
Nicotine, 86
Nicotinic acid. *See* Niacin.
Nicotinic drugs, 740
Nicotinic receptors, 733
Night blindness, 612
Nitrates, for angina pectoris, 196, 252
Nitric oxide
  as central nervous system transmitter, 551
  glomerular filtration rate and, 318
  penile erection and, 978–979
  vasodilation by, 195–196, 196*f*
Nitric oxide synthase, 195, 196*f*
Nitrogen
  dissolved in body fluids, 537, 537*t*. *See also*
      Decompression sickness.
  excretion of, 845
  high partial pressures of, 535
Nitrogen balance, 845
Nitrogen narcosis, 535, 539
Nociceptive reflex, 662
Nociceptors. *See* Pain receptors.
Nodes of Ranvier, 67, 67*f*, 68, 68*f*
Nonalcoholic steatohepatitis (NASH), 838
Nondominant hemisphere, 702
  corpus callosum and, 705
Nonpitting edema, 299
Nonprotein nitrogen
  chronic renal failure and, 406
  placental diffusion of, 1007
Nonshivering thermogenesis, 865, 873
Nonsteroidal antiinflammatory agents, gastric
    mucosa and, 801
Nonvolatile acids, 385, 387, 388, 390
  anion gap and, 395
Norepinephrine
  adrenal medullar secretion of, 736, 884, 921
    basal level of, 737
  of adrenergic nerve endings, 731–732
  adrenergic receptors and, 733
  in basal ganglia, 692–693, 692*f*
  cardiac effects of, 120
  as central nervous system transmitter, 551
  coronary blood flow and, 247, 248
  depression and, 726–727
  drugs blocking release of, 740
  drugs blocking synthesis of, 740
  drugs causing release of, 740
  fatty acid mobilization caused by, 825
  gastrointestinal smooth muscle and, 755,
      756, 757
  glomerular filtration rate and, 318
  metabolic rate and, 867
  molecular structure of, 731
  for shock, 281
  as smooth muscle neurotransmitter,
      95, 96, 97
  sweat glands and, 870
  as sympathomimetic drug, 739
  synthesis of, 732, 884
  thermogenesis and, 873
  as vasoconstrictor, 199, 203, 203*f*, 204
    in skeletal muscle, 244
Norepinephrine system, in brain, 712–713, 713*f*
Nose, 474
Nuclear bag muscle fibers, 657–658, 657*f*
Nuclear chain muscle fibers, 657–658, 657*f*
Nuclear membrane, 11, 11*f*, 13, 17, 17*f*
Nuclear pores, 17, 17*f*
Nucleolus(i), 12*f*, 17, 17*f*, 32
Nucleotides
  deoxyribose, 27–29, 28*f*, 29*f*
  ribose, 29*f*, 30

Nucleus, 11, 11*f*, 17, 17*f*
  evolution of, 18
Nucleus accumbens, Parkinson's disease and,
    693
Nucleus ambiguus, 506
Nucleus parabrachialis, 506
Nucleus retroambiguus, 506
Nucleus tractus solitarius. *See also* Tractus
    solitarius.
  energy expenditure and, 846
  respiration and, 505
  sleep and, 722
Nystagmus, cerebellar, 689

O
Oat bran, 829
Obesity, 850–851
  coronary artery disease and, 829
  cortisol excess causing, 929
  end-stage renal disease associated with, 402
  fat storage in, 825–826
  genetic factors in, 851
    leptin and, 849, 851
    melanocortin system and, 846–847, 851
    in rodents, 826, 847
  hypertension and, 225–226
  left axis deviation in, 135
  sympathetic activation in, 865
  treatment of, 851
  type II diabetes and, 951, 952
Obstructive jaundice, 841–842
Occlusion, of teeth, 969
Oddi, sphincter of, 780–781, 784*f*, 785
Odontoblasts, 970
Odor blindness, 650
Ohm's law, 159, 160, 230–231
Oleic acid, 819
Olfaction. *See also* Smell.
  amygdala and, 719
  hippocampus and, 719
Olfactory bulb, 649*f*, 651, 651*f*
  granule cells in, 650, 652
Olfactory cells, 649, 649*f*, 651
  stimulation of, 649–650, 649*f*
Olfactory cilia, 649, 649*f*
Olfactory membrane, 648–649, 649*f*, 651
Olfactory nerve, 649
Oliguria, 399
Olivocerebellar tract, 670, 683, 683*f*
Oncogenes, 40, 41
Oncotic pressure. *See* Colloid osmotic pressure.
Oocyte
  primary, 987, 1003
  secondary, 1003
Ophthalmoscope, 605–606, 605*f*
Opsins, 614
Opsonization, 19, 425
  phagocytosis and, 439, 439*f*
Optic chiasm, 623, 623*f*
  destruction of, 627
Optic disc, edematous, 748
Optic nerves, 623, 623*f*
  destruction of, 627
  peripheral vs. central retina and, 619
Optic radiation, 623, 623*f*
Optic tracts, 623, 623*f*
  interruption of, 627
Opticokinetic movements, 629
Optics
  of eye, 600–605
  physical principles of, 597–600
Orexigenic substances, 846, 847, 847*t*, 851
Organ of Corti, 634–635, 634*f*, 636–638,
      636*f*, 637*f*
    damage to, 642
    retrograde pathways in, 641–642
Organum vasculosum, 905

Orgasm
  female, 1000
  male, 979
Orlistat, 851
Oscillatory circuits. *See* Reverberatory circuits.
Oscilloscope, for recording membrane
    potentials, 69, 69*f*
Osmolality, 52, 291
  of stomach contents, 767, 768
Osmolar clearance, 354
Osmolarity, 52, 291. *See also* Extracellular fluid
    osmolarity.
  of body fluids, 288*t*, 291
  plasma, 288*t*, 291
    estimated from sodium concentration,
      294, 355
Osmoles, 290–291
Osmoreceptor cells, 355, 356, 356*f*, 358, 905
Osmosis, 51, 51*f*, 290
  active transport combined with, 55–56, 55*f*
  renal reabsorption and, 324, 328
  sodium-potassium pump and, 53
Osmotic coefficient, 291
Osmotic diuresis, 950
Osmotic diuretics, 397, 398*t*
Osmotic equilibrium, of intracellular and
    extracellular fluids, 291–292, 292*f*
Osmotic pressure, 51–52, 51*f*, 291. *See also*
    Colloid osmotic pressure.
  of cerebrospinal fluid, 747
Ossicular system, 633–634, 633*f*
  damage to, 642
Osteitis fibrosa cystica, 968
Osteoblasts, 900, 958, 959–960, 959*f*
  calcitonin and, 966
  of cementum, 971
  fracture repair and, 960
  parathyroid hormone and, 963–964
Osteoclasts, 900, 959–960, 959*f*
  calcitonin and, 966
  of cementum, 971
  estrogen and, 994
  parathyroid hormone and, 963, 964–965
Osteocytes, 958, 959*f*
  parathyroid hormone and, 963, 964
Osteocytic membrane system, 964
  calcitonin and, 966
Osteoid, 958
Osteolysis, 963–964
Osteomalacia, 969
  in renal disease, 406–407, 969
Osteon, 959–960
Osteoporosis, 969
  in postmenopausal women, 969, 994
Osteoprotegerin, 959, 994
Osteoprotegerin ligand, 959, 964
Oval window, 633–634, 633*f*, 635, 635*f*, 636
Ovarian cycle, 988–991. *See also* Female
    hormones; Menstrual cycle.
  follicular phase of, 989–990, 989*f*, 990*f*
  gonadotropic hormones and, 988–989
  hypothalamic-pituitary hormones and,
    996–998, 996*f*, 997*f*
  luteal phase of, 990–991
  ovulation in, 990, 990*f*
  plasma levels of hormones in, 988, 988*f*
  summary of, 991
  suppression of, during nursing, 1015
Ovarian follicle(s), 988*f*
  atretic, 990
  development of, 989–990, 989*f*
  mature, 989*f*, 990
  primary, 989
  primordial, 987, 989, 989*f*
Ovarian hormones, 991–996, 992*f*, 993*f*.
    See also Estrogen(s); Progestins.
  abnormalities of, 999–1000

Ovaries
  anatomy of, 987, 987*f*, 988*f*
  cholesterol used by, 827
Overdrive suppression, 145
Overflow incontinence, 310
Overhydration
  hypernatremia causing, 295*t*, 296
  hyponatremia in, 295, 295*t*
Ovulation, 989*f*, 990, 990*f*, 1003, 1004*f*
  infertility due to failure of, 1001
  preovulatory surge and, 885, 988*f*, 997–998
  suppression of, 1001
  timing of fertilization and, 1000–1001
Ovum(a)
  development of, 987, 989–990, 989*f*
  entry into fallopian tube, 1003, 1004*f*
  fertilized, 1003–1004, 1004*f*
  mature, 1003
  release of. *See* Ovulation.
Oxalate, as anticoagulant, 456, 460
Oxaloacetic acid, in citric acid cycle,
    813, 813*f*
  deficiency of, 824
  starting with fatty acids, 822–823
Oxidases, of peroxisomes, 15–16
Oxidative metabolism. *See also* Aerobic energy.
  at high altitude, 529
  hypoxia caused by defects in, 521
  in skeletal muscle, 78, 79
    for exercise, 1033, 1033*f*, 1033*t*
Oxidative phosphorylation, 814–815, 814*f*
  pentose phosphate pathway and, 816–817
  uncoupled, 865, 873
Oxygen
  brain's special need for, 749
  diffusing capacity for, 491, 492*f*
    carbon monoxide method, 492
  diffusion coefficient of, 487*t*
  diffusion of. *See also* Diffusion, of gases.
    from alveoli to capillaries, 5, 495–496,
      496*f*
    from capillaries to cells, 497, 501
    from capillaries to interstitial fluid,
      496–497, 496*f*
    through capillary membrane, 179, 180
  energy equivalent of, 863
  in extracellular fluid
    normal range of, 7*t*
    regulation of, 6
  lipid solubility of, 46
  in local blood flow control
    acute, 192, 192*f*, 193
    long-term, 197–198
    in skeletal muscle, 243
    smooth muscle and, 97
  placental diffusion of, 1006–1007, 1006*f*
  respiratory control by, 507, 508–510,
    509*f*, 510*f*
  tissue concentration of, capillary blood flow
    and, 178–179
  transport of, 495–502
    from alveoli to capillaries, 495–496, 496*f*
    in blood, 496, 496*f*, 501
    from capillaries to tissue cells, 497, 501
    from capillaries to tissue fluid,
      496–497, 496*f*
    in dissolved state, 498, 501, 521,
      535–536, 536*f*
    during exercise, 498–499
    hemoglobin in, 495, 498–500, 498*f*,
      499*f*, 500*f*
Oxygen consumption
  by brain tissue, 744
  cardiac output and, 230, 230*f*
  in cellular metabolism, 500–501
    ADP concentration and, 500, 501, 501*f*
    blood flow limited, 501

Oxygen consumption, in cellular
    metabolism (*Continued*)
    diffusion limited, 501
    interstitial fluid P_{O_2} and, 496*f*, 497
    intracellular P_{O_2} and, 500–501, 501*f*
  coronary blood flow and, 247, 248
  during exercise, 510, 510*f*, 1036, 1036*f*, 1036*t*
    heat generation and, 1040
    maximal, 1037, 1037*f*, 1039
    work output and, 1038, 1038*f*
  by heart, 109, 249
  metabolic rate determination from, 863
    basal, 863
Oxygen debt, 861, 1034, 1034*f*
Oxygen free radicals, high alveolar P_{O_2} and,
    536–537
Oxygen lack theory, of local blood flow
    regulation, 192, 193, 193*f*
Oxygen partial pressure (P_{O_2})
  alveolar, 488, 488*f*
    altitude and. *See* High altitude, alveolar
      P_{O_2} at.
    high levels of, 499, 535–537, 536*f*
    intracellular, 497
    with oxygen therapy, 521, 521*f*
    solubility coefficient and, 486
    in tissues, hemoglobin buffering of, 499
    ventilation-perfusion ratio and,
      492–494, 493*f*
  arterial
    chemoreceptors and, 208
    during exercise, 1037
    measurement of, 515–516
  atmospheric, 527, 528*t*. *See also* High altitude.
  in tissues
    cerebral blood flow and, 744
    with high alveolar P_{O_2}, 536
Oxygen saturation, arterial, 530
  at different altitudes, 527, 528*f*, 528*t*
  local blood flow and, 192, 192*f*
Oxygen therapy, 520, 521, 521*f*
  in heart failure, with acute pulmonary
    edema, 261
  hyperbaric, 540
  in premature infant, 1027
  for shock, 281
Oxygen toxicity, 501
  at high pressures, 535–537, 539
Oxygen-diffusing capacity, 1037, 1037*t*
Oxygen-hemoglobin dissociation curve, 498,
    498*f*, 499*f*
  fetal, 1006, 1006*f*
  hemoglobin buffering and, 499
  at high pressures, 535–536, 536*f*
  of high-altitude residents, 530, 530*f*
  shift in, factors causing, 499–500, 500*f*
Oxyntic cells. *See* Parietal (oxyntic) cells.
Oxyntic (gastric) glands, 766, 777–778, 777*f*, 779
  hydrogen ion transport in, 54
  peptic cells of, 777, 777*f*, 778, 779
  structure of, 777, 777*f*
Oxyphil cells, 963, 963*f*
Oxytocin, 896, 905–906
  chemical structure of, 904
  copulation and, 1000
  fertilization and, 1003
  hypothalamus and, 716, 904
  labor and, 905
  lactation and, 716, 905–906, 1015–1016
  uterine contraction and, 1012, 1013

P

P wave, 121, 121*f*
  atrial contraction and, 122
  cardiac cycle and, 105, 105*f*
  normal voltage of, 123
  vectorial analysis of, 133*f*

Pacemaker
  cardiac, 118–119
    arrhythmias and, 143
    artificial implanted, 145, 153
    ectopic, 119
    in paroxysmal tachycardia, 148
  gastrointestinal smooth muscle, 754
Pacemaker waves, of smooth muscle, 96
Pacinian corpuscles, 560f, 561–562, 561f, 572
  adaptation of, 562, 562f, 563
  joint angulation and, 580
  stimulus intensity and, 579
  vibrations detected by, 572, 579
Packed red cell volume. See Hematocrit.
Paget disease, calcitonin in, 966
PAH. See Para-aminohippuric acid (PAH).
Pain
  analgesia system of brain and spinal cord,
    586–588, 587f
  brain stem excitatory area and, 711
  in coronary artery disease, 252. See also
    Angina pectoris.
  dual pathways for transmission of,
    584–586, 585f
    surgical interruption of, 586
  electrical stimulation for treatment of, 588
  fast vs. slow, 583
  of headache, 590–592, 591f
  of herpes zoster, 590
  hyperalgesia and, 583–584, 590
  inhibition by tactile signals, 587–588
  of labor, 1013
  parietal, 589–590, 589f
  protective function of, 583
  referred, 588, 588f
    headache as, 591
    from visceral organs, 588, 589, 589f
  of tic douloureux, 590
  tissue damage and, 583, 584
  visceral, 588–590, 589f
Pain fibers, 564
  fast and slow, 584–585
  spatial summation and, 564, 564f
Pain receptors, 559, 560b, 583
  nonadapting nature of, 583–584
  thermal excitation of, 592, 592f
  types of stimuli acting on, 583
Pain reflex, 662
Pain sense, 571
  anterolateral system and, 573
  localization of, 577
Paleocortex, 715
Paleospinothalamic tract, 585, 586
Palmitic acid, 819
Pancreas
  acini of, 773, 780–781, 939, 939f
  physiologic anatomy of, 939, 939f
Pancreatic duct, 780–781
Pancreatic polypeptide, 939
Pancreatic secretions, 780–783, 782f, 783f
  alkalinity of, 800
  amylase, 781, 790
    in neonate, 1025
  deficiency of, 801
  lipases, 781, 792–793, 792f
  proteolytic enzymes, 781, 791, 791f
Pancreatitis, 781, 801
Panhypopituitarism, 902
  in adult, 903
    with gigantism, 903
  dwarfism in, 902–903
Panting, 871
Pantothenic acid, 812–813, 855
Papilla of Vater, 780–781
  blockage at, 801
Papillary muscles, 107, 107f
Papilledema, 748

Para-aminohippuric acid (PAH), 330
  renal plasma flow and, 341–342, 342f
Parachute jumps, deceleratory forces in,
    532–533
Paracrines, 881
Paradoxical sleep, 722
Parafollicular cells, thyroid, 966
Parallax, 605
Parallel fibers, of cerebellum, 684–685
Parasitic infections, eosinophils in, 430
Parasympathetic denervation, 737
Parasympathetic nervous system. See also
    Autonomic nervous system; Vagus
    nerves.
  anatomy of, physiologic, 730–731, 731f
  in arterial pressure control, 206
  bladder and, 308, 308f, 309
  bronchiolar constriction caused by, 473
  cardiac innervation by, 111, 111f, 119,
    201, 202f
  cardiac regulation by, 111, 111f, 119–120
    bradycardia and, 144
    cardiac output and, 231
    vasomotor center and, 203
  circulatory control by, 201, 202f
  coronary blood flow and, 247
  erection and
    in female, 1000
    penile, 978–979
  eye control by, 601, 631, 632, 730–731
  gastric secretions and, 778
  gastrointestinal regulation by, 755, 756–757
    blood flow and, 762
    defecation and, 738, 757, 771, 771f
    large intestine mucus and, 787
    peristalsis and, 759
    psychogenic diarrhea and, 802
  gastrointestinal secretions and, 773–774
  localized activation of, 738
  salivary glands and, 776, 776f
  sexual lubrication and, 979
  ureteral peristalsis and, 309
Parasympathetic tone, 737
Parasympathomimetic drugs, 740
Parathyroid glands, 962–963, 963f
Parathyroid hormone (PTH), 962–966
  bone resorption and, 959
  calcium homeostasis and, 367–369, 368f
    extracellular fluid concentration in,
      963–966, 963f, 965f, 967
    intestinal absorption in, 796, 964
    renal reabsorption in, 339, 964
  chemistry of, 963
  control of secretion of, 965–966, 965f
  deficiency of, 967
  excess of
    in chronic renal failure, 407
    primary, 967–968
    secondary, 968
  phosphate homeostasis and, 369
    extracellular fluid concentration in,
      963–965, 963f
    renal excretion in, 964
  in pregnancy, 1009
  summary of effects of, 965–966, 965f
  vitamin D and, 961–962, 961f
Parathyroid poisoning, 968
Paraventricular nuclei
  food intake and, 846, 849
  pituitary hormones and, 897, 904, 904f,
    905, 906
Parietal (oxyntic) cells, 777, 777f
  ghrelin released by, 848
  hydrochloric acid secretion by, 777–778,
    777f, 778f
    stimulation of, 778, 779
  intrinsic factor secretion by, 778

Parietal lobe, somatosensory signals and, 575
Parietal pain, 589–590, 589f
Parieto-occipitotemporal association area,
    699–700, 699f
  in nondominant hemisphere, 702
  prefrontal association area and, 700
Parkinson's disease, 691, 693–694, 727
Parotid glands, 775, 790
Paroxysmal tachycardia, 148–149
  atrial, 148, 148f
  ventricular, 148–149, 149f
Partial intraventricular block, 145–146, 145f
Partial pressures. See also Carbon dioxide
    partial pressure (Pco$_2$); Oxygen partial
    pressure (Po$_2$).
  of dissolved gases, 485–486
  in gas mixture, 485
  net diffusion and, 486–487
  of water vapor, 486
Parturition, 1011–1014, 1012f
  involution of uterus after, 1013–1014
Passive immunity, 442
Past pointing, 689
Patch-clamp method, 48, 49f
Patent ductus arteriosus, 269–271, 270f, 1023
  aortic pressure pulse associated with,
    169, 169f
  murmur of, 267f, 270
Pco$_2$. See Carbon dioxide partial pressure
    (Pco$_2$).
Pellagra, 854
Pelvic nerves
  bladder and, 308, 309
  parasympathetic fibers in, 731
    defecation reflex and, 771, 771f
    to intestine, 757, 787
Pendrin, 908, 908f
Pendular movements, 687–688
Penetrating arterioles, of brain, 743, 743f
Penile erection, 196, 738, 978–979, 979f
Pentagastrin, 780
Pentose phosphate pathway, 816–817, 816f
Pepsin, 778, 791, 791f
  deficiency of, 800
  excess of, 800
Pepsinogen, 777, 778
  regulation of secretion of, 779
Peptic (chief) cells, 777, 777f, 778, 779
Peptic ulcer, 780, 786, 800, 800f, 801
  obstruction caused by, 804
  treatment of, 801
Peptidases
  of enterocytes, 787, 791
  zinc in, 856
Peptide hormones, 881, 882
  clearance from blood, 886
Peptide linkages, 789, 790, 831
  energy required for, 859, 862
  formation of, 34, 35
Peptide YY, 846f, 848
Peptidyl transferase, 34
Peptones, 783, 783f, 791
Perforins, 441
Periaqueductal gray, pain signals and,
    586–587, 587f
Pericardial effusion, 300
  low-voltage ECG associated with, 137
Perilymph, 637–638
Perimetry, 627, 627f
Periodic breathing, 512–513, 512f
Periodontal membrane, 970
Peripheral chemoreceptor system.
    See Chemoreceptor reflexes;
    Chemoreceptors.
Peripheral circulation, 157
Peripheral membrane proteins, 13f, 14
Peripheral resistance unit (PRU), 162–163

Peripheral vascular resistance. *See* Total peripheral resistance; Vascular resistance.
Peristalsis, 759, 759*f*
  of colon, 771
  of esophagus, 764*f*, 765
  of pharynx, 764, 765
  of rectum, 771
  of small intestine, 769
    of ileum, 769–770, 770*f*
  of stomach, 766
    emptying and, 766, 767
Peristaltic reflex, 759
Peristaltic rush, 769
Peristaltic waves, in small intestine, 769
Peritoneointestinal reflex, 772
Peritonitis
  abdominal muscle spasm in, 665
  intestinal paralysis secondary to, 772
  septic shock secondary to, 280
Peritubular capillaries, 304–305, 305*f*, 306, 307*f*, 311, 311*f*. *See also* Vasa recta.
  reabsorption and, 323–324, 324*f*
    physical forces and, 335–337, 335*f*, 336*t*, 337*f*
Perivascular spaces, of brain, 746, 747, 747*f*
Periventricular nuclei, 586–587, 587*f*
Pernicious anemia, 417, 420, 778, 800, 854
Peroxidases, 536–537
  iodide oxidation by, 908, 908*f*
    deficient, 917
Peroxide radical, high alveolar Po₂ and, 536–537
Peroxisomes, 15–16
  of neutrophils and macrophages, 426
Petit mal epilepsy, 725*f*, 726
pH. *See also* Acid-base regulation; Hydrogen ions.
  bicarbonate buffer system and, 382
  blood
    acid-base disorders and, 393, 394–395, 394*f*
    carbon dioxide transport and, 504
    measurement of, 515–516
    oxygen-hemoglobin dissociation curve and, 499–500, 500*f*
    respiratory control and, 508, 508*f*, 510, 510*f*
  of body fluids, 380, 380*t*
  definition of, 380
  of gastrointestinal secretions, 775*t*
Phagocytes, in spleen, 175
Phagocytosis, 18, 19, 423, 425–426
  after apoptosis, 40
  aqueous humor cleansed by, 607
  bactericidal agents and, 20, 426
  by eosinophils, 430
  in inflammatory response, 428, 429
  innate immunity and, 433
  monocyte-macrophage system and, 426–428
  opsonization and, 439, 439*f*
Phagocytotic vesicle, 19, 19*f*, 425–426
Pharyngoesophageal sphincter, 764
Phasic receptors, 563
Phenylthiocarbamide, 646
Phonation, 474–475
Phonocardiogram, 266, 267*f*
  cardiac cycle and, 105, 105*f*
  of valvular murmurs, 267*f*, 268
Phosphagen energy system, 1033, 1034*b*, 1036
Phosphate, 856. *See also* Hypophosphatemia.
  in bone, 957
    deposition of, 958
    parathyroid hormone and, 963–964
  in extracellular fluid and plasma, 955
    forms of, 955
    level of, 955–956

Phosphate, in extracellular fluid and plasma (*Continued*)
    parathyroid hormone and, 963–965, 963*f*
    in rickets, 968
  fecal excretion of, 957
  fetal accumulation of, 1020, 1020*f*
  intestinal absorption of, 796, 957, 962
    parathyroid hormone and, 964–965
    vitamin D and, 962, 964–965
  phospholipids as donors of, 826
  renal excretion of, 369, 957, 962, 964
    with reduced GFR, 404, 405*f*
  renal failure and, chronic, 407
Phosphate buffer system, 383, 388, 388*f*
Phosphatidylinositol biphosphate (PIP₂), 890
  aldosterone and, 927
Phosphocreatine, 78, 860
  depleted in irreversible shock, 278–279
  in strenuous muscle activity, 860, 861, 1032–1034, 1033*f*
  summary of use of, 861, 861*f*
Phosphodiesterase-5 inhibitors, 196, 986
Phosphofructokinase, inhibition of, 815
Phosphogluconate pathway, 816–817, 816*f*
Phospholipase, pancreatic, 781
Phospholipase A₂, 792–793
Phospholipase C, hormonal activity and, 890, 890*b*, 890*f*
  parathyroid, 965
  thyroid, 914
Phospholipids, 12, 13, 819, 826. *See also* Lecithin.
  chemical structures of, 826, 826*f*
  in chylomicrons, 819
  dietary, 792
  digestion of, 792–793
  insulin and, 944
  in lipoproteins, 821, 821*t*
  second messenger system using, 890, 890*b*, 890*f*
  synthesis of, 826
    in endoplasmic reticulum, 20
    in liver, 822, 839
  thyroid hormones and, 912
  uses of, 826
  structural, 827
Phosphoric acid, as component of DNA, 27, 28*f*
Phosphorus, 856
Phosphorylase, 811, 811*f*
  activation of, 36, 812
Photopsins, 614
Photoreceptors. *See* Cones; Rods.
Physiologic dead space, 471–472, 493, 494
Physiologic shunt, 493, 494
Physiology, 3
Physostigmine, 86
Pia mater, perivascular space and, 747, 747*f*
Pial arteries, 743, 743*f*
Pigment layer, of retina, 609–611, 610*f*
Piloerection, for temperature regulation, 872–873
Piloerector muscles, nerve fibers to, 729–730, 730*f*, 731
Pineal gland, 986
  blood-brain barrier and, 748–749
Pinocytosis, 18–19, 18*f*
  in intestinal epithelium, 794, 794*f*
  of proteins in renal tubule, 326
  in thyroid gland, 908*f*, 909
Pinocytotic vesicle, 18–19, 19*f*
  in intestinal epithelium, 794, 794*f*
PIP₂. *See* Phosphatidylinositol biphosphate (PIP₂).
Pitting edema, 299
Pituicytes, 904
Pituitary gland, 895–906
  adenoma of, 935, 936
  anatomy of, 895, 895*f*

Pituitary gland (*Continued*)
  anterior
    cell types in, 896–897, 896*f*, 896*t*
    hormone deficiencies of, 902–903
    hormones of, 895, 895*f*, 896, 896*t*, 898. *See also specific hormones.*
    hypothalamus and, 716–717, 897–898, 897*f*, 898*t*, 901–902
    pregnancy and, 1009
  embryology of, 895
  intermediate lobe of, 934
  posterior
    hormones of, 895, 896, 897. *See also specific hormones.*
    hypothalamus and, 895, 897, 904, 904*f*, 905, 906
PKC (protein kinase C), 890, 890*f*
Place principle, 638
Placenta, 1005–1007
  anatomy of, 1005–1007, 1006*f*
  blood flow through, 1010
  breaks in membrane of, 1005–1006
  carbon dioxide diffusion through, 1007
  diffusion conductance of, 1005–1006, 1005*f*
  duration in pregnancy and, 1005, 1005*f*
  hormones secreted by, 1007–1009
  nutrient diffusion through, 1007
  oxygen diffusion through, 1006–1007, 1006*f*
  preeclampsia and, 1011
  separation and delivery of, 1013
  waste product diffusion through, 1007
Plaque, dental, 971
Plaques, atheromatous, 827, 828, 828*f*
Plasma. *See also* Extracellular fluid.
  composition of, 287, 288*f*, 288*t*
  as fluid compartment, 4–5, 286, 286*f*, 287
  hypovolemic shock in loss of, 279
    with trauma, 279
  osmolarity of, 288*t*, 291. *See also* Extracellular fluid osmolarity.
    estimated from sodium concentration, 294, 355
  viscosity of, 165
Plasma cells, 423, 424, 437, 441*f*
Plasma colloid osmotic pressure, 181, 181*f*, 184, 184*t*, 185*t*
  albumin and, 184, 184*t*, 833
  lymph flow and, 188
Plasma membrane
  of cell. *See* Cell membrane.
  of skeletal muscle fiber, 71
Plasma proteins. *See also* Albumin.
  as amino acid source, 833, 834*f*
  calcium bound to, 367
  capillaries impermeable to, 4–5
  carbon dioxide transport by, 503
  colloid osmotic pressure and, 184, 184*t*
  of complement system, 438
  cortisol and, 929
  edema caused by decrease in, 297, 298, 300
    in cirrhosis, 377–378, 833
    in nephrotic syndrome, 377
  equilibrium between tissue proteins and, 833–834, 834*f*
  estrogens bound to, 993
  glomerular filtration of, 312, 313, 313*t*. *See also* Proteinuria.
  glucocorticoids and, 835
  hormone transport by, 885–886
    of adrenocortical steroids, 923–924
    of steroids, 885–886
    of testosterone, 980
    of thyroid hormones, 882, 885–886
  immunoglobulins as, 437–438
  in interstitial fluid, 184, 185, 189
  interstitial fluid cations and, 287
  intestinal obstruction and loss of, 279

Plasma proteins (*Continued*)
  lymphatic return of, 186
  magnesium bound to, 369
  major types of, 833
  in neonate, 1025, 1027
  nephrotic syndrome and, 377, 404
  in potential spaces, 300
  progesterone bound to, 993
  synthesis of, 833, 840
  thyroid hormones bound to, 909–910
Plasma substitutes, 281
Plasma transfusion, 280–281
Plasma volume, measurement of, 290
Plasmalemmal vesicles, of capillary endothelial
    cells, 178, 178*f*
Plasmin, 457
Plasminogen, 457
Platelet factor 3, 455
Platelet plug formation, 451–452, 452*f*
Platelets, 423, 424, 451–452
  in clot, 452, 452*f*, 454
  clot retraction and, 454
  concentration of, in blood, 423
  deficiency of, 458
  endothelial surface and, 452, 457
  intrinsic clotting pathway and, 455
  life span of, 425
  prothrombin receptors on, 453
Pleural effusion, 300, 483
  low-voltage ECG associated with, 137
Pleural fluid, 465–466, 483, 483*f*
Pleural pressure, 466, 466*f*
Pleural space, 483
Pluripotential hematopoietic stem cells,
    414–415, 414*f*, 423–424
Pneumonia, 518–519, 518*f*, 519*f*
Pneumotaxic center, 505, 506, 506*f*
Po₂. *See* Oxygen partial pressure (Po₂).
Podocytes, 312–313, 313*f*
Poiseuille's law, 163–164
Poison ivy, 443
Polar body
  first, 1003
  second, 1003
Polarography, 515
Poliomyelitis, macromotor units subsequent to, 82
Polycystic ovary syndrome, 952
Polycythemia, 421
  hematocrit in, 165, 165*f*, 287
Polycythemia vera, 421
  cyanosis in, 521–522
Polymorphonuclear leukocytes, 423, 423*t*,
    424*f*. *See also* Basophils; Eosinophils;
    Neutrophils.
Polypeptide hormones, 881, 882, 885*f*
Polypeptides
  classification into proteins and peptides, 882
  from protein digestion, 791, 791*f*
Polyribosomes, 33
Polysaccharides, 789–790
Pons. *See also* Brain stem.
  respiratory control by, 505, 506, 506*f*
  reticular substance of, 711–712
  swallowing and, 764
Pontine reticular nuclei, 673–674, 673*f*
Pontine reticulospinal tract, 673–674, 674*f*
Pontocerebellar tracts, 670, 682
Pores. *See also* Ion channels.
  in capillaries. *See* Capillaries, pores in.
  in cell membrane, 14
  nuclear, 17, 17*f*
Portal hypertension, 838
Portal vein, 759–760, 759*f*, 837, 837*f*, 838
  blockage in, 838
  colon bacilli in, 839
Portal vessels, hypothalamic-hypophysial,
    897–898, 897*f*

Position senses, 571, 573, 580, 580*f*
Positive and supportive reaction, 663
Positive feedback, 8–9, 8*f*
  in hormone systems, 885
Postcentral gyrus, 575*f*, 576, 577
Posterior parietal cortex
  lesions of, 692
  spatial coordinates of body and, 692, 699, 699*f*
Postganglionic neurons, autonomic
  drugs that block, 740
  drugs that stimulate, 740
  muscarinic receptors of, 733
  parasympathetic, 731
    enteric nervous system and, 757
  sympathetic, 729–730, 730*f*
    adrenal medulla and, 730
    gastrointestinal tract and, 757
  transmitters of, 731, 732
Postsynaptic neuron, 546, 548–549. *See also*
    Neurotransmitters.
  excitatory receptors of, 547, 549–550
  inhibitory receptors of, 547, 549, 550
  second messengers in, 548–549, 549*f*
Postsynaptic potentials, 553–555, 553*f*, 554*f*
  summation of, 553, 554*f*, 555
Postural instability, in Parkinson's disease, 693
Postural reflexes, 663–664
Posture, and baroreceptor reflexes, 206–207.
    See also Equilibrium.
Potassium
  aldosterone secretion and, 921–922
  in bone, 957–958
  cardiac action potential and, 102–103,
    115–116
  in cerebrospinal fluid, 747
  dietary, benefit of, 367
  in extracellular fluid
    aldosterone secretion and, 927
    fibrillation tendency and, 250
    heart function and, 112
    normal range of, 7, 7*t*, 361
    regulation of, 361–362, 362*f*, 362*t*
  gastric acid secretion and, 777–778, 778*f*
  intestinal absorption of, 796
  neuronal somal membrane and, 552–553,
    552*f*
  renal excretion of, 361, 362–363, 363*f*
  renal reabsorption of, 331, 331*f*, 332–333,
    362, 363*f*, 364
  renal secretion of, 311–312, 332, 333, 333*f*,
    362–367, 364*f*
    acidosis and, 364, 367
    aldosterone and, 337–338, 364–366, 364*f*,
      365*f*, 366*f*
    concentration in extracellular fluid and,
      364, 364*f*, 365*f*, 366*f*
    distal tubular flow rate and, 364, 366, 366*f*
  in saliva, 774*f*, 775, 776
  sports-related loss of, 1040
  in sweat, 870
  in skeletal muscle, 243–244
Potassium ion channels, 47, 47*f*, 48, 48*f*
  of cardiac muscle, 66, 115
    in sinus node, 116
    ventricular action potential and,
      115–116
  of cochlear hair cells, 637
  memory and, 708
  of pancreatic beta cells, 945, 945*f*
  in postsynaptic neuron membrane
    excitation and, 549
    G-protein–activated, 549, 549*f*
    inhibition and, 550, 554
  of smooth muscle, 97
  voltage-gated
    in cardiac muscle, 66
    of nerve membrane, 61, 62–63, 62*f*

Potassium leak channels, 59, 59*f*, 60, 63
Potassium-sparing diuretics, 332, 333*f*, 399
Potential energy, of ventricular contraction,
    108*f*, 109
Potential spaces
  fluids in, 300
  pleural, 483
Power law for stimulus intensity, 579, 580*f*
  auditory, 638
P-Q interval, 121*f*, 123
P-R interval, 121*f*, 123
  prolonged, 144–145, 144*f*
Precapillary sphincters, 177
  in local blood flow control, 193, 193*f*
  sympathetic innervation of, 201
  vasomotion of, 178–179, 193
Precordial leads, 126, 126*f*
Prednisolone, 924*t*
Prednisone, 922
Preeclampsia, 1011
  hypertension in, 224
Prefrontal association area, 699*f*, 700, 702–703
Prefrontal cortex
  feeding and, 848
  schizophrenia and, 727
Prefrontal lobotomy, 702, 703
Preganglionic neurons
  as cholinergic neurons, 731
  parasympathetic, 731
  sympathetic, 729, 730*f*
Pregnancy
  circulatory system during, 1010–1011, 1010*f*
  hormones secreted in, 1007–1009, 1007*f*
  maternal body's response to, 1009–1011,
    1010*f*
  metabolism in, 1010
  nutrition in, 1010
  parathyroid enlargement in, 965
  toxemia of, 224
  weight gain in, 1010
Pregnanediol, 993, 1001
Pregnenolone, 922, 923*f*, 932
Prekallikrein, 455
Preload, 109
Prelymphatics, 186
Premature contractions, 146–147
  atrial, 146, 146*f*
  A-V nodal or A-V bundle, 146, 146*f*
  causes of, 146
  definition of, 146
  in long QT syndromes, 147, 148*f*
  ventricular, 146–147, 147*f*
    refractory period and, 103, 103*f*
  in ventricular paroxysmal tachycardia,
    148–149
Premature infant, 1026–1027
  retrolental fibroplasia in, 197–198, 1027
Premotor area, 667–668, 668*f*, 698, 699*f*
  basal ganglia and, 690*f*, 691–692, 691*f*
  Broca's area and, 668–669, 669*f*, 700,
    702, 704
  cerebellar communication with, 682,
    686, 688
  hand skills and, 669
  voluntary eye movement and, 669
Preprohormones, 882
Prerenal acute renal failure, 399–400, 400*b*
Presbyopia, 601
Pressure
  fluid. *See* Hydrostatic pressure; Osmotic
    pressure.
  gas. *See* Partial pressures.
Pressure buffer system, 207, 207*f*
Pressure diuresis, 213–218, 214*f*, 215*f*, 319, 337,
    371–373
  aldosterone oversecretion and, 375, 925
  antidiuretic hormone and, 375–376

Pressure gradient, blood flow and, 159, 160
Pressure natriuresis, 213, 215, 216, 319, 337, 371–373, 371*f*
  aldosterone oversecretion and, 375, 925
  angiotensin II and, 374, 374*f*
  antidiuretic hormone and, 375–376
  obesity and, 225–226
Pressure sensations, 571. *See also* Tactile receptors; Tactile sensations.
  on footpads, equilibrium and, 678
  pathways into central nervous system, 573
Pressure-volume curves, of neonatal lungs, 1021, 1021*f*
Presynaptic facilitation, memory and, 707, 707*f*, 708
Presynaptic inhibition, 554
  by enkephalin, 587
  memory and, 707
Presynaptic membrane, calcium channels in, 548
  memory and, 707, 707*f*, 708
Presynaptic neuron, 546
Presynaptic terminals, 547–548, 547*f*.
    See also Neurotransmitters.
  long-term memory and, 708
  transmitter release from, 548, 550
  transmitter synthesis in, 550–551
Pretectal nuclei, visual fibers to, 623
Prevertebral ganglia, 729
Primary motor cortex, 667, 668*f*
  damage to, 673
Primordial follicle, 987, 989, 989*f*
Primordial germ cells, 973, 974*f*
Principal cells, renal, 332, 332*f*
  aldosterone and, 337
  potassium and, 362–364, 363*f*
Procaine, 69
Procarboxypolypeptidase, 781
Procoagulants, 453
Proelastase, 791
Proerythroblasts, 415, 415*f*. *See also* Erythroblasts.
  erythropoietin and, 416–417
  hemoglobin synthesis in, 417
Progesterone, 987, 988*f*, 991
  adrenal secretion of, 934
  breast development and, 995, 1014
  chemistry of, 992, 992*f*, 993*f*
  in contraceptive drugs, 1001
  degradation of, 993
  endometrial nutrients and, 1005
  excretion of, 993
  fallopian tube relaxation and, 1004
  functions of, 994–995
  gonadotropin inhibition and, 997, 998
  menstrual cycle and, 995–996
  ovarian cycle and, 990, 991
  plasma protein binding of, 993
  in pregnancy, 1007*f*, 1008–1009
  synthesis of, 992, 992*f*, 993*f*
  uterine contractility and, 1011–1012
Progestins, 991, 992, 992*f*. *See also* Progesterone.
  in contraceptive drugs, 1001
Prohormone convertase, 933–934, 933*f*
Prohormones, 882
Prolactin, 896, 896*t*
  lactation and, 1014–1015, 1015*f*
  pregnancy and, 1009
Prolactin inhibitory hormone, 898, 898*t*, 1015
Prometaphase, 38*f*, 39
Promoter, 30, 35–36, 35*f*
Pronucleus
  female, 1003–1004, 1004*f*
  male, 1003–1004, 1004*f*
Proopiomelanocortin, 933–934, 933*f*

Proopiomelanocortin neurons, 846, 847, 847*f*, 849, 933–934
  obesity and, 865
Prophase, 38*f*, 39
Proprioceptive senses, 571. *See also* Position senses.
  equilibrium and, 678
Propriospinal fibers, 656–657, 672*f*
Propulsive movements. *See also* Peristalsis.
  of colon, 770–771
  of small intestine, 769
Propylthiouracil, antithyroid activity of, 915, 917
Prosopagnosia, 700
Prostaglandin(s)
  fertilization and, 1003
  fever and, 876
  glomerular filtration rate and, 318, 319
  platelet synthesis of, 451
  in seminal vesicles, 976
Prostate gland, 307*f*, 973, 973*f*
  cancer of, 985
  function of, 976
  life cycle changes in, 984–985
  testosterone and, 982–983
Protanope, 616
Proteases, in thyroid hormone release, 908*f*, 909
Proteasomes, muscle atrophy and, 82
Protein(s). *See also* Plasma proteins.
  absorption of, 797
  amino acids stored as, 833
  as bases, 379
  as buffers, 383–384
    hemoglobin as, 383, 413
  in cell, 11
  in cell membrane, 13, 13*f*, 14, 45, 46*f*
  chemical structures of, 790, 831
  deposition of
    estrogens and, 994
    testosterone and, 835–836, 982–983, 1031
  in diabetes mellitus, depletion of, 951
  dietary
    complete vs. partial, 835, 843
    deficiency of, 843, 901, 902*f*
    energy available in, 843–844
    gastrin release stimulated by, 779
    glomerular filtration rate and, 321
    metabolic utilization of, 844–845
    recommended intake of, 835, 843
  digestion of, 789, 790–791, 791*f*
    enterogastric reflexes and, 767, 768
    pancreatic enzymes in, 781, 791
  as energy source, 834–835
    in starvation, 835, 843–844
  equilibrium between plasma and tissues, 833–834, 834*f*
  in feces, 798
  in interstitial fluid, 185, 187, 189
  in lipoproteins, 821, 821*t*
  in lymph, 187
  metabolism of, 834–835, 834*f*
    cortisol and, 928–929, 936
    hormonal regulation of, 835–836
    insulin and, 944–945
    liver's functions in, 839–840
  obligatory loss of, 835
  renal reabsorption of, 326
  specific dynamic action of, 864–865
  starvation-related depletion of, 852, 852*f*
  storage of
    insulin and, 835, 945
    in neonate, 1025
  structural, 27
  synthesis of. *See also* Transcription; Translation.
    chemical steps in, 34, 34*f*

Protein(s), synthesis of (*Continued*)
    endoplasmic reticulum and, 20, 20*f*, 33–34, 34*f*
    energy of ATP for, 22, 22*f*, 23, 859
    growth hormone and, 899, 902
    insulin and, 835, 944
    in neonate, 1025
  triglycerides synthesized from, 825
Protein C, 456–457
Protein channels, 45, 46–48, 46*f*, 48*f*. *See also* Ion channels.
  gating of, 47, 48, 48*f*, 49*f*
  selective permeability of, 47, 47*f*
Protein hormones, 881, 882, 885*f*
Protein kinase A, 932
Protein kinase C (PKC), 890, 890*f*
Protein kinases
  calmodulin-dependent, 891
  glucagon and, 948
  hormone action and, 882, 891
Protein sparers, 843–844
Proteinuria, in minimal change nephropathy, 313–314
Proteoglycan filaments, 180–181, 180*f*
  fluid flow and, 299
  of glomerular capillary wall, 312, 313
  interstitial fluid pressure and, 299
  as spacer for cells, 299
Proteoglycans, 14, 20
  of bone, 957, 958
Proteolytic enzymes
  in acrosome, 975, 977
  of phagocytic cells, 426
Proteoses, 783, 791
Prothrombin, 453, 453*f*, 454
Prothrombin activator, 453, 453*f*, 454–456, 455*f*, 456*f*
Prothrombin time, 460–461, 460*f*
Protoplasm, 11
Proximal tubule, 306, 306*f*
  glomerulotubular balance of, 334–335
  reabsorption in, 329–330, 329*f*, 330*f*
    of amino acids, 325–326
    of calcium, 368, 368*f*, 369
    of glucose, 325–326
    of phosphate, 369
    of potassium, 362, 363*f*
    of sodium, 327–328
    of water, 328
  secretion by, 329*f*, 330
  urine concentration and, 346, 346*f*, 348*t*, 352
PRU (peripheral resistance unit), 162–163
Pseudopodium, 23, 23*f*
Psychomotor seizure, 725*f*, 726
Psychosis, 726
  manic-depressive, 727
Pteroylglutamic acid. *See* Folic acid.
PTH. *See* Parathyroid hormone (PTH).
Ptyalin, 774*f*, 775, 790
Puberty
  female, 988, 993, 998–999, 998*f*, 999*f*
    anovulatory cycles at, 998
    gonadotropic hormone levels at, 998–999, 998*f*
    regulation of onset, 984, 999
Pudendal nerve
  external anal sphincter and, 771
  external bladder sphincter and, 308, 308*f*, 310
Pulmonary. *See also* Lungs.
Pulmonary artery(ies), 477
  distensibility of, 167
Pulmonary artery pressure, 158, 159*f*, 477, 478, 478*f*. *See also* Pulmonary hypertension.
  elevated, in mitral valve disease, 269
  during exercise, 480, 481*f*
  left-sided heart failure and, 481
Pulmonary artery stretch receptors, 208
  sodium excretion and, 376

Pulmonary capacities, 469–471, 469f, 470t
Pulmonary capillaries, 489, 490, 490f
  damage to, causing pulmonary edema, 482
  fluid exchange at, 481–483, 482f, 482t
  J receptors adjacent to, 512
  length of time blood stays in, 481
  oxygen therapy and, 521f
  pressure in, 158, 159f, 478, 478f, 481
  as sheet of flow, 481, 489
Pulmonary circulation, 157, 158f, 477–484
  anatomy of, physiologic, 477
  blood flow distribution
    alveolar oxygen concentration and, 479
    hydrostatic pressure zones and,
      479–481, 479f, 480f
    ventilation-perfusion ratio and,
      492–494
  blood volume in, 157, 478–479
  capillary dynamics in, 481–483, 482f
  exercise and, 480, 481f
  left-sided heart failure and, 478–479, 481
  pressures in, 158, 159f, 477–478, 478f
  two components of, 477
Pulmonary congestion
  in heart failure, left-sided, 259
  patent ductus arteriosus with, 270
Pulmonary edema, 482–483, 482f
  in acute mountain sickness, 530
  common causes of, 482
  in decompression sickness, 538
  in heart failure, 256, 298
    as acute edema, 261
    aortic valve lesions and, 268, 269
    decompensated, 258
    left-sided, 259, 482, 483
  after myocardial infarction, 250, 256
  oxygen therapy in, 521, 521f
  in oxygen toxicity, 537
  patent ductus arteriosus with, 270
  in shock, hypovolemic, 277
  in valvular heart disease
    aortic valve, 268, 269
    mitral valve, 269
Pulmonary embolism, 459
Pulmonary function, abbreviations and
  symbols for, 470t
Pulmonary function studies, 469–471, 469f
Pulmonary hypertension. See also Pulmonary
  artery pressure.
  emphysema leading to, 518
  endothelin receptor blockers for, 196
  at high altitude, 530, 531
Pulmonary membrane. See Respiratory
  membrane.
Pulmonary valve, 107
  congenital stenosis of, 136, 136f, 137
  second heart sound and, 107, 266, 266f
Pulmonary vascular resistance
  alveolar oxygen concentration and, 479
  decrease at birth, 1023
  total, 163
Pulmonary veins, 477
Pulmonary venous pressure, 478
Pulmonary ventilation, 465–475
  acid-base disorders and, 392
  alveolar. See Alveolar ventilation.
  definition of, 465
  energy required for, 468
  during exercise, 1037, 1037t
  mechanics of, 465–468, 466f, 467f
  minute respiratory volume in, 471
  respiratory passageways in, 472–475,
    472f
  volume and capacity measurements of,
    469–471, 469f, 470t
Pulmonary volumes, 469–471, 469f, 470t
Pulmonary wedge pressure, 478

Pulp
  of spleen, 175, 175f
  of teeth, 969, 969f, 970
Pulse deficit, premature contractions and, 146
Pulse pressure. See also Arterial pressure pulses.
  definition of, 168
  determinants of, 168–169
Punishment centers, 717–718
  memory and, 709
Pupillary diameter, 601–602, 602f
  autonomic control of, 632, 734t, 735
  dark adaptation by, 615
Pupillary light reflex, 623, 631f, 632, 735
  in central nervous system disease, 632
Pupillary reaction to accommodation, 632
Purines, 27, 37
Purkinje cells, 684–685, 684f, 686
Purkinje fibers, 115, 117–118
  action potentials in, 102f, 103, 117
  blocks in. See also Bundle branch block.
    multiple small, 138
    QRS prolongation caused by, 138
  ectopic pacemaker in, 119–120
  intrinsic rhythmicity of, 119
  synchronous ventricular contraction and, 119
Pursuit movement, 629
Pus, formation of, 430
Putamen, 670, 690, 690f, 691f
  Huntington's disease and, 694
  lesions in, 691
  neurotransmitters in, 692–693, 692f
  Parkinson's disease and, 693
Putamen circuit, 690–691, 690f, 691f
PVCs (premature ventricular contractions),
    146–147, 147f
  refractory period and, 103, 103f
Pyelonephritis, 403–404
Pyloric glands, 777, 778, 779
Pyloric pump, 767, 768
Pyloric sphincter, 756, 767, 768
Pylorus, 767
Pyramidal cells, 697, 698f
  in motor cortex, 669–670, 671, 672
    somatosensory feedback to, 672
Pyramidal tract. See Corticospinal
  (pyramidal) tract.
Pyridoxal phosphate, 854
Pyridoxine, 854–855
  amino acid synthesis and, 834, 854
Pyrimidines, 27, 37
Pyrogens, 875–876
Pyrophosphate, 958
Pyruvic acid, 22
  alanine derived from, 834, 834f
  conversion back to glucose, 816
  conversion to acetyl-CoA, 812–813
  conversion to lactic acid, 816
  from glycolysis, 812, 812f
  production from lactic acid, 816

Q
Q wave, 121, 121f, 132
  after myocardial infarction, 141, 141f
QRS complex, 121, 121f
  bizarre patterns of, 138, 141
  cardiac cycle and, 105, 105f
  current of injury and, 138, 139f
  monophasic action potential and, 122, 122f
  normal voltage of, 123
  prolonged
    definition of, 138
    after myocardial infarctions, 137, 137f, 141
    premature ventricular contractions with, 146
    from Purkinje system blocks, 136f, 138
    in ventricular hypertrophy or dilatation,
      137–138
  vectorial analysis of, 131–132, 132f

QRS complex (*Continued*)
  ventricular contraction and, 122–123
  voltage abnormalities of, 137, 137f
QRS vectorcardiogram, 134, 134f
Q-T interval, 121f, 123
  prolonged, 147, 148f
Quinidine
  for paroxysmal tachycardia, 148
  for ventricular tachycardia, 149

R
R wave, 121, 121f, 132
Radiation, heat loss by, 868–869, 869f
Radioimmunoassay, 891–892, 892f
Rage pattern, 718
  amygdala and, 719
  limbic cortex and, 720
  sympathetic discharge in, 739
RANK ligand, 959
Raphe magnus nucleus, 586–587, 587f
Raphe nuclei
  serotonin system and, 713, 713f
  sleep and, 722
Rapid ejection, period of, 106
Rate of movement sense, 571, 580
Rate receptors, 563
Rathke's pouch, 895
Reabsorption pressure, net, 185, 186
Reactive hyperemia, 194
Reading, 700, 702, 704f, 705
Reagins, 443, 444
Receptor field, of nerve fiber, 564
Receptor potentials, 560–562, 561f
  of cochlear hair cells, 637–638
  of rods, 612–613
  of taste cells, 647
Receptor proteins
  of olfactory cilium, 649, 649f
  postsynaptic, 547f, 548–550, 549f
    down-regulation or up-regulation of,
      569–570
  in taste villus, 647
Receptors, cell membrane, 14
  carbohydrates as, 14
  phagocytosis and, 19
  pinocytosis and, 18–19
Reciprocal inhibition, 566–567, 567f, 663
  flexor reflex and, 662, 662f, 663, 663f
Reciprocal innervation, 663, 672
Recoil pressure, of lungs, 467
Red blood cell count, in neonate, 1024, 1024f
Red blood cells (erythrocytes), 413–420
  A and B antigens on, 445–447, 446f, 446t,
    447t
  concentration of, in blood, 413
  cortisol and, 931
  destruction of, 840, 841
  fetal, 1019, 1020
  functions of, 413
  hemoglobin concentration in, 413. See also
    Hemoglobin.
  life span of, 419–420, 840
  metabolic systems of, 419
  production of, 414–417, 414f, 415f
    regulation of, 416–417, 416f
  radiolabeled, in blood volume
    measurement, 290
  shape and size of, 413, 415f
  spleen as reservoir for, 175
  splenic removal of, 175
  testosterone and, 982
Red muscle, 79
Red nucleus, 670–671, 671f, 678f
  basal ganglia and, 690f
  cerebellar input from, 687, 687f
  cerebellar input to, 684, 687
  dynamic neurons in, 672

Red pulp, of spleen, 175, 427–428
Reduced eye, 600
Re-entry, 149–150
   fibrillation and, 150
Referred pain, 588, 588f
   headache as, 591
   from visceral organs, 588, 589, 589f
Reflexes
   autonomic, 665, 729, 738
      local, 738
   spinal. *See* Spinal cord reflexes.
Reflexive learning, 709
Refraction of light, 597, 597f. *See also* Lenses.
Refractive errors, 602–604, 602f, 603f, 604f
Refractive index, 597
   of parts of eye, 600, 600f
Refractive power, 599f, 600, 600f
   of eye, 600, 600f
Refractory period
   of cardiac muscle, 103, 103f
   of nerve fiber, 69
Regression of tissues, lysosome role in, 19
Regulatory T cells, 442
Regurgitation, valvular, 267
Reinforcement, 718
Reissner's membrane, 634–635, 634f
Relative refractory period, of cardiac action
      potential, 103, 103f
Relaxin, 1009
Release sites, on presynaptic membrane, 548
Renal. *See also* Kidney(s).
Renal artery stenosis, 223–224, 223f, 407
Renal blood flow, 315, 316–317, 317t.
      See also Renal ischemia.
   age-related decrease in, 403
   autoregulation of, 317, 319–321, 319f, 320f
   estimation of, 340t, 341–342, 342f
   filtration fraction calculated from, 342
   medullary, 317, 351–352
   physiologic control of, 317–319
   in pregnancy, 1011
Renal clearance methods, 340–343, 340t, 341f,
      342f, 343t
Renal failure
   acute, 399
      body fluid effects of, 406, 406f
      causes of, 399–401, 400b
      in hypovolemic shock, 277–278
      physiologic effects of, 401
      in transfusion reactions, 448–449
   chronic, 399, 401–407. *See also* End-stage
         renal disease (ESRD).
      anemia in, 406
      body fluid effects of, 406–407, 406f
      causes of, 401, 402b
      glomerulonephritis leading to, 403
      hypertension leading to, 218
      metabolic acidosis in, 393
      nephron function in, 404–405, 405f,
         405t, 406f
      osteomalacia in, 406–407
      progression to end stage, 401–402,
         402f, 402t
      pyelonephritis leading to, 403–404
      transplantation for, 409
      vascular lesions leading to, 403
   dialysis for, 409–410, 409f, 410t
   nephrotic syndrome in, 404
Renal function curves, sodium-loading, 226,
      226f. *See also* Renal output curve.
Renal glycosuria, 408–409
Renal ischemia
   acute renal failure caused by, 399–400,
      400b, 401
   chronic renal failure associated
      with, 403
   hypertension caused by, 407

Renal output curve, 213, 214f
   angiotensin II and, 222, 222f
   chronic, 215–216, 215f
   determinants of pressure and, 214–215, 215f
   infinite feedback gain and, 214, 214f
Renal tubular acidosis, 392, 408
Renal tubules. *See also* Distal tubule; Loop of
      Henle; Proximal tubule.
   active transport in, 55–56, 55f
   hydrogen ion transport in, 54, 55
Renin, 220
   decreased, in primary aldosteronism, 936
   glomerular filtration rate and, 320
   increased, hypertension caused by, 407
Renin-angiotensin system
   aldosterone secretion and, 927
   arterial pressure control and, 220–222, 220f,
      221f, 222f
      in integrated response, 227, 227f, 228
   in cardiac failure, 260
   hypertension and, 223–224, 223f
   in hypovolemic shock, 275
Renointestinal reflex, 772
Renshaw cells, 656–657
Repolarization, in action potential, 61, 61f
Repolarization waves, 121–123, 122f. *See also*
      T wave.
   long QT syndromes and, 147, 148f
Reproduction, homeostatic function of, 6
Residual body, of digestive vesicle, 19, 19f
Residual volume, 469, 469f
   in asthma, 520
   determination of, 471
Resistance, vascular. *See* Vascular resistance.
Respiration. *See also* Breathing.
   artificial, 522–523, 522f
   in athletes, 1035f, 1036–1038, 1037f, 1037t
   functions carried out in, 465
   in neonates, 1021–1022, 1021f, 1024, 1026
   in pregnancy, 1010
   regulation of. *See* Respiratory control.
   thyroid hormones and, 913
Respiratory acidosis. *See* Acidosis, respiratory.
Respiratory alkalosis. *See* Alkalosis, respiratory.
Respiratory bronchiole, 472–473, 489, 489f
Respiratory center, 505–507, 506f
   brain edema and, 512
   chemoreceptor transmission to, 507, 508,
      508f, 509
   Cheyne-Stokes breathing and, 512
   direct chemical control of, 507–508,
      507f, 508f
   exercise-related stimulation of, 510, 511
   high altitude and, 529
   panting and, 871
   sleep apnea and, 513
Respiratory control, 505–513
   anesthesia and, 512
   brain edema and, 512
   in central sleep apnea, 513
   during exercise, 510–511, 510f, 511f
   irritant receptors in, 512
   J receptors in, 512
   in periodic breathing, 512–513, 512f
   peripheral chemoreceptors in, 507, 508–510,
      508f, 509f, 510f
   respiratory center in. *See* Respiratory center.
   voluntary, 512
Respiratory disorders, 515
   constricted, 516, 516f
   hypoxia in, 520
   methods for studying, 515
      blood gases and pH, 515–516
      forced expiratory vital capacity, 517, 517f
      forced expiratory volume, 517, 517f
      maximum expiratory flow, 516–517, 516f
      pulmonary function studies, 469–471, 469f

Respiratory disorders (*Continued*)
   specific pathophysiologies, 517–520
      asthma, 520
      atelectasis, 519, 519f
      emphysema, 517–518, 518f
      pneumonia, 518–519, 518f, 519f
      tuberculosis, 520
Respiratory distress syndrome, neonatal, 468,
      519, 1022, 1026
Respiratory exchange ratio, 504, 844–845
Respiratory membrane, 489–490, 490f
   diffusing capacity of, 491–492
      at high altitude, 529
   diffusion of gases through, 485, 486, 487,
      489–492, 492f
   impaired, hypoxia caused by, 520, 521,
      521f, 522
Respiratory muscles, 465, 466f
Respiratory passages, 472–475, 472f
   humidification in, 487, 487t
Respiratory quotient, 844–845
Respiratory rate, minute respiratory volume
      and, 471
Respiratory tract, insensible water loss through,
      285, 286t
Respiratory unit, 489, 489f
Respiratory waves, 210
Response element. *See* Hormone response
      element.
Resting membrane potential
   of gastrointestinal smooth muscle, 753–754,
      754f, 755
   of nerve fiber, 59–60, 59f, 60f
   of neuronal soma, 552, 552f
   of skeletal muscle fiber, 87
   of smooth muscle, 95
Resuscitators, respiratory, 522–523, 522f
Reticular activating system. *See* Reticular
      substance, excitatory area in.
Reticular lamina, hair cells and, 637–638,
      637f
Reticular nuclei, 673–674, 673f, 678
   alpha waves and, 724
   limbic system and, 715
Reticular substance
   autonomic regulation and, 739
   basal ganglia and, 690f
   cerebellar input to, 684
   excitatory area in, 711–712, 712f
      acetylcholine system and, 713
      auditory pathways and, 639
      sleep and, 722, 723
   hypothalamus and, 715
   inhibitory area in, 712, 712f
   limbic system and, 715
   motor fibers leading to, 670
   pain perception and, 586
   vestibular apparatus and, 678f
Reticulocerebellar tracts, 670, 683, 683f
Reticulocytes, 415, 415f, 417
Reticuloendothelial cells
   of liver sinusoids, 759–760, 837
   of spleen, 175
Reticuloendothelial system, 426–428. *See also*
      Macrophages, tissue.
Reticulospinal tracts, 670, 672f, 673–674, 674f,
      678, 678f
Retina, 609–621
   anatomic and functional elements of,
      609–611, 610f. *See also* Cones;
      Ganglion cells, of retina; Rods.
   blood supply of, 611
   electrotonic conduction in, 617–618
   glucose for, 949
   layers of, 609, 610f
   light and dark adaptation by, 614–615, 614f
   neural function of, 616–621, 617f, 618f, 620f

Retina (*Continued*)
  peripheral vs. central, 619. *See also* Fovea.
  photochemistry of, 611–615, 611*f*, 612*f*, 613*f*.
    See also Color vision.
Retinal, 611–612, 611*f*, 613
  identical in rods and cones, 614
Retinal artery, central, 611
Retinal detachment, 611
Retinal isomerase, 611*f*, 612
Retinitis pigmentosa, 627
Retinoid X receptor, 910, 911*f*, 962
Retinol, 853
Retrograde amnesia, 709
Retrolental fibroplasia, 197–198, 1027
Reverberatory circuits, 567–568, 567*f*, 568*f*
  continuous output from, 568, 568*f*
  in focal epilepsy, 726
  rhythmical output from, 568
Reverse enterogastric reflex, 780
Reverse T$_3$ (RT$_3$), 908*f*, 909, 909*f*
Reverse transcriptase, 41
Reward centers, 717, 718
  memory and, 709
Reynolds' number, 161–162
Rh blood types, 447–449
  erythroblastosis fetalis and, 420, 447–448,
    1024
Rh immunoglobulin globin, 448
Rheumatic fever, 442
  valvular lesions caused by, 266–267
Rhodopsin, 609, 611–614, 611*f*, 613*f*
  absorption curve for, 614, 614*f*
Rhodopsin kinase, 614
Rhythm method of contraception, 1001
Riboflavin (vitamin B$_2$), 854
Ribonucleic acid. *See* RNA (ribonucleic acid).
Ribose, 30
Ribosomal RNA, 31, 32
Ribosomes
  endoplasmic reticulum and, 14, 20, 20*f*,
    33–34, 34*f*
  formation of, 32
  insulin and, 944
  nucleoli and, 17, 32
  protein synthesis on, 32*f*, 33–35, 34*f*
  structure of, 32
Rickets, 968–969
  in hypophosphatemia, 408
  parathyroid enlargement in, 965
  vitamin D–resistant, 969
Rickettsia, 17–18, 18*f*
Right atrial pressure, 172
  cardiac output and, 172. *See also* Cardiac
    output curves.
  exercise and, 245
  in heart failure
    compensated, 257
    decompensated, 258
  measurement of, 174–175, 174*f*
  peripheral venous pressure and, 172
  venous return and. *See* Venous return curves.
Right atrium, stretch of, heart rate increase
    and, 110
Right bundle branch block, right axis deviation
    in, 136–137, 137*f*
Right ventricle
  external work output of, 108
  maximum systolic pressure, 108
Right ventricular dilatation, QRS prolongation
    in, 137–138
Right ventricular hypertrophy
  electrocardiogram with, 136, 136*f*, 137
    QRS prolongation in, 137–138
  in mitral valve disease, 269
Right ventricular pressure curve, 477, 478*f*
Right-handedness, 702
Righting reflex, 664

Right-sided heart failure, emphysema leading
    to, 518
Right-to-left shunt, 269
  in tetralogy of Fallot, 271, 271*f*
Rigor mortis, 82
RISC (RNA-induced silencing complex), 32–33
RNA (ribonucleic acid), 27, 27*f*
  building blocks of, 30
  noncoding, 32–33
  in nucleolus, 17
  synthesis of, 29*f*, 30–31
  types of, 31. *See also specific types.*
  viral, 18
RNA codons, 29*f*, 30, 31–32, 31*t*, 32*f*
RNA polymerase, 29*f*, 30, 35
RNA-induced silencing complex (RISC), 32–33
Rods, 609
  absorption curve for, 614, 614*f*
  dark adaptation by, 614–615
  electrotonic conduction in, 617–618
  ganglion cells excited by, 619
  neural circuitry and, 616–617, 617*f*
    pathway to ganglion cells, 617, 617*f*
  neurotransmitter released by, 617
  number of, 619
  of peripheral retina, 619
  photochemistry of, 611–614, 611*f*, 612*f*, 613*f*
  structure of, 609, 610*f*
Rods of Corti, 637, 637*f*
Root, of tooth, 969, 969*f*
Round window, 635, 635*f*
RT$_3$ (reverse T$_3$), 908*f*, 909, 909*f*
Rubrospinal tract, 670–671, 671*f*, 687, 687*f*
Ruffini's corpuscles, 572
  joint angulation and, 580
Ruffini's endings, 560*f*, 572
Rugae, of bladder mucosa, 308
Ryanodine receptor channels
  in cardiac muscle, 103
  in skeletal muscle, 88

S
S cells, intestinal, 782
S wave, 121, 121*f*, 132
Saccades, 629, 688
Saccule, 674–675, 675*f*, 676–677
Safety factor
  for nerve impulse propagation, 65
    local anesthetics and, 69
  of neuromuscular junction, 85–86
Sagittal sinus, negative pressure in, 173
Saline solutions
  fluid shifts and osmolarities caused by,
    293–294, 293*f*
  isotonic, 291–292, 293, 293*f*
Saliva, 775–776
  daily volume of, 775
  ions in, 775–776
  lingual lipase in, 792
  oral hygiene and, 776
  proteins in, 775
  ptyalin in, 774*f*, 775, 790
Salivary glands, 773, 774*f*, 775
  aldosterone and, 926
  blood supply to, 776
  nervous regulation of, 730–731, 731*f*, 734*t*,
    735, 776, 776*f*
  taste signals and, 648, 776
Salpingitis, infertility secondary to, 1002
Salt appetite, 360
Salt intake. *See also* Sodium; Sodium chloride.
  pressure diuresis and, 217–218. *See also*
    Pressure natriuresis.
  renin-angiotensin system and, 222, 222*f*, 228
Salt sensitivity, 216, 372
  essential hypertension and, 226, 226*f*
Saltatory conduction, 68, 68*f*

Salty taste, 645, 646, 646*t*
Sarcolemma, of skeletal muscle, 71, 87*f*
Sarcomere(s), of skeletal muscle, 71, 72*f*, 73*f*, 74
  addition or subtraction of, 82
  length of, tension and, 77, 77*f*
Sarcoplasm, 73
Sarcoplasmic reticulum
  of cardiac muscle, 103–104, 104*f*
  of skeletal muscle, 73, 73*f*
    in fast fibers, 79
    release of calcium by, 74, 88–89, 88*f*
    T tubules and, 87*f*, 88, 88*f*
    uptake of calcium by, 74, 78, 88–89, 88*f*
  of smooth muscle, 97–98, 98*f*
Satiety, 845
Satiety center, 716, 845, 849
Saturated fat, blood cholesterol and, 827
Saturation diving, 539
Scala media, 634–635, 634*f*, 635*f*, 637
Scala tympani, 634–635, 634*f*, 635*f*, 636, 637
Scala vestibuli, 634–635, 634*f*, 635*f*, 636, 637
Schistosomiasis, 430
Schizophrenia, 727
Schlemm, canal of, 607, 607*f*, 608
Schwann cells, 67, 67*f*
  at neuromuscular junction, 83
  at smooth muscle nerve endings, 95
Scotomata, 627
Scotopsin, 611–612, 611*f*
Scratch reflex, 664
SCUBA diving, 539, 539*f*
Scurvy, 855
Second heart sound, 265–266, 267*f*
Second messengers, 14. *See also* Cyclic
    adenosine monophosphate (cAMP);
    Cyclic guanosine monophosphate
    (cGMP).
  adrenergic or cholinergic receptors and, 733
  hormonal functions and, 888, 889–891
    adenylyl cyclase-cAMP and, 889–890,
      889*b*, 890*f*
    aldosterone and, 927
    calcium-calmodulin and, 891
    phospholipase C and, 890, 890*b*, 890*f*
    thyroid hormones and, 910, 914
  in postsynaptic neurons, 548–549, 549*f*
  in smooth muscle, 97
  in taste cells, 647
Second-degree heart block, 145, 145*f*
Secretin, 758, 758*t*
  bile secretion and, 784, 784*f*, 785
  duodenal mucous glands and, 786
  gastric secretion and, 780
  molecular structure of, 780
  pancreatic secretions and, 782–783, 800
  small intestine motility and, 769
  stomach emptying and, 768
Secretory granules. *See* Secretory vesicles.
Secretory vesicles, 16, 16*f*, 21
  of gastrointestinal glands, 774
  of polypeptide and protein hormones, 882
Segmentation contractions
  of colon, 770
  of small intestine, 768–769, 768*f*
Seizures. *See also* Epilepsy.
  hippocampal, 719
  in oxygen poisoning, 536
Self-antigens, 434–435
Semen, 976–977
  ejaculation of, 979
Semicircular ducts, 674, 675*f*, 676, 676*f*,
    677, 677*f*
  flocculonodular lobes and, 678, 689
Semilunar valves, 106–107, 107*f*. *See also*
    Aortic valve; Pulmonary valve.
  second heart sound and, 107, 265–266
Seminal vesicles, 973, 973*f*, 976

Seminiferous tubules, 973–974, 973*f*, 974*f*
  estrogen in, 980
  injury to, 977
  negative feedback control of, 984
Sensitization, memory and, 706
Sensory areas, of cerebral cortex, 698, 698*f*, 699*f*
Sensory nerve fibers
  classification of, 563–564, 563*f*
  in spinal cord, 655, 655*f*, 656–657, 656*f*
  summation in, 564, 564*f*, 565*f*
Sensory pathways. *See also* Anterolateral system; Dorsal column–medial lemniscal system.
  into central nervous system, 569
  corticofugal, 581–582
  inhibitory feedback in, 569
Sensory receptors, 543, 544*f*. *See also* Tactile receptors.
  adaptation of, 562–563, 562*f*
  differential sensitivity of, 559
  receptor potentials of, 560–562, 561*f*
  types of, 559, 560*b*, 560*f*
Sensory signals
  brain stem excitatory area and, 711–712
  hippocampal activation by, 718–719
Sensory stimulus intensity
  enormous range of, 579
  judgment of, 579, 580*f*
Septic shock, 280
  disseminated intravascular coagulation in, 459
Serotonin
  in basal ganglia, 692–693, 692*f*
  as central nervous system transmitter, 551
  depression and, 726–727
  endogenous analgesia system and, 587
  from mast cells and basophils, 431
  memory and, 707–708
  reticular inhibitory area and, 712
  sleep and, 722
  small intestine peristalsis and, 769
Serotonin system, in brain, 712, 713, 713*f*
Sertoli cells, 974, 974*f*, 975, 976
  estrogen formed by, 980
  follicle-stimulating hormone and, 984
  inhibin secreted by, 984
Serum, 454
Sex chromosomes, 974–975, 981, 1003, 1004
Sex determination, 1004
Sex hormone–binding globulin, 980
Sexual act
  female, 1000
  lubrication for
    by female glands, 1000
    by male glands, 979
  male, 978–979
Sexual behavior
  amygdala and, 720
  hypothalamus and, 717
Sexual function, thyroid hormones and, 914
Sexual reflexes, 738, 978, 1000
Sexual sensation
  anterolateral system and, 573
  male structures associated with, 978
Shaken baby syndrome, 746
Shingles, 590
Shivering, 867
  fever and, 876, 876*f*
  hypothalamic stimulation of, 873
    set-point and, 874, 874*f*
  primary motor center for, 873
  skin receptors and, 872
Shock. *See* Anaphylactic shock; Cardiogenic shock; Circulatory shock; Hypovolemic shock; Septic shock
Shock lung syndrome, 277–278

Short interfering RNA (siRNA), 33
Shunt
  congenital, 269. *See also* Patent ductus arteriosus.
  physiologic, 493, 494
    oxygen therapy and, 521
Shunt flow, 496
Sibutramine, for weight loss, 851
Sickle cell anemia, 415*f*, 420
  hemoglobin structure in, 418
Signal transducer and activator of transcription (STAT) proteins, 888
Silencing RNA (siRNA), 33
Siliconized containers, 460
Simple cells, of visual cortex, 626, 627
Simple spike, 685
Sinoatrial block, 144, 144*f*
Sinoatrial node. *See* Sinus node.
Sinus arrhythmia, 144, 144*f*
Sinus bradycardia, 143–144, 143*f*
Sinus node, 115–116, 116*f*
  action potentials in, 115–116, 116*f*
  atrial stretch and, 229–230
  as pacemaker, 118–119
  parasympathetic stimulation and, 119, 120
  sympathetic stimulation and, 120
Sinus tachycardia, 143, 143*f*
Sinuses, nasal, headache associated with, 591–592, 591*f*
siRNA (silencing RNA), 33
Size principle, 80
Skeletal motor nerve axis, 543–544, 544*f*
Skeletal muscle, 71–82. *See also* Motor functions; Neuromuscular junction.
  action potentials in. *See* Action potential(s), skeletal muscle.
  agonist-antagonist coactivation of, 81
    neuronal circuits and, 566
  in arterial pressure control, 209–210
  in athletes. *See* Sports physiology, muscles in.
  atrophy of, 81, 82
  blood flow in, 191, 192*t*, 243
    control of, 191, 195, 196–197, 198, 243–244
    during exercise, 1038, 1038*f*, 1038*t*
    during rhythmical contractions, 243, 244*f*, 1038*f*
    total body circulation and, 244–245
  capillary pores in, permeability of, 179, 180*t*
  vs. cardiac muscle, 102–104
  central nervous system control of, 543–544, 544*f*
  contraction mechanism of, 74–78, 74*f*, 75*f*, 76*f*
    sequential steps of, 73–74
  contracture of, 82
  decreased mass of, cardiac output and, 234
  denervation of, 82
  different functional types of, 79, 79*f*, 81
  efficiency of, 78–79
  energy sources for, 73, 74, 75, 76, 78–79
    in athletes, 1032, 1033*f*, 1033*t*, 1034*b*, 1035, 1035*f*
  excitation-contraction coupling in, 87, 88–89, 88*f*, 89*f*
  fast and slow fibers in, 79, 1036, 1036*t*
  fatigue in, 80–81
  fatty acid diffusion into, 820
  force of
    vs. length, 77, 77*f*
    vs. velocity of contraction, 77–78, 77*f*
  glucose in, insulin and, 941–942, 946*f*
  glycogen in, 78, 80–81, 811, 941
    during exercise, 1032, 1032*t*, 1035
    recovery of, 1034, 1035*f*
  hyperplasia of, 82

Skeletal muscle (*Continued*)
  hypertrophy of, 81–82
    exercise training and, 1035–1036
  innervation of, 80, 83
  insulin and, 941–942, 946*f*
  isometric vs. isotonic contraction of, 79, 79*f*
  length of
    vs. force, 77, 77*f*
    remodeling of, 82
  lever systems using, 81, 81*f*
  maximum strength of, 80
  motor units of, 80
    after poliomyelitis, 82
  remodeling of, to match function, 81–82
  respiratory, 465, 466*f*
    dyspnea associated with, 522
  sensory receptors in. *See* Golgi tendon organs; Muscle spindles.
  vs. smooth muscle, 91, 92–93, 94
  staircase effect of, 80
  strenuous bursts of activity with, 860–861
  structural organization of, 71–73, 72*f*, 73*f*
  summation in, 80, 80*f*
  sympathetic vasodilator system and, 204
  tension developed in, 77, 77*f*
  testosterone and, 835–836, 982
  tetanization in, 80, 80*f*
  thyroid hormones and, 913
  tone of, 80
  velocity of contraction vs. load on, 77–78, 77*f*
  work output of, 78
Skill learning, 709
Skill memory, 706–707
Skin
  blood flow control in, 195
  cholesterol in, 827
  in defense against infection, 433
  estrogens and, 994
  heat loss through
    blood flow and, 868, 868*f*
    mechanisms of, 868–870, 869*f*
  homeostatic functions of, 6
  insensible water loss through, 285, 286*t*
  testosterone and, 982
  tissue macrophages in, 426
  vitamin D synthesis in, 960
Skin graft, interstitial fluid pressure and, 183
Skin temperature, 867
  local reflexes regulating, 875
  set-point and, 874, 874*f*
Sleep, 721–725
  basic theories of, 722–723
  brain waves in, 723, 724, 725, 725*f*
  cycle between wakefulness and, 722–723
  growth hormone secretion and, 901, 901*f*
  metabolic rate and, 864
  physiologic functions of, 723–724
  rapid eye movement (REM), 712–713, 721–722
    brain waves in, 725, 725*f*
    deprivation of, 723
    possible cause of, 722
  slow-wave, 721–725
    brain waves in, 725, 725*f*
  thyroid hormones and, 913
Sleep apnea, 513
Slit pores, of glomerular capillaries, 312–313, 313*f*
Slow calcium channels, 64
  in cardiac muscle, 102–103
Slow ejection, period of, 106
Slow muscle fibers, 79
Slow pain, 583
Slow sodium-calcium channels, in cardiac muscle, 66, 115
  sinus nodal action potential and, 116
  ventricular action potential and, 115–116

Slow waves, of gastrointestinal smooth muscle, 753–754, 754f, 755
  in small intestine, 769
  in stomach, 766
Slow-chronic pain pathway, 584–585, 585f, 586
Slow-reacting substance of anaphylaxis, 443, 444
  in asthma, 520
  bronchiolar constriction caused by, 473
Slow-twitch muscle fibers, 1036, 1036t
Sludged blood
  in circulatory shock, 277
  in septic shock, 280
Small interfering RNA (siRNA), 33
Small intestine. *See also* Duodenum.
  absorption in
    active transport in, 55–56, 55f
    anatomical basis of, 793–794, 793f, 794f
    of ions, 794–796, 795f
    of nutrients, 796–797
    total area of, 794
    total capacity of, 794
    total volume of, 793
    of water, 794
  carbohydrate digestion in, 790
  digestive enzymes of, 787, 790
  disorders of, 801–802
  fat digestion in. *See* Fats, digestion of.
  malabsorption by, 801–802
  movements of, 768–770, 768f, 770f
  obstruction of, 804, 804f
  peptic ulcer of, 800, 801
  secretions of, 786–787
  secretory cells of, 773, 774f
Smell, 648–652. *See also* Olfaction.
  adaptation of, 650
  affective nature of, 650
  intensities detectable by, 650
  olfactory cell stimulation in, 649–650, 649f
  olfactory membrane in, 648–649, 649f
  primary sensations of, 650
  signal transmission into central nervous system, 651–652, 651f
  taste and, 645
  threshold for, 650
Smoking
  atherosclerosis and, 829
  peptic ulcer and, 801
  pulmonary ventilation in exercise and, 1037–1038
Smooth endoplasmic reticulum, 14, 15f, 20, 20f
Smooth muscle, 91–98
  action potentials in. *See* Action potential(s), smooth muscle.
  autonomic innervation and control of, 94–95, 94f
  contractile mechanism in, 92–93, 92f
    calcium ions and, 93–94, 94f, 97–98
  contraction without action potentials, 96, 97
  energy requirement of, 93
  of gut, stretch-induced excitation of, 96
  hormonal effects on, 97
  junctional potential of, 96
  latch mechanism of, 93, 94
  latent period of, 97–98
  of lymphatic vessels, 188
  maximum force of contraction, 93
  of metarterioles, 177, 193
  multi-unit, 91, 91f, 95, 96
  neuromuscular junctions of, 94–95, 94f
  pacemaker waves of, 96
  peristalsis in, 759
  of precapillary sphincter, 177, 193
  resting membrane potential of, 95
  vs. skeletal muscle, 91, 92–93, 94
  slow wave rhythm of, 95f, 96
  stimulatory factors for, 94, 97

Smooth muscle (*Continued*)
  stress-relaxation of, 93
    reverse, 93
  structural organization of, 91, 91f, 92, 92f
  of trachea, bronchi, and bronchioles, 472–473
  types of, 91, 91f. *See also specific types.*
  vascular. *See also* Blood flow control.
    autoregulation of blood flow and, 194–195
    intrinsic tone of, 737
    local factors controlling, 97
    nitric oxide and, 195, 196f
Sneeze reflex, 473, 512
Sodium. *See also* Hypernatremia; Hyponatremia; Salt intake; Sodium chloride.
  in bone, 957–958
  in cerebrospinal fluid, 747
  dietary intake of
    arterial pressure and, 376
    integrated responses to, 376
    potassium intake and, 367
    recommendations for, 367
  diffusion through capillary pores, 179, 180t
  extracellular fluid, regulation of, 345, 355
    angiotensin II and aldosterone in, 359–360, 359f, 927, 928
    by osmoreceptor-ADH system, 345, 355–357, 358–359, 360
    salt appetite and, 360
    by thirst, 357–360, 358t, 359f
  extracellular fluid volume and, 370–371, 375–376
  intestinal absorption of, 794–795, 795f, 797
    in colon, 795, 797
  intestinal secretion of, 787
  neuronal somal membrane and, 552, 552f
  plasma concentration of
    aldosterone and, 925
    with reduced GFR, 404, 405, 405f
  postsynaptic potentials and, 553, 553f
  renal adaptation to intake of, 303, 304f
  renal excretion of. *See also* Pressure natriuresis.
    angiotensin II and, 374–375, 374f
    balance of intake and, 370
    diuretics and, 397, 398f
    regulation of, 370–371
  renal reabsorption of, 324, 325, 325f
    aldosterone and, 328, 337–338, 375
    angiotensin II and, 338–339, 338f
    arterial pressure and, 337
    atrial natriuretic peptide and, 339
    chloride ions and, 328, 328f
    diuretics and, 397
    estrogen and, 994
    with gradient-time transport, 327–328
    hydrogen ions and, 326, 331, 331f, 390
    oxygen consumption and, 316, 317f
    in pregnancy, 1009, 1011
    by principal cells, 332
    sympathetic activation and, 339
    with transport maximum, 328
    urine concentration and, 353
    water reabsorption and, 328
  in saliva, 774f, 775, 776
  salty taste of ions of, 645
  in sweat gland secretions, 870–871
Sodium bicarbonate. *See also* Bicarbonate.
  for acidosis, 393
  metabolic alkalosis caused by, 393
Sodium channel blockers, 332, 333f, 398t, 399
Sodium chloride. *See also* Chloride; Salt intake; Sodium.
  diarrheal loss of, 796
  mineralocorticoid deficiency and, 924

Sodium chloride (*Continued*)
  renal retention of, angiotensin II and, 221–222, 222f
  renal transport of
    in distal tubule, 331–332, 332f
    urine concentration and, 348–349, 348t, 353
  replacement of, in athletes, 1040
  tubuloglomerular feedback and, 319–320, 320f, 321
Sodium co-transport, 54–55, 55f
  of amino acids and peptides, 54–55, 794–795, 795f, 797
  of glucose, 325–326, 326f, 794–795, 795f, 796, 811
Sodium counter-transport, 55, 55f
Sodium gluconate, for acidosis, 393
Sodium ion channels, 47, 48, 48f. *See also* Calcium-sodium channels.
  acetylcholine-gated, 73–74, 84, 84f, 85, 85f
  epithelial, aldosterone and, 926–927, 926f
  in olfactory cilium, 649, 649f
  of photoreceptors, 612–613, 612f, 613–614, 613f
  of postsynaptic neuronal membrane, 548, 549
  of smooth muscle, 97
  voltage-gated, of muscle fiber, 73–74
  voltage-gated, of nerve membrane, 48, 49f, 61–63, 61f, 62f, 64
    calcium ion concentration and, 64
    local anesthetics and, 69
    propagation of impulse and, 64–65
    refractory period and, 69
Sodium lactate, for acidosis, 393
Sodium space, 289
Sodium-calcium counter-transporter, renal, 368–369, 368f
Sodium-calcium exchanger, in cardiac muscle, 104, 104f
  digitalis activity and, 258
Sodium-chloride co-transport, thiazide diuretics and, 398
Sodium-chloride-potassium co-transport, loop diuretics and, 397–398
Sodium-hydrogen counter-transport, renal, 386–387, 386f
Sodium-iodide symporter, 908, 908f
Sodium-loading renal function curves, 226, 226f
Sodium-potassium ATPase pump, 53–54, 53f
  in cardiac muscle, 104, 104f
    digitalis activity and, 258
  gastric acid secretion and, 777, 778f
  intestinal absorption and, 794–795
  iodide trapping and, 908, 908f
  potassium secretion and, 362, 363–364, 363f, 367
  in re-establishing ionic gradients, 65
  renal reabsorption and, 324, 325, 325f, 327–328
    of bicarbonate, 386–387, 386f
    in collecting tubule, 332, 333f, 337
    in distal tubule, 331–332, 332f, 333f
    in loop of Henle, 331, 331f
  resting membrane potential and, 59, 59f, 60, 60f
  synthesis of, 926–927, 926f
  thyroid hormones and, 912
Solubility coefficients, of gases, 485–486, 486t
Solvent drag, 328
Soma of neuron, 547, 547f
  ion concentration differences and, 552–553, 552f
  resting membrane potential of, 552, 552f
  uniform electrical potential in, 553
Somatic senses. *See also* Sensory pathways.
  classification of, 571
  definition of, 571

Somatomedin C, 900–901
Somatomedins, 900–901
Somatosensory association areas, 577
Somatosensory cortex, 574–577, 575f, 576f
  basal ganglia and, 691, 691f
  cerebellar communication with, 682,
      686, 688
  corticospinal tract and, 669
  motor cortex and, 667, 668f
  thermal signals to, 593
Somatostatin, 898, 898t, 901–902, 949
  gastric secretion and, 780
  pancreatic secretion of, 939
Somatotropes, 896, 896t, 897
Somatotropin. *See* Growth hormone (GH;
  somatotropin).
Sound. *See* Hearing.
Sour taste, 645, 646, 646t
  salivation and, 776
Spacecraft
  acceleratory forces in, 531, 532, 532f
  atmosphere in, 533
  motion sickness in, 533
  weightlessness in, 533–534
Spaces of Disse, 837, 837f, 838
Spasticity, stroke leading to, 673
Spatial coordinates of body
  posterior parietal cortex and, 692, 699, 699f
  prefrontal cortex and, 700
Spatial summation
  in neurons, 555
  in sensory fibers, 564, 564f
    auditory, 638
    thermal, 593
Special senses, definition of, 571
Speech, 474–475, 703–704. *See also* Language.
  articulation in, 704
  Broca's area and, 668–669, 669f,
      702, 704, 704f
  cerebellar lesions and, 689
Sperm count, 978
Spermatids, 974, 974f, 975
Spermatocytes, 974, 974f
Spermatogenesis, 973–976, 974f
  abnormal, 977–978
  estrogen in, 980
  follicle-stimulating hormone and, 975, 983,
      983f, 984
  temperature and, 977, 978
Spermatogonia, 973–976, 974f
Spermatozoa, 974, 974f, 975, 975f. *See also*
    Fertilization.
  abnormal, 978, 978f
  capacitation of, 976–977
  in fallopian tube, 1000, 1003
  maturation of, 975, 976
  mature, physiology of, 976
  in semen, 976–977
  storage of, in testes, 975–976
Spherocytosis, hereditary, 420
Sphincter of Oddi, 780–781, 784f, 785
Sphingolipids, of capillary membrane, 178, 178f
Sphingomyelin, 67
  chemical structure of, 826, 826f
  function of, 826
Spike potentials
  of gastrointestinal smooth muscle,
      753–755, 754f
  of visceral smooth muscle, 95–96, 95f
Spinal anesthesia. *See* Anesthesia, spinal.
Spinal cord
  ascending tracts of, 590f
  cerebellar functions and, 686–687
  cerebellar input from, 683, 683f
  descending tracts of, 590f
  lateral motor system of, 671
  medial motor system of, 671

Spinal cord (*Continued*)
  motor functions of, 655
    excitation by cortex for, 671–673, 672f
    in integrated control system, 694
    organization for, 655–657, 655f, 656f
    pathways from cortex for, 669–671,
        670f, 671f
    reflexes in. *See* Spinal cord reflexes.
    sensory receptors and. *See* Golgi tendon
        organs.
    temperature receptors in, 872
    transection of, 665
Spinal cord injury
  defecation abnormalities in, 803
  micturition abnormalities in, 310
Spinal cord level, 545
Spinal cord reflexes, 694
  autonomic, 665
    defecation reflex, 771, 771f, 803
  cortical input and, 672
  crossed extensor reflex, 663, 663f
  in fetus, 1020
  flexor reflex, 661–663, 662f, 663f
  gastrointestinal, 757
  memory and, 706
  muscle spasm caused by, 664–665
  muscle stretch reflex, 658–659, 658f, 659f
  neuronal organization for, 655–657, 655f, 656f
  postural and locomotive, 663–664
  scratch reflex, 664
  sexual act and, 978, 1000
  spinal shock and, 665
  in temperature regulation, 875
  tendon reflex, 661
Spinal nerves
  dermatomes associated with, 582, 582f
  parasympathetic fibers and, 730–731, 731f
  skeletal motor function and. *See* Motor
      neurons, anterior.
  sympathetic chains and, 729, 730f
Spinal shock, 665
Spindle, mitotic, 17, 38–39
Spinocerebellar tracts, 683, 683f, 687, 687f
  lesions in, 683, 683f, 689
Spinocerebellum, 686, 687–688, 687f
Spino-olivary pathway, 683
Spinoreticular pathway, 683
Spinothalamic tracts, 573f, 575f, 580, 581
Spiral ganglion of Corti, 634f, 636–637,
    636f, 639
Spirometry, 469, 469f, 470–471
  forced vital capacity in, 517, 517f
Spironolactone, 332, 333f, 399
Splanchnic circulation, 759–760, 760f
  vasoconstriction in, in exercise or shock, 762
Spleen
  as blood reservoir, 175, 175f
  macrophages of, 427–428
Sports physiology, 1031–1041. *See also*
    Exercise.
  body fluids and salt in, 1040
  body heat in, 1039–1040
  cardiovascular system in, 1038–1039, 1038f,
      1038t, 1039f, 1039t
  drugs in, 1040
  energy for specific sports in, 1033, 1034b
  female and male athletes in, 1031
  muscles in, 1031–1036
    endurance of, 1032, 1032t, 1033
    metabolic systems in, 1032, 1033f,
        1033t, 1034b
    nutrients used in, 1035, 1035f
    power of, 1032, 1032t, 1033
    strength of, 1031, 1032
    training effect on, 1035–1036, 1035f
  respiration in, 1035f, 1036–1038, 1037f,
      1037t

Sprue, 801–802, 854
  anemia in, 420, 802
Staircase effect, 80
Stapedius muscle, 634
Stapes, 633–634, 633f, 635, 635f, 636
  conduction deafness and, 642
Staphylococcal infection, inflammatory
    response to, 428
Starches
  dietary, 789–790
  digestion of, 790, 790f
    in neonate, 1025
Starling equilibrium, for capillary exchange,
    185–186, 185t
Starling forces, 181
Starvation, 852, 852f. *See also* Malnutrition,
    and metabolic rate.
  fatty acids in blood in, 821
  growth hormone secretion in, 901
  ketosis in, 823
  protein degradation in, 835
  triglycerides in liver in, 822
STAT (signal transducer and activator of
    transcription) proteins, 888
Static position sense, 571, 580
Statins, 829
Statoconia, 675–676, 675f
Stearic acid, 819
  ATP from oxidation of, 823
Steatohepatitis, nonalcoholic (NASH), 838
Steatorrhea
  calcium and vitamin D deficiency in, 969
  in sprue, 802
Stellate cells
  of cerebellum, 685
  of cerebral cortex. *See* Granular cells.
Stem cells
  bone, 960
  pluripotential hematopoietic, 414–415, 414f,
      423–424
Stent, coronary artery, 253
Stepping movements, 664
Stercobilin, 840–841, 841f, 842
Stereocilia
  of cochlea, 637–638
  of vestibular apparatus, 675–676, 675f
Stereopsis, 605, 605f, 625, 630
Sterility. *See* Infertility.
Steroid hormones, 882. *See also* Adrenocortical
    hormones; Androgens; Ovarian
    hormones.
  cholesterol used for, 827, 882
  mechanism of action, 891
  nongenomic actions of, 927
  receptors for, 891
  structures of, 885f
Stimulatory field, 565
Stokes-Adams syndrome, 119, 145
Stomach. *See also* Gastric *entries*.
  absorption in, 793
  anatomy of, 766, 766f
  emptying of. *See* Stomach emptying.
  fat digestion in, 792
  gastrin secretion by, 758, 758t
  mixing function of, 765, 766
  motilin secretion by, 758–759
  peristalsis of, 766
    emptying and, 766, 767
  protein digestion in, 791, 791f
  secretions of. *See* Gastric secretion.
  starch digestion in, 790
  storage function of, 765, 766
  ulcers of. *See* Peptic ulcer.
Stomach emptying, 765, 766–767
  regulation of, 767–768, 780
    peptic ulcer and, 800
Storage colon, 797

Strabismus, 630–631, 630*f*
Streamline flow, 161
Streptococcal infection
  glomerulonephritis secondary to, 400
  inflammatory response to, 428
Streptococcus mutans, 971
Streptokinase, 259
Stress
  ACTH secretion and, 932–933
  arterial pressure increase in, 205
  cortisol and, 929, 930, 930*f*, 932–933
  fat utilization in, 825
Stress response, of sympathetic nervous
    system, 738–739
Stress-relaxation of blood vessels, 227, 227*f*
  increased blood volume and, 238
  intravascular pressure and, 168, 168*f*
  reverse, in hypovolemic shock, 275
Stress-relaxation of smooth muscle, 93
  reverse, 93
Stretch receptors
  atrial. *See* Atrial stretch receptors.
  of bronchi and bronchioles, 506
Stretch reflex. *See* Muscle stretch reflex.
Stria vascularis, 637
Striate cortex, 624
Striated muscle. *See also* Skeletal muscle.
  band structure of, 71
  cardiac muscle as, 101
Stroke
  cerebral circulation and, 745–746
  hypertension and, 218
  motor control system and, 673
Stroke volume output, 106, 109*f*
  aortic valve lesions and, 268
  athletic training and, 1039, 1039*f*
  pulse pressure and, 168–169
Stroke work output, 107–108
Stroke work output curve, 110, 110*f*
Strychnine, 557
Stumble reflex, 664
Subarachnoid space, 747, 747*f*
Subcortical level of nervous system, 545
Subcutaneous tissues, macrophages in, 426
Subendocardial infarction, 249–250
Subliminal zone, 565–566
Sublingual glands, 775
Submandibular glands, 774*f*, 775
Submarines, 540
Submucosal plexus, 755, 756, 756*f*
  parasympathetic neurons in, 757
  of small intestine, 769
Subneural clefts, 83, 84*f*
Substance P, 586
Substantia gelatinosa, 585, 585*f*
Substantia nigra, 690, 690*f*, 691, 691*f*
  dopamine system and, 713, 713*f*
  Huntington's disease and, 694
  neurotransmitters in, 692–693, 692*f*
  Parkinson's disease and, 691, 693–694
Subthalamus, 690, 690*f*, 691, 691*f*
  lesions in, 691, 693–694
Subthreshold stimulus, 565
Subthreshold zone, 565–566
Sucrase, 787, 790
Sucrose, 789–790
Sulfonylurea drugs, 945
Summation
  in neuronal pools, 566
  of postsynaptic potentials, 553, 554*f*, 555,
    556–557
  in sensory fibers, 564, 564*f*, 565*f*
    thermal, 593
  of skeletal muscle contractions, 80, 80*f*
Superior cervical ganglion, 631, 631*f*
Superior colliculus
  involuntary visual fixation and, 629

Superior colliculus (*Continued*)
  turning to visual disturbance and, 630
  visual fibers to, 623
Superior olivary nuclei, 639, 639*f*, 641–642
Superior salivatory nucleus, 648
Superoxide
  high alveolar Po$_2$ and, 536–537
  of neutrophils and macrophages, 426
Superoxide dismutases, 536–537
Supplementary motor area, 668, 668*f*, 669,
    698, 699*f*
  basal ganglia and, 690*f*, 691–692, 691*f*
Suppressor T cells, 441, 441*f*, 442
Suprachiasmatic nucleus, visual fibers to, 623
Supraoptic nucleus, pituitary hormones and,
    897, 904, 904*f*, 905, 906
Suprathreshold stimulus, 565
Supraventricular tachycardias, 148
Surface tension, in alveoli, 467–468
  of premature babies, 468
Surfactant, 468, 490
  neonatal respiratory distress and, 468, 519,
    1022
Surround inhibition, 578–579, 578*f*
Sustentacular cells
  of olfactory membrane, 649, 649*f*
  of taste bud, 646
Swallowing, 763–765, 764*f*
  disorders of, 799
  esophageal secretions and, 776–777
Swallowing center, 764, 764*f*, 765
Swallowing reflex, 764, 765
Sweat
  composition of, 870–871
  water loss in, 285, 286*t*
Sweat glands, 870, 870*f*
  aldosterone and, 926
  autonomic control of, 729–730, 730*f*, 731,
    734*t*, 735, 870–871
Sweating, 870–871. *See also* Evaporative
    heat loss.
  acclimatization to heat and, 871, 877
  hypothalamic control of, 870, 872, 872*f*
    set-point and, 874, 874*f*
  local, 875
  skin receptors and, 872
Sweet taste, 645, 646, 646*t*, 647
Sympathetic chains, 729, 730*f*
Sympathetic denervation, 737
Sympathetic nervous system. *See also*
    Autonomic nervous system.
  adrenal function and. *See* Adrenal medulla.
  alarm response of, 738–739
  anatomy of, physiologic, 729–730, 730*f*
  bladder and, 308, 308*f*
  blood reservoirs and, 175
  bronchiolar dilation and, 473
  in cardiac failure
    acute stage, 255–256, 256*f*, 257, 262
    decline to normal, 257
    decompensated, 262–263
    fluid retention and, 260
  cardiac innervation by, 111, 111*f*,
    119, 201, 202*f*
  cardiac regulation by, 111, 111*f*, 120
    cardiac output and, 231, 238–239, 239*f*
    after myocardial infarction, 251
    tachycardia and, 143
    vasomotor center and, 203
  cerebral blood flow and, 745
  circulatory control by, 201–204, 202*f*
    mean circulatory filling pressure and,
      236, 236*f*
    volume-pressure curves and, 168, 168*f*
  coronary blood flow and, 247, 248
  energy expenditure and, 849
  exercise-related discharge of, 244–245

Sympathetic nervous system (*Continued*)
  eye control by, 631, 632
    Horner's syndrome and, 632
  fatty acid mobilization caused by, 825
  gastrointestinal regulation by, 755, 757
    duodenal mucus and, 786
    glandular secretions and, 774
    ileocecal sphincter and, 770
    reflexes in, 757
    stomach emptying and, 767
    vasoconstriction in, 762
  glomerular filtration rate and, 317–318
  glucose availability and, 812
  heat conduction to skin and, 868
  in hypovolemic shock, 274–275
    vasomotor failure and, 277
  localized activation of, 738
  male sexual act and, 979
  mass discharge of, 738
  metabolic rate and, 867
  nonshivering thermogenesis and, 865
  obesity and, 225
  renal function and, 373–374
    sodium reabsorption in, 339
  salivary glands and, 776
  segmental distribution of fibers in, 730
  sweat glands and, 729–730, 730*f*, 731, 734*t*,
    735, 870–871
  temperature regulation by, 872–873
  ureteral peristalsis and, 309
  vasoconstriction caused by, 165*f*, 166, 166*f*
    norepinephrine and epinephrine in,
      199, 204
    in skeletal muscle, 244
Sympathetic tone, 737
Sympathetic vasoconstrictor tone, 203, 203*f*
Sympathetic vasodilator system, 204, 204*f*
Sympathomimetic drugs, 739–740
  for shock, 281
Synapses, 543, 544*f*, 546–557. *See also*
    Dendrites; Neurotransmitters;
    Postsynaptic neuron; Postsynaptic
    potentials; Presynaptic terminals.
  acid-base abnormalities and, 557
  drug effects on, 557
  facilitation of, 545
  fatigue of, 557
    in reverberatory circuit, 567–568
    stabilizing effect of, 569–570, 569*f*
  hypoxia and, 557
  information processing role of, 545
  memory and, 706, 707, 707*f*
    long-term, 708
  one-way conduction at, 546, 547
  physiologic anatomy of, 547–550, 547*f*
  types of, 546–547
Synaptic afterdischarge, 567
Synaptic body, of rod or cone, 609, 610*f*
Synaptic cleft, 547, 547*f*, 550
  of neuromuscular junction, 83
Synaptic delay, 557
Synaptic space, 83
Synaptic trough, 83, 84*f*
Synaptic vesicles, of neuromuscular junction,
    83, 84*f*, 86
Syncytium
  of cardiac muscle, 101–102, 102*f*
  of gastrointestinal smooth muscle, 753
  of unitary smooth muscle, 91
Synovial spaces, negative pressure in, 183
Systemic circulation, 157. *See also* Circulation.
  blood volume distribution in, 157, 158*f*
  pressures in different portions of,
    158, 159*f*
Systole, 105, 105*f*
  duration of, heart rate and, 105
  emptying of ventricles during, 105*f*, 106

Systolic blood pressure, 158, 168
    age-related increase in, 171, 171*f*
    measurement of, 170–171, 170*f*
Systolic pressure curve, 108, 108*f*
Systolic stretch, 250, 250*f*, 251

T

T$_3$. *See* Triiodothyronine (T$_3$).
T$_4$. *See* Thyroxine (T$_4$).
T lymphocytes, 433, 434. *See also* Lymphocytes.
    activation of, 439–440, 440*f*
    delayed-reaction allergy associated with, 443
    memory cells of, 440
    preprocessing of, 434–435, 435*f*, 442
    specificity of, 435–436
    transfusion of, 442
    types of, 440–442, 441*f*. *See also specific*
        types.
T tubules. *See* Transverse (T) tubules.
T wave, 121, 121*f*, 122–123
    abnormalities in, 141–142, 142*f*
    atrial, 122, 133–134, 133*f*
    cardiac cycle and, 105, 105*f*
    monophasic action potential and, 122, 122*f*
    normal voltage of, 123
    vectorial analysis of, 133, 133*f*
Tabes dorsalis, 310
Tabetic bladder, 310
Tachycardia(s)
    incomplete intraventricular block
        caused by, 145–146
    paroxysmal, 148–149
        atrial, 148, 148*f*
        ventricular, 148–149, 149*f*
    sinus, 143, 143*f*
Tactile receptors, 560*b*, 560*f*, 571–572, 572*f*
    feedback to motor cortex, 672
    flexor reflex and, 662
    nerve fibers from, 564, 572
    position senses and, 580
Tactile sensations, 571–573
    pain inhibition associated with, 587–588
Tactile stimuli, salivation and, 776
Tamponade, cardiac, cardiac output curve and,
        234, 234*f*
Tandem pore domain potassium channel, 59, 59*f*
Tank respirator, 522*f*, 523
Taste, 645–648
    adaptation of, 648
    factors affecting experience of, 645
    preference in, 648
    primary sensations of, 645–648
        thresholds for, 646, 646*t*
    salivation and, 648, 776
    signal transmission into central nervous
        system, 647–648, 648*f*
    taste buds and, 646–647, 647*f*
Taste blindness, 646
Taste cells, 646, 647, 647*f*
Taste hairs, 646
Taste pore, 646, 647*f*
TATA box, 35, 35*f*
Tectorial membrane, 636*f*, 637, 637*f*
Tectospinal tracts, 670, 672*f*
Teeth, 969–972
    abnormalities of, 971–972
    development of, 970–971, 970*f*
    functions of, 969
    mineral exchange in, 971
    parts of, 969, 969*f*
Telophase, 38*f*, 39
Temperature, body, 867–877. *See also* Heat
        loss; Thermogenesis (heat production);
        Thermoreceptors.
    abnormalities of, 875–877, 875*f*, 876*f*.
        See also Fever.
    behavioral control of, 875

Temperature, body (*Continued*)
    core temperature, 867
        range of, 867, 867*f*
        set-point of, 872*f*, 873–874, 874*f*
    food intake and regulation of, 849, 873
    gain of control system for, 8
    heart function and, 112
    heart rate and, 143
    hypothalamic regulation of, 715, 871–875
        anterior hypothalamic-preoptic area
            in, 871, 873
        atmospheric temperature range and,
            871, 871*f*
        deep body receptors and, 872, 874
        fever and, 875–876, 876*f*
        low temperatures and, 877
        neuronal effectors in, 872–873, 872*f*
        posterior hypothalamus in, 872
        set-point in, 872*f*, 873–874, 874*f*, 876, 876*f*
        skin receptors and, 872, 874
        spinal reflexes and, 875
    neonatal regulation of, 873, 1025, 1025*f*
        prematurity and, 1027
    normal range of, 7, 7*t*, 867, 867*f*
    ovulation and, 1001, 1002*f*
    rectal, 867*f*
    skin temperature, 867
        local reflexes regulating, 875
        set-point and, 874, 874*f*
    sympathetic regulation of, 738
Temporal field of vision, 627
Temporal summation
    in neurons, 555
    in sensory fibers, 564, 565*f*
Tendon fibers, muscle fibers and, 71
Tendon receptors. *See* Golgi tendon organs.
Tendon reflex, 661
Teniae coli, 770
Tension-time index, 109
Tensor tympani muscle, 633, 634
Teratoma, 985
Testicular tumors, Leydig cell, 985
Testis(es)
    anatomy of, 973, 973*f*
    cholesterol used by, 827
    descent of, 981
    fetal, human chorionic gonadotropin and,
        984, 1008
    storage of sperm in, 975–976
    temperature of, 977, 978
Testis determining factor, 981
Testosterone
    chemical structure of, 980*f*
    degradation and excretion of, 980
    in fetal development, 980, 981, 981*f*, 984,
        1008
    functions of, 980–982
    luteinizing hormone and, 983, 984
    mechanism of action of, 982–983
    metabolic rate and, 864
    metabolism of, 980
    nongenomic effects of, 983
    ovarian synthesis of, 991, 992, 992*f*
    plasma level of, over life cycle, 980, 981*f*
    protein deposition in tissues and, 835–836,
        982–983, 1031
    secretion of, 979–980, 980*f*
    spermatogenesis and, 975
Tetanization, 80, 80*f*
Tetany, hypocalcemic, 64, 367, 956, 956*f*
    in hypoparathyroidism, 967
    in premature infant, 1027
    in rickets, 968–969
Tetracaine, 69
Tetraethylammonium ion, 63
Tetralogy of Fallot, 271, 271*f*
Tetrodotoxin, 63

Thalamocortical system, 697–698
    alpha waves and, 724
    petit mal epilepsy and, 726
Thalamus. *See also* Ventrobasal complex of
        thalamus.
    alpha waves and, 724
    basal ganglia and, 690, 690*f*, 691–692, 691*f*
        in Parkinson's disease, 693–694
    cerebellar input to, 684
    cerebral cortex and, 697–698, 698*f*, 712
    memory and, 709
    motor cortex input from, 670, 687, 687*f*
    olfactory signals and, 651
    pain pathways to, 585–586, 585*f*
        surgical interruption of, 586
    pain perception and, 586
    reticular excitatory signals and, 711, 712*f*
    sleep and, 722
    somatosensory association areas and, 577
    somatosensory pathways to
        anterolateral, 573, 581, 581*f*
        dorsal column–medial lemniscal, 573,
            574, 574*f*, 576
        joint rotation and, 580, 580*f*
        thermal signals in, 593
    somatosensory role of, 581
    taste signals and, 647–648, 648*f*
    visual pathways in, 623–624, 623*f*
Theca cells, 989, 989*f*, 990
    androgen synthesis in, 992, 993*f*
    of corpus luteum, 990–991
Theobromine, 557
Theophylline, 557
Thermal pain stimuli, 583, 584, 584*f*
Thermode, 871
Thermogenesis (heat production), 867, 873
    during exercise, 1039–1040
    hypothalamic inhibition of, 872, 872*f*
    at low temperatures, 877
    nonshivering, 865, 873
Thermogenic effect of food, 864–865, 867
Thermogenin, 873
Thermoreceptive senses, 571
    anterolateral system and, 573
    localization of, 577
Thermoreceptors, 559, 560*b*, 592–593, 592*f*
    nerve fibers from, 564
    transmission pathways from, 593
Theta waves, 723*f*, 724–725, 725*f*
Thiamine. *See* Vitamin B$_1$ (thiamine).
Thiazide diuretics, 332, 332*f*, 398, 398*t*
Thiocyanate ions
    antithyroid activity of, 915
    in saliva, 776
Third heart sound, 266
Thirst
    extracellular fluid osmolarity and, 357–360,
        358*t*, 359*f*
    hypothalamic control of, 716
Thirst center, 358, 716
Thoracic duct, 186, 186*f*, 819
    rate of flow through, 187
Thoracic duct lymph
    fat in, 187, 760
    protein concentration of, 187
Thought, 705–706
    communication of, 703–704
    elaboration of, 703
    holistic theory of, 706
    prefrontal association area and, 700, 703
    Wernicke area and, 701, 704–705
Threshold for drinking, 358
Thrill, in aortic stenosis, 267
Thrombin, 453, 453*f*, 454
    adsorbed to fibrin fibers, 457
    thrombomodulin binding of, 456–457
Thrombocytes. *See* Platelets.

Thrombocytopenia, 458
Thrombocytopenic purpura, 458
Thromboembolic conditions, 459
Thrombomodulin, 456–457
Thromboplastin, chemical structure of, 826
Thrombosthenin, 451, 454
Thromboxane A$_2$
    platelet aggregation and, 452
    vasoconstriction caused by, 451
Thrombus, 459. *See also* Coronary thrombosis.
Thymine, 27, 28, 28f, 31t
Thymus, T lymphocyte processing in, 434–435, 435f, 442
Thyroglobulin, 882, 907, 908–909, 908f
    cleaving of hormones from, 909, 914
    hypothyroidism and, 917
    organification of, 908–909
    storage of, 909
Thyroid adenoma, 916
Thyroid gland
    anatomy of, 907, 907f
    blood flow in, 907
    calcitonin secretion in, 966
    diseases of, 916–918, 916f, 918f
    histology of, 907, 907f
    inhibitors of, 915
Thyroid hormones, 907–919. *See also*
        Reverse T$_3$ (RT$_3$); Thyroxine (T$_4$);
        Triiodothyronine (T$_3$).
    cold climate and, 873
    daily rate of secretion, 909
    functions of, 910–914
        basal metabolic rate and, 907, 911, 912, 913f
        blood cholesterol and, 827
        body weight and, 912
        carbohydrate metabolism and, 912
        cardiovascular system and, 913
        central nervous system and, 913
        fat metabolism and, 825, 912
        gastrointestinal motility and, 913
        gene transcription and, 910, 911f
        growth and, 912
        liver fats and, 912
        metabolic activity and, 911–912
        muscles and, 913
        nongenomic effects in, 910
        other endocrine glands and, 913–914
        plasma lipids and, 912
        respiration and, 913
        sexual function and, 914
        sleep and, 913
        vitamin requirements and, 912
    long duration of action, 910, 910f
    mechanism of action, 891
    protein binding of, 882, 909–910
    protein metabolism and, 836, 911
    protein synthesis and, 910, 911f
    receptors for, 891, 910, 911f
    regulation of secretion of, 914–915, 915f
    release of
        from thyroid, 909
        to tissues from plasma, 910
    slow onset of, 910, 910f
    structures of, 909f
    synthesis of, 882, 907, 908–909, 908f, 909f
        inhibitors of, 915
    transport of, to tissues, 909–910
Thyroiditis
    autoimmune, 917
    idiopathic goiter and, 917
Thyroid-stimulating hormone (TSH;
        thyrotropin), 896, 896t, 914–915, 915f
    antithyroid substances and, 915
        in foods, 917
    diagnostic measurement of, 916
    endemic goiter and, 917
    hyperthyroidism and, 916

Thyroid-stimulating hormone (TSH;
        thyrotropin) (*Continued*)
    iodide trapping and, 908, 914
    pregnancy and, 1009
    thermogenesis and, 873
Thyroid-stimulating immunoglobulins, 916
Thyrotoxicosis. *See* Hyperthyroidism.
Thyrotropes, 896, 896t
Thyrotropin. *See* Thyroid-stimulating hormone
        (TSH; thyrotropin).
Thyrotropin-releasing hormone (TRH), 898,
        898t, 914–915
    test dose of, 918
    thermogenesis and, 873, 915
Thyroxine (T$_4$), 907. *See also* Thyroid hormones.
    compared to triiodothyronine, 907
    converted to triiodothyronine, 910
    diagnostic measurement of, 916, 918
    heat production and, 873
    mechanism of action, 891
    metabolic rate and, 864, 867
    in pregnancy, 1009
    protein metabolism and, 836
Thyroxine-binding globulin, 882, 909–910
Thyroxine-binding prealbumin, 909–910
Tic douloureux, 590
Tickle sense, 571, 572. *See also* Tactile sensations.
    anterolateral system and, 573
    scratch reflex and, 664
Tidal volume, 469, 469f
    minute respiratory volume and, 471
Tight junctions
    of brain capillaries, 749
    of gastric mucosa, 799–800
    renal tubular, 324, 325f, 327–328
Tissue capillary, high altitude and, 529
Tissue factor, 455, 455f, 456
    prothrombin time and, 461
Tissue gel, 180–181
Tissue plasminogen activator (t-PA)
    for cardiogenic shock, 259
    clot lysis and, 457
    for pulmonary embolism, 459
    for thrombotic occlusion, 459
Tissue thromboplastin. *See* Tissue factor.
Tissue typing, 449
Titin, 73, 73f
Titratable acid, 389–390
TNF (tumor necrosis factor), in inflammation,
        430, 430f
Tolerance, immune, 442
Tone
    muscle. *See* Muscle tone.
    sympathetic and parasympathetic, 737
Tonic contraction, of gastrointestinal smooth
        muscle, 755, 756
Tonic receptors, 562
Tonic seizures, 725
Tonic-clonic seizures, 725
Tonometry, 607, 607f
Tonotopic maps, 640
Torsades de pointes, 147, 148f
Total body water
    measurement of, 289
    regulation of, 345
Total lung capacity, 469, 469f
    determination of, 471
Total peripheral resistance, 163. *See also*
        Vascular resistance.
    cardiac output and, 230–231, 230f
        elevated, 232–233
    in hypovolemic shock, 274
    renal–body fluid system and, 216–217, 216f,
        217f
    renin-angiotensin system and, 223
    volume-loading hypertension and, 219,
        220, 220f

Touch, 571. *See also* Tactile receptors; Tactile
        sensations.
    pathways into central nervous system, 573
Toxic substances
    acute tubular necrosis caused by, 401
    bitter taste of, 646
t-PA. *See* Tissue plasminogen activator (t-PA).
Trace elements, 856–857
Trachea, 472, 472f
Tractus solitarius, 203. *See also* Nucleus tractus
        solitarius.
    autonomic control by, 739
    baroreceptors and, 205, 206
    swallowing and, 764
    taste signals and, 647–648, 648f
Tranquilizers, reward or punishment centers
        and, 718
Transamination
    in amino acid synthesis, 834, 834f, 840
    in deamination, 834–835
Transcellular fluid, 286
Transcortin, 923
Transcription, 27, 27f, 29f, 30–31
    hormonal action and, 888, 889f, 891
        by cortisol, 931
        by growth hormone, 899
        by insulin, 944
        by thyroid hormones, 910, 911f
    in postsynaptic neuron, 549, 549f
    regulation of, 35–36, 35f
Transcription factors, 35–36, 35f
    thyroid hormone receptors as, 891
Transcytosis, in capillary endothelium, 178
Transducin, 613, 613f
Transfer RNA (tRNA), 31, 32, 32f, 34, 34f
Transferrin, 418, 418f, 419–420, 840
Transfusion, for shock, 280–281
    irreversible, 278, 278f
Transfusion reactions, 445, 446, 448–449
    acute renal failure in, 448–449
    Rh blood types and, 447
Translation, 27, 27f, 33–35, 34f. *See also*
        Protein(s), synthesis of.
    growth hormone and, 899
Transmitter substances. *See* Neurotransmitters.
Transmitter vesicles, 547–548, 550
    memory and, 708
    of neuropeptides, 551
    recycling of, 550–551
Transplantation of tissues and organs, 449–450
    kidney transplantation, 409
Transport. *See* Active transport; Diffusion;
        Membrane transport.
Transport maximum, renal tubular, 326–327,
        327f, 327t
Transport proteins, 45, 46f. *See also* Carrier
        proteins; Protein channels.
Transport vesicles, 20–21, 20f
Transpulmonary pressure, 466f, 467
Transverse (T) tubules
    of cardiac muscle, 103–104, 104f
    of skeletal muscle, 73f, 87, 87f, 88–89, 88f
Trauma
    growth hormone secretion in, 901, 902
    hypovolemic shock in, 279
Tremor
    intention tremor, 687–688, 689
    in Parkinson's disease, 693
    thyroid hormones and, 913
Treppe, 80
TRH. *See* Thyrotropin-releasing hormone
        (TRH).
Triamterene, 332, 333f, 399
Trichinosis, 430
Tricuspid valve, 106–107
    first heart sound and, 265, 266, 266f
    as reference level for pressure, 174–175, 174f

Tricyclic antidepressants, 727
Trigeminal nerve, sensory nuclei of, 574
Trigeminal neuralgia, 590
Triglycerides. *See also* Fatty acids.
  in cell, 12
    as neutral fat globules, 14
  chemical structure of, 819
  in chylomicrons, 819–820
  dietary, 791–792, 791*f*
  digestion of, 789, 791*f*
    bile salts and, 792
    emulsification for, 792
    by pancreatic lipase, 792, 792*f*
    in stomach, 792
  energy production from, 822–825. *See also*
    Fats, as energy source.
    regulation of, 825–826
  functions of, 819
  hydrolysis of, 820, 822
  in lipoproteins, 821, 821*t*
  in liver, 821–822
  resynthesis of, in intestinal epithelium,
    797, 819
  storage of, 821–822. *See also* Adipose tissue.
  synthesis of, 821–822
    from carbohydrates, 824–825, 824*f*
    from proteins, 825
  thyroid hormones and, 912
Trigone, 307*f*, 308, 308*f*, 309
Triiodothyronine (T₃), 907. *See also* Reverse T₃
  (RT₃); Thyroid hormones.
  compared to thyroxine, 907
  mechanism of action, 891
  thyroxine converted to, 910
tRNA. *See* Transfer RNA (tRNA).
Trophoblast cells, 1004, 1004*f*, 1005, 1005*f*
  estrogen and progesterone secreted by, 1008
  glucose for fetus and, 1007
  human chorionic gonadotropin secreted by,
    1007–1008, 1007*f*
  nutrition of embryo and, 1005, 1005*f*
  placenta and, 1005, 1006*f*
Tropical sprue, 801
Tropomyosin, in skeletal muscle, 75–76, 75*f*
Troponin
  calmodulin and, 891
  in cardiac muscle, 103
  in skeletal muscle, 75–76, 75*f*
Trypsin, 781, 791
Trypsin inhibitor, 781
Trypsinogen, 781
Tryptophan deficiency, 854
TSH. *See* Thyroid-stimulating hormone (TSH;
  thyrotropin).
Tuber cinereum, 897
Tuberculosis, 520
  bacterial defenses in, 426
Tubular glands, 773, 777*f*. *See also* Oxyntic
  (gastric) glands; Pyloric glands.
Tubulin, 16
Tubuloglomerular feedback, 195, 319–321, 320*f*
Tufted cells, 651, 652
Tumor necrosis factor (TNF), in inflammation,
  430, 430*f*
Turbulent blood flow, 161–162, 161*f*
Twitches, skeletal muscle, 79
Two-point discrimination, 578, 578*f*
Tympanic membrane, 633–634, 633*f*
  damage to, 642
Tyrosine
  hormones derived from, 882–884
  in norepinephrine synthesis, 732
  in thyroid hormone synthesis, 908–909,
    909*f*, 914
Tyrosine kinases
  insulin receptor and, 940–941, 941*f*
  leptin receptor and, 888

U
Ubiquinone, 814
Ubiquitin, muscle atrophy and, 82
Ulcerative colitis, 771, 802–803
Ultimobranchial glands, 966
Ultrafiltration, into peritubular capillary,
  323–324, 325
Ultrasonic flowmeter, 160–161, 161*f*
  for cardiac output measurement, 240
Umami taste, 646
Umbilical arteries, 1005, 1006*f*, 1022, 1022*f*
Umbilical vein, 1005, 1006*f*
Unipolar limb leads, augmented, 126–127, 127*f*
  axes of, 130, 130*f*
  vectorial analysis of potentials in, 131
Unitary (visceral) smooth muscle, 91, 91*f*, 94*f*
  action potentials in, 95, 96
    excited by stretch, 96
    number of fibers in, 96
    spontaneous, 95*f*, 96
Unmyelinated nerve fibers, 67, 67*f*
  classification of, 563, 563*f*, 564
Unsaturated fats
  atherosclerosis prevention and, 829
  blood cholesterol and, 827
  formed in liver, 822
  vitamin E and, 855
Uracil, 30, 31*t*
Urea
  artificial kidney and, 410
  chronic renal failure and, 406
  diffusion through membrane channels, 47
  formation by liver, 835, 839–840
    ATP expended for, 859
  placental diffusion of, 1007
  reabsorption of, in kidney, 328–329, 328*f*,
    333–334
  in sweat, 870
  urine concentration and, 348*t*, 350–351,
    351*f*, 353
Urea recycling, 353
Urea transporters, 328–329, 333–334,
  350, 353
Uremia, 406
  plasma composition in, 410*t*
Ureterorenal reflex, 309
Ureters, 307*f*, 308–309, 308*f*
  pain sensation in, 309
Urethra, 306, 307*f*
  posterior, 307*f*, 308, 308*f*
    micturition reflex and, 309
    voluntary urination and, 310
Urethral glands, 973, 979
Urinary tract infection, septic shock secondary
  to, 280
Urinary tract obstruction
  acute renal failure in, 399, 401
  infection secondary to, 403–404
Urine
  concentration of, 345, 346–353
    basic requirements for, 347–348
    in chronic renal failure, 405, 406*f*
    countercurrent mechanism and, 348–349,
      349*f*, 351–352, 352*f*, 353
    disorders of, 354–355
    distal tubule and collecting ducts and,
      350, 350*f*
    maximal level of, 347
    obligatory volume and, 347, 353
    quantification of, 354
    specific gravity and, 347, 347*f*
    summary of, 352–353, 352*f*
    urea and, 350–351, 351*f*
  dilution of, 345–346, 346*f*
    in chronic renal failure, 405
    disorders of, 354–355
    quantification of, 354

Urine (*Continued*)
  formation of, 310–312, 311*f*. *See also*
    Kidney(s), reabsorption by; Kidney(s),
    secretion by.
  osmolarity of, specific gravity and, 347, 347*f*
  pH of, 380, 380*t*
    minimal, 388
  specific gravity of, 347, 347*f*
  transport from kidney to bladder, 308–309
  volume of
    obligatory, 347, 353
    in pregnancy, 1010
    water loss in, 286, 286*t*
Urine output, arterial blood pressure and, 337
Urobilin, 840–841
Urobilinogen, 840–841, 841*f*, 842
Urogenital diaphragm, 307*f*, 308
Urticaria, 443
Uterine milk, 995, 1004
Uterus, 987, 987*f*, 988*f*. *See also* Implantation;
  Labor.
  contractility of, 1011–1012
    hypothalamus and, 716
  contraction of, oxytocin and, 905
  estrogenic effects on, 993
  involution of, after parturition, 1013–1014
  parturition and, 1011–1013, 1012*f*
  progesterone and, 994
Utilization coefficient, 499
Utricle, 674–675, 675*f*, 676–677
Uvula, of cerebellum, 678

V
Vagal reflex, to stop paroxysmal tachycardia,
  148
Vagina, 987, 987*f*, 988*f*
  estrogenic effects on, 993
Vagovagal reflexes
  gastric muscular tone and, 766
  gastric secretion and, 779
Vagus nerves
  aortic baroreceptors and, 205
  aortic bodies and, 508*f*, 509
  arterial pressure and, 206, 736
  bronchoconstriction and, 473
  cardiac effects of
    atrioventricular block as, 144
    bradycardia as, 144
  cardiac regulation by, 111, 111*f*, 119–120,
    201, 202*f*
    atrial stretch and, 208–209
    sensory signals and, 203
    vasomotor center and, 203, 208
  coronary blood flow and, 247
  duodenal mucous glands and, 786
  food intake and, 846*f*, 848
  gallbladder emptying and, 785
  gastric secretions and, 779, 780, 780*f*
    pepsinogen in, 779
    ulcers and, 801
  gastrointestinal innervation by, 756–757
    reflexes and, 757
  gastrointestinal regulation by, stomach
    emptying and, 767
  pancreatic secretions and, 782
  parasympathetic fibers in, 730, 731*f*
  respiratory control and, 506
  swallowing and, 764*f*, 765
  taste signals and, 647
  in vasovagal syncope, 204
Valvulae conniventes, 793, 793*f*
Valvular heart disease
  cardiac hypertrophy in, 272
  circulatory dynamics in, 268–269
  congenital, 267
  exercise and, 269
  murmurs caused by, 267–268

Valvular heart disease (*Continued*)
  regurgitation in, 267
  rheumatic, 266–267
  stenosis in, 267
van den Bergh reaction, 841–842
van't Hoff's law, 291
Varicose veins, 174
Varicosities
  of postganglionic nerve endings, 732
  of smooth muscle nerve endings, 94*f*, 95
Vas deferens, 973, 973*f*, 975–976
Vasa recta, 306, 307*f*
  blood flow in, 317
  countercurrent exchange in, 348,
    351–352, 352*f*
Vascular capacitance, 167. *See also* Vascular
    compliance.
  sympathetic control of, 168
Vascular compliance, 167. *See also* Vascular
    capacitance.
  arterial, 167
    pressure pulse reduction by, 168, 170
    pressure pulse velocity and, 169–170
    pulse pressure and, 168–169
  venous, 167
Vascular distensibility, 167–168, 168*f*
Vascular endothelial growth factor
    (VEGF), 198
Vascular resistance, 162–165. *See also* Total
    peripheral resistance.
  arterial pressure and, 165, 166
  arterial pressure pulses and, 170
  conductance and, 163, 164
  diameter of vessel and, 164
  hematocrit and, 164–165, 165*f*
  pressure difference and, 159, 160
  pulmonary. *See* Pulmonary vascular
    resistance.
  in series and parallel circuits, 164, 164*f*
  units of, 162–163
  venous pressure and, 172
Vascular smooth muscle. *See also* Blood flow
    control.
  aldosterone and, 927
  autoregulation of blood flow and, 194–195
  local factors controlling, 97
  nitric oxide and, 195, 196*f*
Vascularity of tissues, blood flow regulation
    and, 197–198, 197*f*
Vasoactive intestinal peptide
  gastric secretion and, 780
  penile erection and, 978–979
Vasoconstriction
  cutaneous, for temperature regulation, 872,
    875, 876
  of injured vessel, 451
  ions with effect of, 200
  tissue blood flow and, 165*f*, 166, 166*f*
Vasoconstrictor agent(s), 199
  angiotensin II as, 199, 221
    nitric oxide and, 196
  antidiuretic hormone as, 199, 905
  endothelin as, 196
  limited long-term effect of, 200
Vasoconstrictor area, of medulla, 202,
    202*f*, 203
  baroreceptor signals and, 206
Vasoconstrictor system, sympathetic, 201–204,
    202*f*
  adrenal medullae and, 204
  cerebral ischemia and, 209
  hypothalamus and, 204
Vasoconstrictor tone, sympathetic, 203, 203*f*
Vasodilation
  by carbon dioxide increase, 200
  cutaneous, for temperature regulation,
    872, 875, 877

Vasodilation (*Continued*)
  ions with effect of, 200
  in local blood flow control, 191, 192–193,
    194, 196–197
    nitric oxide and, 195–196, 196*f*
    tissue factors and, 97
  in septic shock, 280
Vasodilator agents, 199–200
  for angina pectoris, 252
  in cardiac muscle, 247
  for essential hypertension, 226
  in gastrointestinal tract, 761
  limited long-term effect of, 200
  in skeletal muscle, 243–244
Vasodilator area, of medulla, 202*f*, 203
Vasodilator system, sympathetic, 204, 204*f*
Vasodilator theory, of local blood flow
    regulation, 192–193
Vasomotion, of precapillary vessels,
    178–179, 193
Vasomotor center of brain stem, 202–204, 204*f*
  baroreceptors and, 6
  chemoreceptors and, 208
  CNS ischemic response and, 209
  exercise and, 244
  progressive shock and, 277
  respiratory waves and, 210
Vasomotor waves, 210–211, 210*f*
Vasopressin. *See* Antidiuretic hormone (ADH;
    vasopressin).
Vasovagal syncope, 204
Vectorcardiogram, 134, 134*f*
Vegetative functions, of brain, 714
VEGF (vascular endothelial growth factor), 198
Veins
  as blood reservoir, 175
  blood volume in, 157, 158
  distensibility of, 167–168, 168*f*
  exercise-related contraction of, 244–245
  functions of, 157, 171, 173–174, 175
  in nervous control of arterial pressure, 205
    in hypovolemic shock, 274
  sympathetic innervation of, 201, 202*f*
  temperature receptors in, 872
Venous admixture, 496, 496*f*
Venous dilation, acute, cardiac output and, 233
Venous plexus, cutaneous, 868, 868*f*
  as blood reservoir, 175
  heat conduction and, 868
Venous pooling of blood, 279
Venous pressures, 172–175. *See also* Blood
    pressure.
  compression points and, 172, 172*f*
  gravity and, 172–173, 173*f*, 174–175, 174*f*
  measurement of, 174–175, 174*f*
  reference level for, 174–175, 174*f*
Venous pump, 171, 173–174
Venous return
  artificial respiration and, 523
  calculation of, 237
  in cardiac failure, 256, 257
  cardiac output and, 110, 112, 229–230
    in pathological conditions, 232–234, 233*f*
  mean filling pressure and, 236–237, 236*f*
  pressure gradient for, 237
  resistance to, 237, 237*f*, 238*f*
    exercise and, 245
    increased blood volume and, 238
    sympathetic stimulation and, 238–239
  shock caused by decrease in, 273, 279, 280
Venous return curves, 234, 235–237
  combinations of patterns of, 237, 238*f*
  exercise and, 245, 245*f*
  in heart failure. *See* Cardiac failure,
    quantitative graphical analysis of.
  mean systemic filling pressure and, 235,
    235*f*, 236–237, 236*f*, 238*f*

Venous return curves (*Continued*)
  normal, 235–236, 235*f*
  resistance to venous return and, 237, 237*f*,
    238*f*
  with simultaneous cardiac output curves,
    238–240, 238*f*
Venous sinuses, of spleen, 175, 175*f*,
    427–428, 427*f*
Venous system
  damming of blood in, after myocardial
    infarction, 250, 255
  lymph emptying into, 186, 186*f*
  volume-pressure curve of, 167–168, 168*f*
Venous thrombosis, femoral, 459
Venous valves, 173–174, 174*f*
  incompetent, 174
Ventilation. *See* Alveolar ventilation;
    Mechanical ventilation; Pulmonary
    ventilation.
Ventilation-perfusion ratio, 492–494
  abnormalities of, 493–494
    atelectasis and, 519
    in emphysema, 494, 518
    in pneumonia, 518–519, 519*f*
    in tuberculosis, 520
  hypoxia and, 520
Ventral lateral geniculate nucleus, 623
Ventral posterior medial nucleus of thalamus,
    647–648, 648*f*
Ventral respiratory group, 505, 506, 506*f*
Ventricles, cardiac
  as pumps, 106
  synchronous contraction of, 119
  transmission of impulse in, 118, 118*f*
Ventricular dilatation
  chemical energy expended and, 109
  circus movement secondary to, 251
  QRS prolongation in, 137–138
Ventricular escape, 119–120, 145
Ventricular fibrillation, 149–151, 150*f*, 151*f*
  circulatory arrest in, 281
  in long QT syndromes, 147
  after myocardial infarction, 250–251
  paroxysmal tachycardia leading to, 149
Ventricular function curves, 110–111,
    110*f*
Ventricular hypertrophy. *See also* Cardiac
    hypertrophy; Left ventricular
    hypertrophy.
  axis deviation in, 135–136, 135*f*, 136*f*
  high voltage in, 136*f*, 137
  QRS prolongation in, 137–138
Ventricular paroxysmal tachycardia,
    148–149, 149*f*
Ventricular pressure, cardiac cycle and, 105,
    105*f*, 106
Ventricular rupture, 251
Ventricular syncytium, 102
Ventricular tachycardia, paroxysmal,
    148–149, 149*f*
Ventricular volume, cardiac cycle and, 105,
    105*f*, 106
Ventricular volume output curve, 110, 110*f*
Ventrobasal complex of thalamus, 574,
    574*f*, 575*f*
  anterolateral pathway and, 581, 581*f*
  joint rotation and, 580*f*
  pain fibers terminating in, 585
  signals to motor cortex from, 670
  thermal signals terminating in, 593
Venules, 177, 178*f*
  function of, 157
Vermis, cerebellar, 681–682, 682*f*, 684, 686
Vertebral fracture, acceleratory forces causing,
    531, 532–533
Very low-density lipoproteins (VLDLs),
    820*f*, 821

Vesicointestinal reflex, 772
Vesicoureteral reflux, 309, 403–404
Vesicular channels, in capillary endothelium, 178
Vesicular follicles, 989
Vestibular apparatus, 674–676, 675f, 676f. See also Equilibrium.
    connections with central nervous system, 678, 678f, 694
    head rotation and, 676, 677, 677f
    linear acceleration and, 676–677
    motion sickness and, 804
    static equilibrium and, 676, 678
Vestibular membrane, 634–635
Vestibular nerve, 676, 678, 678f
Vestibular nuclei, 673f, 674, 678, 678f
    cerebellar input to, 683, 684
    motor fibers leading to, 670
    vomiting and, 804
Vestibulocerebellar tracts, 670, 683, 683f
Vestibulocerebellum, 686–687
Vestibulospinal tracts, 670, 672f, 674, 674f, 678, 678f
Vibration sense, 571, 572. See also Tactile sensations.
    pathways into central nervous system, 573, 579
Villi, intestinal. See also Enterocytes.
    absorption by, of water and electrolytes, 786–787
    central lacteal of, 793f, 794
    contractions of, 769
    epithelium of, 786
    gluten enteropathy and, 801
    pits between. See Crypts of Lieberkühn.
    structure of, 793–794, 793f
    vasculature of, 761, 761f
        countercurrent flow in, 761–762
Villi, placental, 1005, 1006f
    glucose diffusion and, 1007
Virchow-Robin space, 743, 743f
Viruses, 17–18, 18f
    neutralization of, by complement, 439
Viscera
    control of. See Autonomic nervous system.
    insensitive to pain, 589
    temperature receptors in, 872
Visceral pain, 588–590, 589f
Visceral reflexes, 729
Visceral sensations, 571
Visceral smooth muscle, 91. See also Unitary (visceral) smooth muscle.
Viscosity. See Blood, viscosity of.
Visual acuity, 604–605, 604f
    accommodation and, 631
    in central retina, 619
Visual association areas, 624–625
Visual contrast, 618, 626
Visual cortex, 623, 624–626, 624f, 625f
    fusion of two images and, 630
    reading and, 704f, 705
Visual fields, 627, 627f
Visual image(s)
    analysis of
        neuronal patterns in, 626–627, 626f
        two pathways for, 626
    fusion of, 625, 630–631
        lack of, 630–631, 630f
Visual information, interpretation of, 701, 701f
Visual pathways, 623–624, 623f
Visual purple. See Rhodopsin.
Visual receptive aphasia, 703
Vital capacity, 469, 469f
Vitamin(s), 852–855. See also specific vitamins.
    daily requirements of, 852, 853t

Vitamin(s) (Continued)
    deficiencies of
        of B vitamins, vasodilation in, 194
        combined, 854
        in starvation, 852
    in fetus, 1020
    storage in body, 852–853
    thyroid hormones and, 912
Vitamin A, 853
    in retina, 611, 611f, 612
    stored in liver, 840, 852
Vitamin B₁ (thiamine)
    colon bacteria and, 798
    deficiency of, 853. See also Beriberi.
    metabolic function of, 853
Vitamin B₂ (riboflavin), 854
Vitamin B₆ (pyridoxine), 854–855
    amino acid synthesis and, 834, 854
Vitamin B₁₂, 854
    colon bacteria and, 798
    in fetus, 1020
    intrinsic factor and, 778, 800, 854. See also Pernicious anemia.
    red blood cell production and, 417, 420
    stored in liver, 840
Vitamin C, 855
    in fetus, 1020
    neonatal need for, 1025
    osteoporosis secondary to, 969
Vitamin D, 855, 960–962, 961f
    actions of, 962
    calcium absorption and, 796, 855, 962, 964–965
    calcium excretion and, 962
    deficiency of
        hyperparathyroidism secondary to, 968
        rickets in, 968–969
    in fetus, 1020
    for hypoparathyroidism, 967
    neonatal need for, 1025, 1026
    parathyroid hormone and, 961–962, 961f
    phosphate absorption and, 962, 964–965
    phosphate excretion and, 962
    in pregnancy, 1010
    receptors for, 962
    renal calcium reabsorption and, 368–369
    renal hydroxylation of, 304, 961
        impaired in renal failure, 406–407
        parathyroid hormone and, 964–965
    stored in liver, 840, 852
Vitamin D–resistant rickets, 969
Vitamin E, 855
    in fetus, 1020
Vitamin K, 855
    clotting factor deficiencies and, 458, 855
    colon bacteria and, 798, 855
    in fetus, 1020
    hepatic requirement for, 840
    impaired absorption of, 458, 802
    in pregnancy, 1010
    prothrombin activation and, 453
    for surgical patients, 458
    warfarin and, 459–460
Vitreous humor, 606, 606f
VLDLs (very low-density lipoproteins), 820f, 821
Vocal folds, 474–475, 474f
Vocalization, 474–475
Volley principle, 638
Voltage clamp, 62–63, 62f
Voltage-gated channels, 47, 48, 49f.
        See also Calcium ion channels, voltage-gated; Potassium ion channels, voltage-gated; Sodium ion channels, voltage-gated.
    of nerve membrane, 61–63, 61f, 62f

Volume reflex, atrial, 208
Volume-loading hypertension, 218–219, 218f, 220f
Volume-pressure curves, of arterial and venous systems, 167–168, 168f
Volume-pressure diagram, of cardiac cycle, 108–109, 108f, 109f
Volume-pressure work, cardiac, 108
Vomiting, 803–804, 803f
    aversion to foods causing, 651
    hyponatremia caused by, 294–295
    metabolic acidosis caused by, 393
    metabolic alkalosis caused by, 393, 804
    obstruction as cause of, 804, 804f
Vomiting center, 803, 803f, 804
    nausea and, 804
von Willebrand factor, platelets and, 452
von Willebrand's disease, 458

W
W ganglion cells, 619, 630
Walking movements, 664
Warfarin, 459–460
Warmth receptors, 592–593, 592f. See also Thermoreceptive senses.
Waste products, renal excretion of, 303, 311–312, 330
Water
    in cell, 11
    diffusion through capillary pores, 179–180, 180t
    diffusion through cell membrane, 46, 47, 51–52, 51f, 290
    in feces, 798
    in gastrointestinal secretions, 774–775
    intake of, daily, 285, 286t
    intestinal absorption of
        in colon, 797–798
        in small intestine, 794, 795
    intestinal secretion of, 786–787
    loss of, daily, 285–286, 286t
    in pancreatic secretions, 781, 782, 783f
    reabsorption by kidneys, 324, 328, 328f
        angiotensin II and, 338–339, 338f
        antidiuretic hormone and, 339, 339f, 345, 716
        atrial natriuretic peptide and, 339
        estrogen and, 994
        inulin concentration and, 334, 334f
        in loop of Henle, 330–331, 330f
        in pregnancy, 1011
    renal excretion of, hypothalamus and, 716
    renal regulation of, 303
    total body
        measurement of, 289
        regulation of, 345
    vapor pressure of, 486, 487
        altitude and, 527
        in alveoli, 527
Weber-Fechner principle, 579
Weight, body. See also Obesity.
    hypertension and, 225
    thyroid hormones and, 912
Weight loss
    abnormal, 851–852
    in obese patients, 851
Weightlessness, 533–534
Wernicke aphasia, 703, 704
Wernicke area, 699–700, 699f, 701, 701f
    aphasia related to, 703, 704
    auditory areas and, 702, 704–705, 704f
    hemispheric dominance and, 701, 702, 705
    meaning of sounds and, 641
    visual information and, 701, 702, 704f, 705

White blood cell count, in neonate, 1024
White blood cells. *See* Leukocytes (white blood cells).
White muscle, 79
White pulp, of spleen, 175
White ramus(i), 729, 730*f*
Withdrawal reflexes, 662–663
Word blindness, 701, 703
Word deafness, 703
Work, of breathing, 468

Work output
    of heart, 107–109, 108*f*, 109*f*, 110
    of skeletal muscle, 78
Working memory, 703, 706

X
X ganglion cells, 619, 624, 625
Xenograft, 449

Y
Y ganglion cells, 619, 624, 625, 626, 630

Z
Z disc, of skeletal muscle, 71, 72*f*, 73, 73*f*
    contraction mechanism and, 74, 74*f*, 75, 76
Zinc, 856
Zona fasciculata, 921*f*, 922
Zona glomerulosa, 921–922, 921*f*
Zona pellucida, fertilization and, 977, 1003
Zona reticularis, 921*f*, 922

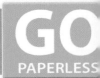
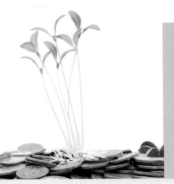
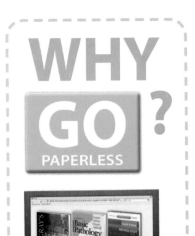
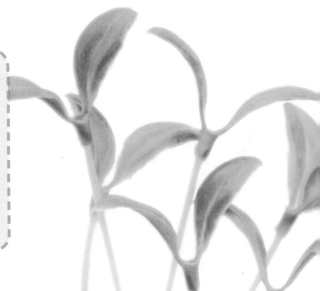